Wolters Kluwer Health
77 Westport Plaza, Suite 450
St. Louis, Missouri 63146
Phone 314/216-2100 ● 800/223-0554
Fax 314/878-5563
FactsandComparisons.com

American
Drug Index 2012

Wolters Kluwer
Health

Facts & Comparisons

American Drug Index

Norman F. Billups, RPh, MS, PhD
Dean and Professor Emeritus
College of Pharmacy
The University of Toledo

Shirley M. Billups, RN, LPC, MEd
Oncology Nurse
Licensed Professional
Counselor

Facts and Comparisons® Publishing Group

Arvind Subramanian, MBA
President & CEO, Clinical Solutions

Scot E. Walker, PharmD, MS, BCPS
Clinical Director

Lauri L. Moore, RPh, MBA
Senior Director, Medi-Span Drug Content, and Facts & Comparisons and Medi-Span Product Management

Paul B. Johnson, RPh
Cathy A. Meives, PharmD
Senior Clinical Managers

Kim S. Dufner, PharmD
Clinical Manager

Andrea L. Williams, RPh
Senior Clinical Editor

Christine M. Cohn, PharmD, BCPS
Esta Razavi, PharmD
Patricia L. Spenard, PharmD
Clinical Editors

Angela J. Bush
Acquisitions Manager

Sarah W. Gremillion
Managing Editor

Michelle M. Polley
Senior Editor

Jennifer A. Besserman
Lesley S. Grissum
Associate Editors

Susan H. Sunderman
Managing Editor, Quality Control

Jennifer M. Love
Senior Composition Specialist

Wendy M. Bell
Managing Technical Editor

Barbara J. Hunter
Inventory Analyst

Facts and Comparisons® Editorial Advisory Panel

Burgunda (Gundy) V. Sweet, PharmD, FASHP

Director, Drug Information and Medication Use Policy
Clinical Associate Professor of Pharmacy
University of Michigan Health System and College of Pharmacy
Ann Arbor, Michigan

David S. Tatro, PharmD

Drug Information Analyst
San Carlos, California

Thomas L. Whitsett, MD

Professor of Medicine and Pharmacology
Vascular Medicine Program
OU Regents Professor
University of Oklahoma Health Sciences Center
Oklahoma City, Oklahoma

Contents

[•] Denotes official name: Generic name or chemical name recognized by the
     USP, NF, or USAN.

Preface

The 56th Edition of the *American Drug Index* (*ADI*) has been prepared for the identification, explanation, and correlation of the many pharmaceuticals available to the medical, pharmaceutical, and allied health professions. The need for this index has become even more acute as the variety and number of drugs and drug products have continued to multiply. *ADI* should be useful to pharmacists, nurses, health care administrators, physicians, medical transcriptionists, dentists, sales personnel, students, and teachers in the fields that incorporate pharmaceuticals.

Special note to medical transcriptionists: Generic names are in lowercase and trade names are in upper/lowercase as appropriate to facilitate transcription. The names for officially designated products (eg, *United States Pharmacopeia* or *USP*) are preceded by a bullet (•) and should appear in lowercase in transcription.

The organization of *ADI* falls into 15 major sections:

Monographs of Drug Products
Standard Medical Abbreviations
Calculations
Common Systems of Weights and Measures
Approximate Practical Equivalents
International System of Units
Normal Laboratory Values
FDA Pregnancy Categories
Controlled Substances Summary
Medical Terminology Glossary
Oral Dosage Forms that Should Not Be Crushed or Chewed
Drug Names that Look Alike and Sound Alike
Discontinued Drugs
Common Abbreviations of Chemotherapy Regimens
Manufacturer and Distributor Listing

MONOGRAPHS: The organization of the monograph section of *ADI* is alphabetical with extensive cross-indexing. Names listed are generic (also called nonproprietary, public name, or common name); brand (also called trademark, proprietary, or specialty); and chemical. Synonyms in general use also are included. All names used for a pharmaceutical appear in alphabetical order, with the pertinent data given under the brand name by which it is made available.

The monograph for a typical brand name product appears in upper/lowercase as appropriate, and consists of the manufacturer, generic name, composition and strength, available pharmaceutic dosage forms, package size, use, and appropriate legend designation (eg, *Rx, OTC, c-v*).

Generic names appear in lowercase in alphabetical order, followed by the pronunciation and the corresponding recognition of the drug to the *USP* (*United States Pharmacopeia*), *NF* (*National Formulary*), and USAN (*USP Dictionary of United States Adopted Names and International Drug Names*). Each of these official generic names is preceded by a bullet (•). The information is in accord with the *USP 34* and *NF 29*, and the 2011 *USP Dictionary of USAN and International Drug Names.*

To minimize medication errors, The Institute for Safe Medication Practices established Tall Man lettering for look-alike pairs. Tall Man lettering was added to generic entries for the drugs involved in the name differentiation project.

Pronunciations have been included for many of the generic drugs. However, not every drug will have a corresponding pronunciation. Some of the most common pronunciations are not listed for every drug. The following list is included as a guide to very common names:

Acetate	ASS-eh-tate	Lactobionate	LACK-toe-BYE-oh-nate
Besylate	BESS-ih-late	Maleate	MAL-ee-ate
Borate	BOE-rate	Mesylate	MEH-sih-LATE
Bromide	BROE-mide	Monosodium	MAHN-oh-SO-dee-uhm
Butyrate	BYOO-tih-rate	Nitrate	NYE-trate
Calcium	KAL-see-uhm	Pendetide	PEN-deh-TIDE
Chloride	KLOR-ide	Pentetate	PEN-teh-tate
Citrate	SIH-trate	Phosphate	FOSS-fate
Dipotassium	die-poe-TASS-ee-uhm	Potassium	poe-TASS-ee-uhm
Disodium	die-SO-dee-uhm	Propionate	PRO-pee-oh-nate
Edetate	eh-deh-TATE	Sodium	SO-dee-uhm
Fosfatex	foss-FAH-tex	Succinate	SUCK-sih-nate
Fumarate	FEW-mah-rate	Sulfate	SULL-fate
Hydrobromide	HIGH-droe-BROE-mide	Tartrate	TAR-trate
Hydrochloride	HIGH-droe-KLOR-ide	Trisodium	try-SO-dee-uhm
Iodide	EYE-oh-dide		

Because of the multiplicity of brand names used for the same therapeutic agent or the same combination of therapeutic agents, some correlation was done. Please turn to aspirin for an example of this. Here under the generic name are listed the various brand names. Following are combinations of aspirin organized in a manner to point out relationships among the many products. Reference then is made to the brand name or names having the indicated composition. Under the brand name are given manufacturer, composition, available forms, sizes, dosage, and use.

The multiplicity of generic names for the same therapeutic agent has complicated the nomenclature of these agents. Examples of multiple generic names for the same chemical substance are:
(1) acetaminophen, N-acetyl-p-aminophenol; (2) guaifenesin, glyceryl guaiacolate, glyceryl guaiacolether, guaianesin, guayanesin; and (3) pyrilamine maleate, pyranilamine maleate, pyraminyl maleate, anisopyradamine.

The cross-indexing feature of *ADI* permits the finding of drugs or drug combinations when only one major ingredient is known. For example, a combination of aluminum hydroxide gel and magnesium trisilicate is available. This combination can be found by looking under the name of either of the two ingredients, and in each case the brand names are given. A second form of cross-indexing lists drugs under various therapeutic and pharmaceutical classes (ie, antacids, antihistamines, diuretics, laxatives).

ABBREVIATIONS: The listing of standard medical abbreviations is included as an aid in interpreting medical orders. The Latin or Greek word and abbreviation are given with the meaning.

CALCULATIONS: A listing of common formulas used to calculate weight, creatinine clearance, ideal body weight, and temperature conversion between Celsius and Farenheit.

WEIGHTS AND MEASURES: Tables containing common systems of weights and measures are included to aid the practitioner in calculating dosages in the metric, apothecary, and avoirdupois systems.

CONVERSION FACTORS: A listing of approximate practical equivalents to aid in calculating and converting dosages among the metric, apothecary, and avoirdupois systems.

INTERNATIONAL SYSTEM OF UNITS: A modernized version of the metric system listed in tables for rapid reference.

NORMAL LABORATORY VALUES: Tables containing normal reference values for commonly requested laboratory tests are included as a guideline for the health care practitioner.

FDA PREGNANCY CATEGORIES: A table summarizing each of the pregnancy categories established by the FDA.

CONTROLLED SUBSTANCES: A brief summary explanation of the key points of the Controlled Substances Act of 1970.

MEDICAL TERMINOLOGY GLOSSARY: Commonly used terms are listed and defined as an aid in interpreting the use given for drug monographs included in *ADI.*

ORAL DOSAGE FORMS THAT SHOULD NOT BE CRUSHED OR CHEWED: This section alerts the health care practitioner about oral dosage forms that should not be crushed, and may serve as an aid in consulting with patients. Examples of products falling into the non-crush category are extended-release, enteric-coated, encapsulated beads, wax matrix, sublingual dosage forms, and encapsulated liquid formulations.

DRUG NAMES THAT LOOK ALIKE AND SOUND ALIKE: A listing of common drugs that look alike and sound alike. Familiarity with this list may prevent the prescriber from making a dispensing error.

DISCONTINUED DRUGS: A combined list of generic and brand products no longer available in the United States because they were withdrawn from the market or discontinued by the manufacturer.

COMMON ABBREVIATIONS OF CHEMOTHERAPY REGIMENS: This section describes the drugs, therapeutic uses, dosages, and dosing schedules of common acronyms used for combination chemotherapy regimens (eg, CHOP). The combination regimens are listed in alphabetical order by acronym.

MANUFACTURER AND DISTRIBUTOR LISTING: The name, address, phone number, and Web site of virtually every American pharmaceutical manufacturer and drug distributor are listed in alphabetical order in this section.

Direct correspondence or communication with reference to a drug or drug product listed in *ADI* to Editorial/Production, Attn: ADI, Wolters Kluwer Health, 77 Westport Plaza, Suite 450, St. Louis, Missouri 63146, or call 1-800-223-0554.

Monographs

Adcetris DS 50mg SDV ... 신 제 시약조

A

AABP. (Brookstone) 0.01% acetic acid, 5.4% antipyrine, 1.4% benzocaine, 0.01% polycosanol 410, glycerin. Soln., Otic. 15 mL w/dropper. *Rx.*
Use: Ophthalmic and otic agent, otic preparation.

A & D Tablets. (Barth's) Vitamins A 10,000 units, D 400 units. Tab. Bot. 100s, 500s. *OTC.*
Use: Vitamin supplement.

•**abacavir succinate.** (ab-ah-KAV-ear SUCK-sih-nate) USAN.
Use: Antiviral.

abacavir sulfate.
Use: Antiviral; nucleoside reverse transcriptase inhibitor.
See: Ziagen.
W/Lamivudine
See: Epzicom.

•**abafilcon A.** (ab-ah-FILL-kahn) USAN.
Use: Contact lens material, hydrophilic.

•**abamectin.** (abe-ah-MEK-tin) USAN.
Use: Antiparasitic.

•**abarelix.** (ab-ah-RELL-ix) USAN.
Use: Gonadotropin-releasing hormone antagonist.

•**abatacept.** (ab-a-TA-sept) USAN.
Use: Immunomodulator, immunologic agent.
See: Orencia.

Abbokinase Open-Cath. (Abbott Diagnostics) Urokinase for catheter clearance gelatin 5 mg, mannitol 15 mg, sodium chloride 1.7 mg, monobasic sodium phosphate anhydrous/mL when reconstituted, preservative free. Single-dose *Univial* 1 mL, 1.8 mL. *Rx.*
Use: Thrombolytic.

Abbott AFP-EIA. (Abbott Diagnostics) Enzyme immunoassay for the quantitative measurement of alpha-fetoprotein (AFP) in human serum and amniotic fluid. Test kits 100s.
Use: Diagnostic aid.

Abbott AFP-EIA Monoclonal. (Abbott Diagnostics) Enzyme immunoassay for the quantitative measurement of alpha-fetoprotein (AFP) in human serum and amniotic fluid.
Use: Diagnostic aid.

Abbott Anti-Delta. (Abbott Diagnostics) Radioimmunoassay for the detection of antibody to hepatitis delta antigen (HDAg) in human serum or plasma.
Use: For research only. Not for use in diagnostic procedures.

Abbott Anti-Delta EIA. (Abbott Diagnostics) Enzyme immunoassay for the detection of antibody to hepatitis delta antigen (HDAg) in human serum or plasma.
Use: For research only. Not for use in diagnostic procedures.

Abbott β-HCG 15/15. (Abbott Diagnostics) Enzyme immunoassay for the quantitative determination of human chorionic gonadotropin (hCG) in human serum.
Use: Diagnostic aid.

Abbott CA125-EIA. (Abbott Diagnostics) Enzyme immunoassay for the quantitative measurement of cancer antigen (CA) 125 in human serum.
Use: For research only. Not for use in diagnostic procedures.

Abbott CEA-EIA Monoclonal. (Abbott Diagnostics) Enzyme immunoassay for the quantitative measurement of carcinoembryonic antigen (CEA) in human serum or plasma to aid in the management of cancer patients and assessing prognosis.
Use: Diagnostic aid.

Abbott CEA-RIA. (Abbott Diagnostics) Solid phase radioimmunoassay for the quantitative measurement of carcinoembryonic antigen (CEA) in human serum or plasma to aid in the management of cancer patients and assessing prognosis.
Use: Diagnostic aid.

Abbott CMV Total AB EIA. (Abbott Diagnostics) Enzyme immunoassay for the detection of antibody to cytomegalovirus in human serum, plasma, and whole blood. Test kits 100s.
Use: Diagnostic aid.

Abbott Diagnostic Reagents. (Abbott Diagnostics) A series of diagnostic tests for cancer, cardiovascular, hepatitis, infectious disease and immunology, metabolic and digestive disease, OB/GYN, rubella, and thyroid.
Use: Diagnostic aid.

Abbott ER-EIA Monoclonal. (Abbott Diagnostics) Enzyme immunoassay for the quantitative measurement of human estrogen receptor in tissue cytosol.
Use: For research only. Not for use in diagnostic procedures.

Abbott ER-ICA Monoclonal. (Abbott Diagnostics) Immunoassay for the detection of estrogen receptor.
Use: For research only. Not for use in diagnostic procedures.

Abbott HB-EIA. (Abbott Diagnostics) Enzyme immunoassay for the detection of hepatitis Be antigen or antibody to hepatitis Be antigen.

Use: Diagnostic aid.

Abbott HBe Test. (Abbott Diagnostics) Radioimmunoassay or enzyme immunoassay for detection of hepatitis Be antigen or antibody to hepatitis Be antigen. Test kits 100s.
Use: Diagnostic aid.

Abbott HIVAB HIV-1 EIA. (Abbott Diagnostics) Enzyme immunoassay for the antibody to human immunodeficiency virus type 1 (HIV-1) in serum or plasma. Test kits 100s, 1000s.
Use: Diagnostic aid.

Abbott HIVAG-1. (Abbott Diagnostics) Enzyme immunoassay for the human immunodeficiency virus type 1 (HIV-1) antigens in serum or plasma. Test kits 100s, 1000s.
Use: Diagnostic aid.

Abbott HTLV I EIA. (Abbott Diagnostics) To detect antibody to Human T-Lymphotropic Virus Type I in serum or plasma. Test kits 100s.
Use: Diagnostic aid.

Abbott HTLV III Antigen EIA. (Abbott Diagnostics) Enzyme immunoassay for the detection of Human T-Lymphotropic Virus Type III (HIV) antigens.
Use: For research only. Not for use in diagnostic procedures.

Abbott HTLV III Confirmatory EIA. (Abbott Diagnostics) Enzyme immunoassay for confirmation of specimens found to be positive to antibody to HTL VIII. Test kits 100s.
Use: Diagnostic aid.

Abbott HTLV III EIA. (Abbott Diagnostics) Enzyme immunoassay for the detection of antibody to Human T-Lymphotropic Virus Type III (HIV) in human serum or plasma. Test kits 1s.
Use: Diagnostic aid.

Abbott IGE EIA. (Abbott Diagnostics) Enzyme immunoassay for quantitative determination of IgE in human serum and plasma. Test kits 100s.
Use: Diagnostic aid.

Abbott PAP-EIA. (Abbott Diagnostics) Enzyme immunoassay for the measurement of prostatic acid phosphatase (PAP) in serum or plasma.
Use: Diagnostic aid.

Abbott RSV-EIA. (Abbott Diagnostics) Enzyme immunoassay for the detection of respiratory syncytial virus (RSV) in nasopharyngeal washes and aspirates.
Use: Diagnostic aid.

Abbott SCC-RIA. (Abbott Diagnostics) Radioimmunoassay for the quantitative measurement of squamous cell carcinoma-associated antigen in human serum.
Use: For research only. Not for use in diagnostic procedures.

Abbott TdT EIA. (Abbott Diagnostics) Enzyme immunoassay for the quantitative measurement of terminal deoxynucleotidyl transferase (TdT), in extracts of human whole blood or isolated mononuclear cells.
Use: Diagnostic aid.

Abbott Testpak hCG-Serum. (Abbott Diagnostics) Monoclonal antibody, enzyme immunoassay for the qualitative determination of human chorionic gonadotropin (hCG) in serum. No instrumentation required.
Use: Diagnostic aid.

Abbott Testpak hCG-Urine. (Abbott Diagnostics) Monoclonal antibody, enzyme immunoassay for the qualitative determination of human chorionic gonadotropin (hCG) in urine. No instrumentation required.
Use: Diagnostic aid.

Abbott Testpack-Strep A. (Abbott Diagnostics) A rapid screening and confirmatory test for the detection of group A beta-hemolytic streptococci from throat swabs. No instrumentation required.
Use: Diagnostic aid.

Abbott Toxo-G EIA. (Abbott Diagnostics) Enzyme immunoassay for the qualitative and quantitative determination of IgG antibody to toxoplasma gondii in human serum and plasma.
Use: Diagnostic aid.

Abbott Toxo-M EIA. (Abbott Diagnostics) Enzyme immunoassay for the qualitative determination of IgM antibody to toxoplasma gondii in human serum.
Use: Diagnostic aid.

•**abciximab.** (ab-SICK-sih-mab) USAN.
Use: Monoclonal antibody; antithrombotic; antiplatelet agent, glycoprotein IIb/IIIa inhibitor.
See: ReoPro.

ABC to Z. (NBTY) Iron 18 mg, Vitamins A 5000 units, D 400 units, E 30 units, B_1 1.5 mg, B_2 1.7 mg, B_3 20 mg, B_5 10 mg, B_6 2 mg, B_{12} 6 mcg, C 60 mg, folic acid 0.4 mg, biotin 30 mcg, Ca, P, I, Mg, Cu, Mn, K, Cl, Cr, Mo, Se, Ni, Si, Sn, V, B, vitamin K, Zn 15 mg. Tab. Bot. 100s. *OTC.*
Use: Mineral, vitamin supplement.

Abelcet. (Enzon) Amphotericin B 100 mg/20 mL (as lipid complex). Susp. for Inj. Single-use Vial w/5-micron filter needles 10 mL, 20 mL. *Rx.*

Use: Antifungal.
- **abetimus sodium.** (a-BE-ti-mus) USAN.
Use: Investigational immunomodulator.
- **abexinostat.** (A-bex-IN-oh-stat) USAN.
Use: Antineoplastic.
Abilify. (Otsuka America) Aripiprazole.
Inj.: 7.5 mg/mL. Single-dose vials. **Oral Soln.:** 1 mg/mL. EDTA, fructose, sucrose, parabens. Orange cream flavor. 150 mL. **Tab.:** 2 mg, 5 mg, 10 mg, 15 mg, 20 mg, 30 mg. Lactose. Pkg. 30s, UD 100s (except 2 mg). *Rx.*
Use: Antipsychotic.
Abilify Discmelt. (Otsuka America) Aripiprazole 10 mg (phenylalanine 1.12 mg), 15 mg (phenylalanine 1.68 mg). Aspartame. Vanilla cream flavor. Orally Disintegrating Tab. Blister 30s. *Rx.*
Use: Antipsychotic.
- **abiraterone acetate.** (A-bir-A-ter-one) USAN.
Use: Antineoplastic.
Abitrexate. (International Pharm) Methotrexate sodium 25 mg/mL. Vial 2 mL, 4 mL, 8 mL. *Rx.*
Use: Antineoplastic.
Ablavar. (Lantheus Medical Imaging) Gadofosveset trisodium 244 mg/mL (also contains fosveset 0.268 mg) (equiv. to 0.25 mmol/mL). Preservative free. Inj., Soln. Single-use vial. 10 mL, 20 mL.
Use: In vivo diagnostic aid.
- **ablukast.** (ab-LOO-kast) USAN.
Use: Antiasthmatic, leukotriene antagonist.
- **ablukast sodium.** (ab-LOO-kast) USAN.
Use: Antiasthmatic, leukotriene antagonist.
See: Ulpax.
- **abobotulinumtoxinA.** (ab-oh-BOT-ue-LYE-num-TOX-in-ay) USAN.
Use: Botulinum toxin.
See: Dysport.
abortifacients.
See: Mifepristone.
Prostaglandins.
Abraxane. (Abraxis Oncology) Paclitaxel 100 mg. With human albumin 900 mg. Pow. for Inj., lyophilized (albumin-bound). Single-use vials. *Rx.*
Use: Antimitotic agent.
Abreva. (GlaxoSmithKline) Docosanol 10%, benzyl alcohol, light mineral oil. Cream. Tube 2 g. *OTC.*
Use: Cold sores; fever blisters.
- **abrineurin.** (aye-bri-NOOR-in) USAN.
Previously brineurin.
Use: Amyotrophic lateral sclerosis (ALS).

absorbable cellulose cotton or gauze.
See: Oxidized Cellulose.
absorbable dusting powder.
Use: Lubricant.
absorbable gelatin film.
Use: Hemostatic, topical.
See: Gelfilm.
Gelfilm Ophthalmic.
absorbable gelatin sponge.
Use: Hemostatic.
See: Gelfoam.
absorbable surgical suture.
Use: Surgical aid.
Absorbase. (Carolina Medical Products) Petrolatum, mineral oil, ceresin wax, wool wax, alcohol. Oint. Tube 114 g, 454 g. *OTC.*
Use: Pharmaceutical aid, emollient base.
absorbent gauze.
Use: Surgical aid.
Absorbent Rub Relief Formula. (DeWitt) Green soap 11.64%, camphor 1.63%, menthol 1.63%, pine tar soap 0.87%, wintergreen oil 0.71%, sassafras oil 0.54%, benzocaine 0.48%, capsicum 0.03%, wormwood oil 0.6%, isopropyl alcohol 75%. Bot. 2 oz. *OTC.*
Use: Analgesic, topical.
Absorbine Jr. (W. F. Young) Menthol 1.27%, absinthium oil, echinacea, iodine, plant extracts of calendula, potassium iodide, thymol, wormwood. Liq., topical. 118 mL w/applicator. *OTC.*
Use: Rub and liniment.
Absorbine Jr. Arthritis Strength. (W. F. Young) Natural menthol 4%, capsaicin 0.025%, acetone, calendula plant extracts, echinacea, wormwood. Liq. *OTC.*
Use: Liniment.
Absorbine Jr. Back Patch. (W.F. Young) Menthol 5%. Aloe barbadensis, camphor, lanolin, zinc oxide. Patch. 22 × 10 cm. 4s. *OTC.*
Use: Rub and liniment.
Absorbine Jr. Extra Strength. (W. F. Young) Natural menthol 4%; plant extracts of calendula, echinacea and wormwood; acetone; chloroxylenol iodine; potassium iodide; thymol; wormwood oil. Liq. Bot. 59 mL, 118 mL. *OTC.*
Use: Liniment.
Absorbine Jr. Ultra Strength. (W.F. Young) Menthol. **Patch:** 5%. Alcohol, camphor, eucalyptus leaf oil, glycerin, kaolin, polysorbate 80, titanium dioxide. 6s. **Spray:** 12%. Alcohol, plant extracts of calendula, echinacea, wormwood, spearmint oil. 118 mL. *OTC.*
Use: Rub and liniment.

Abstral. (ProStrakan) Fentanyl 100 mcg, 200 mcg, 300 mcg, 400 mcg, 600 mcg, 800 mcg. Mannitol. Tab., sublingual. Blister packs. 12s (except 600 mcg, 800 mcg), 32s. *c-II.*
Use: Opioid analgesic.

Abuscreen. (Roche) An immunological and radiochemical assay for morphine and morphine glucuronide in nanogram levels. Utilizes I-125 labeled morphine requiring gamma scintillation equipment. Tests 100s.
Use: Diagnostic aid.

●**acacia syrup.** (ah-KAY-shah) *NF 29.*
Use: Pharmaceutic aid, suspending agent, viscosity agent.

●**acadesine.** (ack-AH-dess-een) USAN.
Use: Platelet aggregation inhibitor.

●**acamprosate calcium.** (a-kam-PROE-sate) USAN.
Use: Antialcoholic agent.
See: Campral.

Acanya. (Valeant) Benzoyl peroxide 2.5%, clindamycin phosphate 1.2%. Kit with benzoyl peroxide gel 40 g and clindamycin phosphate solution 10 g. Gel. *Rx.*
Use: Dermatologic agent, acne treatment.

●**acarbose.** (A-car-bose) USAN.
Use: Alpha-glucosidase inhibitor.
See: Precose.

acarbose. (Various Mfr.) Acarbose 25 mg, 50 mg, 100 mg. Tab. 100s, UD 100s (except 100 mg). *Rx.*
Use: Alpha-glucosidase inhibitor.

Accolate. (AstraZeneca) Zafirlukast 10 mg, 20 mg, lactose, povidone. Tab. Bot. 60s, UD 100s. *Rx.*
Use: Leukotriene receptor antagonist.

Accretropin. (Cangene) Somatropin 5 mg/mL. Sodium chloride 0.75%, phenol 0.34%. Inj. Soln. Multiple-dose vials. *Rx.*
Use: Growth hormone.

AccuHist. (Tiber) Pseudoephedrine hydrochloride 9 mg, chlorpheniramine maleate 0.8 mg/mL. Saccharin, sorbitol. Cherry flavor. Drops. 30 mL with dropper. *Rx.*
Use: Upper respiratory combination, decongestant, antihistamine.

AccuHist DM Pediatric. (Tiber) Pseudoephedrine hydrochloride 15 mg, brompheniramine maleate 1 mg, dextromethorphan HBr 4 mg per 1 mL. Saccharin, sorbitol. Grape flavor. Drops. 30 mL with dropper. *Rx.*
Use: Upper respiratory combination, antitussive combination.

AccuHist PDX. (Tiber) **Drops:** Pseudoephedrine hydrochloride 9 mg, chlorpheniramine maleate 0.8 mg, dextromethorphan HBr 3 mg per 1 mL. Alcohol and sugar free. Saccharin, sorbitol, grape flavor. 30 mL with dropper. **Syrup:** Phenylephrine hydrochloride 5 mg, dextromethorphan HBr 5 mg, guaifenesin 50 mg, brompheniramine maleate 2 mg/ 5 mL. Alcohol free. Sucrose, corn syrup. Grape flavor. 473 mL. *Rx.*
Use: Upper respiratory combination, antitussive combination; antitussive and expectorant combination.

AccuNeb. (Dey) Albuterol sulfate 0.021% (0.63 mg/3 mL), 0.042% (1.25 mg/ 3 mL). Preservative free. Soln. for Inh. UD Vial 3 mL. *Rx.*
Use: Bronchodilator, sympathomimetic.

Accupep HPF. (Sherwood Davis & Geck) Hydrolyzed lactalbumin, maltodextrin, MCT oil, corn oil, mono- and diglycerides, vitamins A, B_1, B_2, B_3, B_5, B_6, B_{12}, C, D, E, K, Ca, Cl, Cu, Fe, I, Mg, Mn, P, Zn, biotin, and choline. Pks. 128 g. *OTC.*
Use: Nutritional supplement.

Accupril. (Pfizer) Quinapril hydrochloride 5 mg, 10 mg, 20 mg, 40 mg. Lactose. Film-coated. Tab. Bot. 90s and UD 100s (except 40 mg). *Rx.*
Use: Antihypertensive; angiotensin-converting enzyme inhibitor.

Accuretic. (Parke-Davis) Quinapril hydrochloride/hydrochlorothiazide 10 mg/12.5 mg, 20 mg/12.5 mg, 20 mg/ 25 mg. Lactose. Film-coated. Tab. Bot. 30s. *Rx.*
Use: Antihypertensive.

Accusens T Taste Function Kit. (Westport Pharmaceuticals, Inc.) Test for ability to distinguish among salty, sweet, sour, and bitter tastants. Kit contains 15 bottles (60 mL) tastants and 30 taste record forms.
Use: Diagnostic aid.

A-C-D Solution. Sodium citrate, citric acid, and dextrose in sterile pyrogen-free solution. (Baxter Pharmaceutical Products, Inc.) Soln. 600 mL Bot. with 70 mL, 120 mL, 300 mL Soln.; 1000 mL Bot. with 500 mL Soln. (Bayer Biological) 500 mL Bot. with 75 mL, 120 mL Soln.; 650 mL Bot. with 80 mL, 130 mL Soln. (The Diamond Co.) 250 mL, 500 mL *Abbo-Vac. Rx.*
Use: Anticoagulant for preparation of plasma or whole blood.

A-C-D Solution Modified. (Bristol-Myers Squibb) Acid citrate dextrose anticoagulant solution modified. *Rx.*

Use: Anticoagulant, radiolabeled.

●**acebutolol hydrochloride.** (ass-cee-BYOO-toe-lahl) *USP 34.*
Use: Antiadrenergic/sympatholytic; beta-adrenergic blocking agent.
See: Sectral.

acebutolol hydrochloride. (Various Mfr.) Acebutolol hydrochloride 200 mg, 400 mg. Cap. Bot. 100s, 1000s. *Rx.*
Use: Antiadrenergic/sympatholytic, beta-adrenergic blocking agent.

●**acecainide hydrochloride.** (ASS-eh-CANE-ide) USAN.
Use: Cardiovascular agent.
See: NAPA.

●**aceclidine.** (ass-ECK-lih-DEEN) USAN.
Use: Cholinergic.

●**acedapsone.** (ASS-eh-DAP-sone) USAN.
Use: Antimalarial; antibacterial, leprostatic.

Acedoval. (Pal-Pak, Inc.) Dover's powder 15 mg, ipecac 1.5 mg, aspirin 162 mg, caffeine anhydrous 8.1 mg. Tab. Bot. 1000s, 5000s. *OTC.*
Use: Analgesic; antispasmodic; antiperistaltic.

●**aceglutamide aluminum.** (AH-see-GLUE-tah-mide ah-LOO-min-uhm) USAN.
Use: Antiulcerative.

acellular pertussis adsorbed, hepatitis B (recombinant) and inactivated poliovirus vaccine combined, diphtheria and tetanus toxoids.
Use: Active immunization, toxoid.
See: Diphtheria and Tetanus Toxoids and Acellular Pertussis Adsorbed, Hepatitis B (Recombinant) and Inactivated Poliovirus Vaccine Combined.

acellular pertussis and Haemophilus influenzae type B conjugate vaccine (DTaP-HIB), diphtheria and tetanus toxoids.
Use: Active immunization, toxoid.
See: Diphtheria and Tetanus Toxoids, Acellular Pertussis and Haemophilus Influenzae Type B Conjugate Vaccine (DTaP-HIB).

acellular pertussis vaccine, adsorbed (DTaP), diphtheria and tetanus toxoids.
Use: Active immunization, toxoid.
See: Diphtheria and Tetanus Toxoids and Acellular Pertussis Vaccine, Adsorbed (DTaP).

●**acemannan.** (ah-see-MAN-an) USAN.
Use: Antiviral; immunomodulator.

acemannan hydrogel.
Use: Mouth and throat product.
See: Oral Wound Rinse.

Aceon. (Solvay Pharm) Perindopril erbumine 4 mg, 8 mg. Lactose. Tab. 100s. *Rx.*
Use: Antihypertensive, angiotensin-converting enzyme inhibitor.

Acephen. (G & W Labs) Acetaminophen 120 mg, 325 mg, 650 mg. Glyceryl stearate (120 mg only), hydrogenated vegetable oil. Supp. 6s (120 mg only); 12s; 50s, 100s, 1000s (except 120 mg); 500s (650 mg only); UD 6s (325 mg only); UD 12s (except 650 mg); UD 50s, UD 100s (120 mg only). *OTC.*
Use: Analgesic.

●**acepromazine maleate.** (ASS-ee-PRO-mah-zeen) *USP 34.*
Use: Anxiolytic.

Acerola-C. (Barth's) Vitamin C 300 mg. Wafer. Bot. 30s, 90s, 180s, 360s. *OTC.*
Use: Vitamin supplement.

Acerola-Plex. (Barth's) Vitamin C 100 mg, bioflavonoids 50 mg. Tab. Bot. 100s, 500s. *OTC.*
Use: Vitamin supplement.

Acetadote. (Cumberland) Acetylcysteine 20% (200 mg/mL). EDTA 0.5 mg/mL. Preservative-free. Inj. Single-dose vials. 30 mL. *Rx.*
Use: Antidote.

Aceta-Gesic. (Rugby) Acetaminophen 325 mg, phenyltoloxamine citrate 30 mg. Tab. Bot. 24s, 1000s. *OTC.*
Use: Upper respiratory combination, analgesic, antihistamine.

●**acetaminophen.** (ass-cet-ah-MEE-noe-fen) *USP 34.* APAP.
Use: Analgesic; antipyretic.
See: Acephen.
Aminofen.
Anacin Aspirin Free Extra Strength.
Apap.
Apra.
Cetafen.
Ed-Apap.
ElixSure.
FeverAll.
Genapap.
Infantaire.
Little Fevers.
Mapap.
Masophen.
Non-Aspirin.
Nortemp.
Ofirmev.
Painaid ESF Extra-Strength Formula.
Pain and Fever.
Pain Relief.
Pain Reliever.
Q-Pap.

Quick Melts.
Silapap.
Triaminic Infants' Fever Reducer/Pain Reliever.
Tylenol.
Tylenol Meltaways Jr.
UN-Aspirin, Extra Strength.
Valorin.
W/Aluminum Hydroxide, Aspirin, Caffeine, Magnesium Hydroxide.
See: Vanquish.
W/Aspirin, Buffered.
See: Excedrin Back & Body Extra Strength.
W/Aspirin, Caffeine.
See: Anacin Advanced Headache.
Excedrin Extra Strength.
Excedrin Migraine.
Goody's Extra Strength.
Goody's Extra Strength Fast Pain Relief.
Summit Extra Strength.
W/Aspirin, Caffeine, Salicylamide.
See: Levacet.
Medi-First Extra Strength Pain Relief.
Painaid.
Saleto.
W/Butalbital.
See: Bupap.
Butalbital, Acetaminophen, and Caffeine.
Cephadyn.
Butex Forte.
Dolgic.
Marten-Tab.
Phrenilin Forte.
Repan CF.
Sedapap.
Tencon.
W/Butalbital, Caffeine.
See: Alagesic LQ.
Americet.
Dolgic Plus.
Esgic.
Esgic-Plus.
Fioricet.
Margesic.
Orbivan.
Repan.
Triad.
W/Butalbital, Caffeine, Codeine.
See: Fioricet with Codeine.
Phrenilin with Caffeine and Codeine.
W/Caffeine.
See: APAP-Plus.
W/Caffeine, Dihydrocodeine Bitartrate.
See: Panlor DC.
Trezix.
W/Caffeine, Isometheptene Mucate.
See: MigraTen.
Prodrin.

W/Caffeine, Magnesium Salicylate, Phenyltoloxamine Citrate.
See: Durabac Forte.
W/Caffeine, Phenyltoloxamine Citrate, Salicylamide.
See: Durabac.
W/Chlorpheniramine Maleate.
See: Coricidin HBP Cold & Flu.
W/Chlorpheniramine Maleate, Codeine Phosphate.
See: Cotabflu.
W/Chlorpheniramine Maleate, Dextromethorphan Hydrobromide.
See: Coricidin HBP Maximum Strength Flu.
Triaminic Flu, Cough & Fever.
Tylenol Plus Children's Cough & Runny Nose.
Vicks Formula 44M Cough, Cold, & Flu Relief.
W/Chlorpheniramine Maleate, Dextromethorphan Hydrobromide, Phenylephrine Hydrochloride.
See: Alka-Seltzer Plus Cold & Cough.
Comtrex Maximum Strength Day & Night Cold & Cough.
Comtrex Maximum Strength Nighttime Cold & Cough.
Robitussin Cough, Cold & Flu Nighttime.
Theraflu Nighttime Severe Cold.
Tylenol Cold Head Congestion Nighttime.
Tylenol Cold Multi-Symptom Nighttime.
Tylenol Plus Children's Flu.
Tylenol Plus Children's Multi-Symptom Cold.
W/Chlorpheniramine Maleate, Phenylephrine Hydrochloride.
See: Alka-Seltzer Plus Fast Crystal Packs.
Comtrex Maximum Strength Day & Night Flu Therapy.
Comtrex Maximum Strength Day & Night Severe Cold and Sinus.
Contac Cold + Flu.
Contac Cold + Flu Night.
Dristan Cold Multi-Symptom Formula.
Dryphen Multi-Symptom Formula.
Medicidin-D.
Pyrroxate Extra Strength.
Sine Off Sinus/Cold.
Tylenol Allergy Multi-Symptom.
Tylenol Allergy Multi-Symptom Convenience Pack.
Tylenol Sinus Congestion & Pain Nighttime.
W/Chlorpheniramine Maleate, Phenylephrine Hydrochloride, Phenyltoloxamine Citrate.
See: Norel SR.

W/Codeine Phosphate.
See: Capital with Codeine.
Cocet.
Vopac.
W/Dexbrompheniramine, Phenylephrine
Hydrochloride.
See: Sinadrin PE.
W/Dextromethorphan Hydrobromide.
See: Triaminic Cough & Sore Throat.
Tylenol Cough & Sore Throat Daytime.
Tylenol Plus Children's Cough & Sore
Throat.
W/Dextromethorphan Hydrobromide,
Diphenhydramine.
See: Diabetic Tussin Cold & Flu.
Diabetic Tussin Night Time Formula
Cold/Flu.
W/Dextromethorphan Hydrobromide,
Diphenhydramine Hydrochloride,
Phenylephrine Hydrochloride.
See: Respa C & C.
W/Dextromethorphan Hydrobromide,
Doxylamine Succinate.
See: Tylenol Cough & Sore Throat
Nighttime.
Vicks NyQuil Cold/Flu Relief.
W/Dextromethorphan Hydrobromide,
Doxylamine Succinate, Phenylephrine
Hydrochloride.
See: Alka-Seltzer Plus Day & Night
Cold.
Alka-Seltzer Plus Night Cold.
Tylenol Cold Multi-Symptom Nighttime.
W/Dextromethorphan Hydrobromide,
Doxylamine Succinate, Pseudoephedrine Hydrochloride.
See: All-Nite.
W/Dextromethorphan Hydrobromide,
Guaifenesin, Phenylephrine Hydrochloride.
See: Phenflu G.
Sine-Off Cough/Cold.
Sudafed PE Multi-Symptom Cold and
Cough.
W/Dextromethorphan Hydrobromide,
Guaifenesin, Pseudoephedrine Hydrochloride.
See: Duraflu.
Flutabs.
Maxiflu DM.
Maxiflu G.
Tylenol Cold Severe Congestion Daytime.
W/Dextromethorphan Hydrobromide,
Phenylephrine Hydrochloride.
See: Alka-Seltzer Plus Day & Night
Cold.
Alka-Seltzer Plus Day Cold.
Alka-Seltzer Plus Day Non-Drowsy
Cold.

Comtrex Maximum Strength Day &
Night Cold & Cough.
Mapap Cold Formula Multi-Symptom.
Theraflu Daytime Severe Cold &
Cough.
Theraflu Warming Relief Daytime
Multi-Symptom Cold.
Tylenol Cold Head Congestion Daytime.
Tylenol Cold Multi-Symptom Daytime.
Vicks DayQuil Multi-Symptom Cold/
Flu Relief.
W/Dextromethorphan Hydrobromide,
Pseudoephedrine Hydrochloride.
See: 666 Cold Preparation Maximum
Strength.
W/Dichloralphenazone, Isometheptene
Mucate.
See: Epidrin.
Midrin.
Migragesic IDA.
Migrazone.
Nodolor.
W/Diphenhydramine Citrate.
See: Goody's PM.
W/Diphenhydramine Hydrochloride.
See: Extra Strength Pain Reliever PM.
Percogesic Extra Strength.
Tylenol Severe Allergy.
Tylenol Sore Throat Nighttime.
Unisom PM Pain.
W/Diphenhydramine Hydrochloride,
Phenylephrine Hydrochloride.
See: Benadryl Allergy & Cold.
Benadryl Allergy & Sinus Headache.
Benadryl Severe Allergy & Sinus
Headache Maximum Strength.
Sudafed PE Multi-Symptom Severe
Cold.
Sudafed PE Nighttime Cold Maximum Strength.
Theraflu Nighttime Severe Cough &
Cold.
Theraflu Sugar-Free Nighttime Severe Cough & Cold.
Theraflu Warming Relief Flu & Sore
Throat.
Tylenol Allergy Multi-Symptom Convenience Pack.
Tylenol Allergy Multi-Symptom Nighttime.
W/Doxylamine Succinate, Phenylephrine
Hydrochloride.
See: Vicks NyQuil Sinex.
W/Guaifenesin.
See: Theraflu Chest Congestion.
Tylenol Chest Congestion.

W/Guaifenesin, Phenylephrine Hydro-
chloride.
See: Coldonyl.
Duratuss A.
Sine-Off Multi Symptom Relief.
Tylenol Sinus Congestion & Pain Se-
vere Daytime.
W/Guaifenesin, Pseudoephedrine Hydro-
chloride.
See: Poly-Vent Plus.
W/Hydrocodone Bitartrate.
See: Anexsia 5/500.
Anexsia 7.5/650.
Anexsia 10/660.
Co-Gesic.
Hycet.
Hydrocodone Bitartrate and Aceta-
minophen.
Hydrogesic.
Liquicet.
Lorcet Plus.
Lorcet 10/650.
Lortab.
Lortab 5/500.
Lortab 7.5/500.
Lortab 10/500.
Margesic H.
Maxidone.
Norco.
Norco 5/325.
Stagesic.
T-Gesic.
Vicodin.
Vicodin ES.
Vicodin HP.
Xodol.
Zamicet.
Zydone.
W/Magnesium Salicylate.
See: Painaid BRF Back Relief Formula.
W/Magnesium Salicylate, Pamabrom.
See: Pamprin Maximum Pain Relief.
W/Oxycodone.
See: Endocet.
Magnacet.
Percocet.
Pimlev.
Tylox.
Xolox.
W/Pamabrom.
See: Painaid PMF Premenstrual For-
mula.
Women's Tylenol Multi-Symptom
Menstrual Relief.
W/Pamabrom, Pyridoxine Hydrochloride.
See: Vitelle Lurline PMS.
W/Pamabrom, Pyrilamine Maleate.
See: Pamprin Multi-Symptom Maximum
Strength.
Prēmsyn PMS.

W/Pentazocine Hydrochloride.
See: Pentazocine Hydrochloride and
Acetaminophen.
Talacen.
W/Pheniramine Maleate, Phenylephrine
Hydrochloride.
See: Theraflu Cold & Sore Throat.
Theraflu Flu & Sore Throat.
Theraflu Nighttime Severe Cold.
W/Phenylephrine Hydrochloride.
See: Alka-Seltzer Plus Sinus.
Comtrex Maximum Strength Day &
Night Flu Therapy.
Comtrex Maximum Strength Day &
Night Severe Cold & Sinus.
Contac Cold + Flu Day.
Dilotab II.
Excedrin Sinus Headache.
Mapap Sinus Congestion and Pain
Maximum Strength.
Sine-Off Non-Drowsy Maximum
Strength.
Sinutab Sinus.
Sudafed PE Sinus Headache.
Vicks DayQuil Sinex.
W/Phenyltoloxamine Citrate.
See: Aceta-Gesic.
BP Poly-650.
Flextra-DS.
Lagesic.
Pain-gesic.
Phenylgesic.
Relagesic.
Staflex.
Zflex.
W/Phenyltoloxamine Citrate, Salicylamide.
See: Duraxin.
Ed-Flex Plus.
W/Propoxyphene Napsalate.
See: Darvocet A500.
Darvocet-N 100.
Trycet.
W/Pseudoephedrine Hydrochloride.
See: Dilotab II.
Mapap Sinus Maximum Strength.
Ornex No Drowsiness.
Ornex No Drowsiness Maximum
Strength.
W/Pseudoephedrine Hydrochloride,
Chlorpheniramine Maleate.
See: BC Allergy, Sinus, Headache.
W/Pseudoephedrine Hydrochloride, Guai-
fenesin.
See: Tylenol Sinus Severe Congestion.
W/Sodium Bicarbonate.
See: Bromo Seltzer.
W/Tramadol Hydrochloride.
See: Ultracet.
acetaminophen. (Various Mfr.) Aceta-
minophen. Cap.: 500 mg. 100s. Liq.:
160 mg/5 mL (May contain methylpara-

ben, saccharin, sorbitol sucrose. 118 mL, 120 mL, 473 mL, 500 mL), 166.6 mg/ 5 mL (237 mL). **Oral Soln.**: 160 mg/ 5 mL. May contain sorbitol, sucrose. 118 mL, 473 mL. **Supp.**: 120 mg, 325 mg, 650 mg. Hydrogenated vegetable oil. 12s. **Tab.**: 325 mg, 500 mg. 25s (500 mg only), 50s (325 mg only), 100s, 700s (500 mg only), 1000s, UD 100s (500 mg only). *OTC.*
Use: Analgesic.
•**acetaminophen and aspirin.** (ass-cet-ah-MEE-noe-fen and ASS-pihr-in) *USP 34.*
Use: Analgesic.
•**acetaminophen and caffeine.** (ass-cet-ah-MEE-noe-fen and KAF-een) *USP 34.*
Use: Analgesic.
acetaminophen and codeine. (Various Mfr.) **Tab.**: Codeine phosphate 15 mg, acetaminophen 300 mg. Bot. 100s, 500s, 1000s. Codeine phosphate 30 mg, acetaminophen 300 mg. Bot. 100s, 500s, 1000s, UD 100s, RN 100s. Codeine phosphate 60 mg, acetaminophen 300 mg. Bot. 100s, 500s, 1000s. *c-iii.* **Soln.**: Codeine phosphate 12 mg, acetaminophen 120 mg/5 mL. Bot. 120 mL, 500 mL, Pt, gal, UD 5 mL, 12.5 mL, 15 mL. *c-v.*
Use: Analgesic combination, narcotic.
•**acetaminophen and codeine phosphate.** (ass-cet-ah-MEE-noe-fen and KOE-deen) *USP 34.*
Use: Analgesic.
•**acetaminophen and diphenhydramine.** (ass-cet-ah-MEE-noe-fen and die-fen-HIGH-druh-meen) *USP 34.*
Use: Analgesic; antihistamine.
•**acetaminophen and pseudoephedrine hydrochloride.** (ass-cet-ah-MEE-noe-fen and SUE-doe-eh-FED-rin) *USP 34.*
Use: Analgesic; decongestant.
•**acetaminophen, aspirin, and caffeine.** (ass-cet-ah-MEE-noe-fen, as-pihr-in, and KAF-een) *USP 34.*
Use: Analgesic.
acetaminophen, caffeine, and dihydrocodeine bitartrate. (Boca) Acetaminophen 712.8 mg, caffeine 60 mg, dihydrocodeine bitartrate 32 mg. Tab. 30s. *c-III.*
Use: Narcotic analgesic.
acetaminophen, children's. (Geri-Care) Acetaminophen 80 mg. Aspartame, dextrose, mannitol, phenylalanine, sugar. Fruit flavor. Chew. Tab. 30s. *OTC.*
Use: Analgesic.

•**acetaminophen, diphenhydramine hydrochloride, and pseudoephedrine hydrochloride.** (ass-cet-ah-MEE-noe-fen, die-fen-HIGH-druh-meen, and SUE-doe-eh-FED-rin) *USP 34.*
Use: Analgesic; antihistamine, decongestant.
acetaminophen extra strength. (Akyma) Acetaminophen 500 mg. Tab. 100s, 700s, 1000s. *OTC.*
Use: Analgesic.
acetaminophenol.
See: Acetaminophen.
acetanilid. (Various Mfr.) Acetylaminobenzene, acetylaniline, antifebrin.
Use: Analgesic (former use).
Acetasol. (Actavis MidAtlantic) Acetic acid 2% with propylene glycol diacetate 3%, benzethonium chloride 0.02%, sodium acetate 0.015%. Soln. Bot. 15 mL. *Rx.*
Use: Otic preparation.
Acetasol HC. (Actavis MidAtlantic) Hydrocortisone 1%, acetic acid 2%, propylene glycol diacetate 3%, sodium acetate 0.015%, benzethonium chloride 0.02%. Citric acid 0.05%. Soln. Bot. 10 mL with dropper. *Rx.*
Use: Anti-infective; corticosteroid, otic.
Aceta w/Codeine. (Century) Acetaminophen 300 mg, codeine phosphate 30 mg. Tab. Bot. 100s. *c-III.*
Use: Analgesic combination, narcotic.
•**acetazolamide.** (uh-seet-uh-ZOLE-uh-mide) *USP 34.*
Tall Man: acetaZOLAMIDE
Use: Carbonic anhydrase inhibitor; anticonvulsant.
See: Diamox Sequels.
acetazolamide. (Bedford Labs) Acetazolamide 500 mg. Pow. for Inj., lyophilized. Preservative-free. Vials. *Rx.*
Use: Anticonvulsant.
acetazolamide. (Various Mfr.) Acetazolamide. **Tab.**: 125 mg, 250 mg. May contain lactose. 100s, 500s (250 mg only), 1,000s (250 mg only). **ER Cap.**: 500 mg. 100s, 1,000s. *Rx.*
Use: Carbonic anhydrase inhibitor; anticonvulsant.
•**acetazolamide sodium, sterile.** (uh-seet-uh-ZOLE-uh-mide SO-dee-uhm) *USP 34.*
Tall Man: acetaZOLAMIDE
Use: Carbonic anhydrase inhibitor.
acet-dia-mer-sulfonamide. Sulfacetamide, sulfadiazine, and sulfamerazine. Susp. *Rx.*
Use: Antibacterial, sulfonamide.

●**acetic acid.** (ah-SEE-tick) *NF 29.*
Use: Pharmaceutic aid, acidifying agent.
See: Otic Domeboro.
W/Antipyrine, Benzocaine, Polycosanol.
See: AABP.
Auralgan.
acetic acid/antipyrine/benzocaine/poly-cosanol 410. (Brookstone) Acetic acid
0.01%, antipyrine 5.4%, benzocaine
1.4%, polycosanol 410 0.01%, glycerin.
Soln.; Otic. 15 mL w/dropper. *Rx.*
Use: Miscellaneous otic preparation.
●**acetic acid, glacial.** (ah-SEE-tick)
USP 34.
Use: Pharmaceutic aid, acidifying
agent.
W/Combinations.
See: Fem ph.
acetic acid irrigation. (Abbott) Acetic
acid 0.25%. Soln. Glass Cont. 250 mL,
1000 mL.
Use: Irrigating solution.
acetic acid otic. (Various Mfr.) Acetic acid
2% with propylene glycol diacetate 3%,
benzethonium chloride 0.02%, and sodium
acetate 0.015%. Soln. Bot. 15 mL. *Rx.*
Use: Otic preparation.
acetic acid, potassium salt. Potassium
Acetate.
**acetic acid 2% and aluminum acetate
otic.** (Bausch & Lomb) Acetic acid 2%
in aluminum acetate solution. Soln.
60 mL. *Rx.*
Use: Otic preparation.
●**acetohydroxamic acid.** (ass-EE-toe-high-drox-AM-ik) *USP 34.*
Use: Enzyme inhibitor, urease.
See: Lithostat.
acetomeroctol.
Use: Antiseptic, topical.
●**acetone.** (ASS-eh-tone) *NF 29.*
Use: Pharmaceutic aid, solvent.
acetone or diacetic acid test.
See: Acetest Reagent.
acetophenetidin.
Use: Analgesic; antipyretic.
See: Phenacetin.
acetorphan.
Use: Enkephalinase inhibitor.
●**acetosulfone sodium.** (ah-SET-oh-SULL-fone SO-dee-uhm) USAN.
Use: Antibacterial, leprostatic.
acetoxyphenylmercury.
See: Phenylmercuric Acetate.
acetylaniline.
See: Acetanilid.
●**acetylcholine chloride.** (ah-SEH-till-KOE-leen KLOR-ide) *USP 34.*
Use: Cardiovascular agent; cholinergic;
miotic; vasodilator, peripheral.

See: Miochol-E.
acetylcholine-like therapeutic agents.
See: Cholinergic agents.
●**acetylcysteine.** (a-se-teel-SIS-teen)
USP 34.
Use: Antidote; mucolytic.
See: Acetadote.
Mucomyst 10.
acetylcysteine. (Various Mfr.) Acetyl-cysteine 10%, 20%. EDTA. Oral Soln.
Vial 4 mL, 10 mL, 30 mL. *Rx.*
Use: Antidote; mucolytic.
●**acetylcysteine and isoproterenol
hydrochloride inhalation solution.**
(ASS-cee-till-SIS-teen and eye-so-pro-TER-uh-nahl) *USP 34.*
Use: Mucolytic.
acetylin.
See: Acetylsalicylic Acid.
N-acetyl-p-aminophenol. Acetaminophen.
acetylphenylisatin.
See: Oxyphenisatin Acetate.
acetylprocainamide-n.
Use: Cardiovascular agent.
See: Acecainide Hydrochloride.
NAPA.
acetylsalicylic acid.
Use: Analgesic; antipyretic; antirheu-matic.
See: Aspirin.
n¹-acetylsulfanilamide.
Use: Sulfonamide therapy.
acetyl sulfisoxazole.
See: Sulfisoxazole Acetyl.
acetyltannic acid. Tannic acid acetate.
Use: Antiperistaltic.
AC Eye. (Walgreen) Tetrahydrozoline
hydrochloride 0.05%, zinc sulfate
0.25%. Ophth. Drops. Bot. 0.75 oz.
OTC.
Use: Decongestant combination, oph-thalmic.
achlorhydria therapy.
See: Glutamic Acid Hydrochloride.
Achol. (Enzyme Process) Vitamin A
4000 units, ketocholanic acids 62 mg.
Tab. Bot. 100s, 250s. *OTC.*
Use: Vitamin supplement.
acid acriflavine.
See: Acriflavine Hydrochloride.
**acid citrate dextrose anticoagulant
solution modified.**
See: A-C-D Solution Modified.
acid citrate dextrose solution.
See: A-C-D Solution.
Acid Gone. (Major Pharmaceuticals) Alu-minum hydroxide 31.7 mg, magnesium
carbonate 119.33 mg per 5 mL. Ben-zyl alcohol, edetate disodium, glycerin,
saccharin, sodium alginate 13 mg,

sorbitol. Liq. 355 mL. *OTC.*
Use: Antacid combination.
acidifiers.
See: Ammonium Chloride.
K-Phos M.F.
Acid Jelly. (Hope Pharm) Oxyquinoline
sulfate 0.025%, ricinoleic acid 0.7%,
glacial acetic acid 0.921%, glycerin 5%,
propylparaben. Jelly. 85 g with applicator. *OTC.*
Use: Vaginal preparation.
acidophilus.
See: Bacid.
Lactinex.
More Dophilus.
acidophilus. (Mason) *Lactobacillus
acidophilus* 20 million units. Sugar 1 g.
Preservative free. Vanilla-banana flavor. Wafers. 100s. *OTC.*
Use: Nutritional supplement.
acidophilus. (Nature's Bounty) *Lactobacillus acidophilus* > 100 million units.
Beeswax/soybean oil mixture, soybean
oil. Cap. 100s. *OTC.*
Use: Nutritional supplement.
acidophilus with bifidus. (Various Mfr.)
Lactobacillus acidophilus 1 billion units,
Lactobacillus bifidus 25 mg. Sugar 1 g.
Strawberry flavor. Wafers. 100s. *OTC.*
Use: Nutritional supplement.
acidophilus with pectin. (Barth's) *Lactobacillus acidophilus* w/natural citrus
pectin 100 mg. Cap. Bot. 100s. *OTC.*
Use: Antidiarrheal.
Acid Reducer 200. (Major) Cimetidine
200 mg. Tab. 30s. *OTC.*
Use: Histamine H$_2$ antagonists.
acid trypaflavine.
See: Acriflavine Hydrochloride.
Acidulated Phosphate Fluoride. (Scherer) Fluoride ion 0.31% in 0.1 molar
phosphate. Soln. Bot. 64 oz. (Office
Product).
Use: Dental caries agent.
Acid-X. (BDI) Acetaminophen 500 mg,
calcium carbonate 250 mg. Tab. Bot.
36s. *OTC.*
Use: Antacid.
• **acifran.** (AYE-si-fran) USAN.
Use: Antihyperlipoproteinemic.
AcipHex. (Eisai) Rabeprazole sodium
20 mg. Mannitol. Enteric coated. DR
Tab. Bot. 30s, 90s, UD 100s. *Rx.*
Use: Proton pump inhibitor.
• **acitretin.** (ASS-ih-TREH-tin) USAN.
Use: Retinoid, second generation.
See: Soriatane.
Soriatane CK.
• **acivicin.** (ace-ih-VIH-sin) USAN.
Use: Antineoplastic.

Aclaro PD. (JSJ Pharmaceuticals)
Hydroquinone 4%. Benzyl alcohol, cetyl alcohol, EDTA, glycerin, methoxycinnamate. Emulsion. Airless pump bot.
44 mL. *Rx.*
Use: Pigment agent.
• **aclarubicin.** (ack-lah-ROO-bih-sin)
USAN. Formerly Aclacinomycin A.
Use: Antineoplastic.
Aclophen. (Nutripharm Laboratories,
Inc.) Phenylephrine hydrochloride
40 mg, chlorpheniramine maleate 8 mg,
acetaminophen 500 mg, dye free. SR
Tab. Bot. 100s. *Rx.*
Use: Analgesic; antihistamine; decongestant.
Aclovate. (Pharmaderm) Alclometasone
dipropionate 0.05%. Cream or Oint.
Tube 15 g, 45 g. *Rx.*
Use: Anti-inflammatory, topical.
A.C.N. (Person and Covey) Vitamin A
25,000 units, ascorbic acid 250 mg, niacinamide 25 mg. Tab. Bot. 100s. *OTC.*
Use: Vitamin supplement.
Acnaveen.
See: Aveenobar Medicated.
Acna-Vite. (Cenci, H.R. Labs, Inc.) Vitamins A 10,000 units, C 250 mg, hesperidin 50 mg, niacinamide 25 mg. Cap.
Bot. 75s. *OTC.*
Use: Dermatologic, acne; vitamin
supplement.
Acne Clear. (Altaire) Benzoyl peroxide
10%. EDTA. Gel. 45 g. *OTC.*
Use: Topical anti-infective.
Acno Cleanser. (Baker Cummins Dermatologicals) Isopropyl alcohol 60%,
laureth-23, tetrasodium EDTA. Bot.
240 mL. *OTC.*
Use: Dermatologic, acne.
Acnomel. (Numark) Sulfur 8%, resorcinol 2%, alcohol 11%. Cream. Tube
28 g. *OTC.*
Use: Keratolytic, acne product.
Acnotex. (C & M Pharmacal) Sulfur 8%,
resorcinol 2%, isopropyl alcohol 20%,
acetone. In lotion base. Bot. 60 mL.
OTC.
Use: Dermatologic, acne.
• **acodazole hydrochloride.** (ah-KOE-dah-ZOLE) USAN.
Use: Antineoplastic.
• **acolbifene hydrochloride.** (aye-KOLE-bi-feen) USAN.
Use: Breast and uterine proliferation or
cancer.
aconiazide. (Lincoln Diagnostics)
Use: Antituberculous. [Orphan Drug]
Acotus. (Whorton Pharmaceuticals, Inc.)
Phenylephrine hydrochloride 5 mg,

guaiacol glyceryl ether 100 mg, menthol 1 mg, alcohol by volume 10%/5 mL. Bot. 4 oz, 12 oz, gal. *OTC.*
Use: Antitussive; decongestant.
ACR. (Western Research) Ammonium chloride 7.5 g. Tab. *Handicount* 28s (36 bags of 28 tab.). *Rx.*
Use: Diuretic.
acriflavine. (Eli Lilly) Acriflavine 1.5 g. Tab. Bot. 100s.
Use: Antiseptic.
acriflavine hydrochloride. (Various Mfr.) Hydrochloride form of acriflavine. Acid acriflavine, acid trypaflavine, flavine, trypaflavine. National Aniline-Pow., Bot. 1 g, 5 g, 10 g, 25 g, 50 g. Tab. 1.5 g. Bot. 50s, 100s. *Rx.*
Use: Anti-infective.
● **acrisorcin.** (ACK-rih-sahr-sin) USAN.
Use: Antifungal.
See: Akrinol.
● **acrivastine.** (ACK-rih-VASS-teen) USAN.
Use: Antihistamine.
acrivastine and pseudoephedrine hydrochloride.
Use: Upper respiratory combination, antihistamine, decongestant.
See: Semprex-D.
● **acronine.** (ACK-row-neen) USAN.
Use: Antineoplastic.
ACT. Dactinomycin.
Use: Antineoplastic.
See: Actinomycin D.
ACT. (J & J Merck Consumer Pharm.)
Rinse: 0.02% (from 0.05% sodium fluoride). **Mint:** Tartrazine, alcohol 8%. **Cinnamon:** Alcohol 7%. Bot. 360 mL, 480 mL. *OTC.*
Use: Dentrifice.
Actacin. (Vangard Labs, Inc.) Triprolidine hydrochloride 2.5 mg, pseudoephedrine hydrochloride 60 mg. Tab. Bot. 100s, 1000s. *Rx-OTC.*
Use: Antihistamine; decongestant.
Actacin-C. (Vangard Labs, Inc.) Codeine phosphate 10 mg, triprolidine hydrochloride 2 mg, pseudoephedrine hydrochloride 20 mg, guaifenesin 100 mg/ 5 mL. Syr. Bot. Pt, gal. *c-v.*
Use: Antihistamine; antitussive; decongestant; expectorant.
Actal Plus. (Sanofi-Synthelabo) Aluminum hydroxide, magnesium hydroxide. Tab. *OTC.*
Use: Antacid.
Actal Suspension. (Sanofi-Synthelabo) Aluminum hydroxide. Susp. *OTC.*
Use: Antacid.

Actal Tablets. (Sanofi-Synthelabo) Aluminum hydroxide. Tab. *OTC.*
Use: Antacid.
Actamin. (Buffington) Acetaminophen 325 mg. Tab. *Dispens-A-Kit* 100s, 200s, 500s. *OTC.*
Use: Analgesic.
Actamine. (H.L. Moore Drug Exchange) **Tab.:** Pseudoephedrine hydrochloride 60 mg, triprolidine hydrochloride 2.5 mg. Bot. 100s, 1000s. **Syr.:** Pseudoephedrine hydrochloride 30 mg, triprolidine hydrochloride 1.25 mg/5 mL. Bot. 120 mL, Pt, gal. *Rx-OTC.*
Use: Antihistamine; decongestant.
Actamin Extra. (Buffington) Acetaminophen 500 mg. Tab. Bot. 100s, 200s, 500s. *OTC.*
Use: Analgesic.
Actamin Super. (Buffington) Acetaminophen 500 mg, caffeine. Sugar, salt, and lactose free. Tab. *Dispens-A-Kit* 500s, *Medipak* 200s. *OTC.*
Use: Analgesic.
Actemra. (Genetech Inc) Tocilizumab 20 mg/mL. Disodium phosphate dodecahydrate, sodium dihydrogen phosphate dehydrate (as a 15 mmol/L phosphate buffer), sucrose 50 mg/mL. Preservative free. Inj., Soln., concentrate. Single-use vial. 4 mL, 10 mL, 20 mL. *Rx.*
Use: Immunologic agent, immunomodulator.
ACTH. Adrenocorticotrophic hormone. Adrenocorticotropin.
Use: Corticosteroid.
See: Corticotropin.
ACTH-Actest. (Forest) Repository corticotropin 40 units or 80 units/mL. Gel. Vial 5 mL. *Rx.*
Use: Corticosteroid.
ActHIB. (Aventis Pasteur) Purified capsular polysaccharide of Haemophilus b 10 mcg, tetanus toxoid 24 mcg/0.5 mL. Sucrose 8.5%. Pow. for Inj., lyophilized. Single-dose vials with 7.5 mL vials of diphtheria and tetanus toxoids and pertussis vaccine as diluents or 0.6 mL vial containing 0.4% sodium chloride diluent. *Rx.*
Use: Agent for active immunization, bacterial vaccine.
ActHIB/DTP. (Aventis Pasteur) Diphtheria and tetanus toxoids and pertussis and *Haemophilus influenzae* type b vaccines. One package consists of one 7.5 mL vial of Connaught's DTwP and 10 single-dose vials of ActHIB vaccine. *Rx.*
Use: Immunization.

Acthrel. (Ferring) Corticorelin ovine triflutata 100 mcg. Cake, lyophilized. 5 mL single-dose vial w/diluent. *Rx.*
Use: Diagnostic aid.

ActiBath. (Andrew Jergens) Colloidal oatmeal 20%. Tab. Effervescent. Pkg. 4s. *OTC.*
Use: Emollient.

Acticin. (Bertek) Permethrin 5%. Coconut oil, lanolin alcohols, light mineral oil. Cream. Tube 60 g. *Rx.*
Use: Scabicide.

Acticort 100. (Baker Cummins Dermatologicals) Hydrocortisone 1%. Lot. Bot. 60 mL. *Rx.*
Use: Corticosteroid, topical.

Actidose. (Paddock) Activated charcoal. 25 g/120 mL or 50 g/240 mL. Soln. *OTC.*
Use: Antidote.

Actidose-Aqua. (Paddock) Activated charcoal. 25 g/120 mL or 50 g/240 mL. Aqueous susp. *OTC.*
Use: Antidote.

Actidose w/Sorbitol. (Paddock) Activated charcoal. 25 g in 120 mL susp. w/sorbitol, 50 g in 240 mL susp. w/sorbitol. Liq. *OTC.*
Use: Antidote.

Actifed Cold & Allergy. (J & J) Phenylephrine hydrochloride 10 mg, chlorpheniramine maleate 4 mg. Tab. Pkg. 12s. *OTC.*
Use: Upper respiratory combination, antihistamine, decongestant.

Actifed Cold & Sinus Maximum Strength. (J & J) Pseudoephedrine hydrochloride 30 mg, chlorpheniramine maleate 2 mg, acetaminophen 500 mg. Tab. Pkg. 20s. *OTC.*
Use: Upper respiratory combination, analgesic, antihistamine, decongestant.

Actigall. (Watson) Ursodiol (Ursodeoxycholic acid) 300 mg. Cap. Bot. 100s. *Rx.*
Use: Gallstone solubilizing agent.

Actimmune. (InterMune) Interferon gamma-1b 100 mcg (2 million units) per 0.5 mL. Mannitol 20 mg, sodium succinate 0.36 mg, polysorbate 20 0.05 mg. Preservative free. Single-dose vials. *Rx.*
Use: Immunologic agent, immunomodulator.

actinomycin C. Name previously used for Cactinomycin.

actinomycin D.
Use: Antineoplastic.
See: Dactinomycin.

•**actinoquinol sodium.** (ack-TIN-oh-kwih-nole SO-dee-uhm) USAN.
Use: Ultraviolet screen.

actinospectacin. *Name previously used for Spectinomycin.*

Actiq. (Cephalon) Fentanyl citrate (as base) 200 mcg, 400 mcg, 600 mcg, 800 mcg, 1,200 mcg, 1,600 mcg. Sugar (each unit contains ≈ 2 g), berry flavor. Loz. on a stick. 30s with carton blister packs. *c-II.*
Use: Opioid analgesic.

•**actisomide.** (ackt-EYE-so-MIDE) USAN.
Use: Cardiovascular agent.

Activase. (Genentech) Alteplase recombinant 50 mg (29 million U), 100 mg (58 million U). L-arginine, phosphoric acid, polysorbate 80. Pow. for Inj., lyophilized. Vials with diluent (50 mL sterile water for injection) and vacuum (50 mg only); vials with diluent (100 mL sterile water for injection) and 1 transfer device (100 mg only). *Rx.*
Use: Thrombolytic.

activated attapulgite. *OTC.*
Use: Dermatologic, acne.
W/Polysorbate 80, colloidal sulfur, salicylic acid, propylene glycol.
See: Sebasorb.

activated charcoal liquid. (Various Mfr.) Activated charcoal 12.5 g, 25 g with propylene glycol. Liq. Bot. 60 mL (12.5 g), 120 mL (25 g). *OTC.*
Use: Antidote.

activated charcoal powder. (Various Mfr.) Activated charcoal 15 g, 30 g, 40 g, 120 g, and 140 g. Pow. *OTC.*
Use: Antidote.

activated charcoal tablets. (Cowley) Activated charcoal 5 g. Tab. Bot. 1000s. *OTC.*
Use: Antidote.

activated ergosterol.
See: Calciferol.

activated 7-dehydrocholesterol.
See: Cholecalciferol.

active immunization agents.
See: Toxoids.
Vaccines, Bacterial.
Vaccines, Viral.

Activella. (Novo Nordisk) Estradiol/norethindrone acetate 0.5 mg/0.1 mg, 1 mg/0.5 mg. Lactose. Film coated. Tab. Dial packs. 28s. *Rx.*
Use: Sex hormone, estrogen and progestin combined.

•**actodigin.** (ACK-toe-dihj-in) USAN.
Use: Cardiovascular agent.

Actonel. (Procter & Gamble) Risedronate sodium 5 mg, 30 mg, 35 mg, 150 mg. Lactose (except 150 mg). Film coated. Tab. 30s (5 mg, 30 mg only), 2000s (5 mg only), dose packs of 1s (150 mg only), dose packs of 3s (150 mg only), dose packs of 4s (35 mg only), dose pack of 12s (35 mg only). *Rx.*

Use: Bisphosphonate.
Actonel with Calcium. (Warner Chilcott)
Risedronate 35 mg. Calcium carbonate
1250 mg (equivalent to elemental cal-
cium 500 mg). Lactose. Film coated.
Tab. 28-day blister packages with 4 rise-
dronate tablets and 24 calcium tab-
lets. *Rx.*
Use: Bisphosphonate.
Actoplus Met. (Takeda) Pioglitazone
hydrochloride and metformin hydro-
chloride 15 mg/500 mg, 15 mg/850 mg.
Film coated. Tab. 60s, 180s. *Rx.*
Use: Antidiabetic combination.
ActoPlus Met XR. (Takeda) Pioglitazone/
ER metformin hydrochloride 15 mg/
1,000 mg, 30 mg/1,000 mg. Film
coated. Lactose, PEG. ER Tab. 30s,
60s, 90s. *Rx.*
Use: Antidiabetic agent.
actoquinol sodium.
Use: Ultraviolet screen.
Actos. (Takeda) Pioglitazone hydrochlo-
ride 15 mg, 30 mg, 45 mg. Lactose.
Tab. Bot. 30s, 90s, 500s. *Rx.*
Use: Antidiabetic, thiazolidinedione.
Acucron. (Seatrace) Acetaminophen
300 mg, salicylamide 200 mg, phenyl-
toloxamine 20 mg. Tab. Bot. 100s,
1000s, 5000s. *OTC.*
Use: Analgesic; antihistamine.
Acu-Dyne. (Acme United Corp.)
Douche: Povidone-iodine. Pkt. 240 mL.
Oint.: Povidone-iodine. Jar. lb. Pkt.
1.2 g, 2.7 g (100s). **Perineal wash
conc.:** Available iodine 1%. Bot. 40 mL.
Prep. Soln.: Povidone-iodine. Bot.
240 mL, Pt, qt, gal. Pkt. 30 mL, 60 mL.
Skin Cleanser: Povidone-iodine. Bot.
60 mL, 240 mL, Pt, qt, gal. **Soln., prep.
swabs:** Available iodine 1%. Bot. 100s.
Soln., swabsticks: Povidone-iodine.
Pkt. 1 or 3 in 25s. **Whirlpool conc.:**
Available iodine 1%. Bot. gal. *OTC.*
Use: Antiseptic; antimicrobial.
Acular. (Allergan) Ketorolac tromethamine 0.5%. Benzalkonium chloride
0.01%, EDTA 0.1%, octoxynol 40, sodium chloride, hydrochloric acid, and/or
sodium hydroxide. Ophth. Soln. Drop.
Bot. 3 mL, 5 mL, 10 mL. *Rx.*
Use: Nonsteroidal anti-inflammatory
drug, ophthalmic.
Acular LS. (Allergan) Ketorolac tromethamine 0.4%. Benzalkonium chloride
0.006%, EDTA 0.015%, sodium chloride, hydrochloric acid, and/or sodium
hydroxide. Ophth. Soln. Drop. Bot.
5 mL. *Rx.*
Use: Nonsteroidal anti-inflammatory
drug, ophthalmic.

Acuvail. (Allergan) Ketorolac tromethamine 0.45%. Sodium chloride, hydrochloric acid, sodium hydroxide. Preservative free. Single-use vial. 0.4 mL. *Rx.*
Use: Ophthalmic and otic agent, nonsteroidal anti-inflammatory drug.
•**acyclovir.** (A-SIKE-low-vir) *USP 34.*
Use: Antiviral.
See: Zovirax.
W/Hydrocortisone.
See: Xerese.
acyclovir. (Various Mfr.) Acyclovir. **Tab.:**
400 mg, 800 mg. Bot. 100s, 500s,
1000s (400 mg only). **Cap.:** 200 mg.
Bot. 100s. **Susp.:** 200 mg/5 mL.
473 mL. *Rx.*
Use: Antiviral.
•**acyclovir sodium.** (A-SIKE-low-vir)
USAN.
Use: Antiviral.
See: Zovirax.
acyclovir sodium. (Various Mfr.) Acyclovir sodium. **Inj.:** 50 mg/mL. Ctns. of 10.
Pow. for Inj.: 500 mg/vial, 1000 mg/
vial. Vials. 10 mL (500 mg only), 20 mL
(1000 mg only). *Rx.*
Use: Antiviral.
Aczone. (Allergan) Dapsone 5%. Methylparaben. Gel, Top. 30 g. *Rx.*
Use: Topical anti-infective.
Adacel. (Aventis Pasteur) Diphtheria toxoid 2 Lf units, tetanus toxoid 5 Lf units,
pertactin 3 mcg, filamentous hemagglutinin (FHA) 5 mcg, detoxified pertussis toxins 2.5 mcg, fimbriae types 2
and 3 5 mcg per 0.5 mL. Formaldehyde,
phenoxyethanol. Inj. Single-dose vials. *Rx.*
Use: Immunization.
Adagen. (Enzon) Pegademase bovine
250 units/mL. Vial 1.5 mL. *Rx.*
Use: Enzyme (ADA) replacement
therapy.
Adalat CC. (Schering) Nifedipine 30 mg,
60 mg, 90 mg. Lactose. Film coated.
ER Tab. Bot. 100s, 1000s (except
90 mg), UD 100s. *Rx.*
Use: Calcium channel blocker.
•**adalimumab.** (ah-dah-LIM-you-mab)
USAN.
Use: Immunomodulator.
See: Humira.
adamantanamine hydrochloride.
See: Amantadine Hydrochloride.
Symmetrel.
•**adapalene.** (ADE-ah-PALE-een) USAN.
Use: Dermatologic, acne, retinoid.
See: Differin.
W/Benzoyl Peroxide.
See: Epiduo.

*Adcica : $2/12 Rovatio. (Viagra)
PAH* (handwritten)

adapalene. (Fougera) Adapalene 0.1%. Edetate disodium, glycerin, parabens, PEG-20, phenoxyethanol, squalane, trolamine. Cream 45 g. *Rx.*
Use: Retinoid.

adapalene. (Various Mfr.) Adapalene. **Cream:** 0.1%. Edetate disodium, glycerin, parabens, PEG-20, phenoxyethanol, squalane, trolamine. 45 g. **Gel:** 0.1%. Disodium edetate, methylparaben, propylene glycol. 45 g. *Rx.*
Use: Retinoid.

Adapettes for Sensitive Eyes. (Alcon) Povidone and other water-soluble polymers, EDTA, sorbic acid. Pkg. 15 mL. *OTC.*
Use: Contact lens care.

Adapin. (Lotus Biochemical) Doxepin hydrochloride **10 mg, 75 mg, 100 mg:** Cap. Bot. 100s, 1000s, UD 100s. **25 mg, 50 mg:** Cap. Bot. 100s, 1000s, 5000s, UD 100s. **150 mg:** Cap. Bot. 50s, 100s. *Rx.*
Use: Antidepressant.

• **adaprolol maleate.** (ad-AH-prole-ole MAL-ee-ate) USAN.
Use: Antihypertensive, β-blocker, ophthalmic.

Adapt. (Alcon) Povidone, EDTA 0.1%, thimerosal 0.004%. Bot. 15 mL. *OTC.*
Use: Contact lens care.

Adapt Wetting Solution. (Alcon) Adsorbobase with thimerosal 0.004%, EDTA 0.1%. Soln. Bot. 15 mL. *OTC.*
Use: Contact lens care.

• **adatanserin hydrochloride.** (ahd-at-AN-ser-in HIGH-droe-KLOR-ide) USAN.
Use: Antidepressant; anxiolytic.

AdatoSil 5000. (Escalon Ophthalmics, Inc.) Polydimethylsiloxane oil. Inj. Vial 10 mL, 15 mL. *Rx.*
Use: Ophthalmic.

Adavite. (Hudson Corp.) Vitamins A 5000 units, D 400 units, E 30 mg, B_1 3 mg, B_2 3.4 mg, B_3 30 mg, B_5 10 mg, B_6 3 mg, B_{12} 9 mcg, C 90 mg, folic acid 0.4 mg, biotin 35 mcg, beta-carotene 1250 units. Tab. Bot. 130s. *OTC.*
Use: Mineral, vitamin supplement.

Adavite-M. (Hudson Corp.) Iron 27 mg, Vitamins A 5000 units, D 400 units, E 30 mg, B_1 3 mg, B_2 3.4 mg, B_3 20 mg, B_5 10 mg, B_6 3 mg, B_{12} 9 mcg, C 190 mg, folic acid 0.4 mg, Ca, Cl, Cr, Cu, I, K, Mg, Mn, Mo, P, Se, Zinc 15 mg, biotin 30 mcg. Tab. Bot. 130s. *OTC.*
Use: Mineral, vitamin supplement.

Adcirca. (Eli Lilly) Tadalafil 20 mg. Film coated. Lactose. Tab. 60s. *Rx.*
Use: Impotence agent, phosphodiesterase type 5 inhibitor.

ADC with Fluoride. (Various Mfr.) Fluoride 0.5 mg, vitamins A 1500 units, D 400 units, C 35 mg, methylparaben/mL. Drops. Bot. 50 mL. *Rx.*
Use: Mineral, vitamin supplement.

Adderall. (Teva) **5 mg:** Dextroamphetamine saccharate 1.25 mg, amphetamine aspartate 1.25 mg, dextroamphetamine sulfate 1.25 mg, amphetamine sulfate 1.25 mg. **7.5 mg:** Dextroamphetamine saccharate 1.875 mg, amphetamine aspartate 1.875 mg, dextroamphetamine sulfate 1.875 mg, amphetamine sulfate 1.875 mg. **10 mg:** Dextroamphetamine sulfate 2.5 mg, dextroamphetamine saccharate 2.5 mg, amphetamine aspartate 2.5 mg, amphetamine sulfate 2.5 mg. **12.5 mg:** Dextroamphetamine saccharate 3.125 mg, amphetamine aspartate 3.125 mg, dextroamphetamine sulfate 3.125 mg, amphetamine sulfate 3.125 mg. **15 mg:** Dextroamphetamine saccharate 3.75 mg, amphetamine aspartate monohydrate 3.75 mg, dextroamphetamine sulfate 3.75 mg, amphetamine sulfate 3.75 mg. **20 mg:** Dextroamphetamine sulfate 5 mg, dextroamphetamine saccharate 5 mg, amphetamine aspartate 5 mg, amphetamine sulfate 5 mg. **30 mg:** Dextroamphetamine saccharate 7.5 mg, amphetamine aspartate 7.5 mg, dextroamphetamine sulfate 7.5 mg, amphetamine sulfate 7.5 mg. Lactose, sucrose. Tab. Bot. 100s. *c-II.*
Use: CNS stimulant, amphetamine.

Adderall XR. (Shire) **5 mg:** Dextroamphetamine saccharate 1.25 mg, amphetamine aspartate monohydrate 1.25 mg, dextroamphetamine sulfate 1.25 mg, amphetamine sulfate 1.25 mg. **10 mg:** Dextroamphetamine saccharate 2.5 mg, amphetamine aspartate monohydrate 2.5 mg, dextroamphetamine sulfate 2.5 mg, amphetamine sulfate 2.5 mg. **15 mg:** Dextroamphetamine saccharate 3.75 mg, amphetamine aspartate monohydrate 3.75 mg, dextroamphetamine sulfate 3.75 mg, amphetamine sulfate 3.75 mg. **20 mg:** Dextroamphetamine saccharate 5 mg, amphetamine aspartate monohydrate 5 mg, dextroamphetamine sulfate 5 mg, amphetamine sulfate 5 mg. **25 mg:** Dextroamphetamine saccharate 6.25 mg, amphetamine aspartate monohydrate 6.25 mg, dextroamphetamine sulfate 6.25 mg, amphetamine sulfate 6.25 mg. **30 mg:** Dextroamphetamine saccharate 7.5 mg, amphet-

amine aspartate monohydrate 7.5 mg,
dextroamphetamine sulfate 7.5 mg,
amphetamine sulfate 7.5 mg. Talc (ex-
cept 10 mg, 20 mg, 30 mg). Sugar
spheres. Cap. Bot. 100s. *c-II.*
Use: CNS stimulant, amphetamine.
Adeecon. (CMC) Vitamins A 5000 units,
D 1000 units. Cap. Bot. 1000s. *OTC.*
Use: Vitamin supplement.
•**adefovir dipivoxil.** (ah-DEF-fah-vihr die-
pih-vox-ill) USAN.
Use: Antiviral, treatment of HIV and
HBV infections.
See: Hepsera.
ADEKs Pediatric. (Scandipharm, Inc.)
Vitamin A 1500 units, D 400 units, E
40 units, K_1 0.1 mg, C 45 mg, B_1
0.5 mg, B_2 0.6 mg, B_3 6 mg, B_5 3 mg,
B_6 0.6 mg, B_{12} 4 mcg, biotin 15 mcg, Zn
5 mg, beta-carotene 1 mg per mL.
Drops. Bot. 60 mL. *OTC.*
Use: Vitamin supplement.
•**adenine.** (A-de-neen) *USP 34.*
Use: Vitamin.
**adeno-associated viral-based vector
cystic fibrosis gene therapy.**
(Targeted Genetics)
Use: Cystic fibrosis. [Orphan Drug]
Adenocard. (Fujisawa) Adenosine 3 mg/
mL, sodium chloride 9 mg/mL. Preser-
vative free. Inj. Vial. 2 mL. Syringe.
2 mL, 5 mL. *Rx.*
Use: Antiarrhythmic.
Adenolin Forte. (Lincoln Diagnostics)
Adenosine-5-monophosphate 25 mg,
methionine 25 mg, niacin 10 mg/mL. Inj.
Vial 15 mL. *Rx.*
Use: Anti-inflammatory.
Adenoscan. (Fujisawa Healthcare)
Adenosine 3 mg/mL. Sodium chloride
9 mg/mL. Preservative free. Inj. Single-
dose vial. 20 mL, 30 mL. *Rx.*
Use: Diagnostic aid.
•**adenosine.** (ah-DEN-oh-seen) *USP 34.*
Use: Antiarrhythmic.
See: Adenocard.
Adenoscan.
adenosine. (Medco Research)
Use: Antineoplastic. [Orphan Drug]
adenosine. (Various Mfr.) Adenosine
3 mg/mL. Sodium chloride 9 mg/mL.
Preservative free. Inj. Vials. 2 mL, 4 mL.
Disposable syringes. 2 mL. *Rx.*
Use: Antiarrhythmic agent.
adenosine in gelatin. (Forest) **Forte:**
Adenosine-5-monophosphate 50 mg/
mL. **Super:** Adenosine-5-monophos-
phate 100 mg/mL. *Rx.*
Use: Varicosity.

Adeno Twelve. (Forest) Adenosine-5-
monophosphate 25 mg, methionine
25 mg, niacin 10 mg/mL. Gel. Inj. Vial
10 mL. *Rx.*
Use: Anti-inflammatory.
adenovirus vaccine type 4. (Wyeth)
Adenovirus vaccine live type 4. At least
32,000 $TCID_{50}$. Tab. Bot. 100s. *Rx.*
Use: Immunization.
adenovirus vaccine type 7. (Wyeth)
Adenovirus vaccine live type 7. At least
32,000 $TCID_{50}$. Tab. Bot. 100s. *Rx.*
Use: Immunization.
adepsine oil.
See: Petrolatum.
AdGVCFTR 10. (GenVec)
Use: Cystic fibrosis. [Orphan Drug]
•**adinazolam.** (AHD-in-AZE-oh-lam)
USAN.
Use: Antidepressant; hypnotic, sedative.
•**adinazolam mesylate.** (AHD-in-AZE-oh-
lam MEH-sih-LATE) USAN.
Use: Antidepressant.
Adipex-P. (Gate) **Cap.:** Phentermine
hydrochloride 37.5 mg, lactose. Bot.
100s. **Tab.:** Phentermine hydrochloride
37.5 mg, lactose, sucrose. Bot. 30s,
100s, 1000s. *c-IV.*
Use: CNS stimulant, anorexiant.
•**adiphenine hydrochloride.** (ah-DIH-feh-
neen HIGH-droe-KLOR-ide) USAN.
Use: Muscle relaxant.
Adisol. (Major) Disulfiram 250 mg,
500 mg. Tab. Bot. 50s (500 mg only),
100s (250 mg only). *Rx.*
Use: Antialcoholic.
Adlerika. (Last) Magnesium sulfate 4 g/
15 mL. Bot. 12 oz. *OTC.*
Use: Laxative.
Adlone. (Forest) Methylprednisolone
acetate 40 mg, 80 mg. Inj. Vial 5 mL.
Rx.
Use: Corticosteroid, topical.
Adolph's Salt Substitute. (Adolphs)
Potassium chloride 2480 mg/5 g, silicon
dioxide, tartaric acid. Gran. Bot. 99.2 g.
OTC.
Use: Salt substitute.
Adolph's Seasoned Salt Substitute.
(Adolphs) Potassium chloride 1360 mg/
5 g, silicon dioxide, tartaric acid. Gran.
Bot. 92.1 g. *OTC.*
Use: Salt substitute.
•**adomiparin.** (A-doe-mi-PAR-in) USAN.
Use: Anticoagulant.
•**adomiparin sodium.** (A-doe-mi-PAR-in)
USAN.
Use: Anticoagulant.
Adonidine. (City Chemical Corp.) Bot. g.
Rx.

Use: Cardiovascular agent.
Adoxa. (Doak) Doxycycline monohydrate. **Cap.:** 150 mg. 60s. **Tab.:** 75 mg, 100 mg, 150 mg. Lactose. Film coated. ADOXA Paks. 30s (150 mg only), 31s (except 150 mg), 60s (100 mg only). *Rx.*
Use: Anti-infective, tetracycline.
•**adozelesin.** (ADE-oh-ZELL-eh-sin) USAN.
Use: Antineoplastic.
Adprin-B. (Pfeiffer) Aspirin 325 mg, calcium carbonate, magnesium carbonate, magnesium oxide. Tab. Bot. 130s. *OTC.*
Use: Analgesic.
ADR.
Use: Antineoplastic.
See: Doxorubicin Hydrochloride.
adrenalin chloride. (JHP Pharmaceuticals) Epinephrine (as hydrochloride) **Soln., intranasal:** 1:1,000 (1 mg/mL). Chlorobutanol, sodium bisulfite. 30 mL. **Inj., Soln.:** 1:1,000 (1 mg/mL) Vial. 1 mL (w/sodium bisulfite), 30 mL (w/ chlorobutanol and sodium bisulfite). *Rx.*
Use: Vasopressor used in shock.
adrenalin(e).
See: Epinephrine.
adrenaline hydrochloride.
See: Epinephrine Hydrochloride.
•**adrenalone.** (ah-DREN-ah-lone) USAN.
Use: Adrenergic, ophthalmic.
adrenamine.
See: Epinephrine.
adrenergic agents.
See: Sympathomimetic agents.
adrenergic-blocking agents.
See: Sympatholytic agents.
adrenine.
See: Epinephrine.
adrenocortical steroids.
See: Corticotropin.
  Corticotropin, repository injection.
  Glucocorticoids.
  Mineralocorticoids.
adrenocorticotrophic hormone. ACTH acts by stimulating the endogenous production of cortisone. *Rx.*
See: ACTH.
  Corticotropin.
Adrenomist Inhalant and Nebulizers. (Nephron) Epinephrine 1%. Bot. 0.5 oz, 1.25 oz. *Rx-OTC.*
Use: Bronchodilator.
Adrenucleo. (Enzyme Process) Vitamin C 250 mg, d-calcium pantothenate 12.5 mg, bioflavonoids 62.5 mg. Tab. Bot. 100s, 250s. *OTC.*
Use: Vitamin supplement.

AdreView. (GE Healthcare) Iobenguane sulfate I 123 74 MBq (2 mCi) per mL at calibration (each mL contains iobenguane sulfate 0.08 mg, sodium dihydrogen phosphate dihydrate 23 mg, disodium hydrogen phosphate dihydrate 2.8 mg, benzyl alcohol 10.3 mg [1% v/v]). Preservative free. Single-use vial. 5 mL. *Rx.*
Use: Radiopharmaceutical.
Adriamycin PFS. (Pharmacia & Upjohn) Doxorubicin hydrochloride 2 mg/mL. Preservative free. Inj. Single-dose vials. 5 mL, 10 mL, 25 mL, 37.5 mL. Multi-dose vials. 100 mL. *Rx.*
Use: Antibiotic, anthracycline.
Adriamycin RDF. (Pharmacia & Upjohn) Doxorubicin hydrochloride 10 mg (lactose 50 mg), 20 mg (lactose 100 mg), 50 mg (lactose 250 mg), 150 mg (lactose 750 mg). Methylparaben. Pow. for Soln., Inj., Lyophilized. Single-dose vial, multiple-dose vial (150 mg only). Rapid dissolution formula. *Rx.*
Use: Antibiotic, anthracycline.
•**adrogolide hydrochloride.** (a-DROEgoe-lide) USAN.
Use: Parkinson disease.
Adrucil. (Gensia Sicor) Fluorouracil 50 mg/mL. Inj. Vial 10 mL, 50 mL, 100 mL. *Rx.*
Use: Antineoplastic; antimetabolite.
Adsorbocarpine. (Alcon) Pilocarpine hydrochloride 1%, 2%, 4%. Bot. 15 mL. *Rx.*
Use: Miotic.
Adsorbotear. (Alcon) Hydroxyethylcellulose 0.4%, povidone 1.67%, water-soluble polymers, thimerosal 0.004%, EDTA 0.1%. Soln. Bot. dropper 15 mL. *OTC.*
Use: Artificial tears.
Adult Acnomel. (Numark) Sulfur 8%. resorcinol 2%, alcohol 15%, propylene glycol. Cream. Tube. 28 g. *OTC.*
Use: Keratolytic, acne product.
Advair Diskus. (GlaxoSmithKline) Fluticasone propionate 100 mcg, salmeterol 50 mcg; fluticasone propionate 250 mcg, salmeterol 50 mcg; fluticasone propionate 500 mcg, salmeterol 50 mcg. Lactose. Pow. for Inh. Disp. device w/28 and 60 blisters. *Rx.*
Use: Respiratory inhalant combination.
Advair HFA. (GlaxoSmithKline) Fluticasone propionate/salmeterol 45 mg/ 21 mcg, 115 mg/21 mcg, 230 mg/ 21 mcg. Inh. Aerosol Spray. 12 g pressurized aluminum canister containing 120 metered inhalations. Boxes. 1s. *Rx.*
Use: Respiratory inhalant combination.

Advance. (Ross) **Ready-to-Feed Infant Formula:** (16 cal/fl oz). Can 13 fl oz. **Conc. Liq:** 32 fl oz. *OTC.*
Use: Nutritional supplement.

Advanced Care Cholesterol Test. (Johnson & Johnson)
Use: At home cholesterol test.

Advanced D5000. (Mason Vitamins) Vitamin D 5,000 units. Soybean oil. Cap., softgel. 50s. *OTC.*
Use: Fat-soluble vitamin.

Advanced Ear Health Formula. (Mason) Vitamin B_1 0.33 mg, B_2 1 mg, B_3 3.33 mg, B_5 1.66 mg, B_6 1.66 mg, B_{12} 300 mcg, Ca, bioflavonoids 300 mg, choline 111.33 mg, inositol 111.33 mg. Sugar free. Tab. 100s. *OTC.*
Use: Multivitamin with minerals.

Advanced Eye Relief. (Bausch & Lomb) Propylene glycol 0.95%, boric acid, edentate disodium, sodium borate, sodium chloride. Preservative free. Soln., Ophth. Single-use container. *OTC.*
Use: Artificial tear solution.

Advanced Eye Relief, Redness Instant Relief. (Bausch & Lomb) Naphazoline hydrochloride 0.012%. 0.2% of polyethylene 300, benzalkonium chloride 0.01%, boric acid, sodium borate, sodium chloride, EDTA. Soln., Ophth. 15 mL. *Rx.*
Use: Ophthalmic and otic agent, ophthalmic decongestant.

Advanced Eye Relief, Redness Maximum Relief. (Bausch & Lomb) Naphazoline hydrochloride 0.03%. Benzalkonium chloride 0.01%, boric acid, EDTA, hydroxypropyl methylcellulose 0.5%, sodium borate, sodium chloride. Soln., Ophth. 15 mL. *OTC.*
Use: Ophthalmic and otic agent, ophthalmic decongestant.

Advanced Formula Centrum Liquid. (Wyeth) Vitamins A 2500 units, E 30 units, C 60 mg, B_1 1.5 mg, B_2 1.7 mg, B_3 20 mg, B_5 10 mg, B_6 2 mg, B_{12} 6 mcg, D 400 units, iron 9 mg, biotin 300 mcg, I, Zn 3 mg, Mn, Cr, Mo, alcohol 6.7%, sucrose. Bot. 236 mL. *OTC.*
Use: Mineral, vitamin supplement.

Advanced Formula Centrum Tablets. (Wyeth) Iron 18 mg, vitamins A 5000 units, D 400 units, E 30 units, B_1 1.5 mg, B_2 1.7 mg, B_3 20 mg, B_5 10 mg, B_6 2 mg, B_{12} 6 mcg, C 60 mg, folic acid 0.4 mg, biotin 30 mcg, B, Ca, Cl, Cr, Cu, I, K, Mg, Mn, Mo, Ni, P, Se, Si, Sn, V, Zn 15 mg, vitamin K. Bot. 60s, 130s, 200s. *OTC.*
Use: Mineral, vitamin supplement.

Advanced Formula Zenate. (Solvay) Fe 65 mg, vitamins A 3000 units, D 400 units, E 10 units, C 70 mg, folic acid 1 mg, B_1 1.5 mg, B_2 1.6 mg, B_3 17 mg, B_6 2.2 mg, B_{12} 2.2 mcg, Ca 200 mg, I 175 mcg, Mg 100 mg, Zn 15 mg. Tab. UD 30s. *Rx.*
Use: Mineral, vitamin supplement.

Advance Pregnancy Test. (Johnson & Johnson) Can be used as early as 3 days after a missed period. Gives results in 30 min. Test kit 1s.
Use: Diagnostic aid.

Advantage 24. (Women's Health Institute) Nonoxynol 93.5%. Gel. 1.5 g (3s, 6s). *OTC.*
Use: Contraceptive, spermicide.

Advate. (Baxter) Antihemophilic factor (recombinant) 250, 500, 1000, 1500, 2000, 3000 units. Glutathione, histidine, sodium, no more than von Willebrand Factor 2 ng/AHF unit. Sodium 108 mEq/L. Plasma/albumin free and preservative-free. Monoclonal purified and solvent-detergent treated. Pow. for Inj. Single-dose vial with 5 mL sterile water for injection. *Rx.*
Use: Antihemophilic agent.

Advera. (Ross) Protein 14.2 g, fat 5.4 g, carbohydrate 51.2 g, l-carnitine 30 mg, taurine 50 mg, vitamins A 2550 units, D 80 units, E 9 units, K 24 mcg, C 90 mg, folic acid 120 mcg, B, 0.75 mg, B_2 0.68 mg, B_6 9.5 mg, B_{12} 12 mcg, niacin 6 mg, choline 50 mg, biotin 50 mcg, B_5 3 mg, sodium 250 mg, potassium 670 mg, chloride 350 mg, Ca 260 mg, Ph 260 mg, Mg 50 mg, I 30 mcg, Mn 1.3 mg, Cu 0.5 mg, Zn 2 mg, Fe 4.5 mg, Se 14 mcg, chromium 17 mcg, Md 54 mcg/240 mL, 1.28 calories/mL, vanilla flavor. Liq. Bot. 273 mL. *OTC.*
Use: Nutritional supplement, enteral.

Advicor. (Abbott Laboratories) Niacin (extended release)/lovastatin 500 mg/20 mg, 750 mg/20 mg, 1,000 mg/20 mg, 1,000 mg/40 mg. PEG. Tab. 90s. *Rx.*
Use: Antihyperlipidemic.

Advil. (Wyeth) Ibuprofen. **Cap.:** 200 mg. Sorbitol. 4s, 20s, 40s, 80s. **Tab.:** 200 mg. Sucrose. Tab. Bot. 8s, 24s, 50s, 72s, 100s, 165s, 250s. *OTC.*
Use: Analgesic; NSAID.

Advil Allergy Sinus. (Pfizer) Pseudoephedrine hydrochloride 30 mg, chlorpheniramine maleate 2 mg, ibuprofen 200 mg. PEG. Tab. 20s, 40s. *OTC.*
Use: Upper respiratory combination, decongestant, antihistamine, analgesic.

Advil, Children's. (Wyeth) Ibuprofen 100 mg/5 mL. Fruit flavor, sorbitol, sucrose, EDTA. Susp. Bot. 119 mL, 473 mL. *OTC.*
Use: Analgesic; NSAID.

Advil Cold & Sinus. (Wyeth) Pseudoephedrine hydrochloride 30 mg, ibuprofen 200 mg. Parabens, sucrose. **Liqui-gels:** Liquid filled. PEG, sorbitol. 16s. **Tab.:** Bot. 20s. *OTC.*
Use: Upper respiratory combination, analgesic, decongestant.

Advil Flu & Body Ache. (Wyeth) Pseudoephedrine hydrochloride 30 mg, ibuprofen 200 mg, parabens, sucrose. Tab. Pkg. 20s. *OTC.*
Use: Upper respiratory combination, analgesic, decongestant.

Advil Liqui-Gels. (Wyeth) Ibuprofen 200 mg. Sorbitol. Cap. Bot. 4s, 20s, 40s, 80s. *OTC.*
Use: Analgesic; NSAID.

Advil Migraine. (Wyeth) Ibuprofen 200 mg. Sorbitol. Cap. Bot. 20s. *OTC.*
Use: Analgesic; NSAID.

Advil Pediatric Drops. (Wyeth) Ibuprofen 100 mg/2.5 mL. Sorbitol, sucrose, EDTA, glycerin, grape flavor. Susp. Bot. 7.5 mL. *OTC.*
Use: Analgesic; NSAID.

Advil PM. (Wyeth) **Cap.:** Diphenhydramine citrate 38 mg, ibuprofen 200 mg. Lactose. 20s, UD 50s. **Tab.:** Diphenhydramine hydrochloride 25 mg, ibuprofen 200 mg. Sorbitol. 38s. *OTC.*
Use: Nonprescription sleep aid.

A.E.R. (Birchwood) Hamamelis water (witch hazel) 50%, glycerin 12.5%, methylparaben, benzalkonium chloride. Pads. Jar 40s. *OTC.*
Use: Dermatologic.

Aerdil. (Econo Med Pharmaceuticals) Triprolidine hydrochloride 1.25 mg, pseudoephedrine hydrochloride 30 mg/ 5 mL. Bot. Pt, gal. *OTC.*
Use: Antihistamine; decongestant.

Aerocell. (Health & Medical Techniques) Exfoliative cytology fixative spray. Bot. 3.5 oz.
Use: Exfoliative cytology fixative spray.

Aerofreeze. (Graham Field) Trichloromonofluoromethane and dichlorodifluoromethane. Spray. Cont. 240 mL. *OTC.*
Use: Anesthetic, local.

AeroHist. (Aero) Chlorpheniramine maleate 8 mg, methscopolamine nitrate 2.5 mg. ER Tab. 100s. *Rx.*
Use: Upper respiratory combination, decongestant, antihistamine, and anticholinergic combination.

AeroHist Plus. (Aero) Phenylephrine hydrochloride 20 mg, chlorpheniramine maleate 8 mg, methscopolamine nitrate 2.5 mg. ER Tab. 100s. *Rx.*
Use: Upper respiratory combination, decongestant, antihistamine, and anticholinergic combination.

AeroKid. (Aero) Phenylephrine hydrochloride 10 mg, chlorpheniramine maleate 4 mg, methscopolamine nitrate 1.25 mg per 5 mL. Sorbitol, saccharin, blue raspberry flavor. Syrup. 20 mL, 120 mL, 473 mL. *Rx.*
Use: Upper respiratory combination, decongestant, antihistamine, and anticholinergic combination.

Aeropin.
Use: Cystic fibrosis. [Orphan Drug]

Aeropure. (Health & Medical Techniques) Isopropanol 7.8%, triethylene glycol 3.9%, essential oils 3%, methyldodecyl benzyl trimethyl ammonium chloride 0.12%, methyldodecylxylene bis (trimethyl ammonium chloride) 0.03%, inert ingredients 85.15%. Bot. 0.8 oz, 4.5 oz.
Use: Antiseptic; deodorant.

Aeroseb-Dex. (Allergan) Dexamethasone 0.01%, alcohol 65.1%. Aerosol 58 g. *Rx.*
Use: Corticosteroid, topical.

Aerosil. (Health & Medical Techniques) Dimethylpolysiloxane. Bot. 4.5 oz.
Use: Lubricant; protectant.

Aerosol OT.
See: Docusate Sodium.

Aerosolv. (Health & Medical Techniques) Isopropyl alcohol, methylene chloride, silicone. Aerosol 5.5 oz.
Use: Adhesive remover.

Aerospan. (Forest) Flunisolide hemihydrate ≈ 80 mcg (flunisolide 78 mcg)/ actuation. Aerosol. Canisters. 5.1 g (60 metered actuations), 8.9 g (120 metered actuations). *Rx.*
Use: Corticosteroid.

AeroTuss 12. (Aero Pharmaceuticals, Inc.) Dextromethorphan HBr 30 mg per 5 mL. Methylparaben, sodium saccharin, sucrose. Grape flavor. Susp. 237 mL. *Rx.*
Use: Nonnarcotic antitussive.

AeroZoin. (Health & Medical Techniques) Benzoin compound tincture 30%, isopropyl alcohol 44.8%. Spray Bot. 3.5 oz. *OTC.*
Use: Dermatologic, protectant.

• **afatinib.** (a-FA-ti-nib) USAN.
Use: Antineoplastic.

• **afatinib dimaleate.** (a-FA-ti-nib) USAN.
Use: Antineoplastic.

Afaxin. (Sanofi-Synthelabo) Vitamin A Palmitate 10,000 units, 50,000 units.

Cap. Bot. *Rx-OTC.*
Use: Vitamin supplement.
Afeditab CR. (Watson) Nifedipine 30 mg,
60 mg. ER Tab. 100s. *Rx.*
Use: Calcium channel blocker.
•**afegostat.** (a-FEG-oh-stat) USAN.
Use: Gaucher disease.
•**afegostat tartrate.** (a-FEG-oh-stat)
USAN.
Use: Gaucher disease.
A-Fil. (PharmaDerm) Methyl anthranilate
5%, titanium dioxide 5% in vanishing
cream base. Tube 45 g. Neutral or dark.
OTC.
Use: Sunscreen.
•**afimoxifene.** (a-fim-OX-i-feen) USAN.
Use: Antineoplastic.
Afinitor. (Novartis) Everolimus 2.5 mg,
5 mg, 10 mg. Butylated hydroxytolu-
ene, lactose. Tab. UD 28s. *Rx.*
Use: Protein-tyrosine kinase inhibitor,
mTOR inhibitor.
Afko-Lube. (A.P.C.) Docusate sodium
100 mg. Cap. Bot. 100s. *OTC.*
Use: Laxative.
Afko-Lube Lax. (A.P.C.) Docusate sodium 100 mg, casanthranol 30 mg.
Cap. Bot. 100s. *OTC.*
Use: Laxative.
•**aflibercept.** (A-fli-BER-sept) USAN.
Use: Angiogenesis inhibitor.
Afluria. (CSL Biotherapies) Hemagglutinin 15 mcg each of A/California/7/2009
NYMC X-181 (H1N1), A/Victoria/210/
2009 NYMC X-187 (H3N2) (an A/Perth/
16/2009-like strain), and B/Brisbane/
60/2008 per 0.5 mL. Mercury 24.5 mcg/
dose. Each dose may contain residual
amounts of sodium taurodeoxycholate
(≤ 10 ppm), ovalbumin (≤ 1 mcg), neomycin sulfate (≤ 0.2 picograms), polymyxin B (≤ 0.03 picograms), and betapropiolactone (< 25 nanograms). Inj.,
Susp. (purified split virus). Preservative-
free 0.5 mL prefilled, single-dose syringe; 5 mL multidose vial with preservative (thimerosal). *Rx.*
Use: Viral vaccine.
•**afovirsen sodium.** (aff-oh-VEER-sen
SO-dee-uhm) USAN.
Use: Antiviral.
Afrin. (Schering-Plough) Oxymetazoline
hydrochloride 0.05%. **Nose Drops:**
Drop. Bot. 20 mL. **Nasal Spray:** Reg.
Bot. 15 mL, 30 mL; Menthol. Bot.
15 mL. **Children's Nose Drops:** Oxy-
metazoline hydrochloride 0.025%.
Drop. Bot. 20 mL. *OTC.*
Use: Decongestant.

Afrin All Night No Drip. (Schering-
Plough) Oxymetazoline hydrochloride
0.05%. Benzalkonium chloride, benzyl
alcohol, edetate disodium, flower oil,
glycerin, PEG. Soln., intranasal. 15 mL.
OTC.
Use: Nasal decongestant, imidazoline.
Afrin Extra Moisturizing. (Schering-
Plough) Oxymetazoline hydrochloride
0.05%. Benzalkonium chloride, edetate
disodium. Soln., Intranasal Spray.
15 mL. *OTC.*
Use: Nasal decongestant, imidazoline.
Afrin Moisturizing Saline Mist.
(Schering-Plough) Sodium chloride
0.64%, benzalkonium chloride, EDTA.
Soln. Bot. 30 mL. *OTC.*
Use: Decongestant.
Afrin No-Drip 12-Hour. (Schering-
Plough) Oxymetazoline hydrochloride
0.05%, carboxymethylcellulose sodium,
microcrystalline cellulose, benzal-
konium chloride, benzyl alcohol, EDTA.
Soln. Spray Bot. 15 mL. *OTC.*
Use: Nasal decongestant, imidazoline.
**Afrin No-Drip 12-Hour Extra Moisturiz-
ing.** (Schering-Plough) Oxymetazoline
hydrochloride 0.05%, carboxymethyl-
cellulose sodium, microcrystalline cellu-
lose, benzalkonium chloride, benzyl
alcohol, EDTA, glycerin, Soln. Spray
Bot. 15 mL. *OTC.*
Use: Nasal decongestant, imidazoline.
Afrinol Repetabs. (Schering-Plough)
Pseudoephedrine sulfate 120 mg. Re-
peat Action Tab. Box 12s, bot. 100s,
dispensary pack 48s. *OTC.*
Use: Decongestant.
**Afrin Severe Congestion with Men-
thol.** (Schering-Plough) Oxymetazoline
hydrochloride 0.05%, benzalkonium
chloride, benzyl alcohol, camphor,
EDTA, eucalyptol, menthol. Soln. Spray
Bot. 15 mL. *OTC.*
Use: Nasal decongestant, imidazoline.
Afrin Sinus. (Schering-Plough) Oxy-
metazoline hydrochloride 0.05%, benzyl
alcohol. Spray. Bot. 15 mL. *OTC.*
Use: Decongestant.
Afrin Sinus 12 Hour Relief. (Schering-
Plough) Oxymetazoline hydrochloride
0.05%. Benzalkonium chloride, benzyl
alcohol, camphor, EDTA, eucalyptol,
menthol. Soln., Intranasal Spray. 15 mL.
OTC.
Use: Nasal decongestant, imidazoline.
Afrin 12-Hour Original. (Schering-
Plough) Oxymetazoline hydrochloride
0.05%, benzalkonium chloride, EDTA.
Soln. Spray Bot. 15 mL. *OTC.*
Use: Nasal decongestant, imidazoline.

After Bite. (Tender) Ammonium hydroxide 3.5% in aqueous solution. Pen-like dispenser. *OTC.*
Use: Analgesic; antipruritic, topical.
After Burn. (Tender) Lidocaine 0.5% in aloe vera 98% solution. *OTC.*
Use: Anesthetic, local.
•**agalsidase alfa.** (aye-GAL-si-days) USAN.
Use: Fabry disease.
•**agalsidase beta.** (aye-GAL-si-days) USAN.
Use: Fabry disease.
See: Fabrazyme.
•**aganepag.** (a-GAN-e-pag) USAN.
Use: Treatment of glaucoma.
•**aganepag ethanediol.** (a-GAN-e-pag) USAN.
Use: Treatment of glaucoma.
•**aganepag isopropyl.** (a-GAN-e-pag) USAN.
Use: Treatment of glaucoma.
•**agar.** (AH-gahr) *NF 29.*
Use: Pharmaceutical aid, suspending agent.
W/Mineral oil.
See: Agoral.
Aggrastat. (Merck) Tirofiban hydrochloride. **Inj.:** 50 mcg/mL. Preservative-free. Single-dose *IntraVia* containers 250 mL (sodium chloride 2.25 g, sodium citrate dihydrate 135 mg), 500 mL (sodium chloride 4.5 g, sodium citrate dihydrate 270 mg). **Conc. Inj.:** 250 mcg/mL. Preservative-free, sodium chloride 8 mg, sodium citrate dihydrate 2.7 mg. Vial 25 mL, 50 mL. *Rx.*
Use: Antiplatelet, glycoprotein IIb/IIIa inhibitor.
aggregation inhibitors.
Use: Antiplatelet agents.
See: Cilostazol.
  Clopidogrel Bisulfate.
  Prasugrel.
Aggrenox. (Boehringer Ingelheim) Dipyridamole 200 mg extended-release, aspirin 25 mg, lactose, sucrose. Cap. Bot. 60s. *Rx.*
Use: Antiplatelet.
agomelatine.
Use: Investigational antidepressant.
Agoral. (Numark) Sennosides A and B 25 mg/15 mL, parabens. Liq. Bot. 473 mL. *OTC.*
Use: Laxative.
A/G-Pro. (Miller Pharmacal Group) Protein hydrolysate 542 mg, L-lysine 50 mg, L-methionine 12.5 mg, vitamin B_6 0.33 mg, C 16.7 mg, iron 1.66 mg, Cu, I, K, Mg, Mn, Zn. Tab. Bot. 180s.

OTC.
Use: Nutritional supplement, amino acid.
Agriflu. (Novartis Vaccines) Hemagglutinin 15 mcg each of A/California/7/2009 NYMC X-181 (H1N1), A/Victoria/210/2009 NYMC X-187 (H3N2) (an A/Perth/16/2009-like virus), and B/Brisbane/60/2008 per 0.5 mL. Each 0.5 mL dose may contain residual amounts of egg proteins (< 0.4 mg), formaldehyde (≤ 10 mcg), polysorbate 80 (≤ 50 mcg), and CTAB (≤ 12 mcg). Inj., Susp. (purified split virus). Preservative-free 0.5 mL prefilled, single-dose syringe. *Rx.*
Use: Viral vaccine.
Agrylin. (Roberts) Anagrelide hydrochloride 0.5 mg. Lactose. Cap. 100s. *Rx.*
Use: Thrombocythemia; polycythemia vera; essential thrombocythemia; thrombocytosis in chronic myelogenous leukemia. [Orphan Drug]
agurin.
See: Theobromine Sodium Acetate.
Ah-Chew. (Dexo Pharma) Phenylephrine tannate equiv. to phenylephrine hydrochloride 10 mg, chlorpheniramine tannate equiv. to chlorpheniramine maleate 2 mg, methscopolamine nitrate 1.5 mg per 5 mL. Parabens, sucralose. Susp. 20 mL, 118 mL. *Rx.*
Use: Upper respiratory combination, anticholinergic, antihistamine, decongestant combination.
Ah-Chew Ultra. (Dexo Pharma) Phenylephrine hydrochloride 10 mg (as phenylephrine tannate), chlorpheniramine maleate 2 mg (as chlorpheniramine tannate), methscopolamine nitrate 1.5 mg. Saccharin, sugar. Chew. Tab. 100s. *Rx.*
Use: Upper respiratory combination, decongestant, antihistamine, and anticholinergic combination.
AHF.
See: Antihemophilic Factor.
A-Hydrocort. (Hospira) Hydrocortisone sodium succinate 100 mg/2 mL or 250 mg/2 mL, 500 mg/4 mL; 1000 mg/8 mL. *Rx.*
Use: Corticosteroid.
AIDS vaccine. (Various Mfr.) Phase I to III AIDS, HIV prophylaxis and treatment. Investigational.
Use: Immunization.
Airacof. (Centurion Labs) Codeine phosphate 7.5 mg, diphenhydramine hydrochloride 12.5 mg, phenylephrine hydrochloride 7.5 mg per 5 mL. Propylene glycol, saccharin, sodium benzoate,

sorbitol. Alcohol free, dye free,' and sugar free. Strawberry flavor. Liq. 473 mL. c-v.
Use: Upper respiratory combination, antitussive combination.
air and surface disinfectant. (Health & Medical Techniques) Aerosol 16 oz.
Use: Antiseptic; deodorant.
•**air, medical.** *USP 34.*
Use: Gas, medicinal.
AK-Beta. (Akorn) Levobunolol hydrochloride 0.25%, 0.5%, polyvinyl alcohol 1.4%, benzalkonium chloride 0.004%, sodium metabisulfite, EDTA, dibasic sodium phosphate, monobasic potassium phosphate, NaCl, hydrochloric acid, sodium hydroxide. Ophth. Soln. Bot. 2 mL, 5 mL, 10 mL, 15 mL. *Rx.*
Use: Antiglaucoma.
AK-Con. (Akorn) Naphazoline hydrochloride 0.1%. Benzalkonium chloride 0.01%, EDTA. Ophth. Soln. Bot. 15 mL. *Rx.*
Use: Ophthalmic decongestant; mydriatic, vasoconstrictor.
AK-Dilate. (Akorn) Phenylephrine hydrochloride 2.5%, 10%. Benzalkonium chloride 0.01%, sodium phosphate mono- and dibasic. Bot. 2 mL (2.5% only), 5 mL (10% only), 15 mL (2.5% only). *Rx.*
Use: Mydriatic, vasoconstrictor; ophthalmic decongestant.
AK-Fluor. (Akorn) Fluorescein sodium 10%. Amp. 5 mL, Vial 5 mL.
Use: Diagnostic aid, ophthalmic.
Akineton Lactate. (Knoll) Biperiden lactate 5 mg in aqueous 1.4% sodium lactate soln/mL. Amp. 1 mL. Box 10s. *Rx.*
Use: Antiparkinsonian.
AK-NaCl. (Akorn) **Oint.:** Sodium chloride hypertonic 5%. Tube 3.5 g. **Soln.:** Sodium chloride hypertonic 5%. Bot. 15 mL. *OTC.*
Use: Ophthalmic.
Akne Drying Lotion. (Alto) Zinc oxide 12%, urea 10%, sulfur 6%, salicylic acid 2%, benzalkonium chloride 0.2%, isopropyl alcohol 70%, in a base containing menthol, silicon dioxide, iron oxide, perfume. Bot. ¾ oz, 2.25 oz. *OTC.*
Use: Dermatologic, acne.
Akne-Mycin. (Coria Laboratories) Erythromycin 2%. Cetostearyl alcohol, petrolatum, mineral oil. Oint. Tubes. 25 g. *Rx.*
Use: Topical anti-infective, antibiotic.
AK-Neo-Dex. (Akorn) Dexamethasone sodium phosphate 0.1%, neomycin sulfate 0.35%. Ophth. Soln. Bot. 5 mL. *Rx.*

Use: Anti-infective; corticosteroid, ophthalmic.
Akne Scrub. (Alto) Povidone-iodine with polyethylene granules. Bot. ¾ oz. *OTC.*
Use: Dermatologic, acne.
AK-Pentolate. (Akorn) Cyclopentolate hydrochloride 1%, benzalkonium chloride 0.01%, EDTA. Soln. Bot. 2 mL, 15 mL. *Rx.*
Use: Cycloplegic, mydriatic.
AK-Poly-Bac. (Akorn) Polymyxin B sulfate 10,000 units, bacitracin zinc 500 units/g, white petrolatum, mineral oil. Oint. Tube 3.5 g. *Rx.*
Use: Anti-infective, ophthalmic.
AK-Ramycin. (Akorn) Doxycycline hyclate 100 mg. Cap. Bot. 50s, 100s, 200s, 250s, 500s, UD 100s. *Rx.*
Use: Anti-infective, tetracycline.
AK-Ratabs. (Akorn) Doxycycline hyclate 100 mg. Tab. Bot. 50s. *Rx.*
Use: Anti-infective, tetracycline.
Akrinol. (Schering-Plough) Acrisorcin.
Use: Antifungal.
AK-Sulf. (Akorn) **Soln.:** Sodium sulfacetamide 10%. Dropper Bot. 2 mL, 5 mL, 15 mL. **Oint.:** Sodium sulfacetamide 10%. Tube 3.5 g. *Rx.*
Use: Anti-infective, ophthalmic.
AK-Taine. (Akorn) Proparacaine hydrochloride 0.5%, glycerin, chlorobutanol, benzalkonium chloride. Dropper bot. 2 mL, 15 mL. *Rx.*
Use: Anesthetic, ophthalmic.
AK-Tate. (Akorn) Prednisolone acetate 1%, benzalkonium chloride, EDTA, polysorbate 80, polyvinyl alcohol, hydroxyethyl cellulose. Susp. Dropper bot. 5 mL, 10 mL, 15 mL. *Rx.*
Use: Corticosteroid, ophthalmic.
Akten. (Akorn) Lidocaine hydrochloride 3.5%. Preservative free. Gel, Ophth. Single-use dropper bottle. 5 mL. *Rx.*
Use: Ophthalmic local anesthetic.
AKTob. (Akorn) Tobramycin 0.3%. Benzalkonium chloride 0.01%, boric acid, sodium sulfate. Soln. Bot. 5 mL. *Rx.*
Use: Anti-infective, ophthalmic.
Ala-Bath. (Del-Ray) Bath oil. Bot. 8 oz. *OTC.*
Use: Emollient.
Alacol. (Ballay) **Drops:** Phenylephrine hydrochloride 1 mg, brompheniramine maleate 0.4 mg per 1 mL. Saccharin, sorbitol. 30 mL with dropper. **Syrup:** Phenylephrine hydrochloride 5 mg, brompheniramine maleate 2 mg per 5 mL. Sugar and alcohol free. Saccharin, sorbitol. Black raspberry flavor. Bot. 473 mL. *Rx.*
Use: Upper respiratory combination, decongestant and antihistamine.

Ala-Cort. (Del-Ray) Hydrocortisone 1%. **Cream:** Tube 1 oz, 3 oz. **Lot.: Bot. 4 oz.** *Rx.*
Use: Corticosteroid, topical.
Ala-Derm. (Del-Ray) Lot. Bot. 8 oz, 12 oz.
Use: Emollient.
Aladrine. (Scherer) Ephedrine sulfate 8.1 mg, secobarbital sodium 16.2 mg. Tab. Bot. 100s. *c-II.*
Use: Decongestant; hypnotic, sedative.
•**alagebrium chloride.** (al-A-je-BREE-um) USAN.
Use: Cardiovascular complications.
Alagesic LQ. (Poly Pharmaceuticals) Acetaminophen 325 mg, butalbital 50 mg, caffeine 40 mg per 15 mL. Alcohol 7.368%, glucose, parabens, saccharin, sorbitol, sucrose. Tropical fruit punch flavor. Soln. 473 mL. *Rx.*
Use: Nonnarcotic analgesic combination, nonnarcotic analgesic with barbiturate.
Alahist AC. (Poly Pharmaceuticals) Codeine phosphate 10 mg, phenylephrine hydrochloride 7.5 mg per 5 mL. Saccharin, sorbitol. Alcohol free. Fruit flavor. Liq. 473 mL. *c-v.*
Use: Upper respiratory combination; antitussive, decongestant.
Alahist DHC. (Poly Pharmaceuticals) Dihydrocodeine bitartrate 3 mg, phenylephrine hydrochloride 7.5 mg per 5 mL. Saccharin, sorbitol. Mango flavor. Liq. 473 mL. *c-v.*
Use: Upper respiratory combination, analgesic, decongestant.
Alahist DM. (Poly Pharmaceuticals) Brompheniramine maleate 4 mg, dextromethorphan HBr 15 mg, phenylephrine hydrochloride 7.5 mg per 5 mL. Saccharin, sorbitol. Alcohol free, dye free, sugar free. Strawberry flavor. Liq. 473 mL. *Rx.*
Use: Upper respiratory combination; antitussive, antihistamine, decongestant.
Alahist IR. (Poly Pharmaceuticals) Dexbrompheniramine maleate 2 mg. Tab. 60s. *Rx.*
Use: Antihistamine, nonselective alkylamine.
Alahist LQ. (Poly Pharmaceuticals) Diphenhydramine hydrochloride 25 mg, phenylephrine hydrochloride 7.5 mg per 5 mL. Saccharin, sorbitol. Alcohol free and sugar free. Fruit candy flavor. Liq. 473 mL. *Rx.*
Use: Upper respiratory combination, decongestant and antihistamine.
Alamag. (Ivax) Aluminum hydroxide 225 mg, magnesium hydroxide 200 mg, sorbitol, sucrose, parabens. Susp. Bot. 355 mL. *OTC.*
Use: Antacid.
Alamag Plus. (Ivax) Magnesium hydroxide 200 mg, aluminum hydroxide 225 mg, simethicone 25 mg/5 mL. Susp. Bot. 355 mL. *OTC.*
Use: Antacid.
Alamast. (Vistakon) Pemirolast potassium 0.1% (1 mg/mL). Lauralkonium chloride 0.005%, glycerin, dibasic and monobasic sodium phosphate, phosphoric acid, and/or sodium hydroxide. Ophth. Soln. 10 mL. *Rx.*
Use: Mast cell stabilizer.
•**alamecin.** (al-ah-MEE-sin) USAN.
Use: Anti-infective.
•**alanine.** (AL-ah-NEEN) *USP 34.*
Use: Amino acid.
•**alaproclate.** (AL-ah-PRO-klate) USAN.
Use: Antidepressant.
Ala-Quin 0.5%. (Del-Ray) Hydrocortisone, iodochlorhydroxyquinoline cream. Tube 1 oz. *Rx-OTC.*
Use: Corticosteroid, topical.
Ala-Scalp HP 2%. (Del-Ray) Hydrocortisone Lot. Bot. 1 oz. *Rx.*
Use: Corticosteroid, topical.
Ala-Seb. (Del-Ray) Shampoo. Bot. 4 oz, 12 oz. *OTC.*
Use: Antiseborrheic.
Ala-Seb T. (Del-Ray) Shampoo **118 mL:** Sulfur 2%, salicylic acid 2%, coal tar 1%, PEG-20. **4 oz:** Coal tar, colloidal sulfur, salicylic acid. **12 oz:** Coal tar, colloidal sulfur, salicylic acid. *OTC.*
Use: Antiseborrheic combination.
Alasulf. (Major) Sulfanilamide 15%, aminacrine hydrochloride 0.2%, allantoin 2%. Vaginal Cream. Tube w/applicator 120 g. *Rx.*
Use: Anti-infective, vaginal.
Alatone. (Major) Spironolactone 25 mg. Tab. Bot. 100s, 250s, 500s, 1000s, UD 100s. *Rx.*
Use: Antihypertensive.
Alavert. (Wyeth) Loratadine 10 mg. Lactose. Orally Disintegrating Tab. 6s, 12s, 15s, 30s, 48s. *OTC.*
Use: Antihistamine, peripherally selective piperidine.
Alavert Allergy & Sinus D-12 Hour. (Wyeth) Pseudoephedrine sulfate 120 mg, loratadine 5 mg. Lactose. ER Tab. 12s, 24s. *OTC.*
Use: Upper respiratory combination, decongestant, antihistamine.
Alavert Children's. (Wyeth) Loratadine 5 mg/5 mL. Sucrose. Syrup. 118 mL. *OTC.*

Use: Antihistamine, peripherally selective piperidine.

Alaway. (Bausch & Lomb) Ketotifen fumarate 0.025%. Benzalkonium chloride 0.01%, glycerin, sodium hydroxide, and/or hydrochloric acid. Soln., Ophth. 10 mL. OTC.
Use: Ophthalmic decongestant.

Alaxin. (Delta Pharmaceutical Group) Oxyethlene oxypropylene polymer 240 mg. Cap. Bot. 100s. OTC.
Use: Laxative.

alazanine triclofenate.
Use: Anthelmintic.

Alazide. (Major) Spironolactone w/hydrochlorothiazide. Tab. Bot. 250s, 1000s. Rx.
Use: Antihypertensive, diuretic.

Alazine. (Major) Hydralazine 10 mg, 25 mg, 50 mg. Cap. Bot. 100s, 1000s. Rx.
Use: Antihypertensive.

• **albaconazole.** (Al-ba-KON-a-zole) USAN.
Use: Antifungal agent.

Albafort. (Baroli) Ferrous fumarate 110 mg, B$_{12}$ 15 mcg, intrinsic factor (as concentrate or from stomach preparations) 240 mg, vitamin C 100 mg, folic acid 0.8 mg. Cap. 100s. Rx.
Use: Trace element, iron.

Albatussin. (Baroli) Carbetapentane citrate 25 mg, guaifenesin 400 mg, phenylephrine hydrochloride 10 mg. Cap. 100s. Rx.
Use: Upper respiratory combination, antitussive and expectorant combination.

Albatussin SR. (Lambda Pharmacal) Dextromethorphan HBr 40 mg, potassium guaiacolsulfonate 600 mg, phenylephrine hydrochloride 20 mg, pyrilamine maleate 25 mg. ER Cap. 100s. Rx.
Use: Antitussive and expectorant combination.

• **albendazole.** (AL-BEND-ah-zole) USP 34.
Use: Anthelmintic.
See: Albenza.

Albenza. (GlaxoSmithKline) Albendazole 200 mg. Lactose, saccharin. Tab. 112s. Rx.
Use: Anthelmintic; hydatid disease. [Orphan Drug]

• **albiglutide.** (al-bi-GLOO-tide) USAN.
Use: Treatment of type 2 diabetes.

• **albinterferon alfa-2b.** (AL-bin-ter-FEER-on) USAN.
Use: Treatment of chronic hepatitis C.

Albolene. (DSE Healthcare) Mineral oil, petrolatum. Fragrance free. Soap. 340 g. OTC.
Use: Emollient.

Albuconn 25%. (Cryosan) Normal serum albumin (human) 12.5 g in 50 mL solution for IV administration. Vial 50 mL. Rx.
Use: Treatment of plasma or blood volume deficit, acute hypoproteinemia, oncotic deficit.

• **albumin, aggregated.** (al-BYOO-min AGG-reh-GAY-tuhd) USAN.
Use: Diagnostic aid, lung-imaging.
See: Technescan MAA.

• **albumin, aggregated iodinated I 131 injection.** (al-BYOO-min AGG-reh-GAY-tuhd) USP 34.
Use: Radiopharmaceutical.

• **albumin, aggregated iodinated I 131 serum.** (al-BYOO-min AGG-reh-GAY-tuhd) USAN. Blood serum aggregates of albumin labeled with iodine-131.
Use: Radiopharmaceutical.
See: Albumotope I-131.

Albuminar-5. (ZLB Behring) Albumin (human) 5%. Soln. with administration set. Bot. 50 mL, 1000 mL. Rx.
Use: Plasma protein fraction.

Albuminar-25. (ZLB Behring) Albumin (human) 25%. Soln. Vials. 20 mL with administration set. Rx.
Use: Plasma protein fraction.

• **albumin, chromated Cr 51 serum.** (al-BYOO-min) USAN. Blood serum albumin labeled with chromium-51.
Use: Radiopharmaceutical.

• **albumin human.** (al-BYOO-MIN) USP 34. Formerly Albumin, Normal Human Serum.
Use: Plasma protein fraction; blood volume supporter.
See: Albuminar-5 and Albuminar-25.
Albunex.
Albutein 5%.
Albutein 25%.
Buminate.
Optison.
Plasbumin-5.
Plasbumin-25.
W/Combinations:
See: Monarc-M.

albumin human, 5%. (Baxter Healthcare) Normal serum albumin 5%. Inj. Vial 250 mL. Rx.
Use: Plasma protein fraction.

albumin human, 25%. (Baxter Healthcare) Normal serum albumin 25%. Inj. Vial 10 mL, 50 mL. Rx.
Use: Plasma protein fraction.

•**albumin, iodinated I 131 injection.** (al-BYOO-min) *USP 34.* Albumin labeled with iodine-131. Inj. *Use:* Diagnostic aid, blood volume determination, intrathecal imaging; radiopharmaceutical.

•**albumin, iodinated I 131 serum.** (al-BYOO-min) *USP 34.* *Use:* Diagnostic aid, blood volume determination, intrathecal imaging; radioactive agent.

•**albumin, iodinated I 125 injection.** (al-BYOO-min) *USP 34.* Albumin labeled with iodine-125. *Use:* Diagnostic aid, blood volume determination; radiopharmaceutical.

•**albumin, iodinated I 125 serum.** (al-BYOO-min) *USP 34.* *Use:* Diagnostic aid, blood volume determination; radiopharmaceutical.

albumin, normal serum 5%. (Baxter Healthcare) Albumin human 5%. Inj. Vial 120 mL. *Rx.* *Use:* Plasma protein fraction.

albumin, normal serum 25%. (Baxter Healthcare) Albumin human 25%. Inj. Vial 10 mL, 50 mL. *Rx.* *Use:* Plasma protein fraction.

albumin-saline diluent. (Bayer Consumer Care) Dilute allergenic extracts and venom products for patient testing and treating. Pre-measured vials 1.8 mL, 4 mL, 4.5 mL, 9 mL, 30 mL. Vial 2 mL, 5 mL, 10 mL, 30 mL. *Use:* Pharmaceutical necessity, diluent.

Albumotope I-131. (Bristol-Myers Squibb) Albumin, iodinated I-131 serum (50 uCi). *Use:* Diagnostic aid.

Albunex. (Mallinckrodt) Albumin (human) 5%, sonicated. Sodium acetyl tryptophanate 0.08 mmol, sodium caprylate 0.08 mmol/g albumin. Inj. Vial. 5 mL, 10 mL, 20 mL. Pkg. 6s. *Rx.* *Use:* Plasma protein fraction.

Albustix Reagent Strips. (Siemens Medical) Firm paper reagent strips impregnated with tetrabromphenol blue, citrate buffer and a protein-adsorbing agent. Bot. 50s, 100s. *Use:* Diagnostic aid.

Albutein 5%. (Grifols Biologicals) Normal serum albumin 5%. Inj. Vial w/IV set 250 mL, 500 mL. *Rx.* *Use:* Plasma protein fraction.

Albutein 25%. (Grifols Biologicals) Normal serum albumin 25%. Inj. Vial w/IV set 50 mL. *Rx.* *Use:* Plasma protein fraction.

•**albuterol.** (al-BYOO-ter-ahl) *USP 34.* *Use:* Bronchodilator, sympathomimetic. *See:* Proventil. Ventolin.

albuterol. (Nephron) Albuterol sulfate 0.042% (1.25 mg/3 mL). Preservative free. Soln. for Inh. 3 mL UD vials. *Rx.* *Use:* Bronchodilator.

albuterol. (Various Mfr.) Albuterol 90 mcg per actuation. Aer. Can. 6.8 g (≥ 80 inhalations), 17 g (≥ 200 inhalations). *Rx.* *Use:* Bronchodilator, sympathomimetic.

albuterol. (Watson) Albuterol sulfate 0.021%. Preservative free. Soln., Inh. 3 mL UD vials. *Rx.* *Use:* Bronchodilator, sympathomimetic.

•**albuterol sulfate.** (al-BYOO-teh-rahl SULL-fate) *USP 34.* *Use:* Bronchodilator, sympathomimetic. *See:* AccuNeb. ProAir HFA. Proventil HFA. Ventolin HFA. VoSpire ER.

albuterol sulfate. (Mylan) Albuterol 4 mg, 8 mg. Polydextrose. Film coated. ER Tab. 100s, 500s. *Rx.* *Use:* Bronchodilator.

albuterol sulfate. (Various Mfr.) Albuterol sulfate. **Tab.:** 2 mg, 4 mg. May contain lactose. Bot. 100s, 500s, 600s. **Syrup:** 2 mg/5 mL. May contain sorbitol. Bot. 473 mL. **Inh. Soln.:** 0.083% (2.5 mg/3 mL), 0.5% (5 mg/mL). UD 3 mL (0.083% only). Vials. 0.5 mL (0.5% only), 20 mL with dropper (0.5% only) *Rx.* *Use:* Bronchodilator, sympathomimetic.

albuterol sulfate and ipratropium bromide. (al-BYOO-ter-ahl SULL-fate and IH-pruh-TROE-pee-uhm BROE-mide) *Use:* Chronic obstructive pulmonary disease (COPD). *See:* Combivent. DuoNeb.

•**albutoin.** (al-BYOO-toe-in) USAN. *Use:* Anticonvulsant.

Albutussin. (AJ Bart) Dextromethorphan hydrobromide 15 mg, phenylephrine hydrochloride 5 mg, pyrilamine maleate 12.5 mg per 5 mL. Menthol, saccharin, sorbitol. Alcohol and sugar free. Peppermint flavor. Liq. 118 mL. *OTC.* *Use:* Upper respiratory combination, antitussive combination.

•**alcaftadine.** (al-KAF-ta deen) USAN. *Use:* Antihistamine. *See:* Lastacaft.

Alcaine. (Alcon) Proparacaine hydrochloride 0.5%. Glycerin, benzalkonium chloride 0.01%. Soln. Bot. 15 mL *Drop-*

Tainers. Rx.
Use: Anesthetic, ophthalmic.
Alcare. (GlaxoSmithKline) Ethyl alcohol 62%. Foam Bot. 210 mL, 300 mL, 600 mL. *OTC.*
Use: Antiseptic.
Alclear Eye. (Walgreen) Sterile isotonic fluid. Lot. Bot. 8 oz. *OTC.*
Use: Anti-irritant, ophthalmic.
•**alclofenac.** (al-KLOE-feh-nak) USAN.
Use: Analgesic; anti-inflammatory.
See: Mervan.
•**alclometasone dipropionate.** (al-kloe-MEH-tah-zone die-PRO-pee-oh-nate) *USP 34.*
Use: Anti-inflammatory, topical.
See: Aclovate.
alclometasone dipropionate. (Taro) Alclometasone dipropionate 0.05%. Hexylene glycol, propylene glycol stearate, petrolatum. Oint. 15 g, 45 g, 60 g. *Rx.*
Use: Anti-inflammatory agent.
alclometasone dipropionate. (Various Mfr.) Alclometasone dipropionate 0.05%. Cream. 15 g, 45 g, 60 g. *Rx.*
Use: Anti-inflammatory agent.
•**alcloxa.** (al-KLOX-ah) USAN.
Use: Astringent; keratolytic.
Alco-Gel. (Tweezerman) Ethyl alcohol 60%. Gel. Tube 60 g, 480 g. *OTC.*
Use: Dermatologic, cleanser.
•**alcohol.** (AL-koe-hol) *USP 34.* Ethanol, ethyl alcohol.
Use: Anti-infective, topical; pharmaceutic aid, solvent.
See: Anbesol.
Anbesol Maximum Strength.
alcohol, dehydrated.
Use: Solvent, vehicle.
•**alcohol, diluted.** (AL-koe-hol) *NF 29.*
Use: Pharmaceutic aid, solvent.
Alcohol 5% and Dextrose 5%. (Abbott Hospital Products) Alcohol 5 mL, dextrose 5 g/100 mL. Bot. 1000 mL. *Rx.*
Use: Nutritional supplement, parenteral.
•**alcohol, rubbing.** (AL-koe-hol) *USP 34.*
Use: Rubefacient.
See: Lavacol.
Alcojet. (Alconox) Biodegradable machine washing detergent and wetting agent. Ctn. 9 × 4 lb, 25 lb, 50 lb, 100 lb, 300 lb. *OTC.*
Use: Detergent, wetting agent.
Alcolec. (American Lecithin) Lecithin w/choline base, cephalin, lipositol. Cap. 100s. Gran. 8 oz, lb. *OTC.*
Use: Nutritional supplement.
Alconefrin 12 and 50. (PolyMedica) Phenylephrine hydrochloride 0.16%

w/benzalkonium chloride. Dropper bot. 30 mL. *OTC.*
Use: Decongestant.
Alconefrin 25. (PolyMedica) Phenylephrine hydrochloride 0.25% w/benzalkonium chloride. Dropper bot. 30 mL. Spray Pkg. 30 mL. *OTC.*
Use: Decongestant.
Alcon Enzymatic Cleaning Tablets for Extended Wear. (Alcon) Pancreatin. Tab. Pkg. 12s. *OTC.*
Use: Contact lens care.
Alcon Opti-Pure Sterile Saline Solution. (Alcon) Sterile unpreserved saline solution. Aerosol 8 oz. *OTC.*
Use: Contact lens care.
Alconox. (Alconox) Biodegradable detergent and wetting agent. Box 4 lb, Container 25 lb, 50 lb, 100 lb, 300 lb. *OTC.*
Use: Contact lens care, detergent; wetting agent.
Alcortin A. (Primus Pharmaceuticals) Hydrocortisone acetate 2%. Aloe polysaccharide 1%, benzyl alcohol, glycerin, iodoquinol 1%, amino methylpropanol, propylene glycol, SD alcohol. Gel. Individual pack. 2 g. *Rx.*
Use: Anti-inflammatory agent, topical corticosteroid.
Alcotabs. (Alconox) Tab. Box 6s, 100s.
Use: Cleanser.
•**alcuronium chloride.** (al-cure-OH-nee-uhm KLOR-ide) USAN. Diallyldinortoxiferin dichloride.
Use: Muscle relaxant.
Aldactazide. (Pfizer US) Spironolactone and hydrochlorothiazide. **25 mg/25 mg:** Bot. 100s, 500s, 1000s, 2500s, UD 100s. **50 mg/50 mg:** Bot. 100s, UD 32s, UD 100s. Tab. *Rx.*
Use: Antihypertensive, diuretic.
Aldactone. (Searle) Spironolactone 25 mg, 50 mg, 100 mg. PEG. Film coated. Tab. 100s, 500s (25 mg only). *Rx.*
Use: Diuretic.
Aldara. (Graceway Pharmaceuticals) Imiquimod 5%. Cetyl alcohol, stearyl alcohol, white petrolatum, benzyl alcohol, parabens. Cream. Boxes. 12s. Single-use packets. *Rx.*
Use: Topical immunomodulator.
•**aldesleukin.** (al-dess-LOO-kin) USAN. Recombinant form of interleukin-2.
Use: Biological response modifier.
See: Proleukin.
Aldex AN. (Zyber) Doxylamine succinate 5 mg. Sucralose. Orange flavor. Chew. Tab. 100s. *Rx.*
Use: Antihistamine, nonselective ethanolamine.

Aldex-CT. (Zyber) Diphenhydramine hydrochloride 12.5 mg, phenylephrine hydrochloride 5 mg. Mannitol, saccharin. Strawberry flavor. Chew. Tab. 100s. *Rx.*
Use: Upper respiratory combination; antihistamine, decongestant.

Aldex DM Tannate. (Zyber) Dextromethorphan HBr 15 mg, pyrilamine maleate 16 mg, phenylephrine hydrochloride 5 mg per 5 mL. Methylparaben, sucralose, sucrose. Grape flavor. Susp. 473 mL. *Rx.*
Use: Upper respiratory combination, antitussive combination.

Aldex GS DM. (Pernix) Dextromethorphan hydrobromide 15 mg, guaifenesin 190 mg, pseudoephedrine hydrochloride 30 mg. Tab. 100s. *Rx.*
Use: Upper respiratory combination, antitussive and expectorant combination.

•**aldioxa.** (al-DIE-ox-ah) USAN. Aluminum dihydroxy allantoinate.
Use: Astringent; keratolytic.

Aldomet Ester Hydrochloride. (Merck & Co.) Methyldopate hydrochloride 250 mg/5 mL, citric acid anhydrous 25 mg, sodium bisulfite 16 mg, disodium edetate 2.5 mg, monothioglycerol 10 mg, sodium hydroxide to adjust pH, methylparaben 0.15%, propylparaben 0.02% w/water for inj. q.s. to 5 mL. Inj. Vial 5 mL. *Rx.*
Use: Antihypertensive.

Aldomet Oral Suspension. (Merck & Co.) Methyldopa 250 mg/5 mL, alcohol 1%, benzoic acid 0.1%, sodium bisulfite 0.2%. Oral Susp. Bot. 473 mL. *Rx.*
Use: Antihypertensive.

Aldomet Tablets. (Merck & Co.) Methyldopa. **125 mg Tab.:** Bot. 100s. **250 mg Tab.:** Bot. 100s, 1000s, UD 100s, unit-of-use 100s. **500 mg Tab.:** Bot. 100s, 500s, UD 100s, unit-of-use 60s, 100s. *Rx.*
Use: Antihypertensive.

Aldosterone RIA Diagnostic Kit. (Abbott Diagnostics) Test kits 50s.
Use: Diagnostic aid.

Aldurazyme. (BioMarin) Laronidase 2.9 mg/5 mL, albumin (human) 0.1% after dilution, NaCl 43.9 mg, sodium phosphate monobasic monohydrate 63.5 mg, sodium phosphate dibasic heptahydrate 10.7 mg, preservative free. Inj. Single-use vials. 5 mL. *Rx.*
Use: Treatment of mucopolysaccharidosis.

ALEC. (Forum Products, Inc.) Dipalmitoyl phosphatidylcholine/phosphatidyl-glycerol.
Use: Neonatal respiratory distress syndrome. [Orphan Drug]

•**alefacept.** (ah-LEE-fah-sept) USAN.
Use: Immunologic agent, immunosuppressive.
See: Amevive.

•**aleglitazar.** (AL-e-GLI-ta-zar) USAN.
Use: Antidiabetic agent.

•**alemcinal.** (al-EM-si-nal) USAN.
Use: Gastrointestinal prokinetic.

•**alemtuzumab.** (al-em-TUE-zue-mab) USAN.
Use: Monoclonal antibody.
See: Campath.

Alenaze-D. (Cypress) Phenylephrine hydrochloride 7.5 mg, brompheniramine maleate 2 mg. Saccharin, sorbitol. Bubble gum flavor. Liq. 473 mL. *Rx.*
Use: Upper respiratory combination, decongestant and antihistamine.

Alenaze-D NR. (Cypress) Phenylephrine hydrochloride 7.5 mg, brompheniramine maleate 4 mg per 5 mL. Saccharin, sorbitol. Bubble gum flavor. Liq. 474 mL. *Rx.*
Use: Upper respiratory combination, decongestant and antihistamine.

•**alendronate sodium.** (al-LEN-droe-nate) *USP 34.*
Use: Bisphosphonate.
See: Fosamax.
W/Cholecalciferol.
See: Fosamax Plus D.

alendronate sodium. (Teva) Alendronate sodium 5 mg, 10 mg, 35 mg, 40 mg, 70 mg. Tab. 30s (except 35 mg and 70 mg), 100s (except 35 mg, 40 mg, 70 mg). Unit-of-use blister packs. 4s, UD 20s (35 mg, 70 mg). *Rx.*
Use: Bisphosphonate.

alendronate sodium. (Various Mfr.) Alendronate sodium 70 mg. May contain mannitol. Tab. Unit-of-use blister packs. 4s, UD 20s. *Rx.*
Use: Bisphosphonate.

Alenic Alka. (Rugby) **Liq.:** Aluminum hydroxide 31.7 mg, magnesium carbonate 137.3 mg, sodium alginate, EDTA, sodium 13 mg. Bot. 355 mL. **Chew. Tab.:** Aluminum hydroxide 80 mg, magnesium trisilicate 20 mg, sodium bicarbonate, calcium stearate, sugar. Bot. 100s. *OTC.*
Use: Antacid.

•**alentemol hydrobromide.** (al-EN-teh-mole HIGH-droe-BROE-mide) USAN.
Use: Antipsychotic; dopamine agonist.

•**aleplasinin.** (al-e-PLAS-in-in) USAN.
Use: Alzheimer disease.

Alersule. (Edwards) Chlorpheniramine maleate 8 mg, phenylephrine hydrochloride 20 mg. Cap. Bot. 100s. *Rx-OTC.*
Use: Antihistamine; decongestant.

Alert-Pep. (Health for Life Brands) Caffeine 200 mg. Cap. Bot. 16s. *OTC.*
Use: CNS stimulant.

Alesse. (Wyeth-Ayerst) Levonorgestrel 0.1 mg, ethinyl estradiol 20 mcg. Lactose. Tab. Pkg. 28s with 7 inert tabs. *Rx.*
Use: Sex hormone, contraceptive hormone.

• **aletamine hydrochloride.** (al-ETT-ahmeen HIGH-droe-KLOR-ide) USAN.
Use: Antidepressant.

Aleve. (Bayer) Naproxen 200 mg (naproxen sodium 220 mg). Tab. Bot. 24s, 50s, 100s, 150s. Cap. Bot. 24s, 50s, 100s, 150s, 200s. Gelcap. Bot. 20s, 40s, 80s. *OTC.*
Use: Nonsteroidal anti-inflammatory agent.

Aleve-D Sinus & Cold. (Bayer) Pseudoephedrine hydrochloride 120 mg, naproxen sodium 220 mg (naproxen 200 mg). Sodium 20 mg, lactose. ER Tab. Pkg. 10s, 20s, 24s, 30s. *OTC.*
Use: Upper respiratory combination, analgesic, decongestant.

• **alexidine.** (ah-LEX-ih-DEEN) USAN.
Use: Anti-infective.

alfa interferon-2a.
See: Roferon A.

alfa interferon-2b.
See: Intron A.

• **alfentanil hydrochloride.** (al-FEN-tuh-NILL HIGH-droe-KLOR-ide) USAN.
Use: Opioid analgesic.

alfentanil hydrochloride. (Abbott) Alfentanil hydrochloride (as base) 500 mcg/mL. Preservative free. Inj. Amps. 2 mL, 5 mL, 10 mL. *c-II.*
Use: Opioid analgesic.

• **alferminogene tadenovec.** (AL-fer-MIN-oh-jeen ta-DEN-oh-vek) USAN.
Use: Gene therapy.

Alferon N. (Hemispherx Biopharma) Interferon Alfa-N3 5 million units/mL, NaCl 8 mg, sodium phosphate dibasic 1.74 mg, potassium phosphate monobasic 0.2 mg, potassium chloride 0.2 mg. Inj. Vial 1 mL. *Rx.*
Use: Immunologic agent.

• **alfimeprase.** (AL-fi-me-prace) USAN.
Use: Thrombolytic.

• **alfuzosin hydrochloride.** (al-FEW-zoe-sin HIGH-droe-KLOR-ide) USAN.
Use: Antihypertensive, alpha-blocker.
See: Uroxatral.

Algel. (Faraday) Magnesium trisilicate 0.5 g, aluminum hydroxide 0.25 g. Tab. Bot. 100s. Susp. Bot. gal. *OTC.*
Use: Antacid.

• **algeldrate.** (AL-jell-drate) USAN.
Use: Antacid.

Algemin. (Thurston) Macrocystis pyrifera alga. Pow. Jar 8 oz. Tab. Bot. 300s. *OTC.*
Use: Dietary aid.

Algenic Alka. (Rugby) Aluminum hydroxide 31.7 mg/mL, magnesium carbonate 137 mg/mL, sodium alginate, sorbitol. Liq. Bot. 355 mL. *OTC.*
Use: Antacid.

Algenic Alka Improved. (Rugby) Aluminum hydroxide 240 mg, magnesium hydroxide 100 mg/Chew. Tab. Bot. 100s, 500s. *OTC.*
Use: Antacid.

• **algenpantucel-L.** (AL-jen-pan-TOO-sel-el) USAN.
Use: Antineoplastic.

• **algestone acetonide.** (al-JESS-tone ah-SEE-toe-nide) USAN.
Use: Anti-inflammatory.

• **algestone acetophenide.** (al-JESS-tone ah-SEE-toe-FEN-ide) USAN.
Use: Hormone, progestin.

Algex. (Health for Life Brands) Menthol, camphor, methylsalicylate, eucalyptus. Liniment. Bot. 4 oz. *OTC.*
Use: Analgesic, topical.

algin.
See: Sodium Alginate.

Algin-All. (Barth's) Sodium alginate from kelp. Tab. Bot. 100s, 500s.

• **alginic acid.** (al-JIN-ik) *NF 29.*
Use: Pharmaceutic aid, tablet binder, emulsifying agent.
W/Combinations.
See: Pretts Diet-Aid.

• **alglucerase.** (al-GLUE-ser-ACE) USAN.
Formerly Macrophage-targeted β-glucocerebrosidase.
Use: Enzyme replacement, type 1 Gaucher disease; enzyme replacement, types 2 and 3 Gaucher disease.
[Orphan Drug]
See: Ceredase.

• **alglucosidase alfa.** (al-gloo-KOSE-i-dase) USAN.
Use: Enzyme replacement therapy.
See: Lumizyme.
Myozyme.

• **alicaforsen sodium.** (a-li-KA-for-sen) USAN.
Use: Anti-inflammatory.

alidine dihydrochloride or phosphate.
See: Anileridine.

•**aliflurane.** (al-IH-flew-rane) USAN.
Use: Anesthetic, inhalation.
Align Daily Probiotic Supplement.
(Procter & Gamble) *Bifidobacterium infantis* 35624 4 mg. Sugar. Lactose
free. Cap. 28s. *OTC.*
Use: Oral nutritional supplement, probiotic.
Alikal. (Sanofi-Synthelabo) Sodium bicarbonate, tartaric acid powder. *OTC.*
Use: Antacid.
Alimentum. (Ross) Casein hydrolysate,
sucrose, tapioca starch, MCT (fractionated coconut oil), safflower oil, soy oil.
Qt. Ready-to-use. *OTC.*
Use: Nutritional supplement-enteral.
Alimta. (Lilly) Pemetrexed 100 mg (mannitol 106 mg), 500 mg (mannitol
500 mg). Inj., Lyophilized, Pow. for Soln.
Single-use vials. *Rx.*
Use: Antimetabolite.
Alinia. (Romark Laboratories)
Nitazoxanide. **Pow. for Oral Susp.:**
100 mg/5 mL (after reconstitution).
Sugar, sucrose 1.48 mg/5 mL, strawberry flavor. Bot. 60 mL. **Tab.:** 500 mg.
Polyvinyl alcohol, sucrose, talc. Film
coated. 60s, UD 6s. *Rx.*
Use: Antiprotozoal.
•**alipamide.** (al-IH-pam-ide) USAN.
Use: Antihypertensive; diuretic.
•**aliskiren.** (a-LIS-kir-EN) USAN.
Use: Renin angiotensin system antagonist; direct renin inhibitor.
See: Tekturna.
W/Amlodipine Besylate.
See: Tekamlo.
W/Hydrochlorothiazide.
See: Tekturna HCT.
•**aliskiren fumarate.** (a-LIS-kir-EN)
USAN.
Use: Cardiovascular agent.
alisobumal.
See: Butalbital.
•**alitame.** (AL-ih-TAME) USAN.
Use: Sweetener.
•**alitretinoin.** (a-li-TRET-i-noyn) USAN.
Use: Retinoid, second generation.
See: Panretin.
alkalinizers, minerals and electrolytes.
See: Bicitra.
Oracit.
Polycitra.
alkalinizers, systemic.
See: Citrate and Citric Acid.
alkalinizers, urinary tract products.
See: Bicitra.
Citrolith.
Polycitra.
Sodium Bicarbonate.
Urocit-K.

Alkalol. (Alkalol) Thymol, eucalyptol,
menthol, camphor, benzoin, potassium
alum, potassium chlorate, sodium bicarbonate, sodium chloride, sweet birch
oil, spearmint oil, pine and cassia oil,
alcohol 0.05%. Bot. Pt. Nasal douche
cup pkg. 1s. *OTC.*
Use: Eyes, nose, throat, and all inflamed mucous membranes.
Alka-Med Liquid. (Halsey Drug) Aluminum hydroxide 200 mg, magnesium
hydroxide 200 mg/5 mL. Bot. 8 oz.
OTC.
Use: Antacid.
Alka-Med Tablets. (Halsey Drug) Magnesium hydroxide, aluminum hydroxide.
Bot. 60s. *OTC.*
Use: Antacid.
Alka-Mints. (Bayer Consumer Care) Calcium carbonate 850 mg (elemental calcium 340 mg). Sorbitol, sugar, sodium
< 5 mg. Assorted flavors and spearmint.
Chew. Tab. 75s. *OTC.*
Use: Mineral supplement; antacid.
Alka-Seltzer Gold. (Bayer Consumer
Care) Citric acid 1,000 mg, potassium
bicarbonate 344 mg, sodium bicarbonate 1,050 mg. Mannitol, sodium
309 mg. Effervescent Tab. 36s. *OTC.*
Use: Antacid combination
Alka-Seltzer Heartburn Relief. (Bayer
Consumer Care) Citric acid 1,000 mg,
sodium bicarbonate 1,940 mg. Acesulfame K, aspartame, phenylalanine
5.6 mg, mannitol. Lemon-lime flavor.
Tab. 36s. *OTC.*
Use: Antacid combination.
Alka-Seltzer Lemon Lime. (Bayer Consumer Care) Citric acid 1,000 mg, aspirin 325 mg, sodium bicarbonate
1,700 mg. Aspartame, phenylalanine
9 mg, sodium 504 mg. Lemon-lime flavor. Tab. 24s. *OTC.*
Use: Antacid combination.
Alka-Seltzer Original. (Bayer Consumer
Care) Aspirin 325 mg, citric acid
1,000 mg, sodium bicarbonate
1,916 mg. Sodium 567 mg. Effervescent Tab. 24s. *OTC.*
Use: Antacid combination.
Alka Seltzer Plus Cold. (Bayer Consumer Care) Aspirin 325 mg, chlorpheniramine maleate 2 mg, phenylephrine bitartrate 7.8 mg. Acesulfame
K, aspartame, mannitol, phenylalanine
8.4 mg (original flavor) or 10 mg
(cherry burst and orange zest flavors),
sodium 474 mg (original flavor) and
476 mg (cherry burst and orange zest
flavors). Effervescent Tab. 20s, 36s,
72s. *OTC.*

Use: Upper respiratory combination; decongestant, antihistamine, and analgesic combination.
Alka-Seltzer Plus Cold & Cough. (Bayer Consumer Care) **Effervescent Tab.:** Aspirin 325 mg, chlorpheniramine maleate 2 mg, dextromethorphan hydrobromide 10 mg, phenylephrine bitartrate 7.8 mg. Acesulfame, aspartame, mannitol, phenylalanine 9 mg, sodium 415. Citrus flavor. 20s. **Liq.:** Acetaminophen 162.5 mg, chlorpheniramine maleate 1 mg, dextromethorphan hydrobromide 5 mg, phenylephrine hydrochloride 2.5 mg per 5 mL. Edetate disodium, PEG 400, sorbitol, sucralose. Alcohol free. 180 mL. **Liqui-Gels:** Dextromethorphan HBr 10 mg, chlorpheniramine maleate 2 mg, phenylephrine hydrochloride 5 mg, acetaminophen 325 mg, Liquid filled. Sorbitol. 12s. *OTC.*
Use: Upper respiratory combination, antitussive combination.
Alka-Seltzer Plus Day & Night Cold. (Bayer Consumer Care) **Effervescent Tab.: Day:** Aspirin 325 mg, dextromethorphan hydrobromide 10 mg, phenylephrine bitartrate 7.8 mg. Acesulfame K, aspartame, mannitol, phenylalanine 9 mg, sodium 416 mg. 10s. **Night:** Aspirin 500 mg, dextromethorphan hydrobromide 10 mg, doxylamine succinate 6.25 mg, phenylephrine bitartrate 7.8 mg. Acesulfame K, aspartame, phenylalanine 5.6 mg, sodium 474 mg, sorbitol. 10s. **Liq. Gels: Day:** Acetaminophen 325 mg, dextromethorphan hydrobromide 10 mg, phenylephrine hydrochloride 5 mg. Mannitol, PEG 400, sorbitol. 10s. **Night:** Acetaminophen 325 mg, dextromethorphan hydrobromide 10 mg, doxylamine succinate 6.25 mg, phenylephrine hydrochloride 5 mg. Mannitol, PEG 400, sorbitol. 10s. *OTC.*
Use: Upper respiratory combination, antitussive combination.
Alka-Seltzer Plus Day Non-Drowsy Cold. (Bayer Consumer Care) **Cap. Liquid filled:** Acetaminophen 325 mg, dextromethorphan HBr 10 mg, phenylephrine hydrochloride 5 mg. Mannitol, PEG 400/600, sorbitol. 12s, 20s. **Liq.:** Acetaminophen 162.5 mg, dextromethorphan hydrobromide 5 mg, phenylephrine hydrochloride 2.5 mg/5 mL. Edetate disodium, PEG 400, sorbitol, sucralose. Alcohol free. 180 mL. *OTC.*
Use: Upper respiratory combination, antitussive combination.

Alka-Seltzer Plus Fast Crystal Packs. (Bayer Consumer Care) Acetaminophen 650 mg, chlorpheniramine maleate 4 mg, phenylephrine hydrochloride 10 mg. Acesulfame K, aspartame, phenylalanine 6 mg, sucralose, sucrose. Taste free. Pow. 10s. *OTC.*
Use: Upper respiratory combination; decongestant, antihistamine, and analgesic combination.
Alka-Seltzer Plus Flu. (Bayer Consumer Care) Dextromethorphan hydrobromide 15 mg, chlorpheniramine maleate 2 mg, aspirin 500 mg. Acesulfame K, aspartame, phenylalanine 6.7 mg, mannitol, saccharin, sodium 381 mg. Honey/orange flavor. Effervescent Tab. Pkg. 20s. *OTC.*
Use: Upper respiratory combination, antitussive, antihistamine, analgesic.
Alka-Seltzer Plus Mucus & Congestion. (Bayer Consumer Care) **Effervescent Tab:** Dextromethorphan HBr 10 mg, guaifenesin 200 mg. Acesulfame K, aspartame, mannitol, phenylalanine 6.7 mg, sodium 296 mg, sucralose. Lemon-lime flavor. 20s. **Cap., liquid filled:** Dextromethorphan hydrobromide 10 mg, guaifenesin 200 mg. Mannitol, PEG 400, PEG 600, sorbitan, sorbitol. 20s. *OTC.*
Use: Upper respiratory combination, expectorant.
Alka-Seltzer Plus Night Cold. (Bayer Consumer Care) **Effervescent Tab.:** Aspirin 500 mg, dextromethorphan HBr 10 mg, doxylamine succinate 6.25 mg, phenylephrine bitartrate 7.8 mg. Acesulfame K, aspartame, phenylalanine 5.6 mg, saccharin, sodium 474 mg, sorbitol. 20s. **Liq.:** Acetaminophen 162.5 mg, dextromethorphan hydrobromide 5 mg, doxylamine succinate 3.125 mg, phenylephrine hydrochloride 2.5 mg per 5 mL. Edetate disodium, PEG 400, sodium 3 mg, sorbitol, sucralose. Alcohol free. 180 mL. **Liquid-Gels:** Dextromethorphan HBr 10 mg, doxylamine succinate 6.25 mg, phenylephrine hydrochloride 5 mg, acetaminophen 325 mg. Sorbitol. 12s. *OTC.*
Use: Upper respiratory combination, antitussive combination.
Alka-Seltzer Plus Sinus. (Bayer Consumer Care) Phenylephrine hydrochloride 5 mg, acetaminophen 250 mg. Acesulfame K, phenylalanine 4.2 mg, saccharin, sodium 477 mg, sorbitol. Effervescent Tab. 20s. *OTC.*
Use: Upper respiratory combination, decongestant and analgesic combination.

Alka-Seltzer Plus Sparkling Original Cold Formula. (Bayer Consumer Care) Aspirin 325 mg, chlorpheniramine maleate 2 mg, phenylephrine bitartrate 5 mg. Acesulfame K, aspartame, mannitol, phenylalanine 8.4 mg, sodium 474 mg, sorbitol. Effervescent Tab. 20s. *OTC.*
Use: Upper respiratory combination, antihistamine and decongestant.
Alka-Seltzer PM. (Bayer Consumer Care) Aspirin 325 mg, diphenhydramine citrate 38 mg. Phenylalanine 4 mg, acesulfame K, aspartame, mannitol. Effervescent Tab. 24s. *OTC.*
Use: Upper respiratory combination, analgesic, antihistamine.
Alka-Seltzer Wake-Up Call. (Bayer Consumer Care) Aspirin 500 mg, caffeine 65 mg. Phenylalanine 9 mg, acesulfame K, aspartame, mannitol. Effervescent Tab. 16s. *OTC.*
Use: Analgesic.
Alkavite. (Vitality) Vitamins A 5000 units, C 250 mg, D 400 units, E 30 units, B_1 100 mg, B_6 3 mg, B_{12} 12 mcg, folic acid 1 mg, B_2 3 mg, niacin 20 mg, biotin 0.03 mg, Ca 68.5 mg, Fe 60 mg, Mg, Zn 4 mg, Se. ER Tab. UD 100s *OTC.*
Use: Vitamin supplement.
Alkeran. (Celgene) Melphalan. **Inj., Lyophilized, Pow. for Reconstitution:** 50 mg (as melphalan hydrochloride). Single-use vials (with povidone 20 mg) with 10 mL of sterile diluent (water for injection with sodium citrate 0.2 g, propylene glycol 6 mL, ethanol 0.52 mL). **Tab.:** 2 mg. Film-coated. Amber Glass Bot. 50s. *Rx.*
Use: Alkylating agent, nitrogen mustard.
alkylamines, nonselective.
Use: Antihistamine.
See: Brompheniramine.
  Chlorpheniramine Maleate.
  Chlorpheniramine Tannate.
  Dexbrompheniramine Maleate.
  Dexchlorpheniramine Maleate.
alkylating agents.
See: Alkyl Sulfonates.
  Estrogen/Nitrogen Mustard.
  Ethylenimines/Methylmelamines.
  Nitrogen Mustards.
  Nitrosoureas.
  Triazenes.
alkylbenzyldimethylammonium chloride. Benzalkonium Chloride.
●**alkyl (C12-15) benzoate.** (al-kil-BEN-zoe-ate) *NF 29.*
Use: Pharmaceutical aid, oleaginous vehicle emollient.

alkyl sulfonates.
Use: Alkylating agents.
See: Busulfan.
●**allantoin.** (al-AN-toe-in) USAN.
Use: Vulnerary, topical.
See: Cutemol Emollient.
  W/Combinations.
See: Anbesol Cold Sore Therapy.
  Nil Vaginal Cream.
  Nose Better Gel.
  Par.
  Tegrin.
AllanVan-DM B.I.D. (Allan) Dextromethorphan tannate 25 mg, pyrilamine tannate 30 mg, phenylephrine tannate 12.5 mg per 5 mL. Methylparaben, saccharin, sucrose. Grape flavor. Susp. 473 mL. *Rx.*
Use: Upper respiratory combination, antitussive combination.
AllanVan-S B.I.D. (Allan) Phenylephrine tannate 12.5 mg, pyrilamine tannate 30 mg per 5 mL. Parabens, saccharin, sucrose. Grape flavor. Susp. 480 mL. *Rx.*
Use: Upper respiratory combination, decongestant and antihistamine.
Allay. (LuChem Pharmaceuticals, Inc.) Acetaminophen 650 mg, hydrocodone bitartrate 7.5 mg. Cap. Bot. 100s. *c-III.*
Use: Analgesic combination; narcotic.
Allbee C-800. (Wyeth) Vitamins E 45 units, C 800 mg, B_1 15 mg, B_2 17 mg, B_3 100 mg, B_5 25 mg, B_{12} 12 mcg. Tab. Bot. 60s. *OTC.*
Use: Vitamin supplement.
Allbee C-800 Plus Iron. (Wyeth) Vitamins E 45 units, C 800 mg, B_1 15 mg, B_2 17 mg, niacin 100 mg, B_6 25 mg, B_{12} 12 mcg, pantothenic acid 25 mg, iron 27 mg, folic acid 0.4 mg. Tab. Bot. 60s. *OTC.*
Use: Mineral, vitamin supplement.
Allbee-T. (Wyeth) Vitamins B_1 15.5 mg, B_2 10 mg, B_6 8.2 mg, B_5 23 mg, B_3 100 mg, C 500 mg, B_{12} 5 mcg. Tab. Bot. 100s, 500s. *OTC.*
Use: Vitamin supplement.
Allbee w/C. (Wyeth) Vitamins B_1 15 mg, B_6 5 mg, B_2 10.2 mg, B_3 50 mg, B_5 10 mg, C 300 mg. Cap. Bot. 30s. *OTC.*
Use: Vitamin supplement.
Allbex. (Health for Life Brands) Vitamins B_1 5 mg, B_2 2 mg, B_6 0.25 mg, calcium pantothenate 3 mg, niacinamide 20 mg, ferrous sulfate 194.4 mg, inositol 10 mg, choline 10 mg, B_{12} (concentrate) 3 mcg. Cap. Bot. 100s, 1000s. *OTC.*
Use: Mineral, vitamin supplement.

All Day Allergy Children's. (Major) Cetirizine hydrochloride 10 mg. Acesulfame K, benzyl alcohol, lactose, maltodextrin, propylene glycol. Tutti frutti flavor. Chew. Tab. 24s. *OTC.* *Use:* Antihistamine, peripherally selective piperazine.

All-Day-C. (Barth's) Vitamin C 200 mg. or 500 mg. Cap (200 mg). Tab (500 mg). with rose hip extract. Bot. 30s, 90s, 180s, 360s. *OTC.* *Use:* Vitamin supplement.

All-Day Iron Yeast. (Barth's) Iron 20 mg, Vitamins B$_1$ 2 mg, B$_2$ 4 mg, niacin 0.57 mg. Cap. Bot. 30s, 90s, 180s. *OTC.* *Use:* Mineral, vitamin supplement.

All-Day-Vites. (Barth's) Vitamins A 10,000 units, D 400 units, B$_1$ 3 mg, B$_2$ 6 mg, niacin 1 mg, C 120 mg, B$_{12}$ 10 mcg, E 30 units. Cap. Bot. 30s, 90s, 180s, 360s. *OTC.* *Use:* Vitamin supplement.

Allegra. (Sanofi-Aventis) **Tab.:** Fexofenadine hydrochloride 30 mg, 60 mg, 180 mg. Film coated. Bot. 100s, 500s, blister pack 100s (60 mg only). **Oral Susp.:** Fexofenadine hydrochloride 6 mg/mL. Parabens, sucrose, xylitol, EDTA. Raspberry cream flavor. 30 mL, 300 mL. *Rx.* *Use:* Antihistamine, peripherally selective piperidine.

Allegra-D 12 Hour. (Sanofi-Aventis) Fexofenadine hydrochloride 60 mg (immediate release), pseudoephedrine hydrochloride 120 mg (extended release). Film coated. ER Tab. Bot. 100s. *Rx.* *Use:* Upper respiratory combination, antihistamine, decongestant.

Allegra-D 24 Hour. (Sanofi-Aventis) Pseudoephedrine hydrochloride 240 mg, fexofenadine hydrochloride 180 mg. PEG, isopropyl and methyl alcohols. Film-coated. ER Tab. 100s. *Rx.* *Use:* Decongestant and antihistamine, upper respiratory combination.

Allegra ODT. (Sanofi Aventis) Fexofenadine hydrochloride 30 mg. Aspartame, mannitol, phenylalanine 5.3 mg. Orally Disintegrating Tab. Orange-cream flavor. 60s. *Rx.* *Use:* Antihistamine, peripherally selective piperidine.

Allegron. Nortriptyline. *Use:* Antidepressant.

Allent. (B.F. Ascher) Pseudoephedrine hydrochloride 120 mg, brompheniramine maleate 12 mg. SR Cap. Bot. 100s. *Rx.* *Use:* Antihistamine; decongestant.

AllePak Dose Pack. (Everton Pharmaceuticals) **Day:** Pseudoephedrine hydrochloride 120 mg, methscopolamine nitrate 2.5 mg. Tab. 10s. **Night:** Chlorpheniramine maleate 8 mg, methscopolamine nitrate 2.5 mg. Tab. 10s. *Rx.* *Use:* Decongestant, antihistamine, and anticholinergic combination.

Allerben. (Forest) Diphenhydramine 10 mg/mL. Inj. Vial 30 mL. *Rx.* *Use:* Antihistamine.

Aller-Chlor. (Rugby) Chlorpheniramine maleate. **Tab.:** 4 mg. Bot. 24s, 100s, 1000s. **Syr.:** 2 mg/5 mL, alcohol 5%, parabens, sugar. Bot. 118 mL. *OTC.* *Use:* Antihistamine, nonselective alkylamine.

Allercon. (Parmed Pharmaceuticals, Inc.) Pseudoephedrine hydrochloride 60 mg, triprolidine hydrochloride 2.5 mg. Tab. Bot. 24s, 100s, 1000s. *OTC.* *Use:* Antihistamine; decongestant.

Allerest. (Insight) **Headache Strength Tab.:** Acetaminophen 325 mg, pseudoephedrine hydrochloride 30 mg, chlorpheniramine maleate 2 mg. Tab. Pkg. 24s. **Nasal Spray:** Oxymetazoline hydrochloride 0.05%. Bot. 0.5 oz. *OTC.* *Use:* Analgesic (Headache Strength Tab. only); antihistamine; decongestant.

Allerest Allergy & Sinus Relief Maximum Strength. (Insight) Pseudoephedrine hydrochloride 30 mg, acetaminophen 325 mg. Tab. 24s. *OTC.* *Use:* Decongestant and analgesic.

Allerest Maximum Strength. (Insight) Pseudoephedrine hydrochloride 30 mg, chlorpheniramine maleate 2 mg. Tab. Bot. 24s. *OTC.* *Use:* Upper respiratory combination, antihistamine, decongestant.

Allerest PE. (Insight) Phenylephrine hydrochloride 10 mg, chlorpheniramine maleate 4 mg. Tab. 8s. *OTC.* *Use:* Upper respiratory combination, decongestant and antihistamine.

Allerfrim. (Rugby) Pseudoephedrine hydrochloride 30 mg, triprolidine hydrochloride 1.25 mg/5 mL. Syr. 118 mL. *OTC.* *Use:* Upper respiratory combination, antihistamine; decongestant.

Allerfrim OTC Syrup. (Rugby) Pseudoephedrine 30 mg, triprolidine 1.25 mg. Syr. Bot. Pt. *OTC.* *Use:* Antihistamine; decongestant.

Allerfrim w/Codeine. (Rugby) Pseudoephedrine hydrochloride 30 mg, triproli-

---

dine hydrochloride 1.25 mg, codeine phosphate 10 mg, alcohol 4.3%. Syr. Bot. 120 mL, Pt, gal. *c-v.*
Use: Antihistamine; antitussive; decongestant.

Allergan Hydrocare Cleaning & Disinfecting Solution. (Allergan) Tris (2-hydroxyethyl) tallow ammonium chloride 0.013%, thimerosal 0.002%, bis (2-hydroxyethyl) tallow ammonium chloride, sodium bicarbonate, dibasic, monobasic and anhydrous sodium phosphate, hydrochloric acid, propylene glycol, polysorbate 80, special soluble polyhema. Bot. 4 oz, 8 oz, 12 oz. *OTC.*
Use: Contact lens care.

Allergan Hydrocare Preserved Saline Solution. (Allergan) Sodium chloride, sodium hexametaphosphate, sodium hydroxide, boric acid, sodium borate, EDTA 0.01%, thimerosal 0.001%. Bot. 8 oz, 12 oz. *OTC.*
Use: Contact lens care.

allergenic extracts. (Various Mfr.) Allergenic extracts of pollens, foods, inhalants, epidermals, fungi, insects, miscellaneous antigens.
Use: Diagnostic aid, allergens.

allergenic extracts, alum-precipitated.
See: Allpyral.
  Center-Al.

Allergen Patch Test Kit. (Healthpoint Medical) Box of tubes of semi-solid pastes or solutions. Allergens are either suspended in 4.5 g petrolatum, USP, or dissolved in 5.5 g water. Kit includes 20 reclosable syringes for topical use only (not for injection), each exuding sufficient allergen to test 150 patients, housed in a plastic case with two drawers. Allergens include benzocaine, mercaptobenzothiazole, colophony, p-phenylenediamine, imidazolidinyl urea (Germall115), cinnamon aldyhyde, lanolin alcohol (woolwax alcohols), carbarubber mix, neomycin sulfate, thiuram rubber mix, formaldehyde, ethylenediamine dihydrochloride, epoxyresin, quaternium 15, p-tert-butylphenol formalde hyderesin, mercapto rubber mix, black rubber p-phenylenediamine mix, potassium dichromate, balsam of Peru and nickel sulfate.

allergen test patches.
Use: Diagnostic aid; allergic dermatitis.
See: T.R.U.E. Test.

Allergex. (Bayer Consumer Care) Silicones, polyethylene and triethylene glycol, antioxidants, mineral oil concentrate. Bot. Pt. Aerosol pt.

ALLERMAX CAPLETS, MAXIMUM STRENGTH   35

Use: Antiallergic.

Allergy. (Major) Chlorpheniramine maleate 4 mg, lactose. Tab. Bot. 24s, 100s. *OTC.*
Use: Antihistamine, nonselective alkylamine.

Allergy-D. (Major) Cetirizine hydrochloride 5 mg, pseudoephedrine hydrochloride 120 mg. Lactose. ER Tab. 12s. *OTC.*
Use: Upper respiratory combination, decongestant and antihistamine.

Allergy DN. (Breckenridge) **Day:** Pseudoephedrine hydrochloride 120 mg, methscopolamine nitrate 2.5 mg. **Night:** Chlorpheniramine maleate 8 mg, methscopolamine nitrate 2.5 mg. Tab. 20s (10 day, 10 night). *Rx.*
Use: Upper respiratory combination, decongestant, antihistamine, and anticholinergic combination.

allergy preparations.
See: Antihistamines.

Allergy Relief. (Zee Medical) Chlorpheniramine maleate 4 mg. Tab. 12s. *OTC.*
Use: Antihistamine.

Allergy Relief & Nasal Decongestant. Loratadine 10 mg, pseudoephedrine sulfate 240 mg. Lactose, PEG. ER Tab. 10s. *OTC.*
Use: Upper respiratory combination, decongestant and antihistamine.

Allergy Tablets. (Major) Chlorpheniramine 4 mg. Tab. Bot. 24s and 100s. *OTC.*
Use: Antihistamine.

Allergy-Time. (Time-Cap Labs) Chlorpheniramine maleate 4 mg. Lactose. Tab. 1,000s. *OTC.*
Use: Antihistamine, nonselective alkylamine.

AllerMax. (Pfeiffer) Diphenhydramine hydrochloride 12.5 mg/5 mL, alcohol 0.5%, glucose, saccharin, sorbitol, sucrose, menthol, raspberry flavor. Liq. Bot. 118 mL. *OTC.*
Use: Antihistamine, nonselective ethanolamine, nonnarcotic antitussive.

AllerMax Allergy & Cough Formula. (Pfeiffer) Diphenhydramine hydrochloride 6.25 mg/5 mL, alcohol 0.5%, raspberry flavor, menthol, sucrose, glucose, saccharin, sorbitol. Bot. 118 mL. *OTC.*
Use: Antihistamine.

AllerMax Caplets, Maximum Strength. (Pfeiffer) Diphenhydramine hydrochloride 50 mg, lactose. Tab. Bot. 24s. *OTC.*
Use: Antihistamine, nonselective ethanolamine.

Allersone. (Roberts) Hydrocortisone 0.5%, diperodon hydrochloride 0.5%, zinc oxide 5%, sodium lauryl sulfate, propylene glycol, cetyl alcohol, petrolatum, methyl- and propylparabens. Oint. Tube 15 g. *Rx-OTC.*
Use: Corticosteroid, topical.

Allersule Forte. (Edwards) Phenylephrine hydrochloride 20 mg, chlorpheniramine maleate 8 mg, methscopolamine nitrate 2.5 mg. Cap. Bot. 100s. *Rx-OTC.*
Use: Anticholinergic; antihistamine; decongestant.

AlleRx. (Cornerstone) Phenylephrine tannate 7.5 mg, chlorpheniramine tannate 3 mg per 5 mL. Methylparaben, saccharin, sucrose. Raspberry flavor. Susp. 473 mL. *Rx.*
Use: Upper respiratory combination.

AlleRx-D. (Cornerstone) Pseudoephedrine hydrochloride 120 mg, methscopolamine nitrate 2.5 mg. ER Tab. Bot. 60s. *Rx.*
Use: Upper respiratory combination, decongestant, anticholinergic combination.

AlleRx DF Dose Pack. (Cornerstone) **Day:** Chlorpheniramine maleate 4 mg, methscopolamine nitrate 2.5 mg. Lactose. **Night:** Chlorpheniramine maleate 8 mg, methscopolamine nitrate 2.5 mg. Lactose.Tab. 20s (10 day, 10 night), 60s (30 day, 30 night). *Rx.*
Use: Upper respiratory combination; decongestant, antihistamine, and anticholinergic combination.

AlleRx Dose Pack. (Cornerstone) **Day:** Pseudoephedrine hydrochloride 120 mg, methscopolamine nitrate 2.5 mg. **Night:** Chlorpheniramine maleate 8 mg, methscopolamine nitrate 2.5 mg, phenylephrine hydrochloride 10 mg. Lactose. CR Tab. Pkg. 20s (10 day, 10 night), 60s (30 day, 30 night). *Rx.*
Use: Upper respiratory combination, anticholinergic, antihistamine, decongestant combination.

Allfen C. (MCR American) Carbetapentane citrate 5 mg, guaifenesin 1000 mg. ER Tab. 100s. *Rx.*
Use: Antitussives with expectorant.

Allfen CDX. (MCR) Codeine phosphate 20 mg, guaifenesin 200 mg. Parabens, sorbitol, sucralose. Liq. 473 mL. *c-III.*
Use: Upper respiratory combination, antitussive with expectorant.

Allfen DM. (MCR American) Dextromethorphan HBr 58 mg, guaifenesin 1000 mg. Dye free. Tab. Bot. 100s. *Rx.*

Use: Upper respiratory combination, antitussive, expectorant.

Alli. (GlaxoSmithKline) Orlistat 60 mg. Cap. 60s, 90s, 120s. *OTC.*
Use: Lipase inhibitor.

All-Nite. (Major) Dextromethorphan HBr 5 mg, doxylamine succinate 2.1 mg, acetaminophen 166.7 mg per 5 mL. Alcohol 10%, saccharin. Liq. Bot. 177 mL. *OTC.*
Use: Upper respiratory combination, antitussive combination.

All-Nite Children's Cold/Cough Relief. (Major) Pseudoephedrine hydrochloride 10 mg, chlorpheniramine maleate 0.67 mg, dextromethorphan HBr 5 mg per 5 mL. Alcohol free. Sucrose. Cherry flavor. Liq. 118 mL. *OTC.*
Use: Antihistamine; antitussive; decongestant.

• **allobarbital.** (AL-low-BAR-bih-tal) USAN. *Formerly Diallybarbituric acid.*
Use: Hypnotic; sedative.

• **allopurinol.** (AL-oh-PURE-ee-nahl) *USP 34.*
Use: Antigout; xanthine oxidase inhibitor; antimetabolite.
See: Aloprim.
Zyloprim.

allopurinol. (Various Mfr.) Allopurinol 100 mg, 300 mg. Tab. Bot. 100s, 500s, 1000s, UD 100s. *Rx.*
Use: Antimetabolite.

allopurinol sodium. (Bedford Labs) Allopurinol sodium 500 mg. Preservative free. Pow. for Inj., lyophilized. Vials with rubber stopper. 30 mL. *Rx.*
Use: Antimetabolite.

Allpyral. (Bayer Consumer Care) Allergenic extracts, alum-precipitated. For subcutaneous inj. pollens, molds, epithelia, house dust, other inhalants, stinging insects.
Use: Diagnostic aid, allergens.

Allres DS. (Allegis) Chlorpheniramine maleate 4 mg (as 8 mg chlorpheniramine tannate), dextromethorphan hydrobromide 30 mg (as 60 mg dextromethorphan tannate), pseudoephedrine hydrochloride 30 mg (as 60 mg pseudoephedrine tannate) per 5 mL. Acesulfame K, aspartame, methylparaben, phenylalanine 25.25 mg, sucralose. Grape bubble gum flavor. Susp. 473 mL. *Rx.*
Use: Upper respiratory combination, antitussive combination.

allylamine antifungal.
Use: Antifungal agent.
See: Terbinafine Hydrochloride.

allylbarbituric acid. Allylisobutylbarbituric acid, butalbital.
Use: Sedative.

W/A.P.C.
See: Anti-Ten.
Fiorinal.
W/Acetaminophen.
See: Panitol.
allyl-isobutylbarbituric acid.
See: Allylbarbituric Acid.
•**allyl isothiocyanate.** (AL-il EYE-soe-THYE-oh-SYE-a-nate) *USP 34.*
Use: Counterirritant in neuralgia.
Almacone. (Rugby) **Chew Tab.**: Aluminum hydroxide 200 mg, magnesium hydroxide 200 mg, simethicone 20 mg. Bot. 100s, 1000s. **Liq.**: Aluminum hydroxide 200 mg, magnesium hydroxide 200 mg, simethicone 20 mg, sodium 0.75 mg/5 mL. Bot. 360 mL, gal. *OTC.*
Use: Antacid.
Almacone II Double Strength Liquid. (Rugby) Aluminum hydroxide 400 mg, magnesium hydroxide 400 mg, simethicone 40 mg/5 mL. Bot. 360 mL, gal. *OTC.*
Use: Antacid.
•**almadrate sulfate.** (AL-ma-drate SULL-fate) USAN. Aluminum magnesium hydroxide-oxide-sulfate-hydrate.
Use: Antacid.
•**almagate.** (AL-mah-gate) USAN.
Use: Antacid.
almagucin. Gastric mucin, dried aluminum hydroxide gel, magnesium trisilicate. *OTC.*
Use: Antacid.
Almebex Plus B₁₂. (Dayton) Vitamins B₁ 1 mg, B₂ 2 mg, B₃ 5 mg, B₆ 0.4 mg, B₁₂ 5 mcg, choline 33 mg/5 mL. Bot. 473 mL (with B₁₂ in separate container). *OTC.*
Use: Vitamin supplement.
•**almond oil.** *NF 29.*
Use: Pharmaceutic aid, emollient, oleaginous vehicle, perfume.
•**almotriptan.** (al-moe-TRIP-tan) USAN.
Use: Antimigraine.
•**almotriptan malate.** (al-moe-TRIP-tan MAL-ee-ate) USAN.
Use: Antimigraine agent, serotonin 5-HT₁ receptor agonist.
See: Axert.
•**alniditan dihydrochloride.** (al-nih-DIH-tan die-HIGH-droe-KLOR-ide) USAN.
Use: Antimigraine.
Alnyte. (Mayer Lab) Scopolamine aminoxide HBr 0.2 mg, salicylamide 250 mg. Tab. Pkg. 16s. *Rx.*
Use: Analgesic; anticholinergic.
Alocass Laxative. (Western Research) Aloin 0.25 g, cascara sagrada 0.5 g,

rhubarb 0.5 g, ginger ⅟₃₂ g, powdered extract of belladonna g. Tab. Bot. 1000s. Pak 28s. *OTC.*
Use: Laxative.
Alocril. (Allergan) Nedocromil sodium 2% (20 mg/mL), benzalkonium chloride 0.01%, NaCl 0.5%, EDTA 0.05%. Ophth. Soln. Bot. 5 mL w/dropper tip. *Rx.*
Use: Ophthalmic agent, mast cell stabilizer.
Alodox Convenience Kit. (OcuSoft) Doxycycline 20 mg (equiv. to doxycycline hyclate 23 mg). Lactose, polydextrose. Tab. 60s. *Rx.*
Use: Tetracycline.
•**aloe.** (AL-oh) *USP 34.*
Use: See Compound Benzoin Tincture.
Aloe Grande Creme. (Gordon Laboratories) Aloe, vitamins E 1500 units, A 100,000 units/oz in cream base. Jar 2.5 oz. *OTC.*
Use: Emollient.
Aloe Vesta. (ConvaTec) **Cloth:** Aloe barbadensis leaf juice, dimethicone, parabens, urea. 24s. **Lot.:** Dimethicone 3%. Alcohols, aloe, glycerin, petrolatum. 60 mL. **Oint:** Miconazole nitrate 2%. Aloe, mineral oil, white petrolatum. 56 g, 141 g. **Spray:** Petrolatum 36%, mineral oil, aloe extract. 60 g. *OTC.*
Use: Emollient.
Aloe Vesta Perineal. (ConvaTec) Solution of sodium C14-16 olefin sulfonate, propylene glycol, aloe vera gel, hydrolyzed collagen. Bot. 118 mL, 236 mL, gal. *OTC.*
Use: Perianal hygiene.
•**alofilcon A.** (AL-oh-FILL-kahn) USAN.
Use: Contact lens material, hydrophilic.
•**alogliptin benzoate.** (AL-oh-GLIP-tin BEN-zoe-ate) USAN.
Use: Antidiabetic.
aloin. (J.T. Baker) A mixture of crystalline pentosides from various aloes. Bot. oz. *OTC.*
Use: Laxative.
Alomide. (Alcon) Lodoxamide tromethamine 0.1%. Soln. *Drop-tainers* 10 mL. *Rx.*
Use: Antiallergic, ophthalmic.
•**alonimid.** (ah-LAHN-ih-mid) USAN.
Use: Hypnotic; sedative.
Alophen. (Numark) Bisacodyl 5 mg, sugar. EC Tab. Bot. 100s. *OTC.*
Use: Laxative.
Aloprim. (Nabi) Allopurinol 500 mg. Preservative free. Pow. for Inj., lyophilized. Vial 30 mL with rubber stoppers. *Rx.*
Use: Antimetabolite.

Aloquin. (Primus Pharma) Aloe polysac-charides 1%, iodoquinol 1.25%, benzyl alcohol, PEG-20, SDA alcohol 40 B. Gel. 60 g. *Rx.*
Use: Miscellaneous topical combination.
Alora. (Watson) Estradiol 0.77 mg (0.025 mg/day), 1.5 mg (0.05 mg/day), 2.3 mg (0.075 mg/day), 3.1 mg (0.1 mg/day). Transdermal System. Calendar packs 8 systems. *Rx.*
Use: Estrogen, sex hormone.
•**alosetron hydrochloride.** (al-OH-seh-trahn HIGH-droe-KLOR-ide) USAN.
Use: Antiemetic.
See: Lotronex.
Alotone. (Major) Triamcinolone 4 mg. Tab. Bot. 100s. *Rx.*
Use: Corticosteroid.
•**alovudine.** (al-OHV-you-deen) USAN.
Use: Antiviral.
Aloxi. (Eisai Inc.) Palonosetron hydro-chloride 0.05 mg/mL. Disodium ede-tate. Inj., Soln. Single-use vials. 1.5 mL (mannitol 83 mg), 5 mL (mannitol 207.5 mg). *Rx.*
Use: 5-HT$_3$ receptor antagonist, anti-emetic/antivertigo agent.
•**alpertine.** (al-PURR-teen) USAN.
Use: Antipsychotic.
l-alpha-acetyl-methadol (LAAM). (Bio Development Corp.) *Rx.*
Use: Treatment of heroin addicts.
[Orphan Drug]
•**alpha amylase.** (AL-fah AM-ih-lace) USAN. A concentrated form of alpha amylase produced by a strain of non-pathogenic bacteria.
Use: Digestive aid; anti-inflammatory.
See: Kutrase Capsules.
Ku-Zyme Capsules.
alpha-amylase w-100. W/Proteinase W-300, cellase W-100, lipase, estrone, testosterone, vitamins, minerals. *Rx.*
Use: Digestive aid.
alpha/beta-adrenergic blocking agent.
See: Carvedilol.
Labetalol Hydrochloride.
alpha-chymotrypsin.
See: Chymotrypsin.
Alphaderm. (Teva) Hydrocortisone 1%. Cream. Tube 30 g, 100 g. *Rx-OTC.*
Use: Corticosteroid, topical.
alpha-d-galactosidase.
Use: Antiflatulent.
Alpha-E. (Barth's) d-Alpha tocopherol.
50 units or 100 units: Cap. Bot. 100s, 500s, 1000s. **200 units:** Cap. Bot. 100s, 250s. **400 units:** Cap. Bot. 100s, 250s, 500s. *OTC.*
Use: Vitamin supplement.

alpha-estradiol. Known as beta-estradiol.
See: Estradiol.
Alpha Fast. (Eastwood) Bath oil. Bot. 16 oz. *OTC.*
Use: Emollient.
alpha-fetoprotein with Tc-99m.
Use: Diagnostic aid.
•**alphafilcon A.** (al-fah-FILL-kahn) USAN.
Use: Contact lens material, hydrophilic.
alpha-galactosidase.
See: Aspergillus niger enzyme.
alpha-galactosidase A.
Use: Fabry disease. [Orphan Drug]
alpha-galactoside A.
Use: Treatment of Fabry disease.
[Orphan Drug]
Alphagan P. (Allergan) Brimonidine tar-trate 0.1%, 0.15%, *Purite* 0.005%, bo-ric acid, potassium chloride, sodium borate, sodium chloride. Hydrochloric acid and/or sodium hydroxide to adjust pH. Soln. Bot. 5 mL, 10 mL, 15 mL. *Rx.*
Use: Agent for glaucoma.
alpha-glucosidase inhibitor.
Use: Antidiabetic agent.
See: Acarbose.
Miglitol.
alpha-glucosidase, recombinant hu-man acid. (Pharmain BV)
Use: Glycogen storage disease type II.
[Orphan Drug]
alpha-hypophamine.
See: Oxytocin.
alpha interferon-2b.
See: Intron A.
•**alpha lipoic acid.** *NF 29.*
Use: Antioxidant.
Alpha-Keri. (Novartis Consumer)
Shower & Bath: Mineral oil, lanolin oil, PEG-4-dilaurate, benzophenone-3, D&C green #6, fragrance. Bot. 4 oz, 8 oz, 16 oz. **Cleansing Bar:** Bar con-taining sodium tallowate, sodium co-coate, water, mineral oil, fragrance, PEG-75, glycerin, titanium dioxide, lanolin oil, sodium chloride, BHT, EDTA, D&C green #5, D&C yellow #10. 120 g. *OTC.*
Use: Emollient.
alpha-methyldopa. *Name previously used for Methyldopa.*
Alphanate. (Grifols) Human antihemo-philic factor ≥ 5 units/mg total protein. Albumin (human) 0.3 to 0.9 g/100 mL, arginine, glycine, heparin, histidine, PEG, sodium. Solvent/detergent treated, heat treated. Inj., lyophilized Pow. for Soln. Kit with single-dose vial and sterile water for Inj. *Rx.*

Use: Antihemophilic agent; treatment for von Willebrand disease. [Orphan Drug]

AlphaNine. (Grifols) Purified heat-treated/solvent preparation of coagulation Factor IX from human plasma. With ≥ 50 units Factor IX per mg protein, < 5 units each Factor II (prothrombin) and Factor VII (proconvertin) per 100 IU Factor IX and < 20 units Factor X (Stuart-Power Factor) per 100 IU Factor IX. In single-dose vials with diluent, double-ended needle, and microaggregated filter. Pow. for Inj. *Rx.*
Use: Antihemophilic.

AlphaNine SD. (Grifols) Factor IX (human) ≥ 150 units/mg protein (solvent/detergent treated). Actual number of units shown on each bottle. Virus filtered. Dextrose, heparin, polysorbate 80, tri(n-butyl) phosphate. Inj., lyophilized Pow. for Soln. Kit with single-dose vial and sterile water for Inj. 10 mL. *Rx.*
Use: Antihemophilic agent.

alpha-1-adrenergic blockers.
Use: Antihypertensives.
See: Alfuzosin.
 Silodosin.
 Tamsulosin Hydrochloride.

alpha-1 antitrypsin. Alpha-1 trypsin inhibitor; human alpha-1 protease inhibitor.
Use: Glycoprotein.

alpha-1-proteinase inhibitor.
Use: Treatment of alpha-1-antitrypsin deficiency.
See: Aralast NP.
 Prolastin.
 Zemaira.

alphasone acetophenide. Name previously used for Algestone acetonide.

alpha-tocopherol.
See: Vitamin E.

alpha-2 adrenergic agonist.
Use: Glaucoma agent.
See: Brimonidine tartrate.

Alpha Vee-12. (Schlucksup) Hydroxocobalamin 1000 mcg/mL. Vial 10 mL. *Rx.*
Use: Vitamin supplement.

Alphosyl. (Schwarz Pharma) Allantoin 1.7%, special crude coal tar extracts 5%. **Lot.:** Bot. 8 fl oz. **Cream:** 2 oz. *OTC.*
Use: Antipruritic.

•**alpidem.** (AL-PIH-dem) USAN.
Use: Antianxiety; anxiolytic.

•**alprazolam.** (al-PRAY-zoe-lam) *USP 34.*
Tall Man: ALPRAZolam
Use: Hypnotic; sedative; antianxiety agent.
See: Niravam.

 Xanax.
 Xanax XR.

alprazolam. (Par Pharmaceuticals) Alprazolam 0.25 mg, 0.5 mg, 1 mg, 2 mg. Aspartame, mannitol, peppermint and vanilla flavoring, phenylalanine, sorbitol, xylitol. Tab. UD 100s. *c-iv.*
Use: Antianxiety agent, benzodiazepine.

alprazolam. (Various Mfr.) Alprazolam. **ER Tab.:** 0.5 mg, 1 mg, 2 mg, 3 mg. May contain lactose. 60s, 500s. **Tab.:** 0.25 mg, 0.5 mg, 1 mg, 2 mg. Bot. 100s, 500s, 1000s (except 2 mg), UD 100s (except 2 mg). *c-iv.*
Use: Management of anxiety disorders.

alprazolam intensol. (Roxane) Alprazolam 1 mg/mL. Flavorless. Oral Soln. 30 mL with calibrated dropper. *c-iv.*
Use: Antianxiety agent.

•**alprenolol hydrochloride.** (al-PREH-nolole HIGH-droe-KLOR-ide) USAN.
Use: Antiadrenergic; β-receptor.

•**alprenoxime hydrochloride.** (al-PRENox-eem) USAN.
Use: Antiglaucoma agent.

•**alprostadil.** (al-PRAHST-uh-dill) *USP 34.*
Formerly Prostaglandin E₁, PGE₁.
Use: Vasodilator; anti-impotence agent; arterial patency agent.
See: Caverject.
 Edex.
 Muse.
 Prostin VR Pediatric.

•**alrestatin sodium.** (AHL-reh-STAT-in SO-dee-uhm) USAN.
Use: Enzyme inhibitor, aldose reductase.

Alrex. (Bausch & Lomb) Loteprednol etabonate 0.2%. Benzalkonium chloride 0.01%, EDTA, glycerin, povidone. Ophth. Susp. Bot. 5 mL, 10 mL. *Rx.*
Use: Corticosteroid, ophthalmic.

AL-721. (Matrix) Phase I/II AIDS, ARC, HIV positive.
Use: Antiviral.

Alsorb Gel. (Standex) Magnesium and aluminum hydroxide. Colloidal Susp. *OTC.*
Use: Antacid.

Alsorb Gel, C.T. (Standex) Calcium carbonate 2 g, glycine 3 g, magnesium trisilicate 3 g. Tab. *OTC.*
Use: Antacid.

Altabax. (GlaxoSmithKline) Retapamulin 1%. White petrolatum. Top. Oint. Tubes. 15 g, 30 g. *Rx.*
Use: Topical anti-infective.

Altacaine. (Altaire) Tetracaine hydrochloride 0.5%. Chlorobutanol, boric acid,

potassium chloride, hydrochloric acid or sodium hydroxide. Soln. 15 mL, 30 mL. *Rx.*
Use: Ophthalmic local anesthetic.

Altace. (Monarch) Ramipril 1.25 mg, 2.5 mg, 5 mg, 10 mg. Cap. Bot. 100s, 500s (except 1.25 mg), 1000s (except 1.25 mg), UD 100s (except 10 mg), bulk pack 5000s (2.5 mg, 5 mg only). *Rx.*
Use: Antihypertensive; renin angiotensin system antagonist.

Altafed. (Altaire Pharmaceuticals) Pseudoephedrine hydrochloride 30 mg, triprolidine hydrochloride 1.25 mg per 5 mL. Methylparaben, sorbitol. Syr. 118 mL. *OTC.*
Use: Upper respiratory combination, decongestant and antihistamine.

Altafrin. (Altaire) Phenylephrine hydrochloride 2.5%, 10%. Ophth. Soln. 5 mL (benzalkonium chloride, sodium phosphate mono- and dibasic), 15 mL (benzalkonium chloride, boric acid, sodium phosphate mono- and dibasic) (except 10%). *OTC.*
Use: Ophthalmic decongestant.

●**altanserin tartrate.** (AL-TAN-ser-in TARtrate) USAN.
Use: Serotonin antagonist.

Altarussin. (Altaire) Guaifenesin 100 mg/5 mL. Alcohol-free. Corn syrup, menthol, saccharin. Syrup. 118 mL. *OTC.*
Use: Expectorant.

Altarussin-PE. (Altaire) Pseudoephedrine hydrochloride 30 mg, guaifenesin 100 mg per 5 mL. Alcohol free. Corn syrup, saccharin. Liq. 118 mL. *OTC.*
Use: Upper respiratory combination, decongestant and expectorant combination.

Altaryl Children's Allergy. (Altaire) Diphenhydramine (as hydrochloride) 12.5 mg per 5 mL. Alcohol free. Sodium 9 mg, glycerin, saccharin, sugar. Cherry flavor. Liq. 118 mL. *OTC.*
Use: Antihistamine.

Altazine. (Altaire) Tetrahydrozoline hydrochloride 0.05%. Soln., Ophth. 15 mL, 30 mL. *OTC.*
Use: Ophthalmic decongestant.

●**alteplase, recombinant.** (AL-teh-PLACE) USAN.
Use: Plasminogen activator.
See: Activase.
Cathflo Activase.

AlternaGEL. (J & J Merck Consumer Pharm.) Aluminum hydroxide 600 mg/5 mL. Liq. Bot. 150 mL, 360 mL. *OTC.*
Use: Antacid.

●**althiazide.** (al-THIGH-azz-ide) USAN.
Use: Antihypertensive; diuretic.

●**altinicline maleate.** (AL-ti-ni-kleen) USAN.
Use: Antiparkinsonian agent.

Altoprev. (Sciele) Lovastatin 10 mg, 20 mg, 40 mg, 60 mg. Sugar, lactose. ER Tab. Bot. 30s. *Rx.*
Use: Antihyperlipidemic.

Altracin. (Alra) Bacitracin.
Use: Antibiotic. [Orphan Drug]

●**altretamine.** (ahl-TRETT-uh-meen) USAN.
Use: Antineoplastic.
See: Hexalen.

al12. (JSJ Pharmaceuticals) Ammonium lactate. **Aer. Foam:** 12%. Butyrospermum parkii, cetyl alcohol, helianthus annuus seed oil. 113.4 g. **Lot:** 12%. Cetyl alcohol, glycerin, mineral oil, PEG-40, PEG-100, parabens. 423 mL. *OTC.*
Use: Emollient.

Al-U-Creme. (MacAllister) Aluminum hydroxide equivalent to 4% aluminum oxide. Susp. Bot. Pt, gal. *OTC.*
Use: Antacid.

Aludrox. (Wyeth) Aluminum hydroxide gel 307 mg, magnesium hydroxide 103 mg/5 mL. Susp. Bot. 355 mL. *OTC.*
Use: Antacid.

alukalin. Activated kaolin.
Use: Antidiarrheal.

Alulex. (Lexington) Magnesium trisilicate 3.25 g, aluminum hydroxide gel 3.5 g, phenobarbital ⅛ g, homatropine methylbromide g. Tab. Bot. 100s. *Rx.*
Use: Agent for peptic ulcer.

alum. Sulfuric acid, aluminum ammonium salt (2:1:1), dodecahydrate. Sulfuric acid, aluminum potassium salt (2:1:1), dodecahydrate.
Use: Astringent.

●**alum, ammonium.** (AL-um) *USP 34.*
Use: Astringent.

Alumate-HC. (Dermco) Hydrocortisone 0.125%, 0.25%, 0.5%, 1%. Cream. Pkg. 0.5 oz, 1 oz, 4 oz. *OTC.*
Use: Corticosteroid, topical.

Alumate Mixture. (Schlicksup) Aluminum hydroxide gel, milk of magnesia/5 mL. Bot. 12 oz, gal. *OTC.*
Use: Antacid.

alumina and magnesia.
Use: Antacid.

alumina and magnesium carbonate.
Use: Antacid.

alumina and magnesium trisilicate.
Use: Antacid.

alumina hydrated. W/Activated attapulgite, pectin. *OTC.*

Use: Antidiarrheal.
alumina, magnesia, and calcium carbonate.
Use: Antacid.
alumina, magnesia, and calcium chloride.
Use: Antacid.
alumina, magnesia, and simethicone.
(Roxane) Aluminum hydroxide 213 mg, magnesium hydroxide 200 mg, simethicone 20 mg, parabens, sorbitol/5 mL. Susp. Bot. UD 15, 30 mL. *OTC.*
Use: Antacid.
alumina, magnesia, calcium carbonate, and simethicone.
Use: Antacid.
alumina, magnesium carbonate, and magnesium oxide.
Use: Antacid.
•**aluminum acetate topical solution.** (ah-LOO-min-uhm) *USP 34.*
Use: Astringent.
See: Buro-Sol Antiseptic.
   Domeboro.
   Domeboro Otic.
aluminum aminoacetate, dihydroxy.
See: Dihydroxyaluminum Aminoacetate.
aluminum chlorhydroxide.
See: Aluminum Chlorohydrate.
•**aluminum chloride.** (ah-LOO-min-uhm KLOR-ide) *USP 34.* Aluminum chloride hexahydrate.
Use: Astringent; drying agent.
See: Drysol.
   Xerac AC.
aluminum chloride (hexahydrate).
(Glades) Aluminum chloride hexahydrate 20% in SD alcohol 40-2 88.5%. Soln. Bot. 37.5 mL, *Dab-O-Matic* applicator bottle 35 mL, 60 mL. *Rx.*
Use: Drying agent.
•**aluminum chlorohydrate.** (ah-LOO-min-uhm) *USP 34.* Formerly *Aluminum chlorhydroxide, aluminum hydroxychloride.*
Use: Anhidrotic.
See: Ostiderm Roll-On.
•**aluminum chlorohydrex.** (ah-LOO-min-uhm) *USAN.* Formerly *Aluminum chlorhydroxide alcohol soluble complex, aluminum chlorohydrol propylene glycol complex.*
Use: Astringent.
•**aluminum chlorohydrex polyethylene glycol.** (ah-LOO-min-uhm) *USP 34.*
Use: Anhidrotic.
•**aluminum chlorohydrex propylene glycol.** (ah-LOO-min-uhm) *USP 34.*
Use: Anhidrotic.

•**aluminum dichlorohydrate.** (ah-LOO-min-uhm) *USP 34.*
Use: Anhidrotic.
•**aluminum dichlorohydrex polyethylene glycol.** (ah-LOO-min-uhm) *USP 34.*
Use: Anhidrotic.
•**aluminum dichlorohydrex propylene glycol.** (ah-LOO-min-uhm) *USP 34.*
Use: Anhidrotic.
aluminum dihydroxyaminoacetate.
(ah-LOO-min-uhm)
See: Dihydroxyaluminum Aminoacetate.
aluminum glycinate, basic.
See: Dihydroxyaluminum Aminoacetate.
aluminum hydroxide.
Use: Antacid.
W/Aspirin, Magnesium Hydroxide.
See: Arthritis Pain Formula.
W/Aspirin, Magnesium Hydroxide, Calcium Carbonate.
See: Ascriptin Maximum Strength.
W/Magnesium Carbonate.
See: Acid Gone.
   Gaviscon Extra Strength Antacid.
W/Magnesium Hydroxide, Simethicone.
See: Maalox Advanced Maximum Strength.
   Maalox Advanced Regular Strength.
   Maalox Regular Strength.
   Mi-Acid Maximum Strength.
   Mylanta Maximum Strength.
   Mylanta Regular Strength.
•**aluminum hydroxide gel.** (ah-LOO-min-uhm) *USP 34.*
Use: Antacid.
See: AlternaGEL.
   Al-U-Creme.
   Amphojel.
W/Aminoacetic acid, magnesium trisilicate.
See: Maracid-2.
W/Calcium carbonate, magnesium carbonate, magnesium trisilicate.
See: Marblen.
W/Magnesium hydroxide.
See: Alsorb Gel.
   Aludrox.
   Delcid.
   Gas Ban DS.
W/Magnesium hydroxide, aspirin.
See: Ascriptin.
   Calciphen.
W/Magnesium hydroxide, simethicone.
See: Di-Gel.
   Gas-Ban DS.
   Maalox Maximum Strength Multi-Symptom.
   Trial AG.

W/Magnesium trisilicilate.
See: Gacid.
Gaviscon.
Maracid 2.
W/Phenindamine tartrate, phenylephrine
hydrochloride, aspirin, caffeine, magnesium carbonate.
See: Dristan.
aluminum hydroxide gel. (Various Mfr.)
Aluminum hydroxide 320 mg/5 mL.
Susp. Bot. 360 mL, 480 mL, UD 15 and
30 mL. OTC.
Use: Antacid.
**aluminum hydroxide gel, concen-
trated.** (Various Mfr.) Aluminum
hydroxide 600 mg/5 mL. Liq. Bot.
30 mL, 180 mL, 480 mL. OTC.
Use: Antacid.
**aluminum hydroxide gel, concen-
trated.** (Roxane) Susp. **450 mg/5 mL:**
Bot. 500 mL, UD 30 mL; **675 mg/5 mL:**
Bot. 180 mL, 500 mL, UD 20 mL and
30 mL. OTC.
Use: Antacid.
aluminum hydroxide gel, dried.
Use: Antacid.
W/Combinations.
See: Aludrox.
Alurex.
Banacid.
Delcid.
Eulcin.
Gaviscon.
Mylanta Maximum Strength.
Mylanta Regular Strength.
Presalin.
aluminum hydroxide glycine.
See: Dihydroxyaluminum aminoace-
tate.
**aluminum hydroxide magnesium
carbonate.**
Use: Antacid.
See: Di-Gel.
•**aluminum monostearate.** (ah-LOO-min-
uhm) NF 29.
Use: Pharmaceutic necessity for prepa-
ration of penicillin G procaine w/alumi-
num stearate suspension.
See: Penicillin G procaine w/aluminum
stearate suspension, sterile.
aluminum paste. (Paddock) Metallic alu-
minum 10%. Oint. Jar lb. OTC.
Use: Dermatologic, protectant.
•**aluminum phosphate gel.** (ah-LOO-min-
uhm FOSS-fate) USP 34.
Use: Antacid.
•**aluminum sesquichlorohydrate.** (ah-
LOO-min-uhm sess-kwih-KLOR-oh-
HIGH-drate) USP 34.
Use: Anhidrotic.

•**aluminum sesquichlorohydrex polyethylene glycol.** (ah-LOO-min-uhm
sess-kwih-KLOR-oh-HIGH-drex poli-
eth-uh-leen gli-cawl) USP 34.
Use: Anhidrotic.
•**aluminum sesquichlorohydrex propylene glycol.** (ah-LOO-min-uhm sess-
kwih-KLOR-oh-HIGH-drex) USP 34.
Use: Anhidrotic.
aluminum sodium carbonate hydroxide.
See: Dihydroxyaluminum sodium
carbonate.
•**aluminum subacetate.** (ah-LOO-min-
uhm sub-AS-e-tate) USP 34.
Use: Astringent.
•**aluminum sulfate.** (ah-LOO-min-uhm
SULL-fate) USP 34.
Use: Pharmaceutic necessity for preparation of aluminum subacetate solution.
See: Aluminum subacetate topical solution.
Ostiderm.
•**aluminum zirconium octachlorohy-
drate.** (ah-LOO-min-uhm zihr-KOE-
nee-uhm) USP 34.
Use: Anhidrotic.
•**aluminum zirconium octachlorohydrex
gly.** (ah-LOO-min-uhm zihr-KOE-nee-
uhm) USP 34.
Use: Anhidrotic.
•**aluminum zirconium pentachlorohy-
drate.** (ah-LOO-min-uhm zihr-KOE-
nee-uhm) USP 34.
Use: Anhidrotic.
•**aluminum zirconium pentachlorohy-
drex gly.** (ah-LOO-min-uhm zihr-KOE-
nee-uhm) USP 34.
Use: Anhidrotic.
•**aluminum zirconium tetrachlorohy-
drate.** (ah-LOO-min-uhm zihr-KOE-
nee-uhm teh-trah-KLOR-oh-HIGH-
drate) USP 34.
Use: Anhidrotic.
•**aluminum zirconium tetrachlorohy-
drex gly.** (ah-LOO-min-uhm zihr-KOE-
nee-uhm teh-trah-KLOR-oh-HIGH-drex
Gly) USP 34.
Use: Anhidrotic.
•**aluminum zirconium trichlorohydrate.**
(ah-LOO-min-uhm zihr-KOE-nee-uhm
try-KLOR-oh-HIGH-drate) USP 34.
Use: Anhidrotic.
•**aluminum zirconium trichlorohydrex
gly.** (ah-LOO-min-uhm zihr-KOE-nee-
uhm try-KLOR-oh-HIGH-drex Gly)
USP 34.
Use: Anhidrotic.
•**alum, potassium.** (AL-um) USP 34.
Use: Astringent.

alum-precipitated allergenic extracts.
See: Allpyral.
Center-Al.
Alurex. (Rexall Group) Magnesium-aluminum hydroxide. **Susp.:** 150 mg, 200 mg/5 mL. Bot. 12 oz. **Tab:** 300 mg, 400 mg. Box 50s. *OTC.*
Use: Antacid.
Aluvea. (Merz Pharmaceutical) Urea 40%. Emulsifying wax, glycerin 99.7%. Cream. 237 mL. *Rx.*
Use: Emollient.
•**alvameline maleate.** (al-va-MEL-een) USAN.
Use: Partial M$_1$ agonist, M$_2$/M$_3$ antagonist.
Alvedil. (Luly-Thomas) Theophylline 4 g, pseudoephedrine hydrochloride 50 mg, butabarbital 15 mg. Cap. Bot. 100s. *Rx.*
Use: Bronchodilator; decongestant; hypnotic; sedative.
•**alverine citrate.** (AL-ver-een SIH-trate) USAN.
Use: Anticholinergic.
Alvesco. (Sepracor) Ciclesonide 80 mcg/actuation, 160 mcg/actuation. Soln., Inhal. 6.1 g canister (60 actuations) w/actuator. *Rx.*
Use: Respiratory inhalant product, intranasal steroid.
•**alvespimycin hydrochloride.** (al-VES-pi-MYE-sin) USAN.
Use: Antineoplastic.
•**alvimopan.** (al-VI-moe-pan) USAN.
Use: Gastrointestinal agent.
See: Entereg.
•**alvircept sudotox.** (AL-vihr-sept SOOD-ah-tox) USAN.
Use: Antiviral.
•**alvocidib.** (al-VOE-si-dib) USAN.
Use: Antineoplastic.
•**alvocidib hydrochloride.** (al-VOE-si-dib) USAN.
Use: Antineoplastic.
Alzapam. (Major) Lorazepam 0.5 mg, 1 mg, 2 mg. Tab. Bot. 100s, 500s. *c-iv.*
Use: Antianxiety.
Ama. (Wampole) Antimitochondrial antibodies test by IFA. Test 48s.
Use: Diagnostic aid.
amacetam sulfate.
See: Pramiracetam sulfate.
•**amadinone acetate.** (aim-AD-ih-nohn ASS-eh-tate) USAN.
Use: Hormone, progestin.
•**amantadine hydrochloride.** (uh-MAN-tuh-deen) *USP 34.*
Use: Antiviral.
See: Symmetrel.

amantadine hydrochloride. (Upsher-Smith) Amantadine hydrochloride 100 mg. Tab. 100s, 500s. *Rx.*
Use: Antiparkinson agent; antiviral agent.
amantadine hydrochloride. (Various Mfr.) **Cap.:** 100 mg. Bot. 100s, 500s, UD 100s. **Syrup:** 50 mg/5 mL. May contain sorbitol and parabens. Bot. 480 mL. *Rx.*
Use: Antiviral; treatment of Parkinson disease.
A-Mantle. (Doak Dermatologics) Water, cetearyl alcohol, sodium lauryl sulfate, sodium cetearyl sulfate, petrolatum, glycerin, synthetic beeswax, mineral oil, methylparaben, aluminum sulfate, calcium acetate, white potato dextrin. Cream. Jar 4 oz. *OTC.*
Use: Ointment, lotion base.
amaranth.
Use: Color (Not for internal use).
Amaryl. (Aventis) Glimepiride 1 mg, 2 mg, 4 mg. Lactose. Tab. Bot. 100s, UD 100s (4 mg only). *Rx.*
Use: Antidiabetic.
Amatine. (Roberts) Midodrine hydrochloride.
Use: Orthostatic hypotension. [Orphan Drug]
•**amatuximab.** (A-ma-TUX-i-mab) USAN.
Use: Antineoplastic.
ambenonium chloride.
Use: Cholinergic for treatment of myasthenia gravis.
See: Mytelase.
Ambenyl Cough. (Forest) Codeine phosphate 10 mg, bromodiphenhydramine hydrochloride 12.5 mg/5 mL, alcohol 5%. Syr. Bot. 4 oz, Pt, gal. *c-v.*
Use: Antihistamine; antitussive.
Amberlite. (Rohm and Haas) I.R.P.-64. Polacrilin.
Ambi 80/780/40. (Ambi) Dextromethorphan HBr 40 mg, guaifenesin 780 mg, pseudoephedrine hydrochloride 80 mg. Dye free. ER Tab. 100s. *Rx.*
Use: Antitussive and expectorant combination.
Ambi 80/700/40. (Ambi) Dextromethorphan HBr 40 mg, guaifenesin 700 mg, pseudoephedrine hydrochloride 80 mg. Dye free. ER Tab. 100s. *Rx.*
Use: Antitussive and expectorant combination.
Ambien. (Sanofi Aventis) Zolpidem tartrate 5 mg, 10 mg. Lactose, PEG. Film coated. Tab. Bot. 100s, 500s, UD 100s. *c-iv.*
Use: Hypnotic/sedative, nonbarbiturate, imidazopyridine.

Ambien CR. (Sanofi Aventis) Zolpidem tartrate 6.25 mg, 12.5 mg. PEG (6.25 mg only), lactose. Coated. ER Tab. 100s, 500s, unit dose 30s, unit dose 100s. *c-iv.*
Use: Nonbarbiturate sedative and hypnotic, imidazopyridine.
Ambifed. (MCR American) Guaifenesin 400 mg, pseudoephedrine hydrochloride 30 mg. Cap. 100s. *Rx.*
Use: Upper respiratory combination, expectorant, decongestant.
Ambifed-G. (MCR American) Guaifenesin 400 mg, pseudoephedrine hydrochloride 20 mg. Cap. 100s. *Rx.*
Use: Upper respiratory combination, expectorant, decongestant.
Ambifed-G DM. (MCR American) **Tab:** Dextromethorphan hydrobromide 20 mg, guaifenesin 400 mg, pseudoephedrine hydrochloride 20 mg. 100s. **ER Tab:** Dextromethorphan hydrobromide 30 mg, guaifenesin 1,000 mg, pseudoephedrine hydrochloride 60 mg. 100s. *Rx.*
Use: Upper respiratory combination, antitussive and expectorant combination.
AMBI 40PSE/400GFN. (AMBI) Guaifenesin 400 mg, pseudoephedrine hydrochloride 40 mg. Cap. 100s. *Rx.*
Use: Upper respiratory combination, expectorant, decongestant.
AMBI 40PSE/400GFN/20DM. (AMBI) Dextromethorphan HBr 20 mg, guaifenesin 400 mg, pseudoephedrine hydrochloride 40 mg. Cap. 100s. *Rx.*
Use: Upper respiratory combination; antitussive, expectorant, decongestant.
AMBI 1000/55. (Ambi) Dextromethorphan HBr 55 mg, guaifenesin 1000 mg. Dye free. ER Tab. 100s. *Rx.*
Use: Antitussive with expectorant, upper respiratory combination.
AMBI 1000/5. (Ambi) Carbetapentane citrate 5 mg, guaifenesin 1000 mg. Tab. 100s. *Rx.*
Use: Antitussive with expectorant, upper respiratory combination.
AMBI 60/580. (Ambi) Pseudoephedrine hydrochloride 60 mg, guaifenesin 580 mg. Tab. 100s. *Rx.*
Use: Decongestant and expectorant combination, upper respiratory combination.
AMBI 60/580/30. (Ambi) Dextromethorphan HBr 30 mg, guaifenesin 580 mg, pseudoephedrine hydrochloride 60 mg. Dye free. ER Tab. 100s. *Rx.*
Use: Antitussive and expectorant combination, upper respiratory combination.

AMBI 60PSE/4CPM. (AMBI) Pseudoephedrine hydrochloride 60 mg, chlorpheniramine maleate 4 mg. Tab. 100s. *OTC.*
Use: Upper respiratory combination, decongestant and antihistamine.
AMBI 60PSE/4CPM/20DM. (AMBI) Pseudoephedrine hydrochloride 60 mg, chlorpheniramine maleate 4 mg, dextromethorphan hydrobromide 20 mg. Tab. 100s. *Rx.*
Use: Upper respiratory combination, decongestant and antihistamine.
AMBI 60PSE/400GFN. (AMBI) Guaifenesin 400 mg, pseudoephedrine hydrochloride 60 mg. Cap. 100s. *Rx.*
Use: Upper respiratory combination, expectorant, decongestant.
AMBI 60PSE/400GFN/20DM. (AMBI) Dextromethorphan HBr 20 mg, guaifenesin 400 mg, pseudoephedrine hydrochloride 60 mg. Cap. 100s. *Rx.*
Use: Upper respiratory combination, antitussive, expectorant, decongestant.
AmBisome. (Astellas) Amphotericin B 50 mg (as liposomal), sucrose. Pow. for Inj. Single-dose Vial w/5-micron filter. *Rx.*
Use: Antifungal.
AMBI 10PEH/4CPM. (AMBI) Phenylephrine hydrochloride 10 mg, chlorpheniramine maleate 4 mg. Tab. 100s. *OTC.*
Use: Upper respiratory combination, decongestant and antihistamine.
AMBI 10PEH/4CPM/20DM. (AMBI) Phenylephrine hydrochloride 10 mg, chlorpheniramine maleate 4 mg, dextromethorphan hydrobromide 20 mg. Tab. 100s. *Rx.*
Use: Upper respiratory combination, antitussive combination.
AMBI 10PEH/400GFN. (AMBI) Guaifenesin 400 mg, phenylephrine hydrochloride 10 mg. Cap. 100s. *Rx.*
Use: Upper respiratory combination, expectorant, decongestant.
AMBI 10PEH/400GFN/20DM. (AMBI) Dextromethorphan HBr 20 mg, guaifenesin 400 mg, phenylephrine hydrochloride 10 mg. Cap. 100s. *Rx.*
Use: Upper respiratory combination, antitussive, expectorant, decongestant.
AMBI 20DM/4CPM. (AMBI) Dextromethorphan hydrobromide 20 mg, chlorpheniramine maleate 4 mg. Tab. 100s. *Rx.*
Use: Upper respiratory combination, decongestant and antihistamine.
•**ambomycin.** (AM-boe-MY-sin) USAN. Isolated from filtrates of *Streptomyces ambofaciens.*
Use: Antineoplastic.

ambrisentan. (am-brih-SEN-tan)
Use: Vasodilator, endothelin receptor antagonist.
See: Letairis.

•**ambruticin.** (am-brew-TIE-sin) USAN.
Use: Antifungal.

ambucaine. Ambutoxate hydrochloride.

•**ambuphylline.** (AM-byoo-fill-in) USAN.
Formerly Bufylline.
Use: Diuretic; muscle relaxant.

•**ambuside.** (AM-buh-SIDE) USAN.
Use: Diuretic.

ambutonium bromide.
Use: Antispasmodic.

AMC. (Schlicksup) Ammonium chloride 7.5 g. Tab. Bot. 1000s. *Rx.*
Use: Diuretic; expectorant.

Amcill. (Parke-Davis) Ampicillin tri-hydrate. **Cap.:** 250 mg, 500 mg. Bot. 100s, 500s, UD 100s. **Oral Susp.:** 125 mg, 250 mg/5 mL. Bot. 100 mL, 200 mL.
Use: Anti-infective, penicillin.

•**amcinafal.** (am-SIN-ah-fal) USAN.
Use: Anti-inflammatory.

•**amcinafide.** (am-SIN-ah-fide) USAN.
Use: Anti-inflammatory.

•**amcinonide.** (am-SIN-oh-nide) *USP 34.*
Use: Corticosteroid, topical.

amcinonide. (Taro) **Cream:** Amcinonide 0.1%. 15 g, 30 g, 60 g. **Oint.:** 0.1%. Benzyl alcohol 2.2%, glycerin, white petrolatum. 15 g, 30 g, 60 g. *Rx.*
Use: Corticosteroid, topical.

•**amdinocillin.** (am-DEE-no-SILL-in) USAN.
Use: Anti-infective.

•**amdinocillin pivoxil.** (am-DEE-no-SILL-in pihv-OX-ill) USAN.
Use: Anti-infective.

•**amdoxovir.** (am-DOX-oh-veer) USAN.
Use: Antiviral; reverse transcriptase inhibitor.

Amdry-D. (Prasco Laboratories) Pseudo-ephedrine hydrochloride 120 mg, meth-scopolamine nitrate 2.5 mg. ER Tab. 60s. *Rx.*
Use: Upper respiratory combination, decongestant and anticholinergic combination.

ameban.
See: Carbarsone.

amebicides.
See: Carbarsone.
  Chiniofon.
  Chloroquine Hydrochloride.
  Chloroquine Phosphate.
  Emetine Hydrochloride.
  Iodoquinol.
  Metronidazole.

Amechol.
Use: Diagnostic aid.
See: Methacholine Chloride.

•**amedalin hydrochloride.** (ah-MEH-dah-lin) USAN.
Use: Antidepressant.

•**ameltolide.** (AH-mell-TOE-lide) USAN.
Use: Anticonvulsant.

Amerge. (GlaxoSmithKline) Naratriptan hydrochloride 1 mg, 2.5 mg, lactose. Tab. Blister pack 9s. *Rx.*
Use: Antimigraine; serotonin 5-HT$_1$ receptor agonist.

Americaine. (Insight Pharmaceuticals) Benzocaine 20%. Polyethylene glycol 300, isobutene, normal butane, propane. Spray. 57 g. *OTC.*
Use: Topical anesthetic.

Americaine Hemorrhoidal. (Insight Pharmaceuticals) Benzocaine 20%. Benzethonium chloride, polyethylene glycol 300, polyethylene glycol 3350. Oint. 28 g. *OTC.*
Use: Anorectal preparation.

Americet. (MCR American) Acetaminophen 325 mg, caffeine 40 mg, butalbital 50 mg. Tab. 100s. *Rx.*
Use: Nonnarcotic analgesic combination with barbiturates.

Amerifed. (Ambi) Pseudoephedrine hydrochloride 80 mg, chlorpheniramine maleate 4 mg per 5 mL. Parabens, aspartame, phenylalanine, alcohol free, sugar free, raspberry flavor. Liq. 30 mL, 473 mL. *Rx.*
Use: Decongestant and antihistamine.

Amerigel. (Amerx Health Care Corp.) **Lot.:** Glycerin, lemon oil, parabens, oak extract (Oakin). Bot. 228 g. **Oint.:** Meadowsweet extract, oakbark extract, polyethylene glycol 400, polyethylene glycol 3350, zinc acetate. Tube. 28.3 g. *OTC.*
Use: Diaper rash product.

Amerituss AD. (Ambi) Dextromethorphan HBr 15 mg, chlorpheniramine maleate 3 mg, phenylephrine hydrochloride 10 mg per 5 mL. Phenylalanine, aspartame, alcohol free, sugar free. Liq. 473 mL. *Rx.*
Use: Upper respiratory combination.

Ames Dextro System Lancets. (Bayer Consumer Care) Sterile disposable lancet. Box 100s.
Use: Diagnostic aid.

•**amesergide.** (am-eh-SIR-jide) USAN.
Use: Serotonin antagonist.

•**ametantrone acetate.** (am-ETT-an-TRONE) USAN.
Use: Antineoplastic.

A-Methapred. (Hospira) Methylprednisolone sodium succinate 40 mg/vial,
125 mg/vial. Inj. Pow. for Soln. *Univial.*
1 mL (40 mg only) with sodium phosphate anhydrous (monobasic 1.6 mg,
dibasic 17.5 mg), lactose 25 mg, benzyl
alcohol 9 mg; 2 mL with sodium phosphate anhydrous (monobasic 1.6 mg,
dibasic 17.4 mg), benzyl alcohol
≈ 18 mg. *Rx.*
Use: Adrenocortical steroid, glucocorticoid.
amethocaine hydrochloride.
Use: Anesthetic, local.
See: Tetracaine hydrochloride.
amethopterin.
Use: Antineoplastic.
See: Methotrexate.
Amevive. (Biogen Idec) Alefacept 15 mg.
Sucrose 12.5 mg, preservative free.
Pow. for Inj., lyophilized. Dose pack. 1s,
4s (in single-use vials with 10 mL
single-use diluent [sterile water for in-
jection]). *Rx.*
Use: Immunologic agent, immunosuppressive.
•**amfenac sodium.** (AM-fen-ack SO-dee-
uhm) USAN.
Use: Anti-inflammatory.
•**amfilcon A.** (AM-FILL-kahn A) USAN.
Use: Contact lens material, hydrophilic.
•**amflutizole.** (am-FLEW-tih-zole) USAN.
Use: Treatment of gout.
amfodyne.
See: Imidecyl iodine.
•**amfonelic acid.** (am-fah-NEH-lick)
USAN.
Use: Central nervous system stimulant.
Amgenal Cough. (Ivax) Bromodiphenhydramine hydrochloride 12.5 mg, codeine phosphate 10 mg/5 mL, alcohol
5%. Syr. Bot. 120 mL, pt, gal. *c-v.*
Use: Antihistamine; antitussive.
AMG 531.
Use: Investigational thrombopoiesis-
stimulating peptibody.
amibiarson.
See: Carbarsone.
Amicar. (Xanodyne) **Tab.:** Aminocaproic
acid 500 mg, 1,000 mg. Bot. 100s.
Soln.: Aminocaproic acid 250 mg/mL,
parabens, EDTA, sorbitol, saccharin,
raspberry flavor. Bot. 473 mL. *Rx.*
Use: Hemostatic, systemic.
•**amicycline.** (AM-ee-SIGH-kleen) USAN.
Use: Anti-infective.
Amidate. (Hospira) Etomidate 2 mg/mL,
propylene glycol 35%. Single-dose
Amp 20 mg/10 mL, 40 mg/20 mL; Abboject syringe 40 mg/20 mL. *Rx.*

Use: Anesthetic, general.
amide local anesthetics.
See: Bupivacaine Hydrochloride.
Bupivacaine Hydrochloride with Epi-
nephrine 1:200,000.
Bupivacaine Spinal.
Carbocaine.
Carbocaine with Neo-Cobefrin.
Chirocaine.
Citanest Forte.
Citanest Plain.
Dibucaine.
Lidocaine and Epinephrine.
Lidocaine Hydrochloride.
Lidocaine Hydrochloride and Epineph-
rine.
Marcaine.
Mepivacaine Hydrochloride.
Mepivacaine Hydrochloride and Levo-
nordefrin.
Naropin.
Octocaine.
Polocaine.
Polocaine MPF.
Polocaine with Levonordefrin.
Prilocaine Hydrochloride.
Ropivacaine Hydrochloride.
Sensorcaine.
Sensorcaine MPF.
Sensorcaine-MPF Spinal.
Septocaine.
Xylocaine.
Xylocaine MPF.
•**amidephrine mesylate.** (AM-ee-DEH-
frin MEH-sih-LATE) USAN.
Use: Adrenergic.
amidofebrin.
See: Aminopyrine.
amidone hydrochloride.
Use: Analgesic; narcotic.
See: Methadone hydrochloride.
amidopyrazoline.
See: Aminopyrine.
amidotrizoate, sodium.
See: Diatrizoate sodium.
•**amifloxacin.** (am-ih-FLOX-ah-SIN)
USAN.
Use: Anti-infective.
•**amifloxacin mesylate.** (am-ih-FLOX-ah-
SIN MEH-sih-LATE) USAN.
Use: Anti-infective.
•**amifostine.** (am-ih-FOSS-teen) USAN.
Formerly Ethiofos.
Use: Cytoprotective agent.
See: Ethyol.
amifostine. (Caraco Pharmaceutical)
Amifostine 500 mg (as amifostine tri-
hydrate). Inj. Pow. for Soln. Single-use
vials. 10 mL. *Rx.*
Use: Cytoprotective agent.

Amigen. (Baxter PPI) Protein hydroly-sate. **5%, 10%:** Bot. 500 mL, 1000 mL; **5% w/dextrose 5%:** Bot. 500 mL, 1000 mL. **5% w/dextrose 5%, alcohol 5%:** Bot. 1000 mL. **5% w/fructose 10%:** Bot. 1000 mL. **5% w/fructose 12.5%, alcohol 2.4%:** Bot. 1000 mL. *Rx.*
Use: Nutritional supplement.
Amigesic. (Amide) Salsalate 500 mg. Cap or Tab. Salsalate 75 mg. Capl. Bot. 100s, 500s. *Rx.*
Use: Analgesic.
●**amikacin.** (am-ih-KAE-sin) *USP 34.*
Use: Anti-infective.
See: Amikin.
amikacin. (Bedford) Amikacin sulfate 250 mg, sodium metabisulfite 0.66%, sodium citrate dihydrate 2.5%/mL. Inj. Vial 2 mL, 4 mL. *Rx.*
Use: Anti-infective.
amikacin. (Various Mfr.) Amikacin 50 mg (as sulfate) per mL, sodium metabisul-fite 0.13%, sodium citrate dihydrate 0.5%. Inj. Vial 2, 4 mL. 10s. *Rx.*
Use: Anti-infective.
●**amikacin sulfate.** (am-ih-KAE-sin) *USP 34.*
Use: Anti-infective.
amikacin sulfate. (Various Mfr.) Ami-kacin sulfate 50 mg/mL. Inj. Vial 2 mL, 4 mL (10s).
Use: Anti-infective.
See: Amikin.
Amikin. (Bristol-Myers Squibb) Amikacin sulfate. Inj. Vial 100 mg, 500 mg, 1 g, disposable syringes 500 mg. *Rx.*
Use: Anti-infective; aminoglycoside.
●**amiloride hydrochloride.** (uh-MILL-oh-ride) *USP 34.*
Tall Man: aMILoride
Use: Diuretic.
See: Midamor.
amiloride hydrochloride and hydro-chlorothiazide.
Use: Antihypertensive; diuretic.
See: Moduretic.
●**amiloxate.** (A-mil-Ox-ate) *USP 34. For-merly isoamyl methoxycinnamate.*
Use: Sunscreen.
●**aminacrine hydrochloride.** (ah-MEE-nah-kreen) USAN.
Use: Anti-infective, topical.
aminarsone.
See: Carbarsone.
Amina-21. (Miller Pharmacal Group) Free-form amino acids 556 mg. Cap. Bot. 100s, 300s. *OTC.*
Use: Dermatologic, wound therapy.

Aminicotin.
Use: Vitamin supplement.
See: Nicotinamide.
aminoacetic acid.
Use: Myasthenia gravis; irrigant.
See: Glycine.
W/Magnesium trisilicate, aluminum hydroxide.
See: Maracid-2.
W/Phenylephrine hydrochloride, chlor-pheniramine maleate, acetaminophen, caffeine.
See: Codimal.
amino acid and protein.
See: Aminoacetic Acid.
Glutamic Acid.
Lysine.
Phenylalanine.
Thyroxine.
amino acid combinations.
See: A/G-Pro.
Amina-21.
Body Fortress Natural Amino.
Dequasine.
EMF.
Jets.
NeuRecover-DA.
NeuRecover-SA.
NeuroSlim.
PDP Liquid Protein.
PowerMate.
PowerSleep.
amino acid derivatives.
See: Carnitor.
L-Carnitine.
Levocarnitine.
amino acids.
Use: Amino acid supplement.
See: Aminosyn.
aminoacridine. (ah-MEE-no-ACK-rih-deen)
See: Aminacrine hydrochloride.
9-aminoacridine hydrochloride. Amina-crine hydrochloride.
Use: Anti-infective, vaginal.
See: Vagisec Plus.
W/Polyoxyethylene nonyl phenol, sodium edetate, docusate sodium.
See: Vagisec Plus.
W/Sulfanilamide, allantoin.
See: Nil Vaginal Cream.
p-aminobenzene-sulfonylacetylimide.
See: Sulfacetamide.
●**aminobenzoate potassium.** (ah-MEE-no-BEN-zoe-ate) *USP 34.*
Use: Analgesic, water-soluble vitamin.
See: Potaba.
W/Potassium salicylate.
See: Pabalate-SF.
aminobenzoate potassium. (Hope Pharm) Aminobenzoate potassium 500 mg. Cap. 250s. *Rx.*

Use: Water-soluble vitamin.

• **aminobenzoate sodium.** (ah-MEE-no-BEN-zoe-ate) *USP 34.*
Use: Analgesic.
See: PABA Sodium.
W/Phenobarbital, colchicine salicylate, vitamin B₁, aspirin.
See: Doloral.
W/Salicylamide, sodium salicylate, ascorbic acid, butabarbital sodium.
See: Bisalate.

• **aminobenzoic acid.** (a-MEE-noe-ben-ZOE-ik) *USP 34. Formerly Paraaminobenzoic acid.*
Use: Ultraviolet screen.

• **aminocaproic acid.** (uh-mee-no-kuh-PRO-ik) *USP 34.*
Use: Hemostatic.
See: Amicar.

aminocaproic acid. (Orphan Medical)
Use: Topical treatment of traumatic hyphema of the eye.

aminocaproic acid. (Various Mfr.)
Aminocaproic acid 250 mg/mL. Inj. Vial 20 mL. *Rx.*
Use: Antifibrinolytic; hemostatic, systemic.

aminocaproic acid. (VersaPharm)
Aminocaproic acid. **Oral Soln.:** 250 mg/mL, saccharin, sorbitol, parabens, raspberry flavor. Bot. 237 mL, 473 mL. **Tab.:** 500 mg. 100s. *Rx.*
Use: Hemostatic.

aminocardol.
Use: Bronchodilator.
See: Aminophylline.

Amino-Cerv. (Cooper Surgical) Urea 8.34%, sodium propionate 0.5%, methionine 0.83%, cystine 0.35%, inositol 0.83%, benzalkonium chloride, water miscible base. Tube with applicator 82.5 g. *Rx.*
Use: Vaginal agent.

2-aminoethanethiol.
Use: Urinary tract agent.

amino-ethyl-propanol.
See: Aminoisobutanol.
W/Bromotheophyllin.
See: Pamabrom.

Aminofen. (Dover Pharmaceuticals) Acetaminophen 325 mg. Tab. 500s. *OTC.*
Use: Analgesic.

Aminofen Max Extra Strength. (Dover Pharmaceuticals) Acetaminophen 500 mg. Tab. 500s. *OTC.*
Use: Analgesic.

aminoform.
Use: Anti-infective, urinary.
See: Methenamine.

Aminogen. (Christina) Vitamin B complex, folic acid. Amp. 2 mL Box 12s, 24s, 100s. Vial 10 mL. *Rx.*
Use: Vitamin supplement.

• **aminoglutethimide.** (ah-MEE-no-glue-TETH-ih-mide) *USP 34.*
Use: Treatment of Cushing syndrome; adrenocortical suppressant; antineoplastic.

aminohippurate sodium. (Merck & Co.)
Aminohippurate sodium 0.2 g/10 mL. Amp 10 mL, 50 mL.
Use: IV diagnostic aid for renal plasma flow and function determination.

• **aminohippurate sodium injection.** (ah-MEE-no-HIP-your-ate) *USP 34.*
Use: Diagnostic aid, renal function determination.

• **aminohippuric acid.** (ah-MEE-no-hip-YOUR-ik) *USP 34.*
Use: Component of aminohippurate sodium (Inj.); diagnostic aid, renal function determination.

aminoisobutanol.
See: Butaphyllamine.
Pamabrom for combinations.

aminoisometradine.
See: Methionine.

• **aminolevulinic acid hydrochloride.** (ah-MEE-no-lev-you-LIN-ik ASS-id HIGH-droe-KLOR-ide) USAN.
Use: Antineoplastic.
See: Levulan Kerastick.

Amino-Min-D. (Tyson) Ca 250 mg, D 100 units, Fe 7.5 mg, Zn 5.6 mg, Mg, I, Mn, Cu, K, Cr, Se, betaine hydrochloride, glutamic acid hydrochloride. Cap. Bot. 100s. *OTC.*
Use: Mineral, vitamin supplement.

Aminonat. Protein hydrolysates (oral).

aminonitrozole.
Use: Antitrichomonal.

Amino-Opti-C. (Tyson) Vitamin C 1000 mg, lemon bioflavonoids 250 mg. Rutin, hesperidin, rose hips powder, dicalcium phosphate, hydrogenated soybean oil. SR Tab. Bot. 100s. *OTC.*
Use: Water-soluble vitamin.

aminopenicillins.
Use: Anti-infective.
See: Amoxicillin.
Amoxicillin and Clavulanate Potassium.
Ampicillin.
Ampicillin Sodium and Sulbactam Sodium.

• **aminopentamide sulfate.** (a-MEE-noe-PEN-ta-mide) *USP 34.*
Use: Anticholinergic.

•aminophylline. (am-in-AHF-ih-lin)
USP 34. Formerly Theophylline ethyl-enediamine.
Use: Muscle relaxant.
W/Combinations.
See: Mudrane.
  Mudrane GG-2.
aminophylline. (Various Mfr.) Amino-phylline. **Inj.:** 25 mg (equivalent to theo-phylline 19.75 mg) per mL. Amps, vi-als. 10 mL, 20 mL. **Tab.:** 100 mg (equivalent to theophylline 79 mg), 200 mg (equivalent to theophylline 158 mg). 100s, UD 100s. *Rx.*
Use: Bronchodilator.
Aminoprel. (Taylor Pharmaceuticals) L-lysine 60 mg, dl-methionine 15 mg, hy-drolyzed protein 750 mg, iron 2 mg, Cu, I, K, Mg, Mn, Zn. Cap. Bot. 180s.
Use: Nutritional supplement.
aminopromazine. (I.N.N.) Proquamezine.
4-aminopyridine.
Use: Relief of symptoms of multiple sclerosis. [Orphan Drug]
aminopyrine.
Use: Antipyretic; analgesic.
See: Dipyrone.
8-aminoquinoline derivatives.
Use: Antimalarial.
See: Primaquine Phosphate.
4-aminoquinoline derivatives.
Use: Antimalarial.
See: Aralen hydrochloride.
  Chloroquine Phosphate.
•aminorex. (am-EE-no-rex) USAN.
Use: Anorexic.
aminosalicylate calcium. (Dumas-Wilson) Aminosalicylate calcium 7.5 g. Bot. 1000s.
Use: Tuberculosis therapy.
aminosalicylate potassium. Monopo-tassium 4-aminosalicylate.
Use: Antibacterial; tuberculostatic.
•aminosalicylate sodium. (uh-MEE-no-suh-LIS-ih-LATE) *USP 34.*
Use: Anti-infective; tuberculostatic.
•aminosalicylic acid. (ah-MEE-no-sal-ih-SILL-ik) *USP 34.*
Use: Antituberculosis agent.
See: Paser.
5-aminosalicylic acid.
See: Mesalamine.
4-aminosalicylic acid.
Use: Treatment of ulcerative colitis in patients intolerant to sulfasalazine. [Orphan Drug]
p-aminosalicylic acid salts.
See: Aminosalicylate Calcium.
  Aminosalicylate Potassium.
  Aminosalicylate Sodium.

aminosidine.
Use: Mycobacterium avium complex; tuberculosis; visceral leishmaniasism (KALA-AZAR). [Orphan Drug]
See: Gabbromicina.
Aminosyn. (Hospira) Crystalline amino acid solution. **3.5%:** 1,000 mL. **5%:** 500 mL, 1,000 mL. **7%:** 500 mL; **8.5%:** 500 mL, 1,000 mL. **10%:** 500 mL, 1,000 mL. **W/Electrolytes: 7%:** 500 mL. **8.5%:** 500 mL. *Rx.*
Use: Nutritional supplement, parenteral.
Aminosyn-HBC 7%. (Hospira) Crystal-line amino acid infusion for high meta-bolic stress. 500 mL, 1,000 mL. *Rx.*
Use: Nutritional supplement, parenteral.
Aminosyn II. (Hospira) Crystalline amino acid. Inj. **3.5%:** 1,000 mL. **5%:** 500 mL, 1,000 mL. **7%:** 500 mL. **8.5%:** 500 mL, 1,000 mL. **10%:** 500 mL, 1,000 mL. **15%:** 2,000 mL. **W/Dextrose: 3.5% in 5% dextrose:** 1,000 mL. **4.25% in 10% dextrose:** 1,000 mL. **4.25% in 20% dextrose:** 500 mL. **4.25% in 25% dextrose:** 500 mL. **W/Electrolytes: 8.5%:** 1,000 mL. *Rx.*
Use: Nutritional supplement, parenteral.
Aminosyn II M. (Hospira) Crystalline amino acid w/electrolytes in dextrose. Inj. **3.5% in 5% dextrose:** 500 mL. **4.25% in 10% dextrose:** 500 mL. *Rx.*
Use: Nutritional supplement, parenteral.
Aminosyn M 3.5%. (Hospira) Crystalline amino acid infusion with electrolytes. 1,000 mL. *Rx.*
Use: Nutritional supplement, parenteral.
Aminosyn-PF. (Hospira) Crystalline amino acid infusions for pediatric use. **7%:** 500 mL. **10%:** 1,000 mL. *Rx.*
Use: Nutritional supplement, parenteral.
Aminosyn-RF. (Hospira) Crystalline amino acid infusion for renal failure pa-tients. 5.2%. Inj. 500 mL. *Rx.*
Use: Nutritional supplement, parenteral.
Amino-Thiol. (Marcen) Sulfur 10 mg, ca-sein 50 mg, sodium citrate 5 mg, phe-nol 5 mg, benzyl alcohol 5 mg/mL. Vial 10 mL, 30 mL. *Rx.*
Use: Treatment of arthritis; neuritis.
aminotrate phosphate. Trolnitratephos-phate.
See: Triethanolamine.
Aminoxin. (Tyson & Assoc.) Pyridoxal-5′-phosphate 20 mg. EC Tab. Bot. 100s. *OTC.*
Use: Water-soluble vitamin.
aminoxytropine tropate hydrochloride. Atropine-N-oxide hydrochloride.
Amio-Aqueous. (Academic Pharmaceu-ticals) Amiodarone.
Use: Antiarrhythmic. [Orphan Drug]

•**amiodarone hydrochloride.** (A-MEE-oh-duh-rone) USAN.
Use: Cardiovascular agent; antiarrhythmic; ventricular.
See: Amio-Aqueous.
Cordarone.
Nexterone.
Pacerone.
amiodarone hydrochloride. (Taro Pharmaceuticals) Amiodarone hydrochloride 400 mg. Lactose. Tab. 30s, 100s, 1000s. *Rx.*
Use: Antiarrhythmic agent.
amiodarone hydrochloride. (Various Mfr.) Amiodarone hydrochloride. **Inj.:** 50 mg/mL, may contain benzyl alcohol. 3 mL vials and amps. **Tab.:** 200 mg. Bot. 60s, 100s, 250s, 500s, UD 100s. *Rx.*
Use: Antiarrhythmic.
Amipaque. (Sanofi-Synthelabo) Metrizamide 18.75%/20 mL Vial.
Use: Radiopaque agent.
•**amiprilose hydrochloride.** (ah-MIH-prih-LOHS) USAN.
Use: Anti-infective; antifungal; anti-inflammatory; antineoplastic; antiviral; immunomodulator.
•**amiquinsin hydrochloride.** (AM-ih-KWIN-sin) USAN. Under study.
Use: Antihypertensive.
Amitin. (Thurston) Vitamin C 200 mg, lemon bioflavonoid 100 mg, niacinamide 60 mg, methionine 100 mg. Tab. Bot. 100s, 500s. *Rx.*
Use: Vitamin supplement.
Amitiza. (Sucampo Pharmaceuticals) Lubiprostone 8 mcg, 24 mcg. Sorbitol. Cap. 60s. *Rx.*
Use: Treatment of chronic constipation.
•**amitraz.** (AM-ih-trazz) *USP 34.*
Use: Scabicide.
•**amitriptyline hydrochloride.** (am-ee-TRIP-tih-leen) *USP 34.*
Use: Antidepressant.
See: Endep.
W/Chlordiazepoxide.
See: Limbitrol.
W/Perphenazine.
See: Etrafon.
amitriptyline hydrochloride. (Various Mfr.) Amitriptyline hydrochloride 10 mg, 25 mg, 50 mg, 75 mg, 100 mg, 150 mg. Tab. Bot. 100s, 500s (75 mg and 100 mg only), 1000s, UD 100s, blister pack 25s (25 mg and 50 mg only), 100s (except 150 mg), 600s (10 mg, 25 mg, 50 mg only). *Rx.*
Use: Antidepressant.

AmLactin. (Upsher-Smith) Ammonium lactate 12%, parabens, light mineral oil. Cream, Lot. 140 g, 225 g, 400 g. *OTC.*
Use: Emollient.
AmLactin Foot Cream Therapy. (Upsher-Smith) Ammonium lactate, emulsifying wax, glycerin, light mineral oil, parabens, potassium lactate, white petrolatum. Cream. 85 g. *OTC.*
Use: Emollient.
AmLactin XL. (Upsher-Smith) Ammonium lactate, potassium lactate, sodium lactate, light mineral oil, white petrolatum, glycerin, xanthan gum, parabens. Lot. 160 g. *OTC.*
Use: Emollient.
•**amlexanox.** (am-LEX-an-ox) USAN.
Use: Mouth and throat product.
See: Aphthasol.
•**amlintide.** (AM-lin-tide) USAN.
Use: Treatment of type I diabetes mellitus; antidiabetic.
amlodipine. (am-LOW-dih-PEEN)
Tall Man: amLODIPine
Use: Calcium channel blocker.
See: Norvasc.
W/Benazepril Hydrochloride.
See: Lotrel.
W/Hydrochlorothiazide/Valsartan.
See: Exforge HCT.
•**amlodipine besylate.** (am-LOW-dih-PEEN) USAN.
Tall Man: amLODIPine
Use: Antianginal; antihypertensive.
See: Norvasc.
W/Aliskiren.
See: Tekamlo.
W/Atorvastatin Calcium.
See: Caduet.
W/Olmesartan Medoxomil.
See: Azor.
W/Valsartan.
See: Exforge.
amlodipine besylate. (Various Mfr.) Amlodipine besylate 2.5 mg, 5 mg, 10 mg. Tab. 90s, 100s, 300s, 500s, 1000s (except 2.5 mg), 2500s (5 mg only), UD 100s, UD 300s (5 mg only). *Rx.*
Use: Calcium channel blocking agent.
amlodipine besylate and benazepril hydrochloride. (Various Mfr.) Amlodipine/benazepril hydrochloride 2.5 mg/10 mg, 5 mg/10 mg, 5 mg/20 mg, 5 mg/40 mg, 10 mg/20 mg, 10 mg/40 mg. May contain lactose. Cap. 100s, 500s (5 mg/40 mg, 10 mg/40 mg). *Rx.*
Use: Antihypertensive combination.

•**amlodipine maleate.** (am-LOW-dih-
PEEN) USAN.
Tall Man: amLODIPine
Use: Antianginal; antihypertensive.
Ammens Medicated. (Bristol-Myers
Squibb) Boric acid 4.55%, zinc oxide
9.10%, talc, starch. Pow. Can 6.25 oz,
11 oz. *OTC.*
Use: Dermatologic; protectant.
ammoidin. Methoxsalen.
Use: Psoralen.
•**ammonia N 13 injection.** (ah-MOE-nee-
ah N13) *USP 34.*
Use: Diagnostic aid, cardiac imaging,
liver imaging; radiopharmaceutical.
•**ammonia solution, strong.** (ah-MOE-
nee-ah) *NF 29.*
Use: Pharmaceutic aid, solvent; source
of ammonia.
•**ammonia spirit, aromatic.** (ah-MOE-
nee-ah) *USP 34.*
Use: Respiratory.
•**ammonio methacrylate copolymer.** (ah-
MOE-nee-oh meth-ah-KRILL-ate koe-
PAHL-ih-mer) *NF 29.*
Use: Pharmaceutic aid, coating agent.
ammonium benzoate.
Use: Antiseptic, urinary.
**ammonium biphosphate, sodium bi-
phosphate, and sodium acid pyrophosphate.**
Use: Genitourinary.
•**ammonium carbonate.** (ah-MOE-nee-
uhm) *NF 29.*
Use: Pharmaceutic aid, source of ammonia.
•**ammonium chloride.** (ah-MOE-nee-
uhm) *USP 34.*
Use: Acidifier; diuretic.
ammonium chloride. (Eli Lilly) Ammonium chloride. 7.5 g. Tab. Enseal Bot.
100s. *Rx.*
Use: Acidifier, urinary.
ammonium chloride. (Hospira) Ammonium chloride 26.75% (5 mEq/mL). To
be diluted before infusion. Inj. Vials.
20 mL (100 mEq) with EDTA 2 mg. *Rx.*
Use: Intravenous nutritional therapy.
ammonium chloride. (Various Mfr.)
Delayed Release Tab.: Plain or E.C.
5 g, 7.5 g. (Bayer Consumer Care)
Inj.: 120 mEq/30 mL. Vial. *Rx.*
Use: Acidifier; diuretic; expectorant;
alkalosis.
•**ammonium lactate.** (ah-MOE-nee-uhm
LACK-tate) USAN.
Use: Antipruritic, topical.
See: al12.
AmLactin.
AmLactin Foot Cream Therapy.
Geri-Hydrolac 12.
Lac-Hydrin.
LAC-Lotion.
ammonium lactate. (Glades) Ammonium lactate (equiv. to 12% lactic acid),
cetyl alcohol, glycerin, glyceryl stearate,
light mineral oil, parabens. Lot. 225 g,
400 g. *Rx.*
Use: Emollient.
ammonium mandelate. Ammonium salt
of mandelic acid 8 g/fl oz. Syr. Bot. Pt,
gal.
Use: Urinary antiseptic, oral.
•**ammonium molybdate.** (ah-MOE-nee-
uhm) *USP 34.*
ammonium nitrate.
See: Reditemp-C.
•**ammonium phosphate.** (ah-MOE-nee-
uhm) *NF 29.* Phosphoric acid diammonium salt. Diammonium phosphate.
Use: Pharmaceutic aid.
•**ammonium sulfate.** (ah-MOE-nee-uhm)
USAN.
Use: Pharmaceutic aid.
ammonium tetrathiomolybdate.
Use: Treatment of Wilson disease.
[Orphan Drug]
ammonium valerate.
Use: Sedative.
Ammonul. (Ucyclyd Pharma) Sodium
benzoate 100 mg and sodium phenylacetate 100 mg per mL. Inj. Single-use
vials. 50 mL. *Rx.*
Use: Hyperammonemia.
ammophyllin.
Use: Bronchodilator.
See: Aminophylline.
Amnesteem. (Mylan) Isotretinoin 10 mg,
20 mg, 40 mg. Cap. 30s, 100s (except
10 mg), UD 30s (10 mg only), UD 100s
(10 mg only). *Rx.*
Use: Retinoid, first generation.
•**amobarbital sodium.** (am-oh-BAR-bih-
tahl) *USP 34.*
Use: Hypnotic; sedative.
amobarbital sodium. (Various Mfr.) **Cap.
1 g:** Bot. 100s, 500s; **3 g:** Bot. 100s,
500s, 1000s. (Various Mfr.) **Tab. 30 mg:**
Bot. 100s; **50 mg:** Bot. 100s. **100 mg:**
Bot. 100s. (Eli Lilly and Co.) Vial
250 mg, 500 mg. (Eli Lilly and Co.)
Use: Sedative; hypnotic.
W/Ephedrine hydrochloride, theophylline,
chlorpheniramine maleate.
See: Amytal Sodium.
W/Secobarbital sodium.
See: Dusotal.
Tuinal.
Amoclan. (West-ward) Amoxicillin/clavu-
lanic acid (as potassium salt) 200 mg/

28.5 mg (potassium 0.143 mEq per
5 mL), 400 mg/57 mg (potassium
0.286 mEq per 5 mL) (after reconstitution) per 5 mL. Phenylalanine 7 mg/
5 mL, aspartame. Golden syrup and orange flavor. Pow. for Oral Susp.
50 mL, 75 mL, 100 mL. *Rx.*
Use: Penicillin, aminopenicillin.
•**amodiaquine.** (am-oh-DIE-ah-kwin)
USP 34.
Use: Antiprotozoal.
•**amodiaquine hydrochloride.** (am-oh-
DIE-ah-kwin) *USP 34.*
Use: Antimalarial.
Amodopa. (Major) Methyldopa 125 mg,
250 mg, 500 mg. Bot. 100s, 500s,
(500 mg only), 1000s (250 mg only),
UD 100s. *Rx.*
Use: Antihypertensive.
Amol. Mono-n-amyl-hydroquinone ether.
See: B-F-I.
Amoline. (Major) Aminophylline 100 mg,
200 mg. Tab. Bot. 100s, 1000s, UD
100s. *Rx-OTC.*
Use: Bronchodilator.
amopyroquin hydrochloride.
See: Propoquin.
•**amorolfine.** (am-OH-role-feen) USAN.
Use: Antimycotic.
Amosan. (Oral-B) Sodium perborate,
saccharin. Single-dose packet box.
1.76 g. 20s, 40s. *OTC.*
Use: Mouth and throat preparation.
•**amotosalen hydrochloride.** (a-moe-
TOE-sa-len) USAN.
Use: Photochemical treatment for
plasma.
Amotriphene. *Rx.*
Use: Coronary vasodilator.
•**amoxapine.** (am-OX-uh-peen) *USP 34.*
Use: Antidepressant.
amoxapine. (Various Mfr.) Amoxapine
25 mg, 50 mg, 100 mg, 150 mg. Tab.
Bot. 30s, 100s, 500s (50 mg only),
1000s, blister pack 100s (25 mg and
50 mg only). *Rx.*
Use: Antidepressant.
•**amoxicillin.** (a-MOX-ih-sil-in) *USP 34.*
Use: Penicillin, aminopenicillin.
See: Amoxil.
DisperMox.
Moxatag.
Trimox.
amoxicillin. (Ranbaxy) Amoxicillin.
Chew. Tab.: 200 mg, 400 mg. Bot. 20s,
100s (400 mg only). **Pow. for Oral
Susp.:** 200 mg/5 mL, 400 mg/5 mL
when reconstituted. Fruit flavor. 50 mL,
75 mL, 100 mL. *Rx.*
Use: Penicillin, aminopenicillin.

amoxicillin. (Various Mfr.) Amoxicillin.
Cap.: 250 mg, 500 mg. 50s (500 mg
only), 100s, 500s, 1000s (250 mg only).
Chew. Tab.: 125 mg, 250 mg. 100s;
250s, 500s (250 mg only). **Pow. for
Susp., Oral:** 125 mg/5 mL, 250 mg/
5 mL when reconstituted. 80 mL,
100 mL, 150 mL. **Tab.:** 500 mg,
875 mg. 20s, 100s, 500s (875 mg only).
Rx.
Use: Penicillin, aminopenicillin.
amoxicillin and clavulanate potassium.
(a-MOX-ih-sil-in and CLAV-you-lon-ate
poe-TASS-ee-uhm)
Use: Aminopenicillin, penicillin.
See: Amoclan.
Augmentin.
Augmentin ES-600.
Augmentin XR.
amoxicillin, clavulanate potassium.
(Geneva) **Chew. Tab.:** Amoxicillin trihydrate 200 mg/clavulanic acid
28.5 mg, amoxicillin trihydrate 400 mg/
clavulanic acid 57 mg. Bot. UD 20s.
Pow. for Oral Susp.: Amoxicillin trihydrate 200 mg/clavulanic acid
28.5 mg, amoxicillin trihydrate 400 mg/
clavulanic acid 57 mg. Vial. 100 mL.
Rx.
Use: Anti-infective, penicillin.
amoxicillin/clavulanate potassium.
(Lek) Amoxicillin/clavulanic acid (as the
potassium salt) 250 mg/125 mg. Tab.
30s. *Rx.*
Use: Penicillin, aminopenicillin.
amoxicillin/clavulanate potassium.
(Sandoz) Amoxicillin 1,000 mg, clavulanic acid 62.5 mg. Film coated. PEG,
potassium 0.31 mEq, sodium 1.25 mEq.
ER Tab. 28s (7-day XR pack) and 40s
(10-day XR pack). *Rx.*
Use: Penicillin, aminopenicillin.
amoxicillin/clavulanate potassium.
(Various Mfr.) **Chew. Tab.:** Amoxicillin/
clavulanic acid (as the potassium salt)
200 mg/28.5 mg, 400 mg/57 mg. 20s,
UD 20s. **Pow. for Oral Susp.:** Amoxi-
cillin/clavulanic acid (as the potassium
salt) 200 mg/28.5 mg, 400 mg/57 mg,
600 mg/42.9 mg per 5 mL after reconstitution. May contain aspartame or
saccharin. 50 mL, 75 mL, 100 mL,
125 mL, 150 mL, 200 mL. **Tab.:** Amoxi-
cillin/clavulanic acid (as the potassium
salt) 500 mg/125 mg, 875 mg/125 mg.
Bot. 20s, 100s, UD 100s. *Rx.*
Use: Anti-infective, penicillin.
amoxicillin intramammary infusion.
Use: Anti-infective; penicillin.

•**amoxicillin sodium.** (a-MOX-ih-sil-in)
USAN.
Use: Antibiotic.
amoxicillin trihydrate. (Various Mfr.)
Amoxicillin trihydrate. **Chew. Tab.:**
125 mg, 250 mg. Bot. 100s, 250s
(250 mg only), 500s (250 mg only).
Tab.: 500 mg, 875 mg. Bot. 20s, 100s,
500s (875 mg only). **Cap.:** 250 mg,
500 mg. Bot. 50s (500 mg only), 100s,
500s, 1000s (250 mg only). **Pow. for**
Oral Susp.: 125 mg/5 mL, 250 mg/mL
when reconstituted. Bot. 80 mL,
100 mL, 150 mL. *Rx.*
Use: Anti-infective; penicillin.
Amoxil. (GlaxoSmithKline) Amoxicillin.
Cap.: 500 mg. Bot. 500s. **Pow. for**
Oral Susp.: 125 mg/5 mL when reconstituted. Sucrose. Strawberry flavor.
80 mL, 150 mL. **Tab.:** 875 mg. Film
coated. Bot. 20s, 100s, 500s. *Rx.*
Use: Aminopenicillin, penicillin.
AMP. Adenosine Phosphate, USAN.
Use: Nutrient.
d-AMP. (Oxypure) Ampicillin trihydrate
500 mg. Cap. Bot. 100s. *Rx.*
Use: Anti-infective; penicillin.
Amperil. (Armenpharm Ltd.) Ampicillin tri-
hydrate 250 mg or 500 mg. Cap. Bot.
100s, 500s. *Rx.*
Use: Anti-infective; penicillin.
Amphadase. (Amphastar) Hyaluronidase
(bovine source) 150 units/mL. Contains
no more than 0.1 mg thimerosal. Soln.
for Inj. Vials. 2 mL. *Rx.*
Use: Physical adjunct.
•**amphecloral.** (AM-feh-klahr-ahl) USAN.
Use: Sympathomimetic; anorexic.
amphenidone.
Use: CNS stimulant.
amphetamine aspartate combinations.
See: Adderall.
Adderall XR.
amphetamine hydrochloride. (Various
Mfr.) Amphetamine hydrochloride
20 mg/mL, 1 mL. Amp. *Rx.*
Use: Vasoconstrictor; CNS stimulant.
amphetamine, levo.
Use: CNS stimulant.
amphetamine phosphate.
Use: CNS stimulant.
amphetamine phosphate, dextro.
(Various Mfr.) Dextroamphetamine
phosphate. Tab.
Use: CNS stimulant.
amphetamine phosphate, dibasic.
(Various Mfr.) Racemic amphetamine
phosphate 5 mg, 10 mg. Cap. or Tab.
Bot. *Rx.*
Use: CNS stimulant.

amphetamines.
See: Amphetamine Sulfate.
Dextroamphetamine Sulfate.
Lisdexamfetamine Dimesylate.
Methamphetamine Hydrochloride.
•**amphetamine sulfate.** (am-FET-a-meen)
USP 34.
Use: CNS stimulant.
W/Combinations.
See: Adderall.
Adderall XR.
amphetamine sulfate. (Various Mfr.)
Amphetamine sulfate 5 mg, 10 mg.
Cap. Tab. Bot. Inj. 20 mg/mL. Vial.
Use: CNS stimulant.
amphetamine sulfate, dextro.
Use: CNS stimulant.
See: Dextroamphetamine Sulfate.
amphetamine with dextroamphetamine
as resin complexes.
Use: Appetite depressant.
Amphocaps. (Halsey Drug) Ampicillin
250 mg, 500 mg. Cap. Bot. 100s. *Rx.*
Use: Anti-infective; penicillin.
Amphojel. (Wyeth) Aluminum hydroxide
gel. 300 mg, 600 mg. Tab. Bot. 100s.
OTC.
Use: Antacid.
•**amphomycin.** (AM-foe-MY-sin) USAN.
An antibiotic produced by *Streptomy-*
ces canus.
Use: Anti-infective.
Amphotec. (Sequus) Amphotericin B (as
cholesteryl) 50 mg, 100 mg. Pow. for
Inj. Single-use Vial 20 mL (50 mg),
50 mL (100 mg). *Rx.*
Use: Antifungal.
•**amphotericin B.** (am-foe-TER-ih-sin B)
USP 34.
Use: Antifungal.
See: Abelcet.
Amphotec.
amphotericin B. (Pharma-Tek) Ampho-
tericin B 50 mg as desoxycholate. Pow.
for Inj. Vial. *Rx.*
Use: Antifungal.
amphotericin B desoxycholate.
Use: Antifungal.
amphotericin B, lipid-based.
Use: Antifungal.
See: Abelcet.
AmBisome.
Amphotec.
amphotericin B lipid complex.
Use: Invasive fungal infections. [Orphan
Drug]
See: Abelcet.
•**ampicillin.** (am-pih-SILL-in) *USP 34.*
Use: Anti-infective.
See: Principen.

•**ampicillin sodium.** (am-pih-SILL-in) *USP 34.*
Use: Anti-infective.
See: Omnipen-N.
ampicillin sodium. (Various Mfr.) Ampicillin sodium 125 mg, 250 mg, 500 mg, 1 g, 2 g, 10 g. Sodium 2.9 mEq/g. Pow. for Inj. Vials. *Rx.*
Use: Anti-infective.
•**ampicillin sodium and sulbactam sodium.** (am-pih-SILL-in and sull-BAK-tam) *USP 34.*
Use: Aminopenicillin, penicillin.
See: Unasyn.
ampicillin/sulbactam. (ESI Lederle) Ampicillin sodium 1 g/sulbactam sodium 0.5 g, ampicillin sodium 2 g/sulbactam sodium 1 g. Inj. Pow. for Soln. Vials. *Rx.*
Use: Aminopenicillin, penicillin.
ampicillin/sulbactam. (Various Mfr.) Ampicillin sodium 10 g/sulbactam sodium 5 g. Inj., Pow. for Soln. Bulk package. *Rx.*
Use: Penicillin, aminopenicillin.
ampicillin trihydrate. (Various Mfr.) Ampicillin (as trihydrate) 250 mg, 500 mg. Cap. Bot. 100s, 500s. *Rx.*
Use: Anti-infective; penicillin.
Amplicor. (Roche) Kits 10s, 96s, 100s. *Rx.*
Use: Diagnostic aid, chlamydia.
Amplicor HIV-1 Monitor. (Roche) Reagent kit for plasma HIV-1 tests. Kit. 24 tests.
Use: Diagnostic aid.
Ampligen. (HEM Research) Poly I: Poly C12U. Phase II/III HIV.
Use: Immunomodulator.
•**amprenavir.** (am-PREN-a-vir) USAN.
Use: Antiviral.
Ampyra. (Acorda) Dalfampridine 10 mg. Film coated. ER Tab. 60s. *Rx.*
Use: Potassium channel blocker.
•**ampyzine sulfate.** (AM-pih-zeen) USAN.
Use: Central nervous system stimulant.
•**amquinate.** (am-KWIN-ate) USAN.
Use: Antimalarial.
•**amrinone.** (AM-rih-nohn) *USP 34.*
Use: Cardiovascular agent.
See: Inocor Lactate.
Amrix. (ECR) Cyclobenzaprine hydrochloride 15 mg, 30 mg. Sugar spheres. ER Cap. 60s. *Rx.*
Use: Skeletal muscle relaxant.
•**amsacrine.** (AM-sah-KREEN) USAN.
Use: Investigational antineoplastic. [Orphan Drug]
•**amuvatinib.** (AM-ue-VA-ti-nib) USAN.
Use: Antineoplastic.

•**amuvatinib hydrochloride.** (AM-ue-VA-ti-nib) USAN.
Use: Antineoplastic.
Amvisc. (Bausch & Lomb) Sodium hyaluronate 12 mg/mL. Inj. Disp. syringe 0.5 mL, 0.8 mL. *Rx.*
Use: Viscoelastic.
Amvisc Plus. (Bausch & Lomb) Sodium hyaluronate 16 mg/mL. Inj. Disp. syringe 0.5 mL, 0.8 mL. *Rx.*
Use: Viscoelastic.
Am-Wax. (AmLab) Urea, benzocaine, propylene glycol, glycerin. Bot. 10 mL. *OTC.*
Use: Otic.
amyl. Phenyl phenol, phenyl mercuric nitrate.
See: Lubraseptic.
amylase.
W/Cellulase, Hyoscyamine Sulfate, Lipase, Phenyltoloxamine Citrate, Protease.
See: Digex.
W/Lipase, protease.
See: Creon.
Palcaps 10.
Pancrelipase.
Tri-Pase 8.
Tri-Pase 16.
Zenpep.
•**amylene hydrate.** (AM-ih-leen HIGH-drate) *NF 29.*
Use: Pharmaceutic aid, solvent.
amylin analog.
Use: Antidiabetic agent.
See: Pramlintide Acetate.
•**amyl nitrite.** (A-mill NYE-trite) *USP 34.*
Use: Vasodilator.
W/Sodium nitrite, sodium thiosulfate.
See: Cyanide Antidote Pkg.
amyl nitrite. (Various Mfr.) Amyl nitrite 0.3 mL. Inh. Covered glass capsules. 12s. *Rx.*
Use: Vasodilator.
amylolytic enzyme.
W/Calcium carbonate, glycine, proteolytic and cellulolytic enzymes.
See: Converspaz.
W/Proteolytic, cellulolytic, lipolytic enzymes.
See: Arco-Lase.
W/Proteolytic, cellulolytic, lipolytic enzymes, iron, ox bile.
See: Ku-Zyme.
Amytal Sodium. (Marathon) Amobarbital sodium. 250 mg, 500 mg. Pow. for Inj. Vial. *c-II.*
Use: Hypnotic; sedative.
Ana. (Wampole) Antinuclear antibodies test by IFA. Test 54s.
Use: Diagnostic aid.

anabolic agents. These agents stimulate constructive processes leading to retention of nitrogen and increasing the body protein.
See: Anadrol-50.
Anavar.
anabolic steroids.
Use: Sex hormone.
See: Nandrolone Decanoate.
Oxandrolone.
Oxymetholone.
Anacaine. (Gordon Laboratories) Benzocaine 10%. Jar oz, lb. *OTC.*
Use: Anesthetic, local.
Anacin. (Insight Pharmaceutical) Aspirin 400 mg, caffeine 32 mg. Tab. Bot. 30s, 50s, 100s, 200s, 300s. Cap. Bot. 100s. *OTC.*
Use: Analgesic.
Anacin Advanced Headache. (Insight Pharmaceutical) Acetaminophen 250 mg, aspirin 250 mg, caffeine 65 mg. Tab. 75s. *OTC.*
Use: Nonnarcotic analgesic.
Anacin Aspirin Free. (Insight Pharmaceutical) Acetaminophen 500 mg. Film coated. Parabens. Tab. 100s. *OTC.*
Use: Analgesic.
Anacin Maximum Strength. (Insight Pharmaceutical) Aspirin 500 mg, caffeine 32 mg. Tab. Bot. 20s, 40s, 75s. *OTC.*
Use: Analgesic.
Anadrol-50. (Alaven) Oxymetholone 50 mg. Lactose. Tab. Bot. 100s. *c-III.*
Use: Anabolic steroid.
anafebrina.
See: Aminopyrine.
Anafranil. (Novartis) Clomipramine hydrochloride 25 mg, 50 mg, 75 mg. Parabens. Cap. Bot. 100s, UD 100s. *Rx.*
Use: Antidepressant.
•**anagestone acetate.** (AN-ah-JEST-ohn) USAN.
Use: Hormone, progestin.
•**anagrelide hydrochloride.** (AN-AGG-reh-lide) USAN.
Use: Antiplatelet agent.
See: Agrylin.
anagrelide hydrochloride. (Mallinckrodt) Anagrelide hydrochloride 0.5 mg, 1 mg. Lactose. Cap. 100s. *Rx.*
Use: Antiplatelet agent.
Ana-Guard. (Bayer Consumer Care) Epinephrine 1:1000. Syr. 1 mL. *Rx.*
Use: Bronchodilator; sympathomimetic.
Ana Hep-2. (Wampole) Antinuclear antibodies test by IFA. Tests 60s.
Use: Diagnostic aid.

•**anakinra.** (an-ah-KIN-rah) USAN.
Use: Immunologic agent, immunomodulator.
See: Kineret.
Ana-Kit. (Bayer Consumer Care) Syringe, epinephrine 1:1000 in 1 mL; four (each 2 mg) chlorpheniramine maleate; two sterilized swabs, tourniquet, instructions/kit. *Rx.*
Use: Anaphylactic therapy.
Analbalm Improved Formula. (Schwarz Pharma) Methyl salicylate 10%, menthol 1.25%, camphor 3%. Liq. Bot. **Green:** 4 oz, gal. **Pink:** 4 oz, Pt, gal. *OTC.*
Use: Counterirritant.
analeptics. Usually a term applied to agents with stimulant action, particularly on the central nervous system.
See: Armodafinil.
Caffeine.
Doxapram Hydrochloride.
Modafinil.
Analgesia. (Rugby) Trolamine sulfate 10%. Cream. Tube 85 g. *OTC.*
Use: Liniment.
analgesic and antihistamine combinations.
Use: Upper respiratory combination.
See: Acetaminophen, Chlorpheniramine Maleate.
Acetaminophen, Diphenhydramine Maleate.
Acetaminophen, Phenyltoloxamine Citrate.
analgesic and decongestant combinations.
Use: Upper respiratory combination.
See: Acetaminophen, Phenylephrine Hydrochloride.
Acetaminophen, Pseudoephedrine Hydrochloride.
Ibuprofen, Pseudoephedrine Hydrochloride.
Naproxen, Pseudoephedrine Hydrochloride.
analgesic, antihistamine, and antitussive combinations.
Use: Upper respiratory combination.
analgesic, antihistamine, and decongestant combinations.
Use: Upper respiratory combination.
analgesic, antihistamine, antitussive, and decongestant combinations.
Use: Upper respiratory combination.
analgesic, antitussive, and decongestant combinations.
Use: Upper respiratory combination.
analgesic, antitussive, decongestant, expectorant combinations.
Use: Upper respiratory combination.

Analgesic Balm. (Various Mfr.) Menthol w/methylsalicylate in a suitable base. *OTC.*
Use: Counterirritant.
Analgesic Balm-GRX. (Geritrex) Methyl salicylate 14%, menthol 6%. Balm. 28 g. *OTC.*
Use: Rub and liniment.
Analgesic Creme Rub. (Major) Trolamine salicylate 10%. Aloe vera, cetyl alcohol, glycerin, mineral oil, parabens, triethanolamine. Cream. 85 g. *OTC.*
Use: Rub and liniment.
Analgesic Liquid. (Weeks & Leo) Triethanolamine salicylate 20% in an alcohol base. Liq. Bot. 4 oz. *OTC.*
Use: Analgesic, topical.
Analgesic Lotion. (Weeks & Leo) Methyl nicotinate 1%, methyl salicylate 10%, camphor 0.1%, menthol 0.1%. Lot. Bot. 4 oz. *OTC.*
Use: Analgesic, topical.
analgesics, central.
See: Clonidine Hydrochloride.
analgesics, miscellaneous.
See: Ziconotide.
analgesics, opioid.
See: Opioid analgesics.
Analpram-E. (Ferndale) Hydrocortisone acetate 2.5%, pramoxine hydrochloride 1%. Cetostearyl alcohol, mineral oil, propylparaben, white petrolatum. Cream. Kit with 4 g single-use tubes of cream and 18 Prax wipes. 30s. *Rx.*
Use: Anti-inflammatory agent; corticosteroid, topical.
Analpram-HC. (Ferndale) **Cream:** Hydrocortisone acetate 1%, 2%, pramoxine hydrochloride 1%. Tube 30 g.
Lot.: Hydrocortisone acetate 2.5%, pramoxine hydrochloride 1%. Hydrophilic. Alcohol, glycerin. 60 mL. *Rx.*
Use: Anesthetic; corticosteroid, local.
Analval. (Pal-Pak, Inc.) Aspirin 227 mg, acetaminophen 162 mg, caffeine 32 mg. Tab. Bot. 1000s. *OTC.*
Use: Analgesic combination.
AnaMantle HC. (Bradley) Hydrocortisone acetate 0.5%, lidocaine hydrochloride 3%, cetyl alcohol, light mineral oil, parabens, glycerin, stearyl alcohol, petrolatum. Cream. Kits. 7 g tubes w/single-use applicators (14s). *Rx.*
Use: Corticosteroid combination.
AnaMantle HC 2.5%. (Bradley) Lidocaine hydrochloride 3%, hydrocortisone acetate 2.5%. Parabens, stearyl alcohol, urea. Gel. 20 single-use 7 g tubes with built-in applicator and single-use cleansing wipes. *Rx.*
Use: Anorectal preparation.

Anamine. (Merz) Pseudoephedrine hydrochloride 30 mg, chlorpheniramine maleate 2 mg/5 mL. Syr. Bot. 473 mL. *Rx.*
Use: Antihistamine; decongestant.
Anamine HD. (Merz) Phenylephrine hydrochloride 5 mg, chlorpheniramine maleate 2 mg, hydrocodone bitartrate 1.67 mg. Syr. Bot. *c-iii.*
Use: Antihistamine; antitussive; decongestant.
Anamine TD. (Merz) Chlorpheniramine maleate 8 mg, pseudoephedrine hydrochloride 120 mg. TD Cap. Bot. 100s. *Rx.*
Use: Antihistamine; decongestant.
• **anamorelin hydrochloride.** (AN-a-moe-REL-in) USAN.
Use: Treatment of cancer anorexia and cancer cachexia.
ananain, comosain.
Use: Burn therapy. [Orphan Drug]
See: Vianain.
Anaplex-DM Cough. (ECR) Dextromethorphan HBr 30 mg, brompheniramine maleate 4 mg, pseudoephedrine hydrochloride 60 mg per 5 mL. Fruit flavor. Alcohol, sugar, and dye free. Syrup. Bot. 473 mL. *Rx.*
Use: Upper respiratory combination, antitussive combination.
Anaprox. (Roche) Naproxen 250 mg (naproxen sodium 275 mg). Tab. Bot. 100s. *Rx.*
Use: Nonsteroidal anti-inflammatory agent.
Anaprox DS. (Roche) Naproxen 500 mg (naproxen sodium 550 mg). Film coated. Tab. Bot. 100s, 500s. *Rx.*
Use: Nonsteroidal anti-inflammatory agent.
anarel. Guanadrel sulfate.
• **anaritide acetate.** (an-NAR-ih-TIDE) USAN.
Use: Antihypertensive; diuretic.
• **anastrozole.** (an-ASS-troe-zole) USAN.
Use: Antineoplastic; hormone.
See: Arimidex.
anastrozole. (Various Mfr.) Anastrozole 1 mg. May contain lactose, PEG, polydextrose. Tab. 30s, 90s, 500s. *Rx.*
Use: Hormone, aromatase inhibitor.
Anatrast. (Mallinckrodt) Barium sulfate 100%. Simethicone, sorbitol, parabens. Paste. Tube 500 g, enema tip assemblies. *Rx.*
Use: Radiopaque agent, GI contrast agent.
Anatuss LA. (Merz) Guaifenesin 400 mg, pseudoephedrine hydrochloride

120 mg. Tab. Bot. 100s. *Rx.*
Use: Decongestant; expectorant.
Anavar. (Pharmacia) Oxandrolone
2.5 mg. Tab. Bot. 100s. *Rx.*
Use: Anabolic steroid.
anayodin.
See: Chiniofon.
•**anazolene sodium.** (an-AZZ-oh-leen)
USAN. Sodium anoxynaphthonate.
Use: Diagnostic aid, blood volume, cardiac output determination.
Anbesol. (Wyeth Consumer Health) **Gel:**
Benzocaine 6.3%, phenol 0.5%, alcohol 70%. Gel. Tube 7.5 g. **Liq.:** Benzocaine 6.3%, phenol 0.5%, povidone-iodine, alcohol 70%, camphor, menthol.
Liq. Bot. 9.3 mL, 22.2 mL. *OTC.*
Use: Anesthetic combination, topical.
Anbesol Baby. (Pfizer) Benzocaine
7.5%. Gel. Tube 0.25 oz. *OTC.*
Use: Anesthetic, local.
Anbesol Cold Sore Therapy. (Wyeth
Consumer Health) Benzocaine 20%, allantoin 1%, camphor 3%, petrolatum
64.9%, aloe, benzyl alcohol, parabens, menthol, vitamin E. Oint. 7.1 g. *OTC.*
Use: Topical local anesthetic, ester local anesthetic.
Anbesol Jr. (Wyeth Consumer Health)
Benzocaine 10%. Acesulfame K, benzyl alcohol, glycerin, methylparaben,
PEG. Bubble gum flavor. Gel. 9 g. *OTC.*
Use: Topical local anesthetic, ester local anesthetic.
Anbesol Maximum Strength. (Wyeth
Consumer Health) **Gel:** Benzocaine
20%, alcohol 60%, carbomer 934P,
polyethylene glycol, saccharin. Tube
7.2 g. **Liq.:** Benzocaine 20%, alcohol
60%, saccharin, polyethylene glycol.
Bot. 9 mL. *OTC.*
Use: Anesthetic, local.
•**ancestim.** (an-SESS-tim) USAN.
Use: Investigational for treatment of anemia; hematopoietic adjuvant, stem cell factor.
Ancid. (Sheryl) Calcium aluminum carbonate, di-amino acetate complex. Tab.
Bot. 100s. Susp. Bot. Pt. *OTC.*
Use: Antacid.
Ancobon. (ICN) Flucytosine 250 mg,
500 mg, lactose, parabens, talc. Cap.
Bot. 100s. *Rx.*
Use: Anti-infective; antifungal.
•**ancriviroc.** (AN-Kri-VIR-ok) USAN.
Use: Antiviral.
•**ancrod.** (AN-krahd) USAN. An active principle obtained from the venom of the Malayan pit viper Agkistrodon rhodostoma.
Use: Anticoagulant.

Andesterone. (Lincoln Diagnostics)
Estrone 2 mg, testosterone 6 mg/mL.
Susp. Vial 15 mL. **Forte:** Estrone 1 mg,
testosterone 20 mg/mL. Inj. Vial 15 mL.
Rx.
Use: Androgen, estrogen combination.
Andrest 90-4. (Seatrace) Testosterone
enanthate 90 mg, estradiol valerate
4 mg/mL. Vial 10 mL. *Rx.*
Use: Androgen, estrogen combination.
Androderm. (Watson) Testosterone
2.5 mg/24 hr (12.2 mg), 5 mg/24 hr
(24.3 mg). Patch. Pkg. 30s (5 mg only),
60s (2.5 mg only). *c-III.*
Use: Sex hormone, androgen.
Andro-Estro 90-4. (Rugby) Estradiol valerate 4 mg, testosterone enanthate
90 mg/mL with chlorobutanol in sesame
oil. Inj. Vial. 10 mL. *Rx.*
Use: Androgen, estrogen combination.
AndroGel-DHT. (Unimed Pharm) Dihydrotestosterone.
Use: AIDS. [Orphan Drug]
AndroGel 1%. (Abbott) Testosterone 1%.
Ethanol 67%. Each packet contains
2.5 or 5 g gel to deliver testosterone
25 or 50 mg. Gel. 30s. Metered-dose
pumps to deliver 75 g or 60 metered
1.25 g doses. *c-III.*
Use: Sex hormone, androgen.
androgen hormone inhibitors.
See: Dutasteride.
Finasteride.
androgens. Substances that possess
masculinizing activities.
Use: Sex hormone.
See: Fluoxymesterone.
Methyltestosterone.
Testosterone.
Testosterone, Buccal.
Testosterone Cypionate.
Testosterone Enanthate.
Testosterone Heptanoate.
Testosterone Phenylacetate.
androgens and estrogens.
Use: Sex hormone.
See: Covaryx.
Covaryx H.S.
Estratest.
Estratest H.S.
Androlin. (Lincoln Diagnostics) Testosterone 100 mg/mL. Vial 10 mL. *c-III.*
Use: Androgen.
Andronaq-50. (Schwarz Pharma) Testosterone 50 mg/mL, sodium carboxymethylcellulose, methylcellulose, povidone, DSS, thimerosal. Inj. Vial.
10 mL. *c-III.*
Use: Androgen.
Andronaq LA. (Schwarz Pharma) Testosterone cypionate 100 mg, benzyl alco-

hol 0.9% in cottonseed oil. Vial 10 mL.
Bot. 12s. *c-III.*
Use: Androgen.
Andronate 100. (Taylor Pharmaceuti-
cals) Testosterone cypionate 100 mg/
mL with benzyl alcohol in cottonseed oil.
Vial 10 mL. *c-III.*
Use: Androgen.
Andronate 200. (Taylor Pharmaceuti-
cals) Testosterone cypionate 200 mg/
mL with benzyl alcohol, benzyl benzo-
ate in cottonseed oil. Vial 10 mL. *c-III.*
Use: Androgen.
Andro 100. (Forest) Testosterone
100 mg/mL. Vial 10 mL. *c-III.*
Use: Androgen.
androstanazole.
See: Stanozold.
androstenopyrazole. Anabolic steroid;
pending release.
Androtest P.
See: Testosterone propionate.
Androvite. (Optimox) Iron 3 mg, vitamins
A 4167 units, D 67 units, E 67 units, B_1
8.3 mg, B_2 8.3 mg, B_3 8.3 mg, B_5
16.7 mg, B_6 16.7 mg, B_{12} 20.8 mcg, C
167 mg, folic acid 0.06 mg, PABA, ino-
sitol, biotin, betaine, B, Cr, Cu, I, Mg,
Mn, Se, Zn 8.3 mg, pancreatin, hesperidin, rutin. Tab. 180s. *OTC.*
Use: Mineral, vitamin supplement.
Androxy. (Upsher-Smith) Fluoxymesterone 10 mg. Lactose. Tab. 100s.
c-III.
Use: Sex hormone.
Andylate. (Vita Elixir) Sodium salicylate
10 g. Tab. *OTC.*
Use: Analgesic.
Andylate Forte. (Vita Elixir) Acetaminophen 3 g, salicylamide 3 g, caffeine
0.25 g. Tab. *OTC.*
Use: Analgesic combination.
Andylate Rub. (Vita Elixir) Methylnicotinate, methyl salicylate, camphor, dipropylene glycol salicylate, oil of cassia,
oleo resin of capsicum, oleo resin of
ginger. *OTC.*
Use: Analgesic, topical.
•**anecortave acetate.** (an-eh-CORE-tave
ASS-eh-tate) USAN.
Use: Angiostatic steroid.
AneCream. (Focus Health Group) Lidocaine hydrochloride 4%. Benzyl alcohol, cholesterol, polysorbate 80, propylene glycol, trolamine. Cream. 15 g,
30 g; 5 g kits w/*Tegaderm* patches 5s
and 10s. *Rx.*
Use: Topical local anesthetic, amide local anesthetic.
Anectine. (GlaxoSmithKline) Succinylcholine chloride. **Soln.:** 20 mg/mL.

Multidose Vial 10 mL. **Sterile Pow.:**
500 mg, 1000 mg. Flo-Pak Box 12s. *Rx.*
Use: Muscle relaxant.
Anefrin Nasal Spray, Long Acting.
(Walgreen) Oxymetazoline hydrochlo-
ride 0.05%. Bot. 0.5 oz. *OTC.*
Use: Decongestant.
Anergan 50. (Forest) Promethazine
hydrochloride 50 mg/mL, EDTA, phenol.
Vial 10 mL. *Rx.*
Use: Antihistamine.
anertan.
See: Testosterone propionate.
Anestacon. (PolyMedica) Lidocaine
hydrochloride 2%. Hydroxypropylmethyl
cellulose 1%, benzalkonium chloride
0.01%. Jelly. Disposable units. 15 mL,
240 mL. *Rx.*
Use: Topical local anesthetic, amide lo-
cal anesthetic.
Anestafoam. (Onset Therapeutics) Lido-
caine 4%. Benzyl alcohol. Top. Foam.
30 g. *OTC.*
Use: Topical local anesthetic, amide local anesthetic.
Anesthesin. (Ethyl-p-aminobenzoate).
Use: Anesthetic, local.
See: Benzocaine.
anesthetics, combination local.
See: Duocaine.
anesthetics, general.
See: Diprivan.
    Droperidol.
    Inapsine.
    Propofol.
    Sevoflurane.
    Ultane.
    Volatile Liquids.
anesthetics, injectable local.
See: Amide Local Anesthetics.
    Anesthetics, Combination Local.
    Bupivacaine Hydrochloride.
    Chloroprocaine Hydrochloride.
    Ester Local Anesthetics.
    Lidocaine Hydrochloride.
    Mepivacaine Hydrochloride.
    Prilocaine Hydrochloride.
    Procaine Hydrochloride.
    Ropivacaine Hydrochloride.
    Tetracaine Hydrochloride.
anesthetics, ophthalmic local.
See: Proparacaine Hydrochloride.
    Tetracaine Hydrochloride.
anesthetics, topical local.
See: Amide Local Anesthetics.
    Benzethonium Chloride w/Lidocaine
    Hydrochloride.
    Benzocaine.
    Ester Local Anesthetics.
    Pramoxine Hydrochloride.

anethaine.
See: Tetracaine Hydrochloride.
•**anethole.** (AN-eh-thole) NF 29.
Use: Pharmaceutic aid, flavor.
aneurine hydrochloride.
See: Thiamine hydrochloride.
Anexsia 5/500. (Mallinckrodt) Hydrocodone bitartrate 5 mg, acetaminophen 500 mg. Tab. Bot. 100s. c-III.
Use: Analgesic combination; narcotic.
Anexsia 7.5/650. (Mallinckrodt) Hydrocodone bitartrate 7.5 mg, acetaminophen 650 mg. Tab. Bot. 100s. c-III.
Use: Analgesic combination, narcotic.
Anexsia 10/660. (Mallinckrodt) Hydrocodone bitartrate 10 mg, acetaminophen 660 mg. Tab. Bot. 100s, 1000s. c-III.
Use: Analgesic combination, narcotic.
Angeliq. (Bayer) Drospirenone 0.5 mg/ estradiol 1 mg per day. Lactose. Film coated. Tab. Blister packs 28s. Rx.
Use: Sex hormone, estrogen and progestin combined.
Angel Sweet. (Garrett) Vitamins A and D$_2$. Cream. Tube 90 g. OTC.
Use: Dermatologic, protectant.
Angen. (Davis & Sly) Estrone 2 mg, testosterone 25 mg/mL. Aqueous Susp. Vial 10 mL. Rx.
Use: Androgen, estrogen combination.
Angerin. (Kingsbay) Nitroglycerin 1 mg. Cap. Bot. 60s. Rx.
Use: Coronary vasodilator.
Angex. (Janssen) Lidoflazine. Rx.
Use: Coronary vasodilator.
Angio-Conray. (Mallinckrodt) Iothalamate sodium 80% (48% iodine), EDTA. Inj. Vial 50 mL.
Use: Radiopaque agent.
Angiomax. (Medicines Company) Bivalirudin 250 mg. Inj., lyophilized. Single-use vial. Rx.
Use: Anticoagulant.
•**angiotensin amide.** (an-JEE-oh-TEN-sin AH-mid) USAN.
Use: Vasoconstrictor.
angiotensin-converting enzyme inhibitors.
Use: Antihypertensive; congestive heart failure.
See: Benazepril Hydrochloride.
Captopril.
Enalapril Maleate.
Fosinopril Sodium.
Lisinopril.
Moexipril Hydrochloride.
Perindopril Erbumine.
Quinapril Hydrochloride.
Ramipril.
Trandolapril.

angiotensin II receptor antagonists.
See: Azilsartan Medoxomil.
Candesartan Cilexetil.
Eprosartan Mesylate.
Irbesartan.
Losartan Potassium.
Telmisartan.
Valsartan.
Angiovist 282. (Berlex) Diatrizoate meglumine 60% (iodine 28%). Vial 50 mL, 100 mL, 150 mL. Box 10s.
Use: Radiopaque agent.
Angiovist 292. (Berlex) Diatrizoate meglumine 52%, diatrizoate sodium 8% (iodine 29.2%). Vial 30 mL, 50 mL, 100 mL. Box 10s.
Use: Radiopaque agent.
Angiovist 370. (Berlex) Diatrizoate meglumine 66%, diatrizoate sodium 10%, (iodine 37%). Vial 50 mL, 100 mL, 150 mL, or 200 mL. Box 10s.
Use: Radiopaque agent.
anhydrohydroxyprogesterone. Ethisterone.
•**anidoxime.** (AN-ih-DOX-eem) USAN.
Use: Analgesic.
•**anidulafungin.** (AN-ih-doo-la-FUN-jin) USAN.
Use: Antifungal.
See: Eraxis.
A-Nil. (Vangard Labs, Inc.) Codeine phosphate 10 mg, bromodiphenhydramine hydrochloride 3.75 mg, diphenhydramine hydrochloride 8.75 mg, ammonium chloride 80 mg, potassium guaiacolsulfonate 80 mg, menthol 0.5 mg/5 mL, alcohol 5%. Bot. Pt. gal. c-v.
Use: Antitussive; expectorant.
•**anileridine.** (an-ih-LURR-ih-deen) USP 34.
Use: Analgesic, narcotic.
•**anileridine hydrochloride.** (an-ih-LURR-ih-deen) USP 34.
Use: Analgesic, narcotic.
•**anilopam hydrochloride.** (AN-ih-low-pam) USAN.
Use: Analgesic.
Animal Shapes. (Major) Vitamin A 2500 units, D 400 units, E 15 units, C 60 mg, B$_1$ 1.05 mg, B$_2$ 1.2 mg, B$_3$ 13.5 mg, B$_6$ 1.05 mg, B$_{12}$ 4.5 mcg, folic acid 0.3 mg. Chew. Tab. Bot. 100s, 250s. OTC.
Use: Vitamin supplement.
Animal Shapes + Iron. (Major) Vitamin A 2500 units, D 400 units, E 15 units, C 60 mg, B$_1$ 1.05 mg, B$_2$ 1.2 mg, B$_3$ 13.5 mg, B$_6$ 1.05 mg, B$_{12}$ 4.5 mcg, folic acid 0.3 mg, iron 15 mg. Chew. Tab.

Bot. 100s, 250s. *OTC.*
Use: Mineral, vitamin supplement.

Animi-3. (PBM Pharm) Omega-3 acids 500 mg (eicosapentaenoic acid [EPA] 35 mg and docosahexaenoic acid [DHA] 350 mg), vitamin B_6 12.5 mg, B_{12} 500 mcg, folic acid 1 mg. Sunflower oil. Cap. 60s. *Rx.*
Use: Dietary supplement.

• **aniracetam.** (AN-ih-RASS-eh-tam) USAN.
Use: Mental performance enhancer.

• **anirolac.** (ah-NIH-role-ACK) USAN.
Use: Analgesic; anti-inflammatory.

• **anise oil.** (AN-is) *NF 29.*
Use: Flavoring.

anisopyradamine.
See: Pyrilamine maleate.

• **anisotropine methylbromide.** (ah-NIH-so-TROE-peen meth-ill-BROE-mide) USAN.
Use: Anticholinergic.

• **anitrazafen.** (AN-ih-TRAY-zaff-en) USAN.
Use: Anti-inflammatory, topical.

• **anivamersen.** (AN-i-va-MER-sen) USAN.
Use: Reversal of pegnivacogin anticoagulation.

anodynon.
See: Ethyl Chloride.

Anodynos. (Buffington) Aspirin 420.6 mg, salicylamide 34.4 mg, caffeine 34.4 mg. Sugar, lactose, and salt free. Tab. Dispens-A-Kit 500s, Bot. 100s, 500s, Medipak 200s. *OTC.*
Use: Analgesic combination.

Anodynos-DHC. (Buffington) Hydrocodone bitartrate 5 mg, acetaminophen 500 mg. Tab. Bot. 100s. *c-III.*
Use: Analgesic combination; narcotic.

Anorex. (Oxypure) Phendimetrazine 35 mg. Tab. Bot. 100s. *c-III.*
Use: Anorexiant.

anorexiants.
Use: Appetite suppressants.
See: Benzphetamine Hydrochloride.
Diethylpropion Hydrochloride.
Phendimetrazine Tartrate.
Phentermine Hydrochloride.
Sibutramine Hydrochloride.

anovlar. Norethindrone plus ethinyl estradiol. *Rx.*
Use: Contraceptive.

• **anoxomer.** (an-OX-ah-MER) USAN.
Use: Pharmaceutic aid, antioxidant; food additive.

anoxynaphthonate sodium. Anazolene sodium.

Anspor. (GlaxoSmithKline) Cephradine (a semisynthetic cephalosporin). **Cap.:** 250 mg, 500 mg. Bot. 20s (500 mg only), 100s, UD 100s. **Oral Susp.:** 125 mg, 250 mg/5 mL. Bot. 100 mL.
Use: Anti-infective; cephalosporin.

Answer. (Carter-Wallace) Reagent in-home pregnancy test kit for urine testing. Test kit box 1s.
Use: Diagnostic aid.

Answer One-Step Pregnancy Test. (Carter-Wallace) Pregnancy test kit for urine testing. Stick. Test kit box 1s. *OTC.*
Use: Diagnostic aid.

Answer Plus. (Carter-Wallace) Reagent in-home pregnancy test kit for urine testing. Test kit box 1s.
Use: Diagnostic aid.

Answer Plus 2. (Carter-Wallace) Reagent in-home pregnancy test kit for urine testing. Test kit box 2s.
Use: Diagnostic aid.

Answer Quick & Simple. (Carter-Wallace) Reagent in-home kit for urine testing. Test kit box 1s.
Use: Diagnostic aid.

Answer 2. (Carter-Wallace) Reagent in-home pregnancy test kit for urine testing. Test kit box 2s.
Use: Diagnostic aid.

Antabuse. (Barr/Duramed) Disulfiram 250 mg, 500 mg. Lactose. Tab. Bot. 50s; 100s, 500s (500 mg only). *Rx.*
Use: Antialcoholic.

Antacid. (Walgreen) Calcium carbonate 500 mg. Tab. Bot. 75s. *OTC.*
Use: Antacid.

Antacid Extra Strength. (Various Mfr.) Calcium carbonate 750 mg. Tab. Bot. 96s. *OTC.*
Use: Antacid.

Antacid M. (Walgreen) Aluminum oxide 225 mg, magnesium hydroxide 200 mg/ 5 mL. Liq. Bot. 12 oz, 26 oz. *OTC.*
Use: Antacid.

Antacid No. 6. (Jones Pharma) Calcium carbonate 0.42 g, glycine 0.18 g. Tab. Bot. 100s. *OTC.*
Use: Antacid.

Antacid #2. (Global Source) Calcium carbonate 5.5 g, magnesium carbonate 2.5 g. Tab. Bot. 100s. *OTC.*
Use: Antacid.

Antacid Relief. (Walgreen) Dihydroxyaluminum sodium carbonate 334 mg. Tab. Bot. 75s. *OTC.*
Use: Antacid.

antacids. Drugs that neutralize excess gastric acid.
See: Alka-Seltzer.

Aluminum Hydroxide.
Aluminum Hydroxide Gel.
Aluminum Hydroxide Gel Dried.
Aluminum Hydroxide Magnesium
 Carbonate.
Aluminum Phosphate Gel.
Calcium Carbonate.
Calcium Carbonate, Precipitated.
Ceo-Two.
Chooz.
Citrocarbonate.
Di-Gel.
Dicarbosil.
Dihydroxyaluminum Aminoacetate.
Dihydroxyaluminum Sodium Carbo-
 nate.
Magaldrate.
Magnesium Carbonate.
Magnesium Hydroxide.
Magnesium Oxide.
Magnesium Trisilicate.
Rolaids.
Romach Antacid.
Simethicone.
Sodium Bicarbonate.
Tums.
Antacid Suspension. (Geneva) Alumi-
 num hydroxide 225 mg, magnesium
 hydroxide 200 mg/5 mL. Bot. 360 mL.
 OTC.
 Use: Antacid.
Antacid Tablets. (Goldline) Calcium
 carbonate 500 mg (elemental calcium
 200 mg). Sucrose, sodium up to 2 mg.
 Assorted flavors. Chew. Tab. Bot.
 150s. *OTC.*
 Use: Mineral supplement; antacid.
Anta-Gel. (Halsey Drug) Aluminum
 hydroxide 200 mg, magnesium hydrox-
 ide 200 mg, simethicone 20 mg/5 mL.
 Bot. 12 oz. *OTC.*
 Use: Antacid; antiflatulent.
antagonists of curariform drugs.
 See: Neostigmine Methylsulfate.
 Tensilon.
Antara. (Reliant) Fenofibrate (micron-
 ized) 43 mg, 130 mg. Sugar spheres.
 Cap. 30s, 100s. *Rx.*
 Use: Antihyperlipidemic agent, fibric
 acid derivatives.
antazoline hydrochloride. Antastan.
•**antazoline phosphate.** (an-TAZ-oh-leen)
 USP 34.
 Use: Antihistamine.
anterior pituitary.
 See: Pituitary, anterior.
Anthelios 40. (La Roche-Posay) Avoben-
 zone 2%, *Mexoryl SX* 3%, octocrylene
 10%, titanium dioxide 5%. PABA free.
 Cream. 50 g. *OTC.*
 Use: Sunscreen.

Anthelios SX. (La Roch-Posay) Avoben-
 zone 2%, ecamsule 2%, octocrylene
 10%. EDTA, glycerin, parabens, stearyl
 alcohol. SPF 15. Cream. 100 g. *OTC.*
 Use: Sunscreen.
anthelmintics.
 Use: A remedy for worms.
 See: Biltricide.
 Carbon Tetrachloride.
 Gentian Violet.
 Ivermectin.
 Mintezol.
 Piperazine.
 Praziquantel.
 Stromectol.
 Tetrachloroethylene.
 Vermox.
•**anthelmycin.** (AN-thell-MY-sin) USAN.
 Use: Anthelmintic.
Anthelvet. Tetramisole hydrochloride.
anthracenedione.
 See: Mitoxantrone Hydrochloride.
 Novantrone.
anthracyclines.
 See: Daunorubicin Citrate Liposomal.
 Daunorubicin Hydrochloride.
 Doxorubicin Hydrochloride.
 Doxorubicin Hydrochloride, Lipo-
 somal.
 Epirubicin Hydrochloride.
 Idarubicin Hydrochloride.
•**anthralin.** (AN-thrah-lin) *USP 34.*
 Use: Antipsoriatic.
 See: Dritho-Scalp.
 Zithranol-RR.
anthralin. (Rising Pharmaceuticals)
 Anthralin 1%. Cream. 50 g. *Rx.*
 Use: Antipsoriatic agent.
•**anthramycin.** (an-THRAH-MY-sin)
 USAN.
 Use: Antineoplastic.
anthraquinone of cascara.
 See: Cascara Sagrada.
anthrax vaccine. (Michigan Biological
 Products Institute) Vial 5 mL. *Rx.*
 Use: Immunization.
•**anthrax vaccine, adsorbed.** (AN-thrax
 VAX-een) *USP 34.*
 Use: Immunization.
 See: BioThrax.
anti-a blood grouping serum.
 Use: Diagnostic aid, blood in vitro.
Antiacid. (Hillcrest North) Aluminum
 hydroxide, magnesium trisilicate, cal-
 cium carbonate. Tab. Bot. 100s. *OTC.*
 Use: Antacid.
antiadrenergic agents, centrally acting.
 See: Clonidine Hydrochloride.
 Guanfacine Hydrochloride.

antiadrenergic agents, peripherally acting.
Use: Antiadrenergic/sympatholytic.
See: Alfuzosin Hydrochloride.
Alpha-1 Adrenergic Blockers.
Doxazosin Mesylate.
Prazosin Hydrochloride.
Reserpine.
Tamsulosin Hydrochloride.
Terazosin Hydrochloride.
antiadrenergics/sympatholytics.
See: Alpha/Beta-Adrenergic Blocking Agents.
Antiadrenergic Agents, Centrally Acting.
Antiadrenergic Agents, Peripherally Acting.
Beta-Adrenergic Blocking Agents.
antialcoholic agents.
See: Acamprosate Calcium.
Disulfiram.
antiandrogens.
See: Bicalutamide.
Eulexin.
Flutamide.
Nilandron.
Nilutamide.
antianginal agents, miscellaneous.
See: Ranolazine.
antianxiety agents.
See: Alprazolam.
Benzodiazepines.
Buspirone Hydrochloride.
Chlordiazepoxide Hydrochloride.
Clonazepam.
Clorazepate Dipotassium.
Diazepam.
Doxepin Hydrochloride.
Hydroxyzine.
Lorazepam.
Meprobamate.
Oxazepam.
antiarrhythmic agents.
See: Adenosine.
Amiodarone Hydrochloride.
Bretylium Tosylate.
Disopyramide.
Dofetilide.
Dronedarone.
Flecainide Acetate.
Ibutilide Fumarate.
Lidocaine Hydrochloride.
Procainamide Hydrochloride.
Propafenone Hydrochloride.
Quinidine.
antiasthmatic combinations.
See: Cromolyn Sodium.
Ephedrine Hydrochloride.
Ephedrine Sulfate.
Isoephedrine Hydrochloride.
Isoetharine.
Isoetharine Hydrochloride.

Isoetharine Mesylate.
Isoproterenol Hydrochloride.
Isoproterenol Sulfate.
Methoxyphenamine Hydrochloride.
Phenylephrine Hydrochloride.
Pseudoephedrine Hydrochloride.
Racephedrine Hydrochloride.
Xanthine Combinations.
antiasthmatic inhalants.
See: AsthmaNefrin.
antibason.
See: Methylthiouracil.
anti-b blood grouping serum.
Use: Diagnostic aid, blood in vitro.
AntibiOtic. (Parnell) **Otic Susp.:** Polymyxin B sulfate 10,000 units, neomycin (as sulfate) 3.5 mg, hydrocortisone 10 mg/mL, thimerosal 0.01%. Bot. 10 mL w/dropper. **Otic Soln.:** Polymyxin B sulfate 10,000 units, neomycin sulfate 5 mg, hydrocortisone 1%. Propylene glycol, glycerin, potassium metabisulfite. Bot. 10 mL. *Rx.*
Use: Anti-infective; anti-inflammatory.
antibiotic and steroid combinations.
See: Ciprofloxacin/Dexamethasone.
Ciprofloxacin/Hydrocortisone.
Dexamethasone Phosphate/Neomycin Sulfate.
Dexamethasone/Tobramycin.
Hydrocortisone Acetate/Chloramphenicol/Polymyxin B.
Hydrocortisone/Neomycin Sulfate.
Hydrocortisone/Neomycin Sulfate/Bacitracin Zinc/Polymyxin B Sulfate.
Loteprednol Etabonate/Tobramycin.
Neomycin and Polymyxin B Sulfates and Dexamethasone.
Neomycin/Polymyxin B Sulfates/Hydrocortisone.
Prednisolone Acetate/Gentamicin Sulfate.
Prednisolone Acetate/Neomycin Sulfate/Polymyxin B Sulfate.
antibiotic combinations.
See: AK-Poly-Bac.
AK-Spore.
Bacitracin Zinc and Polymyxin B Sulfate.
Betadine Plus First Aid Antibiotics and Pain Reliever.
Betadine First Aid Antibiotics Plus Moisturizer.
Double Antibiotic.
Lanabiotic.
Neomycin and Polymyxin B Sulfates and Bacitracin Zinc.
Neomycin and Polymyxin B Sulfates and Gramicidin.
Neosporin.
Neosporin Original.

Neosporin Plus Pain Relief.
Polysporin.
Polytrim.
Terramycin w/Polymyxin B Sulfate.
Tri-Biozene.
Triple Antibiotic.
Antibiotic Ear. (Various Mfr.) **Soln.:**
Hydrocortisone 1%, neomycin sulfate
5 mg, polymyxin B 10,000 units. 10 mL.
Susp.: Hydrocortisone 1%, neomycin
sulfate 5 mg, polymyxin B 10,000 units.
10 mL with dropper. *Rx.*
Use: Steroid and antibiotic combination.
antibiotics/anti-infectives.
See: Amebicides, General.
Amikacin Sulfate.
Amoxicillin.
Amoxicillin and Clavulanate Potassium.
Ampicillin.
Anthelmintics.
Anthracyclines.
Antifungal Agents.
Antimalarial Agents.
Antiprotozoal Agents.
Antituberculosis Agents.
Antiviral Agents.
Azithromycin.
Aztreonam.
Bacampicillin Hydrochloride.
Bacitracin.
Benzoyl Peroxide.
Betadine First Aid Antibiotics Plus
Moisturizer.
Betadine Plus First Aid Antibiotics and
Pain Reliever.
Bicillin C-R.
Blenoxane.
Bleomycin Sulfate.
Capecitabine.
Cefaclor.
Cefadroxil.
Cefazolin Sodium.
Cefditoren Pivoxil.
Cefixime.
Cefmetazole Sodium.
Cefoperazone Sodium.
Cefotaxime Sodium.
Cefotetan Disodium.
Cefoxitin Sodium.
Cefpodoxime Proxetil.
Cefprozil.
Ceftazidime.
Ceftizoxime Sodium.
Ceftriaxone Sodium.
Cefuroxime.
Cephalexin.
Cephalothin Sodium.
Cephradine.
Chloramphenicol.

Ciprofloxacin.
Clarithromycin.
Clindamycin.
Clindamycin Phosphate.
Clioquinol.
Clofazimine.
Cloxacillin Sodium.
Colistimethate Sodium.
Cruex.
Dactinomycin.
Dapsone.
Daunorubicin Hydrochloride.
Demeclocycline.
Desenex.
Dicloxacillin.
Doxycycline.
Enoxacin.
Erythromycin.
Fungicides.
Furazolidone.
Gentamicin Sulfate.
Kanamycin Sulfate.
Lanabiotic.
Levofloxacin.
Lincomycin.
Lomefloxacin Hydrochloride.
Loprox.
Loracarbef.
Lotrimin AF.
Methenamine.
Methicillin Sodium.
Methylene Blue.
Metronidazole.
Minocycline.
Mitomycin.
Mupirocin.
Nafcillin Sodium.
Nalidixic Acid.
Neomycin Sulfate.
Neosporin Original.
Netilmicin Sulfate.
Nitrofurantoin.
Norfloxacin.
Ocuflox.
Ofloxacin.
Oxacillin Sodium.
Oxytetracycline.
Penicillin G Benzathine.
Penicillin G Potassium.
Penicillin G Procaine.
Penicillin G Procaine Combinations.
Penicillin G Sodium.
Penicillin V Potassium.
Penlac Nail Lacquer.
Pentamidine Isethionate.
Phenoxymethyl Penicillin.
Piperacillin Sodium.
Piperacillin Sodium w/Comb.
Polymyxin B Sulfate.
Polysporin.
Pyrimidine Analogs.

Quixin.
Retapamulin.
Rubex.
Sodium Sulfacetamide.
Spectazole.
Spectinomycin.
Spectracef.
Sulfadiazine.
Sulfamethoxazole.
Sulfasalazine.
Sulfisoxazole.
Sulfonamides.
Tetracycline Hydrochloride.
Ticarcillin Disodium.
Tobramycin.
Tobramycin Sulfate.
Tri-Biozene.
Triple Antibiotic.
Trimethoprim.
Vancomycin Hydrochloride.
Xeloda.
antibiotics, ophthalmic.
See: Azithromycin.
Bacitracin.
Chloramphenicol.
Ciprofloxacin Hydrochloride.
Erythromycin.
Gatifloxacin.
Gentamicin Sulfate.
Moxifloxacin Hydrochloride.
Ofloxacin.
Polymyxin B.
Tobramycin.
antibodies, monoclonal.
See: Alemtuzumab.
Campath.
Herceptin.
Rituxan.
Rituximab.
Trastuzumab.
anti-CD45 monoclonal antibodies.
Use: Prevention of graft rejection in organ transplants. [Orphan Drug]
anticholinergic agents.
Use: Antiemetic/antivertigo agents; antiparkinson agents; bronchodilators.
See: Antispasmodics.
Belladonna Alkaloids.
Benztropine Mesylate.
Biperiden.
Buclizine Hydrochloride.
Cyclizine.
Darifenacin Hydrobromide.
Dimenhydrinate.
Diphenhydramine.
Fesoterodine Fumarate.
Flavoxate Hydrochloride.
Glycopyrrolate.
Ipratropium Bromide.
Ipratropium Bromide/Albuterol Sulfate.

Meclizine Hydrochloride.
Mepenzolate Bromide.
Methscopolamine Bromide.
Nabilone.
Oxybutynin Chloride.
Propantheline Bromide.
Scopolamine.
Solifenacin Succinate.
Tiotropium Bromide.
Tolterodine Tartrate.
Trihexyphenidyl Hydrochloride.
Trimethobenzamide Hydrochloride.
Trospium Chloride.
anticholinergic and antitussive combinations.
Use: Upper respiratory combination.
anticholinergic and decongestant combinations.
Use: Upper respiratory combination.
anticholinergic, antihistamine, and decongestant combinations.
Use: Upper respiratory combination.
•**anticoagulant citrate dextrose solution.** (an-tee-koe-ag-ue-lant) *USP 34.*
Use: Anticoagulant for storage of whole blood.
See: A-C-D.
•**anticoagulant citrate phosphate dextrose adenine solution.** *USP 34.*
Use: Anticoagulant for storage of whole blood.
•**anticoagulant citrate phosphate dextrose solution.** *USP 34.*
Use: Anticoagulant for storage of whole blood.
•**anticoagulant heparin solution.** *USP 34.*
Use: Anticoagulant for storage of whole blood.
anticoagulants.
See: Antithrombin Agents.
Heparin.
Low Molecular Weight Heparins.
Selective Factor Xa Inhibitor.
Thrombin Inhibitors.
Warfarin.
•**anticoagulant sodium citrate solution.** *USP 34.*
Use: Anticoagulant for plasma and blood fractionation.
anticonvulsants.
See: Acetazolamide.
Benzodiazepines.
Carbamazepine.
Clonazepam.
Clorazepate Dipotassium.
Diazepam.
Divalproex Sodium.
Felbamate.
Gabapentin.

Hydantoins.
Lacosamide.
Lamotrigine.
Levetiracetam.
Lorazepam.
Magnesium Sulfate.
Mephobarbital.
Methsuximide.
Oxcarbazepine.
Phenobarbital.
Phenytoin.
Phenytoin Sodium.
Pregabalin.
Primidone.
Rufinamide.
Succinimides.
Sulfonamides.
Tiagabine Hydrochloride.
Topiramate.
Valproate.
Valproic Acid.
Vigabatrin.
Zonisamide.
anticytomegalovirus monoclonal antibodies.
Use: Treatment of cytomegalovirus.
antidepressants.
See: Bupropion Hydrochloride.
Monoamine Oxidase Inhibitors.
Nefazodone Hydrochloride.
Selective Serotonin Reuptake Inhibitors.
Serotonin and Norepinephrine Reuptake Inhibitors.
Tetracyclic Compounds.
Trazodone Hydrochloride.
Tricyclic Compounds.
antidiabetic combinations.
See: Glipizide/Metformin Hydrochloride.
Glyburide/Metformin Hydrochloride.
Pioglitazone Hydrochloride/Glimepiride.
Pioglitazone Hydrochloride/Metformin Hydrochloride.
Rosiglitazone Maleate/Glimepiride.
Rosiglitazone Maleate/Metformin Hydrochloride.
Sitagliptin/Metformin Hydrochloride.
antidiabetics.
See: Alpha-Glucosidase Inhibitors.
Amylin Analog.
Antidiabetic Combination Products.
Biguanides.
Dipeptidyl Peptidase-4 Inhibitor.
Glucagon-Like Peptide 1 Receptor Agonists.
Incretin Mimetic Agents.
Insulin.
Meglitinides.
Sulfonylureas.
Thiazolidinediones.

antidiarrheals.
See: Attapulgite, Activated.
Bismuth Subsalicylate.
Cantil.
Diasorb.
Furoxone.
Imodium.
Imodium A-D.
Kaodene Non-Narcotic.
Kaolin.
Kaolin Colloidal.
Kaopectate.
Kao-Spen.
Kapectolin.
K-C.
Lactinex.
Lactobacillus acidophilus and *bulgaricus* mixed culture.
Lactobacillus acidophilus, viable culture.
Logen.
Lomanate.
Lomotil.
Lonox.
Loperamide Hydrochloride.
Milk of Bismuth.
Motofen.
Pepto-Bismol.
Pink Bismuth.
antidiuretics.
See: Pitressin.
Pituitary Posterior Injection.
antidopaminergics.
Use: Antiemetic/antivertigo agents.
See: Chlorpromazine.
Metoclopramide.
Nabilone.
Perphenazine.
Prochlorperazine.
Promethazine.
Thiethylperazine Maleate.
antidotes.
See: Acetylcysteine.
Atropine/Pralidoxime Chloride.
Charcoal, Activated.
Digoxin Immune Fab (Ovine).
Flumazenil.
Fomepizole.
Hydroxocobalamin.
Ipecac.
Methylene Blue.
Methylnaltrexone Bromide.
Nalmefene Hydrochloride.
Naloxone Hydrochloride.
Naltrexone Hydrochloride.
Physostigmine Salicylate.
Pralidoxime Chloride.
Sodium Nitrite.
Sodium Thiosulfate.
antiemetic/antivertigo agents.
See: Anticholinergic Agents.

Antidopaminergics.
Antiemetic/Antivertigo Agents, Miscellaneous.
5-HT$_3$ Receptor Antagonists.
antiemetic/antivertigo agents, miscellaneous.
See: Aprepitant.
Dronabinol.
Fosaprepitant.
Nabilone.
Phosphorated Carbohydrate Solution.
antiepilepsirine.
Use: Treatment for drug-resistant generalized tonic-clonic epilepsy. [Orphan Drug]
antiepileptic agents.
See: Anticonvulsants.
antiestrogens.
Use: Hormone for cancer therapy.
See: Fulvestrant.
Tamoxifen Citrate.
Toremifene Citrate.
antifebrin.
See: Acetanilid.
antiflatulents.
See: Di-Gel.
Simethicone.
Antifoam A Compound. (Hoechst)
Use: Antiflatulent.
See: Simethicone.
antifolic acid.
See: Methotrexate.
Antiformin. Sodium hypochlorite in sodium hydroxide 7.5%, available chlorine 5.2%; may be colored with meta cresol purple.
Use: Antiseptic; antimicrobial.
antifungal agents.
See: Allylamine Antifungals.
Amphotericin B Desoxycholate.
Amphotericin B, Lipid-based.
Anidulafungin.
Butenafine Hydrochloride.
Caspofungin Acetate.
Ciclopirox.
Clioquinol.
Clotrimazole.
Echinocandins.
Econazole Nitrate.
Fluconazole.
Flucytosine.
Fungicides.
Gentian Violet.
Griseofulvin.
Imidazole Antifungals.
Itraconazole.
Ketoconazole.
Micafungin Sodium.
Miconazole Nitrate.
Naftifine Hydrochloride.
Nystatin.

Polyene Antifungals.
Posaconazole.
Sertaconazole Nitrate.
Sulconazol Nitrate.
Terbinafine Hydrochloride.
Tolnaftate.
Triazole Antifungals.
Undecylenic Acid.
Voriconazole.
antiglaucoma agents.
See: AK-Beta.
Betagan Liquifilm.
Betaxolol Hydrochloride.
Betimol.
Betoptic.
Betoptic S.
Bimatoprost.
Carteolol Hydrochloride.
Levobetaxolol Hydrochloride.
Levobunolol Hydrochloride.
Lumigan.
Metipranolol Hydrochloride.
OptiPranolol.
Timolol.
Timolol Maleate.
Timoptic.
Timoptic-XE.
Travatan.
Travoprost.
antihemophilic agents.
See: Antihemophilic Factor (Factor VIII; AHF).
Anti-Inhibitor Coagulant Complex.
Coagulation Factor VIIa, Recombinant.
Factor IX Concentrates.
Factor XIII Concentrate.
Kogenate.
•**antihemophilic factor.** (AN-tee-HEE-moe-FIL-ik) *USP 34.* Factor VIII; AHF.
Use: Antihemophilic.
See: Advate.
Alphanate.
Helixate FS.
Hemofil M.
Koate-DVI.
Kogenate FS.
Monoclate-P.
Recombinate.
ReFacto.
Xyntha.
antihemophilic factor combinations.
See: Antihemophilic Factor/von Willebrand Factor Complex (Factor VIII/VWF; AHF/VWF).
antihemophilic factor, human.
Use: Treatment of von Willebrand disease. [Orphan Drug]
antihemophilic factor (recombinant).
Use: Prophylaxis/treatment of bleeding in hemophilia A. [Orphan Drug]
See: Kogenate FS.

antihemophilic factor/von Willebrand factor complex (factor VIII/VWF; AHF/VWF).
Use: Antihemophilic.
See: Humate-P.
antiheparin.
See: Protamine Sulfate.
antiherpes virus agents.
Use: Antiviral.
See: Acyclovir.
Famciclovir.
Valacyclovir Hydrochloride.
antihistamine, analgesic, and decongestant combinations.
Use: Upper respiratory combination.
antihistamine and analgesic combinations.
Use: Upper respiratory combination.
See: Analgesic and antihistamine combinations.
antihistamine and antitussive combinations.
Use: Upper respiratory combination.
antihistamine and decongestant combinations.
Use: Upper respiratory combination.
antihistamine, anticholinergic, and decongestant combinations.
Use: Upper respiratory combination.
antihistamine, antitussive, analgesic, and decongestant combinations.
Use: Upper respiratory combination.
antihistamine, antitussive, and analgesic combinations.
Use: Upper respiratory combination.
antihistamine, antitussive, and decongestant combinations.
Use: Upper respiratory combination.
antihistamine, antitussive, decongestant, expectorant combinations.
Use: Upper respiratory combination.
Antihistamine Cream. (Towne) Methapyrilene hydrochloride 10 mg, pyrilamine maleate 5 mg, allantoin 2 mg, diperodon hydrochloride 2.5 mg, benzocaine 10 mg, menthol 2 mg/g. Cream. Jar 2 oz. *OTC.*
Use: Antihistamine, topical.
antihistamine, decongestant, and expectorant combinations.
Use: Upper respiratory combination.
See: Acetaminophen, Dextromethorphan Hydrobromide, Guaifenesin, Phenylephrine Hydrochloride.
Chlorpheniramine Maleate, Guaifenesin, Phenylephrine Hydrochloride.
Guaifenesin, Phenylephrine Tannate, Pyrilamine Tannate.
antihistamines.
See: Alkylamines, Nonselective.
Ethanolamines, Nonselective.

Phenothiazines, Nonselective.
Phthalazinones, Peripherally Selective.
Piperazines, Nonselective.
Piperazines, Peripherally Selective.
Piperidines, Nonselective.
Piperidines, Peripherally Selective.
antihistamines, inhalant.
See: Azelastine.
Olopatadine.
Antihist-1. (Various Mfr.) Clemastine fumarate 1.34 mg. Tab. Pkg. 16s. *OTC.*
Use: Antihistamine.
antihyperlipidemic agents.
See: Bile Acid Sequestrants.
Ezetimibe.
Fibric Acid Derivatives.
HMG-CoA Reductase Inhibitors.
Niacin.
antihyperlipidemic combinations.
See: Amlodipine Besylate/Atorvastatin Calcium.
Ezetimibe/Simvastatin.
Niacin/Lovastatin.
Niacin/Simvastatin.
antihypertensives.
See: Acebutolol Hydrochloride.
Adaprolol Maleate.
Alazide.
Alazine.
Aldactazide.
Aldactone.
Alfuzosin Hydrochloride.
Aliskiren/Hydrochlorothiazide.
Alpha$_1$-Adrenergic Blockers.
Althiazide.
Amiquinsin Hydrochloride.
Amlodipine/Benazepril Hydrochloride.
Amlodipine Besylate.
Amlodipine Besylate/Aliskiren.
Amlodipine Maleate.
Amodopa.
Anaritide Acetate.
Atenolol/Chlorthalidone.
Atiprosin Maleate.
Belfosdil.
Bendacalol Mesylate.
Bendroflumethiazide.
Betaxolol Hydrochloride.
Bethanidine Sulfate.
Bevantolol Hydrochloride.
Biclodil Hydrochloride.
Bucindolol Hydrochloride.
Cam-Ap-Es.
Candoxatril.
Candoxatrilat.
Captopril and Hydrochlorothiazide.
Chlorothiazide Sodium.
Chlorthalidone.
Cicletanine.
Cilazapril.
Cithal.

Citrin.
Clentiazem Maleate.
Clonidine.
Clonidine Hydrochloride.
Clonidine Hydrochloride and Chlor-
 thalidone.
Clopamide.
Cyclothiazide.
Debrisoquin Sulfate.
Delapril Hydrochloride.
Diazoxide.
Diazoxide Parenteral.
Dibenzyline.
Dilevalol Hydrochloride.
Ditekiren.
Diuril Sodium.
Doxazosin Mesylate.
Elserpine.
Enalaprilat.
Enalapril Maleate.
Enalapril Maleate/Felodopine.
Enalkiren.
Endralazine Mesylate.
Eprosartan.
Eprosartan Mesylate.
Eserdine.
Eserdine Forte.
Fenoldopam Mesylate.
Flavodilol Maleate.
Flordipine.
Flosequinan.
Forasartan.
Fosinopril.
Fosinopril Sodium.
Guanabenz.
Guanabenz Acetate.
Guanacline Sulfate.
Guanadrel Sulfate.
Guancydine.
Guanethidine Monosulfate.
Guanethidine Sulfate.
Guanfacine Hydrochloride.
Guanisoquin.
Guanisoquin Sulfate.
Guanoclor Sulfate.
Guanoxabenz.
Guanoxan Sulfate.
Guanoxyfen Sulfate.
Harbolin.
H.H.R.
Hiwolfia.
Hydralazine.
Hydralazine Hydrochloride.
Hydralazine Polistirex.
Hydrochloroserpine.
Hydrochlorothiazide/Amlodipine/Vals-
 artan.
Hydrochlorothiazide/Benazepril.
Hydrochlorothiazide/Bisoprolol Fuma-
 rate.
Hydrochlorothiazide/Candesartan Ci-
 lexetil.

Hydrochlorothiazide/Enalapril
 Maleate.
Hydrochlorothiazide/Eprosartan.
Hydrochlorothiazide/Fosinopril So-
 dium.
Hydrochlorothiazide/Hydralazine.
Hydrochlorothiazide/Irbesartan.
Hydrochlorothiazide/Lisinopril.
Hydrochlorothiazide/Losartan Potas-
 sium.
Hydrochlorothiazide/Moexipril Hydro-
 chloride.
Hydrochlorothiazide/Olmesartan Me-
 doxomil.
Hydrochlorothiazide/Propranolol
 Hydrochloride.
Hydrochlorothiazide/Quinapril Hydro-
 chloride.
Hydrochlorothiazide/Telmisartan.
Hydrochlorothiazide/Timolol Maleate.
Hydrochlorothiazide/Valsartan.
Hydroflumethiazide.
Hydropine.
Hydropine H.P.
Hydroxyisoindolin.
Indacrinone.
Indapamide.
Indolapril Hydrochloride.
Indoramin.
Indoramin Hydrochloride.
Indorenate Hydrochloride.
Ingadine.
Inhibace.
Inversine.
Irbesartan.
Ismelin.
Labetalol Hydrochloride.
Leniquinsin.
Levcromakalim.
Lofexidine Hydrochloride.
Losartan Potassium.
Losulazine Hydrochloride.
Mebutamate.
Mecamylamine Hydrochloride.
Medroxalol.
Medroxalol Hydrochloride.
Methalthiazide.
Methyclodine.
Methylclothiazide.
Methyldopa.
Methyldopa and Chlorothiazide.
Methyldopa and Hydrochlorothiazide.
Metipranolol.
Metipranolol Hydrochloride.
Metolazone.
Metoprolol Fumarate.
Metoprolol Succinate.
Metoprolol Tartrate and Hydrochloro-
 thiazide.
Metyrosine.
Moexipril Hydrochloride.

Muzolimine.
Nadolol.
Nadolol and Bendroflumethiazide.
Natrico.
Nebivolol.
Nitrendipine.
Nitroprusside Sodium.
Pargyline Hydrochloride.
Pelanserin Hydrochloride.
Pentolinium Tartrate.
Perindopril Erbumine.
Pheniprazine Hydrochloride.
Phenoxybenzamine Hydrochloride.
Phentolamine Hydrochloride.
Prazosin Hydrochloride.
Prizidilol Hydrochloride.
Quinapril Hydrochloride.
Quinazosin Hydrochloride.
Quinelorane Hydrochloride.
Quinuclium Bromide.
Raunescine.
Rauwolfia/Bendroflumethiazide.
Rauwolfia Serpentina.
Rauwolscine.
Rawfola.
Saprisartan Potassium.
Saralasin Acetate.
Sodium Nitroprusside.
Sulfinalol Hydrochloride.
Teludipine Hydrochloride.
Temocapril Hydrochloride.
Terazosin Hydrochloride.
Tiamenidine Hydrochloride.
Timolol Maleate.
Tipentosin Hydrochloride.
Trandolapril/Verapamil.
Trimazosin Hydrochloride.
Trimethamide.
Trimoxamine Hydrochloride.
Univasc.
Valsartan.
Zankiren Hydrochloride.
Zofenoprilat Arginine.
anti-infectives.
See: Antibiotics/Anti-infectives.
Antiprotozoal Agents.
Antituberculosis Agents.
Antiviral Agents.
Carbapenems.
Cephalosporins and Related Antibiotics.
Fluoroquinolones.
Lipoglycopeptides.
Methenamines.
Metronidazole.
Monobactams.
Sulfonamides.
Tetracyclines.
anti-infectives, miscellaneous.
See: Clindamycin Phosphate.
Metronidazole.
Vancomycin.

anti-infectives, topical.
See: Amphotericin B.
Antibiotic Agents.
Antifungal Agents.
Antiseptics and Germicides.
Antivirals.
Boric Acid.
Burn Preparations.
Chloroxine.
Dapsone.
anti-inflammatory agents.
See: Corticosteroids, Topical.
Nonsteroidal Anti-Inflammatory Drugs,
Topical.
anti-inhibitor coagulant complex.
Use: Antihemophilic agent.
See: Feiba NF.
Anti-Itch. (Taro) Diphenhydramine 2%,
zinc acetate 0.1%. Cetyl alcohol, para-
bens. Cream. 28.4 g. OTC.
Use: Topical antihistamine.
Antilerge. (Merz) Chlorpheniramine
maleate 8 mg, phenylephrine hydro-
chloride 12 mg. Tab. Bot. 30s. OTC.
Use: Antihistamine; decongestant.
antileukemia.
See: Antineoplastic agents.
antimalarial agents.
See: Atovaquone and Proguanil Hydro-
chloride.
Folic Acid Antagonists.
Mefloquine Hydrochloride.
Pyrimethamine.
Sulfadoxine and Pyrimethamine.
antimetabolites.
See: Allopurinol.
Capecitabine.
Cladribine.
Clofarabine.
Cytarabine.
Floxuridine.
Fludarabine Phosphate.
Fluorouracil.
Folic Acid Antagonists.
Gemcitabine Hydrochloride.
Mercaptopurine.
Methotrexate.
Pemetrexed.
Pentostatin.
Purine Analogs and Related Agents.
Pyrimidine Analogs.
Rasburicase.
Thioguanine.
antimigraine agents.
See: Almotriptan Maleate.
Amerge.
Axert.
Frova.
Frovatriptan Succinate.
Imitrex.
Maxalt.

Maxalt-MLT.
Midrin.
Naratriptan Hydrochloride.
Rizatriptan Benzoate.
Serotonin 5-HT$_1$ Receptor Agonists.
Sumatriptan Succinate.
Zolmitriptan.
Zomig.
Zomig ZMT.
antimitotic agents.
See: Epothilones.
Halichondrin B Analogs.
Paclitaxel.
Taxoids.
Vinca Alkaloids.
Vincristine Sulfate.
Vinorelbine Tartrate.
●**antimony potassium tartrate.** (AN-ti-MOE-nee) *USP 34.*
Use: Antischistosomal; leishmaniasis; expectorant; emetic.
W/Guaifenesin, codeine phosphate.
See: Cheracol.
W/Guaifenesin, dextromethorphan HBr.
See: Cheracol D.
antimony preparations.
See: Antimony Potassium Tartrate.
Antimony Sodium Thioglycollate.
Tartar Emetic.
●**antimony sodium tartrate.** *USP 34.*
Use: Antischistosomal.
antimony sodium thioglycollate.
(Various Mfr.). *Rx.*
Use: Schistosomiasis; leishmaniasis; filariasis.
●**antimony trisulfide colloid.** (AN-ti-MOE-nee trye-SUL-fide KOL-oid) USAN.
Use: Pharmaceutic aid.
anti-my9-blocked ricin.
Use: Leukemia treatment.
antinauseants.
See: Antiemetic/antivertigo agents
antineoplastic agents.
See: Adriamycin.
Allopurinol Sodium.
Aloprim.
Amifostine.
Amsacrine.
Antineoplastic Antibiotics.
Arsenic Trioxide.
Azacitidine.
Blenoxane.
Cosmegen.
Elspar.
Emcyt.
Estinyl.
Ethyol.
FUDR.
Gefitinib.
Herceptin.

Hexalen.
Hormones.
Hydrea.
Idamycin PFS.
Leukeran.
Lysodren.
Matulane.
Medroxyprogesterone Acetate.
Megace.
Mercaptopurine.
Methotrexate.
Methotrexate Sodium.
Mitotane.
Monoclonal Antibodies.
Mustargen.
Myleran.
Oncovin.
Oxaliplatin.
Platinum Coordination Complex.
Purinethol.
Tamoxifen Citrate.
Temodar.
Temozolomide.
Thioguanine.
Thiotepa.
Trastuzumab.
Trisenox.
antineoplastic antibiotics.
See: Dactinomycin.
antineoplastics, miscellaneous.
See: Mitotane.
Porfimer Sodium.
Sipuleucel-T.
Talc Powder, Sterile.
antiobesity agents.
See: Adderall.
Adipex-P.
Amphetamines.
Anorex.
Bontril.
Dextroamphetamine.
Didrex.
Diethylpropion Hydrochloride.
Ionamin.
Levo-Amphetamine.
Mazanor.
Phendimetrazine Tartrate.
Phentermine Hydrochloride.
Prelu-2.
Tenuate.
Tenuate Dospan.
Tepanil.
Trimstat.
Xenical.
Antiox. (Merz) Vitamin C 120 mg, vitamin E 100 units, beta-carotene 25 mg. Cap. Bot. 60s. *OTC.*
Use: Vitamin supplement.
Anti-Pak Compound. (Lowitt) Phenylephrine hydrochloride 5 mg, salicylamide 0.23 g, acetophenetidin 0.15 g, caf-

feine 0.03 g, ascorbic acid 50 mg, hesperidin complex 50 mg, chlorprophenpyridamine maleate 2 mg. Tab. Bot. 30s, 100s. *OTC.*
Use: Analgesic; antihistamine; decongestant combination.
antiparasympathomimetics.
See: Parasympatholytic agents.
antiparkinson agents.
See: Amantadine Hydrochloride.
Anticholinergic Agents.
Bromocriptine Mesylate.
Carbidopa.
Carbidopa and Levodopa.
Dopaminergics.
Entacapone.
Pergolide Mesylate.
Rasagiline.
Selegiline Hydrochloride.
Tolcapone.
antipellagra vitamin.
See: Nicotinic acid.
antipernicious anemia principle.
See: Vitamin B$_{12}$.
Antiphlogistine. (Denver Chemical Inc.)
Medicated poultice. Jar 5 oz, lb. Tube 8 oz. Can 5 lb. *OTC.*
Use: Counterirritant.
antiplatelet agents.
See: Aggregation Inhibitors.
Anagrelide Hydrochloride.
Dipyridamole.
Glycoprotein IIb/IIIa Inhibitors.
antiprotozoal agents.
See: Diiodohydroxyquinoline.
Emetine Hydrochloride.
Furazolidone.
Levofuraltadone.
Nitazoxanide.
Quinoxyl.
Sodium Suramin.
Tinidazole.
antipsoriatic agents.
See: Anthralin.
Calcipotriene.
Calcipotriene and Betamethasone Dipropionate.
Methotrexate.
Selenium Sulfide.
antipsychotics.
See: Benzisoxazole Derivatives.
Benzoisothiazol Derivatives.
Dibenzapine Derivatives.
Dihydroindolone Derivatives.
Lithium.
Phenothiazine Derivatives.
Phenylbutylpiperadine Derivatives.
Quinolinone Derivatives.
Thioxanthene Derivatives.
•**antipyrine.** (an-tee-PYE-reen) *USP 34.*
Use: Analgesic; antipyretic.

W/Acetic Acid, Benzocaine, Polycosanol.
See: AABP.
Auralgan.
W/Benzocaine, Chlorobutanol.
See: G.B.A.
W/Benzocaine, Glycerin, Zinc Acetate Dihydrate.
See: Neotic.
W/Benzocaine, Phenylephrine Hydrochloride.
See: Ear-Gesic.
W/Benzocaine, u-Polycosanol 410.
See: Treagan.
W/Carbamide, Benzocaine, Cetyldimethylbenzylammonium Hydrochloride.
See: Auralgesic.
antipyrine and benzocaine.
Use: Anesthetic, local.
See: Auro Ear Drops.
antipyrine and benzocaine otic. (URL)
Benzocaine 1.4%, antipyrine 5.4%, glycerin. Soln. 15 mL with dropper. *Rx.*
Use: Otic preparation.
antipyrine, benzocaine, and phenylephrine hydrochloride.
Use: Anesthetic, local; decongestant eardrop.
antiretroviral agents.
See: Cellular Chemokine Receptor Antagonist.
Fusion Inhibitors.
Integrase Inhibitors.
Non-Nucleoside Reverse Transcriptase Inhibitors.
Nucleoside Analog Reverse Transcriptase Inhibitor Combination.
Nucleoside Reverse Transcriptase Inhibitors.
Nucleotide Analog Reverse Transcriptase Inhibitor.
Protease Inhibitor Combination.
Protease Inhibitors.
antirheumatic agents.
See: Arava.
Azulfidine.
Azulfidine EN-tabs.
Leflunomide.
Plaquenil.
Sulfasalazine.
antirickettsial agents.
See: Chloromycetin.
antiscorbutic vitamin.
See: Ascorbic Acid.
antiseptic, dyes.
See: Acriflavine.
Bismuth Violet.
Crystal Violet.
Fuchsin, Basic.
Gentian Violet.
Methyl Violet.
Pyridium.

antiseptic, mercurials.
See: Merthiolate.
  Phenylmercuric Acetate.
  Phenylmercuric Borate.
  Phenylmercuric Nitrate.
  Phenylmercuric Picrate.
  Thimerosal.
antiseptic, n-chloro compounds.
See: Chloramine-T.
  Chlorazene.
  Dichloramine T.
  Halazone.
antiseptic, phenols.
See: Anthralin.
  Creosote.
  Hexachlorophene.
  Hexylresorcinol.
  Methylparaben.
  Parachlorometaxylenol.
  Phenol.
  o-Phenylphenol.
  Propylparaben.
  Pyrogallol.
  Resorcinol.
  Resorcinol Monoacetate.
  Thymol.
  Trinitrophenol.
antiseptics.
See: Furacin.
  Iodine Products, Anti-infective.
  Phenol.
antiseptics and germicides.
See: Benzalkonium Chloride.
  Benzethonium Chloride w/Menthol.
  Iodine.
  Triclosan.
antiseptic, surface-active agents.
See: Bactine.
  Bactine Pain Relieving Cleansing.
  Benzalkonium Chloride.
  Benzethonium Chloride.
  Ceepryn.
  Diaparene.
  Methylbenzethonium Chloride.
  Zephiran.
Antiseptic Wound & Skin Cleanser.
(MPM Medical) Benzethonium chloride
0.1%, EDTA, glycerin, methylparaben.
Liq. 120 mL. *OTC.*
Use: Topical anti-infective.
antisickling agents.
See: Droxia.
  Hydroxyurea.
Antispasmodic. (Teva) Phenobarbital
16.2 mg, hyoscyamine sulfate
0.1037 mg, atropine sulfate 0.0194 mg,
scopolamine HBr 0.0065 mg. Cap. Bot.
1000s. *Rx.*
Use: Anticholinergic; antispasmodic;
hypnotic; sedative.

Antispasmodic. (Various Mfr.) Atropine
sulfate 0.0194 mg, scopolamine HBr
0.0065 mg, hyoscyamine HBr or sulfate
0.1037 mg, phenobarbital 16.2 mg/mL.
Alcohol 23%, sugar, sorbitol. Elix. Bot.
120 mL, Pt, gal. *Rx.*
Use: GI anticholinergic combination.
antispasmodic agents. Parasympatholytic agents.
See: Anticholinergic Agents.
  Belladonna Alkaloids.
  Dicyclomine Hydrochloride.
  Spasmolytic Agents.
antistreptolysin-O.
Use: Titration procedure.
anti-tac, humanized. (Roche)
Use: Prevention of acute renal allograft
rejection. [Orphan Drug]
Anti-Ten. (Century) Allylisobutylbarbituric
acid ¾ g, aspirin 3 g, phenacetin 2 g,
caffeine g. Tab. Bot. 100s, 1000s. *Rx.*
Use: Analgesic; sedative; stimulant.
antithrombin.
Use: Anticoagulant.
See: ATryn.
antithrombin agents.
Use: Anticoagulant.
See: Antithrombin.
  Antithrombin III (Human).
**antithrombin III (human) concentrate
IV.**
Use: Prophylaxis/treatment of thrombo-
embolic episodes in AT-III deficiency.
[Orphan Drug]
•**antithrombin III human.** *USP 34.*
Use: Thromboembolic.
See: Thrombate III.
antithymocyte globulin (equine).
Use: Immune globulin.
See: Atgam.
antithymocyte globulin (rabbit).
Use: Immunosuppressant.
See: Thymoglobulin.
antithyroid agents.
See: Iothiouracil Sodium.
  Methimazole.
  Methylthiouracil.
  Propylthiouracil.
  Sodium Iodide I 131.
  Tapazole.
antitoxins.
See: Antivenin (Crotalidae) Polyvalent
(Equine Origin).
  Antivenin (Lactrodectus mactans)
(Black Widow Spider Antivenin)
(Equine Origin).
  Botulism Antitoxin.
  Crotalidae Polyvalent Immune Fab
(Ovine Origin).
  Tetanus Immune Globulin.

antitrypsin, alpha-1.
See: Alpha-1 Antitrypsin.
antituberculosis agents.
See: Aminosalicylic Acid.
Capreomycin.
Cycloserine.
Ethambutol Hydrochloride.
Ethionamide.
Isoniazid.
Pyrazinamide.
Rifabutin.
Rifampin.
Rifapentine.
Streptomycin Sulfate.
Anti-Tuss DM. (Century) Guaifenesin 100 mg, dextromethorphan HBr 15 mg/ 5 mL. Syr. Bot. 120 mL, 3.8 L. *OTC.* Use: Antitussive; expectorant.
antitussive, analgesic, antihistamine, and decongestant combinations.
Use: Upper respiratory combination.
antitussive, analgesic, decongestant, expectorant combinations.
Use: Upper respiratory combination.
antitussive and anticholinergic combinations.
Use: Upper respiratory combination.
antitussive and antihistamine combinations.
Use: Upper respiratory combination.
antitussive and decongestant combinations.
Use: Upper respiratory combination.
antitussive and expectorant combinations.
Use: Upper respiratory combination.
antitussive, antihistamine, and decongestant combinations.
Use: Upper respiratory combination.
antitussive, antihistamine, decongestant, expectorant combinations.
Use: Upper respiratory combination.
antitussive combinations.
Use: Upper respiratory combination.
Antitussive Cough Syrup. (Weeks & Leo) Chlorpheniramine 2 mg, phenylephrine hydrochloride 5 mg, dextromethorphan 15 mg, ammonium chloride 50 mg/5 mL. Syr. Bot. *OTC.*
Use: Antihistamine; antitussive; decongestant; expectorant.
Antitussive Cough Syrup with Codeine. (Weeks & Leo) Chlorpheniramine maleate 2 mg, phenylephrine hydrochloride 5 mg, codeine phosphate 10 mg, ammonium chloride 50 mg/ 5 mL. Syr. Bot. 4 oz. *c-v.*
Use: Antihistamine; antitussive; decongestant; expectorant.

antitussive, decongestant, and expectorant combinations.
Use: Upper respiratory combination.
antitussive hydrocodone bitartrate and homatropine methylbromide. (Actavis) Hydrocodone bitartrate 5 mg, homatropine HBr 1.5 mg. Lactose. Tab. 100s, 500s. *c-III.*
Use: Upper respiratory combination, antitussive combination.
antitussives, narcotic.
See: Narcotic antitussive.
antivenin Centruroides sculpturatus. (Arizona State University) Available in Arizona only. 5 mL vials. *Rx.*
Use: Antivenin.
•**antivenin (Crotalidae) polyvalent.** (AN-tee-VEN-in kro-TAL-i-dee POL-ee-VAY-lent) *USP 34.*
Use: Immunization.
antivenin, Crotalidae polyvalent immune fab (ovine).
Use: Bites of North American crotalid snakes. [Orphan Drug]
See: CroFab.
•**antivenin (Latrodectus mactans).** (AN-tee-VEN-in LAT-roe-DEK-tus MAK-tans) *USP 34.* Formerly Widow spider species antivenin (Latrodectus mactans).
Use: Immunization.
antivenin (Latrodectus mactans). (Merck) Black widow spider antivenin (equine origin) ≥ 6000 antivenin units/ vial. Thimerosal 1:10,000. Pow. for Inj. Single-use Vial with 1 vial diluent (Sterile Water for Injection 2.5 mL) and normal horse serum 1 mL (1:10 dilution) for sensitivity testing. *Rx.*
Use: Treatment of black widow spider bites.
•**antivenin (Micrurus fulvius).** (AN-tee-VEN-in mye-KROO-rus FUL-vi-us) *USP 34.*
Use: Immunization.
antivenin (Micrurus fulvius). North American coral snake antivenin (equine origin), phenol 0.25%, thimerosal 0.005%, phenylmercuric nitrate 1:100,000. Pow. for Inj., lyophilized. Single-use Vial with 1 vial diluent (Water for Injection 10 mL). *Rx.*
Use: Bites of North American coral snake and Texas coral snake.
antivenins.
See: Antivenin (Crotalidae) Polyvalent.
Antivenin (Latrodectus mactans).
Antivenin (Micrurus fulvius).
Crotalidae Polyvalent Immune Fab (Ovine origin).

antivenom (Crotalidae) purified (avian). (Ophidian Pharmaceuticals, Inc.) *Use:* Bites of snakes of the Crotalidae family. [Orphan Drug]

Antivert. (Pfizer US) Meclizine hydrochloride 12.5 mg. Tab. Bot. 100s, 1000s, UD 100s. *Rx.*
Use: Antiemetic/antivertigo agent.

Antivert/50. (Pfizer US) Meclizine hydrochloride 50 mg, Tab. Bot. 100s. *Rx.*
Use: Antiemetic/antivertigo agent.

Antivert/25. (Pfizer US) Meclizine hydrochloride 25 mg. Tab. Bot. 100s, 1000s, UD 100s. *Rx.*
Use: Antiemetic/antivertigo agent.

antiviral agents.
See: Abacavir Sulfate.
Acyclovir.
Adefovir Dipivoxil.
Amantadine Hydrochloride.
Antiherpes Virus Agents.
Boceprevir.
Cidofovir.
Entecavir.
Famciclovir.
Foscarnet Sodium.
Ganciclovir.
Oseltamivir Phosphate.
Ribavirin.
Rimantadine Hydrochloride.
Valacyclovir Hydrochloride.
Valganciclovir Hydrochloride.
Zanamivir.

antiviral agents, ophthalmic.
See: Ganciclovir.

antiviral antibodies.
See: Cytomegalovirus Immune Globulin (Human).
Hepatitis B Immune Globulin.
Immune Globulin IV.
Rabies Immune Globulin.
Vaccinia Immune Globulin.
Varicella-Zoster Immune Globulin.

antixerophthalmic vitamin.
See: Vitamin A.

Antizol. (Jazz Pharmaceuticals) Fomepizole 1 g/mL. Preservative free. Inj. Conc. Vial 1.5 mL. *Rx.*
Use: Antidote.

Antril. (Amgen) Interleukin-1 receptor antagonist (human recombinant).
Use: Arthritis; organ rejection. [Orphan Drug]

Antrizine. (Major) Meclizine hydrochloride 12.5 mg. Tab. Bot. 100s, 500s, 1000s. *Rx.*
Use: Antiemetic/antivertigo agent.

Antrocol. (ECR) Atropine sulfate 0.195 mg, phenobarbital 16 mg per 5 mL. Alcohol 20%. Sugar free. Elix. Bot. Pt. *Rx.*

Use: GI anticholinergic combination.

Antrypol. Suramin. *Rx.*
Use: CDC anti-infective agent.

Anucaine. (Calvin) Procaine 50 mg, butyl-p-aminobenzoate 200 mg, benzyl alcohol 265 mg in sweet almond oil/ 5 mL. Amp. 5 mL. Box 6s, 24s, 100s. *OTC.*
Use: Anorectal preparation.

Anucort-HC. (G & W) Hydrocortisone acetate 25 mg in a hydrogenated vegetable oil base. Supp. Box 12s, 24s, 100s. *Rx.*
Use: Anorectal preparation.

Anuject. (Roberts) Procaine. Soln. Vial 5 mL, 10 mL. *Rx.*
Use: Anorectal preparation.

Anu-Med. (Major) Phenylephrine hydrochloride 0.25%, hard fat 88.7%. Corn starch, parabens. Supp. 12. *OTC.*
Use: Anorectal preparation.

Anumed HC. (Major) Hydrocortisone acetate 10 mg. Supp. Box 12s. *Rx.*
Use: Anorectal preparation.

Anuprep HC. (Great Southern) Hydrocortisone acetate 25 mg. Supp. Box 12s.
Use: Anorectal preparation.

Anuprep Hemorrhoidal. (Great Southern) Bismuth subgallate 2.25%, bismuth resorcin compound 1.75%, benzyl benzoate 1.2%, peruvian balsam 1.8%, and zinc oxide 11% in a hydrogenated vegetable oil base. Supp. Box 12s, 24s. *Rx.*
Use: Anorectal preparation.

Anusol-HC. (Salix) Hydrocortisone 2.5%. Cream. Tube 30 g. *Rx.*
Use: Corticosteroid, topical.

Anzemet. (Aventis) Dolasetron mesylate. **Tab.:** 50 mg, 100 mg. Lactose. Film coated. 5s, blister pack 5s, UD 10s. **Inj.:** 20 mg/mL. Mannitol 38.2 mg/mL. Single-use amp. 0.625 mL. 0.625 mL fill in 2 mL *Carpu-ject.* Single-use vial. 5 mL. Multi-dose vial. 25 mL. *Rx.*
Use: Antiemetic; antivertigo.

A1cNow. (Metrika) Reagent kit for blood tests. Box 1s, 2s with lancet(s), monitor, dilution kit. *Rx.*
Use: In vitro diagnostic aid.

AOSEPT. (Ciba Vision) **AODISC Neutralizer:** Platinum-coated tablet. Tab. good for 100 uses or 3 months of daily use. **Disinfecting Soln.:** Hydrogen peroxide 3%, sodium chloride 0.85%, phosphonic acid, phosphate buffer. Soln. Bot. 120 mL, 240 mL, 360 mL. *OTC.*
Use: Contact lens disinfection system.

•**apadenoson.** (a-pa-DEN-oh-son) USAN.
Use: Imaging agent.

•**apafant.** (APP-ah-fant) USAN.
Use: Platelet activating factor antagonist; antiasthmatic.

•**apalcillin sodium.** (APE-al-SIH-lin) USAN.
Use: Anti-infective.

APAP.
See: Acetaminophen.

Apap. (Cypress) Acetaminophen 325 mg, 500 mg. Film coated. Tab. 150s (325 mg only), UD 100s (500 mg only). *OTC.*
Use: Analgesic.

Apap 500. (Cypress) Acetaminophen 500 mg/5 mL. Alcohol and sugar free. Liq. 237 mL. *OTC.*
Use: Analgesic.

Apap Infant's. (Various Mfr.) Acetaminophen 100 mg/mL. May contain butylparaben, saccharin. Oral Soln., Conc. 15 mL. *OTC.*
Use: Analgesic.

•**apaxifylline.** (A-pock-SIH-fih-leen) USAN.
Use: Selective adenosine A_1 antagonist.

•**apaziquone.** (a-PA-zi-kwone) USAN.
Use: Antineoplastic.

•**apazone.** (APP-ah-zone) USAN.
Use: Anti-inflammatory.

Apcogesic. (Apco) Sodium salicylate 5 g, colchicine 1/320 g, calcium carbonate 65 mg, dried aluminum hydroxide gel 130 mg, phenobarbital ⅛ g. Tab. Bot. 100s. *Rx.*
Use: Antigout; hypnotic; sedative.

Apcoretic. (A.P.C) Caffeine anhydrous 100 mg, ammonium chloride 325 mg. Tab. Bot. 90s. *Rx.*
Use: Diuretic.

Ap Creme. (T.E. Williams Pharmaceuticals) Hydrocortisone 0.5%, iodochlorhydroxyquin 3%. Tube. *Rx-OTC.*
Use: Antifungal; corticosteroid, topical.

A.P.C. with gelsemium combinations.
See: Valacet.

ApexiCon. (PharmaDerm) Diflorasone diacetate 0.05%. Oint. 30 g, 60 g. *Rx.*
Use: Anti-inflammatory.

ApexiCon E. (PharmaDerm) Diflorasone diacetate 0.05%. Stearyl alcohol, cetyl alcohol. Cream. 30 g, 60g. *Rx.*
Use: Anti-inflammatory.

APF.
Use: Analgesic.
See: Arthritis Pain Formula.

Aphco Hemorrhoidal Combination.
(A.P.C) Combination package of Aphco Hemorrhoidal ointment 1.5 oz tube, Aphco Hemorrhoidal supp. Box 12s, 1000s. *OTC.*

Use: Anorectal preparation.

Aphen. (Major) Trihexyphenidyl 2 mg, 5 mg. Tab. Bot. 250s, 1000s. *Rx.*
Use: Antiparkinsonian.

Aphrodyne. (Star) Yohimbine hydrochloride 5.4 mg. Tab. Bot. 100s, 1000s. *Rx.*
Use: Anti-impotence agent, alphaadrenergic blocker.

Aphthasol. (Discus Dental) Amlexanox 5%, benzyl alcohol, mineral oil, petrolatum. Paste. Tube. 5 g. *Rx.*
Use: Mouth and throat product.

Apicillin.
See: Ampicillin.

Apidra. (Sanofi Aventis) Insulin glulisine 100 units/mL. Inj. Vials. 10 mL. Cartridge system for use with *OptiClik.* 3 mL. *Rx.*
Use: Antidiabetic agent, insulin.

•**apixaban.** (a-PIX-a-ban) USAN.
Use: Anticoagulant.

•**aplaviroc hydrochloride.** (AP-la-VIR-ok) USAN.
Use: Antiretroviral agent.

Aplenzin. (Sanofi-Aventis) Bupropion hydrobromide 174 mg, 348 mg, 522 mg. Polyethylene glycol. ER Tab. 30s. *Rx.*
Use: Antidepressant.

APL 400-020 V-Beta DNA vaccine.
(Apollon)
Use: Treatment of cutaneous T-cell lymphoma. [Orphan Drug]

•**aplindore fumarate.** (AP-lin-dor) USAN.
Use: Antischizophrenic.

Aplisol. (JHP Pharmaceuticals) Tuberculin purified protein derivative 5 units/ 0.1 mL, polysorbate 80, potassium and sodium phosphates, phenol 0.35%. Vial 1 mL (10 tests), 5 mL (50 tests). *Rx.*
Use: Diagnostic aid.

Aplitest. (Parke-Davis) Purified tuberculin protein derivative buffered with potassium and sodium phosphates, phenol 0.5%/single-use, multipuncture unit. 25s. *Rx.*
Use: Diagnostic aid.

A + D Ointment. (Schering-Plough) Fish liver oil, cholecalciferol. Oint. Tube 1.5 oz, 4 oz. Jar lb. *OTC.*
Use: Emollient.

A + D Zinc Oxide Cream. (ScheringPlough) Dimethicone 1%, zinc oxide 10%. Aloe, benzyl alcohol, coconut oil, cod liver oil, light mineral oil. Cream. 113 g. *OTC.*
Use: Emollient.

Apokyn. (Vernalis) Apomorphine hydrochloride 10 mg/mL. Sodium metabisulfite. Inj. Glass Amps. 2 mL. Cartridges. 3 mL. *Rx.*

Use: Antiparkinson agent, dopaminergic.
- **apolizumab.** (ap-ol-IZ-yoo-mab) USAN.
  Use: Anti-cancer agent.
- **apomorphine hydrochloride.** (ah-poh-MORE-feen) *USP 34.*
  Use: Treatment of Parkinson disease.
  See: Apokyn.
aporphine-10, 11-diol hydrochloride.
  See: Apomorphine hydrochloride.
appetite depressants.
  See: Anorexiants
APPG.
  See: Aqueous Procaine Penicillin G.
Apra Children's. (Altaire) Acetaminophen 160 mg/5 mL. Alcohol-free. Sorbitol, sucrose. Grape and cherry flavor. Elix. 118 mL. *OTC.*
  Use: Analgesic.
- **apraclonidine hydrochloride.** (app-rah-KLOE-nih-deen) *USP 34.*
  Use: Adrenergic, α_2-agonist.
  See: Iopidine.
- **apramycin.** (APP-rah-MY-sin) USAN.
  Use: Anti-infective.
Aprazone. (Major) Sulfinpyrazone 100 mg. Tab. Bot. 100s. *Rx.*
  Use: Antigout agent.
- **aprepitant.** (ap-REH-pih-tant) USAN.
  Use: Antiemetic/antivertigo agent, miscellaneous.
  See: Emend.
Apresodex. (Rugby) Hydrochlorothiazide 15 mg, hydralazine hydrochloride 25 mg. Tab. Bot. 100s, 1000s. *Rx.*
  Use: Antihypertensive.
Apresoline. (Novartis) Hydralazine hydrochloride. **Amp.:** 20 mg w/propylene glycol, methyl and propyl parabens/mL. Pkg. 5s. **Tab.:** 10 mg Bot. 100s, 1200s; 25 mg or 50 mg Bot. 100s, 1000s; 100 mg Bot. 100s. Consumer pack 100s. *Rx.*
  Use: Antihypertensive.
Apresoline-Esidrix. (Novartis) Hydralazine hydrochloride 25 mg, hydrochlorothiazide 15 mg. Tab. Bot. 100s. *Rx.*
  Use: Antihypertensive.
Apri. (Barr) Desogestrel 0.15 mg, ethinyl estradiol 30 mcg. Lactose. Tab. Blister cards 28s with 7 inert tabs. *Rx.*
  Use: Sex hormone, contraceptive hormone.
- **apricoxib.** (AP-ri-KOX-ib) USAN.
  Use: Anti-inflammatory agent.
- **aprindine.** (APE-rin-deen) USAN.
  Use: Cardiovascular agent.
- **aprindine hydrochloride.** (APE-rin-deen) USAN.
  Use: Cardiovascular agent.

- **aprinocarsen sodium.** (ap-ri-NOE-karsen) USAN.
  Use: Protein kinase inhibitor.
Apriso. (Salix) Mesalamine 375 mg. Aspartame, phenylalanine. Enteric coated granules. ER Cap. 4s, 120s. *Rx.*
  Use: Gastrointestinal agent.
Aprobee w/C. (Health for Life Brands) Vitamins B_1 15 mg, B_2 10 mg, B_6 5 mg, niacinamide 50 mg, calcium pantothenate 10 mg, C 250 mg. Cap. Bot. 100s, 1000s. Tab. Bot. 50s, 100s, 1000s. *OTC.*
  Use: Mineral, vitamin supplement.
Aprodine. (Major) **Tab.:** Pseudoephedrine hydrochloride 60 mg, triprolidine hydrochloride 2.5 mg. Lactose, PEG. Bot. 24s. **Syrup:** Pseudoephedrine hydrochloride 30 mg, triprolidine hydrochloride 1.25 mg/5 mL. Methylparaben, saccharin, sucrose. Bot. 118 mL. *OTC.*
  Use: Upper respiratory combination, antihistamine and decongestant.
Aprodine w/Codeine. (Major) Pseudoephedrine hydrochloride 30 mg, triprolidine hydrochloride 1.25 mg, codeine phosphate 10 mg. Syr. Bot. Pt, gal. *c-v.*
  Use: Antihistamine; decongestant.
- **aprotinin.** (app-row-TIE-nin) USAN.
  Use: Enzyme inhibitor, proteinase.
  See: Trasylol.
Aprozide 50/50. (Major) Hydrochlorothiazide 50 mg, hydralazine 50 mg. Cap. Bot. 100s, 250s. *Rx.*
  Use: Antihypertensive.
Aprozide 25/25. (Major) Hydralazine 25 mg, hydrochlorothiazide 25 mg. Cap. Bot. 100s, 250s. *Rx.*
  Use: Antihypertensive.
A.P.S. Aspirin, phenacetin, and salicylamide.
APSAC. Thrombolytic enzyme.
- **aptazapine maleate.** (app-TAZZ-ah-PEEN MAL-ee-ate) USAN.
  Use: Antidepressant.
- **aptiganel hydrochloride.** (app-tih-GAN-ehl) USAN.
  Use: Stroke and traumatic brain injury treatment (NMDA ion channel blocker).
Aptivus. (Boehringer Ingelheim) Tipranavir. **Cap.:** 250 mg. Dehydrated alcohol 7% w/w, polyoxyl 35 castor oil. 120s. **Soln.:** 100 mg/mL. Buttermint-toffee flavor. Unit-of-use w/syringe. 95 mL. *Rx.*
  Use: Antiretroviral, protease inhibitor.
Apyron.
  See: Magnesium acetylsalicylate.
AQ-4B. (Western Research) Trichlormethiazide 4 mg. Tab. Bot. 1000s. *Rx.*

Use: Diuretic.

Aqua-Ban. (Thompson Medical) Caffeine 100 mg, ammonium chloride 325 mg. Tab. Bot. 60s. *OTC.*
Use: Diuretic.

Aqua-Ban, Maximum Strength.
See: Maximum Strength Aqua-Ban.

Aqua-Ban Plus. (Thompson Medical) Ammonium chloride 650 mg, caffeine 200 mg, iron 6 mg. Tab. Bot. 30s. *OTC.*
Use: Diuretic; mineral supplement.

Aquabase. (Pal-Pak, Inc.) Cetyl alcohol, propylene glycol, sodium lauryl sulfate, white wax, purified water. Jar lb. *OTC.*
Use: Pharmaceutic aid; ointment base.

Aquacare. (Numark) Urea 10%. **Cream:** Benzyl alcohol, glycerin, lanolin alcohol, lanolin oil, mineral oil, petrolatum. 75 g. **Lot.:** Mineral oil, parabens, petrolatum. 240 mL. *OTC.*
Use: Emollient.

Aquacillin G. (Armenpharm Ltd.) Penicillin G. *Rx.*
Use: Anti-infective, penicillin.

Aquacycline. (Armenpharm Ltd.) Tetracycline hydrochloride. *Rx.*
Use: Anti-infective, tetracycline.

Aquaderm. (Baker Norton) Octyl methoxycinnamate 7.5%, oxybenzone 6%. SPF 15. Cream. Tube. 105 g. *OTC.*
Use: Sunscreen.

Aquaderm. (C & M Pharmacal) Purified water, glycerin 25%, salicylic acid 0.1%, octoxynol-9 0.03%, FD&C Red #40 0.0001%. Bot. 2 oz. *OTC.*
Use: Emollient.

Aqua-E. (Yasoo) Vitamin E 30 units/mL. PEG 1000. Gluten free and sugar free. Liq. 120 mL, 237 mL. *OTC.*
Use: Fat-soluble vitamin.

Aquaflex Ultrasound Gel Pad. (Parker) Clear, solid, flexible, moist, standoff gel pad for use where transducer movement is impeded by bony or irregular body surfaces. 2 cm × 9 cm.
Use: Ultrasound aid.

Aquafuren. (Armenpharm Ltd.) Nitrofurantoin. *Rx.*
Use: Anti-infective, urinary.

Aquagen. (ALK) Allergenic extracts. Vials.

Aqua Glycolic Face. (Merz) Cetyl ricinoleate, C12-15 alkyl benzoate, glycolic acid, hyaluronic acid, ceresin, ammonium glycolate, glyceryl stearate, PEG-100 stearate, sorbitan stearate, sorbitol, propylene glycol, diazolidinyl urea, parabens, magnesium aluminum silicate, dimethicone, xanthan gum, trisodium EDTA. Cream. 50 mL. *OTC.*
Use: Emollient.

Aqua Glycolic Hand & Body. (Merz) Glycolic acid, ammonium glycolate, cetyl alcohol, glyceryl stearate, PEG-100 stearate, C12-15 alkyl benzoate, mineral oil, stearyl alcohol, magnesium aluminum silicate, xanthan gum, parabens, disodium EDTA. Lot. 117 mL. *OTC.*
Use: Emollient.

Aquakay.
See: Menadione.

Aqua Lacten. (Allergan) Demineralized water, urea, petrolatum, propylene glycol monostearate, sorbitan monostearate, lactic acid. Lot. Bot. 8 oz. *OTC.*
Use: Emollient.

Aqua Mist. (Faraday) Nasal spray. Squeeze Bot. 20 mL.

Aquamycin. (Armenpharm Ltd.) Erythromycin. *Rx.*
Use: Anti-infective, erythromycin.

Aquanil. (Sigma-Tau) Mersalyl 100 mg, theophylline (hydrate) 50 mg, methylparaben 0.18%, propylparaben 0.02%. Vial 10 mL. *OTC.*
Use: Bronchodilator; diuretic.

Aquanil Cleanser. (Person and Covey) Glycerin, cetyl, stearyl, and benzyl alcohol, sodium laureth sulfate, xanthan gum. Lipid free. Lot. Bot. 240 mL, 480 mL. *OTC.*
Use: Dermatologic, cleanser.

Aquanine. (Armenpharm Ltd.) Quinine hydrochloride. *Rx.*
Use: Antimalarial.

Aquaoxy. (Armenpharm Ltd.) Oxytetracycline hydrochloride. *Rx.*
Use: Anti-infective, tetracycline.

Aquaphenicol. (Armenpharm Ltd.) Chloramphenicol. *Rx.*
Use: Anti-infective.

Aquaphilic Ointment. (Medco Lab) Hydrated hydrophilic oint. Jar 16 oz. *OTC.*
Use: Emollient; ointment base.

Aquaphilic Ointment with Carbamide 10% and 20%. (Medco Lab) Stearyl alcohol, white petrolatum, sorbitol, propylene glycol, sodium lauryl sulfate, lactic acid, methylparaben, propylparaben.
Use: Prescription compounding; emollient.

Aquaphor. (Beiersdorf) Cholesterolized anhydrous petrolatum ointment base. Tube 1.75 oz, 3.25 oz, 16 oz, Jar 5 lb, Bar 3 oz. *OTC.*
Use: Pharmaceutic aid; ointment base.
See: Eucerin (Duke).

Aquaphor Antibiotic. (Beiersdorf) Polymyxin B sulfate 10,000 units, bacitracin zinc 500 units/g in a cholesterolized ointment base. Oint. Tube 15 g. *OTC.*

Use: Anti-infective, topical.

Aquaphor Healing Ointment.
(Beiersdorf) Petrolatum, mineral oil, lanolin, alcohol, panthenol, glycerin. Oint. Tubes. 10 g, 50 g. Jars. 99 g, 396 g. *OTC.*
Use: Emollient.

Aquapool Concentrate. (Parker) Color additive for hydrotherapy to control foaming. Bot. Pt, gal.

Aquasol A. (Hospira) Vitamin A palmitate 50,000 IU/mL. Chlorobutanol 0.5%, polysorbate 80, butylated hydroxyanisole, butylated hydroxytoluene. Inj. Vial 2 mL. *Rx.*
Use: Vitamin supplement.

Aquasol E. (Hospira) Vitamin E (as dl-alpha tocopheryl acetate) 15 units per 0.3 mL. Drops. 12 mL, 30 mL. *OTC.*
Use: Fat soluble vitamin.

Aquasonic 100. (Parker) Water-soluble, viscous, contact medium gel for ultrasonic transmission. Bot. 250 mL, 1 L, 5 L.
Use: Ultrasound aid.

Aquasonic 100 Sterile. (Parker) Water-soluble, sterile gel for ultrasonic transmission. Overwrapped Foil Pouches 15 g, 50 g.
Use: Ultrasound aid.

Aquasulf. (Armenpharm Ltd.) Triple sulfa tablet. *Rx.*
Use: Anti-infective.

Aquatab C. (Deston Therapeutics) Carbetapentane citrate 30 mg, guaifenesin 400 mg, phenylephrine hydrochloride 10 mg. Tab. 100s. *Rx.*
Use: Upper respiratory combination, antitussive and expectorant combination.

Aquatab D. (Adams) Guaifenesin 1200 mg, pseudoephedrine hydrochloride 75 mg. ER Tab. Bot. 100s. *Rx.*
Use: Upper respiratory combination, expectorant, decongestant.

Aquatab D Dose Pack. (Adams) Pseudoephedrine hydrochloride 60 mg, guaifenesin 600 mg. SR Tab. Bot. 56s. *Rx.*
Use: Upper respiratory combination, decongestant, expectorant.

Aquatab DM. (Adams) **Syrup:** Guaifenesin 200 mg, dextromethorphan HBr 10 mg per 5 mL. Acesulfame K, aspartame, menthol, methylparaben, phenylalanine. 473 mL. **Tab.:** Guaifenesin 1200 mg, dextromethorphan HBr 60 mg. Bot. 100s. *Rx.*
Use: Upper respiratory combination, expectorant, antitussive.

Aquavite. (Armenpharm Ltd.) Soluble multivitamin.
Use: Vitamin supplement.

Aquavit-E. (Cypress) Dl-alpha tocopheryl acetate 15 IU/0.3 mL. Drops. Bot. 30 mL. *OTC.*
Use: Vitamin supplement.

Aquazide. (Western Research) Trichlormethiazide 4 mg. Tab. Bot. 100s. *Rx.*
Use: Antihypertensive; diuretic.

Aquazide H. (Western Research) Hydrochlorothiazide 50 mg. Tab. Bot. 1000s. *Rx.*
Use: Diuretic.

Aquazol. (Armenpharm Ltd.) Sulfisoxazole.
Use: Anti-infective.

Aqueous Allergens. (Bayer Consumer Care)
Use: Antiallergic.

aquinone.
See: Menadione.

Aquol Bath Oil. (Lamond) Vegetable oil, olive oil. Bot. 4 oz, 6 oz, 16 oz, qt, gal. *OTC.*
Use: Antipruritic; emollient.

ARA-C.
See: Cytarabine.

Aralast NP. (Baxter Healthcare) Alpha-1 proteinase inhibitor (human) 0.5 g, 1 g. Polyethylene glycol, sodium, albumin. Total alpha-1 proteinase inhibitor functional activity in mg is stated on the label of each vial. Preservative free. Inj. lyophilized Pow. for Soln. Single-dose vial. 25 mL of diluent (0.5 g), 50 mL of diluent (1 g). *Rx.*
Use: Respiratory agent, respiratory enzyme.

Aralen Phosphate. (Sanofi-Synthelabo) Chloroquine phosphate 500 mg. Tab. Bot. 25s. *Rx.*
Use: Amebicide; antimalarial.

Aralis. (Sanofi-Synthelabo) Glycobiarsol, chloroquine phosphate. Tab. *Rx.*
Use: Amebicide.

Aranelle. (Barr) **Phase 1:** Norethindrone 0.5 mg, ethinyl estradiol 35 mcg. 7 tabs. **Phase 2:** Norethindrone 1 mg, ethinyl estradiol 35 mcg. 9 tabs. **Phase 3:** Norethindrone 0.5 mg, ethinyl estradiol 35 mcg. Lactose. 5 tabs. Tab. 28s with 7 inert tabs. *Rx.*
Use: Contraceptive hormone, sex hormone.

Aranesp. (Amgen) Darbepoetin alfa 25 mcg/0.42 mL, 25 mcg/mL, 40 mcg/0.4 mL, 40 mcg/mL, 60 mcg/0.3 mL, 60 mcg/mL, 100 mcg/0.5 mL, 100 mcg/mL, 150 mcg/0.3 mL, 150 mcg/0.75 mL, 200 mcg/0.4 mL, 200 mcg/mL, 300 mcg/0.6 mL, 300 mcg/mL, 500 mcg/mL. Preservative-free. In poly-

sorbate or albumin solutions. The polysorbate solution contains polysorbate 80 0.05 mg, sodium phosphate monobasic monohydrate 2.12 mg, sodium phosphate dibasic anhydrous 0.66 mg, sodium chloride 8.18 mg, and water for injection. The albumin solution contains human albumin 2.5 mg, sodium phosphate monobasic monohydrate 2.23 mg, sodium phosphate dibasic anhydrous 0.53 mg, sodium chloride 8.18 mg, and water for injection. Soln. for Inj. Single-dose prefilled *SingleJect* syringe, single-dose prefilled *SureClick* autoinjectors (25 mcg/0.42 mL, 40 mcg/0.4 mL, 60 mcg/0.3 mL, 100 mcg/0.5 mL, 150 mcg/0.3 mL, 200 mcg/0.4 mL, 300 mcg/0.6 mL, 500 mcg/mL only). Single-dose vial 1 mL (25 mcg/mL, 40 mcg/mL, 60 mcg/mL, 100 mcg/mL, 150 mcg/0.75 mL, 200 mcg/mL, 300 mcg/mL, 500 mcg/mL only). *Rx.*
Use: Hematopoietic agent, recombinant human erythropoietin.
• **aranotin.** (AR-ah-NO-tin) USAN.
Use: Antiviral.
Arava. (Hoechst) Leflunomide 10 mg, 20 mg. Film coated. Lactose, PEG. Tab. 30s. *Rx.*
Use: Antirheumatic.
• **arbaclofen.** (ar-BAK-loe-fen) USAN.
Use: CNS agent.
• **arbaprostil.** (ahr-bah-PRAHST-ill) USAN.
Use: Antisecretory, gastric.
Arbinoxa. (Hawthorn Pharmaceuticals) Carbinoxamine maleate. **Tab.:** 4 mg. Lactose. 100s. **Soln.:** 4 mg per 5 mL. Glycerin, parabens, propylene glycol, sorbitol. Bubble gum flavor. 473 mL. *Rx.*
Use: Antihistamine, nonselective ethanolamine.
Arbolic. (Burgin-Arden) Methandriol dipropionate 50 mg/mL. Vial 10 mL. *Rx.*
Use: Anabolic steroid.
Arbutal. (Arcum) Butalbital 0.75 g, phenacetin 2 g, aspirin 3 g, caffeine g. Tab. Bot. 100s, 1000s. *Rx.*
Use: Analgesic; hypnotic; sedative.
• **arbutamine hydrochloride.** (ahr-BYOO-tah-meen) USAN.
Use: Cardiovascular agent.
ARC. (Xttrium Laboratories) Petrolatum 28.5%, zinc oxide 9.14%. Beeswax, lanolin, mineral oil, parabens. Oint. 113 g. *OTC.*
Use: Miscellaneous protectant.
Arcalyst. (Regeneron) Rilonacept 220 mg. Preservative free. PEG 3350, sucrose. Inj., Lyophilized, Pow. for

Soln. Single-use vials. 20 mL. *Rx.*
Use: Immunomodulator, immunologic agents.
Arcet. (Econo Med Pharmaceuticals) Butalbital 50 mg, acetaminophen 325 mg, caffeine 40 mg. Tab. Bot. 100s. *Rx.*
Use: Analgesic; hypnotic; sedative.
• **arcitumomab.** (ahr-sigh-TOO-moe-mab) USAN.
Use: Monoclonal antibody.
See: CEA-Scan.
• **arclofenin.** (AHR-kloe-FEN-in) USAN.
Use: Diagnostic aid for hepatic function determination.
Arcoban. (Arcum) Meprobamate 400 mg. Tab. Bot. 50s, 1000s. *Rx.*
Use: Anxiolytic.
Arcobee w/C. (NBTY) Vitamins B$_1$ 15 mg, B$_2$ 10.2 mg, B$_3$ 50 mg, B$_5$ 10 mg, B$_6$ 5 mg, C 300 mg, tartrazine. Cap. Box 100s. *OTC.*
Use: Vitamin supplement.
Arco-Lase. (Arco) Trizyme 38 mg (amylase 30 mg, protease 6 mg, cellulose 2 mg), lipase 25 mg. Tab. Bot. 50s. *Rx.*
Use: Digestive aid.
Arcosterone. (Arcum) Methyltestosterone. **Oral:** 10 mg, 25 mg. Tab. Bot. 100s, 1000s. **Sublingual Tab.:** 10 mg. Bot. 100s, 1000s. *Rx.*
Use: Androgen.
Arco-Thyroid. (Arco) Thyroid 1.5 g. Tab. Bot. 1000s. *Rx.*
Use: Hormone, thyroid.
Arcotrate. (Arcum) Pentaerythritol tetranitrate 10 mg. Tab. **No. 2:** Pentaerythritol tetranitrate 20 mg. **No. 3:** Pentaerythritol tetranitrate 20 mg, phenobarbital ⅛ g. Bot. 100s, 1000s. *Rx.*
Use: Antianginal.
Arcoval Improved. (Arcum) Vitamin A palmitate 10,000 units, D 400 units, thiamine mononitrate 15 mg, B$_2$ 10 mg, nicotinamide 150 mg, B$_6$ 5 mg, calcium pantothenate 10 mg, B$_{12}$ 5 mcg, C 150 mg, E 5 units. Cap. Bot. 100s, 1000s. *OTC.*
Use: Mineral, vitamin supplement.
Arcum V-M. (Arcum) Vitamin A palmitate 5000 units, D 400 units, B$_1$ 2.5 mg, B$_2$ 2.5 mg, B$_6$ 0.5 mg, B$_{12}$ 2 mcg, C 50 mg, niacinamide 20 mg, calcium pantothenate 5 mg, iron 18 mg. Cap. Bot. 100s, 1000s. *OTC.*
Use: Mineral, vitamin supplement.
A-R-D. (Birchwood) Anatomically shaped dressing. Dispenser 24s.
Use: Antipruritic; counterirritant, rectal.
Ardeben. (Burgin-Arden) Diphenhydramine hydrochloride 10 mg, chlorobutanol 0.5%. Inj. Vial 30 mL. *Rx.*

Use: Antihistamine.

Ardecaine 1%. (Burgin-Arden) Lidocaine hydrochloride 1%. Inj. Vial 30 mL. *Rx.*
Use: Anesthetic, local.

Ardecaine 1% w/Epinephrine. (Burgin-Arden) Lidocaine hydrochloride 1%, epinephrine. Inj. Vial 30 mL. *Rx.*
Use: Anesthetic, local.

Ardecaine 2%. (Burgin-Arden) Lidocaine hydrochloride 2%. Inj. Vial 30 mL. *Rx.*
Use: Anesthetic, local.

Ardecaine 2% w/Epinephrine. (Burgin-Arden) Lidocaine hydrochloride 2%, epinephrine. Inj. Vial 30 mL. *Rx.*
Use: Anesthetic, topical.

Ardefem 40. (Burgin-Arden) Estradiol valerate 40 mg/mL. Vial 10 mL. *Rx.*
Use: Estrogen.

Ardefem 10. (Burgin-Arden) Estradiol valerate 10 mg/mL. Vial 10 mL. *Rx.*
Use: Estrogen.

Ardefem 20. (Burgin-Arden) Estradiol valerate 20 mg/mL. Vial 10 mL. *Rx.*
Use: Estrogen.

●**ardenermin.** (ar-den-ER-min) USAN.
Use: Tumor necrosis factor.

●**ardeparin sodium.** (ahr-dee-PA-rin) USAN.
Use: Anticoagulant.

Ardepred Soluble. (Burgin-Arden) Prednisolone 20 mg, niacinamide 25 mg, disodium edetate 0.5 mg, sodium bisulfite 1 mg, phenol 5 mg/mL. Vial 10 mL. *Rx.*
Use: Corticosteroid combination.

Ardevila. (Sanofi-Synthelabo) Inositol hexanicotinate. Tab. *Rx.*
Use: Vasodilator.

Ardiol 90/4. (Burgin-Arden) Testosterone enanthate 90 mg, estradiol valerate 4 mg/mL. Vial 10 mL. *Rx.*
Use: Androgen, estrogen combination.

Aredia. (Novartis) Pamidronate disodium 30 mg (mannitol 470 mg), 90 mg (mannitol 375 mg). Pow. for Inj., lyophilized. Vial. *Rx.*
Use: Bisphosphonate, antihypercalcemic.

Arestin. (Cord Logistics) Minocycline hydrochloride (as base) 1 mg. ER Dental Pow. Microspheres. UD 12s. *Rx.*
Use: Mouth and throat product; tetracycline.

●**arformoterol tartrate.** (ar-for-MOE-ter-ole) USAN.
Use: Bronchodilator; sympathomimetic.
See: Brovana.

●**argatroban.** (ahr-GAT-troe-ban) USAN.
Use: Anticoagulant.

argatroban. (GlaxoSmithKline) Argatroban 100 mg/mL. D-sorbitol 750 mg, dehydrated alcohol 1000 mg. Inj., Soln., Conc. Single-use vials. 2.5 mL. *Rx.*
Use: Anticoagulant, thrombin inhibitor.

Argesic-SA. (Econo Med Pharmaceuticals) Disalicylic acid 500 mg. Tab. Bot. 100s. *Rx.*
Use: Analgesic, topical.

Arginaid Extra. (Novartis Nutrition) Protein (whey protein isolate, L-arginine, L-cysteine) 25.3 g, carbohydrate (sugar, hydrolyzed corn starch) 219.4 g/L, vitamins A, B_1, B_2, B_3, B_5, B_6, B_{12}, C, D, E, K, biotin, folic acid, Cu, Fe, I, Mn, P, Zn, Na < 295 mg, K < 93 mg/L, 1.05 cal/mL, orange and wild berry flavors. Liq. *Tetra Brik Paks.* OTC.
Use: Enteral nutritional therapy.

●**arginine.** (AHR-jih-neen) *USP 34.*
Use: Ammonia detoxicant; diagnostic aid, pituitary function determination.

arginine butyrate. (AHR-jih-neen)
Use: Sickle cell disease; beta-thalassemia. [Orphan Drug]

●**arginine glutamate.** (AHR-jih-neen GLUE-tah-mate) USAN.
Use: Ammonia detoxicant.

●**arginine hydrochloride.** (AHR-jih-neen) *USP 34.*
Use: Ammonia detoxicant.

arginine hydrochloride. (AHR-jih-neen)
Use: Diagnostic aid.
See: R-Gene 10.

8-arginine-vasopressin.
See: Vasopressin.

●**argipressin tannate.** (AHR-JIH-press-in TAN-ate) USAN.
Use: Antidiuretic.

argyn.
See: Mild Silver Protein.

●**arhalofenate.** (AR-hal-oh-FEN-ate) USAN.
Use: Antidiabetic.

Aricept. (Eisai/Pfizer) Donepezil hydrochloride. **Oral Soln.:** 1 mg/mL. Sodium metabisulfite, sorbitol 70%, methylparaben. Strawberry flavor. 300 mL. **Tab.:** 5 mg, 10 mg, 23 mg. Lactose. Film coated. 30s, 90s, UD blister pack 100s. *Rx.*
Use: Treatment of mild to moderate dementia associated with Alzheimer disease.

Aricept ODT. (Eisai/Pfizer) Donepezil hydrochloride 5 mg, 10 mg. Mannitol. Orally Disintegrating Tab. UD blister pack 30s. *Rx.*
Use: Treatment of mild to moderate dementia associated with Alzheimer disease.

Aridex-D Pediatric. (Gentex) Phenylephrine hydrochloride 2 mg, carbinoxamine maleate 1 mg per 1 mL. Sugar and alcohol free. Sorbitol, sucralose. Bubble gum flavor. Drops. 30 mL. *Rx.*
Use: Pediatric decongestant and antihistamine.

Aridex Pediatric. (Gentex) Phenylephrine hydrochloride 2 mg, carbinoxamine maleate 1 mg, carbetapentane citrate 4 mg per mL. Sorbitol. Sugar free. Bubble gum flavor. Drops. Bot. 30 mL. *Rx.*
Use: Pediatric antitussive combination.

•**arildone.** (AR-ill-dohn) USAN.
Use: Antiviral.

Arimidex. (AstraZeneca) Anastrozole 1 mg, lactose. Tab. Bot. 30s. *Rx.*
Use: Hormone; aromatase inhibitor.

•**aripiprazole.** (a-rih-PIP-ray-zole) USAN.
Tall Man: ARIPiprazole
Use: Antipsychotic; antischizophrenic.
See: Abilify.

Aris Phenobarbital Reagent Strips. (Bayer Consumer Care) Box 25s.
Use: Diagnostic aid.

Aris Phenytoin Reagent Strips. (Bayer Consumer Care) Box 25s.
Use: Diagnostic aid.

Aristocort Acetonide, Sodium Phosphate Salt. (Fujisawa Healthcare)
Use: Corticosteroid, topical.
See: Aristocort.

Aristo-Pak. (Wyeth) Triamcinolone 4 mg. Tab. 16s. *Rx.*
Use: Corticosteroid.

Aristospan Intra-articular. (Sandoz) Triamcinolone hexacetonide 20 mg/mL suspension. Polysorbate 80, sorbitol, benzyl alcohol. Inj. Vials. 1 mL, 5 mL. *Rx.*
Use: Adrenocortical steroid, glucocorticoid.

Aristospan Intralesional. (Sandoz) Triamcinolone hexacetonide 5 mg/mL suspension. Polysorbate 80, sorbitol, benzyl alcohol. Inj. Vials. 5 mL. *Rx.*
Use: Adrenocortical steroid, glucocorticoid.

Arixtra. (GlaxoSmithKline) Fondaparinux sodium 2.5 mg per 0.5 mL, 5 mg per 0.4 mL, 7.5 mg per 0.6 mL, 10 mg per 0.8 mL. Preservative free. Inj. Single-dose prefilled syringes with 27-gauge needle. 10s. *Rx.*
Use: Anticoagulant, selective factor Xa inhibitor.

Arlacel C. (AstraZeneca) Sorbitan sesquioleate. Mixture of oleate esters of sorbitol and its anhydrides.
Use: Surface active agent.

Arlacel 83. (AstraZeneca) Sorbitan sesquioleate.
Use: Surface active agent.

Arlacel 165. (AstraZeneca) Glyceryl monostearate, PEG-100 stearate non-ionic self-emulsifying.
Use: Surface active agent.

Arlamol E. (AstraZeneca) Polyoxypropylene (15), stearyl ether, BHT 0.1%.
Use: Emollient.

Arlatone 507. (AstraZeneca) Padimate O. *OTC.*
Use: Sunscreen.

Arm-a-Med Metaproterenol Sulfate. (Centeon) Metaproterenol sulfate 0.4%, 0.6%, sodium chloride, EDTA. Soln. for nebulization. Vial UD 2.5 mL for use with IPPB device. *Rx.*
Use: Bronchodilator.

Arm-a-Vial. (Centeon) Sterile water, sodium chloride 0.45%, 0.9%. Box 100s. Plastic vial 3 mL, 5 mL.
Use: Electrolyte supplement.

•**armodafinil.** (ar-moe-DAF-in-il) USAN.
Use: Analeptic.
See: Nuvigil.

Armour Thyroid. (Forest) Thyroid desiccated 15 mg (¼ gr), 30 mg (½ gr), 60 mg (1 gr), 90 mg (1 ½ gr), 120 mg (2 gr), 180 mg (3 gr), 240 mg (4 gr), 300 mg (5 gr), dextrose. Tab. Bot. 100s, 1000s (except 15 mg, 90 mg, 240 mg, 300 mg), 5000s (30 mg, 60 mg only), 50,000s (60 mg, 120 mg only), UD 100s (30 mg, 60 mg, 120 mg only). *Rx.*
Use: Thyroid hormone.

Arnica Tincture. (Eli Lilly) Arnica 20% in alcohol 66%. Bot. 120 mL, 480 mL. *OTC.*
Use: Analgesic, topical.

•**arofylline.** (ah-ROE-fih-lin) USAN.
Use: Bronchodilator; asthma prophylactic.

Aromasin. (Pharmacia) Exemestane 25 mg, mannitol, methylparaben, polyvinyl alcohol. Tab. Bot. 30s. *Rx.*
Use: Hormone, breast cancer.

aromatase inhibitors.
See: Anastrozole.
   Arimidex.
   Aromasin.
   Exemestane.
   Femara.
   Letrozole.

Aromatic Ammonia Vaporole. (GlaxoSmithKline) Inhalant. Vial 5 min. Box 10s, 12s, 100s. *Rx.*
Use: Respiratory.

•**aromatic elixir.** (AR-oh-MAT-ik ee-LIX-ir) *NF 29.*
Use: Pharmaceutic aid, vehicle, flavored, sweetened.

aromatic elixir. (Eli Lilly) Alcohol 22%. Bot. 16 fl. oz.
Use: Pharmaceutic aid, flavoring.
AR-121. (Argus) Phase I/II HIV. *Rx.*
Use: Antiviral.
•**arprinocid.** (ahr-PRIN-oh-sid) USAN.
Use: Coccidiostat.
Arranon. (GlaxoSmithKline) Nelarabine 250 mg (5 mg/mL). Sodium chloride 4.5 mg/mL. Inj. Vials. 50 mL. *Rx.*
Use: DNA demethylation agent; antineoplastic.
arseclor.
See: Dichlorophenarsine hydrochloride.
arsenic compounds.
Use: Rarely employed in modern medicine; there are no longer any official compounds.
See: Arsphenamine.
Carbarsone.
Dichlorophenarsine Hydrochloride.
Ferric Cacodylate.
Glycobiarsol.
•**arsenic trioxide.** (AR-se-nik) USAN.
Use: Antineoplastic.
See: Trisenox.
arsenobenzene.
See: Arsphenamine.
arsenphenolamine.
See: Arsphenamine.
Arsobal. Melarsoprol (Mel B).
Use: CDC anti-infective agent.
arsphenamine. Arsenobenzene, arsenobenzol, arsenophenolamine, Ehrlich 606, salvarsan.
Use: Formerly used as antisyphilitic.
arsthinol. Cyclic.
Use: Antiprotozoal.
Artarau. (Archer-Taylor) Rauwolfia serpentina 50 mg, 100 mg. Tab. Bot. 100s, 1000s. *Rx.*
Use: Antihypertensive.
Arta-Vi-C. (Archer-Taylor) Multivitamins with Vitamin C 100 mg. Tab. Bot. 100s. *OTC.*
Use: Vitamin supplement.
Artazyme. (Archer-Taylor) Bot. 13 mL.
Use: Autolyzed proteolytic enzyme.
•**arteflene.** (AHR-teh-fleen) USAN.
Use: Antimalarial.
•**artegraft.** (AHR-teh-graft) USAN. Arterial graft composed of a section of bovine carotid artery that has been subjected to enzymatic digestion with ficin and tanned with dialdehyde starch.
Use: Prosthetic aid, arterial.
•**artemether.** (ar-TEM-ee-ther) USAN.
Use: Antimalarial.
artemether/lumefantrine.
See: Coartem.

arterenol.
See: Norepinephrine bitartrate.
•**artesunate.** (ar-TES-oo-nate) USAN.
Use: Investigational antimalarial agent.
Artha-G. (T.E. Williams Pharmaceuticals) Salsalate 750 mg. Tab. Bot. 120s. *Rx.*
Use: Analgesic.
Arthralgen. (Wyeth) Salicylamide 250 mg, acetaminophen 250 mg. Tab. Bot. 30s, 100s, 500s. *OTC.*
Use: Analgesic combination.
ArthriCare Daytime Formula. (Del) Menthol 1.25%, methyl nicotinate 0.25%, capsaicin 0.025%, with aloe vera gel, carbomer 940, DMDM hydantoin, glyceryl stearate SE, myristyl propionate, propylparaben, triethanolamine. Cream. Jar 90 g. *OTC.*
Use: Analgesic, topical.
Arthritic Pain. (Walgreen) Triethanolamine salicylate 10%. Lot. Bot. 6 oz. *OTC.*
Use: Analgesic, topical.
Arthritis Bayer Timed Release Aspirin. (Bayer Consumer Care) Aspirin 650 mg. TR Tab. Bot. 30s, 72s, 125s. *OTC.*
Use: Analgesic.
Arthritis Hot Creme. (Thompson Medical) Methyl salicylate 15%, menthol 10%, glyceryl stearate, carbomer 934, lanolin, PEG-100 stearate, propylene glycol, trolamine, parabens. Cream. Jar 90 g. *OTC.*
Use: Liniment.
Arthritis Pain Formula. (Whitehall-Robins) Aspirin 500 mg, aluminum hydroxide 27 mg, magnesium hydroxide 100 mg. Tab. Bot. 40s, 100s, 175s. *OTC.*
Use: Salicylate, buffered aspirin.
Arthritis Pain Formula, Aspirin Free. (Whitehall-Robins) Acetaminophen 500 mg. Tab. Bot. 30s, 75s. *OTC.*
Use: Analgesic.
Arthrotec. (Searle) Diclofenac sodium 50 mg/misoprostol 200 mcg, diclofenac sodium 75 mg/misoprostol 200 mcg. Lactose. Film coated. Tab. Bot. 60s, 90s (50 mg only), UD 100s. *Rx.*
Use: Analgesic.
Arthrotin. (Whiteworth Towne) Enteric-coated aspirin 325 mg. Tab. Bot. 100s.
Use: Analgesic.
•**articaine.** (AR-ti-kane) USAN.
Use: Anesthetic, injectable local amide.
Articulose L.A. (Seatrace) Triamcinolone diacetate 40 mg/mL. Vial 5 mL. *Rx.*
Use: Corticosteroid.
artificial tanning agent.
See: Sudden Tan.
artificial tear insert.
See: Lacrisert.

artificial tears. (Rugby) White petrolatum, anhydrous liquid lanolin, mineral oil. Ophth. Oint. Tube 3.5 g. *OTC.*
Use: Lubricant, ophthalmic.

artificial tears. (Various Mfr.) Benzalkonium chloride 0.01%. May also contain EDTA, NaCl, polyvinyl alcohol, hydroxypropyl methylcellulose Soln. Bot. 15 mL, 30 mL. *OTC.*
Use: Lubricant, ophthalmic.

artificial tear solutions.
Use: Lubricant, ophthalmic.
See: Akwa Tears.
  Artificial Tears.
  Artificial Tears Plus.
  Celluvisc.
  Comfort Tears.
  Preservative Free Moisture Eyes.
  Puralube Tears.
  Refresh Plus.
  Systane.
  Teargen.
  Tears Naturale Forte.
  TheraTears.
  Visine Pure Tears.
  Visine Tears.
  Visine Tears Preservative Free.

Artificial Tears Plus. (Various Mfr.) Polyvinyl alcohol 1.4%, povidone 0.6%, chlorobutanol 0.5%, NaCl. Soln. Bot. 15 mL. *OTC.*
Use: Lubricant, ophthalmic.

•**artilide fumarate.** (AHR-tih-lide) USAN.
Use: Cardiovascular agent.

Artiss. (Baxter) Fibrin sealant (human). **Pow. for Soln. Top.:** Total protein 96 to 125 mg/mL, fibrinogen 67 to 106 mg/mL, fibrinolysis inhibitor (synthetic) 2,250 to 3,750 kallikrein-inhibiting units/mL, thrombin (human) 2.5 to 6.5 units/mL, calcium chloride 36 to 44 mcmol/mL (when reconstituted). Single-use vials with or without *Duploject* system. 2 mL, 4 mL, 10 mL. *Artiss Kit* contains the following substances in 4 separate vials: sealer protein concentrate (human), fibrinolysis inhibitor solution (synthetic), thrombin (human), and calcium chloride solution. **Soln. Top.:** Total protein 96 to 125 mg/mL, fibrinogen 67 to 106 mg/mL, thrombin (human) 2.5 to 6.5 units/mL. Single-use prefillled (frozen) syringe with *Duo Set.* 2 mL, 4 mL, 10 mL. *Rx.*
Use: Fibrin agent.

Artra Beauty Bar. (Schering-Plough) Triclocarban 1% in soap base. Cake 3.6 oz. *OTC.*
Use: Dermatologic; cleanser.

Artra Skin Tone Cream. (Schering-Plough) Hydroquinone 2%. Oint. Tube 1 oz (normal only), 2 oz, 4 oz.
Use: Dermatologic.

arylalkylamines.
Use: Nasal decongestant.
See: Adrenalin Chloride.
  Afrin Children's.
  AH-Chew D.
  Cenafed.
  Decofed.
  Dimetapp Decongestant Pediatric.
  Dimetapp, Maximum Strength, Non-Drowsy.
  Dimetapp, Maximum Strength 12-Hour, Non-Drowsy.
  Drixoral 12 Hour Non-Drowsy Formula.
  Efidac 24.
  Ephedrine Sulfate.
  Epinephrine Hydrochloride.
  4-Way Fast Acting.
  Genaphed.
  Kid Kare.
  Little Colds for Infants and Children.
  Little Noses Gentle Formula, Infants & Children.
  Medi-First Sinus Decongestant.
  Nasal Decongestant, Children's Non-Drowsy.
  Nasal Decongestant Oral.
  Neo-Synephrine 4-Hour Extra Strength.
  Neo-Synephrine 4-Hour Mild Formula.
  Neo-Synephrine 4-Hour Regular Strength.
  PediaCare Decongestant, Infants'.
  Phenylephrine Hydrochloride.
  Pretz-D.
  Pseudoephedrine Hydrochloride.
  Pseudoephedrine Sulfate.
  Rhinall.
  Silfedrine, Children's.
  Simply Stuffy.
  Sinustop.
  Sudafed, Children's Non-Drowsy.
  Sudafed Non-Drowsy, Maximum Strength.
  Sudafed Non-Drowsy 12 Hour Long-Acting.
  Sudafed Non-Drowsy 24 Hour Long-Acting.
  Triaminic Allergy Congestion.
  Vicks Sinex.

Arzol Silver Nitrate Applicators. (Arzol) Silver nitrate 75% and potassium nitrate 25%. Applicator. 100s. *Rx.*
Use: Topical anti-infective.

•**arzoxifene hydrochloride.** (ar-ZOX-i-feen) USAN.
Use: Uterine fibroids; endometriosis; dysfunctional uterine bleeding; breast cancer.

5-ASA. Mesalamine.
See: Asacol.
Rowasa.
ASA. (Wampole) Anti-skin antibodies test
by IFA. Test 48s.
Use: Diagnostic aid.
A.S.A. (Eli Lilly) Aspirin. Acetylsalicylic
acid. **Enseal:** 5 g, 10 g. Bot. 100s,
1000s. **Supp.:** 5 g, 10 g. Pkg. 6s, 144s.
OTC.
Use: Analgesic.
Asacol. (Procter & Gamble) Mesalamine
400 mg. Lactose. Tab. DR Bot. 180s.
Rx.
Use: Anti-inflammatory.
Asacol HD. (Warner Chilcott) Mesala-
mine 800 mg. Lactose, PEG. Tab., de-
layed release. 180s. *Rx.*
Use: Gastrointestinal agent.
asafetida, emulsion of. Milk of Asa-
fetida.
Asaped. (Sanofi-Synthelabo) Acetyl-
salicylic acid. Tab. *OTC.*
Use: Analgesic.
Asawin. (Sanofi-Synthelabo) Acetyl-
salicylic acid. Tab. *OTC.*
Use: Analgesic.
A.S.B. (Femco) Calcium carbonate, magnesium carbonate, bismuth subcarbon-
ate, sodium bicarbonate, kaolin. Pow.
Can 3 oz. Tab. Bot. 50s. *OTC.*
Use: Antacid.
Asclerol. (Spanner) Liver injection crude
(2 mcg/mL) 50%, Vitamins B_1 20 mg,
B_2 3 mg, B_6 1 mg, B_{12} 30 mcg, niacin-
amide 100 mg, panthenol 2.8 mg, cho-
line chloride 20 mg, inositol 10 mg/mL.
Multiple dose vial 10 mL. *Rx.*
Use: Vitamin supplement.
ASC Lotionized. (Geritrex) Triclosan
0.3%. Aloe vera gel, sweet almond oil,
parabens, tartrazine. Liq. 8 oz. *OTC.*
Use: Topical anti-infective.
Asco-Caps. (Key) Ascorbic acid 500 mg.
Cap. 100s, 500s. *OTC.*
Use: Water-soluble vitamin.
Ascocid. (Key) Vitamin C (as calcium
ascorbate) 4000 mg/tsp. Gran. 8 oz.
OTC.
Use: Water-soluble vitamin.
Ascomp with Codeine. (Breckenridge)
Codeine phosphate 30 mg, aspirin
325 mg, caffeine 40 mg, butalbital
50 mg. Cap. Bot. 100s, 500s. *c-III.*
Use: Narcotic analgesic combination.
ascorbate sodium. Antiscorbutic vitamin.
•**ascorbic acid.** (ASS-kor-bik) *USP 34.*
Use: Water-soluble vitamin, antiscor-
butic; acidifier, urinary.
See: Asco-Caps.
Ascorbineed.

Ascor L 500.
Cecon.
Cenolate.
Cevi-Bid.
Dull-C.
Neo-Vadrin.
N'Ice.
Sunkist Vitamin C.
Vita-C
ascorbic acid. (Freeda) Ascorbic acid
1000 mg. TR Tab. 100s, 250s, 500s.
OTC.
Use: Water-soluble vitamin.
ascorbic acid. (Humco) Ascorbic acid
60 mg/¼ tsp. Pow. 454 g. *OTC.*
Use: Water-soluble vitamin.
ascorbic acid. (Various Mfr.) Ascorbic
acid 500 mg/mL. Inj. Vials. 50 mL. *Rx.*
Use: Water-soluble vitamin.
ascorbic acid. (Various Mfr.) Ascorbic
acid. **Tab.:** 250 mg, 500 mg, 1000 mg,
1500 mg. Bot. 100s, 250s (500 mg,
1000 mg only), 1000s (500 mg only),
UD 100s (250 mg, 500 mg only).
TR Tab.: 500 mg. Bot. 100s, 250s,
500s. **Cap.:** 500 mg. Bot. 100s.
Liq.: 500 mg/5 mL. Bot. 120 mL,
480 mL. *OTC.*
Use: Water-soluble vitamin.
ascorbic acid and sodium ascorbate.
Use: Water-soluble vitamin.
See: Chewable Vitamin C.
Chew C.
Fruit C 500.
Fruit C 100.
Fruit C 200.
Sunkist Vitamin C.
Vicks Vitamin C.
ascorbic acid injection.
Use: Vitamin supplement.
ascorbic acid salts.
See: Calcium Ascorbate.
Sodium Ascorbate.
Ascorbineed. (Hanlon) Vitamin C
500 mg. T-Cap. Bot. 100s. *OTC.*
Use: Vitamin supplement.
Ascorbin/11. (Taylor Pharmaceuticals)
Lemon bioflavonoids 110 mg, Vitamin
C 1 g, rosehips powder 50 mg, rutin
25 mg. SR Tab. Bot. 100s. *OTC.*
Use: Vitamin supplement.
Ascorbocin. (Paddock) Vitamin C
500 mg, niacin 500 mg, B_1 50 mg, B_6
50 mg, d-α-tocopheryl, polyethylene
glycol 1000 succinate 50 units, lactose/
3 g. Pow. Bot. lb. *OTC.*
Use: Vitamin supplement.
•**ascorbyl palmitate.** (ah-SCORE-bill
PAL-mih-tate) *NF 29.*
Use: Preservative; pharmaceutic aid,
antioxidant.

Ascor L 500. (McGuff) Ascorbic acid 500 mg/mL. EDTA 0.025%, preservative free. Inj. 50 mL. *Rx.*
Use: Water-soluble vitamin.

Ascorvite S.R. (Eon Labs) Vitamin C 500 mg. SR Cap. *OTC.*
Use: Vitamin supplement.

Ascriptin. (Novartis) Aspirin 325 mg, magnesium hydroxide 50 mg, aluminum hydroxide 50 mg. Tab. Bot. 50s, 100s, 225s, 500s. *OTC.*
Use: Analgesic; antacid.

Ascriptin Maximum Strength. (Novartis) Aspirin 500 mg, calcium carbonate 237 mg, magnesium hydroxide 33 mg, aluminum hydroxide 33 mg. Tab. 85s. *OTC.*
Use: Salicylate, buffered aspirin.

asenapine. (a-SEN-a-peen)
Use: Antipsychotic agent.
See: Saphris.

•**asenapine maleate.** (a-SEN-a-peen) USAN.
Use: Serotonin antagonist.

aseptichrome.
See: Merbromin.

Aslum. (Drug Products) Carbolic acid 1%, aluminum acetate, ichthammol, zinc oxide, aromatic oils in a petrolatum-stearin base. Tube. Jar.
Use: Astringent.

Asma. (Wampole) Anti-smooth muscle antibody test by IFA. Test 48.
Use: Diagnostic aid.

AsmalPred Plus. (Tiber Labs) Prednisolone 15 mg per 5 mL (equiv. to prednisolone sodium phosphate 20.2 mg). Alcohol 1.8%, glycerin, sodium benzoate, sorbitol, sucrose. Grape flavor. Soln. 237 mL. *Rx.*
Use: Adrenocortical steroid, glucocorticoid.

Asmanex Twisthaler. (Schering) Mometasone furoate 110 mcg (delivers mometasone fuorate 100 mcg)/actuation, 220 mcg (delivers mometasone furoate 200 mcg)/actuation. Lactose. Pow. for Inh. Inhalation device. 7 units (110 mcg only), 14 units (220 mcg only), 30 units, 60 units (220 mcg only), 120 units (220 mcg only). *Rx.*
Use: Corticosteroid, respiratory inhalant.

Asma-Tuss. (Halsey Drug) Phenobarbital 4 mg, theophylline 15 mg, ephedrine sulfate 12 mg, guaifenesin 50 mg/5 mL. Bot. 4 oz. *Rx.*
Use: Bronchodilator.

Asolectin. (Associated Concentrates) Chemical lecithin 25%, chemical cephalin 22%, inositol phosphatides 16%, soybean oil 2.5%, other miscella-neous sterols and lipids 34.5%. *OTC.*
Use: Diet supplement.

•**asoprisnil.** (as-oh-PRIS-nil) USAN.
Use: Endometriosis.

•**asparaginase.** (ass-PAR-uh-jin-aze) USAN.
Use: Antineoplastic.
See: Elspar.

•**aspartame.** (ass-PAR-tame) *NF 29.*
Use: Sweetener.

•**aspartic acid.** (ass-PAR-tick) *USP 34.*
Aspartic acid; aminosuccinic acid.
Use: Management of fatigue; amino acid.

•**aspartocin.** (ass-PAR-toe-sin) USAN.
Use: Anti-infective.

Aspercreme. (Chattem) Triethanolamine salicylate 10% in cream base. *OTC.*
Use: Analgesic, topical.

Aspercreme Max Roll-On. (Chattem) Menthol 16%, capsaicin, glycerin, propylene glycol, SD alcohol, triethanolamine. Liq. 73 mL. *OTC.*
Use: Rub and liniment.

Aspercreme with Aloe. (Chattem) Trolamine salicylate 10%. Aloe vera, cetyl alcohol, glycerin, mineral oil, parabens. Cream. 85 g. *OTC.*
Use: Rub and liniment.

aspergillus niger enzyme. Alpha-galactosidase. *OTC.*
See: Beano.

aspergillus oryzae enzyme. Diastase.

asperkinase. Proteolytic enzyme mixture derived from aspergillus oryzae.

•**asperlin.** (ASS-per-lin) USAN.
Use: Anti-infective; antineoplastic.

Aspermin. (Buffington) Aspirin 325 mg. Sugar, caffeine, lactose, and salt free. Tab. *Dispens-A-Kit* 500s. *OTC.*
Use: Analgesic.

Aspermin Extra. (Buffington) Aspirin 500 mg. Sugar, caffeine, lactose, and salt free. Tab. *Dispens-A-Kit* 500s. *OTC.*
Use: Analgesic.

•**aspirin.** (ASS-pihr-in) *USP 34.*
Use: Analgesic; antipyretic; antirheumatic. Prophylactic to reduce risk of death or non-fatal MI in patients with a previous infarction or unstable angina pectoris.
See: A.S.A.
Aspirin Low Dose.
Aspir Low.
Bayer Buffered Aspirin.
Bayer Children's Chewable Aspirin.
Bayer, 8-Hour Timed-Release.
Bayer Extra Strength Back & Body Pain.
Bayer Low Adult Strength.

Bayer Women's Aspirin Plus Calcium.
Easprin.
Ecotrin Low Strength.
Ecotrin Regular Strength.
Genprin.
Genuine Bayer Aspirin.
Halfprin 81.
Heartline.
Maximum Bayer Aspirin.
Miniprin Low Dose.
Norwich Extra Strength.
Norwich Regular Strength.
St. Joseph Adult Chewable Aspirin.
St. Joseph Aspirin for Adults.
ZORprin.
W/Acetaminophen, Aluminum Hydroxide, Caffeine, Magnesium Hydroxide.
See: Vanquish.
W/Acetaminophen, Caffeine.
See: Anacin Advanced Headache.
Excedrin Extra Strength.
Excedrin Migraine.
Goody's Extra Strength.
Goody's Extra Strength Fast Pain Relief.
W/Acetaminophen, Caffeine, Phenyltoloxamine Citrate, Salicylamide.
See: Levacet.
W/Acetaminophen, Caffeine, Salicylamide.
See: Medi-First Extra Strength Pain Relief.
Saleto.
W/Aluminum Hydroxide, Calcium Carbonate, Magnesium Hydroxide.
See: Ascriptin.
W/Caffeine.
See: Alka-Seltzer Wake-Up Call.
Anacin.
Anacin Maximum Strength.
Bayer Quick Release Crystals.
BC Fast Pain Relief.
BC Fast Pain Relief Arthritis.
P-A-C Analgesic.
Painaid ESF Extra-Strength Formula.
W/Caffeine, Orphenadrine Citrate.
See: Orphenadrine Compound.
Orphenadrine Compound-DS.
W/Caffeine, Salicylamide.
See: BC Powder Arthritis Strength.
Painaid.
Stanback Headache Powders.
W/Chlorpheniramine Maleate, Dextromethorphan Hydrobromide.
See: Alka-Seltzer Plus Flu.
W/Chlorpheniramine Maleate, Dextromethorphan Hydrobromide, Phenylephrine Bitartrate.
See: Alka-Seltzer Plus Cold & Cough.
W/Chlorpheniramine Maleate, Phenylephrine Bitartrate.
See: Alka-Seltzer Plus Cold.

Alka-Seltzer Plus Sparkling Cold Formula.
W/Citric Acid, Sodium Bicarbonate.
See: Alka-Seltzer Lemon Lime.
Alka-Seltzer Original.
W/Dextromethorphan Hydrobromide, Doxylamine Succinate, Phenylephrine Bitartrate.
See: Alka-Seltzer Plus Day & Night Cold.
Alks-Seltzer Plus Night Cold.
W/Dextromethorphan Hydrobromide, Phenylephrine Bitartrate.
See: Alka-Seltzer Plus Day & Night Cold.
W/Diphenhydramine Citrate.
See: Alka-Seltzer PM.
W/Hydrocodone Bitartrate.
See: Lortab ASA.
W/Magnesium Salicylate, Phenyltoloxamine.
See: Mobigesic.
aspirin, alumina, and magnesia.
Use: Analgesic; antacid.
aspirin, alumina, and magnesium oxide.
Use: Analgesic; antacid.
aspirin and barbiturate combinations.
Use: Analgesic; sedative; hypnotic.
See: BAC.
Butalbital.
Fiorinal.
aspirin and codeine phosphate. (Vintage Pharmaceuticals) Codeine phosphate 15 mg/aspirin 325 mg. Tab. 100s, 500s, 1,000s. *c-III.*
Use: Analgesic, narcotic.
aspirin and dipyridamole.
Use: Antiplatelet.
See: Aggrenox.
aspirin and narcotic combinations.
See: Alor 5/500.
Ascomp with Codeine.
Butalbital, Aspirin, and Caffeine.
Butalbital Compound.
aspirin and oxycodone. (Various Mfr.) Oxycodone hydrochloride 4.5 mg, oxycodone terephthalate 0.38 mg, aspirin 325 mg. Tab. Bot. 100s, 500s, 1000s, UD 25s. *c-II.*
Use: Analgesic combination, narcotic.
aspirin, buffered.
Use: Salicylate.
See: Arthritis Pain Formula.
Ascriptin Maximum Strength.
Bufferin.
Bufferin Extra Strength.
Extra Strength Bayer Plus.
W/Acetaminophen.
See: Excedrin Back & Body Extra Strength.

Aspirin-Free Bayer Select Allergy Sinus. (Bayer Consumer Care) Pseudoephedrine hydrochloride 30 mg, chlorpheniramine maleate 2 mg, acetaminophen 500 mg. Cap. Pkg. 16s. *OTC.*
Use: Analgesic; antihistamine; decongestant.

Aspirin-Free Bayer Select Headache. (Bayer Consumer Care) Acetaminophen 500 mg, caffeine 65 mg. Cap. Bot. 50s. *OTC.*
Use: Analgesic combination.

Aspirin-Free Bayer Select Head & Chest Cold. (Bayer Consumer Care) Pseudoephedrine hydrochloride 30 mg, dextromethorphan HBr 10 mg, guaifenesin 100 mg, acetaminophen 325 mg. Capl. Bot. 16s. *OTC.*
Use: Analgesic; decongestant; expectorant.

Aspirin Free Excedrin. (Bristol-Myers Squibb) Acetaminophen 500 mg, caffeine 65 mg. Tab., Capl. Bot. 20s, 40s, 80s. *OTC.*
Use: Analgesic combination.

Aspirin Low Dose. (Time-Cap Labs) Aspirin 81 mg. Orange flavor. Chew. Tab. 36s. *OTC.*
Use: Salicylate.

Aspirin Plus. (Walgreen) Aspirin 400 mg, caffeine 32 mg. Tab. Bot. 100s. *OTC.*
Use: Analgesic combination.

aspirin salts.
See: Calcium Acetylsalicylate.

Aspirin Uniserts. (Upsher-Smith) Aspirin 125 mg, 300 mg, 650 mg. Supp. Ctn. 12s, 50s. *OTC.*
Use: Analgesic.

aspirin w/codeine no. 4. (Various Mfr.) Codeine phosphate 60 mg, aspirin 325 mg Tab. Bot. 100s, 500s, 1000s. *c-III.*
Use: Analgesic combination, narcotic.

aspirin w/codeine no. 3. (Various Mfr.) Codeine phosphate 30 mg, aspirin 325 mg. Tab. Bot. 100s, 1000s. *c-III.*
Use: Analgesic combination, narcotic.

Aspir Low. (Major) Aspirin 81 mg. Enteric coated. PEG, polydextrose. Tab. 1,000s. *OTC.*
Use: CNS agent, salicylate.

Aspirtab. (Dover Pharmaceuticals) Aspirin 325 mg. Sugar, lactose, and salt free. Tab. UD Box 500s. *OTC.*
Use: Analgesic.

Aspirtab Max. (Dover Pharmaceuticals) Aspirin 500 mg. Sugar, lactose, and salt free. Tab. UD Box 500s. *OTC.*
Use: Analgesic.

Astaril. (Sanofi-Synthelabo) Theophylline anhydrous, ephedrine sulphate. Tab. *Rx.*
Use: Bronchodilator.

Astelin. (Medpointe) Azelastine 137 mcg/ spray. Benzalkonium chloride, EDTA. Nasal Spray. Bot. 17 mg (100 metered sprays) per bottle. 2s. *Rx.*
Use: Antihistamine, peripherally selective phthalazinone.

•**astemizole.** (ASS-TEM-ih-zole) USAN.
Use: Antihistamine; antiallergic.

Astepro. (MEDA Pharmaceuticals) Azelastine 0.15% (205.5 mcg/spray). Equiv. to azelastine base 187.6 mcg. Benzalkonium chloride, edetate disodium. 30 mL (200 metered sprays), 17 mL (106 metered sprays). *Rx.*
Use: Respiratory inhalant, intranasal antihistamine.

asterol.
Use: Antifungal.

Asthmalixir. (Reese) Theophylline 45 mg, ephedrine sulfate 36 mg, guaifenesin 150 mg, phenobarbital 12 mg/ 15 mL, alcohol 19%. Bot. *Rx.*
Use: Bronchodilator; expectorant; hypnotic; sedative.

AsthmaNefrin. (Numark) Racepinephrine hydrochloride 2.25%. Soln. for Inh. Bot. 15 mL. *OTC.*
Use: Sympathomimetic.

AsthmaNefrin Solution & Nebulizer. (Numark) Racepin (racemic epinephrine) as hydrochloride equivalent to epinephrine base 2.25%, chlorobutanol 0.5%. Bot. 0.5 fl oz. With sodium bisulfite. Bot. 1 fl oz. *OTC.*
Use: Bronchodilator.

•**astifilcon A.** (ASS-tih-FILL-kahn) USAN.
Use: Contact lens material, hydrophilic.

Astramorph PF. (APP Pharmaceutical) Morphine sulfate 0.5 mg/mL, 1 mg/mL. Inj. Amp. 2 mL, 10 mL. Single-use vial 10 mL. *c-II.*
Use: Analgesic, narcotic agonist.

Astroglide. (Biofilm) Purified water, glycerin, propylene glycol, parabens. Vaginal gel. Bot 66.5 mL. Travel pks. 5 mL. *OTC.*
Use: Lubricant.

•**astromicin sulfate.** (ASS-troe-MY-sin) USAN.
Use: Anti-infective.

Astro-Vites. (Faraday) Vitamins A 3500 units, D 400 units, C 60 mg, B_1 0.8 mg, B_2 1.3 mg, niacinamide 14 mg, B_6 1 mg, B_{12} 2.5 mcg, folic acid 0.05 mg, pantothenic acid 5 mg, iron 12 mg. Tab. Bot. 100s, 250s. *OTC.*
Use: Mineral, vitamin supplement.

AST/SGOT Reagent Strips. (Bayer Consumer Care) Seralyzer reagent strip. A quantitative strip test for aspartate

transaminase/serum glutamic oxaloacetic transaminase in serum or plasma. Bot. Strip 25s.
Use: Diagnostic aid.

•**astuprotimut-R.** (AS-tu-PROE-ti-mut) USAN.
Use: Immunologic.

Asupirin. (Suppositoria Laboratories, Inc.) Aspirin 60 mg, 120 mg, 200 mg, 300 mg, 600 mg, 1.2 g. Supp. Box 12s, 100s, 1000s. *OTC.*
Use: Analgesic.

Atabee TD. (Defco) Vitamins C 500 mg, B_1 15 mg, B_2 10 mg, B_6 2 mg, nicotinamide 50 mg, calcium pantothenate 10 mg. Cap. Bot. 30s, 1000s. *OTC.*
Use: Vitamin supplement.

Atacand. (AstraZeneca) Candesartan cilexetil 4 mg, 8 mg, 16 mg, 32 mg. Lactose. Tab. Bot. Unit-of-use 30s, 90s (16 mg, 32 mg only); UD 100s (only 16 mg, 32 mg). *Rx.*
Use: Antihypertensive.

Atacand HCT. (AstraZeneca) Candesartan cilexetil/hydrochlorothiazide 16 mg/12.5 mg, 32 mg/12.5 mg, 32 mg/25 mg. Lactose. Tab. UD 100s (16 mg/12.5 mg and 32 mg/12.5 mg only), unit-of-use 90s. *Rx.*
Use: Antihypertensive.

•**atagabalin.** (A-ta-GAB-a-lin) USAN.
Use: CNS agent.

•**ataluren.** (AT-a-LUR-en) USAN.
Use: Genetic mutation disorders.

•**atazanavir sulfate.** (AT-ah-zah-NAH-veer) USAN.
Use: Antiretroviral, protease inhibitor.
See: Reyataz.

Atelvia. (Warner Chilcott) Risedronate sodium 35 mg. Edetate disodium, polysorbate 80. Tab., delayed release. Dose pack 4s. *Rx.*
Use: Bisphosphonate.

•**atenolol.** (ah-TEN-oh-lahl) *USP 34.*
Use: Beta-adrenergic blocker.
See: Tenormin.
W/Combinations.
See: Tenoretic.

atenolol. (Various Mfr.) Atenolol. 25 mg, 50 mg, 100 mg. Tab. 30s, 60s, 90s, 100s, 500s (100 mg only), 1,000s. *Rx.*
Use: Antiadrenergic/sympatholytic; beta-adrenergic blocking agent.

atenolol/chlorthalidone. (Various Mfr.) Atenolol/chlorthalidone 50 mg/25 mg, 100 mg/25 mg. Tab. Bot. 50s, 100s, 250s, 500s, 1000s. *Rx.*
Use: Antihypertensive.

•**atevirdine mesylate.** (at-TEH-vihr-DEEN) USAN.
Use: Antiviral.

Atgam. (Pharmacia) Lymphocyte immune globulin, antithymocyte globulin horse gamma globulin 50 mg/mL. Glycine 0.3 M. Inj. Amps. 5 mL. *Rx.*
Use: Immunosuppressant.

Athlete's Foot. (Walgreen) Zinc undecylenate 20%, undecylenic acid 5%. Oint. Tube 1.5 oz. *OTC.*
Use: Antifungal, topical.

•**atilmotin.** (A-til-MOE-tin) USAN.
Use: Gastrointestinal agent.

•**atipamezole.** (AT-ih-pam-EH-zole) USAN.
Use: Antagonist, α_2-receptor.

•**atiprimod dihydrochloride.** (at-TIH-prih-mahd) USAN.
Use: Antiarthritic, immunomodulator, suppressor cell inducing agent; antiinflammatory; antirheumatic, disease-modifying.

•**atiprimod dimaleate.** (at-TIH-prih-mahd) USAN.
Use: Antiarthritic; anti-inflammatory; immunomodulator; antirheumatic, disease-modifying.

•**atiprosin maleate.** (ah-TIH-pro-SIN) USAN.
Use: Antihypertensive.

Ativan. (Baxter) Lorazepam 2 mg/mL, 4 mg/mL. Inj. Single and 10 mL multidose vials (PEG 400, propylene glycol, benzyl alcohol 2%), boxes of 10 *Tubex. c-IV.*
Use: Anxiolytic.

•**atlafilcon A.** (at-LAH-FILL-kahn A) USAN.
Use: Contact lens material, hydrophilic.

ATnativ. (Bayer) Antithrombin III (human), lyophilized powder/500 units. Inj. Bot. 50 mL w/10 L sterile water. *Rx.*
Use: Thromboembolic. [Orphan Drug]

•**atolide.** (ATE-oh-lide) USAN. Under study.
Use: Anticonvulsant.

•**atomoxetine hydrochloride.** (AT-oh-mox-ah-teen) USAN.
Use: Psychotherapeutic agent.
See: Strattera.

atomoxetine hydrochloride. (Actavis Elizabeth) Atomoxetine 10 mg, 18 mg, 25 mg, 40 mg, 60 mg, 80 mg, 100 mg. Cap. 30s, 90s, 500s (100 mg only), 1,000s (except 100 mg). *Rx.*
Use: Psychotherapeutic agent.

•**atopaxar.** (A-toe-PAX-ar) USAN.
Use: Cardiovascular agent.

• **atopaxar hydrobromide.** (A-toe-PAX-ar) USAN.
Use: Cardiovascular agent.

Atopiclair. (Graceway Pharmaceuticals) Ethylhexyl palmitate, pentylene glycol, shea butter, caprylol glycine, glyceryl, PEG-100, arachidyl glucoside, behenyl alcohol, arachidyl alcohol, bisabolol, tocopheryl acetate (anti-oxidant), glycyrrhetinic acid, carbomer, ethylhexylglycerin, piroctone olamine, sodium hydroxide, allantoin, DMDM hydantoin, vitis vinifer, disodium EDTA, ascorbyl tetraisopalmitate, sodium hyaluronate, propyl gallate, parabens, telmesteine, butylene glycol. Cream. 100 g. *Rx.*
Use: Emollient, miscellaneous.

• **atorvastatin calcium.** (a-TORE-va-statin) USAN.
Use: HMG-CoA reductase inhibitor; antihyperlipidemic agent.
See: Lipitor.
W/Amlodipine Besylate.
See: Caduet.

• **atosiban.** (at-OH-sih-ban) USAN.
Use: Antagonist; oxytocin.

• **atovaquone.** (uh-TOE-vuh-KWONE) *USP 34.*
Use: Antipneumocystic.
See: Mepron.

atovaquone and proguanil hydrochloride.
Use: Antimalarial.
See: Malarone.
Malarone Pediatric.

Atozine. (Major) Hydroxyzine hydrochloride. 10 mg, 25 mg, 50 mg. Tab. Bot. 100s, 250s, 500s (50 mg only), 1000s (except 50 mg), UD 100s. *Rx.*
Use: Anxiolytic.

Atpeg. (AstraZeneca) Polyethylene glycol available as 300, 400, 600, or 4000.
Use: Humectant; surfactant.

• **atracurium besylate.** (AT-rah-CUE-ree-uhm BESS-ih-late) *USP 34.*
Use: Neuromuscular blocker; muscle relaxant.
See: Tracrium.

atracurium besylate. (Bedford Labs) Atracurium besylate 10 mg/mL. Inj. Single-dose vials. 5 mL. Multidose vials (benzyl alcohol 0.9%). 10 mL. *Rx.*
Use: Muscle relaxant.

Atralin. (Coria) Tretinoin 0.05%. Benzyl alcohol, parabens. Gel. 45 g. *Rx.*
Use: First-generation retinoid.

atrasentan.
Use: Investigational selective endothelin-A receptor antagonist.

• **atreleuton.** (at-reh-LOO-tuhn) USAN.
Use: Antiasthmatic.

Atridox. (CollaGenex) Doxycycline 42.5 mg (as hyclate, 10%). Inj. 2-syringe mixing system and blunt cannula. *Rx.*
Use: Mouth and throat product; tetracycline.

Atripla. (Bristol-Myers Squibb/Gilead Sciences) Efavirenz 600 mg, emtricitabine 200 mg, tenofovir disoproxil fumarate 300 mg (equiv. to tenofovir disproxil 245 mg). Film coated. Tab. 30s. *Rx.*
Use: Antiretroviral agent, non-nucleoside reverse transcriptase inhibitor.

Atrocap. (Freeport) Atropine sulfate 0.06 mg, hyoscyamine sulfate 0.3 mg, hyoscine hydrobromide 0.02 mg, phenobarbital 50 mg. TR Cap. Bot. 1000s. *Rx.*
Use: Anticholinergic; antispasmodic; hypnotic; sedative.

Atrocholin. (GlaxoSmithKline) Dehydrocholic acid 130 mg. Tab. Bot. 100s. *OTC.*
Use: Laxative.

Atrofed. (Genetco, Inc.) Pseudoephedrine hydrochloride 60 mg, triprolidine hydrochloride 2.5 mg. Tab. Bot. 24s, 100s, 1000s. *OTC.*
Use: Antihistamine; decongestant.

Atrohist LA. (Medeva) Pseudoephedrine hydrochloride 120 mg, brompheniramine maleate 4 mg, phenyltoloxamine citrate 50 mg. SR Tab with atropine sulfate 0.0242 mg available for immediate release. Bot. 100s. *Rx.*
Use: Antihistamine; decongestant.

Atrohist Pediatric Capsules. (Medeva) Chlorpheniramine maleate 4 mg, pseudoephedrine hydrochloride 60 mg. SR Cap. Bot. 100s. *Rx.*
Use: Antihistamine; decongestant.

Atrohist Pediatric Suspension. (Medeva) Phenylephrine tannate 5 mg, chlorpheniramine tannate 2 mg, pyrilamine tannate 12.5 mg. Susp. Bot. 473 mL. Unit-of-use 118 mL. *Rx.*
Use: Antihistamine; decongestant.

Atrohist Sprinkle. (Medeva) Pseudoephedrine hydrochloride 120 mg, brompheniramine maleate 2 mg, phenyltoloxamine citrate 25 mg. SR Cap. Bot. 100s. *Rx.*
Use: Antihistamine; decongestant.

AtroPen. (Meridian Medical Technologies) Atropine sulfate 0.5 mg, 1 mg, 2 mg. Glycerin, phenol. Inj. Auto-injectors prefilled. *Rx.*
Use: Gastrointestinal anticholinergic/antispasmodic.

•**atropine.** (AT-troe-peen) *USP 34.*
 Use: Anticholinergic.
atropine-hyoscine-hyoscyamine combinations. (Also see Belladonna Products).
 See: Barbella.
 Barbeloid.
 Belbutal No. 2 Kaptabs.
 Brobella-P.B.
 Spabelin.
 Spasmolin.
 Urogesic.
atropine-n-oxide hydrochloride.
 See: Atropine Oxide Hydrochloride.
•**atropine oxide hydrochloride.** (AT-rowpeen OX-ide) USAN.
 Use: Anticholinergic.
atropine/pralidoxime chloride.
 Use: Detoxification agent, antidote.
 See: DuoDote.
•**atropine sulfate.** (AT-row-peen) *USP 34.*
 Use: Anticholinergic/antispasmodic, ophthalmic.
 See: AtroPen.
 Atropine Sulfate S.O.P.
 Bellahist-D LA.
 Sal-Tropine.
 W/Benzoic Acid, Hyoscyamine Sulfate, Methenamine, Methylene Blue, Phenyl Salicylate.
 See: Uritact DS.
 W/Chlorpheniramine Maleate, Hyoscyamine Sulfate, Phenylephrine Hydrochloride, Scopolamine Hydrobromide.
 See: Bellahist-D LA.
 W/Chlorpheniramine Maleate, Hyoscyamine Sulfate, Pseudoephedrine Hydrochloride, Scopolamine Hydrobromide.
 See: Respa A.R.
 Stahist.
 W/Hyoscyamine Hydrobromide or Sulfate, Phenobarbital, Scopolamine Hydrobromide.
 See: Antispasmodic.
 Belladonna Alkaloids with Phenobarbital.
 Bellatal.
 Donnatal.
 Donnatal Extentabs.
 PB-Hyos.
 Quadrapax.
 W/Phenobarbital.
 See: Antrocol.
 Barbeloid.
 Brobella-P.B.
 Donnatal.
 Palbar No. 2.
 Spabelin.
atropine sulfate. (Hospira) Atropine sulfate 0.05 mg/mL, 0.1 mg/mL. *Abboject*

syringes. 5 mL, 10 mL (0.1 mg/mL only). *Rx.*
 Use: Anticholinergic/antispasmodic.
atropine sulfate. (Various Mfr.). Atropine sulfate 0.3 mg/mL. Vial 1 mL, 30 mL; 0.4 mg/mL. Amp. 1 mL, vial 20 mL, 30 mL; 0.5 mg/mL. Vials. 1 mL, 30 mL. Syringes. 5 mL; 0.8 mg/mL. Amp. 0.5 mL, 1 mL. Syringes. 0.5 mL; 1 mg/mL. Amp., vial 1 mL, syringe 10 mL Inj. *Rx.*
 Use: Gastrointestinal anticholinergic/antispasmodic, belladonna alkaloid.
atropine sulfate. (Various Mfr.) Atropine sulfate. **Oint:** 1%. 3.5 g, UD 1 g. **Soln.:** 1%. 2 mL, 5 mL, 15 mL, UD 1 mL. *Rx.*
 Use: Ophthalmic and otic agent, cycloplegic mydriatic.
atropine sulfate and edrophonium chloride. Anticholinesterase muscle stimulant.
 See: Enlon-Plus.
atropine sulfate S.O.P. (Allergan) Atropine sulfate 0.5%, 1%. Oint. Tube 3.5 g. *Rx.*
 Use: Cycloplegic; mydriatic.
Atrosed. (Freeport) Atropine sulfate 0.0195 mg, hyoscine HBr 0.0065 mg, hyoscyamine sulfate 0.104 mg, phenobarbital 0.25 g. Tab. Bot. 1000s, 5000s. *Rx.*
 Use: Anticholinergic; antispasmodic; hypnotic; sedative.
Atrosept. (Geneva) Methenamine 40.8 mg, phenyl salicylate 18.1 mg, atropine sulfate 0.03 mg, hyoscyamine 0.03 mg, benzoic acid 4.5 mg, methylene blue 5.4 mg. Tab. Bot. 100s, 1000s. *Rx.*
 Use: Anti-infective, urinary.
Atrovent. (Boehringer Ingelheim) Ipratropium bromide 0.03% (21 mcg/spray). Nasal Spray. Bot. with spray pump. 30 mL (345 sprays); 0.06% (42 mcg/spray). Bot. with spray pump. 15 mL (165 sprays). *Rx.*
 Use: Bronchodilator.
Atrovent HFA. (Boehringer Ingelheim) Ipratropium bromide 17 mcg per actuation. Aerosol. 12.9 g metered-dose inhaler with mouthpiece (200 inhalations). *Rx.*
 Use: Bronchodilator.
ATryn. (Ovation) Antithrombin 1,750 units (recombinant). Sodium chloride 79 mg, sodium citrate 26 mg. Preservative free. Inj., lyophilized Pow. for Soln. Single-dose vial. *Rx.*
 Use: Anticoagulant, antithrombin agent.
A/T/S. (Medicis) Erythromycin. **Gel:** 2%. Alcohol 92%. Tubes. 30 g. **Top. Soln.:**

2%. Alcohol 66%. Bot. 60 mL. *Rx.*
Use: Topical anti-infective, antibiotic.

AT-Solution. (Sanofi-Synthelabo) Dihydrotachysterol solution.
Use: Antihypocalcemic.

Attain. (Sherwood Davis & Geck) Sodium caseinate, calcium caseinate, maltodextrin, corn oil, soy lecithin. Liq. Can 250 mL and 1000 mL closed system. *OTC.*
Use: Nutritional supplement.

•**attapulgite, activated.** (at-ah-PULL-gyte) *USP 34.*
Use: Antidiarrheal; pharmaceutic aid, suspending agent.
W/Pectin, hydrated alumina.
See: Sebasorb.

A.T. 10.
See: Dihydrotachysterol.

Attenuvax. (Merck & Co.) Measles virus vaccine, live, attenuated $\geq$ 1,000 TCID$_{50}$ (tissue culture infectious doses) per 0.5 mL dose, neomycin 25 mcg, sorbitol 14.5 mg, sucrose 1.9 mg, hydrolyzed gelatin 14.5 mg, human albumin 0.3 mg, fetal bovine serum < 1 ppm per dose, preservative free. Single-dose vial w/diluent, 50-dose vial w/30 mL diluent. *Rx.*
Use: Immunization.
W/Mumpsvax, Meruvax.
See: M-M-R II.

Atuss DS Tannate. (Atley) Dextromethorphan HBr 30 mg (equiv. to dextromethorphan tannate 60 mg), chlorpheniramine maleate 4 mg (equiv. to chlorpheniramine tannate 8 mg), pseudoephedrine hydrochloride 30 mg (equiv. to pseudoephedrine tannate 60 mg) per 5 mL. Acesulfame K, aspartame, methylparaben, phenylalanine 25.25 mg per 5 mL, sucralose. Grape bubblegum flavor. Susp. 473 mL. *Rx.*
Use: Antitussive combination, upper respiratory combination.

Atuss-12 DM. (Atley) Pseudoephedrine hydrochloride (as polistirex) 30 mg, chlorpheniramine maleate (as polistirex) 6 mg, dextromethorphan HBr (as polistirex) 30 mg/5 mL. Corn syrup, parabens. ER Susp. 20 mL, 473 mL. *Rx.*
Use: Pediatric antitussive combination.

Atuss-12 DX. (Atley) Dextromethorphan polistirex (equiv. to dextromethorphan HBr 30 mg), guaifenesin 200 mg/5 mL. Parabens, honey. Honey-lemon flavor. ER Susp. 20 mL, 473 mL. *Rx.*
Use: Antitussive, expectorant.

augmented betamethasone dipropionate.
Use: Corticosteroid, topical.
See: Diprolene.

Augmentin. (GlaxoSmithKline) **Tab.:** Amoxicillin/clavulanic acid (as the potassium salt) 250 mg/125 mg, 500 mg/125 mg, 875 mg/125 mg. PEG, potassium 0.63 mEq. Film coated (except 875 mg). Bot. 20s (except 250 mg), 30s (250 mg only), UD 100s. **Chew. Tab.:** Amoxicillin/clavulanic acid (as the potassium salt) 200 mg/28.5 mg (potassium 0.14 mEq, mannitol, saccharin, aspartame, cherry-banana flavor, phenylalanine 2.1 mg), 400 mg/57 mg (potassium 0.29 mEq, mannitol, phenylalanine 4.2 mg, saccharin, aspartame, cherry-banana flavor). Bot. 20s. **Pow. for Oral Susp.:** Amoxicillin/clavulanic acid (as the potassium salt) 125 mg/31.25 mg per 5 mL (potassium 0.16 mEq/5 mL, mannitol, saccharin, banana flavor), 250 mg/62.5 mg per 5 mL (potassium 0.32 mEq/5 mL, mannitol, saccharin, orange flavor), 400 mg/57 mg per 5 mL (potassium 0.29 mEq/5 mL, mannitol, phenylalanine 7 mg/5 mL, saccharin, aspartame, orange flavor). Bot. 50 mL (except 250 mg/62.5 mg), 75 mL, 100 mL, 150 mL (250 mg/62.5 mg only). *Rx.*
Use: Aminopenicillin, penicillin.

Augmentin ES-600. (GlaxoSmithKline) Amoxicillin 600 mg/clavulanic acid (as the potassium salt) 42.9 mg/5 mL. Potassium 0.23 mEq/5 mL, aspartame, phenylalanine 7 mg/5 mL. Strawberry cream flavor. Pow. for Oral Susp. Bot. 75 mL, 125 mL, 200 mL. *Rx.*
Use: Aminopenicillin, penicillin.

Augmentin XR. (GlaxoSmithKline) Amoxicillin 1000 mg, clavulanic acid 62.5 mg. Potassium 0.32 mEq, sodium 1.27 mEq, PEG. Film coated. ER Tab. Pkg. 28s (7-day XR pack), 40s (10-day XR pack). *Rx.*
Use: Aminopenicillin, penicillin.

Auralgan. (Deston) Antipyrine 5.4%, benzocaine 1.4%, u-polycosanol 410 alcohol 0.0097%. Acetic acid, glycerin. Otic Soln. 14 mL with dropper. *Rx.*
Use: Miscellaneous otic preparation.

Auralgesic. (Wesley) Carbamide 10%, antipyrine 5%, benzocaine 2.5%, cetyldimethylbenzylammonium hydrochloride 0.2%. Bot. 0.5 oz. *Rx.*
Use: Otic.

•**auranofin.** (or-RAIN-oh-fin) *USAN.*
Use: Antirheumatic.
See: Ridaura.

Aureoquin Diamate. *Name previously used for Quinetolate.*

Aurinol Ear Drops. (Various Mfr.) Chloroxylenol and acetic acid, w/benzal-

konium chloride and glycerin. Soln. Bot. 15 mL. *Rx.*
Use: Otic.

Aurocein. (Christina) Gold naphthyl sulfhydryl derivative 5%, 12.5%. Inj. Amp. 10 mL. *Rx.*
Use: Antirheumatic.

Auro-Dri. (Commerce) Boric acid 2.75% in isopropyl alcohol. Soln. 30 mL with dropper. *OTC.*
Use: Otic preparation.

Auro Ear Drops. (Commerce) Carbamide peroxide 6.5% in an anhydrous glycerine base. Soln. 15 mL. *OTC.*
Use: Otic.

Auroguard Otic. (SDA) Benzocaine 1.4%, antipyrine 5.4%, glycerin, oxyquinolone sulfate. Soln. 15 mL. *Rx.*
Use: Otic preparation.

Aurolate. (Taylor Pharmaceuticals) Gold sodium thiomalate 50 mg, benzyl alcohol 0.5%/mL. Inj. Vial 2 mL, 10 mL. *Rx.*
Use: Antirheumatic.

aurolin.
See: Gold sodium thiosulfate.

auropin.
See: Gold sodium thiosulfate.

aurosan.
See: Gold sodium thiosulfate.

•**aurothioglucose.** (or-oh-THIGH-oh-GLUE-kose) *USP 34.*
Use: Antirheumatic.

aurothiomalate, sodium.
See: Gold Sodium Thiomalate.

Ausab. (Abbott Diagnostics) Radioimmunoassay or enzyme immunoassay for detection of antibody to hepatitis B surface antigen. Test kit 100s.
Use: Diagnostic aid.

Ausab EIA. (Abbott Diagnostics) Enzyme immunoassay for the detection of antibody to hepatitis B surface antigen.
Use: Diagnostic aid.

Auscell. (Abbott Diagnostics) Reverse passive hemagglutination test for hepatitis B surface antigen. Test kit 110s, 450s, 1800s.
Use: Diagnostic aid.

Ausria II-125. (Abbott Diagnostics) Radioimmunoassay for detection of hepatitis B surface antigen. Test kit 100s, 500s, 600s, 700s, 800s, 900s, 1000s.
Use: Diagnostic aid.

Auszyme II. (Abbott Diagnostics) Enzyme immunoassay for detection of hepatitis B surface antigen (HBsAg) in human serum or plasma. Test kit 100s, 500s.
Use: Diagnostic aid.

Auszyme Monoclonal. (Abbott Diagnostics) Qualitative third generation enzyme immunoassay for the detection of hepatitis B surface antigen (HBsAg) in human serum or plasma.
Use: Diagnostic aid.

Autoantibody Screen. (Wampole) Autoantibody screening system. To screen serum for the presence of a variety of autoantibodies. Test 48s.
Use: Diagnostic aid.

Autolet Kit. (Bayer Consumer Care) Automatic bloodletting spring-loaded device to obtain capillary blood samples from fingertips, ear lobes, or heels.
Use: Diagnostic aid.

autolymphocyte therapy; ALT. (Cellcor, Inc.)
Use: Treatment of renal cancer. [Orphan Drug]

Autrinic. Intrinsic factor concentrate. *Rx.*
Use: To increase absorption of vitamin B_{12}.

Auxotab Enteric 1 & 2. (Colab) Rapid identification of enteric bacteria and *Pseudomonas.* Test contains capillary units with selective biochemical reagents.
Use: Diagnostic aid.

•**avagacestat.** (A-va-GAY-se-stat) USAN.
Use: CNS agent.

Avage. (Allergan) Tazarotene 0.1%, benzyl alcohol 1%, EDTA, medium chain triglycerides, mineral oil. Cream. 15 g, 30 g. *Rx.*
Use: Retinoid.

Avail. (Menley & James Labs, Inc.) Iron 18 mg, vitamin A 5000 units, D 400 units, E 30 mg, B_1 2.25 mg, B_2 2.55 mg, B_3 20 mg, B_6 3 mg, B_{12} 9 mcg, C 90 mg, folic acid 0.4 mg, Ca, Cr, I, Mg, Se, Zn 22.5 mg. Tab. Bot. 60s. *OTC.*
Use: Mineral, vitamin supplement.

Avalgesic. (Various Mfr.) Methyl salicylate, menthol, camphor, methylnicotinate, dipropylene glycol salicylate, oil of cassia, oleoresins capsicum, ginger. Bot. 120 mL, Pt, gal. *OTC.*
Use: Analgesic, topical.

Avalide. (Bristol-Myers Squibb) Irbesartan/hydrochlorothiazide 150 mg/12.5 mg, 300 mg/12.5 mg, 300 mg/25 mg (film coated). Lactose. Tab. Bot. 30s, 90s; 500s, blister pack 100s (except 300 mg/25 mg). *Rx.*
Use: Antihypertensive.

A-Van. (Stewart-Jackson Pharmacal) Dimenhydrinate 50 mg. Cap. Bot. 100s.
Use: Antivertigo.

•**avanafil.** (av-AN-a-fil) USAN.
Use: Erectile dysfunction.

Avandamet. (GlaxoSmithKline) Rosiglitazone maleate/metformin hydrochloride 2 mg/500 mg, 4 mg/500 mg, 2 mg/1000 mg, 4 mg/1000 mg. Lactose, polyethylene glycol 400. Film coated. Tab. Bot. 60s. *Rx.*
Use: Antidiabetic combination.

Avandaryl. (GlaxoSmithKline) Rosiglitazone (as rosiglitazone maleate) and glimepiride 4 mg/1 mg, 4 mg/2 mg, 4 mg/4 mg, 8 mg/2 mg, 8 mg/4 mg. Lactose, PEG. Tab. 30s. *Rx.*
Use: Antidiabetic combination.

Avandia. (GlaxoSmithKline) Rosiglitazone maleate 2 mg, 4 mg, 8 mg. Lactose, PEG 3000. Film coated. Tab. Bot. 30s (except 2 mg), 60s (2 mg only), 90s (except 2 mg). *Rx.*
Use: Antidiabetic, thiazolidinedione.

Avapro. (Bristol-Myers Squibb Sanofi-Synthelabo Partnership) Irbesartan 75 mg, 150 mg, 300 mg. Lactose. Tab. Bot. 30s, 90s, 500s (except 75 mg), UD 100s (150 mg only). *Rx.*
Use: Renin angiotensin system antagonist, angiotensin II receptor antagonist.

Avar. (Kylemore) **Cleanser:** Sulfur 5%, sodium sulfacetamide 10%, cetyl alcohol, stearyl alcohol. 226.8 g. **Gel:** Sulfur 5%, sodium sulfacetamide 10%, EDTA, benzyl alcohol. 45 g. *Rx.*
Use: Keratolytic agent.

Avar-e Emollient. (Kylemore) Sulfur 5%, sodium sulfacetamide 10%, glycerin, EDTA, benzyl alcohol, cetyl alcohol. Cream. 45 g. *Rx.*
Use: Acne product.

Avar-e Green. (Kylemore) Sulfur 5%, sodium sulfacetamide 10%, glycerin, EDTA, benzyl alcohol, cetyl alcohol. For color correction. Cream. 45 g. *Rx.*
Use: Acne product.

Avar-e LS. (Kylemore) Sodium sulfacetamide 10%, sulfur 2%. Benzyl alcohol, cetyl alcohol, disodium EDTA, glycerin, glyceryl, PEG 100, phenoxyethanol, polawax, zinc oxide. Cream. 45 g. *Rx.*
Use: Acne product combination.

Avar LS Cleanser. (Kylemore) Sodium sulfacetamide 10%, sulfur 2%. Benzyl alcohol, cetyl alcohol, phenoxyethanol, propylene glycol, stearyl alcohol. Soap. 226.8 g. *Rx.*
Use: Acne production combination.

• **avasimibe.** (av-ASS-ih-mibe) USAN.
Use: Antiatherosclerotic; hypolipidemic (acylCoA: Cholesterol acyltransferase [ACAT] inhibitor).

Avastin. (Genentech) Bevacizumab 25 mg/mL. Preservative-free. Inj., Soln.,
Conc. Single-use vials. 4 mL (with α, α-trehalose dihydrate 240 mg, sodium phosphate [monobasic] 23.3 mg, sodium phosphate [dibasic] 4.8 mg), 16 mL (with α, α-trehalose dihydrate 960 mg, sodium phosphate [monobasic] 92.8 mg, sodium phosphate [dibasic] 19.2 mg). *Rx.*
Use: Monoclonal antibody.

Aveeno Anti-Itch. (J & J Consumer) Calamine 3%, pramoxine hydrochloride 1%. Camphor, cetyl alcohol, petrolatum. Cream. 28 g. *OTC.*
Use: Poison ivy treatment.

Aveeno Baby. (J & J Consumer) Dimethicone 1.2%. Benzyl alcohol, cetyl alcohol, glycerin, petrolatum. Lot. 227 mL. *OTC.*
Use: Emollient.

Aveenobar Medicated. (Rydelle) Aveeno colloidal oatmeal 50%, sulfur 2%, salicylic acid 2%, in soap-free cleansing bar. *Formerly Acnaveen.* Bar 3.5 oz. *OTC.*
Use: Antipruritic.

Aveenobar Oilated. (Rydelle) Vegetable oils, lanolin derivative, glycerine 29%, aveeno colloidal oatmeal 30% in soap-free base. *Formerly Emulave.* Bar. 3 oz. *OTC.*
Use: Emollient.

Aveenobar Regular. (Rydelle) Colloidal oatmeal 50%, an ionic sulfonate, hypoallergenic lanolin. *Formerly Aveeno Bar.* Bar 3.2 oz., 4.4 oz. *OTC.*
Use: Dermatologic; cleanser.

Aveeno Bath. (J & J Consumer) Colloidal oatmeal. Box 1 lb, 4 lb. *OTC.*
Use: Emollient.

Aveeno Cleansing Bar. (Rydelle) **Combination Skin:** Soap free. Colloidal oatmeal 51%, sodium cocoyl isethionate, glycerin, lactic acid, sodium lactate, petrolatum, magnesium aluminum silicate, potassium sorbate, titanium dioxide, PEG 14M. Bar 90 g. **Dry Skin:** Soap free. Colloidal oatmeal 51%, sodium cocoyl isethionate, vegetable oil and shortening, glycerin, PEG-75, lauramide DEA, lactic acid, sodium lactate, sorbic acid, titanium dioxide. Bar 90 g. *OTC.*
Use: Dermatologic; cleanser.

Aveeno Colloidal Oatmeal. (Rydelle) Colloidal oatmeal. Box 1 lb, 4 lb. *OTC.*
Use: Emollient.

Aveeno Daily Moisturizing. (J & J Consumer) Dimethicone 1.25%. Benzyl alcohol, cetyl alcohol, glycerin, petrolatum. Lot. 354 mL. *OTC.*
Use: Emollient.

Aveeno Dry. (Rydelle) Dry skin formula, soap free, emollient colloidal oatmeal, vegetable oils, lanolin derivative, and glycerin 29% in mild surfactant base. Cleansing bar 90 g. *OTC.*
Use: Dermatologic; cleanser.

Aveeno Lotion. (J & J Consumer) Colloidal oatmeal 1%, glycerin, petrolatum, dimethicone, phenylcarbinol. Lot. Bot. 354 mL. *OTC.*
Use: Emollient.

Aveeno Moisturizing Cream. (J & J Consumer) Colloidal oatmeal, glycerin, petrolatum, dimethicone, phenylcarbinol. Cream. Tube 120 g. *OTC.*
Use: Emollient.

Aveeno Normal. (J & J Consumer) Normal to oily skin formula, soap free. Colloidal oatmeal 50%, lanolin derivative and mild surfactant. Cleansing bar 96 g, 132 g. *OTC.*
Use: Dermatologic; cleanser.

Aveeno Oilated. (Rydelle) Aveeno colloidal oatmeal impregnated with 35% liquid petrolatum, refined olive oil. Box 8 oz, 2 lb. *OTC.*
Use: Emollient.

Aveeno Shave. (J & J Consumer) Oatmeal flour. Gel. Can 210 g. *OTC.*
Use: Emollient.

Aveeno Shower & Bath. (J & J Consumer) Colloidal oatmeal, 5% mineral oil, laureth-4, silica benzaldehyde. Oil. Bot. 240 mL. *OTC.*
Use: Emollient.

Avelox. (Schering-Plough) Moxifloxacin hydrochloride 400 mg, lactose. Tab. Bot. 30s, UD 50s, *ABC* Packs of 5. *Rx.*
Use: Anti-infective; fluoroquinolone.

Avelox I.V. (Schering-Plough) Moxifloxacin hydrochloride 400 mg per 250 mL. Sodium chloride 0.8%. Preservative free. Premix Inj. Flexible bag (latex free) 250 mL. *Rx.*
Use: Anti-infective, fluoroquinolone.

Aventyl Hydrochloride Pulvules. (Eli Lilly) Nortriptyline hydrochloride 25 mg. Cap. Bot. 100s, 500s. *Rx.*
Use: Antidepressant.

Aviane. (Barr) Ethinyl estradiol 20 mcg, levonorgestrel 0.1 mg. Lactose. Tab. Pkg. 28s with 7 inert tabs. *Rx.*
Use: Sex hormone, contraceptive hormone.

•**avilamycin.** (ah-VILL-ah-MY-sin) USAN.
Use: Anti-infective.

Avinar. Uredepa.
Use: Antineoplastic.

Avinza. (King Pharmaceuticals) Morphine sulfate 30 mg, 45 mg, 60 mg, 75 mg, 90 mg, 120 mg (for use only in opioid-tolerant patients). Sugar starch spheres, fumaric acid. ER Pellets Cap. 100s. *c-ii.*
Tall Man: AVINza
Use: Opioid analgesic.

Avita. (Bertek) Tretinoin. **Cream:** 0.025%, stearyl alcohol. Tube 20 g, 45 g. **Gel:** 0.025%, ethanol 83%. Tube. 20 g, 45 g. *Rx.*
Use: Dermatologic, retinoid.

•**avitriptan fumarate.** (av-ih-TRIP-tan FEW-mah-rate) USAN.
Use: Antimigraine.

•**avobenzone.** (AV-ah-BENZ-ohn) USAN.
Use: Sunscreen.
W/Combinations.
See: PreSun Ultra.
  TI-Screen Sports.
W/Ecamsule, Octocrylene.
See: Anthelios SX.
  UV Protective.
W/Ecamsule, Octocrylene, Titanium Dioxide.
See: Capital Soleil 20.
W/Homosalate, Octisalate, Octocrylene, Oxybenzone.
See: Neutrogena Ultra Sheer Dry-Touch Sunblock.
W/Mexoryl SX, Octocrylene, Titanium Dioxide.
See: Anthelios 40.

Avodart. (GlaxoSmithKline) Dutasteride 0.5 mg. Cap. 30s, 90s. *Rx.*
Use: Sex hormone, androgen hormone inhibitor.

Avonex. (Biogen Idec) **Pow. for Inj., lyophilized:** Interferon beta-1A 33 mcg (6.6 million units [30 mcg/vial when reconstituted]). Albumin human 16.5 mg, sodium chloride 6.4 mg, dibasic sodium phosphate 6.3 mg, monobasic sodium phosphate 1.3 mg/vial. Preservative free. In Administration Dose Packs (single-use vial w/diluent [Sterile Water for Injection], alcohol wipes, gauze pad, syringe, *MicroPin* vial access pin, needle, and bandage). **Prefilled Syringe:** 30 mcg/0.5 mL. Albumin-free. Sodium acetate trihydrate 0.79 mg, glacial acetic acid 0.25 mg, arginine hydrochloride 15.8 mg, polysorbate 20 0.025 mg in water for injection. Administration dose packs (single-use syringe, needle, reclosable accessory pouch, alcohol wipes, gauze pads, and bandages). *Rx.*
Use: Immunologic agent, immunomodulator.

Avonique. (Armenpharm Ltd.) Vitamins A 4000 units, D 400 units, B$_1$ 1 mg, B$_2$ 1.2 mg, B$_6$ 2 mg, B$_{12}$ 2 mcg, calcium pantothenate 5 mg, B$_3$ 10 mg, C 30 mg, calcium 100 mg, phosphorus 76 mg,

iron 10 mg, manganese 1 mg, magnesium 1 mg, zinc 1 mg. *OTC.*
Use: Mineral, vitamin supplement.

•**avoparcin.** (AVE-oh-PAR-sin) USAN.
Use: Anti-infective.

Avosil. (Avocet) BHT 0.2%, parabens 0.3%, PEG, sodium salicylate 2%. Oint. 56.7 g. *OTC.*
Use: Dermatological agent.

•**avridine.** (AV-rih-deen) USAN.
Use: Antiviral.

Awake. (Walgreens) Caffeine 100 mg. Tab. Bot. 36s. *OTC.*
Use: CNS stimulant.

axerophthol.
See: Vitamin A.

Axert. (Ortho-McNeil) Almotriptan malate 6.25 mg, 12.5 mg. Mannitol. Tab. UD 6s (6.25 mg), 12s (12.5 mg). *Rx.*
Use: Antimigraine agent, serotonin 5-HT$_1$ receptor agonist.

Axid. (Braintree) Nizatidine 15 mg/mL. Parabens, saccharin, sucrose. Bubble gum flavor. Oral Soln. 480 mL. *Rx.*
Use: Histamine H$_2$ antagonist.

Axid AR. (Wyeth Consumer) Nizatidine 75 mg. Tab. Bot. 12s, 30s. *OTC.*
Use: Histamine H$_2$ antagonist.

Axid Pulvules. (GlaxoSmithKline) Nizatidine 150 mg. Cap. 60s. *Rx.*
Use: Histamine H$_2$ antagonist.

Axiron. (Lilly) Testosterone 30 mg per 1.5 mL. Ethanol, isopropyl alcohol. Soln. 110 mL metered-dose pump w/ applicator (each metered-dose pump delivers 60 metered 30 mg doses). *c-III.*
Use: Sex hormone, androgen.

•**axitinib.** (AX-i-TI-nib) USAN.
Use: Antineoplastic.

•**axitirome.** (ax-i-TYE-rome) USAN.
Use: Hypolipidemic.

•**axomadol.** (ax-OH-ma-dole) USAN.
Use: Analgesic.

Axona. (Accera) Caprylidene 40 g (20 g medium-chain triglycerides). Acesulfame potassium, sucralose. Vanilla flavor. 40 g packets. 30s (also contains potassium caseinate [milk-derived protein]), maltodextrin, whey protein [milk-derived], sugar, sunflower oil, dimagnesium phosphate, tricalcium phosphate, dipotassium phosphate, soy lecithin, distilled monoglyceride, sodium ascorbate [vitamin C], silicon dioxide, natural vanilla bean extract, vitamin E acetate, vitamin A palmitate, zinc sulfate, pyridoxine hydrochloride [vitamin B$_6$], folic acid, and chromium chloride). *Rx.*
Use: Nutritional supplement.

Axsain. (Rodlen Labs) Capsaicin 0.25% in an emollient base, lidocaine, alcohols, white petrolatum. Cream. 60 g. *OTC.*
Use: Counterirritant.

Aygestin. (Duramed) Norethindrone acetate 5 mg. Lactose. Tab. Bot. 50s, blister pack 10s. *Rx.*
Use: Sex hormone, progestin.

Ayr Saline. (B.F. Ascher) Sodium chloride 0.65%, benzalkonium chloride, EDTA. Soln. **Drops:** Bot. 5 mL. **Gel:** Aloe vera gel, glycerin, parabens. Tube. 14 g. **Mist:** Bot. 50 mL. *OTC.*
Use: Dermatologic; moisturizer.

•**azabon.** (AZE-ah-bahn) USAN.
Use: CNS stimulant.

•**azacitidine.** (AZE-ah-SIGH-tih-deen) USAN. *Formerly Ladakamycin.*
Tall Man: azaCITIDine
Use: DNA demethylation agent.
See: Vidaza.

•**azaclorzine hydrochloride.** (AZE-ah-KLOR-zeen) USAN. *Formerly Nonachlazine.*
Use: Coronary vasodilator.

•**azaconazole.** (AZE-ah-CONE-ah-zole) USAN. *Formerly Azoconazole.*
Use: Antifungal.

AZA-CR. NCI Investigational agent.
See: Azacitidine.

Azactam. (Bristol-Myers Squibb) Aztreonam 500 mg, 1 g, 2 g (≈ 780 mg L-arginine/g of aztreonam). Pow. for Inj. (lyophilized cake). Single-dose vial 15 mL (500 mg, 1 g), 30 mL (2 g only); Single-dose infusion bot. 100 mL (1 g and 2 g). *Rx.*
Use: Anti-infective.

•**azalanstat dihydrochloride.** (aze-ah-LAN-stat) USAN.
Use: Hypolipidemic.

Azaline. (Major) Sulfasalazine 500 mg. Tab. Bot. 100s, 500s, 1000s.
Use: Anti-inflammatory.

•**azaloxan fumarate.** (aze-ah-LOX-ahn) USAN.
Use: Antidepressant.

•**azanator maleate.** (AZE-an-nay-tore) USAN.
Use: Bronchodilator.

•**azanidazole.** (AZE-ah-NIH-dah-zole) USAN.
Use: Antiprotozoal.

•**azaperone.** (AZE-app-eh-RONE) USP 34.
Use: Antipsychotic.

•**azaribine.** (aze-ah-RYE-bean) USAN.
Use: Dermatologic.

•**azarole.** (AZE-ah-role) USAN.
Use: Immunoregulator.

Azasan. (Various Mfr.) Azathioprine
25 mg, 50 mg, 75 mg, 100 mg. Lactose.
Tab. 100s. *Rx.*
Use: Immunosuppressant.

•**azaserine.** (AZE-ah-SER-een) USAN.
Use: Antifungal.

AzaSite. (Inspire) Azithromycin 1%.
EDTA, benzalkonium chloride 0.003%,
sodium chloride, sodium citrate, po-
loxamer 407, polycarbophil. Ophth.
Soln. 2.5 mL. *Rx.*
Use: Ophthalmic antibiotic.

•**azatadine maleate.** (aze-AT-ad-EEN)
USP 34.
Use: Antihistamine.
See: Optimine.
W/Combinations.
See: Rynatan.

•**azathioprine.** (AZE-uh-THIGH-oh-preen)
USP 34.
Tall Man: azaTHIOprine
Use: Immunosuppressant.
See: Azasan.
Imuran.

azathioprine. (aaiPharma) Azathioprine
50 mg. Tab. 100s. *Rx.*
Use: Immunosuppressant.

azathioprine sodium. (Various Mfr.) Aza-
thioprine sodium 100 mg. Pow. for Inj.
Vial. 20 mL. *Rx.*
Use: Antileukemic.

•**azathioprine sodium for injection.**
(AZE-uh-THIGH-oh-preen) *USP 34.*
Use: Immunosuppressant.

5-aza-2′-deoxycytidine.
Use: Treatment of acute leukemia.
[Orphan Drug]

5-AZC.
See: Azacitidine.

Azdone. (Schwarz Pharma) Hydro-
codone bitartrate 5 mg, aspirin 500 mg.
Tab. Bot. 100s, 1000s. *c-III.*
Use: Analgesic combination, narcotic.

•**azelaic acid.** (aze-eh-LAY-ik) USAN.
Use: Dermatologic; acne.
See: Azelex.
Finacea.
Finevin.

•**azelastine.** (ah-ZELL-ass-teen) USAN.
Use: Antiallergic, antiasthmatic, anti-
histamine, peripherally selective
phthalazinone.
See: Astelin.
Astepro.
Optivar.

azelastine hydrochloride. (Apotex) Azelastine hydrochloride 0.1%. Benzalkonium chloride, edetate disodium.

Spray, Soln., intranasal. 137 mcg
(200 metered sprays). *Rx.*
Use: Respiratory inhalant, intranasal
antihistamine.

azelastine hydrochloride. (Various Mfr.)
Azelastine hydrochloride 0.05% (equiv.
to azelastine 0.457 mg). Benzalkonium
chloride 0.25 mg, disodium edetate dihydrate, hydroxypropylmethylcellulose,
sodium hydroxide. Soln., Ophth. 6 mL
w/dropper. *Rx.*
Use: Ophthalmic antihistamine.

Azelex. (Allergan) Azelaic acid 20%, gly-
cerin, cetearyl alcohol, benzoic acid.
Cream. Tube 30 g, 50 g. *Rx.*
Use: Dermatologic, acne.

•**azepindole.** (AZE-eh-PIN-dole) USAN.
Use: Antidepressant.

•**azetepa.** (AZE-eh-teh-pah) USAN.
Use: Antineoplastic.

•**azficel-T.** (az-FYE-sel) USAN.
Use: Treatment of nasolabial fold
wrinkles.

azidothymidine.
See: Zidovudine.

•**3-azido-2, 3 dideoxyuridine.** USAN.
Use: Antiviral, HIV.

Azidouridine. (Berlex) Phase I HIV-posi-
tive symptomatic, ARC, AIDS. *Rx.*
Use: Antiviral.

Azilect. (Teva) Rasagiline (as base)
0.5 mg, 1 mg. Mannitol. Tab. 30s. *Rx.*
Use: Antiparkinson agent.

•**azilsartan medoxomil.** (AY-zil-SAR-tan
me-DOX-oh-mil) USAN.
Use: Angiotensin II receptor antagonist.
See: Edarbi.

•**azimilide dihydrochloride.** (azz-IM-ih-
lide die-HIGH-droe-KLOR-ide) USAN.
Use: Cardiovascular agent.

•**azipramine hydrochloride.** (aze-IPP-
RAH-meen) USAN.
Use: Antidepressant.

•**azithromycin.** (UHZ-ith-row-MY-sin)
USP 34.
Use: Anti-infective, macrolide; ophthal-
mic antibiotic.
See: AzaSite.
Zithromax.
ZMax.

azithromycin. (Baxter) Azithromycin
500 mg. Pow. for Inj., lyophilized. Vials.
10 mL. *Rx.*
Use: Macrolide, anti-infective.

azithromycin. (Greenstone) Azithromycin (as azithromycin dihydrate)
100 mg/5 mL and 200 mg/5 mL when
reconstituted, 1 g/packet. Sucrose.
Cherry/banana/creme de vanilla flavors
(100 mg/5 mL and 200 mg/5 mL),

cherry/banana flavor (1 g/packet). Pow.
for Susp. 15 mL, 22.5 mL (200 mg/mL),
30 mL (200 mg/mL). Single-dose
packet. 3s, 10s (1 g/packet). *Rx.*
Use: Macrolide.
azithromycin. (Various Mfr.) Azithromycin 250 mg, 500 mg, 600 mg. May
contain lactose. Tab. 1s (250 mg); 3s,
6s (250 mg and 500 mg); 30s; UD 9s
(500 mg); UD 18s (250 mg); UD 50s
(250 mg and 500 mg); UD 100s
(250 mg). *Rx.*
Use: Macrolide.
•**azlocillin.** (AZZ-low-SILL-in) USAN.
Use: Anti-infective.
Azma-Aid. (Purepac) Theophylline
118 mg, ephedrine 24 mg, phenobarbital 8 mg. Tab. Bot. 100s, 250s, 1000s.
Rx.
Use: Bronchodilator.
Azmacort. (Kos) Triamcinolone acetonide 75 mcg/actuation. Aerosol Susp.
Inhalation. 20 g w/actuator (≥ 240 me-
tered doses). *Rx.*
Use: Respiratory inhalant, corticoste-
roid.
azoconazole.
See: Azaconazole.
Azodyne Hydrochloride.
See: Pyridium.
•**azolimine.** (aze-OLE-ih-meen) USAN.
Use: Diuretic.
AZO Negacide. (Sanofi-Synthelabo)
Nalidixic acid, phenazopyridine hydro-
chloride. Tab. *Rx.*
Use: Anti-infective, urinary.
AZO-100. (Scruggs) Phenylazodiamino-
pyridine hydrochloride 100 mg. Tab.
Bot. 100s, 1000s. *OTC.*
Use: Analgesic, urinary.
Azopt. (Alcon) Brinzolamide 1%. Benzal-
konium chloride 0.01%, mannitol, car-
bomer 974P tyloxapol, sodium chloride,
hydrochloric acid and/or sodium
hydroxide, and EDTA. Ophth. Susp.
Drop-Tainers 2.5 mL, 5 mL, 10 mL,
15 mL. *Rx.*
Use: Glaucoma treatment.
Azor. (Daiichi Sankyo) Amlodipine
besylate/olmesartan medoxomil 5 mg/
20 mg, 5 mg/40 mg, 10 mg/20 mg,
10 mg/40 mg. Tab. 30s, 90s, 1000s,
blister 100s. *Rx.*
Use: Antihypertensive combination.
•**azosemide.** (AZE-oh-SEH-mide) USAN.
Use: Diuretic.

AZO Standard. (Amerifit Brands) Phen-
azopyridine hydrochloride 95 mg. Tab.
Bot. 30s. *OTC.*
Use: Interstitial cystitis agent.
AZO Standard Maximum Strength.
(Amerifit Brands) Phenazopyridine
hydrochloride 97.5 mg. PEG. Tab. 12s
OTC.
Use: Interstitial cystitis agent.
Azostix Reagent Strips. (Bayer Con-
sumer Care) Bromthymol blue, urease,
buffers. Colorimetric test for blood urea
nitrogen level. Bot 25 strips.
Use: Diagnostic aid.
•**azotomycin.** (aze-OH-toe-MY-sin)
USAN. Antibiotic isolated from broth fil-
trates of *Streptomyces ambofaciens.*
Use: Antineoplastic.
Azovan Blue.
See: Evans Blue Dye (City Chemical;
Harvey).
AZO Wintomylon. (Sanofi-Synthelabo)
Nalidixic acid, phenazopyridine hydro-
chloride. *Rx.*
Use: Anti-infective, urinary.
AZT.
See: Zidovudine.
AZT-P-ddi. (Baker Norton) Phase I AIDS.
Investigational.
Use: Antiviral.
•**aztreonam.** (AZZ-TREE-oh-nam)
USP 34.
Use: Antimicrobial.
See: Azactam.
aztreonam. (APP Pharmaceutical)
Aztreonam 500 mg, 1 g, 2 g. L-arginine
(≈ 780 mg per gram aztreonam). Inj.,
lyophilized cake for Soln. Single-dose
vial. *Rx.*
Use: Anti-infective agent, monobactam.
Azulfidine. (Pfizer) Sulfasalazine
500 mg. Tab. Bot. 100s, 300s, UD 100s.
Rx.
Use: Anti-inflammatory, antirrheumatic.
Azulfidine EN-tabs. (Pfizer) Sulfasala-
zine 500 mg. Enteric coated. DR Tab.
Bot. 100s, 300s. *Rx.*
Use: Anti-inflammatory, antirheumatic.
•**azumolene sodium.** (AH-ZUH-moe-
leen) USAN.
Use: Muscle relaxant.
Azurette. (Watson) Desogestrel 0.15 mg,
ethinyl estradiol 20 mcg. Lactose. Tab.
Blister pack 21s w/2 inert green tab-
lets and 5 ethinyl estradiol 10 mcg blue
tablets. *Rx.*
Use: Oral monophasic contraceptive.

B

B₁. Thiamine hydrochloride.
B₂. Riboflavin.
B₃. Niacin, nicotinamide.
B₅. Calcium pantothenate.
B₆. Pyridoxine hydrochloride.
B₆ 50. (Western Research) Vitamin B₆ 50 mg. Tab. Bot. 1000s. *OTC.*
Use: Vitamin supplement.
B₁₂. Cyanocobalamin. *OTC.*
Babee Teething. (Pfeiffer) Benzocaine 2.5%, cetalkonium Cl 0.02%, alcohol, eucalyptol, menthol, camphor. Soln. Bot. 15 mL. *OTC.*
Use: Anesthetic, local.
Baby Anbesol. (Whitehall-Robins) Benzocaine 7.5%, saccharin. Gel. Tube 7.2 g. *OTC.*
Use: Mouth and throat preparation.
BabyBIG. (California Dept. of Health Sciences) Botulism immune globulin IV (human) 100 ± 20 mg (50 mg/mL when reconstituted). Sucrose 5%, albumin (human) 1%. Solvent/detergent-treated. Preservative free. Pow. for Inj., lyophilized. Single-dose vial with 2 mL vial of diluent. *Rx.*
Use: Infant botulism, immune globulin.
Baby Ddrops. (J.R. Carlson Labs) Vitamin D₃ (cholecalciferol) 400 units per 0.03 mL. Gluten free, preservative free, and sugar free. Drops. 11 mL. *OTC.*
Use: Fat-soluble vitamin.
Baby Gas-X Infant. (Novartis Consumer Health) Simethicone 20 mg/0.3 mL. Mannitol. Alcohol free. Drops. 30 mL. *OTC.*
Use: Antiflatulent.
Baby Orajel. (Del) Benzocaine. **Gel:** 7.5%. Saccharin, sorbitol, alcohol free. Tube 9.45 g. **Liq.:** 7.5%. Parabens, saccharin, sorbitol. Berry flavor. 13.3 mL. *OTC.*
Use: Mouth and throat preparation.
Baby Orajel Nighttime Formula. (Del) Benzocaine 10%, saccharin, sorbitol, alcohol free. Gel. Tube 6 g. *OTC.*
Use: Mouth and throat preparation.
Baby Orajel Teeth & Gum Cleanser. (Del) Poloxamer 407 2%, simethicone 0.12%, parabens, saccharin, sorbitol. Gel. Tube 14.2 g. *OTC.*
Use: Mouth and throat preparation.
Baby Vitamin. (Ivax) Vitamins A 1500 units, D 400 units, E 5 units, B₁ 0.5 mg, B₂ 0.6 mg, B₃ 8 mg, B₆ 0.4 mg, B₁₂ 2 mcg, C 35 mg/mL. Drop. Bot. 50 mL. *OTC.*
Use: Vitamin supplement.

Baby Vitamin Drops with Iron. (Ivax) Iron 10 mg, vitamins A 1500 units, D 400 units, E 5 units, B₁ 0.5 mg, B₂ 0.6 mg, B₃ 8 mg, B₆ 0.4 mg, C 35 mg/mL. Bot. 50 mL. *OTC.*
Use: Mineral, vitamin supplement.
BAC. Benzalkonium Chloride.
•**bacampicillin hydrochloride.** (BACK-am-PIH-sill-in) *USP 34.*
Use: Anti-infective.
See: Spectrobid.
Bacco-Resist. (Vita Elixir) Lobeline sulfate ¹⁄₆₄ g.
Use: Smoking deterrent.
Bacid. (Novartis) A specially cultured strain of human *Lactobacillus acidophilus,* sodium carboxymethylcellulose 100 mg, sodium 0.5 mEq. Cap. Bot. 50s, 100s. *OTC.*
Use: Antidiarrheal; nutritional supplement.
Bacillus Calmette-Guérin.
See: BCG vaccine.
•**bacitracin.** (bass-ih-TRAY-sin) *USP 34.*
Use: Anti-infective.
See: Altracin.
W/Neomycin, Polymyxin B Sulfate.
See: Mycitracin.
Neosporin Original.
Neo-Thrycex.
Tigo.
W/Neomycin Sulfate.
See: Bacitracin-Neomycin.
W/Polymyxin B sulfate
See: Polysporin.
W/Polymyxin B Sulfate and Neomycin Sulfate.
See: Trimixin.
bacitracin. (Various Mfr.) An antibiotic produced by a strain of *Bacillus subtilis.* Diagnostic Tabs., Oint., Ophth. Oint. 500 units/g. Tube 3.5 g, 3.75 g. Soluble Tab., Systemic Use, Vial, Topical Use, Vial, Troche. Vaginal Tab.
Use: Anti-infective. [Orphan Drug]
bacitracin. (Various Mfr.) Bacitracin 500 units/g. Oint. 3.5 g, 3.75 g. *Rx.*
Use: Anti-infective, ophthalmic.
bacitracin-neomycin ointment. (Various Mfr.) Neomycin sulfate equivalent to 3.5 mg base, bacitracin 500 units/g. Topical Oint. Tube 0.5 oz, 1 oz, Ophth. Oint. ⅛ oz. *OTC.*
Use: Anti-infective, topical.
bacitracin/neomycin/polymyxin B ointment. (Various Mfr.) Polymyxin B sulfate 10,000 units/g, neomycin sulfate 3.5 mg/g, bacitracin zinc 400 units/g. Tube 3.5 g. *Rx.*
Use: Anti-infective, ophthalmic.

• **bacitracin zinc.** (bass-ih-TRAY-sin) *USP 34. Rx.*
Use: Anti-infective.
W/Hydrocortisone Acetate, Neomycin Sulfate, Polymyxin B.
See: Coracin.
W/Neomycin Sulfate, Polymyxin B Sulfate.
See: Bacitracin Zinc and Polymyxin B Sulfate.
Neomycin and Polymyxin B sulfates and Bacitracin Zinc.
Neosporin Original.
Neotal.
Ocutricin.
Triple Antibiotic.
W/Polymyxin B sulfate.
See: AK-Poly-Bac.
Double Antibiotic.
Polysporin.
W/Polymyxin B Sulfate, Lidocaine, Neomycin.
See: Lanabiotic.
W/Polymyxin B Sulfate, Neomycin, Pramoxine Hydrochloride.
See: Neosporin Plus Pain Relief.
Tri-Biozene.
bacitracin zinc. (Pharmacia) Bacitracin zinc 10,000 units, 50,000 units. Sterile pow. Vial. *Rx.*
Use: Anti-infective.
bacitracin zinc and polymyxin B sulfate. (Roerig) Polymyxin B sulfate 10,000 units, bacitracin zinc 500 units/ g, white petrolatum, mineral oil. Ophth. Oint. Tube 3.5 g. *Rx.*
Use: Antibiotic.
bacitracin zinc/neomycin sulfate/polymyxin B sulfate/hydrocortisone.
(Various Mfr.) Hydrocortisone 1%, neomycin sulfate 0.35%, bacitracin zinc 400 units, polymyxin B sulfate 10,000 units. Tube 3.5 g. *Rx.*
Use: Anti-infective; corticosteroid ophthalmic.
bacitracin zinc ointment. (Alpharma) Bacitracin zinc is an anhydrous ointment base. Polymyxin B sulfate 10,000 units, bacitracin zinc 500 units. Oint. Tube 3.5 g. *OTC.*
Use: Anti-infective, topical.
Bacit White. (Whiteworth Towne) Bacitracin. Oint. Tube 0.5 oz, 1 oz. *OTC.*
Use: Anti-infective, topical.
Backache Maximum Strength Relief. (Bristol-Myers Squibb) Magnesium salicylate anhydrous (as tetrahydrate) 467 mg. Cap. Bot. 24s, 50s. *OTC.*
Use: Analgesic.
• **baclofen.** (BACK-low-fen) *USP 34. Rx.*
Use: Muscle relaxant.

See: Gablofen.
Lioresal.
W/Phenylalanine
See: Kemstro.
baclofen. (Various Mfr.) Baclofen 10 mg, 20 mg. Tab. Bot. 30s, 100s, 250s, 500s, 1000s, UD 100s. *Rx.*
Use: Muscle relaxant.
baclofen. *Rx.*
Use: Treatment of muscle spasticity; dystonia. [Orphan Drug]
l-baclofen. *Rx.*
Use: Trigeminal neuralgia. [Orphan Drug]
Bacmin. (Marnel) Iron 27 mg, Vitamin A 5000 units, E 30 units, C 500 mg, B_1 20 mg, B_2 20 mg, B_3 100 mg, B_5 25 mg, B_6 25 mg, B_{12} 50 mcg, biotin 0.15 mg, folic acid 0.8 mg, Cr, Cu, Mg, Mn, Zn 22.5 mg. Tab. Bot. 100s. *Rx.*
Use: Mineral, vitamin supplement.
Bac-Neo-Poly. (Burgin-Arden) Bacitracin 400 units, neomycin sulfate 5 mg, polymyxin B sulfate 5000 units/g. Oint. Tube 5 oz. *OTC.*
Use: Anti-infective, topical.
Bactal Soap. (Whittaker General) Triclosan 0.5%, anhydrous soap 10%. Liq. Bot. 240 mL, ½ gal. *OTC.*
Use: Antiseptic; cleaner.
• **bacteriostatic water for injection.** *USP 34.*
Use: Pharmaceutic aid, diluting and dissolving drugs for injection.
bacteriostatic water for injection. (Abbott) 30 mL. Multiple-dose fliptop vial (plastic).
Use: Pharmaceutic aid, diluting and dissolving drugs for injection.
bacteriuria tests. In vitro diagnostic aids.
See: Microstix-3.
Uricult.
Bacti-Cleanse. (Pedinol Pharmacal) Benzalkonium chloride, mineral oil, isopropyl palmitate, cetyl alcohol, glycerine, glyceryl stearate, PEG-100 stearate, dimethicone, diazolidinyl urea, parabens, DMDM hydantoin, EDTA. Liq. Bot. 453.6 g. *OTC.*
Use: Dermatologic cleanser.
Bacticort. (Rugby) Hydrocortisone 1%, neomycin sulfate equivalent to 0.35% neomycin base, polymyxin B sulfate 10,000 units/mL, benzalkonium Cl, cetyl alcohol, glyceryl monostearate, mineral oil, polyoxyl 40 stearate, propylene glycol. Ophth. Soln. Bot. 7.5 mL. *Rx.*
Use: Anti-infective; corticosteroid, ophthalmic.
Bactigen Group A Streptococcus. (Wampole) Latex agglutination slide test

for the qualitative detection of group A streptococcal antigen directly from throat swabs. Test kit 60s.
Use: Diagnostic aid.

Bactigen Group A Streptococcus with Gast Trak Slides. (Wampole) Latex agglutination slide test for qualitative detection of group A streptococcal antigen directly from throat swabs. Test 24s. Kit 48s.
Use: Diagnostic aid.

Bactigen H. Influenzae. (Wampole) Rapid latex agglutination slide test for the qualitative detection of *Haemophilus influenzae* type b antigen in cerebrospinal fluid, serum, and urine. Test kit 15s, 30s.
Use: Diagnostic aid.

Bactigen Meningitis Panel. (Wampole) Rapid latex agglutination slide test for the qualitative detection of *Haemophilus influenzae* type b, *Neisseria meningitidis* A/B/C/Y/W135, and *Streptococcus pneumoniae* antigens in cerebrospinal fluid, serum, and urine. Test kit 18s.
Use: Diagnostic aid.

Bactigen Salmonella-Shigella. (Wampole) Latex agglutination slide test for the qualitative detection of *Salmonella* or *Shigella* from cultures. Test kit 96s.
Use: Diagnostic aid.

Bactine Antiseptic Anesthetic. (Bayer Consumer Care) Benzalkonium Cl 0.13%, lidocaine 2.5%, EDTA, alcohol 3.17%. **Spray:** 60 mL, 120 mL, 480 mL. **Aerosol:** 90 g. *OTC.*
Use: Topical local anesthetic.

Bactine First Aid Antibiotic. (Bayer Consumer Care) Polymyxin B sulfate 5000 units, bacitracin 500 units, neomycin sulfate 5 mg/g in mineral oil, white petrolatum. Oint. Tube 15 g. *OTC.*
Use: Anti-infective, topical.

Bactine Hydrocortisone Skin Cream. (Bayer Consumer Care) Hydrocortisone 0.5%. Tube 0.5 oz. *OTC.*
Use: Corticosteroid, topical.

Bactine Maximum Strength. (Bayer Consumer Care) Hydrocortisone 1%, glycerin, mineral oil, methylparaben, white petrolatum. Cream. Tube 30 g. *OTC.*
Use: Corticosteroid, topical.

Bactine Pain Relieving Cleansing. (Bayer Consumer Care) Lidocaine 2.5%, benzalkonium chloride 0.13%. EDTA. Spray. 150 mL. *OTC.*
Use: Topical local anesthetic.

Bactocill. (GlaxoSmithKline) Oxacillin sodium 500 mg, 1 g, 2 g, 4 g, 10 g. Pow. for Inj. Vial (except 10 g); piggyback and *ADD-Vantage* vial (only 1 g and 2 g); Bulk vial (10 g only). *Rx.*
Use: Anti-infective; penicillin.

Bacto Shield Foam. (Steris) Chlorhexidine gluconate 4%, isopropyl alcohol 4%. Foam. Aerosol. 180 mL. *OTC.*
Use: Dermatologic, cleanser.

Bacto Shield Solution. (Steris) Chlorhexidine gluconate 4%, isopropyl alcohol 4%. Soln. Bot. 960 mL. *OTC.*
Use: Dermatologic, cleanser.

Bacto Shield 2. (Steris) Chlorhexidine gluconate 2%, isopropyl alcohol 4%. Soln. Bot. 960 mL. *OTC.*
Use: Preoperative skin preparation, cleanser.

Bactrim. (Roche) Sulfamethoxazole 400 mg, trimethoprim 80 mg. Tab. 100s, 500s. *Rx.*
Use: Anti-infective.

Bactrim DS. (Roche) Trimethoprim 160 mg, sulfamethoxazole 800 mg. Tab. 100s, 500s. *Rx.*
Use: Anti-infective.

Bactrim Suspension. (Roche) Sulfamethoxazole 200 mg, trimethoprim 40 mg/5 mL. Susp. Bot. 16 oz. *Rx.*
Use: Anti-infective.

Bactroban. (GlaxoSmithKline) Mupirocin. **Oint.:** 2% (20 mg/g). Polyethylene glycol base. Tube 22 g. **Cream:** Mupirocin 2% (as calcium 2.15%). Oil/water base, benzyl alcohol, cetyl alcohol, stearyl alcohol. Tubes. 15 g, 30 g. *Rx.*
Use: Topical local anesthetic antibiotic.

Bactroban Nasal. (GlaxoSmithKline) Mupirocin 2% (as calcium 2.15%). Glycerin esters. Oint. 1 g. *Rx.*
Use: Anti-infective used in adult patients and health care workers during institutional outbreaks.

Bacturcult. (Wampole) A urinary bacteria culture medium diagnostic urine culture system for urine collection, bacteriuria screening, and presumptive bacterial identification. Test kit 10s, 100s.
Use: Diagnostic aid.

•**bafetinib.** (ba-FE-ti-nib) USAN. Antineoplastic.

B.A. Gradual. (Federal) Theophylline 260 mg, pseudoephedrine hydrochloride 50 mg, butabarbital 15 mg. Gradual. Bot. 50s, 1000s. *Rx.*
Use: Bronchodilator; decongestant; hypnotic; sedative.

Bain de Soleil All Day For Kids SPF 30. (Procter & Gamble) Ethylhexyl p-methoxycinnamate, 2-ethylhexyl 2-cyano-3, 3-diphenyl acrylate, oxyben-

zone, titanium dioxide, stearyl alcohol, tocopheryl acetate, EDTA. PABA free. Waterproof. Lot. Bot. 120 mL. *OTC.*
Use: Sunscreen.

Bain de Soleil All Day Waterproof Sunblock. (Procter & Gamble) SPF 15, 30. Ethylhexyl p-methoxycinnamate, 2-ethylhexyl 2-cyano-3, 3-diphenyl acrylate, oxybenzone, titanium dioxide, stearyl alcohol, vitamin E, EDTA. Lot. Bot. 120 mL. *OTC.*
Use: Sunscreen.

Bain de Soleil All Day Waterproof Sunfilter. (Procter & Gamble) SPF 4, 8. 2-ethylhexyl 2-cyano-3, 3-diphenyl acrylate, ethylhexyl p-methoxycinnamate, titanium dioxide, stearyl alcohol, vitamin E, EDTA. Lot. Bot. 120 mL. *OTC.*
Use: Sunscreen.

Bain de Soleil Body Silkening Creme. (Procter & Gamble) Padimate O, ethylhexyl p-methoxycinnamate, oxybenzone, benzyl alcohol. Waterproof. Cream. Bot. 94 g. *OTC.*
Use: Sunscreen.

Bain de Soleil Body Silkening Spray. (Procter & Gamble) Padimate O, oxybenzone, ethylhexyl p-methoxycinnamate. Waterproof. Lot. Bot. 240 mL. *OTC.*
Use: Sunscreen.

Bain de Soleil Body Silkening Stick. (Procter & Gamble) Padimate O, ethylhexyl p-methoxycinnamate, oxybenzone, dioxybenzone. Stick 53 g. *OTC.*
Use: Sunscreen.

Bain de Soleil Face Creme. (Procter & Gamble) Padimate O, ethylhexyl p-methoxycinnamate, oxybenzone. Waterproof. Cream. Bot. 60 g. *OTC.*
Use: Sunscreen.

Bain de Soleil Kids Sport. (Procter & Gamble) SPF 25. Ethylhexyl p-methoxycinnamate, 2-ethylhexyl 2-cyano-3, 3-diphenyl acrylate, titanium dioxide, PVP/eicosene copolymer, dimethicone, cyclomethicone, triethanolamine, glyceryl tribehenate, tocopheryl acetate, carbomer, EDTA, DMDM hydantoin. PABA free. Waterproof, all day protection. Lot. Bot. 120 mL. *OTC.*
Use: Sunscreen.

Bain de Soleil Lip Protecteur. (Procter & Gamble) Ethylhexyl p-methoxycinnamate, oxybenzone, 2-ethylhexyl salicylate, oleyl alcohol, petrolatum. PABA free. Lip balm 3 g. *OTC.*
Use: Sunscreen.

Bain de Soleil Megatan. (Procter & Gamble) Ethylhexyl p-methoxycinnamate, 2-ethylhexyl salicylate, lanolin, cocoa butter, palm oil, aloe, DMDM hydantoin, xanthan gum, shea butter, EDTA. Lot. Bot. 120 mL. *OTC.*
Use: Sunscreen.

Bain de Soleil Orange Gelee SPF 4. (Procter & Gamble) Ethylhexyl p-methoxycinnamate, 2-ethylhexyl salicylate. PABA free. Gel. Tube 93.75 g. *OTC.*
Use: Sunscreen.

Bain de Soleil SPF 8+ Color. (Procter & Gamble) Octyl methoxycinnamate, octocrylene, mineral oil, cetyl alcohol, EDTA. Lot. Bot. 118 mL. *OTC.*
Use: Sunscreen.

Bain de Soleil SPF 15+ Color. (Procter & Gamble) Octyl methoxycinnamate, octocrylene, oxybenzone, mineral oil, cetyl alcohol, EDTA. Lot. Bot. 118 mL. *OTC.*
Use: Sunscreen.

Bain de Soleil SPF 30+ Color. (Procter & Gamble) Octocrylene, octyl methoxycinnamate, oxybenzone, mineral oil, cetyl alcohol, EDTA. Lot. Bot. 118 mL. *OTC.*
Use: Sunscreen.

Bain de Soleil Sport. (Procter & Gamble) SPF 15. 2-ethylhexyl 2-cyano-3, 3-diphenyl acrylate, ethylhexyl p-methoxycinnamate, titanium dioxide, dimethicone, cyclomethicone, panthenol, tocopheryl acetate, carbomer, EDTA, DMDM hydantoin. PABA free. Waterproof, sweatproof, all day protection. Lot. Bot. 180 mL. *OTC.*
Use: Sunscreen.

Bain de Soleil Tropical Deluxe SPF 4. (Procter & Gamble) Ethylhexyl p-methoxycinnamate, 2-ethylhexyl salicylate, cetyl alcohol, EDTA. PABA free. Waterproof. Lot. Bot. 240 mL. *OTC.*
Use: Sunscreen.

Bain de Soleil Under Eye. (Procter & Gamble) Ethylhexyl p-methoxycinnamate, oxybenzone, 2-ethylhexyl salicylate. Stick 1.5 g. *OTC.*
Use: Sunscreen.

Bakers Best. (Scherer) Water, alcohol 38%, propylene glycol, extract of capsicum, glycerin, boric acid, Tween 80, diethylphthalate, rose oil, pyrilamine maleate, glacial acetic acid, Uvinul MS 40, hexetidine, benzalkonium Cl 50%, sodium hydroxide 76%. Bot. 8 oz. *OTC.*
Use: Antipruritic; antiseborrheic, topical.

Balacall DM. (Centurion Labs) Brompheniramine maleate 2 mg, dextromethorphan HBr 10 mg, phenylephrine hydrochloride 5 mg per 5 mL. Saccharin. Alcohol free, dye free, sugar free.Syr. 473 mL. *Rx.*

Use: Upper respiratory combination, antihistamine, antitussive, decongestant.

•**balafilcon A.** (ba-lah-FILL-kahn A) USAN.
Use: Contact lens material, hydrophilic.

Balamine DM. (Ballay) **Oral Drops:** Pseudoephedrine hydrochloride 25 mg, carbinoxamine maleate 2 mg, dextromethorphan HBr 3.5 mg per 1 mL. Menthol, grape flavor. Bot. 30 mL w/dropper. **Syr.:** Dextromethorphan HBr 12.5 mg, carbinoxamine maleate 4 mg, pseudoephedrine hydrochloride 60 mg per 5 mL. Menthol, grape flavor. Bot. 473 mL. *Rx.*
Use: Upper respiratory combination, antitussive combination.

Balanced B$_{100}$. (Fibertone) Vitamins B$_1$ 100 mg, B$_2$ 100 mg, B$_3$ 100 mg, B$_5$ 100 mg, B$_6$ 100 mg, B$_{12}$ 100 mcg, folic acid 0.1 mg, PABA 100 mg, inositol 100 mg, d-biotin 100 mcg. SR Tab. Bot. 50s. *OTC.*
Use: Mineral, vitamin supplement.

Balanced Salt Solution. (Various Mfr.) Sodium Cl 0.64%, potassium Cl 0.075%, calcium Cl 0.048%, magnesium Cl 0.03%, sodium acetate 0.39%, sodium citrate 0.17%, sodium hydroxide or hydrochloric acid. Soln. *Drop-Tainer* 18 mL, 500 mL.
Use: Irrigant, ophthalmic.

•**balapiravir.** (BAL-a-PIR-a-vir) USAN.
Use: Anti-infective.

•**balapiravir hydrochloride.** (BAL-a-PIR-a-vir) USAN.
Use: Anti-infective.

Baldex Ophthalmic. (Bausch & Lomb) Dexamethasone phosphate. **Oint.:** 0.05%. Tube 3.75 g. **Soln.:** 0.01%. Dropper Bot. 5 mL. *Rx.*
Use: Corticosteroid, ophthalmic.

BAL in Oil. (Becton Dickinson & Co.) 2, 3-dimercaptopropanol 100 mg, benzylbenzoate 210 mg, peanut oil 680 mg/mL. Amp. 3 mL. Box 10s. *Rx.*
Use: Antidote.

Balmex. (Block Drug) Zinc oxide. **Cream:** 11.3%. Mineral oil, parabens, soybean oil. 118 g. **Oint.:** 11.3%, aloe vera gel, parabens, mineral oil. Tubes. 30 g, 60 g, 120 g, 454 g. *OTC.*
Use: Emollient.

Balmex Baby Powder. (Block Drug) Specially purified balsam Peru, zinc oxide, starch, calcium carbonate. Shaker top can. 4 oz. *OTC.*
Use: Adsorbent, emollient.

Balneol. (Alaven) Glyceryl, lanolin oil, mineral oil, methylparaben, PEG-4,

PEG-40, PG-100, propylene glycol. Lot. 88 mL. *OTC.*
Use: Anorectal preparation, perianal hygiene product.

Balneol For Her. (Alaven) Glyceryl, lanolin oil, mineral oil, methylparaben, PEG-4, PEG-40, PEG-100, propylene glycol. Lot. 89 mL. *OTC.*
Use: Anorectal preparation, perianal hygiene product.

Balneol For Her Convenience Packets. (Alaven) Glyceryl, hydrocortisone 0.25%, lanolin oil, methylparaben, mineral oil, PEG-4, PEG-40, PEG-100, propylene glycol. Lot. 20s. *OTC.*
Use: Anorectal preparation, perianal hygiene product.

Balneol Hygienic Cleansing. (Alaven) Mineral oil, lanolin oil, methylparaben. Bot. 120 mL. *Formerly Balneol Perianal Cleansing. OTC.*
Use: Anorectal preparation.

Balnetar. (Westwood Squibb) Coal tar 2.5% in mineral oil, lanolin oil. Liq. 221 mL. *OTC.*
Use: Dermatologic.

•**balsalazide disodium.** (bahl-SAL-ah-zide) USAN.
Use: Anti-inflammatory, gastrointestinal agent.
See: Colazal.

balsalazide disodium. (Various Mfr.) Balsalazide disodium 750 mg. Sodium ≈ 79 to 86 mg. Cap. 30s, 280, 350s, 500s, UD 100s. *Rx.*
Use: Anti-inflammatory, gastrointestinal agent.

balsam Peru.
W/Combinations.
See: Vasolex.
Xenaderm-T.

Balsan. Specially purified balsam Peru.
See: Balmex Baby Powder.

Balziva. (Barr Laboratories) Ethinyl estradiol 35 mcg, norethindrone 0.4 mg. Lactose. Tab. 28s with 7 inert tablets. *Rx.*
Use: Contraceptive hormone, sex hormone.

•**bambermycins.** (BAM-ber-MY-sinz) USAN.
Use: Anti-infective.

•**bamethan sulfate.** (BAM-eth-an) USAN.
Use: Vasodilator.

•**bamifylline hydrochloride.** (BAM-ih-FILL-in) USAN.
Use: Bronchodilator.

•**bamnidazole.** (bam-NIH-DAH-zole) USAN.
Use: Antiprotozoal, trichomonas.

Banacid. (Buffington) Magnesium trisilicate 220 mg. Tab. Bot. 100s, 200s, 500s. *OTC.*
Use: Antacid.

Banadyne-3. (Norstar Consumer) Lidocaine 4%, menthol 1%, alcohol 45%. Soln. Bot. 7.5 mL. *OTC.*
Use: Mouth and throat preparation.

B & A. (Eastern Research) Sodium bicarbonate, potassium, aluminum, borax. Hygienic pow. Jar 8 oz, 5 lb. *Rx.*
Use: Vaginal agent.

• **bandage, adhesive.** *USP 34.*
Use: Surgical aid.

• **bandage, gauze.** *USP 34.*
Use: Surgical aid.

B and O Supprettes No. 15A & No. 16A. (Amerifit) Opium 30 mg, 60 mg, belladonna extract 16.2 mg. Supp. Jar 12s. *c-II.*
Use: Analgesic; antispasmodic; narcotic.

Banflex. (Forest Pharm) Orphenadrine citrate 30 mg/mL. Inj. Vial 10 mL. *Rx.*
Use: Muscle relaxant.

Bangesic. (H.L. Moore Drug Exchange) Menthol, camphor, methyl salicylate, eucalyptus oil in nongreasy base. Bot. 2 oz, gal. *OTC.*
Use: Analgesic, topical.

Banocide.
See: Diethylcarbamazine citrate.

Banophen. (Major) Diphenhydramine hydrochloride. **Tab.:** 25 mg. Bot. 24s, 100s. **Cap.:** 25 mg. Bot. 24s, 100s. *OTC.*
Use: Antihistamine, nonselective ethanolamine.

Banophen Allergy. (Major) Diphenhydramine hydrochloride 12.5 mg/5 mL, sugar. Elixir. Bot. 118 mL. *OTC.*
Use: Antihistamine, nonselective ethanolamine.

Banophen Decongestant. (Major) Diphenhydramine 25 mg, pseudoephedrine 60 mg. Cap. Bot. 24s. *OTC.*
Use: Antihistamine; decongestant.

Bansmoke. (Thompson Medical) Benzocaine 6 mg, corn syr., dextrose, lecithin, sucrose. Gum. Pack 24s. *OTC.*
Use: Smoking deterrent.

Banzel. (Eisai) Rufinamide. **Tab.:** 200 mg, 400 mg. Film coated. Lactose, PEG. 30s (200 mg), 120s (400 mg). **Susp.:** 40 mg/mL. Parabens, potassium sorbate, propylene glycol. Orange flavor. 460 mL. *Rx.*
Use: Anticonvulsant.

• **bapineuzumab.** (BAP-ee-NUE-zoo-mab) USAN.
Use: Alzheimer disease.

Baraclude. (Bristol-Myers Squibb Company) Entecavir. **Oral Soln.:** 0.05 mg/mL. Parabens. Orange flavor. 210 mL. **Tab.:** 0.5 mg, 1 mg. Lactose. Film-coated. 30s. *Rx.*
Use: Antiviral agent.

Barbased. (Major) **Tab.:** Butabarbital 0.25 g, 0.5 g. Tab. Bot. 1000s. **Elix.:** Butabarbital 30 mg/5 mL, alcohol 7%. Bot. 480 mL. *Rx.*
Use: Hypnotic; sedative.

Barbatose No. 2. (Pal-Pak, Inc.) Barbital 64.8 mg, hyoscyamus sulfate, passiflora, valerian. Tab. Bot. 1000s. *Rx.*
Use: Sedative.

Barbella Elixir. (Forest) Phenobarbital 0.25 g, hyoscyamine sulfate 0.1037 mg, atropine sulfate 0.0194 mg, scopolamine HBr 0.0065 mg, alcohol 24%/5 mL. Elix. Bot. 4 oz, gal. *Rx.*
Use: Anticholinergic; antispasmodic; hypnotic; sedative.

Barbella Tablets. (Forest) Phenobarbital 16.2 mg, atropine sulfate 0.0194 mg, hyoscyamine sulfate 0.1037 mg, hyoscine HBr 0.0065 mg. Tab. Bot. 100s, 1000s, 5000s. *Rx.*
Use: Anticholinergic; antispasmodic; hypnotic; sedative.

Barbeloid. (Pal-Pak, Inc.) Phenobarbital 16.2 mg, hyoscyamine sulfate 0.1037 mg, atropine sulfate 0.0194 mg, scopolamine HBr 0.0065 mg. Tab. Bot. 100s, 1000s. *Rx.*
Use: Anticholinergic; antispasmodic; hypnotic; sedative.

Barbenyl.
See: Phenobarbital.

Barbiphenyl.
See: Phenobarbital.

barbital. Barbitone, Deba, Dormonal, Hypnogene, Malonal, Sedeval, Uronal, Veronal, Vesperal, diethylbarbituric acid, diethylmalonylurea.
Use: Hypnotic; sedative.

barbital sodium. Barbitone sodium, diethylbarbiturate monosodium, diethylmalonylurea sodium, Embinal, Medinal, Veronal sodium.
Use: Hypnotic; sedative.

barbitone.
See: Barbital.

barbitone sodium.
See: Barbital Sodium.

barbiturate-aspirin combinations.
See: Aspirin-barbiturate combinations.

barbiturates.
See: Methohexital Sodium.

barbiturates, intermediate duration.
See: Butabarbital.
barbiturates, long duration.
See: Barbital.
Mebaral.
Mephobarbital.
Phenobarbital.
Phenobarbital Sodium.
barbiturates, short duration.
See: Amobarbital.
Amobarbital Sodium.
Butalbital.
Pentobarbital Salts.
Secobarbital.
barbiturates, ultrashort duration.
See: Pentothal Sodium.
Thiopental Sodium.
•**bardoxolone.** (bar-DOX-oh-lone) USAN.
Use: Anti-inflammatory.
•**bardoxolone methyl.** (bar-DOX-oh-lone)
USAN.
Use: Anti-inflammatory.
Baricon. (Mallinckrodt) Barium sulfate
98%. Simethicone, sorbitol, sucrose,
lemon-vanilla flavor. Pow. for Susp.
UD 340 g. *Rx.*
Use: Radiopaque agent, GI contrast
agent.
Baridium. (Pfeiffer) Phenazopyridine
hydrochloride 100 mg. Tab. Bot. 32s.
OTC.
Use: Interstitial cystitis agent.
Bari-Stress M. (Alpharma) Vitamins B₁
10 mg, B₂ 10 mg, niacinamide 100 mg,
C 300 mg, B₆ 2 mg, B₁₂ 4 mcg, folic
acid 1.5 mg, calcium pantothenate
20 mg. **Cap.:** Bot. 30s, 100s, 1000s.
Tab.: Bot. 100s, 1000s. *Rx.*
Use: Mineral, vitamin supplement.
•**barium hydroxide lime.** (BA-ree-uhm)
USP 34.
Use: Carbon dioxide absorbent.
•**barium sulfate.** (BA-ree-uhm) *USP 34.*
Paste; For suspension; Suspension;
Tablets.
Use: Radiopaque agent, miscellaneous
GI contrast agent.
See: Anatrast.
Baricon.
Barobag.
Baro-cat.
Barosperse.
Bar-test.
Bear-E-Yum CT.
Bear-E-Yum GI.
Cheetah.
Enecat CT.
Enhancer.
Entero VU.
Entrobar.

Epi-C.
E-Z-HD.
E-Z-Paque.
E-Z-Paque Liquid.
E-Z-Paste.
Flo-Coat.
HD 85.
HD 200 Plus.
Imager ac.
Intropaste.
Liqui-Coat HD.
Liquid Barosperse.
Liquid Polibar.
Liquid Polibar Plus.
Medebar Plus.
MedeScan.
Prepcat.
Readi-Cat.
Readi-Cat 2.
Tomocat.
Tonopaque.
Varibar Honey.
Varibar Nectar.
Varibar Pudding.
Varibar Thin Honey.
Varibar Thin Liquid.
barium sulfate preparation.
See: Fleet.
Barlevite. (Barth's) Vitamins B₆ 0.6 mg,
B₁₂ 3 mcg, pantothenic acid 0.6 mg, D
3 units, l-lysine 20 mg/0.6 mL. 100-day
supply. *OTC.*
Use: Vitamin, mineral supplement.
•**barmastine.** (BAR-mast-een) USAN.
Use: Antihistamine.
**BarnesHind Cleaning and Soaking
Solution.** (PBH Wesley Jessen) Clean-
ing and buffering agents, benzalkonium
chloride 0.01%, disodium edetate
0.2%. Soln. Bot. 1.2 oz, 4 oz. *OTC.*
Use: Contact lens care.
**BarnesHind Wetting & Soaking Solu-
tion.** (PBH Wesley Jessen) Polyvinyl
alcohol, povidone, hydroxyethyl cellulose, octylphenoxy (oxyethylene) ethanol, benzalkonium chloride, edetate disodium. Soln. Bot. 4 oz. *OTC.*
Use: Contact lens care.
BarnesHind Wetting Solution. (PBH
Wesley Jessen) Polyvinyl alcohol, edetate disodium 0.02%, benzalkonium
chloride 0.004%. Soln. Bot. 35 mL,
60 mL. *OTC.*
Use: Contact lens care.
Barobag. (Mallinckrodt) Barium sulfate
95%. Simethicone. Vanilla flavor. Pow.
for Susp. Enema kit. 340 g, 454 g. UD
bot. 225 g, 900 g. Bulk. 25 lb. *Rx.*
Use: Radiopaque agent, GI contrast
agent.

Baro-Cat. (Mallinckrodt) Barium sulfate 1.5%. Simethicone, sorbitol, pineapple-banana flavor. Susp. Bot. 300 mL, 900 mL, 1900 mL. *Rx.*
Use: Radiopaque agent, GI contrast agent.

Baroset. (Lafayette) Air contrast stomach. Unit-of-use kit. Case 12s.
Use: Radiopaque agent.

barosmin.
See: Diosmin.

Barosperse. (Mallinckrodt) Barium sulfate 95%. Simethicone, sorbitol, cherry flavor. Pow. for Susp. UD Bot. 180 g, 1200 g. Container. 25 lb. *Rx.*
Use: Radiopaque agent, GI contrast agent.

Bar-test. (Glenwood) Barium sulfate 650 mg. Tab. 100s. *Rx.*
Use: Radiopaque agent, GI contrast agent.

Basa. (Freeport) Acetylsalicylic acid 324 mg. Tab. Bot. 1000s. *OTC.*
Use: Analgesic.

basic aluminum carbonate.
See: Basaljel.

basic aluminum glycinate.
See: Dihydroxyaluminum aminoacetate.

basic bismuth carbonate.
See: Bismuth subcarbonate.

basic bismuth gallate.
See: Bismuth subgallate.

basic bismuth nitrate.
See: Bismuth subnitrate.

basic bismuth salicylate.
See: Bismuth subsalicylate.

basic fuchsin.
See: Carbol-Fuchsin.

●**basifungin.** (bass-ih-FUN-jin) USAN.
Use: Antifungal.

●**basiliximab.** (bass-ih-LICK-sih-mab) USAN.
Use: Immunosuppressant.
See: Simulect.

Basis, Glycerin Soap. (Beiersdorf) Tallow, coconut oil, glycerin. Sensitive and normal to dry. Bar 90 g, 150 g. *OTC.*
Use: Dermatologic, cleanser.

Basis, Superfatted Soap. (Beiersdorf) Sodium tallowate, sodium cocoate, petrolatum, glycerin, zinc oxide, sodium Cl, titanium dioxide, lanolin, alcohol, beeswax, BHT, EDTA. Bar 99 g, 225 g. *OTC.*
Use: Dermatologic, cleanser.

●**batabulin sodium.** (bat-a-BUE-lin) USAN.
Use: Antineoplastic agent.

●**batanopride hydrochloride.** (bah-TAN-oh-pride) USAN.
Use: Antiemetic.

●**batelapine maleate.** (bat-EH-lap-EEN) USAN.
Use: Antipsychotic.

●**batimastat.** (bat-IM-ah-stat) USAN.
Use: Antineoplastic.

●**bavisant.** (BAV-i-sant) USAN.
Use: CNS agent.

●**bavisant dihydrochloride.** (BAV-i-sant) USAN.
Use: CNS agent.

●**bavituximab.** (bav-i-TUX-i-mab) USAN.
Use: Antineoplastic.

Baycadron. (Wockhardt) Dexamethasone 0.5 mg per 5 mL. Alcohol 5.1%, benzoic acid 0.1%, sugar. Raspberry flavor. Elix. 237 mL.
Use: Corticosteroid.

Bayer Aspirin, Genuine. (Bayer Consumer Care) Aspirin 325 mg. Tab. Bot. 50s, 100s, 200s, 300s. Pkg. 12s, 24s. *OTC.*
Use: Analgesic.

Bayer Aspirin, Maximum. (Bayer Consumer Care) Aspirin 500 mg. Tab. Bot. 30s, 60s, 100s. *OTC.*
Use: Analgesic.

Bayer Buffered Aspirin. (Bayer Consumer Care) Buffered aspirin 325 mg. Tab. Bot. 100s. *OTC.*
Use: Analgesic.

Bayer Children's Chewable Aspirin. (Bayer Consumer Care) Aspirin 1.25 g (81 mg). Chew. Tab. Bot. 30s. *OTC.*
Use: Analgesic.

Bayer 8-Hour Timed-Release Aspirin. (Bayer Consumer Care) Aspirin 10 g (650 mg). TR Tab. Bot. 30s, 72s, 125s. *OTC.*
Use: Analgesic.

Bayer Enteric Coated Caplets, Regular Strength. (Bayer Consumer Care) Aspirin 325 mg. EC Tab. Bot. 50s, 100s. *OTC.*
Use: Analgesic.

Bayer Enteric 500 Aspirin, Extra Strength. (Bayer Consumer Care) Aspirin 500 mg. EC Tab. Bot. 60s. *OTC.*
Use: Analgesic.

Bayer Extra Strength Back & Body Pain. (Bayer Consumer Care) Aspirin 500 mg, caffeine 32.5 mg. Tab. 50s, 100s. *OTC.*
Use: Analgesic; CNS stimulant.

Bayer Low Adult Strength. (Bayer Consumer Care) Aspirin 81 mg, lactose. DR Tab. Bot. 120s. *OTC.*
Use: Analgesic.

Bayer Muscle & Joint Cream. (Bayer Consumer Care) Menthol 10%, camphor 4%, methyl salicylate 30%. EDTA, glyceryl, lanolin, stearyl alcohol. Cream 56 g, 114 g. *OTC.*
Use: Rub and liniment.

Bayer PM Extra Strength Aspirin Plus Sleep Aid. (Bayer Consumer Care) Aspirin 500 mg, diphenhydramine hydrochloride 25 mg. Cap. Bot. 24s. *OTC.*
Use: Analgesic.

Bayer Quick Release Crystals. (Bayer Consumer Care) Aspirin 850 mg, caffeine 65 mg. Acesulfame K, aspartame, phenylalanine 6 mg per packet, sucralose. Crystals. 20s. *OTC.*
Use: Nonnarcotic analgesic combination.

Bayer Select Chest Cold. (Bayer Consumer Care) Dextromethorphan HBr 15 mg, acetaminophen 500 mg. Cap. Pkg. 16s. *OTC.*
Use: Analgesic; antitussive.

Bayer Select Maximum Strength Backache. (Bayer Consumer Care) Magnesium salicylate tetrahydrate 580 mg. Cap. Bot. 24s, 50s. *OTC.*
Use: Analgesic.

Bayer Select Maximum Strength Night Time Pain Relief. (Bayer Consumer Care) Acetaminophen 500 mg, diphenhydramine hydrochloride. Tab. Bot. 24s, 50s. *OTC.*
Use: Antihistamine.

Bayer Select Maximum Strength Sinus Pain Relief. (Bayer Consumer Care) Acetaminophen 500 mg, pseudoephedrine hydrochloride 30 mg. Tab. Bot. 50s. *OTC.*
Use: Analgesic; decongestant.

Bayer Women's Aspirin Plus Calcium. (Bayer Consumer Care) Aspirin 81 mg, calcium 300 mg, lactose, mineral oil, polydextrose. Tab. 60s, 90s. *OTC.*
Use: Analgesic; mineral supplement.

Baylocaine 4%. (Bay Labs) Lidocaine 4% w/methylparaben. Soln. Bot. 50 mL, 100 mL.
Use: Anesthetic, local.

Baylocaine 2% Viscous. (Bay Labs) Lidocaine 2% w/sodium carboxymethylcellulose. Soln. Bot. 100 mL. *OTC.*
Use: Local anesthetic, topical.

BayRho-D. (Bayer) $Rh_o(D)$ immune globulin (human). Prefilled single-dose syringe. Single-dose syringe. Single-dose vial. *Rx.*
Use: Immunization.

BayRho-D Full Dose Pharmaceutical. (Bayer) $Rh_o(D)$ immune globulin 15% to 18% protein. Glycine 0.21 to 0.32 M, solvent/detergent treated, preservative free. Soln. for Inj. Individual and multiple-pack single-dose syringes w/attached needles and vials. *Rx.*
Use: Immune globulin.

•**bazedoxifene acetate.** (bay-ze-DOX-i-feen) USAN.
Use: Osteoporosis; estrogen receptor modulator.

BCAD 2. (Mead Johnson Nutritionals) Protein 24 g (L-glutamine, potassium aspartate, L-lysine hydrochloride, L-tyrosine, L-proline, L-alanine, L-arginine, L-phenylalanine, L-threonine, L-serine, glycine, L-histidine, L-methionine, L-tryptophan, L-cystine, L-carnitine, taurine), carbohydrate 57 g (corn syr. solids, sugar, modified corn starch), fat 8.5 g (soy oil)/100 g, vitamins, A, B_1, B_2, B_3, B_5, B_6, B_{12}, C, D, E, K, biotin, choline, folic acid, inositol, Ca, chloride, Cr, Cu, Fe, I, Mg, Mn, Mo, P, Se, Zn, Na 610 mg, K 1220 mg/g, 410 cal/100 g. Pow. Can 1 lb. *OTC.*
Use: Enteral nutritional therapy.

BC Allergy, Sinus, Headache. (GlaxoSmithKline Consumer Healthcare) Pseudoephedrine hydrochloride 60 mg, chlorpheniramine maleate 4 mg, acetaminophen 650 mg. Pow. 6s, 12s. *OTC.*
Use: Decongestant, antihistamine, and analgesic combination, upper respiratory combination.

BC Arthritis Strength. (Block Drug) Aspirin 742 mg, salicylamide 222 mg, caffeine 36 mg. Pow. Bot. 6s, 24s, 50s. *OTC.*
Use: Analgesic combination.

BC Fast Pain Relief. (GlaxoSmithKline Consumer Healthcare) Aspirin 845 mg, caffeine 65 mg. Lactose, potassium 55 mg per packet. Pow. 2s, 6s, 24s. *OTC.*
Use: Analgesic combination.

BC Fast Pain Relief Arthritis. (GlaxoSmithKline Consumer Health Care) Aspirin 1,000 mg, caffeine 65 mg. Potassium 65 mg per packet, lactose. Pow. 2s, 6s, 50s. *OTC.*
Use: Nonnarcotic analgesic combination.

BCG, live.
Use: Biological response modifier.
See: TheraCys.
    Tice BCG.

•**BCG vaccine.** *USP 34.*
Use: Active immunization, bacterial vaccine.
See: BCG vaccine.
    TheraCys.

BCG vaccine. (Organon) Tice strain (1 to 8 × 10^8 CFU equiv. to ≈ 50 mg). Preservative free. Pow. for Inj., lyophilized. Vials. *Rx.*
Use: Active immunization, bacterial vaccine.

BCNU.
Use: Antineoplastic.
See: BiCNU.

BCO. (Western Research) Vitamins B$_1$ 10 mg, B$_2$ 2 mg, B$_6$ 1.5 mg, B$_{12}$ 25 mcg, niacinamide 50 mg. Tab. Bot. 1000s. *OTC.*
Use: Vitamin supplement.

B-Com. (Century) Vitamins B$_1$ 3 mg, B$_2$ 3 mg, B$_6$ 0.5 mg, niacinamide 20 mg, calcium pantothenate 5 mg, B$_{12}$ 1 mcg, desiccated liver (undefatted) 60 mg, debittered brewer's dried yeast 60 mg. Cap. Bot. 100s, 1000s. *OTC.*
Use: Mineral, vitamin supplement.

B-Complex and B$_{12}$. (NBTY) Vitamins B$_1$ 7 mg, B$_2$ 14 mg, B$_3$ 4.5 mg, B$_{12}$ 25 mcg, protease 10 mg. Tab. Bot. 90s. *OTC.*
Use: Vitamin supplement.

B-Complex Capsules. (Arcum) Vitamins B$_1$ 1.5 mg, B$_2$ 2 mg, niacinamide 10 mg, B$_6$ 0.1 mg, calcium pantothenate 1 mg, desiccated liver 70 mg, dried yeast 100 mg. Cap. Bot. 100s, 1000s. *OTC.*
Use: Mineral, vitamin supplement.

B-Complex Capsules J.F. (Bryant) Vitamins B$_1$ 1 mg, B$_2$ 0.3 mg, nicotinic acid 0.3 mg, B$_6$ 0.25 mg, desiccated liver 0.15 g, yeast powder, dried 0.15 g. Cap. Bot. 100s, 1000s. *OTC.*
Use: Mineral, vitamin supplement.

B-Complex Elixir. (Nion Corp.) B$_1$ 2.3 mg, B$_2$ 1 mg, B$_3$ 6.7 mg, B$_6$ 0.3 mg, alcohol 10%. Elix. Bot. 240 mL, 480 mL. *OTC.*
Use: Mineral, vitamin supplement.

B-Complex-50. (Nion Corp.) Vitamins B$_1$ 50 mg, B$_2$ 50 mg, B$_3$ 50 mg, B$_5$ 50 mg, B$_6$ 50 mg, B$_{12}$ 50 mcg, FA 0.4 mg, biotin 50 mcg, PABA 50 mg, choline bitartrate 50 mg, inositol 50 mg. SR Tab. Bot. 100s. *OTC.*
Use: Mineral, vitamin supplement.

B-Complex "50". (Vitaline) Vitamins B$_1$ 50 mg, B$_2$ 50 mg, B$_3$ 50 mg, B$_4$ 50 mg, B$_5$ 50 mg, B$_6$ 50 mg, B$_{12}$ 50 mcg, FA 0.1 mg, PABA 30 mg, inositol 50 mg, biotin 50 mcg, choline bitartrate 50 mg. Reg. or TR Tab. Bot. 90s, 1000s. *OTC.*
Use: Vitamin supplement.

B-Complex 100. (Rabin-Winters) Vitamins B$_1$ 100 mg, B$_2$ 2 mg, B$_6$ 2 mg, niacinamide 125 mg, panthenol 10 mg/mL. Inj. Vial 30 mL. *Rx.*
Use: Vitamin supplement.

B-Complex-150. (Nion Corp.) Vitamins B$_1$ 150 mg, B$_2$ 150 mg, B$_3$ 150 mg, B$_5$ 150 mg, B$_6$ 150 mg, B$_{12}$ 1 mcg, FA 0.4 mg, biotin 150 mcg, PABA 100 mg, choline bitartrate 150 mg, inositol 150 mg. SR Tab. Bot. 30s. *OTC.*
Use: Mineral, vitamin supplement.

B-Complex 100/100. (Sandia) Vitamins B$_1$ 100 mg, B$_2$ 2 mg, B$_6$ 2 mg, niacinamide 100 mg/mL. Inj. Vial 30 mL. *Rx.*
Use: Vitamin supplement.

B Complex + C. (Various Mfr.) Vitamins B$_1$ 15 mg, B$_2$ 10 mg, B$_3$ 100 mg, B$_5$ 20 mg, B$_6$ 5 mg, B$_{12}$ 10 mcg, C 500 mg. Tab. Bot. 100s. *OTC.*
Use: Vitamin supplement.

B-Complex + C. (NBTY) Vitamins C 200 mg, B$_1$ 10 mg, B$_2$ 10 mg, B$_3$ 50 mg, B$_5$ 10 mg, B$_6$ 5 mg. Tab. Bot. 100s. *OTC.*
Use: Vitamin supplement.

B-Complex 25-25. (Forest) Niacinamide 100 mg, vitamins B$_1$ 25 mg, B$_2$ 1 mg, B$_6$ 2 mg, pantothenic acid 2 mg/mL. Inj. Vial 30 mL. *Rx.*
Use: Vitamin supplement.

B-Complex/Vitamin C Caplets. (Geneva) Vitamins B$_1$ 15 mg, B$_2$ 10.2 mg, B$_3$ 50 mg, B$_5$ 10 mg, B$_6$ 5 mg, C 300 mg. Cap. Bot. 100s. *OTC.*
Use: Vitamin supplement.

B-Complex with B-12. (Ivax) B$_1$ 1.5 mg, B$_2$ 1.7 mg, B$_3$ 20 mg, B$_5$ 10 mg, B$_6$ 2 mg, B$_{12}$ 6 mcg, FA 0.4 mg. Tab. Bot. 100s. *OTC.*
Use: Mineral, vitamin supplement.

B Complex with B$_{12}$ Capsules. (Bryant) Vitamins B$_1$ 2 mg, B$_2$ 2 mg, B$_6$ 0.5 mg, niacinamide 10 mg, B$_{12}$ 2 mcg, biotin 10 mcg, calcium pantothenate 1.5 mg, choline dihydrogen citrate 40 mg, inositol 30 mg, desiccated liver 1 g, brewer's yeast 3 g. Cap. Bot. 100s, 1000s. *OTC.*
Use: Mineral, vitamin supplement.

B Complex with C and B-12. (Ivax) Vitamins B$_1$ 50 mg, B$_2$ 5 mg, B$_3$ 125 mg, B$_5$ 6 mg, B$_6$ 5 mg, B$_{12}$ 1000 mcg, C 50 mg. Inj. Vial 10 mL. *Rx.*
Use: Vitamin supplement.

B-Complex with Vitamin C and B$_{12}$-10,000. (Fujisawa Healthcare) Vitamins B$_1$ 20 mg, B$_2$ 3 mg, B$_3$ 75 mg, B$_5$ 5 mg, B$_6$ 5 mg, B$_{12}$ 1000 mcg, C 100 mg. Covial. 10 mL multiple dose. *Rx.*
Use: Vitamin supplement.

BC-1000. (Solvay) Vitamins B$_1$ 50 mg, B$_2$ 5 mg, B$_{12}$ 1000 mcg, B$_6$ 5 mg, d-panthenol 6 mg, niacinamide 125 mg, ascorbic acid 50 mg, benzyl alcohol 1%/mL. Vial 10 mL. *OTC.*
Use: Vitamin supplement.

BC Powder, Arthritis Strength. (Glaxo-SmithKline Consumer Healthcare) Aspirin 742 mg, salicylamide 222 mg, caffeine 38 mg. Lactose. Pow. Pkg. 50s. *OTC.*
Use: Analgesic combination.

BC Tablets. (Block Drug) Aspirin 325 mg, salicylamide 95 mg, caffeine 16 mg. Tab. Pkg 4s. Bot. 50s, 100s. *OTC.*
Use: Analgesic combination.

B-C w/Folic Acid. (Geneva) Vitamins B_1 15 mg, B_2 15 mg, B_3 100 mg, B_5 18 mg, B_6 4 mg, B_{12} 5 mcg, C 500 mg, folic acid 0.5 mg. Tab. Bot. 100s. *Rx.*
Use: Mineral, vitamin supplement.

B-C w/Folic Acid Plus. (Geneva) Fe 27 mg, vitamins A 5000 units, E 30 units, B_1 20 mg, B_2 20 mg, B_3 100 mg, B_5 25 mg, B_6 25 mg, B_{12} 50 mcg, C 500 mg, FA 0.8 mg, biotin 0.15 mg, Cr, Cu, Mg, Mn, Zn 22.5 mg. Tab. Bot. 100s. *Rx.*
Use: Mineral, vitamin supplement.

B-Day. (Barth's) Vitamins B_1 7 mg, B_2 14 mg, niacin 4.67 mg, B_{12} 5 mcg. Tab. Bot. 100s, 500s. *OTC.*
Use: Vitamin supplement.

B-D Glucose. (Becton Dickinson & Co.) Glucose 5 g. Chew. Tab. Bot. 36s. *OTC.*
Use: Hyperglycemic.

B Dozen. (Standex) Vitamin B_{12} 25 mcg Tab. Bot. 1000s. *OTC.*
Use: Vitamin supplement.

B-Dram w/C Computabs. (Dram) Vitamins B_1 5 mg, B_2 10 mg, B_6 5 mg, nicotinamide 50 mg, calcium pantothenate 20 mg. Tab. Bot. 100s. *OTC.*
Use: Mineral, vitamin supplement.

Beano. (AKPharma) Alpha-D-galactosidase derived from *Aspergillus niger*, a fungal source in carrier of water and glycerol. Liq. Bot. 75 serving size at 5 drops per dose. Tab. Pkg. 12s. Bot. 30s, 100s. *OTC.*
Use: Antiflatulent.

Bear-E-Yum CT. (Mallinckrodt) Barium sulfate 1.5%. Simethicone, sorbitol. Susp. Bot. 200 mL, 1900 mL. *Rx.*
Use: Radiopaque agent, GI contrast agent.

Bear-E-Yum GI. (Mallinckrodt) Barium sulfate 60%. Simethicone. Susp. Bot. 200 mL. *Rx.*
Use: Radiopaque agent, GI contrast agent.

Bebatab No. 2. (Freeport) Belladonna ⅙ g, phenobarbital 0.25 g. Tab. Bot. 1000s. *Rx.*
Use: Anticholinergic; antispasmodic; hypnotic; sedative.

Bebulin VH. (Baxter) Factor IX, II, X, and low amounts of VII (human). Vapor-treated. Actual number of units shown on each bottle. Heparin, dry natural rubber latex. Inj., Pow. for Soln. Single-dose vials with sterile water for injection. *Rx.*
Use: Antihemophilic agent.

•**becanthone hydrochloride.** (BEE-kan-thone) USAN.
Use: Antischistosomal.

•**becaplermin.** (beh-kah-PLER-min) USAN.
Use: Chronic dermal ulcers treatment.
See: Regranex.

•**becatecarin.** (BE-Ka-TEK-ar-in) USAN.
Use: Antineoplastic.

Beceevite. (Halsey Drug) Vitamins C 300 mg, B_1 15 mg, B_2 10 mg, niacin 50 mg, B_6 5 mg, pantothenic acid 10 mg. Cap. Bot. 100s. *OTC.*
Use: Vitamin supplement.

•**beclomethasone dipropionate.** (BEK-low-METH-uh-zone die-PRO-peo-uh-NATE) *USP 34.*
Use: Corticosteroid; intranasal steroid.
See: Beconase AQ.
QVAR.
Vanceril.
Vanceril Double Strength.

beclomycin dipropionate.
Use: Corticosteroid.

Beclovent. Beclomethasone dipropionate. *Rx.*
Use: Respiratory inhalant, corticosteroid.

•**becocalcidiol.** (BE-koe-KAL-si-DYE-ol) USAN.
Use: Psoriasis.

Becomp-C. (Cenci, H.R. Labs, Inc.) Vitamins C 250 mg, B_1 25 mg, B_2 10 mg, nicotinamide 50 mg, B_6 2 mg, calcium pantothenate 10 mg, hesperidin complex 50 mg. Cap. Bot. 100s, 500s. *OTC.*
Use: Mineral, vitamin supplement.

Beconase AQ. (GlaxoSmithKline) Beclomethasone dipropionate 0.042% (42 mcg/actuation), dextrose, polysorbate 80, benzalkonium chloride, 0.25% w/w phenylethyl alcohol. Spray. Bot. 25 g (180 metered doses per bottle) with metering pump and nasal adaptor. *Rx.*
Use: Corticosteroid; intranasal steroid.

Becotin-T. (Eli Lilly) Vitamins B_1 15 mg, B_2 10 mg, B_6 5 mg, niacinamide 100 mg, pantothenic acid 20 mg, B_{12} 4 mcg, C 300 mg. Tab. Bot. 100s, 1000s, Blister pkg. 10 × 10s. *OTC.*
Use: Vitamin supplement.

• **bectumomab.** (beck-TYOO-moe-mab)
USAN.
Use: Monoclonal antibody, diagnosis of
non-Hodgkin lymphoma and detection of AIDS-related lymphoma.

• **bedaquiline.** (bed-AK-wi-leen) USAN.
Use: Treatment of tuberculosis.

• **bedaquiline fumarate.** (bed-AK-wi-leen)
USAN.
Use: Treatment of tuberculosis.

• **bederocin.** (be-DER-oh-sin) USAN.
Use: Antibacterial agent.

Bedoce. (Lincoln Diagnostics) Crystalline anhydrous vitamin B_{12} 1000 mcg/
mL. Vial 10 mL. *Rx.*
Use: Vitamin supplement.

Bedoce-Gel. (Lincoln Diagnostics) Vitamin B_{12} 1000 mcg/mL in 17% gelatin
soln. Vial 10 mL. *Rx.*
Use: Vitamin supplement.

• **bedoradrine sulfate.** (bed-OR-a-dreen)
USAN.
Use: Tocolytic agent.

Bedside Care. (Sween) Bot. 8 oz, gal.
Use: Dermatologic.

beechwood creosote.
See: Creosote.

Bee-Forte w/C. (Rugby) Vitamins B_1
25 mg, B_2 12.5 mg, B_3 50 mg, B_5
10 mg, B_6 3 mg, B_{12} 2.5 mcg, C
250 mg. Cap. Bot. 100s. *OTC.*
Use: Vitamin supplement.

beef peptones. (Sandia) Water-soluble
peptones derived from beef 20 mg/
2 mL. Inj. Vial 30 mL. *Rx.*
Use: Nutritional supplement, parenteral.

Beelith. (Beach) Pyridoxine hydrochlo-
ride 20 mg, magnesium oxide 600 mg.
Tab. Bot. 100s. *OTC.*
Use: Mineral, vitamin supplement.

Beepen-VK. (GlaxoSmithKline) Penicillin
V. **Tab.:** 250 mg, Bot. 1000s; 500 mg,
Bot. 500s. **Pow. for Oral Soln.:**
125 mg/5 mL; 250 mg/5 mL. Bot.
100 mL, 200 mL. *Rx.*
Use: Anti-infective; penicillin.

Bee-Thi. (Burgin-Arden) Cyanocobalamin 1000 mcg, thiamine hydrochloride 100 mg in isotonic soln. of sodium
chloride/mL. Vial 10 mL, 20 mL. *Rx.*
Use: Vitamin supplement.

Bee-Twelve 1000. (Burgin-Arden)
Cyanocobalamin 1000 mcg/mL. Vial
10 mL, 30 mL. *Rx.*
Use: Vitamin supplement.

Bee-Zee. (Rugby) Vitamins E 45 mg,
B_1 15 mg, B_2 10.2 mg, B_3 100 mg, B_5
25 mg, B_6 10 mg, B_{12} 6 mcg, C 600 mg,
zinc 5.2 mg. Tab. Bot. 60s. *OTC.*
Use: Mineral, vitamin supplement.

• **befetupitant.** (BEF-et-UE-pi-tant) USAN.
Use: CNS agent.

Behepan.
See: Cyanocobalamin.

• **belagenpumatucel-L.** (BEL-a-JEN-pum-
a-too-sel) USAN.
Use: Antineoplastic.

• **belatacept.** (bel-a-TA-sept) USAN.
Use: Immunosuppressive agent.

Belatol. (Cenci, H.R. Labs) **No. 1:** Belladonna leaf extract ⅛ g, phenobarbital
0.25 g. Tab. Bot. 100s, 1000s. **No. 2:**
Belladonna leaf extract, phenobarbital
0.5 g. Tab. Bot. 100s, 1000s. *Rx.*
Use: Anticholinergic; antispasmodic;
hypnotic; sedative.

Belatol Elixir. (Cenci, H.R. Labs, Inc.)
Phenobarbital 20 mg, belladonna
6.75 mg/5 mL w/alcohol 45%. Bot. Pt,
gal. *Rx.*
Use: Anticholinergic; antispasmodic;
hypnotic; sedative.

Belbutal No. 2 Kaptabs. (Churchill)
Phenobarbital 32.4 mg, hyoscyamine
sulfate 0.1092 mg, atropine sulfate
0.0215 mg, hyoscine HBr 0.0065 mg.
Tab. Bot. 100s. *Rx.*
Use: Anticholinergic; antispasmodic;
hypnotic; sedative.

Beldin. (Halsey Drug) Diphenhydramine
hydrochloride 12.5 mg/5 mL w/alcohol
5%. Bot. Gal. *OTC.*
Use: Antihistamine.

Belexal. (Pal-Pak, Inc.) Vitamins B_1
1.5 mg, B_2 2 mg, B_6 0.167 mg, calcium
pantothenate 1 mg, niacinamide
10 mg, brewer's yeast. Tab. Bot. 1000s,
5000s. *OTC.*
Use: Mineral, vitamin supplement.

Belexon Fortified Improved. (A.P.C.)
Liver fraction No. 2, 3 g, yeast extract
3 g, vitamins B_1 5 mg, B_2 6 mg, niacinamide 10 mg, calcium pantothenate
2 mg, cyanocobalamin 1 mcg, iron
10 mg. Cap. Bot. 100s. *OTC.*
Use: Mineral, vitamin supplement.

Belfer. (Forest) Vitamins B_1 2 mg, B_2
2 mg, B_{12} 10 mcg, B_6 2 mg, C 50 mg,
iron 17 mg. Tab. Bot. 100s. *OTC.*
Use: Mineral, vitamin supplement.

• **belfosdil.** (bell-FOSE-dill) USAN.
Use: Antihypertensive; calcium channel
blocker.

Belganyl.
See: Suramin.

• **belimumab.** (bel-LIM-oo-mab) USAN.
Use: Monoclonal antibody.
See: Benlysta.

• **belladonna.** (bell-a-DON-a) *USP 34.*
Use: Gastrointestinal anticholinergic/an-
tispasmodic.

belladonna alkaloids.
Use: Anticholinergic; antispasmodic.
See: Hyoscyamine Sulfate.
W/Chlorpheniramine Maleate, Pseudo-
ephedrine Hydrochloride.
See: Respa A.R.
W/Combinations.
See: Atropine Sulfate.
Belladonna.
L-Hyoscyamine Sulfate.
**belladonna alkaloids with phenobarbi-
tal.** (Various Mfr.) Atropine sulfate
0.0194 mg, scopolamine HBr
0.0065 mg, hyoscyamine HBr or sul-
fate 0.1037 mg, phenobarbital 16.2 mg.
Tab. Bot. 50s, 100s, 1000s, UD 100s.
Rx.
Use: GI anticholinergic combination.
**belladonna and phenobarbital combi-
nations.**
Use: Anticholinergic; antispasmodic;
hypnotic; sedative.
See: Bebatab No. 2.
Belatol.
Chardonna-2.
Spabelin No. 2.
•**belladonna extract.** (bell-a-DON-a)
USP 34. Rx.
Use: Antispasmodic.
W/Butabarbital Sodium.
See: Butibel.
belladonna extract. (Eli Lilly) Belladonna
extract 15 mg (0.187 mg belladonna).
Tab. *Rx.*
Use: Antispasmodic.
belladonna extract combinations.
Use: Anticholinergic; antispasmodic.
See: B & O Supprettes.
•**belladonna leaf.** (bell-a-DON-a) *USP 34.*
Use: Antispasmodic.
**belladonna leaf, phenobarbital, and
benzocaine.**
Use: Anticholinergic.
•**belladonna tincture.** (bell-a-DON-a)
USP 34.
Use: Antispasmodic.
Bellahist-D LA. (Cypress) Phenylephrine
hydrochloride 20 mg, chlorpheniramine
maleate 8 mg, hyoscyamine sulfate
0.19 mg, atropine sulfate 0.04 mg,
scopolamine HBr 0.01 mg. Alcohol and
dye free. ER Tab. 100s. *Rx.*
Use: Upper respiratory combination, decongestant, antihistamine, anticholinergic combination.
Bellaneed. (Hanlon) Belladonna, phenobarbital 16 mg. Cap. Bot. 100s. *Rx.*
Use: Anticholinergic; antispasmodic;
hypnotic; sedative.

Bell/ans. (C.S. Dent & Co.) Sodium bicarbonate 520 mg (sodium content
144 mg). Tab. Bot. 30s, 60s. *OTC.*
Use: Antacid.
Bellastal. (Wharton) Atropine sulfate
0.0194 mg, scopolamine HBr
0.0065 mg, hyoscyamine HBr or
SO_4 0.1037 mg, phenobarbital 16.2 mg.
Cap. Bot. 1000s. *Rx.*
Use: Anticholinergic; antispasmodic.
Bellatal. (Richwood Pharmaceuticals)
Phenobarbital 16.2 mg, hyoscyamine
sulfate 0.1037 mg, atropine sulfate
0.0194 mg, scopolamine HBr
0.0065 mg, lactose. Tab. Bot. 100s,
500s. *Rx.*
Use: Hypnotic; sedative.
•**belotecan hydrochloride.** (BEL-oh-TEE-
kan) USAN.
Use: Antineoplastic.
•**beloxamide.** (bell-OX-ah-mid) USAN.
Use: Antihyperlipoproteinemic.
•**beloxepin.** (beh-LOX-eh-pin) USAN.
Use: Antidepressant.
•**bemarinone hydrochloride.** (BEH-mah-
rih-NOHN) USAN.
Use: Cardiovascular agent, positive inotropic, vasodilator.
•**bemesetron.** (beh-meh-SET-rone)
USAN.
Use: Antiemetic.
Beminal 500. (Whitehall-Robins) Vita-
mins B_1 25 mg, B_2 12.5 mg, B_3
100 mg, B_6 10 mg, B_5 20 mg, C
500 mg, B_{12} 5 mcg. Tab. Bot. 100s.
OTC.
Use: Vitamin supplement.
•**bemitradine.** (beh-MIH-trah-DEEN)
USAN.
Use: Antihypertensive; diuretic.
•**bemoradan.** (beh-MOE-rah-DAN) USAN.
Use: Cardiovascular agent.
•**bemotrizinol.** (be-MOE-trye-zi-nol)
USAN.
Use: Sunscreen.
Benacen. (Cenci, H.R. Labs, Inc.) Pro-
benecid 0.5 g. Tab. Bot. 100s, 1000s.
Rx.
Use: Antigout.
Benacol. (Cenci, H.R. Labs, Inc.) Di-
cyclomine hydrochloride 20 mg. Tab.
Bot. 100s, 1000s. *Rx.*
Use: Anticholinergic; antispasmodic.
benactyzine hydrochloride. 2-Diethyl-
aminoethyl benzilate hydrochloride.
Use: Anxiolytic.
benactyzine/meprobamate. Psycho-
therapeutic combination.
Benadryl. (McNeil) Diphenhydramine
hydrochloride. **Cream:** 1%. Tube 1 oz.

Elix. (w/alcohol 14%): 12.5 mg/5 mL. Bot. 4 oz, pt, gal, UD 5 mL (100s). **Spray:** 1%. Bot. 2 oz. **Tab.:** 25 mg. Bot. 100s. *OTC.*
Use: Antihistamine.

Benadryl. (Pfizer) Diphenhydramine hydrochloride 50 mg/mL. Amps 1 mL; *Steri-vials* (with benzethonium chloride) 1 mL, 10 mL; *Steri-dose* syringe 1 mL. *Rx.*
Use: Antihistamine.

Benadryl Allergy. (McNeil) Diphenhydramine hydrochloride. **Chew. Tab.:** 12.5 mg, aspartame, phenylalanine 4.2 mg, grape flavor. Pkg. 24s. **Tab.:** 25 mg. Pkg. 24s. Bot. 100s. **Liq.:** 12.5 mg/5 mL. Bot. 118 mL. *OTC.*
Use: Antihistamine, nonselective ethanolamine.

Benadryl Allergy & Cold. (McNeil) Phenylephrine hydrochloride 5 mg, diphenhydramine hydrochloride 12.5 mg, acetaminophen 325 mg. Tab. Pkg. 24s. *OTC.*
Use: Upper respiratory combination, decongestant, antihistamine, analgesic.

Benadryl Allergy Kapseals. (McNeil) Diphenhydramine hydrochloride 25 mg, lactose. Cap. Pkg. 24s, 48s. *OTC.*
Use: Antihistamine, nonselective ethanolamine.

Benadryl Allergy Plus Sinus Headache. (McNeil) Phenylephrine hydrochloride 5 mg, diphenhydramine hydrochloride 12.5 mg, acetaminophen 325 mg. PEG. Tab. 24s, 48s. *OTC.*
Use: Decongestant, antihistamine, and analgesic, upper respiratory combination.

Benadryl Allergy Quick Dissolve. (McNeil) Diphenhydramine hydrochloride 25 mg. Sucralose. Vanilla mint flavor. Orally Disintegrating Strips. 10s, 20s. *OTC.*
Use: Antihistamine.

Benadryl Allergy Ultratabs. (McNeil) Diphenhydramine hydrochloride 25 mg. Tab. Bot. 24s, 48s, 100s. *OTC.*
Use: Antihistamine, nonselective ethanolamine.

Benadryl Children's Allergy. (McNeil) **Liq.:** Diphenhydramine hydrochloride 12.5 mg/5 mL, sugar, cherry flavor. Bot. 118 mL, 236 mL. **Orally Disintegrating Tab.:** Diphenhydramine citrate 19 mg, phenylalanine 4.5 mg. Aspartame. 20s. *OTC.*
Use: Antihistamine, nonselective ethanolamine.

Benadryl Children's Allergy & Cold. (McNeil) Pseudoephedrine hydrochloride 30 mg, diphenhydramine citrate 19 mg (equiv. to diphenhydramine hydrochloride 12.5 mg). Phenylalanine 4.6 mg, aspartame, lactose, mannitol. *Fastmelt* Tab. Pkg. 20s. *OTC.*
Use: Upper respiratory combination, decongestant, antihistamine.

Benadryl Children's Anti-Itch. (Johnson & Johnson) Camphor 0.45%. Benzyl alcohol, EDTA, menthol, SD alcohol. Gel. 85 g. *OTC.*
Use: Miscellaneous topical combination.

Benadryl Children's Dye-Free Allergy. (McNeil) Diphenhydramine 12.5 mg/ 5 mL, saccharin, sorbitol, alcohol free, bubble-gum flavor. Liq. Bot. 118 mL. *OTC.*
Use: Antihistamine, nonselective ethanolamine.

Benadryl-D Allergy & Sinus. (McNeil) Phenylephrine hydrochloride 10 mg, diphenhydramine hydrochloride 25 mg. PEG. Tab. 24s. *OTC.*
Use: Upper respiratory combination, decongestant and antihistamine.

Benadryl-D Children's Allergy & Sinus. (McNeil) Pseudoephedrine hydrochloride 30 mg, diphenhydramine hydrochloride 12.5 mg per 5 mL. Alcohol and sugar free. Saccharin, sorbitol. Grape flavor. Liq. 118 mL. *OTC.*
Use: Upper respiratory combination, decongestant and antihistamine.

Benadryl Dye-Free Allergy. (McNeil) Diphenhydramine hydrochloride 25 mg, sorbitol. Cap. Bot. 24s. *OTC.*
Use: Antihistamine, nonselective ethanolamine.

Benadryl Elixir. (McNeil) Diphenhydramine hydrochloride 12.5 mg/5 mL w/ alcohol 14%. Bot. 4 oz, pt, gal, UD (5 mL) 100s. *OTC.*
Use: Antihistamine.

Benadryl Injection. (Pfizer) Diphenhydramine hydrochloride 50 mg/mL. Amp. 1 mL, *Steri-Vials* 10 mL, *Steri-dose* syringe 1 mL. *Rx.*
Use: Antihistamine.

Benadryl Itch Relief. (McNeil) Diphenhydramine hydrochloride 1%, zinc acetate 0.1%, alcohol 73.6%, aloe vera. Spray. Bot. 59 mL. *OTC.*
Use: Antihistamine.

Benadryl Itch Relief Children's. (McNeil) **Cream:** Diphenhydramine hydrochloride 1%, zinc acetate 0.1%, aloe vera, cetyl alcohol, parabens. Jar 14.2 g. **Spray:** Diphenhydramine hydrochloride 1%, zinc acetate 0.1%, alcohol 73.6%, aloe vera, povidone.

Can. 59 mL. *OTC.*
Use: Antihistamine.

Benadryl Itch Relief, Maximum Strength. (McNeil) **Cream:** Diphenhydramine hydrochloride 2%, zinc acetate 0.1%, parabens, aloe vera. Tube 14.2 g. **Stick:** Diphenhydramine hydrochloride 2%, zinc acetate 0.1%, alcohol 73.5%, aloe vera. Tube 14 mL. *OTC.*
Use: Antihistamine.

Benadryl Itch Stopping Gel Children's Formula. (McNeil) Diphenhydramine hydrochloride 1%, zinc acetate 1%, camphor, parabens. Gel. Tube 118 mL. *OTC.*
Use: Antihistamine.

Benadryl Itch Stopping Gel, Maximum Strength. (McNeil) Diphenhydramine hydrochloride 2%, zinc acetate 1%, camphor, parabens. Tube 118 g. *OTC.*
Use: Antihistamine.

Benadryl Itch Stopping Spray, Extra Strength. (McNeil) Diphenhydramine hydrochloride 2%, zinc acetate 0.1%, alcohol 73.5%, glycerin, tromethamine. Spray. Bot. 59 mL. *OTC.*
Use: Antihistamine.

Benadryl Itch Stopping Spray, Original Strength. (McNeil) Diphenhydramine hydrochloride 1%, zinc acetate 0.1%, alcohol 73.6%, glycerin, tromethamine. Spray. Bot. 59 mL. *OTC.*
Use: Antihistamine.

Benadryl Severe Allergy & Sinus Headache, Maximum Strength. (McNeil) Phenylephrine hydrochloride 5 mg, diphenhydramine hydrochloride 25 mg, acetaminophen 325 mg. PEG. Tab. 20s. *OTC.*
Use: Upper respiratory combination, decongestant, antihistamine, and analgesic combination.

Benahist 50. (Keene Pharmaceuticals) Diphenhydramine 50 mg/mL. Vial 10 mL. *Rx.*
Use: Antihistamine.

Benahist 10. (Keene Pharmaceuticals) Diphenhydramine 10 mg/mL. Vial 30 mL. *Rx.*
Use: Antihistamine.

benanserin hydrochloride.
Use: Serotonin antagonist.

Benaphen Caps. (Major) Diphenhydramine 25 mg, 50 mg. Cap. Bot. 100s, 1000s. *OTC.*
Use: Antihistamine.

•**benapryzine hydrochloride.** (BEN-ah-PRY-zeen) USAN.
Use: Anticholinergic.

Benase. (Ferndale) Proteolytic enzymes extracted from Carica papaya 20,000 units enzyme activity. Tab. Bot. 1000s. *Rx.*
Use: Reduction of edema, relief of episiotomy.

•**benazeprilat.** (BEN-AZE-eh-prill-at) USAN.
Use: Angiotensin-converting enzyme inhibitor.

•**benazepril hydrochloride.** (BEN-AZE-eh-prill) USAN.
Use: Angiotensin-converting enzyme inhibitor, renin angiotensin system antagonist.
See: Lotensin.
W/Combinations.
See: Lotensin HCT.
Lotrel.

benazepril hydrochloride. (Various Mfr.) Benazepril hydrochloride 5 mg, 10 mg, 20 mg, 40 mg. May contain lactose, maltodextrin. Tab. 30s, 100s, 500s, 1,000s. *Rx.*
Use: Angiotensin-converting enzyme inhibitor, renin angiotensin system antagonist.

benazepril hydrochloride/hydrochlorothiazide. (Sandoz) Hydrochlorothiazide/benazepril hydrochloride 6.25 mg/ 5 mg, 12.5 mg/10 mg, 12.5 mg/20 mg, 25 mg/20 mg. Lactose. Tab. 100s. *Rx.*
Use: Antihypertensive.

Bencort. (River's Edge) Benzoyl peroxide 5%, hydrocortisone 0.5%. Acetylated lanolin alcohol, cetyl alcohol, EDTA, lanolin oil, mineral oil, parabens, tetrasodium EDTA. Lot. 25 g. *Rx.*
Use: Acne product, combination.

•**bendacalol mesylate.** (ben-DACK-ah-LOLE) USAN.
Use: Antihypertensive.

•**bendamustine hydrochloride.** (BEN-da-MUS-teen) USAN.
Use: Mechlorethamine derivative, ethylenimine/methylmelamine; alkylating agent.
See: Treanda.

•**bendazac.** (BEN-dah-ZAK) USAN.
Use: Anti-inflammatory.

•**bendroflumethiazide.** (ben-droe-floo-meth-EYE-a-zide) *USP 34.*
Use: Antihypertensive; diuretic.
W/Combinations.
See: Corzide.

bendroflumethiazide and rauwolfia.
See: Rauwolfia/Bendroflumethiazide.

Benefiber. (Novartis) Fiber. **Chew. Tab.:** 1 g. Acesulfame K, aspartame, dextrates, phenylalanine, sorbitol, sucra-

lose, wheat dextrin. Gluten free and sugar free. Assorted fruit and orange crème flavors. 100s. **Pow.:** 1.5 g per teaspoon. Wheat dextrin. Gluten free and sugar free. 70 g, 133 g, 217 g, 315 g, 437.5 g, 665 g. *OTC.*
Use: Laxative, bulk-producing laxative.

Benefiber Drink Mix. (Novartis) Fiber 3 g per packet. Acesulfame K, aspartame, maltodextrin, phenylalanine, potassium citrate, wheat dextrin. Sugar free. Cherry pomegranate, citrus punch, kiwi strawberry, and raspberry tea flavors. Pow. 8s, 16s. *OTC.*
Use: Laxative, bulk-producing laxative.

Benefiber for Children. (Novartis) Fiber 1.5 g per teaspoon. Wheat dextrin. Gluten free and sugar free. Pow. 153 g. *OTC.*
Use: Laxative, bulk-producing laxative.

Benefiber Plus Calcium. (Novartis) Fiber. **Tab.:** 1 g. Acesulfame K, aspartame, calcium 100 mg, dextrates, maltodextrin, phenylalanine, sorbitol, sucralose, wheat dextrin. Gluten free and sugar free. Berry flavor. Chew. 90s. **Pow.:** 3 g per tablespoon. Calcium 300 mg, wheat dextrin. Gluten free and sugar free. 423.8 g. *OTC.*
Use: Laxative, bulk-producing laxative.

Benefiber Plus Heart Health. (Novartis) Fiber. **Tab.:** 1 g. Folic acid 44.7 mcg, vitamin B_6 0.23 mg, B_{12} 0.67 mcg, wheat dextrin. Gluten free and sugar free. 60s. **Pow.:** 1.5 g per teaspoon. Folic acid 67 mg, vitamin B_6 0.35 mg, B_{12} 1 mcg, wheat dextrin. Gluten free and sugar free. 181.4 g. *OTC.*
Use: Laxative, bulk-producing laxative.

Benefiber Sticks. (Novartis) Fiber 3 g per packet. Acesulfame K, aspartame, maltodextrin, phenylalanine (all except unflavored), tartrazine (citrus punch flavor), wheat dextrin. Sugar free. Unflavored, cherry pomegranate, citrus punch, kiwi strawberry, and raspberry tea flavors. Pow. 8s, 16s, 28s. *OTC.*
Use: Laxative, bulk-producing laxative.

Benefiber Ultra. (Novartis) Fiber 3 g. Wheat dextrin. Sugar free and gluten free. Tab. 72s, 114s. *OTC.*
Use: Laxative, bulk-producing laxative.

BeneFIX. (Wyeth) Factor IX (recombinant) 250 units, 500 units, 1,000 units, 2,000 units. Actual number of units shown on each bottle. Glycine, L-histidine, polysorbate 80, sucrose. Preservative free. Inj., lyophilized Pow. for Soln. Kit w/single-dose vial and diluent. *Rx.*
Use: Antihemophilic agent.

Benemid. (Merck & Co.) Probenecid 0.5 g. Tab. Bot. 100s, 1000s, UD 100s. *Rx.*
Use: Antigout.

Benepro Tabs. (Major) Probenecid 500 mg. Tab. Bot. 100s, 1000s. *Rx.*
Use: Antigout.

bengal gelatin.
See: Agar.

Bengay Children's Vaporizing Rub. (Pfizer) Camphor, menthol, w/oils of turpentine, eucalyptus, cedar leaf, nutmeg, thyme in stainless white base. Jar 1.125 oz. *OTC.*
Use: Analgesic, topical.

Bengay Extra Strength. (Pfizer) Methyl salicylate 30%, menthol 8%. Balm. Jar 3.75 oz. *OTC.*
Use: Analgesic, topical.

Bengay Extra Strength Sports. (Pfizer) Methyl salicylate 28%, menthol 10%. Balm. Tube 1.25 oz, 3 oz. *OTC.*
Use: Analgesic, topical.

Bengay Gel. (Pfizer) Methyl salicylate 15%, menthol 7%, alcohol 40%. Gel. Tube 1.25 oz, 3 oz. *OTC.*
Use: Analgesic, topical.

Bengay Greaseless. (Pfizer) Methyl salicylate 18.3%, menthol 16%. Oint. Tube 1.25 oz, 3 oz, 5 oz. *OTC.*
Use: Analgesic, topical.

Bengay Lotion. (Pfizer) Methyl salicylate 15%, menthol 7% in lotion base. Lot. Bot. 2 oz, 4 oz. *OTC.*
Use: Analgesic, topical.

Bengay Ointment. (Pfizer) Methyl salicylate 15%, menthol 10% in ointment base. Oint. Tube 1.25 oz, 3 oz, 5 oz. *OTC.*
Use: Analgesic, topical.

Bengay Original. (Pfizer) Methyl salicylate 18.3%, menthol 16%. Oint. Tube. 37.5 g, 90 g, 150 g. *OTC.*
Use: Analgesic, topical.

Bengay Patch. (Pfizer) Menthol 1.4%. Glycerin. Patch, regular and large size. 1s. *OTC.*
Use: Liniment.

Bengay Sports Gel. (Pfizer) Methyl salicylate, menthol, alcohol 40%. Gel. Tube 1.25 oz, 3 oz. *OTC.*
Use: Analgesic, topical.

Benicar. (Sankyo Pharm) Olmesartan medoxomil 5 mg, 20 mg, 40 mg. Lactose. Film-coated. Tab. Bot. 30s, 90s (except 5 mg), blister card 100s (except 5 mg). *Rx.*
Use: Antihypertensive.

Benicar HCT. (Sankyo Pharma) Hydrochlorothiazide/olmesartan medoxomil. 12.5 mg/20 mg, 12.5 mg/40 mg, 25 mg/

40 mg. Lactose. Film-coated. Tab. 30s, 90s, 1000s, blister card 10s. *Rx.*
Use: Antihypertensive.

Benlysta. (Human Genome Sciences) Belimumab 120 mg, 400 mg. Polysorbate 80, sucrose 80 mg/mL. Latex free, preservative free. Inj., lyophilized Pow. for Soln. Single-use vial. 20 mL. *Rx.*
Use: Monoclonal antibody.

•**benorterone.** (bee-NAHR-ter-ohn) USAN.
Use: Antiandrogen.

•**benoxaprofen.** (ben-OX-ah-PRO-fen) USAN.
Use: Anti-inflammatory; analgesic.

•**benoxinate hydrochloride.** (ben-OX-ih-nate) *USP 34.*
Use: Anesthetic, topical.
See: Fluress.

•**benperidol.** (BEN-peh-rih-dahl) USAN.
Use: Antipsychotic.

•**benralizumab.** (BEN-ra-LIZ-oo-mab) USAN.
Use: Respiratory agent.

•**bensalan.** (BEN-sal-an) USAN.
Use: Disinfectant.

Bensal HP. (7 Oaks) Benzoic acid 6%, salicylic acid 3%, extract of oak bark. Oint. Tube 15 g, 30 g. Jar 30 g, 60 g. *Rx.*
Use: Anti-infective, topical.

•**benserazide.** (ben-SER-ah-zide) USAN.
Use: Inhibitor, decarboxylase; antiparkinson.

Benson's Bottom Paint. (Benson's Bottom Paint) Cetyl alcohol, emulsifying wax, glycerin, paraffin, petrolatum, stearyl alcohol, triethanolamine, zinc oxide. Oint. 56.7 g. *OTC.*
Use: Diaper rash product.

•**bentazepam.** (BEN-tay-zeh-pam) USAN.
Use: Hypnotic; sedative.

Bentical. (Lamond) Bentonite, zinc oxide, zinc carbonate, titanium dioxide. Bot. 4 oz, 6 oz, 8 oz, 16 oz, 32 oz, 0.5 gal, gal.
Use: Emollient.

•**bentiromide.** (ben-TEER-oh-mide) USAN.
Use: Diagnostic aid, pancreas function determination.

•**bentonite.** (BEN-tun-ite) *NF 29.*
Use: Pharmaceutic aid, suspending agent.

bentonite magma.
Use: Pharmaceutic aid, suspending agent.

bentonite, purified.
Use: Pharmaceutic aid.

•**bentoquatam.** (BEN-toe-KWAH-tam) USAN.
Use: Barrier for prevention of allergic contact dermatitis.
See: Ivy Block.

Bentyl. (Axcan Scandipharm) Dicyclomine hydrochloride. **Cap.:** 10 mg. Bot. 100s, 500s, UD 100s. **Tab.:** 20 mg. Bot. 100s, 500s, 1000s, UD 100s. **Syr.:** 10 mg/5 mL. Saccharin. Bot. Pt. **Inj.:** 10 mg/mL. Amps. 2 mL. Vials. 10 mL. *Rx.*
Use: GI anticholinergic/antispasmodic.

•**benurestat.** (BEN-YOU-reh-stat) USAN.
Use: Enzyme inhibitor, urease.

Benylin Expectorant. (Warner Lambert) Dextromethorphan HBr 5 mg, guaifenesin 100 mg per 5 mL. Saccharin, sorbitol, raspberry flavor, alcohol free, sugar free. Bot. Liq. 118 mL. *OTC.*
Use: Upper respiratory combination, antitussive, expectorant.

Benza. (Century) Benzalkonium chloride 1:5000, 1:750. Bot. 2 oz, 4 oz.
Use: Antimicrobial; antiseptic.

Benzac AC 5 & 10. (Galderma) Benzoyl peroxide 5%, 10%, glycerine and EDTA in water base. Gel. Tube 60 g, 90 g. *Rx.*
Use: Antiacne.

Benzac AC Wash 5 & 10. (Galderma) Benzoyl peroxide 5%, 10%, glycerin. Liq. 240 mL. *Rx.*
Use: Antiacne.

Benzac 5 & 10. (Galderma) Benzoyl peroxide 5%, 10%, alcohol 12%. Tube 60 g, 90 g. *Rx.*
Use: Antiacne.

BenzaClin. (Dermik) Clindamycin 1%, benzoyl peroxide 5%. Gel. 25 g, 50 g. Pump. 35 g, 50 g. *BenzaClin Care Kit* w/ 50 g pump and 20 topical ampules of viscontour serum. *Rx.*
Use: Anti-infective, antibiotic, topical.

Benzac W Wash 5 & 10. (Galderma) Benzoyl peroxide 5%, 10%, Bot. 120 mL (5% only), 240 mL. *Rx.*
Use: Antiacne.

Benzagel Wash. (Dermik) Benzoyl peroxide 10%, alcohol 14%. Gel. 60 g. *Rx.*
Use: Dermatologic, acne.

•**benzalkonium chloride.** (benz-al-KOE-nee-uhm) USAN.
Use: Surface antiseptic; pharmaceutical aid, preservative.
See: Bacti-Cleanse.
Eye-Stream.
Germicin.
Mycocide NS.
Otrivin.

Remedy.
Ultra Tears.
Zephiran.
W/Benzocaine, Butamben, Tetracaine Hydrochloride.
See: Cetacaine.
W/Chloroxylenol, Hydrocortisone, Pramoxine Hydrochloride.
See: Cortic-ND.
Mediotic-HC.
W/Lidocaine.
See: Bactine Pain Relieving Cleansing.
W/Lidocaine Hydrochloride.
See: Bactine Antiseptic Anesthetic.
Medi-Quik.
W/Other Combinations.
See: Bite Rx.
Cortane-B Lotion.
Cydonol Massage Lotion.
Dacriose.
Garamycin.
Ionax Foam.
Isopto Plain & Tears.
Mycomist.
Oxyzal Wet Dressing.
SalineX.
Tearisol.
Benzamycin. (Dermik) Benzoyl peroxide 5%, erythromycin 3%, alcohol 20%. Gel. 8 g, 23 g, 46 g. *Rx.*
Use: Anti-infective, topical.
Benzamycin Pak. (Dermik) Benzoyl peroxide 5%, erythromycin 3%, SD alcohol 40B. Gel. 0.8 g pouches. 60s. *Rx.*
Use: Anti-infectives, topical.
•**benzbromarone.** (BENZ-brome-ah-rone) USAN.
Use: Uricosuric.
Benzedrex. (B.F. Ascher) Propylhexedrine 250 mg, menthol, lavender oil. Inhaler. *OTC.*
Use: Nasal decongestant.
BenzEFoam. (Onset Therapeutics) Benzoyl peroxide 5.3%. Cetearyl alcohol, disodium EDTA, glycerin, parabens. Foam. 60 g. *Rx.*
Use: Anti-infective, topical; antibiotic agent.
•**benzethonium chloride.** (benz-eth-OH-nee-uhm) *USP 34.* Topical solution; Tincture.
Use: Anti-infective, topical; pharmaceutic aid, preservative.
See: Antiseptic Wound & Skin Cleanser.
W/Combinations.
See: Dermoplast Antibacterial.
W/Diphenhydramine Hydrochloride, Zinc Acetate.
See: Calagel Maximum Strength.
W/Lidocaine Hydrochloride.
See: StaphAseptic.

W/Menthol.
See: Gold Bond Antiseptic First Aid Quick Spray.
•**benzetimide hydrochloride.** (benz-ETT-ih-mide) USAN.
Use: Anticholinergic.
•**benzilonium bromide.** (BEN-zill-oh-nih-uhm) USAN.
Use: Anticholinergic.
•**benzindopyrine hydrochloride.** (BENZ-in-doe-pie-reen) USAN.
Use: Antipsychotic.
Benziq. (Graceway Pharmaceuticals) Benzoyl peroxide 5.25%. Benzyl alcohol, disodium EDTA, glycerin. Gel. 50 g. *Rx.*
Use: Anti-infective, topical; antibiotic agent.
Benziq LS. (Graceway Pharmaceuticals) Benzoyl peroxide 2.75%. Benzyl alcohol, disodium EDTA, glycerin. Gel. 50 g. *Rx.*
Use: Anti-infective, topical; antibiotic agent.
Benziq Wash. (Graceway Pharmaceuticals) Benzoyl peroxide 5.25%. Benzyl alcohol, cetyl alcohol, disodium EDTA, glycerin, PEG-100. Soap. 175 g. *Rx.*
Use: Anti-infective, topical; antibiotic agent.
benzisoxazole derivatives.
Use: Antipsychotic.
See: Iloperidone.
Paliperidone.
Risperidone.
Ziprasidone.
benzoate and phenylacetate.
Use: Treatment of hyperammonemia. [Orphan Drug]
Benzo-C. (Freeport) Benzocaine 5 mg, cetalkonium Cl 5 mg, ascorbic acid 50 mg. Troche. Bot. 1000s, cello-packed boxes 1000s. *OTC.*
Use: Anesthetic, local.
•**benzocaine.** (BEN-zoe-kane) *USP 34.* Ethyl-p-aminobenzoate. Anesthesin, orthesin, parathesin.
Use: Anesthetic, topical.
See: Americaine.
Americaine Hemorrhoidal.
Anbesol Cold Sore Therapy.
Anbesol Jr.
Bansmoke.
Benz-O-Sthetic.
Boil-Ease.
Cēpacol Sore Throat Lozenges.
Dent-O-Kain/20.
Dermoplast.
Dermoplast Antibacterial.
Detane.

Foille Medicated First Aid.
Hurricaine.
Lanacane.
Maximum Strength Anbesol.
Orabase.
Orajel.
Orajel D.
Orajel Mouth-Aid.
Orajel P.M. Nighttime Formula Tooth-
ache Pain Relief.
Orajel Regular Strength.
OraMagic Plus.
SensoGARD.
Solarcaine.
Solarcaine Medicated First Aid.
Trocaine.
W/Acetic Acid, Antipyrine, Polycosanol.
See: AABP.
Auralgan.
W/Antipyrine, Glycerin, Zinc Acetate Dihy-
drate.
See: Neotic.
W/Antipyrine, Phenylephrine Hydrochlo-
ride.
See: Ear-Gesic.
W/Antipyrine, u-Polycosanol 410.
See: Treagan.
W/Benzalkonium Chloride, Butamben,
Tetracaine Hydrochloride.
See: Cetacaine.
W/Camphor, Menthol.
See: Chiggerex.
W/Chloroxylenol, Hydrocortisone Ace-
tate.
See: TriOxin.
W/Dextromethorphan Hydrobromide.
See: Cēpacol Sore Throat Plus Cough
Relief.
Cough-X.
Tetra-Formula.
W/Glycerin.
See: Cēpacol Dual Relief Sore Throat
& Coating Spray.
W/Menthol.
See: Cēpacol Maximum Numbing Sore
Throat.
Cēpacol Sore Throat Pain Relief
Maximum Numbing.
Sting-Kill.
W/Menthol, Methyl Salicylate.
See: Dendracin Neurodendtraxin.
W/Pectin.
See: Cēpacol Sore Throat & Coating
Relief Maximum Numbing.
W/Phenol.
See: Anbesol.
W/Resorcinol.
See: Unguentine Maximum Strength.
Vagisil.
Vagisil Maximum Strength.

W/Sulfur.
See: Chigg Away.
W/Combinations.
See: Anacaine.
Anbesol Cold Sore Therapy.
Auralgesic.
Benzo-C.
Benzodent.
Bicozene.
Boil-Ease Salve.
Chloraseptic Children's.
Chloraseptic Kids Sore Throat.
Chloraseptic Sore Throat.
Chloraseptic Sore Throat Relief.
Culminal.
Dent's Extra Strength Toothache
Gum.
Dent's Lotion-Jel.
Dent's Maximum Strength Toothache
Drops.
Dent's Toothache Gum.
Denture Orajel.
Dent-Zel-Ite.
Dermoplast.
Dermoplast Antibacterial.
Foille.
Foille Medicated First Aid.
Foille Plus.
Hurricaine.
Jiffy.
Lanacane.
Orabase B.
Orabase Baby.
Orabase Lip.
Orabase with Benzocaine.
Orajel Mouth-Aid.
Rectal Medicone.
Rectal Medicone Unguent.
Solarcaine.
Spec-T Sore Throat Anesthetic.
Tanac Liquid.
Tanac Stick.
Toothache.
Zilactin-B Medicated.
benzocaine. (Various Mfr.) Benzocaine
5%. Cream. 480 g. *OTC.*
Use: Topical local anesthetic, ester lo-
cal anesthetic.
benzochlorophene sodium. Sodium salt
of ortho-benzyl-para-chlorophenol.
•**benzoctamine hydrochloride.** (benz-
OCK-tah-meen) USAN.
Use: Hypnotic; muscle relaxant; sedative.
Benzodent. (Procter & Gamble) Benzo-
caine 20%. Tube 30 g. *OTC.*
Use: Anesthetic, local.
•**benzodepa.** (BEN-zoe-DEH-pah) USAN.
Use: Antineoplastic.
benzodiazepines.
Use: Antianxiety agents; anticonvulsants; sedative/hypnotics, nonbarbi-
turates.

See: Alprazolam.
Clonazepam.
Clorazepate Dipotassium.
Chlordiazepoxide Hydrochloride.
Diazepam.
Estazolam.
Flurazepam Hydrochloride.
Lorazepam.
Oxazepam.
Quazepam.
Temazepam.
Triazolam.
● **benzoic acid.** (ben-ZOE-ik) *USP 34.*
Use: Pharmaceutic aid, antifungal.
W/Atropine Sulfate, Hyoscyamine Sulfate, Methenamine, Methylene Blue, Phenyl Salicylate.
See: Uritact DS.
W/Boric acid, zinc oxide, zinc stearate.
See: Whitfield's.
benzoic acid. (Various Mfr.) Benzoic acid. Pkg. 0.25 lb, 1 lb. *OTC.*
Use: Antifungal; fungistatic.
benzoic acid, 2-hydroxy. Salicylic acid.
benzoic and salicylic acids.
Use: Antifungal, topical.
See: Whitfield's.
● **benzoin.** (BEN-zoyn) *USP 34.*
Use: Protectant, topical; expectorant.
See: Sprayzoin.
W/Podophyllum resin.
See: Podoben.
benzoin. (Morton International) Benzoin, tolu balsam, styrax, alcohol w/propellant. Aerosol. Can 7 oz. *OTC.*
Use: Skin protectant.
benzoisothiazol derivatives.
See: Lurasidone Hydrochloride.
benzol. Usually refers to benzene.
Benzo-Menth. (Pal-Pak, Inc.) Benzocaine 2.2 mg. Tab. Bot. 1000s. *OTC.*
Use: Anesthetic, topical.
● **benzonatate.** (ben-ZOE-nah-tate) *USP 34.*
Use: Nonnarcotic antitussive.
See: Tessalon.
Tessalon Perles.
Zonatuss.
benzonatate softgels. (Various Mfr.) Benzonatate 100 mg, 200 mg. Cap. Bot. 100s, 500s. *Rx.*
Use: Nonnarcotic antitussive.
benzoquinonium chloride.
Use: Muscle relaxant.
Benz-O-Sthetic. (Geritrex) Benzocaine 20%. Spray. 56 g. *OTC.*
Use: Local anesthetic, topical.
benzosulfimide.
See: Saccharin.

benzosulphinide sodium. *Name previously used for Saccharin sodium.*
● **benzoxiquine.** (benz-OX-ee-kwine) USAN.
Use: Disinfectant.
● **benzoylpas calcium.** (benz-oe-ILL-pass) USAN.
Use: Anti-infective, tuberculostatic.
● **benzoyl peroxide.** (BEN-zoyl per-OX-ide) *USP 34.*
Use: Keratolytic.
See: Acne Clear.
Benzac AC Wash.
Benzac W Wash.
BenzEFoam.
Benziq.
Benziq LS.
Benziq Wash.
BP 5.25%.
BP 4.25%.
BP 7% Wash.
Brevoxyl Cleansing.
Brevoxyl-8 Acne Wash Kit.
Brevoxyl-4 Acne Wash Kit.
Clearasil Maximum Strength Acne Treatment.
Clinac BPO.
Delos.
Desquam-E.
Desquam-X.
Inova Easy Pad.
NeoBenz Micro.
NeoBenz Micro SD.
NeoBenz Micro Wash.
Neutrogena Clear Pore.
Oxy Oil-Free Maximum Strength Acne Wash.
Pacnex HP.
Pacnex LP.
PanOxyl.
PanOxyl AQ.
RE Benzoyl Peroxide.
SE BPO.
SE BPO 7%.
Soluclenz Rx.
Theroxide.
Triaz.
ZoDerm.
W/Adapalene.
See: Epiduo.
W/Chlorhydroxyquinoline, Hydrocortisone.
See: Vanoxide-HC.
W/Clindamycin.
See: Acanya.
Duac CS.
W/Hydrocortisone.
See: Bencort.
Vanoxide HC.
W/Polyoxyethylene Lauryl Ether.
See: Benzac 5 & 10.

Desquam-X 5.
Desquam-X 10.
W/Salicylic Acid, Tocopherol.
See: Inova 8/2 Acne Control Therapy.
Inova 4/1 Acne Control Therapy.
W/Sulfur.
See: NuOx.
Sulfoxyl.
benzoyl peroxide. (Fougera) Benzoyl peroxide 4.5%, 6.5%, 8.5%. Cetyl alcohol, disodium EDTA, glycerin, glyceryl stearate, PEG-100, urea 10%. Cleanser. 400 mL. *Rx.*
Use: Anti-infective, topical; antibiotic agent.
benzoyl peroxide. (Kylemore Pharmaceuticals) Benzoyl peroxide 4%. Alcohol, propylene glycol. Lot. 297 g. *Rx.*
Use: Topical anti-infective, antibiotic.
benzoyl peroxide. (River's Edge) Benzoyl peroxide. **5.75%:** Cetyl alcohol, disodium EDTA, glycerin, urea 10%. **7%:** Alcohols, aloe, glycerin, green tea extract, PEG, propylene glycol, triethanolamine. Soap. 473 mL (5.75%), 180 g (7%). *Rx.*
Use: Anti-infective, topical; antibiotic agent.
benzoyl peroxide. (Various Mfr.) Benzoyl peroxide. **Mask:** 5%. In 30 mL. **Lot.:** 5%, 10%. Bot. 30 mL. **Gel:** 2.5%, 4%, 5%, 8%, 10%. Tube 42.5 g (4%, 8%), 60 g (2.5%, 5%, 10%), 90 g (except 2.5%). *Rx.*
Use: Anti-infective, topical; antibiotic agent.
benzoyl peroxide wash. (Various Mfr.) Benzoyl peroxide 2.5%, 5%, 10%. Liq. Bot. 118 mL (5% only) 148 mL (except 2.5%), 237 mL. *Rx.*
Use: Keratolytic.
n'-benzoylsulfanilamide.
See: Sulfabenzamide.
benzphetamine hydrochloride. (benz-FET-uh-meen)
Use: CNS stimulant, anorexiant.
See: Didrex.
benzphetamine hydrochloride. (Various Mfr.) Benzphetamine hydrochloride 50 mg. May contain lactose, polydextrose, sorbitol. Tab. 30s, 90s, 100s, 500s. *Rx.*
Use: CNS stimulant, anorexiant.
•**benzquinamide.** (benz-KWIN-ah-mid) USAN.
Use: Antiemetic.
•**benztropine mesylate.** (BENZ-troe-peen) *USP 34.*
Use: Parasympatholytic, antiparkinsonian.
benztropine mesylate. (West-Ward) Benztropine mesylate 1 mg/mL. Inj.,

Soln. Amp. 2 mL. *Rx.*
Use: Antiparkinson agent, anticholinergic.
benztropine mesylate. (Various Mfr.) Benztropine mesylate 0.5 mg, 1 mg, 2 mg. Tab. 100s, 1000s (except 0.5 mg), UD 100s. *Rx.*
Use: Antiparkinson agent, anticholinergic.
benztropine methanesulfonate.
See: Benztropine mesylate.
•**benzydamine hydrochloride.** (ben-ZIH-dah-meen) USAN.
Use: Analgesic; anti-inflammatory; antipyretic.
benzydroflumethiazide.
See: Bendroflumethiazide.
•**benzyl alcohol.** (BEN-zil) *NF 29.* Phenylcarbinol.
Use: Anesthetic; antiseptic, topical; pharmaceutic aid, antimicrobial.
See: Topic.
Zilactin-L.
•**benzyl benzoate.** (BEN-zil) *USP 34.*
Use: Pharmaceutical necessity for Dimercaprol Inj.
benzyl benzoate saponated. (Various Mfr.) Triethanolamine 20 g, oleic acid 80 g, benzyl benzoate q.s. 1000 mL.
Use: Scabicide, pediculicides.
benzyl carbinol.
See: Phenylethyl alcohol.
benzylpenicillin, benzylpenicilloic, benzylpenilloic acid. (Kremers Urban)
Use: Assessment of penicillin sensitivity. [Orphan Drug]
See: Pre-Pen/MDM.
benzyl penicillin-C-14. (Nuclear-Chicago) Carbon-14 labelled penicillin. Vacuum-sealed glass vial 50 microcuries, 0.5 millicuries.
Use: Radiopharmaceutical.
benzyl penicillin G, potassium.
See: Penicillin G potassium.
benzyl penicillin G, sodium.
See: Penicillin G sodium.
•**benzylpenicilloyl polylysine concentrate.** (BEN-zil-PEN-i-SIL-oh-il POL-ee-LYE-seen) *USP 34.*
Use: In vivo diagnostic aid.
See: Pre-Pen.
Bepanthen.
See: Panthenol.
Bephedin. Benzyl ephedrine.
bephenium hydroxynaphthoate.
Use: Anthelmintic, hookworms.
•**bepotastine.** (BEP-oh-TAS-teen) USAN.
Use: Mast cell stabilizer.
•**bepotastine besilate.** (BEP-oh-TAS-teen) USAN.

Use: Mast cell stabilizer.
See: Bepreve.

Bepreve. (ISTA Pharmaceuticals) Bepotastine besilate 1.5% (equiv. to bepotastine 10.7 mg base). Benzalkonium chloride 0.005%, monobasic sodium phosphate dihydrate, sodium chloride, sodium hydroxide. Soln., Ophth. Bot. 10 mL. *Rx.*
Use: Ophthalmic and otic agent, mast cell stabilizer.

•**beractant.** (ber-ACT-ant) USAN.
Use: Lung surfactant; respiratory distress syndrome. Respiratory failure; pulmonary hypertension; pneumonia; sepsis. [Orphan Drug]
See: Survanta.

•**beraprost.** (BEH-reh-prahst) USAN.
Use: Platelet aggregation inhibitor, improves ischemic syndromes.

•**beraprost sodium.** (BEH-reh-prahst) USAN.
Use: Platelet aggregation inhibitor, improves ischemic action.

berberine sulfate. (BUR-bur-een)
Use: Antimicrobial.

•**berefrine.** (BEH-reh-FREEN) USAN. *Formerly* Burefrine.
Use: Mydriatic.

Ber-Ex. (Dolcin) Calcium succinate 2.8 g, acetyl salicylic acid 3.7 g. Tab. Bot. 100s, 500s. *OTC.*
Use: Antiarthritic; antirheumatic.

Berinert P. (Aventis Behring) C1-Esterase-inhibitor, human, pasteurized.
Use: Hereditary angioedema. [Orphan Drug]

Berocca Plus. (Roche) Vitamins A 5000 units, E 30 units, C 500 mg, B_1 20 mg, B_2 20 mg, B_3. Tab. Bot. 100s. *Rx.*
Use: Iron, vitamin supplement.

Berri-Freez. (Geritrex) Menthol 3.5%, camphor, glycerin, isopropyl alcohol, parabens, triethanolamine. Gel. 473 g. *OTC.*
Use: Rub and liniment.

•**berythromycin.** (beh-RITH-row-MY-sin) USAN.
Use: Antiamebic; anti-infective.

Beserol. (Sanofi-Synthelabo) Acetaminophen, chlormezanone. Tab. *Rx.*
Use: Analgesic; tranquilizer; muscle relaxant.

•**besifloxacin hydrochloride.** (BE-si-FLOX-a-sin) USAN.
Use: Ophthalmic and otic agent, antibiotic.
See: Besivance.

•**besipirdine hydrochloride.** (beh-SIH-pihr-deen) USAN.
Use: Cognition enhancer; Alzheimer disease.

Besivance. (Bausch & Lomb) Besifloxacin 0.6%. Besifloxacin hydrochloride 6.63 mg equiv. to 6 mg base. Benzalkonium chloride 0.01%, edetate disodium dihydrate. Susp.; Ophth. Bot. 5 mL. *Rx.*
Use: Ophthalmic and otic agent, antibiotic.

•**besonprodil.** (be-son-PROE-dil) USAN.
Use: Parkinson disease.

Besta. (Roberts) Vitamins B_1 20 mg, B_2 15 mg, niacinamide 100 mg, calcium pantothenate 20 mg, E 50 units, magnesium sulfate 70 mg, zinc 18.4 mg, B_{12} 4 mcg, B_6 25 mg, C 300 mg. Cap. Bot. 100s. *OTC.*
Use: Vitamin, mineral supplement.

Best C. (Roberts) Ascorbic acid 500 mg. TR Cap. Bot. 100s. *OTC.*
Use: Vitamin supplement.

Bestrone. (Bluco) Estrone in aqueous susp. 2 mg/mL, 5 mg/mL. Inj. Vial 10 mL. *Rx.*
Use: Hormone, estrogen.

beta-adrenergic blockers, ophthalmic.
See: AKBeta.
  Betagan Liquifilm.
  Betaxolol Hydrochloride.
  Betimol.
  Betoptic.
  Betoptic S.
  Levobunolol Hydrochloride.
  Metipranolol Hydrochloride.
  OptiPranolol.
  Timolol.
  Timolol Maleate.
  Timoptic.
  Timoptic in Ocudose.
  Timoptic-XE.

beta-adrenergic blocking agents.
See: Acebutolol Hydrochloride.
  Atenolol.
  Betaxolol Hydrochloride.
  Bisoprolol Fumarate.
  Carteolol Hydrochloride.
  Esmolol Hydrochloride.
  Metoprolol.
  Nadolol.
  Nebivolol.
  Penbutolol Sulfate.
  Pindolol.
  Propranolol Hydrochloride.
  Sotalol Hydrochloride.
  Timolol Maleate.

beta alethine.
Use: Antineoplastic. [Orphan Drug]
See: Betathine.

• **beta carotene.** (BAY-tah CARE-oh-teen) *USP 34.*
Use: Ultraviolet screen.
See: Lumitene.

beta carotene. (Various Mfr.) Beta carotene 15 mg (vitamin A 25,000 units). Softgel cap. Bot. 60s, 100s. *OTC.*
Use: Vitamin supplement.

• **beta cyclodextrin.** (BAY-tah sigh-kloe-DEX-trin) *NF 29.*
See: Betadex.

• **betadex.** (BAY-tah-dex) USAN. *Formerly beta cyclodextrin.*
Use: Pharmaceutical aid.

Betadine. (Purdue) Povidone-iodine.
Available as: Aerosol Spray, Bot. 3 oz. Antiseptic Gz. Pads 3" × 9". Box 12s. Antiseptic Lubricating Gel, Tube 5 g. Disposable Medicated Douche, concentrated packette w/cannula and 6 oz water. Douche, Bot. 1 oz, 4 oz, 8 oz. Douche Packette, 0.5 oz (6 per carton). *Helafoam* Solution Canister 250 g. Mouthwash/Gargle, Bot. 6 oz. Oint. Tube 1 oz. Jar 1 lb, 5 lb. Oint., Packette. Perineal Wash Conc. Kit, Bot. 8 oz w/dispenser. Skin Cleanser, Bot. 1 oz, 4 oz. Skin Cleanser Foam, Canister 6 oz. Solution, 0.5 oz, 8 oz, 16 oz, 32 oz, gal. Solution Packette, oz. Solution Swab Aid, 100s. Solution Swabsticks, 1s Box 200s; 3s Box 50s. Surgical Scrub, Bot. Pt w/dispenser, qt, gal, packette 0.5 oz. Surgi-prep Sponge-Brush 36s. Vaginal Suppositories, Box 7s w/vaginal applicator. Viscous Formula Antiseptic Gauze Pads: 3" × 9", 5" × 9". Box 12s. Whirlpool Concentrate, Bot. Gal. *OTC.*
Use: Antiseptic.

Betadine Cream. (Purdue) Povidone-iodine 5% mineral oil, polyoxyethylene stearate, polysorbate, sorbitan monostearate, white petrolatum. Cream. Tube 14 g. *OTC.*
Use: Antimicrobial; antiseptic.

Betadine 5% Sterile Ophthalmic Prep Solution. (Alcon) Povidone-iodine 5%. Soln. Bot. 50 mL. *Rx.*
Use: Antiseptic, ophthalmic.

Betadine Medicated Disposable Douche. (Purdue) Povidone-iodine 10%. Soln (0.3% when diluted). Vial 5.4 mL with 180 mL bot. Sanitized water. 1 and 2 packs. *OTC.*
Use: Vaginal agent.

Betadine Medicated Douche. (Purdue) Povidone-iodine 10% (0.3% when diluted). Soln. In 15 mL (6s) packettes and 240 mL. *OTC.*
Use: Vaginal agent.

Betadine Medicated Premixed Disposable Douche. (Purdue) Povidone-iodine 10%. Soln. (0.3% when diluted). Bot. 180 mL. 1s, 2s. *OTC.*
Use: Vaginal agent.

Betadine Medicated Suppositories. (Purdue) Povidone-iodine 10%. Supp. In 7s w/applicator. *OTC.*
Use: Vaginal agent.

Betadine PrepStick. (Purdue) Povidone-iodine 10%. Soln. Prep Swab. Box 150s, 600s. *OTC.*
Use: Anti-infective, topical.

Betadine PrepStick Plus. (Purdue) Povidone-iodine 10%, alcohol. Soln. Prep Swab. Box 150s, 600s. *OTC.*
Use: Anti-infective, topical.

Betadine Shampoo. (Purdue) Povidone-iodine 7.5%. Shampoo. Bot. 118 mL. *OTC.*
Use: Antiseborrheic.

beta-estradiol.
See: Estradiol.

beta eucaine hydrochloride. *Name previously used for Eucaine hydrochloride.*

Betagan Liquifilm. (Allergan) Levobunolol hydrochloride 0.25%, 0.5%. Liquifilm. Bot. 2 mL (0.5%), 5 mL, 10 mL, 15 mL (0.5%) w/B.I.D. C Cap and Q.D. C Cap (0.5%). *Rx.*
Use: Antiglaucoma, beta-adrenergic blocker.

Betagen. (Enzyme Process) Vitamins B_1 1 mg, B_2 1.2 mg, niacin 15 mg, B_6 18 mg, pantothenic acid 18 mg, choline 1.8 g, betaine 96 mg. 6 Tab. Bot. 100s, 250s. *OTC.*
Use: Mineral, vitamin supplement.

Betagen Surgical Scrub. (Ivax) Povidone-iodine. Bot. Pt, gal. *OTC.*
Use: Antiseptic.

• **betahistine hydrochloride.** (BEE-tah-HISS-teen) USAN.
Use: Vasodilator, Meniere disease; diamine oxidase inhibitor, increase microcirculation.

beta-hypophamine.
See: Vasopressin.

betaine. (Orphan Medical)
Use: Treatment of homocystinuria. [Orphan Drug]
See: Cystadane.

• **betaine hydrochloride.** (BEE-tane) *USP 34.* Acidol hydrochloride, lycine hydrochloride.
Use: Replenisher adjunct, electrolytes.
W/Ferrous fumarate, docusate sodium, desiccated liver, vitamins, minerals.
See: Hemaferrin.

Betalin S. (Eli Lilly) Thiamine hydrochloride 50 mg, 100 mg. Tab. Bot. 100s.

OTC.
Use: Vitamin supplement.
• **betamethasone.** (BAY-tuh-METH-uh-zone) *USP 34.*
Use: Adrenocortical steroid, glucocorticoid.
See: Celestone.
• **betamethasone acetate.** (BAY-tuh-METH-uh-zone) *USP 34.*
Use: Corticosteroid, topical.
• **betamethasone dipropionate.** (BAY-tuh-METH-uh-zone) *USP 34.*
Use: Corticosteroid, topical.
See: Diprolene.
Diprosone.
Psorion.
W/Calcipotriene.
See: Taclonex.
Taclonex Scalp.
W/Clotrimazole.
See: Clotrimazole and Betamethasone Dipropionate.
betamethasone dipropionate, augmented. (Various Mfr.) Betamethasone (augmented). **Cream:** 0.05%, propylene glycol, sorbitol solution, white petrolatum. 15 g, 50 g. **Gel:** 0.05%, propylene glycol. 15 g, 50 g. *Rx.*
Use: Anti-inflammatory.
betamethasone dipropionate (augmented). (Fougera) Betamethasone dipropionate 0.05%. Hydroxypropylcellulose, isopropyl alcohol 30%, propylene glycol. Lot. 30 mL, 60 mL. *Rx.*
Use: Anti-inflammatory agent, topical corticosteroid.
betamethasone sodium phosphate and betamethasone acetate.
Use: Adrenocortical steroid, glucocorticoid.
See: Celestone Soluspan.
• **betamethasone valerate.** (BAY-tuh-METH-uh-zone) *USP 34.*
Use: Corticosteroid, topical.
See: Beta-Val.
Luxiq.
Valisone.
Valnac.
• **betamicin sulfate.** (bay-tah-MY-sin) USAN.
Use: Anti-infective.
betanaphthol. 2-Naphthol.
Use: Parasiticide.
Betapace. (Bayer) Sotalol hydrochloride 80 mg, 120 mg, 160 mg, 240 mg, lactose. Tab. Bot. 100s, UD 100s. *Rx.*
Use: Antiadrenergic/sympatholytic, beta-adrenergic blocker.
Betapace AF. (Bayer) Sotalol hydrochloride 80 mg, 120 mg, 160 mg, lactose.

Tab. UD 60s, 100s. *Rx.*
Use: Antiadrenergic/sympatholytic, beta-adrenergic blocker.
Betapen-VK. (Bristol-Myers Squibb) Penicillin V potassium. **Oral Soln.:** 125 mg/mL, 250 mg/5 mL Bot. 100 mL, 200 mL (250 mg/5mL only). **Tab.:** 250 mg, 500 mg. Tab. Bot. 100s, 1000s (250 mg only). *Rx.*
Use: Anti-infective, penicillin.
beta-phenyl-ethyl-hydrazine. Phenelzine dihydrogen sulfate.
See: Nardil.
beta-pyridyl-carbinol. Nicotinyl alcohol. Alcohol corresponding to nicotinic acid.
BetaRx. (VivoRx, Inc.) Encapsulated porcine islet preparation.
Use: Type I diabetic patients already on immunosuppression. [Orphan Drug]
Betasept. (Purdue) Chlorhexidine gluconate 4%, isopropyl 4%, alcohol. Liq. Bot. 946 mL. *OTC.*
Use: Dermatologic.
Betaseron. (Bayer) Interferon beta-1b 0.3 mg. Albumin human 15 mg, mannitol 15 mg per vial. Preservative free. Pow. for Inj., lyophilized. Single-use vial (capacity 3 mL) w/1.2 mL prefilled syringe of diluent (sodium chloride 0.54%), alcohol prep pads, and vial adaptor with attached needle for each drug vial. Blister units. 15s. *Rx.*
Use: Immunologic agent, immunomodulator.
Betathine. (Dovetail Technologies, Inc.) Beta alethine.
Use: Antineoplastic. [Orphan Drug]
Beta-2. (Nephron) Isoetharine hydrochloride 1% with glycerin, sodium bisulfite, parabens. Liq. Bot. 10 mL, 30 mL. *Rx.*
Use: Respiratory product.
Beta-Val. (Teva) Betamethasone valerate equivalent to 0.1% betamethasone base in cream base. Cream. Tube 15 g, 45 g. *Rx.*
Use: Corticosteroid, topical.
BetaVent. (Wraser) Carbetapentane citrate 20 mg, guaifenesin 100 mg per 5 mL. Alcohol free. Grape flavor. Syr. 473 mL. *Rx.*
Use: Antitussive with expectorant, upper respiratory combination.
Beta XMA. (Beta Dermaceuticals) Aloe, C14-22 alcohols, castor oil, cetyl alcohol, *butyrospermum parkii*, dimethicone, emu oil, methylparaben, PEG-40, PEG-100, triethanolamine. Cream. 118 g. *OTC.*
Use: Emollient.

betaxolol. (KVK-Tech) Betaxolol hydrochloride 10 mg, 20 mg. Lactose, PEG. Film coated. Tab. 100s. *Rx.*
Use: Antiadrenergic/sympatholytic, beta-adrenergic blocking agent.

•**betaxolol hydrochloride.** (BAY-TAX-oh-lahl) *USP 34.*
Use: Antiadrenergic/sympatholytic, beta-adrenergic blocking agent.
See: Betoptic S.
Kerlone.

betaxolol hydrochloride. (Various Mfr.) Betaxolol hydrochloride 5.6 mg (equiv. to 5 mg base)/mL (0.5%). Ophth. Soln. Bot. 2.5 mL, 5 mL, 10 mL, 15 mL. *Rx.*
Use: Antiglaucoma, beta-adrenergic blocker.

•**bethanechol chloride.** (beth-AN-ih-kole) *USP 34.*
Use: Cholinergic.
See: Myotonachol.
Urabeth.
Urecholine.

bethanechol chloride. (Various Mfr.) Bethanechol chloride 5 mg, 10 mg, 25 mg, 50 mg. Tab. Bot. 100s, 250s (10 mg, 25 mg only), 500s (50 mg only), 1000s, UD 100s. *Rx.*
Use: Urinary cholinergic.

•**bethanidine sulfate.** (beth-AN-ih-deen) USAN.
Use: Antihypertensive.

Bethaprim. (Major) Trimethoprim 40 mg, sulfamethoxazole 200 mg/5 mL, alcohol 0.26%, saccharin, sorbitol. Susp. *Rx.*
Use: Anti-infective.

Bethaprim DS Tabs. (Major) Trimethoprim 160 mg, sulfamethoxazole 800 mg. Tab. Bot. 100s, 500s, UD 100s. *Rx.*
Use: Anti-infective.

Bethaprim SS Tabs. (Major) Trimethoprim 80 mg, sulfamethoxazole 400 mg. Tab. Bot. 100s, 500s. *Rx.*
Use: Anti-infective.

•**betiatide.** (BEH-tie-ah-tide) USAN.
Use: Pharmaceutic aid.

Betimol. (Novartis Ophthalmics) Timolol maleate (as hemihydrate) 0.25%, 0.5%, benzalkonium Cl 0.01%, monosodium and disodium phosphate dihydrate. Soln. Bot. 2.5 mL, 5 mL, 10 mL, 15 mL. *Rx.*
Use: Antiglaucoma, beta-adrenergic blocker.

Betoptic S. (Alcon) Betaxolol hydrochloride 2.8 mg (equiv. to 2.5 mg base) per mL (0.25%), benzalkonium chloride 0.01%, mannitol, polysulfonic acid, hydrochloric acid or sodium hydroxide,

EDTA. Susp. *Drop-Tainer* dispenser 2.5 mL, 5 mL, 10 mL, 15 mL. *Rx.*
Use: Antiglaucoma, beta-adrenergic blocker.

•**bevacizumab.** (beh-vuh-SIZ-uh-mab) USAN.
Use: Antiangiogenic; monoclonal antibody.
See: Avastin.

•**bevantolol hydrochloride.** (beh-VAN-toe-LOLE) USAN.
Use: Antianginal; antihypertensive; cardiac depressant, antiarrhythmic.

•**bevirimat dimeglumine.** (be-VIR-i-mat) USAN.
Use: Antiretroviral.

•**bexarotene.** (bex-AIR-oh-teen) USAN.
Use: Antineoplastic; antidiabetic; rexinoid.
See: Targretin.

•**bexlosteride.** (bex-LOW-ster-ide) USAN.
Use: Prostate cancer.

Bexomal-C. (Roberts) Vitamins B_1 6 mg, B_2 7 mg, B_3 80 mg, B_5 10 mg, B_6 5 mg, B_{12} 6 mcg, C 250 mg. Tab. Bot. 50s. *OTC.*
Use: Vitamin supplement.

Bexxar Dosimetric Packaging. (Corixa/GlaxoSmithKline) **Nonradioactive Component:** Tositumomab 14 mg/mL. Maltose (w/v) 10%. Preservative free. Inj. Single-use vials 35 mg, 225 mg. **Radioactive Component:** Iodine I 131 tositumomab 0.1 mg/mL (0.61 mCi/mL at calibration). Preservative free. Inj. Single-use vials (contains povidone 5% to 6%, maltose 1 to 2 mg/mL, sodium chloride 0.85 to 0.95 mg/mL, ascorbic acid 0.9 to 1.3 mg/mL). *Rx.*
Use: Monoclonal antibody.

Bexxar Therapeutic Packaging. (Corixa/GlaxoSmithKline) **Nonradioactive Component:** Tositumomab 14 mg/mL. Maltose (w/v) 10%. Preservative free. Inj. Single-use vials 35 mg, 225 mg. **Radioactive Component:** Iodine I 131 tositumomab 1.1 mg/mL (5.6 mCi/mL at calibration). Preservative-free. Inj. Single-use vials (contains povidone 5% to 6%, maltose 9 to 15 mg/mL, sodium chloride 0.85 to 0.95 mg/mL, ascorbic acid 0.9 to 1.3 mg/mL). *Rx.*
Use: Monoclonal antibody.

Beyaz. (Bayer Healthcare) **Drospirenone/ethinyl estradiol Tab.:** 3 mg/0.02 mg. Film coated. Lactose, PEG. 24s. **Levomefolate calcium Tab.:** 0.451 mg. Film coated. Lactose, PEG. 4s. *Rx.*

Use: Oral contraceptive, oral monophasic contraceptive.

•**bezafibrate.** (BEH-zah-FIE-brate) USAN.
Use: Antihyperlipoproteinemic.

Bezon. (Whittier) Vitamins B_1 5 mg, B_2
3 mg, niacinamide 20 mg, pantothenic
acid 3 mg, B_6 0.5 mg, C 50 mg, B_{12}
1 mcg. Cap. Bot. 30s, 100s. *OTC.*
Use: Vitamin supplement.

Bezon Forte. (Whittier) Vitamins B_1
25 mg, B_2 12.5 mg, niacinamide 50 mg,
pantothenic acid 10 mg, B_6 5 mg, C
250 mg. Cap. Bot. 30s, 100s. *OTC.*
Use: Vitamin supplement.

B-F-I. (Numark Labs) Bismuth-formic-
iodide, zinc phenolsulfonate, bismuth
subgallate, amol, potassium alum, boric acid, menthol, eucalyptol, thymol,
and inert diluents. Pow. Can. 0.25 oz,
1.25 oz, 8 oz. *OTC.*
Use: Antiseptic, topical.

B-50. (NBTY) Vitamins B_1 50 mg, B_2
50 mg, B_3 50 mg, B_5 50 mg, B_6 50 mg,
B_{12} 50 mcg, folic acid 0.1 mg, d-
biotin 50 mcg, PABA, choline bitartrate,
inositol. Tab. Bot. 50s, 100s. *OTC.*
Use: Mineral, vitamin supplement.

B-50 Time Release. (NBTY) Vitamins B_1
50 mg, B_2 50 mg, B_3 50 mg, B_5 50 mg,
B_6 50 mg, B_{12} 50 mcg, folic acid
0.1 mg, d-biotin 50 mcg, PABA 50 mg,
choline bitartrate 50 mg, inositol 50 mg,
lecithin. Tab. Bot. 100s. *OTC.*
Use: Mineral, vitamin supplement.

B.G.O. (Calotabs) Iodoform, salicylic
acid, sulfur, zinc oxide, phenol (liquefied) 1%, calamine, menthol, petrolatum, lanolin, mineral oil, undecylenic
acid 1%. Jar ⅞ oz, Tube 1 oz. *OTC.*
Use: Antifungal, topical; antiseptic.

Biafine. (OrthoNeutrogene) Avocado oil,
parabens. Emulsion. 45 g, 90 g. *Rx.*
Use: Flexible hydroactive dressings and
granules.

•**bialamicol hydrochloride.** (bye-AH-lam-
IH-KAHL) USAN.
Use: Antiamebic.

•**biapenem.** (bye-ah-PEN-en) USAN.
Use: Anti-infective.

biaphasic insulin. A suspension of insulin crystals in a solution of insulin buffered at pH 7. Insulin Novo Rapitard. Inj.

Biaxin. (Abbott) **Gran. for Oral Susp.:**
Clarithromycin 125 mg/5 mL, 250 mg/
5 mL. Sucrose, fruit punch flavor. Bot.
50 mL, 100 mL. **Tab.:** Clarithromycin
250 mg, 500 mg. Film-coated. 60s,
ABBO-PAC UD 100s. *Rx.*
Use: Anti-infective, macrolide.

Biaxin XL. (Abbott) Clarithromycin
500 mg. Lactose. Film-coated. ER Tab.
Bot. 60s, *BIAXIN XL PAC* blister pack
4 × 14s. *Rx.*
Use: Anti-infective, macrolide.

•**bibapcitide.** (bib-APP-sih-tide) USAN.
Use: Radionuclide carrier; detection
and localization of deep vein thrombosis.

•**bicalutamide.** (bye-kah-LOO-tah-mide)
USAN.
Use: Antineoplastic; antiandrogen.
See: Casodex.

bicalutamide. (Various Mfr.) Bicalutamide 50 mg. May contain lactose,
PEG. Tab. 30s, 100s, 500s, 1,000s, UD
30s. *Rx.*
Use: Hormone, antiandrogen.

Bicarsim. (Kramer-Novis) Simethicone
80 mg. Sugar. Tab. 60s. *OTC.*
Use: Antiflatulent.

Bicarsim Forte. (Kramer-Novis) Simethicone 125 mg. Sugar. Tab. 60s. *OTC.*
Use: Antiflatulent.

•**bicifadine hydrochloride.** (bye-SIGH-
fah-deen) USAN.
Use: Analgesic.

Bicillin C-R. (Monarch) **600,000 units/
dose:** Penicillin G benzathine
300,000 units, penicillin G procaine
300,000 units. *Tubex* 1 mL.
1,200,000 units/dose: Penicillin G
benzathine 600,000, penicillin G procaine 600,000. *Tubex* 2 mL. Inj. *Rx.*
Use: Anti-infective.

Bicillin C-R 900/300. (Monarch)
1,200,000 units/dose (penicillin G
benzathine 900,000, penicillin G procaine 300,000), parabens, lecithin, povidone. *Tubex* 2 mL. *Rx.*
Use: Anti-infective.

Bicillin L-A. (Monarch) Penicillin G
benzathine 600,000 units/dose,
1,200,000 units/dose, 2,400,000 units/
dose, povidone, parabens. Inj. *Tubex*
1 mL (600,000 only), 2 mL (1,200,000
only); Prefilled syringes 4 mL
(2,400,000 only). *Rx.*
Use: Anti-infective.

•**biciromab.** (bye-SIH-rah-mab) USAN.
Use: Monoclonal antibody, antifibrin.

•**biclodil hydrochloride.** (BYE-kloe-DILL)
USAN.
Use: Antihypertensive, vasodilator.

BiCNU. (Bristol Labs Oncology) Carmustine (BCNU) 100 mg, sterile diluent
3 mL. Pow. for Inj., lyophilized. Preservative free. Single-dose vial. *Rx.*
Use: Antineoplastic, alkylating agent.

Bicycline. (Knight) Tetracycline hydrochloride 250 mg. Cap. Bot. 100s. *Rx.*
Use: Anti-infective.

Bidex-A. (SJ Pharmaceuticals) Dextromethorphan HBr 25 mg, guaifenesin 600 mg. Dye free. ER. Tab. 100s. *Rx.*
Use: Antitussive with expectorant, upper respiratory combination.

Bidhist-D. (Cypress) Pseudoephedrine hydrochloride 45 mg, brompheniramine maleate 6 mg. ER Tab. 100s. *Rx.*
Use: Decongestant and antihistamine, upper respiratory combination.

BiDil. (NitroMed) Isosorbide dinitrate 20 mg, hydralazine hydrochloride 37.5 mg. Lactose. Film-coated. Tab. 180s. *Rx.*
Use: Vasodilator.

•**bidisomide.** (bye-DIH-so-mide) USAN.
Use: Cardiovascular agent, antiarrhythmic.

•**bifeprunox.** (bye-fee-PRUE-nox) USAN.
Use: Antipsychotic agent.

•**bifeprunox mesylate.** (bye-fee-PRUE-nox) USAN.
Use: Antipsychotic agent.

BiferaRx. (Alaven) Fe 28 mg (as polysaccharide iron complex 22 mg and heme iron polypeptide [bovine source] 6 mg), B_{12} 25 mcg, folate 1 mg. Film coated. PEG. Tab. 90s. *Rx.*
Use: Multivitamin with iron.

Bifidobacterium infantis 35624.
See: Align Daily Probiotic Supplement.

•**bifonazole.** (BYE-FONE-ah-zole) USAN.
Use: Antifungal.

biguanides.
Use: Antidiabetic agent.
See: Metformin Hydrochloride.

bile acid sequestrants.
See: Cholestyramine.
Colesevelam Hydrochloride.
Colestipol Hydrochloride.

bile acids, oxidized. Note also dehydrocholic acid.
W/Atropine methyl nitrate, ox and hog bile extract, phenobarbital.
See: G.B.S.

bile extract.
W/Combinations
See: Biloric.
Enzobile Improved.

bile extract, ox. (Eli Lilly) Purified ox gall. Enseal 5 g, Bot. 100s, 500s, 1000s. (C.D. Smith) Tab. 5 g, Bot. 1000s. (Stoddard) Tab. 3 g, Bot. 100s, 500s, 1000s.
Use: Digestive enzymes.

bilein. Bile salts obtained from ox bile.

bile-like products. Bile products.
See: Bile salts.
Dehydrocholic acid.

bile salts. (Eli Lilly) Sodium glycocholate and taurocholate.

bile salts and belladonna. (Various Mfr.) Belladonna, nux vomica compound bile salts 60 mg, belladonna leaf extract 5 mg, nux vomica extract 2 mg, phenolphthalein 30 mg, sodium salicylate 15 mg, aloin 15 mg. Tab. Bot. 1000s. *Rx.*
Use: Laxative; antispasmodic.

Bili-Labstix SG Reagent Strips. (Bayer Consumer Care) Urinalysis reagent strip test for specific gravity, pH, protein, glucose, ketone, bilirubin, and blood. Bot. 100s.
Use: Diagnostic aid.

Bilirubin Reagent Strips. (Bayer Consumer Care) Seralyzer reagent strip. Quantitative strip test for total bilirubin serum or plasma. Bot. 25s.
Use: Diagnostic aid.

bilirubin test.
See: Ictotest.

Bilivist. (Berlex) Ipodate sodium 500 mg. Cap. Bot. 120s. *Rx.*
Use: Radiopaque agent.

Biloric. (Arcum) Pepsin 9 mg, ox bile 160 mg. Cap. Bot. 100s, 1000s. *OTC.*
Use: Antispasmodic.

Bilstan. (Standex) Bile salts 0.5 g, cascara sagrada powder extract 0.5 g, phenolphthalein 0.5 g, aloin ⅛ g, podophyllin g. Tab. Bot. 100s. *OTC.*
Use: Laxative.

Biltricide. (Schering) Praziquantel 600 mg. Tab. Bot. 6s. *Rx.*
Use: Anthelmintic.

•**bimatoprost.** (bi-MA-toe-prost) USAN.
Use: Antiglaucoma; prostaglandin agonist.
See: Latisse.
Lumigan.

•**bimosiamose disodium.** (bye-moh-SYE-a-mose) USAN.
Use: Anti-inflammatory agent.

•**bindarit.** (BIN-dah-rit) USAN.
Use: Antirheumatic.

•**binetrakin.** (bih-NEH-trah-kin) USAN.
Use: Gastrointestinal carcinoma; rheumatoid arthritis; dendritic cell activation; immunomodulatory.

•**biniramycin.** (bih-NEER-ah-MY-sin) USAN.
Use: Anti-infective.

•**binodenoson.** (bi-NOE-den-oh-son) USAN.
Use: Vasodilator.

•**binospirone mesylate.** (bih-NO-spy-rone) USAN.
Use: Anxiolytic.

Bintron. (Madland) Liver fraction 4.6 g, ferrous sulfate 5 g, vitamins B_1 3 mg, B_2 0.5 mg, B_6 0.15 mg, C 20 mg, calcium pantothenate 0.3 mg, niacinamide 10 mg. Tab. Bot. 100s, 1000s. *OTC.*
Use: Mineral, vitamin supplement.

Biobrane. (Sanofi-Synthelabo) Temporary skin substitute available in various sizes. *OTC.*
Use: Dermatologic.

Biobron SF. (Advanced Generic) Dextromethorphan hydrobromide 15 mg, guaifenesin 350 mg, phenylephrine hydrochloride 10 mg per 5 mL. Parabens, propylene glycol, saccharin. Alcohol free and sugar free. Cherry flavor. Liq. 473 mL. *OTC.*
Use: Upper respiratory combination, antitussive and expectorant combination.

Biocal 500. (Bayer Consumer Care) Calcium 500 mg. Tab. Bot. 75s. *OTC.*
Use: Mineral supplement.

Biocal 250. (Bayer Consumer Care) Calcium 250 mg. Chew. Tab. Bot. 75s. *OTC.*
Use: Calcium supplement.

Biocult-GC. (Orion) Swab test for gonorrhea. For endocervical, urethral, rectal, and pharyngeal cultures. Box 1 test per kit.
Use: Diagnostic aid.

bioflavonoid compounds.
See: Amino-Opti-C.
  Bioflex.
  C Factors "1000" Plus.
  Ester-C Plus 500 mg Vitamin C.
  Ester-C Plus Multi-Mineral.
  Ester-C Plus 1000 mg Vitamin C.
  Flavons.
  Flavons-500.
  Pan C-500.
  Peridin-C.
  Quercetin.
  Span C.
  Tri-Super Flavons 1000.

Bioflex. (Advanced Generic) Vitamin C 500 mg, citrus bioflavonoids 50 mg, hawthorn berry extract 25 mg, horse chestnut extract 25 mg, hesperidin complex 25 mg, rutin 40 mg, witch hazel extract 25 mg. Tab. 60s. *OTC.*
Use: Water-soluble vitamin.

BioGaia. (Nutraceutics) 100 million *Lactobacillus reuteri* Protectis per 5 drops. Medium chain triglyceride oil, sunflower oil. Preservative free and sugar free. Soln., Conc. 5 mL. *OTC.*

Use: Oral nutritional supplement, probiotic product.

Biogastrone.
See: Carbenoxolone.

Biogil. (Advanced Generic) Dextromethorphan hydrobromide 15 mg, guaifenesin 300 mg, phenylephrine hydrochloride 10 mg. Parabens, sorbitol. Alcohol free and sugar free. Grape flavor. Liq. 473 mL. *Rx.*
Use: Upper respiratory combination, antitussive and expectorant combination.

BioGlo. (Hub Pharmaceuticals) Fluorescein sodium 1 mg. Strip. 100s. *OTC.*
Use: Diagnostic aid, ophthalmic.

BioGtuss. (Advanced Generics) Dextromethorphan hydrobromide 15 mg, guaifenesin 300 mg, phenylephrine hydrochloride 10 mg. Aspartame, glycerin, parabens, phenylalanine 17 mg per 5 mL, propylene glycol. Alcohol free and sugar free. Grape flavor. Liq. 473 mL. *Rx.*
Use: Upper respiratory combination, antitussive and expectorant combination.

Biohist-LA. (IVAX) Chlorpheniramine maleate 12 mg, pseudoephedrine hydrochloride 120 mg. SR Tab. Bot. 100s. *Rx.*
Use: Upper respiratory combination, antihistamine, decongestant.

•**biological indicator for dry-heat sterilization, paper strip.** *USP 34.*
Use: Biological indicator, sterilization.

•**biological indicator for ethylene oxide sterilization, paper strip.** *USP 34.*
Use: Biological indicator, sterilization.

•**biological indicator for steam sterilization, paper strip.** *USP 34.*
Use: Biological indicator, sterilization.

•**biological indicator for steam sterilization, self-contained.** *USP 34.*
Use: Biological indicator, sterilization.

biological response modifiers.
See: Aldesleukin.
  BCG, Live.
  Denileukin Diftitox.
  Ontak.
  TheraCys.
  TICE BCG.

Bionate 50-2. (Seatrace) Testosterone cypionate 50 mg, estradiol cypionate 2 mg/mL. Vial 10 mL. *Rx.*
Use: Androgen; estrogen combination.

Bionect. (JSJ Pharmaceuticals) Hyaluronic acid. **Cream:** 0.2%. As sodium salt. Parabens, PEG. 25 g. **Gel:** 0.2%. As sodium salt. Parabens. 30 g. **Spray:**

0.2%. As sodium salt. Parabens. 20 mL. *Rx.*
Use: Physical adjunct.

Bionel. (Advanced Generic) Dextromethorphan hydrobromide 15 mg, guaifenesin 200 mg, pseudoephedrine hydrochloride 30 mg per 5 mL. Aspartame, glycerin, parabens, phenylalanine 19 mg per 5 mL. Alcohol free, dye free, and sugar free. Liq. 473 mL. *OTC.*
Use: Upper respiratory combination, antitussive and expectorant combination.

Bionel Pediatric. (Advanced Generic) Dextromethorphan hydrobromide 5 mg, guaifenesin 50 mg, pseudoephedrine hydrochloride 15 mg per 5 mL. Aspartame, parabens, phenylalanine 14 mg. Alcohol free. Liq. 473 mL. *Rx.*
Use: Upper respiratory combination antitussive and expectorant combination.

Bion Tears. (Alcon) Dextran 70 0.1%, hydroxypropyl methylcellulose 2910 0.3%, NaCl, KCl, sodium bicarbonate. Preservative free. Soln. In single-use 0.45 mL containers (28s). *OTC.*
Use: Artificial tears.

Bioral.
See: Carbenoxolone.

Bio-Rescue. (Biomedical Frontiers) Dextran and deferoxamine.
Use: Acute iron poisoning. [Orphan Drug]

Bios I.
See: Inositol.

Biospec DMX. (Deliz Pharmaceutical) Dextromethorphan hydrobromide 15 mg, guaifenesin 25 mg. Glucose, saccharin. Alcohol free. Cherry flavor. Liq. 473 mL. *OTC.*
Use: Upper respiratory combination, antitussive with expectorant.

Biosynject. (Chembiomed, Inc.) Trisaccharides A and B.
Use: Hemolytic disease of the newborn. [Orphan Drug]

Bio-Tab. (International Ethical Labs) Doxycycline hyclate 100 mg. Tab. Bot. 50s, 100s, 500s. *Rx.*
Use: Anti-infective, tetracycline.

Biotect Plus. (Advanced Generic) Vitamins A 1,666.67 units, D 133.33 units, E 33.33 units, B_1 16.67 mg, B_2 16.67 mg, B_3 16.67 mg, B_5 16.67 mg, B_6 16.67 mg, B_{12} 16.67 mcg, C 166.67 mg, Fe 3.33 mg, folate 0.33 mg, Cr, Cu, Mg, Mn, Mo, Se, Zn, biotin, choline, inositol, lysine. Acesulfame K, glycerin, methylparaben, polysorbate 80, xylitol. Alcohol free, dye free, and sugar free. Strawberry flavor.

Liq. 473 mL. *OTC.*
Use: Multivitamin with minerals.

Biotel U.T.I. (Biotel Corp.) In vitro diagnostic home test to detect urinary tract infections by screening for nitrate in urine. Test kit 12s.
Use: Diagnostic aid.

Biotène Dry Mouth. (GlaxoSmithKline) Sodium monofluorophosphate. Glucose, glycerin, lactoferrin, lactoperoxidase, sodium benzoate, sorbitol, xylitol. Fresh mint flavor. Paste; dental. 127.6 g. *OTC.*
Use: Mouth and throat product, preparation for sensitive teeth.

Biotène with Calcium. (Laclede) Propylene glycol, xylitol, poloxamer 407, hydroxyethylcellulose, sodium benzoate, peppermint, benzoic acid, zinc gluconate, aloe vera, calcium lactate, lactoferrin, lysozyme, lactoperoxidase, potassium thiocyanate, glucose oxidase. Alcohol free. Mouthwash. 474 mL. *OTC.*
Use: Mouth and throat products.

Biothesin. (Pal-Pak, Inc.) Phosphorated carbohydrate solution ceriumoxalate 120 mg, bismuth subnitrate 120 mg, benzocaine 15 mg, aromatics. Tab. 1000s. *OTC.*
Use: Antiemetic; antivertigo.

BioThrax. (Emergent BioDefense Operations Lansing) Anthrax vaccine. *Bacillus antracis* 83 kDa. Aluminum 1.2 mg/mL, benzethonium chloride 25 mcg/mL, formaldehyde 100 mcg/mL. Inj., Susp. Multidose vial. 5 mL. *Rx.*
Use: Active immunization agent, bacterial vaccine.

Bio-Throid. (Bio-Tech) Thyroid desiccated 7.5 mg (⅛ g), 15 mg (¼ g), 30 mg (½ g), 60 mg (1 g), 90 mg (1½ g), 120 mg (2 g), 150 mg (2½ g), 180 mg (3 g), 240 mg (4 g). Cap. Bot. 100s, 1,000s. *Rx.*
Use: Hormone, thyroid.

Bio T Pres. (Advanced Generic) Dextromethorphan hydrobromide 10 mg, guaifenesin 200 mg, phenylephrine hydrochloride 5 mg. Aspartame, glycerin, parabens, phenylalanine 17 mg per 5 mL, propylene glycol. Alcohol free and sugar free. Cherry flavor. Liq. 473 mL. *Rx.*
Use: Upper respiratory combination, antitussive and expectorant combination.

Bio T Pres Pediatric. (Advanced Generics) Dextromethorphan hydrobromide 5 mg, guaifenesin 75 mg, phenylephrine hydrochloride 2.5 mg. Aspartame, glycerin, parabens, phenyl-

alanine 5 mg per 5 mL, propylene glycol. Alcohol free, dye free, and sugar free. Orange flavor. Liq. 473 mL. *Rx.*
Use: Upper respiratory combination, antitussive and expectorant combination.

Biotuss. (GIL) Dextromethorphan HBr 15 mg, guaifenesin 300 mg, phenylephrine hydrochloride 10 mg per 5 mL. Phenylalanine 3.75 mg/5 mL. Alcohol and sugar free. Grape flavor. Liq. 473 mL. *Rx.*
Use: Upper respiratory combination, antitussive and expectorant combination.

Bio-Tussi. (Advanced Generic) Dextromethorphan hydrobromide 10 mg, guaifenesin 200 mg, phenylephrine hydrochloride 5 mg per 5 mL. Aspartame, glycerin, parabens, phenylalanine 19 mg per 5 mL, propylene glycol. Alcohol free and sugar free. Cherry flavor. Liq. 473 mL. *OTC.*
Use: Upper respiratory combination, antitussive and expectorant combination.

Bio-Tytra. (Health for Life Brands) Neomycin sulfate 2.5 mg, gramicidin 0.25 mg, benzocaine 10 mg. Troche. Box 10s. *Rx.*
Use: Anti-infective.

•**bipenamol hydrochloride.** (bye-PEN-ah-MAHL) USAN.
Use: Antidepressant.

•**biperiden.** (by-PURR-ih-den) *USP 34.*
Use: Anticholinergic; antiparkinson.

•**biperiden hydrochloride.** (by-PURR-ih-den) *USP 34.*
Use: Anticholinergic; antiparkinson.
See: Akineton.

•**biperiden lactate, injection.** (by-PURR-ih-den) *USP 34.*
Use: Anticholinergic; antiparkinsonian.

biphasic oral contraceptives.
See: Jenest-28.
LoSeasonique.
Mircette.
Necon 10/11.
Ortho-Novum 10/11.

•**biphenamine hydrochloride.** (bye-FEN-ah-meen) USAN.
Use: Anesthetic, local; anti-infective; antimicrobial.

Bipole-S. (Spanner) Testosterone 25 mg, estrone 2 mg/mL. Inj. Vial. 10 mL. *Rx.*
Use: Androgen, estrogen combination.

•**biricodar dicitrate.** (BYE-rih-koe-dahr die-SIH-trate) USAN.
Use: Chemotherapy agent, multidrug resistance inhibitor.

Bisac-Evac. (G & W) Bisacodyl. **EC Tab.:** 5 mg. Bot. 25s. **Supp.:** 10 mg. Pkg. 8s, 12s, 50s, 100s, 500s, 1000s. *OTC.*
Use: Laxative.

•**bisacodyl.** (BISS-uh-koe-dill) *USP 34.*
Use: Laxative, irritant or stimulant laxative.
See: Alophen.
Bisac-Evac.
Bisacodyl Uniserts.
Bisa-Lax.
Correctol.
Dacodyl.
Deficol.
Delco-Lax.
Doxidan.
Dulcagen.
Dulcolax.
Dulcolax Bowel Prep Kit.
Ex-Lax Ultra.
Feen-a-mint.
Fleet Laxative.
Modane.
Reliable Gentle Laxative.
Women's Gentle Laxative.

bisacodyl. (Various Mfr.) Bisacodyl. **Enteric-coated Tab.:** 5 mg. Bot. 25s, 50s, 100s, 1000s, UD 100s. **Supp.:** 10 mg. Pkg. 12s, 16s, 100s. *OTC.*
Use: Laxative.

•**bisacodyl tannex.** (BISS-uh-koe-dill) USAN.
Use: Laxative.

Bisacodyl Uniserts. (Upsher-Smith) Bisacodyl 10 mg. Supp. Pack. 12s. *OTC.*
Use: Laxative.

Bisalate. (Allison) Sodium salicylate 5 g, salicylamide 2.5 g, sodium paraminobenzoate 5 g, ascorbic acid 50 mg, butabarbital sodium ⅛ g. Tab. Bot. 100s, 1000s. *Rx.*
Use: Antirheumatic.

Bisa-Lax. (Bergen Brunswig) **Supp.:** Bisacodyl 10 mg. Hydrogenated vegetable oil. 50s. **EC Tab.:** Bisacodyl 5 mg. 25s, 50s. *OTC.*
Use: Laxative.

•**bisantrene hydrochloride.** (BISS-an-TREEN) USAN.
Use: Antineoplastic.

bisatin.
See: Oxyphenisatin.

•**bisdisulizole disodium.** (bis-dye-SU-li-zole) USAN.
Use: Dermatologic agent; sunscreen.

bishydroxycoumarin.
See: Dicumarol.

Bismapec. (Pal-Pak, Inc.) Bismuth hydroxide 137.7 mg, colloidal kaolin

648 mg, citrus pectin 129.6 mg. Tab. Bot. 1000s. *OTC.*
Use: Antidiarrheal.
Bismatrol Maximum Strength. (Major) Bismuth subsalicylate 525 mg per 15 mL. Saccharin, sodium 6 mg. Liq. 237 mL. *OTC.*
Use: Antidiarrheal.
bismuth. (Contract Pharmacal Corporation) Bismuth subsalicylate 262 mg. Cherry flavoring, mannitol, saccharin, sorbitol, wintergreen oil flavoring. Sugar free. Chew. Tab. 30s. *OTC.*
Use: Antidiarrheal.
•**bismuth aluminate.** (BISS-muth) USAN. Aluminum bismuth oxide.
•**bismuth carbonate.** (BISS-muth) USAN.
Use: Protectant, topical.
•**bismuth citrate.** (BISS-muth) *USP 34.*
bismuth glycolylarsanilate.
Use: Antiamebic.
See: Glycobiarsol.
bismuth hydroxide.
See: Bismuth, Milk of.
bismuth, insoluble products.
See: Bismuth subgallate.
Bismuth subsalicylate.
Bismuth tribromophenate.
bismuth magma. *Name previously used for Milk of Bismuth.*
•**bismuth, milk of.** (BISS-muth) *USP 34.*
Formerly Bismuth Magma.
Use: Astringent; antacid.
bismuth oxycarbonate.
See: Bismuth subcarbonate.
bismuth potassium tartrate. Basic bismuth potassium bismuthotartrate. (Brewer) 25 mg/mL. Amp. 2 mL. (Miller Pharmacal Group) 0.016 g/mL. Amp. 2 mL. Box 12s, 100s; Bot. 30 mL, 60 mL. (Raymer) 2.5%. Amp. 2 mL. Box 12s, 100s. *Rx.*
Use: Agent for syphilis.
bismuth resorcin compound.
W/Bismuth subgallate, balsam Peru, benzocaine, zinc oxide, boric acid.
See: Bonate.
bismuth sodium tartrate.
Use: Syphilis.
bismuth subbenzoate.
Use: Dusting powder for wounds.
•**bismuth subcarbonate.** (BISS-muth sub-KAR-bo-nate) *USP 34.*
Use: Protectant, topical.
bismuth subcarbonate.
Use: Gastroenteritis; diarrhea.
W/Hydrocortisone acetate, belladonna extract, ephedrine sulfate, zinc oxide, boric acid, balsam Peru, cocoa butter.
See: K-C.

bismuth subcitrate potassium.
W/Metronidazole, Tetracycline Hydrochloride.
See: Pylera.
•**bismuth subgallate.** (BISS-muth sub-GAL-ate) *USP 34.*
Use: Topically for skin conditions; orally as an antidiarrheal.
See: Devrom.
W/Balsam Peru, Bismuth Resorcin Compound, Zinc Oxide.
See: Versal.
W/Opium Powder, Pectin, Kaolin, Zinc Phenolsulfonate.
See: Paregoric.
Pectin.
•**bismuth subnitrate.** (BISS-muth sub-NYE-trate) *USP 34.*
Use: Pharmaceutic necessity; gastroenteritis; amebic dysentery; locally for wounds.
•**bismuth subsalicylate.** (BISS-muth sub-sa-LIS-i-late) *USP 34.* Basic bismuth salicylate. Agent for syphilis. Used in combination with metronidazole and tetracycline hydrochloride to treat active duodenal ulcer associated with *Helicobacter pylori* infection.
Use: Antidiarrheal; antacid; antiulcerative.
See: Bismatrol Maximum Strength.
Kaopectate.
Kaopectate Children's.
Kaopectate Extra Strength.
Kao-Tin.
Maalox Total Relief.
Peptic Relief.
W/Calcium Carbonate.
See: Pepto-Bismol.
W/Pectin, Salol, Kaolin, Zinc Sulfocarbolate, Aluminum Hydroxide.
See: Pepto-Bismol.
bismuth tannate. (Various Mfr.) Tan bismuth. *OTC.*
Use: Astringent and protective in GI disorders.
bismuth tribromophenate.
Use: Intestinal antiseptic.
bismuth, water-soluble products.
See: Bismuth potassium tartrate.
•**bisnafide dimesylate.** (BISS-nah-fide die-MEH-sih-late) USAN.
Use: Antineoplastic.
•**bisobrin lactate.** (BISS-oh-brin LACK-tate) USAN.
Use: Fibrinolytic.
•**bisoctrizole.** (bis-OK-trye-zole) USAN.
Use: Sunscreen.
•**bisoprolol.** (bih-SO-pro-lahl) *USP 34.*
Use: Antiadrenergic/sympatholytic, beta-adrenergic blocking agent.

•**bisoprolol fumarate.** (bih-SO-pro-lahl) *USP 34.*
Use: Antiadrenergic/sympatholytic, beta-adrenergic blocking agent.
See: Zebeta.
W/Combinations.
See: Ziac.
bisoprolol fumarate. (Eon) Bisoprolol fumarate 5 mg, 10 mg. Tab. Bot. 30s, 100s. *Rx.*
Use: Antiadrenergic/sympatholytic, beta-adrenergic blocking agent.
bisoprolol fumarate and hydrochlorothiazide. (Various Mfr.) Bisoprolol fumarate/hydrochlorothiazide 2.5 mg/6.25 mg, 5 mg/6.25 mg, 10 mg/6.25 mg. Tab. Bot. 30s (10 mg/6.25 mg only), 100s, 500s, 1000s. *Rx.*
Use: Antihypertensive, diuretic.
•**bisoxatin acetate.** (biss-OX-at-in) USAN.
Use: Laxative.
bisphosphonates.
Use: Antihypercalcemic; bone resorption inhibitor.
See: Alendronate Sodium.
Alendronate Sodium/Vitamin D₃.
Etidronate Disodium.
Ibandronate Sodium.
Pamidronate Disodium.
Risedronate/Calcium Carbonate.
Risedronate Sodium.
Tiludronate Disodium.
Zoledronic Acid.
•**bispyrithione magsulfex.** (BISS-PIHR-ih-thigh-ohn mag-sull-fex) USAN.
Use: Antidandruff; anti-infective; antimicrobial.
bis-tropamide. Tropicamide.
See: Mydriacyl.
Bi-Tann DP. (Midland Healthcare) Pseudoephedrine tannate 75 mg, dexchlorpheniramine tannate 2.5 mg per 5 mL. Methylparaben, saccharin, sucrose. Strawberry-banana flavor. Susp. 118 mL, 473 mL. *Rx.*
Use: Upper respiratory combination, decongestant and antihistamine.
Bite & Itch Lotion. (Weeks & Leo) Pramoxine hydrochloride 1%, pyrilamine maleate 2%, pheniramine maleate 0.2%, chlorpheniramine maleate 0.2%. Bot. 4 oz. *OTC.*
Use: Dermatologic, topical.
Bite Rx. (International Lab. Tech.) Aluminum acetate 0.5%, benzalkonium chloride. Soln. Bot. 120 mL. *OTC.*
Use: Astringent.
bithionol. (bye-THYE-oh-nole)
Use: Anti-infective.

•**bithionolate, sodium.** (bye-THIGH-oh-noe-late) USAN.
Use: Topical anti-infective.
Bitin. CDC anti-infective agent.
See: Bithionol.
•**bitolterol mesylate.** (by-TOLE-tor-ole) USAN.
Use: Bronchodilator, sympathomimetic.
Bitrate. (Arco) Phenobarbital 15 mg, pentaerythritol tetranitrate 20 mg. Tab. Bot. 100s. *Rx.*
Use: Antianginal; hypnotic; sedative.
•**bivalirudin.** (bye-VAL-ih-ruh-din) USAN.
Use: Anticoagulant; antithrombotic.
See: Angiomax.
•**bixalomer.** (bix-AL-oh-mer) USAN.
Use: Hyperphosphatemia.
•**bizelesin.** (bye-ZELL-eh-sin) USAN.
Use: Antineoplastic.
Black and White Bleaching Cream. (Schering-Plough) Hydroquinone 2%. Cream. Tube 0.75 oz, 1.5 oz. *Rx.*
Use: Dermatologic.
Black and White Ointment. (Schering-Plough) Resorcinol 3%. Oint. Tube 0.62 oz, 2.25 oz.
Use: Antiseptic; dermatologic, topical.
Black Draught. (Lee Pharmaceuticals) Sennosides. **Chew. Tab.:** 10 mg. Sugar. Bot. 30s. **Tab.:** 6 mg, sucrose. Bot. 30s. **Gran.:** 20 mg/5 mL, tartrazine, sucrose. Bot. 22.5 g. *OTC.*
Use: Laxative.
black widow spider, antivenin.
See: Antivenin (Latrodectus mactans).
Blairex Hard Contact Lens Cleaner. (Blairex) Anionic detergent. Liq. Bot. 60 mL. *OTC.*
Use: Contact lens care.
Blairex Sterile Saline Solution. (Blairex) Sodium Cl, boric acid, sodium borate. Soln. Bot. Aerosol. 90 mL, 240 mL, 360 mL. *OTC.*
Use: Contact lens care.
Blairex System. (Blairex) Sodium Cl 135 mg. Tab. 200s, 365s w/15 mL bot. *OTC.*
Use: Contact lens care.
Blairex System II. (Blairex) Sodium Cl 250 mg. Tab. 90s, 180s w/27.7 mL bot. *OTC.*
Use: Contact lens care.
Blaud Strubel. (Strubel) Ferrous sulfate 5 g. Cap. Bot. 100s. *OTC.*
Use: Mineral supplement.
Blefcon. (Madland) Sodium sulfacetamide 30%. Oint. Tube ⅛ oz. *Rx.*
Use: Anti-infective, ophthalmic.
•**bleomycin.** (Various Mfr.) Bleomycin 15 units, 30 units. Pow. for Inj. Vial. *Rx.*

Use: Antineoplastic; antibiotic.
bleomycin sulfate. (Various Mfr.) Bleomycin sulfate 15 units, 30 units. Pow.
for Inj. Vial. *Rx.*
Use: Antineoplastic.
• **bleomycin sulfate, sterile.** (BLEE-oh-
MY-sin) *USP 34.* Antibiotic obtained from
cultures of *Streptomyces verticillus.*
Use: Antineoplastic; antibiotic.
Blephamide. (Allergan) Sulfacetamide
sodium 10%, prednisolone acetate
0.2%. Susp. Bot. 2.5 mL, 5 mL, 10 mL.
Rx.
Use: Anti-inflammatory; anti-infective,
ophthalmic.
Blephamide Ophthalmic Ointment.
(Allergan) Prednisolone acetate 0.2%,
sulfacetamide sodium 10%. Ophth.
Oint. Tube 3.5 g. *Rx.*
Use: Anti-inflammatory; anti-infective,
ophthalmic.
Bleph-10. (Allergan) Sulfacetamide so-
dium 10%. Polyvinyl alcohol 1.4%,
benzalkonium chloride 0.005%, poly-
sorbate 80, sodium thiosulfate, EDTA.
Soln. 2.5 mL, 5 mL, 15 mL. *Rx.*
Use: Ophthalmic and otic agent, antibi-
otic.
Bleph-10 Sterile Ophthalmic Ointment.
(Allergan) Sulfacetamide sodium 10%.
Tube 3.5 g. *Rx.*
Use: Anti-infective, ophthalmic.
• **blinatumomab.** (BLIN-a-toom-oh-mab)
USAN.
Use: Antineoplastic agent.
Blis. (Del) Boric acid 47.5%, salicylic acid
17%. Bot. 7 oz. *OTC.*
Use: Antifungal, topical.
BlisterGard. (Medtech) Alcohol 6.7%, py-
roxylin solution, oil of cloves, B-hydroxy-
quinolone. Liq. Bot. 30 mL. *OTC.*
Use: Dermatologic, protectant.
Blistex. (Blairex) Camphor 0.5%, phenol
0.5%, allantoin 1%, lanolin, mineral oil.
Tube 4.2 g, 10.5 g. *OTC.*
Use: Lip protectant.
Blistex Lip Balm. (Blairex) SPF 10.
Camphor 0.5%, phenol 0.5%, allantoin
1%, dimethicone 2%, pamidate 0.25%,
oxybenzone, parabens, petrolatum.
Tube 4.5 g. *OTC.*
Use: Lip protectant.
Blistex Ultra Protection. (Blairex) Octyl
methoxycinnamate, oxybenzone, octyl-
salicylate, menthylanthranilate, homo-
salate, dimethicone. Tube 4.2 g. *OTC.*
Use: Lip protectant.
Blistik. (Blairex) Padimate O 6.6%, oxy-
benzone 2.5%, dimethicone 2%. Lip-
balm stick 4.5 g. *OTC.*
Use: Lip protectant.

Blis-To-Sol. (Oakhurst) **Liq.:** Tolnaftate
1%. Bot. 30 mL. **Pow.:** Zinc undecy-
lenate 12%. Bot. 60 g. **Soln.:** Tolnaftate
1%. Bot. 30 mL, 55.5 mL. *OTC.*
Use: Antifungal, topical.
BLM.
See: Bleomycin Sulfate.
Blocadren. (Merck & Co.) Timolol
maleate 5 mg, 20 mg. Tab. Bot. 100s.
Rx.
Use: Antiadrenergic/sympatholytic,
beta-adrenergic blocker.
Block Out by Sea & Ski. (Carter-
Wallace) Padimate O, octyl methoxycin-
namate, oxybenzone. Cream. Tube
120 g. *OTC.*
Use: Sunscreen.
Block Out Clear by Sea & Ski. (Carter-
Wallace) Padimate O, octyl methoxy-
cinnamate, octyl salicylate, SD alcohol
40. Lot. Bot. 120 mL. *OTC.*
Use: Sunscreen.
blood, anticoagulants.
See: Anticoagulants.
• **blood cells, red.** *USP 34.* Formerly
Blood cells, human red.
Use: Blood replenisher.
blood coagulation.
See: Hemostatics.
blood glucose concentrator.
See: Glucagon.
blood glucose test.
See: Chemstrip bG.
First Choice.
Glucostix.
• **blood grouping serum, anti-A.** *USP 34.*
Use: Diagnostic aid, blood, in vitro.
• **blood grouping serum, anti-B.** *USP 34.*
Use: Diagnostic aid, blood, in vitro.
• **blood grouping serums anti-D, anti-C,
anti-E, anti-c, anti-e.** *USP 34.* Formerly *Anti-Rh typing serums.*
Use: Diagnostic aid, blood, in vitro.
**blood group specific substances A, B
and AB.** Formerly *Blood Grouping specific substances A and B.*
Use: Blood neutralizer.
Blood Sugar Balance. (Mason) Magnesium 200 mg (magnesium content expressed in mg elemental magnesium),
biotin 600 mcg, bitter melon 200 mg,
chromium 48 mcg, ginkgo 120 mg,
gymnema 300 mg, iron oxide, lipoic
acid 150 mg, mineral oil, quercetin
50 mg, vanadium 40 mcg, zinc 30 mg.
PEG. Gluten free, lactose free, preservative free, and sugar free. Tab. 60s.
OTC.
Use: Nutritional supplement, multimineral.

•**blood, whole.** *USP 34. Formerly Blood, whole human.*
Use: Blood replenisher.

Bludex. (Burlington) Methenamine 40.8 mg, methylene blue 5.4 mg, phenylsalicylate 18.1 mg, atropine sulfate 0.03 mg, hyoscyamine 0.03 mg, benzoic acid 4.5 mg. Tab. Bot. 100s, 1000s. *Rx.*
Use: Antiseptic; antispasmodic, urinary.

Blue. (Various Mfr.) Pyrethrins 0.3%, piperonyl butoxide 3%, petroleum distillate 1.2%. Gel. Bot. 30 g, 480 g. *OTC.*
Use: Pediculicide.

Blue-Emu Maximum Strength. (NFI Consumer Products) Menthol 2.5%. Aloe vera gel, balm mint extract, boswella extract, citrus extract, emu oil, eucalyptus oil, ginger extract, isopropyl alcohol, nettle leaf extract, peppermint extract, rosemary oil, urea. Spray. 59.15 mL. *OTC.*
Use: Topical analgesic.

Blue Gel Muscular Pain Reliever. (Rugby) Menthol in a specially formulated base. Gel. Tube 240 g. *OTC.*
Use: Liniments.

Blue Ice. (Geritrex) Menthol 2%, isopropyl alcohol. Gel. 227 g. *OTC.*
Use: Rub and liniment.

Blue Star. (McCue Labs.) Salicylic acid, benzoic acid, methyl salicylate, camphor, lanolin, petrolatum. Oint. Jar 2 oz. *OTC.*
Use: Dermatologic, counterirritant.

Blu-12 100. (Bluco) Cyanocobalamin 100 mcg/mL. Vial 30 mL. *Rx.*
Use: Vitamin supplement.

Blu-12 1000. (Bluco) Cyanocobalamin 1000 mcg/mL. Vial 30 mL. *Rx.*
Use: Vitamin supplement.

B-Major. (Barth's) Vitamins B_1 7 mg, B_2 14 mg, niacin 2.35 mg, B_{12} 7.5 mcg, B_6 0.15 mg, pantothenic acid 0.37 mg, choline 85 mg, inositol 6 mg, biotin, folic acid, aminobenzoic acid. Cap. Bot. 1s, 3s, 6s, 12s. *Rx-OTC.*
Use: Mineral, vitamin supplement.

B-N. (Eric, Kirk & Gary) Bacitracin 500 units, neomycin sulfate 5 mg. Oint. Tube 0.5 oz. *OTC.*
Use: Anti-infective, topical.

b-naphthyl salicylate. Betol, naphthosalol, salinaphthol.
Use: gastrointestinal and genitourinary, antiseptic.

•**boceprevir.** (boe-SE-pre-vir) USAN.
Use: Treatment of hepatitis C infection.
See: Victrelis.

Bodi Kleen. (Geritrex) Triethanolamine lauryl sulfate, 2-phenoxy-ethanol, hexy-lene glycol, aloe vera gel. Spray. 8 oz. *OTC.*
Use: Anorectal preparation.

Body Fortress Natural Amino. (Nature's Bounty) Protein 1.67 g, lactalbumin hydrolysate 1500 mg, yeast and preservative free. Tab. Bot. 150s. *OTC.*
Use: Amino acid.

Boil-Ease. (Del) Benzocaine 20% with camphor, lanolin, eucalyptus oil, menthol, petrolatum, phenol. Oint. 30 g. *OTC.*
Use: Topical local anesthetic, ester local anesthetic.

BoilnSoak. (Alcon) Sodium Cl 0.7%, boric acid, sodium borate, thimerosal 0.001%, disodium edetate 0.1%. Bot. 8 oz, 12 oz. *OTC.*
Use: Contact lens care.

•**bolandiol dipropionate.** (bole-AN-die-ole die-PRO-pee-oh-nate) USAN.
Use: Anabolic.

•**bolasterone.** (BOLE-ah-STEE-rone) USAN.
Use: Anabolic.

Bolax. (Boyd) Docusate sodium 240 mg, phenolphthalein 30 mg, dihydrocholic acid ¾ g. Cap. Bot. 100s. *OTC.*
Use: Laxative.

•**boldenone undecylenate.** (BOLE-deen-ohn uhn-deh-sih-LEN-ate) USAN. Parenabol. Under study.
Use: Anabolic.

•**bolenol.** (BOLE-ee-nahl) USAN.
Use: Anabolic.

•**bolmantalate.** (BOLE-MAN-tah-late) USAN.
Use: Anabolic.

Bonacal Plus. (Kenwood) Vitamins A 5000 units, D 400 units, C 100 mg, B_1 3 mg, B_2 3 mg, B_6 10 mg, B_{12} 4 mcg, niacinamide 20 mg, d-calcium pantothenate 3.3 mg, iron 42 mg, calcium 350 mg, manganese 0.33 mg, zinc 0.1 mg, magnesium 1.67 mg, potassium 1.67 mg. Tab. Bot. 100s. *OTC.*
Use: Mineral, vitamin supplement.

Bonamil Infant Formula with Iron. (Wyeth) Protein 2.3 g (from nonfat milk, taurine), fat 5.4 g (from soybean and coconut oils, soy lecithin), carbohydrate 10.7 g (from lactose), linoleic acid 1300 mg, vitamin A 300 units, D 60 units, E 2.85 units, K 8 mcg, B_1 100 mcg, B_2 150 mcg, B_6 63 mcg, B_{12} 0.2 mcg, B_3 750 mcg, folic acid 7.5 mcg, B_5 315 mcg, biotin 2.2 mcg, vitamin C 8.3 mg, choline 15 mg, Ca 69 mg, P 54 mg, Mg 6 mg, Fe 1.8 mg, Zn 0.75 mg, Mn 15 mcg, Cu 70 mcg,

l 5 mcg, Na 27 mg, K 93 mg, Cl 63 mg/ 100 cal (5.3 cal/g). Conc., Liq. Bot. 453 g. Conc. 384 mL. Ready-to-feed liq. 946 mL. *OTC.*
Use: Nutritional supplement, enteral.

Bonate. (Suppositoria Laboratories, Inc.) Bismuth subgallate, balsam Peru, benzocaine, zinc oxide. Supp. Box 12s, 100s, 1000s. *OTC.*
Use: Anorectal preparation.

Bonefos. (Leiras) Disodium clodronate tetrahydrate.
Use: Bone resorption inhibitor. [Orphan Drug]

B 100. (Fibertone) Vitamins B_1 100 mg, B_2 100 mg, B_3 100 mg, B_5 100 mg, B_6 100 mg, B_{12} 100 mcg, FA 0.4 mg, biotin 50 mcg, PABA 100 mg, choline bitartrate 100 mg, inositol 100 mg. SR Tab. Bot. 100s. *OTC.*
Use: Vitamin supplement.

B-100. (NBTY) Vitamins B_1 100 mg, B_2 100 mg, B_3 100 mg, B_5 100 mg, B_6 100 mg, B_{12} 100 mcg, folic acid 0.1 mg, d-biotin 100 mcg, PABA 100 mg, choline bitartrate, inositol, lecithin. Tab. Bot. 50s, 100s. *OTC.*
Use: Mineral, vitamin supplement.

B150. (NBTY) Vitamins B_1 150 mg, B_2 150 mg, B_3 150 mg, B_5 150 mg, B_6 150 mg, B_{12} 150 mcg, folic acid 0.1 mg, d-biotin 150 mcg, PABA 150 mg, choline bitartrate 150 mg, inositol 150 mg, lecithin. Tab. Bot. 100s. *OTC.*
Use: Mineral, vitamin supplement.

B125. (NBTY) Vitamins B_1 125 mg, B_2 125 mg, B_3 125 mg, B_5 125 mg, B_6 125 mg, B_{12} 125 mcg, folic acid 0.1 mg, d-biotin 125 mcg, PABA 125 mg, choline bitartrate 125 mg, inositol 125 mg, lecithin. Tab. Bot. 100s. *OTC.*
Use: Mineral, vitamin supplement.

Bone Meal w/Vitamin D. (Nature's Bounty) Calcium 220 mg, vitamin D 100 units, phosphorus 100 mg, iron 0.45 mg, copper 3.25 mg, zinc 20 mcg, manganese 2.75 mcg, magnesium 0.925 mg. Tab. Bot. 100s, 250s. *OTC.*
Use: Mineral, vitamin supplement.

Bonine. (Insight) Meclizine hydrochloride 25 mg. Lactose, saccharin. Raspberry flavor. Chew. Tab. 8s. *OTC.*
Use: Antiemetic/antivertigo agent, anticholinergic.

Bonine for Kids. (Insight) Cycliziine hydrochloride 25 mg. Mannitol, sorbitol, sucralose. Berry flavor. Chew. Tab. 8s. *OTC.*
Use: Antiemetic/antivertigo agent, antidopaminergic.

Boniva. (Roche) Ibandronate sodium (as base). **Inj.:** 1 mg/mL. Single-use pre-filled syringe. 5 mL. **Tab.:** 150 mg. Lactose. Film coated. UD 1s. *Rx.*
Use: Bisphosphonate.

Bontril PDM. (Valeant) Phendimetrazine tartrate 35 mg, sugar, isopropyl alcohol, lactose. Tab. Bot. 100s, 1000s. *c-iii.*
Use: CNS stimulant, anorexiant.

Bontril Slow Release. (Valeant) Phendimetrazine tartrate 105 mg. SR Cap. Bot. 100s. *c-iii.*
Use: CNS stimulant, anorexiant.

Boost. (Nestle Nutrition) Protein 41.7 g (milk protein), carbohydrate 171 g (corn syr., sugar), fat 16.7 g (soy lecithin, vegetable oil), Na 542.1 mg, K 1,668 mg, vitamin A, B_1, B_2, B_3, B_5, B_6, B_{12}, C, D, E, K, Ca, Cl, Cr, Cu, Fe, I, Mg, Mo, Mn, P, Se, Zn, biotin, choline, folic acid. Lactose free. Butter pecan, chocolate, strawberry, and vanilla flavors. Liq. 240 mL. *OTC.*
Use: Defined formula diet, supplemental nutritional formula.

Boost Glucose Control. (Nestle Nutrition) Protein 66.72 g (Ca caseinate, Na caseinate, L-arginine, milk protein), carbohydrate 66.72 g (fructose, maltodextrin, sucralose, tapioca dextrin), fat 29.9 g (soy lecithin, vegetable oil), Na 750.6 mg, K 271.05 mg, vitamin A, B_1, B_2, B_3, B_5, B_6, B_{12}, C, D, E, K, Ca, Cl, Cr, Cu, Fe, I, Mg, Mo, Mn, P, Se, Zn, biotin, choline, folic acid. Lactose free. Chocolate, strawberry, and vanilla flavors. Liq. 240 mL. *OTC.*
Use: Defined formula diet, supplemental nutritional formula.

Boost High Protein. (Nestle Nutrition) Protein 70.5 g (Ca caseinate, Na caseinate, milk protein), carbohydrate 137.61 g (corn syr., sugar), fat 25.02 g (soy lecithin, vegetable oil, Na 708.9 mg, K 1,584.6 mg, vitamin A, B_1, B_2, B_3, B_5, B_6, B_{12}, C, D, E, K, Ca, Cl, Cr, Cu, Fe, I, Mg, Mo, Mn, P, Se, Zn, biotin, choline, folic acid. Lactose free. Chocolate, strawberry, and vanilla flavors. Liq. 240 mL. *OTC.*
Use: Defined formula diet, supplemental nutritional formula.

Boost Kid Essentials. (Nestle Nutrition) Protein 28.68 g (L-carnitine, Ca caseinate, Na caseinate, taurine, whey protein), carbohydrate 135.25 g (fructose, maltodextrin, sugar), fat 36.89 g (medium chain triglycerides, soybean oil, soy lecithin, sunflower oil) Na 737.7 mg, K 1,106.6 mg, vitamin A, B_1, B_2, B_3, B_5, B_6, B_{12}, C, D, E, K, Ca, Cl, Cr, Cu,

Fe, I, Mg, Mn, Mo, P, Se, Zn, biotin, choline, folic acid, inositol. Lactose free. Chocolate, strawberry, and vanilla flavors. Liq. 244 mL w/probiotic straw. *OTC.*
Use: Defined formula diet, supplemental nutritional formula.

Boost Kid Essentials 1.5. (Nestle Nutrition) Protein 42.19 g (Ca caseinate, L-carnitine, M-inositol, Na caseinate, taurine, whey protein) carbohydrate 164.56 g (maltodextrin, sugar), fat 75.11 g (medium chain triglycerides, soybean oil, soy lecithin, sunflower oil), Na 691.98 mg, K 1,303.8 mg, vitamin A, B_1, B2, B_3, B_5, B_6, B_{12}, C, D, E, K, Ca, Cl, Cr, Cu, Fe, I, Mg, Mn, Mo, P, Se, Zn, biotin, choline, folic acid. Lactose free. Vanilla flavor. Liq. 237 mL. *OTC.*
Use: Defined formula diet, supplemental nutritional formula.

Boost Kid Essentials 1.5 with Fiber. (Nestle Nutrition) Protein 42.19 g (Ca caseinate, L-carnitine, M-inositol, Na caseinate, taurine, whey protein), carbohydrate 164.56 g (maltodextrin, sugar), fat 75.11 g (medium chain triglycerides, soybean oil, soy lecithin, sunflower oil), Na 691.98 mg, K 1,303.8 mg, vitamin A, B_1, B_2, B_3, B_5, B_6, B_{12}, C, D, E, K, Ca, Cl, Cr, Cu, Fe, I, Mg, Mn, Mo, P, Se, Zn, biotin, choline, folic acid. Lactose free. Vanilla flavor. Liq. 237 mL. *OTC.*
Use: Defined formula diet, supplemental nutritional formula.

Boost Nutritional Pudding. (Nestle Nutrition) Protein 7 g, fat 9 g, carbohydrate 32 g, sodium 120 mg, potassium 320 mg, calories 240/serving, vitamins A, C, D, E, K, B_6, B_{12}, B_1, B_2, B_3, B_5, Ca, Fe, folic acid, biotin, P, I, Mg, Zn, Se, Cu, Mn, Cr, Mo, sugar. Pudding Cont. 142 g. *OTC.*
Use: Nutritional supplement.

Boost Plus. (Nestle Nutrition) Protein 58.38 g (Ca caseinate, Na caseinate, milk protein), carbohydrate 187.65 g (corn syr., sugar), fat 58.38 g (soy lecithin, vegetable oil), Na 708.9 mg, K 1,584.6 mg, vitamins A, B_1, B_2, B_3, B_5, B_6, B_{12}, C, D, E, K, Ca, Cl, Cr, Cu, Fe, I, Mg, Mo, Mn, P, Se, Zn, biotin, choline, folic acid. Lactose free. Chocolate, strawberry, and vanilla flavors. Liq. 240 mL. *OTC.*
Use: Defined formula diet, supplemental nutritional formula.

Boostrix. (GlaxoSmithKline) Diphtheria toxoid 2.5 Lf units, tetanus toxoid 5 Lf units, pertactin 2.5 mcg, FHA (filamentous hemagglutinin) 8 mcg, inactivated pertussis toxins 8 mcg per 0.5 mL. Sodium chloride, formaldehyde. Inj. Single-dose vials, disposable prefilled Tip-Lok syringes. *Rx.*
Use: Agent for active immunization.

Bopen-VK. (Boyd) Potassium phenoxymethyl penicillin 400,000 units. Tab. Bot. 100s.
Use: Anti-infective, penicillin.

borax. Sodium borate.

•**boric acid.** (BOR-ik) *NF 29.*
Use: Antiseptic, pharmaceutic necessity; topical anti-infective.
W/Combinations.
See: Saratoga.

2-bornanone. Camphor.

•**bornelone.** (BORE-neh-LONE) USAN.
Use: Ultraviolet screen.

•**bornyl acetate.** (BOR-nil) USAN.
Use: Flavoring agent.

•**borocaptate sodium B 10.** (bore-oh-CAP-tate) USAN.
Use: Antineoplastic; radiopharmaceutical.

Borocell. (Neutron Technology) Sodium monomercaptoundecahdroclosododecaborate.
Use: Boron neutron capture therapy (BNCT) in glioblastoma multiforme.

boroglycerin. (Emerson) Glycerol borate. Bot. Pt.
Use: Agent for dermatitis.

boroglycerin glycerite. Boric acid 31 parts, glycerin 96 parts.
Use: Agent for dermatitis.

borotannic complex. Boric acid 31 mg, tannic acid 50 mg.
Use: Dermatologic agent.

•**bortezomib.** (bore-TEZZ-oh-mib) USAN.
Use: Antineoplastic.
See: Velcade.

•**bosentan.** (boe-SEN-tan) USAN.
Use: Vasodilator, endothelin receptor antagonist.
See: Tracleer.

Boston Advance Cleaner. (Polymer Technology) Concentrated homogenous surfactant with friction-enhancing agents. Soln. Bot. 30 mL. *OTC.*
Use: Contact lens care.

Boston Advance Comfort Formula. (Polymer Technology) Buffered, slightly hypertonic. Polyaminopropyl biguanide 0.00015%, EDTA 0.05%, cationic cellulose derivative polymer. Soln. Bot. 120 mL. *OTC.*
Use: Contact lens care.

Boston Advance Conditioning Solution. (Polymer Technology) Sterile, buf-

fered, slightly hypertonic. Polyaminopro-
pyl biguanide 0.0015%, EDTA 0.05%.
Soln. Bot. 120 mL or with cleaner in a
convenience pack. *OTC.*
Use: Contact lens care.
Boston Advance Rewetting Drops.
(Polymer Technology) Buffered, slightly
hypertonic. Polyaminopropyl biguanide
0.0015%, EDTA 0.05%. Drops. Bot.
10 mL. *OTC.*
Use: Contact lens care.
Boston Cleaner. (Bausch & Lomb) Concentrated homogeneous surfactant with
friction-enhancing agents, sodium Cl.
Soln. Bot. 30 mL. *OTC.*
Use: Contact lens care.
Boston Conditioning Solution. (Poly-
mer Technology) Sterile, buffered,
slightly hypertonic, low viscosity. EDTA
0.05%, chlorhexidine gluconate
0.006%. Soln. Bot. 120 mL. *OTC.*
Use: Contact lens care.
Boston Reconditioning Drops. (Polymer Technology) Hydrophilic polyelec-
trolyte, polyvinyl alcohol, hydroxyethylcellulose, chlorhexidine gluconate,
EDTA. Soln. Bot. 120 mL. *OTC.*
Use: Contact lens care.
Boston Rewetting Drops. (Polymer
Technology) Buffered, slightly hypertonic. Chlorhexidine gluconate 0.006%,
EDTA 0.05%, cationic cellulose derivative polymer. Soln. Bot. 10 mL. *OTC.*
Use: Contact lens care.
Boston Simplicity Multi-Action. (Polymer Technology) PEO sorbitan monolaurate, silicone glycol copolymer, cellulosic viscosifier, derivatized PEG, chlorhexidine gluconate, polyaminopropyl
biguanide, EDTA. 0.05%. Soln. Bot.
60 mL, 90 mL, 120 mL. *OTC.*
Use: Contact lens product.
•**bosutinib.** (boe-SUE-ti-nib) USAN.
Use: Antineoplastic.
Botox. (Allergan) OnabotulinumtoxinA
100 units (one unit corresponds to the
calculated median lethal intraperitoneal
dose [LD$_{50}$] in mice). Human albumin
0.5 mg, sodium chloride 0.9 mg. Preservative free. Pow. for Inj. (vacuum
dried). Single-use vial. *Rx.*
Use: Ophthalmic; treatment of cervical
dystonia; axillary hyperhidrosis, strabismus and blepharospasm.
Botox Cosmetic. (Allergan) OnabotulinumtoxinA 100 units (one unit corresponds to the calculated median lethal
intraperitoneal dose [LD$_{50}$] in mice).
Human albumin 0.5 mg, sodium chloride 0.9 mg. Preservative free. Pow. for
Inj. (vacuum dried). Single-use vial. *Rx.*

Use: Treatment of glabellar lines.
botulinum toxins.
See: AbobotulinumtoxinA.
Botulinum toxin type A.
Botulinum toxin type B.
Botulinum toxin type F.
IncobotulinumtoxinA.
Myobloc.
OnabotulinumtoxinA.
botulinum toxin type A.
Use: Ophthalmic; treatment of cervical
dystonia, glabellar lines; axillary hy-
perhidrosis, strabismus and blepharo-
spasm.
See: Botox.
Botox Cosmetic.
botulinum toxin type B.
Use: Cervical dystonia.
See: Myobloc.
botulinum toxin type F. (Porton Product
Limited)
Use: Cervical dystonia; essential
blepharospasm. [Orphan Drug]
•**botulism antitoxin.** (BOT-yoo-lism)
USP 34.
Use: Prophylaxis and treatment of the
toxins of *Clostridium botulinum*, types
A or B; passive immunizing agent.
botulism immune globulin.
Use: Infant botulism.
See: BabyBIG.
Bounty Bears. (NBTY) Vitamins A
2500 units, D 400 units, E 15 units,
C 60 mg, B$_1$ 1.05 mg, B$_2$ 1.2 mg, B$_3$
13.5 mg, B$_6$ 1.05 mg, B$_{12}$ 4.5 mcg, folic
acid 0.3 mg. Tab. Bot. 100s. *OTC.*
Use: Mineral, vitamin supplement.
Bounty Bears Plus Iron. (NBTY) Vita-
mins A 2500 units, D 400 units, E
15 units, C 60 mg, B$_1$ 1.05 mg, B$_2$
1.2 mg, B$_3$ 13.5 mg, B$_6$ 1.05 mg, B$_{12}$
4.5 mcg, folic acid 0.3 mg, iron 15 mg.
Tab. Bot. 100s. *OTC.*
Use: Mineral, vitamin supplement.
bourbonal.
See: Ethyl Vanillin.
bovine colostrum.
Use: AIDS-related diarrhea. [Orphan
Drug]
**bovine immunoglobulin concentrate,
Cryptosporidium parvum.**
Use: Anti-infective. [Orphan Drug]
bovine whey protein concentrate.
Use: Treatment of cryptosporidiosis.
[Orphan Drug]
See: Immuno-C.
bowel evacuants.
Use: Laxative.
See: CoLyte.
Fleet Prep Kit 1.
Fleet Prep Kit 3.

Fleet Prep Kit 2.
GoLYTELY.
HalfLytely.
MiraLax.
NuLYTELY.
OCL.
Polyethylene Glycol.
Polyethylene Glycol and Electrolytes.
Tridrate Bowel Cleansing System.
X-Prep Bowel Evacuant Kit-1.

Bowman's Poison Antidote Kit. (Jones Pharma) Syr. of ipecac 1 oz, 1 bottle; activated charcoal liquid 2 oz, 3 bottles. *OTC.*
Use: Antidote.

Bowsteral. (Jones Pharma) Isopropanol 60%. Bot. Pt, gal.
Use: Disinfectant.

•**boxidine.** (BOX-ih-deen) USAN.
Use: Adrenal steroid blocker; antihyperlipoproteinemic.

Boylex. (Health for Life Brands) Diperodon, hexachlorophene, rosin cerate, ichthammol, carbolic acid, thymol, camphor, juniper tar. Tube oz. *OTC.*
Use: Drawing salve.

BP Allergy Junior. (Brookstone) Chlorpheniramine tannate 4 mg, phenylephrine tannate 20 mg per 5 mL. Aspartame, methylparaben, phenylalanine 5 mg per 5 mL, prosweet, saccharin, sorbitol. Alcohol free. Bubble gum flavor. Susp. 473 mL. *Rx.*
Use: Upper respiratory combination, decongestant and antihistamine.

B-Pap. (Wren) Acetaminophen 120 mg, sodium butabarbital 15 mg/5 mL. Bot. Pt, gal. *Rx.*
Use: Analgesic; sedative.

b-pas.
See: Calcium Benzoyl PAS.

BP Cleansing Wash. (Brookstone) Sodium sulfacetamide 10%, sulfur 4%. Cetyl alcohol, disodium EDTA, glyceryl stearate, parabens, PEG 100 stearate, stearyl alcohol, urea 10%. Soap. 473 mL. *Rx.*
Use: Acne product, combination.

BP 8 Cough. (Brookstone) Dextromethorphan hydrobromide 15 mg, guaifenesin 175 mg, pseudoephedrine hydrochloride 30 mg per 5 mL. Parabens, saccharin, sorbitol. Alcohol free. Grape flavor. Susp. 473 mL. *Rx.*
Use: Upper respiratory combination, antitussive and expectorant combination.

BP-50. (Brookstone) Urea 50%. Cetyl alcohol, disodium EDTA, glycerin, lactic acid, PEG-6, titanium dioxide, vitamin E. Emulsion. 284 g. *Rx.*
Use: Emollient.

BP 5.25%. (River's Edge Pharmaceuticals) Benzoyl peroxide 5.25%. Alcohols, aloe, glycerin, PEG, propylene glycol, triethanolamine. Soap. 175 g. *Rx.*
Use: Topical anti-infective, antibiotic agent.

BP 4.25%. (River's Edge Pharmaceuticals) Benzoyl peroxide 4.25%. Alcohols, aloe, glycerin, green tea extract, PEG, propylene glycol, triethanolamine. Soap. 473 mL. *Rx.*
Use: Topical anti-infective, antibiotic agent.

B-Plex. (Ivax) Vitamins B_1 15 mg, B_2 15 mg, B_3 100 mg, B_5 18 mg, B_6 4 mg, B_{12} 5 mcg, C 500 mg, folic acid 0.5 mg. Tab. Bot. 100s. *Rx.*
Use: Mineral, vitamin supplement.

BPM PE DM. (Boca Pharmaceuticals) Brompheniramine maleate 2 mg, dextromethorphan hydrobromide 10 mg, phenylephrine hydrochloride 5 mg per 5 mL. Glycerin, sorbitol, saccharin, sodium benzoate. Alcohol free, sugar free. Raspberry flavor. Syr. 473 mL. *Rx.*
Use: Upper respiratory combination, antitussive combination.

BPM Pseudo 6/45 mg. (Boca Pharmacal) Pseudoephedrine hydrochloride 45 mg, brompheniramine maleate 6 mg. ER Tab. 30s, 100s. *Rx.*
Use: Decongestant and antihistamine, upper respiratory combination.

BP Poly-650. (Brookstone) Acetaminophen 650 mg, phenyltoloxamine citrate 60 mg. Tab. 100s. *Rx.*
Use: Nonnarcotic antitussive.

BP 7% Wash. (River's Edge) Benzoyl peroxide 7%. Aloe barbadensis, benzyl alcohol, camellia oleifera leaf (green tea) extract, cetyl alcohol, glycerin, PEG-100. Soap. 473 mL. *Rx.*
Use: Anti-infective, topical; antibiotic agent.

Brace. (GlaxoSmithKline) Denture adhesive. Tube 1.4 oz, 2.4 oz.

Bradosol Bromide. (Novartis) Domiphen bromide.
Use: Antiseptic.

branched chain amino acids.
Use: Nutritional supplement; amyotrophic lateral sclerosis agent. [Orphan Drug]

Brasivol Fine, Medium, and Rough. (GlaxoSmithKline) Aluminum oxide scrub particles in a surfactant cleansing base. **Fine:** Jar 153 g. **Medium:** Jar 180 g. **Rough:** Jar 195 g. *OTC.*
Use: Scrub cleanser.

•**brasofensine maleate.** (brah-so-FEN-seen) USAN.
Use: Antiparkinsonian.

Bravelle. (Ferring) Urofollitropin 75 units FSH activity. Contains up to 2% luteinizing hormone activity. Pow. for Inj., lyophilized. Vials with NaCl 2 mL as diluent and lactose monohydrate 23 mg. *Rx.*
Use: Ovulation stimulant.

Breatheasy. (Pascal Co. Inc.) Racemic epinephrine hydrochloride 2.2%. Soln. inhaled by use of nebulizer. Bot. 0.25 oz, 0.5 oz, 1 oz. *OTC.*
Use: Bronchodilator.

Breathe Free. (Thompson Medical) Sodium chloride 0.65%, benzalkonium chloride. Soln. Spray Bot. 45 mL. *OTC.*
Use: Nasal decongestant.

Breathe Right Cold Nasal Strips. (GlaxoSmithKline) Menthol. Strip. Pkg. 10s. *OTC.*
Use: Upper respiratory combination, topical.

Breathe Right Colds Nasal Strips. (GlaxoSmithKline) Menthol. Strip. Pkg. 10s. *OTC.*
Use: Upper respiratory combination, topical.

•**brecanavir.** (bre-KAN-a-vir) USAN.
Use: Antiretroviral.

Breezee Mist. (Pedinol Pharmacal) Aluminum chlorhydrate, undecylenic acid, menthol. Aerosol. Bot. 4 oz. *OTC.*
Use: Antifungal; deodorant; antiperspirant; foot powder.

Breezee Mist Foot Powder. (Pedinol Pharmacal) Isobutane, talc, aluminum chlorhydrate, cyclomethicone, isopropyl myristate, propylene carbonate, stearalkonium hectorite, undecylenic acid, menthol. Pow. Aerosol can. 113 g. *OTC.*
Use: Antifungal, topical.

•**bremelanotide.** (BRE-mel-AN-oh-tide) USAN.
Use: Melanocortin agent.

•**brentuximab vedotin.** (bren-TUK-see-mab ve-DOE-tin) USAN.
Use: Antineoplastic.

•**brequinar sodium.** (BREh-kwih-NAHR) USAN.
Use: Antineoplastic.

•**bretazenil.** (bret-AZZ-eh-nill) USAN.
Use: Anxiolytic.

Brethancer. (Novartis)
Use: Inhaler, complete unit to be used with *Brethaire.*

•**bretylium tosylate.** (bre-TILL-ee-uhm TAH-sill-ate) *USP 34.*
Use: Hypotensive; antiadrenergic; cardiovascular agent, antiarrhythmic.

Brevibloc. (Baxter) Esmolol hydrochloride 10 mg/mL, 250 mg/mL. Inj. **10 mg/ mL:** Vial 10 mL. **250 mg/mL:** Amp

10 mL, propylene glycol 25%, alcohol 25%. *Rx.*
Use: Antiadrenergic/sympatholytic, beta-adrenergic blocker.

Brevibloc Double Strength. (Baxter) Esmolol hydrochloride 20 mg/mL. Preservative free. Inj. Ready-to-use 5 mL vials. 100 mL bags. *Rx.*
Use: Beta-adrenergic blocking agent.

Brevicon. (Watson) Norethindrone 0.5 mg, ethinyl estradiol 35 mcg. Lactose. Tab. *Wallette* 28s with 7 inert tabs. *Rx.*
Use: Sex hormone, contraceptive.

Brevital Sodium. (JHP Pharm) Methohexital sodium. **Vial:** 2.5 g/250 mL. **Amp.:** 2.5 g. *Rx.*
Use: Anesthetic, general.

Brevoxyl-8. (GlaxoSmithKline) Benzoyl peroxide 8%. Cetyl alcohol, stearyl alcohol. Gel. Tube 42.5 g, 90 g. *Rx.*
Use: Anti-infective; antibiotic, topical.

Brevoxyl-8 Acne Wash Kit. (GlaxoSmithKline) Benzoyl peroxide 8%. Castor oil, glycerin, mineral oil, parabens. Cream. 170 g. Kit w/SFC lotion (106.6 mL). *Formerly Brevoxyl Creamy Wash. Rx.*
Use: Anti-infective; antibiotic, topical.

Brevoxyl-8 Cleansing. (GlaxoSmithKline) Benzoyl peroxide 8%. Cetyl alcohol. Lot. Bot. 297 g. *Rx.*
Use: Anti-infective, antibiotic, topical.

Brevoxyl-4. (GlaxoSmithKline) Benzoyl peroxide 4%. Cetyl alcohol, stearyl alcohol. Gel. Tube 42.5 g, 90 g. *Rx.*
Use: Antiacne.

Brevoxyl-4 Acne Wash Kit. (GlaxoSmithKline) Benzoyl peroxide 4%. Glycerin, castor oil, parabens, mineral oil. Cream. 170 g. Kit w/SFC lotion (106.6 mL). *Formerly Brevoxyl Creamy Wash. Rx.*
Use: Anti-infective; antibiotic, topical.

Brevoxyl-4 Cleansing. (GlaxoSmithKline) Benzoyl peroxide 4%. Cetyl alcohol. Lot. Bot. 297 g. *Rx.*
Use: Anti-infective, antibiotic, topical.

brewer's yeast. (NBTY) Vitamins B_1 0.06 mg, B_2 0.02 mg, B_3 0.2 mg. Tab. Bot. 250s. *OTC.*
Use: Vitamin supplement.

Brexin EX. (Savage) **Liq.:** Pseudoephedrine hydrochloride 30 mg, guaifenesin 200 mg/5 mL. **Tab.:** Pseudoephedrine hydrochloride 60 mg, guaifenesin 400 mg. Bot. 100s. *OTC.*
Use: Decongestant, expectorant.

•**briakinumab.** (BRYE-a-kin-ue-mab) USAN.
Use: Immunomodulator.

•**brifentanil hydrochloride.** (brih-FEN-tah-NILL) USAN.
Use: Analgesic; narcotic.

Brigen-G. (Grafton) Chlordiazepoxide 5 mg, 10 mg, 25 mg. Tab. Bot. 500s. *c-iv.*
Use: Anxiolytic.

Brij 96 and 97. (ICI) Polyoxyl 10 oleyl ether available as 96 and 97.
Use: Surface active agent.

Brij-721. (ICI) Polyoxyethylene 21 stearyl ether (100% active).
Use: Surface active agent.

•**brimonidine tartrate.** (brih-MOE-nih-DEEN) USAN.
Use: Agent for glaucoma.
See: Alphagan P.

brimonidine tartrate. (Various Mfr.) Brimonidine tartrate 0.2%. Soln. 5 mL, 10 mL, 15 mL. *Rx.*
Use: Agent for glaucoma.

brimonidine tartrate/timolol maleate.
Use: Agent for glaucoma.
See: Combigan.

brineurin.
See: Abrineurin.

•**brinolase.** (BRIN-oh-laze) USAN. Fibrinolytic enzyme produced by *Aspergillus oryzae.*
Use: Fibrinolytic.

•**brinzolamide.** (brin-ZOE-lah-mide) *USP 34.*
Use: Antiglaucoma agent.
See: Azopt.

Bristoject. (Bristol-Myers Squibb) Prefilled disposable syringes w/needle.
Available with: Aminophylline: 250 mg/10 mL. Atropine sulfate: 5 mg/5 mL or 1 mg/mL. 10s. Calcium Cl: 10%. 10 mL. 10s. Dexamethasone: 20 mg/5 mL. Dextrose: 50%. 50 mL. 10s. Diphenhydramine: 50 mg/5 mL. Dopamine hydrochloride: 200 mg/5 mL, 400 mg/10 mL. Ephedrine: 50 mg/10 mL. Epinephrine: 1:10,000. 10 mL. 10s. Lidocaine hydrochloride: 1%: 5 mL, 10 mL; 2%: 5 mL; 4%: 25 mL, 50 mL; 20%: 5 mL, 10 mL. Magnesium sulfate: 5 g/10 mL, 10s. Metaraminol: 1%. 10 mL. Sodium bicarbonate: 75%: 50 mL; 84%: 50 mL. 10s.
Use: Medical device.

British anti-Lewisite. Dimercaprol.
See: BAL.

•**brivanib.** (bri-VAN-ib) USAN.
Use: Antineoplastic.

•**brivaracetam.** (BRIV-a-RA-se-tam) USAN.
Use: Anticonvulsant.

Brobella-P.B. (Brothers) Atropine sulfate 0.0195 mg, hyoscine HBr 0.0065 mg, hyoscyamine sulfate 0.1040 mg, phenobarbital 0.25 g. Tab. Bot. 100s, 1000s. *Rx.*
Use: Anticholinergic; antispasmodic; hypnotic; sedative.

•**brocresine.** (broe-KREE-seen) USAN.
Use: Histidine decarboxylase inhibitor.

•**brocrinat.** (BROE-krih-NAT) USAN.
Use: Diuretic.

Brocycline. (Brothers) Tetracycline hydrochloride 250 mg. Cap. Bot. 100s, 1000s. *Rx.*
Use: Anti-infective, tetracycline.

•**brodalumab.** (broe-DAL-ue-mab) USAN.
Use: Immunomodulator.

Brofed. (Marnel) Pseudoephedrine hydrochloride 30 mg, brompheniramine maleate 4 mg/5 mL, parabens, saccharin, sorbitol, sucrose, corn syr., menthol, mint flavor. Liq. Bot. 473 mL. *Rx.*
Use: Upper respiratory combination, antihistamine, decongestant.

•**brofoxine.** (BROE-fox-een) USAN.
Use: Antipsychotic.

•**bromadoline maleate.** (BROE-mah-DOE-leen) USAN.
Use: Analgesic.

bromaleate.
See: Pamabrom.

Bromaline. (Rugby) Brompheniramine maleate 1 mg, pseudoephedrine hydrochloride 15 mg per 5 mL. Corn syrup, glycerin, propylene glycol, saccharin, sodium 5 mg, sorbitol. Alcohol free. Grape flavor. Soln. 118 mL, 473 mL. *OTC.*
Use: Upper respiratory combination, decongestant and antihistamine.

Bromaline DM. (Rugby) Brompheniramine maleate 1 mg, dextromethorphan hydrobromide 5 mg, pseudoephedrine hydrochloride 15 mg. Fructose, saccharin, sorbitol. Alcohol free. Grape flavor. Elix. 473 mL. *OTC.*
Use: Upper respiratory combination, antitussive combination.

Bromanate. (Alpharma) Brompheniramine maleate 1 mg/5 mL, pseudoephedrine hydrochloride 15 mg, alcohol free, grape flavor. Elix. Bot. 118 mL, 237 mL, 473 mL, gal. *OTC.*
Use: Upper respiratory combination, antihistamine, decongestant.

Bromanate DM Cold & Cough. (Alpharma) Pseudoephedrine hydrochloride 15 mg, brompheniramine maleate 1 mg, dextromethorphan HBr 5 mg per 5 mL. Alcohol free, grape flavor. Elixir.

Bot. 118 mL. *OTC.*
Use: Upper respiratory combination, decongestant, antihistamine, antitussive.

Bromanyl. (Various Mfr.) Bromodiphenhydramine hydrochloride 12.5 mg, codeine phosphate 10 mg, alcohol 5%. Syr. Bot. Pt, gal. *c-v.*
Use: Antihistamine; antitussive.

Bromarest DX. (Warner Chilcott) Pseudoephedrine hydrochloride 30 mg, brompheniramine maleate 2 mg, dextromethorphan HBr 10 mg, alcohol 0.95%. Butterscotch flavor. Syr. Bot. 480 mL. *Rx.*
Use: Antihistamine; antitussive; decongestant.

Bromatan Plus. (Cypress) Dextromethorphan tannate 30 mg, dexchlorpheniramine tannate 3.5 mg, pseudoephedrine tannate 45 mg per 5 mL. Aspartame, parabens, phenylalanine 7 mg/5 mL. Orange-pineapple flavor. Susp. 473 mL. *Rx.*
Use: Upper respiratory combination, antitussive combination.

Bromatap. (Ivax) Brompheniramine maleate 2 mg, phenylephrine hydrochloride 12.5 mg, alcohol 2.3%/5 mL. Liq. Bot. 4 oz, 8 oz, pt, gal. *OTC.*
Use: Antihistamine; decongestant.

bromauric acid. Hydrogen tetrabromoaurate.

•**bromazepam.** (broe-MAY-zeh-pam) USAN.
Use: Anxiolytic.

Brombay. (Rosemont) Brompheniramine maleate 2 mg/5 mL, alcohol 3%. Elix. Bot. 4 oz, pt, gal. *OTC.*
Use: Antihistamine.

•**bromchlorenone.** (brome-KLOR-ee-nohn) USAN.
Use: Anti-infective, topical.

Bromdex D. (Breckenridge) Brompheniramine maleate 3 mg, dextromethorphan hydrobromide 30 mg, pseudoephedrine hydrochloride 50 mg. Saccharin, sorbitol. Alcohol free and sugar free. Berry vanilla flavor. Syr. 473 mL. *Rx.*
Use: Upper respiratory combination, antitussive combination.

•**bromelains.** (BROE-meh-lanes) USAN.
Use: Anti-inflammatory.
See: Dayto-Anase.

Brometane DX Cough. (Hi-Tech) Pseudoephedrine hydrochloride 30 mg, brompheniramine maleate 2 mg, dextromethorphan HBr 10 mg per 5 mL. Alcohol, saccharin, sorbitol. Sugar free.

Syr. Bot. 473 mL. *Rx.*
Use: Upper respiratory combination, antitussive combination.

Bromfed DM. (Wockhardt) Brompheniramine maleate 2 mg, dextromethorphan hydrobromide 10 mg, pseudoephedrine hydrochloride 30 mg. Alcohol 0.95%, methylparaben, sugar. Butterscotch flavor. Syr. 118 mL, 473 mL. *Rx.*
Use: Upper respiratory combination, antitussive combination.

•**bromfenac.** (BROME-fen-ak) USAN.
Use: Nonsteroidal anti-inflammatory agent, ophthalmic.
See: Xibrom.

bromhexine. (Boehringer Ingelheim)
Use: Mild/moderate keratoconjunctivitis sicca. [Orphan Drug]

•**bromhexine hydrochloride.** (brome-HEX-een) USAN.
Use: Expectorant; mucolytic.

Bromhist-DM. (Cypress) Brompheniramine maleate 1 mg, dextromethorphan HBr 4 mg, pseudoephedrine hydrochloride 15 mg per mL. Alcohol, sugar, and dye free. Maltitol, saccharin, sorbitol. Grape flavor. Drops. 30 mL. *Rx.*
Use: Upper respiratory combination, antitussive combination.

Bromhist-DM Pediatric. (Cypress) Pseudoephedrine hydrochloride 30 mg, brompheniramine maleate 2 mg, dextromethorphan hydrobromide 5 mg, guaifenesin 50 mg per 5 mL. Alcohol free, dye free. Saccharin, sorbitol. Grape flavor. Syr. 473 mL. *Rx.*
Use: Upper respiratory combination, antitussive and expectorant combination.

Bromhist-NR. (Cypress) Pseudoephedrine hydrochloride 12.5 mg, brompheniramine maleate 1 mg per 1 mL. Alcohol and sugar free. Saccharin, sorbitol. Cherry flavor. Drops. 30 mL with dropper. *Rx.*
Use: Upper respiratory combination, decongestant and antihistamine.

Bromhist Pediatric. (Cypress) Pseudoephedrine hydrochloride 15 mg, brompheniramine maleate 1 mg per 1 mL. Alcohol, sugar, and dye free. Saccharin, sorbitol. Cherry flavor. Drops. 30 mL with dropper. *Rx.*
Use: Upper respiratory combination, decongestant and antihistamine.

Bromhist PDX. (Cypress) Phenylephrine hydrochloride 5 mg, dextromethorphan hydrobromide 5 mg, guaifenesin 50 mg, brompheniramine maleate 2 mg/5 mL. Alcohol free. Parabens,

sugar. Grape flavor. Syr. 473 mL. *Rx.*
Use: Upper respiratory combination, antitussive combination, antitussive and expectorant.

bromides.
See: Peacock's Bromides.

bromide salts.
See: Ferrous Bromide.
Strontium Bromide.

Bromi-Lotion. (Gordon Laboratories) Aluminum hydroxychloride 20%, emollient base. Lot. Bot. 1.5 oz, 4 oz. *OTC.*
Use: Antiperspirant.

•**bromindione.** (BROME-in-die-ohn) USAN.
Use: Anticoagulant.

Bromi-Talc. (Gordon Laboratories) Potassium alum, bentonite, talc. Shaker can 3.5 oz, 1 lb, 5 lb. *OTC.*
Use: Bromidrosis; hyperhidrosis.

•**bromocriptine.** (BROE-moe-KRIP-teen) USAN.
Use: Enzyme inhibitor, prolactin.

•**bromocriptine mesylate.** (BROE-moe-KRIP-teen) *USP 34.*
Use: Enzyme inhibitor, prolactin.
See: Cycloset.
Parlodel.

bromocriptine mesylate. (Mylan) Bromocriptine mesylate. **Cap.:** 5 mg. 30s, 100s. **Tab.:** 2.5 mg. May contain lactose, EDTA. 30s, 100s. *Rx.*
Use: Enzyme inhibitor, prolactin; antiparkinson agent.

bromodiethylacetylurea.
See: Carbromal.

•**bromodiphenhydramine hydrochloride.** (BROE-moe-die-fen-HIGH-drah-meen) *USP 34.*
Use: Antihistamine.

•**bromodiphenhydramine hydrochloride/codeine phosphate.** (BROE-moe-die-fen-HIGH-drah-meen) *USP 34.* Antitussive combination.

bromodiphenhydramine hydrochloride/codeine phosphate. (Rosemont) Bromodiphenhydramine hydrochloride 12.5 mg, codeine phosphate 10 mg. Syr. Bot. 480 mL. *c-v.*
Use: Antitussive combination.

bromoform. Tribromomethane.

bromoisovaleryl urea. Alpha, bromoisovaleryl urea.

Bromophin.
See: Apomorphine Hydrochloride.

Bromo Seltzer. (Warner Lambert) Acetaminophen 325 mg, sodium bicarbonate 2.78 g, citric acid 2.22 g (when dissolved, forms sodium citrate 2.85 g)/dose. Large (2 ⅝ oz), King (4.25 oz),

Giant (9 oz), Foil pack, single-dose 48s. *OTC.*
Use: Antacid; analgesic.

bromotheophyllinate aminoisobutanol.
See: Pamabrom.

bromotheophyllinate pyranisamine.
See: Pyrabrom.

bromotheophyllinate pyrilamine.
See: Pyrabrom.

8-bromotheophylline.
See: Pamabrom.

Bromotuss w/Codeine. (Rugby) Bromodiphenhydramine hydrochloride 12.5 mg, codeine phosphate 10 mg, alcohol 5%. Syr. Bot. 120 mL, pt, gal. *c-v.*
Use: Antihistamine; antitussive.

•**bromoxanide.** (broe-MOX-ah-nide) USAN.
Use: Anthelmintic.

Brom/PE/DM. (Brighton Pharmaceuticals) Brompheniramine maleate 2 mg, dextromethorphan hydrobromide 10 mg, phenylephrine hydrochloride 5 mg per 5 mL. Glycerin, prosweet, saccharin, sodium benzoate, sorbitol. Strawberry flavor. Syr. 473 mL. *Rx.*
Use: Upper respiratory combination, antitussive combination.

•**bromperidol.** (brome-PURR-ih-dahl) USAN.
Use: Antipsychotic.

•**bromperidol decanoate.** (brome-PURR-ih-dole deh-KAN-oh-ate) USAN.
Use: Antipsychotic.

Bromphen DX. (Rugby) Pseudoephedrine hydrochloride 30 mg, brompheniramine maleate 2 mg, dextromethorphan HBr 10 mg, alcohol 0.95%. Syr. Bot. 480 mL. *Rx.*
Use: Antihistamine; antitussive; decongestant.

Bromphenex DM. (Breckenridge) Dextromethorphan HBr 30 mg, brompheniramine maleate 4 mg, pseudoephedrine hydrochloride 60 mg per 5 mL. Alcohol, sugar, and dye free. Sorbitol, saccharin. Fruit flavor. Liq. 473 mL. *Rx.*
Use: Antitussive combination, upper respiratory combination.

brompheniramine.
Use: Antihistamine, nonselective alkylamine.
See: Bidhist.
BrōveX.
BrōveX CT.
Lodrane D.
Lodrane 24.
Lodrane XR.
LoHist 12 Hour.
VaZol.

Brompheniramine Cough. (Geneva)
Pseudoephedrine hydrochloride 30 mg,
brompheniramine maleate 2 mg, dextromethorphan HBr 10 mg, alcohol
0.95%. Syr. Bot. 480 mL. *Rx.*
Use: Antihistamine; antitussive; decongestant.
brompheniramine/hydrocodone/PSE.
(Varsity) Hydrocodone bitartrate
2.5 mg, brompheniramine maleate
3 mg, pseudoephedrine hydrochloride
30 mg per 5 mL. Alcohol and sugar free.
Saccharin, sorbitol. Bubble gum fla-
vor. Liq. 473 mL. *c-III.*
Use: Upper respiratory combination, an-
titussive combination.
•**brompheniramine maleate.** (brome-fen-
AIR-uh-meen) *USP 34.*
Use: Antihistamine.
See: Lodrane 12 Hour.
W/Carbetapentane Citrate, Phenyl-
ephrine Hydrochloride
See: Vazotan.
V-Cof.
W/Chlophedianol Hydrochloride, Pseudo-
ephedrine Hydrochloride.
See: Dicel CD.
W/Codeine Phosphate.
See: Brōvex CB.
Brōvex CBX.
EndaCof-AC.
Nalex AC.
W/Codeine Phosphate, Phenylephrine
Hydrochloride.
See: Brōvex PB C.
Brōvex PB CX.
M-End PE.
Poly-Tussin AC.
W/Codeine Phosphate, Pseudoephed-
rine Hydrochloride.
See: CPB WC.
Mar-Cof BP.
M-END WC.
Mesehist WC.
W/Dextromethorphan Hydrobromide,
Guaifenesin, Phenylephrine Hydrochlo-
ride.
See: AccuHist PDX.
Bromhist-PDX.
W/Dextromethorphan Hydrobromide,
Guaifenesin, Pseudoephedrine Hydro-
chloride.
See: Bromhist DM Pediatric.
Histacol DM Pediatric.
Pediahist DM.
W/Dextromethorphan Hydrobromide,
Phenylephrine Hydrochloride.
See: Alahist DM.
Balacall DM.
BPM PE DM.
BROM/PE/DM.

Brōvex PB DM.
Brōvex PEB DM.
Children's Dimaphen DM.
LoHist-DM.
Phenylephrine Complex.
TGQ 7.5PEH/4BRM/15DM.
TL-Hist DM.
Tusdec-DM.
W/Dextromethorphan Hydrobromide,
Pseudoephedrine Hydrochloride.
See: AccuHist DM Pediatric.
Anaplex-DM Cough.
Bromaline DM.
Bromdex D.
Brometane-DX Cough.
Bromfed DM.
Bromhist-DM.
Bromhist PDX.
Bromphenex DM.
Brotapp DM.
BrōveX PSB DM.
Dallergy DM.
Dimaphen DM Cough, Cold & Allergy.
Dimetane DX.
DM/PSE/BPM.
Myphetane DX Cough.
Neo DM.
PBM Allergy.
Pediahist DM.
Prohist DM.
PSE Brom DM.
Q-Tapp DM Cold and Cough.
Sildec-DM.
TGQ 50PSE/3BRM/30DM.
W/Dihydrocodeine Bitartrate, Phenyl-
ephrine Hydrochloride.
See: Poly-Tussin DHC.
W/Dihydrocodeine Bitartrate, Pseudo-
ephedrine Hydrochloride.
See: J-COF DHC.
W/Phenylephrine Hydrochloride.
See: Alacol.
Alenaze-D.
Alenaze-D NR.
Brōvex PB.
Cenhist.
Dimetapp Children's Cold & Allergy.
Dimetapp Cold & Allergy.
LoHist PEB.
Respahist-II.
Seradex-LA.
Tanabid SR.
VaZol-D.
Vazotab.
Zotex-PE.
W/Pseudoephedrine Hydrochloride.
See: Bidhist-D.
BPM Pseudo 6/45 mg.
Bromaline.
Bromhist-NR.
Bromhist Pediatric.

Brotapp.
Brövex PSB.
BröveX SR.
Histex SR.
J-Tan D PD.
Lodrane.
Lodrane 12 D.
Lodrane 24 D.
LoHist-LQ.
LoHist PSB.
LoHist 12D.
PSE-BPM.
Q-Tapp.
Respahist.
Sildec.
Sinuhist.
SymPak II.
Touro Allergy.
ULTRAbrom.

brompheniramine maleate. (River's Edge) Brompheniramine maleate 1 mg. Saccharin. Alcohol free, dye free, and sugar free. Strawberry-banana flavor. Drops. 30 mL. *Rx.*
Use: Antihistamine; alkylamine, nonselective.

brompheniramine maleate/pseudoephedrine hydrochloride. (Cypress) Pseudoephedrine hydrochloride 60 mg, brompheniramine maleate 4 mg/5 mL. Saccharin, sorbitol, raspberry flavor. Syrup. 473 mL. *Rx.*
Use: Upper respiratory combination, decongestant, antihistamine.

brompheniramine maleate/pseudoephedrine hydrochloride. (Kylemore Pharmaceuticals) Brompheniramine maleate 1 mg, pseudoephedrine hydrochloride 7.5 mg. Glycerin, sorbitol, propylene glycol, saccharin, parabens. Alcohol free, dye free, and sugar free. Cotton candy flavor. Drops. 30 mL w/ dropper. *Rx.*
Use: Upper respiratory combination, decongestant and antihistamine.

brompheniramine maleate/pseudoephedrine hydrochloride. (River's Edge Pharmaceuticals) Brompheniramine maleate 1 mg, pseudoephedrine hydrochloride 7.5 mg. Saccharin, sorbitol. Alcohol free, dye free, and sugar free. Cotton candy flavor. Soln., Conc. 30 mL w/dropper. *Rx.*
Use: Upper respiratory combination, decongestant and antihistamine.

brompheniramine/phenylephrine tannate. (ANI Pharmaceuticals) Brompheniramine tannate 12 mg, phenylephrine tannate 20 mg per 5 mL. Acesulfame K, aspartame, methylparaben, phenylalanine 6 mg per 5 mL. Bubble gum flavor. Susp. 473 mL. *Rx.*
Use: Upper respiratory combination, decongestant and antihistamine.

brompheniramine tannate.
See: J-Tan.
P-Tex.
W/Carbetapentane Tannate, Phenylephrine Tannate.
See: Vazotan Tannate.
W/Dextromethorphan Tannate, Phenylephrine Tannate.
See: Dur-Tann DM.
Neo DM.
W/Phenylephrine Tannate.
See: Brövex ADT.
C-Tan D Plus Oral Suspension.
J-Tan D.
Relhist.
W/Pseudoephedrine Tannate.
See: BröveX PD.
B-Vex PD
Lodrane D.

brompheniramine tannate. (Ani Pharmaceuticals, Inc.) Brompheniramine tannate. **Chew. Tab.:** 12 mg. Sugar. Banana flavor. 60s. **Oral Susp.:** 12 mg per 5 mL. Methylparaben, sucrose, tartrazine. Banana flavor. 118 mL. *Rx.*
Use: Antihistamine.

brompheniramine tannate. (Various Mfr.) Brompheniramine tannate 12 mg. Chew. Tab. 60s. *Rx.*
Use: Antihistamine.

Brompton's cocktail. Heroin or morphine 10 mg, cocaine 10 mg, alcohol, chloroform water, syr. *c-ii.*
Use: Analgesic, narcotic.

bronchodilators.
See: Anticholinergics.
Sympathomimetics.
Xanthine Derivatives.

Broncholate. (Sanofi Synthelabo) Ephedrine hydrochloride 12.5 mg, guaifenesin 200 mg. **Cap.:** Bot. 100s, 1000s. **Softgels:** Bot. 100s. **Syr.:** Ephedrine hydrochloride 6.25 mg, guaifenesin 100 mg/5 mL, orange flavor. Bot. 473 mL. *Rx.*
Use: Bronchodilator; expectorant.

Broncotron-D. (Seyer Pharmatec) Dextromethorphan HBr 20 mg, guaifenesin 200 mg, phenylephrine hydrochloride 5 mg per 5 mL. Phenylalanine, aspartame, sorbitol. Cherry flavor. Susp. 30 mL, 473 mL. *Rx.*
Use: Antitussive and expectorant combination, upper respiratory combination.

Brondecon. (Parke-Davis) **Tab.:** Oxtriphylline 200 mg, guaifenesin 100 mg. Bot. 100s. **Elix.:** Oxtriphylline 100 mg,

guaifenesin 50 mg/5 mL w/alcohol 20%. Bot. 8 oz, 16 oz. *Rx.*
Use: Bronchodilator; expectorant.

Bronitin. (Whitehall-Robins) Theophylline hydrous 120 mg, guaifenesin 100 mg, ephedrine hydrochloride 24.3 mg, pyrilamine maleate 16.6 mg. Tab. Bot. 24s, 60s. *OTC.*
Use: Bronchodilator.

Bronitin Mist. (Whitehall-Robins) Epinephrine bitartrate in inhalation aerosol. Each spray releases 0.3 mg epinephrine bitartrate equivalent to 0.16 mg epinephrine base. Bot. 15 mL or 15 mL refills. *OTC.*
Use: Bronchodilator.

Bronkaid Dual Action. (Bayer Consumer Care) Ephedrine sulfate 25 mg, guaifenesin 400 mg. Tab. Bot. 24s. *OTC.*
Use: Bronchodilator; upper respiratory combination, decongestant, expectorant.

Bronkids. (Great Southern Laboratories) Chlorpheniramine maleate 0.6 mg, dextromethorphan HBr 2.75 mg, phenylephrine hydrochloride 1.5 mg/mL. Alcohol and sugar free. Saccharin, sorbitol. Bubble gum flavor. Drops, Oral. 30 mL. *Rx.*
Use: Upper respiratory combination, antitussive combination.

Bronkometer. (Sanofi-Synthelabo) Isoetharine mesylate 0.61%, saccharin, menthol, alcohol 30%. Metered dose of 340 mcg isoetharine in fluorohydrocarbon propellant. Bot. w/nebulizer 10 mL, 15 mL. Refill 10 mL, 15 mL. *Rx.*
Use: Bronchodilator.

Bronkosol. (Sanofi-Synthelabo) Isoetharine hydrochloride 1% w/glycerin, sodium bisulfite, parabens for oral inhalation. Bot. 10 mL, 30 mL. *Rx.*
Use: Bronchodilator.

Bronkotuss. (Hyrex) Chlorpheniramine maleate 4 mg, guaifenesin 100 mg, ephedrine sulfate 8.216 mg, hydriodic acid syr. 1.67 mg/5 mL w/alcohol 5%. Bot. Pt, gal. *Rx.*
Use: Antihistamine; decongestant; expectorant.

Brontex Liquid. (Procter & Gamble) Codeine phosphate 2.5 mg, guaifenesin 75 mg/5 mL, methylparaben, saccharin, sucrose. Liq. Bot. 473 mL. *c-v.*
Use: Antitussive expectorant; narcotic.

Brontex Tablets. (Procter & Gamble) Codeine phosphate 10 mg, guaifenesin 300 mg. Tab. Bot. 100s. *c-III.*
Use: Antitussive expectorant; narcotic.

Brontuss DX. (Portal) Dextromethorphan hydrobromide 20 mg, guaifenesin 200 mg, phenylephrine hydrochloride 10 mg. Cherry flavoring, maltitol, propylene glycol, saccharin, sorbitol. Alcohol free, dye free, gluten free, and sugar free. Liq. 118 mL. *OTC.*
Use: Upper respiratory combination, antitussive and expectorant combination.

• **broperamole.** (BROE-PURR-ah-mole) USAN.
Use: Anti-inflammatory.

• **bropirimine.** (broe-PIE-rih-MEEN) USAN.
Use: Antineoplastic; antiviral.

Broserpine. (Brothers) Reserpine 0.25 mg. Tab. Bot. 250s, 100s.
Use: Antihypertensive.

Brotapp. (Silarx) Brompheniramine maleate 1 mg, pseudoephedrine hydrochloride 15 mg. Grape flavoring, propylene glycol, saccharin, sodium benzoate, sorbitol. Alcohol free and sugar free. Liq. 118 mL, 237 mL, 437 mL. *OTC.*
Use: Upper respiratory combination, decongestant and antihistamine.

Brotapp DM. (Silarx) Brompheniramine maleate 1 mg, dextromethorphan hydrobromide 5 mg, pseudoephedrine hydrochloride 15 mg. Saccharin, sorbitol. Alcohol free and sugar free. Grape flavor. Liq. 118 mL, 237 mL. *OTC.*
Use: Upper respiratory combination, antitussive combination.

• **brotizolam.** (broe-TIE-zoe-LAM) USAN.
Use: Hypnotic; sedative.

Bro-T's. (Brothers) Bromisovalum 0.12 g, carbromal 0.2 g. Tab. Bot. 100s, 1000s. *Rx.*
Use: Sedative; anxiolytic.

Bro-Tuss. (Brothers) Dextromethorphan HBr 15 mg, chlorpheniramine maleate 2 mg, phenylephrine hydrochloride 5 mg, ammonium Cl 100 mg, sodium citrate 150 mg, vitamin C 30 mg/10 mL. Bot. 4 oz, pt, gal. *OTC.*
Use: Antihistamine; antitussive; decongestant; expectorant.

Bro-Tuss A.C. (Brothers) Acetaminophen 120 mg, codeine phosphate 10 mg, phenylephrine hydrochloride 5 mg, chlorpheniramine maleate 2 mg, menthol 1 mg, alcohol 10%/5 mL. Bot. Pt, gal. *c-v.*
Use: Analgesic; antihistamine; antitussive; decongestant.

Brovana. (Sepracor) Arformoterol (as base) 7.5 mcg/mL. Soln. for Inh. Unit-dose vials. 2 mL. *Rx.*
Use: Bronchodilator, sympathomimetic.

BröveX. (MCR American) Brompheniramine tannate 12 mg/5 mL. Methylparaben, saccharin, sucrose, tartrazine. Banana flavor. Oral Susp. Bot. 20 mL, 118 mL. *Rx.*
Use: Antihistamine, nonselective alkylamine.

BröveX ADT. (MCR American) Brompheniramine tannate 12 mg, phenylephrine tannate 10 mg per 5 mL. Aspartame, parabens, phenylalanine 7 mg per 5 mL. Bubble gum flavor. Susp. 473 mL. *Rx.*
Use: Upper respiratory combination, decongestant and antihistamine.

BröveX CB. (MCR American) Brompheniramine maleate 4 mg, codeine phosphate 10 mg. Tab. 100s. *c-III.*
Use: Upper respiratory combination, antitussive combination.

BröveX CBX. (MCR American) Brompheniramine maleate 4 mg, codeine phosphate 20 mg. Tab. 100s. *c-III.*
Use: Upper respiratory combination, antitussive combination.

BröveX CT. (MCR American) Brompheniramine tannate 12 mg, sucrose, banana flavor. Chew. Tab. Bot. 60s. *Rx.*
Use: Antihistamine, nonselective alkylamine.

BröveX-D. (MCR American) Phenylephrine tannate 20 mg, brompheniramine tannate 12 mg per 5 mL. Aspartame, parabens. Bubble gum flavor. Susp. 473 mL. *Rx.*
Use: Decongestant and antihistamine.

BröveX PB. (MCR American) Brompheniramine maleate 4 mg, phenylephrine hydrochloride 10 mg. Tab. 100s. *Rx.*
Use: Upper respiratory combination, decongestant and antihistamine.

BröveX PB C. (MCR American) Brompheniramine maleate 4 mg, codeine phosphate 10 mg, phenylephrine hydrochloride 10 mg. Tab. 100s. *c-III.*
Use: Upper respiratory combination, antitussive combination.

BröveX PB CX. (MCR American) Brompheniramine maleate 4 mg, codeine phosphate 20 mg, phenylephrine hydrochloride 10 mg. Tab. 100s. *c-III.*
Use: Upper respiratory combination, antitussive combination.

BröveX PB DM. (MCR American) Brompheniramine maleate 4 mg, dextromethorphan hydrobromide 20 mg, phenylephrine hydrochloride 10 mg. Tab. 100s. *Rx.*
Use: Upper respiratory combination, antitussive combination.

BröveX PD. (MCR American) Pseudoephedrine tannate 30 mg, brompheniramine tannate 6 mg per 5 mL. Aspartame, parabens, phenylalanine 7 mg per 5 mL. Cotton candy flavor. Oral Susp. 480 mL. *Rx.*
Use: Upper respiratory combination, decongestant and antihistamine.

BröveX PEB DM. (MCR American) Brompheniramine maleate 4 mg, dextromethorphan hydrobromide 20 mg, phenylephrine hydrochloride 10 mg per 5 mL. Parabens, sorbitol, sucralose. Alcohol free. Bubble gum flavor. Liq. 473 mL. *Rx.*
Use: Upper respiratory combination, antitussive combination.

BröveX PSB. (MCR American) Brompheniramine maleate 4 mg, pseudoephedrine hydrochloride 20 mg per 5 mL. Saccharin, sorbitol. Cotton candy flavor. Liq. 473 mL. *Rx.*
Use: Upper respiratory combination, decongestant and antihistamine.

BröveX PSB DM. (MCR American) Brompheniramine maleate 4 mg, dextromethorphan hydrobromide 20 mg, pseudoephedrine hydrochloride 20 mg per 5 mL. Saccharin, sorbitol. Alcohol free. Cotton candy flavor. Liq. 473 mL. *Rx.*
Use: Upper respiratory combination, antitussive combination.

BröveX SR. (MCR American) Pseudoephedrine hydrochloride 90 mg, brompheniramine maleate 9 mg. Sucrose. ER Cap. 100s. *Rx.*
Use: Decongestant and antihistamine, upper respiratory combination.

Bryrel. (Sanofi-Synthelabo) Piperazine citrate anhydrous 110 mg/mL. Syr. Bot. oz. *Rx.*
Use: Anthelmintic.

B-Scorbic. (Pharmics) Vitamins C 300 mg, B_1 25 mg, B_2 10 mg, calcium pantothenate 10 mg, niacinamide 50 mg, lemon flavored complex 200 mg. Tab. Bot. 100s, 1000s. *OTC.*
Use: Mineral, vitamin supplement.

BSS. (Alcon) Sodium Cl 0.64%, potassium Cl 0.075%, magnesium Cl 0.03%, calcium Cl 0.048%, sodium acetate 0.39%, sodium citrate 0.17%, sodium hydroxide or hydrochloric acid. Bot. 15 mL, 30 mL, 250 mL, 500 mL. *Rx.*
Use: Irrigant, ophthalmic.

BSS Plus. (Alcon) **Part I:** Sodium Cl 7.44 mg, potassium Cl 0.395 mg, dibasic sodium phosphate 0.433 mg, sodium bicarbonate 2.19 mg, hydrochloric acid, or sodium hydroxide/mL. Soln.

Bot. 240 mL. **Part II:** Calcium chloride dihydrate 3.85 mg, magnesium chloride hexahydrate 5 mg, dextrose 24 mg, glutathione disulfide 4.5 mg/mL. Soln. Bot. 10 mL. *Rx.*
Use: Irrigant, ophthalmic.

BTA Rapid Urine Test. (Bard) Reagent kit for detection of bladder tumor associated analytes in urine to aid in management of bladder cancer. Kits of 15 and 30 tests.
Use: Diagnostic aid.

B-12. (Mason Natural) Vitamin B_{12} (cyanocobalamin) 1,500 mcg. Gluten free, preservative free, and sugar free. ER Tab. 60s. *OTC.*
Use: Water-soluble vitamin.

B₂-400. (Bio-Tech) Riboflavin 400 mg. Preservative free and dye free. Cap. 100s. *OTC.*
Use: Water-soluble vitamin.

●**bucainide maleate.** (byoo-CANE-ide) USAN.
Use: Cardiovascular agent, antiarrhythmic.

buchu.
See: Diosmin.

●**bucindolol hydrochloride.** (BYOO-SIN-doe-lole) USAN.
Use: Investigative; antihypertensive.

Buckley's Chest Congestion. (Novartis) Guaifenesin 100 mg/5 mL. Alcohol and sugar free. Acesulfame potassium, menthol, parabens. Liq. 118 mL. *OTC.*
Use: Expectorant.

Buckley's Cough Mixture. (Novartis) Dextromethorphan HBr 12.5 mg/5 mL. Alcohol and sugar free. Menthol, parabens, pine needle oil. Liq. 118 mL. *OTC.*
Use: Nonnarcotic antitussive.

●**buclizine hydrochloride.** (BYOO-klih-zeen) USAN.
Use: Antiemetic; antinauseant.

●**bucromarone.** (byoo-KROE-mah-rone) USAN.
Use: Cardiovascular agent, antiarrhythmic.

●**bucrylate.** (BYOO-krih-late) USAN.
Use: Surgical aid, tissue adhesive.

Budeprion SR. (Teva) Bupropion hydrochloride 100 mg, 150 mg. SR Tab (12 hour). 60s, 100s. *Rx.*
Use: Antidepressant.

Budeprion XL. (Teva) Bupropion hydrochloride 150 mg, 300 mg. Lactose and tartrazine (300 mg only). Film-coated. ER Tab. (24 hour). 30s, 500s. *Rx.*
Use: Antidepressant.

●**budesonide.** (BYOO-DESS-oh-nide) USAN.

Use: Anti-inflammatory; adrenocortical steroid, glucocorticoid; corticosteroid, intranasal steroid.
See: Entocort EC.
Pulmicort Flexhaler.
Pulmicort Respules.
Rhinocort Aqua.
W/Formoterol.
See: Symbicort.

budesonide. (Teva) Budesonide 0.25 mg per 2 mL, 0.5 mg per 2 mL. Disodium edetate. Susp., Inhal. Single-dose vial. 30s. *Rx.*
Use: Respiratory inhalant product, corticosteroid.

●**budiodarone.** (BUE-di-OH-da-rone) USAN.
Use: Antiarrhythmic.

●**budiodarone tartrate.** (BUE-di-OH-da-rone) USAN.
Use: Antiarrhythmic.

Buf Acne Cleansing Bar. (3M) Salicylic acid 1%, sulfur 1%. Bar. 3.5 oz. *OTC.*
Use: Antiacne.

Buf-Bar. (3M) Sulphur 3% and titanium dioxide. Bar 105 g. *OTC.*
Use: Antiacne.

Buf Body Scrub. (3M) Round cleansing sponge on plastic handles. *OTC.*
Use: Cleansing sponge.

Buff-A. (Merz) Aspirin acid 5 g buffered w/magnesium hydroxide, aluminum hydroxide dried gel. Tab. Bot. 100s, 1000s. *OTC.*
Use: Analgesic; antacid.

Buffaprin. (Buffington) Aspirin 325 mg buffered with magnesium oxide. Sugar, caffeine, lactose, salt free. Tab. *Dispense-A-Kit* 500s. *OTC.*
Use: Analgesic.

Buffasal. (Dover Pharmaceuticals) Aspirin 325 mg, magnesium oxide. Sugar, lactose, salt free. Tab. UD Box 500s. *OTC.*
Use: Analgesic.

Buffasal Max. (Dover Pharmaceuticals) Aspirin 500 mg, magnesium oxide. Sugar, lactose, salt free. Tab. *OTC.*
Use: Analgesic.

Buffered Aspirin. (Various Mfr.) Aspirin 325 mg with buffers. Tab. Bot. 100s, 500s, 1000s, UD 100s and 200s. *OTC.*
Use: Analgesic.

buffered intrathecal electrolyte/dextrose injection.
Use: Diluent. [Orphan Drug]
See: Elliot's B.

Bufferin. (Novartis) Aspirin 325 mg with calcium carbonate 158 mg, magnesium oxide 63 mg, magnesium carbonate 34 mg. Coated. Tab. 12s, 36s, 60s,

100s, 200s, UD 150s. *OTC.*
Use: Salicylate, aspirin, buffered.
Bufferin Extra Strength. (Novartis) Aspirin 500 mg with calcium carbonate, magnesium carbonate, and magnesium oxide. Tab. 130s. *OTC.*
Use: Salicylate, aspirin, buffered.
Buffex. (Roberts) Aspirin 325 mg w/ dihydroxyaluminum aminoacetate. Tab. Bot. 1000s, *Sanipack* 1000s. *OTC.*
Use: Analgesic.
Buf Foot Care Kit. (3M) Cleansing system for the feet. *OTC.*
Use: Foot preparation.
Buf Foot Care Lotion. (3M) Moisturizing lotion for feet. *OTC.*
Use: Foot preparation.
Buf Foot Care Soap. (3M) Bar 3.5 oz. *OTC.*
Use: Foot preparation.
•**bufilcon A.** (BYOO-fill-kahn A) USAN.
Use: Contact lens material, hydrophilic.
Buf Kit for Acne. (3M) Cleansing sponge, cleansing bar 3.5 oz w/booklet, holding tray. *OTC.*
Use: Antiacne.
Buf Lotion. (3M) Moisturizing lotion. *OTC.*
Use: Emollient.
•**buformin.** (BYOO-FORE-min) USAN.
Use: Antidiabetic.
Bufosal. (Table Rock) Sodium salicylate 15 g/dram w/calcium carbonate, sodium bicarbonate as granulated effervescent powder. Bot. 4 oz. *OTC.*
Use: Analgesic; antacid.
Buf-Ped Non-Medicated Cleansing Sponge. (3M) Abrasive cleansing sponge. *OTC.*
Use: Cleansing skin or feet.
Buf-Puf Bodymate. (3M) Oval two-sided cleansing sponge. Abrasive/gentle. *OTC.*
Use: Cleansing all areas of the body.
Buf-Puf Medicated. (3M) Water-activated. Salicylic acid 0.5% (reg. strength), alcohols, benzoate, EDTA, triethanolamine, and vitamin E acetate. Salicylic acid 2% (max. strength). Pads. Jar 30s. *OTC.*
Use: Antiacne.
Buf-Puf Non-Medicated Cleansing Sponge. (3M) Abrasive cleansing sponge. *OTC.*
Use: Skin cleansing.
Buf-Sul. (Sheryl) Sulfacetamide 167 mg, sulfadiazine 167 mg, sulfamerazine 167 mg. Tab. Bot. 100s. Susp. Bot. Pt. *Rx.*
Use: Anti-infective, sulfonamide.

Buf-Tabs. (Halsey Drug) Aspirin 5 g. Tab. w/aluminum hydroxide, glycine magnesium carbonate. Bot. 100s. *OTC.*
Use: Analgesic; antacid.
Bugs Bunny Chewable Vitamins and Minerals. (Bayer Consumer Care) Vitamins A 5000 units, D 400 units, E 30 units, C 60 mg, folic acid 0.4 mg, B_1 1.5 mg, B_2 1.7 mg, niacin 20 mg, B_6 2 mg, B_{12} 6 mcg, biotin 40 mcg, pantothenic acid 10 mg, iron 18 mg, calcium 100 mg, phosphorus 100 mg, iodine 150 mcg, magnesium 20 mg, copper 2 mg, zinc 15 mg. Chew. Tab. Bot. 60s. *OTC.*
Use: Mineral, vitamin supplement.
Bugs Bunny Complete. (Bayer Consumer Care) Ca 100 mg, iron 18 mg, vitamins A 5000 units, D 400 units, E 30 mg, B_1 1.5 mg, B_2 1.7 mg, B_3 20 mg, B_5 10 mg, B_6 2 mg, C 60 mg, folic acid 0.4 mg, biotin 40 mcg, Cu, I, Mg, P, aspartame, phenylalanine, Zn 15 mg. Tab. Bot. 60s. *OTC.*
Use: Mineral, vitamin supplement.
Bugs Bunny Plus Iron. (Bayer Consumer Care) Vitamins A 2500 units, E 15 units, C 60 mg, folic acid 0.3 mg, B_1 1.05 mg, B_2 1.2 mg, niacin 13.5 mg, B_6 1.05 mg, B_{12} 4.5 mcg, D 400 units, iron 15 mg. Chew. Tab. Bot. 60s. *OTC.*
Use: Mineral, vitamin supplement.
Bugs Bunny With Extra C. (Bayer Consumer Care) Vitamins A 2500 units, D 400 units, E 15 units, C 250 mg, folic acid 0.3 mg, B_1 1.05 mg, B_2 1.2 mg, niacin 13.5 mg, B_6 1.05 mg, B_{12} 4.5 mcg. Tab. Bot. 60s. *OTC.*
Use: Mineral, vitamin supplement.
Bulk Forming Fiber Laxative. (Goldline Consumer) Calcium polycarbophil 625 mg (equiv. to polycarbophil 500 mg). Tab. Bot. 60s. *OTC.*
Use: Laxative.
bulkogen. A mucin extracted from the seeds of Cyanopsis tetragonaloba.
bulk-producing laxatives.
See: Bulk Forming Fiber Laxative.
Citrucel.
Citrucel Sugar Free.
Equalactin.
Fiber.
Fiberall Orange Flavor.
Fiberall Tropical Fruit Flavor.
FiberCon.
Fiber-Lax.
FiberNorm.
Genfiber.
Genfiber, Orange Flavor.
Hydrocil Instant.
Konsyl.

Konsyl-D.
Konsyl Easy Mix Formula.
Konsyl Fiber.
Konsyl-Orange.
Maltsupex.
Metamucil.
Metamucil Orange Flavor, Original Texture.
Metamucil Orange Flavor, Smooth Texture.
Metamucil Original Texture.
Metamucil, Sugar Free, Orange Flavor, Smooth Texture.
Metamucil, Sugar Free, Smooth Texture.
Modane.
Natural Fiber Laxative.
Perdiem Fiber Therapy.
Polycarbophil.
Psyllium.
Reguloid.
Reguloid, Orange.
Reguloid, Sugar Free Orange.
Reguloid, Sugar Free Regular.
Serutan.
Syllact.
Unifiber.

Bullfrog. (Chattem) Benzophenone-3, octyl methoxycinnamate, isostearyl alcohol, aloe, hydrogenated vegetable oil, vitamin E. Waterproof. Stick 16.5 g. *OTC.*
Use: Sunscreen.

Bullfrog Extra Moisturizing. (Chattem) Benzophenone-3, octocrylene, octyl methoxycinnamate, vitamin E, aloe. SPF 18. Gel. Tube 90 g. *OTC.*
Use: Sunscreen.

Bullfrog for Kids. (Chattem) SPF 18. Octocrylene, octyl methoxycinnamate, octyl salicylate, vitamin E, aloe, alcohols, benzoate. Gel. Tube 60 g. *OTC.*
Use: Sunscreen.

Bull Frog Marathon Mist With UV Extender. (Chattem) Avobenzone 3%, homosalate 15%, octisalate 5%, octocrylene 10%, oxybenzone 6%. Aloe, glycerin, propylene glycol, SD alcohol. SPF 50. Spray. 177 mL. *OTC.*
Use: Sunscreen.

Bull Frog Quik Gel With UV Extender. (Chattem) Avobenzone 3%, homosalate 15%, octisalate 5%, octocrylene 10%, oxybenzone 6%. Aloe, glycerin, propylene glycol, SD alcohol. SPF 50. Gel. 147 mL. *OTC.*
Use: Sunscreen.

Bullfrog Sport. (Chattem) SPF 18. Benzophenone-3, octocrylene, octyl methoxycinnamate, octyl salicylate, titanium dioxide, diazolidinyl urea, EDTA,

parabens, vitamin E, aloe. Lot. Bot. 120 mL. *OTC.*
Use: Sunscreen.

Bullfrog Sunblock. (Chattem) SPF 18, 36. Benzophenone-3, octocrylene, octyl methoxycinnamate, aloe, vitamin E, isostearyl alcohol. PABA free. Waterproof. Gel. Tube 120 g. *OTC.*
Use: Sunscreen.

•**bumetanide.** (BYOO-MET-uh-hide) *USP 34.*
Use: Loop diuretic.

bumetanide. (Teva) Bumetanide 0.5 mg, 1 mg, 2 mg. Lactose. Tab. 100s, 1000s (except 0.5 mg). *Rx.*
Use: Loop diuretic.

bumetanide. (Various Mfr.) Bumetanide. **Tab:** 0.5 mg, 1 mg, 2 mg. Bot. 100s. **Inj.:** 0.25 mg/mL. Amp. 2 mL. Vial 2 mL, 4 mL, 10 mL; 4 mL fill in 5 mL. *Rx.*
Use: Loop diuretic.

•**bumetrizole.** (BYOO-meh-TRY-zole) USAN.
Use: Ultraviolet screen.

Buminate. (Baxter PPI) Normal serum albumin (human). **25%:** Soln. in 20 mL w/o administration set; 50 mL and 100 mL w/administration set. **5%:** Soln. in 250 mL, 500 mL w/administration set. *Rx.*
Use: Albumin replacement.

•**bunamidine hydrochloride.** (BYOO-NAM-ih-deen) USAN.
Use: Anthelmintic.

bunamiodyl sodium.
Use: Diagnostic aid, radiopaque medium.

•**bunaprolast.** (BYOO-nah-PROLE-ast) USAN.
Use: Antiasthmatic.

•**bunolol hydrochloride.** (BYOO-no-lole) USAN.
Use: Antiadrenergic, β-receptor.

Bun Reagent Strips. (Bayer Consumer Care) *Seralyzer* reagent strips. A quantitative strip test for BUN in serum or plasma. Bot. 25s.
Use: Diagnostic aid.

Bupap. (ECR) Butalbital 50 mg, acetaminophen 650 mg. Tab. Bot. 100s. *Rx.*
Use: Analgesic.

Buphenyl. (Medicis) Sodium phenylbutyrate. **Tab.:** 500 mg. Bot. 250s, 500s. **Pow.:** 3.2 g (3 g sodium phenylbutyrate)/tsp and 9.1 g (8.6 g sodium phenylbutyrate)/tsp. Bot. 500 mL, 950 mL. *Rx.*
Use: Antihyperammonemic.

•**bupicomide.** (byoo-PIH-koe-mide) USAN.
Use: Antihypertensive.

bupivacaine and epinephrine.
Use: Anesthetic, local.
See: Marcaine w/Epinephrine.
•**bupivacaine hydrochloride.** (byoo-PIH-vah-cane) *USP 34.*
Use: Anesthetic, local.
See: Bupivacaine Hydrochloride.
  Bupivacaine Hydrochloride with Epinephrine 1:200,000.
  Bupivacaine Spinal.
  Marcaine.
  Marcaine w/Epinephrine.
  Sensorcaine.
  Sensorcaine MPF.
  Sensorcaine MPF Spinal.
bupivacaine hydrochloride. (Abbott)
  Bupivacaine hydrochloride 0.25%, 0.5%, 0.75%. Inj. Amp. 20 mL, 30 mL, 50 mL (0.25% only). Vial 10 mL, 30 mL. Multidose vial 50 mL (except 0.75%) with methylparaben 1 mg/mL. *Abboject* 30 mL (0.5% only), 50 mL (0.25% only). *Rx.*
Use: Anesthetic, local.
bupivacaine hydrochloride with epinephrine 1:200,000. (Hospira) Bupivacaine hydrochloride 0.25%, 0.5%, 0.75% with epinephrine 1:200,000. Inj. Amp. 30 mL (except 0.25%), 50 mL (0.25% only). Vial 10 mL, 30 mL (except 0.75%). Fliptop multidose vial 50 mL (except 0.75%). *Rx.*
Use: Anesthetic, local.
bupivacaine in dextrose.
Use: Anesthetic, local.
Bupivacaine Spinal. (Abbott) Bupivacaine hydrochloride 0.75% in dextrose 8.25%. Preservative free. Inj. Amp. 2 mL. *Rx.*
Use: Anesthetic, local.
Buprenex. (Reckitt & Benckiser) Buprenorphine hydrochloride 0.3 mg/mL w/ 50 mg anhydrous dextrose. Inj. Amp. 1 mL. *c-III.*
Use: Analgesic; narcotic.
buprenorphine. (Roxane Labs) Buprenorphine hydrochloride 2 mg, 8 mg. Lactose, mannitol. Tab., sublingual. 30s. *c-III.*
Use: Opioid agonist-antagonist analgesic.
•**buprenorphine hydrochloride.** (BYOO-preh-NAHR-feen) *USP 34.*
Use: Analgesic.
See: Buprenex.
  Butrans.
  Subutex.
W/Naloxone.
See: Suboxone.
buprenorphine hydrochloride.
  (Hospira) Buprenorphine hydrochloride 0.3 mg/mL with anhydrous dextrose

50 mg. Inj. *Carpu-ject* 1 mL. *c-III.*
Use: Analgesic.
•**bupropion hydrobromide.** (bue-PRO-pee-ahn) USAN.
Use: CNS agent.
•**bupropion hydrochloride.** (byoo-PRO-pee-ahn) USAN.
Tall Man: buPROPion.
Use: Antidepressant; smoking deterrent.
See: Aplenzin.
  Budeprion SR.
  Wellbutrin.
  Wellbutrin SR.
  Wellbutrin XL.
  Zyban.
bupropion hydrochloride. (Reckitt & Colman)
Use: Treatment of opiate addiction. [Orphan Drug]
bupropion hydrochloride. (Various Mfr.) **ER Tab. (24 hour):** 150 mg, 300 mg. 30s, 60s, 90s, 500s. **ER Tab (12 hour):** 100 mg, 150 mg, 200 mg. 60s, 100s, 180s (200 mg only), 250s (150 mg only), 500s, 1,000s (200 mg only). **Tab.:** Bupropion hydrochloride 75 mg, 100 mg. 30s, 100s, 500s, 1,000s. *Rx.*
Use: Antidepressant.
•**buramate.** (BYOO-rah-mate) USAN.
Use: Anticonvulsant; antipsychotic; anxiolytic.
Burdeo. (Hill Dermaceuticals) Aluminum subacetate 100 mg, boric acid 300 mg/oz. Bot. 3 oz. Roll-on 8 oz. *OTC.*
Use: Deodorant.
Burn-a-Lay. (Ken-Gate) Chlorobutanol 0.75%, oxyquinoline benzoate 0.025%, zinc oxide 2%, thymol 0.5%. Cream. Tube oz. *OTC.*
Use: Burn therapy.
Burnate. (Burlington) Vitamins A 4000 units, D_2 400 units, thiamine hydrochloride 3 mg, riboflavin 2 mg, niacinamide 10 mg, pyridine hydrochloride 2 mg, cyanocobalamin 5 mcg, calcium pantothenate 0.5 mg, folic acid 0.4 mg, ascorbic acid 50 mg, ferrous fumarate 300 mg, calcium 200 mg, iodine 0.15 mg, copper 1 mg, magnesium 5 mg, zinc 1.5 mg. Tab. Bot. 100s. *OTC.*
Use: Mineral, vitamin supplement.
Burn-O-Jel. (S.S.S. Company) Lidocaine hydrochloride 0.5%. Aloe vera gel, EDTA, glycerin, ethyl alcohol. Gel. 85 g. *OTC.*
Use: Topical local anesthetic, amide local anesthetic.
burn preparations.
Use: Topical anti-infective.

See: Mafenide.
Nitrofurazone.
Silver Sulfadiazine.
Burn-Quel. Halperin aerosol dispenser 1 oz, 2 oz.
Use: Burn therapy.
burn therapy.
See: Burn-A-Lay.
Burn-Quel.
Foille.
Nupercainal.
Silvadene.
Solarcaine.
Sulfamylon.
Unguentine.
Buro-Sol Antiseptic. (Doak Dermatologics) Contents make a diluted Burow's Solution. Aluminum acetate topical soln. plus benzethonium Cl. Pow. Pkg. (2.36 g) 12s, 100s. Bot. Pow. 4 oz, 1 lb, 5 lb. OTC.
Use: Astringent.
Burow's Otic. (Rugby) Acetic acid 2% in aluminum acetate solution. Soln. 60 mL. Rx.
Use: Otic preparation.
Bursul. (Burlington) Sulfamethizole 500 mg. Tab. Bot. 100s. Rx.
Use: Anti-infective; sulfonamide.
Bur-Zin. (Lamond) Aluminum acetate solution 2%, zinc oxide 10%. Bot. 4 oz, 8 oz, pt, qt, gal. Also w/o lanolin. OTC.
Use: Antipruritic, counterirritant.
•**buserelin acetate.** (BYOO-seh-REH-lin ASS-eh-tate) USAN.
Use: Gonad-stimulating principle.
•**buspirone hydrochloride.** (byoo-SPY-rone) USP 34.
Tall Man: busPIRone.
Use: Anxiolytic.
buspirone hydrochloride. (Mylan) Buspirone hydrochloride 30 mg. Tab. Bot. 60s, 100s, 180s. Rx.
Use: Anxiolytic.
buspirone hydrochloride. (Par) Buspirone hydrochloride 7.5 mg. May contain lactose. Tab. 100s, 500s. Rx.
Use: Anxiolytic.
buspirone hydrochloride. (Various Mfr.) Buspirone hydrochloride 5 mg, 10 mg, 15 mg. May contain lactose. Tab. Bot. 100s, 500s. Rx.
Use: Anxiolytic.
•**busulfan.** (bue-SUL-fan) USP 34.
Use: Alkylating agent.
See: Busulfex.
Myleran.
Busulfex. (Ben Venue Labs) Busulfan 6 mg/mL. Inj. Single-use ampules 10 mL w/syringe filters. Rx.
Use: Alkylating agent.

•**butabarbital.** (byoo-tah-BAR-bih-tahl) USP 34.
Use: Hypnotic; sedative.
See: Butisol.
Da-Sed.
Expansatol.
W/Combinations
See: Dapco.
Monosyl.
Petn.
Phenazopyridine Plus.
Pyridium Plus.
Quibron Plus.
Sedapap.
•**butabarbital sodium.** (byoo-tah-BAR-bih-tahl) USP 34.
Use: Hypnotic; sedative.
See: Butalan.
Butisol Sodium.
Quiebar.
Renbu.
W/Belladonna Extract.
See: Butibel.
W/Combinations.
See: Bisalate.
Eulcin.
Indogesic.
Monosyl.
Phrenilin.
Quiebel.
butabarbital sodium. (Various Mfr.) Butabarbital sodium 15 mg, 30 mg. Tab. Bot. 100s (30 mg only), 1000s.
Use: Sedative; hypnotic.
butacaine.
Use: Anesthetic, local.
•**butacetin.** (byoot-ASS-ih-tin) USAN.
Use: Analgesic; antidepressant.
•**butaclamol hydrochloride.** (byoo-tah-KLAM-ole) USAN.
Use: Antipsychotic.
Butagen Caps. (Ivax) Phenylbutazone 100 mg. Cap. Bot. 100s, 500s. Rx.
Use: Antirheumatic; hypnotic; sedative.
Butalan. (Lannett) Sodium butabarbital 0.2 g/30 mL. Elix. Bot. Pt, gal.
Use: Hypnotic; sedative.
•**butalbital.** (BYOO-TAL-bih-tuhl) USP 34.
Formerly Allybarbituric acid.
Use: Hypnotic; sedative.
W/Acetaminophen
See: Bupap.
Butex Forte.
Cephadyn.
Dolgic.
Marten-Tab.
Phrenilin Forte.
Promacet.
Repan CF.
Sedapap.

Tencon.
W/Acetaminophen, Caffeine.
See: Alagesic LQ.
Americet.
Arbutal.
Arcet.
Dolgic LQ.
Dolgic Plus.
Esgic.
Esgic-Plus.
Fioricet.
Margesic.
Medigesic Plus.
Orbivan.
Repan.
Triad.
W/Acetaminophen, Caffeine, Codeine
Phosphate.
See: Phrenilin w/Caffeine and Codeine.
W/Aspirin, Caffeine.
See: Butalbital Compound.
Fiorinal.
Medigesic Plus.
W/Aspirin, Caffeine, Codeine Phosphate.
See: Ascomp with Codeine.
Butalbital, Aspirin, Caffeine with Co-
deine Phosphate.
Fiorinal with Codeine.
Floricet with Codeine.
W/Aspirin, Caffeine, Phenacetin.
See: Arbutal.
W/Hyoscyamine Hydrobromide, Phen-
azopyridine Hydrochloride.
See: PhenazoForte Plus.
**butalbital, acetaminophen, and caf-
feine.** (Various Mfr.) Acetaminophen
325 mg, 500 mg, caffeine 40 mg, butal-
bital 50 mg, Tab. Bot. 30s, 50s, 100s,
500s, 1000s, UD 100s. *Rx.*
Use: Analgesic.
**butalbital, acetaminophen, caffeine,
and codeine phosphate.** (Breckenridge) Codeine phosphate 30 mg, acetaminophen 325 mg, caffeine 40 mg, butalbital 50 mg. Cap. 100s, 500s. *c-III.*
Use: Narcotic analgesic.
butalbital and aspirin.
Use: Analgesic; sedative.
butalbital, aspirin, and caffeine.
(Various Mfr.) **Tab.:** Aspirin 325 mg,
caffeine 40 mg, butalbital 50 mg. Bot.
30s, 50s, 100s, 500s, 1000s, UD 100s.
Cap.: Aspirin 325 mg, caffeine 40 mg,
butalbital 50 mg. Bot. 100s, 1000s. *c-III.*
Use: Analgesic combination.
**butalbital, aspirin, caffeine with co-
deine phosphate.** (Watson) Aspirin
325 mg, butalbital 50 mg, caffeine
40 mg, codeine phosphate 30 mg. Cap.
100s, 500s. *c-III.*
Use: Opioid analgesic combination.

butalbital compound. (Various Mfr.) As-
pirin 325 mg, caffeine 40 mg, butalbital
50 mg. Tab., Cap. Bot. 100s, 1000s
(Tab. only). *c-III.*
Use: Analgesic.
butalgin.
See: Methadone hydrochloride.
•**butamben.** (BYOO-tam-ben) *USP 34.*
Formerly Butyl aminobenzoate.
Use: Anesthetic, local.
W/Benzocaine, Tetracaine Hydrochloride,
Bezalkonium Chloride.
See: Cetacaine.
•**butamirate citrate.** (byoo-tah-MY-rate
SIH-trate) USAN.
Use: Antitussive.
•**butane.** (BUE-tane) *NF 29.*
Use: Aerosol propellant.
•**butaperazine.** (BYOO-tah-PURR-ah-
zeen) USAN.
Use: Antipsychotic.
•**butaperazine maleate.** (BYOO-tah-
PURR-ah-zeen) USAN.
Use: Antipsychotic.
butaphyllamine. Ambuphylline. Theo-
phylline aminoisobutanol. Theophyl-
line with 2-amino-2-methyl-1-propanol.
Butapro. (Health for Life Brands) Buta-
barbital sodium 0.2 g/30 mL. Elix. Bot.
Pt, gal. *c-v.*
Use: Hypnotic; sedative.
•**butaprost.** (BYOO-tah-PRAHST) USAN.
Use: Bronchodilator.
Butazone. (Major) Phenylbutazone
100 mg. Cap. Tab. Bot. 100s (Cap.
only), 500s. *Rx.*
Use: Antirheumatic.
•**butedronate tetrasodium.** (BYOO-teh-
DROE-nate TET-rah-SO-dee-uhm)
USAN.
Use: Diagnostic aid, bone imaging.
butelline.
See: Butacaine Sulfate.
•**butenafine hydrochloride.** (byoo-TEN-
ah-feen) USAN.
Use: Topical anti-infective, antifungal.
See: Lotrimin Ultra.
Mentax.
butenafine hydrochloride. (Penederm)
Use: Treatment of interdigital tinea pe-
dis, athlete's foot.
•**buterizine.** (byoo-TER-ih-ZEEN) USAN.
Use: Vasodilator, peripheral.
butethanol.
See: Tetracaine.
Butex Forte. (Athlon) Acetaminophen
650 mg, butalbital 50 mg, benzyl al-
cohol, EDTA, parabens. Cap. Bot. 100s.
Rx.
Use: Analgesic.

•**buthiazide.** (byoo-THIGH-azz-IDE) USAN.
Use: Antihypertensive; diuretic.
Butibel. (Wallace) Butabarbital sodium 15 mg, belladonna extract 15 mg. **Tab.:** Bot. 100s. **Elix.:** Per 5 mL. Alcohol 7%, sucrose, saccharin. Orange flavor. Bot. Pt. *Rx.*
Use: GI anticholinergic combination.

•**butikacin.** (BYOO-tih-KAY-sin) USAN.
Use: Anti-infective.

•**butilfenin.** (BYOO-till-FEN-in) USAN.
Use: Diagnostic aid, hepatic function determination.

•**butirosin sulfate.** (byoo-TIHR-oh-sin) USAN. A mixture of the sulfates of the A and B forms of an antibiotic produced by *Bacillus circularis.*
Use: Anti-infective.

Butisol Sodium. (Medpointe) Butabarbital sodium. **Elix.:** 30 mg/5 mL. Bot. Pt, gal. **Tab.:** 30 mg, 50 mg. Bot. 100s, 1000s (30 mg only). *c-III.*
Use: Hypnotic; sedative.

•**butixirate.** (BYOO-TIX-ih-rate) USAN.
Use: Analgesic; antirheumatic.

•**butoconazole nitrate.** (BYOO-toe-KOE-nuh-zole) USP 34.
Use: Antifungal.
See: Gynazole-1.
    Mycelex-3.

butolan. Benzylphenyl carbamate.

•**butonate.** (BYOO-tahn-ate) USAN.
Use: Anthelmintic.

•**butopamine.** (BYOO-TOE-pah-meen) USAN.
Use: Cardiovascular agent.

•**butoprozine hydrochloride.** (byoo-TOE-pro-ZEEN) USAN.
Use: Cardiovascular agent, antiarrhythmic; antianginal.

butopyronoxyl. (Indalone) Butylmesityl oxide.
Use: Insect repellant.

•**butorphanol.** (BYOO-TAR-fan-ahl) USAN.
Use: Analgesic; antitussive.

•**butorphanol tartrate.** (BYOO-TAR-fan-ahl) USP 34.
Use: Analgesic; antitussive.
See: Stadol.

butorphanol tartrate. (Various Mfr.) Butorphanol tartrate. **Inj.:** 1 mg/mL, 2 mg/mL. Vials 1 mL (1 mg/mL only), 2 mL. **Nasal Spray:** 10 mg/mL. Vials 2.5 mL. *c-IV.*
Use: Analgesic; antitussive.

•**butoxamine hydrochloride.** (byoo-TOX-ah-meen) USAN.
Use: Antidiabetic; antihyperlipoproteinemic.

Butrans. (Purdue) Buprenorphine 5 mcg/h, 10 mcg/h, 20 mcg/h. Patch. Carton of 4 individually packaged systems and a pouch containing 4 patch-disposal units. *c-III.*
Use: Opioid agonist-antagonist analgesic.

•**butriptyline hydrochloride.** (BYOO-TRIP-till-een) USAN.
Use: Antidepressant.

•**butyl alcohol.** (BUE-til AL-ka-hol) NF 29. Butyl alcohol is n-butyl alcohol.
Use: Pharmaceutic aid, solvent.

butyl aminobenzoate. n-butyl p-aminobenzoate. Scuroforme.
Use: Anesthetic, local.
W/Benzocaine, Tetracaine Hydrochloride.
See: Cetacaine.
W/Benzyl Alcohol, Phenylmercuric Borate, Benzocaine.
See: Dermathyn.
W/Procaine, Benzyl Alcohol, in Sweet Almond Oil.
See: Anucaine.

•**butylated hydroxyanisole.** (BUE-ti-LAY-ted hye-drox-ee-AN-i-sole) NF 29.
Use: Pharmaceutic aid, antioxidant.

•**butylated hydroxytoluene.** (BUE-ti-LAY-ted hye-drox-ee-TOL-yoo-een) NF 29.
Use: Pharmaceutic aid, antioxidant.

•**butylparaben.** (byo-till-PAR-ah-ben) NF 29.
Use: Pharmaceutic aid, antifungal.

butylphenylsalicylamide.
See: Butylphenamide.

butyrophenone. Class of antipsychotic agents. *Rx.*
See: Haloperidol.

butyrylcholinesterase. (Pharmavene)
Use: Treat cocaine overdose; postsurgical apnea. [Orphan Drug]

B-Vex PD. (Midlothian Laboratories) Brompheniramine tannate 6 mg, pseudoephedrine tannate 30 mg per 5 mL. Aspartame, methylparaben, phenylalanine 5 mg per 5 mL, prosweet, saccharin, sorbitol. Cotton candy flavor. Susp. 473 mL. *Rx.*
Use: Upper respiratory combination, decongestant and antihistamine.

B vitamins with vitamin C, oral.
See: Dialyvite Multi-Vitamins for Dialysis Patients.
    Dialyvite with Zinc.

B vitamins with vitamin C, parenteral.
See: Neurodep.
   Vicam.
B-Vite Injection. (Bluco) Vitamins B_1
   50 mg, B_2 5 mg, B_6 5 mg, niacinamide
   125 mg, B_{12} 1000 mcg, dexpanthenol
   6 mg, C 50 mg/10 mL. Mono vial w/ben-
   zyl alcohol 1% in water for injection.
   Rx.
   Use: Vitamin supplement.
Byetta. (Amylin Pharmaceuticals, Inc.)
   Exenatide 250 mg/mL. Inj. Soln. Prefilled pens. 1.2 mL (60 doses) (provides
   5 mcg/dose), 2.4 mL (60 doses) (provides 10 mcg/dose). *Rx.*
   Use: Antidiabetic agent; incretin mimetic agent.
Bystolic. (Forest Laboratories) Nebivolol
   (as nebivolol hydrochloride) 2.5 mg,
   5 mg, 10 mg, 20 mg. Lactose. Tab. 30s,
   100s, UD 100s (except 2.5 mg). *Rx.*
   Use: Antiadrenergic/sympatholytic,
   beta-adrenergic blocking agent.

C

- **cabazitaxel.** (ka-BAZ-i-TAX-el) USAN.
  Use: Taxoid.
  See: Jevtana.
- **cabergoline.** (cab-ERR-go-leen) USAN.
  Use: Antidyskinetic; antihyperprolactin-
  emic; antiparkinsonian; dopamine
  agonist; hyperprolactinemic disorders
  treatment.
  cabergoline. (Various Mfr.) Cabergoline
  5 mg. May contain lactose. Tab. 8s. *Rx.*
  Use: Agent for gout.
- **cabozantinib.** (KA-boe-ZAN-ti-nib)
  USAN.
  Use: Antineoplastic.
- **cabufocon A.** (cab-YOU-FOE-kahn A)
  USAN.
  Use: Contact lens material, hydrophobic.
- **cabufocon B.** (cab-YOU-FOE-kahn B)
  USAN.
  Use: Contact lens material.
  Cachexon. (Telluride) L-Glutathione.
  Use: AIDS-associated cachexia.
  [Orphan Drug]
  cacodylic acid. Dimethylarsinic acid.
- **cactinomycin.** (KACK-tih-no-MY-sin)
  USAN. Antibiotic produced by *Strepto-
  myces chrysomallus. Formerly Actino-
  mycin C.*
  Use: Antineoplastic.
  cade oil.
  See: Juniper Tar.
- **cadexomer iodine.** (kad-EX-oh-mer)
  USAN.
  Use: Antiseptic; antiulcerative.
  Caduet. (Pfizer) Amlodipine besylate/
  atorvastatin calcium (as base) 2.5 mg/
  10 mg, 2.5 mg/20 mg, 2.5 mg/40 mg,
  5 mg/10 mg, 5 mg/20 mg, 5 mg/40 mg,
  5 mg/80 mg, 10 mg/10 mg, 10 mg/
  20 mg, 10 mg/40 mg, 10 mg/80 mg.
  Calcium carbonate. Film-coated. Tab.
  30s. *Rx.*
  Use: Antihyperlipidemic.
  Cafatine-PB. (Major) Ergotamine tartrate
  2 mg, caffeine 100 mg, belladonna alkaloids 0.25 mg, pentobarbital 60 mg.
  Supp. Box foil 10s. *Rx.*
  Use: Antimigraine.
  Cafcit. (Bedford) Caffeine citrate. **Oral
  Soln.:** 20 mg/mL. **Inj.:** 20 mg/mL (caffeine citrate 2 mg equivalent to caffeine
  base 1 mg). Preservative free. Vial
  3 mL. *Rx.*
  Use: CNS stimulant.
  Cafenol. (Sanofi-Synthelabo) Aspirin,
  caffeine. *OTC.*
  Use: Analgesic combination.

Cafergot P-B Suppositories. (Novartis)
Ergotamine tartrate 2 mg, caffeine
100 mg, bellafoline 0.25 mg, pentobarbital 60 mg. Supp. Box 12s. *Rx.*
Use: Antimigraine.
Cafergot P-B Tablets. (Novartis) Ergotamine tartrate 1 mg, caffeine 100 mg,
bellafoline 0.125 mg, pentobarbital so-
dium 30 mg. Tab. *SigPak* dispensing
pkg. of 90s, 250s. *c-iv.*
Use: Antimigraine.
Cafergot Tablets. (Novartis) Ergotamine
tartrate 1 mg, caffeine 100 mg. Sugar
coated. Parabens, sugar. Tab. 100s.
SigPak dispensing pkg. of 90s. *Rx.*
Use: Antimigraine.
Caffedrine. (Various Mfr.) Caffeine
200 mg. Tab. Pkg. 16s. *OTC.*
Use: CNS stimulant.
- **caffeine.** (ka-FEEN) *USP 34.*
  Use: CNS stimulant; apnea of prematu-
  rity.
  See: Cafcit.
  Caffedrine.
  Enerjets.
  Fastlene.
  .44 Magnum.
  Keep Alert.
  Keep Going.
  Lucidex.
  Maximum Strength NoDoz.
  Overtime.
  Stay Alert.
  Stay Awake.
  357 HR Magnum.
  20-20.
  Valentine.
  Vivarin.
  W/Acetaminophen.
  See: APAP-Plus.
  Excedrin Tension Headache.
  W/Acetaminophen, Aluminum Hydroxide,
  Aspirin, Magnesium Hydroxide.
  See: Vanquish.
  W/Acetaminophen, Aspirin.
  See: Anacin Advanced Headache.
  Excedrin Extra Strength.
  Excedrin Migraine.
  Goody's Extra Strength.
  Goody's Extra Strength Fast Pain Re-
  lief.
  Painaid ESF Extra-Strength Formula.
  W/Acetaminophen, Aspirin, Salicylamide.
  See: Medi-First Extra Strength Pain Re-
  lief.
  Painaid.
  Saleto.
  W/Acetaminophen, Butalbital.
  See: Alagesic LQ.
  Americet.
  Butalbital, Acetaminophen, and Caf-
  feine.

Dolgic Plus.
Esgic.
Esgic-Plus.
Margesic.
Orbivan.
Triad.
W/Acetaminophen, Butalbital, Codeine
Phosphate.
See: Butalbital, Acetaminophen, Caffeine, and Codeine Phosphate.
Phrenilin w/Caffeine and Codeine.
W/Acetaminophen, Dihydrocodeine Bitartrate.
See: Panlor DC.
Trezix.
W/Acetaminophen, Isometheptene Mucate.
See: Prodrin.
W/Acetaminophen, Magnesium Salicylate, Phenyltoloxamine Citrate.
See: Durabac Forte.
W/Acetaminophen, Phenyltoloxamine, Salicylamide.
See: Durabac.
Levacet.
W/Acetaminophen, Pyrilamine Maleate.
See: Midol Menstrual Complete.
W/Aspirin.
See: Alka-Seltzer Wake-Up Call.
Anacin.
Anacin Maximum Strength.
Bayer Quick Release Crystals.
BC Fast Pain Relief.
BC Fast Pain Relief Arthritis.
Summit Extra Strength.
W/Aspirin, Butalbital.
See: Butalbital, Aspirin, and Caffeine.
Butalbital Compound.
Fiorinal.
W/Aspirin, Butalbital, Codeine Phosphate.
See: Butalbital, Aspirin, Caffeine w/Codeine Phosphate.
W/Aspirin, Orphenadrine Citrate.
See: Orphenadrine Compound.
Orphenadrine Compound-DS.
W/Aspirin, Salicylamide.
See: BC Powder Arthritis Strength.
Stanback Headache Powders.
W/Butalbital, Codeine Phosphate.
See: Fiorinal with Codeine.
W/Isometheptene Mucate, Acetaminophen.
See: MigraTen.
caffeine and sodium benzoate. (Bedford, American Regent) Caffeine and sodium benzoate 250 mg/mL (caffeine 121 mg, sodium benzoate 129 mg). Inj. Single-use vial. 2 mL. Rx.
Use: CNS stimulant.

•**caffeine citrate.** (ka-FEEN) USP 34.
Use: CNS stimulant.
W/Phenylephrine Hydrochloride, Pheniramine Maleate, Sodium Salicylate.
See: Scot-Tussin Original Multi-Action Cold and Allergy Formula.
W/Sodium Citrate, Phenylephrine Hydrochloride, Pheniramine Maleate, Sodium Salicylate, Codeine Phosphate.
See: Tussirex.
Tussirex Sugar Free.
caffeine citrate. (Paddock) Caffeine citrate. Inj.: 20 mg/mL. Preservative free. Vials. 3 mL. Oral Soln.: 20 mg/mL. Preservative free. Vials. 3 mL. Rx.
Use: Analeptic, central nervous system stimulant.
caffeine citrated.
Use: CNS stimulant.
caffeine sodio-benzoate.
See: Caffeine Sodium Benzoate.
caffeine sodium salicylate. (Various Mfr.) Caffeine sodium salicylate. Bot. 1 oz; Pkg. 0.25 lb, 1 lb. OTC.
Use: CNS stimulant.
Cagol. (Harvey) Guaiacol 0.1 g, eucalyptol 0.08 g, iodoform 0.2 g, camphor 0.05 g/2 mL in olive oil. Vial 30 mL. Rx.
Use: Expectorant.
Caladryl. (Pfizer) Calamine 8%, pramoxine hydrochloride 1%, alcohol, camphor, diazolidinyl urea, parabens. Lot. Bot. 177 mL. OTC.
Use: Antipruritic, topical; poison ivy treatment.
Caladryl Clear. (Pfizer) Pramoxine hydrochloride 1%, zinc acetate 0.1%, alcohol, camphor, diazolidinyl urea, parabens. Lot. Bot. 177 mL. OTC.
Use: Antipruritic, topical; poison ivy treatment.
Calafol. (Alaven) Vitamin B_6 25 mg, vitamin B_{12} 425 mg, FA 1.6 mg, Ca 400 mg, D_3 400 units. Tab. 90s. Rx.
Use: Nutritional product.
Calaformula. (Eric, Kirk & Gary) Ferrous gluconate 130 mg, calcium lactate 130 mg, vitamins A 1000 units, D 400 units, B_1 2 mg, B_2 2 mg, niacinamide 5 mg, ascorbic acid 20 mg, folic acid 0.13 mg, Mg 0.25 mg, Cu 0.25 mg, Zn 0.25 mg, Mn 0.25 mg, K 0.075 mg. Cap. Bot. 50s, 100s, 500s, 1000s, 5000s. OTC.
Use: Mineral, vitamin supplement.
Calaformula F. (Eric, Kirk & Gary) Calaformula plus fluorine 0.333 mg. Tab. Bot. 100s. Rx.
Use: Mineral, vitamin supplement; dental caries agent.
Calagel Maximum Strength. (Tec Labs) Benzethonium chloride 0.15%, diphen-

hydramine hydrochloride 2%, zinc acetate 0.215%. Disodium edetate, menthol. Gel. 177.44 mL. *OTC.*
Use: Antihistamine preparation, topical.
Calahist. (Walgreen) Diphenhydramine hydrochloride 1%, calamine 8.1%, camphor 0.1%. Lot. Bot. 6 oz. *OTC.*
Use: Antipruritic, topical.
•**calamine.** (kal-a-MINE) *USP 34.*
Use: Protectant, topical.
W/Diphenhydramine Hydrochloride.
See: Ivarest Maximum Strength.
W/Pramoxine Hydrochloride.
See: Aveeno Anti-Itch.
Caladryl.
calamine. (Various Mfr.) Calamine 6.97%, zinc oxide 6.97%, glycerin. Lot. Bot. 118 mL, 240 mL, 480 mL. *OTC.*
Use: Antiseptic; astringent; poison ivy treatment.
calamine, phenolated. (Humco) Calamine, zinc oxide, glycerin, liquefied phenol 1%. Lot. Bot. 177 mL. *OTC.*
Use: Antiseptic; astringent; poison ivy treatment.
Calamycin. (Pfeiffer) Pyrilamine maleate, zinc oxide 10%, calamine 10%, benzocaine, chloroxylenol, zirconium oxide, isopropyl alcohol 10%. Lot. Bot. 120 mL. *OTC.*
Use: Antipruritic, topical.
Calan SR. (Pfizer) Verapamil hydrochloride 120 mg, 180 mg, 240 mg. Film-coated. ER Tab. Bot. 100s, 500s (240 mg only), UD 100s. *Rx.*
Use: Calcium channel blocker.
Cal-Bid. (Roberts) Elemental calcium 250 mg, ascorbic acid 100 mg, vitamin D 125 units. Tab. Bot. 100s. *OTC.*
Use: Mineral, vitamin supplement.
Cal-Carb Forte. (Vitaline) Calcium carbonate. **Cap.:** 1250 mg (elemental calcium 500 mg). Bot. 100s. **Chew Tab.:** 1250 mg (elemental calcium 500 mg). Mint flavor. Bot. 100s. *OTC.*
Use: Mineral supplement.
Calcarb 600 with Vitamin D. (Ivax) Calcium carbonate 1.5 g (elemental calcium 600 mg), vitamin D 125 units. Tab. Bot. 60s. *OTC.*
Use: Vitamin, mineral supplement.
Cal-C-Caps. (Key) Elemental calcium (as calcium citrate) 180 mg. Cap. 100s. *OTC.*
Use: Mineral supplement.
Cal-Cee. (Key) Calcium citrate 1150 mg (elemental calcium 250 mg). Tab. 100s. *OTC.*
Use: Mineral supplement.
Calcet. (Mission) Calcium 150 mg, vitamin D_3 100 units. Tab. Bot. 100s. *OTC.*
Use: Mineral, vitamin supplement.

Calcet Plus. (Mission Pharmacal) Elemental calcium 152.8 mg, elemental iron 18 mg, vitamins A 5000 units, D 400 units, E 30 mg, B_1 2.25 mg, B_2 2.55 mg, B_3 30 mg, B_5 15 mg, B_6 3 mg, B_{12} 9 mcg, C 500 mg, folic acid 0.8 mg, zinc 15 mg, sugar. Tab. Bot 60s. *OTC.*
Use: Mineral, vitamin supplement.
Calcibind. (Mission) Inorganic phosphate content 31% to 36%, sodium content $\approx$ 11%. Pow. 300 g bulk pack. *Rx.*
Use: Antiurolithic.
CalciCaps. (Nion Corp.) Calcium (dibasic calcium phosphate, calcium gluconate, calcium carbonate) 125 mg, vitamin D 67 units, phosphorus 60 mg. Tab. Bot. 100s, 500s. *OTC.*
Use: Mineral, vitamin supplement.
CalciCaps M-Z. (Nion Corp.) Ca 400 mg, Mg 133 mg, Zn 5 mg, vitamin A 1667 mg, D 133 units, Se. Tab. Bot. 90s. *OTC.*
Use: Mineral, vitamin supplement.
CalciCaps, Super. (Nion Corp.) Calcium 400 mg, phosphorus 41.7 mg, vitamin D 100 units. Tab. Bot. 90s. *OTC.*
Use: Mineral, vitamin supplement.
CalciCaps with Iron. (Nion Corp.) Calcium 125 mg, phosphorus 60 mg, vitamin D 67 units, ferrous gluconate 7 mg, tartrazine. Tab. Bot. 100s, 500s. *OTC.*
Use: Mineral, vitamin supplement.
Calci-Chew. (Watson) Calcium carbonate 1250 mg (elemental calcium 500 mg). Sugar. Cherry and assorted flavors. Chew. Tab. Bot. 100s. *OTC.*
Use: Mineral supplement.
Calcidrine. (Abbott) Codeine 8.4 mg, calcium iodide anhydrous 152 mg, alcohol 6%/5 mL. Syr. Bot. 120 mL, 480 mL. *c-v.*
Use: Antitussive; expectorant.
Calciferol. (Schwarz Pharma) Ergocalciferol (vitamin D_2) 8000 units/mL in propylene glycol. Liq. 60 mL. *OTC.*
Use: Refractory rickets; familial hypophosphatemia; hypoparathyroidism.
Calcijex. (Abbott) Calcitriol 1 mcg/mL, polysorbate 20 4 mg, sodium chloride 1.5 mg, sodium ascorbate 10 mg, dibasic sodium phosphate 7.6 mg, anhydrous, EDTA. Inj. Amp. 1 mL. *Rx.*
Use: Antihypocalcemic; antihypoparathyroid; vitamin.
Calci-Mix. (Watson) Calcium carbonate 1250 mg (elemental calcium 500 mg). Cap. Bot. 100s. *OTC.*
Use: Mineral supplement.
Calcionate. (Various Mfr.) Calcium glubionate 1.8 g/5 mL. Syr. Bot. 473 mL. *OTC.*
Use: Mineral supplement.

•**calcipotriene.** (kal-sih-POE-try-een) USAN.
Use: Antipsoriatic.
See: Dovonex.
  Sorilux.
W/Betamethasone Dipropionate.
See: Taclonex.
  Taclonex Scalp.
calcipotriene. (Taro Pharmaceuticals) Calcipotriene 0.005%. Alpha tocopherol, edetate disodium, mineral oil, petrolatum, propylene glycol. Oint. 60 g. *Rx.*
Use: Antipsoriatic agent.
calcipotriene. (Various Mfr.) Calcipotriene 0.005%. Soln. 60 mL. *Rx.*
Use: Antipsoriatic.
Calciquid. (Breckenridge) Calcium glubionate 1.8 g/5 mL. Syr. Bot. 473 mL. *OTC.*
Use: Mineral supplement.
•**calcitonin.** (kal-sih-TOE-nin) USAN.
Use: Treatment of Paget disease, calcium regulator.
See: Calcimar.
  Cibacalcin.
  Miacalcin.
  Osteocalcin.
calcitonin-human for injection.
Hormone from thyroid gland.
Use: Plasma hypocalcemic hormone; symptomatic Paget disease of bone. [Orphan Drug]
See: Cibacalcin.
calcitonin-salmon.
Use: Antihypercalcemic.
See: Fortical.
  Miacalcin.
calcitonin-salmon. (Various Mfr.) Calcitonin-salmon 200 units per 0.09 mL spray. Soln., Intranasal. Glass bottle. 3.7 mL. *Rx.*
Use: Endocrine and metabolic agent.
Cal-Citrate. (Bio-Tech) Elemental calcium. **Tab.:** 250 mg. Bot. 250s. **Cap.:** 225 mg. 100s, 250s. *OTC.*
Use: Mineral supplement.
•**calcitriol.** (KAL-sih-TRY-ole) USAN.
Use: Antihypocalcemic, calcium regulator; vitamin.
See: Calcijex.
  Rocaltrol.
  Vectical.
calcitriol. (Roxane) Calcitriol 1 mcg/mL. Oral Soln. 15 mL with single-use graduated oral dispensers. *Rx.*
Use: Antihypocalcemic, calcium regulator; vitamin.
calcitriol. (Teva) Calcitriol 0.25 mcg, 0.5 mcg. Mannitol, sorbitol. Cap. 100s. *Rx.*
Use: Vitamin.

calcitriol injection. (aaiPharma) Calcitriol 1 mcg/mL, 2 mcg/mL, sodium chloride, EDTA. Inj. 1 mL vial. *Rx.*
Use: Antihypocalcemic, calcium regulator; vitamin.
calcium.
Use: Mineral.
See: Calcium Acetate.
  Calcium Ascorbate.
  Calcium Carbonate.
  Calcium Citrate.
  Calcium Gluconate.
  Calcium Lactate.
  Tricalcium Phosphate.
•**calcium acetate.** (KAL-see-um) *USP 34.*
Use: Pharmaceutic aid, buffering agent; hyperphosphatemia; mineral.
See: Calphron.
  Eliphos.
  PhosLo.
calcium acetylsalicylate. Kalmopyrin, kalsetal, soluble aspirin, tylcalsin.
Use: Analgesic.
calcium aluminum carbonate.
W/Dl-Amino Acetate Complex.
See: Ancid.
•**calcium aminosalicylate.** (KAL-see-um) *NF 29.* Aminosalicylate calcium.
calcium amphomycin.
See: Amphomycin.
calcium and magnesium carbonates.
Use: Mineral; antacid.
•**calcium and vitamin D with minerals.** (KAL-see-um) *USP 34.*
Use: Mineral, vitamin supplement.
Calcium Antacid Extra Strength.
(Various Mfr.) Calcium carbonate 750 mg (elemental calcium 300 mg). Chew. Tab. Bot. 96s. *OTC.*
Use: Mineral supplement; antacid.
•**calcium ascorbate.** (KAL-see-uhm a-skor-bate) *USP 34.*
Use: Water-soluble vitamin.
See: Ascocid.
calcium ascorbate. (Freeda) **Tab.:** Calcium ascorbate 500 mg. Calcium 75 mg. Sugar free. Buffered. Bot. 100s, 250s, 500s. **Pow.:** Calcium ascorbate 814 mg per ¼ tsp. Calcium 100 mg per ¼ tsp. Sugar free. Buffered. Bot. 120 g, 1 lb. *OTC.*
Use: Water-soluble vitamin.
calcium benzoyl-p-aminosalicylate.
See: Benzoylpas Calcium.
calcium benzoylpas.
See: Benzoylpas Calcium.
calcium bis-dioctyl sulfosuccinate.
See: Dioctyl Calcium Sulfosuccinate.
calcium carbimide. Calcium cyanamide. Sulfosuccinate.

•**calcium carbonate.** (KAL-see-um KAR-bo-nate) *USP 34. Formerly calcium carbonate, precipitated.*
Use: Antacid; mineral; hyperphosphatemia.
See: Alka-Mints.
  Antacid Tablets.
  Cal-Carb Forte.
  Calci-Chew.
  Calci-Mix.
  Calcium Antacid Extra Strength.
  Calcium 600.
  Cal•Gest.
  Caltrate 600.
  Chooz.
  Dicarbosil.
  Equilet.
  Maalox Children's.
  Maalox Regular Strength.
  Mylanta Children's.
  Nephro-Calci.
  Os-Cal 500.
  Oysco 500.
  Oyst-Cal 500.
  Oyster Shell Calcium.
  Pepto Children's.
  Rolaids Extra Strength Softchews.
  Surpass.
  Surpass Extra Strength.
  Titralac.
  Trial Antacid.
  Tums Calcium for Life Bone Health.
  Tums Calcium for Life PMS.
  Tums E-X.
  Tums Kids.
  Tums Quik Pak.
  Tums Smooth Dissolve.
  Tums Ultra.
W/Aspirin, Magnesium Hydroxide, Aluminum Hydroxide.
See: Ascriptin Maximum Strength.
W/Aspirin, Magnesium Oxide, Magnesium Carbonate.
See: Bufferin.
  Bufferin Extra Strength.
  Extra Strength Bayer Plus.
W/Combinations.
See: Acid-X.
  Actonel with Calcium.
  Calcarb 600 with Vitamin D.
  Ca-Plus-Protein.
  Gas Ban.
  Gas-X with Maalox Extra Strength.
  MagneBind 400 Rx.
  MagneBind 300.
  MagneBind 200.
  Mylanta Gelcaps.
  Mylanta Supreme.
  Mylanta Ultra Tabs.
  Natabec.
  Pepcid Complete.

  Rolaids.
  Rolaids Calcium Rich.
  Rolaids Extra Strength.
  Rolaids Multi-Symptom.
  Titralac Plus.
  Tums Plus.
W/Famotidine, Magnesium Hydroxide.
See: Dual Action Complete.
  Tums Dual Action.
W/Sodium Fluoride.
See: Florical.
W/Simethicone.
See: Maalox Advanced Maximum Strength.
  Maalox Junior.
  Rolaids Extra Strength Plus Gas Relief.
calcium carbonate. (Various Mfr.) Calcium carbonate. **Tab.:** 500 mg (elemental calcium 200 mg). 100, 120s, UD 100s. 600 mg (elemental calcium 240 mg). 60s, 72s, 150s, UD 100s. 648 to 650 mg (elemental calcium 260 mg). 100s, 250s, 500s, 1,000s. 1,250 mg (elemental calcium 500 mg). 100s. 1,500 mg (elemental calcium 600 mg). 60s, 150s. **Chew. Tab.:** 1,250 mg (elemental calcium 500 mg). 60s. **Oral Susp.:** 1,250 mg per 5 mL (elemental calcium 500 mg per 5 mL). 500 mL, UD 5 mL. **Pow.:** 454 g. *OTC.*
Use: Mineral supplement; antacid.
calcium carbonate. (Various Mfr.) Precipitated chalk; carbonic acid, calcium salt (1:1).
Use: Antacid; calcium supplement.
calcium carbonate, aromatic. (Eli Lilly) Calcium carbonate 10 g. Tab. Bot. 100s, 1000s. *OTC.*
Use: Antacid.
Calcium Carbonate 600 mg + Vitamin D. (Major) Ca 600 mg, D 125 units. Tab. Bot. 60s. *OTC.*
Use: Mineral, vitamin supplement.
calcium carbonate, sodium chloride, and potassium chloride.
Use: Salt replacement.
See: Sustain.
calcium caseinate.
Use: Mineral supplement.
calcium channel blockers.
Use: Angina pectoris; vasospastic and unstable angina.
See: Amlodipine.
  Clevidipine Butyrate.
  Diltiazem Hydrochloride.
  Felodipine.
  Isradipine.
  Nicardipine Hydrochloride.
  Nifedipine.
  Nimodipine.

Nisoldipine.
Verapamil Hydrochloride.
Calcium Chel 330. (Novartis)
Use: Antidote, heavy metals.
See: Calcium Trisodium Pentetate.
•**calcium chloride.** (KAL-see-um)
USP 34.
Use: Electrolyte, calcium replenisher.
W/Dibasic Sodium Phosphate, Monobasic
Sodium Phosphate, Sodium Chloride.
See: Cephosol.
W/Dibasic Sodium Phosphate, Monoba-
sic Sodium Phosphate, Silicon Diox-
ide, Sodium Chloride, Sodium Bicarbo-
nate.
See: NeutraSal.
calcium chloride. (Pharmacia) Calcium
chloride. 1 g. Inj. Amp. 10 mL, 25s. (To-
rigian) 1 g. Inj. Amp. 10 mL 12s, 25s,
100s. (Trent) 10%. Inj. Amp. 10 mL.
(Bayer Consumer Care) 13.6 mEq/
10 mL Inj. Vial.
Use: Antihypocalcemic.
•**calcium chloride Ca 45.** (KAL-see-um)
USAN.
Use: Radiopharmaceutical.
•**calcium chloride Ca 47.** (KAL-see-um)
USAN.
Use: Radiopharmaceutical.
•**calcium citrate.** (KAL-see-um) USP 34.
Use: Mineral supplement.
See: Cal-C-Caps.
Cal-Cee.
Cal-Citrate.
Citracal.
Citrus Calcium.
calcium citrate. (Various Mfr.) **Tab.:** Elemental calcium 250 mg. Bot. 100s,
120s, 250s, 500s, 1000s. Calcium citrate 950 mg. Bot. 100s. **Pow. for
Susp.:** Elemental calcium 760 mg/
5 mL. Pow. Bot. 454 g. *OTC.*
Use: Mineral supplement.
calcium cyclamate. Calcium cyclohexanesulfamate.
calcium cyclobarbital.
Use: Central depressant.
calcium cyclohexanesulfamate.
See: Calcium Cyclamate.
•**calcium dioctyl sulfosuccinate.** (KAL-
see-uhm die-OC-tuhl sul-foe-SUCK-
sih-nate) USP 34. Docusate calcium.
See: Surfak.
•**calcium disodium edathamil.** (KAL-see-
uhm die-SO-dee-uhm eh-DA-tha-mill)
USP 34.
•**calcium disodium edetate.** (KAL-see-
uhm die-SO-dee-uhm ed-deh-TATE)
USP 34. Edetate calcium disodium.
Use: Antidote for acute and chronic lead

poisoning, lead encephalopathy.
See: Calcium Disodium Versenate.
calcium disodium versenate. (Graceway) Calcium disodium edetate
200 mg/mL. Inj. Amp 5 mL. *Rx.*
Use: IV or IM for lead poisoning and
lead encephalopathy.
•**calcium dl-pantothenate.** (KAL-see-
uhm dl pan-toe-THEH-nate) USP 34.
Calcium Pantothenate, Racemic.
calcium edetate sodium.
See: Calcium Disodium Edetate.
calcium EDTA.
See: Calcium Disodium Edetate.
Calcium 500. (Rugby) Vitamin D 100 units
(as cholecalciferol), calcium 500 units (as
calcium carbonate). Malted milk powder,
nonfat dried milk, sugar. Vanilla flavor.
Chew. Tab. 60s. *OTC.*
Use: Nutritional combination product.
Calcium 500+D. (21st Century) Vitamin
D 800 units (as cholecalciferol), calcium 1,000 mg (as oyster shell). Preservative free. Tab. 200s. *OTC.*
Use: Nutritional combination product.
Calcium-Folic Acid Plus D. (Brookstone) Vitamin D_3 300 units, B_6 10 mg,
B_{12} 125 mcg, folate 100 mcg B, Ca,
Mg. fructose. Chocolate flavor. Wafers,
chewable. 60s. *Rx.*
Use: Multivitamin with minerals.
calcium 4-benzamidosalicylate. Cal-
cium aminacyl B-PAS. Benzoylpas calcium.
•**calcium glubionate.** (KAL-see-uhm
glue-BYE-oh-nate) USP 34.
Use: Calcium replenisher.
See: Calcionate.
Calciquid.
calcium glucoheptonate. (Various Mfr.)
Cal. D-glucoheptonate O. *OTC.*
Use: Nutritional supplement.
•**calcium gluconate.** (KAL-see-uhm glue-
KAHN-nate) USP 34.
Use: Mineral supplement.
See: Cal-G.
calcium gluconate. (Bio-Tech) Calcium
gluconate 500 mg. Cap. 100s. *OTC.*
Use: Mineral supplement.
calcium gluconate. (Freeda) Elemental
calcium 346.7 mg/15 mL. Pow. Bot.
448 g. *OTC.*
Use: Mineral supplement.
calcium gluconate. (Various Mfr.) Calcium gluconate ≈ 555.6 mg (elemental calcium 50 mg). Tab. 100s, 500s.
Calcium gluconate 500 mg (elemental
calcium 45 mg). Tab. 100s, 1,000s,
UD 100s. Calcium gluconate 648 to
650 mg (elemental calcium 58.5 to

60 mg). Tab. 100s, 1,000s. Calcium gluconate 972 to 975 mg (elemental calcium 87.75 to 90 mg). Tab. 1,000s, UD 100s. *OTC.*
Use: Mineral supplement.

calcium gluconate. (Various Mfr.) Calcium gluconate 650 mg. Chew. Tab. 30s, 60s, 90s, 100s, 120s. *OTC.*
Use: Mineral supplement.

calcium gluconate. (Various Mfr.) Calcium gluconate 10% (elemental calcium 0.465 mEq/mL [9.3 mg]). Inj. Soln. Preservative free. 10 mL and 50 mL single-dose vials and 100 mL and 200 mL pharmacy bulk vials. *Rx.*
Use: Mineral supplement.

calcium gluconate gel 2.5%. (LTR Pharmaceuticals, Inc.)
Use: Topical treatment of hydrogen fluoride burns. [Orphan Drug]
See: H-F.

calcium glycerophosphate. Neurosin. W/Phosphorus.
See: Prelief.

•**calcium hydroxide.** (KAL-see-uhm) *USP 34.*
Use: Astringent; pharmaceutic necessity for calamine lotion.

calcium hydroxide. (Eli Lilly) Calcium hydroxide. Pow. Bot. 4 oz.
Use: Lime water.

calcium hydroxylapatite.
Use: Physical adjunct.
See: Radiesse.

calcium hypophosphite.
Use: Mineral supplement.

calcium iodide.
W/Codeine Phosphate.
See: Calcidrine.

calcium iodized.
See: Cal-Lime-1.

calcium iodobehenate. Calioben.

•**calcium ipodate.** (KAL-see-uhm ip-OH-date) *USP 34.* Ipodate calcium.
See: Oragrafin Calcium.

calcium kinate gluconate. Kinate is hexahydrotetrahydroxybenzoate. Calcium quinate.

•**calcium lactate.** (KAL-see-um LAK-tate) *USP 34.*
Use: Mineral supplement.
See: Cal-Lac.
W/Calcium Glycerophosphate.
See: Calphosan.
W/Niacinamide, Folic Acid, Ferrous Gluconate, Vitamins.
See: Pergrava No. 2.

calcium lactate. (Various Mfr.) Calcium lactate 648 to 650 mg (elemental calcium 84.5 mg). Tab. Bot. 100s, 1000s.

Elemental calcium 100 mg. Tab. Bot. 100s, 250s. *OTC.*
Use: Mineral supplement.

•**calcium lactobionate.** (KAL-see-um) *USP 34.*
Use: Mineral supplement.

calcium lactophosphate. Lactic acid hydrogen phosphate calcium salt.

calcium leucovorin.
Use: For overdosage of folic acid antagonists; megaloblastic anemias.
See: Leucovorin Calcium.

•**calcium levulinate.** (KAL-see-uhm LEV-you-lih-nate) *USP 34.*
Use: Calcium replenisher.

calcium/magnesium. (Windmill) Ca 1,000 mg (calcium content expressed in mg elemental calcium), Mg 500 mg (magnesium content expressed in mg elemental magnesium). Preservative free and sugar free. Tab. 60s. *OTC.*
Use: Nutritional supplement, multimineral.

Calcium Magnesium Chelated. (NBTY) Ca 500 mg, Mg 250 mg. Tab. Bot. 50s, 100s. *OTC.*
Use: Mineral supplement.

Calcium Magnesium Zinc. (NBTY) Ca 333 mg, Mg 133 mg, Zn 8.3 mg. Tab. Bot. 100. *OTC.*
Use: Mineral supplement.

calcium microcrystalline hydroxyapatite. (Pure Encapsulations) Calcium microcrystalline hydroxyapatite 150 mg, 300 mg. Bovine, vitamin C. Cap. 90s, 180s. *OTC.*
Use: Mineral.

calcium novobiocin. Calcium salt of an antibacterial substance produced by *Streptomyces niveus.*
Use: Anti-infective.

•**calcium oxytetracycline.** (KAL-see-uhm ox-EE-tet-rah-SYE-kleen) *NF 29.* Oxytetracycline calcium.

•**calcium pantothenate.** (KAL-see-uhm pan-toe-THEH-nate) *USP 34.*
Use: Pantothenic acid (B_5) deficiency; coenzyme A precursor; vitamin, enzyme cofactor.
W/Combinations.
See: Arcum-VM.
Maintenance Vitamin Formula.
Mulvidren-F.
Probec-T.
Uplex.
Vicon-C.
Vicon Forte.
W/Zinc Sulfate, Niacinamide, Magnesium Sulfate, Manganese Sulfate, Vitamin Complex.
See: Vicon Plus.

calcium pantothenate. (Various Mfr.) Calcium pantothenate 100 mg (equiv. to 92 mg pantothenic acid), 218 mg (equiv. to 200 mg pantothenic acid), 545 mg (equiv. to 500 mg pantothenic acid). Tab. Bot. 100s, 250s. OTC.
Use: Pantothenic acid deficiency, water-soluble vitamin.

•calcium pantothenate, racemic. (KAL-see-uhm pan-toe-THEH-nate, ray-SEE-mik) USP 34.
Use: Vitamin B, enzyme cofactor.

•calcium phosphate, dibasic. (KAL-see-um) USP 34.
Use: Calcium replenisher; pharmaceutic aid, tablet base.

calcium phosphate, monocalcium.
See: Dicalcium Phosphate.

•calcium phosphate, tribasic. (KAL-see-um) NF 29. Tricalcium phosphate.
Use: Mineral supplement.
See: Posture.

•calcium polycarbophil. (KAL-see-uhm PAHL-ee-CAR-boe-fill) USP 34.
Use: Laxative.
See: Equalactin.
  Fibercon.
  FiberNorm.
  Konsyl Fiber.

calcium polysulfide.
Use: Wet dressing, soak.

calcium quinate.
See: Calcium Kinate Gluconate.

calcium receptor agonists.
See: Cinacalcet Hydrochloride.

•calcium saccharate. (KAL-see-uhm SACK-uh-rate) USP 34.
Use: Pharmaceutic aid, sweetener, stabilizer.

calcium saccharin. Saccharin calcium.
Use: Pharmaceutic aid, sweetener.

•calcium silicate. (KAL-see-uhm SILL-eh-cate) NF 29.
Use: Pharmaceutic aid, tablet excipient.

Calcium 600. (Various Mfr.) Calcium carbonate 1500 mg (elemental calcium 600 mg). Tab. Bot. 60s, 100s. OTC.
Use: Mineral supplement.

Calcium 600-D. (Rugby) Vitamin D 400 units (as cholecalciferol), calcium 600 mg (as calcium carbonate). Maltodextrin, propylene glycol, sodium 5 mg. Tab. 60s. OTC.
Use: Nutritional combination product.

Calcium 600 + D. (NBTY) Calcium 600 mg, vitamin D 125 units. Film-coated. Tab. Bot. 60s. OTC.
Use: Mineral, vitamin supplement.

Calcium 600/Vitamin D. (Schein) Ca 600 mg, D 125 units. Tab. Bot. 60s. OTC.
Use: Mineral, vitamin supplement.

•calcium stearate. (KAL-see-uhm STEE-uh-rate) NF 29.
Use: Pharmaceutic aid, tablet and capsule lubricant.

calcium succinate.
W/Aspirin.
See: Ber-Ex.
  Dolcin.

•calcium sulfate. (KAL-see-um) NF 29.
Use: Pharmaceutic aid, tablet and capsule diluent.

calcium thiosulfate.
Use: Wet dressing, soak.

calcium trisodium pentetate.
Use: Antidote, heavy metals.
See: Calcium Chel 330.

•calcium undecylenate. (KAL-see-uhm un-DES-eye-lie-nate) USP 34.
Use: Antifungal.
See: Caldesene.
  Cruex Squeeze Powder.

calcium with vitamin D. (Rexall Sundown) Vitamin D 400 units (as cholecalciferol), calcium 1,000 mg (as oyster shell). Sodium 10 mg. Gluten free, preservative free. Tab. 250s. OTC.
Use: Nutritional combination product.

Caldecort. (Novartis) Hydrocortisone 0.5%. Spray. Aerosol Can 1.5 oz. OTC.
Use: Corticosteroid, topical.

Caldesene. (Insight) Calcium undecylenate 10%. Pow. 60 g, 120 g. OTC.
Use: Antifungal agent.

Caldesene. (Insight) Cod liver oil (vitamins A and D), zinc oxide 15%, lanolin oil, petrolatum 54%, parabens, talc. Oint. 37.5 g. OTC.
Use: Emollient.

Caldesene. (Insight) Talc 81%, zinc oxide 15%. Pow., Top. 142 g. OTC.
Use: Diaper rash product, topical.

•caldiamide sodium. (KAL-DIE-ah-MIDE) USAN.
Use: Pharmaceutic aid.

Cal-D-Mint. (Enzyme Process) Ca 800 mg, Mg 150 mg, Fe 18 mg, iodine 0.1 mg, Cu 2 mg, vitamin D 200 units. Tab. Bot. 100s, 250s. OTC.
Use: Mineral, vitamin supplement.

Caldolor. (Cumberland Pharmaceuticals) Ibuprofen 100 mg/mL. Arginine 78 mg/mL. Inj., Soln. Single-dose vial. 4 mL, 8 mL. Rx.
Use: Nonsteroidal anti-inflammatory agent.

Cal-D-Phos. (Archer-Taylor) Dicalcium phosphate 4.5 g, calcium gluconate 3 g, vitamin D. Tab. Bot. 1000s. *OTC.*
Use: Mineral, vitamin supplement.

calfactant.
Use: Lung surfactant.
See: Infasurf.

Cal-G. (Key) Calcium gluconate 700 mg (as elemental calcium 50 mg). Cap. 100s, 250s. *OTC.*
Use: Mineral supplement.

Cal•Gest. (Rugby) Calcium carbonate 500 mg (elemental calcium 200 mg). Dextrose. Assorted flavors. Chew. Tab. 150s. *OTC.*
Use: Mineral supplement.

Calicylic. (Gordon Laboratories) Salicylic acid 10%, mineral oil, cetyl alcohol, propylene glycol, white wax, sodium lauryl sulfate, oleic acid, methyl- and propylparabens, triethanolamine. Cream. Tube. 60 g. *OTC.*
Use: Keratolytic.

Cal-Im. (Standex) Calcium glycerophosphate 1%, calcium levulinate 1.5%. Vial 30 mL. *Rx.*
Use: Mineral supplement.

Calinate-FA. (Solvay) Ca 250 mg, vitamins A 4000 units, D 400 units, B_1 3 mg, B_2 3 mg, B_6 5 mg, B_{12} 1 mcg, folic acid 1 mg, C 50 mg, B_3 (niacinamide) 20 mg, B_5 (d-panthenol) 1 mg, Fe 60 mg, I 0.02 mg, Mn 0.2 mg, Mg 0.2 mg, Zn 0.1 mg, Cu 0.15 mg. Tab. Bot. 100s. *Rx.*
Use: Mineral, vitamin supplement.

calioben.
See: Calcium Iodobehenate.

Calivite. (Apco) Calcium carbonate 885 mg, ferrous sulfate 199 mg, vitamins A 3600 units, D 400 units, C 75 mg, B_1 1.5 mg, B_2 1.95 mg, B_6 0.75 mg, nicotinic acid 15 mg, B_{12} activity 0.025 mcg, choline 1500 mcg, inositol 2500 mcg, pantothenic acid 75 mcg, folic acid 25 mcg, p-aminobenzoic acid 12 mcg, K 10 mg, Mg 1 mg, Zn 0.075 mg, Mn 0.02 mg, Cu 0.01 mg, cobalt 0.02 mcg. Tab. Bot. 100s. *OTC.*
Use: Mineral, vitamin supplement.

Cal-Lac. (Bio-Tech) Calcium lactate 500 mg (elemental calcium 96 mg). Cap. Bot. 100s. *OTC.*
Use: Mineral supplement.

Cal-Lime-1. (Scrip) Calcium iodized 1 g. Tab. Bot. 1000s.

Calmol 4. (Mentholatum Co.) Cocoa butter 80%, zinc oxide 10%, parabens. Supp. Box 12s, 24s. *OTC.*
Use: Anorectal preparation.

Calmoseptine. Menthol 0.44%, zinc oxide 20.625%. Glycerin, lanolin. Top. Oint. 71 g, 113 g. *OTC.*
Use: Protectant.

Calmosin. (Spanner) Calcium gluconate, strontium bromide. Amp. 10 mL. 100s.

Cal-Nor. (Vortech Pharmaceuticals) Calcium glycerophosphate 100 mg, calcium levulinate 150 mg/10 mL. Inj. Vial 100 mL. *Rx.*
Use: Mineral supplement.

Calocarb. (Pal-Pak, Inc.) Calcium carbonate 648 mg, cinnamon flavor. Tab. Bot. 1000s. *OTC.*
Use: Antacid.

calomel. Mercurous chloride.
Use: Cathartic.

CaloMist. (Fleming) Cyanocobalamin 25 mcg/0.1 mL. Benzyl alcohol, benzalkonium chloride. Spray, Intranasal. 18 mL (60 sprays). *Rx.*
Use: Water-soluble vitamin.

Calotabs. (Calotabs) Docusate sodium 100 mg, casanthranol 30 mg. Tab. Box 10s. *OTC.*
Use: Laxative.

caloxidine (iodized calcium).
See: Calcium Iodized.

Calphosan. (Glenwood) Calcium glycerophosphate 50 mg, calcium lactate 50 mg/10 mL sodium chloride solution. Contains calcium 0.08 mEq/mL. Inj. Amp. 10 mL, Vial 60 mL. *Rx.*
Use: Mineral supplement.

Calphron. (Nephro-Tech) Calcium acetate 667 mg (elemental calcium 169 mg). Tab. 200s. *Rx.*
Use: Mineral supplement.

Calsan. (Burgin-Arden) Calcium glycerophosphate 10 mg, calcium levulinate 15 mg, chlorobutanol 0.5% mL. Inj. Vial 100 mL. *Rx.*
Use: Calcium supplement.

Cal Sup Instant 1000. (3M) Elemental calcium 1000 mg, vitamins D 400 units, C 60 mg. Pow. Packet 12s. *OTC.*
Use: Mineral, vitamin supplement.

Cal Sup 600 Plus. (3M) Elemental calcium 600 mg, vitamins D 200 units, C 30 mg. Tab. Bot. 60s. *OTC.*
Use: Mineral, vitamin supplement.

•calteridol calcium. (KAL-TER-ih-dahl KAL-see-uhm) USAN.
Use: Pharmaceutic aid.

Caltrate Plus. (Wyeth) Vitamin D 200 units, Ca 600 mg, Zn 7.5 mg, Mg, Cu, Mn, B. Sugar free. Tab. Bot. 60s. *OTC.*
Use: Mineral, vitamin supplement.

Caltrate 600. (Wyeth) Calcium carbonate 1500 mg (elemental calcium

600 mg). Preservative free. Tab. Bot. 60s. *OTC.*
Use: Mineral supplement.

Caltrate 600 + D. (Wyeth) Vitamin D 200 units, Ca 600 mg. Sugar free. Tab. Bot. 60s. *OTC.*
Use: Mineral, vitamin supplement.

Caltrate 600 + Iron. (Wyeth) Calcium carbonate 600 mg, iron 18 mg, vitamin D 125 units. Tab. Bot. 60s. *OTC.*
Use: Mineral, vitamin supplement.

Caltro. (Geneva) Elemental calcium 250 mg, vitamin D 125 units. Tab. Bot. 100s, 1000s. *OTC.*
Use: Mineral, vitamin supplement.

•**calusterone.** (kal-YOO-ster-ohn) USAN.
Use: Antineoplastic.

Cam-Ap-Es. (Camall) Hydrochlorothiazide 15 mg, reserpine 0.1 mg, hydralazine hydrochloride 25 mg. Tab. Bot. 100s. *Rx.*
Use: Antihypertensive.

•**cambendazole.** (kam-BEND-ah-zole) USAN.
Use: Anthelmintic.

Cambia. (Mipharm) Diclofenac 50 mg. Aspartame, mannitol, saccharin. Pow. for Soln. Boxes of 9 individual packets. *Rx.*
Use: CNS agent, nonsteroidal anti-inflammatory agent.

Camellia. (O'Leary) Moisturizer for face, hands and body. For normal to oily skin. Lot. Bot. 4 oz. *OTC.*
Use: Emollient.

Cameo. (Medco Lab) Mineral oil, isopropyl myristate, lanolin oil, PEG-8-Dioleate. Oil. Plastic Bot. 8 oz, 16 oz, 32 oz. *OTC.*
Use: Emollient.

•**camiglibose.** (kah-mih-GLIE-bose) USAN.
Use: Antidiabetic, glucohydrolase inhibitor.

Camila. (Barr) Norethindrone 0.35 mg. Lactose. Tab. 28s. *Rx.*
Use: Sex hormone, contraceptive hormone.

•**camobucol.** (kam-oh-BUE-kol) USAN.
Use: Anti-inflammatory.

Camouflage Crayon. (O'Leary) Coverup for minor skin discolorations, under eye concealer, lipstick fixer. Available in 6 shades. Crayon 0.05 oz. *OTC.*
Use: Skin coverup.

Campath. (Bayer HealthCare) Alemtuzumab 30 mg/mL. Sodium chloride 8 mg, dibasic sodium phosphate 1.44 mg, potassium chloride 0.2 mg, monobasic potassium phosphate 0.2 mg, EDTA 0.0187 mg. Preservative

free. Inj., Soln. Conc. Single-use vials. *Rx.*
Use: Monoclonal antibody.

Campho-Phenique. (Bayer) Camphor 10.8%, phenol 4.7%. **Liq.:** Bot. 22.5 mL, 45 mL, 120 mL. **Gel:** Tube. 6.9 g, 15 g. *OTC.*
Use: Analgesic; antiseptic, local.

Campho-Phenique Cold Sore Treatment and Scab Relief. (Bayer Consumer) Pramoxine hydrochloride 1%. Petrolatum 30%, alcohols, EDTA, glycerin, parabens, ureas. Mint flavor. Cream. 6.5 g. *OTC.*
Use: Local anesthetics, topical.

•**camphor.** (KAM-fore) *USP 34.*
Use: Topical antipruritic; anti-infective; pharmaceutic necessity for camphorated phenol; paregoric and flexible collodion; antitussive; expectorant, local counterirritant; nasal decongestant.
See: Benadryl Children's Anti-Itch. Itch Relief Gel Spritz.
W/Menthol.
See: Tiger Balm.
W/Combinations.
See: Anbesol Cold Sore Therapy.
Bayer Muscle & Joint Cream.
Chiggerex.
Ivy-Dry Super.
Mentholatum.
Mentholatum Cherry Chest Rub for Kids.
Nose Better Gel.
Söltice Quick-Rub.
TheraPatch Vapor Patch for Kids Cough Suppressant.
Tom's of Maine Natural Cough & Cold Rub Cough Suppressant.
Vicks Sinex.
Vicks Vapor Inhaler.
Vicks VapoRub.
Vicks VapoSteam.

camphorated, parachlorophenol.
Use: Anti-infective, dental.

camphoric acid ester. Ester of p-Tolylmethylcarbinal as Diethanolamine Salt.

Campral. (Forest) Acamprosate calcium 333 mg. DR Tab. 180s, 1,080s. Dose pak 180s. *Rx.*
Use: Antialcoholic agent.

Camptosar. (Pharmacia) Irinotecan hydrochloride 20 mg/mL, sorbitol 45 mg. Inj. Vial. 2 mL, 5 mL. *Rx.*
Use: Antineoplastic, DNA topoisomerase inhibitor.

•**canagliflozin.** (KAN-a-gli-FLOE-zin) USAN.
Use: Antidiabetic.

•**canakinumab.** (KAN-a-KIN-ue-mab) USAN.
Use: Immunomodulator.
See: Ilaris.

Canasa. (Axcan Scandipharm) Mesalamine 1000 mg (in base of hard fat). Supp. 30s. *Rx.*
Use: Anti-inflammatory.

Cancidas. (Merck) Caspofungin acetate 50 mg, 70 mg. Pow. for Inj., lyophilized. Single-use Vial. *Rx.*
Use: Antifungal, echinocandins.

C & E Capsules. (NBTY) Vitamins C 500 mg, E 400 mg. Cap. Bot. 50s, 100s. *OTC.*
Use: Vitamin supplement.

•**candesartan.** (kan-deh-SAHR-tan) USAN.
Use: Antagonist, angiotensin II receptor; antihypertensive.

•**candesartan cilexetil.** (kan-deh-SAHR-tan sigh-LEX-eh-till) USAN.
Use: Antagonist, angiotensin II receptor; antihypertensive.
See: Atacand.
W/Hydrochlorothiazide.
See: Atacand HCT.

C & E Softgels. (NBTY) Vitamins E 400 mg, C 500 mg. Cap. Bot. 50s.
Use: Vitamin supplement.

•**candicidin.** (KAN-dih-SIDE-in) *USP 34.*
An antifungal antibiotic derived from *Strepomyces griseus.*
Use: Antifungal.

candida albicans skin test antigen.
Use: Diagnostic aid.
See: Candin.

candida test. (SmithKline Diagnostics) Culture test for *Candida.* Box 4s.
Use: Diagnostic aid.

Candin. (ALK) *Candida albicans* skin test antigen prepared from the culture filtrate and cells of 2 strains of *Candida albicans.* Vial 1 mL. *Rx.*
Use: Evaluation of cell-mediated immunity; diagnostic aid.

•**candoxatril.** (kan-DOXE-at-trill) USAN.
Use: Antihypertensive.

•**candoxatrilat.** (kan-DOXE-at-trill-at) USAN.
Use: Antihypertensive.

Candycon. (Allison) Chlorprophenpyridamine maleate 2 mg, phenylephrine hydrochloride 5 mg. Tab. Bot. 50s. *OTC.*
Use: Antihistamine; decongestant.

•**canertinib dihydrochloride.** (can-ER-tin-ib) USAN.
Use: Epithelial tumors.

•**canfosfamide hydrochloride.** (kan-FOS-fa-mide) USAN.
Use: Antineoplastic.

•**cangrelor.** (KAN-grel-or) USAN.
Use: Antiplatelet.

•**cangrelor tetrasodium.** (KAN-grel-or) USAN.
Use: Antiplatelet.

Cankaid Liquid. (Dickinson) Carbamide peroxide 10% in anhydrous glycerol, EDTA. Soln. 22.5 mL. *OTC.*
Use: Mouth and throat product.

cannabinoids.
Use: Antiemetic; antivertigo agent.
See: Dronabinol.

cannabis.
Use: Antiemetic; antivertigo.
See: Dronabinol.

•**canrenoate potassium.** (kan-REN-oh-ate) USAN.
Use: Aldosterone antagonist.

•**canrenone.** (kan-REN-ohn) USAN.
Use: Aldosterone antagonist.

cantharidin.
Use: Keratolytic.

Cantil. (Hoechst Marion Roussel) Mepenzolate bromide 25 mg. Tab. Bot. 100s. *Rx.*
Use: Anticholinergic; antispasmodic.

•**cantuzumab mertansine.** (can-TUE-zue-mab mer-TAN-seen) USAN.
Use: Colorectal and pancreatic cancer.

•**cantuzumab ravtansine.** (kan-TOOZ-ue-mab rav-TAN-seen) USAN.
Use: Antineoplastic.

Ca-Orotate. (Miller Pharmacal Group) Calcium (as calcium orotate) 50 mg. Tab. Bot. 100s. *OTC.*
Use: Mineral supplement.

C-A-P. (Eastman Kodak) Cellulose acetate phthalate.

Capastat Sulfate. (Akorn) Capreomycin 1 g/10 mL. Vial 10 mL. *Rx.*
Use: Antituberculosis agent.

•**capecitabine.** (cap-eh-SITE-ah-bean) USAN.
Use: Antineoplastic, antimetabolite.
See: Xeloda.

Capex. (Galderma) Fluocinolone acetonide 0.01%, dibasic calcium phosphate dihydrate 5.48 mg. Shampoo. In 12 mg capsule with shampoo base to be mixed by pharmacist before dispensing. *Formerly Fs Shampoo (Hill) Rx.*
Use: Anti-inflammatory; corticosteroid, topical.

Caphosol. (EUSA Pharma) Dibasic sodium phosphate 3.2 g, monobasic sodium phosphate 0.9 g, calcium chloride 5.2 g, sodium chloride 56.9 g. Vanilla

flavor. Soln. Dose box. 30s, 120s (1 dose = two 15 mL amps mixed together). *Rx.*
Use: Mouth and throat product, saliva substitute.

•**capimorelin tartrate.** (CAP-eh-mohr-lyn) USAN.
Use: Prevention of frailty; congestive heart failure; catabolic illness.

Capital Soleil 20. (Vichy) Avobenzone 2%, ecamsule 2%, octocrylene 10%, titanium dioxide 2%. SFP 20. Cream. 100 g. *OTC.*
Use: Sunscreen.

Capital with Codeine. (Carnrick) **Susp.:** Acetaminophen 120 mg, codeine phosphate 12 mg/5 mL. Bot. 473 mL. *c-v.*
Tab.: Codeine phosphate 30 mg, acetaminophen 325 mg. Bot. 100s. *c-III.*
Use: Analgesic combination, narcotic.

Ca-Plus-Protein. (Miller Pharmacal Group) Calcium (as contained in a calcium-protein complex made with specially isolated soy protein) 280 mg. Tab. Bot. 100s. *OTC.*
Use: Mineral supplement.

Capmist DM. (Capital) Dextromethorphan hydrobromide 30 mg, guaifenesin 400 mg, pseudoephedrine hydrochloride 30 mg. Maltodextrin. Tab. 30s. *OTC.*
Use: Upper respiratory combination, antitussive and expectorant combination.

Capnitro. (Freeport) Nitroglycerin 6.5 mg. TR Cap. Bot. 100s. *Rx.*
Use: Antianginal agent.

•**capobenate sodium.** (CAP-oh-BEN-ate) USAN.
Use: Cardiovascular agent, antiarrhythmic.

•**capobenic acid.** (CAP-oh-BEN-ik) USAN.
Use: Cardiovascular agent, antiarrhythmic.

Capoten. (Par) Captopril 12.5 mg, 25 mg, 50 mg, 100 mg. Lactose. Tab. Bot 100s, 1,000s (except 12.5 mg and 100 mg), UD 100s (except 100 mg). *Rx.*
Use: Renin angiotensin system antagonist, angiotensin-converting enzyme inhibitor.

•**capravirine.** (cap-ruh-VYE-reen) USAN.
Use: Antiviral.

•**capreomycin.** (CAP-ree-oh-MY-sin) *USP 34.* An antibiotic derived from *Streptomyces capreolus.* Caprocin.
Use: Antituberculosis agent.
See: Capastat Sulfate.

•**capromab pendetide.** (KAP-row-mab PEN-deh-TIDE) USAN.

Use: Monoclonal antibody; in vivo diagnostic aid.
See: ProstaScint.

•**capromorelin tartrate.** (kap-roe-moor-lyn) USAN.
Use: Prevention of frailty; congestive heart failure; carabolic illness.

caprylate, salts.
See: Caprylate Sodium.

caprylate sodium. (Ingram) Caprylate sodium 33%. Inj. Amp. 1 mL. Pkg. 12s, 25s, 100s.
Use: Antifungal.

caprylidene.
Use: Nutritional supplement.
See: Axona.

•**capsaicin.** (kap-SAY-uh-sin) *USP 34.*
Use: Analgesic, topical; antineuralgic; specific pain syndromes, topical.
See: Axsain.
Capsin.
Capzasin-P.
Icy Hot PM.
No Pain-HP.
Pain Doctor.
Qutenza.
Rid-a-Pain-HP.
Zostrix.
Zostrix Diabetic Foot Pain.
Zostrix Maximum Strength.
W/Lidocaine, Menthol, Methyl Salicylate.
See: Terocin.
W/Menthol.
See: Capzasin Quick Relief.
W/Menthol, Methyl Salicylate.
See: Medi-Derm.
Medrox.

capsaicin. (Various Mfr.) Capsaicin 0.025%, 0.075%. Cream. Tube. 45 g (0.025% only), 60 g. *OTC.*
Use: Analgesic, topical; antineuralgic; specific pain syndromes, topical.

•**capsicum.** (KAP-see-kum) *USP 34.*
Use: Carminative; counterirritant, external; stomachic.

•**capsicum oleoresin.** (KAP-see-kum OH-lee-oh-RES-in) *USP 34.*
Use: Carminative; counterirritant, external; stomachic.

Capsin. (Fleming & Co.) Capsaicin 0.025%, 0.075%, benzyl alcohol, propylene glycol, denatured alcohol. Lot. Bot. 59 mL. *OTC.*
Use: Analgesic, topical.

capsules, empty gelatin. (Eli Lilly) Lilly markets clear empty gelatin capsules in sizes 000, 00, 0, 1, 2, 3, 4, 5.

•**captamine hydrochloride.** (KAP-tam-een) USAN.
Use: Depigmentor.

•**captopril.** (KAP-toe-prill) *USP 34.*
Use: Angiotensin-converting enzyme inhibitor, renin angiotensin system antagonist.
See: Capoten.
captopril. (Various Mfr.) Captopril 12.5 mg, 25 mg, 50 mg, 100 mg. Tab. Bot. 100s, 500s, 1000s, 5000s (except 100 mg), UD 100s, blister 600s. *Rx.*
Use: Angiotensin-converting enzyme inhibitor, renin angiotensin system antagonist.
captopril and hydrochlorothiazide.
(Teva) Hydrochlorothiazide/captopril 15 mg/25 mg, 15 mg/50 mg, 25 mg/25 mg, 25 mg/50 mg. Tab. Bot. 100s, 1000s. *Rx.*
Use: Antihypertensive; diuretic.
•**capuride.** (CAP-you-ride) USAN.
Use: Hypnotic; sedative.
Capzasin. (Chattem) Capsaicin 0.025%, menthol 10%. Aloe barbadensis leaf juice, glycerin, parabens, SD alcohol 15%. Gel. 42.5 g. *OTC.*
Use: Counterirritant.
Capzasin•HP. (Chattem) Capsaicin 0.1%. Alcohols, petrolatum. Cream. 42.5 g. *OTC.*
Use: Counterirritant.
Capzasin•P. (Chattem) Capsaicin 0.035%. Alcohols, petrolatum. Cream. Tube 42.5 g. *OTC.*
Use: Analgesic, topical.
Carac. (Dermik) Fluorouracil 0.5%. Glycerin, parabens. Cream. Tubes. 30 g. *Rx.*
Use: Pyrimidine antagonist, topical.
•**caracemide.** (car-ASS-eh-MIDE) USAN.
Use: Antineoplastic.
Carafate. (Axcan Scandipharm) **Tab.:** Sucralfate 1 g. Bot. 100s, 120s, 500s. **Susp.:** Sucralfate 1 g/10 mL, sorbitol, methylparaben. Bot. 415 mL. *Rx.*
Use: Antiulcerative.
•**caramel.** (KAR-uh-mel) *NF 29.*
Use: Pharmaceutic aid, color.
caramiphen hydrochloride.
Use: Proposed antiparkinson.
•**caraway.** (KAR-uh-way) *NF 29.*
Use: Flavoring.
•**caraway oil.** (KAR-uh-way) *NF 29.*
Use: Flavoring.
•**carbachol.** (KAR-bah-kole) *USP 34.*
Use: Parasympathomimetic; cholinergic, ophthalmic.
See: Miostat Intraocular.
W/Methylcellulose.
See: Isopto Carbachol.
carbacrylamine resins.
Use: Cation-exchange resin.

•**carbadox.** (KAR-bah-dox) USAN.
Use: Anti-infective.
Carbaglu. (Accredo Health Group Inc) Carglumic acid 200 mg. Tab., dispersible. 5s, 60s. *Rx.*
Use: Endocrine and metabolic agent.
•**carbamazepine.** (KAR-bam-AZE-uh-peen) *USP 34.*
Tall Man: carBAMazepine
Use: Analgesic; anticonvulsant.
See: Carbatrol.
Epitol.
Equetro.
Tegretol.
Tegretol-XR.
carbamazepine. (Taro) Carbamazepine. **Chew. Tab.:** 200 mg. Sorbitol. Cherry flavor. 100s, 400s. **ER Tab.:** 100 mg, 200 mg, 400 mg. Lactose. 30s, 100s, 1,000s. *Rx.*
Use: Anticonvulsant.
carbamazepine. (Various Mfr.) Carbamazepine. **Chew. Tab.:** 100 mg. May contain lactose, sorbitol, sucrose. Bot. 100s, 500s, UD 50s, UD 100s. **Tab.:** 200 mg. May contain lactose. Bot. 100s, 500s, 1000s, UD 25s, UD 50s, UD 100s. **Susp.:** 100 mg/5 mL. May contain sorbitol, sucrose. Bot. 450 mL, UD 5 mL, UD 10 mL. *Rx.*
Use: Anticonvulsant.
carbamide.
Use: Emollient.
See: Urea.
carbamide compounds.
See: Acetylcarbromal.
Carbromal.
•**carbamide peroxide.** (CAR-bah-mide purr-ox-ide) *USP 34.* Urea compound w/hydrogen peroxide (1:1).
Use: Anti-inflammatory; mouth and throat product.
See: Cankaid Liquid.
Gly-Oxide.
Orajel Perioseptic.
carbamide peroxide 6.5% in glycerin.
Use: Otic.
See: Murine Ear Drops.
Murine Ear Wax Removal System.
carbamylcholine chloride.
See: Carbachol.
carbamylmethylcholine chloride.
See: Urecholine.
•**carbantel lauryl sulfate.** (CAR-ban-tell LAH-ruhl) USAN.
Use: Anthelmintic.
carbapenem.
Use: Anti-infective.
See: Doripenem.
Ertapenem.

Imipenem-Cilastatin.

Meropenem.

Carbaphen 12. (GIL) Carbetapentane tannate 60 mg, chlorpheniramine tannate 8 mg, phenylephrine tannate 20 mg per 5 mL. Alcohol and sugar free. Acesulfame K, aspartame, methylparaben, phenylalanine 1 mg. Blueberry-banana flavor. Liq. 473 mL. *Rx.*
Use: Upper respiratory combination, antitussive combination.

carbarsone. (Various Mfr.) N-carbamoylarsanilic acid. Amabevan, ameban, amibiarson, arsambide, fenarsone, leucarsone, aminarsone, amebarsone. p-Ureidobenzenearsonic acid. Caps.
Use: Acute and chronic amebiasis and trichomoniasis.

●**carbaspirin calcium.** (kar-ba-SPEER-in) USAN.
Use: Analgesic.

Carbatab-12. (GM) Carbetapentane citrate 60 mg, guaifenesin 600 mg, phenylephrine hydrochloride 15 mg. ER Tab. 100s. *Rx.*
Use: Antitussive and expectorant combination, upper respiratory combination.

Carbatrol. (Shire) Carbamazepine 100 mg, 200 mg, 300 mg. Lactose. ER Cap. 120s. *Rx.*
Use: Anticonvulsant.

Carbatuss. (GM Pharmaceuticals) Carbetapentane citrate 20 mg, guaifenesin 100 mg, phenylephrine hydrochloride 10 mg per 5 mL. Alcohol free. Spearmint flavor. Liq. 15 and 473 mL. *Rx.*
Use: Upper respiratory combination; antitussive, expectorant, decongestant.

Carbatuss CL. (GM Pharmaceuticals) Carbetapentane citrate 20 mg, potassium guaiacolsulfonate 100 mg, phenylephrine hydrochloride 10 mg per 5 mL. Sugar free. Saccharin, sorbitol, menthol. Liq. 15 mL, 473 mL. *Rx.*
Use: Antitussive and expectorant combination.

Carbaxefed RF. (Morton Grove) Pseudoephedrine hydrochloride 15 mg, carbinoxamine maleate 1 mg per 1 mL. Sugar and alcohol free. Saccharin, sorbitol. Cherry flavor. Oral Drops. 30 mL bottle with dropper. *Rx.*
Use: Pediatric decongestant and antihistamine.

●**carbazeran.** (KAR-BAY-zeh-ran) USAN.
Use: Cardiovascular agent.

●**carbenicillin disodium, sterile.** (KAR-ben-ih-SILL-in die-SO-dee-uhm,

STEER-ill) *USP 34.*
Use: Anti-infective.
See: Geopen.

●**carbenicillin indanyl sodium.** (car-BEN-ih-SILL-in IN-duh-nil) *USP 34.*
Use: Extended-spectrum penicillin.

●**carbenicillin phenyl sodium.** (CAR-ben-ih-SILL-in FEN-ill) USAN.
Use: Anti-infective.

●**carbenicillin potassium.** (CAR-ben-ih-SILL-in) USAN.
Use: Anti-infective.

●**carbenoxolone sodium.** (CAR-ben-ox-ah-lone) USAN.
Use: Corticosteroid, topical.

carbetapentane citrate.
Use: Antitussive.
W/Brompheniramine Maleate, Phenylephrine Hydrochloride.
See: V-Cof.
W/Brompheniramine Tannate, Carbetapentane Tannate, Phenylephrine Tannate.
See: Vazotan.
W/Dexchlorpheniramine Maleate, Phenylephrine Hydrochloride.
See: Corzall-PE.
W/Guaifenesin.
See: AMBI 1000/5.
   BetaVent.
   Duratuss CS.
   Dynex VR.
   Tusso-ZMR.
   Tusso-ZMR.
   XPect-AT.
W/Guaifenesin, Phenylephrine Hydrochloride.
See: Albatussin.
   Carbatab-12.
   Extendryl GCP.
   Gentex 30.
   Levall.
   Phencarb GG.
   Zinx GCP.
W/Guaifenesin, Pseudoephedrine Hydrochloride.
See: Exall-D.
W/Pseudoephedrine Hydrochloride.
See: Corzall.
W/Pseudoephedrine Hydrochloride, Pyrilamine Maleate.
See: Corzall Plus.

carbetapentane tannate.
Use: Nonnarcotic antitussive.
W/Brompheniramine Tannate, Phenylephrine Tannate.
See: Vazotan Tannate.
W/Chlorpheniramine Tannate.
See: Tannic-12.
   Tannic-12 S.

Trionate.
Tussi-12.
Tussi-12 S.
Tussizone-12 RF.
Tustan 12S.
W/Chlorpheniramine Tannate, Ephedrine
Tannate, Phenylephrine Tannate.
See: Quad-Tus Tannate Pediatric.
Rynatuss.
Rynatuss Pediatric.
W/Chlorpheniramine Tannate, Phenyl-
ephrine Tannate.
See: D-Tann CT.
Dytan CS.
XiraTuss.
W/Diphenhydramine Tannate.
See: D-Tann AT.
W/Diphenhydramine Tannate, Phenyl-
ephrine Tannate.
See: D-Tann CD.
D-Tann CT.
Dytan-CS.
W/Guaifenesin, Phenylephrine Hydro-
chloride.
See: Carbatuss.
W/Phenylephrine Tannate.
See: Levall 12.
Zinx D-Tuss.
W/Phenylephrine Tannate, Pyrilamine
Tannate.
See: C-Tanna 12D.
Tannate-12D S.
Tannihist-12 D.
Tussi-12D.
Tussi-12D S.
W/Pseudoephedrine Tannate.
See: Carb Pseudo-Tan.
Respi-Tann.
Respi-Tann Pd.
Carbetaplex. (Breckenridge Pharma-
ceutical) Carbetapentane citrate 20 mg,
guaifenesin 100 mg, phenylephrine
hydrochloride 15 mg per 5 mL. Sugar,
alcohol, and dye free. Saccharin. Straw-
berry flavor. Liq. 480 mL. *Rx.*
Use: Antitussive and expectorant com-
bination.
•**carbetimer.** (kar-BEH-tih-MER) USAN.
Use: Antineoplastic.
•**carbidopa.** (KAR-bih-doe-puh) *USP 34.*
Use: Decarboxylase inhibitor.
See: Lodosyn.
W/Levodopa.
See: Carbidopa and Levodopa.
Parcopa.
Sinemet CR.
Sinemet-10/100.
Sinemet-25/100.
Sinemet-25/250.
W/Levodopa and Entacapone.
See: Stalevo 50.

Stalevo 100.
Stalevo 150.
Stalevo 125.
Stalevo 75.
Stalevo 200.
carbidopa and levodopa. (Various Mfr.)
ER Tab.: Carbidopa 25 mg, levodopa
100 mg. 100s, 500s. **Tab.:** Carbidopa
10 mg, levodopa 100 mg; carbidopa
25 mg, levodopa 100 mg; carbidopa
25 mg, levodopa 250 mg; carbidopa
50 mg, levodopa 200 mg. Bot. 100s,
500s, 1000s. **Orally disintegrating
Tab.:** Carbidopa 10 mg, levodopa
100 mg; carbidopa 25 mg, levodopa
100 mg; carbidopa 25 mg, levodopa
250 mg. Aspartame, mannitol, phenyl-
alanine 3.37 mg (10 mg/100 mg, 25 mg/
100 mg), phenylalanine 8.42 mg
(25 mg/250 mg), sorbitol. Peppermint
flavor. 100s, 500s. *Rx.*
Use: Antiparkinsonian.
•**carbinoxamine maleate.** (KAR-bin-OX-
a-meen) *USP 34.*
Use: Antihistamine.
See: Arbinoxa.
Histex CT.
Histex I/E.
Histex Pd.
Palgic.
Pediatex.
Pediatex 12.
W/Dextromethorphan Hydrobromide,
Phenylephrine Hydrochloride.
See: XiraHist DM Pediatric.
W/Dextromethorphan Hydrobromide,
Pseudoephedrine Hydrochloride.
See: Balamine DM.
Cordron-DM NR.
Pseudo Carb DM Pediatric.
W/Phenylephrine Hydrochloride.
See: Histamax D.
XiraHist Pediatric.
W/Pseudoephedrine Hydrochloride.
See: Cordron-D.
Cordron-D NR.
Pseudo Carb Pediatric.
Sildec.
carbinoxamine maleate. (Boca) Car-
binoxamine maleate. **Tab.:** 4 mg. Lac-
tose 100s. **Soln.:** 4 mg per 5 mL.
Parabens, sorbitol. Bubble gum flavor.
118 mL, 473 mL. *Rx.*
Use: Antihistamine.
**carbinoxamine maleate and carbinox-
amine tannate.** (Brighton) Carbinox-
amine maleate 2 mg, carbinoxamine
tannate 6 mg/5 mL. Alcohol, dye, and
sugar free. Saccharin, sorbitol, parabens. Bubble-gum flavor. Oral Susp.
118 mL, 473 mL. *Rx.*

Use: Antihistamine.

carbinoxamine maleate, pseudoephedrine hydrochloride, dextromethorphan HBr. (Cypress) **Syrup:** Carbinoxamine maleate 4 mg, pseudoephedrine hydrochloride 60 mg, dextromethorphan HBr 15 mg/5 mL. Bot. 120 mL, pt, gal. **Drops:** Carbinoxamine maleate 2 mg, pseudoephedrine hydrochloride 25 mg, dextromethorphan HBr 4 mg/mL. Bot. 30 mL w/dropper. *Rx.*
Use: Antihistamine; decongestant; antitussive.

carbinoxamine oral drops. (Morton Grove) Carbinoxamine maleate 2 mg, pseudoephedrine hydrochloride 25 mg/mL, sorbitol, parabens, alcohol free, raspberry, fruit flavors. Bot. 30 mL w/calibrated dropper. *Rx.*
Use: Upper respiratory combination, antihistamine, decongestant.

carbinoxamine syrup. (Morton Grove) Carbinoxamine maleate 4 mg, pseudoephedrine hydrochloride 60 mg/5 mL, sorbitol, parabens, alcohol free, raspberry, fruit flavors. Bot. 118 mL, 237 mL, 473 mL. *Rx.*
Use: Upper respiratory combination, antihistamine, decongestant.

carbinoxamine tannate.
Use: Antihistamine.
W/Combinations.
See: Pediatex 12 D.
W/Dextromethorphan Tannate, Pseudoephedrine Tannate.
See: Carb PSE 12 DM.

•**carbiphene hydrochloride.** (KAR-bih-FEEN) USAN.
Use: Analgesic.

Carbiset. (Nutripharm Laboratories, Inc.) Pseudoephedrine 60 mg, carbinoxamine maleate 4 mg. Tab. Bot. 100s, 500s. *Rx.*
Use: Antihistamine; decongestant.

Carbiset-TR. (Nutripharm Laboratories, Inc.) Pseudoephedrine hydrochloride 120 mg, carbinoxamine maleate 8 mg. Tab. Bot. 100s. *Rx.*
Use: Antihistamine; decongestant.

Carbocaine. (Hospira) Mepivacaine hydrochloride. **1%:** Methylparaben. Inj. Multidose vial 50 mL. **1.5%:** Inj. Single-dose vial 30 mL. **2%:** Inj. Single-dose vial 20 mL. Multidose vial 50 mL, methylparaben. **3%:** Acetone sodium bisulfite. Inj. Dental Cartridge 1.8 mL. *Rx.*
Use: Anesthetic, local amide, injectable.

Carbocaine with Neo-Cobefrin. (Eastman-Kodak) Mepivacaine hydrochloride 2% with levonordefrin 1:20,000, acetone sodium bisulfite. Inj. Dental cartridge 1.8 mL. *Rx.*
Use: Anesthetic, local amide, injectable.

•**carbocloral.** (KAR-boe-KLOR-uhl) USAN.
Use: Hypnotic; sedative.
See: Chloralurethane.

•**carbocysteine.** (kar-boe-SIS-teen) USAN.
Use: Mucolytic.

Carbodec DM. (Rugby) **Syr.:** Pseudoephedrine hydrochloride 60 mg, carbinoxamine maleate 4 mg, dextromethorphan HBr 15 mg, alcohol < 0.6%/5 mL. Bot. 30 mL, 120 mL, pt, gal. **Drops:** (Pediatric Pharmaceuticals) Pseudoephedrine hydrochloride 25 mg, carbinoxamine maleate 2 mg, dextromethorphan HBr 4 mg, alcohol 0.6%/mL. Bot. 30 mL. *Rx.*
Use: Antihistamine, antitussive, decongestant.

Carbodec Syrup. (Rugby) Pseudoephedrine hydrochloride 60 mg, carbinoxamine maleate 4 mg/5 mL. Syr. Bot. 473 mL. *Rx.*
Use: Antihistamine, decongestant.

Carbodec Tablets. (Rugby) Pseudoephedrine hydrochloride 60 mg, carbinoxamine maleate 4 mg. Tab. Bot. 100s. *Rx.*
Use: Antihistamine, decongestant.

Carbodec TR. (Rugby) Pseudoephedrine hydrochloride 120 mg, carbinoxamine maleate 8 mg. Tab. Bot. 100s. *Rx.*
Use: Antihistamine, decongestant.

Carbodex DM. (Tri-Med) **Drops:** Carbinoxamine maleate 2 mg, pseudoephedrine hydrochloride 15 mg, dextromethorphan HBr 4 mg per 1 mL. Bot. 30 mL. **Syrup:** Dextromethorphan HBr 15 mg, brompheniramine maleate 4 mg, pseudoephedrine hydrochloride 45 mg per 5 mL. Menthol, sorbitol. Bot. 473 mL. *Rx.*
Use: Upper respiratory combination, antihistamine, antitussive, decongestant.

Carbofed DM. (Hi-Tech) **Drops:** Pseudoephedrine hydrochloride 15 mg, carbinoxamine maleate 1 mg, dextromethorphan HBr 4 mg per 1 mL. Alcohol and sugar free. Bot. 30 mL w/dropper. *Rx.*
Use: Upper respiratory combination, antitussive combination.

Carb-O-Lac HP. (Geritrex) Ammonium lactate 10%, urea 20%, lactic acid, petrolatum, propylene glycol, stearyl alcohol. Cream. 277 g. *OTC.*
Use: Emollient.

carbol-fuchsin paint. Original fuchsin formula known as Castellani's Paint. Basic Fuchsin 0.3%, phenol 4.5%, resorcinol 10%, acetone 5%, alcohol 10%. Paint. Bot. 30 mL, 120 mL, 480 mL.
Use: Antifungal, topical.
See: Castellani's Paint.

•**carbol-fuchsin, topical solution.** (KAR-buhl-FOOK-sin) *USP 34.*
Use: Antifungal.

•**carbomer.** (KAR-boe-mer) *NF 29.* A polymer of acrylic acid, crosslinked with a polyfunctional agent.
Use: Pharmaceutic aid, emulsifying, suspending agent.

•**carbomer copolymer.** (KAR-boe-mer) *NF 29.*
Use: Pharmaceutic aid.

•**carbomer interpolymer.** (KAR-boe-mer) *NF 29.*
Use: Pharmaceutic aid; emulsifying, suspending agent.

•**carbomer 940.** (KAR-boe-mer 940) *NF 29.*
Use: Pharmaceutic aid, emulsifying, suspending agent.

•**carbomer 941.** (KAR-boe-mer 941) *NF 29.*
Use: Pharmaceutic aid, emulsifying, suspending agent.

•**carbomer 910.** (KAR-boe-mer 910) *NF 29.*
Use: Pharmaceutic aid, emulsifying, suspending agent.

•**carbomer 934.** (KAR-boe-mer 934) *NF 29.*
Use: Pharmaceutic aid, emulsifying, suspending agent.

•**carbomer 934p.** (KAR-boe-mer 934) *NF 29. Formerly carpolene.*
Use: Pharmaceutic aid, emulsifying, suspending, viscosity, thickening agent.

•**carbomer 1342.** (KAR-boe-mer 1342) *NF 29.*
Use: Pharmaceutic aid, emulsifying, suspending agent.

carbomycin. An antibiotic from *Streptomyces halstedii.*
Use: Anti-infective.

•**carbon dioxide.** (KAR-bahn dye-OX-ide) *USP 34.*
Use: Inhalation, respiratory.

•**carbonic acid, dilithium salt.** (KAR-bahn-ik acid, dye-LITH-ee-uhm) *USP 34.* Lithium Carbonate.

•**carbonic acid, disodium salt.** (KAR-bahn-ik) *USP 34.* Sodium Carbonate.

•**carbonic acid, monosodium salt.** (KAR-bahn-ik) *USP 34.* Sodium Bicarbonate.

carbonic anhydrase inhibitors.
See: Acetazolamide.
  Brinzolamide.
  Dorzolamide Hydrochloride.
  Methazolamide.

Carbonis Detergens, Liquor.
See: Coal Tar Topical Solution.

•**carbon monoxide c 11.** (KAR-bahn moe-NOX-ide C11) *USP 34.*
Use: Diagnostic aid, blood volume determination; radiopharmaceutical.

•**carbon tetrachloride.** (KAR-bahn teh-truh-KLOR-ide) *NF 29.* Benzinoform.
Use: Pharmaceutic aid, solvent.

carbonyl diamide.
See: Chap Cream.

carbonyl iron.
Use: Trace element.
See: Feosol.
  Ferralet 90.
  Icar.
  Ircon.
  Iron Chews.
  Wee Care.

Carb-O-Philic/10. (Geritrex) DMDM hydantoin, lactic acid, lemon oil, petrolatum, propylene glycol, urea. Cream. 454 g. *OTC.*
Use: Emollient.

Carb-O-Philic/20. (Geritrex) DMDM hydantoin, lactic acid, lemon oil, petrolatum, propylene glycol, urea. Cream. 454 g. *OTC.*
Use: Emollient.

•**carboplatin.** (kar-boe-PLATT-in) *USP 34.*
Tall Man: CARBOplatin
Use: Antineoplastic.
See: Paraplatin.

carboplatin. (Mayne) Carboplatin 10 mg/mL. Inj. Single-use vials. 5 mL, 15 mL, 45 mL. *Rx.*
Use: Antineoplastic.

carboplatin. (Various Mfr.) Carboplatin 50 mg, 150 mg, 450 mg. Mannitol. Pow. for Inj., lyophilized. Single-dose vials. *Rx.*
Use: Antineoplastic.

•**carboprost.** (KAR-boe-prahst) USAN.
Use: Oxytocic.

•**carboprost methyl.** (KAR-boe-prahst METH-ill) USAN.
Use: Oxytocic.

•**carboprost tromethamine.** (KAR-boe-prahst troe-METH-ah-meen) *USP 34.*
Use: Oxytocic.

carbose D.
See: Carboxymethylcellulose Sodium.

carbowax. Polyethylene glycol 300, 400, 1540, 4000.

carboxymethylcellulose.
Use: Ocular lubricant.
See: Refresh Tears.

•**carboxymethylcellulose calcium.** (kar-BOX-ee-meth-ill-SELL-you-lohs) *NF 29.*
Use: Pharmaceutic aid, tablet disintegrant.

carboxymethylcellulose salt of dextroamphetamine. Carboxyphen.

•**carboxymethylcellulose sodium.** (kar-BOX-ee-meth-ill-SELL-you-lohs) *USP 34.*
Use: Pharmaceutic aid, suspending agent, tablet excipient, viscosity-increasing agent; cathartic.
W/Combinations.
See: Clear Eyes for Dry Eyes.
 Ex-Caloric Wafers.
 Foxalin.
 Refresh.
W/Glycerin.
See: Optive.

•**carboxymethylcellulose sodium 12.** (car-BOX-ee-meth-ill-SELL-you-lohs) *NF 29.*
Use: Pharmaceutic aid, suspending, viscosity-increasing agent; mucolytic agent.

Carb PSE 12 DM. (River's Edge) Dextromethorphan tannate 27.5 mg, carbinoxamine tannate 3.2 mg, pseudoephedrine tannate 45.2 mg per 5 mL. Methylparaben, saccharin, sorbitol. Candy apple flavor. Susp. Bot. 473 mL. *Rx.*
Use: Antitussive combination, upper respiratory combination.

Carb Pseudo-Tan. (Hi-Tech) Carbetapentane tannate 25 mg, pseudoephedrine tannate 75 mg per 5 mL. Dye free. Methylparaben, saccharin, sucrose. Cherry flavor. Susp. 473 mL. *Rx.*
Use: Antitussive combination, upper respiratory combination.

Carbromal. (Various Mfr.) Bromodiethylacetylurea, bromadel, nyctal, planadalin, uradal. *Rx.*
Use: Sedative; hypnotic.
W/Bromisovalum (Bromural).
See: Bro-T's.

carbutamide.
Use: Hypoglycemic.

•**carbuterol hydrochloride.** (kar-BYOO-ter-ole) USAN.
Use: Bronchodilator.

•**cardamon.** (KAR-duh-mohn) *NF 29.* Oil, seed, Cpd. Tincture.
Use: Flavoring.

Cardene I.V. (EKR Therapeutics) Nicardipine hydrochloride 0.1 mg/mL, 0.2 mg/mL. Inj., Soln. 200 mL premixed, single-use *Galaxy* container in either dextrose 4.8% or sodium chloride 0.86% (0.1 mg/mL), 200 mL premixed single-use *Galaxy* container in either dextrose 5% or sodium chloride 0.83% (0.2 mg/mL). *Rx.*
Use: Calcium channel blocker.

Cardene SR. (Roche) Nicardipine hydrochloride 30 mg, 45 mg, 60 mg. Lactose. ER Cap. Bot. 60s, 200s (except 60 mg). *Rx.*
Use: Calcium channel blocker.

Cardenz. (Miller Pharmacal Group) Vitamins C 25 mg, E 5 mg, inositol 30 mg, p-aminobenzoic acid 9 mg, A 2000 units, B_6 1.5 mg, B_{12} 1 mcg, D 100 units, niacinamide 20 mg, Mg 23 mg, I 0.05 mg, K 8 mg. Tab. Bot. 100s. *OTC.*
Use: Mineral, vitamin supplement.

cardiac glycosides.
Use: Inotropic agent.
See: Digoxin.

Cardilate. (GlaxoSmithKline) Erythrityl tetranitrate 10 mg. Tab. Bot. 100s.
Use: Antianginal.

Cardio-Green Disposable Unit. (Becton Dickinson & Co.) Cardio-Green 10 mg. Vial. Amp. Aqueous solvent and calibrated syringe.
Use: Diagnostic aid.

Cardi-Omega 3. (Thompson Medical) EPA 180 mg, DHA 120 mg, cholesterol 5 mg, < 2% RDA of vitamins A, B_1, B_2, B_3, C, D, Fe, Ca. Cap. Bot. 60s. *OTC.*
Use: Mineral, vitamin supplement.

cardioplegic solution.
Use: During open heart surgery.
See: Plegisol.

Cardiotek Rx. (Stewart-Jackson) Vitamin B_6 50 mg, B_{12} 500 mcg, FA 2 mg. With L-arginine hydrochloride. Coated. Tab. 30s. *Rx.*
Use: Nutritional product.

Cardiotrol-CK. (Roche) Lyophilized human serum containing 3 CK isoenzymes from human tissue source. 10 × 2 mL.
Use: Diagnostic aid, quality control.

Cardiotrol-LD. (Roche) Lyophilized human serum containing all LD isoenzymes from human tissue source. 10 × 1 mL.
Use: Diagnostic aid, quality control.

Cardizem. (Biovail) **Tab.:** Diltiazem hydrochloride 30 mg, 60 mg, 90 mg, 120 mg. Lactose, methylparaben. Bot. 100s, 500s (30 mg, 60 mg only), UD 100s. **Pow. for Inj.:** 25 mg. Single-use

containers. Cartons. 6 *Lyo-Ject* syringes with diluent. *Rx.*
Use: Calcium channel blocker.

Cardizem CD. (Biovail) Diltiazem hydrochloride 120 mg, 180 mg, 240 mg, 300 mg, 360 mg. Sucrose. ER Cap. Bot. 30s (except 360 mg), 90s, UD 100s (except 360 mg). *Rx.*
Use: Calcium channel blocker.

Cardizem LA. (Abbott) Diltiazem hydrochloride 120 mg, 180 mg, 240 mg, 300 mg, 360 mg, 420 mg. Sucrose. ER Tab. Bot. 7s, 30s, 90s, 1000s. *Rx.*
Use: Calcium channel blocker.

Cardoxin. (Vita Elixir) Digoxin 0.25 mg. Tab. *Rx.*
Use: Cardiovascular agent.

Cardura. (Pfizer) Doxazosin mesylate (as base) 1 mg, 2 mg, 4 mg, 8 mg. Lactose. Tab. Bot. 100s, UD 100s. *Rx.*
Use: Antihypertensive.

Cardura XL. (Pfizer) Doxazosin mesylate (as base) 4 mg, 8 mg. ER Tab. 30s. *Rx.*
Use: Antiadrenergic agent, peripherally acting.

Ca-Rezz. (FNC Medical Corporation) Triclosan. **Soap: 0.2%:** Alcohol, aloe vera, parabens, polysorbate 80, propylene glycol, urea. 237 mL. **0.25%:** Alcohol, aloe vera, parabens, polysorbate 80, propylene glycol. 361 mL. **0.3%:** Disodium EDTA, parabens, propylene glycol, urea. 355 mL. **Cream:** 0.3%. Alcohol, aloe vera, glyceryl, mineral oil, parabens, PEG, propylene glycol, safflower oil, triethanolamine, urea, vitamins A, D, and E. 275 g. *OTC.*
Use: Topical anti-infective, antiseptic and germicide.

•**carfentanil citrate.** (kar-FEN-tah-NILL SIH-trate) USAN.
Use: Analgesic; narcotic.

Cargentos.
See: Silver protein, mild.

•**carglumic acid.** (kar-GLOO-mik) USAN.
Use: Treatment of hyperammonemia due to N-acetylglutamate synthase deficiency.

Carimune NF. (ZLB Bioplasma) Immune globulin IV 3 g, 6 g, 12 g. Preservative-free. With 1.67 g sucrose/g protein. Pow. for Inj., lyophilized. Vials. 3 g, 6 g, 12 g. *Rx.*
Use: Immune globulin.

•**cariporide mesylate.** (kar-ee-POR-ide) USAN.
Use: Cardiovascular agent.

•**cariprazine.** (kar-IP-ra-zeen) USAN.
Use: CNS agent.

•**cariprazine hydrochloride.** (kar-IP-ra-zeen) USAN.
Use: CNS agent.

•**carisoprodol.** (car-eye-so-PRO-dole) *USP 34.*
Use: Muscle relaxant.
See: Soma.

carisoprodol. (Various Mfr.) Carisoprodol 350 mg. Tab. Bot. 30s, 60s, 100, 500s, 1000s, UD 100s.
Use: Muscle relaxant.

carisoprodol. (Wallace) Carisoprodol 250 mg. Potassium sorbate. Tab. 100s. *Rx.*
Use: Skeletal muscle relaxant, centrally acting.

carisoprodol, aspirin, and codeine phosphate. (Amide) Carisoprodol 200 mg, aspirin 325 mg, codeine phosphate 16 mg. Tab. 100s, 500s. *c-III.*
Use: Skeletal muscle relaxant.

carisoprodol compound. (Various Mfr.) Carisoprodol 200 mg, aspirin 325 mg. Tab. Bot. 15s, 30s, 40s, 100s, 500s, 1000s. *Rx.*
Use: Analgesic; muscle relaxant.

Cari-Tab. (Jones Pharma) Fluoride 0.5 mg, vitamins A 2000 units, D 200 units, C 75 mg. Softab. Bot. 100s. *Rx.*
Use: Vitamin supplement; dental caries agent.

•**carlumab.** (KAR-lue-mab) USAN.
Use: Immunomodulator.

•**carmantadine.** (kar-MAN-tah-deen) USAN.
Use: Antiparkinsonian.

•**carmegliptin.** (kar-mee-GLIP-tin) USAN.
Use: Antidiabetic.

•**carmegliptin dihydrochloride.** (kar-mee-GLIP-tin) USAN.
Use: Antidiabetic.

Carmol 40. (Pharmaderm) Urea 40%. **Cream:** Mineral oil, petrolatum, cetyl alcohol. Tube. 28.35 g, 85 g. **Gel:** Glycerin, EDTA. Tube. 15 mL *Rx.*
Use: Emollient.

Carmol HC Cream 1%. (Doak Dermatologics) Micronized hydrocortisone acetate 1%, urea 10% in water-washable base. Tube 1 oz, Jar 4 oz. *Rx.*
Use: Corticosteroid, topical.

Carmol Scalp Treatment. (Doak Dermatologics) Sulfacetamide sodium 10%. EDTA, methylparaben, urea 10%. Lot. 85 g. *Rx.*
Use: Topical anti-infective, antibiotic.

Carmol 10. (Pharmaderm) Urea (carbamide) 10% in hypoallergenic water-washable lotion base. Bot. 6 fl oz. *OTC.*
Use: Emollient.

Carmol 20. (Pharmaderm) Urea (carbamide) 20% in hypoallergenic vanishing cream base. Tube 3 oz, Jar lb. *OTC.*
Use: Emollient.

•**carmustine.** (KAR-muss-teen) USAN. BCNU.
Use: Antineoplastic, alkylating agent.
See: BiCNU.
Gliadel.

Carnation Follow-Up. (Carnation) Protein (from nonfat milk) 18 g, carbohydrate (from lactose and corn syrup) 89.2 g, fat 27.7 g, vitamins A, D, E, K, C, B_1, B_2, B_3, B_6, B_{12}, B_5, biotin, choline, Ca, P, Cl, Mg, I, Mn, Cu, Zn, Fe 13 mg, inositol, cholesterol 11.4 mg, taurine, Na 264 mg, K 913 mg. Pow. 360 g. Conc. 390 mL. *OTC.*
Use: Nutritional supplement.

Carnation Good-Start. (Carnation) Protein 16 g, carbohydrate 74.4 g, fat 34.5 g, vitamins A, D, E, K, B_1, B_2, B_3, B_5, B_6, B_{12}, C, biotin, choline, inositol, cholesterol 68 mg, taurine, Ca, P, Mg, Fe 10 mg, Zn, Mn, Cu, I, Cl, Na 162 mg, K 663 mg. Pow 360 g. Conc. 390 mL. *OTC.*
Use: Nutritional supplement.

Carnation Instant Breakfast. (Carnation) Nonfat instant breakfast containing 280 K calories w/15 g protein and 8 oz whole milk. Pkt. 35 g, Ctn. 6s. Six flavors. *OTC.*
Use: Nutritional supplement.

•**carnidazole.** (kar-NIH-dah-zole) USAN. Methylnitroimidazole.
Use: Antiparasitic; antiprotozoal.

Carnitor. (Sigma-Tau) Levocarnitine. **Soln.:** 100 mg/mL, sucrose, parabens, cherry flavor. Bot. 118 mL. **Tab.:** 330 mg. Bot. 90s. **Inj.:** 200 mg/mL, preservative-free. Single-dose vial, amp. *Rx.*
Use: Amino acid derivative.

•**caroxazone.** (kar-OX-ah-zone) USAN.
Use: Antidepressant.

•**carphenazine maleate.** (kar-FEN-azz-een) USAN.
Use: Antipsychotic.

•**carprofen.** (car-PRO-fen) USAN.
Use: Investigational analgesic, NSAID.

•**carrageenan.** (ka-rah-GEE-nan) *NF 29.*
Use: Pharmaceutic aid, suspending, viscosity-increasing agent.

Carrasyn. (Carrington) Phase I AIDS, ARC. *Rx.*
Use: Antiviral, immunomodulator.

•**carsatrin succinate.** (car-SAT-rin) USAN.
Use: Cardiovascular agent.

•**cartazolate.** (kar-TAZZ-oh-late) USAN.
Use: Antidepressant.

•**carteolol hydrochloride.** (KAR-tee-oh-lahl) *USP 34.*
Use: Antiadrenergic/sympatholytic, beta-adrenergic blocking agent; antiglaucoma.
See: Cartrol.

carteolol hydrochloride. (Various Mfr.) Carteolol hydrochloride 1%. Soln. Bot. 5 mL, 10 mL, 15 mL. *Rx.*
Use: Antiglaucoma; beta-adrenergic blocker.

Carter's Little Pills. (Carter-Wallace) Bisacodyl 5 mg. Bot. 30s, 85s. *OTC.*
Use: Laxative.

Cartia XT. (Andrx Pharmaceuticals) Diltiazem hydrochloride 120 mg, 180 mg, 240 mg, 300 mg. Sucrose. ER Cap. Box 30s, 90s, 500s, 1000s. *Rx.*
Use: Calcium channel blocker.

Cartrol. (Abbott) Carteolol hydrochloride 2.5 mg, 5 mg. Lactose. Tab. Bot. 100s. *Rx.*
Use: Antiadrenergic, sympatholytic, beta-adrenergic blocker.

•**carubicin hydrochloride.** (kah-ROO-bih-sin) USAN. *Formerly carminomycin hydrochloride.*
Use: Antineoplastic.

•**carumonam sodium.** (kah-roo-MOE-nam) USAN.
Use: Anti-infective.

•**carvedilol.** (CAR-veh-DILL-ole) USAN.
Use: Antianginal; antihypertensive; antiadrenergic/sympatholytic.
See: Coreg.

carvedilol. (Various Mfr.) Carvedilol 3.125 mg, 6.25 mg, 12.5 mg, 25 mg. May contain lactose, mannitol, sucrose. Tab. 28s, 30s, 100s, 500s, 1000s, UD 100s, blister 100s. *Rx.*
Use: Antiadrenergic/sympathomimetic, alpha/beta-adrenergic blocking agent.

carvedilol phosphate.
Use: Antiadrenergic/sympatholytic.
See: Coreg CR.

Car-Vit. (Mericon Industries) Ascorbic acid 60 mg, vitamins A acetate 4000 units, D-2 400 units, ferrous fumarate 90 mg (elemental iron 30 mg), oyster shell 600 mg (calcium 230 mg). Cap. Bot. 90s, 1000s. *OTC.*
Use: Mineral, vitamin supplement.

•**carvotroline hydrochloride.** (car-VAH-trah-leen) USAN.
Use: Antipsychotic.

•**carzelesin.** (car-ZELL-eh-sin) USAN.
Use: Antineoplastic, site-selective DNA binding.

carzenide.
Use: Carbonic anhydrase inhibitor.

casa-dicole. (Halsey Drug) Docusate sodium 100 mg, casanthrol 30 mg. Cap. Bot. 100s. OTC.
Use: Laxative.

•**casanthranol.** (kass-AN-thrah-nole) USP 34. A purified mixture of the anthranol glycosides derived from cascara sagrada.
Use: Laxative.
W/Docusate Sodium.
See: Calotabs.
Dio-Soft.
Docusate with Casanthranol.
Easy-Lax Plus.
Laxative & Stool Softener.

Cascara. (Eli Lilly) Cascara 150 mg. Tab. Bot. 100s. OTC.
Use: Laxative.

Cascara Aromatic. (Humco Holding Group) Cascara sagrada, alcohol 18%. Liq. Bot. 120 mL, 473 mL. OTC.
Use: Laxative.

cascara fluid extract, aromatic.
Use: Laxative.

cascara glycosides.
Use: Laxative.

•**cascara sagrada.** (kass-KA-rah sah-GRAH-dah) USP 34.
Use: Cathartic.
See: Bilstan.
Cascara Aromatic.
Nature's Remedy.

cascara sagrada fluid extract.
(Intramed) Alcohol 18%/5 mL. Bot. Pt, gal, UD 5 mL.
Use: Laxative. [Orphan Drug]

cascarin.
See: Casanthranol.

Casodex. (AstraZeneca) Bicalutamide 50 mg, lactose. Tab. Bot. 30s, 100s, UD 30s. Rx.
Use: Antineoplastic; hormone, antimutagenic.

•**casopitant mesylate.** (KAS-oh-pi-tant) USAN.
Use: CNS agent.

•**caspofungin acetate.** (KASS-poe-FUN-jin) USAN.
Use: Antifungal.
See: Cancidas.

CAST. (Biomerica) Reagent test for immunoglobulin E in serum. Tube Kit 25s.
Use: Diagnostic aid.

Castellani Paint Modified. (Pedinol Pharmacal) Basic fuchsin, phenol resorcinol, acetone. Bot. 30 mL, 120 mL, 480 mL. Also available as colorless solution without basic fuchsin.

Bot. 30 mL, 120 mL, 480 mL. Rx.
Use: Antifungal, topical.

Castellani's Paint. (Penta) Carbolfuchsin solution. Fuchsin 0.3%, phenol 4.5%, resorcinol 10%, acetone 1.5%, alcohol 13%. Bot. 1 oz, 4 oz, pt. Rx.
Use: Antifungal, topical.

•**castor oil.** (KASS-ter) USP 34.
Use: Laxative; pharmaceutic aid, plasticizer.
See: Emulsoil.
W/Combinations.
See: Xenaderm.

castor oil. (Various Mfr.) Castor oil. Liq. Bot. 60 mL, 120 mL, 480 mL. OTC.
Use: Laxative; pharmaceutic aid, plasticizer.

castor oil, hydrogenated.
Use: Laxative.

Cataflam. (Novartis) Diclofenac 50 mg (as potassium). Sucrose. Tab. Bot. 100s, UD 100s. Rx.
Use: Analgesic, NSAID.

Catapres. (Boehringer Ingelheim) Clonidine hydrochloride 0.1 mg, 0.2 mg, 0.3 mg. Lactose. Tab. 100s. Rx.
Use: Antiadrenergic/sympatholytic; antiadrenergic agent, centrally acting.

Catapres-TTS-1. (Boehringer Ingelheim) Clonidine hydrochloride 0.1 mg/24 h (surface area, 3.5 cm^2) (total clonidine content, 2.5 mg). Mineral oil. Transdermal patch. 12s. Rx.
Use: Antiadrenergic/sympatholytic; antiadrenergic agent, centrally acting.

Catapres-TTS-3. (Boehringer Ingelheim) Clonidine hydrochloride 0.3 mg/24 h (surface area, 10.5 cm^2) (total clonidine content, 7.5 mg). Mineral oil. Transdermal patch. 4s. Rx.
Use: Antiadrenergic/sympatholytic; antiadrenergic agent, centrally acting.

Catapres-TTS-2. (Boehringer Ingelheim) Clonidine hydrochloride 0.2 mg/24 h (surface area, 7 cm^2) (total clonidine content, 5 mg). Mineral oil. Transdermal patch. 12s. Rx.
Use: Antiadrenergic/sympatholytic; antiadrenergic agent, centrally acting.

Catatrol. (AstraZeneca) Viloxazine.
Use: Antidepressant.

catechins.
Use: Treatment of external genital and perianal warts.
See: Kunecatechins.

Cathflo Activase. (Genentech) Alteplase 2 mg, L-arginine, phosphoric acid, polysorbate 80. Pow. for Inj., lyophilized. Vials. Rx.
Use: Thrombolytic.

cathomycin calcium. Calcium novobiocin.
Use: Anti-infective.

cathomycin sodium. Novobiocin sodium.
Use: Anti-infective.

cationic resins.
See: Sodium-Removing Resins.

•**catramilast.** (ka-TRA-mil-ast) USAN.
Use: Dermatologic.

Caverject. (Pharmacia & Upjohn) Alprostadil. **Inj., aqueous:** 10 mcg/mL, 20 mcg/mL, 40 mcg/2 mL Amps. 1 mL and kit with 2 mL *Luer-lock* syringe, 2½-inch needles (one 27-gauge and one 30-gauge) alcohol swab. **Pow. for Inj., lyophilized:** 5 mcg/mL, 10 mcg/mL, 20 mcg/mL, 40 mcg/mL, benzyl alcohol 8.4 mg, lactose. Vials, vials with diluent syringes (except 40 mcg/mL). *Rx.*
Use: Anti-impotence agent.

Caverject Impulse. (Pharmacia & Upjohn) Alprostadil 10 mcg/0.5 mL, 20 mcg/0.5 mL, benzyl alcohol 4.45 mg, lactose. Blister tray containing 1 dual chamber syringe system, 1 needle, 2 alcohol swabs. *Rx.*
Use: Anti-impotence agent.

Cav-X Fluoride Treatment. (Palisades Pharmaceuticals) Stannous fluoride 0.4%. Gel. Bot. 121.9 g. *Rx.*
Use: Dental caries agent.

Cayston. (Gilead Sciences) Aztreonam 75 mg. Lysine 46.7 mg. Preservative free and arginine free. Pow. for Soln., lyophilized; Inhal. Single-dose vial. 2 mL w/1 mL ampule of sodium chloride 0.17% diluent. *Rx.*
Use: Anti-infective agent, monobactam.

Caziant. (Watson) **Phase 1:** Desogestrel 0.1 mg, ethinyl estradiol 25 mcg. **Phase 2:** Desogestrel 0.125 mg, ethinyl estradiol 25 mcg. **Phase 3:** Desogestrel 0.15 mg, ethinyl estradiol 25 mcg.Lactose. 28-day blister card w/7 green inert tablets. Tab. *Rx.*
Use: Oral contraceptive, oral triphasic contraceptive.

C-Bio. (Barth's) Vitamin C 150 mg, citrus bioflavonoid complex 100 mg, rutin 50 mg. Tab. Bot. 100s, 500s, 1000s. *OTC.*
Use: Vitamin supplement.

C-B Time. (Arco) Vitamins C 300 mg, B_1 15 mg, B_2 10 mg, B_3 100 mg, B_5 20 mg, B_6 5 mg, B_{12} 5 mcg. Liq. Bot. 120 mL. *OTC.*
Use: Vitamin supplement.

CC-Galactosidase. Alpha-galactosidase A.
Use: Fabry disease. [Orphan Drug]

CCNU. Lomustine.
Use: Antineoplastic.
See: CeeNU.

C-Crystals. (NBTY) Vitamin C 5000 mg/tsp. Crystals. Bot. 180 g. *OTC.*
Use: Vitamin supplement.

CDDP.
Use: Antineoplastic.
See: Cisplatin.

C.D.P. (Ivax) Chlordiazepoxide hydrochloride 5 mg, 10 mg, 25 mg. Cap. Bot. 100s, 500s, 1000s. *c-iv.*
Use: Anxiolytic.

Cea. (Abbott Diagnostics) Radioimmunoassay or enzyme immunoassay for quantitative measurement of carcinoembryonic antigen in human serum or plasma. Test Kit 100s.
Use: Diagnostic aid.

Cea-Roche. (Roche) Radioimmunoassay capable of detecting and measuring plasma levels of CEA in the nanogram range. Sensitivity-0.5 ng/mL of CEA.
Use: Diagnostic aid.

Cea-Roche Test Kit. (Roche) Carcinoembryonic antigen, a glycoprotein which is a constituent of the glycocalyx of embryonic entodermal epithelium. Test Kit.
Use: Diagnostic aid.

CEA-Scan. (Immunomedics; Mallinckrodt-Baker) Arcitumomab 1.25 mg. Reconstitute with Tc 99m sodium pertechnetate in NaCl for Inj. Inj. Single-dose Vial. *Rx.*
Use: For detection of recurrent or metastatic colorectal carcinoma of the liver, extrahepatic abdomen and pelvis; radioimmunoscintigraphy.

Ceb Nuggets. (Scot-Tussin) Vitamins B_1 15 mg, B_2 15 mg, B_6 5 mg, B_{12} 5 mcg, C 600 mg, niacinamide 100 mg, E 40 units, calcium pantothenate 20 mg, folic acid 0.1 mg. Nugget. Bot. 60s. *OTC.*
Use: Mineral, vitamin supplement.

Cebo-Caps. (Forest) Placebo capsules. *OTC.*
Use: Vitamin supplement.

Ceclor. (Eli Lilly) Cefaclor 125 mg/5 mL, 187 mg/5 mL, 250 mg/5 mL, 375 mg/5 mL. Sucrose, strawberry flavor. Pow. for Oral Susp. Bot. 50 mL (187 mg/5 mL, 375 mg/mL), 75 mL (125 mg/5 mL, 250 mg/5 mL), 100 mL (187 mg/5 mL, 375 mg/5 mL), 150 mL (125 mg/5 mL, 250 mg/5 mL). *Rx.*
Use: Anti-infective, cephalosporin.

Ceclor Pulvules. (Eli Lilly) Cefaclor 250 mg. Cap. Bot. 15s, 100s, UD 100s. *Rx.*
Use: Anti-infective, cephalosporin.

Cecon. (Abbott) Ascorbic acid 100 mg/mL. Soln. Bot. w/dropper 50 mL. *OTC.*
Use: Water-soluble vitamin.

Cedax. (Pernix Therapeutics) **Cap.:** Ceftibuten 400 mg. Parabens. Bot. 20s. **Pow. for Oral Susp.:** Ceftibuten 90 mg/5 mL, 180 mg/5 mL. Polysorbate 80, sodium benzoate, sucrose. Cherry flavor. 30 mL (180 mg/5 mL only); 60 mL; 90 mL, 120 mL (90 mg/5 mL only). *Rx.*
Use: Anti-infective, cephalosporin.

• **cedefingol.** (seh-deh-FIN-gole) USAN.
Use: Antineoplastic, adjunct; antipsoriatic.

• **cedelizumab.** (sed-eh-LIE-zoo-mab) USAN.
Use: Monoclonal antibody; immunosuppressant.

Ceebevim. (NBTY) Vitamins B_1 15 mg, B_2 10.2 mg, B_3 50 mg, B_5 10 mg, B_6 5 mg, C 300 mg. Cap. Bot. 100s, 300s. *OTC.*
Use: Vitamin supplement.

CeeNU. (Bristol Labs Oncology) Lomustine (CCNU) 10 mg, 40 mg, 100 mg, mannitol. Cap. 20s, dose pk. of 2 cap. each of all 3 strengths. *Rx.*
Use: Antineoplastic, alkylating agent.

Ceepa. (Geneva) Theophylline 130 mg, ephedrine hydrochloride 24 mg, phenobarbital 8 mg. Tab. Bot. 100s, 1000s. *Rx.*
Use: Bronchodilator; decongestant; hypnotic; sedative.

Ceepryn. Cetylpyridinium chloride. *OTC.*
Use: Antiseptic.
See: Cēpacol.

Cee with Bee. (Wesley) Vitamins B_1 15 mg, B_2 10.2 mg, B_3 50 mg, B_5 10 mg, B_6 5 mg, C 300 mg, tartrazine. Bot. 100s, 1000s. *OTC.*
Use: Vitamin supplement.

• **cefaclor.** (SEFF-uh-klor) *USP 34.*
Use: Anti-infective, cephalosporin.
See: Ceclor.
Raniclor.

cefaclor. (Various Mfr.) Cefaclor. **Cap.:** 250 mg, 500 mg. Bot. 15s (500 mg), 30s (250 mg), 100s, 500s, 1000s (250 mg). **Pow. for Oral Susp.:** 125 mg/5 mL, 187 mg/5 mL, 250 mg/5 mL, 375 mg/5 mL. Bot. 50 mL (187 mg/5 mL, 375 mg/5 mL only), 75 mL (125 mg/5 mL, 250 mg/5 mL only), 100 mL (187mg/5 mL, 375 mg/5 mL only), 150 mL (125 mg/5 mL, 250 mg/5 mL only). *Rx.*
Use: Anti-infective.

cefaclor. (Zenith Goldline) Cefaclor 375 mg, 500 mg. ER Tab. Bot. 100s. *Rx.*
Use: Anti-infective.

• **cefadroxil.** (SEFF-uh-DROX-ill) *USP 34.*
Use: Anti-infective, cephalosporin.

cefadroxil. (Various Mfr.) Cefadroxil (as monohydrate). **Cap.:** 500 mg. Bot 100s. **Tab.:** 1 g. Bot 24s, 50s, 100s, 500s. *Rx.*
Use: Anti-infective, cephalosporin.

• **cefamandole.** (SEFF-ah-MAN-dole) USAN.

• **cefamandole sodium for injection.** (SEFF-ah-MAN-dole) *USP 34.*
Use: Anti-infective, cephalosporin.

Cefanex. (Apothecon) Cephalexin monohydrate 250 mg, 500 mg. Cap. Bot. 100s.
Use: Anti-infective, cephalosporin.

• **cefaparole.** (SEFF-ah-pah-ROLE) USAN.
Use: Anti-infective.

• **cefatrizine.** (SEFF-ah-TRY-zeen) USAN.
Use: Anti-infective, cephalosporin.

• **cefazaflur sodium.** (seff-AZE-ah-flure) USAN.
Use: Anti-infective, cephalosporin.

• **cefazolin sodium.** (seff-AH-zoe-lin) USAN.
Tall Man: ceFAZolin
Use: Anti-infective, cephalosporin.

cefazolin sodium. (Apothecon) Cefazolin sodium 500 mg, 1 g, 5 g, 10 g, 20 g. Sodium 2.1 mEq/g. Pow. for Inj. Vials, piggyback vials (except 10 g, 20 g); pharmacy bulk packages (10 g, 20 g only). *Rx.*
Use: Anti-infective.

• **cefbuperazone.** (SEFF-byoo-PURR-ah-zone) USAN.
Use: Anti-infective, cephalosporin.

• **cefdinir.** (SEFF-dih-ner) USAN.
Use: Anti-infective, cephalosporin.
See: Omnicef.

cefdinir. (Various Mfr.) Cefdinir. **Cap.:** 300 mg. 60s, 100s, UD 10s, UD 50s. **Susp.:** 125 mg/5 mL, 250 mg/5 mL. May contain sucrose. Strawberry or cherry flavor. 60 mL, 100 mL. *Rx.*
Use: Anti-infective, cephalosporin.

• **cefditoren pivoxil.** (SEFF-dih-TOR-en pih-VOX-ill) USAN.
Use: Anti-infective.
See: Spectracef.

cefditoren pivoxil. (Aristos) Cefditoren (as cefditoren pivoxil) 200 mg, 400 mg. May contain mannitol, sodium cassinate. Tab. Blister pack. 20s, 28s (400 mg only). *Rx.*
Use: Anti-infective agent, cephalosporin and related antibiotic.

• **cefepime.** (SEFF-eh-pim) USAN.
Use: Anti-infective.

cefepime. (Baxter) Cefepime. Inj., Soln. **1 g:** Dextrose 1.03 g. 50 mL single-dose *Galaxy* containers. **2 g:** Dextrose 2.06 g. 100 mL single-dose *Galaxy* containers. *Rx.*
Use: Anti-infective agent, cephalosporin and related antibiotic.

•**cefepime hydrochloride.** (SEFF-eh-pim) USAN.
Use: Anti-infective.

cefepime hydrochloride. (Apotex USA) Cefepime hydrochloride 500 mg, 1 g, 2 g. Inj., Pow. for Soln. Vials. 1s, 10s. *Rx.*
Use: Anti-infective.

•**cefetecol.** (seff-EH-teh-kahl) USAN.
Use: Antibacterial, cephalosporin.

Cefinal II. (Alto) Salicylamide 150 mg, acetaminophen 250 mg, doxylamine succinate 25 mg. Tab. Bot. 100s. *OTC.*
Use: Analgesic combination.

•**cefixime.** (sef-IX-eem) *USP 34.*
Use: Anti-infective, cephalosporin.
See: Suprax.

Cefizox. (Fujisawa) Ceftizoxime sodium. **Pow. for Inj. (sodium 2.6 mEq/g, as sodium):** 500 mg (single-dose fliptop vials 10 mL); 1 g, 2 g (single-dose flip-top vials 20 mL, piggyback vial 100 mL); 10 g (pharmacy bulk pkg). **Inj. (as sodium):** 1 g, 2 g. Frozen, premixed, single-dose plastic containers 50 mL. *Rx.*
Use: Anti-infective, cephalosporin.

•**cefmenoxime hydrochloride, sterile.** (SEFF-men-ox-eem) *USP 34.*
Use: Anti-infective, cephalosporin.

•**cefmetazole.** (seff-MET-ah-zole) *USP 34.*
Use: Anti-infective, cephalosporin.

•**cefmetazole for injection.** (seff-MET-ah-zole) *USP 34.*
Use: Anti-infective, cephalosporin.

•**cefmetazole sodium.** (seff-MET-ah-zole) *USP 34.*
Use: Anti-infective, cephalosporin.

•**cefonicid monosodium.** (seh-FAHN-ih-SID MAHN-oh-SO-dee-uhm) USAN.
Use: Anti-infective, cephalosporin.

•**cefoperazone sodium.** (SEFF-oh-PUR-uh-zone) *USP 34.*
Use: Anti-infective, cephalosporin.

•**ceforanide for injection.** (seh-FAR-ah-NIDE) *USP 34.*
Use: Anti-infective, cephalosporin.

cefotaxime. (Cura) Cefotaxime 1 g, 2 g. Sodium 2.2 mEq/g. Inj. Infusion bottles. Packages of 25. *Rx.*
Use: Antibiotic.

cefotaxime. (Various Mfr.) Cefotaxime 500 mg, 1 g, 2 g, 10 g. Sodium 2.2 mEq/ g. Pow. for Inj. Vials. Packages of 10 (500 mg only), packages of 25 (1 g, 2 g only), bottles (10 g only). *Rx.*
Use: Antibiotic.

•**cefotaxime sodium.** (seff-oh-TAX-eem) *USP 34.*
Use: Anti-infective, cephalosporin.
See: Claforan.

•**cefotetan.** (SEFF-oh-tee-tan) *USP 34.*
Tall Man: cefoTEtan
Use: Anti-infective, cephalosporin.

•**cefotetan disodium.** (SEFF-oh-tee-tan die-SO-dee-uhm) *USP 34.*
Use: Anti-infective.

cefotetan disodium. (Abraxis) Cefotetan 1 g, 2 g, 10 g. Sodium 3.5 mEq/mL. Inj., Pow. for Soln. Vials (1 g only), 20 mL (2 g and 10 g only). *Rx.*
Use: Anti-infective, cephalosporin.

•**cefotiam hydrochloride sterile.** (SEFF-oh-TIE-am) *USP 34.*
Use: Anti-infective, cephalosporin.

•**cefovecin sodium.** (sef-OH-vee-sin) USAN.
Use: Antibacterial (veterinary).

•**cefoxitin.** (seff-OX-ih-tin) USAN.
Tall Man: cefOXitan
Use: Anti-infective, cephalosporin.

cefoxitin. (American Pharmaceutical Partners) Cefoxitin (as sodium) 1 g, 2 g, 10 g. Pow. for Inj. Vials and infusion bottles (1 g, 2 g); pharmacy bulk packages (10 g). *Rx.*
Use: Anti-infective, cephalosporin.

cefoxitin and dextrose. (B. Braun Mc-Gaw) Cefoxitin sodium 1 g, 2 g. Dextrose 50 mL. Preservative free. Inj., Pow. for Soln. Single-use *Duplex* drug delivery system container. *Rx.*
Use: Anti-infective agent, cephalosporin and related antibiotic.

•**cefoxitin sodium.** (seff-OX-ih-tin) *USP 34.*
Tall Man: cefOXitan
Use: Anti-infective, cephalosporin.

•**cefpimizole.** (seff-PIH-mih-zole) USAN.
Use: Anti-infective, cephalosporin.

•**cefpimizole sodium.** (seff-PIH-mih-zole) USAN.
Use: Anti-infective, cephalosporin.

•**cefpiramide.** (SEFF-PIHR-am-ide) USAN.
Use: Anti-infective, cephalosporin.

•**cefpiramide sodium.** (SEFF-PIHR-am-ide) USAN.
Use: Anti-infective, cephalosporin.

•**cefpirome sulfate.** (SEFF-pihr-ome) USAN.
Use: Anti-infective, cephalosporin.

•**cefpodoxime proxetil.** (SEFF-pode-OX-eem PROX-uh-til) *USP 34.*
Use: Anti-infective, cephalosporin.
See: Vantin.

cefpodoxime proxetil. (Aurobindo) Cefpodoxime proxetil. **Tab.:** 100 mg, 200 mg. Lactose. Film-coated. 20s. **Susp.:** 50 mg/5 mL, 100 mg/5 mL. Lactose, sucrose. 50 mL, 75 mL, 100 mL. *Rx.*
Use: Cephalosporin.

•**cefprozil.** (SEFF-pro-zill) *USP 34.*
Use: Anti-infective, cephalosporin.

cefprozil. (Various Mfr.) **Pow. for Oral Susp.:** Cefprozil (as anhydrous when reconstituted) 125 mg per 5 mL, 250 mg per 5 mL. May contain aspartame, sucrose, phenylalanine. 50 mL, 75 mL, 100 mL. **Tab.:** Cefprozil (as anhydrous) 250 mg, 500 mg. 50s (500 mg only), 100s. *Rx.*
Use: Anti-infective.

•**cefroxadine.** (SEFF-ROX-ah-deen) USAN.
Use: Anti-infective, cephalosporin.

•**cefsulodin sodium.** (SEFF-SULL-oh-din) USAN.
Use: Anti-infective, cephalosporin.

•**ceftaroline fosamil.** (sef-TAR-oh-leen FOS-a-mil) USAN.
Use: Anti-infective, cephalosporin.
See: Teflaro.

•**ceftazidime.** (seff-TAZE-ih-deem) *USP 34.*
Tall Man: cefTAZidime
Use: Anti-infective, cephalosporin.
See: Ceptaz.
Fortaz.
Tazicef.
Tazidime.

ceftazidime. (Sandoz) Ceftazidime 1 g, 2 g, 6 g. Sodium 2.3 mEq/g. Pow. for Inj. Vials (except 6 g). Bulk packages (6 g only). *Rx.*
Use: Antibiotic.

•**ceftibuten.** (seff-TIE-byoo-ten) USAN.
Use: Anti-infective.
See: Cedax.

Ceftin. (GlaxoWellcome) Cefuroxime (as axetil). **Tab.:** 125 mg, 250 mg, 500 mg. Film-coated. Bot. 10s (250 mg only), 20s, 60s (except 125 mg), UD 50s (500 mg only), 100s (except 500 mg). **Susp.:** 125 mg/5 mL, 250 mg/5 mL. Sucrose. Tutti-frutti flavor. Bot. 50 mL, 100 mL. *Rx.*
Use: Anti-infective, cephalosporin.

•**ceftizoxime sodium.** (SEFF-tih-ZOX-eem) *USP 34.*
Use: Anti-infective, cephalosporin.
See: Cefizox.

•**ceftobiprole.** (sef-TOE-bye-prole) USAN.
Use: Antibiotic.

•**ceftobiprole medocaril.** (sef-TOE-bye-prole me-DOK-a-ril) USAN.
Use: Antibiotic.

•**ceftriaxone sodium.** (SEFF-TRY-AXE-own) *USP 34.*
Tall Man: cefTRIAXone
Use: Anti-infective, cephalosporin.
See: Rocephin.

✓ **ceftriaxone sodium.** (Various Mfr.) Ceftriaxone sodium (as base). **Inj.:** 1 g, 2 g. May contain dextrose. Sodium 3.6 mEq/g. 50 mL *ADD-Vantage* vials. **Pow. for Inj.:** 250 mg, 500 mg, 1 g, 2 g, 10 g. Sodium 3.6 mEq per g. Vials (except 10 g), bulk containers (10 g only). *Rx.*
Use: Anti-infective.

•**cefuroxime.** (SEFF-yur-OX-eem) USAN.
Use: Anti-infective, cephalosporin.

•**cefuroxime axetil.** (SEFF-your-OX-eem ACK-seh-TILL) *USP 34.*
Use: Anti-infective, cephalosporin.
See: Ceftin.

cefuroxime axetil. (Ranbaxy) Cefuroxime (as axetil). **Oral Susp.:** 125 mg/5 mL, 250 mg/5 mL when reconstituted. Aspartame, mannitol, phenylalanine 4.5 mg/5 mL, sucrose. Fruit flavor. 50 mL, 100 mL. **Tab.:** 125 mg, 250 mg, 500 mg. 20s (250 mg, 500 mg), 60s, 100s. *Rx.*
Use: Anti-infective, cephalosporin.

•**cefuroxime pivoxetil.** (SEFF-your-OX-eem pih-VOX-eh-till) USAN.
Use: Anti-infective, cephalosporin.

•**cefuroxime sodium.** (SEFF-your-OX-eem) *USP 34.*
Use: Anti-infective, cephalosporin.
See: Zinacef.

cefuroxime sodium. (Various Mfr.) Cefuroxime sodium 750 mg, 1.5 g, 7.5 g. Sodium 2.4 mEq/g. Pow. for Inj. Vials. 10 mL (750 mg only), 20 mL (1.5 g only), 100 mL piggyback vials (750 mg, 1.5 g only), pharmacy bulk package (7.5 g only). *Rx.*
Use: Anti-infective, cephalosporin.

Celebrex. (Searle) Celecoxib 50 mg, 100 mg, 200 mg, 400 mg. Lactose. Cap. Bot. 60s (50 mg, 400 mg only); 100s, 500s (except 50 mg, 400 mg); UD 100s (except 50 mg). *Rx.*
Tall Man: CeleBREX
Use: Nonsteroidal anti-inflammatory agent.

•**celecoxib.** (cell-ih-COX-ib) USAN.
Use: Nonsteroidal anti-inflammatory agent.
See: Celebrex.

Celestone. (Schering) Betamethasone 0.6 mg/5 mL. Alcohol, sorbitol, sugar. Soln. Bot. 118 mL. *Rx.*
Use: Adrenocortical steroid, glucocorticoid.

Celestone Soluspan. (Schering) Betamethasone sodium phosphate 3 mg, betamethasone acetate 3 mg/mL, EDTA, benzalkonium chloride. Multidose vials. 5 mL. *Rx.*
Use: Adrenocortical steroid, glucocorticoid.

Celexa. (Forest) Citalopram hydrobromide. **Tab.:** 10 mg, 20 mg, 40 mg, lactose. Bot. 100s, UD 100s (except 10 mg). **Oral Soln.:** 10 mg/5 mL, sorbitol, parabens, peppermint flavor. Bot. 240 mL. *Rx.*
Tall Man: CeleXA
Use: Antidepressant, SSRI.

•**celgosivir hydrochloride.** (sell-GO-sih-vihr) USAN.
Use: Antiviral; inhibitor, alpha-glucoside.

•**celiprolol hydrochloride.** (SEE-lih-PRO-lahl) USAN.
Use: Investigational beta-adrenergic blocking agent.

Cellaburate. (Eastman Kodak) Cellulose acetate butyrate.
Use: Pharmaceutic aid, plastic-filming agent.

cellacefate.
Use: Pharmaceutic aid, tablet coating agent.
See: Cellulose Acetate Phthalate.

CellCept. (Roche) Mycophenolate mofetil. **Cap.:** 250 mg. Bot. 100s, 120s, 500s. **Pow. for Soln., Inj., lyophilized:** 500 mg (as mycophenolate mofetil hydroxide). Preservative free. Vials. 20 mL. **Pow. for Oral Susp.:** 200 mg/mL (when reconstituted). Aspartame, methylparaben, sorbitol, phenylalanine 0.56 mg/mL, mixed fruit flavor. Bot. 225 mL. **Tab.:** 500 mg. Alcohols, PEG. Film-coated. Bot. 100s, 500s. *Rx.*
Use: Immunosuppressant.

Cellepacbin. (Arthrins) Vitamins A 1200 units, B_1 1.5 mg, B_2 1.5 mg, B_6 0.75 mg, niacinamide 7.5 mg, panthenol 3 mg, C 20 mg, B_{12} 2 mcg, E 1 units. Cap. Bot. 180s. *OTC.*
Use: Vitamin supplement.

Cellothyl. (Numark) Methylcellulose 0.5 g. Tab. Bot. 100s, 1000s. *OTC.*
Use: Laxative.

cellular chemokine receptor (CCR5) antagonist.
Use: Antiretroviral agent.
See: Maraviroc.

•**cellulase.** (SELL-you-lace) USAN. A concentrate of cellulose-splitting enzymes derived from *Aspergillus niger* and other sources.
Use: Enzyme, digestive adjunct.
W/Amylase, Hyoscyamine Sulfate, Lipase, Phenyltoloxamine Citrate, Protease.
See: Digex.

cellulolytic enzyme.
See: Cellulase.

cellulose.
W/Combinations.
See: Zeasorb.

•**cellulose acetate.** (SELL-you-lohs) *NF 29.*
Use: Pharmaceutic aid, coating agent; polymer membrane, insoluble.

•**cellulose acetate phthalate.** (SELL-you-lohs ASS-eh-tate THAL-ate) *NF 29.*
Use: Pharmaceutic aid, tablet coating agent.
See: Cellacefate.

•**cellulose, carboxymethyl, sodium salt.** (SELL-you-lohs kar-BOX-ee-meth-ill) *USP 34.* Carboxymethylcellulose sodium.

•**cellulose, hydroxypropyl methyl ether.** (SELL-you-lohs, hi-DROX-ee-pro-pill meth-ill E-thur) *USP 34.* Hydroxypropyl methylcellulose.

cellulose methyl ether.
See: Methylcellulose.

•**cellulose microcrystalline.** (SELL-you-lohs my-KROE-cris-tahl-een) *NF 29.*
Use: Pharmaceutic aid, tablet and capsule diluent.

cellulose, nitrate. Pyroxylin.

•**cellulose, oxidized.** (SELL-you-lohs, OX-ih-dized) *USP 34.*
Use: Hemostatic.

•**cellulose, oxidized regenerated.** (SELL-you-lohs, OX-ih-dized) *USP 34.*
Use: Hemostatic.

cellulose, powdered.
Use: Tablet and capsule diluent.

•**cellulose sodium phosphate.** (SELL-you-lohs) *USP 34.*
Use: Antiurolithic.
See: Calcibind.

cellulosic acid.
See: Oxidized Cellulose.

Celluvisc. (Allergan) Carboxymethylcellulose 1%, NaCl, KCl, sodium lactate. Ophth. Soln. Single-use containers 0.3 mL (UD 30s). *OTC.*
Use: Artificial tears.

Celontin. (Pfizer US) Methsuximide 300 mg. Cap. 100s. *Rx.*
Use: Anticonvulsant.

Cena-K. (Century) Potassium and chloride 20 mEq/15 mL (10% KCl), saccharin. Bot. Pt, gal. *Rx.*
Use: Electrolyte supplement.

Cenalax. (Century) Bisacodyl. **Tab.:** 5 mg. Bot. 100s, 1000s. **Supp.:** 10 mg. Pkg. 12s, 1000s. *OTC.*
Use: Laxative.

●**cenderitide.** (sen-DER-i-tide) USAN.
Use: Cardiovascular agent.

Cenestin. (Barr/Duramed) Synthetic conjugated estrogens, A, 0.3 mg, 0.45 mg, 0.625 mg, 0.9 mg, 1.25 mg. Lactose. Film-coated. Tab. Bot. 30s, 100s, 1000s. *Rx.*
Use: Estrogen, sex hormone.

Cenhist. (Centurion Labs) Brompheniramine maleate 6 mg, phenylephrine hydrochloride 15 mg, Saccharin, sucralose, xylitol. Orange flavor. Chew. Tab. 60s. *OTC.*
Use: Upper respiratory combination, decongestant and antihistamine.

●**cenicriviroc.** (SEN-i-kri-VIR-ok) USAN.
Use: Treatment of HIV infection and arthritis.

●**cenicriviroc mesylate.** (SEN-i-kri-VIR-ok) USAN.
Use: Treatment of HIV infection and arthritis.

●**cenplacel-L.** (SEN-pla-sel-el) USAN.
Use: Immunomodulator.

Centany. (Medimetriks Pharmaceuticals) Mupirocin 2%. Alcohol, carylic/capric/myristic/stearic triglyceride, castor oil, propylene glycol. Oint. 30 g; kits w/ gauze pads and latex-free cloth tape strips. *Rx.*
Use: Topical anti-infective, antibiotic.

Centeon Thyroid. (Aventis) Desiccated animal thyroid glands (active thyroid hormones) T-4 thyroxine, T-3 thyronine 0.25 g, 0.5 g, 1 g, 1.5 g, 2 g, 3 g, 4 g, 5 g. Tab. Bot. 100s, 1000s. Handy Hundreds, Carton Strip 100s. *Rx.*
Use: Hormone, thyroid.

Center-Al. (Center) Allergenic extracts, alum precipitated 10,000 PNU/mL, 20,000 PNU/mL. Vial 10 mL, 30 mL. *Rx.*
Use: Antiallergic.

Centergy DM. (Centurion Labs) Chlorpheniramine maleate 1 mg, dextromethorphan hydrobromide 3 mg, phenylephrine hydrochloride 2 mg per mL. Glycerin, sorbitol. Strawberry flavor. Drops. 30 mL. *Rx.*
Use: Upper respiratory combination, antitussive combination.

Centoxin. (Centocor) Nebacumab.
Use: Antibacterial. [Orphan Drug]

Centrafree. (NBTY) Iron 27 mg, vitamins A 5000 units, D 400 units, E 30 units, B_1 2.25 mg, B_2 2.6 mg, B_3 20 mg, B_5 10 mg, B_6 3 mg, B_{12} 9 mcg, C 90 mg, folic acid 0.4 mg, biotin 45 mcg, Ca, Cl, Cr, Cu, I, K, Mg, Mn, Mo, P, Se, Zn. Tab. Bot. 100s. *OTC.*
Use: Mineral, vitamin supplement.

central nervous system depressants.
See: Sedative/Hypnotic Agents.

central nervous system stimulants.
See: Amphetamines.
Analeptics.
Anorexiants.
Dexmethylphenidate Hydrochloride.
Methylphenidate Hydrochloride.

Centrovite Advanced Formula. (Rugby) Fe 18 mg, A 5000 units, D 400 units, E 30 units, B_1 1.5 mg, B_2 1.7 mg, B_3 20 mg, B_5 10 mg, B_6 2 mg, B_{12} 6 mcg, C 60 mg, Fa 0.4 mg, biotin 30 mcg, Ca, Cl, Cr, Cu, I, vitamin K, Mg, Mn, Mo, Ni, P, Se, Si, Sn, V, Zn, K. Tab. Bot. 100s. *OTC.*
Use: Mineral, vitamin supplement.

Centrovite Jr. (Rugby) Iron 18 mg, vitamins A 5000 units, D 400 units, E 15 units, B_1 1.5 mg, B_2 1.7 mg, B_3 20 mg, B_5 10 mg, B_6 2 mg, B_{12} 6 mcg, C 60 mg, folic acid 0.4 mg, biotin 45 mcg, Cr, Cu, I, Mg, Mn, Mo, Zn. Chew. Tab. Bot. 60s. *OTC.*
Use: Mineral, vitamin supplement.

Centrum. (Wyeth) Vitamins A 5000 units, E 30 units, C 90 mg, folic acid 400 mcg, B_1 2.25 mg, B_2 2.6 mg, B_6 3 mg, niacinamide 20 mg, B_{12} 9 mcg, D 400 units, biotin 45 mcg, pantothenic acid 10 mg, Ca 162 mg, P 125 mg, I 150 mcg, Fe 27 mg, Mg 100 mg, K 30 mg, Mn 5 mg, chromium 25 mcg, Se 25 mcg, Mo 25 mcg, Zn 15 mg, Cu 2 mg, vitamin K 25 mcg, Cl 27.2 mg. Tab. *OTC.*
Use: Mineral, vitamin supplement.

Centrum, Advanced Formula. (Wyeth) Vitamins A 2500 units, E 30 units, C 60 mg, B_1 1.5 mg, B_2 1.7 mg, B_3 20 mg, B_5 10 mg, B_6 2 mg, B_{12} 6 mcg, D_2 400 units, Fe 9 mg, biotin 300 mcg per 15 mL. With I, Zn, Mn, Cr, Mo, alcohol. 6.6%. Liq. Bot. 236 mL. *OTC.*
Use: Mineral, vitamin supplement.

Centrum Jr. (Wyeth) Vitamins A 5000 units, D 400 units, E 30 units, C 60 mg, folic acid 400 mcg, B_1 1.5 mg, B_6 2 mg, B_{12} 6 mcg, riboflavin 1.7 mg, niacinamide 20 mg, Fe 18 mg, Mg 25 mg, Cu 2 mg, Zn 10 mg, biotin 45 mcg, panthothenic acid 10 mg, Mo 20 mcg, chromium 20 mcg, I 150 mcg,

Mn 1 mg. Chew. Tab. Bot. 60s. *OTC.*
Use: Mineral, vitamin supplement.

Centrum Performance. (Wyeth) Ca 100 mg, Fe 18 mg, A 5000 units, D 400 units, E 60 units, B_1 4.5 mg, B_2 5.1 mg, B_3 40 mg, B_5 10 mg, B_6 6 mg, B_{12} 18 mcg, C 120 mg, folic acid 400 mcg, K 25 mcg, biotin 40 mcg, chloride 72 mcg, Ginkgo biloba leaf 60 mg, ginseng root 50 mg, B, Cr, Cu, I, K, Mg, Mn, Mo, Ni, P, Se, Si, Sn, V, Zn 15 mg, glucose, lactose, maltodextrin, sucrose. Tab. Bot. 120s. *OTC.*
Use: Mineral, vitamin supplement.

Centrum Silver. (Wyeth) Vitamin A 3500 units, D 400 units, E 45 units, B_1 1.5 mg, B_2 1.7 mg, B_3 20 mg, B_5 10 mg, B_6 3 mg, B_{12} 25 mcg, C 60 mg, folic acid 400 mcg, Zn 15 mg, vitamin K 10 mcg, biotin 30 mcg, chloride, lutein 250 mcg, B, Ca, Cr, Cu, I, K, Mg, Mn, Mo, Ni, P, Se, Si, V, sucrose, glucose. Tab. Bot. 220s. *OTC.*
Use: Mineral, vitamin supplement.

Centrum Silver Gel-Tabs. (Wyeth) Vitamins A 6000 units, D 400 units, E 45 units, B_1 1.5 mg, B_2 1.7 mg, B_3 20 mg, B_5 10 mg, B_6 3 mg, B_{12} 25 mcg, C 60 mg, K 10 mcg, biotin 30 mcg, folic acid 200 mcg, Fe 9 mg. With Ca 200 mg, Cu, I, Mg, P, Zn, Cl, Cr, Mn, Mo, Ni, K, Se, Si, V. Tab. Bot. 60s. *OTC.*
Use: Mineral, vitamin supplement.

Centrum Silver Ultra Women's. (Pfizer Consumer Healthcare) Vitamins A (43% as beta-carotene) 3,500 units, B_1 1.1 mg, B_2 1.1 mg, B_3 14 mg, B_5 5 mg, B_6 5 mg, B_{12} 50 mcg, C 100 mg, D 800 units, E 35 units, K, folic acid 400 mcg, biotin 30 mcg, Ca, Fe 8 mg, P, I, Mg, Zn, Se, Cu, Mn, Cr, Mo, Cl, potassium, Ni, Si, V, boron, lutein 300 mcg. Gelatin, hydrogenated palm oil, MCTs, PEG, polyvinyl alcohol, sucrose, maltodextrin, sunflower oil, soy. Tab. 100s. *OTC.*
Use: Nutritional supplement.

Centurion A-Z. (Mission Pharmacal) Fe 27 mg, A 5000 units, D 400 units, E 30 units, B_1 2.25 mg, B_2 2.6 mg, B_3 20 mg, B_5 10 mg, B_6 3 mg, B_{12} 9 mcg, C 90 mg, FA 0.4 mg, biotin 0.45 mg, Ca, Cl, Cr, Cu, I, K, Mg, Mn, Mo, P, Se, Zn, vitamin K. Tab. Bot. 130s. *OTC.*
Use: Mineral, vitamin supplement.

Ceo-Two. (Beutlich) Potassium bitartrate, sodium bicarbonate in polyethylene glycol base. Supp. Box 10s. *OTC.*
Use: Laxative.

Cēpacol. (Combe) Cetylpyridinium chloride 0.05%, alcohol denatured 14%, di-

sodium EDTA, glycerin, polysorbate 80, saccharin. Mouthwash. 24 oz, 32 oz. *OTC.*
Use: Mouth and throat product.

Cēpacol Dual Relief Sore Throat + Coating Spray. (Combe) Benzocaine 5%, glycerin 33%. Acesulfame K, PEG, SD alcohol 38B. Sugar free. Cherry flavor. Spray 22.2 mL. *OTC.*
Use: Topical anesthetic.

Cēpacol Fizzlers. (Combe) Benzocaine 6 mg. Corn syrup, mannitol, sodium bicarbonate, sucralose. Grape flavor. Tab., orally disintegrating. 12s. *OTC.*
Use: Mouth and throat product.

Cēpacol Maximum Numbing Sore Throat. (Combe) **Cherry flavor:** Benzocaine 15 mg, menthol 3.6 mg. Glucose, acesulfame K, propylene glycol, sucrose. Loz. 18s. **Citrus flavor:** Benzocaine 15 mg, menthol 2.1 mg. Maltitol, sucrose. Loz. 18s. **Honey-lemon flavor:** Benzocaine 15 mg, menthol 2.6 mg. Maltitol, sucrose. Loz. 18s. *OTC.*
Use: Mouth and throat product.

Cēpacol Menthol Regular Strength. (Combe) Menthol 3 mg. Glucose, peppermint oil, propylene glycol, sucrose. Loz. Blister 648s. *OTC.*
Use: Mouth and throat product.

Cēpacol Sore Throat From Post Nasal Drip. (Combe) Menthol 5.4 mg. Glucose, sucrose. Cherry flavor. 18s. *OTC.*
Use: Mouth and throat product.

Cēpacol Sore Throat Pain Relief Maximum Numbing. (Combe) Benzocaine 15 mg, menthol 4 mg. Acesulfame K, maltitol. Sugar free. Cherry flavor. Loz. 16s. *OTC.*
Use: Mouth and throat product.

Cēpacol Sore Throat + Coating Relief Maximum Numbing. (Combe) Benzocaine 15 mg, pectin 5 mg. Acesulfame K. Sugar free. Lemon lime flavor. Loz.18s. *OTC.*
Use: Mouth and throat product.

Cēpacol Sore Throat Plus Cough Relief. (Combe) Benzocaine 7.5 mg, dextromethorphan HBr 5 mg. Glucose, sucrose. Mixed berry flavor. Loz. 18s. *OTC.*
Use: Nonnarcotic antitussive.

Cēpastat Cherry Lozenges. (GlaxoSmithKline) Phenol 14.5 mg, menthol, sorbitol, saccharin. Sugar free. Loz. Box 18s. *OTC.*
Use: Anesthetic.

Cēpastat Extra Strength. (GlaxoSmithKline) Phenol 29 mg, menthol, sorbitol, eucalyptus oil. Sugar free. Loz. Pkg. 18s. *OTC.*

Use: Anesthetic.

•**cephacetrile sodium.** (SEFF-ah-seh-TRILE) USAN.
Use: Anti-infective, cephalosporin.

Cephadyn. (Atley Pharmaceuticals) Acetaminophen 650 mg, butalbital 50 mg. Tab. 100s, 500s. *Rx.*
Use: Nonnarcotic analgesic combination, nonnarcotic analgesic with barbiturate.

•**cephalexin.** (SEFF-ah-LEX-in) *USP 34.*
Use: Anti-infective, cephalosporin.
See: Keflex.

cephalexin. (Various Mfr.) Cephalexin.
Cap.: 250 mg, 500 mg. Bot. 100s, 250s (500 mg), 500s, 1000s, UD 20s, 100s. **Tab.:** 250 mg, 500 mg. Bot. 20s, 100s, 500s. **Pow. for Oral Susp.:** 125 mg/5 mL, 250 mg/5 mL. Bot. 100 mL, 200 mL. *Rx.*
Use: Anti-infective, cephalosporin.

cephalin.
W/Lecithin with Choline Base, Lipositol.
See: Alcolec.

•**cephaloglycin.** (SEFF-ah-low-GLIE-sin) USAN.
Use: Anti-infective.

•**cephaloridine.** (SEFF-ah-lor-ih-deen) USAN.
Use: Anti-infective, cephalosporin.

cephalosporins and related antibiotics.
Use: Antibiotics.
See: Cefaclor.
   Cefadroxil.
   Cefazolin Sodium.
   Cefdinir.
   Cefditoren Pivoxil.
   Cefepime Hydrochloride.
   Cefixime.
   Cefmetazole Sodium.
   Cefoperazone Sodium.
   Cefotaxime Sodium.
   Cefotetan Disodium.
   Cefoxitin Sodium.
   Cefpodoxime Proxetil.
   Cefprozil.
   Ceftaroline Fosamil.
   Ceftazidime.
   Ceftibuten.
   Ceftizoxime Sodium.
   Ceftriaxone Sodium.
   Cefuroxime Axetil.
   Cephalexin.
   Cephradine.

•**cephalothin sodium.** (seff-AY-low-thin) *USP 34.*
Use: Anti-infective, cephalosporin.

•**cephapirin benzathine.** (SEFF-uh-PIE-rin BEN-zuh-theen) *USP 34.*

•**cephapirin sodium.** (SEFF-uh-PIE-rin) *USP 34.*
Use: Anti-infective.

cephazolin sodium.
See: Cefazolin Sodium.

•**cephradine.** (SEFF-ruh-deen) *USP 34.*
Use: Anti-infective, cephalosporin.

Cephulac. (Hoechst) Lactulose 10 g/15 mL (< galactose 1.6 g, lactose 1.2 g, other sugars 1.2 g). Soln. Bot. 473 mL, 1.9 L, UD 30 mL. *Rx.*
Use: Laxative.

Ceprotin. (Baxter) Protein C concentrate (human) 500 units, 1,000 units. Inj. Lyophilized Pow. for Soln. Single-dose vials. Each vial contains human albumin 8 mg/mL, trisodium citrate dihydrate 4.4 mg/mL, sodium chloride 8.8 mg/mL when reconstituted. *Rx.*
Use: Thrombolytic agent, human protein C.

Ceptaz. (GlaxoWellcome) Ceftazidime pentahydrate with L-arginine 1 g, 2 g. Vial. Infusion packs (1 g, 2 g). *Rx.*
Use: Anti-infective, cephalosporin.

ceramide trihexosidase/alpha-galactosidase A. (Genzyme)
Use: Fabry disease. [Orphan Drug]

Cerapon. (Purdue) Triethanolamine polypeptide oleate condensate.

CeraVe. (Coria Labs) Caprylic/capric triglyceride, cetyl alcohol, cetearyl alcohol, dimethicone, disodium EDTA, glycerin, parabens, petrolatum. Cream. 453 g. *OTC.*
Use: Emollient.

CeraVe AM. (Coria Labs) Homosalate 12%, octinoxate 7.5%, octocrylene 2%, zinc oxide 3.5%, cetearyl alcohol, dimethicone, disodium EDTA, glycerin, hyaluronic acid, parabens. SPF 30. Lot. 89 mL. *OTC.*
Use: Sunscreen.

CeraVe PM. (Coria Labs) Caprylic/capril triglyceride, ceramide, cetearyl alcohol, cholesterol, dimethicone, disodium EDTA, glycerin, glyceryl, hyaluronic acid, methosulfate, niacinamide, parabens. Lot., controlled-release. 89 mL. *OTC.*
Use: Emollient.

Cerebyx. (Parke-Davis) Fosphenytoin sodium 75 mg/mL (equivalent to phenytoin sodium 50 mg/mL). Inj., Soln.; concentrate. Vial. 2 mL. *Rx.*
Use: Anticonvulsant, hydantoin.

Ceredase. (Genzyme Corporation) Alglucerase 80 units/mL. Preservative free. Soln. for Inj. 5 mL with albumin 1%. *Rx.*
Use: Enzyme replacement for type 1 Gaucher disease.

Cerefolin. (Pan American Labs) Vitamin B_2 5 mg, vitamin B_6 50 mg, vitamin B_{12} 1 mg. L-methylfolate 5.635 mg. Tab. 90s. *Rx.*
Use: Nutritional product.

Cerefolin NAC. (Pan American) Vitamin B_{12} 2,000 mcg (as methylcobalamin), folate 5.6 mg (as L-methylfolate), N-acetylcysteine 600 mg. PEG, saccharin. Gluten free, lactose free, and sugar free. Tab. 90s, 500s. *Rx.*
Use: Nutritional supplement, multivitamin.

cerelose.
See: Glucose.

Ceretex. (Enzyme Process) Iron 15 mg, vitamins B_{12} 10 mcg, B_1 2 mg, B_6 1 mg, niacinamide 1 mg, pantothenic acid 0.15 mg, B_2 2 mg, iodine 15 mg/2 mL. Bot. 60 mL, 240 mL. *OTC.*
Use: Mineral, vitamin supplement.

Cerezyme. (Genzyme) Imiglucerase 212 units (equiv. to a withdrawal dose of 200 units) (mannitol 170 mg, sodium citrate 70 mg [trisodium citrate 52 mg, disodium hydrogen citrate 18 mg] per vial), 424 units (equiv. to a withdrawal dose of 400 units) (mannitol 340 mg, sodium citrate 140 mg [trisodium citrate 104 mg, disodium hydrogen citrate 36 mg] per vial). Preservative free. Pow. for Inj., lyophilized. Vials. *Rx.*
Use: Treatment for Gaucher disease.

Cerisa. (Stratus Pharmaceuticals) Sodium sulfacetamide 10%, sulfur 1%. Cetyl alcohol, disodium EDTA, glyceryl stearate, lactic acid, parabens, PEG-100, stearyl alcohol, white petrolatum. Wash. 170.1 g. *Rx.*
Use: Acne product combination.

Cernevit-12. (Baxter Healthcare) Vitamin A 3500 units, D_3 200 units, E (as dl-alpha tocopheryl) 11.2 units, C 125 mg, B_3 46 mg, B_5 17.25 mg, B_6 4.53 mg, B_2 4.14 mg, B_1 3.51 mg, folic acid 414 mcg, d-biotin 60 mcg, B_{12} 5.5 mcg. Pow. for Inj., lyophilized. Single-dose vial 5 mL. *Rx.*
Use: Vitamin supplement.

Ceron. (Cypress) Phenylephrine hydrochloride 12.5 mg, chlorpheniramine maleate 4 mg. Saccharin, sorbitol. Alcohol free and sugar free. Raspberry flavor. Syrup. 473 mL. *Rx.*
Use: Upper respiratory combination, decongestant and antihistamine.

•**ceronapril.** (seh-ROE-nap-rill) USAN.
Use: Antihypertensive.

Ceron-DM. (Cypress) **Syrup:** Dextromethorphan Hbr 15 mg, chlorpheniramine maleate 4 mg, phenylephrine hydrochloride 12.5 mg per 5 mL. Alcohol and sugar free. Saccharin, sorbitol. Grape flavor. 118 mL, 473 mL. *Rx.*
Use: Upper respiratory combination, antitussive combination.

Cerovite. (Rugby) Iron 18 mg, vitamins A 5000 units, D 400 units, E 30 units, B_1 1.5 mg, B_2 1.7 mg, B_3 20 mg, B_5 10 mg, B_6 2 mg, B_{12} 6 mcg, C 60 mg, folic acid 0.4 mg, Ca, Cl, Cr, Cu, I, Mg, Mn, Mo, Ni, P, Se, Si, SN, V, biotin 30 mcg, vitamin K, Zn 15 mg. Tab. Bot. 130s. *OTC.*
Use: Mineral, vitamin supplement.

Cerovite Advanced Formula. (Rugby) Iron (as ferrous fumarate) 18 mg, A 3500 units, D 400 units, E 30 units, B_1 1.5 mg, B_2 1.7 mg, B_3 20 mg, B_5 10 mg, B_6 2 mg, B_{12} 6 mcg, C 60 mg, folic acid 0.4 mg, biotin 30 mcg, B, Ca, P, I, Mg, Cu, Mn, K, Cl, Cr, Mo, Se, Ni, Si, Sn, V, vitamin K, Zn 15 mg, vitamin K_1, lutein, lycopene. Tab. Bot. 130s. *OTC.*
Use: Iron with vitamin supplement.

Cerovite Jr. (Rugby) Iron 18 mg, vitamins A 3,500 units, D 400 units, E 30 units, B_1 1.5 mg, B_2 1.7 mg, B_3 20 mg, B_5 10 mg, B_6 2 mg, B_{12} 6 mcg, C 60 mg, Ca 108 mg, folic acid 0.4 mg, Cu, I, K 10 mcg, Mg, Zn, Mn, Mo, P, biotin 45 mcg, Cr. Aspartame, maltodextrin, mannitol, phenylalanine 4.5 mg, various flavorings. Chew. Tab. 60s. *OTC.*
Use: Mineral, vitamin supplement.

Cerovite Senior. (Rugby) Vitamins A 6000 units, D 400 units, E 45 units, B_1 1.5 mg, B_2 1.7 mg, B_3 20 mg, B_5 10 mg, B_6 3 mg, B_{12} 25 mcg, C 60 mg, iron 9 mg, folic acid 0.2 mg, Ca 200 mg, Zn 15 mg, biotin 30 mcg, Cu, I, Mg, P, Cl, Cr, Mn, Mo, Ni, Se, Si, V, vitamin K. Tab. Bot. 60s. *OTC.*
Use: Mineral, vitamin supplement.

Certagen Liquid. (Ivax) Vitamins A 2500 units, B_1 1.5 mg, B_2 1.7 mg, B_3 20 mg, B_5 10 mg, B_6 2 mg, B_{12} 6 mcg, C 60 mg, D_3 400 units, E 30 units, biotin 300 mcg, iron 9 mg, Zn 3 mg, Cr, I, Mn, Mo/15 mL. Alcohol 6.6%. Liq. Bot. 237 mL. *OTC.*
Use: Mineral, vitamin supplement.

Certagen Tablets. (Ivax) Iron 18 mg, A 5000 units, D 400 units, E 30 units, B_1 1.5 mg, B_2 1.7 mg, B_3 20 mg, B_5 10 mg, B_6 2 mg, B_{12} 6 mcg, C 60 mg, folic acid 0.4 mg, biotin 30 mcg, Ca, P, I, Mg, Cu, Mn, K, Cl, Cr, Mo, Se, Ni, Si, Sn, V, vitamin K, Zn 15 mg. Tab. Bot. 130s, 1000s. *OTC.*
Use: Mineral, vitamin supplement.

•**certolizumab pegol.** (SER-toe-LIZ-oo-mab PEG-ol)
Use: Immunologic agent, immunomodulator.
See: Cimzia.
Cerubidine. (Bedford) Daunorubicin hydrochloride 21.4 mg (equivalent to daunorubicin 20 mg), mannitol 100 mg. Pow. for Inj., lyophilized. Single-dose vial. *Rx.*
Use: Antibiotic, anthracycline.
•**ceruletide.** (seh-ROO-leh-tide) USAN.
Use: Stimulant, gastric secretory.
•**ceruletide diethylamine.** (seh-ROO-leh-tide die-ETH-ill-ah-meen) USAN.
Use: Stimulant, gastric secretory.
Cervarix. (GlaxoSmithKline) Human papillomavirus (types 16, 18) bivalent vaccine, recombinant ≈ 20 mcg of HPV 16 L1 protein, 20 mcg of HPV 18 L1 protein per 0.5 mL (each 0.5 mL dose contains approximately 50 mcg of 3-O-desacyl-4'-monophosphoryl lipid A [MPL], aluminum hydroxide 0.5 mg, sodium chloride 4.4 mg, sodium dihydrogen phosphate dihydrate 0.624 mg). Preservative free. Inj., Susp. Single-dose vial and prefilled *TIP-LOK* syringes (tip cap and rubber plunger of the needleless prefilled syringes contain dry natural latex rubber). *Rx.*
Use: Agent for active immunization, viral vaccine.
cervical ripening agents.
See: Dinoprostone.
Cervidil. (Forest) Dinoprostone 10 mg. Insert. 1s. *Rx.*
Use: Cervical ripening.
Ces. (ICN) Conjugated estrogens 0.625 mg, 1.25 mg, 2.5 mg. Tab. *Rx.*
Use: Estrogen.
Cesamet. (Meda) Nabilone 1 mg. Corn starch. Cap. 20s. *c-II.*
Use: Antiemetic/antivertigo agent.
Cesia. (Prasco) **Phase 1:** Desogestrel 0.1 mg, ethinyl estradiol 25 mcg. 7 tabs. **Phase 2:** Desogestrel 0.125 mg, ethinyl estradiol 25 mcg. 7 tabs. **Phase 3:** Desogestrel 0.15 mg, ethinyl estradiol 25 mcg. 7 tabs. Lactose, talc. Tab. 28s with 7 inert tabs. *Rx.*
Use: Contraceptive hormone, sex hormone.
•**cesium chloride Cs 131.** (SEE-zee-uhm KLOR-ide) USAN.
Use: Radiopharmaceutical agent.
Ceta. (C & M Pharmacal) Soap-free. Propylene glycol, hydroxyethylcellulose, cetyl and cetearyl alcohols, sodium lauryl sulfate, parabens. Liq. Bot. 240 mL. *OTC.*
Use: Dermatologic cleanser.

•**cetaben sodium.** (SEE-tah-ben) USAN.
Use: Antihyperlipoproteinemic.
Cetacaine. (Cetylite) Benzocaine 14%, tetracaine hydrochloride 2%, butamben 2%, benzalkonium chloride 0.5%, cetyl dimethyl ethyl ammonium bromide 0.005% in a bland water-soluble base. **Aerosol:** 56 g. **Liq.:** 56 mL. **Oint.:** 37 g. **Gel:** 29 g. *Rx.*
Use: Topical local anesthetic.
Cetacort. (Galderma) Hydrocortisone 0.25%, 0.5%, 1% w/cetyl alcohol, propylene glycol, stearyl alcohol, sodium lauryl sulfate, butylparaben, methylparaben, propylparaben, purified water. Bot. 120 mL (0.25% only), 60 mL (0.5%, 1% only). *Rx.*
Use: Corticosteroid, topical.
Cetafen. (Hart Health & Safety) Acetaminophen 325 mg. Sugar free. Film-coated. Tab. UD 100s, UD 250s. *OTC.*
Use: Analgesic.
Cetafen Extra. (Hart Health & Safety) Acetaminophen 500 mg. Sugar free. Film-coated. Tab. UD 100s. *OTC.*
Use: Analgesic.
Cetaklenz. (Geritrex) Cetyl alcohol, propylene glycol, sodium lauryl sulfate, stearyl alcohol, DMDM hydantoin, parabens. Fragrance free. Cleanser. 120 mL. *OTC.*
Use: Cleanser.
•**cetalkonium chloride.** (SEET-al-KOE-nee-uhm) USAN.
Use: Anti-infective, topical.
•**cetamolol hydrochloride.** (SEET-AM-oh-lahl) USAN.
Use: Anti-adrenergic, beta-receptor.
Cetaphil. (Galderma) **Cream, Lot.:** Cetyl alcohol, stearyl alcohol, propylene glycol (cream only), sodium lauryl sulfate, methylparaben, propylparaben, butylparaben. Bot. 480 g (cream), 120 mL, 240 mL, 480 mL (lotion). **Antibacterial Bar:** Triclosan, petrolatum. Soap-free. 127 g. **Bar:** Petrolatum. Soap-free. 127 g. **Cleanser:** Cetyl alcohol, stearyl alcohol, parabens. Bot. 236 mL. *OTC.*
Use: Dermatologic cleanser.
Cetaphil Daily Advance. (Galderma) Benzyl alcohol, butyrospermum parkii, cetearyl alcohol, glycerin, macadamia seed oil, stearyl alcohol. Lot. 226 g. *OTC.*
Use: Emollient.
Cetazol. (Professional Pharmacal) Acetazolamide 250 mg. Tab. Bot. 100s. *Rx.*
Use: Anticonvulsant; diuretic.
•**cethromycin.** (ceth-roe-MYE-sin) USAN.
Use: Antibacterial.

●**cetiedil citrate.** (see-TIE-eh-DILL SIH-trate) *USAN.*
Use: Vasodilator, peripheral.

●**cetilistat.** (ce-tye-LI-stat) *USAN.*
Use: Treatment of obesity.

cetirizine. (Apotex) Cetirizine hydrochloride 5 mg. Lactose. Tab. 100s. *OTC.*
Use: Antihistamine, peripherally selective piperazine.

cetirizine. (Various Mfr.) Cetirizine hydrochloride 10 mg. May contain lactose, polydextrose. Tab. 100s, 300s. *OTC.*
Use: Antihistamine, peripherally selective piperazine.

●**cetirizine hydrochloride.** (seh-TIH-rih-zeen) *USAN.*
Use: Antihistamine, peripherally selective piperazine.
See: All Day Allergy Children's.
Zyrtec Allergy.
Zyrtec Children's Allergy.
Zyrtec Children's Hives Relief.
Zyrtec Hives Relief.
W/Pseudoephedrine Hydrochloride.
See: All Day Allergy-D.
Zyrtec-D 12 Hour.

cetirizine hydrochloride. (Various Mfr.) Cetirizine hydrochloride 1 mg/mL. May contain parabens, saccharin, sucrose. Syr. 118 mL, 473 mL. *OTC.*
Use: Antihistamine, peripherally selective piperazine.

●**cetocycline hydrochloride.** (SEE-toe-SIGH-kleen) *USAN. Formerly cetotetrine hydrochloride.*
Use: Anti-infective.

●**cetophenicol.** (see-toe-FEN-ih-kole) *USAN.*
Use: Antibacterial.

●**cetostearyl alcohol.** (SEE-toe-STEER-il) *NF 29.*
Use: Pharmaceutic aid, emulsifying agent.

Cetraxal. (WraSer Pharmaceuticals) Ciprofloxacin 0.2%. Preservative free. Soln., Otic. Single-use container. 14s. *Rx.*
Use: Otic preparation, otic antibiotic.

●**cetraxate hydrochloride.** (seh-TRAX-ate) *USAN.*
Use: Antiulcerative; gastrointestinal.

cetrorelix acetate.
Use: Sex hormone; gonadotropin-releasing hormone antagonist.
See: Cetrotide.

Cetrotide. (Serono) Cetrorelix acetate 0.25 mg, 3 mg. Inj. Trays containing 1 vial of 0.26 to 0.27 mg or 3.12 to 3.24 mg cetorelix acetate, 1 mL or 3 mL syr. of Sterile Water for Inj., 20-gauge needle, 27-gauge needle, alcohol swabs. 1s, 7s (0.25 mg only). *Rx.*
Use: Sex hormone; gonadotropin-releasing hormone antagonist.

●**cetuximab.** (seh-TUCKS-ih-mab) *USAN.*
Use: Monoclonal antibody.
See: Erbitux.

●**cetyl alcohol.** (SEE-till) *NF 29.*
Use: Pharmaceutic aid, emulsifying and stiffening agent.

Cetylcide Solution. (Cetylite Industries) Cetyldimethylethyl ammonium bromide 6.5%, benzalkonium chloride 6.5%, isopropyl alcohol 13%. Inert ingredients 74%, including sodium nitrite. Bot. 16 oz, 32 oz.
Use: Disinfectant.

●**cetyl esters wax.** (SEE-till ess-ters) *NF 29. Formerly synthetic spermacet.*
Use: Pharmaceutic aid, stiffening agent.

●**cetylpyridinium chloride.** (SEE-till-pihr-ih-DIH-nee-uhm) *USP 34.*
Use: Anti-infective, topical; pharmaceutic aid, preservative.
See: Cēpacol.

cetyltrimethyl ammonium bromide. (Bioline Labs) Cetrimide B.P., Cetavlon, CTAB.
Use: Antiseptic.

Cevi-Bid. (Lee) Ascorbic acid 500 mg. Tab. Bot. 100s, 500s, UD 12s, 96s. *OTC.*
Use: Water-soluble vitamin.

●**cevimeline hydrochloride.** (seh-vih-MEH-leen) *USAN.*
Use: Treatment of Alzheimer disease, adjunct; dry mouth.
See: Evoxac.

cevitamic acid.
See: Ascorbic Acid.

cevitan.
See: Ascorbic Acid.

Cewin. (Sanofi-Synthelabo) Ascorbic acid. *OTC.*
Use: Vitamin supplement.

Ceylon gelatin.
See: Agar.

Cezin. (Forest) Vitamins B_1 20 mg, B_2 10 mg, B_3 100 mg, B_5 20 mg, B_6 5 mg, C 300 mg, magnesium sulfate 70 mg, zinc sulfate 80 mg. Cap. Bot. 100s. *OTC.*
Use: Vitamin supplement.

Cezin-S. (Forest) Vitamins A 10,000 units, D 50 units, E 50 units, B_1 10 mg, B_2 5 mg, B_3 50 mg, B_5 10 mg, B_6 2 mg, C 200 mg, folic acid 0.5 mg, Zn 18 mg, Mg, Mn. Cap. Bot. 100s. *Rx.*
Use: Vitamin supplement.

C Factors "1000" Plus. (Solgar) Vitamin C 1000 mg, rose hips 25 mg, citrus bioflavonoids complex 250 mg, rutin 50 mg, hesperidin 25 mg. Sodium free, sugar free. Tab. Bot. 50s. *OTC.*
Use: Water-soluble vitamin.

C.G. (Sigma-Tau) Chorionic gonadotropin (lyophilized) 10,000 units, mannitol 100 mg, supplied with diluent. Univial 10 mL. *Rx.*
Use: Hormone, chorionic gonadotropin.

CG Disposable Unit.
See: Cardio Green.

CG Ria. (Abbott Diagnostics) Radioimmunoassay for the quantitative measurement of total circulating serum cholylglycine.
Use: Diagnostic aid.

CGU WC. (Elge) Codeine phosphate 6.3 mg, guaifenesin 100 mg per 5 mL. Alcohol and sugar free. PEG, saccharin, sorbitol. Liq. 473 mL. *c-v.*
Use: Upper respiratory combination, antitussive with expectorant.

Chantel Vitamin E. (National Vitamin) dl-alpha tocopheryl acetate, ergocalciferol, cetyl alcohol, panthenol, parabens, safflower oil, urea, vegetable oil. Cream. 454 g. *OTC.*
Use: Emollient.

Chantix. (Pfizer) Varenicline tartrate 0.5 mg (as base), 1 mg (as base). Film-coated. Tab. First-month packs (1 card of eleven 0.5-mg Tab. and 3 cards of fourteen 1-mg Tab.), Continuing-therapy packs (4 cards of fourteen 1-mg Tab.), Bot. 56s. *Rx.*
Use: Smoking cessation.

Chap Cream. (Ar-Ex) Carbonyl diamide. Cream. Tube 1.5 oz, 3.25 oz. Jar 4 oz, 9 oz, 18 oz. *OTC.*
Use: Emollient.

Chapoline Cream Lotion. (Wade) Glycerin, boric acid, chlorobutanol 0.5%, alcohol 10%. Lot. Bot. 4 oz, pt, gal. *OTC.*
Use: Emollient.

Chapstick Medicated Lip Balm. (Wyeth) **Jar:** Petrolatum 60%, camphor 1%, menthol 0.6%, phenol 0.5%, microcrystalline wax, mineral oil, cocoa butter, lanolin, paraffin wax, parabens 7 g. **Squeezable tube:** Petrolatum 67%, camphor 1%, menthol 0.6%, phenol 0.5%, microcrystalline wax, mineral oil, cocoa butter, lanolin, parabens 10 g. **Stick:** Petrolatum 41%, camphor 1%, menthol 0.6%, phenol 0.5%, paraffin wax, mineral oil, cocoa butter, 2-octyl dodecanol, arachidyl propionate, polyphenyl methylsiloxane 556, white wax,oleyl alcohol, isopropyl lanolate, carnuba wax, isopropyl myristate, lanolin, cetyl alcohol, parabens. 4.2 g. *OTC.*
Use: Mouth and throat preparation.

Chapstick Sunblock 15. (Wyeth) Padimate O 0.7%, oxybenzone 3%. Stick 4.25 g. *OTC.*
Use: Lip protectant.

Chapstick Sunblock 15 Petroleum Jelly Plus. (Wyeth) White petrolatum 89%, padimate O 7%, oxybenzone 3%, aloe, lanolin. Stick 10 g. *OTC.*
Use: Lip protectant.

CharcoAid. (Requa, Inc.) Activated charcoal 15 g/120 mL, 30 g/150 mL, sorbitol. Susp. Bot. *OTC.*
Use: Antidote.

CharcoAid 2000. (Requa, Inc.) Activated charcoal 15 g/120 mL, 50 g/240 mL with and without sorbitol. Liq. 15 g/240 mL. Granules. Bot. *OTC.*
Use: Antidote.

charcoal. (Various Mfr.) Cap., Tab. *OTC.*
Use: Antiflatulent.

• **charcoal, activated.** (CHAR-kole) *USP 34.*
Use: Antidote, general purpose; pharmaceutic aid, adsorbent.
See: Actidose-Aqua.
   CharcoAid.
   Charcoal Plus.
   Charcocaps.

Charcoal Plus. (Kramer) Activated charcoal 250 mg, sugar. EC Tab. Bot. 120s. *OTC.*
Use: Antiflatulent.

CharcoCaps. (Requa, Inc.) Activated charcoal 260 mg. Cap. Bot. 36s. *OTC.*
Use: Antiflatulent.

Charo Scatter-Paks. (Requa, Inc.) Activated charcoal 5 g. Packet.
Use: Odor absorbent.

Chaz Scalp Treatment Dandruff Shampoo. (Revlon) Zinc pyrithione 1% in liquid shampoo. *OTC.*
Use: Antiseborrheic.

Chealamide. (Vortech Pharmaceuticals) Disodium edetate 150 mg/mL. Inj. Vial. 20 mL. *Rx.*
Use: Chelating agent.

Checkmate. (Oral-B) Acidulated phosphate fluoride 1.23%. Bot. 2 oz, 16 oz. *Rx.*
Use: Dental caries agent.

Cheetah. (Mallinckrodt) Barium sulfate 2.2%. Simethicone, sorbitol, saccharin, sodium benzoate. Susp. Bot. 250 mL, 450 mL, 900 mL, 1900 mL. *Rx.*
Use: Radiopaque agent, GI contrast agent.

Chek-Stix Urinalysis Control Strips.
(Bayer Consumer Care) Bot. 25s.
Use: Diagnostic aid.

chelafrin.
See: Epinephrine.

Chelated Calcium Magnesium. (NBTY)
Ca^{++} 500 mg, Mg 250 mg. Tab. Protein
coated. Bot. 50s. *OTC.*
Use: Mineral supplement.

Chelated Calcium Magnesium Zinc.
(NBTY) Ca^{++} 333 mg, Mg 133 mg,
Zn 8.3 mg. Tab. Bot. 100s. *OTC.*
Use: Mineral supplement.

Chelated Manganese. (Freeda) Manganese 20 mg, 50 mg. Tab. Bot. 100s,
250s, 500s. *OTC.*
Use: Mineral supplement.

chelating agents.
See: Deferasirox.
Deferoxamine Mesylate.
Dimercaprol.
Edetate Calcium Disodium.
Pentetate Calcium Trisodium.
Pentetate Zinc Trisodium.
Prussian Blue Oral.
Succimer.
Trientine Hydrochloride.

chelen.
See: Ethyl Chloride.

Chemet. (Ovation) Succimer 100 mg.
Cap. Bot. 100s. *Rx.*
Use: Chelating agent.

Chemipen. Potassium phenethicillin.
Use: Anti-infective, penicillin.

Chemovag. (Forest) Sulfisoxazole 0.5 g.
Supp. Bot. 12s w/applicators. *Rx.*
Use: Anti-infective, sulfonamide.

Chemozine. (Tennessee Pharmaceutic)
Sulfadiazine, 0.167 g, sulfamerazine
0.167 g, sulfamethazine 0.167 g. Tab.
Bot. 100s, 1000s. Susp. Bot. Pt, gal. *Rx.*
Use: Anti-infective, sulfonamide.

Chemstrip K. (Boehringer Mannheim)
Reagent papers for ketones in urine.
Paper Bot. 25s, 100s.
Use: Diagnostic aid.

Chemstrip Micral. (Boehringer Mannheim) In vitro reagent strips to detect
albumin in urine. Strip Pkg. 5s, 30s.
Use: Diagnostic aid.

Chemstrip Mineral. (Boehringer Mannheim) In vitro reagent strips used to
detect albumin in urine. Strip Pkg. 5s,
30s.
Use: In vitro diagnostic aid.

Chemstrip 9. (Boehringer Mannheim)
Broad range test for glucose, protein,
pH, blood, ketones, bilirubin, urobilino-
gen, nitrite, leukocytes in urine. Strip
Bot. 100s.
Use: Diagnostic aid.

Chemstrip 7. (Boehringer Mannheim)
Broad range test for glucose, protein,
pH, blood, ketones, bilirubin, leukocytes. Strip Bot. 100s.
Use: Diagnostic aid.

Chemstrip 10 SG. (Boehringer Mannheim) Broad range test for glucose,
protein, pH, blood, ketones, bilirubin,
urobilinogen, nitrite, leukocytes in urine.
Strip Bot. 100s.
Use: Diagnostic aid.

Chemstrip 2 GP. (Boehringer Mannheim)
Broad range test for glucose and pro-
tein. Strip Bot. 100s.
Use: Diagnostic aid.

Chemstrip 2 LN. (Boehringer Mannheim)
Broad range test for nitrite and leuko-
cytes. Strip Bot. 100s.
Use: Diagnostic aid.

Chemstrip uGK. (Boehringer Mannheim)
Broad range test for glucose and ke-
tones. Strip Bot. 50s, 100s.
Use: Diagnostic aid.

Chenatal. (Miller Pharmacal Group) Calcium 580 mg, Mg 200 mg, vitamins C
100 mg, folic acid 0.4 mg, A 5000 units,
D 400 units, B_1 3 mg, B_2 3 mg, B_6
5 mg, B_{12} 9 mcg, niacinamide 30 mg,
pantothenic acid 5 mg, tocopherols
(mixed) 10 mg, Fe 20 mg, Cu 1 mg,
Mn 2 mg, K 10 mg, Zn 25 mg, I 0.1 mg.
2 Tabs. Bot. 100s. *OTC.*
Use: Mineral, vitamin supplement.

Chenix. (Solvay) Chenodil.
Use: Anticholelithogenic. [Orphan Drug]

Chenodal. (Manchester Pharmaceuti-
cals) Chenodiol 250 mg. Film coated.
Tab. 100s. *Rx.*
Use: Gallstone solubilizing agent.

chenodeoxycholic acid.
Use: Urolithic.
See: Chenodiol.

•**chenodiol.** (KEEN-oh-DIE-ahl) USAN.
Formerly chenic acid.
Use: Anticholelithogenic.
See: Chenodal.

Cheracol. (Lee Pharmaceuticals) Codeine phosphate 10 mg, guaifenesin
100 mg/5 mL, alcohol 4.75%. Bot. 2 oz,
4 oz, pt. *c-v.*
Use: Antitussive; expectorant.

Cheracol Cough. (Lee Pharmaceuticals)
Codeine phosphate 10 mg, guaifenesin
100 mg per 5 mL. Alcohol 4.75%, fructose, sucrose. Syr. Bot. 60 mL, 120 mL,
480 mL. *c-v.*
Use: Upper respiratory combination, antitussive, expectorant.

Cheracol D Cough Formula. (Lee Pharmaceuticals) Dextromethorphan HBr
10 mg, guaifenesin 100 mg per 5 mL.

Alcohol 4.75%, fructose, sucrose. Syrup. Bot. 118 mL, 180 mL. *OTC.*
Use: Upper respiratory combination, antitussive with expectorant.

Cheracol Plus. (Lee Pharmaceuticals) Dextromethorphan HBr 10 mg, guaifenesin 100 mg per 5 mL. Alcohol 4.75%, fructose, sucrose. Liq. Bot. 118 mL. *OTC.*
Use: Upper respiratory combination, antitussive with expectorant.

Cheracol Sore Throat. (Lee Pharmaceuticals) Phenol 1.4%, saccharin, sorbitol, alcohol 12.5%. Spray Bot. 180 mL. *OTC.*
Use: Mouth and throat product.

Cheratussin AC Expectorant Cough Suppressant. (Qualitest Pharmaceuticals) Codeine phosphate 10 mg, guaifenesin 100 mg per 5 mL. Sugar free. Alcohol 3.5%, saccharin, sorbitol. Syrup. 118 mL, 236 mL, 473 mL, 3785 mL. *c-v.*
Use: Antitussive with expectorant, upper respiratory combination.

Cheratussin DAC. (Qualitest) Codeine phosphate 10 mg, guaifenesin 100 mg, pseudoephedrine hydrochloride 30 mg per 5mL. Alcohol 2.1%. Menthol, saccharin, sorbitol. Sugar free. Soln. 473 mL. *c-v.*
Use: Upper respiratory combination; analgesic, expectorant, decongestant.

Chero-Trisulfa-V. (Vita Elixir) Sulfadiazine 0.166 g, sulfacetamide 0.166 g, sulfamerazine 0.166 g, sodium citrate 0.5 g/5 mL. Susp. Bot. Pt.
Use: Anti-infective, sulfonamide.

•**cherry juice.** *NF 29.*
Use: Flavoring.

•**cherry syrup.** *NF 29.*
Use: Pharmaceutic aid, vehicle.

Chest Throat. (Lane) Eucalyptol, anise, horehound, tolu balsam, benzoin tincture, sugar, corn syrup. Loz. Pkg. 30s. *OTC.*
Use: Antiseptic.

Chewable Multivitamins w/Fluoride. (H.L. Moore Drug Exchange) Fluoride 1 mg, vitamins A 2500 units, D 400 units, E 15 units, B_1 1.05 mg, B_2 1.2 mg, B_3 13.5 mg, B_6 1.05 mg, B_{12} 4.5 mcg, C 60 mg, folic acid 0.3 mg, sucrose. Tab. Bot. 100s. *Rx.*
Use: Mineral, vitamin supplement; dental caries agent.

Chewable Vitamin C. (Various Mfr.) Vitamin C (as sodium ascorbate and ascorbic acid) 250 mg, 500 mg. Chew. Tab. Bot. 100s. *OTC.*
Use: Water-soluble vitamin.

Chew-C. (Key Company) Vitamin C (as ascorbic acid and sodium ascorbate) 500 mg. Sugar. Orange flavor. Chew. Tab. 100s. *OTC.*
Use: Water-soluble vitamin.

Chew-Vims. (Barth's) Vitamins A 5000 units, D 400 units, B_1 3 mg, B_2 6 mg, niacin 1.71 mg, C 100 mg, B_{12} 5 mcg, E 5 units. Tab. Bot. 30s, 90s, 180s, 360s. *OTC.*
Use: Water-soluble vitamin.

Chew-Vi-Tab. (Halsey Drug) Vitamins A 2500 units, D 400 units, E 15 units, C 60 mg, folic acid 0.3 mg, B_1 1.05 mg, B_2 1.2 mg, niacin 13.5 mg, B_6 1.05 mg, B_{12} 4.5 mcg. Tab. Bot. 100s. *OTC.*
Use: Vitamin supplement.

Chew-Vi-Tab with Iron. (Halsey Drug) Vitamins A 5000 units, C 60 mg, E 15 units, folic acid 0.4 mg, $B_1$1.5 mg, B_2 1.7 mg, niacin 20 mg, B_6 2 mg, B_{12} 6 mcg, D 400 units, iron 18 mg. Tab. Bot. 100s. *OTC.*
Use: Mineral, vitamin supplement.

chicken pox vaccine.
See: Varivax.

Chigg Away. (Pierson Labs) Benzocaine 5%, sulfur 10%. Cetyl alcohol, glycerin, glyceryl, isopropyl alcohol, parabens, petrolatum, triethanolamine. Lot. 118 mL. *OTC.*
Use: Local anesthetic, topical combination.

Chiggerex. (Scherer) Benzocaine with camphor, menthol. Oint. 50 g. *OTC.*
Use: Topical local anesthetic.

Children's Advil. (Wyeth) Ibuprofen 100 mg/5 mL. Sorbitol, sucrose, EDTA, fruit flavor. Susp. Bot. 119 mL, 473 mL. *OTC.*
Use: Analgesic, NSAID.

Children's Advil. (Wyeth) Ibuprofen 50 mg. Aspartame, phenylalanine 2.1 mg, fruit and grape flavor. Chew. Tab. Bot. 24s, 50s. *OTC.*
Use: Analgesic, NSAID.

Children's Advil Cold. (Wyeth) Pseudoephedrine hydrochloride 15 mg, ibuprofen 100 mg per 5 mL. Sorbitol, sucrose. Alcohol free. Grape flavor. Susp. 120 mL. *OTC.*
Use: Decongestant and analgesic.

Children's Benadryl Allergy Fastmelt. (Pfizer) Diphenhydramine 12.5 mg (equiv. to 19 mg citrate). Aspartame, mannitol, phenylalanine 4.5 mg. Orally Disintegrating Tab. 20s. *OTC.*
Use: Antihistamine.

Children's Dimaphen DM. (Major) Brompheniramine maleate 1 mg, dextromethorphan hydrobromide 5 mg, phenyl-

ephrine hydrochloride 2.5 mg. Sodium 3 mg, sorbitol, sucralose. Alcohol free. Grape flavor. Elix. 118 mL. *OTC.*
Use: Upper respiratory combination, antitussive combination.

Children's Elixir DM Cough & Cold. (AmerisourceBergen) Pseudoephedrine hydrochloride 15 mg, brompheniramine maleate 1 mg, dextromethorphan HBr 5 mg per 5 mL. Saccharin, sorbitol, grape flavor, alcohol free. Elixir. Bot. 118 mL. *OTC.*
Use: Upper respiratory combination, decongestant, antihistamine, antitussive.

Children's Formula Cough. (Pharmakon) Guaifenesin 50 mg, dextromethorphan HBr 5 mg/5 mL, sucrose, corn syrup. Alcohol free. Grape flavor. Syr. Bot. 118 mL, 236 mL. *OTC.*
Use: Expectorant; antitussive.

Children's Ibuprofen Cold. (Major) Pseudoephedrine hydrochloride 15 mg, ibuprofen 100 mg/5 mL. Alcohol-free. Corn syrup. Berry flavor. Susp. 120 mL. *OTC.*
Use: Decongestant, analgesic.

Children's Kaopectate. (Pharmacia) Attapulgite 600 mg/5 mL. Liq. Bot. 180 mL. *OTC.*
Use: Antidiarrheal.

Children's Loratadine. (Taro) Loratadine 5 mg per 5 mL. Fruit flavor. Syrup. 120 mL. *OTC.*
Use: Antihistamine, peripherally selective piperidine.

Children's Motrin. (McNeil Consumer) Ibuprofen. **Chew. Tab.:** 50 mg. Aspartame, phenylalanine 3 mg, orange flavor. Bot. 24s. **Susp.:** 100 mg/5 mL. Sucrose. Grape and bubble gum flavors. Bot. 60 mL, 120 mL. *OTC.*
Use: Analgesic, NSAID.

Children's Motrin Cold. (McNeil Consumer) Ibuprofen 100 mg, pseudoephedrine hydrochloride 15 mg/5 mL. Dye free. Acesulfame K, sucralose, sucrose. Berry, grape, or tropical punch flavors. Susp. 118 mL. *OTC.*
Use: Analgesic and decongestant, upper respiratory combination.

Children's NasalCrom. (Pharmacia) Cromolyn sodium 40 mg/mL (cromolyn sodium 5.2 mg/spray), benzalkonium chloride 0.01%, EDTA 0.01%. Spray. Bot. 13 mL, 26 mL. *OTC.*
Use: Analgesic; prophylactic.

Children's No Aspirin Elixir. (Walgreen) Acetaminophen 80 mg/2.5 mL. Nonalcoholic. Elix. Bot. 4 oz. *OTC.*
Use: Analgesic.

Children's No-Aspirin Tablets. (Walgreen) Acetaminophen 80 mg. Tab. Bot. 30s. *OTC.*
Use: Analgesic.

Children's Silfedrine. (Silarx) Pseudoephedrine hydrochloride 30 mg/5 mL. Liq. Bot. 118 mL. *OTC.*
Use: Decongestant, nasal.

Children's Sunkist Multivitamins Complete. (Novartis) Iron 18 mg, vitamin A 5000 units, D_3 400 units, E 30 units, B_1 1.5 mg, B_2 1.7 mg, B_3 20 mg, B_5 10 mg, B_6 2 mg, B_{12} 6 mcg, C 60 mg, folic acid 0.4 mg, Ca, Cu, I, K, Mg, Mn, P, Zn 10 mg, biotin 40 mcg, vitamin K, sorbitol, aspartame, phenylalanine, tartrazine. Chew. Tab. Bot. 60s. *OTC.*
Use: Mineral, vitamin supplement.

Children's Sunkist Multivitamins + Extra C. (Novartis) Vitamin A 2500 units, E 15 units, D_3 400 units, B_1 1.05 mg, B_2 1.2 mg, B_3 13.5 mg, B_6 1.05 mg, B_{12} 4.5 mcg, C 250 mg, folic acid 0.3 mg, vitamin K_1 5 mcg, sorbitol, aspartame, phenylalanine, tartrazine. Chew. Tab. Bot. 60s. *OTC.*
Use: Mineral, vitamin supplement.

Children's Ty-Tabs. (Major) Acetaminophen 80 mg. Tab. Bot. 100s, 1000s. *OTC.*
Use: Analgesic.

Chinese gelatin.
See: Agar.

Chinese isinglass.
Use: Amebicide.

chiniofon.
Use: Amebicide.

Chinositol. (Vernon) 8-Hydroxyquinoline sulfate 7.5 g. Tab. Vial 6s. Trit. Tab. (600 mg) Bot. 50s. Vial 110s. Pow. 1 oz.
Use: Antiseptic.

ChiRhoStim. (ChiRhoClin) Secretin 16 mcg, 40 mcg. Mannitol 20 mg (16 mcg), 50 mg (40 mcg), L-cysteine 1.5 mg (16 mcg), 3.75 mg (40 mcg). Inj. lyophilized Pow. for Soln. Vial. *Rx.*
Use: Diagnostic aid, gastrointestinal function test.

chlamydia trachomatis test.
Use: Diagnostic aid.
See: MicroTrak.

Chlamydiazyme. (Abbott Diagnostics) Enzyme immunoassay for detection of *Chlamydia trachomatis* from urethral or urogenital swabs. Test Kit 100s.
Use: Diagnostic aid.

Chlo-Amine. (Hollister-Stier) Chlorpheniramine maleate 2 mg, sugar, orange flavor. Chew. Tab. Bot. 96s. *OTC.*
Use: Antihistamine, nonselective alkylamine.

• **chlophedianol hydrochloride.** (KLOE-fee-DIE-ah-nole) USAN.
Use: Antitussive.
W/Brompheniramine Maleate, Pseudo-ephedrine Hydrochloride.
See: Dicel CD.
W/Guaifenesin, Pseudoephedrine Hydro-chloride.
See: Vanacof Dx.
W/Pseudoephedrine Hydrochloride.
See: Clofera.
W/Triprolidine Hydrochloride.
See: ProHist CF.

Chloracol 0.5%. (Horizon) Chlor-amphenicol 5 mg/mL with chlorobuta-nol, hydroxypropyl methylcellulose.
Dropper bot. 7.5 mL. *Rx.*
Use: Anti-infective, ophthalmic.

Chlorafed. (Roberts) Chlorpheniramine maleate 2 mg, pseudoephedrine hydro-chloride 30 mg/5 mL, alcohol, dye, sugar, and corn free. Liq. Bot. 120 mL, 480 mL. *OTC.*
Use: Antihistamine; decongestant.

Chlorafed H.S. Timecelles. (Roberts) Chlorpheniramine maleate 4 mg, pseudoephedrine hydrochloride 60 mg. SR Cap. Bot. 100s. *Rx.*
Use: Antihistamine; decongestant.

Chlorafed Timecelles. (Roberts) Chlor-pheniramine maleate 8 mg, pseudo-ephedrine hydrochloride 120 mg. SA Timecelles. Bot. 100s. *Rx.*
Use: Antihistamine; decongestant.

Chlorahist. (Evron) Chlorpheniramine maleate. **Tab:** 4 mg. Bot. 100s, 1000s. **Cap:** 8 mg, 12 mg. Bot. 250s, 1000s. **Syr:** 2 mg/4 mL. Bot. qt. *Rx-OTC.*
Use: Antihistamine.

• **chloral betaine.** (KLOR-uhl BEE-tah-een) USAN.
Use: Hypnotic; sedative.

• **chloral hydrate.** (KLOR-uhl HIGH-drate) *USP 34.*
Use: Hypnotic/sedative, nonbarbiturate.
See: Somnote.

chloral hydrate. (Various Mfr.) Chloral hydrate. **Cap.:** 500 mg. 100s, 500s, 1,000s, UD 100s. **Syrup:** 250 mg/5 mL, 500 mg/5 mL. Pt., gal., UD 5 mL (100s) (500 mg/5 mL only); UD 10 mL (40s and 100s). *c-IV.*
Use: Hypnotic/sedative, nonbarbiturate.

chloral hydrate betaine (1:1) com-pound. Chloral Betaine.

chloralpyrine dichloralpyrine.
See: Dichloralantipyrine.

chloralurethane. *Name used for Carbo-chloral.*

• **chlorambucil.** (klor-AM-byoo-sill) *USP 34.*
Use: Antineoplastic; alkylating agent; nitrogen mustard.
See: Leukeran.

Chloramine-T. Sodium paratoluenesul-fan chloramide, chloramine, chloro-zone. **Eli Lilly:** Tab. (0.3 g), Bot. 100s, 1000s. **Robinson:** Pow., 1 oz.
Use: Antiseptic; deodorant.
See: Chlorazene.

• **chloramphenicol.** (KLOR-am-FEN-ih-kole) *USP 34.*
Use: Anti-infective; antirickettsial; treat-ment of superficial ocular infections involving the conjunctiva or cornea caused by susceptible organisms.
W/Hydrocortisone Acetate.
See: Chloromycetin/Hydrocortisone.

• **chloramphenicol palmitate.** (KLOR-am-FEN-ih-kahl pal-mih-tate) *USP 34.*
Use: Anti-infective; antirickettsial.

• **chloramphenicol pantothenate com-plex.** (KLOR-am-FEN-ih-kahl PAN-toe-THEH-nate) USAN.
Use: Anti-infective; antirickettsial.

• **chloramphenicol sodium succinate.** (KLOR-am-FEN-ih-kahl) *USP 34.*
Use: Anti-infective; antirickettsial.
See: Mychel-S.

chloramphenicol sodium succinate. (Various Mfr.) Chloramphenicol sodium succinate 100 mg/mL. Inj. Vial. 1 g in 15 mL.
Use: Anti-infective; antirickettsial.

Chloraseptic Children's. (Prestige) Benzocaine 5 mg. Loz. Pkg. 18s. *OTC.*
Use: Anesthetic, local.

Chloraseptic Kids' Sore Throat. (Pres-tige) Benzocaine 2 mg, menthol 2 mg. Glycerin, sucralose. Strips. 20s. *OTC.*
Use: Mouth and throat products.

Chloraseptic Kids' Sore Throat. (Pres-tige) Phenol 0.5%. Sugar and alcohol free. Saccharin. Grape flavor. Spray. Bot. 177 mL. *OTC.*
Use: Mouth and throat product.

Chloraseptic Liquid. (Prestige) Total phenol 1.4% as phenol and sodium phenolate, saccharin. Menthol and cherry flavors. Liq. Bot. 180 mL, 360 mL (mouthwash/gargle); 45 mL, 240 mL, 360 mL (throat spray). *OTC.*
Use: Anesthetic; antiseptic, local.

Chloraseptic Lozenge. (Prestige) Total phenol 32.5 mg as phenol and sodium phenolate. Menthol and cherry flavors. Pkg. 18s, 36s. *OTC.*
Use: Anesthetic; antiseptic.

Chloraseptic Sore Throat. (Prestige)
Acetaminophen 166.6 mg per 5 mL.
Corn syrup, menthol, saccharin, sorbitol. Cherry flavor. Liq. 283 mL. *OTC.*
Use: Analgesic.
Chloraseptic Sore Throat. (Prestige)
Loz.: Benzocaine 6 mg, menthol 10 mg.
Pkg. 18s. **Spray:** Phenol 1.4%. Saccharin. Alcohol free. Cherry, mint, menthol, and citrus flavors. 177 mL. *OTC.*
Use: Mouth and throat product.
Chloraseptic Sore Throat Relief. (Prestige) Benzocaine 3 mg, menthol 3 mg.
Acesulfame, sucralose. Cherry and citrus flavors. Strips. 40s. *OTC.*
Use: Mouth and throat products.
Chlorazene. (Badger) Chloramine-T, sodium p-toluene-sulfonchloramide. **Pow.:**
UD Pkg. 20 g, 38 g, 50 g, 88 g, 200 g,
240 g, 320 g, Bot. 1 lb, 5 lb. **Aromatic
Pow. (5%):** Bot. 1 lb, 5 lb. **Tab. (0.3 g):**
Bot. 20s, 100s, 1000s, 5000s. *OTC.*
Use: Antiseptic; deodorant.
chlorazepate dipotassium.
See: Clorazepate Dipotassium.
chlorazepate monopotassium.
See: Clorazepate Monopotassium.
Chlorazine. (Major) Prochlorperazine
5 mg, 10 mg. Tab. Bot. 100s.
Use: Antiemetic; antipsychotic; antivertigo.
chlorbutanol.
See: Chlorobutanol.
chlorbutol.
See: Chlorobutanol.
•**chlorcyclizine hydrochloride.** (klor-SIK-lih-zeen) *NF 29.*
Use: Antihistamine.
W/Codeine Phosphate.
See: Notuss NX.
W/Codeine Phosphate, Phenylephrine
Hydrochloride.
See: Nasotuss.
W/Codeine Phasphate, Pseudoephedrine Hydrochloride.
See: Notuss NxD.
•**chlordantoin.** (KLOR-dan-toe-in) USAN.
Use: Antifungal.
Chlordex GP. (Cypress) Dextromethorphan HBr 7.5 mg, guaifenesin 100 mg,
phenylephrine hydrochloride 10 mg,
chlorpheniramine maleate 2 mg per
5 mL. Alcohol and sugar free. Saccharin, sorbitol. Grape flavor. Syrup.
473 mL. *Rx.*
Use: Upper respiratory combination, antitussive and expectorant combination.
•**chlordiazepoxide.** (klor-DIE-aze-ee-POX-side) *USP 34.*
Tall Man: chlordiazePOXIDE
Use: Anxiolytic.
See: Brigen-G.
W/Amitriptyline.
See: Limbitrol.
Limbitrol DS.
•**chlordiazepoxide hydrochloride.** (klor-DIE-aze-ee-POX-ide) *USP 34.*
Tall Man: chlordiazePOXIDE
Use: Hypnotic; sedative; anxiolytic.
W/Clidinium Bromide.
See: Librax.
RE Chlordiazepoxide/Clidinium.
chlordiazepoxide hydrochloride.
(Various Mfr.) Chlordiazepoxide hydrochloride 5 mg, 10 mg, 25 mg. Cap.
20s, 100s, 500s, 1000s, UD 100s. *c-iv.*
Use: Anxiolytic.
chlordiazepoxide with clidinium bromide. (Various Mfr.) Clidinium 2.5 mg,
chlordiazepoxide hydrochloride 5 mg.
Cap. Bot. 100s, 500s, 1000s, UD 100s.
Rx.
Use: Gastrointestinal anticholinergic
combination.
Chlordrine S.R. (Rugby) Pseudoephedrine hydrochloride 120 mg, chlorpheniramine maleate 8 mg. SR Cap. Bot.
100s. *Rx.*
Use: Antihistamine; decongestant.
Chloren 8 T.D. (Wren) Chlorpheniramine
maleate 8 mg. Tab. Bot. 100s, 1000s.
OTC.
Use: Antihistamine.
Chloren 12 T.D. (Wren) Chlorpheniramine maleate 12 mg. Tab. Bot. 100s,
1000s. *Rx-OTC.*
Use: Antihistamine.
Chloresium Tooth Paste. (Rystan)
Chlorophyllin copper complex. Tube
3.25 oz. *OTC.*
Use: Deodorant, oral.
chlorethyl.
See: Ethyl Chloride.
chlorguanide hydrochloride.
See: Chloroguanide Hydrochloride.
•**chlorhexidine gluconate.** (klor-HEX-ih-deen GLUE-koe-nate) USAN.
Use: Antimicrobial.
See: Bacto Shield.
Bacto Shield 2.
Hibistat.
Peridex.
PerioChip.
PerioGard.
Surgilube.
chlorhexidine gluconate. (Various Mfr.)
Chlorhexidine gluconate. **Oral rinse:**
0.12%. 473 mL. **Cloth:** 2%. Aloe vera,
glycerin. Alednol free. 6s. *Rx.*
Use: Mouth and throat product.

chlorhexidine gluconate mouthrinse.
Use: Amelioration of oral mucositis associated with cytoreductive therapy for conditioning patients for bone marrow transplantation. [Orphan Drug]
See: Peridex.
PerioGard.

•**chlorhexidine hydrochloride.** (klor-HEX-ih-deen) USAN.
Use: Anti-infective, topical.

•**chlorhexidine phosphanilate.** (klor-HEX-ih-deen FOSS-fah-nih-LATE) USAN.
Use: Anti-infective.

chlorinated and iodized peanut oil.
Chloriodized oil.

•**chlorindanol.** (klor-IN-dah-nahl) USAN.
Use: Antiseptic, spermaticide.

chlorine compound, antiseptic. Antiseptic, chlorine.

chloriodized oil. Chlorinated and iodized peanut oil.

•**chlormadinone acetate.** (klor-MAD-ih-nohn) USAN.
Use: Hormone, progestin.

Chlor Mal w/Sal + APAP S.C. (Global Source) Chlorpheniramine maleate 2 mg, acetaminophen 150 mg, salicylamide 175 mg. Tab. Bot. 1000s. *OTC.*
Use: Analgesic; antihistamine.

chlormerodrin. Mercloran. *Rx.*
Use: Diuretic.

•**chlormerodrin Hg 197.** (klor-MER-oh-drin) USAN.
Use: Diagnostic aid, renal function determination; radiopharmaceutical.

•**chlormerodrin Hg 203.** (klor-MER-oh-drin) USAN.
Use: Diagnostic aid, renal function determination; radiopharmaceutical.

chlormezanone. Chlormethazanone.
Use: Anxiolytic.

Chlor-Niramine Allergy Tabs. (Whiteworth Towne) Chlorpheniramine maleate 4 mg. Tab. Bot. 24s, 100s. *OTC.*
Use: Antihistamine.

chloroacetic acids.
See: Monochloroacetic Acid.

•**chlorobutanol.** (Klor-oh-BYOO-tah-nole) *NF 29.*
Use: Anesthetic; antiseptic; hypnotic; pharmaceutic aid, antimicrobial.
W/Combinations.
See: Ardeben.
Depo-Testadiol.
Efedron NaSal.
Lacril.
Lacri-Lube.
Minirin.
Pred-G.

•**chlorocresol.** (KLOR-oh-KREE-sole) *NF 29.*
Use: Antiseptic; disinfectant.

chloroethane.
Use: Anticholinergic; antispasmodic; topical anesthetic.
See: Ethyl Chloride.

Chlorofair. (Bausch & Lomb) **Soln.:** Chloramphenicol 5 mg/mL. Bot. 7.5 mL. **Oint.:** Chloramphenicol 10 mg/g in white petrolatum base with mineral oil, polysorbate 60. Tube 3.5 g. *Rx.*
Use: Anti-infective, ophthalmic.

chloroguanide hydrochloride. (Various Mfr.) Proguanil hydrochloride. *Rx.*
Use: Antimalarial.

Chlorohist-LA. (Roberts) Xylometazoline hydrochloride 0.1%. Soln. Spray 15 mL. *OTC.*
Use: Decongestant.

Chloromag. (Merit) Magnesium chloride hexahydrate 200 mg/mL (1.97 mEq/mL). Benzyl alcohol 1%, sodium chloride 9 mg. Inj., Soln. Multiple-dose vials. 50 mL. *Rx.*
Use: Intravenous nutritional therapy, mineral.

chloromethapyrilene citrate.
See: Chlorothen Citrate.

Chloromycetin/Hydrocortisone. (Parke-Davis) Hydrocortisone acetate 0.5% (2.5% as powder), chloramphenicol 0.25% (1.25% as powder). Pow. Bot. with dropper 5 mL. *Rx.*
Use: Anti-infective, ophthalmic.

chlorophenothane.
Use: Pediculicide.

chlorophyll. (Freeda) Chlorophyll 20 mg, sugar free. Tab. Bot. 100s, 250s, 500s. *OTC.*
Use: Deodorant, oral.

chlorophyll derivatives, systemic.
See: Chlorophyll.
Derifil.

chlorophyllin.
Use: Deodorant; healing agent.

•**chlorophyllin copper complex.** (KLOR-oh-FILL-in KAHP-uhr) USAN.
Use: Deodorant.
See: Chloresium.
Derifil.
PALS.

•**chlorophyllin copper complex sodium.** (KLOR-oh-FILL-in KAHP-uhr) *USP 34.*
Use: Deodorant.

•**chloroprocaine hydrochloride.** (klor-oh-PRO-cane) *USP 34.*
Use: Anesthetic, local ester, injectable.
See: Nesacaine.
Nesacaine-MPF.

chloroprocaine hydrochloride. (Bedford) Chloroprocaine hydrochloride 2%, 3%, preservative-free. Inj. Single-dose vials. 20 mL. *Rx.*
Use: Anesthetic, local ester, injectable.

•**chloroquine.** (KLOR-oh-kwin) *USP 34.*
Use: Antiamebic; antimalarial.

•**chloroquine phosphate.** (KLOR-oh-kwin) *USP 34.*
Use: Antiamebic; antimalarial; lupus erythematosus agent.
See: Aralen Phosphate.

chloroquine phosphate. (Various Mfr.) Chloroquine phosphate 250 mg (equiv. to 150 mg base), 500 mg (equiv. to 300 mg base). May contain lactose (500 mg only). Tab. Bot. 20s, 22s (250 mg only); 25s (500 mg only); 30s (250 mg only); 100s; 500s (500 mg only); 1000s, UD 100s (250 mg only). *Rx.*
Use: Amebicide.

chlorothen.
Use: Antihistamine.

chlorothen citrate. (Whittier) Chlorothen citrate. Tab. Bot. 100s.
Use: Antihistamine.

W/Pyrilamine, Thenylpyramine.
See: Derma-Pax.

chlorothenylpyramine. Chlorothen.

•**chlorothiazide.** (KLOR-oh-THIGH-uh-zide) *USP 34.*
Use: Diuretic.
See: Diuril.

W/Methyldopa.
See: Aldoclor.

chlorothiazide. (Various Mfr.) Chlorothiazide 250 mg, 500 mg. Tab. 100s. *Rx.*
Use: Diuretic.

•**chlorothiazide sodium for injection.** (KLOR-oh-THIGH-uh-zide) *USP 34.*
Use: Antihypertensive; diuretic.

chlorothymol.
Use: Anti-infective.

•**chlorotrianisene.** (klor-oh-try-AN-ih-seen) *USP 34.*
Use: Estrogen.

•**chloroxine.** (KLOR-ox-een) USAN.
Use: Topical anti-infective.

•**chloroxylenol.** (KLOR-oh-ZIE-len-ole) *USP 34.*
Use: Antibacterial.

W/Benzalkonium Chloride, Hydrocortisone, Pramoxine Hydrochloride.
See: Cortic-ND.
  Mediotic-HC.

W/Benzocaine, Hydrocortisone Acetate.
See: TriOxin.

W/Glycerin, Pramoxine Hydrochloride, Zinc Acetate Dihydrate.
See: Zinotic.
  Zinotic ES.

W/Hydrocortisone, pramoxine.
See: Oto-End 10.
  Otomar-HC.
  Zoto-HC.

W/Methyl Salicylate, Menthol, Camphor, Thymol, Eucalyptus Oil, Isopropyl Alcohol.
See: Gordobalm.

W/Pramoxine Hydrochloride, Zinc Acetate Dihydrate.
See: ZinOtic ES.

chlorozone.
See: Chloramine-T.

Chlorpazine. (Major) Prochlorperazine maleate 5 mg, 10 mg, 25 mg. Tab. Bot. 100s, UD 100s (5 mg, 10 mg only). *Rx.*
Use: Antipsychotic.

Chlorphed. (Roberts) Brompheniramine maleate 10 mg/mL. Inj. Vial 10 mL. *Rx.*
Use: Antihistamine.

Chlorphed-LA. (Roberts) Oxymetazoline 0.05%. Soln. Spray 15 mL. *OTC.*
Use: Decongestant.

Chlorphedrine SR. (Ivax) Chlorpheniramine maleate 8 mg, pseudoephedrine hydrochloride 120 mg. Cap. Bot. 100s. *Rx.*
Use: Antihistamine; decongestant.

•**chlorphenesin carbamate.** (KLOR-fen-ee-sin CAR-bah-mate) USAN.
Use: Muscle relaxant.

chlorpheniramine. (KVK Tech) Chlorpheniramine maleate 12 mg. Calcium 28 mg, lactose, propyl parahydroxybenzoate, sodium benzoate, sucrose, sugar. ER Tab. 24s, 60s. *OTC.*
Use: Antihistamine; alkylamine, nonselective.

chlorpheniramine/codeine. (Breckenridge) Chlorpheniramine maleate 2 mg, codeine phosphate 10 mg per 5 mL. Glycerin, parabens, saccharin, sorbitol. Alcohol free, dye free, and sugar free. Grape flavor. Liq. 473 mL. c-v.
Use: Upper respiratory combination, antitussive combination.

•**chlorpheniramine maleate.** (klor-fen-IHR-ah-meen) *USP 34.*
Use: Antihistamine, nonselective alkylamine.
See: Aller-Chlor.
  Allergy.
  Allergy Relief.
  Allergy-Time.
  Chlo-Amine.
  Chlor-Trimeton Allergy 8 Hour.

Chlor-Trimeton Allergy 12 Hour.
ED Chlorped Jr.
Efidac 24.
Pediox-S.
QDALL AR.
W/Acetaminophen.
See: Coricidin HBP Cold & Flu.
W/Acetaminophen, Codeine Phosphate.
See: Cotabflu.
W/Acetaminophen, Dextromethorphan
Hydrobromide.
See: Coricidin HBP Maximum Strength
Flu.
Theraflu Nighttime Severe Cold.
Triaminic Flu, Cough & Fever.
Tylenol Plus Children's Cough &
Runny Nose.
Vicks Formula 44M Cough, Cold, &
Flu Relief.
W/Acetaminophen, Dextromethorphan
Hydrobromide, Phenylephrine Hydro-
chloride.
See: Alka-Seltzer Plus Cold & Cough.
Comtrex Maximum Strength Day &
Night Cold & Cough.
Comtrex Maximum Strength Night-
time Cold & Cough.
Robitussin Cough, Cold & Flu Night-
time.
Theraflu Nighttime Severe Cold.
Tylenol Cold Head Congestion Night-
time.
Tylenol Cold Multi-Symptom Nighttime.
Tylenol Plus Children's Flu.
Tylenol Plus Children's Multi-
Symptom Cold.
W/Acetaminophen, Phenylephrine Hydro-
chloride.
See: Alka-Seltzer Plus Fast Crystal
Packs.
Comtrex Maximum Strength Day &
Night Flu Therapy.
Comtrex Maximum Strength Day &
Night Severe Cold & Sinus.
Contac Cold + Flu.
Contac Cold + Flu Night.
Dristan Cold Multi-Symptom Formula.
Dryphen Multi-Symptom Formula.
Medicidin-D.
Onset Forte Micro-Coated.
Pyrroxate Extra Strength.
Sine Off Sinus/Cold.
Tylenol Allergy Multi-Symptom.
Tylenol Allergy Multi-Symptom Conve-
nience Pack.
Tylenol Plus Children's Cold.
Tylenol Sinus Congestion & Pain
Nighttime.
W/Acetaminophen, Pseudoephedrine
Hydrochloride.
See: BC Allergy, Sinus, Headache.

W/Aspirin, Dextromethorphan Hydrobro-
mide.
See: Alka-Seltzer Plus Flu.
W/Aspirin, Phenylephrine Bitartrate.
See: Alka-Seltzer Plus Cold.
Alka-Seltzer Plus Sparkling Original
Cold Formula.
W/Belladonna Alkaloids, Pseudoephed-
rine Hydrochloride.
See: Respa A.R.
W/Codeine Phosphate.
See: Cotab A.
Cotab AX.
EndaCof-C.
Lexuss 210.
Notuss-AC
TL-Hist CM.
Zodryl AC 80.
Zodryl AC 50.
Zodryl AC 40.
Zodryl AC 60.
Zodryl AC 30.
Zodryl AC 35.
Zodryl AC 25.
Z-Tuss AC.
W/Codeine Phosphate, Phenylephrine
Hydrochloride.
See: Endal CD.
W/Codeine Phosphate, Pseudoephed-
rine Hydrochloride.
See: Phenylhistine DH.
Zodryl DAC 80.
Zodryl DAC 50.
Zodryl DAC 40.
Zodryl DAC 60.
Zodryl DAC 30.
Zodryl DAC 35.
Zodryl DAC 25.
W/Dextromethorphan Hydrobromide.
See: AMBI 20 DM/4CPM.
Coricidin HBP Cough & Cold.
Dimetapp Long Acting Cough Plus
Cold.
Robitussin Pediatric Cough & Cold
Long Acting.
Scot-Tussin DM.
Triaminic Cough & Runny Nose.
Tricodene Sugar Free Cough & Cold.
Vicks Children's NyQuil Cold &
Cough Relief.
Vicks Formula 44m Pediatric Cough
& Cold Relief.
W/Dextromethorphan Hydrobromide, Guai-
fenesin, Phenylephrine Hydrochloride.
See: Chlordex GP.
DM/CPM/PE/GG.
Donatussin.
W/Dextromethorphan Hydrobromide,
Methscopolamine Nitrate.
See: Extendryl DM.

W/Dextromethorphan Hydrobromide,
Phenylephrine Hydrochloride.
 See: AMBI 10PEH/4CPM/20DM.
  Amerituss AD.
  Bronkids.
  Centergy DM.
  Ceron-DM.
  Corfen-DM.
  CP DEC-DM.
  C-Phen DM.
  DM/PE/CPM.
  Donatussin DM.
  Ed-A-Hist DM.
  Father John's Medicine Plus.
  Maxichlor PEH DM.
  Nasohist DM.
  Neo DM.
  NoHist DMX.
  NoHist-PDX.
  P Chlor DM.
  PE-Hist DM.
  Phenabid DM.
  Relahist-DM.
  Rondec-DM.
  Rondex-DM.
  Sonahist DM.
  TGQ 15DM/5PEH/2CPM.
  Trigofen DM.
  Trital DM.
  Z-Dex 120.
  ZoDen DM.
W/Dextromethorphan Hydrobromide,
Pseudoephedrine Hydrochloride.
 See: AccuHist PDX.
  Allres DS.
  AMBI 60PSE/4CPM/20DM.
  Atuss DS.
  CPM/PSE DM.
  Dicel DM.
  Esocor P.
  KidKare Children's Cough/Cold.
  Mesehist DM.
  Neutrahist PDX.
  Pedia Relief Cough-Cold.
  Pediatric Cough & Cold.
  Pediatric Cough & Cold Medicine.
  Rescon DM.
  Triaminic-D Children's.
W/Dihydrocodeine Bitartrate, Phenyl-
ephrine Hydrochloride.
 See: DiHydro-PE.
  Duohist DH.
W/Dihydrocodeine Bitartrate, Pseudo-
ephedrine Hydrochloride.
 See: DiHydro-CP.
W/Guaifenesin, Hydrocodone Bitartrate,
Pseudoephedrine Hydrochloride.
 See: ZTuss Expectorant.
W/Guaifenesin, Phenylephrine Hydro-
chloride.
 See: P Chlor GG.

W/Hydrocodone Bitartrate
 See: Hydro-PC.
  TussiCaps Full Strength.
  TussiCaps Half Strength.
W/Hydrocodone Bitartrate, Phenylephrine
Hydrochloride.
 See: Histinex HC.
  Neo HC.
  Notuss-Forte.
  Relacon-HC.
  Vanex-HD.
W/Hydrocodone Bitartrate, Pseudo-
ephedrine Hydrochloride.
 See: Notuss-Forte.
W/Methscopolamine Nitrate.
 See: AeroHist.
  AllePak Dose Pack.
  Allergy ND.
  AlleRx DF Dose Pack.
  AlleRx Dose Pack.
  NoHist EXT.
  RelCof CPM.
W/Methscopolamine Nitrate, Phenyl-
ephrine Hydrochloride.
 See: AeroHist Plus.
  AeroKid.
  CPM 8/PE 20/MSC 1.25.
  Dallergy.
  Dallergy PE.
  Dehistine.
  Denaze.
  DriHist SR.
  Drysec.
  Duradryl.
  Extendryl.
  NoHist-Plus.
  OMNIhist II LA.
  PCM.
  PE-CPM-MSN 8-2-0.75.
  PE HCL-CPM-MSN 10-2-0.75.
  Phenylephrine CM.
  QV Allergy.
  Ralix.
  Relcof PSE.
  Rescon.
  Rescon-MX.
  SymPak.
  SymPak PDX.
  Zinx PCM.
W/Methscopolamine Nitrate, Pseudo-
ephedrine Hydrochloride.
 See: CPM 8/PSE 90/MSC 2.5.
  DryMax.
  Relcof PSE.
  Time-Hist QD.
W/Phenylephrine Hydrochloride.
 See: Actifed Cold & Allergy.
  AMBI 10PEH/4CPM.
  Allerest PE.
  Ceron.
  C-Phen.

Dallergy.
Dallergy-Jr.
Ed A-Hist.
Extendryl PEM.
Nasohist.
NoHist.
NoHist LQ.
Phenabid.
Rescon-Jr.
Sonahist.
W/Phenylephrine Hydrochloride, Phenyl-
toloxamine Citrate.
See: Nalex-A.
NoHist-A.
Rhinacon A.
W/Phenylephrine Hydrochloride, Pyril-
amine Maleate.
See: MyHist-PD.
Polyhist PD.
Pyrichlor PE.
W/Pseudoephedrine Hydrochloride.
See: AccuHist.
Allerest Maximum Strength.
AMBI 60PSE/4CPM.
Colfed-A.
CPM PSE.
Deconamine.
Deconomed SR.
Duratuss DA.
Genaphed Plus.
Histex.
LoHist-D.
Neutrahist.
PSE CPM.
PSE 15/CPM 2.
RE2+30.
Sudafed Sinus & Allergy.
SudaHist.
Sudal-12 Tannate.
SudoGest Sinus & Allergy Maximum
Strength.
Zinx Chlor-D.
d-chlorpheniramine maleate.
See: Polaramine Expectorant.
chlorpheniramine maleate. (Various
Mfr.) Chlorpheniramine maleate 4 mg.
Tab. Bot. 24s, 100s, 1000s. OTC.
Use: Antihistamine, nonselective alkyl-
amine.
chlorpheniramine maleate. (Various
Mfr.) Chlorpheniramine maleate 8 mg,
10 mg. SR Cap. Bot. 100s, 1000s. Rx.
Use: Antihistamine, nonselective alkyl-
amine.
chlorpheniramine maleate. (Various
Mfr.) Chlorpheniramine maleate 10 mg/
mL, benzyl alcohol 1.5%. Inj. Multidose
vial. Rx.
Use: Antihistamine, nonselective alkylamine.

**chlorpheniramine maleate/phenyl-
ephrine hydrochloride.** (Silarx) **Liq.:**
Phenylephrine hydrochloride 3.5 mg,
chlorpheniramine maleate 1 mg per
5 mL. Alcohol and sugar free. Saccharin, sorbitol. Raspberry flavor. 30 mL
with dropper. **Syrup:** Phenylephrine
hydrochloride 12.5 mg, chlorpheniramine maleate 4 mg per 5 mL. Alcohol
and sugar free. Saccharin, sorbitol.
Raspberry flavor. 118 mL, 473 mL. Rx.
Use: Upper respiratory combination,
decongestant and antihistamine.
**chlorpheniramine maleate/pseudo-
ephedrine hydrochloride.** (Various
Mfr.) Pseudoephedrine hydrochloride
120 mg, chlorpheniramine maleate
8 mg. May contain parabens, sucrose.
ER Cap. Bot. 100s, 250s, 500s, 1000s.
OTC.
Use: Antihistamine and decongestant,
upper respiratory combination.
**chlorpheniramine maleate/pseudo-
ephedrine hydrochloride LA.** (River's
Edge) Pseudoephedrine hydrochloride
120 mg, chlorpheniramine maleate
12 mg. Lactose. ER Tab. 100s. Rx.
Use: Upper respiratory combination, de-
congestant and antihistamine.
• **chlorpheniramine maleate with
pseudoephedrine hydrochloride.**
(klor-fen-IHR-ah-meen MAL-ee-ate with
SOO-do-ee-fed-rin) USP 34.
Use: Antihistamine, decongestant.
• **chlorpheniramine polistirex.** (klor-fen-
IHR-ah-meen pahl-ee-STIE-rex) USAN.
Use: Antihistamine.
W/Combinations.
See: Atuss-12 DM.
Codeprex.
W/Hydrocodone Polistirex.
See: Tussionex PennKinetic.
**chlorpheniramine polistirex/hydro-
codone polistirex.** (Various Mfr.)
Chlorpheniramine maleate (as chlor-
pheniramine polistirex) 8 mg, hydro-
codone bitartrate (as hydrocodone
polistirex) 10 mg. May contain corn
syrup, parabens, polysorbate 80, pro-
pylene glycol, sucrose. ER Susp.
473 mL. c-III.
Use: Upper respiratory combination, an-
titussive combination.
chlorpheniramine tannate.
See: Ed-Chlor-Tan.
Pediatan.
TanaHist PD.
W/Carbetapentane Tannate.
See: Tannic-12.
Tannic-12 S.
Trionate.

Tussi-12.
Tussi-12 S.
Tussizone-12 RF.
Tustan 12S.
W/Carbetapentane Tannate, Ephedrine
Tannate, Phenylephrine Tannate.
See: Quad-Tus Tannate Pediatric.
Rynatuss.
Rynatuss Pediatric.
W/Carbetapentane Tannate, Phenyl-
ephrine Tannate.
See: D-Tann CT.
Dytan CS.
XiraTuss.
W/Dextromethorphan Tannate, Pseudo-
ephedrine Tannate.
See: Atuss DS Tannate.
W/Methscopolamine Nitrate.
See: Dexodryl.
W/Methscopolamine Nitrate, Phenyl-
ephrine Tannate.
See: AH-Chew.
AH-Chew Ultra Tannate.
Redur-PCM.
W/Phenylephrine Tannate.
See: AlleRx.
BP Allergy Junior.
Ed Chlor-PED D.
Ny-Tannic.
PediaPhyl D.
PE Tann/CP Tann.
Phenyl Chlor-Tan Pediatric.
R-Tanna.
Rynatan.
Rynatan Pediatric.
Ry-Tann.
TanaHist-D Pediatric.
Tannate Pediatric.
W/Phenylephrine Tannate, Pyrilamine
Tannate.
See: Conal.
Nalex-A 12.
Triotann Pediatric.
Triple Tannate Pediatric.
**chlorpheniramine tannate and pseudo-
ephedrine tannate.** (Various Mfr.)
Pseudoephedrine tannate 75 mg,
chlorpheniramine tannate 4.5 mg/5 mL,
strawberry/banana flavor, alcohol free.
Susp. Bot. 118 mL, 473 mL. *Rx.*
Use: Upper respiratory combination, de-
congestant, antihistamine.
•**chlorphentermine hydrochloride.** (klor-
FEN-ter-meen) USAN.
Use: Anorexic.
chlorphthalidone.
See: Chlorthalidone.
•**chlorpromazine.** (klor-PRO-muh-zeen)
USP 34.
Tall Man: chlorproMAZINE
Use: Antiemetic; antipsychotic.

•**chlorpromazine hydrochloride.** (klor-
PRO-muh-zeen) *USP 34.*
Tall Man: chlorproMAZINE
Use: Antiemetic; antipsychotic.
See: Promachlor.
**chlorpromazine hydrochloride injec-
tion.** (Various Mfr.) Chlorpromazine
hydrochloride 25 mg/mL. sodium metabisulfite, sodium sulfite. Amp. 1 mL,
2 mL. *Rx.*
Use: Antipsychotic.
chlorpromazine hydrochloride tablets.
(Various Mfr.) Chlorpromazine hydrochloride 10 mg, 25 mg, 50 mg, 100 mg,
200 mg. Tab. Bot. 100s, 1000s, UD
100s. *Rx.*
Use: Antipsychotic.
•**chlorpropamide.** (klor-PRO-puh-mide)
USP 34.
Tall Man: chlorproPAMIDE
Use: Antidiabetic.
chlorpropamide. (Various Mfr.) Chlorpropamide 100 mg, 250 mg. Tab. Bot.
100s, 250s (250 mg only), 500s, 1000s,
UD 100s, UD 600s. *Rx.*
Use: Antidiabetic.
chlorprophenpyridamine maleate.
See: Chlorpheniramine maleate.
Chlor-Pro 10. (Schein) Chlorpheniramine
maleate 10 mg/mL, benzyl alcohol. Inj.
Vial 30 mL. *Rx.*
Use: Antihistamine.
chlorquinol. Mixture of the chlorinated
products of 8-hydroxyquinoline containing about 65% of 5,7-dichloro-8-
hydroxyquinoline.
**chlortetracycline and sulfamethazine
bisulfates.**
Use: Anti-infective.
•**chlortetracycline bisulfate.** (klor-the-
trah-SIGH-kleen) *USP 34.*
Use: Anti-infective; antiprotozoal.
•**chlorthalidone.** (klor-THAL-ih-dohn)
USP 34.
Use: Diuretic.
See: Thalitone.
W/Combinations.
See: Clorpress.
Tenoretic.
chlorthalidone. (Various Mfr.) Chlorthalidone 25 mg, 50 mg, 100 mg. Tab. Bot.
100s, 250s (50 mg only), 500s (100 mg
only). *Rx.*
Use: Diuretic.
Chlor-Trimeton Allergy. (Schering-
Plough) Chlorpheniramine maleate
4 mg, lactose. Tab. Box. 24s. *OTC.*
Use: Antihistamine.
Chlor-Trimeton Allergy•D 4 Hour.
(Schering-Plough) Pseudoephedrine

sulfate 60 mg, chlorpheniramine maleate 4 mg, lactose. Tab. Box. 24s. *OTC.*
Use: Upper respiratory combination, decongestant, antihistamine.

Chlor-Trimeton Allergy•D 12 Hour.
(Schering-Plough) Pseudoephedrine sulfate 120 mg, chlorpheniramine maleate 8 mg, butylparaben, sugar, lactose. Tab. Bot. 24s. *OTC.*
Use: Upper respiratory combination, decongestant, antihistamine.

Chlor-Trimeton Allergy 8 Hour.
(Schering-Plough) Chlorpheniramine maleate 8 mg. ER Tab. Box. 15s. *OTC.*
Use: Antihistamine, nonselective alkylamine.

Chlor-Trimeton Allergy 12 Hour.
(Schering-Plough Healthcare) Chlorpheniramine maleate 12 mg. ER Tab. Box. 10s. *OTC.*
Use: Antihistamine, nonselective alkylamine.

Chlor-Trimeton 4 Hour Relief.
(Schering-Plough) Chlorpheniramine maleate 4 mg, pseudoephedrine sulfate 60 mg. Tab. Box 24s, 48s. *OTC.*
Use: Antihistamine; decongestant.

Chlor-Trimeton 12 Hour Allergy.
(Schering-Plough) Chlorpheniramine maleate 8 mg, pseudoephedrine sulfate 120 mg. SR Tab. Box 24s, 48s. UD 96s. *OTC.*
Use: Antihistamine; decongestant.

Chlor-Trimeton 12 Hour Relief.
(Schering-Plough) Chlorpheniramine 8 mg, pseudoephedrine sulfate 120 mg. Tab. Box 12s. Bot. 36s. *OTC.*
Use: Antihistamine; decongestant.

•**chlorzoxazone.** (klor-ZOX-uh-zone) *USP 34.*
Use: Muscle relaxant.
See: Paraflex.
  Parafon Forte DSC.
  Remular-S.

chlorzoxazone. (Various Mfr.) Chlorzoxane 250 mg, 500 mg. Tab. Bot. 100s, 500s (500 mg only), 1000s.
Use: Muscle relaxant.

chlorzoxazone and acetaminophen.
Use: Analgesic; muscle relaxant.

•**chocolate.** (CHOK-a-lat) *NF 29.*
Use: Flavoring.

Choice DM. (Bristol-Myers Squibb) Protein 38.1 g, carbohydrate 101.5 g, fat 42.3 g, Na 846 mg, K 1818.9 mg per liter, 0.93 Cal/mL; vitamins A, D, E, K, C, B_1, B_2, B_3, B_5, B_6, FA, biotin, Ca, P, I, Mg, Zn, Mn, Cl, K, Na, Se, Cr, Mo, sucrose. Vanilla and chocolate flavors. Liq. 237 mL ready-to-use cans. *OTC.*

Use: Enteral nutrition therapy.

Choice DM AlC Home Blood Test.
(Bristol-Myers Squibb) Kit for blood samples. 1 single-use test kit. *OTC.*
Use: In vitro diagnostic aid.

Choice DM Daily Moisturizing. (Bristol-Myers Squibb) Petrolatum, glycerin, dimethicone, steareth-2, alcohols, laureth-23, magnesium aluminum silicate, carbomer, potassium sorbate, sodium hydroxide, aloe. Fragrance free. Lot. 226.8 mL. *OTC.*
Use: Emollient.

Choice DM Gentle Care. (Bristol-Myers Squibb) Sorbitol, poloxamer 407, sodium, saccharin, cetylpyridinium chloride, citric acid. Alcohol and sugar free. Fresh mint flavor. Mouthwash. 500 mL. *OTC.*
Use: Mouth and throat product.

Choice DM Sugar Free Shakes. (Bristol-Myers Squibb) **Mocha cappuccino flavor:** Protein 30.7 g, carbohydrate 33.8 g, fat 7.7 g, Na 460.5 mg. K 1043.8 mg per liter, 0.38 Cal/mL; vitamins A, D, E, K, B_1, B_2, B_3, B_5, B_6, B_{12}, Ca, Fe, FA, biotin, P, I, Mg, Zn, Se, Cu, Cr, Mo. Liq. 325 mL. **Chocolate fudge flavor:** Protein 30.7 g, carbohydrate 36.8 g, fat 6.1 g, Na 460.5 mg. K 1043.8 mg per liter, 0.38 Cal/mL; vitamins A, D, E, K, B_1, B_2, B_3, B_5, B_6, B_{12}, Ca, Fe, FA, biotin, P, I, Mg, Zn, Se, Cu, Cr, Mo. Liq. 325 mL. **French vanilla flavor:** Protein 30.7 g, carbohydrate 24.6 g, fat 6.1 g, Na 399.1 mg. K 337.7 mg per liter, 0.31 Cal/mL; vitamins A, D, E, K, B_1, B_2, B_3, B_5, B_6, B_{12}, Ca, Fe, FA, biotin, P, I, Mg, Zn, Se, Cu, Cr, Mo. Liq. 325 mL. **Strawberries'n cream flavor:** Protein 30.7 g, carbohydrate 21.5 g, fat 7.7 g, Na 399.1 mg. K 337.7 mg per liter, 0.31 Cal/mL; vitamins A, D, E, K, B_1, B_2, B_3, B_5, B_6, B_{12}, Ca, Fe, FA, biotin, P, I, Mg, Zn, Se, Cu, Cr, Mo. Liq. 325 mL. *Rx.*
Use: Enteral nutrition therapy.

Choice 10. (Whiteworth Towne) Potassium chloride 10%. Soln., unflavored. Bot. Gal. *Rx.*
Use: Electrolyte supplement.

Choice 20. (Whiteworth Towne) Potassium chloride 20%. Soln., unflavored. Bot. Gal. *Rx.*
Use: Electrolyte supplement.

cholacrylamine resin. Anion exchange resin consisting of a water-soluble polymer having a molecular weight equivalent between 350 and 360 in which aliphatic quaternary amine groups are attached to an acrylic backbone by ester linkages.

cholalic acid. Cholic acid.
Cholan-DH. (Medeva) Dehydrocholic acid 250 mg. Tab. Bot. 100s.
Use: Laxative.
cholanic acid. Dehydrodesoxycholic acid.
Cholebrine. (Mallinckrodt) Iocetamic acid (62% iodine) 750 mg. Tab. Bot. 100s, 150s.
Use: Radiopaque agent.
• **cholecalciferol.** (kole-eh-kal-SIH-fer-ole) *USP 34.* Formerly 7-Dehydrocholesterol, activated.
Use: Vitamin D_3 (antirachitic).
See: A and D Ointment.
    Advanced D5000.
    Baby Ddrops.
    Ddrops.
    Delta-D.
    D-5000 Super Strength.
    D400.
    D1000.
    D_3-50.
    D_3 Healthy Kids.
    High Potency D-1000.
    Maximum D3.
    Maximum Strength D-2000.
    Super Strength D-2000 IU.
    Ultra Strength D2000.
    Ultra Strength Vitamin D_3.
    Vitamin D_3.
W/Alendronate Sodium.
See: Fosamax Plus D.
choleretic. Bile salts.
See: Bile Preps and Forms.
    Dehydrocholic Acid.
    Tocamphyl.
cholesterin.
See: Cholesterol.
• **cholesterol.** (koe-LESS-ter-all) *NF 29.*
Use: Pharmaceutic aid, emulsifying agent.
cholesterol reagent strips. (Bayer Consumer Care) A quantitative strip test for cholesterol in serum. Seralyzer reagent strips. Bot. 25s.
Use: Diagnostic aid.
cholestyramine. (Various Mfr.) Anhydrous cholestyramine resin 4 g/9 g powder. May contain sucrose, sorbitol. Pow. for Oral Susp. 9 g Packet. 42s, 60s. Cans. 378 g. *Rx.*
Use: Antihyperlipidemic; bile acid sequestrant.
cholestyramine light. (Various Mfr.) Anhydrous cholestyramine resin 4 g/5.7 g powder. May contain aspartame. Pow. for Oral Susp. 5 g and 5.7 g Packets. 60s. Cans. 210 g, 231 g, 239 g. *Rx.*
Use: Antihyperlipidemic; bile acid sequestrant.

• **cholestyramine resin.** (koe-less-TEER-uh-meen) *USP 34.*
Use: Antihyperlipidemic; ion-exchange resin, bile acid sequestrants.
See: Cholestyramine Light.
    Prevalite.
    Questran.
    Questran Light.
Choletec. (Bracco) Mebrofenin 45 mg (when sodium pertechnetate Tc-99m injection is added to the vial, the diagnostic agent technetium Tc-99m mebrofenin is formed containing up to 3,700 MBq [100 millicuries] of Tc-99m). Parabens. Also contains stannous fluoride dihydrate (minimum) and total tin 1.03 mg maximum (as stannous fluoride dihydrate). Inj., Lyophilized Pow. for Soln. Kits of 10 multidose vials. *Rx.*
Use: Radiopaque agent.
Cholidase. (Freeda) Choline 450 mg, inositol 150 mg, vitamins B_6 2.5 mg, B_{12} 5 mcg, E 7.5 mg. Tab. Bot. 100s, 250s, 500s. *OTC.*
Use: Lipid, vitamin supplement.
choline. (Various Mfr.) Choline 650 mg. Tab. 90s, 100s. *OTC.*
Use: Lipotropic.
• **choline bitartrate.** (koe-leen bye-TAR-trait) *USP 34.*
• **choline chloride.** (koe-leen) *USP 34.* (Various Mfr.)
Use: Liver supplement. [Orphan Drug]
choline chloride, carbamate. Carbachol.
choline chloride succinate.
See: Succinylcholine Chloride.
choline dihydrogen citrate. 2-Hydroxyethyl trimethylammonium citrate US vitamin 0.5 g. Bot. 100s, 500s.
Use: Lipotropic.
choline magnesium trisalicylate. (Sidmak) Choline magnesium trisalicylate 500 mg, 750 mg, 1000 mg. Tab. Bot. 100s, 500s. *Rx.*
Use: Analgesic.
cholinergic agents.
Use: Parasympathomimetic agents.
See: Mecholyl Ointment.
    Mestinon.
    Mytelase.
    Pilocarpine.
    Tensilon.
    Urecholine.
    Urinary Cholinergics.
cholinergic blocking agents.
See: Parasympatholytic Agents.
• **choline salicylate.** (koe-leen suh-lih-sih-late) USAN.
Use: Analgesic.

cholinesterase inhibitors. Agents that inhibit the enzyme cholinesterase and enhance the effects of endogenous acetylcholine.
Use: Glaucoma therapy; Alzheimer disease; muscle stimulant.
See: Donepezil Hydrochloride.
Eserine Salicylate.
Eserine Sulfate.
Galantamine Hydrobromide.
Neostigmine Methylsulfate.
Rivastigmine Tartrate.
Tacrine Hydrochloride.

choline theophyllinate.
See: Oxtriphylline.

Cholinoid. (Ivax) Choline 111 mg, inositol 111 mg, vitamins B_1 0.33 mg, B_2 0.33 mg, B_3 3.33 mg, B_5 1.7 mg, B_6 0.33 mg, B_{12} 1.7 mcg, C 100 mg, lemon bioflavonoid complex 100 mg. Cap. Bot. 100s. *OTC.*
Use: Lipid, vitamin supplement.

Chol Meth in B. (Esco) Choline bitartrate 235 mg, inositol 112 mg, methionine 70 mg, betaine anhydrous 50 mg, vitamins B_{12} 6 mcg, B_1 6 mg, B_6 3 mg, niacin 10 mg. Cap. Bot. 500s, 1000s. *OTC.*
Use: Vitamin supplement.

Cholografin Meglumine. (Bracco Diagnostics) Iodipamide meglumine 520 mg, iodine 257 mg/mL. EDTA. Inj. Vials. 20 mL. *Rx.*
Use: Radiopaque agent; parenteral agent.

cholylglycine.
See: CG RIA.

chondodendron tomentosum.
See: Curare.

•**chondroitin sulfate and sodium hyaluronate.** (kon-DRO-ih-tin SULL-fate and SO-dee-uhm HIGH-ah-loo-rohn-ate) *USP 34.* Surgical aid in anterior segment procedures including cataract extraction and intraocular lens implantation. *Rx.*
See: DisCoVisc.
Viscoat.

•**chondroitin sulfate sodium.** (kon-DRO-ih-tin SULL-fate SO-dee-uhm) *NF 29.*
Use: Dietary supplement.

chondrus. Irish Moss.
See: Kondremul.

Chooz. (Schering-Plough) Calcium carbonate 500 mg (elemental calcium 200 mg). Sucrose, glucose. Mint flavor. Gum Tab. Pkg. 16s. *OTC.*
Use: Mineral supplement; antacid.

•**choriogonadotropin alfa.** (kore-ee-oh-goe-NAD-oh-troe-pin) USAN.

Use: Sex hormone, ovulation stimulant.
See: Ovidrel.

chorionic gonadotropin.
Use: Ovulation stimulant.
See: Pregnyl.

chorionic gonadotropin. (Various Mfr.) Chorionic gonadotropin 5,000 units per vial with 10 mL diluent (500 units per mL), 10,000 units per vial with 10 mL diluent (1,000 units per mL), 20,000 units per vial with 10 mL diluent (2,000 units per mL). Pow. for Inj. Vials. 10 mL. *Rx.*
Use: Ovulation stimulant.

Chromagen FA. (Ther-Rx) Elemental iron (from ferrous asparto glycinate) 70 mg, succinic acid 75 mg, vitamin C (as calcium ascorbate and calcium threonate) 152 mg, folic acid 1 mg, vitamin B $_{12}$ 10 mcg. Lactose. Film-coated. Tab. 90s. *Rx.*
Use: Mineral, vitamin supplement.

Chromagen Forte. (Ther-Rx) Elemental iron (from ferrous asparto glycinate and ferrous fumarate) 151 mg, succinic acid 50 mg, vitamin C (as calcium ascorbate and calcium threonate) 60.8 mg, folic acid 1 mg, B_{12} 10 mcg. Lactose. Film-coated. Tab. 90s. *Rx.*
Use: Mineral, vitamin supplement.

Chromagen OB. (Savage) Ca 200 mg, Cu, folic acid 1 mg, Fe 28 mg, Mn, B_2 1.8 mg, B_1 1.6 mg, B_6 20 mg, C 60 mg, D 400 units, Zn 25 mg, E 30 units, niacinamide 5 mg, B_{12} 12 mcg, docusate calcium 25 mg. Cap. Bot. 100s. *Rx.*
Use: Vitamin supplement.

chromargyre.
See: Merbromin.

chromated. Solution (Cr^{51}).
See: Chromitope Sodium.

Chromelin Complexion Blender. (Summers) Dihydroxyacetone 5%, isopropyl alcohol, propylene glycol. Susp. 30 mL. *OTC.*
Use: Hyperpigmenting.

chromic acid, disodium salt. Sodium Chromate Cr^{51}.

•**chromic chloride.** (kroe-MIK) *USP 34.*
Use: Supplement, trace mineral.

chromic chloride. (American Regent) Chromium 4 mcg/mL (as chromic chloride 20.5 mcg/mL). Preservative free. Inj., Soln. Single-use vial. 10 mL. *Rx.*
Use: Trace metal.

chromic chloride. (Hospira) Chromium 4 mcg/mL (as chromic chloride 20.5 mcg/mL). Preservative free. Inj., Soln. Vial. 10 mL. *Rx.*
Use: Trace metal.

•**chromic chloride Cr 51.** (kroe-MIK) USAN.
Use: Radiopharmaceutical.

•**chromic phosphate Cr 51.** (kroe-MIK) USAN.
Use: Radiopharmaceutical.

•**chromic phosphate P 32 suspension.** (kroe-MIK) *USP 34.*
Use: Radiopharmaceutical.

Chromitope Sodium. (Bristol-Myers Squibb) Chromate Cr^{51}, sodium for Inj. 0.25 mCi.
Use: Radiopharmaceutical.

chromium. A trace metal used in IV nutritional therapy that helps maintain normal glucose metabolism and peripheral nerve function.
See: Chromic Chloride.

•**chromium Cr 51 edetate.** (KRO-me-um) *USP 34.*
Use: Radiopharmaceutical.

•**chromonar hydrochloride.** (kroe-moe-NAHR) USAN.
Use: Coronary vasodilator.

Chronulac. (Hoechst) Lactulose 10 g/ 15 mL (< galactose 1.6 g, lactose 1.2 g, other sugars 1.2 g). Soln. Bot. 240 mL, 960 mL. *Rx.*
Use: Laxative.

Chur-Hist. (Churchill) Chlorpheniramine 4 mg. Kaptab. Bot. 100s.
Use: Antihistamine.

•**chymotrypsin.** (kye-moe-TRIP-sin) *USP 34.*
Use: Proteolytic enzyme.

Cialis. (Lilly) Tadalafil 2.5 mg, 5 mg, 10 mg, 20 mg. Lactose. Film-coated. 30s (except 2.5 mg), blisters of 2 × 15 (2.5 mg, 5 mg). *Rx.*
Use: Erectile dysfunction.

Cibacalcin. (Novartis) Calcitonin-human for injection.
Use: Paget disease. [Orphan Drug]

CI basic violet 3. Gentian Violet.

Ciba Vision Cleaner. (Ciba Vision) Cocoamphocarboxyglycinate, sodium lauryl sulfate, sorbic acid 0.1%, hexylene glycol, EDTA 0.2%. Soln. 5 mL, 15 mL. *OTC.*
Use: Contact lens care.

Ciba Vision Saline. (Ciba Vision) Buffered, isotonic with NaCl, boric acid. Soln. Bot. 90 mL, 240 mL, 360 mL. *OTC.*
Use: Contact lens care, rinsing, storage.

cibenzoline.
See: Cifenline Succinate.

•**ciclafrine hydrochloride.** (SIK-lah-freen) USAN.
Use: Antihypotensive.

•**ciclazindol.** (sigh-CLAY-zin-dole) USAN.
Use: Antidepressant.

•**ciclesonide.** (sye-KLES-oh-nide) USAN.
Use: Respiratory inhalant, intranasal steroid.
See: Alvesco.
Omnaris.

•**cicletanine.** (sik-LET-ah-neen) USAN.
Use: Antihypertensive.

•**ciclopirox.** (sigh-kloe-PEER-ox) USAN.
Use: Antifungal agent, topical anti-infective.
See: CNL8 Nail Kit.
Loprox.
Penlac Nail Lacquer.

ciclopirox. (Fougera) Ciclopirox 0.77%. Isopropyl alcohol. **Gel:** 30 g, 45 g. *Rx.*
Use: Antifungal agent, topical anti-infective.

ciclopirox. (Paddock) Ciclopirox 1%. Shampoo, Susp. 120 mL. *Rx.*
Use: Topical anti-infective, antifungal agent.

ciclopirox. (Perrigo) Ciclopirox 0.77%. Benzyl alcohol, cetyl alcohol, myristyl alcohol, stearyl alcohol, lactic acid, mineral oil. Lot. 30 mL, 60 mL. *Rx.*
Use: Antifungal agent, topical anti-infective.

ciclopirox. (Various Mfr.) Ciclopirox 0.77%. Top. Susp. 30 mL, 60 mL. *Rx.*
Use: Antifungal agent, topical anti-infective.

ciclopirox nail laquer. (Various Mfr.) Ciclopirox 8%. May contain isopropyl alcohol. Top. Soln. 3.3 mL, 6.6 mL with brushes. *Rx.*
Use: Topical anti-infective, antifungal agent.

•**ciclopirox olamine.** (sigh-kloe-PEER-ox OLE-ah-meen) *USP 34.*
Use: Antifungal.

•**cicloprofen.** (SIK-low-pro-fen) USAN.
Use: Anti-inflammatory.

•**cicloprolol hydrochloride.** (SIGH-kloe-PRO-lahl) USAN.
Use: Antiadrenergic, beta-receptor.

Cidex Plus. (Johnson & Johnson) Glutaraldehyde 3.2%. Soln. Gal.
Use: Disinfectant, sterilizing.

Cidex-7. (Johnson & Johnson) Glutaraldehyde 2% and vial of activator with aqueous potassium salt as buffer and sodium nitrite as a corrosive inhibitor. Soln. Bot. Qt., gal., 5 gal.
Use: Disinfectant, sterilizing.

C.I. direct blue 53 tetrasodium salt. Evans Blue. *Rx.*

•**cidofovir.** (sigh-DAH-fah-vihr) USAN.
Use: Antiviral.
See: Vistide.

• **cidoxepin hydrochloride.** (sih-DOX-eh-PIN) USAN.
Use: Antidepressant.

• **cifenline.** (sigh-FEN-leen) USAN. *Formerly cibenzoline.*
Use: Cardiovascular, antiarrhythmic.

• **cifenline succinate.** (sigh-FEN-leen) USAN.
Use: Cardiovascular agent, antiarrhythmic.

• **ciglitazone.** (sigh-GLIE-tah-ZONE) USAN.
Use: Antidiabetic.

cignolin.
See: Anthralin.

• **ciladopa hydrochloride.** (SIGH-lah-doe-pah) USAN.
Use: Antiparkinsonian, dopaminergic.

• **cilansetron.** (sil-an-SE-tron) USAN.
Use: Gastrointestinal agent; irritable bowel syndrome.

• **cilansetron hydrochloride.** (sil-an-SE-tron) USAN.
Use: Gastrointestinal agent; irritable bowel syndrome.

cilastatin-imipenem. A formulation of imipenem, a thienamycin antibiotic, and cilastatin sodium, the inhibitor of the renal dipeptidase, dehydropeptidase-1.
Use: Anti-infective.
See: Primaxin I.M.
Primaxin I.V.

• **cilastatin sodium.** (SIGH-lah-STAT-in) *USP 34.*
Use: Enzyme inhibitor.
W/Imipenem.
See: Primaxin.

• **cilazapril.** (sile-AZE-ah-PRILL) USAN.
Use: Investigational antihypertensive.

• **cilengitide.** (sye-LEN-gi-tide) USAN.
Use: Angiogenesis inhibitor.

• **cilexetil.** (sigh-LEX-eh-till) USAN.
Use: Anti-infective.

Cilfomide. (Sanofi-Synthelabo) Inositol hexanicotinate. Tab. *Rx.*
Use: Hypolipidimic, peripheral vasodilator.

Cillium. (Whiteworth Towne) Psyllium seed husk 4.94 g, 14 calories/rounded tsp. Pow. Bot. 420 g, 630 g. *OTC.*
Use: Laxative.

• **cilmostim.** (SILL-moe-stim) USAN. *Formerly rhM-CSF, M-CSF, CSF-1.*
Use: Hematopoietic, macrophage colony-stimulating factor.

• **cilobamine mesylate.** (SIGH-low-BAM-een) USAN. *Formerly clobamine mesylate.*
Use: Antidepressant.

• **cilofungin.** (SIGH-low-FUN-jin) USAN.
Use: Antifungal.

• **cilomilast.** (sill-OH-mih-last) USAN.
Use: Investigational drug for asthma; COPD; arthritis; atopic dermatitis; multiple sclerosis.

• **cilostazol.** (sill-OH-stah-zole) USAN.
Use: Antithrombotic; platelet inhibitor; vasodilator.
See: Pletal.

cilostazol. (Various Mfr.) Cilostazol 50 mg, 100 mg. Tab. 60s, 500s (100 mg only). *Rx.*
Use: Antiplatelet agent.

Ciloxan. (Alcon) Ciprofloxacin. **Oint.:** 3.33 mg (equivalent to 3 mg base)/g. Mineral oil, white petrolatum. Tube. 3.5 g. **Soln.:** 3.5 mg/mL (equiv. to 3 mg base). Benzalkonium chloride 0.006%, mannitol 4.6%, EDTA 0.05%. Drop-Tainers 2.5 mL, 5 mL. *Rx.*
Use: Anti-infective.

• **ciluprevir.** (sigh-loo-PRAH-veer) USAN.
Use: Hepatitis C.

• **cimaterol.** (sigh-MAH-teh-role) USAN.
Use: Repartitioning agent.

• **cimetidine.** (sigh-MET-ih-deen) *USP 34.*
Use: Histamine H_2 antagonist.
See: Acid Reducer 200.
Tagamet.
Tagamet HB 200.

cimetidine. (Various Mfr.) Cimetidine. **Inj.:** 150 mg/mL. Vial single-dose. 2 mL, Multidose vial. 8 mL (may contain benzyl alcohol 9 mg/mL as a preservative). **Oral Soln.:** 300 mg (as hydrochloride)/5 mL. May contain alcohol, parabens, saccharin, sorbitol. Bot. 240 mL, 480 mL, UD 5 mL. **Tab.:** 200 mg, 300 mg, 400 mg, 800 mg. Tab. Bot. 30s (800 mg only); 60s (400 mg only); 100s; 250s (800 mg only); 500s, 1,000s (except 800 mg). *Rx.*
Use: Histamine H_2 receptor antagonist.

cimetidine. (Various Mfr.) Cimetidine 200 mg. Tab. Bot. 30s, 50s. *OTC.*
Use: Histamine H_2 receptor antagonist.

• **cimetidine hydrochloride.** (sigh-MET-ih-deen) USAN.
Use: Histamine H_2 receptor antagonist.

cimetidine in 0.9% sodium chloride. (Hospira) Cimetidine hydrochloride 6 mg/mL. Inj. (premixed). Single-dose flexible container. 50 mL. *Rx.*
Use: Histamine H_2 antagonist.

Cimzia. (UCB) Certolizumab pegol. **Inj., lyophilized Pow. for Soln:** 200 mg. Preservative free. Single-use vials. **Inj., Soln:** 200 mg/mL. Preservative free. Single-use prefilled syringe. 1 mL. *Rx.*
Use: Immunologic agent, immunomodulator.

• **cinacalcet hydrochloride.** (sin-a-KAL-set) USAN.
Use: Hyperparathyroidism agent.
See: Sensipar.

Cinacort Span. (Foy Laboratories) Triamcinolone acetonide 40 mg/mL. Vial 5 mL. *Rx.*
Use: Corticosteroid.

• **cinalukast.** (sin-ah-LOO-kast) USAN.
Use: Antiasthmatic; leukotriene antagonist.

• **cinanserin hydrochloride.** (sin-AN-ser-in) USAN.
Use: Serotonin inhibitor.

cinchona alkaloid.
Use: Antimalarial.

cinchona bark. (Various Mfr.).
Use: Antimalarial, tonic.
W/Anhydrous Quinine, Cinchonidine, Cinchonine, Quinidine, Quinine.
See: Totaquine.

cinchonine salts. (Various Mfr.).
Use: Quinine dihydrochloride.

cinchophen.
Use: Analgesic.

• **cinepazet maleate.** (SIN-eh-PAZZ-ett) USAN.
Use: Antianginal.

• **cinflumide.** (SIN-flew-mide) USAN.
Use: Muscle relaxant.

• **cingestol.** (sin-JESS-tole) USAN.
Use: Hormone, progestin.

• **cinnamedrine.** (sin-am-ED-reen) USAN.
Use: Muscle relaxant.

cinnamic aldehyde. *Name previously used for Cinnamaldehyde.*

cinnamon.
Use: Flavoring.

cinnamon oil. (Various Mfr.).
Use: Pharmaceutic aid.

• **cinnarizine.** (sin-NAHR-ih-zeen) USAN.
Use: Antihistamine.

cinnopentazone. INN for Cintazone.

Cinobac. (Oclassen) Cinoxacin 250 mg. Cap. Bot. 40s. *Rx.*
Use: Anti-infective, urinary.

• **cinoxate.** (sin-OX-ate) USAN.
Use: Ultraviolet screen.

• **cinperene.** (SIN-peh-reen) USAN.
Use: Antipsychotic.

Cin-Quin. (Solvay) Quinidine sulfate. (Contains 83% anhydrous quinidine alkaloid.) **Tab.:** 100 mg, 200 mg, 300 mg. Bot. 100s, 1000s, UD 100s. **Cap.:** 200 mg. Bot. 100s. 300 mg. Bot. 100s, 1000s, UD 100s. *Rx.*
Use: Antiarrhythmic.

• **cinromide.** (SIN-row-mide) USAN.
Use: Anticonvulsant.

Cinryze. (Lev Pharmaceuticals) C1 inhibitor (human) 500 units. Preserva-tive free. Inj., lyophilized Pow. for Soln. Single-use vial. *Rx.*
Use: Hematological agent, protein C1 inhibitor.

• **cintazone.** (SIN-tah-zone) USAN.
Use: Anti-inflammatory.

• **cintriamide.** (sin-TRY-ah-mid) USAN.
Use: Antipsychotic.

• **cioteronel.** (SIGH-oh-TEH-row-nell) USAN.
Use: Dermatologic, acne; androgenic alopecia and keloid, antimutagenic.

• **cipamfylline.** (sigh-PAM-fih-lin) USAN.
Use: Antiviral.

Cipralan. (Roche) Cifenline succinate. *Formerly cibenzoline. Rx.*
Use: Antiarrhythmic.

• **cipralisant maleate.** (ci-PRAL-is-ant) USAN.
Use: Histamine H_3 antagonist; ADHD.

• **ciprefadol succinate.** (sih-PREH-fah-dahl) USAN.
Use: Analgesic.

Cipro. (Schering-Plough) Ciprofloxacin. **Tab.:** As ciprofloxacin hydrochloride 250 mg, 500 mg, 750 mg. Film-coated. Bot. 50s, 100s, UD 100s. **Microcapsules for Oral Susp.:** 250 mg/5 mL (5%), 500 mg/5 mL (10%) when reconstituted. Sucrose, strawberry flavor. Bot. 100 mL with diluent. *Rx.*
Use: Anti-infective, fluoroquinolone.

• **ciprocinonide.** (sih-PRO-SIN-oh-nide) USAN.
Use: Adrenocortical steroid.

Ciprodex. (Alcon) Ciprofloxacin 0.3%, dexamethasone 0.1%. Benzalkonium chloride, boric acid, EDTA. Susp. 5 mL, 7.5 mL. *Drop-Tainer. Rx.*
Use: Steroid and antibiotic combination.

• **ciprofibrate.** (sip-ROW-FIE-brate) USAN.
Use: Antihyperlipoproteinemic.

• **ciprofloxacin.** (sip-ROW-FLOX-ah-sin) USP 34.
Use: Anti-infective, fluoroquinolone.
See: Cetraxal.
Ciloxan.
Cipro.
Cipro I.V.
Proquin XR.
W/Dexamethasone.
See: Ciprodex.

ciprofloxacin. (Barr) Ciprofloxacin 250 mg/5 mL (5%), 500 mg/5mL (10%) (when reconstituted). Sucrose, strawberry flavor. Pow. for Oral Susp. Bot. of microcapsules, diluent, and a teaspoon. *Rx.*

Use: Anti-infective, fluoroquinolone.

ciprofloxacin. (Dr. Reddy's) Ciprofloxacin (as ciprofloxacin hydrochloride) 100 mg. Film-coated. Tab. 6s. *Rx.*
Use: Fluoroquinolone.

ciprofloxacin. (Sandoz) Ciprofloxacin 200 mg, 400 mg. Lactic acid. Inj. Soln. 100 mL dextrose 5% flexible container (0.2%) (200 mg only), 200 mL dextrose 5% flexible container (0.2%) (400 mg only). *Rx.*
Use: Anti-infective, fluoroquinolone.

ciprofloxacin. (Various Mfr.) Ciprofloxacin. **ER Tab.:** As ciprofloxacin hydrochloride. 500 mg, 1000 mg. 30s (1000 mg only), 50s, 100s, 250s (1000 mg only), 500s, UD 10s (1000 mg only). **Soln.:** 3.5 mg/mL (equiv. to 3 mg base). Benzalkonium chloride 0.006%, mannitol, and EDTA. Dropper Bot. 2.5 mL, 5 mL, 10 mL. **Inj. Conc.:** 200 mg, 400 mg. May contain lactic acid. Vials. 20 mL (1%) (200 mg), 40 mL (1%) (400 mg). **Tab.:** As ciprofloxacin hydrochloride. 250 mg, 500 mg, 750 mg. 50s, 100s, 500s, UD 10s. *Rx.*
Use: Ophthalmic antibiotic; fluoroquinolones.

• **ciprofloxacin hydrochloride.** (sip-ROW-FLOX-ah-sin) *USP 34.*
Use: Anti-infective, ophthalmic.
See: Ciloxan.

ciprofloxacin in 5% dextrose. (Various Mfr.) Ciprofloxacin 200 mg, 400 mg. May contain lactic acid. Dextrose 5%. Inj., Soln. Flexible cont. (0.2%). 100 mL (200 mg only), 200 mL (400 mg only). *Rx.*
Use: Anti-infective, fluoroquinolone.

Cipro HC Otic. (Alcon) Ciprofloxacin 0.2%, hydrocortisone 1%/mL. Benzyl alcohol. Susp. Bot. 10 mL. *Rx.*
Use: Steroid and antibiotic combination.

Cipro I.V. (Schering-Plough) Ciprofloxacin. **Inj., Conc.:** 200 mg, 400 mg. Lactic acid. Vials. 20 mL (1%) (200 mg only), 40 mL (1%) (400 mg only). **Inj.:** 200 mg, 400 mg. Lactic acid. Dextrose 5%. Flexible cont. (0.2%). 100 mL (200 mg only), 200 mL (400 mg only). *Rx.*
Use: Anti-infective, fluoroquinolone.

• **ciprostene calcium.** (sigh-PRAHS-teen) USAN.
Use: Platelet aggregation inhibitor.

• **ciramadol.** (sihr-AM-ah-dole) USAN.
Use: Analgesic.

• **ciramadol hydrochloride.** (sihr-AM-ah-dole) USAN.
Use: Analgesic.

Circavite-T. (Circle) Iron 12 mg, vitamins A 10,000 units, D 400 units, E 15 mg, B_1 10.3 mg, B_2 10 mg, B_3 100 mg, B_5 18.4 mg, B_6 4.1 mg, B_{12} 5 mcg, C 200 mg, Cu, I, Mg, Mn, Zn 1.5 mg. Bot. 100s. *OTC.*
Use: Mineral, vitamin supplement.

• **cirolemycin.** (sih-ROW-leh-MY-sin) USAN.
Use: Anti-infective; antineoplastic.

• **cisapride.** (SIS-uh-PRIDE) USAN.
Note: Withdrawn from US market. Available from the manufacturer on a limited-access protocol.
Use: Gastrointestinal; stimulant, peristaltic.

• **cisatracurium besylate.** (sis-ah-trah-CURE-ee-uhm BESS-ih-late) USAN.
Use: Nondepolarizing neuromuscular blocking agent; muscle relaxant.
See: Nimbex.

• **cisconazole.** (SIS-KOE-nah-zahl) USAN.
Use: Antifungal.

• **cisplatin.** (SIS-plat-in) *USP 34. Formerly cis-Platinum II.*
Tall Man: CISplatin
Use: Antineoplastic.

cisplatin. (Various Mfr.) Cisplatin 1 mg/mL. Inj. Multidose vial 50 mL, 100 mL, 200 mL. *Rx.*
Use: Antineoplastic.

cis-retinoic acid. (13-cis-Retinoic Acid).
Use: Antiacne.
See: Accutane.
Isotretinoin.

9-cis retinoic acid. (Allergan)
Use: Promyelocytic leukemia treatment; prevention of retinal detachment caused by proliferative vitreoretinopathy. [Orphan Drug]

• **citalopram hydrobromide.** (sih-TAHL-oh-pram) USAN.
Use: Antidepressant.
See: Celexa.

citalopram hydrobromide. (Roxane) Citalopram (as hydrobromide) 10 mg per 5 mL. Sorbitol, parabens. Peppermint flavor. Oral Soln. 240 mL. *Rx.*
Use: Antidepressant.

citalopram hydrobromide. (Various Mfr.) Citalopram hydrobromide 10 mg, 20 mg, 40 mg. May contain lactose. Tab. 30s, 100s, 500s, 1,000s, UD 100s (except 10 mg). *Rx.*
Use: Antidepressant.

Citanest Forte. (Dentsply Pharm) Prilocaine hydrochloride 4% with epinephrine 1:200,000, sodium metabisulfite. Inj. Dental cartridge 1.8 mL. *Rx.*
Use: Anesthetic, local amide, injectable.

Citanest Plain. (Dentsply Pharm) Prilocaine hydrochloride 4%. Inj. Dental Cartridge. 1.8 mL. *Rx.*
Use: Anesthetic, local amide, injectable.

•**citenamide.** (sigh-TEN-ah-MIDE) USAN.
Use: Anticonvulsant.

Cithal. (Table Rock) Watermelon seed extract 2 g, theobromine 4 g, phenobarbital 0.25 g. Cap. Bot. 100s, 500s. *Rx.*
Use: Antihypertensive.

•**citicoline sodium.** (SIGH-tih-koe-leen) USAN.
Use: Poststroke and posthead trauma treatment.

Citracal. (Mission) Elemental calcium 200 mg. Tab. Bot. 100s. *OTC.*
Use: Calcium supplement.

Citracal 1500 + D. (Mission) Calcium citrate 1500 mg, vitamin D 200 units. Tab. Bot. 60s. *OTC.*
Use: Mineral, vitamin supplement.

Citracal + D₃ Maximum. (Bayer) Calcium 315 mg, vitamin D 200 units. PEG, propylene glycol. Coated. Tab. 240s. *OTC.*
Use: Nutritional supplement.

Citracal Plus with Magnesium. (Mission) Ca 250 mg, vitamin D 125 units, B₆ 5 mg, B, Cu, Mg, Mn, Zn. Tab. Bot. 150s. *OTC.*
Use: Mineral, vitamin supplement.

Citracal Prenatal 90 + DHA. (Mission) **Cap.:** Docosahexaenoic acid 250 mg. 6 blister packs of 5s. **Tab.:** Calcium 200 mg, iron 90 mg, vitamin A 2700 units, D₃ 400 units, E 30 units, thiamin 30 mg, riboflavin 3.4 mg, niacinamide 20 mg, B₆ 20 mg, B₁₂ 12 mcg, C 120 mg, folic acid 1 mg, iodine 150 mcg, zinc 25 mg, copper 2 mg, docusate sodium 50 mg. 6 blister packs of 5s. *Rx.*
Use: Prenatal vitamin.

Citracal Prenatal + DHA. (Mission) **Cap.:** Docosahexaenoic acid 250 mg. 6 blister packs of 5s. **Tab.:** Calcium 125 mg, iron 27 mg, vitamin A 2700 units, D₃ 400 units, E 30 units, thiamin 3 mg, riboflavin 3.4 mg, niacinamide 20 mg, B₆ 20 mg, C 120 mg, folic acid 1 mg, iodine 150 mcg, zinc 25 mg, copper 2 mg, docusate sodium 50 mg. 6 blister packs of 5s. *Rx.*
Use: Prenatal vitamin.

Citra Forte. (Boyle and Co. Pharm.) Hydrocodone bitartrate 5 mg, ascorbic acid 30 mg, pheniramine maleate 2.5 mg, pyrilamine maleate 3.33 mg, potassium citrate 150 mg/5 mL. Bot. Pt, gal. *c-III.*
Use: Antihistamine; antitussive; vitamin supplement.

Citranox. (Alconox)
Use: Liquid acid detergent for manual and ultrasonic washers.

Citra pH. (ValMed, Inc.) Sodium citrate dihydrate 450 mg/30 mL. Soln. 30 mL. *OTC.*
Use: Antacid.

Citrasan B. (Sandia) Lemon bioflavonoid complex 300 mg, vitamins C 300 mg, B₁ 30 mg, B₂ 10 mg, B₆ 5 mg, B₁₂ 4 mcg, calcium pantothenate 10 mg, niacinamide 50 mg. Tab. Bot. 100s, 1000s. *OTC.*
Use: Mineral, vitamin supplement.

Citrasan K. (Sandia) Vitamins C 125 mg, K 0.66 mg, lemon bioflavonoid complex 125 mg/5 mL. Liq. Bot. Pt, gal. *OTC.*
Use: Vitamin supplement.

Citrasan K-250. (Sandia) Vitamins C 250 mg, K 1 mg, lemon bioflavonoid 250 mg. Tab. Bot. 100s, 1000s. *OTC.*
Use: Vitamin supplement.

citrate acid.
Use: Systemic alkalinizer.

citrate and citric acid.
Use: Alkalinizer.
See: Oracit.
  Polycitra.
  Polycitra K.
  Polycitra LC.
  Taron-Crystals.

citrated normal human plasma.
See: Plasma, Normal Human.

Citresco-K. (Esco) Vitamins C 100 mg, K 0.7 mg, citrus bioflavonoid complex 100 mg. Cap. Bot. 100s, 500s, 1000s. *OTC.*
Use: Vitamin supplement.

•**citric acid.** (SI-trik) *USP 34.*
Use: Component of anticoagulant solutions and drug products.
W/Aspirin, Sodium Bicarbonate.
See: Alka-Seltzer Lemon Lime.
  Alka-Seltzer Original.
W/Potassium Bicarbonate, Sodium Bicarbonate.
See: Alka-Seltzer Gold.
W/Sodium Bicarbonate.
See: Alka-Seltzer Heartburn Relief.
W/Simethicone, Sodium Bicarbonate.
See: E-Z Gas II.

citric acid, glucono-delta-lactone and magnesium carbonate.
Use: Renal and bladder calculi of the apatite or struvite variety. [Orphan Drug]

citric acid, magnesium oxide, and sodium carbonate irrigation.
Use: Irrigant, ophthalmic.

citric acid monohydrate.
W/Potassium Citrate Monohydrate.
See: Taron-Crystals.
citrin.
See: Vitamin P.
Citrin Capsules. (Table Rock) Watermelon seed extract 4 g. Bot. 100s, 500s. *Rx.*
Use: Antihypertensive.
Citrocarbonate. (Lee) Sodium bicarbonate 0.78 g, sodium citrate anhydrous 1.82 g/3.9 g. Bot. 4 oz, 8 oz. *OTC.*
Use: Antacid.
Citrocarbonate Effervescent Granules. (Lee) Sodium bicarbonate 780 mg, sodium citrate anhydrous 1820 mg, sodium 700.6 mg/5 mg. Bot. 150 g. *OTC.*
Use: Analgesic; antacid.
Citro Cee, Super. (Marlyn Nutraceuticals) Bioflavonoids 500 mg, rutin 50 mg, vitamin C 500 mg, rose hips powder 500 mg. Tab. Bot. 50s, 100s. *OTC.*
Use: Vitamin supplement.
Citrolith. (Beach) Potassium citrate 50 mg, sodium citrate 950 mg. Tab. Bot. 100s, 500s. *Rx.*
Use: Alkalinizer, urinary.
Citroma. (Century) Magnesium citrate. Oral Soln. Bot. 10 oz. *OTC.*
Use: Laxative.
Citroma Low Sodium. (National Magnesia) Magnesium citrate, lemon or cherry flavor in sugar-free vehicle. Oral soln. Bot. 10 oz. *OTC.*
Use: Laxative.
Citrotein. (Novartis) Sucrose, pasteurized egg white solids, amino acids, maltodextrin, citric acid, natural and artificial flavors, mono- and diglycerides, partially hydrogenated soybean oil, 0.66 cal/mL, protein 40.7 g, carbohydrate 120.7 g, fat 1.55 g, Na 698 mg, K 698 mg/L. Tartrazine (orange flavor only). Orange, grape, and punch flavors. Pow. 1.57 oz. Pkt., Can 14.16 oz. *OTC.*
Use: Nutritional supplement, enteral.
•**citrovorum factor.** (sih-troe-VOHR-uhm) *USP 34.*
See: Leucovorin calcium.
Citrucel. (GlaxoSmithKline) Methylcellulose. **Pow.:** 2 g/heaping tbsp., sucrose, orange flavor. Can. 480 g, 846 g. **Tab.:** 500 mg. Maltodextrin. 164s. *OTC.*
Use: Laxative
Citrucel Fiber Shake. (GlaxoSmithKline) Methylcellulose 2 g per packet. Sugar free. Phenylalanine 49 mg, aspartame. Chocolate flavor. Pow. Packets. 10.7 g. *OTC.*
Use: Laxative.

Citrucel Sugar Free. (GlaxoSmithKline) Methylcellulose 2 g, aspartame, phenylalanine 52 mg/levelled scoop. Pow. Can. 245 g, 480 g. *OTC.*
Use: Laxative.
citrus bioflavonoid compound.
See: Bioflavonoid Compounds.
Vitamin P.
Citrus Calcium. (Rugby) Calcium citrate 200 mg. Lactose free. Coated Tab. 100s. *OTC.*
Use: Mineral supplement.
Citrus Calcium + D. (Rugby) Vitamin D (as cholecalciferol)/calcium (as calcium citrate) 250 units/200 mg, 250 units/315 mg. Lactose free. PEG. Tab. 60s (250 units/315 mg), 100s (250 units/200 mg). *OTC.*
Use: Nutritional combination product.
•**cixutumumab.** (SIKS-ue-TUE-mue-mab) USAN.
Use: Antineoplastic.
CKA Canker Aid. (Pannett Prod.) Benzocaine, aluminum hydrate, magnesium trisilicate, sodium acid carbonate. Pow. *OTC.*
Use: Cancer; cold sores.
CK (CPK) Reagent Strips. (Bayer Consumer Care) Seralyzer reagent strips for creatinine phosphokinase in serum or plasma. Bot. 25s.
Use: Diagnostic aid.
•**cladribine.** (KLAD-rih-BEAN) USAN.
Use: Antineoplastic.
See: Leustatin.
cladribine. (Bedford) Cladribine 1 mg/mL, sodium chloride 9 mg/mL. Soln. for Inj. Single-use Vial 20 mL w/10 mL fill. *Rx.*
Use: Antineoplastic.
Claforan. (Hoechst Marion Roussel) Cefotaxime sodium. **Pow. for Inj. (sodium 2.2 mEq/g):** 500 mg. Vial Pkg. 10s. 1 g, 2 g. Vial. Pkg. 10s, 25s, 50s. Infusion bot. 10s, *ADD-Vantage* system Vial 25s, 50s. 10 g. Bot. **Inj. (sodium 2.2 mEq/g):** 1 g, 2 g. Premixed, frozen. 50 mL Pkg. 12s. *Rx.*
Use: Anti-infective, cephalosporin.
•**clamoxyquin hydrochloride.** (KLAM-OX-ee-kwin) USAN.
Use: Amebicide.
Claravis. (Teva) Isotretinoin 10 mg, 20 mg, 30 mg, 40 mg. EDTA. Cap. Blister packs. 30s, 100s (except 30 mg). *Rx.*
Use: Retinoid, first generation.
Clarifoam EF. (Onset) Sodium sulfacetamide 10%, sulfur 5%. Cetyl alcohol, parabens. Aer. Foam. 60 g. *Rx.*

Use: Dermatological agent, acne combination product.

Clarinex. (Schering) Desloratadine. **Syrup:** 2.5 mg/5 mL. Sugar, EDTA. Bubble gum flavor. 480 mL. **Tab.:** 5 mg. Lactose. Film-coated. Bot. 100s, 500s, unit-of-use 30s, UD hospital pack 100s. *Rx.*
Use: Antihistamine, peripherally selective piperidine.

Clarinex-D 12 Hour. (Schering) Pseudoephedrine sulfate 120 mg, desloratadine 2.5 mg. EDTA. ER Tab. 100s. *Rx.*
Use: Decongestant and antihistamine.

Clarinex-D 24 Hour. (Schering) Pseudoephedrine sulfate 240 mg, desloratadine 5 mg. EDTA. ER Tab. 100s. *Rx.*
Use: Decongestant and antihistamine, upper respiratory combination.

Clarinex RediTabs. (Schering) Desloratadine 2.5 mg (phenylalanine 1.4 mg), 5 mg (phenylalanine 2.9 mg). Mannitol, aspartame, tutti frutti flavor. Rapidly disintegrating Tab. Blister packs. 30s. *Rx.*
Use: Antihistamine, peripherally selective piperidine.

Claris. (Stratus) Sodium sulfacetamide 10%, sulfur 1%. Cetyl alcohol, disodium EDTA, glyceryl stearate, parabens, PEG-100, stearyl alcohol, urea. Soap. 473 mL. *Rx.*
Use: Acne product, combination.

•**clarithromycin.** (kluh-RITH-row-MY-sin) *USP 34.*
Use: Anti-infective.
See: Biaxin.
  Biaxin XL.

clarithromycin. (Teva) Clarithromycin. **ER Tab.:** 500 mg. Lactose. Filmcoated. 60s. **Tab.:** 250 mg, 500 mg. Film-coated. Tab. 60s. *Rx.*
Use: Macrolide, anti-infective.

clarithromycin. (Dava) Clarithromycin 125 mg/5 mL, 250 mg/5 mL (after reconstitution). Maltodextrin, sucrose. Fruit punch flavor. Gran. for Susp., Oral. 50 mL, 100 mL. *Rx.*
Use: Macrolide, anti-infective.

Claritin. (Schering-Plough) Loratadine 5 mg/5 mL. Sugar, sucrose, EDTA. Fruit flavor. Syrup. Bot. 120 mL. *OTC.*
Use: Antihistamine, peripherally selective piperidine.

Claritin Allergy, Children's. (Schering-Plough) **Chew. Tab.:** Loratadine 5 mg. Phenylalanine 1.4 mg, aspartame, mannitol. Grape flavor. 5s, 10s. **Syrup:** Loratadine 5 mg/5 mL. Maltitol, sorbitol, sucralose. Grape flavor. 60 mL, 120 mL. *OTC.*

Use: Antihistamine, peripherally selective piperidine.

Claritin-D. (Schering-Plough) Loratadine 5 mg, pseudoephedrine sulfate 120 mg. Tab, SR Tab. Bot. 30s (except Tab.), 100s, unit-of-use 10s, 30s (except SR Tab.), UD 100s. *OTC.*
Use: Antihistamine, decongestant.

Claritin-D 12-Hour. (Schering-Plough) Pseudoephedrine sulfate 120 mg, loratadine 5 mg. Lactose. ER Tab. Bot. 10s, 20s, 30s. *OTC.*
Use: Upper respiratory combination, decongestant, antihistamine.

Claritin-D 24-Hour. (Schering-Plough) Loratadine 10 mg, pseudoephedrine sulfate 240 mg. PEG, sugar. ER Tab. Bot. 15s. *OTC.*
Use: Upper respiratory combination, antihistamine, decongestant.

Claritin Eye. (Schering-Plough) Ketotifen fumarate 0.025%. Glycerol, sodium hydroxide and/or hydrochloric acid, benzalkonium chloride 0.01%. Soln., Ophth. 5 mL. *OTC.*
Use: Ophthalmic and otic agent, ophthalmic antihistamine.

Claritin Hives Relief. (Schering-Plough) Loratadine 10 mg. Lactose. Tab. 10s. *OTC.*
Use: Antihistamine, peripherally selective piperidine.

Claritin Non-Drowsy Liqui-Gels. (Schering-Plough) Loratadine 10 mg. Sorbitol. Cap., Liquid filled. 70s. *OTC.*
Use: Antihistamine; piperidine, peripherally selective.

Claritin Reditabs. (Schering-Plough) Loratadine 5 mg, 10 mg. Mannitol, mint flavor. Orally Disintegrating Tab. 4s (10 mg only), 10s, 20s (10 mg only), 30s, 40s (5 mg only). *OTC.*
Use: Antihistamine, peripherally selective piperidine.

Claritin 24-Hour Allergy. (Schering-Plough) Loratadine 10 mg. Lactose. Tab. 1s, 2s, 5s, 10s, 20s, 30s, 40s. *OTC.*
Use: Antihistamine, peripherally selective piperidine.

•**clavulanate potassium.** (CLAV-you-lah-nate) *USP 34.*
Use: Inhibitor, β-lactamase.

clavulanate potassium/amoxicillin.
Use: Penicillin, aminopenicillin.
See: Amoclan.
  Augmentin.
  Augmentin ES-600.
  Augmentin XR.

clavulanate/ticarcillin.
Use: Extended-spectrum penicillin.

See: Timentin.
clavulanic acid/amoxicillin.
Use: Penicillin, aminopenicillin.
See: Amoclan.
  Augmentin.
  Augmentin ES-600.
  Augmentin XR.
clavulanic acid/ticarcillin.
Use: Extended-spectrum penicillin.
See: Timentin.
•**clazolam.** (CLAY-zoe-lam) USAN.
Use: Anxiolytic.
•**clazolimine.** (clay-ZOLE-ih-meen) USAN.
Use: Diuretic.
Clean and Clear Foaming Facial Cleanser. (Johnson & Johnson) Triclosan 0.25%. BHT, glycerin, parabens, triethanolamine. Oil free. Soap. 240 mL. *OTC.*
Use: Topical anti-infective, antiseptic and germicide.
Clearasil Adult Care Cream. (Procter & Gamble) Sulfur, resorcinol, alcohol 10%, parabens. Cream. Tube. 17 g. *OTC.*
Use: Dermatologic, acne.
Clearasil Adult Care Medicated Blemish Stick. (Procter & Gamble) Sulfur 8%, resorcinol 1%, bentonite 4%, laureth-4, titanium dioxide. Stick ⅛ oz. *OTC.*
Use: Dermatologic, acne.
Clearasil Antibacterial Soap. (Procter & Gamble) Triclosan 0.75%. Bar 92 g. *OTC.*
Use: Dermatologic, acne.
Clearasil Clearstick for Sensitive Skin, Maximum Strength. (Procter & Gamble) Salicylic acid 2%, alcohol 39%, aloe vera gel, menthol, EDTA. Liq. 35 mL. *OTC.*
Use: Dermatologic, acne.
Clearasil Clearstick, Maximum Strength. (Procter & Gamble) Salicylic acid 2%, alcohol 39%, menthol, EDTA. Liq. 35 mL. *OTC.*
Use: Dermatologic, acne.
Clearasil Clearstick, Regular Strength. (Procter & Gamble) Salicylic acid 1.25%, alcohol 39%, aloe vera gel, menthol, EDTA. Liq. 35 mL. *OTC.*
Use: Dermatologic, acne.
Clearasil Daily Face Wash. (Procter & Gamble) Triclosan 0.3%, glycerin, aloe vera gel, EDTA. Liq. Bot. 135 mL. *OTC.*
Use: Dermatologic, acne.
Clearasil Double Clear. (Procter & Gamble) **Pads, maximum strength:** Salicylic acid 2%, alcohol 40%, witch hazel distillate, menthol. Jar 32s. **Pads,**

regular strength: Salicylic acid 1.25%, alcohol 40%, witch hazel distillate, menthol. Jar 32s. *OTC.*
Use: Dermatologic, acne.
Clearasil Double Textured Pads. (Procter & Gamble) **Pads, regular strength:** Salicylic acid 2%, alcohol 40%, glycerin, aloe vera gel, EDTA. Pkg. 32s, 40s. **Pads, maximum strength:** Salicylic acid 2%, alcohol 40%, menthol, aloe vera gel, EDTA. Pkg. 32s, 40s. *OTC.*
Use: Dermatologic, acne.
Clearasil Maximum Strength Acne Treatment. (Procter & Gamble) Benzoyl peroxide 10%, parabens in vanishing base. Cream. Tube 18 g. *OTC.*
Use: Dermatologic, acne.
Clearasil Medicated Deep Cleanser. (Procter & Gamble) Salicylic acid 0.5%, alcohol 42%, menthol, EDTA, aloe vera gel, hydrogenated castor oil. Liq. Bot. 229 mL. *OTC.*
Use: Dermatologic, acne.
Clearasil 10%. (Procter & Gamble) Benzoyl peroxide 10%. Bot. oz. *OTC.*
Use: Dermatologic, acne.
Clear-Atadine Children's. (Major) Loratadine 5 mg/5 mL. Alcohol free. Sucrose. Fruit flavor. Syrup. 120 mL. *OTC.*
Use: Antihistamine, peripherally selective piperidine.
Clear-Atadine D. (Major) Pseudoephedrine sulfate 240 mg, loratadine 10 mg. Lactose, PEG. ER Tab. 10s, 15s. *OTC.*
Use: Decongestant and antihistamine, upper respiratory combination.
Clear Away. (Schering-Plough) Salicylic acid 40%. Disc Pck. 18s. *OTC.*
Use: Dermatologic, acne.
Clear Away Plantar. (Schering-Plough) Salicylic acid 40%. Disc (for feet) Pck. 24s. *OTC.*
Use: Dermatologic, acne.
Clearblue Easy Ovulation Test. (Iverness) For urine test. Kit. Contains 7 test sticks. *OTC.*
Use: Ovulation test.
Clearblue Easy Pregnancy Test. (Iverness) Dip stick for pregnancy test. Kit 2s. *OTC.*
Use: Diagnostic aid.
Clearex Acne. (Health for Life Brands) Allantoin, sulfur, resorcinol, d-panthenol, isopropanol. Cream. Tube 1.5 oz. *OTC.*
Use: Dermatologic, acne.
Clear Eyes ACR Seasonal Relief. (Medtech) Naphazoline hydrochloride 0.012%. Benzalkonium chloride, EDTA,

zinc sulfate 0.25%, glycerin 0.2%, boric acid, sodium citrate, sodium chloride. Ophth. Soln. Bot. 15 mL. *OTC.*
Use: Mydriatic, vasoconstrictor; ophthalmic decongestant.

Clear Eyes Contact Lens Relief. (Medtech) Sorbic acid 0.25%, EDTA 0.1%, sodium chloride, hypromellose, glycerin. Drops. 15 mL. *OTC.*
Use: Artificial tears.

Clear Eyes Eye Drops. (Ross) Naphazoline hydrochloride 0.012%. Bot. 15 mL, 30 mL. *OTC.*
Use: Mydriatic, vasoconstrictor.

Clear Eyes for Dry Eyes. (Medtech) Carboxymethylcellulose sodium 1%, glycerin 0.25%. Boric acid, EDTA. Soln. 15 mL. *OTC.*
Use: Artificial tears.

Clear Eyes for Redness Relief. (Medtech) Naphazoline hydrochloride 0.012%. Glycerin 0.2%, benzalkonium chloride, boric acid, EDTA, sodium borate. Ophth. Soln. 6 mL, 15 mL, 30 mL. *OTC.*
Use: Ophthalmic decongestant.

Clear Eyes Tears Plus Redness Relief. (Medtech) Naphazoline hydrochloride 0.012%. Hypromellose 0.8%, glycerin 0.25%, benzalkonium chloride, EDTA, boric acid, calcium chloride, magnesium chloride, potassium chloride, sodium borate, sodium chloride. Ophth. Soln. 15 mL. *OTC.*
Use: Ophthalmic decongestant.

Clearly CalaGel. (Tec) Diphenhydramine hydrochloride, zinc acetate, menthol, EDTA. Gel. Tube. 180 g. *OTC.*
Use: Antipruritic, topical.

•**clebopride.** (KLEH-boe-PRIDE) USAN.
Use: Antiemetic.

Cleeravue-M. (Stonebridge) Minocycline 50 mg. Lactose. Film-coated. Tab. 60s. *Rx.*
Use: Tetracycline.

•**clemastine.** (KLEM-ass-teen) USAN.
Use: Antihistamine.

•**clemastine fumarate.** (KLEM-ass-teen) *USP 34.*
Use: Antihistamine, nonselective ethanolamine.
See: Antihist-D.
  Dayhist-1.
  Tavist.
  Tavist Allergy.
  W/Combinations.
  See: Tavist Allergy/Sinus/Headache.

clemastine fumarate. (Various Mfr.) Clemastine fumarate. 0.67 mg/5 mL, may contain alcohol. Syr. Bot. 118 mL,

120 mL. *Rx.*
Use: Antihistamine, nonselective ethanolamine.

clemastine fumarate. (Various Mfr.) Clemastine fumarate 1.34 mg, 2.68 mg. Tab. Bot. 100s. *OTC.*
Use: Antihistamine, nonselective ethanolamine.

Clenia. (Upsher-Smith) Sodium sulfacetamide 10%, sulfur 5%, parabens, EDTA. **Cream:** Tube. 28 g. **Foam:** Bot. 170 mg, 340 mg. *Rx.*
Use: Keratolytic.

Clens. (Alcon) Cleansing agent with benzalkonium chloride 0.02%, EDTA 0.1%. Soln. Bot. 60 mL. *OTC.*
Use: Contact lens care.

•**clentiazem maleate.** (klen-TIE-ah-zem) USAN.
Use: Antianginal; antihypertensive; antagonist, calcium channel.

Cleocin. (Pfizer) Clindamycin phosphate 2%. Benzyl alcohol, cetostearyl alcohol, mineral oil. Vag. Cream. Tube. 40 g with 7 disposable applicators. *Rx.*
Use: Vaginal preparation; anti-infective.

Cleocin HCl. (Pfizer) Clindamycin hydrochloride 75 mg, 150 mg, 300 mg, tartrazine, lactose. Cap. 100s (75 mg); 100s, UD 100s (150 mg, 300 mg). *Rx.*
Use: Anti-infective.

Cleocin Pediatric. (Pfizer) Clindamycin palmitate 75 mg/5 mL. Ethylparaben, sucrose. Gran. for Oral Soln. 100 mL. *Rx.*
Use: Anti-infective.

Cleocin Phosphate. (Pfizer) Clindamycin phosphate 150 mg/mL. Benzyl alcohol, disodium edetate. Vial 2 mL, 4 mL, 6 mL; *ADD-Vantage* Vial 4 mL, 6 mL. *Rx.*
Use: Anti-infective.

Cleocin Phosphate IV. (Pfizer) Clindamycin phosphate 300 mg, 600 mg, 900 mg. Disodium edetate. Inj. *Galaxy* container w/dextrose 5%. *Rx.*
Use: Anti-infective agent, lincosamide.

Cleocin T. (Pfizer) Clindamycin phosphate. **Gel:** 1%. Methylparaben. 30 g, 60 g. **Lotion:** 1%. Cetostearyl alcohol 2.5%, glycerin, isostearyl alcohol 2.5%, methylparaben 0.3%. 60 mL. **Top. Susp.:** 1%. Isopropyl alcohol 50%. 30 mL, 60 mL, single-use pledget applicators. *Rx.*
Use: Anti-infective.

Cleocin Vaginal Ovules. (Pfizer) Clindamycin phosphate 100 mg (as base). Vag. Supp. Cartons of 3s with applicator. *Rx.*
Use: Anti-infective, vaginal.

Clerz Drops for Hard Lenses. (Alcon) Hypertonic solution with hydroxyethylcellulose, sorbic acid, poloxamer 407, EDTA 0.1%, thimerosal 0.001%. Soln. Bot. 25 mL. *OTC.*
Use: Contact lens care.

Clerz Drops for Soft Lenses. (Alcon) Hypertonic solution with hydroxyethylcellulose, sodium borate, poloxamer 407, sorbic acid, thimerosal 0.001%, EDTA 0.1%. Soln. Bot. 25 mL. *OTC.*
Use: Contact lens care.

Clerz Plus. (Alcon) Buffered, isotonic, citrate buffer, NaCl, EDTA 0.05%, polyquaternium-1 0.001%, PEG-11. Drops. Bot. 5 mL, 8 mL, 10 mL. *OTC.*
Use: Contact lens product.

Clerz 2 for Hard Lenses. (Alcon) Isotonic solution with hydroxyethylcellulose, poloxamer 407, sodium chloride, potassium chloride, sodium borate, boric acid, sorbic acid, EDTA. Soln. Bot. 5 mL, 15 mL, 30 mL. *OTC.*
Use: Contact lens care.

●**clevidipine.** (klev-ID-i-peen) USAN.
Use: Cardiovascular agent.

●**clevidipine butyrate.** (klev-ID-i-peen) USAN.
Use: Cardiovascular agent, calcium channel blocking agent.
See: Cleviprex.

Cleviprex. (The Medicines Company) Clevidipine butyrate 0.5 mg/mL. Glycerin 22.5 mg/mL, purified egg yolk phospholipids 12 mg/mL, soybean oil 200 mg/mL. Inj., Emulsion. Single-use vial. 50 mL, 100 mL. *Rx.*
Use: Cardiovascular agent, calcium channel blocking agent.

●**clevudine.** (cleh-VOO-deen) USAN.
Use: Antiviral.

clidinium bromide.
Use: Anticholinergic.
W/Chlordiazepoxide Hydrochloride.
See: Librax.
See: RE Chlordiazepoxide/Clidinium.

Climara. (Bayer Healthcare) Estradiol 2 mg (0.025 mg/day), 2.85 mg (0.0375 mg/day), 3.8 mg (0.05 mg/day), 4.55 mg (0.06 mg/day), 5.7 mg (0.075 mg/day), 7.6 mg (0.1 mg/day). Transdermal System. Box 4s. *Rx.*
Use: Estrogen, sex hormone.

ClimaraPro. (Bayer Healthcare) Estradiol 0.045 mg/levonorgestrel 0.015 mg/day. Transdermal Patch (22 cm²). 4s. *Rx.*
Use: Sex hormone, estrogen and progestin combined.

Clinac BPO. (Ferndale) Benzoyl peroxide 7%, EDTA. Gel. Tube. 45 g, 90 g. *Rx.*
Use: Anti-infective, topical.

●**clinafloxacin hydrochloride.** (klin-ah-FLOX-ah-sin) USAN.
Use: Anti-infective.

Clindagel. (Galderma) Clindamycin phosphate 1%, methylparaben. Gel. Tube. 7.5 g, 42 g, 77 g. *Rx.*
Use: Anti-infective, topical.

ClindaMax. (PharmaDerm) Clindamycin phosphate. **Cream:** 2%. Benzyl alcohol, cetostearyl alcohol, mineral oil. 40 g tube with 7 disposable applicators. **Gel:** 1%, methylparaben. 30 g, 60 g. **Lot.:** 1%, cetostearyl alcohol 2.5%, glycerin, isostearyl alcohol 2.5%, methylparaben 0.3%. 60 mL. *Rx.*
Use: Anti-infective, topical.

●**clindamycin.** (KLIN-dah-MY-sin) USAN.
Use: Anti-infective; dermatologic, acne. Oral as antibiotic. Vaginal as anti-infective. AIDS-associated pneumonia. [Orphan Drug]
See: BenzaClin.
Evoclin.
W/Benzoyl Peroxide.
See: Duac CS.

●**clindamycin hydrochloride.** (KLIN-dah-MY-sin) *USP 34.*
Use: Anti-infective.
See: Cleocin HCl.

clindamycin hydrochloride. (Various Mfr.) Clindamycin hydrochloride 150 mg, 300 mg. May contain lactose. Cap. 16s (300 mg only), 100s, UD 25s (150 mg only), UD 50s (300 mg only). *Rx.*
Use: Lincosamide.

clindamycin 1%/benzoyl peroxide 5%. (Mylan) Benzoyl peroxide 5%, clindamycin 1%. Gel. 50 g. *Rx.*
Use: Acne product combination.

●**clindamycin palmitate.** (KLIN-dah-MY-sin PAL-mih-tate) *USP 34.*
Use: Anti-infective.
See: Cleocin Pediatric.

clindamycin palmitate hydrochloride. (Paddock) Clindamycin palmitate hydrochloride 75 mg per 5 mL. May contain cherry flavoring, dextrin, ethylparaben, sucrose. Granules for Soln. 100 mL. *Rx.*
Use: Anti-infective agent, lincosamide.

●**clindamycin phosphate.** (KLIN-dah-MY-sin) *USP 34.*
Use: Anti-infective.
See: Cleocin.
Cleocin Phosphate.

Cleocin T.
Cleocin Vaginal Ovules.
Clindagel.
ClindaMax.
Clindesse.
PledgaClin.
W/Combinations.
See: Ziana.
clindamycin phosphate. (Greenstone)
Clindamycin phosphate 2%. Cream.
Tube. 40 g with 7 disposable applica-
tors. *Rx.*
Use: Anti-infective.
clindamycin phosphate. (VersaPharm)
Clindamycin phosphate 1%. Isopropyl
alcohol 50%, propylene glycol. Pledget,
topical. 60s. *Rx.*
Use: Topical anti-infective, antibiotic.
clindamycin phosphate. (Various Mfr.)
Clindamycin phosphate. **Inj.:** 150 mg/
mL. May contain benzyl alcohol, di-
sodium edetate. Vial. 2 mL, 4 mL, 6 mL.
ADD-Vantage vial. 2 mL, 4 mL, 6 mL.
Top. Susp.: 1%. Bot. 30 mL, 60 mL.
Gel: 1%. Tube 30 g, 60 g. **Lot.:** 1%.
Bot. 60 mL. *Rx.*
Use: Lincosamide; dermatologic, acne.
Clindesse. (KV Pharma) Clindamycin
phosphate 2%. EDTA, mineral oil,
parabens. Cream. Carton of 1 single-
dose, prefilled, disposable applicator.
Rx.
Use: Vaginal preparation.
Clindex.
See: Chlordiazepoxide and Clidinium
Bromide.
clinocaine hydrochloride.
See: Procaine Hydrochloride.
Clinoril. (Merck) Sulindac 200 mg. Tab.
100s. *Rx.*
Use: Analgesic; NSAID.
Clinoxide. (Geneva) Clidinium bromide
2.5 mg, chlordiazepoxide hydrochlo-
ride, 5 mg. Cap. Bot. 100s, 500s. *c-iv.*
Use: Gastrointestinal; anticholinergic.
•**clioquinol.** (KLYE-oh-KWIN-ole) *USP 34.*
Formerly Iodochlorhydroxyquin.
Use: Antiamebic; anti-infective, topical.
W/Hydrocortisone.
See: Hysone.
•**clioxanide.** (klie-OX-ah-nide) USAN.
Use: Anthelmintic.
Clipoxide. (Schein) Clidinium bromide
2.5 mg, chlordiazepoxide hydrochlo-
ride 5 mg. Cap. Bot. 100s, 500s. *c-v.*
Use: Anticholinergic; antispasmodic.
•**cliprofen.** (klih-PRO-fen) USAN.
Use: Anti-inflammatory.
clobamine mesylate. *Name previously
used for cilobamine mesylate.*

Use: Antidepressant.
•**clobazam.** (KLOE-bazz-am) USAN.
Use: Investigational anxiolytic.
•**clobetasol propionate.** (kloe-BEE-tah-
sahl PRO-ee-oh-nate) *USP 34.*
Use: Anti-inflammatory.
See: Clobex.
Cormax.
Olux.
Olux-E.
Temovate.
clobetasol propionate. (Glades Pharmaceutical) Clobetasol propionate
0.05%. Cetyl alcohol, ethanol 60%,
stearyl alcohol. Top. Foam. 50 g, 100 g.
Rx.
Use: Anti-inflammatory agent, topical
corticosteroid.
clobetasol propionate. (Taro) Clobetasol propionate 0.05%. Soln. 25 mL,
50 mL. *Rx.*
Use: Anti-inflammatory agent.
clobetasol propionate. (Various Mfr.)
Clobetasone propionate 0.05%. **Gel:**
Tube. 15 g, 30 g, 60 g. **Cream:** Tube.
15 g, 30 g, 45 g. **Ointment:** White
petrolatum. Tube. 15 g, 30 g, 45 g. *Rx.*
Use: Anti-inflammatory; corticosteroid,
topical.
•**clobetasone butyrate.** (kloe-BEE-tih-
sone BYOO-tah-rate) USAN.
Use: Corticosteroid; anti-inflammatory.
Clobex. (Galderma) Clobetasol propionate 0.05%. **Lot.:** Mineral oil. 15 mL,
30 mL, 59 mL, 118 mL. **Shampoo:** Alcohol. 118 mL. **Spray:** 0.05%. Alcohol. 60 mL. *Rx.*
Use: Anti-inflammatory; corticosteroid,
topical.
•**clocortolone acetate.** (kloe-CORE-toe-
lone) USAN.
Use: Corticosteroid, topical.
•**clocortolone pivalate.** (kloe-CORE-toe-
lone PIH-vah-late) *USP 34.*
Use: Corticosteroid, topical.
Clocream. (Pharmacia) Vitamins A and
D in vanishing base. Tube oz. *OTC.*
Use: Emollient.
•**clodanolene.** (Kloe-DAN-oh-leen)
USAN.
Use: Muscle relaxant.
•**clodazon hydrochloride.** (KLOE-dah-
zone) USAN.
Use: Antidepressant.
Cloderm. (Valeant) Clocortolone pivalate
0.1%. Cream. Tube 15 g, 45 g. *Rx.*
Use: Corticosteroid, topical.
•**clodronate disodium.** (kloe-DRAHN-
ate) USAN.
Use: Bone calcium regulator.

• **clodronic acid.** (kloe-DRAHN-ik) USAN.
Use: Calcium regulator.

• **clofarabine.** (kloe-FAR-a-bine) USAN.
Use: Antimetabolite.
See: Clolar.

• **clofazimine.** (kloe-FAZZ-ih-meen)
USP 34.
Use: Investigational tuberculostatic, leprostatic. [Orphan Drug]

Clofera. (Centrix) Chlophedianol hydrochloride 12.5 mg, pseudoephedrine hydrochloride 30 mg. Saccharin, sorbitol. Alcohol free, dye free, gluten free, and sugar free. Grape flavor. Liq. 473 mL. *OTC.*
Use: Upper respiratory combination, antitussive combination.

• **clofilium phosphate.** (KLOE-FILL-ee-uhm) USAN.
Use: Cardiovascular agent, antiarrhythmic.

• **cloflucarban.** (KLOE-flew-CAR-ban) USAN.
Use: Antiseptic; disinfectant.

• **clogestone acetate.** (kloe-JESS-tone) USAN. Under study.
Use: Hormone, progestin.

Clolar. (Genzyme Corporation) Clofarabine 1 mg/mL. Preservative free. Soln. for Inj. Vials. 20 mL. *Rx.*
Use: Antimetabolite.

• **clomacran phosphate.** (KLOE-mah-KRAN) USAN. Under study.
Use: Antipsychotic.

• **clomegestone acetate.** (KLOE-meh-JESS-tone) USAN. Under study.
Use: Hormone, progestin.

• **clometherone.** (kloe-METH-ehr-OHN) USAN.
Use: Antiestrogen.

Clomid. (Aventis Pasteur) Clomiphene citrate 50 mg. Tab. Bot. 30s. *Rx.*
Use: Sex hormone, ovulation stimulant.

• **clominorex.** (kloe-MEE-no-rex) USAN.
Use: Anorexic.

• **clomiphene citrate.** (KLOE-mih-feen SIH-trate) *USP 34.*
Tall Man: clomiPHENE
Use: Antiestrogen; sex hormone, ovulation stimulant.
See: Clomid.
  Milophene.
  Serophene.

clomiphene citrate. (Various Mfr.) Clomiphene citrate 50 mg. Tab. Bot. 10s, 30s. *Rx.*
Use: Sex hormone, ovulation stimulant.

• **clomipramine hydrochloride.** (kloe-MIH-pruh-meen) USAN.
Tall Man: clomiPRAMINE
Use: Antidepressant.
See: Anafranil.

clomipramine hydrochloride. (Various Mfr.) Clomipramine hydrochloride 25 mg, 50 mg, 75 mg. Cap. Bot. 100s, 1000s. *Rx.*
Use: Antidepressant.

• **clonazepam.** (kloe-NAY-ze-pam)
USP 34.
Tall Man: clonazePAM
Use: Anticonvulsant; antianxiety agent.
See: Klonopin.

clonazepam. (Barr) Clonazepam 0.125 mg, 0.25 mg, 0.5 mg, 1 mg, 2 mg. Phenylalanine 2.4 mg, aspartame, mannitol, xylitol. Strawberry flavor. Orally Disintegrating Tab. Blister pack. 60s. *c-IV.*
Use: Antianxiety agent; anticonvulsant.

clonazepam. (Various Mfr.) Clonazepam 0.5 mg, 1 mg, 2 mg. May contain lactose. Tab. Bot. 100s, 500s, 1000s, UD 100s. *c-IV.*
Use: Anticonvulsant; antianxiety agent.

• **clonidine.** (KLOE-nih-DEEN) USAN.
Tall Man: cloNIDine
Use: Antihypertensive.
See: Catapres.

clonidine. (Par Pharmaceutical) Clonidine hydrochloride 0.1 mg/24 h (surface area, 10.8 cm^2) (total clonidine content, 3.67 mg); 0.2 mg/24 h (surface area, 21.6 cm^2) (total clonidine content, 7.34 mg); 0.3 mg/24 h (surface area, 32.4 cm^2) (total clonidine content, 11.02 mg). Transdermal patch. 4s. *Rx.*
Use: Antiadrenergic/sympatholytic; antiadrenergic agent, centrally acting.

clonidine. (Various Mfr.) Clonidine hydrochloride 0.1 mg, 0.2 mg, 0.3 mg. May contain lactose. Tab. 30s, 100s, 500s, 1,000s, UD 25s (except 0.3 mg), UD 100s, UD 300s (0.2 mg only). *Rx.*
Use: Antiadrenergic/sympatholytic; antiadrenergic agent, centrally acting.

• **clonidine hydrochloride.** (KLOE-nih-DEEN) *USP 34.*
Tall Man: cloNIDine
Use: Antihypertensive. Epidural use for pain in cancer patients.
See: Catapres.
  Duraclon.
  Jenloga.
  Kapvay.
  Nexiclon XR.
W/Chlorthalidone
  See: Clorpress.

clonidine hydrochloride. (American Reagent) Clonidine hydrochloride. **Inj., Soln.:** 100 mcg/mL. Preservative free. Single-dose vial. 10 mL. **Inj., Soln., concentrate:** 500 mcg/mL. Preservative free. Vial. 10 mL. *Rx.*
Use: Central analgesic.

•**clonitrate.** (KLOE-nye-trate) USAN.
Use: Coronary vasodilator.

•**clonixeril.** (kloe-NIX-ehr-ill) USAN.
Use: Analgesic.

•**clonixin.** (kloe-NIX-in) USAN.
Use: Analgesic.

•**clopamide.** (kloe-PAM-id) USAN.
Use: Antihypertensive; diuretic.

•**clopenthixol.** (KLOE-pen-THIX-ole) USAN.
Use: Antipsychotic.

•**cloperidone hydrochloride.** (KLOE-per-ih-dohn) USAN.
Use: Hypnotic; sedative.

clophenoxate hydrochloride.
Use: Cerebral stimulant.

•**clopidogrel bisulfate.** (kloe-PIH-doe-grell bye-SULL-fate) *USP 34.*
Use: Platelet inhibitor.
See: Plavix.

clopidogrel bisulfate. (Apotex) Clopidogrel bisulfate (as base) 75 mg. Lactose. Film-coated. Tab. 30s, 90s, 1000s, UD 100s. *Rx.*
Use: Antiplatelet agent; aggregation inhibitor.

•**clopimozide.** (KLOE-PIM-oh-zide) USAN.
Use: Antipsychotic.

•**clopipazan mesylate.** (KLOE-pip-ah-ZAN) USAN.
Use: Antipsychotic.

•**clopirac.** (KLOE-pih-rack) USAN.
Use: Anti-inflammatory.

•**cloprednol.** (kloe-PRED-nahl) USAN.
Use: Corticosteroid, topical.

•**cloprostenol sodium.** (kloe-PROSTE-een-ole) USAN.
Use: Prostaglandin.

•**clorazepate dipotassium.** (klor-AZE-eh-PATE DIE-poe-TASS-ee-uhm) *USP 34.*
Use: Anxiolytic; anticonvulsant.
See: Tranxene.

clorazepate dipotassium. (Various Mfr.) Clorazepate dipotassium 3.75 mg, 7.5 mg, 15 mg. Tab. Bot. 20s (7.5 mg only), 100s, 500s, 1000s, UD 100s, UD 500s (7.5 mg only). *c-iv.*
Use: Anxiolytic; anticonvulsant.

•**clorazepate monopotassium.** (clor-AZE-eh-PATE MAHN-oh-poe-TASS-ee-uhm) USAN.

Use: Anxiolytic.

•**clorethate.** (klahr-ETH-ate) USAN.
Use: Hypnotic; sedative.

•**clorexolone.** (KLOR-ex-oh-LONE) USAN.
Use: Diuretic.

Clorfed Capsules. (Stewart-Jackson Pharmacal) Chlorpheniramine 8 mg, pseudoephedrine 120 mg. Bot. 100s. *Rx-OTC.*
Use: Antihistamine; decongestant.

Clorfed Expectorant. (Stewart-Jackson Pharmacal) Pseudoephedrine 30 mg, guaifenesin 100 mg, codeine 10 mg/ 5 mL. Bot. Pt. *c-v.*
Use: Antitussive; decongestant; expectorant.

Clorfed II. (Stewart-Jackson Pharmacal) Chlorpheniramine 4 mg, pseudoephedrine 60 mg. Tab. Bot. 100s. *OTC.*
Use: Antihistamine; decongestant.

•**cloroperone hydrochloride.** (KLOR-oh-PURR-ohn) USAN.
Use: Antipsychotic.

•**clorophene.** (KLOR-oh-feen) USAN.
Use: Disinfectant.

Clorpactin WCS-90. (Guardian Laboratories) Sodium oxychlorosene 2 g. Bot. 5s.
Use: Antiseptic.

•**clorprenaline hydrochloride.** (klor-PREN-ah-leen) USAN.
Use: Bronchodilator.

Clorpress. (Mylan) Clonidine hydrochloride/chlorthalidone. 0.1 mg/15 mg, 0.2 mg/15 mg, 0.3 mg/15 mg. Tab. 100s. *Rx.*
Use: Antihypertensive.

•**clorsulon.** (KLOR-sull-ahn) *USP 34.*
Use: Antiparasitic; fasciolicide.

•**clortermine hydrochloride.** (klor-TER-meen) USAN.
Use: Anorexic.

•**closantel.** (KLOSE-an-tell) USAN.
Use: Anthelmintic.

•**closiramine aceturate.** (kloe-SIH-rah-meen ah-SEE-tur-ate) USAN.
Use: Antihistamine.

clostridial collagenase.
Use: Dupuytren disease. [Orphan Drug]

•**clothiapine.** (KLOE-THIGH-ah-peen) USAN.
Use: Antipsychotic.

•**clothixamide maleate.** (kloe-THIX-ah-mid) USAN.
Use: Antipsychotic.

•**cloticasone propionate.** (kloe-TIK-ah-SONE PRO-pee-oh-nate) USAN.
Use: Anti-inflammatory.

•**clotrimazole.** (kloe-TRIM-uh-zole) *USP 34.*
Use: Antifungal.
See: Cruex.
  Desenex.
  Fungi Cure Intensive.
  Gyne-Lotrimin 3.
  Gyne-Lotrimin 3 Combination Pack.
  Lotrimin AF.
  Mycelex.
  Mycelex-7.
  Mycelex-7 Combination Pack.
clotrimazole. (Alra) Clotrimazole 1%, benzyl alcohol. Vaginal cream. In 45 g with 7 disposable applicators. *OTC.*
Use: Antifungal, vaginal.
clotrimazole. (Roxane) Clotrimazole 10 mg. Troches. 70s, 140s, 500s, UD 70s. *Rx.*
Use: Mouth and throat product.
clotrimazole. (Various Mfr.) Clotrimazole. **Cream:** 1%. Vanishing base, benzyl alcohol 1%, cetostearyl alcohol. Tubes. 15 g, 30 g, 45 g, 2 × 45 g. **Top. Soln.:** 1%, PEG 400. Bot. 30 mL. *Rx-OTC.*
Use: Antifungal, topical anti-infective.
clotrimazole. (Various Mfr.) Clotrimazole. **Vaginal Insert.:** 200 mg. Box 3s with applicator. **Vaginal Cream:** 2%. Tube 21 g with 3 disp. applicators. 1%. Tube 15 g, 30 g. 45 g with applicators. *Rx-OTC.*
Use: Antifungal, *Candida* infections.
clotrimazole and betamethasone dipropionate. (Fougera) Clotrimazole 1%, betamethasone dipropionate 0.05%, mineral oil, white petrolatum, cetearyl alcohol, benzyl alcohol. Cream. 15 g. 45 g. *Rx.*
Use: Antifungal; anti-inflammatory.
clotrimazole and betamethasone dipropionate. (Various Mfr.) Betamethasone (as dipropionate) 0.05%, clotrimazole 1%. Lot. 30 mL. *Rx.*
Use: Anti-inflammatory agent.
clotrimazole combination pack. (Various Mfr.) Clotrimazole. **Vag. Supp.:** 200 mg. 3s w/applicator. **Top. Cream:** 1%. Tube. Pack. *OTC.*
Use: Antifungal.
•**clove oil.** (klove) *NF 29.*
Use: Pharmaceutic aid, flavor.
Cloverine. (Medtech) White salve. Tin Oz. *OTC.*
Use: Dermatologic, counterirritant.
•**clover, red.** ((KLOE-ver)) *NF 29.*
Use: Dietary supplement.
Clovocain. (Vita Elixir) Benzocaine, oil of cloves. *OTC.*
Use: Anesthetic, local.

•**cloxacillin benzathine.** (KLOX-ah-SILL-in BENZ-ah-theen) *USP 34.*
Use: Anti-infective.
•**cloxacillin sodium.** (KLOX-ah-SILL-in) *USP 34.*
Use: Anti-infective, penicillin.
See: Cloxapen.
cloxacillin sodium. (Various Mfr.) Cloxacillin sodium. **Cap.:** 250 mg, 500 mg. Bot. 100s, UD 100s (250 mg only). **Pow. for Oral Soln.:** 125 mg/5 mL when reconstituted. Bot. 100 mL, 200 mL. *Rx.*
Use: Anti-infective, penicillin.
Cloxapen. (GlaxoSmithKline) Cloxacillin sodium 250 mg, 500 mg. Cap. Bot. 30s (500 mg only), 100s, UD 100s (500 mg only). *Rx.*
Use: Anti-infective, penicillin.
•**cloxyquin.** (KLOX-ee-kwin) *USAN.*
Use: Anti-infective.
•**clozapine.** (KLOE-zuh-PEEN) *USP 34.*
Tall Man: cloZAPine
Use: Antipsychotic.
See: Clozaril.
  Fazalco.
clozapine. (Teva) Clozapine 200 mg. Tab. 100s, 500s, UD 100s. *Rx.*
Use: Antipsychotic agent.
clozapine. (Various Mfr.) Clozapine 12.5 mg, 25 mg, 50 mg, 100 mg. Tab. Bot. 30s (12.5 mg only), 100s, 500s (except 12.5 mg), UD 100s (except 12.5 mg). *Rx.*
Use: Antipsychotic.
Clozaril. (Novartis) Clozapine 25 mg, 100 mg. Lactose, talc. Tab. 100s, 500s, UD 100s. *Rx.*
Use: Antipsychotic.
C-Max. (Bio-Technology General) Vitamin C 1000 mg, Mg 40 mg, Zn 5 mg, K 10 mg, Mn 1 mg, pectin 10 mg. Gradual release Tab. Bot. 100s. *OTC.*
Use: Mineral, vitamin supplement.
C.M.C. Cellulose Gum.
See: Carboxymethylcellulose Sodium.
CMV. (Wampole) Cytomegalovirus antibody test system for the qualitative and semi-quantitative detection of CMV antibody in human serum. Test 100s.
Use: Diagnostic aid.
CMV-IGIV.
Use: Immunization.
See: Cytogam.
  Cytomegalovirus Immune Globulin Intravenous.
CNL8 Nail Kit. (JSJ Pharmaceuticals) Ciclopirox 8%. Isopropyl alcohol. Top. Soln. Kit w/nail lacquer, remover swabs, emery board, 28 topical vitamin E 5%

capsules. 5 mL. 3s. *Rx.*
Use: Anti-infective, topical; antifungal agent.
CNS stimulants.
See: Amphetamines.
Central Nervous System Stimulants.
Methylphenidate Hydrochloride.
Coadvil. (Whitehall-Robins) Ibuprofen 200 mg, pseudoephedrine hydrochloride 30 mg. Tab. Bot. 100s. *OTC.*
Use: Analgesic; decongestant.
CoaguChek PT. (Roche) In vitro. PT/INR. Test strips. 48s. *OTC.*
Use: Diagnostic aid.
coagulants.
See: Heparin Antagonists.
coagulation factor IX.
Use: Antihemophilic. [Orphan Drug]
See: Factor IX Complex, Vapor Heated Bebulin VH Immuno.
Mononine.
coagulation factor IX (human).
Use: Antihemophilic. [Orphan Drug]
See: AlphaNine.
coagulation factor IX (recombinant).
Use: Antihemophilic. [Orphan Drug]
See: BeneFix.
coagulation factor VIIa, recombinant.
Use: Antihemophilic agent.
See: NovoSeven RT.
•**coal tar.** (kole tar) *USP 34.*
Use: Topical antieczematic; antipsoriatic.
See: Balnetar.
Creamy Tar.
Ionil T.
L.C.D. Compound.
MG217 Medicated Tar.
PC-Tar.
Polytar Soap.
PsoriGel.
PsoriNail.
Psovent.
Tera-Gel.
Zetar.
W/Allantoin.
See: Alphosyl.
W/Salicylic Acid.
See: Ionil T.
coal tar, distillate.
Use: Dermatologic, topical.
See: Doak Tar.
Doak Tar Oil Forte.
Lavatar.
W/Hydrocortisone, Zinc Oxide.
See: Tarpaste.
coal tar extract.
Use: Dermatologic, topical.
W/Salicylic Acid.
See: Neutrogena T/Sal.

coal tar paste.
Use: Dermatologic, topical.
W/Zinc Paste.
See: Tarpaste.
coal tar topical solution. Liquor Carbonis Detergens. L.C.D.
Use: Antieczematic, topical.
Co-Apap. (Various Mfr.) Pseudoephedrine hydrochloride 30 mg, chlorpheniramine maleate 2 mg, dextromethorphan HBr 15 mg, acetaminophen 325 mg. Tab. Bot. 24s, 50s, 1000s. *OTC.*
Use: Analgesic; antihistamine; antitussive; decongestant.
Coartem. (Novartis) Artemether 20 mg/lumefantrine 120 mg. Tab. 24s. *Rx.*
Use: Anti-infective agent, antimalarial preparation.
•**cobalamine concentrate.** (koe-BALL-uh-meen kahn-SEN-trate) *USP 34.*
Use: Hematopoietic vitamin.
See: Vitamin B_{12}.
cobalt gluconate.
W/Ferrous Gluconate, Vitamin B_{12} Activity, Desiccated Stomach Substance, Folic Acid.
See: Chromagen.
cobalt-labeled vitamin B_{12}.
See: Rubratope-57.
•**cobaltous chloride Co 57.** (koe-BALL-tuss) USAN.
Use: Radiopharmaceutical.
See: Cobatope-57
•**cobaltous chloride Co 60.** (koe-BALL-tuss) USAN.
Use: Radiopharmaceutical.
cobalt standards for vitamin B_{12}.
See: Cobatope-57.
Cobatope-57. (Bristol-Myers Squibb) Cobaltous Chloride Co 57.
•**cobicistat.** (koe-BIS-i-stat) USAN.
Use: Treatment of HIV infection.
Co-Bile. (Western Research) Hog bile 64.8 mg, pancreas substance 64.8 mg, papain-pepsin complex 97.2 mg, diatase malt 16.2 mg, papain 48.6 mg, pepsin 48.6 mg. Tab. Bot. 1000s. *Rx-OTC.*
Use: Digestive enzyme.
•**cocaine.** (koe-CANE) *USP 34.*
Use: Topical local anesthetic, ester local anesthetic.
•**cocaine hydrochloride.** (koe-KANE) *USP 34.*
Use: Anesthetic, local.
cocaine hydrochloride. (Roxane) **Top. Soln.:** Cocaine hydrochloride 4%, 10%. Bot. Multidose 10 mL. UD 4 mL. **Pow.:** (Mallinckrodt). Cocaine hydrochloride 5 g, 25 g. *c-II.*

Use: Topical local anesthetic, ester local anesthetic.

cocaine viscous. (Roxane) Cocaine viscous 4%, 10%. Soln. Top. Bot. Multidose 10 mL. UD 4 mL. *c-II.*
Use: Topical local anesthetic, ester local anesthetic.

• **coccidioidin.** (cox-id-ee-OY-din) *USP 34.*
Use: Diagnostic aid, dermal reactive indicator.

cocculin.
See: Picrotoxin.

Cocet. (Poly Pharmaceuticals) Acetaminophen 650 mg, codeine phosphate 30 mg. Tab. 100s, 500s. c-iii.
Use: Opioid analgesic combination.

Cocilan. (Health for Life Brands) Euphorbia, wild lettuce, cocillana, squill, senega, cascarin (bitterless). Syr. Bot. Gal. Available w/codeine. Bot. Gal.

cocoa.
Use: Pharmaceutic aid, flavored vehicle.

• **cocoa butter.** (koe-koe) *NF 29.*
Use: Pharmaceutic aid, suppository base.

Codal-DM. (Cypress) Dextromethorphan HBr 10 mg, pyrilamine maleate 8.33 mg, phenylephrine hydrochloride 5 mg per 5 mL. Alcohol, sugar, and dye free. Syrup. Bot. 473 mL. *OTC.*
Use: Upper respiratory combination, antitussive combination.

Codanol. (A.P.C.) Vitamins A, D, hexachlorophene, zinc oxide. Oint. Tube 1.5 oz, 4 oz. Jar lb. *OTC.*
Use: Dermatologic, counterirritant.

Codap. (Solvay) Codeine phosphate 32 mg, acetaminophen 325 mg. Tab. Bot. 250s. *c-III.*
Use: Analgesic combination.

Codehist DH. (Geneva) Pseudoephedrine 30 mg, chlorpheniramine maleate 2 mg, codeine phosphate 10 mg/5 mL, alcohol 5.7%. Elix. Bot. 120 mL, 480 mL. *c-v.*
Use: Antihistamine; antitussive; decongestant.

• **codeine.** (KOE-deen) *USP 34.*
Use: Opioid analgesic.
See: Codeine Phosphate.
Codeine Sulfate.

codeine methylbromide. Eucodin.
Use: Antitussive.

• **codeine phosphate.** (KOE-deen) *USP 34.*
Use: Analgesic; antitussive, narcotic.
W/Acetaminophen.
See: Acetaminophen and Codeine Phosphate.

Capital w/Codeine.
Cocet.
Tylenol with Codeine.
Vopac.
W/Acetaminophen, Caffeine, Butalbital.
See: Fioricet with Codeine.
Phrenilin w/Caffeine and Codeine.
W/Acetaminophen, Chlorpheniramine Maleate.
See: Cotabflu.
W/Aspirin.
See: Aspirin and Codeine Phosphate.
W/Aspirin, Butalbital, Caffeine.
See: Ascomp with Codeine.
Butalbital, Aspirin, Caffeine w/Codeine Phosphate.
Fiorinal with Codeine.
W/Brompheniramine Maleate.
See: Brōvex CB.
Brōvex CBX.
EndaCof AC.
Nalex AC.
W/Brompheniramine Maleate, Phenylephrine Hydrochloride.
See: Brōvex PB C.
Brōvex PB CX.
M-End PE.
Poly-Tussin AC.
W/Brompheniramine Maleate, Pseudoephedrine Hydrochloride.
See: CPB WC.
Mar-Cof BP.
M-END WC.
Mesehist WC.
W/Chlorcyclizine Hydrochloride.
See: Notuss NX.
W/Chlorcyclizine Hydrochloride, Phenylephrine Hydrochloride.
See: Nasotuss.
W/Chlorcyclizine Hydrochloride, Pseudoephedrine Hydrochloride.
See: Notuss NXD.
W/Chlorpheniramine Maleate.
See: Cotab A.
Cotab AX.
EndaCof-C.
Lexus 210.
Notuss-AC.
TL-Hist CM.
Zodryl AC 80.
Zodryl AC 50.
Zodryl AC 40.
Zodryl AC 60.
Zodryl AC 30.
Zodryl AC 35.
Zodryl AC 25.
Z-Tuss AC.
W/Chlorpheniramine Maleate, Phenylephrine Hydrochloride.
See: Endal CD.

W/Chlorpheniramine Maleate, Pseudo-
ephedrine Hydrochloride.
See: Phenylhistine DH.
Zodryl DAC 80.
Zodryl DAC 50.
Zodryl DAC 40.
Zodryl DAC 60.
Zodryl DAC 30.
Zodryl DAC 35.
Zodryl DAC 25.
W/Dexchlorpheniramine Maleate, Phenyl-
ephrine Hydrochloride.
See: Dexphen W/C.
W/Diphenhydramine Hydrochloride,
Phenylephrine Hydrochloride.
See: Airacof.
W/Guaifenesin.
See: Allfen CDX.
Brontex.
CGU WC.
Cheratussin AC Expectorant Cough
Suppressant.
Dex-Tuss.
ExeClear-C.
Gani-Tuss NR.
Guiatuss AC.
Iophen C-NR.
Mar-Cof-CG.
M-Clear.
M-Clear WC.
Myci-GC.
Mytussin AC Cough.
Pro-Clear.
Romilar AC.
Tussi-Organidin NR.
Tussi-Organidin-S NR.
Tusso-C.
W/Guaifenesin, Phenylephrine Hydro-
chloride.
See: Giltuss Ped-C.
W/Guaifenesin, Pseudoephedrine Hydro-
chloride.
See: Guiatuss DAC.
Lortuss EX.
Mytussin DAC.
Tusnel C.
Zodryl DEC 80.
Zodryl DEC 50.
Zodryl DEC 40.
Zodryl DEC 60.
Zodryl DEC 30.
Zodryl DEC 35.
Zodryl DEC 25.
W/Phenylephrine Hydrochloride.
See: Alahist AC.
Cheratussin DAC.
Notuss-PE.
W/Phenylephrine Hydrochloride, Pro-
methazine Hydrochloride.
See: Promethazine VC w/Codeine.
W/Phenylephrine Hydrochloride, Pyril-
amine Maleate.

See: Pro-Red AC.
Zotex-C.
W/Pseudoephedrine Hydrochloride.
See: EndaCof-DC.
Notuss-DC.
Nucofed.
W/Pseudoephedrine Hydrochloride,
Triprolidine Hydrochloride.
See: Poly Hist NC.
codeine phosphate. (Various Mfr.) Co-
deine phosphate 15 mg/mL, 30 mg/mL.
May contain sulfites. Inj. *Carpuject* sy-
ringe system. 2 mL. *c-ii.*
Use: Opioid analgesic.
codeine phosphate and aspirin.
See: Aspirin and Codeine Phosphate.
codeine phosphate and guaifenesin.
(Ethex) Codeine phosphate 10 mg,
guaifenesin 300 mg. Sugar, PEG. Tab.
Bot. 100s. *c-iii.*
Use: Upper respiratory combination, an-
titussive combination.
•**codeine polistirex.** (KOE-deen pahl-ee-
STIE-rex) USAN.
Use: Antitussive.
W/Combinations.
See: Codeprex.
codeine resin complex combinations.
See: Omni-Tuss.
•**codeine sulfate.** (KOE-deen) *USP 34.*
Use: Analgesic; antitussive, narcotic.
See: Golacol.
codeine sulfate. (Various Mfr.) Codeine
sulfate 15 mg, 30 mg, 60 mg. Tab. Bot.
100s (except 15 mg), UD 100s (ex-
cept 60 mg). *c-ii.*
Use: Opioid analgesic.
codelcortone.
See: Prednisolone.
Codeprex. (Celltech Pharmaceuticals)
Codeine polistirex 20 mg, chlorpheniramine polistirex 4 mg per 5 mL. EDTA,
parabens, sucrose, vegetable oil.
Cherry-cream flavor. ER Susp. 473 mL.
c-iii.
Use: Antitussive combination.
Codimal. (Schwarz Pharma) Chlorpheniramine maleate 2 mg, pseudoephedrine hydrochloride 30 mg, acetaminophen 325 mg. Cap.Tab. Bot. 24s,
100s, 1000s. *OTC.*
Use: Antihistamine, decongestant, analgesic.
Codimal DM. (Victory) Dextromethorphan HBr 10 mg, phenylephrine hydrochloride 5 mg, pyrilamine maleate
8.33 mg per 5 mL. Saccharin, sorbitol,
menthol. Alcohol, sugar, and dye free.
Syrup. Bot. 118 mL, 473 mL. *OTC.*
Use: Upper respiratory combination, antitussive combination.

Codimal-L.A. (Schwarz Pharma) Chlorpheniramine maleate 8 mg, pseudoephedrine hydrochloride 120 mg. SR Cap. Bot. 100s, 1000s. *Rx.*
Use: Antihistamine, decongestant.

Codimal-L.A. Half Capsules. (Schwarz Pharma) Pseudoephedrine hydrochloride 60 mg, chlorpheniramine maleate 4 mg, sucrose. Cap. Bot. 100s. *Rx.*
Use: Antihistamine; decongestant.

cod liver oil. Emulsion.
Use: Vitamin A and D therapy.
See: Cod Liver Oil Concentrate.
W/Zinc Oxide.
See: Caldesene.
Desitin.

cod liver oil concentrate. (Schering-Plough) Concentrate of cod liver oil with vitamins A and D added. **Cap.:** Bot. 40s, 100s. **Tab.:** Bot. 100s, 240s. Also w/vitamin C. Bot. 100s. *OTC.*
Use: Vitamin supplement.

codorphone hydrochloride. *Name previously used for Conorphone hydrochloride.*
Use: Analgesic.
See: Conorphone Hydrochloride.

•**codoxime.** (CODE-ox-eem) USAN.
Use: Antitussive.

Codoxy. (Halsey Drug) Oxycodone hydrochloride 4.5 mg, oxycodone terephthalate 0.38 mg, aspirin 325 mg. Tab. Bot. 100s. *c-II.*
Use: Analgesic combination.

Coease. (Advance Medical) Sodium hyaluronate 12 mg/mL, NaCl 9 mg/mL. Inj. Disp. syringe. 0.5 mL, 0.8 mL. *Rx.*
Use: Ophthalmic surgical adjunct.

Cogentin. (Merck & Co.) Benztropine mesylate. **Tab.:** 0.5 mg Bot. 100s; 1 mg Bot. 100s, UD 100s; 2 mg Bot. 100s, 1000s, UD 100s. **Inj.:** Benztropine mesylate 1 mg/mL w/sodium chloride 9 mg and water for injection q.s. to 1 mL Amp. 2 mL, Box 6s. *Rx.*
Use: Antiparkinsonian.

Co-Gesic. (Schwarz Pharma) Hydrocodone bitartrate 5 mg, acetaminophen 500 mg. Tab. Bot. 100s, 500s. *c-III.*
Use: Analgesic combination.

Cognex. (Parke-Davis) Tacrine hydrochloride 10 mg, 20 mg, 30 mg, 40 mg. Lactose. Cap. Bot. 120s, UD 100s. *Rx.*
Use: Psychotherapeutic.

Co-Hep-Tral. (Davis & Sly) Folic acid 10 mg, vitamin B_{12} 100 mcg, liver injection q.s./mL. Vial 10 mL. *Rx.*
Use: Mineral, vitamin supplement.

Co-Hist. (Roberts) Pseudoephedrine hydrochloride 30 mg, chlorpheniramine 2 mg, acetaminophen 325 mg. Tab.

Bot. 500s, 1000s. *OTC.*
Use: Analgesic; antihistamine; decongestant.

Colabid. (Major) Probenecid 500 mg, colchicine 0.5 mg. Tab. Bot. 100s, 1000s. *Rx.*
Use: Antigout.

Colace. (Purdue) Docusate sodium. **Cap.:** 50 mg, 100 mg. Bot. 30s, 60s, 250s (100 mg only), 1000s (100 mg only), UD 100s. **Syr.:** 60 mg/15 mL with alcohol less than 1%, menthol, parabens, sucrose. Bot. 237 mL, 473 mL. **Liq.:** 150 mg/15 mL, parabens. Bot. 30 mL, 480 mL. *OTC.*
Use: Laxative.

Colace. (Purdue) Glycerin. Supp. Bot. 12s, 24s, 48s, 100s. *OTC.*
Use: Laxative.

Colace Infant/Child Suppositories. (Purdue) Glycerin. Supp. 12s, 24s. *OTC.*
Use: Laxative.

Colagyn. (Smith & Nephew) Zinc sulfocarbolate, potassium, oxyquinoline sulfate, lactic acid, boric acid. Jelly. Tube w/applicator and refill 6 oz. Douche Pow. 3 oz, 7 oz, 14 oz. *OTC.*

Colana. (Hance) Euphorbia pilulifera tincture 8 mL, wild lettuce syrup 8 mL, cocillana tincture 2.5 mL, squill compound syrup 1.5 mL, cascara 0.25 g, menthol 4.8 mg/fl oz. Bot. 4 fl oz, gal. Also w/Dionin 15 mg/fl oz. Syr. Bot. gal.

Colazal. (Salix) Balsalazide disodium 750 mg (equiv. to mesalamine 267 mg). Sodium ≈ 86 mg. Cap. Bot. 280s, 500s.
Use: Treatment of ulcerative colitis.

•**colchicine.** (KOHL-chih-seen) *USP 34.*
Use: Gout suppressant. Treat multiple sclerosis; familial Mediterranean fever; Behçet syndrome [Orphan Drug].
See: Colcrys.
W/Sodium Salicylate, Calcium Carbonate, Dried Aluminum Hydroxide Gel, Phenobarbital.
See: Apcogesic.

colchicine. (Various Mfr.) Colchicine 0.6 mg (1/100 g). Tab. Bot. 30s, 60s, 100s, 100s. *Rx.*
Use: Gout suppressant. Treat multiple sclerosis; familial Mediterranean fever; Behçet syndrome [Orphan Drug].

colchicine salicylate.
W/Phenobarbital, Sodium Para-Aminobenzoate, Vitamin B_1, Aspirin.
See: Doloral.

Colcrys. (AR Scientific) Colchicine 0.6 mg. Film coated. Lactose, polydex-

trose. Tab. 30s, 60s, 100s, 250s, 500s, 1,000s. *Rx.*
Use: Agent for gout.

Cold & Cough Tussin. (Amerisource Bergen) Dextromethorphan HBr 10 mg, guaifenesin 200 mg, pseudoephedrine hydrochloride 30 mg. Sorbitol. Softgels. Pkg. 12s. *OTC.*
Use: Upper respiratory combination, antitussive, expectorant, decongestant.

Cold & Hot Pain Relief Therapy Patch. (Major Pharmaceuticals) Menthol 5%. Aloe vera, disodium EDTA, methylparaben. Patch. 8 × 12 cm. 5s. *OTC.*
Use: Rub and liniment.

•**cold cream.** *USP 34.*
Use: Emollient; water in oil emulsion ointment base.

Coldec D. (Breckenridge) Pseudoephedrine hydrochloride 80 mg, carbinoxamine maleate 8 mg. Tab. Bot. 100s. *Rx.*
Use: Upper respiratory combination, decongestant, antihistamine.

Coldec DM. (Silarx) Dextromethorphan HBr 15 mg, brompheniramine maleate 4 mg, pseudoephedrine hydrochloride 60 mg per 5 mL. Saccharin, sorbitol, grape flavor, alcohol free, sugar free. Syrup. Bot. 480 mL. *Rx.*
Use: Upper respiratory combination, antitussive, antihistamine, decongestant.

Cold-Gest Cold. (Major) Chlorpheniramine maleate 8 mg, pseudoephedrine hydrochloride 75 mg. Cap. Pkg. 10s, 20s. *OTC.*
Use: Antihistamine, decongestant.

Coldmist JR. (Breckenridge) Pseudoephedrine hydrochloride 48 mg, guaifenesin 595 mg. ER Tab. Bot. 100s. *Rx.*
Use: Upper respiratory combination, decongestant and expectorant.

Coldmist LA. (Breckenridge) Pseudoephedrine hydrochloride 85 mg, guaifenesin 795 mg. ER Tab. Bot. 100s. *Rx.*
Use: Upper respiratory combination, decongestant, expectorant.

Coldonyl. (Dover) Acetaminophen 325 mg, phenylephrine hydrochloride 5 mg, guaifenesin 100 mg. Sugar free. Tab. UD 500s. *OTC.*
Use: Upper respiratory combination, decongestant and expectorant combination.

Coldran. (Halsey Drug) Phenylephrine hydrochloride 5 mg, chlorpheniramine maleate 2 mg, salicylamide 1.5 g, acetaminophen 0.5 g, caffeine. Tab. Bot. 30s. *OTC.*
Use: Decongestant, analgesic, antihistamine.

Coldrine. (Roberts) Acetaminophen 325 mg, pseudoephedrine hydrochloride 30 mg, sodium metabisulfite. Tab. Bot. 1000s, 500s (packets), 4-dose boxes. *OTC.*
Use: Analgesic, decongestant.

Cold Sore. (Purepac) Camphor, benzoin, aluminum chloride. Lot. Bot. 0.5 oz. *OTC.*
Use: Cold sores, fever blisters.

Cold Symptoms Relief. (Major) Pseudoephedrine hydrochloride 30 mg, chlorpheniramine maleate 2 mg, dextromethorphan HBr 10 mg, acetaminophen 325 mg. Tab. Bot. 50s. *OTC.*
Use: Decongestant, antihistamine, antitussive, analgesic.

Cold Symptoms Relief Maximum Strength. (Major) Dextromethorphan HBr 15 mg, chlorpheniramine maleate 2 mg, pseudoephedrine hydrochloride 30 mg, acetaminophen 500 mg. Tab. Pkg. 24s. *OTC.*
Use: Upper respiratory combination, antitussive, antihistamine, decongestant, analgesic.

Cold Tablets. (Walgreen) Phenylephrine hydrochloride 5 mg, chlorpheniramine maleate 2 mg, acetaminophen 325 mg. Tab. Bot. 50s. *OTC.*
Use: Decongestant, analgesic, antihistamine.

Cold Tablets Multiple Symptom. (Walgreen) Acetaminophen 500 mg, pseudoephedrine hydrochloride 30 mg, chlorpheniramine maleate 2 mg, dextromethorphan HBr 10 mg. Tab. Bot. 50s. *OTC.*
Use: Analgesic, decongestant, antihistamine, antitussive.

•**coleneuramide.** (COL-e-NURE-a-mide) USAN.
Use: Diabetic neuropathy.

•**colesevelam hydrochloride.** (koe-leh-SEH-veh-lam) USAN.
Use: Antihyperlipidemic; bile acid sequestrant.
See: Welchol.

Colestid. (Pharmacia) Colestipol hydrochloride 5 g/7.5 g granules. Gran. for Oral Susp. **Unflavored Gran.:** Bot. 300 g, 500 g. Packets. 5 g (30s, 90s). **Flavored Gran.:** Aspartame, mannitol, orange flavor. Bot. 450 g (60 doses). Packets. 7.5 g (60s). **Tab.:** 1 g. Bot. 120s, 500s. *Rx.*
Use: Antihyperlipidemic; bile acid sequestrant.

•**colestilan chloride.** (koe-LES-ti-lan)
USAN.
Use: Hyperphosphatemia/hypercholes-
terolemia.

•**colestipol hydrochloride.** (koe-LESS-
tih-pole) *USP 34.*
Use: Antihyperlipidemic.
See: Colestid.

colestipol hydrochloride. (Global) Co-
lestipol hydrochloride 5 mg. Gran. for
Oral Susp. Packets. 5 g (30s and 90s).
Bot. 500 g. *Rx.*
Use: Antihyperlipidemic agent, bile acid
sequestrant.

colestipol hydrochloride. (Various Mfr.)
Colestipol hydrochloride 1 g. Tab. 120s,
500s. *Rx.*
Use: Antihyperlipidemic agent, bile acid
sequestrant.

•**colestolone.** (koe-LESS-toe-LONE)
USAN.
Use: Hypolipidemic.

Col-Evac. (Forest) Potassium bitartrate,
bicarbonate of soda and a blended
base of polyethylene glycols. Supp.
Box. 2s, 12s.
Use: Laxative.

•**colforsin.** (kole-FAR-sin) USAN.
Use: Antiglaucoma agent.

**colfosceril palmitate, cetyl alcohol,
tyloxapol.**
Use: Hyaline membrane disease; adult
respiratory distress syndrome.
[Orphan Drug]

colimycin sodium methanesulfonate.
(Parke-Davis)
See: Colistimethate Sodium.

colimycin sulfate.
See: Coly-Mycin.

•**colistimethate sodium.** (koe-LISS-tih-
METH-ate) *USP 34.*
Use: Anti-infective.
See: Coly-Mycin M Parenteral.

colistimethate sodium. (Paddock) Colistin base as colistimethate sodium or
pentasodium colistimethanesulfonate
150 mg. Lyophilized Cake for Inj. Vials.
Rx.
Use: Anti-infective.

**colistin and neomycin sulfates and
hydrocortisone acetate.**
Use: Anti-infective; anti-inflammatory.

colistin base.
W/Neomycin and Hydrocortisone.
See: Cortisporin-TC.
W/Neomycin Base, Hydrocortisone Ace-
tate, Thonzonium Bromide, Polysor-
bate 80, Acetic Acid, Sodium Acetate.
See: Coly-Mycin S Otic Drops.

colistin methanesulfonate.
See: Colistimethate Sodium.

Co-Liver. (Standex) Folic acid 1 mg, vita-
min B$_{12}$ 100 mcg, liver 10 mcg/mL. Inj.
Vial 10 mL. *Rx.*
Use: Mineral, vitamin supplement.

Colladerm. (C & M Pharmacal) Glycerin,
soluble collagen, hydrolysed elastin, allantoin, ethylhydroxycellulose, sorbic,
octoxynol-9. Bot. 2.3 oz. *OTC.*
Use: Emollient.

collagenase.
Use: Enzyme preparation.
See: Collagenase Santyl.

collagenase ABC. (Advance Biofactures)
Collagenase 250 units/g in white petro-
latum. Oint. Tube. 25 g, 50 g. *OTC.*
Use: Enzyme, topical.

•**collagenase clostridium histolyticum.**
(kol-AJ-e-nase klos-TRID-ee-um HIS-
toe-LIT-ik-um) USAN.
Use: Enzyme; Dupuytren contracture.
See: Xiaflex.

collagenase (lyophilized) for injection.
Use: Peyronie disease. [Orphan Drug]

Collagenase Santyl. (Ross) Collagenase
enzyme 250 units/g, white petrolatum.
Oint. Tube. 15 g, 30 g. *Rx.*
Use: Enzyme preparation.

collagen implant. (Lacrimedics) Colla-
gen 0.2 mm, 0.3 mm, 0.4 mm, 0.5 mm,
0.6 mm. Box 12s. *Rx.*
Use: Collagen implant, ophthalmic.
See: Zyderm I.
Zyderm II.

•**collodion.** (kah-LOW-dee-uhm) *USP 34.*
Use: Topical protectant.

colloidal aluminum hydroxide.
See: Aluminum Hydroxide Gel.

colloidal oatmeal.
Use: Emollient.
See: Actibath.
Aveeno.

colloidal sulfur.
Use: Antiseborrheic.
W/Combinations.
See: MG217 Medicated Tar-Free.

Colloral. (AutoImmune) Purified type II
collagen.
Use: Juvenile rheumatoid arthritis.
[Orphan Drug]

Collyrium for Fresh Eyes Wash.
(Wyeth-Ayerst) Boric acid, sodium borate, benzalkonium chloride. Soln. Bot.
120 mL. *OTC.*
Use: Irrigant, ophthalmic.

ColoCARE. (Helena Laboratories) In-
home fecal test. Kit. 3s.
Use: Diagnostic aid.

Colocort. (Paddock Laboratories) Hydrocortisone 100 mg/60 mL. Methylpara-

ben. Rectal Susp. Single-dose bot. with lubricated rectal applicator tips. 60 mL. *Rx.*
Use: Anorectal preparation.

Coloctyl. (Eon Labs) Docusate sodium 100 mg. Cap. Bot. 100s, 1000s, UD 1000s. *OTC.*
Use: Laxative.

Cologel. (Eli Lilly) Methylcellulose 450 mg/5 mL, alcohol 5%, saccharin. Bot. 16 fl oz. *OTC.*
Use: Laxative.

colony-stimulating factor.
Use: Hematopoietic agent.
See: Filgrastim.
  Pegfilgrastim.
  Sargramostim.

color allergy screening test.
See: CAST.

ColoScreen. (Helena Laboratories) Occult blood screening test. Kit 12s, 25s, 50s. 3 tests per kit.
Use: Diagnostic aid.

ColoScreen/VPI. (Helena Laboratories) Occult blood screening test. Box 100s, 1000s.
Use: Diagnostic aid.

Coltab Children's. (Roberts) Phenylephrine hydrochloride 2.5 mg, chlorpheniramine maleate 1 mg. Chew. Tab. Bot. 30s. *OTC.*
Use: Antihistamine; decongestant.

•**colterol mesylate.** (KOLE-ter-ole) USAN.
Use: Bronchodilator.

Columbia Antiseptic Powder. (F.C. Sturtevant) Zinc oxide, talc, carbolic acid, boric acid. Pow. 30 g, 420 g. *OTC.*
Use: Topical combination.

Coly-Mycin M Parenteral. (JHP Pharmaceuticals) Colistimethate sodium equivalent to 150 mg colistin base. Inj. Vial. *Rx.*
Use: Anti-infective.

Coly-Mycin S Otic. (JHP Pharmaceuticals) Hydrocortisone 1%, neomycin sulfate 4.71 mg. Colistin sulfate 3 mg, thonzonium bromide 0.05%/mL, polysorbate 80, acetic acid, sodium acetate, thimerosal. Susp. Dropper bot. 5 mL, 10 mL. *Rx.*
Use: Steroid and antibiotic combination.

Colyte. (Alaven Pharmaceuticals) Polyethylene glycol-electrolyte 3350. **Gal:** PEG 3350 227.1 g, sodium sulfate 21.5 g, sodium bicarbonate 6.36 g, sodium chloride 5.53 g, potassium chloride 2.82 g. **4 L:** PEG 3350 240 g, sodium sulfate 22.72 g, sodium bicarbonate 6.72 g, sodium chloride 5.84 g,

potassium chloride 2.98 g. Soln. Bot. 1 gal, 4 L. *Rx.*
Use: Bowel evacuant.

Combichole. (Trout) Dehydrocholic acid 2 g, desoxycholic acid 1 g. Tab. Bot. 100s, 1000s. *Rx.*
Use: Hydrocholeretic.

Combigan. (Allergan) Brimonidine tartrate 0.2%, timolol 0.5% (as timolol maleate 6.8 mg/mL). Benzalkonium chloride 0.005%. Soln., Ophth. 5 mL, 10 mL, 15 mL. *Rx.*
Use: Agent for glaucoma.

CombiPatch. (Novartis) **Transdermal Patch 9 cm^2:** Estradiol 0.05 mg/norethindrone acetate 0.14 mg per day. **Transdermal Patch 16 cm^2:** Estradiol 0.05 mg/norethindrone acetate 0.25 mg per day. Box. 8s. *Rx.*
Use: Sex hormone, estrogen and progestin combination.

Combistix. (Bayer Consumer Care) Urine test for glucose, protein and pH. In 100s.
Use: Diagnostic aid.

Combistix Reagent Strips. (Siemans Medical) Protein test area: tetrabromphenol blue, citrate buffer, protein-absorbing agent; glucose test area: glucose oxidase, orthotolidin and a catalyst; pH test area methyl red and bromthymol blue. Strip Box 100s.
Use: Diagnostic aid.

Combivent. (Boehringer Ingelheim) Ipratropium bromide 18 mcg, albuterol sulfate 103 mcg/actuation (equivalent to albuterol base 90 mcg). Aer. Metered dose inhaler 14.7 g (200 inhalations) w/mouthpiece. *Rx.*
Use: Bronchodilator, anticholinergic.

Combivir. (GlaxoSmithKline) Lamivudine 150 mg, zidovudine 300 mg. Tab. Bot. 60s, UD 120s. *Rx.*
Use: Antiviral, nucleoside analog reverse transcriptase inhibitor combination.

•**comfilcon A.** (kom-FIL-kon) USAN.
Use: Contact lens material, hydrophilic.

ComfortCare GP Wetting & Soaking. (PBH Wesley Jessen) Buffered, isotonic. Chlorhexidine gluconate 0.005%, EDTA 0.02%, octylphenoxy (oxyethylene) ethanol, povidone, polyvinyl alcohol, propylene glycol, hydroxyethylcellulose, NaCl. Soln. Bot. 120 mL, 240 mL. *OTC.*
Use: Contact lens care.

Comfort Drops. (PBH Wesley Jessen) Isotonic solution containing naphazoline 0.03%, benzalkonium chloride 0.005%, edetate disodium 0.02%. Bot. 15 mL. *OTC.*
Use: Contact lens care.

Comfort Gel Liquid. (Walgreen) Aluminum hydroxide compressed gel 200 mg, magnesium hydroxide 200 mg, simethicone 20 mg/5 mL. Gel. Bot. 12 oz. *OTC.*
Use: Antacid; antiflatulent.

Comfort Gel Tablets. (Walgreen) Magnesium hydroxide 85 mg, simethicone 25 mg, aluminum hydroxide-magnesium carbonate co-dried gel 282 mg. Tab. Bot. 100s. *OTC.*
Use: Antacid; antiflatulent.

Comfort Tears. (Allergan) Hydroxyethylcellulose, benzalkonium chloride 0.005%, edetate disodium 0.02%. Soln. Bot. 15 mL. *OTC.*
Use: Artificial tear solution.

Comhist. (Roberts) Phenylephrine hydrochloride 10 mg, chlorpheniramine maleate 2 mg, phenyltoloxamine citrate 25 mg. Tab. Bot. 100s. *Rx.*
Use: Antihistamine; decongestant.

Comhist L.A. (Roberts) Phenylephrine hydrochloride 20 mg, chlorpheniramine maleate 4 mg, phenyltoloxamine citrate 50 mg. Cap. Bot. 100s. *Rx.*
Use: Antihistamine; decongestant.

Compal. (Solvay) Dihydrocodeine 16 mg, acetaminophen 356.4 mg, caffeine 30 mg. Cap. Bot. 100s. *c-III.*
Use: Analgesic combination.

Compat Nutrition Enteral Delivery System. (Novartis) Top fill feeding containers 600 mL, 1400 mL. Gravity delivery set. Pump delivery set. Compat enteral feeding pump.
Use: Nutritional supplement.

Compete. (Mission Pharmacal) Iron 27 mg, vitamins A 5000 units, D 400 units, E 45 units, B_1 2 mg, B_2 2.6 mg, B_3 30 mg, B_6 20.6 mg, B_{12} 9 mcg, C 90 mg, folic acid 0.4 mg, Zn 22.5 mg. Tab. Bot. 100s. *OTC.*
Use: Mineral, vitamin supplement.

Compleat. (Nestle Nutrition) Protein 48 g (Na caseinate), carbohydrate 128 g (corn syrup, maltodextrin), fat 40 g (canola oil, chicken puree), sodium 1,000 mg, potassium 1,720 mg. Vitamin A, B_1, B_2, B_3, B_5, B_6, B_{12}, C, D, E, K, Ca, Cl, Cr, Cu, Fe, I, Mg, Mo, Mn, P, Se, Zn, biotin, choline, folic acid. Chocolate and vanilla flavors. Liq. 1,000 mL, 1,500 mL. *OTC.*
Use: Milk-based formula.

Compleat B Meat Base Formula. (Novartis) Beef, nonfat milk, hydrolyzed cereal solids, maltodextrin, pureed fruits and vegetables, corn oil, mono- and diglycerides. Bot. 250 mL, Can 250 mL. *OTC.*
Use: Nutritional supplement, eternal.

Compleat Modified Formula Meat Base. (Novartis) Hydrolyzed cereal solids, calcium caseinate, pureed fruits and vegetables, corn oil, beef puree, mono- and diglycerides. Can 250 mL. *OTC.*
Use: Enteral nutritional supplement.

Compleat Regular Formula. (Novartis) Deionized water, beef puree, hydrolyzed cereal solids, green bean puree, pea puree, nonfat milk, corn oil, maltodextrin, peach puree, orange juice, mono- and diglycerides, carrageenan, vitamins, minerals. Bot. 250 mL, Can 250 mL. *OTC.*
Use: Nutritional supplement, eternal.

Complete Vitamins. (Mission Pharmacal) Vitamins A 5000 units, D 400 units, E 45 units, C 90 mg, B_1 2.25 mg, folic acid 0.4 mg, B_2 2.6 mg, B_3 30 mg, B_6 25 mg, B_{12} 9 mcg, ferrous gluconate 233 mg, zinc 22.5 mg. Tab. Bot. 100s, 1000s. *OTC.*
Use: Mineral, vitamin supplement.

Completone Elixir Fort. (Sanofi-Synthelabo) Ferrous gluconate.
Use: Mineral supplement.

Complex 15 Cream. (Baker Cummins Dermatologicals) Jar 4 oz. *OTC.*
Use: Emollient.

Complex 15 Lotion. (Baker Cummins Dermatologicals) Bot. 8 oz. *OTC.*
Use: Emollient.

Complex Zinc Carbonates.
Use: Mineral supplement.

Comply Liquid. (Sherwood Davis & Geck) sodium caseinate, calcium caseinate, hydrolyzed cornstarch, sucrose, corn oil, soy lecithin, vitamins A, B_1, B_2, B_3, B_5, B_6, B_{12}, C, D, E, K, folic acid, biotin, choline, Ca, Cl, Cu, Fe, I, Mg, Mn, P, Zn. Can 250 mL, Bot. 200 mL. *OTC.*
Use: Nutritional supplement, enteral.

compound cb3025.
See: Alkeran.

compound E.
See: Cortisone Acetate.

compound F.
See: Hydrocortisone.

compound 42.
See: Warfarin.

compound Q.
Use: Antiviral.

compound S.
Use: Antiviral.
See: Retrovir.
Zidovudine.

Compound 347. (Minrad) Enflurane. Liq. for Inh. 250 mL. *Rx.*
Use: General anesthetic.

Compound W. (Medtech) Salicylic acid 17% w/w in flexible collodion vehicle w/ether 63.5%. Bot. 0.31 oz. *OTC.*
Use: Keratolytic.

Compound W for Kids. (Medtech) Salicylic acid 40% in a plaster vehicle, lanolin, rubber. Pad. Box. 12s. *OTC.*
Use: Keratolytic.

Compound W Freeze Off. (Medtech) Dimethyl ether, propane, isobutane. Spray. 80 mL with 12 applicators. *OTC.*
Use: Removal of warts.

Compound W One Step Wart Remover for Kids. (Medtech) Salicylic acid 40% in a plaster vehicle, lanolin, rubber. Pad. Box 12s. *OTC.*
Use: Keratolytic.

Compoz. (Medtech) **Tab.:** Diphenhydramine hydrochloride 50 mg. Pkg. 12s, 24s. **Cap.:** Diphenhydramine hydrochloride 25 mg. Pkg. 16s. *OTC.*
Use: Sleep aid.

Compro. (Paddock) Prochlorperazine 25 mg. Supp. Box 12s. *Rx.*
Use: Antiemetic; antipsychotic.

Comtan. (Novartis) Entacapone 200 mg, mannitol, sucrose. Tab. Bot. 10s, 100s, 500s. *Rx.*
Use: Antiparkinsonian.

Comtrex Maximum Strength Day & Night Cold & Cough. (Novartis Consumer) **Day:** Dextromethorphan HBr 10 mg, phenylephrine hydrochloride 5 mg, acetaminophen 325 mg. **Night:** Dextromethorphan HBr 10 mg, chlorpheniramine maleate 2 mg, phenylephrine hydrochloride 6 mg, acetaminophen 325 mg. Tab. 20s (10 day, 10 night). *OTC.*
Use: Upper respiratory combination, antitussive combination.

Comtrex Maximum Strength Day & Night Flu Therapy. (Novartis Consumer) **Day:** Phenylephrine hydrochloride 5 mg, acetaminophen 325 mg. PEG. **Night:** Phenylephrine hydrochloride 5 mg, chlorpheniramine maleate 2 mg, acetaminophen 325 mg. PEG. Tab. 20s (10 day, 10 night). *OTC.*
Use: Upper respiratory combination, decongestant, antihistamine, analgesic.

Comtrex Maximum Strength Day & Night Severe Cold & Sinus. (Novartis Consumer) **Day:** Phenylephrine hydrochloride 5 mg, acetaminophen 325 mg. PEG. **Night:** Phenylephrine hydrochloride 5 mg, chlorpheniramine maleate 2 mg, acetaminophen 325 mg. PEG. Tab. 20s (10 day, 10 night). *OTC.*
Use: Upper respiratory combination, decongestant, antihistamine, and analgesic combination.

Comtrex Maximum Strength Nighttime Cold & Cough. (Novartis Consumer) **Liq.:** Dextromethorphan 5 mg, chlorpheniramine maleate 0.67 mg, pseudoephedrine hydrochloride 10 mg, acetaminophen 166.7 mg per 5 mL. Alcohol 10%, saccharin, sucrose. 240 mL. **Tab.:** Dextromethorphan HBr 10 mg, chlorpheniramine maleate 2 mg, phenylephrine hydrochloride 6 mg, acetaminophen 325 mg. 20s. *OTC.*
Use: Antitussive combination, upper respiratory combination.

Comtrex Multi-Symptom Deep Chest Cold. (Novartis Consumer) Guaifenesin 200 mg, acetaminophen 325 mg. PEG, polyvinyl alcohol. Cap. 24s. *OTC.*
Use: Expectorant with analgesic combination, upper respiratory combination.

Comvax. (Merck) *Haemophilus* b PRP 7.5 mcg, *Neisseria meningitidis* OMPC 125 mcg, hepatitis B surface antigen 5 mcg, aluminum hydroxide $\approx$ 225 mcg, sodium borate decahydrate 35 mcg/ 0.5 mL, sodium chloride 0.9%. Inj. Single-dose vials. 0.5 mL *Rx.*
Use: Agent for active immunization, bacterial vaccine.

Conal. (Cypress) Phenylephrine tannate 15 mg, chlorpheniramine tannate 8 mg, pyrilamine tannate 12.5 mg per 5 mL. Aspartame, parabens, phenylalanine 7 mg/5 mL. Raspberry flavor. Susp. 473 mL. *Rx.*
Use: Upper respiratory combination, decongestant and antihistamine.

Concentraid. (Ferring) Desmopressin acetate 0.1 mg/mL (0.1 mg equals 400 units arginine vasopressin). Soln. Disposable intranasal pipettes containing 20 mcg/2 mL. *Rx.*
Use: Hormone.

Concentrated Cleaner. (Bausch & Lomb) Anionic sulfate surfactant with friction-enhancing agents and sodium chlorine. Soln. Bot. 30 mL. *OTC.*
Use: Contact lens care.

Concentrated Milk of Magnesia. (Roxane) Magnesium hydroxide 2,400 mg per 10 mL. Benzyl alcohol, lemon oil, sorbitol, sugar. Lemon flavor. Susp., Conc. 400 mL. *OTC.*
Use: Antacid; Laxative.

Concentrated Milk of Magnesia-Cascara. (Roxane) Milk of magnesia-cascara 15 mL equivalent to milk of magnesia 30 mL and aromatic cascara fluid extract 5 mL, alcohol 7%. *OTC.*
Use: Laxative.

Concentrated Multiple Trace Element.
(American Regent) Zinc (as sulfate) 5 mg, copper (as sulfate) 1 mg, manganese (as sulfate) 0.5 mg, chromium (as chloride) 10 mcg. Vial. 10 mL. *Rx.*
Use: Trace element supplement.

concentrated oleovitamin A and D.
See: Oleovitamin A & D.

Concentrated Phillips' Milk of Magnesia. (Roxane) Magnesium hydroxide 800 mg/5 mL, sorbitol, and sugar. Strawberry and orange vanilla creme flavors. Liq. 8 fl. oz. *OTC.*
Use: Antacid; laxative.

Concentrin. (Parke-Davis) Dextromethorphan HBr 15 mg, pseudoephedrine hydrochloride 30 mg, guaifenesin 100 mg. Cap. Bot. 12s. *OTC.*
Use: Antitussive; decongestant; expectorant.

Conceptrol Disposable Contraceptive. (Johnson & Johnson) Nonoxynol-9 4%. Vaginal gel. Tube. 2.7 mL (6s, 10s). *OTC.*
Use: Contraceptive, spermicide.

Concerta. (McNeil) Methylphenidate hydrochloride 18 mg, 27 mg, 36 mg, 54 mg, lactose. ER Tab. Bot. 100s. *c-II.*
Use: Central nervous system stimulant.

Condol Suspension. (Sanofi-Synthelabo) Dipyrone, chlormezanone. *Rx.*
Use: Analgesic; muscle relaxant.

Condol Tablets. (Sanofi-Synthelabo) Dipyrone, chlormezanone. *Rx.*
Use: Analgesic; muscle relaxant.

Condylox. (Watson) Podofilox 0.5%, alcohol 95%. Soln. Bot. 3.5 mL. *Rx.*
Use: Keratolytic.

C1-esterase-inhibitor, human, pasteurized.
Use: Prevention, treatment of angioedema.
See: Berinert P.

C1-esterase-inhibitor, human, pasteurized. (Alpha Therapeutic)
Use: Prevention, treatment of angioedema. [Orphan Drug]

C1-inhibitor. (Osterreichisches Baxter Healthcare)
Use: Treatment of angioedema. [Orphan Drug]

C1-inhibitor (human).
See: Cinryze.

C1-inhibitor (human) vapor heated. (Immuno Therapeutics)
Use: Treatment of angioedema. [Orphan Drug]

Conest. (Grafton) Conjugated estrogens 0.625 mg, 1.25 mg, 2.5 mg. Tab. Bot. 100s, 1000s. *Rx.*
Use: Estrogen.

Confident. (Block Drug) Carboxymethylcellulose gum, ethylene oxide polymer, petrolatum/mineral oil base. Tube 0.7 oz, 1.4 oz, 2.4 oz. *OTC.*
Use: Denture adhesive.

Congess. (Fleming & Co.) **Sr.:** Guaifenesin 250 mg, pseudoephedrine hydrochloride 120 mg. SR Cap. **Jr.:** Guaifenesin 125 mg, pseudoephedrine hydrochloride 60 mg. TR Cap. Bot. 100s, 1000s. *Rx-OTC.*
Use: Decongestant; expectorant.

Congestac. (B.F. Ascher) Pseudoephedrine hydrochloride 60 mg, guaifenesin 400 mg. Tab. Bot. 12s, 24s. *OTC.*
Use: Upper respiratory combination, decongestant, expectorant.

Congesta DM. (TriMarc Labs) Dextromethorphan hydrobromide 20 mg, guaifenesin 400 mg. Maltodextrin. Tab. 90s. *OTC.*
Use: Upper respiratory combination, antitussive with expectorant.

Congestaid. (Zee Medical) Pseudoephedrine hydrochloride 30 mg. Tab. 24s. *OTC.*
Use: Decongestant.

congo red. Injection.
Use: Hemostatic in hemorrhagic disorders.

•**conivaptan hydrochloride.** (kahn-ih-VAP-tahn) USAN.
Use: Hyponatremia; vasopressin receptor antagonist.
See: Vaprisol Premixed in Dextrose 5%.

conjugated estrogens.
Use: Estrogen.
See: Estrogens, Conjugated.

•**conorphone hydrochloride.** (KOE-nahr-fone) USAN. *Formerly Codorphone.*
Use: Analgesic.

Conray. (Mallinckrodt) Iothalamate meglumine 600 mg, iodine 282 mg/mL. EDTA. Inj. Vials. 30 mL, 50 mL, 100 mL. Bot. 100 mL, 150 mL, 200 mL. Prefilled power injector syringes. 50 mL, 125 mL. *Rx.*
Use: Radiopaque agent.

Conray 43. (Mallinckrodt) Iothalamate meglumine 430 mg, iodine 202 mg/mL. EDTA. Inj. Vials. 50 mL, 100 mL. Bot. 150 mL, 200 mL, 250 mL. Prefilled syringes. 50 mL. *Rx.*
Use: Radiopaque agent.

Conray 30. (Mallinckrodt) Iothalamate meglumine 300 mg, iodine 141 mg/mL. EDTA. Inj. Vials. 50 mL. Bot. 150 mL, 300 mL. *Rx.*
Use: Radiopaque agent.

Consin Compound Salve. (Wisconsin Pharmacal Co.) Carbolic acid ointment. Jar 2 oz, lb. *OTC.*
Use: Minor skin irritations.

Constonate 60. Docusate sodium 100 mg, 250 mg. Cap. Bot. 100s, 1000s. *OTC.*
Use: Laxative.

Constulose. (Alra) Lactulose 10 g/15 mL (< galactose 1.6 g, lactose 1.2 g, other sugars). Soln. Bot. 237 mL, 946 mL. *Rx.*
Use: Analgesic; laxative.

Contac Cold + Flu. (GlaxoSmithKline Consumer Healthcare) Phenylephrine hydrochloride 5 mg, chlorpheniramine maleate 7 mg, acetaminophen 500 mg. Tab. 24s, 36s. *OTC.*
Use: Upper respiratory combination, decongestant, antihistamine, and analgesic combination.

Contac Cold + Flu Day & Night. (GlaxoSmithKline Consumer Healthcare) **Day:** Phenylephrine hydrochloride 5 mg, acetaminophen 500 mg. **Night:** Phenylephrine hydrochloride 5 mg, chlorpheniramine maleate 2 mg, acetaminophen 500 mg. Tab. 28s (16 day and 12 night). *OTC.*
Use: Upper respiratory combination, decongestant, antihistamine, and analgesic combination.

Contac Cough & Chest Cold. (GlaxoSmithKline) Pseudoephedrine hydrochloride 15 mg, dextromethorphan HBr 5 mg, guaifenesin 50 mg, acetaminophen 125 mg/5 mL, alcohol 10%, saccharin, sorbitol. Liq. Bot. 4 fl. oz. *OTC.*
Use: Analgesic; antitussive; decongestant; expectorant.

Contac Cough and Sore Throat Formula. (GlaxoSmithKline) Dextromethorphan HBr 5 mg, acetaminophen 125 mg/5 mL, alcohol 10%. Bot. 120 mL. *OTC.*
Use: Analgesic; antitussive.

Contac Day & Night Allergy/Sinus Relief. (GlaxoSmithKline) **Day:** Pseudoephedrine hydrochloride 60 mg, acetaminophen 650 mg. Capl. **Night:** Pseudoephedrine hydrochloride 60 mg, diphenhydramine hydrochloride 50 mg, acetaminophen 650 mg. Tab. Pkg. 20 (15 day; 5 night). *OTC.*
Use: Upper respiratory combination, decongestant, antihistamine, analgesic.

Contac Day & Night Cold & Flu. (GlaxoSmithKline) **Day:** Pseudoephedrine hydrochloride 60 mg, dextromethorphan HBr 30 mg, acetaminophen 650 mg. **Night:** Pseudoephedrine hydrochloride 60 mg, diphenhydramine hydrochloride 50 mg, acetaminophen 650 mg. Tab. Pkg. 20s (15 day, 5 night). *OTC.*
Use: Upper respiratory combination, decongestant, antihistamine, antitussive, analgesic.

Contac Nighttime Cold. (GlaxoSmithKline) Acetaminophen 167 mg, dextromethorphan HBr 5 mg, pseudoephedrine hydrochloride 10 mg, doxylamine succinate 1.25 mg/5 mL, alcohol 25%. Bot. 177 mL. *OTC.*
Use: Analgesic, decongestant, antitussive, antihistamine.

Contac Non-Drowsy Formula Sinus. (GlaxoSmithKline) Pseudoephedrine hydrochloride 30 mg, acetaminophen 500 mg. Capl. Tab. Pkg. 24s. *OTC.*
Use: Decongestant, analgesic.

Contac Severe Cold & Flu Maximum Strength. (GlaxoSmithKline) Dextromethorphan HBr 15 mg, chlorpheniramine maleate 2 mg, pseudoephedrine hydrochloride 30 mg, acetaminophen 500 mg. Tab. Bot. 30s. *OTC.*
Use: Upper respiratory combination, antitussive, antihistamine, decongestant, analgesic.

Contac Severe Cold & Flu Nighttime. (GlaxoSmithKline) Pseudoephedrine hydrochloride 10 mg, chlorpheniramine maleate 0.67 mg, dextromethorphan HBr 5 mg, acetaminophen 167 mg, alcohol 18.5%, saccharin, sorbitol, glucose. Liq. Bot. 180 mL. *OTC.*
Use: Antihistamine; antitussive; decongestant.

contact lens products, disinfectant. *OTC.*
See: Allergan Hydrocare Cleaning and Disinfecting.
Aosept.
Disinfecting Solution.
Flex-Care.
Hydrocare.
Lensept.
Lens Plus Oxysept.
Opti-Free.
Opti-One.
Oxysept.
ReNu MultiPurpose.
Ultra-Care.

contact lens products, enzymatic cleaners. *OTC.*
See: Ultrazyme Enzymatic Cleaner.

contact lens products, rewetting solutions. *OTC.*
See: Adapettes for Sensitive Eyes.
Clerz.
Clerz 2.
Comfort Tears.
Lens Fresh.
Lens-Wet.
Opti-Free.
Opti-One.

Sensitive Eyes Drops.
Sterile Lens Lubricant.
contact lens products, soft. *OTC.*
Use: Contact lens care, rinsing,
storage.
See: Allergan Hydrocare Preserved Sa-
line.
Blairex Sterile Saline Solution.
BoilnSoak.
Ciba Vision Saline.
Hypoclear.
Lens Plus Preservative Free.
Lensrins.
Opti-Soft.
ReNu Saline.
Saline Solution.
Sensitive Eyes Plus.
Sensitive Eyes Saline.
Sterile Saline.
Unisol.
Unisol 4.
**contact lens products, surfactant
cleaning solutions.** *OTC.*
See: Ciba Vision Cleaner.
Daily Cleaner.
LC-65 Daily Contact Lens Cleaner.
Lens Clear.
MiraFlow Extra Strength.
Pliagel.
Preflex Daily Cleaning Especially for
Sensitive Eyes.
Sensitive Eyes Saline/Cleaning Solu-
tion.
Sof/Pro-Clean.
contraceptive hormones.
Use: Sex hormone.
See: Biphasic Oral Contraceptives.
Contraceptives, Emergency.
Etonogestrel.
Etonogestrel/Ethinyl Estradiol.
Levonorgestrel.
Levonorgestrel/Ethinyl Estradiol.
Levonorgestrel-Releasing Intrauterine
System.
Medroxyprogesterone.
Medroxyprogesterone Acetate/Estra-
diol Cypionate.
Monophasic Oral Contraceptives.
Norelgestromin/Ethinyl Estradiol.
Norethindrone.
Norgestrel.
Oral Contraceptives.
Progestin-Only Products.
Triphasic Oral Contraceptives.
Ulipristal Acetate.
contraceptives, emergency.
See: Levonorgestrel.
Plan B.
Preven.
contraceptives, intrauterine system.
See: Mirena.

contraceptives, miscellaneous.
See: Depo-Provera.
Oral Contraceptives.
VCF.
contraceptives, monophasic oral.
Use: Sex hormone, contraceptive hor-
mone.
See: Alesse.
Apri.
Aviane.
Azurette.
Balziva.
Beyaz.
Brevicon.
Cryselle.
Desogen.
Femcon Fe.
Jolessa.
Junel Fe 1/20.
Junel Fe 1.5/30.
June 21 Day 1/20.
Junel 21 Day 1.5/30.
Kariva.
Kelnor 1/35.
Lessina.
Levlen.
Levlite.
Levora.
Loestrin Fe 1/20.
Loestrin Fe 1.5/30.
Loestrin 24 Fe.
Loestrin 21 1/20.
Loestrin 21 1.5/30.
Lo/Ovral.
Low-Ogestrel.
Lutera.
Lybrel.
Microgestin Fe 1/20.
Microgestin Fe 1.5/30.
Mircette.
Modicon.
MonoNessa.
Necon 1/50.
Necon 1/35.
Necon 0.5/35.
Nordette-28.
Norinyl 1 + 50.
Norinyl 1 + 35.
Nortrel 1/35.
Nortrel 0.5/35.
Ogestrel 0.5/50.
Ortho-Cept.
Ortho-Cyclen.
Ortho-Novum 1/50.
Ortho-Novum 1/35.
Ovcon-50.
Ovcon-35.
Ovral.
Portia.
Quasense.
Reclipsen.

Safyral.
Seasonale.
Solia.
Sprintec.
Sronyx.
Yasmin.
YAZ.
Zenchent.
Zovia 1/50E.
Zovia 1/35E.
contraceptives, oral.
See: Oral Contraceptives.
contraceptives, vaginal foams.
See: Delfen.
contraceptives, vaginal jellies and creams.
See: Colagyn.
Conceptrol.
Ortho-Gynol.
Contrin. (Geneva) Iron (from ferrous fumarate) 110 mg, B_{12} 15 mcg, IFC (intrinsic factor as concentrate or from stomach preparations) 240 mg, C 75 mg, folic acid 0.5 mg. Cap. Bot. 100s. Rx.
Use: Mineral, vitamin supplement.
ControlRx. (Omnii Oral) Neutral sodium fluoride 1.1%, Microdent (emulsion of dimethicone and poloxamer 407) 2%. Sorbitol, saccharin. Berry and vanilla mint flavors. Paste. 56 g. Rx.
Use: Prevention of dental caries.
Converspaz. (B.F. Ascher) Cellulase 5 mg, protease 10 mg, amylase 30 mg, lipase 13 mg, l-hyoscamine sulfate 0.0625 mg. Cap. Bot. 100s. Rx.
Use: Decongestant; expectorant.
Cool-Mint Listerine. (Warner Lambert) Thymol, eucalyptol, methyl salicylate, menthol, alcohol 21.6%. Liq. Bot. 90 mL, 180 mL, 360 mL, 540 mL, 720 mL, 960 mL. OTC.
Use: Mouthwash.
CooperVision Balanced Salt. (Ciba Vision) Sterile intraocular irrigation soln. Bot. 15 mL, 500 mL.
Use: Irrigant, ophthalmic.
Copavin Pulvules. (Eli Lilly) Codeine sulfate 15 mg, papaverine hydrochloride 15 mg. Cap. Bot. 100s. c-v.
Use: Antitussive.
Copaxone. (Teva) Glatiramer acetate 20 mg/mL, mannitol 40 mg. Preservative free. Inj. Single-use premixed prefilled syringes. Rx.
Use: Multiple sclerosis agent; immunosuppressant.
COPE. (Mentholatum Co.) Aspirin 421 mg, magnesium hydroxide 50 mg, aluminum hydroxide 25 mg, caffeine 32 mg. Tab. Bot. 36s, 60s. OTC.
Use: Analgesic; antacid.

Copegus. (Genentech) Ribavirin 200 mg. Film-coated. Tab. 168s. Rx.
Use: Antiviral agent.
copper. (Hospira) Copper 0.4 mg/mL (as 1.07 mg of cupric chloride). Inj. Vial. 10 mL. Rx.
Use: Trace metal.
•**copper gluconate.** (KAHP-er GLUE-kohn-ate) USP 34.
Use: Supplement, trace mineral.
copperhead bite therapy.
See: Antivenin, (Crotalidae) Polyvalent.
Copperin. (Vernon) Iron ammonium citrate, copper (6 g). "A" adult dose, "B" children dose. Bot. 30s, 10s, 500s.
Use: Mineral supplement.
Coppertone. (Schering-Plough) A series of sun-care products marketed under the Coppertone name including Waterproof Lotions SPF 4, 6, 8, 15, and 25. Bot. 4 fl oz, 8 fl oz. Oil SPF 2: Bot. 4 fl oz, 8 fl oz; Lite Formula Oil SPF 2: Bot. 4 fl oz; Lite Lotion SPF 4: Bot. 4 fl oz; Dark Tanning Body Mousse SPF 4: Tube 4 oz; Suntanning Gel SPF 4: Tube 3 oz; Noskote SPF 8: Tube 0.44 oz, Jar 1 oz; Noskote SPF-15, Jar 1 oz. Contain one or more of the following ingredients: Padimate O, oxybenzone, homosalate, ethylhexyl p-methocinnamate. OTC.
Use: Sunscreen.
Coppertone Bug and Sun Adult Formula. (Schering-Plough) Ethylhexyl p-methoxynnamate, oxybenzone, 2-ethylhexyl salicylate, homosalate. SPF 15.Waterproof. PABA-free. Aloe vera. Lot. Bot. 237 mL. OTC.
Use: Sunscreen; insect repellant.
Coppertone Bug and Sun Kid's Formula. (Schering-Plough) Octocrylene, ethylhexyl p-methoxycinnamate, oxybenzone. SPF 30. Waterproof. PABA-free. Hypoallergenic. Aloe vera. Lot. Bot. 237 mL. OTC.
Use: Sunscreen; insect repellant.
Coppertone Dark Tanning. (Schering-Plough) Padimate O in spray base (SPF 2). Spray. Bot. 8 fl oz. OTC.
Use: Sunscreen.
Coppertone Face. (Schering-Plough) A series of sunscreen lotions with SPF 2, 4, 6 and 15 in a nongreasy base with padimate O, oxybenzone (SPF 15 only). OTC.
Use: Sunscreen.
Coppertone Kids Sunblock. (Schering-Plough) **SPF 15:** Ethylhexyl p-methoxy-cinnamate, oxybenzone, 2-ethylhexyl salicylate, homosalate. Lot. Bot. 120 mL, 240 mL. **SPF 30:** Octocrylene,

ethylhexyl p-methoxycinnamate, oxybenzone, 2-ethylhexyl salicylate. Lot. Bot. 120 mL, 240 mL. *OTC.*
Use: Sunscreen.

Coppertone Lipkote. (Schering-Plough) Ethylhexyl p-methoxycinnamate, oxybenzone. SPF 15. Stick 4.5 g. *OTC.*
Use: Sunscreen.

Coppertone Moisturizing Sunblock. (Schering-Plough) **SPF 45:** Ethylhexyl p-methoxycinnamate, 2-ethylhexyl salicylate, octocrylene, oxybenzone. Lot. Bot. 120 mL, 300 mL. **SPF 25, 30:** Ethylhexyl p-methoxycinnamate, oxybenzone, 2-ethylhexyl salicylate, homosalate. Lot. Bot. SPF 30: 120 mL, 240 mL; SPF 25: 120 mL. **SPF 15:** Ethylhexyl p-methoxycinnamate, oxybenzone. Lot. Bot. 120 mL, 240 mL, 300 mL. *OTC.*
Use: Sunscreen.

Coppertone Moisturizing Sunscreen. (Schering-Plough) Ethylhexyl p-methoxycinnamate, oxybenzone, benzyl alcohol, vitamin E, aloe. PABA free. SPF 6, 8. Waterproof. Lot. Bot. 120 mL, 240 mL. *OTC.*
Use: Sunscreen.

Coppertone Moisturizing Suntan. (Schering-Plough) **SPF 2:** Homosalate, vitamin E, aloe. PABA free. Waterproof. Oil. Bot. 120 mL. **SPF 4:** Ethylhexyl p-methoxycinnamate, oxybenzone, benzyl alcohol, vitamin E, aloe. PABA free. Waterproof. Lot. Bot. 120 mL, 240 mL. *OTC.*
Use: Sunscreen.

Coppertone Noskote. (Schering-Plough) Homosalate 8%, oxybenzone 3%. (SPF 8) Oint. Jar 13.2 g, 30 g. *OTC.*
Use: Sunscreen.

Coppertone SPF-25 Sunblock Lotion. (Schering-Plough) Ethylhexyl p-methoxycinnamate, oxybenzone, padimate O in lotion base (SPF 25). Bot. 120 mL. *OTC.*
Use: Sunscreen.

Coppertone Sport. (Schering-Plough) Ethylhexyl p-methoxycinnamate, oxybenzone. SPF 4, 8, 15, 30. Lot. Bot. 120 mL. *OTC.*
Use: Sunscreen.

Coppertone Tan Magnifier Suntan. (Schering-Plough) **SPF 2:** Triethanolamine salicylate. Oil Bot. 120 mL. **SPF 4 Lotion:** Ethylhexyl p-methoxycinnamate. Bot. 120 mL. **Gel:** 2-phenylbenzimidazole-5-sulfonic acid. Tube 120 g. *OTC.*
Use: Sunscreen.

Coppertone Water Babies. (Schering-Plough) SPF 30, SPF 45. Ethylhexyl p-methoxycinnamate, 2-ethylhexyl salicylate, oxybenzone, homosalate, alcohol, aloe, parabens. PABA free. Waterproof. Lot. Bot. 118 mL. *OTC.*
Use: Sunscreen.

copper trace metal additive. (I.M.S., Ltd.) Copper 1 mg. Inj. Vial 10 mL. *Rx.*
Use: Copper supplement.

•**copper undecylenate.** (KAHP-er undeh-sil-EN-ate) USAN.
Use: Copper supplement.

Co-Pyronil 2. (Eli Lilly) Chlorpheniramine maleate 4 mg, pseudoephedrine hydrochloride 60 mg. Pulvule. Bot. 100s. *OTC.*
Use: Antihistamine, decongestant.

Corab. (Abbott Diagnostics) Radioimmunoassay for detection of antibody to hepatitis B core antigen. Test kit 100s.
Use: Diagnostic aid.

Corab-M. (Abbott Diagnostics) Radioimmunoassay for the qualitative determination of specific Ig antibody to hepatitis B virus core antigen (Anti-HBc Ig) in human serum or plasma and may be used as an aid in the diagnosis of acute or recent hepatitis B infection.
Use: Diagnostic aid.

Corace. (Forest) Cortisone acetate 50 mg/mL. Inj. Vial 10 mL. *Rx.*
Use: Corticosteroid, topical.

Coracin. (Roberts) Hydrocortisone acetate 1%, neomycin sulfate 0.5%, bacitracin zinc 400 units, polymyxin B sulfate 10,000 units/g in white petrolatum and mineral oil base. Oint. Tube 3.5 g. *Rx.*
Use: Anti-infective; corticosteroid, ophthalmic.

Coral. (Young Dental) Fluoride ion 1.23%, 0.1 molar phosphate. Jar 250 g, Coral II: 180 disposable cup units/carton. *Rx.*
Use: Fluoride, dental.

Coral Calcium Plus Vitamin D & Magnesium. (Mason) Ca, Mg, vitamin D_3 200 units. Gluten free, preservative free, and soy free. Cap. 60s. *OTC.*
Use: Nutritional supplement.

Coral/Plus. (Young Dental) Free fluoride ion 2.2%, recrystallized kaolinite. Tube 250 g. *Rx.*

coral snake antivenin. (NABI)
See: Antivenin (*Micrurus fulvius*).

Cordarone. (Wyeth-Ayerst) Amiodarone hydrochloride. **Tab.:** 200 mg. Lactose. Bot. 60s, UD 100s. **Inj.:** 50 mg/mL. Benzyl alcohol 20.2 mg/mL. Amp. 3 mL. *Rx.*
Use: Antiarrhythmic.

228 CORDRAN

Cordran. (Aqua Pharmaceuticals) Flurandrenolide 0.05%, 0.025%. White petrolatum. Tube 15 g (0.05% only), 30 g, 60 g. *Rx.*
Use: Corticosteroid, topical.

Cordran Lotion. (Aqua Pharmaceuticals) Flurandrenolide 0.05%, cetyl alcohol, benzyl alcohol, stearic acid, glyceryl monostearate, polyoxyl 40 stearate, glycerin, mineral oil, menthol, purified water. Squeeze bot. 15 mL, 60 mL. *Rx.*
Use: Corticosteroid, topical.

Cordran SP. (Aqua Pharmaceuticals) Flurandrenolide 0.05%, 0.025% in emulsified base w/cetyl alcohol, mineral oil. Tube 15 g (0.05% only), 30 g, 60 g. *Rx.*
Use: Corticosteroid, topical.

Cordran Tape. (Watson) Flurandrenolide 4 mcg/sq. cm. Roll 7.5 cm × 60 cm, 7.5 cm × 200 cm. *Rx.*
Use: Corticosteroid, topical.

Cordrol. (Vita Elixir) Prednisolone 5 mg, 10 mg, 20 mg. Tab. Bot. 100s. *Rx.*
Use: Corticosteroid.

Cordron-D. (Cypress) Pseudoephedrine hydrochloride 17.5 mg, carbinoxamine maleate 2 mg per 5 mL. Sugar, alcohol, and dye free. Saccharin, sorbitol. Liq. 473 mL. *Rx.*
Use: Decongestant and antihistamine, upper respiratory combination.

Cordron-DM NR. (Cypress) Dextromethorphan HBr 15 mg, carbinoxamine maleate 3 mg, pseudoephedrine hydrochloride 12.5 mg per 5 mL. Alcohol, dye, and sugar free. Saccharin, sorbitol. Liq. 473 mL. *Rx.*
Use: Antitussive combination, upper respiratory combination.

Cordron-D NR. (Cypress) Pseudoephedrine hydrochloride 12.5 mg, carbinoxamine maleate 2 mg per 5 mL. Alcohol, sugar, and dye free. Saccharin, sorbitol. Liq. 473 mL. *Rx.*
Use: Upper respiratory combination, decongestant and antihistamine.

Coreg. (GlaxoSmithKline) Carvedilol 3.125 mg, 6.25 mg, 12.5 mg, 25 mg. Lactose, sucrose. Tab. Bot. 100s. *Rx.*
Use: Antihypertensive.

Coreg CR. (GlaxoSmithKline) Carvedilol (as phosphate) 10 mg, 20 mg, 40 mg, 80 mg. ER Cap. (contains immediate- and controlled-release microparticles). 30s, 90s. *Rx.*
Use: Antiadrenergic/sympatholytic.

Corfen-DM. (Cypress) Chlorpheniramine maleate 4 mg, dextromethorphan hydrobromide 15 mg, phenylephrine hydrochloride 10 mg. Saccharin, sorbitol. Alcohol free, dye free, and sugar free. Grape flavor. Liq. 473 mL. *Rx.*
Use: Upper respiratory combination, antitussive combination.

Corgard. (Monarch) Nadolol 20 mg, 120 mg, 160 mg. Tab. Bot. 100s, 1000s (except 20 mg, 160 mg), *Unimatic* 100s (except 120 mg, 160 mg). *Rx.*
Use: Antiadrenergic/sympatholytic, beta-adrenergic blocker.

•**coriander oil.** (kor-ee-ANN-der oil) *NF 29.*
Use: Pharmaceutic aid, flavor.

Coricidin HBP Chest Congestion & Cough. (Schering-Plough) Dextromethorphan HBr 10 mg, guaifenesin 200 mg. Softgel Cap. 20s. *OTC.*
Use: Upper respiratory combination, antitussive with expectorant.

Coricidin HBP Cold & Flu. (Schering-Plough) Chlorpheniramine maleate 2 mg, acetaminophen 325 mg. Tab. Bot. 12s. *OTC.*
Use: Upper respiratory combination, antihistamine, analgesic.

Coricidin HBP Cough & Cold. (Schering-Plough) Dextromethorphan HBr 30 mg, chlorpheniramine maleate 4 mg. Sugar. Tab. Pkg. 16s. *OTC.*
Use: Upper respiratory combination, antitussive combination.

Coricidin HBP Maximum Strength Flu. (Schering-Plough) Dextromethorphan HBr 15 mg, chlorpheniramine maleate 2 mg, acetaminophen 500 mg. Lactose. Tab. Pkg. 20s. *OTC.*
Use: Upper respiratory combination, antitussive combination.

Corifact. (CSL Behring) Factor XIII concentrate (human) 1,000 to 1,600 units (the actual units of potency of factor XIII are stated on each vial label and carton). Preservative free. Inj., lyophilized Pow. for Soln. Kit w/single-dose vial (each vial contains human albumin 120 to 200 mg, total protein 120 to 320 mg, and glucose 80 to 120 mg) and diluent. *Rx.*
Use: Antihemophilic agent.

Corlopam. (Hospira) Fenoldopam mesylate 10 mg/mL. Sodium metabisulfite 1 mg. Inj. Concentrate. Single-dose Amp. 1 mL, 2 mL. *Rx.*
Use: Antihypertensive.

Cormax. (Oclassen) Clobetasol propionate. **Cream:** 0.05%. White petrolatum, cetyl alcohol, stearyl alcohol, lanolin oil, parabens. 30 g, 45 g. **Oint.:** 0.05%. White petrolatum, sorbitan sesquioleate. Tube. 15 g, 45 g. **Soln.:** 0.05%. Alcohol 40%. 25 mL, 50 mL. *Rx.*
Use: Corticosteroid, topical.

•**cormethasone acetate.** (core-METH-ah-sone) USAN.
Use: Anti-inflammatory, topical.

Corn Huskers. (Warner Lambert) Glycerin 6.7%, SD alcohol, algin, TEA-oleoyl sarcosinate, guar gum, methylparaben, calcium sulfate, calcium chloride, TEA-fumarate, TEA-borate. Bot. 4 oz, 7 oz. *OTC.*
Use: Emollient.

•**corn oil.** (korn) *NF 29.*
Use: Pharmaceutic aid, solvent, oleaginous vehicle.

Corotrope. (Sanofi-Synthelabo) Milrinone for IV use. *Rx.*
Use: Cardiovascular agent.

corpus luteum, extract (water soluble).
See: Progesterone.

Corque. (Geneva) Hydrocortisone 1%, iodochlorhydroxyquin 3%. Cream. Tube 20 g. *Rx.*
Use: Corticosteroid, topical.

Correctol. (Schering-Plough) Bisacodyl 5 mg, talc, lactose, sugar. EC Tab. Bot. 30s, 60s, 90s. *OTC.*
Use: Laxative.

Cortaid, Maximum Strength. (J&J Consumer) Hydrocortisone in parabens 1%, cetyl and stearyl alcohols, glycerin, white petrolatum. Cream. Tube 15 g, 30 g. *OTC.*
Use: Corticosteroids, topical.

Cortaid Maximum Strength Spray. (J&J Consumer) Hydrocortisone 1%, alcohol 55%, glycerin, methylparaben. Liq. Pump spray 45 mL. *OTC.*
Use: Corticosteroid, topical.

Cortan. (Halsey Drug) Prednisone 5 mg. Tab. Bot. 1000s. *Rx.*
Use: Corticosteroid.

Cortane-B. (Blansett) Hydrocortisone 1%, pramoxine hydrochloride 1%, chloroxylenol 0.1%, benzalkonium chloride. Lot. 60 mL. *Rx.*
Use: Corticosteroid, topical.

Cortane-B Aqueous. (Blansett) Hydrocortisone 1%, pramoxine hydrochloride 1%, chloroxylenol 0.1%. Drops. 10 mL. *Rx.*
Use: Otic preparation.

Cortane-B Otic. (Blansett) Hydrocortisone 1%, pramoxine hydrochloride 1%, chloroxylenol 0.1%. Drops. 10 mL. *Rx.*
Use: Otic preparation.

Cort-Dome. (Bayer Consumer Care) Hydrocortisone alcohol. **Cream:** 0.25%: 1 oz, 4 oz; 0.5%, 1%: 1 oz. **Lot.:** 0.25%, 0.5%: 4 oz; 1%: 1 oz. *Rx.*
Use: Corticosteroid, topical.

Cort-Dome High Potency. (Bayer Consumer Care) Hydrocortisone acetate

25 mg in a monoglyceride base. *Rx.*
Use: Corticosteroid, topical.

Cortef. (Pfizer) Hydrocortisone. Tab. **5 mg:** Bot. 50s. **10 mg, 20 mg:** Bot. 100s. *Rx.*
Use: Corticosteroid.

cortenil.
See: Desoxycorticosterone Acetate.

cortical hormone products.
See: Aristocort.
Betamethasone.
Betamethasone Sodium Phosphate.
Betamethasone Sodium Phosphate and Betamethasone Acetate.
Budesonide.
Celestone.
Celestone Phosphate.
Celestone Soluspan.
Corticotropin.
Cortisone Acetate.
Decadron.
Desoxycorticosterone Acetate.
Dexamethasone.
Entocort EC.
Fludrocortisone Acetate.
Hydrocortisone.
Hydrocortone Acetate.
Hydrocortone Phosphate.
Medrol.
Methylprednisolone.
Prednisolone.
Prednisone.
Triamcinolone.

Cortic-ND. (Everett) Hydrocortisone 1%, pramoxine hydrochloride 1%, chloroxylenol 0.1%, benzalkonium chloride. Drops. 15 mL. *Rx.*
Use: Otic preparation.

•**corticorelin acetate.** (core-tih-kah-REH-lin) USAN.
Use: Hormone

•**corticorelin ovine triflutate.** (core-tih-kah-REH-lin OH-vine TRY-flew-TATE) USAN.
Use: Hormone, corticotropin-releasing; diagnostic aid, adrenocortical insufficiency; Cushing syndrome. [Orphan Drug]
See: Acthrel.

corticosteroid/mydriatic combination, ophthalmic. Prednisolone acetate 0.25%, atropine sulfate 1%. *Rx.*
Use: Treatment of anterior uveitis.

corticosteroids.
Use: Respiratory inhalant; ophthalmic conditions.
See: Beclomethasone Dipropionate.
Budesonide.
Dexamethasone.
Difluprednate.
Flunisolide.

Fluocinolone Acetonide.
Fluorometholone.
Fluticasone Propionate.
Loteprednol Etabonate.
Mometasone Furoate.
Prednisolone.
Rimexolone.
Triamcinolone Acetonide.

corticosteroids, topical.
See: Desonide.
Halobetasol Propionate.
Hydrocortisone.
Hydrocortisone Acetate.
Mometasone furoate.
Prednicarbate.
Triamcinolone Acetonide.

•**corticotropin.** (core-tih-koe-TROE-pin)
USP 34.
Use: Adrenocortical steroids.
See: Corticotropin Injection, Repository.
Cosyntropin.

•**corticotropin, repository, injection.**
(core-tih-koe-TROE-pin) USP 34.
Use: Hormone, adrenocorticotrophic;
corticosteroid, topical; diagnostic aid,
adrenocortical insufficiency.
See: H.P. Acthar Gel.

Cortifoam. (Schwarz Pharma) Hydrocortisone acetate 10% in an aerosol
foam w/propylene glycol, emulsifying
wax, stearenth 10, cetyl alcohol, methylparaben, propylparaben, trolamine, inert propellants. Container 20 g w/rectal
applicator for 14 applicatorsful. Rx.
Use: Corticosteroid, topical.

cortisol.
Note: Cortisol was the official published name for hydrocortisone in
USP 24. The name was changed back
to Hydrocortisone, USP. in Supplement 1 to the USP 24.
See: Hydrocortisone.

cortisol cyclopentylpropionate.
See: Cortef Fluid.

cortisone.
Use: Adrenocortical steroid, glucocorticoid.
See: Cortisone Acetate.

•**cortisone acetate.** (CORE-tih-sone)
USP 34.
Use: Corticosteroid, topical.
See: Cortistan.
Cortone Acetate.

cortisone acetate. (Various Mfr.) Cortisone acetate 25 mg. Tab. 8s, 100s,
500s, 1,000s, UD 100s. Rx.
Use: Adrenocortical steroid, glucocorticoid.

Cortisporin. (Monarch) Polymyxin B sulfate 10,000 units/g, neomycin sulfate
3.5 mg as base, hydrocortisone acetate
0.5%. Methylparaben 0.25%, white, liquid petrolatum. Cream. Tube 7.5 g. Rx.
Use: Anti-infective; corticosteroid, topical.

Cortisporin-TC. (Monarch) Neomycin
sulfate 3.3 mg, hydrocortisone 1%, colistin sulfate 3 mg, thonzonium bromide
0.5 mg. Susp. Bot. 10 mL w/dropper. Rx.
Use: Steroid and antibiotic combination, otic.

Cortistan. (Standex) Cortisone 25 mg/
10 mL. Rx.
Use: Corticosteroid.

•**cortivazol.** (core-TIH-vah-zole) USAN.
Use: Corticosteroid, topical.

Cortizone•5. (Pfizer Consumer Healthcare) Hydrocortisone 0.5%. White
petrolatum. Oint. Tube 30 g. OTC.
Use: Corticosteroid, topical.

Cortizone Kids. (Pfizer Consumer
Healthcare) Hydrocortisone 0.5%,
parabens, cetearyl alcohol, glycerin,
white petrolatum. Cream. Tube 14 g.
OTC.
Use: Corticosteroid, topical.

Cortizone 10. (Chattem) Hydrocortisone
1%. Aloe, disodium EDTA, glycerin,
PEG-8, SD alcohol 2%. Liq. 36 mL.
OTC.
Use: Anti-inflammatory agent, topical
corticosteroid.

Cortizone•10. (Pfizer Consumer Healthcare) Hydrocortisone 1%. Aloe, cetearyl alcohol, glycerin, mineral oil,
parabens, petrolatum. Oint. 28 g, 57 g.
Cream. 14 g, 28 g, 57 g. OTC.
Use: Anti-inflammatory agent.

Cortizone•10 External Anal Itch Relief.
(Pfizer Consumer Healthcare) Hydro-
cortisone 1%. Cetearyl alcohol, glycerin,
mineral oil, parabens, petrolatum.
Cream. 28 g. OTC.
Use: Anti-inflammatory agent.

Cortizone•10 Plus. (Pfizer Consumer
Healthcare) Hydrocortisone 1%. Alcohol,
aloe, glycerin, mineral oil, parabens,
petrolatum. Cream. 28 g, 57 g. OTC.
Use: Anti-inflammatory agent.

Cortizone•10 Quick Shot. (Pfizer Con-
sumer Healthcare) Hydrocortisone 1%.
Alcohols. Spray. 44 mL. OTC.
Use: Anti-inflammatory agent.

•**cortodoxone.** (CORE-toe-dox-OHN)
USAN.
Use: Anti-inflammatory.

Cortone Acetate. (Merck & Co.) Cortisone acetate 50 mg/mL, sodium chloride, sodium carboxymethylcellulose,
benzyl alcohol. Susp. Inj. Vial 10 mL. Rx.
Use: Corticosteroid.

Cortril Topical Ointment 1%. (Pfizer)
Hydrocortisone 1%, cetyl and stearyl
alcohol, propylene glycol, sodium lauryl

sulfate, petrolatum, cholesterol, mineral oil, methyl- and propylparabens in ointment base. Oint. Tube 0.5 oz.
Use: Corticosteroid, topical.

Cortrosyn. (Amphastar) Cosyntropin 0.25 mg, mannitol 10 mg, Pow. for Inj., lyophilized. Vials with diluent. *Rx.*
Use: Corticosteroid.

Corubeen. (Spanner) Vitamin B_{12} crystalline 1000 mcg/mL. Vial 10 mL. *Rx.*
Use: Vitamin supplement.

Corvert. (Pharmacia) Ibutilide fumarate 0.1 mg/mL. Soln. Vial. 10 mL. *Rx.*
Use: Antiarrhythmic.

Corvite Free. (Vertical Pharmaceuticals) Vitamin D_3 400 units, E 125 units, C 500 mg, B_1 25 mg, B_2 3.4 mg, B_3 35 mg, B_5 5 mg, B_6 35 mg, B_{12} 70 mcg, folic acid 1.25 mcg, biotin 75 mcg, alpha-lipoic acid 10 mg, coenzyme Q_{10} 35 mg, lutein 400 mcg, lycopene 125 mcg. Dye free, gluten free, lactose free, sugar free. Tab. 100s. *Rx.*
Use: Multivitamin with minerals.

Corzall. (Hawthorn) Carbetapentane citrate 20 mg, pseudoephedrine hydrochloride 30 mg. Saccharin, sorbitol. Alcohol free, dye free, and sugar free. Grape flavor. Liq. 473 mL. *Rx.*
Use: Upper respiratory combination, antitussive combination.

Corzall-PE. (Hawthorn) Carbetapentane citrate 20 mg, dexchlorpheniramine maleate 1 mg, phenylephrine hydrochloride 10 mg. Glycerin, propylene glycol, saccharin, sorbitol. Alcohol free, dye free, and sugar free. Cherry flavor. Liq. 473 mL. *Rx.*
Use: Upper respiratory combination, antitussive combination.

Corzall Plus. (Hawthorn) Carbetapentane citrate 20 mg, pseudoephedrine hydrochloride 30 mg, pyrilamine maleate 7.5 mg. Saccharin, sorbitol. Alcohol free, dye free, and sugar free. Fruit gum flavor. Liq. 473 mL.
Use: Upper respiratory combination, antitussive combination.

Corzide. (King Pharma) Nadolol/bendroflumethiazide 40 mg/5 mg, 80 mg/5 mg. Lactose. Tab. Bot. 100s. *Rx.*
Use: Antihypertensive.

Corzyme. (Abbott Diagnostics) Enzyme immunoassay for detection of antibody to hepatitis B core antigen in serum or plasma. Test kit 100s.
Use: Diagnostic aid.

Corzyme-M. (Abbott Diagnostics) Enzyme immunoassay for the detection of Ig antibody to hepatitis B core antigen (Anti-HBc Ig). In human serum or plasma. Test kit 100s.
Use: Diagnostic aid.

•**cositecan.** (COS-eye-TEE-kan) USAN.
Use: Antineoplastic agent.

Cosmegen. (Merck) Actinomycin D (dactinomycin) 500 mcg. Mannitol 20 mg. Pow. for Inj., lyophilized. Vials. *Rx.*
Use: Antineoplastic; antibiotic.

Cosmoline.
See: Petrolatum.

Cosopt. (Merck) Dorzolamide 2%, timolol 0.5%. Benzalkonium chloride 0.0075%, mannitol. Soln. *Ocumeters.* 5 mL, 10 mL. *Rx.*
Use: Antiglaucoma agent.

Cosulid. (Novartis) Sulfachloropyridazine.

•**cosyntropin.** (koe-sin-TROE-pin) USAN.
Use: Hormone, adrenocorticotrophic.
See: Cortrosyn.

cosyntropin. (Sandoz) Cosyntropin 0.25 mg/mL. Mannitol 10 mg, sodium chloride 6.4 mg. Preservative free. Inj., Soln. Vial. 1 mL. *Rx.*
Use: Adrenocortical steroid, corticotropin (ACTH).

Cotab A. (MCR American) Chlorpheniramine maleate 4 mg, codeine phosphate 10 mg. Cap. 100s. *c-III.*
Use: Upper respiratory combination, antitussive, antihistamine.

Cotab AX. (MCR American) Chlorpheniramine maleate 4 mg, codeine phosphate 20 mg. Tab. 100s. *c-III.*
Use: Upper respiratory combination, antitussive combination.

Cotabflu. (MCR American) Acetaminophen 500 mg, chlorpheniramine maleate 4 mg, codeine phosphate 20 mg. Tab. 100s. *c-III.*
Use: Upper respiratory combination, antitussive combination.

Cotaphylline. (Major) Oxtriphylline 100 mg, 200 mg. Tab. Bot. 100s, 500s. *Rx.*
Use: Bronchodilator.

cotarnine chloride. Cotarnine hydrochloride.
Use: Astringent.

cotarnine hydrochloride.
See: Cotarnine Chloride.

•**cotinine fumarate.** (koe-TIH-neen) USAN.
Use: Antidepressant; psychomotor stimulant.

Cotolate. (Major) Benztropine 1 mg, 2 mg. Tab. Bot. 100s, 1000s. *Rx.*
Use: Antiparkinsonian.

•**cotton, purified.** (KAHT-uhn) *USP 34.*
Use: Surgical aid.

•**cottonseed oil.** (KAHT-uhn-seed) *NF 29.*
Use: Pharmaceutic aid; solvent, oleaginous vehicle.

Co-Tuss V. (Rugby) Hydrocodone bitartrate 5 mg, guaifenesin 100 mg. Liq. Bot. 480 mL. *c-III.*
Use: Antitussive; expectorant.

CO₂-releasing suppositories.
See: Ceo-Two.

Cotylenol Children's Chewable Cold Tablet. (McNeil Consumer) Acetaminophen 80 mg, chlorpheniramine maleate 0.5 mg, pseudoephedrine hydrochloride 7.5 mg. Chew. Tab. Bot. 24s. *OTC.*
Use: Analgesic; antihistamine; decongestant.

Cotylenol Children's Liquid Cold Formula. (McNeil Consumer) Acetaminophen 160 mg, chlorpheniramine maleate 1 mg, pseudoephedrine hydrochloride 15 mg, sorbitol/5 mL. Bot. 4 oz. *OTC.*
Use: Analgesic; antihistamine; decongestant.

Cotylenol Cold Formula. (McNeil Consumer) Chlorpheniramine maleate 2 mg, dextromethorphan HBr 15 mg, pseudoephedrine hydrochloride 30 mg, acetaminophen 325 mg. **Tab.:** Box 24s, Bot. 50s, 100s. **Capl.:** Bot. 24s, 50s. *OTC.*
Use: Analgesic; antihistamine; antitussive; decongestant.

Cotylenol Liquid Cold Formula. (McNeil Consumer) Acetaminophen 650 mg, chlorpheniramine maleate 4 mg, pseudoephedrine hydrochloride 60 mg, dextromethorphan hydrochloride 30 mg/30 mL, alcohol 7.5%, sorbitol. Bot. 5 oz. *OTC.*
Use: Analgesic; antihistamine; antitussive; decongestant.

Cough Formula Comtrex. (Bristol-Myers Squibb) Pseudoephedrine hydrochloride 15 mg, dextromethorphan HBr 7.5 mg/5 mL, guaifenesin, saccharin, sucrose. Liq. Bot. 120 mL, 240 mL. *OTC.*
Use: Antitussive; expectorant.

Cough Syrup. (Ivax) Phenylephrine hydrochloride 5 mg, dextromethorphan HBr 10 mg, guaifenesin 100 mg, alcohol free. Bot. 120 mL. *OTC.*
Use: Antitussive; decongestant; expectorant.

Coumadin. (Bristol-Myers Squibb) Warfarin sodium. **Tab.:** 1 mg, 2 mg, 2.5 mg, 3 mg, 4 mg, 5 mg, 6 mg, 7.5 mg, 10 mg. Dye-free (10 mg only). Lactose. Bot. 100s, 1000s (except 7.5 mg, 10 mg), UD 100s. **Pow. for Soln., Inj., lyophilized:** Warfarin sodium 5.4 mg (2 mg/mL when reconstituted). Mannitol, preservative-free.

Single-use vials. 5 mg. *Rx.*
Use: Anticoagulant.

coumarin.
Use: Anticoagulant; treat renal cell carcinoma. [Orphan Drug]

coumarin and indandione derivatives.
Use: Anticoagulant.
See: Coumadin.
   Warfarin Sodium.

•**coumermycin.** (KOO-mer-MY-sin) USAN.
Use: Anti-infective.

•**coumermycin sodium.** (KOO-mer-MY-sin) USAN.
Use: Anti-infective.

counterirritants.
See: Capsaicin.

Counterpain Rub. (Bristol-Myers Squibb) Methylsalicylate, eugenol, menthol. Oint. Tube 1 oz. *OTC.*
Use: Analgesic, topical.

Covaryx. (Centrix) Esterified estrogens 1.25 mg, methyltestosterone 2.5 mg. Lactose, tartrazine. Film-coated. Tab. 100s. *Rx.*
Use: Estrogen and androgen combination, sex hormone.

Covaryx H.S. (Centrix) Esterified estrogens 0.625 mg, methyltestosterone 1.25 mg. Lactose, tartrazine. Film-coated. Tab. 100s. *Rx.*
Use: Estrogen and androgen combination, sex hormone.

Covera-HS. (Pfizer) Verapamil hydrochloride 180 mg, 240 mg. Film-coated. ER Tab. Bot. 100s, UD 100s. *Rx.*
Use: Calcium channel blocker.

Covermark. (O'Leary) Neutral cream, hypoallergenic, opaque, greaseless. Jar 1 oz, 3 oz, available in 11 shades. *OTC.*
Use: Conceals birthmarks and skin discolorations.

Covermark Stick. (O'Leary) For normal to oily skin, available in 7 shades. *OTC.*
Use: Conceals birthmarks and skin discolorations.

Co-Xan. (Schwarz Pharma) Theophylline anhydrous 150 mg, ephedrine hydrochloride 25 mg, guaifenesin 100 mg, codeine phosphate 15 mg, alcohol 10%/15 mL. Syr. Bot. Pt. *Rx.*
Use: Antitussive; bronchodilator; decongestant; expectorant.

Cozaar. (Merck) Losartan potassium 25 mg (potassium 2.12 mg), 50 mg (potassium 4.24 mg), 100 mg (potassium 8.48 mg). Lactose. Film-coated. Tab. Bot. 1000s, unit-of-use 30s (except 25 mg), 90s, 100s, UD 100s. *Rx.*
Use: Renin angiotensin system antagonist, angiotensin II receptor antagonist.

CPB WC. (Elge) Brompheniramine maleate 1.3 mg, codeine phosphate 6.3 mg, pseudoephedrine hydrochloride 10 mg per 5 mL. Saccharin, sorbitol. Cherry flavor. Liq. 473 mL. *c-v.*
Use: Upper respiratory combination, antitussive combination.

CP DEC-DM. (Hi-Tech) **Syrup:** Dextromethorphan HBr 15 mg, chlorpheniramine maleate 4 mg, phenylephrine hydrochloride 12.5 mg per 5 mL. Alcohol and sugar free. Saccharin, sorbitol. Grape flavor. 118 mL, 473 mL. *Rx.*
Use: Upper respiratory combination, antitussive combination.

C.P.-DM. (Hi-Tech) Pseudoephedrine hydrochloride 15 mg, carbinoxamine maleate 1 mg, dextromethorphan HBr 4 mg per 1 mL. Saccharin, sorbitol, grape flavor. Drops. Bot. 30 mL w/dropper. *Rx.*
Use: Upper respiratory combination, decongestant, antihistamine, antitussive.

C-Phed Tannate. (Morton Grove) Pseudoephedrine tannate 75 mg, chlorpheniramine tannate 4.5 mg/5 mL, strawberry/banana flavor. Susp. Bot. 118 mL. *Rx.*
Use: Upper respiratory combination, decongestant, antihistamine.

C-Phen. (Boca Pharmacal) **Drops:** Phenylephrine hydrochloride 3.5 mg, chlorpheniramine maleate 1 mg per 1 mL. Alcohol and sugar free. Sorbitol. 30 mL with dropper. **Syrup:** Phenylephrine hydrochloride 12.5 mg, chlorpheniramine maleate 4 mg per 5 mL. Alcohol and sugar free. Sorbitol. 118 mL, 473 mL. *Rx.*
Use: Upper respiratory combination, decongestant and antihistamine.

C-Phen DM. (Boca Pharmacal) **Drops:** Dextromethorphan HBr 3 mg, chlorpheniramine maleate 1 mg, phenylephrine hydrochloride 3.5 mg per 1 mL. Alcohol and sugar free. Sorbitol. Grape flavor. 30 mL with dropper. **Syrup:** Dextromethorphan HBr 15 mg, chlorpheniramine maleate 4 mg, phenylephrine hydrochloride 12.5 mg per 5 mL. Alcohol and sugar free. Sorbitol. Grape flavor. 118 mL, 473 mL. *Rx.*
Use: Upper respiratory combination, antitussive combination.

Cplex. (Arcum) Vitamins B_1 10 mg, B_2 10 mg, B_6 5 mg, B_{12} 10 mcg, niacinamide 100 mg, calcium pantothenate 25 mg, C 150 mg, liver 50 mg, dried yeast 50 mg. Cap. Bot. 100s, 1000s. *OTC.*
Use: Mineral, vitamin supplement.

C.P.M. (Ivax) Chlorpheniramine 4 mg. Tab. Bot. 1000s. *OTC.*
Use: Antihistamine.

CPM 8/PE 20/MSC 1.25. (Cypress) Phenylephrine hydrochloride 20 mg, chlorpheniramine maleate 8 mg, methscopolamine nitrate 1.25 mg. Lactose. ER Tab. 100s. *Rx.*
Use: Decongestant, antihistamine, and anticholinergic, upper respiratory combination.

CPM 8/PSE 90/MSC 2.5. (Cypress) Pseudoephedrine hydrochloride 90 mg, chlorpheniramine maleate 8 mg, methscopolamine nitrate 2.5 mg. Dye free. ER Tab. Bot. 100s. *Rx.*
Use: Upper respiratory combination, decongestant, antihistamine, anticholinergic.

CPM PSE. (Boca Pharmacal) Chlorpheniramine maleate 2 mg, pseudoephedrine hydrochloride 30 mg per 5 mL. Sorbitol. Alcohol and dye free. Grape flavor. Syr.473 mL. *Rx.*
Use: Upper respiratory combination, decongestant and antihistamine.

CPM/PSE DM. (Trigen Laboratories) Chlorpheniramine maleate 0.8 mg, dextromethorphan hydrobromide 3 mg, pseudoephedrine hydrochloride 9 mg per 5 mL. Glycerin, parabens, potassium sorbate, propylene glycol, sorbitol, sucralose. Grape flavor. Drops. 30 mL. *Rx.*
Use: Upper respiratory combination, antitussive combination.

CP-TANNIC. (Cypress) Pseudoephedrine tannate 75 mg, chlorpheniramine tannate 4.5 mg/5 mL, strawberry/banana flavor. Susp. Bot. 473 mL. *Rx.*
Use: Upper respiratory combination, decongestant, antihistamine.

Crantex. (Breckenridge) Phenylephrine hydrochloride 7.5 mg, guaifenesin 100 mg/5 mL. Alcohol, sugar, and dye free. Saccharin, sorbitol. Liq. 473 mL. *Rx.*
Use: Upper respiratory combination, decongestant and expectorant combination.

Crantex ER. (Breckenridge) Phenylephrine hydrochloride 10 mg, guaifenesin 300 mg. Sugar. ER Cap. 100s. *Rx.*
Use: Decongestant and expectorant.

Cream Camellia. (O'Leary) Jar 2 oz. *OTC.*
Use: Emollient.

•**creatinine.** (kree-OT-ih-nihn) *NF 29.*
Use: Bulking agent for freeze drying.

creatinine reagent strips. (Bayer Consumer Care) Seralyzer reagent strips.

A quantitative strip test for creatinine in serum or plasma. Bot. 25s.
Use: Diagnostic aid.

Cremagol. (Cremagol) Emulsion of liquid petrolatum, agar agar, acacia, glycerin. Bot. 14 oz. W/cascara 11 g/oz, Bot. 14 oz. W/phenolphthalein 2 g/oz, Bot. 14 oz. *OTC.*
Use: Laxative.

Creomulsion Adult Formula. (Summit) Dextromethorphan HBr 20 mg/15 mL. Alcohol free. Sucrose. Syrup. 118 mL. *OTC.*
Use: Nonnarcotic antitussive.

Creomulsion for Children. (Summit) Dextromethorphan HBr 5 mg/5 mL. Alcohol free. Sucrose. Cherry flavor. Syrup. 118 mL. *OTC.*
Use: Nonnarcotic antitussive.

Creon. (Abbott) Lipase 8000 units, amylase 30,000 units, protease 13,000 units, pancreatin 300 mg. Cap. Bot. 100s, 250s. *Rx.*
Use: Digestive enzyme.

Creon Delayed Release. (Solvay) Lipase/protease/amylase 6,000 units/19,000 units/30,000 units; 12,000 units/38,000 units/60,000 units; 24,000 units/76,000 units/120,000 units. Enteric-coated spheres. Cap., delayed release. 100s, 250s. *Rx.*
Use: Digestive enzyme.

creosote. Wood creosote, creosote, beechwood creosote.

Creo-Terpin. (Lee) Dextromethorphan HBr 10 mg/15 mL (3.33 mg/5 mL). Tartrazine, alcohol 25%, saccharin, corn syrup. Liq. Bot. 120 mL. *OTC.*
Use: Nonnarcotic antitussive.

Crescormon. (Pharmacia) Somatotropin 4 units. Vial. IM administration. *Rx.*
Note: Crescormon will be available only for patients who qualify for treatment. Apply to Kabi Group Inc. for approval.
Use: Hormone, growth.

•**cresol.** (KREE-sole) *NF 29.*
Use: Antiseptic; disinfectant.

cresol preparations.
Use: Antiseptic; disinfectant.
See: Saponated Cresol.

Crestor. (AstraZeneca) Rosuvastatin calcium (as base) 5 mg, 10 mg, 20 mg, 40 mg. Lactose. 30s (40 mg only), 90s (except 40 mg), UD 100s (except 5 mg). *Rx.*
Use: HMG-CoA reductase inhibitors, antihyperlipidemic agent.

m-cresyl-acetate.
See: Cresylate.

Cresylate. (Recsei) M-cresyl-acetate 25%, isopropanol 25%, chlorobutanol 1%, benzyl alcohol 1%, castor oil 5%, propylene glycol. Bot. 15 mL with dropper, pt. *Rx.*
Use: Otic preparation.

cresylic acid. Same as Cresol.

•**crilvastatin.** (krill-vah-STAT-in) USAN.
Use: Antihyperlipidemic.

Crinone. (Watson Labs) Progesterone 8% (90 mg). Glycerin, mineral oil, palm oil. Vaginal Gel. Single-use, prefilled, disposable applicator delivering 1.125 gel. 6s, 18s. *Rx.*
Use: Assisted reproductive technology treatment.

•**crisnatol mesylate.** (KRISS-nah-tole) USAN.
Use: Antineoplastic.

Criticare HN. (Bristol-Myers Squibb) High nitrogen elemental diet. Protein 14%, fat 4.3%, carbohydrate 81.5%. Bot. 8 oz. *OTC.*
Use: Nutritional supplement, enteral.

Crixivan. (Merck) Indinavir sulfate 100 mg, 200 mg, 333 mg, 400 mg (corresponding to 125 mg, 250 mg, 416.3 mg, 500 mg indinavir sulfate, respectively). Lactose. Cap. Unit-of-use 18s, 90s, 120s (400 mg only); 135s (333 mg only); 180s (100 mg, 400 mg only); 360s (200 mg only); unit dose 42s (400 mg only). *Rx.*
Use: Antiretroviral agent, protease inhibitor.

•**crizotinib.** (kriz-OH-ti-nib) USAN.
Use: Antineoplastic.

CroFab. (Altana) Crotalidae polyvalent immune fab (ovine origin). Total protein 1 g, thimerosal (mercury 0.11 mg)/vial. Single-use Vial. Diluent not included. *Rx.*
Use: Antivenin.

Croferrin. (Forest) Iron peptonate 50 mg, liver injection 2.5 mcg, vitamin B_{12} 12.5 mcg, lidocaine hydrochloride 1%, phenol 0.5%, sodium citrate 0.125%, sodium bisulfite 0.009%/mL. Vial 10 mL, 30 mL. *Rx.*
Use: Mineral, vitamin supplement.

•**crofilcon A.** (kroe-FILL-kahn A) USAN.
Use: Contact lens material, hydrophilic.

•**crolibulin.** (KROE-li-BUE-lin) USAN.
Use: Antineoplastic.

Cro-Man-Zin. (Freeda) Cr 200 mcg, Mn 5 mg, Zn 25 mg, kosher, sugar free. Tab. Bot. 100s, 250s. *OTC.*
Use: Electrolyte, mineral supplement.

•**cromitrile sodium.** (KROE-mih-TRILE) USAN.
Use: Antiasthmatic.

•**cromolyn sodium.** (KROE-moe-lin) *USP 34.*
Use: Antiasthmatic; prophylactic; mastocytosis. [Orphan Drug]
See: Children's NasalCrom.
Gastrocrom.
Intal.
NasalCrom.

cromolyn sodium. (Major Pharmaceuticals) Cromolyn sodium 40 mg/mL (5.2 mg/spray). Soln., Nasal. 26 mL. *OTC.*
Use: Respiratory inhalant, mast cell stabilizer.

cromolyn sodium. (Various Mfr.) Cromolyn sodium. **Inhalation:** 20 mg/2 mL. Vial or Amps. 60 mL, 120 mL. **Soln. for Nebulization:** 20 mg. Vial. 2 mL. *Rx.*
Use: Antiasthmatic; prophylactic.

cromolyn sodium. (Various Mfr.) Cromolyn sodium 4%. Soln. 10 mL, 15 mL. *Rx.*
Use: Ophthalmic mast cell stabilizer.

Cronetal.
See: Disulfiram.

•**croscarmellose sodium.** (KRAHS-CAR-mell-ose) *NF 29. Formerly Cross-linked Carboxymethylcellulose Sodium and Modified Cellulose Gum.*
Use: Pharmaceutic aid, tablet disintegrant.

•**crospovidone.** (krahs-PAV-ih-dohn) *NF 29.*
Use: Pharmaceutic aid, tablet excipient.

Cross Aspirin. (Cross) Aspirin 325 mg. Sugar, salt and lactose free. Tab. Bot. 100s, 1000s. *OTC.*
Use: Analgesic.

CroTAb. (CroFab)

Crotalidae antivenin polyvalent. (Wyeth) 1 vial of lyophilized serum, 1 vial of bacteriostatic water 10 mL, USP, 1 vial normal horse serum. Inj. Vial Combination Pkg. *Rx.*
Use: Antivenin.

Crotalidae polyvalent immune fab (ovine origin).
Use: Antivenin.
See: CroFab.

•**crotaline antivenin, polyvalent.** (kroe-TAHL-een an-tee-VEH-nen pahl-ee-VAY-lent) *USP 34.* Antivenin Crotalidae Polyvalent, North and South American antisnakebite serum. *Rx.*
Use: Immunizing agent.

•**crotamiton.** (kroe-TAM-ih-tuhn) *USP 34.*
Use: Scabicide.
See: Eurax.

CRPA Latex Test. (Laboratory Diagnostics) Rapid latex agglutination test for the qualitative determination of C-reactive protein. CRPA, 1 mL CRP Positest Control, 0.5 mL CRPA Latex Test Kit.
Use: Diagnostic aid.

Cruex. (Novartis) **Aer., Pow:** Miconazole nitrate 2%. Aloe, SD alcohol 10%. 85 g. **Cream:** Clotrimazole 1%. Benzyl alcohol 1%, cetostearyl alcohol. Tube. 15 g. *OTC.*
Use: Anti-infective, topical; antifungal agent.

Cruex Spray Powder. (Novartis Consumer Health) Undecylenic acid 2% and zinc undecylenate 20%. Pow. Aerosol can 1.8 oz, 3.5 oz, 5.5 oz. *OTC.*
Use: Antifungal, topical.

Cruex Squeeze Powder. (Novartis Consumer Health) Calcium undecylenate 10%. Pow. Plastic squeeze bot. 1.5 oz. *OTC.*
Use: Antifungal, topical.

cryptosporidium hyperimmune bovine colostrum IgG concentrate. (Immucell)
Use: Treat diarrhea in AIDS patients. [Orphan Drug]

Cryselle. (Barr) Norgestrel 0.3 mg, ethinyl estradiol 30 mcg. Packs. 21s. 28s with 7 inert tabs. *Rx.*
Use: Sex hormone, contraceptive hormone.

crystalline trypsin. Highly purified preparation of enzyme as derived from mammalian pancreas glands.

crystal violet.
See: Methylrosaniline Chloride.

Crysti-Liver. (Roberts) Liver injection (equivalent to B_{12} 10 mcg), crystalline B_{12} 100 mcg, folic acid 0.4 mg. Inj. Vial 10 mL. *Rx.*
Use: Mineral, vitamin supplement.

Crystodigin. (Eli Lilly) Digitoxin 0.05 mg, 0.1 mg. Tab. Bot. 100s. *Rx.*
Use: Cardiovascular agent.

CTab.
See: Cetyl Trimethyl Ammonium Bromide.

C-Tan D Plus Oral Suspension. (Centurion Labs) Brompheniramine tannate 5 mg, phenylephrine tannate 5 mg per 5 mL. Raspberry flavor. Susp., Oral. 473 mL. *Rx.*
Use: Upper respiratory combination, decongestant and antihistamine.

C-Tanna 12D. (Prasco) Carbetapentane tannate 30 mg, pyrilamine tannate 30 mg, phenylephrine tannate 5 mg per 5 mL. Methylparaben, sucrose, saccharin, tartrazine. Strawberry-currant flavor. Susp. 118 mL. *Rx.*

Use: Antitussive combination, upper respiratory combination.

C-Tussin. (Century) Codeine phosphate 10 mg, pseudoephedrine hydrochloride 30 mg, guaifenesin 100 mg/5 mL, alcohol 7.5%. Bot. 120 mL, gal. *c-iv.*
Use: Antitussive; decongestant; expectorant.

Cubicin. (Cubist) Daptomycin 500 mg. Preservative free. Pow. for Inj., lyophilized Cake. Single-use vials. 10 mL. *Rx.*
Use: Anti-infective.

Culminal. (Culminal) Benzocaine 3% in water-miscible cream base. Tube 1 oz. *OTC.*
Use: Anesthetic, local.

Culturelle for Kids. (Amerfit) Lactobacillus GG 1 billion live cells. Gluten free, lactose free, and preservative free. Inulin, mannitol. Pow. 30s. *OTC.*
Use: Oral nutritional supplement, probiotic.

Culturelle with Lactobacillus GG. (Amerfit) Lactobacillus GG 10 billion live cells. Cap. 10s. *OTC.*
Use: Oral nutritional supplement, probiotic.

Culturette 10 Minute Group A Step ID. (Hoechst) Latex slide agglutination test for group A streptococcal antigen on throat swabs. Kit 55 determinations.
Use: Diagnostic aid.

•**cupric acetate Cu 64.** (koo-PRIK) USAN.
Use: Radioactive agent.

•**cupric chloride.** (koo-PRIK) *USP 34.*
Use: Supplement, trace mineral.

•**cupric sulfate.** (koo-PRIK) *USP 34.*
Use: Antidote to phosphorus.

cupric sulfate. (American Regent) Copper 0.4 mg/mL (as 1.57 mg of sulfate). Inj. Vial 10 mL. *Rx.*
Use: Trace metal.

Cuprid. (Merck & Co.) Trientine hydrochloride 250 mg. Cap. Bot. 100s. *Rx.*
Use: Chelating agent.

Cuprimine. (Aton Pharma) Penicillamine 250 mg. Cap. 100s. *Rx.*
Use: Chelating agent.

•**cuprimyxin.** (KUH-prih-mix-in) USAN.
Use: Antifungal.

Cupri-Pak. (SoloPak Pharmaceuticals, Inc.) Copper. **0.4 mg/mL:** Vial 10 mL, 30 mL. **2 mg/mL:** Vial 5 mL. *Rx.*
Use: Nutritional supplement, parenteral.

curare.
Use: Muscle relaxant.

curare antagonist.
See: Neostigine Methylsulfate. Tensilon.

Curel. (Bausch & Lomb) Glycerin, petrolatum, dimethicone, parabens. Lot. 180, 300, 390 mL. Cream. Tube. 90 g. *Rx-OTC.*
Use: Emollient.

Curity Sponge Sticks. (Kendall) Iodine 1%. Latex free. Stick, topical. 2s. *OTC.*
Use: Topical anti-infective, antiseptic and germicide.

Curity Wet Skin Scrub Pack. (Kendall) Iodine 0.75% to 1%. Latex free. Soln. Kit w/2 large winged rib sponges, 2 sponge sticks, wrap, gloves, applicators, and towels. *OTC.*
Use: Topical anti-infective, antiseptic and germicide.

Curosurf. (Cornerstone Biopharma) Poractant alfa (porcine origin). Phospholipids 80 mg/mL (including phosphatidylcholine 54 mg, of which 30.5 mg is dipalmitoyl phosphatidylcholine and 1 mg of protein, including 0.3 mg of SP-B), preservative free. Intratracheal Susp. Single-use vials. 1.5 mL, 3 mL. *Rx.*
Use: Lung surfactant; respiratory distress syndrome.

curral.
See: Diallyl Barbituric Acid.

Cutar Emulsion. (Summers) LCD 7.5% (coal tar 1.5%) in mineral oil, lanolin alcohols extract, parabens. Liq. 177 mL, 1 gal. *OTC.*
Use: Dermatologic.

Cutemol Emollient. (Summers) Allantoin 0.2%, liquid petrolatum, acetylated lanolin, lanolin alcohols extract, isopropyl myristate, water. Cream. Jar 2 oz. *OTC.*
Use: Emollient.

Cutivate. (Pharmaderm) Fluticasone propionate. **Cream:** 0.05%. Jar 15 g, 30 g, 60 g. **Lot.:** 0.05%. Cetostearyl alcohol, parabens. 60 mL. **Oint.:** 0.005%. Jar 15 g, 30 g, 60 g. *Rx.*
Use: Corticosteroid, topical.

Cutter Insect Repellent. (Bayer Consumer Care) N,N-Diethyl-meta-toluamide 28.5%, other isomers 1.5%. Vial 1 oz; Foam, Can 2 oz; Spray 7 oz, Aerosol can 14 oz; Assortment Pack; First Aid Kits, Trial Pack, 6s; Marine Pack 3s; Camp Pack 4s; Pocket Pack, Travel Pack. *OTC.*
Use: Insect repellent.

Cuvposa. (Shionogi Pharma) Glycopyrrolate 1 mg per 5 mL. Parabens, propylene glycol, saccharin, sorbitol. Cherry flavor. Soln. 16 oz. *Rx.*
Use: Gastrointestinal anticholinergic/antispasmodic, quaternary anticholinergic.

C vitamin.
See: Ascorbic Acid.
CY 1899. (Cytel Corp.)
Use: Antiviral, hepatitis B. [Orphan Drug]
CY 1503. (Cytel Corp.)
Use: Antithromboembolic. [Orphan Drug]
Cyanide Antidote Package. (Various Mfr.) 2 amp. (300 mg/10 mL) sodium nitrite; 2 vials (12.5 g/50 mL), sodium thiosulfate; 12 amps amyl nitrite inhalant 5 minim/0.3 mL, disposable syringes, stomach tube, tourniquet, and instructions. *Rx.*
Use: Antidote, cyanide poisoning.
Cyanocob. (Paddock) Vitamin B_{12} 1000 mcg/mL. Bot. 1000 mL, Vial 10 mL. *Rx.*
Use: Vitamin supplement.
•**cyanocobalamin.** (sigh-an-oh-koe-BAL-uh-min) *USP 34. Formerly Vitamin B_{12}.*
Use: Water-soluble vitamin, hematopoietic.
See: B-12.
   CaloMist.
   Nascobal.
   Rapid B-12 Energy.
   Twelve Resin-K.
   Vitamin B_{12}.
W/Combinations.
See: Folgard.
   FOLTX.
•**cyanocobalamin Co 58.** (sigh-an-oh-koe-BAL-uh-min) *USP 34.*
Use: Diagnostic aid, pernicious anemia; radioactive agent.
•**cyanocobalamin Co 57.** (sigh-an-oh-koe-BAL-uh-min) *USP 34.*
Use: Diagnostic aid, pernicious anemia; radioactive agent.
•**cyanocobalamin Co 60.** (sigh-an-oh-koe-BAL-uh-min) *USP 34.*
Use: Diagnostic aid, pernicious anemia; radioactive agent.
cyanocobalamin crystalline. *Rx-OTC.*
Use: Vitamin B_{12} supplement.
See: Cyomin.
   Vitamin B_{12}.
Cyanokit. (King Pharma) Hydroxocobalamin 25 mg/mL (after reconstitution). Inj., lyophilized Pow. for Soln. 5 g kit. In two 250-mL colorless glass vials (2.5 g per vial), 2 sterile transfer spikes, 1 sterile IV infusion set. *Rx.*
Use: Detoxification agent, antidote.
Cyanover. (Research Supplies) Cyanocobalamin 100 mcg, liver injection 10 mcg, folic acid 10 mg/mL. *Lyo-layer* vial 10 mL with vial of diluent 10 mL. *Rx.*

Use: Mineral, vitamin supplement.
•**cyclacillin.** (SIGH-klah-SILL-in) *USP 34.*
Use: Anti-infective.
cyclamate sodium. Cyclohexanesulfamate dihydrate salt.
•**cyclamic acid.** (sigh-KLAM-ik) USAN.
Use: Sweetener, nonnutritive.
•**cyclazocine.** (SIGH-CLAY-zoe-seen) USAN. Under study.
Use: Analgesic.
Cyclessa. (Organon) **Phase 1:** Desogestrel 0.1 mg, ethinyl estradiol 25 mcg. 7 tabs. **Phase 2:** Desogestrel 0.125 mg, ethinyl estradiol 25 mcg. 7 tabs. **Phase 3:** Desogestrel 0.15 mg, ethinyl estradiol 25 mcg. 7 tabs. Lactose, talc. Tab. 28s with 7 inert tabs. *Rx.*
Use: Sex hormone, contraceptive hormone.
•**cyclindole.** (sigh-KLIN-dole) USAN.
Use: Antidepressant.
Cyclinex-1. (Ross) Protein 7.5 g (from carnitine, cystine, histidine, isoleucine, leucine, lysine, methionine, phenylalanine, taurine, threonine, tryptophan, tyrosine, valine), fat 27 g (from palm oil, hydrogenated coconut oil, soy oil), carbohydrate 52 g (from hydrolyzed corn starch), linoleic acid 2000 mg, Fe 10 mg, Na 215 mg, K 760 mg, Ca, vitamins A, B_1, B_2, B_3, B_5, B_6, B_{12}, C, D, E, K, biotin, choline, folic acid, inositol, Cl, Cu, I, Mg, Mn, P, Se, Zn and 515 Cal per 100 g. Nonessential amino acid free. Pow. Can 350 g. *OTC.*
Use: Nutritional supplement.
Cyclinex-2. (Ross) Protein 15 g (from carnitine, cystine, histidine, isoleucine, leucine, lysine, methionine, phenylalanine, taurine, threonine, tryptophan, tyrosine, valine), fat 20.7 g (from palm oil, hydrogenated coconut oil, soy oil), carbohydrate 40 g (from hydrolyzed cornstarch), Fe 17 mg, Na 1175 mg, K 1830 mg, Ca, vitamins A, B_1, B_2, B_3, B_5, B_6, B_{12}, C, D, E, K, biotin, choline, folic acid, inositol, Cl, Cu, I, Mg, Mn, P, Se, Zn and 480 Cal per 100 g. Nonessential amino acid free. Pow. Can 325 g. *OTC.*
Use: Nutritional supplement.
•**cycliramine maleate.** (SIGH-klih-rah-meen) USAN.
Use: Antihistamine.
•**cyclizine.** (SIGH-klih-zeen) *USP 34.*
Use: Antihistamine.
•**cyclizine hydrochloride.** (SIGH-klih-zeen) *USP 34.*
Use: Antiemetic.
See: Bonine for Kids.
   Marezine.

•**cyclizine lactate injection.** (SIGH-klih-zeen LACK-tate) *USP 34.*
Use: Antihistamine; antinauseant.

cyclobarbital.
Use: Central depressant.

cyclobarbital calcium.
Use: Hypnotic; sedative.

•**cyclobendazole.** (SIGH-kloe-BEN-dah-zole) USAN.
Use: Anthelmintic.

•**cyclobenzaprine hydrochloride.** (SIGH-kloe-BEN-zuh-preen) *USP 34.*
Use: Muscle relaxant.
See: Amrix.
 Fexmid.
 Flexeril.

cyclobenzaprine hydrochloride. (Various Mfr.) Cyclobenzaprine hydrochloride 5 mg, 10 mg. May contain lactose. Tab. Bot. 30s, 100s, 500s, 1000s, UD 30s (5 mg only). *Rx.*
Use: Muscle relaxant.

cyclobenzaprine hydrochloride. (Watson) Cyclobenzaprine hydrochloride 7.5 mg. Tab. 30s, 100s, 1000s. *Rx.*
Use: Muscle relaxant.

cyclocumarol.
Use: Anticoagulant.

•**cyclofilcon A.** (SIGH-kloe-FILL-kahn A) USAN.
Use: Contact lens material, hydrophilic.

Cyclogen. (Schwarz Pharma) Dicyclomine hydrochloride 10 mg, sodium chloride 0.9%, chlorobutanol hydrate 0.5%. Vial 10 mL, Box 12s. *Rx.*
Use: Antispasmodic.

•**cycloguanil pamoate.** (SIGH-kloe-GWAHN-ill PAM-oh-ate) USAN.
Use: Antimalarial.

Cyclogyl. (Alcon) Cyclopentolate hydrochloride 0.5%, 1%, 2%. Soln. *Drop-tainer* 2 mL, 5 mL, 15 mL. *Rx.*
Use: Cycloplegic; mydriatic.

•**cycloheximide.** (sigh-KLOE-HEX-ih-mid) USAN.
Use: Antipsoriatic.

•**cyclomethicone.** (sigh-kloe-METH-ih-cone) *NF 29.*
Use: Pharmaceutic aid, wetting agent.

cyclomethycaine and methapyrilene.
Use: Anesthetic, local.

cyclomethycaine sulfate.
Use: Anesthetic, local.

Cyclomydril. (Alcon) Phenylephrine hydrochloride 1%, cyclopentolate hydrochloride 0.2%. Droptainer 2 mL, 5 mL. *Rx.*
Use: Mydriatic.

Cyclonil. (Seatrace) Dicyclomine hydrochloride 10 mg/mL. Vial 10 mL. *Rx.*

Use: Anticholinergic; antispasmodic.

Cyclopar. (Parke-Davis) Tetracycline hydrochloride. Cap. **250 mg:** Bot. 100s, 1000s. **500 mg:** Bot. 100s, UD 100s. *Rx.*
Use: Anti-infective, tetracycline.

•**cyclopentamine hydrochloride.** (SIGH-kloe-PEN-teh-meen) *USP 34.*
Use: Adrenergic, vasoconstrictor.

•**cyclopenthiazide.** (SIGH-kloe-pen-THIGH-ah-zide) USAN.
Use: Antihypertensive; diuretic.

•**cyclopentolate hydrochloride.** (sigh-kloe-PEN-toe-tate) *USP 34.*
Use: Anticholinergic, ophthalmic.
See: AK-Pentolate.
 Cyclogyl.
W/Phenylephrine Hydrochloride.
See: Cyclomydril.

cyclopentolate hydrochloride. (Various Mfr.) Cyclopentolate hydrochloride 1% Soln. Bot. 2 mL, 15 mL. *Rx.*
Use: Anticholinergic, ophthalmic.

8 cyclopentyl 1,3-dipropylxanthine. (SciClone)
Use: Cystic fibrosis. [Orphan Drug]

cyclopentylpropionate.
See: Depo-Testosterone.

•**cyclophenazine hydrochloride.** (SIGH-kloe-FEH-nazz-een) USAN.
Use: Antipsychotic.

•**cyclophosphamide.** (sigh-kloe-FOSS-fuh-mide) *USP 34.*
Use: Antineoplastic, immunosuppressant; alkylating agent; nitrogen mustard.
See: Cytoxan.

cyclophosphamide. (Baxter) Cyclophosphamide (as monohydrate) 500 mg, 1 g, 2 g. Inj., Pow. for Soln. Single-dose vial. *Rx.*
Use: Alkylating agent, nitrogen mustard.

cyclophosphamide. (Roxanne) Cyclophosphamide 25 mg, 50 mg. Lactose. Tab. 100s. *Rx.*
Use: Alkylating agent, nitrogen mustard.

cycloplegic mydriatics.
See: Atropine Sulfate.
 Tropicamide.

•**cyclopropane.** (sigh-kloe-PRO-pane) *USP 34.*
Use: Anesthetic, general.

•**cycloserine.** (sigh-kloe-SER-een) *USP 34.*
Tall Man: cycloSERINE
Use: Antituberculosis agent.
See: Seromycin Pulvules.

l-cycloserine.
Use: Treat Gaucher disease. [Orphan Drug]

Cycloset. (Santarus) Bromocriptine mesylate 0.8 mg. Lactose. Tab. Unit of use. 200s, 600s. *Rx.*
Use: Antiparkinson agent.

cyclosporin A.
Use: Immunosuppressant.
See: Cyclosporine.

•**cyclosporine.** (SIGH-kloe-spore-EEN) *USP 34. Formerly Cyclosporin A.*
Tall Man: cycloSPORINE
Use: Immunosuppressant.
See: Gengraf.
  Neoral.
  Sandimmune.

cyclosporine. (Apotex) Cyclosporine 100 mg. Alcohol. Cap. UD 30s. *Rx.*
Use: Immunologic agent, immunosuppressive.

cyclosporine. (Ivax) Cyclosporine 50 mg. Sorbitol. Soft. Gel. Cap. UD 30s. *Rx.*
Use: Immunologic agent.

cyclosporine. (Pliva) Cyclosporine 100 mg/mL. Oral Soln. Bot. 50 mL. *Rx.*
Use: Immunosuppressant.

cyclosporine. (Various Mfr.) Cyclosporine 25 mg, 100 mg, castor oil, sorbitol, alcohol. Soft gelatin Cap. UD 30s. *Rx.*
Use: Immunosuppressant.

cyclosporine injection. (Bedford Labs) Cyclosporine 50 mg/mL. Inj. Single-use vials. 5 mL. *Rx.*
Use: Immunosuppressant.

cyclosporine ophthalmic.
Use: Severe keratoconjunctivitis sicca; graft rejection following keratoplasty. [Orphan Drug]

cyclosporine ophthalmic emulsion.
Use: Immunologic agent.
See: Restasis.

cyclosporine 2% ophthalmic ointment. (Allergan)
Use: Treatment of graft rejection after keratoplasty and corneal melting syndromes. [Orphan Drug]

•**cyclothiazide.** (SIGH-kloe-thigh-AZZ-ide) USAN.
Use: Antihypertensive; diuretic.

Cycofed. (Cypress) Codeine phosphate 20 mg, pseudoephedrine hydrochloride 60 mg per 5 mL. Spearmint flavor. Syr. Bot. 473 mL. *c-III.*
Use: Upper respiratory combination, antitussive, decongestant.

Cycofed Pediatric. (Cypress) Codeine phosphate 10 mg, pseudoephedrine hydrochloride 30 mg, guaifenesin

100 mg/5 mL, alcohol 6%. Syrup. Bot. 480 mL. *c-v.*
Use: Antitussive, decongestant, expectorant.

Cydec Oral. (Cypress) Pseudoephedrine hydrochloride 25 mg, carbinoxamine maleate 2 mg/mL, raspberry flavor. Drops. Bot. 30 mL. *Rx.*
Use: Upper respiratory combination, decongestant, antihistamine.

Cydonol Massage Lotion. (Gordon Laboratories) Isopropyl alcohol 14%, methyl salicylate, benzalkonium chloride. Lot. Bot. 4 oz, gal. *OTC.*
Use: Counterirritant.

•**cyheptamide.** (sigh-HEP-tah-mid) USAN.
Use: Anticonvulsant.

Cyklokapron. (Pfizer) Tranexamic acid. Inj. 100 mg/mL. Amp. 10 mL. *Rx.*
Use: Hemostatic.

Cylex Sugar Free. (Pharmakon) Benzocaine 15 mg, cetylpyridinium chloride 5 mg, sorbitol. Loz. Pkg. 12s. *OTC.*
Use: Antiseptic; analgesic, topical.

Cylex Throat. (Pharmakon) Benzocaine 15 mg, cetylpyridinium chloride 5 mg, sorbitol. Loz. Pkg. 12s. *OTC.*
Use: Antiseptic; analgesic, topical.

Cymbalta. (Eli Lilly) Duloxetine 20 mg, 30 mg, 60 mg. Sucrose, sugar spheres. Enteric-coated pellets. DR Cap. 30s (except 20 mg), 60s (20 mg only), 90s (except 20 mg), 1,000s (except 20 mg), UD 30s (60 mg only), UD 100s (except 20 mg). *Rx.*
Use: Antidepressant.

Cynobal. (Arcum) Cyanocobalamin 10 mcg, 1000 mcg/mL. Inj. Vial 10 mL (1000 mcg only), 30 mL. *Rx.*
Use: Vitamin supplement.

•**cypenamine hydrochloride.** (sigh-PEN-ah-meen) USAN.
Use: Antidepressant.

•**cyprazepam.** (sigh-PRAY-zeh-pam) USAN.
Use: Hypnotic; sedative.

•**cyproheptadine.** (sip-row-HEP-tuh-deen) USAN.
Use: Antihistamine, nonselective piperidine; antipruritic.

cyproheptadine. (Various Mfr.) Cyproheptadine. **Tab.:** 4 mg. Bot. 100s, 1,000s, UD 100s. **Syr.:** 2 mg/5 mL. May contain alcohol. Bot. 473 mL. *Rx.*
Use: Antihistamine, nonselective piperidine; antipruritic.

•**cyprolidol hydrochloride.** (sigh-PRO-lih-dahl) USAN.
Use: Antidepressant.

•**cyproterone acetate.** (sigh-PRO-ter-ohn) USAN.
Use: Antiandrogen.

•**cyproximide.** (sigh-PROX-ih-MIDE) USAN.
Use: Antidepressant; antipsychotic.

Cyren A.
See: Diethylstilbestrol.

Cyronine. (Major) Liothyronine sodium 25 mcg. Tab. Bot. 100s. *Rx.*
Use: Hormone, thyroid.

Cystadane. (Rare Disease Therapeutics) Betaine anhydrous 1 g/1.7 mL. Pow. for Inj. Bot. 180 g. *Rx.*
Use: Treatment of homocystinuria.

Cystagon. (Mylan) Cysteamine bitartrate 50 mg, 150 mg. Cap. Bot. 100s, 500s. *Rx.*
Use: Urinary tract agent.

Cystamin.
See: Methenamine.

Cystamine. (Tennessee Pharmaceutic) Methenamine 2 g, phenyl salicylate 0.5 g, phenazopyridine hydrochloride 10 mg, benzoic acid ⅛ g, hyoscyamine sulfate g, atropine sulfate g. SC Tab. Bot. 100s, 1000s. *Rx.*
Use: Anti-infective, urinary.

•**cysteamine.** (sis-TEE-ah-MEEN) USAN.
Use: Antiurolithic, cystine calculi; nephropathic cystinosis. [Orphan Drug]

•**cysteamine hydrochloride.** (sis-TEE-ah-MEEN) USAN.
Use: Antiurolithic, cystine calculi; nephropathic cystinosis.
See: Cystagon.

Cystex. (Numark) Methenamine 162 mg, sodium salicylate 162.5 mg, benzoic acid 32 mg. Tab. Bot. 40s, 100s. *OTC.*
Use: Anti-infective, urinary.

cystic fibrosis gene therapy. (Genzyme)
Use: Cystic fibrosis. [Orphan Drug]

cystic fibrosis TR gene therapy (recombinant adenovirus). (Gerac)
Use: Cystic fibrosis. [Orphan Drug]
See: AdGVCFTR 10.

•**cystine.** (SIS-TEEN) USAN.
Use: Amino acid replacement therapy, an additive for infants on TPN.

Cysto. (Freeport) Methenamine 40.8 mg, methylene blue 5.4 mg, phenyl salicylate 18.1 mg, atropine sulfate 0.03 mg, hyoscyamine 0.03 mg, benzoic acid 4.5 mg. Tab. Bot. 1000s. *Rx.*
Use: Anti-infective, urinary.

Cystografin. (Bracco Diagnostics) Diatrizoate meglumine 300 mg, iodine 141 mg/mL. EDTA. Inj. Bot. 100 mL in 200 mL, 300 mL fill in 400 mL. *Rx.*
Use: Radiopaque agent.

Cystografin Dilute. (Bracco Diagnostics) Diatrizoate meglumine 180 mg, iodine 85 mg/mL. EDTA. Inj. Bot. 300 mL w/or without administration sets. *Rx.*
Use: Radiopaque agent.

Cystospaz. (PolyMedica) l-hyoscyamine 0.15 mg. Tab. Bot. 100s. *Rx.*
Use: Anticholinergic; antispasmodic.

Cysview. (GE Healthcare Inc) Hexaminolevulinate hydrochloride 100 mg (equiv. to hexaminolevulinate base 85 mg). Pow. for Soln.; intravesical. Kit w/100 mg vial, diluents (50 mg vial), and 1 *Luer-Lock* catheter adapter. *Rx.*
Use: In vivo diagnostic aid.

•**cytarabine.** (SIGH-tar-ah-bean) *USP 34.*
Use: Antineoplastic; antiviral.
See: DepoCyt.
Tarabine PFS.

cytarabine. (Abraxis) Cytarabine 100 mg/mL. Inj. Soln. Single-dose vials *Rx.*
Use: Antimetabolite, pyrimidine analog.

cytarabine. (Mayne Pharma) Cytarabine 20 mg/mL, preservative free. Inj. Single and multidose vials 5 mL, bulk pkg. vial 50 mL. *Rx.*
Use: Antineoplastic; antiviral.

cytarabine. (Various Mfr.) Cytarabine 100 mg, 500 mg, 1 g, 2 g. Pow. for Inj. Vials. *Rx.*
Use: Antineoplastic; antiviral.

•**cytarabine hydrochloride.** (SITE-ah-rah-been) USAN. *Formerly Cytosine Arabinoside Hydrochloride.*
Use: Antiviral management of acute leukemias.
See: Cytosar-U.

Cyto B2. (Solace Nutrition) Riboflavin 343 mg per 1 g. Pow. 100 g. *OTC.*
Use: Water-soluble vitamin.

CytoGam. (CSL Behring) Cytomegalovirus immune globulin IV (human) 50 ± 10 mg/mL. Sucrose 5%, human albumin 1%, preservative free, solvent/detergent treated. Soln. for Inj. Vial 20 mL, 50 mL. *Rx.*
Use: Antiviral, cytomegalovirus; immune globulin.

cytomegalovirus immune globulin (human) intravenous.
Use: Immune globulin.
See: CytoGam.

cytomegalovirus immune globulin intravenous (human). (Bayer)
Use: With ganciclovir sodium for the treatment of CMV pneumonia in bone marrow transplant patients. [Orphan Drug]

Cytomel. (Monarch) Liothyronine sodium 5 mcg, 25 mcg, 50 mcg, sucrose. Tab. Bot. 100s. *Rx.*
Use: Hormone, thyroid.

cytoprotective agents.
See: Allopurinol sodium.
Amifostine.
Dexrazoxane.
Mesna.

cytosine arabinoside hydrochloride.
Cytarabine hydrochloride.

Cytosol. (Cytosol) Calcium chloride 48 mg, magnesium chloride 30 mg, potassium chloride 75 mg, sodium acetate 390 mg, sodium chloride 640 mg, sodium citrate 170 mg/100 mL. Soln. Bot. 200 mL, 500 mL. *Rx.*
Use: Irrigant.

Cytotec. (Pfizer) Misoprostol 100 mcg, 200 mcg. Tab. Bot. UD 100s, unit-of-use 60s, 100s (200 mcg only), 120s (100 mg only). *Rx.*
Use: Prostaglandins, antiulcerative.

Cytovene. (Roche) Ganciclovir 500 mg, sodium 46 mg. Inj. (as sodium). Pow, lyophilized. Vial. 10 mL. *Rx.*
Use: Antiviral.

Cytox. (MPL) Cyanocobalamin 500 mcg, vitamins B_6 20 mg, B_1 100 mg, benzyl alcohol 2% in isotonic solution of sodium chloride/mL. Inj. Vial 10 mL. *Rx.*
Use: Vitamin supplement.

Cytra-K. (Cypress) Potassium citrate monohydrate 1100 mg, citric acid monohydrate 334 mg/5 mL. Soln. Bot. 473 mL. *Rx.*
Use: Alkalinizer, systemic.

Cytra-LC. (Cypress) Potassium citrate monohydrate 550 mg, sodium citrate dihydrate 500 mg, citric acid monohydrate 334 mg/5 mL. Soln. Bot. 473 mL. *Rx.*
Use: Alkalinizer, systemic.

Cytra-3. (Cypress) Potassium citrate monohydrate 550 mg, sodium citrate dihydrate 500 mg, citric acid monohydrate 334 mg/5 mL. Syr. Bot. 480 mL. *Rx.*
Use: Alkalinizer, systemic.

Cytra-2. (Cypress) Sodium citrate dihydrate 500 mg, citric acid monohydrate 334 mg/5 mL. Soln. Bot. 16 oz. *Rx.*
Use: Alkalinizer, systemic.

D

DAA.
See: Dihydroxy Aluminum Aminoacetate.

DAB$_{389}$ IL-2. (Seragen)
Use: Cutaneous T-cell lymphoma.
[Orphan Drug]

•**dabigatran.** (da-bye-GAT-ran) USAN.
Use: Deep vein thrombosis; stroke prevention.

•**dabigatran etexilate.** (da-bye-GAT-ran ee-TEKS-i-late) USAN.
Use: Deep vein thrombosis; stroke prevention.
See: Pradaxa.

•**dabigatran etexilate mesylate.** (da-bye-GAT-ran ee-TEKS-i-late) USAN.
Use: Deep vein thrombosis; stroke prevention.

•**dabrafenib.** (da-BRAF-e-nib) USAN.
Use: Antineoplastic.

•**dabuzalgron hydrochloride.** (da-bue-ZAL-gron) USAN.
Use: Urinary agent.

•**dacarbazine.** (da-CAR-buh-zeen) USP 34.
Use: Antineoplastic.
See: DTIC-Dome.

dacarbazine. (Various Mfr.) Dacarbazine 100 mg, 200 mg. May contain mannitol. Pow. for Inj. Vials. Rx.
Use: Alkylating agent, antineoplastic.

Dacex-A. (Cypress Pharmaceutical) Phenylephrine hydrochloride 2 mg, carbinoxamine maleate 1 mg, dextromethorphan HBr 2 mg per 1 mL. Sugar and alcohol free. Saccharin, sorbitol. Cherry flavor. Oral Drops. Bot. 30 mL with calibrated dropper. Rx.
Use: Pediatric antitussive.

Dacex DM. (Cypress) Dextromethorphan HBr 25 mg, guaifenesin 175 mg, phenylephrine hydrochloride 12.5 mg per 5 mL. Alcohol and sugar free. Saccharin, sorbitol. Strawberry flavor. Syrup. 473 mL. Rx.
Use: Upper respiratory combination, antitussive and expectorant combination.

Dacex-PE. (Cypress) Dextromethorphan HBr 30 mg, guaifenesin 600 mg, phenylephrine hydrochloride 10 mg. Sugar, gluten, and dye free. ER Tab. 100s. Rx.
Use: Antitussive and expectorant combination, upper respiratory combination.

•**daclatasvir.** (dak-LAT-as-vir) USAN.
Use: Treatment of hepatitis C.

•**daclizumab.** (dac-KLYE-zue-mab) USAN.
Use: Immunosuppressant.

Dacodyl. (Major) **Tab.:** Bisacodyl 5 mg. Bot. 100s, 250s, 1000s. UD 100s. **Supp.:** Bisacodyl 10 mg. Box 12s, 100s. OTC.
Use: Laxative.

Dacogen. (Eisai) Decitabine 50 mg. Pow. for Inj., lyophilized. Single-dose vials. Rx.
Use: Antineoplastic; DNA demethylation agent.

•**dacomitinib.** (DAK-oh-MI-ti-nib) USAN.
Use: Antineoplastic.

•**dactinomycin.** (DAK-tih-no-MY-sin) USP 34.
Tall Man: DACTINomycin
Use: Antineoplastic; antibiotic.
See: Cosmegen.

dactinomycin. (Bedford Labs) Dactinomycin 500 mcg. Mannitol 20 mg. Inj., lyophilized Pow. for Soln. Single-dose vial. Rx.
Use: Antineoplastic antibiotic.

Daily Betic. (Optimum) Vitamin A (as beta carotene) 2,500 units, C 60 mg, D 200 units, E 30 units, B$_1$ 1.5 mg, B$_2$ 1.7 mg, B$_3$ 20 mg, B$_5$ 10 mg, B$_6$ 2.5 mg, B$_{12}$ 5 mcg, folic acid 200 mcg, biotin 75 mcg, lutein 250 mcg, alphalipoic acid 50 mg, Ca, Cr, I, K, Mg, Mn, Se, V, Zn. PEG. Tab. 60s. OTC.
Use: Multivitamin with minerals (except iron).

Daily Cleaner. (Bausch & Lomb) Isotonic solution with sodium Cl, sodium phosphate, tyloxapol, hydroxyethylcellulose, polyvinyl alcohol with thimerosal 0.004%, EDTA 0.2%. Soln. Bot. 45 mL. OTC.
Use: Contact lens care.

Daily Conditioning Treatment. (Blairex) Padimate O 7.5%, oxybenzone 3.5%, petrolatum. Stick 11.4 g. SPF 15. OTC.
Use: Lip protectant.

Daily Vitamins. (Rugby) Vitamins A 2500 units, D 400 units, E 15 units, C 60 mg, B$_1$ 1.2 mg, B$_2$ 1.2 mg, B$_6$ 1.05 mg, B$_{12}$ 4.5 mcg, niacinamide 13.5 mg/5 mL. Bot. 273 mL, 473 mL. OTC.
Use: Vitamin supplement.

Daily Vitamins Tablets. (Kirkman) Vitamins A 5000 units, D 400 units, C 50 mg, B$_1$ 3 mg, B$_2$ 2.5 mg, B$_6$ 1 mg, B$_{12}$ 1 mcg, niacinamide 20 mg, d-calcium pantothenate 1 mg. Tab. Bot. 100s. OTC.
Use: Vitamin supplement.

Daily Vitamins w/Iron. (Kirkman) Vitamins A 5000 units, D 400 units, B_1 2 mg, B_2 2.5 mg, B_6 1 mg, B_{12} 1 mcg, niacinamide 20 mg, d-calcium pantothenate 1 mg, iron 18 mg. Tab. Bot. 100s. *OTC.*
Use: Vitamin supplement.

Daily-Vite. (Rugby) Vitamins A 5,000 units, C 60 mg, D 400 units, E 30 units, B_1 1.5 mg, B_2 1.7 mg, B_3 20 mg, B_5 10 mg, B_6 2 mg, B_{12} 6 mcg, folic acid 400 mcg, Fe 18 mg. Dextrose, glyceryl, PEG, sucrose, soy. Tab. 100s, 1,000s. *OTC.*
Use: Multivitamin.

Daily-Vite w/Iron & Minerals. (Rugby) Iron 18 mg, vitamins A 5000 units, D 400 units, E 30 mg, B_1 1.5 mg, B_2 1.7 mg, B_3 20 mg, B_5 10 mg, B_6 2 mg, B_{12} 6 mcg, C 60 mg, folic acid 0.4 mg, Ca, Cl, Cr, Cu, I, K, Mg, Mn, Mo, P, Se, zinc 15 mg, biotin, vitamin K. Tab. Bot. 100s. *OTC.*
Use: Mineral, vitamin supplement.

Dairy Ease. (Blistex) Lactase 3300 FCC units, mannitol, sucrose. Tab. Bot. 60s, 100s. *OTC.*
Use: Digestive enzyme.

Dakin's Solution.
See: Sodium Hypochlorite Solution.

Dakin's Solution Full Strength. (Century) Sodium hypochlorite 0.5%. Soln. Bot. Pt, gal. *OTC.*
Use: Anti-infective, topical.

Dakin's Solution Half Strength. (Century) Sodium hypochlorite 0.25%. Soln. Bot. Pt. *OTC.*
Use: Anti-infective, topical.

Dalalone. (Forest) Dexamethasone sodium phosphate 4 mg/mL. Parabens, sodium bisulfite. Vial 5 mL. *Rx.*
Use: Corticosteroid.

d-ala-peptide t.
Use: Antiviral.

•**dalbavancin.** (dal-ba-VAN-sin) USAN.
Use: Investigational antibiotic.

•**daledalin tosylate.** (dah-LEH-dah-lin TAH-sill-ate) USAN.
Use: Antidepressant.

•**dalfampridine.** (dal-FAM-pri-deen) USAN.
Use: Potassium channel blocker.
See: Ampyra.

•**dalfopristin.** (dal-FOE-priss-tin) USAN.
Use: Anti-infective.
W/Quinupristin.
See: Synercid.

Daliresp. (Forest Pharmaceuticals) Roflumilast 500 mcg. Lactose. Tab. 30s, 90s. *Rx.*

Use: Selective phosphodiesterase 4 inhibitor.

Dallergy. (Laser) **Oral Drops:** Phenylephrine hydrochloride 2 mg, chlorpheniramine maleate 1 mg per 1 mL. Saccharin, sorbitol. Alcohol free and sugar free. Peach flavor. 30 mL with dropper. **Syrup:** Chlorpheniramine maleate 2 mg, phenylephrine hydrochloride 8 mg, methscopolamine nitrate 0.75 mg/5 mL. Bot. 473 mL. **Tab.:** Chlorpheniramine maleate 4 mg, phenylephrine hydrochloride 10 mg, methscopolamine nitrate 1.25 mg. Bot. 100s. *Rx.*
Use: Upper respiratory combination, anticholinergic, antihistamine, decongestant combination.

Dallergy. (Palmetto Pharmaceuticals) Chlorpheniramine maleate 2 mg, methscopolamine nitrate 1.25 mg, phenylephrine hydrochloride 10 mg. Mannitol, saccharin, sugar. Grape flavor. Chew. Tab. 100s. *Rx.*
Use: Upper respiratory combination; decongestant, antihistamine, and anticholinergic combination.

Dallergy-D. (Laser) Chlorpheniramine maleate 2 mg, phenylephrine hydrochloride 5 mg/5 mL. Bot. 118 mL. *OTC.*
Use: Antihistamine, decongestant.

Dallergy DM. (Laser) Dextromethorphan HBr 15 mg, brompheniramine maleate 3 mg, pseudoephedrine hydrochloride 30 mg per 5 mL. Alcohol and sugar free. Saccharin, sorbitol. Berry vanilla flavor. Syrup. 30 mL, 473 mL. *Rx.*
Use: Upper respiratory combination, antitussive combination.

Dallergy-Jr. (Laser) **ER Cap.:** Phenylephrine hydrochloride 20 mg, chlorpheniramine maleate 4 mg. Sucrose. Bot. 100s. **Susp.:** Phenylephrine tannate 20 mg, chlorpheniramine tannate 4 mg per 5 mL. Alcohol free. Magnasweet, methylparaben, saccharin, sucrose. Peaches and cream flavor. 473 mL. *Rx.*
Use: Upper respiratory combination, antihistamine, decongestant.

Dallergy PE. (Palmetto Pharmaceuticals) Chlorpheniramine maleate 8 mg, methscopolamine nitrate 2.5 mg, phenylephrine hydrochloride 20 mg. ER cap. 100s. *Rx.*
Use: Upper respiratory combination; decongestant, antihistamine, and anticholinergic combination.

•**dalotuzumab.** (DAL-oh-TOOZ-oo-mab) USAN.
Use: Antineoplastic.

d'Alpha E 1000 Softgels. (Naturally) Vitamin E (as d-alpha tocopherol) 1000 IU. Cap. 30s, 60s. *OTC.*
Use: Vitamin supplement.

•**dalteparin sodium.** (dal-TEH-puh-rin) USAN.
Use: Anticoagulant; antithrombotic; low molecular weight heparin.
See: Fragmin.

•**daltroban.** (DAL-troe-ban) USAN.
Use: Platelet aggregation inhibitor; immunosuppressant.

•**dalvastatin.** (DAL-vah-STAT-in) USAN.
Use: Antihyperlipidemic.

Damacet-P. (Mason) Hydrocodone bitartrate 5 mg, acetaminophen 500 mg. Tab. Bot. 100s, 500s. *c-III.*
Use: Analgesic combination; narcotic.

Dambose.
See: Inositol.

Danatrol. (Sanofi-Synthelabo) Danazol. Cap. *Rx.*
Use: Gonadotropin inhibitor.

•**danazol.** (DAN-uh-ZOLE) *USP 34.*
Use: Anterior pituitary suppressant, sex hormone.

danazol. (Various Mfr.) Danazol 50 mg, 100 mg, 200 mg. Cap. Bot. 60s (200 mg only), 100s, 500s (200 mg only). *Rx.*
Use: Anterior pituitary suppressant, sex hormone.

Dandruff Shampoo. (Walgreen) Zinc pyrithione 2 g/100 mL. Bot. 11 oz. Tube 7 oz. *OTC.*
Use: Antiseborrheic.

•**danegaptide.** (dan-e-GAP-tide) USAN.
Use: Cardiovascular agent.

•**daniplestim.** (dan-ih-PLEH-stim) USAN.
Use: Antineutropenic; hematopoietic stimulant; treatment of chemotherapy-induced bone marrow suppression.

Danogar Tablets. (Sanofi-Synthelabo) Danazol. *Rx.*
Use: Gonadotropin inhibitor.

Danol Capsules. (Sanofi-Synthelabo) Danazol. *Rx.*
Use: Gonadotropin inhibitor.

•**danoprevir.** (dan-OH-pre-vir) USAN.
Use: Treatment of hepatitis C.

•**danoprevir sodium.** (dan-OH-pre-vir) USAN.
Use: Treatment of hepatitis C.

Dantrium. (Procter & Gamble) Dantrolene sodium. Cap. **25 mg:** Bot. 100s, 500s, UD 100s; **50 mg:** Bot. 100s; **100 mg:** Bot. 100s, UD 100s. *Rx.*
Use: Muscle relaxant.

Dantrium IV. (Procter & Gamble) Dantrolene sodium 20 mg. Vial. 70 mL. *Rx.*
Use: Muscle relaxant.

•**dantrolene.** (dan-troe-LEEN) USAN.
Use: Muscle relaxant.

•**dantrolene sodium.** (dan-troe-LEEN) USAN.
Use: Muscle relaxant.
See: Dantrium.
Revonto.

dantrolene sodium. (Actavis Totowa) Dantrolene sodium 25 mg, 50 mg, 100 mg. Lactose. Cap. 100s, 500s, UD 100s. *Rx.*
Use: Direct acting skeletal muscle relaxants.

Dapa Extra Strength Tablets. (Ferndale) Acetaminophen 500 mg. Bot. 50s, 100s, 1000s, UD 100s. *OTC.*
Use: Analgesic.

•**dapagliflozin.** (dap-A-gli-FLOE-zin) USAN.
Use: Investigational antidiabetic agent.

Dapco. (Schlicksup) Salicylamide 300 mg, butabarbital 15 mg. Tab. Bot. 100s, 1000s. *c-III.*
Use: Analgesic; hypnotic; sedative.

•**dapiclermin.** (DA-pi-kler-min) USAN.
Use: Dietary aid.

•**dapiprazole hydrochloride.** (DAP-ih-PRAY-zole) USAN.
Use: Alpha-adrenergic blocker; anti-glaucoma agent; neuroleptic; psycho-therapeutic agent.

•**dapoxetine hydrochloride.** (dap-OX-eh-teen) USAN.
Use: Antidepressant.

•**dapsone.** (DAP-sone) *USP 34.* Formerly Diaminodiphenylsulfone.
Use: Leprostatic; topical anti-infective.
See: Aczone.

dapsone. (Jacobus) Dapsone 25 mg, 100 mg. Tab. Bot. 100s. *Rx.*
Use: Leprostatic.

Daptacel. (Aventis Pasteur) Diphtheria toxoid 15 Lf, tetanus toxoid 5 Lf, pertussis toxoid 10 mcg, hemagglutinin 5 mcg, pertactin 3 mcg, fimbriae types 2 and 3 5 mcg/0.5 mL. Formaldehyde, phenoxyethanol. Inj. Single-dose vials. *Rx.*
Use: Immunization.

•**daptomycin.** (DAP-toe-MY-sin) USAN.
Tall Man: DAPTOmycin
Use: Anti-infective.
See: Cubicin.

Daragen. (Galderma) Collagen polypeptide, benzalkonium Cl in a mild amphoteric base. Shampoo. Bot. 8 oz. *OTC.*
Use: Dermatologic.

•**darapladib.** (dar-AP-la-dib) USAN.
Use: Lp-PLA2 inhibitor.

Daraprim. (Amedra Pharmaceuticals) Pyrimethamine 25 mg. Lactose. Tab. Bot. 100s. *Rx.*
Use: Antimalarial.

Dara Soapless Shampoo. (Galderma) Purified water, potassium coco hydrolyzed protein, sulfated castor oil, pentasodium triphosphate, sodium benzoate, sodium lauryl sulfate, fragrance. Shampoo. Bot. 8 oz, 16 oz. *OTC.*
Use: Dermatologic, scalp.

•**darbepoetin alfa.** (DAR-be-POE-e-tin) USAN.
Use: Hematopoietic agent, recombinant human erythropoietin.
See: Aranesp.

•**darbufelone mesylate.** (DAR-byoo-feh-lone) USAN.
Use: Anti-inflammatory; antiarthritic.

Darco G-60. (AstraZeneca) Activated carbon from lignite.
Use: Purifier.

•**darglitazone sodium.** (dahr-GLIH-tah-zone) USAN.
Use: Oral hypoglycemic.

•**darifenacin.** (dare-ee-FEN-a-sin) USAN.
Use: Treatment of overactive bladder.

•**darifenacin hydrobromide.** (dar-ih-FEN-ah-sin)
Use: Treatment of overactive bladder.
See: Enablex.

•**darodipine.** (DA-row-dih-PEEN) USAN.
Use: Antihypertensive; bronchodilator; vasodilator.

•**darunavir.** (dar-UE-na-vir) USAN.
Use: Antiretroviral.

darunavir ethanolate.
Use: Antiretroviral.
See: Prezista.

Darvon Compound 65 Pulvules. (Eli Lilly) Propoxyphene hydrochloride 65 mg, aspirin 389 mg, caffeine 32.4 mg. Pulv. Bot. 100s, *Rx Pak* 500s. *c-IV.*
Use: Analgesic combination; narcotic.

•**dasantafil.** (da-SAN-ta-fil) USAN.
Use: Erectile dysfunction.

•**dasatinib.** (da-SA-ti-nib) USAN.
Use: Protein-tyrosine kinase inhibitor; treatment of leukemia.
See: Sprycel.

Da-Sed. (Sheryl) Butabarbital 0.5 g. Tab. Bot. 100s. *c-III.*
Use: Hypnotic; sedative.

Dasin. (GlaxoSmithKline) Ipecac 3 mg, acetylsalicylic acid 130 mg, camphor 15 mg, caffeine 8 mg, atropine sulfate 0.13 mg. Cap. Bot. 100s, 500s. *Rx.*
Use: Analgesic; anticholinergic; antispasmodic.

DaTscan. (GE Healthcare) Ioflupane I 123 74 MBq (2 mCi) per mL at calibration (each mL contains ioflupane 0.07 to 0.13 mcg, acetic acid 5.7 mg, sodium acetate 7.8 mg, and ethanol 0.05 mL [5%]). Preservative free. Inj., Soln. Single-use vial. 2.5 mL. *c-II.*
Use: In vivo diagnostic aid.

daturine hydrobromide.
See: Hyoscyamine Salts.

daunorubicin citrate liposomal.
Use: Antibiotic.
See: DaunoXome.

daunorubicin citrate liposome.
Use: Treatment of advanced HIV-associated Kaposi sarcoma. [Orphan Drug]
See: DaunoXome.

•**daunorubicin hydrochloride.** (DAW-no-RUE-bih-sin) *USP 34.*
Tall Man: DAUNOrubicin
Use: Antineoplastic.
See: Cerubidine

daunorubicin hydrochloride. (Various Mfr.) Daunorubicin hydrochloride 20 mg, 50 mg, mannitol 100 mg (20 mg), 250 mg (50 mg). Pow. for Inj., lyophilized. Single-dose vial 10 mL (20 mg only), 20 mL (50 mg only). *Rx.*
Use: Antineoplastic.

daunorubicin hydrochloride for injection. (Various Mfr.) Daunorubicin hydrochloride for Injection 5 mg/mL (equivalent to 5.34 mg daunorubicin hydrochloride), preservative free. Single-use vial. 4 mL, 10 mL. *Rx.*
Use: Antibiotic.

DaunoXome. (Gilead Sciences) Daunorubicin citrate liposomal 2 mg/mL (equivalent to daunorubicin base 50 mg). Inj. Single-use vials and single-unit packs. *Rx.*
Use: Antibiotic; treatment of advanced HIV-associated Kaposi sarcoma.

•**davalintide.** (DA-va-LIN-tide) USAN.
Use: Treatment of obesity.

•**davalintide acetate.** (DA-va-LIN-tide) USAN.
Use: Treatment of obesity.

Davosil. (Colgate Oral) Silicon carbide in glycerin base. Jar 8 oz, 10 oz. *OTC.*
Use: Agent for oral hygiene.

•**davunetide.** (dav-u-NE-tide) USAN.
Use: Alzheimer disease.

Dayalets + Iron. (Abbott) Vitamins B_1 1.5 mg, B_2 1.7 mg, B_6 2 mg, B_{12} 6 mcg, C 60 mg, A 5000 units, D 400 units, E 30 units, iron 18 mg, folic acid 0.4 mg, niacinamide 20 mg. Filmtab. Bot. 100s.

OTC.
Use: Mineral, vitamin supplement.

Daycare. (Procter & Gamble) Pseudo-ephedrine hydrochloride 10 mg, dex-tromethorphan HBr 3.3 mg, guaifenesin 33.3 mg, acetaminophen 108 mg. Alcohol 10%, saccharin. Expectorant Liq. Bot. 180 mL, 300 mL. *OTC.*
Use: Analgesic, antitussive, decongestant, expectorant.

Dayhist-1. (Major) Clemastine fumarate 1.34 mg (equivalent to clemastine 1 mg). Lactose. Tab. Pkg. 8s. *OTC.*
Use: Antihistamine, nonselective ethanolamine.

Daypro. (Searle) Oxaprozin 600 mg. Film-coated. Capl. Bot. 100s, 500s, UD 100s. *Rx.*
Use: Nonsteroidal anti-inflammatory agent.

Daypro ALTA. (Pharmacia) Oxaprozin potassium 678 mg (equivalent to 600 mg oxaprozin). Film-coated. Tab. Bot. 100s, 500s, UD 100s. *Rx.*
Use: Nonsteroidal anti-inflammatory agent.

DayQuil.
See: Vicks DayQuil.

Day Tab. (Towne) Vitamins A 5000 units, D 400 units, B_1 15 mg, B_2 10 mg, B_6 5 mg, B_{12} 5 mcg, folic acid 400 mcg, pantothenic acid 10 mg, zinc 15 mg, copper 2 mg, C 600 mg, niacinamide 20 mg. Tab. Bot. 100s, 200s. *OTC.*
Use: Mineral, vitamin supplement.

Day Tab Essential. (Towne) Vitamins A 5000 units, D 400 units, E 15 units, C 60 mg, folic acid 0.4 mg, B_1 1.5 mg, B_2 1.7 mg, B_6 2 mg, B_{12} 6 mcg, niacin 20 mg. Tab. Bot. 200s. *OTC.*
Use: Vitamin supplement.

Day Tab Plus Iron. (Towne) Iron 18 mg, vitamins A 5000 units, D 400 units, B_1 1.5 mg, B_2 1.7 mg, B_6 2 mg, B_{12} 6 mcg, pantothenic acid 10 mg, folic acid 0.1 mg, niacinamide 20 mg, C 60 mg. Tab. Bot. 100s. *OTC.*
Use: Mineral, vitamin supplement.

Day Tabs, New. (Towne) Vitamins A 5000 units, E 15 units, D 400 units, C 60 mg, folic acid 0.4 mg, B_1 1.5 mg, B_2 1.7 mg, B_6 20 mg, B_{12} 6 mcg, niacin 20 mg. Tab. Bot. 100s, 250s. *OTC.*
Use: Vitamin supplement.

Day Tabs Plus Iron, New. (Towne) Vitamins A 5000 units, E 15 units, D 400 units, C 60 mg, folic acid 0.4 mg, B_1 1.5 mg, B_2 1.7 mg, B_6 20 mg, B_{12} 6 mcg, niacin 20 mg, iron 18 mcg. Tab. Bot. 250s. *OTC.*
Use: Mineral, vitamin supplement.

Day Tab Stress Complex. (Towne) Vitamins A 5000 units, C 600 mg, B_1 15 mg, B_2 10 mg, B_6 5 mg, B_{12} 6 mcg, niacin 100 mg, D 400 units, E 30 units, folic acid 400 mcg, pantothenic acid 20 mg, iron 18 mg, zinc 15 mg, copper 2 mg. Tab. Bot. 60s. *OTC.*
Use: Mineral, vitamin supplement.

Day Tab with Iron. (Towne) Vitamins A 5000 units, D 400 units, E 15 units, C 60 mg, folic acid 1.5 mg, B_1 15 mg, B_2 1.7 mg, B_6 2 mg, B_{12} 6 mcg, niacin 20 mg, iron 18 mg. Tab. Bot. 200s. *Rx.*
Use: Mineral, vitamin supplement.

Daytime Sinus Relief Non-Drowsy Maximum Strength. (Akyma) Pseudo-ephedrine hydrochloride 30 mg, acetaminophen 500 mg. Tab. 24s. *OTC.*
Use: Decongestant and analgesic.

Dayto-Anase. (Dayton) Bromelains 50,000 units (protease activity). Tab. Bot. 60s. *OTC.*
Use: Enzyme.

Dayto Himbin. (Dayton) Yohimbine 5.4 mg. Tab. Bot. 60s. *Rx.*
Use: Alpha-adrenergic blocker.

Daytrana. (Shire) Methylphenidate hydrochloride 10 mg, 15 mg, 20 mg, 30 mg. Transdermal Patch. 10s, 30s. *c-II.*
Use: Central nervous system stimulant.

•**dazadrol maleate.** (DAY-zah-drole) USAN.
Use: Antidepressant.

•**dazepinil hydrochloride.** (dahz-EH-pih-NILL) USAN.
Use: Antidepressant.

•**dazmegrel.** (DAZE-meh-grell) USAN.
Use: Inhibitor (thromboxane synthetase).

•**dazopride fumarate.** (DAY-zoe-PRIDE) USAN.
Use: Peristaltic stimulant.

•**dazoxiben hydrochloride.** (DAZE-OX-ih-ben) USAN.
Use: Antithrombotic.

Dbed. Dibenzylethylenediamine dipenicillin G.
Use: Anti-infective; penicillin.

DB Electrode Paste. (Day-Baldwin) Tube 5%.

DCA.
See: Desoxycorticosterone Acetate.

DCF.
Use: Anti-infective.
See: Nipent.

DCP. (Towne) Calcium 180 mg, phosphorus 105 mg, vitamins D 66.7 units. Tab. Bot. 100s. *OTC.*
Use: Mineral, vitamin supplement.

DC Softgels. (Ivax) Docusate calcium 240 mg. Softgel Cap. Bot. 100s, 500s. *OTC.*
Use: Laxative.

DC 240. (Ivax) Docusate calcium 240 mg. Cap. Bot. 100s, 500s. *OTC.*
Use: Laxative.

DDAVP. (Sanofi-Aventis) Desmopressin acetate. **Tab.:** 0.1 mg, 0.2 mg, lactose. 100s. **Spray Soln., Intranasal:** 0.1 mg/mL. 5 mL (50 sprays of 10 mcg). Rhinal tube delivery system. 2.5 mL w/2 applicator tubes. **Inj.:** 4 mcg/mL. Single-dose amp. 1 mL, multidose vial 10 mL. *Rx.*
Use: Posterior pituitary hormone.

ddI. Didanosine.
Use: Antiviral.

Ddrops. (J.R. Carlson Labs) Vitamin D_3 (cholecalciferol) 1,000 units per 0.03 mL, 2,000 units per 0.03 mL. Gluten free, preservative free, and sugar free. Drops. 11 mL. *OTC.*
Use: Fat-soluble vitamin.

DDS.
See: Dapsone.

DDT.
See: Chlorophenothane.

deacetyllanatoside C.
See: Deslanoside.

deadly nightshade leaf.
See: Belladonna Leaf.

1-deamino-8-d-arginine vasopressin. Desmopressin acetate.
Use: Hormone.
See: Concentraid.
DDAVP.

deba.
See: Barbital.

Debacterol. (Epien Medical) Sulfuric acid 30%, sulfonated phenolics 50%. Liq. 1.5 mL *Rx.*
Use: Mouth and throat product.

•**debrisoquin sulfate.** (deb-RICE-oh-kwin) USAN.
Use: Antihypertensive.

Debrox. (GlaxoSmithKline) Carbamide peroxide 6.5%, glycerin, propylene glycol, sodium stannate. Drops. 30 mL with dropper. *OTC.*
Use: Otic preparation.

Deca-Bon. (Barrows) Vitamins A 3000 units, D 400 units, C 60 mg, B_1 1 mg, B_2 1.2 mg, B_6 1 mg, B_{12} 1 mcg, niacinamide 8 mg, panthenol 3 mg, biotin 30 mcg/0.6 mL. Drops. Bot. 50 mL. *OTC.*
Use: Vitamin supplement.

Decaderm. (Merck & Co.) Dexamethasone 0.1% w/isopropyl myristate gel, wood alcohols, refined lanolin alcohol, microcrystalline wax, anhydrous citric acid, anhydrous sodium phosphate dibasic. Tube 30 g. *Rx.*
Use: Corticosteroid.

Decagen. (Ivax) Iron 18 mg, vitamins A 5000 units, D 400 units, E 30 units, B_1 1.7 mg, B_2 2 mg, B_3 20 mg, B_5 10 mg, B_6 3 mg, B_{12} 6 mcg, C 60 mg, folic acid 0.4 mg, Ca, Cl, Cr, Cu, B, I, K, Mg, Mn, Mo, Ni, P, Se, Si, Sn, V, Zn 15 mg, vitamin K, biotin 30 mcg. Tab. Bot. 130s. *OTC.*
Use: Mineral, vitamin supplement.

Decaject. (Merz) Dexamethasone sodium phosphate 4 mg/mL. Vial 5 mL, 10 mL. *Rx.*
Use: Corticosteroid.

Decalix. (Pharmed) Dexamethasone 0.5 mg/5 mL. Bot. 100 mL. *Rx.*
Use: Corticosteroid.

Decameth. (Foy Laboratories) Dexamethasone sodium phosphate injection 4 mg/5 mL Inj. Vial. *Rx.*
Use: Corticosteroid.

Decameth L.A. (Foy Laboratories) Dexamethasone sodium phosphate injection 8 mg/mL. Inj. Vial 5 mL. *Rx.*
Use: Corticosteroid.

Decameth Tablets. (Foy Laboratories) Dexamethasone 0.75 mg. Bot. 1000s. *Rx.*
Use: Corticosteroid.

Decapryn. (Hoechst) Doxylamine succinate 12.5 mg. Tab. Bot. 100s. *OTC.*
Use: Antihistamine.

Decasone Injection. (Forest) Dexamethasone sodium phosphate equivalent to dexamethasone phosphate 4 mg/mL. Vial 5 mL. *Rx.*
Use: Corticosteroid.

Decavac. (Aventis Pasteur) Diphtheria 2 Lf units and tetanus 5 Lf units per 0.5 mL dose. Preservative free. Inj. 0.5 mL *Luer-Lok* syringe (with not more than 0.28 mg of aluminum and trace thimerosal [up to 0.3 mcg mercury/dose]). *Rx.*
Use: Agent for active immunization.

decavitamin. (Various Mfr.) Vitamins A 4000 units, D 400 units, C 70 mg, calcium pantothenate 10 mg, B_1 2 mg, B_2 2 mg, B_6 2 mg, B_{12} 5 mcg, folic acid 100 mcg, nicotinamide 20 mg. Cap. or Tab. *OTC.*
Use: Vitamin supplement.

De-Chlor HD. (Cypress) Hydrocodone bitartrate 2.5 mg, chlorpheniramine maleate 4 mg, phenylephrine hydrochloride 10 mg per 5 mL. Alcohol and sugar free. Saccharin, sorbitol. Cherry flavor. Liq. 473 mL. *c-III.*

Use: Upper respiratory combination, antitussive combination.

Decholin. (Bayer Consumer Care) Dehydrocholic acid 250 mg. Tab. Bot. 100s, 500s. *OTC.*
Use: Hydrocholeretic.

Decicain. Tetracaine hydrochloride.

•**decitabine.** (deh-SIGH-tah-BEAN) USAN.
Use: Antineoplastic; DNA demethylation agent.
See: Dacogen.

declaben. (DEH-klah-BEN) *Formerly Lodelaben.*
Use: Antiarthritic; emphysema therapy adjunct.

Declomycin. (ESP Pharma) Demeclocycline hydrochloride 150 mg, 300 mg. Tab. Bot. 100s (150 mg only), 48s (300 mg only). *Rx.*
Use: Anti-infective; tetracycline.

Decodult. (Wesley Pharmacal) Phenylephrine hydrochloride 5 mg, chlorpheniramine maleate 2 mg, acetaminophen 300 mg. Tab. Bot. 1000s. *OTC.*
Use: Upper respiratory combination, decongestant, antihistamine, analgesic.

Decohistine DH. (Morton Grove) Pseudoephedrine hydrochloride 30 mg, chlorpheniramine maleate 2 mg, codeine phosphate 10 mg per 5 mL. Alcohol 5.8%, sugar, menthol, parabens, sorbitol, grape/honey flavor. Liq. Bot. 118 mL, 473 mL, 3.8 L. *c-v.*
Use: Upper respiratory combination, antihistamine, antitussive, decongestant.

Decolate. (Wesley) Phenylephrine hydrochloride 5 mg, chlorpheniramine maleate 4 mg, guaifenesin 100 mg. Tab. Bot. 1000s. *Rx.*
Use: Upper respiratory combination, decongestant, antihistamine, expectorant.

Deconamine. (Kenwood) **Syrup:** Chlorpheniramine maleate 2 mg, pseudoephedrine hydrochloride (as d-pseudoephedrine) 30 mg/5 mL. Sorbitol, sucrose, grape flavor. Alcohol and dye free. Bot. 473 mL. **Tab.:** Chlorpheniramine maleate 4 mg, pseudoephedrine hydrochloride 60 mg, lactose. Bot. 100s. *Rx.*
Use: Upper respiratory combination, antihistamine and decongestant.

Deconex. (Poly Pharmaceuticals) Guaifenesin 390 mg, phenylephrine hydrochloride 10 mg. Cap. 60s. *Rx.*
Use: Upper respiratory combination, decongestant and expectorant combination.

Deconex DM. (Poly) Dextromethorphan HBr 30 mg, guaifenesin 900 mg, phenylephrine hydrochloride 30 mg. ER Tab. 100s. *Rx.*
Use: Antitussive and expectorant combination, upper respiratory combination.

Deconex DMX. (Poly Pharmaceuticals) Dextromethorphan HBr 15 mg, guaifenesin 380 mg, phenylephrine hydrochloride 10 mg. Maltodextrin. Cap. 60s. *OTC.*
Use: Upper respiratory combination; antitussive, expectorant, decongestant.

decongestant, analgesic, antihistamine, antitussive combinations.
Use: Upper respiratory combination.

decongestant, analgesic, antihistamine combinations.
Use: Upper respiratory combination.

decongestant, analgesic, antitussive, expectorant combinations.
Use: Upper respiratory combination.

decongestant and analgesic combinations.
Use: Upper respiratory combination.

decongestant and antihistamine combinations.
Use: Upper respiratory combination.

decongestant and expectorant combinations.
Use: Upper respiratory combination.

decongestant, anticholinergic, and antihistamine combinations.
Use: Upper respiratory combination.

decongestant, anticholinergic, antihistamine, and antitussive combinations.
Use: Upper respiratory combination.

decongestant, antihistamine, and analgesic combinations.
Use: Upper respiratory combination.

decongestant, antihistamine, and antitussive combinations.
Use: Upper respiratory combination.

decongestant, antihistamine, and expectorant combinations.
Use: Upper respiratory combination.

decongestant, antihistamine, antitussive, and expectorant combinations.
Use: Upper respiratory combination.

decongestant, antitussive, and expectorant combinations.
Use: Upper respiratory combination.

Decongestant Formula Mediquell. (Parke-Davis) Dextromethorphan HBr 30 mg, pseudoephedrine hydrochloride 60 mg. Square.
Use: Antitussive, decongestant.

decongestant, nasal.
See: Nasal Decongestants.

Deconomed SR. (Iopharm) Chlorpheniramine maleate 8 mg, pseudoephedrine
hydrochloride 120 mg. Sucrose, parabens. ER Cap. Bot. 100s, 500s. *Rx.*
Use: Upper respiratory combination, antihistamine and decongestant.

Deconsal CT. (Cornerstone) Phenylephrine hydrochloride 10 mg, pyrilamine maleate 16 mg. Saccharin,
sugar. Dye free. Grape flavor. Chew.
Tab. 100s. *Rx.*
Use: Upper respiratory combination, decongestant and antihistamine.

Deconsal II. (Cornerstone) Phenylephrine hydrochloride 25 mg, guaifenesin 275 mg. ER Tab. Bot. 100s. *Rx.*
Use: Upper respiratory combination, decongestant and expectorant combination.

•**dectaflur.** (DECK-tah-flure) USAN.
Use: Dental caries agent.

Decubitex. (I.C.P. Pharmaceuticals)
Oint.: Biebrich scarlet red sulfonated
0.1%, balsam Peru, castor oil, zinc oxide, starch, sodium propionate, parabens. Jar 15 g, 60 g, 120 g, lb. **Pow.:**
Biebrich scarlet red sulfonated 0.1%,
starch, zinc oxide, sodium propionate,
parabens. Bot. 30 g, UD 1 g. *OTC.*
Use: Antipruritic; dermatologic, wound
therapy; emollient.

Decylenes. (Rugby) Undecylenic acid,
zinc undecylenate. Oint. Tube 30 g,
lb. *OTC.*
Use: Antifungal, topical.

Deep-Down Pain Relief Rub. (Glaxo-
SmithKline) Methyl salicylate 15%,
menthol 5%, camphor 0.5%. Tube
1.25 oz, 3 oz. *OTC.*
Use: Analgesic, topical.

Deep Strength Musterole. (Schering-
Plough) Methyl salicylate 30%, menthol 3%, methyl nicotinate 0.5%. Tube
1.25 oz, 3 oz. *OTC.*
Use: Analgesic, topical.

•**deferasirox.** (de-FER-a-sir-ox) USAN.
Use: Chelating agent.
See: Exjade.

•**deferiprone.** (de-FER-ip-rone) USAN.
Use: Iron overload.

•**deferitrin.** (de-FER-i-trin) USAN.
Use: Chelating agent.

•**deferoxamine.** (DEE-fer-OX-ah-meen)
USAN.
Use: Chelating agent (iron).

•**deferoxamine hydrochloride.** (DEE-fer-
OX-ah-meen) USAN.
Use: Chelating agent for iron.

•**deferoxamine mesylate.** (DEE-fer-OX-
ah-meen) *USP 34.*

Use: Iron depleter; antidote to iron poisoning; chelating agent.
See: Desferal.

deferoxamine mesylate. (Hospira)
Deferoxamine mesylate 500 mg, 2 g.
Pow. for Inj., lyophilized. Vials. *Rx.*
Use: Detoxification agent, chelating
agent.

defibrotide. (Crinos International)
Use: Thrombotic thrombocytopenic purpura. [Orphan Drug]

Deficol. (Vangard Labs, Inc.) Bisacodyl
5 mg. Tab. Bot. 100s, 1000s. *OTC.*
Use: Laxative.

Definity. (Bristol-Myers Squibb) Octafluoropropane 6.52 mg/mL in lipid-coated
microspheres. Preservative free. Inj.
Single-use vials. 2 mL. Requires activation with a *Vialmix* (not included). *Rx.*
Use: Radiopaque agent, parenteral
agent.

•**deflazacort.** (deh-FLAZE-ah-cart) USAN.
Use: Anti-inflammatory.

•**degarelix.** (DEG-a-REL-ix) USAN.
Use: Antineoplastic.

•**degarelix acetate.** (DEG-a-REL-ix)
USAN.
Use: Treatment of prostate cancer.
See: Firmagon.

Dehistine. (Cypress) Phenylephrine
hydrochloride 10 mg, chlorpheniramine
maleate 2 mg, methscopolamine nitrate 1.25 mg/5 mL. Root beer flavor, alcohol free, sugar free. Syrup. Bot.
473 mL. *Rx.*
Use: Upper respiratory combination, decongestant, antihistamine, anticholinergic.

Dehydrex. (Holles)
Use: Recurrent corneal erosion.
[Orphan Drug]

•**dehydrocholate sodium injection.**
USP 34.
Use: Relief of liver congestion; diagno-
sis of cardiac failure.
See: Decholin Sodium.

7-dehydrocholesterol, activated.
(Various Mfr.) Vitamin D-3.
Use: Vitamin supplement.
See: Cholecalciferol.

•**dehydrocholic acid.** (dee-HIGH-droe-
KOLE-ik) *USP 34.*
Use: Orally, hydrocholeretic and chole-
retic.
See: Atrocholin.
Cholan-DH.
Decholin.
W/Bile, Homatropine Methylbromide,
Pepsin.
See: Biloric.

W/Desoxycholic Acid.
See: Combichole.
W/Docusate Sodium, Phenolphthalein.
See: Bolax.
dehydrocholin.
Use: Hydrocholeretic.
See: Dehydrocholic Acid.
dehydrodesoxycholic acid.
See: Cholanic Acid.
dehydroepiandrosterone. (Genelabs Technologics, Inc.)
Use: Treatment of systemic lupus erythematosus (SLE). [Orphan Drug]
dehydroepiandrosterone sulfate sodium. (Pharmadigm)
Use: Treat serious burns; accelerate re-epithelialization of donor sites in autologous skin grafting. [Orphan Drug]
DEKA. (Dayton) Dextromethorphan hydrobromide 15 mg, guaifenesin 100 mg, pseudoephedrine hydrochloride 15 mg, dexbrompheniramine maleate 0.5 mg per 5 mL. Saccharin, sucrose, parabens. Grape flavor. Liq. 120 mL. *Rx.*
Use: Antitussive and expectorant.
DEKA Pediatric. (Dayton) Pseudoephedrine hydrochloride 12.5 mg, dextromethorphan hydrobromide 4 mg, guaifenesin 40 mg, dexbrompheniramine maleate 0.5 mg per 1 mL. Alcohol free. EDTA, parabens, saccharin, sucrose. Grape flavor. Drops. 30 mL with calibrated dropper. *Rx.*
Use: Pediatric antitussive and expectorant.
Dekasol. (Seatrace) Dexamethasone phosphate 4 mg/mL. Vial 5 mL, 10 mL. *Rx.*
Use: Corticosteroid.
Dekasol L.A. (Seatrace) Dexamethasone acetate 8 mg/mL. Vial 5 mL. *Rx.*
Use: Corticosteroid.
De-Koff. (Whiteworth Towne) Terpin hydrate w/dextromethorphan. Elix. Bot. 4 oz. *OTC.*
Use: Antitussive, expectorant.
Delacort Lotion. (Mericon Industries) Hydrocortisone 0.5%. Bot. 4 oz. *OTC.*
Use: Corticosteroid, topical.
•**delafloxacin.** (DEL-a-FLOX-a-sin) USAN.
Use: Antibacterial.
•**delafloxacin meglumine.** (DEL-a-FLOX-a-sin ME-gloo-meen) USAN.
Use: Antibacterial.
•**delamanid.** (DEL-a-MAN-id) USAN.
Use: Treatment of tuberculosis.
•**delapril hydrochloride.** (DELL-ah-prill) USAN.

Use: Antihypertensive; angiotensin-converting enzyme inhibitor.
Del Aqua-10. (Del-Ray) Benzoyl peroxide 10%. 42.5 g. *Rx.*
Use: Dermatologic, acne.
Delaquin. (Schlicksup) Hydrocortisone 0.5%, iodoquin 3%. Lot. Bot. 3 oz. *Rx.*
Use: Antifungal; corticosteroid.
Delatestadiol. (Dunhall Pharmaceuticals, Inc.) Testosterone enanthate 90 mg, estradiol valerate 4 mg/mL, chlorobutanol in sesame oil. Amp. 10 mL. *Rx.*
Use: Androgen, estrogen combination.
Delatestryl. (Indevus Pharmaceuticals) Testosterone enanthate 200 mg/mL. Sesame oil, chlorobutanol 5 mg. Inj. Multidose vials. 5 mL. Single-dose syringe w/needle. 1 mL. *c-III.*
Use: Sex hormone, androgen.
•**delavirdine mesylate.** (de-la-VIR–deen) USAN.
Use: Antiretroviral, non-nucleoside reverse transcriptase inhibitor.
See: Rescriptor.
Delazinc. (Mericon) Zinc oxide 25%. Mineral oil petrolatum. Oint. 454 g. *OTC.*
Use: Skin protectant.
Delcid. (GlaxoSmithKline) Aluminum hydroxide 600 mg, magnesium hydroxide 665 mg/5 mL. Alcohol 0.3%, saccharin. Bot. 8 oz. *OTC.*
Use: Antacid.
Del-Clens. (Del-Ray) Soapless cleanser. Bot. 8 oz. *OTC.*
Use: Dermatologic, cleanser.
Delco-Lax. (Delco) Bisacodyl 5 mg. Tab. Bot. 1000s. *OTC.*
Use: Laxative.
Delcozine. (Delco) Phendimetrazine tartrate 70 mg. Tab. Bot. 1000s, 5000s. *c-III.*
Use: Anorexiant.
•**delequamine hydrochloride.** (deh-LEH-kwah-meen) USAN.
Use: Anti-impotence agent.
Delestrec. Estradiol 17-undecanoate. *Rx.*
Use: Estrogen.
Delestrogen. (JHP) Estradiol valerate. **10 mg/mL:** In sesame oil, chlorobutanol. Multidose Vial 5 mL. **20 mg/mL, 40 mg/mL:** In castor oil, benzyl benzoate, benzyl alcohol. Multidose Vial 5 mL. *Rx.*
Use: Estrogen, sex hormone.
Delfen Contraceptive Foam. (Johnson & Johnson) Nonoxynol-9 12.5% in an oil-in-water emulsion at pH 4.5 to 5. Starter can with applicator 20 g. Refill 20 g, 42 g. *OTC.*
Use: Contraceptive, spermicide.

•**deligoparin sodium.** (de-li-GOE-pa-rin) USAN.
Use: Inflammatory bowel disease.
delinal. Propenzolate hydrochloride.
•**delmadinone acetate.** (del-MAD-ih-nohn ASS-eh-tate) USAN.
Use: Antiandrogen; antiestrogen; hormone, progestin.
•**delmitide acetate.** (DEL-mi-tide) USAN.
Use: Antidiarrheal.
Del-Mycin. (Del-Ray) Erythromycin 2%, ethyl alcohol 66%. Topical Soln. Bot. 60 mL. *Rx.*
Use: Dermatologic, acne.
Delos. (Rochester Pharmaceuticals) Benzoyl peroxide 3.5%. Alcohols, aloe, caprylic/capric triglyceride, edetate disodium, glycerin, parabens, soya sterols. Lot. 45 g. *Rx.*
Use: Topical anti-infective, antibiotic.
Del-Stat. (Del-Ray) Abradant cleaner. Jar. 2 oz. *OTC.*
Use: Dermatologic, acne.
Delsym. (Adams Respiratory Therapeutics) Dextromethorphan HBr (as polistirex) 30 mg/5 mL. EDTA, corn syrup, sucrose, parabens. Orange flavor, grape flavor. ER Oral Susp. Bot. 89 mL, 148 mL. *OTC.*
Use: Nonnarcotic antitussive.
Deltacortone. Prednisone.
Use: Corticosteroid.
Delta-Cortril. Prednisolone.
Use: Corticosteroid.
Delta-D. (Freeda) Cholecalciferol (vitamin D_3) 400 IU. Sugar free. Tab. Bot. 250s, 500s. *OTC.*
Use: Vitamin supplement.
•**deltafilcon A.** (DELL-tah-FILL-kahn A) USAN.
Use: Contact lens material, hydrophilic.
•**deltafilcon B.** (DELL-tah-FILL-kahn B) USAN.
Use: Contact lens material, hydrophilic.
delta-1-cortisone.
Use: Corticosteroid.
delta-1-hydrocortisone.
Use: Corticosteroid.
See: Prednisolone.
•**deltibant.** (DELL-tih-bant) USAN.
Use: Antagonist (bradykinin).
Del-Trac. (Del-Ray) Acne lotion. Bot. 2 oz. *OTC.*
Use: Dermatologic, acne.
•**delucemine hydrochloride.** (de-LOO-se-meen) USAN.
Use: Neuroprotector.
Delysid. Lysergic acid diethylamide.
Use: Potent psychotogenic.
Demadex. (Roche) Torsemide 5 mg,

10 mg, 20 mg, 100 mg. Tab. UD 100s. *Rx.*
Use: Diuretic.
•**demeclocycline.** (DEH-meh-kloe-SIGH-kleen) *USP 34.* Formerly Demethyl-chlortetracycline.
Use: Anti-infective.
See: Declomycin.
•**demeclocycline hydrochloride.** (DEH-meh-kloe-SIGH-kleen) *USP 34.*
Use: Anti-infective, tetracycline.
See: Declomycin.
demeclocycline hydrochloride. (Impax) Demeclocycline hydrochloride 150 mg, 300 mg. Lactose. Tab. 48s (300 mg only), 100s, 500s. *Rx.*
Use: Anti-infective.
demeclocycline hydrochloride and nystatin tablets.
Use: Anti-infective.
•**demecycline.** (DEH-meh-SIGH-kleen) USAN.
Use: Anti-infective.
Demerol. (Abbott) Meperidine hydrochloride 25 mg/mL, 50 mg/mL, 75 mg/mL, 100 mg/mL. Inj. Amp (preservative free). 0.5 mL (50 mg only), 1 mL (50 mg and 100 mg only); 1.5 mL and 2 mL (50 mg only). Multidose vial (contains metocresol as preservative) 20 mL (100 mg only), 30 mL (50 mg only). *Carpuject* syringe (preservative free). 1 mL. *c-II.*
Use: Opioid analgesic, narcotic agonist.
Demerol. (Sanofi-Synthelabo) Meperidine hydrochloride. **Syrup:** 50 mg/ 5 mL. Alcohol free. Glucose, saccharin. Banana flavor. Bot. 473 mL. **Tab.:** 50 mg, 100 mg. Bot. 100s; 500s, UD 25s (50 mg only). *c-II.*
Use: Opioid analgesic.
demethylchlortetracycline hydrochloride.
Use: Anti-infective; tetracycline.
See: Demeclocycline hydrochloride.
•**demoxepam.** (dem-OX-eh-pam) USAN.
Use: Anxiolytic.
Demser. (Aton Pharma) Metyrosine 250 mg. Cap. Bot. 100s. *Rx.*
Use: Antihypertensive.
•**denagliptin tosylate.** (den-a-GLIP-tin) USAN.
Use: Antidiabetic agent.
Denalan Denture Cleanser. (Whitehall-Robins) Sodium percarbonate 30%. Bot. 7 oz., 13 oz. *OTC.*
Use: Agent for oral hygiene.
•**denatonium benzoate.** (DEE-nah-TOE-nee-uhm BEN-zoh-ate) *NF 29.*

Use: Pharmaceutic aid (flavor, alcohol denaturant).

Denavir. (GlaxoSmithKline) Penciclovir 10 mg/g. Cream. Tube 2 g. *Rx.*
Use: Cold sores.

Denaze. (Cypress) Phenylephrine hydrochloride 10 mg, chlorpheniramine maleate 4 mg, methscopolamine nitrate 1.25 mg per 5 mL. Saccharin, sorbitol. Sugar, alcohol, and dye free. Blue raspberry flavor. Liq. 473 mL. *Rx.*
Use: Decongestant, antihistamine, and anticholinergic combination, upper respiratory combination.

Dencorub. (Last) Methyl salicylate 20%, menthol 0.75%, camphor 1%, eucalyptus oil 0.5%. Tube 1.25 oz, 2.75 oz. *OTC.*
Use: Analgesic, topical.

Dencorub Analgesic Liquid. (Last) Oleoresin capsicum suspension in aqueous vehicle. Bot. 6 oz. *OTC.*
Use: Analgesic, topical.

Dendracin Neurodendtraxcin. (Physicians' Science and Nature) Capsaicin 0.0375%, methyl salicylate 30%, menthol 10%. Aloe gel, benzocaine, borage oil, cetyl alcohol, parabens, PEG 100. Lot. 60 mL. *OTC.*
Use: Topical local anesthetic.

•**denenicokin.** (DEN-en-i-KOE-kin) USAN.
Use: Antineoplastic agent.

•**denibulin hydrochloride.** (den-i-BUE-lin) USAN.
Use: Antineoplastic.

•**denileukin diftitox.** (deh-nih-LOO-kin DIFF-tih-tox) USAN.
Use: Treatment of proliferative malignant diseases and autoimmune diseases expressing interleukin 2 receptors. Biological response modifier; antineoplastic.
See: Ontak.

•**denofungin.** (DEE-no-FUN-jin) USAN.
Use: Antifungal; antibacterial.

Denorex Everyday Dandruff. (Prestige) Pyrithione zinc 2%. Propylene glycol, menthol. Shampoo. 118 mL, 240 mL. *OTC.*
Use: Dermatologic agent.

Denorex Mountain Fresh. (Prestige) Coal tar solution 9%, menthol 1.5%. Bot. 4 oz, 8 oz. *OTC.*
Use: Antiseborrheic.

Denorex with Conditioners. (Prestige) Coal tar solution 9%, menthol 1.5%. Bot 4 oz, 8 oz. *OTC.*
Use: Antiseborrheic.

•**denosumab.** (den-o-SUE-mab) USAN.

Use: Osteoporosis.
See: Prolia.
Xgeva.

Denquel. (Procter & Gamble) Potassium nitrate 5%, calcium carbonate, glycerin, flavors. Tube 1.6 oz, 3 oz, 4.5 oz. *OTC.*
Use: Dentifrice.

Denta 5000 Plus. (Rising Pharmaceuticals) Sodium fluoride 1.1%, spearmint flavor. Cream. 51 g (2s). *Rx.*
Use: Dental caries agent.

DentaGel. (Rising Pharmaceuticals) Sodium fluoride 1.1%, saccharin, parabens, sorbitol, fresh mint flavor. Gel. 56 g. *Rx.*
Use: Dental caries agent.

Dental Caries Preventive. (Colgate Oral) Fluoride ion 1.2%, alumina abrasive. 2 g Box 200s, Jar 9 oz. *Rx.*
Use: Dental caries agent.

Dentiva. (Nuvora) Eucalyptus oil, menthol, peppermint oil, sucralose, wintergreen oil, xylitol, zinc. Alcohol free and sugar free. Loz. 12s. *OTC.*
Use: Mouth and throat product.

Dent-O-Kain/20. (Geritrex) Benzocaine 20%. Benzyl alcohol, saccharin. Liq. 9 mL. *OTC.*
Use: Mouth and throat product.

Dentrol. (Block Drug) Carboxymethylcellulose, polyethylene oxide homopolymer, peppermint and spearmint in mineral oil base. Bot. 0.9 oz, 1.8 oz. *OTC.*
Use: Denture adhesive.

Dent's Dental Poultice. (C.S. Dent & Co.) Glycerin, mineral oil, polyoxyethylene sorbitan monooleate. Bot. 0.125 oz, 0.25 oz. *OTC.*
Use: Dental poultice.

Dent's Ear Wax Drops. (C.S. Dent & Co.) Glycerin, mineral oil, polyoxyethylene sorbitan monooleate. Bot. 0.125 oz, 0.25 oz. *OTC.*
Use: Otic.

Dent's Extra Strength Toothache Gum. (C.S. Dent & Co.) Benzocaine 20%. Gum. Box. 1 g. *OTC.*
Use: Anesthetic, local.

Dent's Lotion-Jel. (C.S. Dent & Co.) Benzocaine in special base. Tube 2 oz. *OTC.*
Use: Anesthetic, local.

Dent's Maximum Strength Toothache Drops. (C.S. Dent & Co.) Benzocaine 20%, alcohol 74%, eugenol chlorobutanol anhydrous 0.09%. Liq. Bot. 3.7 mL. *OTC.*
Use: Anesthetic, local.

Dent's Toothache Drops Treatment. (C.S. Dent & Co.) Alcohol 60%, chlorobutanol anhydrous (chloroform deriva-

tive) 0.09%, propylene glycol, eugenol. Bot. 3.75 mL. *OTC.*
Use: Anesthetic, local.

Dent's Toothache Gum. (C.S. Dent & Co.) Benzocaine, eugenol, petrolatum in base of cotton and wax. Box 1.05 g. *OTC.*
Use: Anesthetic, local.

Denture Orajel. (Del) Benzocaine 10%, saccharin. Gel. Tube. 9.45 g. *OTC.*
Use: Anesthetic, local.

Dent-Zel-Ite. (Last) Oral Mucosal Analgesic: Benzocaine 5%, alcohol, glycerin. Bot. 1.875 g. **Temporary Dental Filling:** Sandarac gum, alcohol. Bot. 1 oz. **Toothache Drops:** Eugenol 85% in alcohol. Bot. 1 oz. *OTC.*
Use: Anesthetic, local.

•**denufosol tetrasodium.** (den-ue-FOE-sol) USAN.
Use: Investigational for cystic fibrosis.

denyl sodium.
Use: Anticonvulsant.
See: Diphenylhydantoin Sodium.

deodorizers, systemic. Chlorophyll derivatives (chlorophyllin). *OTC.*
Use: Oral: Control of fecal and urinary odors in colostomy, ileostomy, or incontinence. Topical: Reduce pain and inflammation (wounds, burns, surface ulcers, skin irritation).
See: Chloresium.
  Chlorophyll.
  Derifil.

2′deoxycoformycin. Pentostatin.
Use: Antibiotic; antineoplastic.
See: Nipent.

deoxynojirimycin. (Pharmacia) Butyl-DNJ. *Rx.*
Use: Antiviral.

Depacon. (Abbott) Valproate 100 mg/mL. EDTA, preservative free. Inj. Single-dose vials. 5 mL. *Rx.*
Use: Anticonvulsant.

Depakene. (Abbott) Valproic acid. **Cap.:** 250 mg. Parabens, corn oil. Bot. 100s. **Syrup:** 250 mg/5 mL. Sorbitol, parabens, sucrose. Bot. 473 mL. *Rx.*
Use: Anticonvulsant.

Depakote. (Abbott) Divalproex sodium. **DR Tab.:** 125 mg, 250 mg, 500 mg. Talc. Bot. 100s, 500s (except 125 mg), *Abbo-Pac* UD 100s. **Sprinkle Cap.:** 125 mg. Coated particles. Bot. 100s, *Abbo-Pac* UD 100s. *Rx.*
Use: Anticonvulsant.

Depakote ER. (Abbott) Divalproex sodium 250 mg, 500 mg. Lactose, polydextrose (500 mg only). ER Tab. Bot. 60s (250 mg only), 100s, 500s, *Abbo-Pac* UD 100s. *Rx.*
Use: Anticonvulsant.

Depa-Syrup. (Alra) Valproic acid syrup 250 mg/5 mL. Bot. 4 oz, 16 oz. *Rx.*
Use: Anticonvulsant.

•**depelestat.** (dep-EL-e-stat) USAN.
Use: Cystic fibrosis.

Depen. (Wallace) Penicillamine 250 mg. Tab. Bot. 100s. *Rx.*
Use: Chelating agent.

depepsen. Amylosulfate sodium.
Use: Digestive aid.

depGynogen. (Forest) Estradiol cypionate in cottonseed oil 5 mg/mL, cottonseed oil, chlorobutanol. Inj. Vial 10 mL. *Rx.*
Use: Estrogen.

Deplin. (Pamlab) Folic acid (as L-methylfolate) 7.5 mg, 15 mg. Gluten free, lactose free, and sugar free. Tab. 30s (7.5 mg only), 90s, 500s (7.5 mg only). *Rx.*
Use: Vitamin.

DepoCyt. (Enzon) Cytarabine, liposomal 10 mg/mL, preservative free, sodium chloride 0.9%. Inj. Vial. 5 mL. *Rx.*
Use: Antimetabolite.

DepoDur. (EKR Therapeutics) Morphine sulfate 10 mg/mL. ER Liposomal Inj. Single-use vials in cartons of 5. 1 mL, 1.5 mL, 2 mL. *c-II.*
Use: Opioid analgesic.

Depoestra. (Tennessee Pharmaceutic) Estradiol cypionate 5 mg/mL. Vial 10 mL. *Rx.*
Use: Estrogen.

Depo-Estradiol. (Pfizer) Estradiol cypionate 5 mg/mL. Chlorobutanol 5.4 mg, cottonseed oil. Inj. Vial 5 mL. *Rx.*
Use: Estrogen, sex hormone.

DepoGen. (Hyrex) Estradiol cypionate 5 mg/mL, cottonseed oil, chlorobutanol. Inj. Vial 10 mL. *Rx.*
Use: Estrogen.

Depo-Medrol. (Pfizer) Methylprednisolone acetate 20 mg/mL, 40 mg/mL, 80 mg/mL. Polyethylene glycol, myristyl-gamma-picolinium chloride. Inj. Vials. 1 mL (excpet 20 mg/mL), 5 mL, 10 mL (40 mg/mL only). *Rx.*
Use: Adrenocortical steroid, glucocorticoid.

Depo-Provera. (Pfizer) Medroxyprogesterone acetate 400 mg/mL, polyethylene glycol 3350, sodium sulfate anhydrous, myristyl-gamma-picolinium Cl. Vial 2.5 mL, 10 mL, 1 mL *U-Ject.* *Rx.*
Use: Hormone, progestin.

Depo-Provera Contraceptive Injection. (Pfizer) Medroxyprogesterone acetate 150 mg/mL, with PEG-3350 28.9 mg, polysorbate 80 2.41 mg, sodium Cl

8.68 mg, methylparaben 1.37 mg, propylparaben 0.15 mg. Vial. 1 mL. *Rx.*
Use: Contraceptive.

Depo-Sub Q Provera 104. (Pfizer) Medroxyprogesterone acetate 104 mg (160 mg/mL). Sodium chloride 5.2 mg, parabens, polyethylene glycol. Inj. Prefilled single-use syringes. 0.65 mL. *Rx.*
Use: Contraceptive hormone.

Depo-Testadiol. (Pfizer) Testosterone cypionate 50 mg, estradiol cypionate 2 mg/mL, chlorobutanol in cottonseed oil. Inj. (in oil). Vial 10 mL. *Rx.*
Use: Androgen, estrogen combination.

Depo-Testosterone. (Pfizer) Testosterone cypionate. Inj. Soln. **100 mg/mL:** In benzyl alcohol 9.45 mg, cottonseed oil 736 mg. Benzyl benzoate 0.1 mL. Vials. 10 mL. **200 mg/mL:** In benzyl benzoate 0.2 mL, benzyl alcohol 9.45 mg, cottonseed oil 560 mg. Vials. 1 mL, 10 mL. *c-III.*
Use: Sex hormone, androgen.

deprenyl. Selegiline hydrochloride.
See: Eldepryl.

•**depreotide.** (deh-PREE-oh-tide) USAN.
Use: Diagnostic aid.

Deproist Expectorant/Codeine. (Geneva) Pseudoephedrine hydrochloride 30 mg, codeine phosphate 10 mg, guaifenesin 100 mg/5 mL. Bot. 120 mL, 480 mL. *c-v.*
Use: Antitussive, decongestant, expectorant.

•**deprostil.** (deh-PRAHST-ill) USAN.
Use: Antisecretory, gastric.

Dequasine. (Miller Pharmacal Group) L-lysine 20 mg, l-cysteine 50 mg, DL-methionine 150 mg, N-acetyl cysteine 50 mg, vitamin C 200 mg, Ca 40 mg, Cu 1 mg, Fe 5 mg, I 0.015 mg, K 20 mg, Mg 40 mg, Mn 5 mg, Mo 150 mcg, Zn 5 mg. Tab. Bot. 100s. *OTC.*
Use: Amino acid; vitamin, mineral supplement.

•**deracoxib.** (der-ah-KOX-ib) USAN.
Use: Anti-inflammatory; analgesic.

Derifil. (Rystan) Chlorophyllin copper complex 100 mg. Tab. Bot. 30s, 100s, 1000s. *OTC.*
Use: Deodorant, oral.

Dermabase. (Paddock) Mineral oil, petrolatum, cetostearyl alcohol, propylene glycol, sodium lauryl sulfate, isopropyl palmitate, imidazolidinyl urea, methyl- and propylparabens. Cream. Jar 1 lb. *OTC.*
Use: Emollient.

Dermacort. (Solvay) Hydrocortisone. **Cream:** 0.5%, 1% in a water soluble cream of stearyl alcohol, cetyl alcohol, isopropyl palmitate, citric acid, polyoxyethylene 40 stearate, sodium phosphate, propylene glycol, water, benzyl alcohol, buffered to pH 5. 0.5% in 30 g tube, 1% in 1 lb jar. **Lot.:** 1% in lotion base, buffered to pH 5. Paraben free. Bot. 120 mL. *Rx.*
Use: Corticosteroid, topical.

Derma-Cover. (Scrip) Sulfur, salicylic acid, hyamine 10x, isopropyl alcohol 22%, in powder film forming base. Bot. 2 oz. *OTC.*
Use: Keratolytic.

Dermadrox. (Geritrex) Aluminum hydroxide gel, zinc chloride, lanolin, calcium carbonate, vitamin A in a hydrophilic ointment base. Oint. 113 g. *OTC.*
Use: Topical combination.

Derma-Guard. (Greer) Protective adhesive pow. Can w/sifter top, 4 oz. Spray Top Bot. 4 oz, pkg. 1 lb. Rings. Pkg. 5s, 10s. *OTC.*
Use: Dermatologic, protectant.

Dermal Therapy Finger Care. (Bayer) Urea 20%. Beeswax, cetyl alcohol, disodium EDTA, emulsifying wax, parabens, PEG, petrolatum, lactic acid, triethanolamine. Lot. 18 mL. *OTC.*
Use: Emollient.

Dermamycin. (Pfeiffer) **Cream:** Diphenhydramine hydrochloride 2% in a base of parabens, polyethylene glycol monostearate and propylene glycol. Tube 28.35 g. **Spray:** Diphenhydramine hydrochloride 2%, menthol 1%, alcohol, methylparaben. Bot. 60 mL. *OTC.*
Use: Antihistamine, topical.

Dermaneed. (Hanlon) Zirconium oxide 4.5%, calamine 6%, zinc oxide 4%, actamer 0.1% in bland lotionized base. Bot. 4 oz. *OTC.*
Use: Antipruritic, topical.

Derma-Pax. (Recsei) Diphenhydramine hydrochloride 0.5%. Benzyl alcohol. Lot. 118 mL. *OTC.*
Use: Antihistamine, topical; corticosteroid, topical.

Derma-Pax HC. (Recsei) Hydrocortisone 0.5%, pyrilamine maleate 0.2%, pheniramine 0.06%, benzyl alcohol 1%. Liq. Bot. 60 mL, 120 mL, 480 mL. *OTC.*
Use: Antihistamine, topical; corticosteroid, topical.

DermaPhor. (DermaRite) Petrolatum 44%, lanolin alcohol, mineral oil, paraffin wax. Oint. 228 g. *OTC.*
Use: Emollient.

Dermarest. (Del) Diphenhydramine hydrochloride 2%, resorcinol 2%, aloe vera gel, benzalkonium chloride, EDTA,

menthol, methylparaben, propylene glycol. Gel. Tube 29.25 g, 56.25 g. *OTC.*
Use: Antihistamine, topical.

Dermarest Dricort. (Del) Hydrocortisone 1%, white petrolatum. Cream. Bot. 14 g. *OTC.*
Use: Corticosteroid, topical.

Dermarest Plus. (Del) **Gel:** Diphenhydramine hydrochloride 2%, menthol 1%, aloe vera gel, benzalkonium chloride, isopropyl alcohol, methylparaben, propylene glycol. Tube 15 g, 30 g.
Spray: Diphenhydramine hydrochloride 2%, menthol 1%, aloe vera gel, benzalkonium chloride, methylparaben propylene glycol, SDA 40 alcohol, EDTA. Bot. 60 mL. *OTC.*
Use: Antihistamine, topical.

Dermasept Antifungal. (Pharmakon) Tannic acid 6.098%, zinc Cl 5.081%, benzocaine 2.032%, methylbenzethonium hydrochloride, tolnaftate 1.017%, undecylenic acid 5.081%, ethanol 38B 58.539%, phenol, benzyl alcohol, benzoic acid, coal tar, camphor, menthol. Liq. Bot. 30 mL. *OTC.*
Use: Antifungal, topical.

Dermasil. (Chesebrough-Ponds USA) Glycerin and dimethicone in a base containing cyclomethicone, sunflower oil, petrolatum, borage oil, lecithin, vitamin E acetate, vitamin A palmitate, vitamin D$_3$, corn oil, EDTA, methylparaben. Lot. Bot. 120 mL, 240 mL. *OTC.*
Use: Emollient.

Derma-Smoothe/FS Oil. (Hill Dermaceuticals) Fluocinolone acetonide 0.01%. Oil. Bot. 4 oz. *Rx.*
Use: Antipsoriatic; antiseborrheic, topical.

Derma-Smoothe Oil. (Hill Dermaceuticals) Refined peanut oil, mineral oil in lipophilic base. *OTC.*
Use: Antipruritic; dermatologic, protectant.

Derma Soap. (Ferndale) Dowicil 0.1%. 4 oz w/dispenser. *OTC.*
Use: Antiseptic.

Derma-Soft. (Vogarell) Salicylic acid, castor oil, triethanolamine. Medicated cream. Tube ¾ oz. *OTC.*
Use: Keratolytic.

Derma-Sone 1%. (Hill Dermaceuticals) Hydrocortisone 1%, pramoxine hydrochloride 1%, cetyl alcohol, glyceryl monostearate, isopropyl myristate, potassium sorbate, furcelleran. *Rx-OTC.*
Use: Anesthetic; corticosteroid, local.

Dermasorcin. (Lamond) Resorcin 2%, sulfur 5%. Bot. 1 oz, 2 oz, 4 oz, 8 oz, pt, 32 oz, 0.5 gal. *OTC.*
Use: Dermatologic, acne; antiseborrheic, topical.

Dermastringe. (Lamond) Bot. 4 oz, 6 oz, 8 oz, pt, 32 oz, gal. *OTC.*
Use: Dermatologic, cleanser.

Dermasul. (Lamond) Sulfur 5%. Bot. 1 oz, 2 oz, 4 oz, 8 oz, pt, 32 oz, 0.5 gal, gal. *OTC.*
Use: Dermatologic, acne; antiseborrheic, topical.

Dermathyn. (Davis & Sly) Benzyl alcohol 3%, benzocaine 3.5%, butyl-p-aminobenzoate 1%, phenylmercuric borate. Tube 1 oz. *OTC.*
Use: Anesthetic, local.

Dermatic Base. (Whorton Pharmaceuticals, Inc.) Compounding cream base. Bot. 16 oz.
Use: Pharmaceutical aid, emollient base.

Dermatol.
See: Bismuth Subgallate.

Dermatop E. (Dermik) Prednicarbate 0.1%. **Cream:** White petrolatum, lanolin alcohols, mineral oil, cetostearyl alcohol, EDTA, lactic acid. Tube. 15 g, 60 g.
Oint.: Glycerin. Tube. 15 g, 60 g. *Rx.*
Use: Corticosteroid, topical.

DermaVite. (GlaxoSmithKline) Vitamin A 3500 units (29% as beta carotene), E 60 units, B$_2$ 8.5 mg, B$_6$ 10 mg, C 120 mg, folate 400 mcg, Zn 45 mg, biotin 600 mcg, lycopene 5 mg, Ca, Cr, Cu, Mn, Se, Si, sucrose. Tab. Bot. 60s. *OTC.*
Use: Vitamin, mineral supplement.

DermaZinc. (Dermalogix) Zinc pyrithione 0.25%, aloe vera, cetyl alcohol, dimethicone, lanolin, methylparaben, mineral oil, PEG-75. Cream. 114 g. *OTC.*
Use: Emollient.

Dermazine. (Dermalogix) Pyrithione zinc 0.25%. Parabens. Shampoo. 240 mL. *OTC.*
Use: Dermatologic agent.

Dermed. (Holloway) Vitamins A and D with hydrogenated vegetable oil. Cream. Tube 60 g, 120 g. *OTC.*
Use: Emollient.

Dermeze. (Premo) Thenylpyramine hydrochloride 2%, benzocaine 2%, tyrothricin 0.25 mg/g. Massage Lot. Bot. 5¾ oz. *OTC.*
Use: Anesthetic; antihistamine; anti-infective.

Dermolate Anti-Itch. (Schering-Plough) Hydrocortisone 0.5% petrolatum, mineral oil, chlorocresol. Cream. Tube 15 g, 30 g. *OTC.*
Use: Corticosteroid, topical.

Dermol HC. (Dermol Pharmaceuticals, Inc.) **Cream:** Hydrocortisone 1%, 2.5%. Tube 30 g. **Oint.:** Hydrocortisone

1%. Tube 30 g. *Rx.*
Use: Anorectal preparation.
Dermolin. (Roberts) Menthol racemic, methyl salicylate, camphor, mustard oil, isopropyl alcohol 8%. Bot. 3 oz, pt, gal. *OTC.*
Use: Liniment.
Dermoplast. (Prestige) Benzocaine 20%. Menthol 0.5%, methylparaben, aloe, lanolin. Spray. Bot. 59 mL. *OTC.*
Use: Topical local anesthetic, ester local anesthetic.
Dermoplast. (Prestige) Benzocaine 8%. Menthol 0.5%, aloe, glycerin, parabens, lanolin. Lot. Bot. 90 mL. *OTC.*
Use: Topical local anesthetic, ester local anesthetic.
Dermoplast Antibacterial. (Medtech) Benzocaine 20%. Benzethonium chloride 0.2%, menthol, methylparaben, aloe, lanolin. Spray. 59 mL. *OTC.*
Use: Topical local anesthetic, ester local anesthetic.
DermOtic. (Hill Dermaceuticals) Fluocinolone acetonide oil 0.01%. Otic Drops. 20 mL. *Rx.*
Use: Otic preparation.
Dermovan. (Galderma) Glyceryl stearate, spermaceti, mineral oil, glycerin, cetyl alcohol, butylparaben, methylparaben, propylparaben, purified water. Vanishing-type base, Jar 1 lb. *OTC.*
Use: Dermatologic, protectant.
Dermtex HC. (Pfeiffer) Hydrocortisone 0.5% in a glycerin base. Tube 15 g. *OTC.*
Use: Corticosteroid, topical.
Dermuspray. (Warner Chilcott) Trypsin 0.1 mg, balsam Peru 72.5 mg, castor oil 650 mg/0.82 mL. Aer. Bot. 120 g. *Rx.*
Use: Enzyme, topical.
DES.
See: Diethylstilbestrol.
desacchromin. A nonprotein bacterial colloidal dispersion of polysaccharide.
•**desciclovir.** (DESS-sigh-kloe-veer) USAN.
Use: Antiviral.
•**descinolone acetonide.** (DESS-SIN-ole-ohn ah-SEE-toe-nide) USAN.
Use: Corticosteroid, topical.
Desenex. (Novartis) Miconazole nitrate. **Spray, Liq.:** 2%. PEG 300, SD alcohol 40-B. 133 g. **Pow.:** 2%. Talc. 43 g, 85 g. *OTC.*
Use: Topical antifungal agent.
Desenex. (Novartis) Clotrimazole 1%. Benzyl alcohol 1%, cetostearyl alcohol. Cream. Tube. 15 g, 30 g. *OTC.*
Use: Antifungal, topical.

Desenex Foot & Sneaker Spray. (Novartis) Aluminum chlorhydrex w/alcohol 89.3%. Aerosol Can 2.7 oz. *OTC.*
Use: Foot deodorant; antiperspirant.
Desenex Liquid Spray. (Novartis) Miconazole nitrate 2%. PEG 300, SD alcohol 40-B. Spray, Liq. 133 g. *OTC.*
Use: Anti-infective, antifungal agent.
De Serpa. (de Leon) Reserpine 0.25 mg, 0.5 mg. Tab. Bot. 100s, 500s, 1000s (0.25 mg only). *Rx.*
Use: Antihypertensive.
deserpidine.
Use: Antihypertensive.
W/Methyclothiazide.
See: Enduronyl.
Desert Pure Calcium. (CalWhite Mineral Co.) Calcium (from mineral calcite) 500 mg, vitamin D 125 units. Tab. Bot. 200s. *OTC.*
Use: Mineral, vitamin supplement.
Desferal. (Novartis) Deferoxamine mesylate 500 mg/5 mL. Amp. 4s. *Rx.*
Use: Antidote.
•**desflurane.** (dess-FLEW-rane) *USP 34.*
Use: Anesthetic.
See: Suprane.
•**desipramine hydrochloride.** (dess-IPP-ruh-meen) *USP 34.*
Use: Antidepressant.
See: Norpramin.
desipramine hydrochloride. (Various Mfr.) Desipramine hydrochloride 10 mg, 25 mg, 50 mg, 75 mg, 100 mg, 150 mg. May contain lactose. Tab. 50s (150 mg only), 100s, 500s (except 10 mg, 150 mg), 1,000s (25 mg, 50 mg only). *Rx.*
Use: Antidepressant.
•**desirudin.** (deh-SIHR-uh-din) USAN.
Use: Anticoagulant.
See: Iprivask.
Desitin. (Pfizer) Cod liver oil, zinc oxide 40%, talc, petrolatum, lanolin. Oint. 30 g, 60 g, 120 g, 240 g, 270 g. *OTC.*
Use: Astringent; skin protectant.
Desitin Clear. (Pfizer) White petrolatum 60.4%. Cocoa butter, light mineral oil, mineral oil, modified lanolin, sunflower seed oil, vitamin A, vitamin D, vitamin E. Top. Oint. 50 g, 99 g. *OTC.*
Use: Diaper rash product.
Desitin Creamy. (Pfizer) Zinc oxide 10%, mineral oil, white petrolatum, parabens. Oint. Tube 57 g. *OTC.*
Use: Antifungal, topical.
Desitin with Zinc Oxide. (Pfizer) Cornstarch 88.2%, zinc oxide 10%. Pow. Bot. 28 g, 397 g. *OTC.*
Use: Diaper rash preparation.

●**deslanoside.** (dess-LAN-oh-side)
USP 34.
Use: Cardiovascular agent.

●**desloratadine.** (dess-lore-AT-ah-deen)
USAN.
Use: Antihistamine, peripherally selective piperidine.
See: Clarinex.
Clarinex RediTabs.
W/Pseudoephedrine Sulfate.
See: Clarinex-D 12 Hour.
Clarinex-D 24 Hour.

●**deslorelin.** (DESS-low-REH-lin) USAN.
Use: Gonadotropin inhibitor; LHRH agonist. [Orphan Drug]
See: Somagard (as acetate).

Desma. (Tablicaps) Diethylstilbestrol
25 mg. Tab. Patient dispenser 10s. *Rx.*
Use: Estrogen.

●**desmopressin acetate.** (DESS-moe-PRESS-in) USAN.
Use: Posterior pituitary hormone.
See: DDAVP.
Stimate.
W/Chlorobutanol.
See: Minirin.

desmopressin acetate. (Various Mfr.)
Desmopressin acetate. **Tab.:** 0.1 mg,
0.2 mg. May contain lactose. 100s. **Inj.,**
Soln.: 4 mcg/mL. Single-dose Amp.
1 mL, multidose vial 10 mL. **Spray,**
Soln., intranasal: 0.1 mg/mL (10 mcg/
spray). Bot. 5 mL (50 sprays), rhinal
tube delivery system. 2.5 mL (2 applicators per carton). *Rx.*
Use: Posterior pituitary hormone.

●**desmoteplase.** (des-moe-TE-plase)
USAN.
Use: Cardiovascular agent.

Desogen. (Organon) Desogestrel
0.15 mg, ethinyl estradiol 30 mcg. Lactose. Tab. Pack. 28s with 7 inert tabs.
Rx.
Use: Sex hormone, contraceptive hormone.

●**desogestrel.** (DESS-oh-JESS-trell)
USP 34.
Use: Hormone, progestin.
W/Ethinyl Estradiol.
See: Apri.
Azurette.
Caziant.
Cesia.
Desogen.
Mircette.
Ortho-Cept.
Reclipsen.
Velivet.

Desonate. (Intendis) Desonide 0.05%.
Edetate disodium dihydrate, parabens.

Gel. 15 g, 30 g, 60 g. *Rx.*
Use: Anti-inflammatory agent, topical corticosteroid.

●**desonide.** (DESS-oh-nide) USAN.
Use: Anti-inflammatory.
See: Desonate.
LoKara.
Verdeso.

desonide. (Fougera) Desonide 0.05%,
light mineral oil, cetyl alcohol, stearyl
alcohol, parabens, EDTA. Lot. 59 mL,
118 mL. *Rx.*
Use: Anti-inflammatory; corticosteroid,
topical.

desonide. (Various Mfr.) Desonide
0.05%. Oint. Cream. Tube 15 g, 60 g.
Rx.
Use: Anti-inflammatory; corticosteroid,
topical.

desonide cream. (Galderma) Desonide
0.05% in cream base. Tube 15 g, 60 g.
Rx.
Use: Corticosteroid, topical.

DesOwen. (Galderma) Desonide 0.05%.
Cream. Tube 15 g, 60 g. *Rx.*
Use: Corticosteroid, topical.

●**desoximetasone.** (dess-OX-ee-MET-ah-
sone) *USP 34.*
Use: Anti-inflammatory; corticosteroid,
topical.
See: Topicort.

desoximetasone. (Perrigo) Desoximetasone. **Gel.:** 0.05%. SD alcohol
20%, docusate sodium, EDTA, trolamine. Tubes. 15 g, 60 g. **Oint.:** 0.25%.
Sorbitan sesquioleate, white petrolatum. Tubes. 15 g, 60 g. *Rx.*
Use: Anti-inflammatory; topical corticosteroid.

●**desoxycorticosterone acetate.** (dess-
OX-ee-core-tih-koe-STURR-ohn)
USP 34.
Use: Adrenocortical steroid (salt-
regulating).

●**desoxycorticosterone pivalate.** (dess-
OX-ee-core-tih-koe-STURR-ohn)
USP 34.
Use: Adrenocortical steroid (salt-
regulating).

●**desoxycorticosterone trimethylac-
etate.** (dess-OX-ee-core-tih-koe-
STURR-ohn) *USP 34.*
Use: Adrenocortical steroid (salt-
regulating).

desoxyephedrine hydrochloride.
(Various Mfr.) *c-II.*
Use: CNS stimulant.
See: Methamphetamine Hydrochloride.

Desoxyn. (Ovation Pharm) Methamphetamine hydrochloride 5 mg. Lactose.

Tab. Bot. 100s. *c-II*.
Use: CNS stimulant, amphetamine.
desoxy norephedrine.
Use: CNS stimulant.
See: Amphetamine Hydrochloride.
desoxyribonuclease.
Use: Enzyme, topical.
Despec. (International Ethical) Phenyl-ephrine hydrochloride 5 mg, guaifene-sin 100 mg per 5 mL. Alcohol, sugar, and dye free. Saccharin, sorbitol. Grape flavor. Liq. 15 mL, 120 mL, 240 mL. *OTC.*
Use: Antitussive and expectorant com-bination, decongestant and expecto-rant combination, upper respiratory combination.
Despec DM. (International Ethical) **ER Tab.:** Dextromethorphan HBr 60 mg, guaifenesin 800 mg, pseudoephedrine hydrochloride 120 mg. 100s. **Liq.:** Dex-tromethorphan HBr 15 mg, guaifenesin 100 mg, phenylephrine hydrochloride 5 mg per 5 mL. Saccharin, sorbitol. Grape flavor. 15 mL, 473 mL. *Rx.*
Use: Antitussive and expectorant com-bination.
Despec-EXP. (International Ethical) Dihydrocodeine bitartrate 7.5 mg, guai-fenesin 100 mg, pseudoephedrine hydrochloride 15 mg per 5 mL. Sac-charin, sorbitol. Alcohol free, dye free, and sugar free. Vanilla mint flavor. Syrup. 473 mL. *c-III.*
Use: Upper respiratory combination, an-titussive and expectorant combination.
Despec NR. (International Ethical) Dex-tromethorphan hydrobromide 4 mg, guaifenesin 20 mg, phenylephrine hydrochloride 1.5 mg per mL. Saccha-rin, sorbitol. Grape flavor. Drops. 15 mL, 30 mL w/dropper. *Rx.*
Use: Upper respiratory combination; an-titussive, decongestant, expectorant.
Despec-Tab. (International Ethical) Guai-fenesin 400 mg, pseudoephedrine hydrochloride 40 mg. Maltodextrin. Tab. 60s. *Rx.*
Use: Upper respiratory combination, de-congestant and expectorant combina-tion.
Desquam-E 5 & 10. (Westwood Squibb) Benzoyl peroxide 10%, EDTA. Gel. Tube 42.5 g. *Rx.*
Use: Dermatologic, acne.
Desquam-X 10. (Westwood Squibb) Ben-zoyl peroxide 10%. Lactic acid, EDTA, sorbitol. Bar 106 g. *Rx.*
Use: Dermatologic, acne.
de-Stat. (Sherman Pharmaceuticals, Inc.) Surfactant cleaner, benzalkonium Cl

0.01%, EDTA 0.25%. Soln. Bot. 118 mL. *OTC.*
Use: Contact lens care.
destructive agents.
See: Chloroacetic Acids.
•**desvenlafaxine succinate.** (des-VEN-la-fax-een) USAN.
Use: Antidepressant, serotonin and nor-epinephrine reuptake inhibitor.
See: Pristiq.
Detachol. (Ferndale) Bland, nonirritating liquid for removing adhesive tape. Pkg. 4 oz.
Use: Adhesive remover.
Detane. (Del) Benzocaine 7.5%. Car-bomer 940, PEG 400. Gel. Tubes. 15 g. *OTC.*
Use: Topical local anesthetic.
•**deterenol hydrochloride.** (dee-TEER-eh-nahl) USAN.
Use: Adrenergic, ophthalmic.
detergents. Surface-active.
See: pHisoDerm.
pHisoHex.
Zephiran.
detigon hydrochloride.
See: Chlophedianol hydrochloride.
•**detirelix acetate.** (DEH-tih-RELL-ix) USAN.
Use: Antagonist (LHRH).
•**detomidine hydrochloride.** (deh-TOE-mih-deen) USAN.
Use: Hypnotic; sedative.
detoxification agents.
See: Antidotes.
Chelating Agents.
Detrol. (Pfizer) Tolterodine tartrate 1 mg, 2 mg. Tab. Bot. 60s, 500s, UD 140s. *Rx.*
Use: Anticholinergic.
Detrol LA. (Pfizer) Tolterodine tartrate 2 mg, 4 mg. Sucrose. ER Cap. Bot. 30s, 90s, 500s, UD blisters 100s. *Rx.*
Use: Anticholinergic.
Detussin Expectorant. (Various Mfr.) Pseudoephedrine hydrochloride 60 mg, hydrocodone bitartrate 5 mg, guaifenesin 200 mg, alcohol. Liq. Bot. 480 mL. *c-III.*
Use: Antitussive, decongestant, expec-torant.
•**deuterium oxide.** (doo-TEER-ee-uhm) USAN.
Use: Radiopharmaceutical.
•**devazepide.** (dev-AZE-eh-PIDE) USAN.
Use: Antagonist (cholecystokinin); anti-spasmodic, gastrointestinal.
Devrom. (Parthenon) Bismuth subgallate 200 mg, lactose, sugar. Chew. Tab. Bot. 100s.
Use: Deodorant, systemic.

Dexacort Phosphate Respihaler.
(Medeva) Dexamethasone sodium phosphate equivalent to 0.1 mg dexamethasone phosphate ($\approx$ 0.084 mg dexamethasone) w/fluorochlorohydrocarbons as propellants, alcohol 2%. Aerosol for oral inhalation, 170 sprays in 12.6 g pressurized container.
Use: Bronchodilator.

Dexacort Phosphate Turbinaire.
(Medeva) Dexamethasone sodium phosphate 0.1 mg equivalent to dexamethasone 0.084 mg w/fluorochlorohydrocarbons as propellants and alcohol 2%. Aerosol w/nasal applicator. Container 170 sprays; refill package without nasal applicator.
Use: Nasal corticosteroid.

Dexafed. (Roberts) Phenylephrine hydrochloride 5 mg, dextromethorphan HBr 10 mg, guaifenesin 100 mg/5 mL. Syr. Bot. 120 mL. *OTC.*
Use: Antitussive, decongestant, expectorant.

DexAlone. (DexGen) Dextromethorphan HBr 30 mg. Sorbitol. Cap., Liquid-filled. Pkg. 30s. *OTC.*
Use: Nonnarcotic antitussive.

•**dexamethasone.** (DEX-uh-METH-uh-sone) *USP 34.*
Use: Adrenocortical steroid, glucocorticoid; corticosteroid, topical.
See: Aeroseb-Dex.
Baycadron.
Decaderm.
Decameth.
Decameth L.A.
Dexaport.
DexPak Jr. 10 Day TaperPak.
DexPak 6 Day TaperPak.
DexPak Taperpak.
DexPak 13 Day TaperPak.
Maxidex.
Ozurdex.
TobraDex.
Zema-Pak 10 Day.
Zema-Pak 13 Day.
W/Ciprofloxacin.
See: Ciprodex.
W/Neomycin Sulfate, Polymyxin B Sulfate.
See: Dexasporin.
Maxitrol Ointment.
Neomycin and Polymyxin B Sulfates and Dexamethasone Ophthalmic Ointment.

dexamethasone. (Roxane) Dexamethasone 1 mg, 2 mg. Tab. 100s, UD 100s. *Rx.*
Use: Adrenocortical steroid, glucocorticoid.

dexamethasone. (Steris) Dexamethasone 0.1%. Susp., Ophth. 5 mL. *Rx.*
Use: Corticosteroid, ophthalmic.

dexamethasone. (Various Mfr.) Dexamethasone. **Elix.:** 0.5 mg/5 mL. May contain alcohol. 100 mL, 237 mL. **Oral Soln.:** 0.5 mg/5 mL. May contain sorbitol. Sugar free. 500 mL, UD 5 mL, UD 20 mL, 237 mL. **Tab.:** 0.25 mg, 0.5 mg, 0.75 mg, 1.5 mg, 4 mg, 6 mg. 50s (1.5 mg, 4 mg, 6 mg only), 100s, 500s (0.75 mg, 1.5 mg, 4 mg only), 1,000s (except 6 mg), UD 100s (except 0.25 mg). *Rx.*
Use: Adrenocortical steroid, glucocorticoid.

•**dexamethasone acefurate.** (DEX-ah-METH-ah-sone ASS-eh-fer-ate) USAN.
Use: Anti-inflammatory; topical steroid.

•**dexamethasone acetate.** (DEX-ah-METH-ah-sone) *USP 34.*
Use: Adrenocortical steroid (anti-inflammatory).

•**dexamethasone beloxil.** (DEX-ah-METH-ah-sone bel-OX-il) USAN.
Use: Anti-inflammatory.

•**dexamethasone dipropionate.** (DEX-ah-METH-ah-sone die-PRO-pee-oh-nate) USAN.
Use: Anti-inflammatory; steroid.

Dexamethasone Intensol. (Roxane) Dexamethasone 1 mg/mL. Alcohol 30%. Concentrated oral soln. Bot. 30 mL w/dropper. *Rx.*
Use: Glucocorticoid, adrenocortical steroid.

•**dexamethasone sodium phosphate.** (DEX-ah-METH-ah-sone) *USP 34.*
Use: Adrenocortical steroid (anti-inflammatory); corticosteroid, topical.
See: Dalalone.
Decaject.
Decameth.
Dexone.
Solurex.

dexamethasone sodium phosphate. (Various Mfr.) Dexamethasone sodium phosphate. **Inj.: 4 mg/mL:** 1 mL, 5 mL, 10 mL, 30 mL vials and 1 mL disp. syringe and 1 mL fill in 2 mL vials. **10 mg/mL:** 1 mL and 10 mL vials and 1 mL disp. syringe. **Soln., otic:** 0.1%. Sodium citrate, sodium borate, polysorbate 80, edetate disodium dihydrate, sodium bisulfite 0.1%, phenylethyl alcohol 0.25%, benzalkonium chloride 0.02%. Bot. 5 mL. **Ophth. Soln.:** 0.1%. 5 mL. *Rx.*
Use: Adrenocortical steroid (anti-inflammatory); corticosteroid, topical; ophthalmic corticosteroid.

•**dexamisole.** (DEX-AM-ih-sole) USAN.
Use: Antidepressant.

dexamphetamine.
See: Dextroamphetamine.

Dexaphen-S.A. Tablets. (Major) Pseudoephedrine sulfate 120 mg, dexbrompheniramine maleate 6 mg. Bot.
100s, 500s. *Rx.*
Use: Antihistamine, decongestant.

Dexaport. (Freeport) Dexamethasone
0.75 mg. Tab. Bot. 1000s. *Rx.*
Use: Corticosteroid.

Dexasone. (Various Mfr.) Dexamethasone sodium phosphate 4 mg/mL,
parabens, sodium bisulfite. Vial 5 mL,
10 mL, 30 mL. *Rx.*
Use: Corticosteroid.

Dexasone Injection. (Roberts) Dexamethasone sodium phosphate 4 mg/
mL. Vial 5 mL, 30 mL. *Rx.*
Use: Corticosteroid.

Dexasporin Ointment. (Bausch & Lomb)
Dexamethasone 0.1%, neomycin sul-
fate equivalent to 0.35% neomycin base
and 10,000 units polymyxin B sulfate.
Ophth. Oint. Tube 3.5 g. *Rx.*
Use: Steroid; anti-infective, ophthalmic.

Dexasporin Suspension. (Various Mfr.)
Dexamethasone 0.1%, neomycin sulfate equivalent to 0.35%, neomycin
base and 10,000 units polymyxin B sul-
fate/mL, hydroxypropyl methylcellulose,
polysorbate 20, benzalkonium chloride.
Drops. Bot. 5 mL. *Rx.*
Use: Anti-infective; corticosteroid, ophthalmic.

**Dexatrim Max Daytime Appetite Con-
trol.** (Chattem) Asian ginseng root
standardized extract 250 mg, Ca, caffeine 200 mg, Cr, epigallocatechin gallate 90 mg, vitamins B_1 15 mg, B_2
17 mg, B_3 20 mg, B_5 25 mg, B_6 10 mg,
B_{12} 60 mcg. Film-coated. ER Tab. 60s.
OTC.
Use: Dietary aid.

**Dexatrim Natural Caffeine Free
Caplets.** (Chattem) Chromium
250 mcg, heartleaf 120 mg, thermonu-
trient blend 100 mg, vanadium
100 mcg. Box. Blister pak 30s. *OTC.*
Use: Dietary aid.

•**dexbrompheniramine maleate.** (DEX-
brom-fen-IR-a-meen) *USP 34.*
Use: Antihistamine.
See: Ala-hist IR.
W/Acetaminophen, Phenylephrine Hydro-
chloride.
See: Sinadrin PE.
W/Dextromethorphan Hydrobromide,
Phenylephrine Hydrochloride.
See: Panatuss DXP.

Tussall.
Tussall-ER.
Y-Cof DM.
W/Pseudoephedrine Sulfate.
See: Drixoral Cold & Allergy.

dexbrompheniramine tannate.
W/Dextromethorphan Tannate, Phenyl-
ephrine Tannate, Pyrilamine Maleate.
See: Poly Tan DM.

•**dexchlorpheniramine maleate.** (DEX-
klor-fen-IR-a-meen) *USP 34.*
Use: Antihistamine, nonselective alkyl-
amine.
See: Polaramine.
Polaramine Repetabs.
W/Carbetapentane Citrate, Phenyl-
ephrine Hydrochloride.
See: Corzall-PE.
W/Codeine Phosphate, Phenylephrine
Hydrochloride.
See: Dexphen W/C.
W/Dextromethorphan Hydrobromide,
Phenylephrine Hydrochloride, Pyril-
amine Maleate.
See: P-Hist.
Resperal.
W/Methscopolamine Nitrate, Phenyl-
ephrine Hydrochloride.
See: Extendryl.
Dexphen M.
W/Methscopolamine Nitrate, Pseudo-
ephedrine Hydrochloride.
See: D-Hist D.
Histatab D.
W/Phenylephrine Hydrochloride.
See: NalDex.

dexchlorpheniramine maleate. (Morton
Grove) Dexchlorpheniramine maleate
2 mg/5 mL. Alcohol, orange flavor.
Syrup. 473 mL. *Rx.*
Use: Antihistamine.

dexchlorpheniramine maleate. (Various
Mfr.) Dexchlorpheniramine maleate
4 mg, 6 mg. ER Tab. Bot. 100s, 1000s.
Rx.
Use: Antihistamine, non-selective alkyl-
amine.

dexchlorpheniramine tannate.
W/Dextromethorphan Tannate, Phenyl-
ephrine Tannate.
See: Dextromethorphan Tannate,
Phenylephrine Tannate, Dexchlor-
pheniramine Tannate.
W/Dextromethorphan Tannate, Pseudo-
ephedrine Tannate.
See: Bromatan Plus.
Dur-Tann Forte.
Indamix DM.
W/Pseudoephedrine Tannate, Pyrilamine
Tannate.
See: Nalfrx.

•**dexclamol hydrochloride.** (DEX-clay-mahl) USAN.
Use: Hypnotic; sedative.

Dexcon-DM. (Cypress Pharmaceutical) Dextromethorphan HBr 20 mg, guaifenesin 100 mg, phenylephrine hydrochloride 10 mg per 5 mL. Sugar and alcohol free. Saccharin, sorbitol. Strawberry flavor. Syrup. 473 mL. *Rx.*
Use: Antitussive and expectorant combination.

Dexedrine Spansules. (Amedra) Dextroamphetamine sulfate 5 mg, 10 mg, 15 mg. Sugar spheres. ER. Cap. 100s. *c-II.*
Use: CNS stimulant, amphetamine.

•**dexelvucitabine.** (DEX-el-vue-SYE-tabeen) USAN.
Use: Antiretroviral.

•**dexetimide.** (dex-ETT-ih-mid) USAN.
Use: Anticholinergic; antiparkinsonian.

DexFerrum. (American Regent) Iron 50 mg/mL (as dextran). Inj. Single-dose vial. 1 mL, 2 mL. *Rx.*
Use: Hematinic, trace element.

DexFol. (Rising) Vitamin B$_1$ 1.5 mg, B$_2$ 1.5 mg, B$_3$ 20 mg, B$_5$ 10 mg, B$_6$ 50 mg, B$_{12}$ 1 mg, C 60 mg, FA 5 mg, biotin 300 mcg. Tab. 90s. *Rx.*
Use: Nutritional product.

Dex4 Glucose. (Can-Am Care) Glucose, lemon, orange, raspberry, grape flavors. Chew. Tab. Bot. 10s, 50s. *OTC.*
Use: Glucose-elevating agent.

Dex GG TR. (Boca Pharmacal) Dextromethorphan HBr 60 mg, guaifenesin 1000 mg. ER Tab. Bot. 100s. *Rx.*
Use: Upper respiratory combination, antitussive, expectorant.

•**dexibuprofen.** (dex-EYE-byoo-PRO-fen) USAN.
Use: Analgesic; anti-inflammatory.

•**dexibuprofen lysine.** (dex-EYE-byoo-PRO-fen LIE-seen) USAN.
Use: Analgesic (cyclooxygenase inhibitor); anti-inflammatory.

Dexilant. (Takeda Pharmaceuticals America) Dexlansoprazole 30 mg, 60 mg. PEG, sucrose, sugar spheres. Cap., delayed release. 30s, 90s, 1,000s, UD 100s. *Rx.*
Use: GI agent, proton pump inhibitor.

•**deximafen.** (dex-IH-mah-fen) USAN.
Use: Antidepressant.

•**dexivacaine.** (dex-IH-vah-CANE) USAN.
Use: Anesthetic.

•**dexlansoprazole.** (dex-lan-SOE-prazole) USAN.
Use: Gastrointestinal agent.
See: Dexilant.

•**dexmedetomidine.** (DEX-meh-dih-TOE-mih-deen) USAN.
Use: Anxiolytic.

•**dexmedetomidine hydrochloride.** (DEX-meh-dih-TOE-mih-deen)
Use: Sedative/hypnotic, nonbarbiturate.
See: Precedex.

•**dexmethylphenidate hydrochloride.** (dex-meth-il-FEN-i-date) USAN.
Use: Central nervous system stimulant.
See: Focalin.
Focalin XR.

dexmethylphenidate hydrochloride. (Teva) Dexmethylphenidate hydrochloride 2.5 mg, 5 mg, 10 mg. Lactose. Tab. 100s. *c-II.*
Use: Central nervous system stimulant.

Dexodryl. (Dexo Pharma) **Chew Tab.:** Chlorpheniramine maleate (as chlorpheniramine tannate) 2 mg, methscopolamine nitrate 1.5 mg. Saccharin, sugar. 100s. **Susp.:** Chlorpheniramine maleate (as chlorpheniramine tannate) 2 mg, methscopolamine nitrate 1.5 mg per 5 mL. Parabens, sucralose. 118 mL. *Rx.*
Use: Upper respiratory combination, decongestant, antihistamine, and anticholinergic combination.

Dexone. (Keene Pharmaceuticals) Dexamethasone sodium phosphate 4 mg/mL. Sodium sulfate, benzyl alcohol. Inj. Vial 5 mL, 10 mL. *Rx.*
Use: Glucocorticoid.

•**dexormaplatin.** (DEX-ore-mah-PLAT-in) USAN.
Use: Antineoplastic.

•**dexoxadrol hydrochloride.** (dex-OX-ah-drole) USAN.
Use: Antidepressant; stimulant (central); analgesic.

DexPak Jr. 10 Day TaperPak. (ECR) Dexamethasone 1.5 mg. Lactose. Tab. 10-day pack. 35s. *Rx.*
Use: Adrenocortical steroid, glucocorticoid.

DexPak 6 Day TaperPak. (ECR) Dexamethasone 1.5 mg. Lactose. Tab. 6-day pack. 21s. *Rx.*
Use: Adrenocortical steroid, glucocorticoid.

DexPak TaperPak. (ECR) Dexamethasone 1.5 mg. Tab. 51s. *Rx.*
Use: Adrenocortical steroid, glucocorticoid.

DexPak 13 Day TaperPak. (ECR) Dexamethasone 1.5 mg. Lactose. Tab. 13-day pack. 51s. *Rx.*
Use: Adrenocortical steroid, glucocorticoid.

•**dexpanthenol.** (DEX-PAN-theh-nahl)
USP 34.
Use: Treatment of paralytic ileus and
postoperative distention; cholinergic.
See: Ilopan.
Panthoderm.

•**dexpemedolac.** (dex-peh-MED-oh-lack)
USAN.
Use: Analgesic.

Dexphen M. (Boca Pharmacal) Dexchlorpheniramine maleate 1 mg, methscopolamine nitrate 1.25 mg, phenylephrine hydrochloride 10 mg per 5 mL.
Sorbitol. Root beer flavor. Oral Soln.
473 mL. *Rx.*
Use: Upper respiratory combination, decongestant, antihistamine, and anticholinergic combination.

Dexphen w/C. (Breckenridge) Codeine
phosphate 10 mg, dexchlorpheniramine
maleate 1 mg, phenylephrine hydrochloride 5 mg per 5 mL. Grape flavoring, propylene glycol, saccharin, sodium
benzoate, sorbitol. Alcohol free, dye
free, gluten free, and sugar free. Liq.
473 mL. *c-v.*
Use: Upper respiratory combination, antitussive combination.

•**dexpramipexole.** (DEX-pram-i-PEX-ole)
USAN.
Use: Treatment of amyotrophic lateral
sclerosis.

•**dexpramipexole dihydrochloride.**
(DEX-pram-i-PEX-ole) USAN.
Use: Treatment of amyotrophic lateral
sclerosis.

•**dexpropanolol hydrochloride.** (DEX-
pro-PRAN-oh-lole) USAN.
Use: Antiadrenergic (β-receptor); cardiovascular agent (antiarrhythmic).

•**dexrazoxane.** (dex-ray-ZOX-ane) USAN.
Use: Cytoprotective agent.
See: Totect.
Zinecard

dexrazoxane. (Bedford) Dexrazoxane
(as dexrazoxane hydrochloride)
250 mg, 500 mg. Pow. for Soln., Inj.,
lyophilized. Single-use vials with 25 mL
sodium lactate injection (250 mg) or
50 mL sodium lactate injection
(500 mg). *Rx.*
Use: Cytoprotective agent.

•**dexsotalol hydrochloride.** (dex-SOE-ta-
lol) USAN.
Use: Cardiovascular agent (antiarrhythmic).

•**dextofisopam.** (dex-toe-FIS-oh-pam)
USAN.
Use: Crohn disease

dextran adjunct. *Rx.*
Use: Plasma expander.
See: Promit.

dextran and deferoxamine.
Use: Acute iron poisoning. [Orphan
Drug]
See: Bio-Rescue.

•**dextran 40.** (DEX-tran 40) USAN. Polysaccharide (m.w. 40,000) produced by
the action of *Leuconostoc mesenteroides* on sucrose.
Use: Blood flow adjuvant; plasma volume extender.
See: 10% LMD.
Gentran 40.
Rheomacrodex.

dextran 40. (McGaw) Dextran 40 10%
with 0.9% sodium chloride or in 5%
dextrose. Inj. 500 mL. *Rx.*
Use: Plasma expander.

dextran 45, 75. Polysaccharide (m.w.
45,000, 75,000) produced by the action
of *Leuconostoc mesenteroides* on sac-
charose. Rheotran (45). *Rx.*
Use: Blood volume expander.

•**dextran 1.** (DEX-tran 1) *USP 34.*
Use: Plasma volume extender.

•**dextran 70.** (DEX-tran 70) USAN. Poly-
saccharide (m.w. 70,000) produced by
the action of *Levconostoc mesenteroi-
des* on sucrose.
Use: Plasma volume extender.
See: Gentran 70.
Hyskon.
Macrodex.

dextran 70. (McGaw) Dextran 70 6% in
0.9% sodium chloride. Inj. 500 mL. *Rx.*
Use: Plasma expander.

•**dextran 75.** (DEX-tran 75) USAN. Polysaccharide (m.w. 75,000) produced by
the action of *Leuconostoc mesenteroides* on sucrose.
Use: Plasma volume extender.
See: Macrodex.

dextran 6%. (Abbott) *Rx.*
See: Dextran 75.

dextran sulfate, inhaled aerosolized.
Use: Antiviral. [Orphan Drug]
See: Uendex.

dextran sulfate sodium. (Ueno Fine
Chemicals Industry)
Use: AIDS drug. [Orphan Drug]

•**dextrates.** (DEX-traytz) *NF 29.* Mixture
of sugars (≈ 92% dextrose monohydrate and 8% higher saccharides;
dextrose equivalent is 95% to 97%) resulting from the controlled enzymatic
hydrolysis of starch.
Use: Pharmaceutic aid (tablet binder, diluent).

•**dextrin.** *NF 29.*
  Use: Pharmaceutic aid (suspending, viscosity-increasing agent; tablet binder; tablet, capsule diluent).
•**dextroamphetamine.** (DEX-troe-am-FET-ah-meen) USAN.
  Use: Stimulant (central).
dextroamphetamine. (Various Mfr.) Dextroamphetamine sulfate. **Tab:** 5 mg, 10 mg. May contain sucrose. Bot. 100s. **ER Cap:** 5 mg, 10 mg, 15 mg. May contain sucrose. Bot. 100s. *c-II.*
  Use: CNS stimulant, amphetamine.
dextroamphetamine phosphate. Monobasic d-a-methylphenethlyamine phosphate. (+)-α-Methylphenethylamine phosphate.
  Use: CNS stimulant.
dextroamphetamine saccharate.
  Use: CNS stimulant.
  W/Combinations.
  See: Adderall.
    Adderall XR.
dextroamphetamine saccharate/ amphetamine aspartate/dextro- amphetamine sulfate/amphetamine sulfate. (Barr) Dextroamphetamine saccharate/amphetamine aspartate/ dextroamphetamine sulfate/amphet- amine sulfate 5 mg (1.25 mg/1.25 mg/ 1.25 mg/1.25 mg), 10 mg (2.5 mg/ 2.5 mg/2.5 mg/2.5 mg), 15 mg (3.75 mg/ 3.75 mg/3.75 mg/3.75 mg), 20 mg (5 mg/5 mg/5 mg/5 mg), 25 mg (6.25 mg/6.25 mg/6.25 mg/6.25 mg), 30 mg (7.5 mg/7.5 mg/7.5 mg/7.5 mg). ER Cap. 100s. c-ii.
  Use: Amphetamine mixture.
•**dextroamphetamine sulfate.** (DEX-troe-am-FET-uh-meen) *USP 34.*
  Use: CNS stimulant, amphetamine.
  See: Dexedrine Spansules.
    Dextrostat.
    ProCentra.
  W/Combinations.
  See: Adderall.
    Adderall XR.
Dextro-Chek Normal Control. (Bayer Consumer Care) Clear liquid containing measured amount of glucose 0.1%.
  Use: Glucometer calibration aid.
Dextro-Chek Calibrators. (Bayer Consumer Care) Clear liquid soln. containing measured amounts of glucose. Low calibrator contains 0.05% w/v glucose. High calibrator contains 0.3% w/v glucose.
  Use: Glucometer calibration aid.
Dextro-Chlorpheniramine Maleate.
  Use: Antihistamine.
  See: Polaramine.

•**dextromethorphan.** (DEX-troe-meth-OR-fan) *USP 34.*
  Use: Cough suppressant; antitussive.
  W/Combinations.
  See: DMax Pediatric.
•**dextromethorphan hydrobromide.** (DEX-troe-meth-OR-fan) *USP 34.*
  Use: Antitussive.
  See: AeroTuss 12.
    Buckley's Cough.
    Creomulsion Adult Formula.
    Creomulsion for Children.
    Creo-Terpin.
    Delsym.
    DexAlone.
    ElixSure Children's Cough.
    Hold DM.
    Little Colds Cough Formula.
    PediaCare Children's Long-Acting Cough.
    Robitussin Cough Gels.
    Robitussin Pediatric Cough.
    Scot-Tussin DM Cough Chasers.
    Silphen DM.
    Simply Cough.
    Sucrets DM.
    Sucrets DM Cough Formula.
    Sucrets DM Cough Suppressant.
    Theraflu Thin Strips Long Acting Cough.
    Triaminic Long Acting Cough.
    Trocal.
    Vicks 44 Cough Relief.
  W/Acetaminophen.
  See: Triaminic Cough & Sore Throat.
    Tylenol Cough & Sore Throat Daytime.
    Tylenol Plus Children's Cough & Sore Throat.
  W/Acetaminophen, Chlorpheniramine Maleate.
  See: Coricidin HBP Maximum Strength Flu.
    Triaminic Flu, Cough & Fever.
    Tylenol Plus Children's Cough & Runny Nose.
    Vicks Formula 44M Cough, Cold, & Flu Relief.
  W/Acetaminophen, Chlorpheniramine Maleate, Phenylephrine Hydrochloride.
  See: Alka-Seltzer Plus Cold & Cough.
    Theraflu Nighttime Severe Cold.
  W/Acetaminophen, Diphenhydramine.
  See: Diabetic Tussin Cold & Flu.
    Diabetic Tussin Night Time Formula Cold/Flu.
  W/Acetaminophen, Diphenhydramine Hydrochloride, Phenylephrine Hydrochloride.
  See: Respa C & C.

W/Acetaminophen, Doxylamine Succinate.
See: Tylenol Cough & Sore Throat
Nighttime.
Vicks NyQuil Cold/Flu Relief.
W/Acetaminophen, Doxylamine Succinate, Phenylephrine Hydrochloride.
See: Alka-Seltzer Plus Day & Night
Cold.
Alka-Seltzer Plus Night Cold.
Tylenol Cold Multi-Symptom Nighttime.
W/Acetaminophen, Doxylamine Succinate, Pseudoephedrine Hydrochloride.
See: All-Nite.
W/Acetaminophen, Guaifenesin.
See: Comtrex Multi-Symptom Deep
Chest Cold.
Phenflu G.
Sine-Off Cough/Cold.
Sudafed PE Multi-Symptom Cold and
Cough.
W/Acetaminophen, Guaifenesin, Pseudoephedrine Hydrochloride.
See: Duraflu.
Flutabs.
Maxiflu DM.
Maxiflu G.
Tylenol Cold Severe Congestion.
W/Acetaminophen, Phenylephrine Hydrochloride.
See: Alka-Seltzer Plus Day & Night
Cold.
Alka-Seltzer Plus Day Cold.
Alka-Seltzer Plus Day Non-Drowsy
Cold.
Comtrex Maximum Strength Day &
Night Cold & Cough.
Mapap Cold Formula Multi-Symptom.
Theraflu Daytime Severe Cold &
Cough.
Theraflu Warming Relief Daytime
Multi-Symptom Cold.
Tylenol Cold Head Congestion Daytime.
Tylenol Cold Multi-Symptom Daytime.
Vicks DayQuil Multi-Symptom Cold/
Flu Relief.
W/Acetaminophen, Pseudoephedrine
Hydrochloride.
See: 666 Cold Preparation Maximum
Strength.
W/Aspirin, Chlorpheniramine Maleate.
See: Alka-Seltzer Plus Flu.
W/Aspirin, Doxylamine Succinate,
Phenylephrine Bitartrate.
See: Alka-Seltzer Plus Day & Night
Cold.
Alka-Seltzer Plus Night Cold.
W/Aspirin, Phenylephrine Bitartrate.
See: Alka-Seltzer Plus Day & Night
Cold.

W/Benzocaine.
See: Cēpacol Sore Throat Plus Cough
Relief.
W/Brompheniramine Maleate, Guaifenesin, Phenylephrine Hydrochloride.
See: AccuHist PDX.
Bromhist-PDX.
W/Brompheniramine Maleate, Guaifenesin, Pseudoephedrine Hydrochloride.
See: Bromhist DM Pediatric.
Histacol DM Pediatric.
Pediahist DM.
W/Brompheniramine Maleate, Phenylephrine Hydrochloride.
See: Alahist DM.
Balacall DM.
BPM PE DM.
BROM/PE/DM.
BröveX PB DM.
BröveX PEB DM.
Children's Dimaphen DM.
LoHist-DM.
Phenylephrine Complex.
TGQ 7.5PEH/4BRM/15DM.
TL-Hist DM.
Tusdec-DM.
W/Brompheniramine Maleate, Pseudoephedrine Hydrochloride.
See: AccuHist DM Pediatric.
Anaplex-DM Cough.
Bromaline DM.
Bromdex D.
Brometane-DX Cough.
Bromfed DM.
Bromhist-DM.
Bromhist PDX.
Bromphenex DM.
Brotapp DM.
BröveX PSB.
BröveX PSB DM.
Dallergy DM.
Dimaphen DM Cough, Cold & Allergy.
Dimetane DX.
DM/PSE/BPM.
Myphetane DX Cough.
Neo DM.
PBM Allergy.
Pediahist DM.
Prohist DM.
PSE Brom DM.
Q-Tapp DM Cold and Cough.
Sildec-DM.
TGQ 50PSE/3BRM/30DM.
TGQ 40PSE/4BRM/20DM.
TGQ 30PSE/3BRM/15DM.
W/Carbinoxamine Maleate, Phenylephrine Hydrochloride.
See: TriTuss-A.
W/Carbinoxamine Maleate, Pseudoephedrine Hydrochloride.
See: Cordron-DM.

W/Chlorpheniramine Maleate.
  See: AMBI 20DM/4CPM.
    Coricidin HBP Cough & Cold.
    Dimetapp Long Acting Cough Plus
     Cold.
    Robitussin Pediatric Cough & Cold
     Long Acting.
    Scot-Tussin DM.
    Triaminic Cough & Runny Nose.
    Tricodene Sugar Free Cough & Cold.
    Vicks Formula 44m Pediatric Cough
     & Cold Relief.
    Vicks Children's NyQuil Cold & Cough
     Relief.
W/Chlorpheniramine Maleate, Guaifene-
  sin, Phenylephrine Hydrochloride.
  See: Chlordex GP.
    DM/CPM/PE/GG.
    Donatussin.
    Genelan-NF.
W/Chlorpheniramine Maleate, Meth-
  scopolamine Nitrate.
  See: Extendryl DM.
W/Chlorpheniramine Maleate, Phenyl-
  ephrine Hydrochloride.
  See: AMBI 10PEH/4CPM/20DM.
    Amerituss AD.
    Bronkids.
    Centergy DM.
    Ceron-DM.
    Corfen-DM.
    CP DEC-DM.
    C-Phen DM.
    DM/PE/CPM.
    Donatussin DM.
    Ed-A-Hist DM.
    Father John's Medicine Plus.
    Maxichlor PEH DM.
    Nasohist DM.
    Neo DM.
    NoHist DMX.
    NoHist-PDX.
    P Chlor DM.
    PE-Hist DM.
    Phenabid DM.
    Relahist-DM.
    Rondec-DM.
    Rondex-DM.
    Sonahist DM.
    TGQ 15DM/5PEH/2CPM.
    Trigofen DM.
    Trital DM.
    Z-Dex 12D.
    ZoDen DM.
W/Chlorpheniramine Maleate, Pseudo-
  ephedrine Hydrochloride.
  See: AccuHist PDX.
    Allres DS.
    AMBI 60PSE/4CPM/20DM.
    CPM/PSE DM.
    Dicel DM.

    Esocor P.
    KidKare Children's Cough/Cold.
    Mesehist DM.
    Neutrahist PDX.
    Pedia Relief Cough-Cold.
    Pediatric Cough & Cold.
    Pediatric Cough & Cold Medicine.
    Rescon DM.
    Triaminic-D Children's.
W/Dexbrompheniramine Maleate,
  Phenylephrine Hydrochloride.
  See: Panatuss DXP.
    Tussall.
    Tussall-ER.
    Y-Cof DM.
W/Dexchlorpheniramine Maleate, Phenyl-
  ephrine Hydrochloride, Pyrilamine
  Maleate.
  See: P-Hist.
    Resperal.
W/Diphenhydramine Tannate, Phenyl-
  ephrine Tannate.
  See: Duratuss AC.
W/Doxylamine Succinate.
  See: Vicks NyQuil Cough.
W/Doxylamine Succinate, Pseudoephed-
  rine Hydrochloride.
  See: Lortuss DM.
W/Guaifenesin.
  See: Alka-Seltzer Plus Mucus & Con-
    gestion.
    AMBI 1000/55.
    Bidex-A.
    Biospec DMX.
    Cheracol D Cough Formula.
    Cheracol Plus.
    Congesta DM.
    Coricidin HBP Chest Congestion &
     Cough.
    Dex-Tuss DM.
    Diabetic Tussin DM.
    Diabetic Tussin Maximum Strength
     DM.
    Extra Action Cough.
    Fenesin DM IR.
    Gan-Tuss DM NR.
    Genatuss DM.
    Geri-Tussin DM.
    GFN 1000/DM 60.
    GFN 1200/DM 60.
    GUAI 800 mg/DM 30 mg.
    Guaifenesin DM.
    Guaifenesin-DM NR.
    Guaifenesin DM 1000/60.
    Guaifenex DM.
    Guiatuss DM.
    Iobid DM.
    Iophen DM-NR.
    Kolephrin GG/DM.
    Mucinex Cough for Kids.
    Mucinex Cough Mini-Melts for Kids.

Mucinex DM Maximum Strength.
MucusRelief DM.
Mucinex DM.
NeoTuss.
Respa-DM.
Robafen DM Max.
Robitussin Cough & Congestion.
Robitussin Cough DM.
Robitussin Cough Sugar-Free DM.
Robitussin-DM.
Safe Tussin DM.
Scot-Tussin Senior Clear.
Siltussin-DM.
Touro DM.
TUSSI-bid.
Tussi-Organidin DM-S NR.
Vicks 44E Cough & Chest Congestion Relief.
Vicks Formula 44e Pediatric Cough & Chest Congestion Relief.
Zotex-EX.
W/Guaifenesin, Phenylephrine Hydrochloride.
　See: AMBI 10PEH/400GFN/20DM.
　Biobron SF.
　Biogil.
　BioGtuss.
　Bio T Pres.
　Bio T Pres Pediatric.
　Biotuss.
　Bio-Tussi.
　Broncotron-D.
　Brontuss DX.
　Dacex DM.
　Dacex PE.
　Deconex DM.
　Deconex DMX.
　Despec NR.
　Dynatuss EX.
　Endacon.
　ExeCof.
　ExeTuss-DM.
　GFN 1200/DM 20/PE 40.
　Giltuss.
　Giltuss Pediatric.
　Giltuss TR.
　Guaifen.
　Maxiphen DM.
　NeoTuss-D.
　Phlemex Forte.
　Phlemex-PE.
　Robitussin Children's Cough & Cold CF.
　Robitussin Pediatric Cough/Cold CF.
　SINUtuss DM.
　TriTuss.
　TriTuss ER.
　Tussi-Pres.
　Tussi-Pres Pediatric.
　Tusso DM.
　Tusso DMR.

Tusso XR.
Z-Dex.
Z-Dex Pediatric.
Zotex.
Zotex-D.
Zotex Pediatric.
W/Guaifenesin, Potassium Citrate
　See: Sorbutuss NR.
W/Guaifenesin, Pseudoephedrine Hydrochloride.
　See: Aldex GS DM.
　Ambifed-G DM.
　AMBI 40PSE/400GFN/20DM.
　AMBI 60/580/30.
　AMBI 60PSE/400GFN/20DM.
　Bionel.
　Bionel Pediatric.
　Capmist DM.
　Despec.
　Donatussin DM.
　ExeFen DMX.
　GFN 600/PSE 60/DM 30.
　Liquicough DM.
　Maxifed DM.
　Maxifed DMX.
　Medent-DMI.
　Poly-Vent DM.
　Pseudo Cough.
　Q-Tussin CF.
　Relacon DM NR.
　Relasin DM.
　Robafen CF.
　Robitussin Cough & Cold D.
　Sudafed Multi-Symptom Cold & Cough.
　TGQ 30PSE/150GFN/15DM.
　Tidafen DM.
　TL-DEX DM.
　Touro CC-LD.
　Tusnel.
　Tusnel-DM Pediatric.
　Tusnel Pediatric.
　Z-Cof DMX.
　Z-Cof 8 DM.
　Z-Cof I.
W/Pheniramine Maleate, Phenylephrine Hydrochloride.
　See: Theraflu Cold & Cough.
W/Phenylephrine Hydrochloride.
　See: Dimetapp Toddler's Decongestant Plus Cough.
　Little Colds Decongestant Plus Cough.
　PediaCare Children's Multi-Symptom Cold.
　Safetussin CD.
　Theraflu Thin Strips Daytime Cough & Cold.
　Triaminic Children's Thin Strips Day Time Cold & Cough.
　Triaminic Daytime Cold & Cough.

Vicks Formula 44D Cough & Head
Congestion Relief.
W/Phenylephrine Hydrochloride, Pyril-
amine Maleate.
See: Albutussin.
Aldex DM Tannate.
Codal-DM.
Codimal DM.
MyHist-DM.
Poly Hist DM.
Pyril DM.
Reme Hist DM.
Triplex DM.
W/Potassium Guaiacolsulfonate.
See: Prolex DM.
Prolex DMX.
W/Promethazine Hydrochloride.
See: Promethazine w/Dextromethor-
phan Cough.
W/Pseudoephedrine Hydrochloride, Pyril-
amine Maleate.
See: Viravan-PDM.
**dextromethorphan hydrobromide/
benzocaine.**
Use: Nonnarcotic antitussive.
See: Cēpacol Ultra Sore Throat Plus
Cough.
Cough-X.
Tetra Formula.
**dextromethorphan hydrobromide/
guaifenesin.** (URL) Dextromethorphan
HBr 30 mg, guaifenesin 500 mg. Dye-
free. ER Tab. 100s. *Rx.*
Use: Antitussive with expectorant, upper respiratory combination.
**dextromethorphan hydrobromide,
pseudoephedrine hydrochloride,
chlorpheniramine maleate 30-30-
4 mg tannate.** (Acella Pharmaceuticals) Chlorpheniramine maleate 4 mg,
dextromethorphan hydrobromide
30 mg, pseudoephedrine hydrochloride
30 mg per 5 mL. Parabens, saccharin. Grape bubble gum flavor. Susp.
473 mL. *Rx.*
Use: Upper respiratory combination, antitussive combination.
•**dextromethorphan polistirex.** (DEX-
troe-meth-OR-fan pahl-ee-STIE-rex)
USAN.
Use: Antitussive.
W/Combinations.
See: Atuss-12 DM.
Atuss-12 DX.
dextromethorphan tannate.
Use: Antitussive.
W/Brompheniramine Tannate, Phenylephrine Tannate.
See: Dur-Tan DM.
Neo DM.

W/Chlorpheniramine Tannate, Pseudo-
ephedrine Tannate.
See: Atuss DS Tannate.
W/Combinations.
See: TanaCof-DM.
Tanafed DMX.
Viravan-DM.
W/Dexbrompheniramine Tannate,
Phenylephrine Tannate, Pyrilamine
Maleate.
See: Poly Tan DM.
W/Dexchlorpheniramine Tannate,
Pseudoephedrine Tannate.
See: Atuss DS Tannate.
Bromatan Plus.
Dur-Tann Forte.
Indamix DM.
W/Diphenhydramine Tannate, Phenyl-
ephrine Tannate.
See: D-Tann DM.
W/Guaifenesin, Pseudoephedrine Tan-
nate.
See: Z-Cof 12 DM.
W/Phenylephrine Tannate, Pyrilamine
Tannate.
See: AllanVan-DM B.I.D.
ViraTan-DM B.I.D.
**dextromethorphan tannate, phenyl-
ephrine tannate, dexchlorphenir-
amine tannate.** (River's Edge)
Dexchlorpheniramine tannate 2 mg,
dextromethorphan tannate 30 mg,
phenylephrine tannate 20 mg per 5 mL.
Saccharin. Alcohol free and sugar free.
Cotton candy or strawberry flavor.
Susp., Oral. 473 mL. *Rx.*
Use: Upper respiratory combination, antitussive combination.
**dextromethorphan tannate, phenyl-
ephrine tannate, pyrilamine tannate.**
(River's Edge) Dextromethorphan tannate 25 mg, phenylephrine tannate
15.5 mg, pyrilamine tannate 15.5 mg
per 5 mL. Saccharin. Alcohol free and
sugar free. Cherry flavor. Susp., Oral.
473 mL. *Rx.*
Use: Upper respiratory combination, antitussive combination.
dextromoramide tartrate.
Use: Analgesic; narcotic.
dextro-pantothenyl alcohol.
See: Ilopan.
Panthenol.
dextropropoxyphene hydrochloride.
Use: Analgesic.
See: Propoxyphene Hydrochloride.
•**dextrorphan hydrochloride.** (DEX-trore-
fan) USAN.
Use: Treatment of cerebral ischemia;
vasospastic therapy adjunct.

•**dextrose.** (DEX-trose) *USP 34.*
Use: Fluid and nutrient replenisher.
W/Fructose, Phosphoric Acid.
See: Emetrol.
Nausatrol.
Nausea Relief.
Nausetrol.
dextrose-alcohol injection. *Rx.*
Use: Nutritional supplement, parenteral.
See: 5% Alcohol and 5% Dextrose in
Water.
dextrose and Isolyte combinations.
Use: Intravenous nutritional therapy,
intravenous replenishment solution.
See: Isolyte M in 5% Dextrose.
Isolyte H in 5% Dextrose.
Isolyte P in 5% Dextrose.
Isolyte S with 5% Dextrose.
Isolyte R in 5% Dextrose.
dextrose and Normosol combinations.
Use: Intravenous nutritional therapy,
intravenous replenishment solution.
See: Normosol-M and 5% Dextrose.
Normosol-R and 5% Dextrose.
dextrose and Plasmalyte combinations.
Use: Intravenous nutritional therapy,
intravenous replenishment solution.
See: Plasma-Lyte 56 and 5% Dextrose.
Plasma-Lyte M and 5% Dextrose.
Plasma-Lyte 148 and 5% Dextrose.
Plasma-Lyte R and 5% Dextrose.
dextrose and Ringer's combinations.
Use: Intravenous nutritional therapy,
intravenous replenishment solution.
See: Half-Strength Lactated Ringer's in
2.5% Dextrose.
Lactated Ringer's in 5% Dextrose.
Ringer's in 5% Dextrose.
dextrose-electrolyte solutions. *Rx.*
Use: Intravenous nutritional therapy,
intravenous replenishment solutions.
See: Dextrose 2.5% with 0.45% Sodium
Chloride.
Dextrose 3.3% and 0.3% Sodium
Chloride.
Dextrose 5% and Electrolyte No. 48.
Dextrose 5% and Electrolyte No. 75.
Dextrose 5% with 0.2% Sodium
Chloride.
Dextrose 5% and 0.225% Sodium
Chloride.
Dextrose 5% with 0.3% Sodium
Chloride.
Dextrose 5% with 0.33% Sodium
Chloride.
Dextrose 5% with 0.45% Sodium
Chloride.
Dextrose 5% with 0.9% Sodium
Chloride.
Dextrose 10% and Electrolyte No. 48.

Dextrose 10% with 0.2% Sodium
Chloride.
Dextrose 10% with 0.225% Sodium
Chloride.
Dextrose 10% with 0.45 Sodium
Chloride.
Dextrose 10% and 0.9% Sodium
Chloride.
Dianeal Low Calcium w/4.25% Dextrose.
Dianeal Low Calcium w/1.5% Dextrose.
Dianeal Low Calcium w/2.5% Dextrose.
Dianeal PD-2 w/4.25% Dextrose.
Dianeal PD-2 w/1.5% Dextrose.
Dianeal PD-2 w/3.5% Dextrose.
Dianeal PD-2 w/2.5% Dextrose.
Half-Strength Lactated Ringer's in
2.5% Dextrose.
Ionosol B and 5% Dextrose.
Ionosol-T and 5% Dextrose.
Isolyte H in 5% Dextrose.
Isolyte M in 5% Dextrose.
Isolyte P in 5% Dextrose.
Isolyte R in 5% Dextrose.
Isolyte S with 5% Dextrose.
Lactated Ringer's in 5%% Dextrose.
Normosol-M and 5%% Dextrose.
Normosol-R and 5% Dextrose.
Plasma-Lyte 56 and 5% Dextrose.
Plasma-Lyte M and 5% Dextrose.
Plasma-Lyte 148 and 5% Dextrose.
Plasma-Lyte R and 5% Dextrose.
Potassium Chloride in 5% Dextrose
and Lactated Ringer's.
Potassium Chloride in 5% Dextrose.
Potassium Chloride in 3.3% Dextrose
and 0.3% Sodium Chloride.
Potassium Chloride in 5% Dextrose
and 0.2% Sodium Chloride.
Potassium Chloride in 5% Dextrose
and 0.33% Sodium Chloride.
Potassium Chloride in 5% Dextrose
and 0.45% Sodium Chloride.
Potassium Chloride in 5% Dextrose
and 0.9% Sodium Chloride.
Potassium Chloride in 10% Dextrose
and 0.2% Sodium Chloride.
Ringer's in 5% Dextrose.
UltraBag Dianeal PD-2 w/4.25% Dextrose.
UltraBag Dianeal PD-2 w/1.5% Dextrose.
UltraBag Dianeal PD-2 w/2.5% Dextrose.
•**dextrose excipient.** (DEX-trose) *NF 29.*
Use: Pharmaceutic aid (tablet excipient).
dextrose 5% and electrolyte No. 48.
(Baxter PPI) Dextrose 50 g, calories

180/L with Na$^+$ 25 mEq, K$^+$ 20 mEq, Mg^{++} 3 mEq, Cl$^-$ 24 mEq, phosphate 3 mEq, acetate 23 mEq with osmolarity 348 mOsm/L. Soln. Bot. 250 mL. *Rx.*
Use: Intravenous nutritional therapy, intravenous replenishment.

dextrose 5% and electrolyte No. 75.
(Baxter PPI) Dextrose 50 g, calories 180/L with Na$^+$ 40 mEq, K$^+$ 35 mEq, Cl$^-$ 48 mEq, phosphate 15 mEq, and lactate 20 mEq with osmolarity 402 mOsm/L. Soln. Bot. 250 mL, 500 mL, 1000 mL. *Rx.*
Use: Intravenous nutritional therapy, intravenous replenishment.

dextrose 5% and lactated ringer's and potassium chloride.
Use: Intravenous nutritional therapy, intravenous replenishment solution.
See: Potassium Chloride in 5% Dextrose and Lactated Ringer's.

dextrose 5% and potassium chloride.
Use: Intravenous nutritional therapy, intravenous replenishment solution.
See: Potassium Chloride in 5% Dextrose.

dextrose 5% and sodium chloride 0.45% and potassium chloride.
Use: Intravenous nutritional therapy, intravenous replenishment solution.
See: Potassium Chloride in 5% Dextrose and 0.45% Sodium Chloride.

dextrose 5% and sodium chloride 0.9% and potassium chloride.
Use: Intravenous nutritional therapy, intravenous replenishment solution.
See: Potassium Chloride in 5% Dextrose and 0.9% Sodium Chloride.

dextrose 5% and sodium chloride 0.33% and potassium chloride.
Use: Intravenous nutritional therapy, intravenous replenishment solution.
See: Potassium Chloride in 5% Dextrose and 0.33% Sodium Chloride.

dextrose 5% and sodium chloride 0.2% and potassium chloride.
Use: Intravenous nutritional therapy, intravenous replenishment solution.
See: Potassium Chloride in 5% Dextrose and 0.2% Sodium Chloride.

dextrose 5% and 0.225% sodium chloride. (Abbott) Dextrose 50 g, calories 170/L, Na $^+$ 38.5 mEq, Cl$^-$ 38.5 mEq, osmolarity 329 mOsm/L. Soln. Bot. 250 mL, 500 mL, 1000 mL. *Rx.*
Use: Intravenous nutritional therapy, intravenous replenishment solution.

dextrose 5% with 0.45% sodium chloride. (Various Mfr.) Dextrose 50 g, calories 170/L, Na$^+$ 77 mEq, Cl$^-$ 77 mEq, osmolarity ≈ 405 mOsm/L. Soln. Bot.

250 mL, 500 mL, 1000 mL. *Rx.*
Use: Intravenous nutritional therapy, intravenous replenishment solution.

dextrose 5% with 0.9% sodium chloride. (Various Mfr.) Dextrose 50 g, calories 170/L, Na$^+$ 154 mEq, Cl$^-$ 154 mEq, osmolarity ≈ 560 mOsm/L. Soln. Bot. 250 mL, 500 mL, 1000 mL. *Rx.*
Use: Intravenous nutritional therapy, intravenous replenishment solution.

dextrose 5% with 0.3% sodium chloride. (Abbott) Dextrose 50 g, calories 170/L, Na$^+$ 51 mEq, Cl$^-$ 51 mEq, osmolarity 355 mOsm/L. Soln. Bot. 250 mL, 500 mL, 1000 mL. *Rx.*
Use: Intravenous nutritional therapy, intravenous replenishment solution.

dextrose 5% with 0.33% sodium chloride. (Various Mfr.) Dextrose 50 g, calories 170/L, Na$^+$ 56 mEq, Cl$^-$ 56 mEq, osmolarity 365 mOsm/L. Soln. Bot. 250 mL, 500 mL, 1000 mL. *Rx.*
Use: Intravenous nutritional therapy, intravenous replenishment solution.

dextrose 5% with 0.2% sodium chloride. (Various Mfr.) Dextrose 50 g, calories 170/L, Na$^+$ 34 mEq, Cl$^-$ 34 mEq, osmolarity ≈ 320 mOsm/L. Soln. Bot. 250 mL, 500 mL, 1000 ML. *Rx.*
Use: Intravenous nutritional therapy, intravenous replenishment solution.

dextrose large volume parenterals.
(Abbott Hospital Products) *Rx.*
Use: Nutritional supplement, parenteral.

dextrose small volume parenterals.
(Abbott Hospital Products) **Dextrose 5%:** 50 mL, 100 mL pressurized pintop vial. **Dextrose 10%:** 5 mL amp. **Dextrose 25%:** 10 mL syringe. **Dextrose 50%:** 50 mL Abboject syringe (18 g × 1.5″), 50 mL Fliptop vial. **Dextrose 70%:** 70 mL pressurized pintop vial. *Rx.*
Use: Nutritional supplement, parenteral.

dextrose-sodium chloride injection.
(Abbott) 10% dextrose and 0.225% sodium chloride. Inj. Single-dose container. 500 mL.
Use: Nutritional supplement, parenteral.

dextrose 10% and electrolyte no. 48.
(Baxter Healthcare) Dextrose 100 g, calories 350/L, Na$^+$ 25 mEq, K$^+$ 20 mEq, Mg^{++} 3 mEq, Cl$^-$ 24 mEq, phosphate 3 mEq, lactate 23 mEq, osmolarity 600 mOsm/L, sodium bisulfite Soln. Bot. 250 mL. *Rx.*
Use: Intravenous nutritional therapy, intravenous replenishment solution.

dextrose 10% and 0.9% sodium chloride. (Various Mfr.) Dextrose 100 g, calories 340/L, Na$^+$ 154 mEq, Cl$^-$

154 mEq, osmolarity 813–815 mOsm/L. Soln. Bot. 500 mL, 1000 mL. *Rx.*
Use: Intravenous nutritional therapy, intravenous replenishment solution.

dextrose 10% and 0.2% sodium chloride and potassium chloride.
Use: Intravenous nutritional therapy, intravenous replenishment solution.
See: Potassium Chloride in 10% Dextrose and 0.2% Sodium Chloride.

dextrose 10% with 0.45% sodium chloride. (B. Braun) Dextrose 100 g, calories 340/L, Na$^+$ 77 mEq, Cl$^-$ 77 mEq, osmolarity 660 mOsm/L. Soln. Bot. 1000 mL. *Rx.*
Use: Intravenous nutritional therapy, intravenous replenishment solution.

dextrose 10% with 0.2% sodium chloride. (Various Mfr.) Dextrose 100 g, calories 340/L, Na$^+$ 34 mEq, Cl$^-$ 34 mEq, osmolarity 575 mOsm/L. Soln. Bot. 250 mL. *Rx.*
Use: Intravenous nutritional therapy, intravenous replenishment solution.

dextrose 10% with 0.225% sodium chloride. (Abbott) Dextrose 100 g, calories 340/L, Na$^+$ 38.5 mEq, Cl$^-$ 38.5 mEq, osmolarity 582 mOsm/L. Soln. Bot. 250 mL, 500 mL. *Rx.*
Use: Intravenous nutritional therapy, intravenous replenishment solution.

dextrose 3.3% and 0.3% sodium chloride. (B. Braun) Dextrose 33 g, calories 110/L, Na$^+$ 51 mEq, Cl$^-$ 51 mEq, osmolarity 270 mOsm/L. Soln. Bot. 250 mL, 500 mL, 1000 mL. *Rx.*
Use: Intravenous nutritional therapy, intravenous replenishment solution.

dextrose 3.3% dextrose and 0.3% sodium chloride and potassium chloride.
Use: Intravenous nutritional therapy, intravenous replenishment solution.
See: Potassium chloride in 3.3% Dextrose and 0.3% Sodium Chloride.

dextrose 2.5% with 0.45% sodium chloride. (Various Mfr.) Dextrose 25 g, calories 85/L, Na$^+$ 77 mEq, Cl$^-$ 77 mEq, osmolarity 280 mOsm/L. Soln. Bot. 500 mL, 1000 mL. *Rx.*
Use: Intravenous nutritional therapy, intravenous replenishment solution.

DextroStat. (Shire Richwood) Dextroamphetamine sulfate 5 mg, 10 mg. Sucrose, lactose, tartrazine. Tab. Bot. 100s. *c-II.*
Use: CNS stimulant, amphetamine.

Dex-Tuss. (Cypress) Codeine phosphate 10 mg, guaifenesin 300 mg per 5 mL. Alcohol, sugar, and gluten free. Saccharin, sorbitol. Grape flavor. Liq. 473 mL. *c-v.*

Use: Upper respiratory combination, antitussive with expectorant.

Dex-Tuss DM. (Cypress) Dextromethorphan HBr 10 mg, guaifenesin 100 mg per 5 mL. Alcohol, sugar, and gluten free. Saccharin, sorbitol. Grape flavor. Liq. 473 mL. *Rx.*
Use: Upper respiratory combination, antitussive with expectorant.

Dexule. (Health for Life Brands) Vitamins A 1333 units, D 133 units, B$_1$ 0.33 mg, B$_2$ 0.4 mg, C 10 mg, niacinamide 3.3 mg, iron 3.3 mg, calcium 29 mg, phosphorus 15 mg, methylcellulose 100 mg, benzocaine 3 mg. Cap. Bot. 21s, 90s. *OTC.*
Use: Mineral, vitamin supplement.

Dexyl. (Pinex) Dextromethorphan HBr 15 mg, vitamin C 20 mg. Tab. Box 20s. *OTC.*
Use: Antitussive; vitamin supplement.

•**dezaguanine.** (DEH-zah-GWAHN-een) USAN.
Use: Antineoplastic.

•**dezaguanine mesylate.** (DEE-zah-GWAHN-een) USAN.
Use: Antineoplastic.

•**dezinamide.** (deh-ZIN-ah-mide) USAN.
Use: Anticonvulsant.

D-Film. (Ciba Vision) Poloxamer 407, EDTA 0.25%, benzalkonium Cl 0.025%. Gel. Tube 25 g. *OTC.*
Use: Contact lens care.

D-5000 Super Strength. (21st Century) Cholecalciferol 5,000 units. Calcium 180 mg. Gluten free. Tab. 110s. *OTC.*
Use: Fat-soluble vitamin.

DFMO. Eflornithine hydrochloride. *Rx.*
Use: Anti-infective.
See: Ornidyl.

D400. (Mason) Cholecalciferol (D$_3$). **Chew. Tab.:** 400 units. Fructose, sucrose, sunflower oil, xylitol. Vanilla flavor. 100s. **Cap., softgel:** 400 units. Glycerin, soybean oil. 100s. *OTC.*
Use: Vitamin, fat-soluble vitamin.

d4T.
Use: Antiviral.
See: Stavudine.

DFP. Disopropyl fluorophosphate (Various Mfr.)

d-Glucose. Dextrose. *Rx.*
Use: Nutritional supplement, parenteral.
See: D-10-W.

DHC Plus. (Purdue) Dihydrocodeine bitartrate 16 mg, acetaminophen 356.4 mg, caffeine 30 mg. Cap. Bot. 100s. *c-III.*
Use: Analgesic combination; narcotic.

DHEA. (Athena Neurosciences) EL10. *Rx.*
Use: Antiviral; immunomodulator.
D.H.E. 45. (Xcel) Dihydroergotamine mesylate 1 mg/mL, alcohol 6.2%, glycerin 15%. Inj. Amp. 1 mL. *Rx.*
Use: Antimigraine, ergotamine derivative.
D-Hist D. (Midlothian) Pseudoephedrine hydrochloride 45 mg, dexchlorpheniramine maleate 3.5 mg, methscopolamine nitrate 1 mg. ER Tab. 100s. *Rx.*
Use: Upper respiratory combination, decongestant, antihistamine, and anticholinergic combination.
DHPG. Ganciclovir sodium. *Rx.*
Use: Antiviral.
See: Cytovene.
DHS Conditioning Rinse. (Person and Covey) Conditioning ingredients. Bot. 8 oz. *OTC.*
Use: Dermatologic, hair.
DHS Shampoo. (Person and Covey) Blend of cleansing surfactants and emulsifiers. Plastic bot. w/dispenser 8 oz, 16 oz. *OTC.*
Use: Dermatologic, hair, and scalp.
DHS Tar Gel Shampoo. (Person and Covey) Coal tar 0.5% Bot. 240 g. *OTC.*
Use: Antipsoriatic; antiseborrheic.
DHS Tar Shampoo. (Person and Covey) Coal tar 0.5%. Liq. Bot. 120 mL, 240 mL, 480 mL. *OTC.*
Use: Antipsoriatic; antiseborrheic.
DHS Zinc. (Person and Covey) Pyrithione zinc 2%. Shampoo. Bot. 240 mL, 360 mL. *OTC.*
Use: Dermatologic agent.
DiaBeta. (Hoechst Marion Roussel) Glyburide 1.25 mg, 2.5 mg, 5 mg. Tab. 50s (1.25 mg only), 100s (2.5 mg only), 500s (except 1.25 mg), 1000s (5 mg only). *Rx.*
Use: Antidiabetic.
Diabetic Tussin. (Health Care Products) Guaifenesin 100 mg/5 mL. Alcohol and dye free. Aspartame, menthol, methylparaben, phenylalanine 8.4 mg/5 mL. Liq. Bot. 118 mL. *Rx.*
Use: Antitussive, decongestant, expectorant.
Diabetic Tussin Cold & Flu. (Health Care Products) Acetaminophen 325 mg, dextromethorphan hydrobromide 10 mg, diphenhydramine 12.5 mg. Acesulfame K, aspartame, menthol, methylparaben, orange flavoring, PEG, phenylalanine 8.4 mg, potassium sorbate, propylene glycol. Alcohol free, dye free, and sugar free. Liq. 118 mL,
237 mL. *OTC.*
Use: Upper respiratory combination, antitussive combination.
Diabetic Tussin DM. (Health Care Products) Dextromethorphan HBr 10 mg, guaifenesin 100 mg per 5 mL. Methylparaben, menthol, aspartame, phenylalanine 8.4 mg per 5 mL. Alcohol, sugar, and dye free. Liq. Bot. 118 mL. *OTC.*
Use: Upper respiratory combination, antitussive with expectorant.
Diabetic Tussin Maximum Strength DM. (Health Care Products) Dextromethorphan HBr 10 mg, guaifenesin 200 mg per 5 mL. Aspartame, phenylalanine 8.4 mg per 5 mL, menthol, methylparaben, PEG. Sugar, alcohol, and dye free. Liq. Bot. 237 mL. *OTC.*
Use: Upper respiratory combination, antitussive with expectorant.
Diabetic Tussin Night Time Formula Cold/Flu. (Health Care Products) Acetaminophen 325 mg, dextromethorphan hydrobromide 10 mg, diphenhydramine 12.5 mg. Acesulfame K, aspartame, menthol, methylparaben, PEG, phenylalanine 8.4 mg per 5 mL. Alcohol free, dye free, and sugar free. Liq. 118 mL. *OTC.*
Use: Upper respiratory combination, antitussive combination.
DiabetiDerm. (Health Care Products) Undecylenic acid 10%. Aloe, cetyl alcohol, clotrimazole, disodium EDTA, glyceryl, lavender oil, parabens, PEG-100, tea tree oil, triethanolamine, urea. Cream. 42 g. *OTC.*
Use: Anti-infective, topical; antifungal agent.
diacetic acid test.
See: Acetest Reagent.
Diaceto w/Codeine. (Archer-Taylor) Codeine 0.25 g, 0.5 g. Tab. or Cap. Bot. 500s, 1000s. *c-II.*
Use: Analgesic; narcotic.
Diaceto w/Gelsemium. (Archer-Taylor) Phenobarbital 0.5 g, gelsemium 3 min. Tab. Bot. 1000s. *c-IV.*
Use: Hypnotic; sedative.
•**diacetolol hydrochloride.** (DIE-ah-SEET-oh-lahl) USAN.
Use: Antiadrenergic (β-receptor).
diacetrizoate, sodium.
See: Diatrizoate.
diacetylated monoglycerides.
Use: Pharmaceutic aid (plasticizer).
diacetylcholine chloride. Succinylcholine Cl.
See: Anectine Chloride.
diacetyl-dihydroxydiphenylisatin.
See: Oxyphenisatin Acetate.

diacetyldioxyphenylisatin.
See: Oxyphenisatin Acetate.
diacetylmorphine salts. Heroin. Illegal
in USA by federal statute because of
its addiction potential.
Di-Ademil.
See: Hydroflumethiazide.
diagnostic agents.
See: Aplisol.
Aplitest.
Candida Albicans Skin Test Antigen.
Candin.
Cardio-Green Disposable Unit.
Cea-Roche.
Cholecystography Agents.
Cholografin Meglumine.
Coccidioidin.
Evans Blue Dye.
EZ Detect Strep-A Test.
Fertility Tape.
First Choice.
Fluor-I-Strip.
Fluor-I-Strip A.T.
Fluress.
Hema-Combistix Reagent Strips.
Histolyn-CYL.
Histoplasmin.
HIVAB HIV-1/HIV-2 (rDNA) EIA.
Immunex CRP.
Indigo Carmine.
Kidney Function Agents.
Liver Function Agents.
Mannitol.
Mono-Latex.
Mono-Plus.
MSTA.
Mumps Skin Test Antigen.
Persantine IV.
Pharmalgen Hymenoptera Venoms.
Pharmalgen Standardized Allergenic
Extracts.
Phentolamine Methanesulfonate.
Radiopaque Agents.
Rheumatex.
Rheumaton.
Spherulin.
SureCell Herpes (HSV) Test.
SureCell Strep A Test.
Tine Test.
True Test.
Tubersol.
Urography Agents.
Venomil.
diagnostic agents for urine.
See: Acetest Reagent.
Albustix Reagent Strips.
Biotel Diabetes.
Biotel U.T.I.
Chemstrip Micral.
Clinistix Reagent Strips.
Clinitest.

Fortel Midstream.
Fortel Plus.
HCG-Nostick.
Hema-Combistix Reagent Strips.
Hemastix Reagent Strips.
Hematest Reagent Strips.
Ictotest Reagent Tablets.
Ketostix Reagent Strips.
SureCell hCG-Urine Test.
Uristix.
Wampole One-Step hCG.
diallylamicol. Diallyl-diethylaminoethyl
phenol di hydrochloride.
diallylbarbituric acid. Allobarbital, Allo-
barbitone, Curral.
dialminate. Mixture of magnesium carbo-
nate and (aluminate) dihydroxyalumi-
num glycinate.
Dialyte Pattern LM w/4.25% Dextrose.
(Gambro) Dextrose 42.5 g/L, Na^+
131.5, Ca^{++} 3.5, Mg^{++} 0.5, Cl⁻ 94, and
lactate 40 with osmolarity 485 mOsm/
L. Soln. Bot. 1000 mL, 2000 mL,
4000 mL. *Rx.*
Use: Peritoneal dialysis solution.
Dialyte Pattern LM w/1.5% Dextrose.
(Gambro) Dextrose 15 g/L, Na^+
131 mEq, Ca^{++} 3.5 mEq, Mg^{++} 0.5 mEq,
Cl⁻ 94 mEq, and lactate 40 mEq with
osmolarity 345 mOsm/L. Soln. Bot.
1000 mL, 2000 mL, 4000 mL. *Rx.*
Use: Peritoneal dialysis solution.
Dialyte Pattern LM w/2.5% Dextrose.
(Gambro) Dextrose 25 g/L, Na^+
131.5 mEq, Ca^{++} 3.5 mEq, Mg^{++}
0.5 mEq, Cl⁻ 94 mEq, and lactate
40 mEq with osmolarity 395 mOsm/L.
Soln. Bot. 1000 mL, 2000 mL, 4000 mL.
Rx.
Use: Peritoneal dialysis solution.
**Dialyvite Multi-Vitamins for Dialysis
Patients.** (Hillestad) Vitamin B_6 10 mg,
vitamin B_{12} 6 mcg, vitamin C 100 mg,
folic acid 1 mg, d-biotin 300 mcg, panto-
thenic acid 10 mg, thiamine 1.5 mg,
riboflavin 1.7 mg, niacinamide 20 mg.
Tab. 100s. *Rx.*
Use: Nutritional combination product.
Dialyvite 3000. (Hillestad) Vitamin C
100 mg, B_1 1.5 mg, B_2 1.7 mg, B_3
20 mg, B_5 10 mg, B_6 25 mg, B_{12} 1 mg,
FA 3 mg, biotin 300 mcg, E 30 units,
Se 70 mcg, Zn 15 mg. Tab. 90s. *OTC.*
Use: Nutritional combination product.
Dialyvite with Zinc. (Hillestad) Vitamin
B_1 1.5 mg, vitamin B_2 1.7 mg, vitamin
B_3 20 mg, vitamin B_5 10 mg, vitamin
B_6 10 mg, vitamin B_{12} 6 mcg, C 100 mg,
d-biotin 300 mcg, folic acid 1 mg, Zn
50 mg. Tab. 100s. *Rx.*
Use: Nutritional combination, B vitamin
with vitamin C.

diaminodiphenylsulfone.
Use: Antimalarial.
See: Dapsone.
diaminopropyl tetramethylene.
See: Spermine.
3,4-diaminopyridine. (Jacobus)
Use: Lambert-Eaton myasthenic syndrome. [Orphan Drug]
•**diamocaine cyclamate.** (die-AM-oh-CANE SIH-klah-mate) USAN.
Use: Anesthetic, local.
Diamox Squels. (Barr) Acetazolamide 500 mg. ER Cap. 100s. *Rx.*
Use: Diuretic, carbonic anhydrase inhibitor.
diamthazole dihydrochloride. (DYE-am-tha-ZOLE)
Use: Antifungal.
Dianeal Low Calcium w/4.25% Dextrose. (Baxter) Dextrose 4.25 g/L, Na$^+$132 mEq/L, Ca^{++} 2.5 mEq/L, Mg^{++} 0.5 mEq/L, Cl$^-$ 95 mEq/L, lactate 40 mEq/L, osmolarity 483 mOsm/L. Preservative free. Inj., Soln. *AMBU-FLEX II* and *AMBU-FLEX III* containers. 2,000 mL, 2,500 mL, 3,000 mL, 5,000 mL, 6,000 mL. *Rx.*
Use: Electrolyte, peritoneal dialysis solution.
Dianeal Low Calcium w/1.5% Dextrose. (Baxter) Dextrose 1.5 g/L, Na$^+$ 132 mEq/L, Ca^{++} 2.5 mEq/L, Mg^{++} 0.5 mEq/L, Cl$^-$ 95 mEq/L, lactate 40 mEq/L, osmolarity 344 mOsm/L. Preservative free. Inj., Soln. *AMBU-FLEX II* container. 2,000 mL, 2,500 mL, 3,000 mL, 5,000 mL, 6,000 mL. *Rx.*
Use: Electrolyte, peritoneal dialysis solution.
Dianeal Low Calcium w/2.5% Dextrose. (Baxter) Dextrose 2.5 g/L, Na$^+$ 132 mEq/L, Ca^{++} 2.5 mEq/L, Mg^{++} 0.5 mEq/L, Cl$^-$ 95 mEq/L, lactate 40 mEq/L, osmolarity 395 mOsm/L. Preservative free. Inj., Soln. *AMBU-FLEX II* and *AMBU-FLEX III* containers. 2,000 mL, 2,500 mL, 3,000 mL, 5,000 mL, 6,000 mL. *Rx.*
Use: Electrolyte, peritoneal dialysis solution.
Dianeal 137 w/4.25% Dextrose. (Baxter) Dextrose 42.5 g/L, Na$^+$ 132 mEq, Ca^{++} 3.5 mEq, Mg^{++} 1.5 mEq, Cl$^-$ 102 mEq, lactate 35 mEq with osmolarity 486 mOsm/L. Soln. 2,000 mL. *Rx.*
Use: Peritoneal dialysis solution.
Dianeal 137 w/1.5% Dextrose. (Baxter) Dextrose 15 g/L, Na$^+$ 132 mEq, Ca^{++} 3.5 mEq, Mg^{++} 1.5 mEq, Cl$^-$ 102 mEq, lactate 35 mEq with osmolarity

347 mOsm/L. Soln. 2,000 mL. *Rx.*
Use: Peritoneal dialysis solution.
Dianeal PD-2 w/4.25% Dextrose. (Baxter) Dextrose 4.25 g/L, Na$^+$ 132 mEq/L, Ca^{++} 3.5 mEq/L, Mg^{++} 0.5 mEq/L, Cl$^-$ 96 mEq/L, lactate 40 mEq/L, osmolarity 485 mOsm/L. Preservative free. Inj., Soln. *AMBU-FLEX II* container. 1,000 mL, 2,000 mL, 2,500 mL, 3,000 mL, 5,000 mL, 6,000 mL. *AMBU-FLEX III* container. 500 mL, 1,000 mL, 2,000 mL, 2,500 mL, 3,000 mL, 5,000 mL, 6,000 mL. *Rx.*
Use: Electrolyte, peritoneal dialysis solution.
Dianeal PD-2 w/1.5% Dextrose. (Baxter) Dextrose 1.5 g/L, Na$^+$ 132 mEq/L, Ca^{++} 3.5 mEq/L, Mg^{++} 0.5 mEq/L, Cl$^-$ 96 mEq/L, lactate 40 mEq/L, osmolarity 346 mOsm/L. Preservative free. Inj., Soln. *AMBU-FLEX II* container. 1,000 mL, 2,000 mL, 2,500 mL, 3,000 mL, 5,000 mL, 6,000 mL. *AMBU-FLEX III* container. 250 mL, 500 mL, 1,000 mL, 2,000 mL, 2,500 mL, 3,000 mL, 5,000 mL, 6,000 mL. *Rx.*
Use: Electrolyte, peritoneal dialysis solution.
Dianeal PD-2 w/3.5% Dextrose. (Baxter) Dextrose 3.5 g/L, Na$^+$ 132 mEq/L, Ca^{++} 3.5 mEq/L, Mg^{++} 0.5 mEq/L, Cl$^-$ 96 mEq/L, lactate 40 mEq/L, osmolarity 447 mOsm/L. Preservative free. Inj., Soln. *AMBU-FLEX III* container. 2,500 mL. *Rx.*
Use: Electrolyte, peritoneal dialysis solution.
Dianeal PD-2 w/2.5% Dextrose. (Baxter) Dextrose 2.5 g/L, Na$^+$ 132 mEq/L, Ca^{++} 3.5 mEq/L, Mg^{++} 0.5 mEq/L, Cl$^-$ 96 mEq/L, lactate 40 mEq/L, osmolarity 396 mOsm/L. Preservative free. Inj., Soln. *AMBU-FLEX II* container. 1,000 mL, 2,000 mL, 2,500 mL, 3,000 mL, 5,000 mL, 6,000 mL. *AMBU-FLEX III* container. 250 mL, 500 mL, 1,000 mL, 2,000 mL, 2,500 mL, 3,000 mL, 5,000 mL, 6,000 mL. *Rx.*
Use: Electrolyte, peritoneal dialysis solution.
Dianeal peritoneal dialysis solution with 1.1% amino acid.
Use: Nutritional supplement for dialysis patients. [Orphan Drug]
Dianeal w/4.25% Dextrose. (Baxter PPI) Dextrose 42.5 g/L, Na$^+$ 141 mEq, Ca^{++} 3.5 mEq, Mg^{++} 1.5 mEq, Cl$^-$ 101 mEq, lactate 45 mEq with osmolarity 503 mOsm/L. Soln. Bot. 2000 mL. *Rx.*
Use: Peritoneal dialysis solution.

Dianeal w/1.5% Dextrose. (Baxter PPI) Dextrose 15 g/L, Na+ 141 mEq, Ca++ 3.5 mEq, Mg++1.5 mEq, Cl- 101 mEq, lactate 45 mEq with osmolarity 364 mOsm/ L. Soln. Bot. 1000 mL, 2000 mL. *Rx.*
Use: Peritoneal dialysis solution.

•**diapamide.** (die-APP-am-ide) USAN.
Use: Antihypertensive; diuretic.

Diapantin. (Janssen) Isopropamide bromide. *Rx.*
Use: Anticholinergic.

Diaparene. (Bayer Consumer Care) Methylbenzethonium chloride. Pow. Bot. 4 oz, 9 oz, 12.5 oz, 14 oz.
Use: Disinfectant; surface active agent.

Diaparene Ointment. (Bayer Consumer Care) Methylbenzethonium chloride 0.1% w/petrolatum, glycerin. Tube 1 oz, 2 oz, 4 oz. *OTC.*
Use: Antimicrobial, topical.

Diaparene Peri-Anal Cream. (Bayer Consumer Care) Methylbenzethonium chloride 1:1000, zinc oxide, starch, cod liver oil, white petrolatum, lanolin, calcium caseinate. Cream. Tube 1 oz, 2 oz, 4 oz. *OTC.*
Use: Antimicrobial; astringent.

Diaper Guard. (Del) Dimethicone 1%, white petrolatum 66%, cocoa butter, parabens, vitamins A, D_3, E, zinc oxide. Oint. Tube 49.6 g, 99.2 g. *OTC.*
Use: Diaper rash preparation.

Diaper Rash. (Various Mfr.) Zinc oxide, cod liver oil, lanolin, methylparaben, petrolatum, talc. Oint. Tube 113 g. *OTC.*
Use: Diaper rash preparation.

diaphenylsulfone. Dapsone.
Use: Leprostatic.

•**diaplasinin.** (dye-a-PLAS-in-in) USAN.
Use: Hematologic agent.

Di-Ap-Trol. (Foy Laboratories) Phendimetrazine tartrate 35 mg. Tab. Bot. 100s, 1000s. *c-III.*
Use: Anorexiant.

Diarrest. (Dover Pharmaceuticals) Calcium carbonate, pectin. Tab. Sugar, lactose, salt free. UD box 500s. *OTC.*
Use: Antidiarrheal.

diarrhea therapy.
See: Antidiarrheal.

Diaserp. (Major) Chlorothiazide 250 mg, 500 mg, w/reserpine. Tab. Bot. 100s. *Rx.*
Use: Antihypertensive.

Diasorb. (Columbia) Activated nonfibrous attapulgite. **Liq.:** 750 mg per 5 mL. Bot. 120 mL. **Tab.:** 750 mg. Pkg. 24s. *OTC.*
Use: Antidiarrheal.

Diasporal. (Doak Dermatologics) *Formerly Sulfur Salicyl Diasporal.* Sulfur 3%, salicylic acid 2%, isopropyl alcohol in diasporal base. Cream. Jar 3¾ oz. *OTC.*
Use: Antiseptic, topical.

Diastase.
See: Aspergillus oryzae enzyme.

Diastat. (Xcel) Diazepam 2.5 mg. Benzyl alcohol 1.5%, ethyl alcohol 10%. Rectal gel. Twin pack. Includes lubricating jelly, plastic applicator with flexible, molded tip in two lengths.
Use: Anticonvulsant.

Diastat AcuDial. (Xcel) Diazepam 2.5 mg, 10 mg, 20 mg. Benzyl alcohol 1.5%, ethyl alcohol 10%. Rectal Gel. Twin packs. Includes lubricating jelly and plastic applicator. *c-IV.*
Use: Anticonvulsant; antianxiety agent.

•**diatrizoate meglumine.** (die-ah-TRIH-zoe-ate meh-GLUE-meen) *USP 34.*
Use: Radiopaque agent, parenteral agent.
See: Angiovist 282.
    Cystografin.
    Cystografin Dilute.
W/Sodium diatrizoate.
See: Renovist.

diatrizoate meglumine 52% and diatrizoate sodium 8%.
Use: Radiopaque agent, parenteral agent.
See: Renografin-60.

diatrizoate meglumine 52.7% and iodipamide meglumine 26.8% (38% iodine).
Use: Radiopaque agent.
See: Sinografin.

diatrizoate meglumine 66% and diatrizoate sodium 10%.
Use: Radiopaque agent, iodinated GI contrast agent.
See: Gastrografin.
    Hypaque-76.
    MD-76 R.
    RenoCal-76.

diatrizoate methylglucamine.
Use: Diagnostic aid (radiopaque medium).
See: Diatrizoate Meglumine.

diatrizoate methylglucamine sodium.
Use: Diagnostic aid (radiopaque medium).

•**diatrizoate sodium.** (DYE-a-trye-ZOE-ate) *USP 34.*
Use: Diagnostic aid (radiopaque medium).
See: Hypaque.
    Urovist Sodium 300.
W/Methylglucamine diatrizoate, sodium citrate, disodium ethylenediamine tetraacetate dihydrate, methylparaben, propylparaben.
See: Renovist.

diatrizoate sodium (59.87% iodine).
Use: Radiopaque agent, iodinated GI
contrast agent.
See: Hypaque Sodium.

•**diatrizoate sodium I 131.** (DYE-a-trye-
ZOE-ate) USAN.
Use: Radiopharmaceutical.

•**diatrizoate sodium I 125.** (DYE-a-trye-
ZOE-ate) USAN.
Use: Radiopharmaceutical.

•**diatrizoic acid.** (DIE-at-rih-ZOE-ik)
USP 34.
Use: Diagnostic aid (radiopaque me-
dium).
See: Hypaque Sodium Salt.

Diatx. (Pan American) Vitamin B_1 1.5 mg,
B_2 1.5 mg, B_3 20 mg, B_5 10 mg, B_6
50 mg, B_{12} 1 mg, C 60 mg, folic acid
5 mg, D-biotin 300 mcg, dye free. Tab.
Bot. 90s. *Rx.*
Use: Vitamin supplement.

DiatxFe. (Pan American) Fe (as ferrous
fumarate) 100 mg, B_1 1.5 mg, B_2
1.5 mg, B_3 20 mg, B_5 10 mg, B_6 50 mg,
B_{12} 1 mg, C 60 mg, folic acid 5 mg, D-
biotin 300 mcg, dye free. Tab. Bot. 90s.
Rx.
Use: Vitamin supplement.

•**diaveridine.** (DIE-ah-ver-ih-deen) USAN.
Use: Anti-infective.

•**diazepam.** (DIE-aze-uh-pam) *USP 34.*
Use: Agent for control of emotional dis-
turbances; anxiolytic; hypnotic; seda-
tive.
See: Diastat.
Diastat AcuDial.
Diazepam Intensol.
Valium.

diazepam. (Roxane) Diazepam 5 mg/
5 mL. Sorbitol, wintergreen spice flavor.
Oral Soln. 500 mL, 5 mg patient cups,
10 mg patient cups. *c-IV.*
Use: Agent for control of emotional disturbances; anxiolytic; hypnotic; sedative; anticonvulsant.

diazepam. (Teva) Diazepam 2.5 mg,
10 mg, 20 mg. Benzyl alcohol 1.5%,
ethyl alcohol 10%, benzoic acid, propylene glycol. Gel, rectal. Prefilled unit-
dose rectal delivery system 2s. Includes lubricating jelly and plastic applicator with flexible, molded tip 4.4 cm
(2.5 mg, 10 mg) or 6 cm (20 mg) in
length. *c-IV.*
Use: Antianxiety agent, benzodiazepine.

diazepam. (Various Mfr.) **Tab.:** 2 mg,
5 mg, 10 mg. May contain lactose. Bot.
100s, 500s, 1000s, 5000s. **Inj.:** 5 mg/
mL. Propylene glycol 40%, ethyl alcohol

10%, sodium benzoate 5%, benzoic
acid, benzyl alcohol 1.5%. 2 mL *Carpuject* cartridges. *c-IV.*
Use: Agent for control of emotional disturbances; anxiolytic; hypnotic; sedative; anticonvulsant.

Diazepam Intensol. (Roxane) Diazepam
5 mg/mL. Alcohol 19%. Oral Soln. Concentrate. 30 mL with dropper. *c-IV.*
Use: Anxiolytic; anticonvulsant.

**diazepam viscous solution for rectal
administration.** (Athena Neurosciences)
Use: To treat acute repetitive seizures.
[Orphan Drug]

•**diaziquone.** (DIE-azz-ih-kwone) USAN.
Use: Antineoplastic.

diazomycins a, b, and c. Antibiotic obtained from *Streptomyces ambofaciens.* Under study.

•**diazoxide.** (DIE-aze-OX-ide) *USP 34.*
Use: Antihypertensive.
See: Proglycem.

dibasic calcium phosphate dihydrate.
Use: Replenisher (calcium); pharma-
ceutic aid (tablet base).
See: Diostate D.

Dibatrol. (Lexis Laboratories) Chlorpropamide 100 mg, 250 mg. Tab. Bot.
100s, 1000s. *Rx.*
Use: Antidiabetic.

dibenzapine derivatives.
Use: Antipsychotic.
See: Asenapine.
Clozapine.
Loxapine.
Olanzapine.
Quetiapine Fumarate.

•**dibenzepin hydrochloride.** (die-BEN-
zeh-pin) USAN.
Use: Antidepressant.

•**dibenzothiophene.** (die-BEN-zoe-
THIGH-oh-feen) USAN.
Use: Keratolytic.

Dibenzyline. (Wellspring) Phenoxybenzamine hydrochloride 10 mg. Cap.
Bot. 100s. *Rx.*
Use: Pheochromocytoma agent; antihypertensive.

•**dibotermin alfa.** (dye-BOE-ter-min)
USAN.
Use: Osteoinductive agent.

•**dibromsalan.** (die-BROME-sah-lan)
USAN.
Use: Antimicrobial; disinfectant.

•**dibucaine.** (DIE-byoo-cane) *USP 34.*
Use: Topical local anesthetic, amide lo-
cal anesthetic.
See: Nupercainal.

W/Sodium bisulfite.
See: Nupercainal.
W/Zinc oxide, bismuth subgallate, acetone sodium bisulfite.
See: Nupercainal.
dibucaine. (Various Mfr.) Dibucaine 1%. Oint. 30 g. *OTC.*
Use: Topical local anesthetic, amide local anesthetic.
•**dibucaine hydrochloride.** (DIE-byoo-cane) *USP 34.*
Use: Anesthetic, local.
W/Antipyrine, hydrocortisone, polymyxin B sulfate, neomycin sulfate.
See: Otocort.
W/Colistin sodium methanesulfonate, citric acid, sodium citrate.
See: Coly-Mycin M Parenteral.
dibutoline sulfate. Ethyl (2-hydroxyethyl)-dimethylammonium sulfate (2:1) bis (dibutyl-carbam-ate).
Use: Anticholinergic; antispasmodic.
•**dibutyl sebacate.** (dye-BUE-til SEB-a-kate) *NF 29.*
Use: Pharmaceutic aid (plasticizer).
Dical. (Rugby) Calcium 116 mg, vitamin D 133 units, phosphorus 90 mg. Captab. Bot. 1000s. *OTC.*
Use: Mineral, vitamin supplement.
dicalcium phosphate. (Various Mfr.) Dibasic calcium phosphate, monocalcium phosphate. **Cap.:** 7.5 g, 10 g. **Tab.:** 7.5 g, 10 g, 15 g. **Wafer:** 15 g. *OTC.*
Use: Mineral supplement.
W/Calcium Gluconate and Vitamin D.
See: CalciCaps.
Dical-Dee. (Alpharma) Vitamin D 350 units, dibasic calcium phosphate 4.5 g, calcium gluconate 3 g. Cap. Bot. 100s, 1000s. *OTC.*
Use: Mineral, vitamin supplement.
Dicaldel. (Faraday) Dibasic calcium phosphate 300 mg, calcium gluconate 200 mg, vitamin D 33 units. Cap. Bot. 100s, 250s, 500s, 1000s. *OTC.*
Use: Mineral, vitamin supplement.
Dical-D with Vitamin C. (Abbott) Dibasic calcium phosphate containing calcium 116.7 mg, phosphorus 90 mg, vitamin D 133 units, ascorbic acid 15 mg. Cap. Bot. 100s.
Use: Mineral, vitamin supplement.
Dicaltabs. (Faraday) Dibasic calcium phosphate 108 mg, calcium gluconate 140 mg, vitamin D 35 units. Tab. Bot. 100s, 250s, 1000s. *OTC.*
Use: Mineral, vitamin supplement.
Dicarbosil. (BIRA) Calcium carbonate 500 mg (elemental calcium 200 mg). Sodium < 2 mg, ANC 10 mEq. Pepper-

mint flavor. Chew. Tab. Roll 12s. *OTC.*
Use: Mineral supplement; antacid.
Dicel CD. (Centrix) Brompheniramine maleate 2 mg, chlophedianol hydrochloride 12.5 mg, pseudoephedrine hydrochloride 30 mg. Glycerin, grape flavoring, propylene glycol, saccharin, sorbitol. Alcohol free, dye free, and sugar free. Liq. 473 mL. *OTC.*
Use: Upper respiratory combination, antitussive combination.
Dicel DM. (Centrix) Chlorpheniramine maleate 2 mg, dextromethorphan hydrobromide 10 mg, pseudoephedrine hydrochloride 30 mg. Maltodextrin, glycyrrhizic, vegetable oil, PEG, soy lecithin, sucralose, sugar. Alcohol free. Cotton candy flavor. Chew. Tab. 20s. *Rx.*
Use: Upper respiratory combination, antitussive combination.
Di-Cet. (Sanford & Son) Methylbenzethonium Cl 24.4 g, sodium carbonate monohydrate 48.8 g, sodium nitrite 24.4 g, trisodium ethylenediamine tetra-acetate monohydrate 2.4 g. Pow. Pkg. 2.4 g. Box 24s.
Use: Disinfectant.
dichloralantipyrine. Dichloralphenazone. Chloralpyrine. A complex of 2 mol. chloral hydrate with 1 mol. antipyrine. Sominat.
W/Isometheptene mucate, acetaminophen.
See: Midrin.
•**dichloralphenazone.** (die-klor-al-FEN-ah-zone) *USP 34.*
Use: Hypnotic; sedative.
W/Acetaminophen, Isometheptene Mucate.
See: Epidrin.
Midrin.
Migragesic IDA.
Migrazone.
Nodolor.
Dichloramine T. (Various Mfr.) (1% to 5% in chlorinated paraffin). P-Toluenesulfone-dichloramine.
Use: Antiseptic.
dichloren.
See: Mechlorethamine Hydrochloride.
dichloroacetic acid. *Rx.*
Use: Cauterizing agent.
•**dichlorodifluoromethane.** (die-KLOR-oh-die-flure-oh-METH-ane) *NF 29.*
Use: Pharmaceutic aid (aerosol propellant).
W/Trichloromonofluroromethane.
See: Gebauer's Spray and Stretch.
dichlorodiphenyl trichloroethane.
See: Chlorophenothane.

dichlorophenarsine hydrochloride. (Chlorarsen, Clorarsen, Fontarsol, Halarsol).

dichlorophene. Related to hexachlorophene.

•**dichlorotetrafluoroethane.** (die-KLOR-oh-teh-trah-flur-oh-ETH-ane) *NF 29.*
Use: Pharmaceutic aid (aerosol propellant).
W/Ethyl Chloride.
See: Fluro-Ethyl.

•**dichlorvos.** (DIE-klor-vahs) USAN.
Use: Anthelmintic.

•**dicirenone.** (die-sigh-REN-ohn) USAN.
Use: Hypotensive; aldosterone antagonist.

Dickey's Old Reliable Eye Wash. (Dickey Drug) Berberine sulfate, boric acid, parabens. Plastic dropper bot. 8 mL, 12 mL, 1 oz. *OTC.*
Use: Counterirritant, ophthalmic.

diclofenac epolamine.
Use: Nonsteroidal anti-inflammatory agent, topical.

•**diclofenac potassium.** (die-KLOE-fen-ak) USAN.
Use: Analgesic; NSAID.
See: Cambia.
Cataflam.
Zipsor.

diclofenac potassium. (Various Mfr.) Diclofenac potassium 50 mg. Tab. Bot. 100s, 500s. *Rx.*
Use: Analgesic; NSAID.

•**diclofenac sodium.** (die-KLOE-fen-ak) *USP 34.*
Use: Analgesic; NSAID.
See: Solaraze.
Voltaren.
Voltaren-XR.

diclofenac sodium. (Akorn) Diclofenac sodium 0.1%. EDTA. Soln., Ophth. 2.5 mL, 5 mL. *Rx.*
Use: Nonsteroidal anti-inflammatory drug.

diclofenac sodium. (Various Mfr.) Diclofenac sodium. **ER Tab.:** 100 mg. Bot. 100s. **DR Tab.:** 25 mg, 50 mg, 75 mg. May be enteric coated. Bot. 42s (except 25 mg), 60s, 100s, 500s (except 25 mg), 1000s (except 25 mg), UD 100s (50 mg only). *Rx.*
Use: Analgesic; NSAID.

diclofenac sodium and misoprostol.
Use: Arthritis treatment, antiulcerative.
See: Arthrotec.

diclofenac sodium ophthalmic solution 0.1%. Diclofenac sodium 0.1%, mannitol. Soln. Bot. 5 mL. *Rx.*
Use: Analgesic; NSAID, ophthalmic.

Dicloxacil. (Ivax) Dicloxacillin sodium 250 mg, 500 mg. Cap. Bot. 100s. *Rx.*
Use: Anti-infective; penicillin.

•**dicloxacillin.** (DIE-klox-uh-SILL-in) USAN.
Use: Anti-infective.
See: Dynapen.
Pathocil.

•**dicloxacillin sodium.** (DIE-klox-uh-SILL-in) *USP 34.*
Use: Anti-infective.

dicloxacillin sodium. (Various Mfr.) Dicloxacillin sodium 250 mg, 500 mg. Cap. Bot. 30s (500 mg only), 40s, 50s (500 mg only), 100s, 500s, UD 100s. *Rx.*
Use: Anti-infective

Dicole. (Halsey Drug) Docusate sodium 100 mg. Cap. Bot. 100s. *OTC.*
Use: Laxative.

Dicomal-DM. (Econolab) Dextromethorphan HBr 10 mg, pyrilamine maleate 8.33 mg, phenylephrine hydrochloride 5 mg per 5 mL. Menthol, saccharin, sorbitol. Alcohol, sugar, and dye free. Syrup. Bot. 473 mL. *OTC.*
Use: Upper respiratory combination, antitussive, antihistamine, decongestant.

dicophane.
Use: Pediculicide.
See: Chlorophenothane.
DDT.

•**dicumarol.** (dye-KOO-ma-role) USAN.
Use: Anticoagulent.

•**dicyclomine hydrochloride.** (die-SIGH-kloe-meen) *USP 34.*
Use: Anticholinergic; antispasmodic.
See: Bentyl.

dicyclomine hydrochloride. (Various Mfr.) Dicyclomine hydrochloride. **Cap.:** 10 g, 20 mg. 30s (10 mg only), 100s, 120s (10 mg only), 1000s, UD 100s (10 mg only). **Tab.:** 20 mg. 15s, 20s, 30s, 100s, 120s, 250s, 1000s, UD 100s. **Syrup:** 10 mg/5 mL. 118 mL, pt, gal. **Inj.:** 10 mg/mL. Vials. 2 mL, 10 mL. *Rx.*
Use: Gastrointestinal antispasmodic/anticholinergic.

Dicynene. (Baxter PPI) *Rx.*
Use: Hemostatic.
See: Ethamsylate.

dicysteine.
See: Cystine.

•**didanosine.** (die-DAN-oh-SEEN) USAN.
Use: Antiretroviral, nucleoside reverse transcriptase inhibitor.
See: Videx.
Videx EC.

didanosine. (Barr) Didanosine 125 mg,

200 mg, 250 mg, 400 mg. Dextrose, talc. Enteric-coated pellets. DR Cap. 30s, 500s (125 mg only); UD 30s (except 125 mg). *Rx.*
Use: Nucleoside reverse transcriptase inhibitor.

didanosine. (Mylan) Didanosine 125 mg. Cap., delayed release. 30s, 500s. *Rx.*
Use: Antiretroviral agent, nucleoside reverse transcriptase inhibitor.

didehydrodideoxythymidine.
Use: Antiviral.
See: Stavudine.

Di-Delamine. (Del) Tripelennamine hydrochloride 0.5%, diphenhydramine hydrochloride 1%, benzalkonium chloride 0.12%. **Gel:** In clear gel. Tube 1.25 oz. **Spray:** Spray pump 4 oz. *OTC.*
Use: Antipruritic, topical.

dideoxycytidine.
Use: Antiviral.

2,3 dideoxycytidine.
Use: Antiviral (AIDS).

dideoxyinisine.
Use: Antiviral.

Didrex. (Pharmacia) Benzphetamine hydrochloride 50 mg. Lactose, sorbitol. Tab. Bot. 100s, 500s. *c-III.*
Use: CNS stimulant, anorexiant.

Didronel. (Procter & Gamble Pharm) Etidronate disodium 200 mg, 400 mg. Tab. Bot. 60s. *Rx.*
Use: Bisphosphonate.

•**dienestrol.** (die-en-ESS-trole) *USP 34.*
Use: Estrogen therapy; atrophic vaginitis.
See: D V. Cream.
Ortho Dienestrol Vaginal Cream.

dienestrol. (Ortho-McNeil) Dienestrol 0.01%. Tube 78 g w/applicator.
Use: Estrogen.

•**dienogest.** (dye-EN-oh-jest) USAN.
Use: Oral contraceptive; hormone replacement therapy.

diet aids, nonprescription.
Use: Dietary aid.

•**diethanolamine.** (DYE-eth-a-NOL-a-meen) *NF 29.*
Use: Pharmaceutic acid (alkalizing agent).
See: Diolamine.

diethazine hydrochloride.
Use: Antiparkinsonian.

diethoxin. Intracaine hydrochloride.

•**diethylcarbamazine citrate.** (die-ETH-ill-car-BAM-ah-zeen) *USP 34.*
Use: Anthelmintic.

diethyldithiocarbamate.
Use: Trial drug for AIDS. [Orphan Drug]
See: Imuthiol.

diethylenediamine citrate. Piperazine Citrate, Piperazine Hexahydrate.

diethylmalonylurea.
See: Barbital.

•**diethyl phthalate.** (dye-ETH-il THAL-ate) *NF 29.*
Use: Pharmaceutic aid (plasticizer).

diethylpropion. (Various Mfr.) **Tab.:** Diethylpropion 25 mg. Bot. 100s, 500s, 1000s. **SR Tab.:** Diethylpropion 75 mg. Bot. 100s, 250s, 500s, 1000s. *c-IV.*
Use: Anorexiant.

•**diethylpropion hydrochloride.** (die-ETH-uhl-PRO-pee-ahn) *USP 34.*
Use: Anorexic.
See: Tepanil.
Tepanil Ten-Tab.

diethylpropion hydrochloride. (Various Mfr.) Diethlpropion hydrochloride. **Tab.:** 25 mg. Bot. 100s. **CR Tab.:** 75 mg. Bot. 100s. *c-IV.*
Use: CNS stimulant, anorexiant.

diethylstilbestrol dipropionate. (Various Mfr.) Diethylstilbestrol dipropionate. **Amp.:** In oil, 0.5 mg, 1 mg, 5 mg/mL. **Tab.:** 0.5 mg, 1 mg, 5 mg.
Use: Estrogen.

•**diethyltoluamide.** (die-ETH-ill-toe-LOO-ah-mide) *USP 34.*
Use: Repellent (arthropod).

n, n-diethylvanillamide.
See: Ethamivan.

Diet-Tuss. (Health for Life Brands) Dextromethorphan 30 mg, thenylpyramine hydrochloride, pyrilamine maleate 80 mg, sodium salicylate 200 mg, sodium citrate 600 mg, ammonium Cl 100 mg/fl oz. Sugar free. Bot. 4 oz. *OTC.*
Use: Analgesic, antihistamine, antitussive, expectorant.

•**difenoximide hydrochloride.** (dye-fen-OX-i-mide) USAN.
Use: Antiperistaltic.

•**difenoxin.** (DIE-fen-OX-in) USAN.
Use: Antidiarrheal; antiperistaltic.
W/Atropine sulfate.
See: Motofen.

Differin. (Galderma) Adapalene. **Gel:** 0.1%. EDTA, methylparaben. Tube. 45 g. **Cream:** 0.1%. EDTA, glycerin, parabens. Tube. 45 g. **Lot:** 0.1%. EDTA, parabens, phenoxyethanol, propylene alcohol, stearyl alcohol, triglycerides. 56.6 g. **Soln.:** 0.1%. Alcohol 30%, PEG-400. 30 mL glass bottles with applicator and 60 unit-of-use pledgets. *Rx.*
Use: Dermatologic, acne; retinoid.

Difil-G. (Stewart-Jackson) Dyphylline

200 mg, guaifenesin 300 mg. Tab. 100s. *Rx.*
Use: Antiasthmatic combination, xanthine combination.

Difil-G Forte. (Stewart-Jackson) Dyphylline 100 mg, guaifenesin 100 mg per 5 mL. Menthol flavor. Liq. 237 mL. *Rx.*
Use: Antiasthmatic combination, xanthine combination.

Difil-G 400. (SJ Pharmaceuticals) Dyphylline 200 mg, guaifenesin 400 mg. Maltodextrin. Tab. 100s. *Rx.*
Use: Antiasthmatic combination, xanthine combination.

• **diflorasone diacetate.** (die-FLORE-ah-sone) *USP 34.*
Use: Anti-inflammatory, topical; antipruritic.
See: ApexiCon.
ApexiCon E.
Florone.
Maxiflor.
Psorcon E.

diflorasone diacetate. (Various Mfr.) Diflorasone diacetate 0.05%. Cream. Oint. Tube. 15 g, 30 g, 60 g. *Rx.*
Use: Anti-inflammatory, topical; antipruritic.

• **difloxacin hydrochloride.** (die-FLOX-ah-SIN) USAN.
Use: Anti-infective (DNA gyrase inhibitor).

• **difluanine hydrochloride.** (die-FLEW-an-EEN) USAN.
Use: CNS stimulant.

Diflucan. (Pfizer) Fluconazole. **Tab.:** 50 mg, 100 mg, 150 mg, 200 mg. Bot. 30s (except 150 mg), UD 100s (100 mg, 200 mg only), UD 1s (150 mg only). **Pow. for Oral Susp.:** 10 mg/mL when reconstituted, sucrose, orange flavor. Bot. 350 mg; 40 mg/mL when reconstituted, sucrose, orange flavor. Bot. 1,400 mg. *Rx.*
Use: Antifungal.

• **diflucortolone.** (die-flew-CORE-toe-lone) USAN.
Use: Corticosteroid, topical.

• **diflucortolone pivalate.** (die-flew-CORE-toe-lone) USAN.
Use: Corticosteroid, topical.

• **diflumidone sodium.** (die-FLEW-mih-DOHN) USAN.
Use: Anti-inflammatory.

• **diflunisal.** (die-FLOO-nih-sal) *USP 34.*
Use: Salicylate.

diflunisal. (Teva) Diflunisal 500 mg. Tab. Bot. 100s, 500s, unit-of-use 60s. *Rx.*
Use: Salicylate.

• **difluprednate.** (DIE-flew-PRED-nate) USAN.
Use: Corticosteroid, ophthalmic.
See: Durezol.

• **diftalone.** (DIFF-tah-lone) USAN.
Use: Anti-inflammatory; analgesic.

• **digalloyl trioleate.** (dye-GAL-loe-il trye-OH-lee-ate) USAN.

Di-Gel. (Schering-Plough) Aluminum hydroxide (equivalent to dried gel) 200 mg, magnesium hydroxide 200 mg, simethicone 20 mg/5 mL. Saccharin, sorbitol. Liq. Bot. 180 mL, 360 mL. *OTC.*
Use: Antacid; antiflatulent.

Di-Gel, Advanced. (Schering-Plough) Magnesium hydroxide 128 mg, calcium carbonate 280 mg, simethicone 20 mg. Tab. Bot. 30s, 60s, 90s. *OTC.*
Use: Antacid; antiflatulent.

Digestamic. (Lexis Laboratories) Pancrelipase 300 mg, pepsin 100 mg. Tab. Bot. 50s. *Rx-OTC.*
Use: Digestive aid.

Digestamic Liquid. (Lexis Laboratories) Belladonna leaf fluid extract 0.64 min/5 mL. Bot. 8 oz. *Rx-OTC.*
Use: Anticholinergic; antispasmodic.

Digestant. (Canright) Pancreatin 5.25 g, ox bile extract 2 g, pepsin 5 g, betaine hydrochloride 1 g. Tab. Bot. 100s, 1000s. *Rx-OTC.*
Use: Digestive aid.

Digestive Compound. (Thurston) Betaine hydrochloride 3.25 g, pepsin 1 g, papain 2 g, mycozyme 2 g, ox bile 2 g. 2 Tab. Bot. 100s, 500s. *Rx-OTC.*
Use: Digestive aid.

digestive enzymes.
See: Amylase.
Kutrase Capsules.
Ku-Zyme Capsules.
Lipase.
Lipram.
Pancrease.
Pancrecarb.
Pancrelipase.
Panokase Tablets.
Plaretase 800.
Protease.
Ultrase.
Viokase.

digestive products, miscellaneous.
Use: Digestive enzyme supplement.
See: Arco-Lase.
Enzobile Improved.
Ku-Zyme Capsules.

Digex. (Pronoval) Amylase 30 mg, cellulase 2 mg, hyoscyamine sulfate 0.0625 mg, lipase 1,200 units, phenyltoloxamine citrate 15 mg, protease 6 mg. Cap. 100s. *Rx.*
Use: Gastrointestinal anticholinergic/

antispasmodic, gastrointestinal anticholinergic combination.

Digex NF. (Pronova) Hyoscyamine sulfate 0.0625 mg, phenyltoloxamine citrate 15 mg. Lactose. Cap. 100s. *Rx.*
Use: Gastrointestinal anticholinergic/antispasmodic, gastrointestinal anticholinergic combination.

Digibind. (GlaxoSmithKline) Digoxin immune Fab (ovine) 38 mg/vial, sodium chloride 28 mg, preservative free. Each vial will bind ≈ digoxin 0.5 mg. Pow. for Inj., lyophilized. Vial. *Rx.*
Use: Antidote.

Digidote. (Boehringer Mannheim)
Use: Antidote. [Orphan Drug]

DigiFab. (Savage) Digoxin immune Fab (ovine) 40 mg/vial, sodium acetate 2 mg, preservative free. Each vial will bind ≈ 0.5 mg digoxin. Pow. for Inj., lyophilized. Vial. *Rx.*
Use: Antidote.

•**digitalis.** (dih-jih-TAL-iss) *USP 34.*
Use: Cardiovascular agent.
See: Crystodigin.
Deslanoside.
Digoxin.
Lanoxin.

digitalis leaf, powdered.
Use: Cardiovascular agent.

digitalis tincture.
Use: Cardiovascular agent.

•**digoxin.** (dih-JOX-in) *USP 34.*
Use: Cardiovascular agent.
See: Lanoxin.

digoxin. (Various Mfr.) Digoxin. **Tab.:** 0.125 mg, 0.25 mg. Bot. 1000s **Ped. Elix.:** 0.05 mg/mL. Bot. 60 mL; UD 2.5 mL, 5 mL. **Inj.:** 0.25 mg/mL, alcohol 10%, propylene glycol 40% per mL. *Tubex* or *Carpuject* 1 mL, 2 mL. *Rx.*
Use: Inotropic agent; cardiac glycoside.

digoxin. (Elkins-Sinn) Digoxin 0.25 mg/ mL, alcohol 0.1 mL, propylene glycol 0.4 mL per mL. Inj. Amp. 2 mL. *Rx.*
Use: Inotropic agent; cardiac glycoside.

digoxin antibody.
See: Digibind.

digoxin immune Fab (ovine).
Use: Antidote.
See: Digibind.
Digidote.
DigiFab.

digoxin injection, pediatric. (Abbott) Digoxin 0.1 mg/mL, propylene glycol 40%, alcohol 10%. Ped. Inj. Amp. 1 mL. *Rx.*
Use: Inotropic agent; cardiac glycoside.

digoxin I-125 immunoassay. (Abbott Diagnostics) Digoxin diagnostic kit for the quantitative determination of serum digoxin. 100s, 300s.
Use: Diagnostic aid.

Digoxin Riabead. (Abbott Diagnostics) Solid-phase radioimmunoassay for quantitative measurement of serum digoxin. Test kit 100s, 300s.
Use: Diagnostic aid.

•**dihexyverine hydrochloride.** (die-HEX-ih-ver-een) USAN.
Use: Anticholinergic.

Dihistine Elixir. (Various Mfr.) Phenylephrine hydrochloride 5 mg, chlorpheniramine maleate 2 mg/5 mL. Bot. Pt, gal. *OTC.*
Use: Antihistamine, decongestant.

Dihistine Expectorant. (Alpharma) Pseudoephedrine hydrochloride 30 mg, codeine phosphate 10 mg, guaifenesin 100 mg per 5 mL. Alcohol 7.5%, saccharin, sorbitol, sucrose. Liq. Bot. 473 mL. *c-v.*
Use: Upper respiratory combination, antitussive, decongestant, expectorant.

dihydan soluble.
See: Phenytoin Sodium.

dihydrocodeine. Paracodin. Drocode.
Use: Analgesic, antitussive.

•**dihydrocodeine bitartrate.** (die-high-droe-KOE-deen bye-TAR-trate) *USP 34.*
Use: Analgesic.
See: Hydrocodone Bitartrate.
W/Acetaminophen, Caffeine.
See: Trezix.
W/Brompheniramine Maleate, Phenylephrine Hydrochloride.
See: Poly-Tussin DHC.
W/Brompheniramine Maleate, Pseudoephedrine Hydrochloride.
See: J-Cof DHC.
W/Caffeine, Aspirin.
See: Synalgos-DC.
W/Chlorpheniramine Maleate, Phenylephrine Hydrochloride.
See: DiHydro-PE.
Duohist DH.
Pancof PD.
W/Chlorpheniramine Maleate, Pseudoephedrine Hydrochloride.
See: DiHydro-CP.
W/Combinations.
See: Novahistine DH.
Pancof.
Pancof EXP.
Tricof.
Tricof EXP.
Tricof PD.
WellTuss EXP.
W/Guaifenesin.
See: J-Max DHC.

W/Guaifenesin, Phenylephrine Hydro-
chloride.
See: Donatuss DC.
Poly-Tussin EX.
W/Guaifenesin, Pseudoephedrine Hydro-
chloride.
See: Despec-EXP.
W/Phenylephrine Hydrochloride.
See: Alahist DHC.
W/Phenylephrine Hydrochloride, Pyril-
amine Maleate.
See: Poly Hist DHC.
dihydrocodeinone resin complex.
W/Phenyltoloxamine resin complex.
See: Tussionex.
**dihydrocodeine 3 mg/BPM 4 mg/
phenylephrine hydrochloride 7.5 mg.**
(Kylemore) Brompheniramine maleate
4 mg, dihydrocodeine bitartrate 3 mg,
phenylephrine hydrochloride 7.5 mg.
Glycerin, propylene glycol, saccharin,
sorbitol. Grape flavor. Liq. 473 mL. *c-v.*
Use: Upper respiratory combination,
antitussive combination.
DiHydro-CP. (Cypress Pharmaceutical)
Chlorpheniramine maleate 2 mg,
dihydrocodeine bitartrate 7.5 mg,
pseudoephedrine hydrochloride 15 mg
per 5 mL. Saccharin, sorbitol. Alcohol
free, dye free, and sugar free. Grape
flavor. Syr. 473 mL. *c-iii.*
Use: Upper respiratory combination, antitussive combination.
dihydroergocornine. Ergot alkaline
component of hydergine.
dihydroergocristine. Ergot alkaloid component of hydergine.
dihydroergocryptine. Ergot alkaloid
component of hydergine.
dihydroergotamine. (Sandoz) (D.H.E. 45)
Dihydroergotamine mesylate. Amp. *Rx.*
Use: Agent for migraine; antiadrenergic.
•**dihydroergotamine mesylate.** (DIE-
high-droe-err-GOT-uh-meen) *USP 34.*
Dihydroergotamine methanesulfonate.
Use: Antiadrenergic; antimigraine.
See: D.H.E. 45.
Migranal.
dihydroergotamine mesylate. (Various
Mfr.) Dihydroergotamine mesylate
1 mg/mL. Alcohol 6.2%, glycerin 15%.
Inj. Vial. 1 mL. *Rx.*
Use: Migraine agent.
dihydroergotoxine. Ergoloid mesylate. *Rx.*
Use: Psychotherapeutic agent.
See: Ergoloid Mesylates.
Gerimal.
Hydergine.
5,6-dihydro-5-azacytidine. (Ilex
Oncology)
Use: Antineoplastic. [Orphan Drug]

dihydrofollicular hormone.
See: Estradiol.
dihydrofolliculin.
See: Estradiol.
dihydrohydroxycodeinone.
Use: Analgesic; narcotic.
See: Oxycodone. (Eucodal, Eukodal).
dihydroindolone derivatives.
Use: Antipsychotic.
See: Molindone Hydrochloride.
dihydromorphinone hydrochloride.
See: Dilaudid.
DiHydro-PE. (Cypress Pharmaceutical)
Chlorpheniramine maleate 2 mg,
dihydrocodeine bitartrate 3 mg, phenyl-
ephrine hydrochloride 7.5 mg per 5 mL.
Saccharin, sorbitol. Grape flavor. Syr.
118 mL. *c-v.*
Use: Upper respiratory combination, an-
titussive combination.
•**dihydrostreptomycin sulfate.** (die-
HIGH-droe-strep-toe-MY-sin) *USP 34.*
Use: Anti-infective.
dihydrotachysterol. (die-HIGH-droe-
tack-ISS-ter-ole)
Use: Vitamin.
dihydrotestosterone.
Use: AIDS. [Orphan Drug]
See: Androgel-DHT.
dihydrotheelin.
See: Estradiol.
dihydroxyacetone.
See: Chromelin Complexion Blender.
•**dihydroxyaluminum aminoacetate.**
(die-hye-DROX-ee-ah-LOO-mi-num ah-
MEE-no-ASS-eh-tate) *USP 34.*
Use: Antacid.
•**dihydroxyaluminum sodium carbonate.** (die-hye-DROX-ee-ah-LOO-mi-
num ah-MEE-no-ASS-eh-tate) *USP 34.*
Use: Antacid.
See: Rolaids.
dihydroxycholecalciferol.
See: Rocaltrol.
24,25 dihydroxycholecalciferol.
(Lemmon)
Use: Uremic osteodystrophy. [Orphan
Drug]
dihydroxyestrin.
See: Estradiol.
dihydroxyfluorane. Fluorescein.
dihydroxyphenylisatin.
See: Oxyphenisatin Acetate.
dihydroxyphenyloxindol.
See: Oxyphenisatin Acetate.
dihydroxypropyl theophylline. Dyphylline.
See: Neothylline
•**dihydroxy (stearato) aluminum.** *NF 29.*
Aluminum monostearate.

diiodohydroxyquin.
Use: Amebicide.
See: Iodoquinol.

diiodohydroxyquinoline.
See: Iodoquinol.

diisopromine hydrochloride. (Lab. for Pharmaceutical Development, Inc.)
See: Desquam-X.

diisopropyl phosphorofluoridate.
See: Floropryl.

diisopropyl sebacate.
Use: Moisturizing agent.

dilaminate. Mixture of magnesium carbide and dihydroxyaluminum glycinate. *OTC.*
Use: Antacid.

Dilantin. (Parke-Davis) Phenytoin 30 mg, 100 mg. Lactose, sugar. ER Cap. 100s, 1,000s, UD 100s. *Rx.*
Use: Anticonvulsant, hydantoin.

Dilantin Infatab. (Pfizer) Phenytoin 50 mg. Saccharin, sucrose. Chew. Tab. 100s, UD 100s. *Rx.*
Use: Anticonvulsant.

Dilantin-125. (Pfizer) Phenytoin 125 mg per 5 mL. Alcohol ≤ 0.6%, glycerin, sodium benzoate, sucrose. Orange-vanilla flavor. Susp. 240 mL. *Rx.*
Use: Anticonvulsant.

Dilantin Sodium w/Phenobarbital Kapseal. (Parke-Davis) Phenytoin sodium 100 mg, phenobarbital 16 mg, 32 mg. Cap. Bot. 100s, 1000s, UD 100s (32 mg only). *Rx.*
Use: Anticonvulsant; hypnotic; sedative.

Dilantin-30 Pediatric. (Parke-Davis) Phenytoin 30 mg/5 mL, alcohol 0.6%. Susp. Bot. 240 mL, 5 mL. *Rx.*
Use: Anticonvulsant.

Dilatrate-SR. (Schwarz Pharma) Isosorbide dinitrate 40 mg. Lactose, sucrose. SR Cap. Bot. 100s. *Rx.*
Use: Vasodilator.

Dilaudid. (Purdue Pharma) Hydromorphone hydrochloride. **Inj., Soln.:** 1 mg/mL, 2 mg/mL, 4 mg/mL. Amps. 1 mL. Multidose vials (with EDTA and methyl- and propylparabens, vial stopper contains latex). 20 mL (2 mg/mL only). **Liq.:** 1 mg/1 mL. Parabens, sucrose, glycerin. May contain sodium metabisulfite. 473 mL. **Supp.:** 3 mg. Cocoa butter. Box 6s. **Tab.:** 2 mg, 4 mg, 8 mg (may contain sodium metabisulfite). Lactose. Bot. 100s, 500s (except 8 mg), UD 100s (except 8 mg). *c-II.*
Use: Opioid analgesic.

Dilaudid-HP. (Purdue Pharma) Hydromorphone hydrochloride. **Inj. Soln., Conc.:** 10 mg/mL. Amps. 1 mL, 5 mL.

Single-dose vials. 50 mL. **Inj., Lyophilized Pow. for Soln., Conc.:** 250 mg (10 mg/mL after reconstitution). Preservative free. Single-dose vials. *c-II.*
Use: Opioid analgesic.

•**dilevalol hydrochloride.** (DIE-LEV-ah-lole) USAN.
Use: Antihypertensive; antiadrenergic (β-receptor).

Dilex-G. (Poly) Dyphylline 100 mg, guaifenesin 100 mg per 5 mL. Alcohol free. Parabens, saccharin, sucrose, sorbitol. Menthol flavor. Syrup. 473 mL. *Rx.*
Use: Antiasthmatic combination, xanthine combination.

Dilex-G 400. (Poly) Dyphylline 200 mg, guaifenesin 400 mg. Tab. 100s. *Rx.*
Use: Antiasthmatic combination, xanthine combination.

Dilex-G 200. (Poly) Dyphylline 100 mg, guaifenesin 200 mg per 5 mL. Sugar free. Syrup. 473 mL. *Rx.*
Use: Antiasthmatic combination, xanthine combination.

dilithium carbonate. Lithium carbonate, USP.
Use: Antipsychotic.

•**dilmapimod.** (dil-MAP-i-mod) USAN.
Use: Respiratory agent.

•**dilmapimod tosylate.** (dil-MAP-i-mod) USAN.
Use: Respiratory agent.

Dilotab II. (Zee Medical) Acetaminophen 325 mg, phenylephrine hydrochloride 5 mg. Tab. 100s, 250s. *OTC.*
Use: Analgesic, decongestant, upper respiratory combination.

•**diloxanide furoate.** (dye-LOX-a-nide FUR-oh-ate) *USP 34.*
Use: Anti-infective.

Dilt-CD. (Apotex USA) Diltiazem hydrochloride 120 mg, 180 mg, 240 mg, 300 mg. Sucrose. ER Cap. 30s, 90s, 500s. *Rx.*
Use: Calcium channel blocker.

Diltia XT. (Andrx Pharmaceuticals) Diltiazem hydrochloride 120 mg, 180 mg, 240 mg. Lactose. ER Cap. Bot. 100s, 500s, 1000s. *Rx.*
Use: Calcium channel blocker.

•**diltiazem hydrochloride.** (dill-TIE-uh-zem) *USP 34.*
Use: Vasodilator (coronary), calcium channel blocker.
See: Cardizem.
Cardizem CD.
Cardizem LA.
Cartia XT.
Dilt-CD.
Diltia XT.

Dilt-XR.
Diltzac.
Matzim LA.
Taztia XT.
Tiazac.

diltiazem hydrochloride. (Various Mfr)
Diltiazem hydrochloride 360 mg,
420 mg. May contain sucrose. ER Cap.
30s (420 mg only), 90s, 1000s. *Rx.*
Use: Calcium channel blocker.

diltiazem hydrochloride. (Various Mfr.)
Diltiazem. **Inj.:** 5 mg/mL. Vials. 5 mL,
10 mL, 25 mL. **Tab.:** 30 mg, 60 mg,
90 mg, 120 mg. May contain lactose or
methylparaben. Bot. 100s, 500s,
1000s. *Rx.*
Use: Calcium channel blocker.

**diltiazem hydrochloride extended-
release.** (Various Mfr.) Diltiazem hydrochloride 60 mg, 90 mg, 120 mg,
180 mg, 240 mg, 300 mg. May contain
sucrose or sugar spheres. ER Cap.
Bot. 30s (except 60 mg, 90 mg), 90s
(except 60 mg, 90 mg), 100s (except
300 mg), 500s (except 60 mg, 90 mg),
1000s (except 60 mg, 90 mg). *Rx.*
Use: Calcium channel blocking agent.

•**diltiazem maleate.** (dill-TIE-ah-zem
MAL-ate) USAN.
Use: Calcium channel blocker; antihy-
pertensive.

Dilt-XR. (Apotex USA) Diltiazem hydro-
chloride 120 mg, 180 mg, 240 mg. ER
Cap. 100s. *Rx.*
Use: Calcium channel blocker.

Diltzac. (Apotex) Diltiazem hydrochloride
120 mg, 180 mg, 240 mg, 300 mg,
360 mg. ER Cap. 30s, 90s, 100s, 500s,
1,000s (120 mg only). *Rx.*
Use: Cardiovascular agent, calcium
channel blocking agent.

diluent.
See: Broncho Saline.
Sodium Chloride.
Sodium Chloride 0.45%.
Sodium Chloride 0.9%.

Dimaphen DM. (Major) Pseudoephedrine hydrochloride 15 mg, brompheniramine maleate 1 mg, dextromethorphan HBr 5 mg per 5 mL. Saccharin,
sorbitol, grape flavor, alcohol free. Elix.
Bot. 118 mL. *OTC.*
Use: Upper respiratory combination, antitussive combination.

•**dimefadane.** (DIE-meh-fah-dane) USAN.
Use: Analgesic.

•**dimefilcon A.** (DIE-meh-FILL-kahn A)
USAN.
Use: Contact lens material (hydrophilic).

•**dimefline hydrochloride.** (DIE-meh-
fleen) USAN.
Use: Respiratory.

•**dimefocon A.** (DIE-meh-FOE-kahn A)
USAN.
Use: Contact lens material (hydrophobic).

Dimenest. (Forest) Dimenhydrinate
50 mg/mL. Vial 10 mL. *Rx.*
Use: Antiemetic; antivertigo.

•**dimenhydrinate.** (die-men-HIGH-drih-
nate) USP 34.
Tall Man: dimenhyDRINATE
Use: Antiemetic; antihistamine.
See: Dimenest.
Dimentabs.
Dramamine.
Dymenate.
Signate.
Traveltabs.

Dimentabs. (Jones Pharma) Dimenhydrinate 50 mg. Tab. Bot. 100s. *OTC.*
Use: Antiemetic; antivertigo.

•**dimepranol acedoben.** (DIE-MEH-prah-
nahl ah-SEE-doe-BEN) USAN.
Use: Immunomodulator.

•**dimercaprol.** (die-mer-CAP-role)
USP 34. Formerly BAL.
Use: Antidote to gold, arsenic, and mer-
cury poisoning; metal complexing
agent.
See: BAL in Oil.

Dimetane Decongestant. (Wyeth Consumer Healthcare) **Capl.:** Brompheniramine maleate 4 mg, phenylephrine
hydrochloride 10 mg. Capl. Bot. 24s,
48s. **Elix.:** Brompheniramine maleate
2 mg, phenylephrine hydrochloride
5 mg/5 mL, alcohol 2.3%. Bot. 120 mL.
OTC.
Use: Antihistamine, decongestant.

Dimetane DX. (Creekwood Pharmaceutical) Brompheniramine maleate
2 mg, dextromethorphan hydrobromide
10 mg, pseudoephedrine hydrochloride 30 mg per 5 mL. Berry flavoring,
glycerin, propylene glycol, saccharin,
sorbitol. Alcohol free, dye free, gluten
free, and sugar free. Liq. 118 mL. *Rx.*
Use: Upper respiratory combination, antitussive combination.

Dimetapp Children's Cold & Allergy.
(Wyeth Consumer Healthcare) Phenylephrine hydrochloride 2.5 mg, brompheniramine maleate 1 mg per 5 mL. Alcohol free. Sorbitol, sucralose. Grape
flavor. Elix. 237 mL with dosage cup.
OTC.
Use: Upper respiratory combination, decongestant and antihistamine.

Dimetapp Children's Cold & Fever. (Wyeth Consumer Healthcare) Pseudoephedrine hydrochloride 15 mg, ibuprofen 100 mg per 5 mL. Alcohol free. Sorbitol, sucrose. Grape flavor. Susp. 120 mL. *OTC.*
Use: Pediatric decongestant and analgesic.

Dimetapp Children's ND Non-Drowsy Allergy. (Wyeth Consumer Healthcare) Loratadine. **Orally Disintegrating Tab.:** 10 mg. Aspartame, corn syrup, mannitol, phenylalanine 8.4 mg. 6s, 12. **Syrup:** 5 mg/5 mL. Sucrose. 118 mL. *OTC.*
Use: Antihistamine, peripherally selective piperidine.

Dimetapp Children's Nighttime Flu. (Wyeth Consumer Healthcare) Pseudoephedrine hydrochloride 15 mg, brompheniramine maleate 1 mg, dextromethorphan HBr 5 mg, acetaminophen 160 mg per 5 mL. Corn syrup, saccharin, sorbitol, bubble gum flavor, alcohol free. Syr. Bot. 118 mL. *OTC.*
Use: Upper respiratory combination, decongestant, antihistamine, antitussive, analgesic.

Dimetapp Children's Non-Drowsy Flu. (Wyeth Consumer Healthcare) Pseudoephedrine hydrochloride 15 mg, dextromethorphan HBr 5 mg, acetaminophen 160 mg per 5 mL. Corn syrup, saccharin, sorbitol, fruit flavor, alcohol free. Syrup. Bot. 118 mL. *OTC.*
Use: Upper respiratory combination, decongestant, antitussive, analgesic.

Dimetapp Cold & Allergy Elixir. (Wyeth Consumer Healthcare) Pseudoephedrine hydrochloride 15 mg, brompheniramine maleate 1 mg/5 mL, corn syrup, saccharin, sorbitol, grape flavor, alcohol free. Elix. Bot. 118 mL, 237 mL. *OTC.*
Use: Upper respiratory combination, decongestant, antihistamine.

Dimetapp DM Children's Cold & Cough. (Wyeth Consumer Healthcare) Pseudoephedrine hydrochloride 15 mg, brompheniramine maleate 1 mg, dextromethorphan HBr 5 mg per 5 mL. Sorbitol, saccharin, corn syrup, grape flavor, alcohol free. Elix. Bot. 118 mL, 237 mL. *OTC.*
Use: Upper respiratory combination, decongestant, antihistamine, antitussive.

Dimetapp Long Acting Cough Plus Cold. (Wyeth Consumer Healthcare) Dextromethorphan HBr 7.5 mg, chlorpheniramine maleate 1 mg per 5 mL. Sodium 3 mg/5 mL, sorbitol, sucralose.

Fruit punch flavor. Syrup. 118 mL. *OTC.*
Use: Antitussive combination, upper respiratory combination.

Dimetapp, Maximum Strength 12-Hour Non-Drowsy. (Wyeth Consumer Healthcare) Pseudoephedrine hydrochloride 120 mg. ER Tab. Pkg. 10s. *OTC.*
Use: Nasal decongestant, arylalkylamine.

Dimetapp Sinus. (Wyeth Consumer Healthcare) Pseudoephedrine hydrochloride 30 mg, ibuprofen 200 mg. Cap. Bot. 20s, 40s. *OTC.*
Use: Antihistamine, decongestant.

Dimetapp Toddler's Decongestant Plus Cough. (Wyeth Consumer Healthcare) Phenylephrine hydrochloride 2.5 mg, dextromethorphan HBr 1.25 mg per 0.8 mL. Glycerin, sorbitol, sucralose. Grape flavor, alcohol free. Drops. Bot. 15 mL w/dropper. *OTC.*
Use: Upper respiratory combination, antitussive combination.

•**dimethadione.** (DIE-meth-ah-DIE-ohn) USAN.
Use: Anticonvulsant.

•**dimethicone.** (DIE-meth-ih-cone) *NF 29.*
Use: Prosthetic aid (soft tissue); component of barrier creams; lubricant; hydrophobic agent.
See: Aloe Vesta.
  Aveeno Baby.
  Aveeno Daily Moisturizing.
  Gold Bond Medicated Triple Action Relief.
  Pro-Q.
  Silicone.
W/Combinations.
See: Soothe & Cool.
W/Pramoxine Hydrochloride.
See: Gold Bond Intensive Healing.
W/Zinc Oxide.
See: A & D Zinc Oxide Cream.

•**dimethicone 350.** (DIE-meth-ih-cone 350) USAN.
Use: Prosthetic aid for soft tissue.

•**dimethindene maleate.** (DIE-METH-indeen) *USP 34.*
Use: Antihistamine.

•**dimethisoquin hydrochloride.** (diemeh-THIGH-so-kwin) USAN.
Use: Antibiotic, topical.

•**dimethisterone.** (DIE-meth-ISS-ter-ohn) *NF 29.*
Use: Hormone, progestin.

dimethoxyphenyl penicillin sodium.
Use: Anti-infective.
See: Methicillin Sodium.

dimethpyridene maleate. Dimethindene Maleate.

dimethylaminophenazone.
See: Aminopyrine.
dimethylamino pyrazine sulfate.
See: Ampyzine Sulfate.
dimethylcarbamate.
See: Mestinon.
dimethylhexestrol dipropionate.
Promethestrol Dipropionate.
•**dimethyl fumarate.** (dye-METH-il)
USAN.
Use: Immunomodulator.
dimethyl polysiloxane.
See: Dimethicone.
•**dimethyl sulfoxide.** (die-METH-uhl sull-FOX-ide) *USP 34.*
Use: Interstitial cystitis agent.
See: Rimso-50.
dimethyl sulfoxide. (Bioniche) Dimethyl sulfoxide in a 50% aqueous solution.
50 mL. *Rx.*
Use: Interstitial cystitis agent.
dimethyl sulfoxide. (Pharma 21)
Use: Increased intracranial pressure.
[Orphan Drug]
dimethyl-tubocurarine iodide.
Use: Muscle relaxant.
dimethylurethimine.
See: Meturedepa.
•**dimoxamine hydrochloride.** (die-MOX-AH-meen) USAN.
Use: Memory adjuvant.
Dimycor. (Standard Drug Co.) Penta-erythritol tetranitrate 10 mg, pheno-barbital 15 mg. Tab. Bot. 1000s. *Rx.*
Use: Antianginal; hypnotic; sedative.
•**dinaciclib.** (din-a-SYE-klib) USAN.
Use: Antineoplastic.
Dinacrin. (Sanofi-Synthelabo) Isonico-tinic acid, hydrazide. *Rx.*
Use: Antituberculosal.
•**dinoprost.** (DIE-no-proste) USAN.
Use: Oxytocic; prostaglandin.
•**dinoprostone.** (DIE-no-PROSTE-ohn)
USP 34.
Use: Abortifacient; agent for cervical rip-ening; oxytocic; prostaglandin.
See: Cervidil.
Prepidil.
Prostin E$_2$.
•**dinoprost tromethamine.** (DIE-no-proste troe-METH-ah-meen) *USP 34.*
Use: Oxytocic; prostaglandin.
Diocto. (Various Mfr.) Docusate sodium.
Syr.: 60 mg/15 mL. Bot. 480 mL. **Liq.:**
150 mg/15 mL. Bot. 480 mL. *OTC.*
Use: Laxative.
Dioctolose. (Ivax) Docusate potassium
100 mg. Cap. Bot. 100s, 1000s.
Use: Laxative.

dioctyl calcium sulfosuccinate. (die-OCK-till SULL-foe-SUCK-sih-nate)
Docusate Calcium.
Use: Laxative.
dioctyl sodium sulfosuccinate.
Use: Non-laxative fecal softener.
See: Docusate Sodium.
Dioctyn Softgels. (Dixon-Shane) Docu-sate sodium 100 mg. Sorbitol. Cap.
1000s. *OTC.*
Use: Fecal softener.
diodone injection.
See: Iodopyracet injection.
•**diohippuric acid I 125.** (dye-oh-hip-YOOR-ik) USAN.
Use: Radiopharmaceutical.
•**diohippuric acid I 131.** (dye-oh-hip-YOOR-ik) USAN.
Use: Radiopharmaceutical.
Dio-Hist. (Health for Life Brands) Dextro-methorphan 30 mg, thenylpyramine hydrochloride 80 mg, phenylephrine hydrochloride 20 mg, potassium tartrate
$\frac{1}{24}$ g/oz. Bot. 4 oz. *OTC.*
Use: Antihistamine.
diolamine. Diethanolamine.
diolostene.
See: Methandriol.
Dionex. (Henry Schein) Docusate so-dium 100 mg, 250 mg. Cap. Bot. 100s,
250s, 1000s. *OTC.*
Use: Laxative.
dionin. Ethylmorphine hydrochloride.
Use: Cough depressant, oral; ocular lymphagogue.
Dionosil Oily. (GlaxoSmithKline) Propyl-iodone 60% in peanut oil. Inj. Vial
20 mL.
Use: Radiopaque agent.
diophyllin.
See: Aminophylline.
diopterin. Pteroylglutamic acid, PDGA,
Pteroyl-alpha-glutamylglutamic acid.
Use: Antineoplastic.
Diorapin. (Standex) **Tab.:** Estrogenic conjugate 0.625 mg, methyltestos-terone 5 mg. Bot. 100s. **Inj.:** Estrone
2 mg, testosterone 25 mg/mL. Vial
10 mL. *Rx.*
Use: Androgen, estrogen combination.
Diosmin. Buchu resin obtained from lvs. of barosma serratifolia and alliedruta-ceae.
Dio-Soft. (Standex) Docusate sodium
100 mg, casanthranol 30 mg. Cap. Bot.
100s. *OTC.*
Use: Laxative.
Diostate D. (Pharmacia) Vitamin D
400 units, calcium 343 mg, phosphorus
265 mg. 3 Tab. Bot. 100s. *OTC.*
Use: Mineral, vitamin supplement.

•**diotyrosine I 125.** (die-oh-TIE-row-seen) USAN.
Use: Radiopharmaceutical.
•**diotyrosine I 131.** (die-oh-TIE-row-seen) USAN.
Use: Radiopharmaceutical.
Diovan. (Novartis) Valsartan 40 mg, 80 mg, 160 mg, 320 mg. Polyethylene glycol 8000. Tab. Bot. 30s (40 mg only), 90s (except 40 mg), UD 100s (except 320 mg). *Rx.*
Use: Renin angiotensin system antagonist.
Diovan HCT. (Novartis) Valsartan/hydrochlorothiazide 80 mg/12.5 mg, 160 mg/12.5 mg, 160/25 mg, 320 mg/12.5 mg, 320 mg/25 mg. Tab. Bot. 90s, UD 100s. *Rx.*
Use: Antihypertensive.
•**dioxadrol hydrochloride.** (die-OX-ah-drole) USAN.
Use: Antidepressant.
dioxindol. Diacetylhydroxyphenylisatin.
dioxyanthranol.
See: Anthralin.
•**dioxybenzone.** (die-ox-ee-BEN-zone) *USP 34.*
Use: Ultraviolet screen.
W/Oxybenzone.
See: Solbar Plus 15.
dipalmitoylphosphatidylcholine.
Colfosceril palmitate.
Use: Synthetic lung surfactant.
dipalmitoylphosphatidylcholine/phosphatidylglycerol.
Use: Neonatal respiratory distress syndrome. [Orphan Drug]
See: ALEC.
diparcol hydrochloride. Diethazine.
Dipegyl.
See: Nicotinamide.
Dipentum. (UCB) Osalazine sodium 250 mg. Cap. Bot. 100s, 500s. *Rx.*
Use: Gastrointestinal agent.
dipeptidyl peptidase-4 inhibitor.
Use: Antidiabetic agent.
See: Linagliptin.
Saxagliptin.
Sitagliptin Phosphate.
diperodon hydrochloride.
Use: Anesthetic.
W/Methapyrilene Hydrochloride, Pyrilamine Maleate, Allantoin, Benzocaine, Menthol.
See: Antihistamine.
diphenadione.
Use: Anticoagulant.
Diphen AF. (Morton Grove) Diphenhydramine hydrochloride 12.5 mg/5 mL, saccharin, sugar, cherry flavor. Liq. Bot.

118 mL, 237 mL, 473 mL. *OTC.*
Use: Antihistamine, nonselective ethanolamine.
Diphenatol. (Rugby) Diphenoxylate hydrochloride 2.5 mg, atropine sulfate 0.025 mg. Tab. Bot. 100s, 500s, 1000s.
Use: Antidiarrheal.
Diphenhist. (Rugby) Diphenhydramine hydrochloride. **Cap.:** 25 mg. Benzyl alcohol, butylparaben, EDTA, lactose, parabens. 100s. **Oral Soln.:** 12.5 mg/5 mL. Saccharin sucrose. Bot. 120 mL, 473 mL. *OTC.*
Use: Antihistamine.
Diphenhist Captabs. (Rugby) Diphenhydramine hydrochloride 25 mg. Tab. Bot. 100s. *OTC.*
Use: Antihistamine, nonselective ethanolamine.
diphenhydramine. (Various Mfr.) Diphenhydramine hydrochloride 25 mg. Tab. Bot. 24s, 100s. *OTC.*
Use: Antihistamine, nonselective ethanolamine.
diphenhydramine and pseudoephedrine capsules.
Use: Antihistamine, decongestant.
•**diphenhydramine citrate.** (die-fen-HIGH-druh-meen) *USP 34.*
Tall Man: diphenhydrAMINE
Use: Antihistamine.
W/Acetaminophen.
See: Goody's PM.
W/Aspirin.
See: Alka-Seltzer PM.
W/Pseudoephedrine Hydrochloride.
See: Benadryl Children's Allergy & Cold.
Benadryl-D Children's Allergy & Sinus.
•**diphenhydramine hydrochloride.** (die-fen-HIGH-druh-meen) *USP 34.*
Tall Man: diphenhydrAMINE
Use: Antihistamine, nonselective ethanolamine, antitussive.
See: Altaryl Children's Allergy.
Benadryl Allergy Quick Dissolve.
Benadryl Itch Stopping Spray, Extra Strength.
Benadryl Itch Stopping Spray, Original Strength.
Benahist.
Clearly CalaGel.
Dermamycin.
Dermarest.
Fenylhist.
40 Winks.
Histine.
Hydramine Cough.
Hyrexin-50.
Nighttime Sleep Aid.
PediaCare Children's NightTime Cough.

Q-dryl.
Silphen Cough.
Simply Sleep.
Snooze Fast.
Theraflu Thin Strips Multi Symptom.
Triaminic Children's Allergy.
Triaminic Cough & Runny Nose.
Triaminic Thin Strips Long Acting
  Cough.
Tusstat.
Unisom SleepGels.
Unisom SleepMelts.
W/Acetaminophen.
  See: Excedrin PM.
  Extra Strength Pain Reliever PM.
  Legatrin PM.
  Percogesic Extra Strength.
  Tylenol PM.
  Tylenol Severe Allergy.
  Tylenol Sore Throat Nighttime.
  Unisom PM Pain.
W/Acetaminophen, Dextromethorphan
  Hydrobromide.
  See: Diabetic Tussin Cold & Flu.
  Diabetic Tussin Night Time Formula
  Cold/Flu.
W/Acetaminophen, Dextromethorphan
  Hydrobromide, Phenylephrine Hydro-
  chloride.
  See: Respa C & C.
W/Acetaminophen, Phenylephrine Hydro-
  chloride.
  See: Benadryl Allergy & Cold.
  Benadryl Allergy & Sinus Headache.
  Benadryl Severe Allergy & Sinus
  Headache Maximum Strength.
  Sudafed PE Multi-Symptom Severe
  Cold.
  Sudafed PE Nighttime Cold Maxi-
  mum Strength.
  Theraflu Nighttime Severe Cough &
  Cold.
  Theraflu Sugar-Free Nighttime Se-
  vere Cough & Cold.
  Theraflu Warming Relief Flu & Sore
  Throat.
  Tylenol Allergy Multi-Symptom Conve-
  nience Pack.
  Tylenol Allergy Multi-Symptom Night-
  time.
W/Benzethonium Chloride, Zinc Acetate.
  See: Calagel Maximum Strength.
W/Calamine.
  See: Ivarest Maximum Strength.
W/Codeine Phosphate, Phenylephrine
  Hydrochloride.
  See: Airacof.
W/Dextromethorphan Hydrobromide,
  Phenylephrine Hydrochloride.
  See: Duratuss AC.

W/Hydrocortisone, Nystatin.
  See: First Duke's Mouthwash.
W/Hydrocortisone, Nystatin, Tetracycline
  Hydrochloride.
  See: First Mary's Mouthwash.
W/Ibuprofen.
  See: Advil PM.
W/Phenylephrine Hydrochloride.
  See: Alahist LQ.
  Aldex-CT.
  Benadryl-D Allergy & Sinus.
  PediaCare Children's NightRest Multi-
  Symptom Cold.
  Pediatex-CT.
  Robitussin Pediatric Cough & Cold
  Nighttime.
  Sudafed PE Day & Night.
  Sudafed PE Nighttime Nasal Decon-
  gestant.
  Theraflu Thin Strips Nighttime Cold &
  Cough.
  Triaminic Children's Thin Strips Night
  Time Cold & Cough.
  Triaminic Night Time Cold & Cough.
W/Pseudoephedrine Hydrochloride.
  See: Respa-SA.
  Tekral.
W/Zinc Acetate.
  See: Anti-Itch.
diphenhydramine hydrochloride.
  (Various Mfr.) Diphenhydramine hydro-
  chloride 25 mg, 50 mg. Cap. Bot. 24s
  (25 mg only), 100s, 1000s. *Rx-OTC.*
  Use: Antihistamine.
diphenhydramine hydrochloride.
  (Various Mfr.) Diphenhydramine hydro-
  chloride 50 mg/mL. Inj. 1 mL fill in
  2 mL cartridges. *Rx.*
  Use: Antihistamine.
diphenhydramine hydrochloride.
  (Various Mfr.) Diphenhydramine hydrochloride 25 mg, 50 mg. Tab. 24s
  (25 mg), 50s (50 mg), 100s (25 mg).
  OTC.
  Use: Antihistamine.
**diphenhydramine hydrochloride,
  acetaminophen, and pseudoephedrine hydrochloride combinations.**
  Use: Upper respiratory combination, antihistamine, analgesic, decongestant.
**diphenhydramine hydrochloride,
  acetaminophen, dextromethorphan
  hydrobromide, pseudoephedrine
  hydrochloride combinations.**
  Use: Upper respiratory combination, antihistamine, analgesic, antitussive, decongestant.
**diphenhydramine hydrochloride and
  acetaminophen combinations.**
  Use: Upper respiratory combination, antihistamine, analgesic.

diphenhydramine hydrochloride and pseudoephedrine hydrochloride combinations.
Use: Upper respiratory combination, antihistamine, decongestant.

diphenhydramine tannate.
See: Dytan.
W/Carbetapentane Tannate, Phenylephrine Tannate.
See: D-Tann CD.
W/Dextromethorphan Tannate, Phenylephrine Tannate.
See: D-Tann DM.
W/Phenylephrine Tannate.
See: D-Tann.
Dytan-D.

•**diphenidol hydrochloride.** (die-FEN-ih-dahl) USAN.
Use: Antiemetic

•**diphenidol pamoate.** (die-FEN-ih-dahl) USAN.
Use: Antiemetic.

•**diphenoxylate hydrochloride.** (die-fen-OX-ih-late) *USP 34.*
Use: Antiperistaltic to treat diarrhea.
W/Atropine.
See: Lomotil.

diphenylhydantoin. Phenytoin.
Use: Anticonvulsant.

diphenylhydantoin sodium. Phenytoin sodium.
Use: Anticonvulsant.

diphenylhydroxycarbinol. Benzhydrol hydrochloride.

diphenylisatin.
See: Oxyphenisatin Acetate.

diphosphonic acid.
See: Etidronic acid.

diphosphopyridine (DPN).
Use: Antialcoholic. Under study.

diphosphothiamin. Cocarboxylase.

diphtheria and tetanus toxoids, adult.
(Merck) Diphtheria 2 Lf units, tetanus 2 Lf units/0.5 mL dose. Aluminum ≤ 0.53 mg, formaldehyde < 100 mcg (0.02%), trace thimerosal (mercury ≤ 0.3 mcg/dose). Inj., Susp. Single-dose vial. 0.5 mL. *Rx.*
Use: Active immunization, toxoid.

diphtheria and tetanus toxoids, adsorbed (for adult use).
Use: Active immunization, toxoid.
See: Decavac.
Diphtheria & Tetanus Toxoids, Adult.

diphtheria and tetanus toxoids, adsorbed (for pediatric use).
Use: Active immunization, toxoid.
See: Diphtheria & Tetanus Toxoids, Pediatric.

diphtheria and tetanus toxoids and acellular pertussis adsorbed, hepatitis B (recombinant) and inactivated poliovirus vaccine combined.
Use: Active immunization, toxoid.
See: Pediarix.

diphtheria and tetanus toxoids and acellular pertussis vaccine, adsorbed.
Use: Prevention against diphtheria, tetanus, and pertussis; immunizing agent.
See: Adacel.
Boostrix.
Daptacel.
Infanrix.
Tripedia.

diphtheria and tetanus toxoids, pediatric. (Aventis Pasteur) Diphtheria 6.7 Lf units, tetanus 5 Lf units/0.5 mL dose, aluminum potassium sulfate, thimerosal. Inj. Multidose vial 5 mL. *Rx.*
Use: Active immunization, toxoid.

diphtheria equine antitoxin. *Rx.*
Use: Prophylaxis and treatment of diphtheria.

•**diphtheria toxin for Schick Test.** (diff-THEER-ee-uh) *USP 34. Formerly Diphtheria Toxin, Diagnostic.*
Use: Diagnostic aid (dermal reactivity indicator).

Dipimol. (Everett) Dipyridamole 25 mg, 50 mg, 75 mg. Tab. Bot. 100s, 500s, 1000s.
Use: Antianginal.

dipivalyl epinephrine.
See: Propine Sterile Ophthalmic.

•**dipivefrin.** (die-PIHV-eh-FRIN) USAN.
Formerly Dipivalyl Epinephrine.
Use: Adrenergic, ophthalmic.

•**dipivefrin hydrochloride.** (die-PIHV-eh-FRIN) *USP 34.*
Use: Antiglaucoma agent.

Diprivan. (AstraZeneca) Propofol 10 mg/mL, soybean oil 100 mg, glycerol 22.5 mg, egg lecithin 12 mg, EDTA 0.005%, ph = 7 to 8.5. Inj. Single-use amp. 20 mL. Single-use infusion vial 50 mL, 100 mL. Prefilled single-use syr. 50 mL. *Rx.*
Use: Anesthetic, general.

Diprolene. (Schering-Plough) Betamethasone dipropionate 0.05%.
Cream: In cream base. Tube 15 g.
Oint.: In ointment base. Tube 15 g, 45 g. *Rx.*
Use: Anti-inflammatory; antipruritic, topical.

Diprolene AF Cream. (Schering-Plough) Betamethasone dipropionate cream

equivalent to 0.05% betamethasone. Tube 15 g, 45 g. *Rx.*
Use: Corticosteroid, topical.

dipropylacetic acid.
See: Valproic Acid.

Diprosone. (Schering-Plough) Betamethasone dipropionate 0.64 mg (equiv. to 0.5 mg betamethasone).
Cream: W/mineral oil, white petrolatum, polyethylene glycol 1000 monocetyl ether, cetostearyl alcohol, phosphoric acid, monobasic sodium phosphate with 4-chloro-m-cresol as preservative. Tube 15 g, 45 g. **Lot.:** W/isopropyl alcohol (46.8%). Bot. 20 mL, 60 mL.
Oint.: In white petrolatum and mineral oil base. Tube 15 g, 45 g. *Rx.*
Use: Corticosteroid, topical.

Diprosone Aerosol 0.1%. (Schering-Plough) Betamethasone dipropionate 6.4 mg (equiv. to 5 mg betamethasone) in vehicle of mineral oil, caprylic-capric triglyceride w/isopropyl alcohol 10%, inert hydrocarbon propellants (propane and isobutane). Can 85 g. *Rx.*
Use: Corticosteroid, topical.

•**dipyridamole.** (DIE-pih-RID-uh-mole) *USP 34.*
Use: Coronary vasodilator; antiplatelet agent.
See: Persantine.
W/Aspirin.
See: Aggrenox.

dipyridamole. (Various Mfr.) **Tab.:**
25 mg: 90s, 100s, 500s, 1,000s, 5,000s, UD 100s. **50 mg, 75 mg:** 100s, 500s, 1,000s, UD 100s. **Inj.:** 5 mg/mL. 50 mg of polyethylene glycol 600, tartaric acid 2 mg. Vial. 2 mL, 10 mL. *Rx.*
Use: Coronary vasodilator; antiplatelet agent.

•**dipyrithione.** (DIE-pihr-ih-THIGH-ohn) USAN.
Use: Antifungal; anti-infective.

•**dipyrone.** (DIE-pie-rone) USAN. *Formerly Methampyrone.*
Use: Analgesic; antipyretic.

•**diquafosol tetrasodium.** (dye-kwa-FOS-ol) USAN.
Use: Dry eye.

•**dirithromycin.** (die-RITH-row-MY-sin) USAN.
Use: Anti-infective, macrolide.

•**dirucotide.** (dye-RUK-oh-tide) USAN.
Use: Multiple sclerosis.

•**dirucotide acetate.** (dye-RUK-oh-tide) USAN.
Use: Multiple sclerosis.

disaccharide tripeptide glycerol dipalmitoyl.
Use: Antineoplastic. [Orphan Drug]
See: ImmTher.

Disalcid. (3M) Salsalate. **Tab.:** 500 mg, 750 mg. Bot. 100s, 500s, UD 100s.
Cap.: 500 mg. Bot. 100s. *Rx.*
Use: Analgesic.

Discase. (Omnis Surgical) Chymopapain 5 units/2 mL. Vial 5 mL. *Rx.*
Use: Intradiscal injection for herniated lumbar intervertebral discs.

DisCoVisc. (Alcon) Sodium hyaluronate 17 mg and sodium chondroitin sulfate 40 mg per mL. Soln. Single-use disposable syringe with 27-gauge cannula and cannula locking ring delivering 0.5 mL or 1 mL packaged in a blister tray. *Rx.*
Use: Ophthalmic surgical adjunct.

Disinfecting Solution. (Bausch & Lomb) Buffered, isotonic. Sodium chloride, sodium borate, boric acid, chlorhexidine 0.005%, EDTA 0.1%, thimerosal 0.001%. Bot. 355 mL. *OTC.*
Use: Contact lens disinfection system.

•**disiquonium chloride.** (die-SIH-CONE-ee-uhm) USAN.
Use: Antiseptic.

Diskets. (Cebert) Methadone hydrochloride 40 mg. Orange-pineapple flavor. Dispersible Tab. 100s. *c-II.*
Use: Opioid analgesic.

Dismiss Douche. (Schering-Plough) Sodium Cl, sodium citrate, citric acid, cetearyl octoate, ceteareth-27, fragrance. Pow. for dilution. Pkg. 2s.
Use: Vaginal agent.

Disobrom. (Geneva) Pseudoephedrine sulfate 120 mg, dexbrompheniramine maleate 6 mg. Tab. Bot 100s, 1000s. *Rx.*
Use: Antihistamine, decongestant.

•**disobutamide.** (DIE-so-BYOO-tam-ide) USAN.
Use: Cardiovascular agent (antiarrhythmic).

disodium carbonate.
See: Sodium Carbonate.

disodium chromate. Sodium Chromate Cr 51 Injection.

disodium chromoglycate.
See: Intal.
Nasalcrom.

disodium clodronate. (Discovery)
Use: Antihypercalcemic. [Orphan Drug]

disodium clodronate tetrahydrate.
Use: Increased bone resorption due to malignancy. [Orphan Drug]
See: Bonefos.

disodium edathamil.
See: Edathamil Disodium.
disodium edetate. Disodium ethylenedi-aminetetra acetate.
See: Edetate disodium.
disodium phosphate.
See: Sodium phosphate.
disodium phosphate heptahydrate.
See: Sodium phosphate.
disodium thiosulfate pentahydrate.
See: Sodium thiosulfate.
di-sodium versenate.
See: Edathamil Disodium.
•**disofenin.** (DIE-so-FEN-in) USAN.
Use: Diagnostic aid (carrier agent).
Disophrol. (Schering-Plough) Pseudo-ephedrine sulfate 60 mg, dex-brompheniramine maleate 2 mg. Tab. Bot. 100s. *OTC.*
Use: Antihistamine, decongestant.
Disophrol Chronotabs. (Schering-Plough) Dexbrompheniramine maleate 6 mg, pseudoephedrine sulfate 120 mg. SA Tab. Bot. 100s. *OTC.*
Use: Antihistamine, decongestant.
•**disopyramide.** (DIE-so-PIR-uh-mide) USAN.
Use: Cardiovascular agent (antiar-rhythmic).
•**disopyramide phosphate.** (DIE-so-PIHR-ah-mide) *USP 34.*
Use: Cardiovascular agent; antiar-rhythmic.
See: Norpace.
Norpace CR.
disopyramide phosphate. (Various Mfr.) Disopyramide phosphate. **Cap.:** 100 mg, 150 mg. Bot. 100s, 500s. **ER Cap.:** 150 mg. Bot. 100s. *Rx.*
Use: Antiarrhythmics.
•**disoxaril.** (die-SOX-ar-ILL) USAN.
Use: Antiviral.
DisperMox. (Ranbaxy) Amoxicillin 200 mg, 400 mg. Aspartame, phenyl-alanine 5.6 mg. Strawberry flavor. Tab. for Oral Susp. 20s, 60s, 500s (400 mg only), 1000s (200 mg only), UD 100s. *Rx.*
Use: Penicillin, aminopenicillin.
Dispos-a-Med. (Parke-Davis) Isoetha-rine hydrochloride 0.5%, 1%. Can of prefilled sterile tubes 0.5 mL. 50s. *Rx.*
Use: Bronchodilator.
distaquaine.
See: Penicillin V.
distigmine bromide. Hexamarium bro-mide.
•**disufenton sodium.** (dye-soo-FEN-ton) USAN.
Use: Neuroprotectant.

•**disulfiram.** (die-SULL-fih-ram) *USP 34.*
Use: Alcohol deterrent.
See: Antabuse.
Ditate DS. (Savage) Testosterone enan-thate 360 mg, estradiol valerate 16 mg, benzyl alcohol 2% in sesame oil. Sy-ringe 2 mL. Box 10s. Vial 2 mL. *Rx.*
Use: Androgen, estrogen combination.
•**ditekiren.** (DIE-teh-KIE-ren) USAN.
Use: Antihypertensive.
dithranol.
See: Anthralin.
D.I.T.I. Creme. (Dunhall Pharmaceuti-cals, Inc.) Iodoquinol 100 mg, sulfa-nilamide 500 mg, diethylstilbestrol 0.1 mg/g. Jar. 4 oz. *Rx.*
Use: Anti-infective, vaginal.
D.I.T.I.-2 Creme. (Dunhall Pharmaceuti-cals, Inc.) Sulfanilamide 15%, amina-crine hydrochloride 0.2%, allantoin 2%. Tube 142 g. *Rx.*
Use: Anti-infective, vaginal.
•**ditiocade sodium.** (DIT-ee-oh-kade) USAN.
Use: Radiopharmaceutical.
Ditropan XL. (Janssen) Oxybutynin chloride 5 mg, 10 mg, 15 mg, lactose. ER Tab. Bot. 100s *Rx.*
Use: Anticholinergic.
Diulo. (Pharmacia) Metolazone 2.5 mg, 5 mg, 10 mg. Tab. Bot. 100s. *Rx.*
Use: Antihypertensive, diuretic.
diuretic combinations.
See: Alazide.
Aldactazide.
Dyazide.
Maxzide.
Maxzide-25 MG.
Moduretic.
Spironazide.
Spironolactone w/Hydrochlorothiazide.
Spirozide.
Triamterene w/Hydrochlorothiazide.
diuretics.
See: Diuretics, Loop.
Diuretics, Thiazides and Related.
diuretics, loop.
See: Bumex.
Edecrin.
Edecrin Sodium Intravenous.
Furosemide.
Lasix.
Luramide.
diuretics, osmotic.
See: Ismotic.
Mannitol.
Osmitrol.
diuretics, potassium-sparing.
See: Amiloride Hydrochloride.
Spironolactone.
Triamterene.

diuretics, thiazides and related.
See: Chlorthiazide.
　　Chlorthalidone.
　　Hydrochlorothiazide.
　　Indapamide.
　　Methyclothiazide.
　　Metolazone.
Diuretic Tablets. (Faraday) Buchu
　　leaves 150 mg, uva ursi leaves 150 mg,
　　juniper berries 120 mg, bone meal,
　　parsley, asparagus. Bot. 100s. *Rx.*
Use: Diuretic.
Diuril. (Ovation) Chlorothiazide (as
　　chlorothiazide sodium) 500 mg. Preser-
　　vative free. Inj., Lyophilized, Pow. for
　　Soln. Single-use vials. *Rx.*
Use: Diuretic.
Diuril. (Salix) Chlorothiazide 250 mg/
　　5 mL. Alcohol 0.5%. Parabens, saccha-
　　rin, sucrose. Oral Susp. 237 mL. *Rx.*
Use: Antihypertensive; diuretic.
•**divalproex sodium.** (die-VAL-pro-ex)
　　USAN.
Use: Anticonvulsant.
See: Depakote.
　　Depakote ER.
divalproex sodium. (Various Mfr.) Dival-
　　proex sodium 125 mg, 250 mg, 500 mg.
　　Enteric coated. May contain lactose.
　　Delayed-release Tab. 30s, 100s, 500s,
　　1,000s, UD 100s. *Rx.*
Use: CNS agent, anticonvulsant.
Divigel. (Upsher-Smith) Estradiol 0.1%.
　　Ethanol. Gel. Single-dose packets
　　(30s). 0.25 g, 0.5 g, 1 g. *Rx.*
Use: Sex hormone, estrogen.
divinyl oxide. Vinyl ether, divinyl ether.
Use: Inhalation anesthetic.
Dizac. (Ohmeda) Diazepam 5 mg/mL,
　　preservative free. Inj. Vial 3 mL. *c-iv.*
Use: Anxiolytic; anticonvulsant; muscle
　　relaxant.
Dizmiss. (Jones Pharma) Meclizine
　　hydrochloride 25 mg. Tab. Bot. 100s,
　　1000s. *OTC.*
Use: Antiemetic; antivertigo.
•**dizocilpine maleate.** (die-ZOE-sill-
　　PEEN) USAN.
Use: Neuroprotective.
dl-desoxyephedrine hydrochloride.
See: dl-Methamphetamine hydrochlo-
　　ride.
dl-methamphetamine hydrochloride.
　　dl-Desoxyephedrine hydrochloride.
dl-norephedrine hydrochloride.
DMax. (Great Southern) Dextromethor-
　　phan HBr 15 mg, phenylephrine hydro-
　　chloride 8 mg, carbinoxamine maleate
　　4 mg per 5 mL. Berry flavor. Syrup.
　　30 mL, 473 mL. *Rx.*
Use: Antitussive, antihistamine, decon-
　　gestant.

DMax Pediatric. (Great Southern) Dex-
　　tromethorphan HBr 4 mg, phenyl-
　　ephrine 2 mg, carbinoxamine maleate
　　2 mg per 1 mL. Purple. Berry flavor.
　　Drops. 30 mL bot. with 1 mL dropper.
　　Rx.
Use: Antitussive, antihistamine, decon-
　　gestant.
DM Cough. (Rosemont) Dextromethor-
　　phan HBr 10 mg/5 mL, alcohol 5%.
　　Syrup. Bot. 120 mL, pt, gal. *OTC.*
Use: Antitussive.
DM/CPM/PE/GG. (Kylemore Pharmaceu-
　　ticals) Dextromethorphan hydrobromide
　　15 mg, guaifenesin 100 mg, phenyl-
　　ephrine hydrochloride 10 mg, chlor-
　　pheniramine maleate 2 mg per 5 mL.
　　Fruit gum flavoring, glycerin, parabens,
　　propylene glycol, saccharin, sorbitol.
　　Syrup. 473 mL. *Rx.*
Use: Upper respiratory combination, an-
　　titussive and expectorant combina-
　　tion.
DMCT. (Wyeth) Demethylchlortetracy-
　　cline. *Rx.*
Use: Anti-infective; tetracycline.
See: Declomycin hydrochloride.
d-methorphan hydrobromide.
See: Dextromethorphan Hydrobromide.
d-methylphenylamine sulfate.
See: Dextroamphetamine Sulfate.
**DML Dermatological Moisturizing Lo-
　　tion.** (Person and Covey) Purified wa-
　　ter, petrolatum, glycerin, methyl glu-
　　cose sesquisterate, dimethicone,
　　methyl gluceth-20 sesquisterate, ben-
　　zyl alcohol, volatile silicone, glyceryl
　　stearate, stearic acid, palmitic acid, ce-
　　tyl alcohol, xanthan gum, magnesium
　　aluminum silicate carbomer 941, so-
　　dium hydroxide. Bot. 8 oz. *OTC.*
Use: Emollient.
DML Facial Moisturizer. (Person and
　　Covey) Octyl methoxycinnamate 8%,
　　oxybenzone 4%, benzyl alcohol, petro-
　　latum, EDTA. SPF 15. Cream. Tube
　　45 g. *OTC.*
Use: Sunscreen.
DML Forte. (Person and Covey) Petrola-
　　tum, PPG-2 myristyl ether propionate,
　　glyceryl stearate, glycerin, stearic acid,
　　d-panthenol, DEA-cetyl phosphate, si-
　　methicone, PVP eicosene copolymer,
　　benzyl alcohol, cetyl alcohol, silica, di-
　　sodium EDTA, BHA, magnesium alumi-
　　num silicate, sodium carbomer 1342.
　　Tube 113 g. *OTC.*
Use: Emollient.
DM/PE/CPM. (Kylemore Pharmaceuti-
　　cals) Chlorpheniramine maleate 1 mg,
　　dextromethorphan hydrobromide 3 mg,

phenylephrine hydrochloride 1.5 mg. Glycerin, parabens, propylene glycol, saccharin, sorbitol. Alcohol free and sugar free. Fruit gum flavor. Drops. 30 mL w/dropper. *Rx.*
Use: Upper respiratory combination, antitussive combination.

DM/PSE/BPM. (Kylemore Pharmaceuticals) Brompheniramine maleate 3 mg, dextromethorphan hydrobromide 30 mg, pseudoephedrine hydrochloride 50 mg per 5 mL. Glycerin, parabens, propylene glycol, saccharin, sorbitol. Berry-vanilla flavor. Syrup. 473 mL. *Rx.*
Use: Upper respiratory combination, antitussive combination.

DMP 777. (DuPont)
Use: Cystic fibrosis. [Orphan Drug]

DMSO.
See: Dimethyl sulfoxide.

DNA demethylation agents.
See: Azacitidine.
 Decitabine.
 Nelarabine.

DNA topoisomerase inhibitors.
See: Irinotecan hydrochloride.
 Topotecan.

Doak Tar. (Doak Dermatologics) **Lot.:** Tar distillate 5%. Bot. 118 mL. **Oil:** Tar distillate 2%. Mineral oil. Bot. 237 mL. **Shampoo:** Coal tar 1.2%, isopropyl alcohol. Bot. 237 mL. *OTC.*
Use: Antiseborrheic.

Doak Tar Oil Forte. (Doak Dermatologics) Tar distillate 5%. Bot. 4 oz.
Use: Antiseborrheic.

Doak Tersaseptic. (Doak Dermatologics) Liquid cleanser, pH 6.8. Bot. 4 oz, pt, gal. *OTC.*
Use: Detergent.

Doan's. (Novartis Consumer Health) Magnesium salicylate 377 mg (as tetrahydrate, equiv. to magnesium salicylate anhydrous 303.7 mg). Tab. 24s. *OTC.*
Use: Analgesic.

Doan's Backache Spray. (Novartis Consumer Health) Methyl salicylate 15%, menthol 8.4%, methyl nicotinate 0.6%. Aerosol Can 4 oz. *OTC.*
Use: Analgesic, topical.

Doan's Pills. (Novartis Consumer Health) Magnesium salicylate 325 mg. Tab. Ctn. 24s, 48s. *OTC.*
Use: Analgesic.

Doan's PM, Extra Strength.
See: Extra Strength Doan's PM.

dobutamine. (Various Mfr.) Dobutamine hydrochloride 12.5 mg/mL. May contain sulfites. Inj., Soln., Conc. Single-use vial 20 mL, 40 mL, 100 mL pharmacy bulk packages. *Rx.*
Use: Cardiovascular agent.

•**dobutamine hydrochloride.** (doe-BYOOT-ah-meen) *USP 34.*
Tall Man: DOBUTamine
Use: Cardiovascular agent.

dobutamine hydrochloride in 5% dextrose injection. (Baxter) Dobutamine 250 mg per 250 mL (1 mg/mL), 500 mg per 500 mL (1 mg/mL), 500 mg per 250 mL (2 mg/mL), 1,000 mg per 250 mL (4 mg/mL). Sodium bisulfite. Preservative free. Inj., Soln. Single-use Viaflex Plus plastic container. 250 mL (except 500 mg/500 mL), 500 mL (500 mg/500 mL). *Rx.*
Use: Vasopressor.

•**dobutamine in dextrose for injection.** (doe-BYOOT-ah-meen) *USP 34.*
Tall Man: DOBUTamine
Use: Cardiovascular agent.

•**dobutamine lactobionate.** (doe-BYOOT-ah-meen) USAN.
Tall Man: DOBUTamine
Use: Cardiovascular agent.

•**dobutamine tartrate.** (doe-BYOOT-ah-meen) USAN.
Tall Man: DOBUTamine
Use: Cardiovascular agent.

•**docebenone.** (dah-SEH-beh-nohn) USAN.
Use: Inhibitor (5-lipoxygenase).

•**docetaxel.** (doe-seh-TAX-ehl) USAN.
Tall Man: DOCEtaxel
Use: Antineoplastic, antimitotic.
See: Taxotere.

docetaxel. (Winthrop) Docetaxel 20 mg/mL. Alcohol, polysorbate 80 (in 50/50 [v/v] ratio polysorbate 80/dehydrated alcohol). Inj., Soln.; concentrate. Single-use vial. *Rx.*
Use: Antimitotic agent, taxoid.

•**doconazole.** (doe-KOE-nah-zole) USAN.
Use: Antifungal.

•**docosanol.** (doe-KOE-sah-nole) USAN.
Use: Antiviral.
See: Abreva.

Doctase. (Purepac) Docusate sodium 100 mg, casanthranol 30 mg. Cap. Bot. 100s. *OTC.*
Use: Laxative.

Doctyl. (Health for Life Brands) Docusate sodium 100 mg. Tab. Bot. 40s, 100s, 1000s. *OTC.*
Use: Laxative.

Doctylax. (Health for Life Brands) Docusate sodium 100 mg, acetophenolisatin 2 mg, prune conc. ¾ mg. Tab. Bot. 40s, 100s, 1000s. *OTC.*
Use: Laxative.

Docu. (Hi-Tech Pharmacal) Docusate sodium. **Syrup:** 20 mg/5 mL, alcohol 5%. Bot. 480 mL. **Liq.:** 150 mg/15 mL. Bot. 480 mL. *OTC.*
Use: Laxative.
•**docusate calcium.** (DOCK-you-sate) *USP 34. Formerly Dioctyl Calcium Sulfosuccinate.*
Use: Laxative; stool softener.
See: DC Softgels.
Stool Softner.
Stool Softner DC.
Surfak.
Surfak Stool Softener.
docusate calcium. (Various Mfr.) Docusate calcium 240 mg. Cap. Bot. 100s, 500s, UD 100s, 300s. *OTC.*
Use: Laxative.
•**docusate potassium.** (DOCK-you-sate) *USP 34.*
Use: Laxative; stool softener.
•**docusate sodium.** (DOCK-you-sate) *USP 34. Formerly Dioctyl Sodium Sulfosuccinate.*
Use: Pharmaceutical aid (surfactant); stool softener.
See: Colace.
Coloctyl.
Diocto.
Dioctyn Softgels.
Docu.
DocuSol Mini.
DOK.
D.O.S.
D-S-S.
Dulcolax Stool Softener.
Duosol.
Easy-Lax.
ex-lax Stool Softener.
Konsto.
Non-Habit Forming Stool Softner.
Phillips' Liqui-Gels.
Silace.
Sof-lax.
Stool Softner.
Stulex.
W/Betaine Hydrochloride, Zinc, Manganese, Molybdenum.
See: Hemaferrin.
W/Casanthranol.
See: Calotabs.
Dio-Soft.
DOK-Plus.
Easy-Lax Plus.
Laxative and Stool Softener.
W/Ferrous Fumarate, Betaine Hydrochloride, Desiccated Liver, Vitamins, Minerals.
See: Hemaferrin.
W/Phenolphthalein.
See: Feen-A-Mint Dual Formula.

Phillips' LaxCaps.
W/Phenolphthalein, Dehydrocholic Acid.
See: Bolax.
W/Polyoxyethylene-Nonyl-Phenol, Sodium Edetate, 9-Aminoacridine Hydrochloride.
See: Vagisec Plus.
W/Senna Concentrate.
See: DOK Plus.
PeriColace.
Senna Plus.
Senokot S.
W/Sennosides.
See: ex-lax Gentle Strength.
Senna-S.
docusate sodium. (Roxane) Docusate sodium 50 mg/15 mL, 100 mg/30 mL, saccharin, sucrose, parabens. Syr. UD 15 mL, 30 mL (100s). *OTC.*
Use: Laxative.
docusate sodium. (UDL) Docusate sodium 50 mg. Softgel cap. Bot. 100s, UD 100s *OTC.*
Use: Laxative.
docusate sodium. (Various Mfr.) Docusate sodium. **Cap.:** 250 mg. Bot. 100s, 1000s, UD 100s. **Softgel Cap.:** 100 mg, 250 mg. Bot. 100s, 1000s, UD 100s, 300s (100 mg only). *OTC.*
Use: Laxative.
docusate with casanthranol. (Various Mfr.) Docusate sodium 100 mg, casanthranol 30 mg. Cap. Bot. 100s, 1000s, UD 100s, 300s, 600s. *OTC.*
Use: Laxative; stool softener.
DocuSol Mini. (Alliance Labs) Docusate sodium 283 mg. PEG, glycerin. Enema, rectal. 5s. *OTC.*
Use: Laxative.
•**dofetilide.** (doe-FEH-till-ide) USAN.
Use: Cardiovascular agent; antiarrhythmic.
See: Tikosyn.
Dofus. (Miller Pharmacal Group) Freeze-dried *Lactobacillus acidophilus* minimum of 1 billion organisms. Cap. w/*Lactobacillus bifidus* organisms added. Bot. 60s. *OTC.*
Use: Nutritional supplement; antidiarrheal.
DOK. (Major) Docusate sodium 250 mg. Cap. 100s. *OTC.*
Use: Laxative.
DOK Plus. (Major) Docusate 50 mg (as sodium), senna concentrate 8.6 mg (as sennosides). PEG-400. Tab. 100s. *OTC.*
Use: Laxative combination.
Doktors Spray. (Scherer) Phenylephrine hydrochloride 0.25%, chlorobutanol, sodium bisulfite, benzalkonium chloride.

Soln. Bot. 30 mL. *OTC.*
Use: Decongestant.

Dolacet. (Roberts) Hydrocodone bitartrate 5 mg, acetaminophen 500 mg. Cap. Bot. 100s. *c-III.*
Use: Analgesic combination, narcotic.

Dolamide Tabs. (Major) Chlorpropamide 100 mg, 250 mg. Bot. 100s, 500s, 1000s. *Rx.*
Use: Antidiabetic.

Dolamin. (Harvey) Ammonium sulfate 0.75% with sodium chloride, benzyl alcohol. Amp. 10 mL. In 12s, 25s, 100s. *Rx.*
Use: Antineuralgic.

dolantin.
See: Meperidine hydrochloride.

•**dolasetron mesylate.** (dahl-AH-setrahn) *USP 34.*
Use: Antiemetic; antimigraine.
See: Anzemet.

Dolcin. (Dolcin) Aspirin 3.7 g, calcium succinate 2.8 g. Tab. Bot. 100s, 200s. *OTC.*
Use: Analgesic.

Doldram. (Dram) Salicylamide 7.5 g. Tab. Bot. 100s.
Use: Analgesic.

Dolene AP-65. (Wyeth) Propoxyphene hydrochloride 65 mg, acetaminophen 650 mg. Tab. Bot. 100s, 500s. *c-IV.*
Use: Analgesic combination; narcotic.

Dolene Compound-65. (Wyeth) Propoxyphene hydrochloride 65 mg, aspirin 389 mg, caffeine 32.4 mg. Cap. Bot. 100s, 500s. *c-IV.*
Use: Analgesic combination; narcotic.

Dolene Plain. (Wyeth) Propoxyphene hydrochloride 65 mg. Cap. Bot. 100s, 500s. *c-IV.*
Use: Analgesic; narcotic.

Dolgic. (Athlon) Acetaminophen 650 mg, butalbital 50 mg. Tab. Bot. 100s. *Rx.*
Use: Analgesic.

Dolgic LQ. (Athlon) Acetaminophen 108.3 mg, caffeine 13.3 mg, butalbital 16.6 mg/5 mL, alcohol 7.368%, orange, tropical fruit punch flavors. Soln. 473 mL. *Rx.*
Use: Analgesic, nonnarcotic.

Dolgic Plus. (Victory Pharma) Butalbital 50 mg, acetaminophen 750 mg, caffeine 40 mg. Film-coated. Tab. 100s. *Rx.*
Use: Nonnarcotic analgesic combination.

Dolomite. (Halsey Drug) Calcium 426 mg, magnesium 246 mg. Tab. w/ guar and acacia gum. Bot. 250s. *OTC.*
Use: Mineral supplement.

Dolomite. (NBTY) Magnesium 78 mg, calcium 130 mg. Tab. Bot. 100s, 250s.

OTC.
Use: Mineral supplement.

Dolomite Plus Capsules. (Barth's) Magnesium 37 mg, calcium 187 mg, phosphorus 50 mg, iodine 0.25 mg. Bot. 100s, 500s, 1000s. *OTC.*
Use: Mineral supplement.

Dolomite Tablets. (Faraday) Calcium 150 mg, magnesium 90 mg. Bot. 250s. *OTC.*
Use: Mineral supplement.

Dolonil. (Parke-Davis)
See: Pyridium Plus.

Dolono. (R.I.D.) Acetaminophen 160 mg/5 mL, sorbitol, sucrose, alcohol free, cherry flavor. Elixir. Bot. 120 mL. *OTC.*
Use: Analgesic.

Dolophine Hydrochloride. (Roxane) Methadone hydrochloride 5 mg, 10 mg. Tab. Bot. 100s. *c-II.*
Use: Opioid analgesic.

Dolopirona Tablets. (Sanofi-Synthelabo) Dipyrone with chlormezanone. *Rx.*
Use: Analgesic; anxiolytic; muscle relaxant.

Doloral. (Progressive Enterprises) Colchicine salicylate 0.1 mg, phenobarbital 8 mg, sodium para-aminobenzoate 15 mg, vitamins B₁ 25 mg, aspirin 325 mg. Tab. Bot. 100s, 1000s. *Rx.*
Use: Antiarthritis, antigout.

dolosal.
See: Meperidine hydrochloride.

•**dolutegravir.** (DOE-loo-TEG-ra-vir) USAN.
Use: Treatment of HIV infection.

dolvanol.
Use: Analgesic; narcotic.
See: Meperidine Hydrochloride.

•**domazoline fumarate.** (DOME-AZE-ohleen) USAN.
Use: Anticholinergic.

Domeboro. (Bayer Consumer Care) Aluminum sulfate and calcium acetate when added to water gives therapeutic effect of Burow's. One pkg. or Tab./pt water approximately equivalent to 1:40 dilution. **Pkg.:** 2.2 g, 12s, 100s. **Effervescent Tab.:** Box 12s, 100s, 1000s. *OTC.*
Use: Anti-inflammatory, topical.

Domeboro Otic. (Bayer Consumer Care) Acetic acid 2% (in aluminum acetate solution). Soln. Bot. 60 mL with dropper. *Rx.*
Use: Otic.

Dome-Paste Bandage. (Bayer Consumer Care) Zinc oxide, calamine and gelatin bandage. Pkg. 4" × 10 yd. and 3" × 10 yd. impregnated gauze bandage. *OTC.*
Use: Dermatologic, wound therapy.

domestrol.
See: Diethylstilbestrol.
D.O.M.F.
Use: Antimicrobial.
See: Merbromin (Mercurochrome).
•**domiodol.** (dome-EYE-oh-DOLE) USAN.
Use: Mucolytic.
•**domiphen bromide.** (DOE-mih-fen) USAN.
Use: Antiseptic; anti-infective, topical.
Domol Bath and Shower Oil. (Bayer Consumer Care) D₁-isopropyl sebacate, isopropyl myristate with mineral oil. Bot. 240 mL. *OTC.*
Use: Emollient.
•**domperidone.** (dome-PEH-rih-dohn) USAN.
Use: Investigational antiemetic.
Donatuss DC. (Laser) Dihydrocodeine bitartrate 7.5 mg, guaifenesin 50 mg, phenylephrine hydrochloride 7.5 mg per 5 mL. Saccharin, sucrose. Alcohol free and gluten free. Grape flavor. Syr. 473 mL. c-iii.
Use: Upper respiratory combination, antitussive and expectorant combination.
Donatussin. (Laser) **Drops:** Phenylephrine hydrochloride 1.5 mg, guaifenesin 20 mg per 1 mL. Raspberry flavor. Drops. 30 mL with dropper. **Syrup:** Phenylephrine hydrochloride 10 mg, chlorpheniramine maleate 2 mg, dextromethorphan HBr 15 mg, guaifenesin 100 mg per 5 mL. Bot. 473 mL. *Rx.*
Use: Upper respiratory combination, antitussive and expectorant combination, decongestant and expectorant combination.
Donatussin DM. (Laser) **Drops:** Dextromethorphan HBr 3 mg, chlorpheniramine maleate 1 mg, phenylephrine hydrochloride 1.5 mg per 1 mL. Bubble gum flavor. 30 mL with dropper. **Syrup:** Dextromethorphan HBr 15 mg, guaifenesin 150 mg, pseudoephedrine hydrochloride 30 mg per 5 mL. Alcohol and sugar free. Saccharin, sorbitol. Cool-mint flavor. 30 mL, 473 mL. *Rx.*
Use: Antitussive combination, antitussive and expectorant combination, upper respiratory combination.
Dondril. (Whitehall-Robins) Dextromethorphan HBr 10 mg, phenylephrine hydrochloride 5 mg, chlorpheniramine maleate 1 mg. Tab. Bot. 24s. *OTC.*
Use: Antihistamine; antitussive; decongestant.
donepezil. (Teva) Donepezil hydrochloride 5 mg, 10 mg. Aspartame, manni-

tol, phenylalanine, strawberry flavoring, xylitol. Tab., orally disintegrating. UD 30s. *Rx.*
Use: Cholinesterase inhibitor.
donepezil. (UDL) Donepezil hydrochloride 5 mg, 10 mg. Film coated. Lactose. Tab. UD blister pack 300s. *Rx.*
Use: Cholinesterase inhibitor.
•**donepezil hydrochloride.** (doe-NEPP-eh-zill) USAN.
Use: Treatment of mild to moderate dementia of the Alzheimer type.
See: Aricept.
Aricept ODT.
D1000. (Mason) Cholecalciferol 1,000 units. Fructose, sucrose, sunflower oil, xylitol. Preservative free. Peach vanilla flavor. Chew. Tab. 50s. *OTC.*
Use: Fat-soluble vitamin, vitamin D.
D1000 Plus. (Mason) Vitamin D₃ 1,000 units, B₆ 10 mg, B₁₂ 200 mcg, folic acid 400 mcg, PEG. Tab. 60s. *OTC.*
Use: Multivitamin with minerals.
•**donetidine.** (doe-NEH-tih-DEEN) USAN.
Use: Antiulcerative.
Donna. (Arcum) Menthol, thymol, eucalyptol, exsiccated alum, boric acid. 4 oz, 14 oz. *Rx.*
Use: Vaginal agent.
Donnaphen. (Health for Life Brands) Phenobarbital 16.2 mg, hyoscyamine sulfate 0.1037 mg, atropine sulfate 0.0194 mg, hyoscine HBr 0.0065 mg/ 5 mL. Elix. Bot. Pt, gal. *Rx.*
Use: Anticholinergic; antispasmodic.
Donna-Sed Elixir. (Vortech Pharmaceuticals) Atropine sulfate 0.0194 mg, scopolamine HBr 0.0065, hyoscyamine HBr, or SO₄ 0.1037 mg, phenobarbital 16.2 mg, alcohol 23%. Liq. Bot. 118 mL, gal. *Rx.*
Use: Gastrointestinal; anticholinergic.
Donnatal. (PBM Pharm) **Elix.:** Atropine sulfate 0.0194 mg, scopolamine hydrobromide 0.0065 mg, hyoscyamine hydrobromide or sulfate 0.1037 mg, phenobarbital 16.2 mg per 5 mL. Ethyl alcohol 95%, saccharin, sucrose, sorbitol. Grape flavor. 118 mL, 473 mL. **Tab.:** Atropine sulfate 0.0194 mg, scopolamine hydrobromide 0.0065 mg, hyoscyamine hydrobromide or sulfate 0.1037 mg, phenobarbital 16.2 mg. Lactose. 100s, 1,000s. *Rx.*
Use: Gastrointestinal anticholinergic combination.
Donnatal Extentabs. (PBM Pharm) Atropine sulfate 0.0582 mg, scopolamine hydrobromide 0.0195 mg, hyoscyamine

sulfate 0.3111 mg, phenobarbital 48.6 mg. Lactose, polydextrose. Film-coated. ER Tab. 100s, 500s. *Rx.*
Use: Gastrointestinal anticholinergic combination.

Don't. (Del) Sucrose octa acetate 5%, isopropyl alcohol 54%. Bot. 0.45 oz. *OTC.*
Use: Nail-biting deterrent.

•**dopamantine.** (DOE-pah-MAN-teen) USAN.
Use: Antiparkinsonian.

dopamine. (AstraZeneca) Dopamine. **Amp.:** 200 mg/5 mL, Box 10s; 400 mg/10 mL, Box 5s. **Additive Syringe:** 200 mg/5 mL, Box 1s; 400 mg/10 mL, Box 1s. *Rx.*
Use: Inotropic agent.

•**dopamine hydrochloride.** (DOE-puh-meen) *USP 34.*
Tall Man: DOPamine
Use: Adrenergic; vasopressor.

dopamine hydrochloride. (Various Mfr.) Dopamine hydrochloride 40 mg/mL, 80 mg/mL, 160 mg/mL. May contain sodium metabisulfate. Inj. Vials. 5 mL, 10 mL (except 160 mg/mL). *Rx.*
Use: Vasopressor.

dopamine hydrochloride and dextrose injection.
Use: Adrenergic; emergency treatment of low blood pressure.

dopamine hydrochloride in dextrose 5% injection. (Various Mfr.) Dopamine 200 mg/250 mL (0.8 mg/mL), 400 mg/500 mL (0.8 mg/mL), 400 mg/250 mL (1.6 mg/mL), 800 mg/500 mL (1.6 mg/mL), 800 mg/250 mL (3.2 mg/mL). May contain sulfites. Inj., Soln. Premixed single-use container. 250 mL (200 mg/250 mL, 400 mg/250 mL, 800 mg/250 mL), 500 mL (400 mg/500 mL, 800 mg/500 mL). *Rx.*
Use: Vasopressor.

dopamine receptor agonists, nonergot.
Use: Antiparkinson agents.
See: Pramipexole Dihydrochloride.

dopaminergics.
Use: Antiparkinson agents.
See: Apomorphine Hydrochloride.
Dopamine Receptor Agonists, Nonergot.
Ropinirole Hydrochloride.

•**dopexamine.** (doe-PEX-ah-MEEN) USAN.
Use: Cardiovascular agent.

•**dopexamine hydrochloride.** (doe-PEX-ah-MEEN) USAN.
Use: Cardiovascular agent.

Dopram. (Baxter Healthcare Corp.) Doxapram hydrochloride 20 mg/mL, 0.9% benzyl alcohol. Inj. Multiple-dose vial 20 mL. *Rx.*
Use: CNS stimulant, analeptic.

Doral. (Questcor) Quazepam 7.5 mg, 15 mg. Tab. Bot. 100s, 500s, UD 100s. *c-IV.*
Use: Sedative/hypnotic, nonbarbiturate.

•**doramapimod.** (dore-a-MAP-i-mod) USAN.
Use: Crohn disease; RA; psoriasis.

•**dorastine hydrochloride.** (DAHR-ass-teen) USAN.
Use: Antihistamine.

•**doretinel.** (DOE-REH-tin-ell) USAN.
Use: Antikeratinizing agent.

Doribax. (Janssen) Doripenem 500 mg. Preservative free. Inj., Pow. for Soln., Conc. Single-use vials. *Rx.*
Use: Carbapenem, antibiotic.

Doriglute Tabs DEA. (Major) Glutethimide 0.5 g. Tab. Bot. 100s, 250s, 1000s. *c-II.*
Use: Hypnotic.

•**doripenem.** (dore-i-PEN-em) USAN.
Use: Antibiotic, carbapenem.
See: Doribax.

Dormeer. (Taylor Pharmaceuticals) Scopolamine aminoxide HBr 0.2 mg. Cap. Bot. 100s, 1000s. *Rx.*
Use: Hypnotic; sedative.

dormethan.
See: Dextromethorphan Hydrobromide

Dormin Capsules. (Randob) Diphenhydramine hydrochloride 25 mg, lactose. Bot. 32s, 72s. *OTC.*
Use: Sleep aid.

Dormin Sleeping Caplets. (Randob) Diphenhydramine hydrochloride 25 mg. Bot. 32s. *OTC.*
Use: Sleep aid.

dormiral.
See: Phenobarbital.

dormonal.
See: Barbital.

Dormutol. (Health for Life Brands) Scopolamine aminoxide HBr 0.2 mg. Cap. Bot. 24s, 60s. *Rx.*
Use: Hypnotic; sedative.

•**dornase alfa.** (DOR-nace AL-fuh) USAN.
Use: Cystic fibrosis. [Orphan Drug]
See: Pulmozyme.

Doryx. (Warner Chilcott) Doxycycline hyclate. **Cap., coated pellets:** 75 mg, 100 mg. Bot. 50s (100 mg only), 60s (75 mg only). **DR Tab.:** 75 mg, 100 mg, 150 mg. Lactose. 60s (75 mg and 150 mg), 100s (75 mg and 100 mg). *Rx.*
Use: Anti-infective; tetracycline.

dorzolamide. (Prasco Laboratories) Dorzolamide 2% (as dorzolamide hydrochloride). Benzalkonium chloride 0.0075%, hydroxyethyl cellulose, sodium hydroxide, sodium citrate. Soln., Ophth. *Ocumeter Plus.* 10 mL. *Rx.*
Use: Agent for glaucoma, carbonic anhydrase inhibitor.

•**dorzolamide hydrochloride.** (dore-ZOLE-lah-mide) *USP 34.*
Use: Carbonic anhydrase inhibitor.
See: TruSopt.

dorzolamide hydrochloride and timolol maleate.
Use: Agents for glaucoma.
See: Cosopt.

dorzolamide hydrochloride and timolol maleate. (Various Mfr.) Dorzolamide hydrochloride 2%, timolol maleate 0.5%. May contain benzalkonium chloride 0.0075%, mannitol. Soln., Ophth. 5 mL, 10 mL. *Rx.*
Use: Agent for glaucoma.

D.O.S. (Goldline Consumer) Docusate sodium 100 mg, 250 mg, parabens. Softgel Cap. Bot. 100s, 500s (250 mg only), 1000s (100 mg only). *OTC.*
Use: Laxative.

Dosaflex. (Richwood Pharmaceuticals) Senna fruit extract, parabens, sucrose, alcohol 7%. Syrup. Bot. 237 mL. *OTC.*
Use: Laxative.

Doss Syrup. (Rosemont) Docusate sodium 20 mg/5 mL. Bot. Pt, gal. *OTC.*
Use: Laxative; stool softener.

•**dothiepin hydrochloride.** (DOE-THIGH-eh-pin) USAN.
Use: Antidepressant.

Dotirol. (Sanofi-Synthelabo) Ampicillin trihydrate available in Cap, Susp., Inj. (IV, IM). *Rx.*
Use: Anti-infective; penicillin.

Double-Action Toothache Kit. (C.S. Dent & Co.) **Liq.:** Benzocaine, alcohol 74%, chlorobutanol anhydrous 0.09%. Bot. 3.7 mL. **Maronox Pain Relief Tablets:** Acetaminophen 325 mg. Tab. Box. 8s. *OTC.*
Use: Analgesic, topical.

Double Antibiotic. (Fougera) Polymyxin B sulfate 10,000 units, bacitracin zinc 500 units per g. Oint. Tubes. $\approx$ 15 g, $\approx$ 30 g, UD 0.9 g (144s). *OTC.*
Use: Topical anti-infective, antibiotic.

Double Sal. (Pal-Pak, Inc.) Sodium salicylate 648 mg. EC Tab. Bot. 1000s. *OTC.*
Use: Analgesic.

Double Strength Gaviscon-2. (Glaxo-SmithKline) Aluminum hydroxide 160 mg, magnesium trisilicate 40 mg, alginic acid, calcium stearate, sodium bicarbonate, sucrose. Tab. Bot. 48s. *OTC.*
Use: Antacid.

Dovacet Capsules. (Pal-Pak, Inc.) Dover's powder 24.3 mg, aspirin 324 mg, caffeine 32.4 mg. Bot. 1000s.
Use: Analgesic.

Dover's Powder. Ipecac 1 part, opium 1 part, lactose 8 parts.
Use: Analgesic; diaphoretic; sedative.
W/Atropine Sulfate, A.P.C., Camphor.
See: Dasin.

Dovonex. (LeoPharma) Calcipotriene. **Cream:** 0.005%. Tube 30 g, 60 g, 100 g. **Oint.:** 0.005%. Tube 30 g, 60 g, 100 g. **Soln.:** 0.005%. Menthol. Bot. 60 mL. *Rx.*
Use: Dermatologic; antipsoriatic.

Dowicil 200.
Use: Antibacterial.
See: Derma Soap.

Dow-Isoniazid. (Hoechst) Isoniazid 300 mg. Tab. Bot. 30s. *Rx.*
Use: Antituberculosal.

Doxamin. (Forest) Thiamine hydrochloride 100 mg, vitamin B_6 100 mg/mL. Vial 10 mL. *Rx.*
Use: Vitamin supplement.

Doxapap-N. (Major) Propoxyphene napsylate 100 mg, acetaminophen 650 mg. Tab. Bot. 100s, 500s. *c-IV.*
Use: Analgesic combination, narcotic.

Doxaphene Capsules. (Major) Propoxyphene hydrochloride 65 mg. Cap. Bot. 1000s. *c-IV.*
Use: Analgesic; narcotic.

Doxaphene Compound 65 Caps. (Major) Propoxyphene hydrochloride, acetaminophen. Cap. Bot. 1000s. *c-IV.*
Use: Analgesic combination, narcotic.

•**doxapram hydrochloride.** (DOX-uh-pram) *USP 34.*
Use: Respiratory and CNS stimulant, analeptic.
See: Dopram.

doxapram hydrochloride. (Bedford) Doxapram hydrochloride 20 mg/mL. Benzyl alcohol 0.9%. Inj. Multiple-dose vial. 20 mL.
Use: Respiratory and CNS stimulant.

•**doxaprost.** (DOX-ah-proste) USAN.
Use: Bronchodilator.

Doxate. Docusate sodium. *OTC.*
Use: Laxative.

•**doxazosin mesylate.** (DOX-uh-ZOE-sin) USAN.
Use: Antihypertensive, antiadrenergic.
See: Cardura.
Cardura XL.

doxazosin mesylate. (Various Mfr.) Doxazosin mesylate (as base) 1 mg, 2 mg, 4 mg, 8 mg. May contain lactose. Tab. Bot. 100s, 500s, 1000s, UD 100s. *Rx.*
Use: Antihypertensive, antiadrenergic.

•**doxepin hydrochloride.** (DOX-uh-pin) *USP 34.*
Use: Psychotherapeutic agent; antidepressant.
See: Prudoxin.
Silenor.
Sinequan.

doxepin hydrochloride. (Various Mfr.) Doxepin hydrochloride. **Cap.:** 10 mg, 25 mg, 50 mg, 75 mg, 100 mg, 150 mg. Bot. 50s (150 mg only), 100s, 500s, 1000s, blister pack 25s (25 mg, 50 mg only), blister pack 100s (except 150 mg). **Oral Conc.:** 10 mg/mL. Bot. 120 mL. *Rx.*
Use: Antidepressant.

•**doxercalciferol.** (dox-ehr-kal-SIFF-eh-role) USAN.
Use: Secondary hyperparathyroidism associated with end-stage renal disease.
See: Hectorol.

Doxidan. (Pharmacia) Bisacodyl 5 mg. DR Tab. 10s, 30s, 90s. *OTC.*
Use: Laxative.

Doxil. (Ortho Biotech) Doxorubicin hydrochloride 2 mg/mL. Sucrose. Preservative free. Inj., Susp., Liposomal Conc. Single-use vials. 10 mL, 30 mL. *Rx.*
Use: Antibiotic, anthracycline.

•**doxofylline.** (DOX-oh-fill-een) USAN.
Use: Bronchodilator.

•**doxorubicin.** (DOX-oh-ROO-bih-sin) USAN.
Tall Man: DOXOrubicin
Use: Antineoplastic; antibiotic, anthracycline.

•**doxorubicin hydrochloride.** (DOX-oh-ROO-bih-sin) *USP 34.*
Tall Man: DOXOrubicin
Use: Antineoplastic; antibiotic, anthracycline.
See: Adriamycin PFS.
Adriamycin RDF.
Doxil.

doxorubicin hydrochloride. (Bedford Labs) Doxorubicin hydrochloride. **Inj., Lyophilized, Pow. for Soln.:** 10 mg (lactose 50 mg), 20 mg (lactose 100 mg), 50 mg (lactose 250 mg). Single-dose flip-top vials. **Inj.:** 2 mg/mL. Sodium chloride 0.9%, hydrochloric acid. Vials. 5 mL, 10 mL, 25 mL, 100 mL. *Rx.*
Use: Antibiotic, anthracycline.

•**doxpicomine hydrochloride.** (DOX-PIH-koe-meen) USAN. *Formerly Doxpicodin Hydrochloride.*
Use: Analgesic.

Doxy. (APP) **100:** Doxycycline hyclate 100 mg. Mannitol 300 mg. Pow. for Inj., lyophilized. Vial. **200:** Doxycycline hyclate 200 mg. Mannitol 600 mg. Pow. for Inj., lyophilized. Vial. *Rx.*
Use: Anti-infective; tetracycline.

•**doxycycline.** (DOX-ee-SIGH-kleen) *USP 34.*
Use: Anti-infective, tetracycline; mouth and throat product.
See: Adoxa.
Alodox Convenience Kit.
Atridox.
Doryx.
Doxy.
Monodox.
Nutridox.
Oracea.
Oraxyl.
Periostat.
Vibramycin.
Vibra-Tabs.

doxycycline. (Eon) Doxycyline (as hyclate) 75 mg, 100 mg. Sugar spheres. Coated pellets, Cap. 50s (100 mg only), 60s (75 mg only), 100s. *Rx.*
Use: Anti-infective.

doxycycline. (Ivax) Doxycycline (as hyclate) 20 mg. Lactose. Film-coated. Tab. 100s, 500s, 1000s. *Rx.*
Use: Mouth and throat product.

doxycycline. (Mylan) Doxycycline hyclate 75 mg, 100 mg. Lactose. Tab., delayed release. 60s (75 mg), 100s (100 mg), 500s. *Rx.*
Use: Anti-infective agent, tetracycline.

doxycycline. (Par) Doxycycline (as monohydrate) 75 mg. Lactose. Film-coated. Tab. 100s, 500s. *Rx.*
Use: Anti-infective.

doxycycline. (Teva) Doxycycline 25 mg per 5 mL (as monohydrate). Maltodextrin, parabens, sucrose. Raspberry flavor. Pow. for Susp. 60 mL. *Rx.*
Use: Anti-infective agent, tetracycline.

doxycycline. (Various Mfr.) Doxycycline hyclate. **Tab.:** 20 mg (may contain lactose) (film-coated), 100 mg. Bot. 50s (100 mg only); 60s (20 mg only); 100s; 200s, 500s, UD 100s (100 mg only); 1000s (20 mg only). **Cap.:** 50 mg, 100 mg. Bot. 50s, 500s, UD 100s (100 mg only). **Pow. for Inj., lyophilized:** 100 mg. Vials. *Rx.*
Use: Anti-infective, tetracycline.

doxycycline. (Various Mfr.) Doxycycline (as monohydrate) 50 mg, 100 mg,

150 mg (polydextrose). May contain corn starch, lactose. Tab. Film-coated. 30s (150 mg only), 50s (100 mg only), 100s (50 mg, 150 mg only), 250s (100 mg only), 500s (150 mg only). *Rx.*
Use: Tetracycline.
doxycycline monohydrate. (Watson) Doxycycline (as monohydrate) 50 mg, 100 mg. Cap. 50s (100 mg only), 100s (50 mg only), 250s (100 mg only). *Rx.*
Use: Tetracycline.
•**doxylamine succinate.** (dox-IL-a-meen) *USP 34.*
Use: Antihistamine, nonselective ethanolamine.
See: Aldex AN.
Decapryn.
Doxytex.
Unisom Nighttime Sleep-Aid.
W/Acetaminophen, Dextromethorphan Hydrobromide.
See: Tylenol Cough & Sore Throat Nighttime.
Vicks NyQuil Cold/Flu Relief.
W/Acetaminophen, Dextromethorphan Hydrobromide, Phenylephrine Hydrochloride.
See: Alka-Seltzer Plus Day & Night Cold.
Alka-Seltzer Plus Night Cold.
Tylenol Cold Multi-Symptom Nighttime.
W/Acetaminophen, Phenylephrine Hydrochloride.
See: Vicks NyQuil Sinex.
W/Aspirin, Dextromethorphan Hydrobromide, Phenylephrine Bitartrate.
See: Alka-Seltzer Plus Day & Night Cold.
Alka-Seltzer Plus Night Cold.
W/Dextromethorphan Hydrobromide.
See: Vicks NyQuil Cough.
W/Dextromethorphan Hydrobromide, Pseudoephedrine Hydrochloride.
See: All-Nite.
Lortuss DM.
W/Pseudoephedrine Hydrochloride.
See: Lortuss LQ.
doxylamine succinate, acetaminophen, and pseudoephedrine hydrochloride combinations.
Use: Upper respiratory combination, antihistamine, analgesic, decongestant.
See: Acetaminophen, Doxylamine Succinate, and Pseudoephedrine Hydrochloride Combinations.
Doxy-Lemmon. (Teva) **Cap.:** Doxycycline hyclate equivalent to 100 mg of doxycycline base. Cap. Bot. 50s, 500s, UD 100s. **Tab.:** Doxycycline hyclate equivalent to 100 mg doxycycline base.

Tab. Bot. 50s, 500s, UD 100s. *Rx.*
Use: Anti-infective; tetracycline.
Doxy-Tabs. (Houba) Doxycycline hyclate 100 mg. FC Tab. Bot. 50s, 500s. *Rx.*
Use: Anti-infective; tetracycline.
Doxy-Tabs-50. (Houba) Doxycycline hyclate 50 mg. Tab. Bot. 50s. *Rx.*
Use: Anti-infective; tetracycline.
Doxytex. (Centurion Labs) Doxylamine succinate 2.5 mg per 2.5 mL. Alcohol free, sugar free. Apple sauce flavor. Liq. 473 mL. *Rx.*
Use: Antihistamine; ethanolamine, nonselective.
D-Phen 1000. (Midlothian) Phenylephrine hydrochloride 30 mg, guaifenesin 1000 mg. ER Tab. 100s. *Rx.*
Use: Upper respiratory combination, decongestant and expectorant combination.
DPPC. Colfosceril palmitate. *Rx.*
Use: Lung surfactant.
•**draflazine.** (DRAFF-lah-ZEEN) USAN.
Use: Cardioprotectant.
Dramamine. (Pharmacia) Dimenhydrinate 50 mg. Tab. 36s, 100s, 1,000s, blister pkg. 12s, UD 100s. *OTC.*
Use: Antiemetic; antivertigo.
Dramamine Less Drowsy Formula. (McNeil Consumer) Meclizine hydrochloride 25 mg, lactose. Tab. Pkg. 8s. *OTC.*
Use: Antiemetic; antivertigo.
Dramamine II. (Pharmacia) Meclizine hydrochloride 25 mg, lactose. Tab. Pkg. 8s. *OTC.*
Use: Antiemetic; antivertigo.
Dramanate. (Taylor Pharmaceuticals) Dimenhydrinate 50 mg/mL. Inj. Vial 10 mL. *Rx.*
Use: Antiemetic; antivertigo.
dramarin.
See: Dramamine.
dramyl.
See: Dramamine.
Drawing Salve. (Whiteworth Towne) Tube oz. *OTC.*
Use: Dermatologic, wound therapy.
Drawing Salve with Triquinodin. (Whiteworth Towne) Tube 2 oz. *OTC.*
Use: Dermatologic, wound therapy.
Dr. Berry's Skin Toner. (Last) Hydroquinone 2%. Jar oz. *Rx.*
Use: Dermatologic.
Dr. Brown's Home Drug Testing System. (Personal Health and Hygiene) 1 urine specimen collection kit for detecting drugs of abuse (marijuana, cocaine, amphetamine, methamphetamine, phencyclidine, codeine, morphine, heroin). Kit 1s. *OTC.*
Use: Diagnostic aid.

DRC Peri-Anal Cream. (Xttrium) Lassar's paste 37.5%, anhydrous lanolin, 37.5%, cold cream 25%. Tube 5 oz. OTC.
Use: Dermatologic protectant, perianal.

Dr. Dermi-Heal. (Quality Formulations, Inc.) Zinc oxide 25%, allantoin 1%, peruvian balsam, castor oil, white petrolatum. Oint. Tube 75 g. OTC.
Use: Astringent.

Dr. Drake's Cough Medicine. (Last) Dextromethorphan HBr 10 mg/5 mL. Bot. 2 oz. OTC.
Use: Antitussive.

Dr. Edwards' Olive. (Oakhurst) Sennosides (from senna concentrate) 8.6 mg. Tab. 75s. OTC.
Use: Laxative.

Dri-A Caps. (Barth's) Vitamin A 10,000 units. Cap. Bot. 100s, 500s. OTC.
Use: Vitamin supplement.

Dri A & D Caps. (Barth's) Vitamins A 10,000 units, D 400 units. Cap. Bot. 100s, 500s. OTC.
Use: Vitamin supplement.

•**dribendazole.** (dry-BEN-dah-ZOLE) USAN.
Use: Anthelmintic.

Dri-E. (Barth's) Vitamin E. Cap.
100 units: Bot. 100s, 500s, 1000s.
200 units: Bot. 100s, 250s, 500s.
400 units: Bot. 100s, 250s. OTC.
Use: Vitamin supplement.

Dri/Ear. (Pfeiffer) Isopropyl alcohol 95%, glycerin 5%. Liq. 30 mL. OTC.
Use: Otic preparation.

dried aluminum hydroxide gel.
Use: Antacid.
See: Aluminum Hydroxide Gel, dried.

dried yeast.
See: Yeast, dried.

DriHist SR. (Prasco) Phenylephrine hydrochloride 20 mg, chlorpheniramine maleate 8 mg, methscopolamine nitrate 2.5 mg. ER Tab. 100s. Rx.
Use: Upper respiratory combination, decongestant, antihistamine, anticholinergic combination.

Driminate Tabs. (Major) Dimenhydrinate 50 mg. Tab. Bot. 100s, 1000s. OTC.
Use: Antiemetic; antivertigo.

•**drinidene.** (DRIH-nih-deen) USAN.
Use: Analgesic.

Drisdol. (Sanofi Pharm) Ergocalciferol (Vitamin D₂). **Cap.:** 50,000 units. Tartrazine. Bot. 50s. **Drops:** 8000 units/mL in propylene glycol. Liq. Bot. 60 mL. Rx-OTC.
Use: Refractory rickets; hypophosphatemia; hypoparathyroidism.

Dristan Cold Multi-Symptom Formula. (Wyeth Consumer) Phenylephrine hydrochloride 5 mg, chlorpheniramine maleate 2 mg, acetaminophen 325 mg. PEG. Tab. 20s. OTC.
Use: Upper respiratory combination; decongestant, antihistamine, and analgesic.

Dristan 12-Hr Nasal. (Wyeth Consumer) Oxymetazoline hydrochloride 0.05%, benzalkonium chloride, benzyl alcohol, edetate sodium, sodium chloride. Spray. 15 mL. OTC.
Use: Nasal decongestant, imidazoline.

Dritho-Scalp. (Summers Lab) Anthralin 0.5%. White petrolatum, cetostearyl alcohol. Cream. Tube 50 g. Rx.
Use: Antipsoriatic.

Drixoral. (Schering-Plough) Dexbrompheniramine maleate 6 mg, pseudoephedrine sulfate 120 mg. SA Tab. Box 10s, 20s, 40s. Bot. 48s, 100s. OTC.
Use: Antihistamine, decongestant.

Drixoral. (Schering-Plough) Pseudoephedrine sulfate 30 mg, brompheniramine maleate 2 mg. Sorbitol, sugar. Syrup. Bot. 118 mL. OTC.
Use: Antihistamine, decongestant.

Drixoral Allergy Sinus. (Schering-Plough Healthcare) Pseudoephedrine sulfate 60 mg, dexbrompheniramine maleate 3 mg, acetaminophen 500 mg. Parabens. ER Tab. Pkg. 12s. OTC.
Use: Upper respiratory combination, decongestant, antihistamine, analgesic.

Drixoral Cold & Allergy. (Schering-Plough Healthcare) Dexbrompheniramine maleate 6 mg, pseudoephedrine sulfate 120 mg. Sugar, lactose, butylparaben. Tab. Pkg. 20s. OTC.
Use: Upper respiratory combination, antihistamine, decongestant.

Drixoral Cough & Congestion Liquid Caps. (Schering-Plough) Pseudoephedrine hydrochloride 60 mg, dextromethorphan HBr 30 mg. Cap. Pkg. 10s. OTC.
Use: Antihistamine, decongestant.

Drixoral Non-Drowsy Formula. (Schering-Plough) Pseudoephedrine sulfate 120 mg. Sugar. Tab. Pkg. 10s, 20s. OTC.
Use: Decongestant.

Drixoral Plus. (Schering-Plough) Pseudoephedrine sulfate 60 mg, dexbrompheniramine maleate 3 mg, acetaminophen 500 mg. TR Tab. Bot. 12s, 24s. OTC.
Use: Analgesic, antihistamine, decongestant.

Drixoral Sustained-Action. (Schering-Plough) Pseudoephedrine sulfate 120 mg, dexbrompheniramine maleate 6 mg. Sugar, lactose. Tab. Pkg. 10s. Bot. 20s, 40s. *OTC.*
Use: Antihistamine; decongestant.

●**drobuline.** (DROE-byoo-leen) USAN.
Use: Cardiovascular agent (antiar-rhythmic).

●**drocinonide.** (droe-SIN-oh-nide) USAN.
Use: Anti-inflammatory.

drocode.
See: Dihydrocodeine.

●**droloxifene.** (drole-OX-ih-feen) USAN.
Use: Antineoplastic.

●**droloxifene citrate.** (drole-OX-ih-feen) USAN.
Use: Antineoplastic.

●**drometrizole.** (DROE-meh-TRY-zole) USAN.
Use: Ultraviolet screen.

●**dromostanolone propionate.** (DRAHM-oh-STAN-oh-lone) *USP 34.*
Use: Antineoplastic.

●**dronabinol.** (droe-NAB-ih-nahl) *USP 34.*
Use: Antiemetic; antivertigo.
See: Marinol.

dronabinol. (Watson) Dronabinol 2.5 mg, 5 mg, 10 mg. Sesame oil. Cap. 60s. *c-III.*
Use: Antiemetic; antivertigo.

dronedarone. (DROE-ne-da-rone)
Use: Antiarrhythmic.
See: Multaq.

drop chalk. (Various Mfr.) Calcium carbonate, prepared. Prepared chalk.

●**droperidol.** (dro-PER-i-dahl) *USP 34.*
Use: Antipsychotic; anxiolytic; general anesthetic.

droperidol. (Various Mfr.) Droperidol 2.5 mg/mL. Inj. Vial 2 mL. *Rx.*
Use: Anesthetic, general.

●**droprenilamine.** (droe-preh-NILL-ah-meen) USAN.
Use: Vasodilator (coronary).

●**drospirenone.** (droe-SPYE-reh-nohn) USAN.
Use: Sex hormone, contraceptive, hormone.
See: Yasmin.
W/Estradiol.
See: Angeliq.
W/Ethinyl Estradiol.
See: Gianvi.
Ocella.
YAZ.
W/Ethinyl Estradiol, Levomefolate Calcium.
See: Beyaz.

drotrecogin alfa (activated).
Use: Thrombolytic agent, recombinant human activated protein C.
See: Xigris.

●**droxacin sodium.** (DROX-ah-sin) USAN.
Use: Anti-infective.

Droxia. (Bristol-Myers Squibb Oncology/Virology) Hydroxyurea 200 mg, 300 mg, 400 mg. Lactose. Cap. Bot. 60s. *Rx.*
Use: Antisickling agent.

●**droxidopa.** (droks-eye-DOE-pa) USAN.
Use: Neurogenic hypotension.

●**droxifilcon A.** (DROX-ih-fill-kahn A) USAN.
Use: Contact lens material (hydrophilic).

●**droxinavir hydrochloride.** (drox-IN-ah-veer) USAN.
Use: Antiviral.

●**drozitumab.** (droe-ZIT-ue-mab) USAN.
Use: Antineoplastic.

Dr. Scholl's Advanced Pain Relief Corn Removers. (Schering-Plough) Salicylic acid 40% in a rubber-based vehicle. Disc. 6s. *OTC.*
Use: Keratolytic.

Dr. Scholl's Athlete's Foot. (Schering-Plough) **Pow.:** Tolnaftate 1%. Talc. Bot. 63 g. **Spray Liq.:** Tolnaftate 1%, alcohol 36%. Bot. 113 mL. *OTC.*
Use: Antifungal, topical.

Dr. Scholl's Athlete's Foot Cream. (Schering-Plough) Tolnaftate 1%. Tube 0.5 oz. *OTC.*
Use: Antifungal, topical.

Dr. Scholl's Callus Removers. (Schering-Plough) Salicylic acid 40% in a rubber-based vehicle. 6 pads, 4 discs. Extra thick in 4 discs. *OTC.*
Use: Keratolytic.

Dr. Scholl's Clear Away. (Schering-Plough) Salicylic acid 40% in a rubber-based vehicle. Disc 18s. *OTC.*
Use: Keratolytic.

Dr. Scholl's Clear Away One Step. (Schering-Plough) Salicylic acid 40% in a rubber-based vehicle. Strip 14s. *OTC.*
Use: Keratolytic.

Dr. Scholl's Clear Away Plantar. (Schering-Plough) Salicylic acid 40% in a rubber-based vehicle. Disc 24s. *OTC.*
Use: Keratolytic.

Dr. Scholl's Corn/Callus Remover. (Schering-Plough) Salicylic acid 12.6% in a flexible collodion, alcohol 18%, ether 55%, hydrogenated vegetable oil. Liq. 10 mL with 3 cushions. *OTC.*
Use: Keratolytic.

Dr. Scholl's Corn/Callus Salve. (Schering-Plough) Salicylic acid 15%. Tube 0.4 oz. *OTC.*
Use: Keratolytic.

Dr. Scholl's Corn Remover. (Schering-Plough) Salicylic acid 40% in a rubber-based vehicle. Discs: 6s as wrap-arounds, 9s as ultra thin, small, waterproof, regular, soft, and extra-thick. *OTC.*
Use: Keratolytic.

Dr. Scholl's Corn Salve. (Schering-Plough) Salicylic acid 15%. Jar 0.4 oz. *OTC.*
Use: Keratolytic.

Dr. Scholl's Cracked Heel Relief. (Schering-Plough) Lidocaine 2%, benzethonium chloride 0.13%. Aloe. Cream. Tubes. 89 mL. *OTC.*
Use: Anesthetic, local.

Dr. Scholl's Ingrown Toenail Reliever. (Schering-Plough) Sodium sulfide 1%. Bot. 0.33 oz. *OTC.*
Use: Foot preparation.

Dr. Scholl's Maximum Strength Tritan. (Schering-Plough) Tolnaftate 1%. **Pow.:** Talc. Bot. 56 g. **Spray Pow.:** SD alcohol 40 14%. Bot. 85 g. *OTC.*
Use: Antifungal, topical.

Dr. Scholl's Moisturizing Corn Remover Kit. (Schering-Plough) Salicylic acid 40% in a rubber-based vehicle, moisturizing cream, pain relief cushions. Disc 6s. *OTC.*
Use: Keratolytic.

Dr. Scholl's One Step Corn Removers. (Schering-Plough) Salicylic acid 40% in a rubber-based vehicle. Strips 6s. *OTC.*
Use: Keratolytic.

Dr. Scholl's Pro Comfort Jock Itch Spray. (Schering-Plough) Tolnaftate 1%. Aerosol Can 3.5 oz. *OTC.*
Use: Antifungal, topical.

Dr. Scholl's Wart Remover Kit. (Schering-Plough) Salicylic acid 17% in a flexible collodion, alcohol 17%, ether 52%. Liq. 10 mL with brush and 6 adhesive pads. *OTC.*
Use: Keratolytic.

Dr. Scholl's Zino Pads with Medicated Disks. (Schering-Plough) Salicylic acid 20%, 40%. Protective pads designed for use with and without salicylic acid-impregnated disks. *OTC.*
Use: Keratolytic.

Dr. Smith's Adult Care. (Beta Dermaceuticals) Zinc oxide 10%, petrolatum, lanolin, mineral oil, olive oil. Oint. Tube. 85 g. *OTC.*
Use: Topical protectant.

Dr. Smith's Diaper. (Beta Dermaceuticals) Zinc oxide 10%, petrolatum, lanolin, mineral oil, olive oil. Oint. Tube. 85 g. *OTC.*
Use: Topical protectant.

Drucon C R. (Standard Drug Co.) Phenylephrine hydrochloride 25 mg, chlorpheniramine maleate 4 mg. Tab. Bot. 100s. *OTC.*
Use: Antihistamine, decongestant.

Drucon with Codeine. (Standard Drug Co.) Codeine phosphate 10 mg, phenylephrine hydrochloride 10 mg, chlorpheniramine maleate 2 mg, menthol 1 mg, alcohol 5%/5 mL. Bot. Pt. *c-v.*
Use: Antihistamine, antitussive, decongestant.

Dry Eyes. (Bausch & Lomb) White petrolatum, mineral oil, lanolin. Oint. Tube 3.5 g. *OTC.*
Use: Lubricant, ophthalmic.

Dry Eye Therapy. (Bausch & Lomb) Glycerin 0.3%, potassium chloride, sodium chloride, sodium citrate, sodium phosphate, zinc chloride. Drop. Single-use Bot. 0.3 mL (UD 32s). *OTC.*
Use: Ophthalmic.

drying agents.
See: Aluminum Chloride (Hexahydrate). Formaldehyde.

DryMax. (Jaymac Pharmaceutical) Chlorpheniramine maleate 4 mg, methscopolamine nitrate 1.25 mg, pseudoephedrine hydrochloride 30 mg. Glycerin, propylene glycol, saccharin, sucrose. Alcohol free and gluten free. Grape flavor. Syrup. 118 mL. *Rx.*
Use: Upper respiratory combination; decongestant, antihistamine, and anticholinergic combination.

Dryphen Multi-Symptom Formula. (Major) Phenylephrine hydrochloride 5 mg, chlorpheniramine maleate 2 mg, acetaminophen 325 mg. Tab. Bot. 40s. *OTC.*
Use: Upper respiratory combination, decongestant, antihistamine, analgesic.

Drysec. (A.G. Marin) Phenylephrine hydrochloride 20 mg, chlorpheniramine maleate 8 mg, methscopolamine nitrate 2.5 mg. ER Tab. 100s. *Rx.*
Use: Decongestant, antihistamine, and anticholinergic combination, upper respiratory combination.

Dry Skin Creme. (Gordon Laboratories) Cetyl alcohol, lubricating oils in a water-soluble base. Jar 2 oz, 1 lb, 5 lb. *OTC.*
Use: Emollient.

Drysol. (Person & Covey) Aluminum chloride hexahydrate 20% in 93% SD alcohol 40. Bot. 37.5 mL; 35 mL, 60 mL w/*Dab-O-Matic* applicator. *Rx.*
Use: Drying agent.

Drysum Shampoo. (Summers) Alcohol 15%, acetone 6%. Plastic bot. 4 oz.

OTC.
Use: Dermatologic, hair.

Drytergent. (C & M Pharmacal) TEA-dodecylbenzenesulfonate, boric acid, lauramide DEA, propylene glycol, tartrazine, purified water, color, fragrance. Liq. Bot. 240 mL, 480 mL. *OTC.*
Use: Dermatologic, acne.

Drytex. (C & M Pharmacal) Salicylic acid 2%, benzalkonium chloride 0.1%, acetone 10%, isopropyl alcohol 40%, tartrazine. Lot. Bot. 240 mL. *OTC.*
Use: Dermatologic, acne.

DSS. (Dioctyl sodium sulfosuccinate) Docusate sodium. *OTC.*
Use: Laxative.
See: Colace.
　Docusate Sodium.
　DOK.
　DOS.
　D-S-S.

D-S-S. (Magno-Humphries) Docusate sodium 100 mg. Cap. Bot. 100s. *OTC.*
Use: Laxative; stool softener.

DST. Dihydrostreptomycin.
See: Dihydrostreptomycin Sulfate.

D-Tab. (Palm) Phenylephrine hydrochloride 40 mg, guaifenesin 1200 mg. Film-coated. ER Tab. 100s. *Rx.*
Use: Upper respiratory combination, decongestant and expectorant combination.

D-Tann. (Midlothian) **Chew. Tab.:** Phenylephrine tannate 10 mg, diphenhydramine tannate 25 mg. Phenylalanine. Berry flavor. 60s. **Susp.:** Phenylephrine tannate 7.5 mg, diphenhydramine tannate 25 mg per 5 mL. Methylparaben, saccharin, sucrose. Bubble gum flavor. Susp.118 mL. *Rx.*
Use: Decongestant and antihistamine, upper respiratory combination.

D-Tann AT. (Midlothian) Carbetapentane tannate 30 mg, diphenhydramine tannate 25 mg per 5 mL. Aspartame, parabens, phenylalanine 7 mg per 5 mL. Cotton candy flavor. Susp. 118 mL. *Rx.*
Use: Upper respiratory combination, antitussive combination.

D-Tann CD. (Midlothian) Carbetapentane tannate 30 mg, diphenhydramine tannate 25 mg, phenylephrine tannate 15 mg per 5 mL. Parabens, PEG, saccharin. Strawberry flavor. Susp. 118 mL. *Rx.*
Use: Upper respiratory combination, antitussive, antihistamine, decongestant.

D-Tann CT. (Midlothian) **Susp.:** Carbetapentane tannate 30 mg, diphenhydramine tannate 25 mg, phenylephrine tannate 7.5 mg per 5 mL. Methylparaben, sucrose, saccharin. Strawberry-banana flavor. 118 mL. **Tab.:** Carbetapentane tannate 30 mg, diphenhydramine tannate 25 mg, phenylephrine tannate 10 mg. Lactose. 60s. *Rx.*
Use: Antitussive combination, upper respiratory combination.

D-Tann DM. (Midlothian) Dextromethorphan tannate 75 mg, diphenhydramine tannate 25 mg, phenylephrine tannate 7.5 mg per 5 mL. Aspartame, parabens, phenylalanine 7 mg per 5 mL. Black cherry flavor. Susp. 118 mL. *Rx.*
Use: Upper respiratory combination, antitussive combination.

D-10-W. (Various Mfr.) Dextrose in water injection 10% (amps 3 mL); vials 250 mL, 500 mL, 1000 mL; 17 mL fill in 20 mL, 500 mL fill in 1000 mL, 1000 mL fill in 2000 mL vials. *Rx.*
Use: Carbohydrate supplement.

D-3. D vitamin.
See: Cholecalciferol.

D3-50. (Bio-Tech) Vitamin D_3 50,000 units. Dye free, preservative free, sugar free, yeast free. Cap. 100s. *OTC.*
Use: Fat-soluble vitamin.

DTIC. Dacarbazine.
Use: Antineoplastic.
See: DTIC-Dome.

DTIC-Dome. (Bayer) Dacarbazine 100 mg, 200 mg. May contain mannitol. Inj. Vials. *Rx.*
Use: Antineoplastic.

DTP. Diphtheria and tetanus toxoids and pertussis vaccine, adsorbed. *Rx.*
Use: Immunization.
See: Infanarix.
　Tripedia.

D_3 Healthy Kids. (Mason Vitamins) Vitamin D_3 400 units. Fructose, sucrose, sunflower oil. Chew. Tab. 60s. *OTC.*
Use: Fat-soluble vitamin.

D-2. D vitamin.
See: Ergocalciferol.

Duac CS. (GlaxoSmithKline) Benzoyl peroxide 5%, clindamycin 1%, EDTA, glycerin, methylparaben. Gel 45 g. *Formerly Duac. Rx.*
Use: Anti-infective, topical.

Dual Action Complete. (Major Pharmaceuticals) Calcium carbonate 800 mg, famotidine 10 mg, magnesium hydroxide 165 mg. Aspartame, dextrates, lactose, phenylalanine 2.2 mg. Chew Tab. 25s. *OTC.*
Use: Histamine H_2 antagonist combination.

Dual-Wet. (Alcon) Polyvinyl alcohol, duasorb water-soluble polymetric system, benzalkonium chloride 0.01%, disodium edetate 0.05%. Bot. 2 oz. *OTC.*
Use: Contact lens care.

•**duazomycin.** (doo-AZE-oh-MY-sin) USAN. Antibiotic isolated from broth filtrates of *Streptomyces ambofaciens.*
Use: Antineoplastic.

duazomycin A. *Name used for Duazomycin.*
Use: Antineoplastic.

duazomycin B. *Name used for Azotomycin.*
Use: Antineoplastic.

duazomycin C. *Name used for Ambomycin.*
Use: Antineoplastic.

Duet. (Xanodyne) Vitamin A 3000 units, B_1 1.8 mg, B_2 4 mg, B_3 30 mg, B_6 25 mg, B_{12} 12 mcg, C 120 mg, D 400 units, E 30 mg, folic acid 1 mg, Ca 100 mg, Cu 2 mg, Fe 29 mg, Mg 25 mg, Zn 25 mg. Aspartame, mannitol, sorbitol, sucrose. Phenylalanine 9 mg per tablet. Vanilla flavor. Chew. Tab. 90s. *Rx.*
Use: Multivitamin with calcium and iron.

Duetact. (Takeda) Pioglitazone hydrochloride/glimepiride 30 mg/2 mg, 30 mg/4 mg. Lactose. Tab. 30s, 90s. *Rx.*
Use: Antidiabetic combination.

Duet DHA. (Xanodyne) **Cap.:** Purified omega-3 fatty acids 300 mg including docosahexaenoic acid ≥ 200 mg. 5 blister packs of 6s. **Tab.:** Vitamin A 3000 units, B_1 1.8 mg, B_2 4 mg, B_3 20 mg, B_6 25 mg, B_{12} 12 mcg, C 120 mg, D 400 units, E 30 mg, folic acid 1 mg, Ca 200 mg, Cu 2 mg, Fe 29 mg, Mg 25 mg, Zn 25 mg. Sucrose. 5 blister packs of 6s. *Rx.*
Use: Multivitamin with calcium and iron.

Duet DHA^{EC}**.** (Xanodyne) **Cap.:** Purified omega-3 fatty acids 300 mg including ≥ 200 mg docosahexaenoic acid. Enteric coated. 5 blister packs of 6s. **Tab.:** Vitamin A 3000 units, B_1 1.8 mg, B_2 4 mg, B_3 20 mg, B_6 25 mg, B_{12} 12 mcg, C 120 mg, D 400 units, E 30 mg, folic acid 1 mg, Ca 200 mg, Cu 2 mg, Fe 24 mg, Mg 25 mg, Zn 25 mg. Sucrose. 5 blister packs of 6s. *Rx.*
Use: Multivitamin with calcium and iron.

•**dulaglutide.** (DOO-la-GLOO-tide) USAN.
Use: Antidiabetic agent.

Dulcagen Suppositories. (Ivax) Bisacodyl 10 mg. Box 12s, 100s. *OTC.*
Use: Laxative.

Dulcolax. (Boehringer Ingelheim) **EC Tab.:** Bisacodyl 5 mg, lactose, sucrose,

parabens. Bot. 10s, 25s, 50s, 100s. **Liq.:** Magnesia (magnesium hydroxide) 400 mg per 5 mL. Original flavor. Sugar free. 355 mL. *OTC.*
Use: Laxative; antacid.

Dulcolax Balance. (Boehringer Ingelheim) PEG 3350 17 g. Pow. for Soln. 238 g. *OTC.*
Use: Laxative, bowel evacuant.

Dulcolax Bowel Prep Kit. (Boehringer Ingelheim) Bisacodyl 5 mg. Docusate sodium, lactose, parabens, sucrose. Tab. 4s. *OTC.*
Use: Laxative.

Dulcolax Stool Softener. (Boehringer Ingelheim) Docusate sodium 100 mg. Glycerin, sorbitol. Soft Gel Cap. 25s. *OTC.*
Use: Laxative.

DuLeek-Dp 15. (Seton Pharmaceuticals) Folate 15 mg. Tab. 90s. *Rx.*
Use: Water-soluble vitamin.

DuLeek-Dp 7.5. (Seton Pharmaceuticals) Folate 7.5 mg. Tab. 30s, 90s. *Rx.*
Use: Water-soluble vitamin.

Dulera. (Schering) Mometasone furoate/formoterol fumarate 100 mcg/5 mcg, 200 mcg/5 mcg per actuation. Aer. Canister w/actuator. 13 g. *Rx.*
Use: Respiratory inhalant combination.

Dull-C. (Freeda) Ascorbic acid 1060 mg/¼ tsp. Sugar free. Pow. Bot. 120 g, 1 lb. *OTC.*
Use: Vitamin supplement.

•**duloxetine.** (doo-LOX-eh-teen) USAN.
Tall Man: DULoxetine
Use: Antidepressant.
See: Cymbalta.

Dulphalac. (Solvay) Lactulose 10 g/5 mL. Syr. Bot. 240 mL, 480 mL, 960 mL, UD 30 mL. *Rx.*
Use: Laxative.

Duo. (GlaxoSmithKline) Tube 0.5 oz.
Use: Adhesive.

Duocaine. (Amphastar) Lidocaine hydrochloride 10 mg/mL, bupivacaine hydrochloride 3.75 mg/mL. Preservative free. Inj. 10 mL single-dose vials. Cartons of 25. *Rx.*
Use: Anesthetic, injectable local.

Duocet. (Mason) Hydrocodone bitartrate 5 mg, acetaminophen 500 mg. Tab. Bot. 100s. *c-III.*
Use: Analgesic combination; narcotic.

DuoDERM. (ConvaTec) **Sterile dressing:** 10 cm × 10 cm. Pack 5s. 20 cm × 20 cm. Pack 3s. **Sterile gran.:** Packet 4 g. Pack 5s. *OTC.*
Use: Dermatologic, wound therapy.

DuoDERM Extra Thin. (ConvaTec) Flexible hydroactive sterile dressings. 4″ ×

4", 6" × 6". Pck. 10s. *OTC.*
Use: Dressing, topical.
DuoDote. (Survival Technology) Atropine 2.1 mg/0.7 mL, pralidoxime chloride 600 mg/2 mL. Benzyl alcohol 40 mg. Inj. Soln. Single-use dual chamber prefilled auto-injectors. *Rx.*
Use: Antidote.
Duofilm. (Stiefel) Salicylic acid 16.7%, lactic acid 16.7% in flexible collodion. Bot. 15 mL w/applicator. *OTC.*
Use: Keratolytic.
Duo-Flow. (Ciba Vision) Poloxamer 188, benzalkonium Cl 0.013%, EDTA 0.25%. Soln. Bot. 120 mL. *OTC.*
Use: Contact lens care.
Duohist DH. (Breckenridge) Chlorpheniramine maleate 2 mg, dihydrocodeine bitartrate 7.25 mg, phenylephrine hydrochloride 5 mg per 5 mL. Alcohol, sugar, and dye free. Saccharin, sorbitol. Strawberry flavor. Liq. 473 mL. *c-III.*
Use: Upper respiratory combination, antitussive combination.
Duo-K. (Various Mfr.) Potassium 20 mEq, chloride 3.4 mEq/15 mL (from potassium gluconate and potassium chloride). Bot. Pt, gal. *Rx.*
Use: Mineral supplement.
Duolube. (Bausch & Lomb) White petrolatum, mineral oil. Sterile, preservative and lanolin free. Oint. Tube 3.5 g. *OTC.*
Use: Lubricant, ophthalmic.
Duonate-12. (URL) Phenylephrine tannate 5 mg, pyrilamine tannate 30 mg/5 mL. Susp. Unit of use 118 mL w/oral syr. *Rx.*
Use: Upper respiratory combination, decongestant, antihistamine.
DuoNeb. (Dey) Ipratropium bromide 0.5 mg, albuterol sulfate 3 mg (equivalent to albuterol base 2.5 mg). Inhalation soln. Unit-dose vial 3 mL. Box 30s, 60s. *Rx.*
Use: Bronchodilator, anticholinergic.
•**duoperone fumarate.** (DOO-oh-per-OHN) USAN.
Use: Neuroleptic.
DuoPlant. (Stiefel) Salicylic acid 27%, alcohol 50%, flexible collodion, hydroxypropyl cellulose, lactic acid. Liq. Bot. 14 g. *OTC.*
Use: Ketatolytic (wart removal).
Duosol. (Kirkman) Docusate sodium 100 mg, 250 mg. Cap. Bot. 100s, 1000s. *OTC.*
Use: Laxative.
Duotal. (Health for Life Brands) **1.5 g.:** Secobarbital sodium ¾ g, amobarbital g. Cap. **3 g.:** Secobarbital sodium 1.5 g, amobarbital 1.5 g. Cap. Bot.

100s, 500s, 1000s. *c-II.*
Use: Hypnotic; sedative.
duotal.
See: Guaiacol Carbonate.
Duotan PD. (Scientific Laboratories) Pseudoephedrine tannate 75 mg, dexchlorpheniramine tannate 2.5 mg per 5 mL. Methylparaben, saccharin, sucrose. Strawberry-banana flavor. Susp. 118 mL, 473 mL. *Rx.*
Use: Pediatric decongestant and antihistamine.
Duotrate 45. (Jones Pharma) Pentaerythritol tetranitrate 45 mg. SR Cap. Bot. 100s. *Rx.*
Use: Antianginal.
Duotrate 30. (Jones Pharma) Pentaerythritol tetranitrate 30 mg. SR Cap. Bot. 100s. *Rx.*
Use: Antianginal.
Duovin-S. (Spanner) Estrone 2.5 mg, progesterone 25 mg/mL. Vial 10 mL. *Rx.*
Use: Estrogen, progestin combination.
Duo-WR, No. 1 & No. 2. (Whorton Pharmaceuticals, Inc.) **No. 1:** Salicylic acid, compound tincture benzoin. **No. 2:** Compound tincture benzoin, formaldehyde. Bot. 0.25 oz. *OTC.*
Use: Keratolytic.
Duphalac. (Solvay) Lactulose 10 g/15 mL (1.6 g galactose, 1.2 g lactose, 1.2 g or less of other sugars). Soln. Bot. 240 mL, 480 mL, 960 mL, UD 30 mL. *Rx.*
Use: Laxative.
Duplast. (Beiersdorf) Adhesive coated elastic cloth. 8" × 4" Strip. Box 10s. 10" × 5" Strip. Box 8s, 10s.
Duplex Shampoo. (C & M Pharmacal) Sodium lauryl sulfate 15%, lauramide DEA, purified water. Bot. Pt, gal. *OTC.*
Use: Dermatologic.
duponol.
See: Gardinol type detergents (Sodium Lauryl Sulfate).
Durabac. (Poly Pharmaceuticals) Acetaminophen 325 mg, caffeine 50 mg, phenyltoloxamine citrate 20 mg, salicylamide 250 mg. Cap. 100s. *Rx.*
Use: Nonnarcotic analgesic combination.
Durabac Forte. (Poly Pharm) Acetaminophen 500 mg, magnesium salicylate 500 mg, caffeine 50 mg, phenyltoloxamine citrate 20 mg. Tab. 100s. *Rx.*
Use: Nonnarcotic analgesic.
DURAcare. (Blairex) Buffered hypertonic salt solution, non-ionic detergents with thimerosal 0.004%, EDTA 0.1%. Soln. Bot. 30 mL. *OTC.*
Use: Contact lens care.

Duraclon. (Bioniche Pharma) Clonidine hydrochloride 100 mcg/mL, 500 mcg/mL. Preservative free. Inj. Vials. 10 mL. *Rx.*
Use: Analgesic.

DuraDEX. (ProEthic Pharmaceuticals) Dextromethorphan HBr 20 mg, guaifenesin 1200 mg. Dye free. ER Tab. 100s. *Rx.*
Use: Antitussive with expectorant.

Duradryl. (Breckenridge Pharm.) Phenylephrine hydrochloride 10 mg, chlorpheniramine maleate 2 mg, methscopolamine nitrate 1.25 mg/5mL. Alcohol and sugar free. Sorbitol. Cherry flavor. Syrup. Bot. 473 mL. *Rx.*
Use: Upper respiratory combination, decongestant, antihistamine, anticholinergic.

Dura-Estrin. (Roberts) Estradiol cypionate in oil 5 mg/mL. Inj. Vial 10 mL. *Rx.*
Use: Estrogen.

Duraflex Comfort. (Trimarc Labs) Aloe, capsicum, glucosamine, menthol, methyl salicylate, methyl sulfonyl methane, methylparaben, sorbitol, urea. Gel. 59.14 g. *OTC.*
Use: Rub and liniment.

Duraflu. (Kowa Pharmaceuticals) Dextromethorphan HBr 20 mg, guaifenesin 200 mg, pseudoephedrine hydrochloride 60 mg, acetaminophen 500 mg. Dye free. Tab. 100s. *Rx.*
Use: Upper respiratory combination, antitussive and expectorant combination.

Duragen. (Roberts) Estradiol valerate in oil 20 mg, 40 mg/mL. Inj. Vial 10 mL. *Rx.*
Use: Estrogen.

Duragesic-50. (Janssen) Fentanyl 5 mg (50 mcg/h). Transdermal System. Alcohol < 0.2 mL released during use. Cartons containing 5 individually packaged systems. For use only in opioid-tolerant patients. *c-II.*
Use: Opioid analgesic.

Duragesic-100. (Janssen) Fentanyl 10 mg (100 mcg/h). Transdermal System. Alcohol < 0.2 mL released during use. Cartons containing 5 individually packaged systems. For use only in opioid-tolerant patients. *c-II.*
Use: Opioid analgesic.

Duragesic-75. (Janssen) Fentanyl 7.5 mg (75 mcg/h). Transdermal System. Alcohol < 0.2 mL released during use. Cartons containing 5 individually packaged systems. For use only in opioid-tolerant patients. *c-II.*
Use: Opioid analgesic.

Duragesic-12. (Janssen) Fentanyl 1.25 mg (12.5 mcg/h). Transdermal System. Alcohol < 0.2 mL released during use. Cartons containing 5 individually packaged systems. *c-II.*
Use: Opioid analgesic.

Duragesic-25. (Janssen) Fentanyl 2.5 mg (25 mcg/h). Transdermal System. Alcohol < 0.2 mL released during use. Cartons containing 5 individually packaged systems. *c-II.*
Use: Opioid analgesic.

Duralex. (American Urologicals, Inc.) Pseudoephedrine hydrochloride 120 mg, chlorpheniramine maleate 8 mg. SR Cap. Bot. 100s, 1000s. *Rx.*
Use: Antihistamine, decongestant.

Dura-Meth. (Foy Laboratories) Methylprednisolone 40 mg/mL. Vial 5 mL, 10 mL. *Rx.*
Use: Corticosteroid.

Duramist Plus 12–Hr Decongestant. (Pfeiffer) Oxymetazoline hydrochloride 0.05%, benzalkonium chloride, EDTA, sodium chloride. Spray. Bot. 15 mL. *OTC.*
Use: Nasal decongestant, imidazoline.

Duramorph. (Baxter) Morphine sulfate 0.5 mg/mL, 1 mg/mL. Inj. Single-use amp. 10 mL. *c-II.*
Use: Opioid analgesic.

Durapam. (Major) Flurazepam hydrochloride 15 mg, 30 mg. Cap. Bot. 100s, 500s. *c-IV.*
Use: Hypnotic; sedative.

•**durapatite.** (der-APP-ah-tite) USAN.
Use: Prosthetic aid.

Duraphen Forte. (ProEthic Laboratories) Dextromethorphan HBr 30 mg, guaifenesin 1200 mg, phenylephrine hydrochloride 30 mg. Dye free. ER Tab. 100s. *Rx.*
Use: Antitussive and expectorant combination.

Duraphen II DM. (ProEthic Laboratories) Dextromethorphan HBr 20 mg, guaifenesin 800 mg, phenylephrine hydrochloride 20 mg. Dye free. ER Tab. 100s. *Rx.*
Use: Antitussive and expectorant combination.

DuraProxin. (Pharmaceutica North America) Camphor 3%, menthol 1.25%. Disodium ethylenediaminetetraacetate, glycerin, polysorbate 80. Patch. 30s. *OTC.*
Use: Rub and liniment, patch.

DuraProxin ES. (Pharmaceutica North America) Camphor 3%, menthol 1.25%, methyl salicylate 10%. Disodium ethylenediaminetetraacetate, glycerin,

polysorbate 80. Patch. 30s. *OTC.*
Use: Rub and liniment, patch.
Duraquin. (Parke-Davis) Quinidine gluconate 330 mg. SR Tab. Bot. 100s, UD 100s. *Rx.*
Use: Cardiovascular agent.
Durasal II. (Prasco) Pseudoephedrine hydrochloride 60 mg, guaifenesin 600 mg. SR Tab. 100s. *Rx.*
Use: Upper respiratory combination, decongestant, expectorant.
DuraScreen. (Schwarz Pharma) SPF 30. Octyl methoxycinnamate, octyl salicylate, oxybenzone, 2-phenylbenzimidazole-sulfonic acid, titanium dioxide, cetearyl alcohol, diazolidinyl urea, parabens, shea butter. Lot. Bot. 105 mL. *OTC.*
Use: Sunscreen.
DuraScreen SPF 15. (Schwarz Pharma) SPF 15. Ethylhexyl p-methoxycinnamate, 2-ethylhexyl salicylate, oxybenzone, parabens, titanium dioxide. Lot. Bot. 105 mL. *OTC.*
Use: Sunscreen.
Dura-Tap/PD. (Dura) Pseudoephedrine hydrochloride 60 mg, chlorpheniramine maleate 4 mg. Cap. Bot. 100s. *Rx.*
Use: Antihistamine, decongestant.
Duratears Naturale. (Alcon) White petroleum, anhydrous liquid lanolin, mineral oil. Oint. Tube 3.5 g. *OTC.*
Use: Lubricant, ophthalmic.
Duration. (Schering-Plough Healthcare) Oxymetazoline hydrochloride 0.05%, benzalkonium chloride, EDTA. Soln. Spray Bot. 30 mL. *OTC.*
Use: Nasal decongestant, imidazoline.
Duration Mentholated Vapor Spray. (Schering-Plough) Oxymetazoline hydrochloride 0.05%, aromatics. Squeeze bot. 15 mL. *OTC.*
Use: Decongestant.
Duration Mild Nasal Spray. (Schering-Plough) Phenylephrine hydrochloride 0.5%. Bot. 15 mL. *OTC.*
Use: Decongestant.
Duratuss. (Victory) Phenylephrine hydrochloride 25 mg, guaifenesin 900 mg. ER Tab. 100s. *Rx.*
Use: Decongestant and expectorant combination, upper respiratory combination.
Duratuss A. (Victory) Phenylephrine hydrochloride 20 mg, guaifenesin 600 mg, acetaminophen 650 mg. ER Tab. 100s. *Rx.*
Use: Decongestant and expectorant combination, upper respiratory combination.

Duratuss CS. (Victory) Carbetapentane citrate 60 mg, guaifenesin 900 mg. ER Tab. 100s. *Rx.*
Use: Antitussive with expectorant, upper respiratory combination.
Duratuss DA. (Victory Pharma) Chlorpheniramine maleate 12 mg, pseudoephedrine hydrochloride 100 mg. Sugar. Cap. 100s. *Rx.*
Use: Upper respiratory combination, decongestant and antihistamine.
Duratuss GP. (Victory) Phenylephrine hydrochloride 25 mg, guaifenesin 1,200 mg. ER Tab. 100s. *Rx.*
Use: Decongestant and expectorant, upper respiratory combination.
Duraxin. (Portal) Phenyltoloxamine citrate 25 mg, acetaminophen 325 mg, salicylamide 200 mg. Cap. 30s. *Rx.*
Use: Antihistamine and analgesic.
Durazyme. (Blairex) Nonionic detergent preserved w/thimerosal 0.004%, EDTA 0.1% in sterile buffered hypertonic salt soln. Bot. 30 mL. *OTC.*
Use: Contact lens care.
Durezol. (Alco Vision) Difluprednate 0.05%. Sodium EDTA, boric acid, glycerin, polysorbate 80, sodium acetate, sodium hydroxide, sorbic acid 0.1%. Ophth. Emulsion. Bot. 2.5 mL, 5 mL. *Rx.*
Use: Corticosteroid, ophthalmic.
Dur-Tann DM. (Midlothian) Dextromethorphan tannate 20 mg, brompheniramine tannate 8 mg, phenylephrine tannate 20 mg per 5 mL. Alcohol free. Methylparaben, phenylalanine, saccharin, bubble gum flavor. Susp. 473 mL. *Rx.*
Use: Upper respiratory combination, antitussive combination.
Dur-Tann Forte. (Midlothian) Dextromethorphan tannate 30 mg, dexchlorpheniramine tannate 3.5 mg, pseudoephedrine tannate 45 mg per 5 mL. Methylparaben, saccharin, sucrose. Grape flavor. Susp. 473 mL. *Rx.*
Use: Upper respiratory combination, antitussive combination.
Dusotal. (Harvey) Sodium amobarbital ¾ g, sodium secobarbital g. Cap. Bot. 1000s. (3 g) Bot. 1000s. *c-II.*
Use: Hypnotic; sedative.
•**dusting powder, absorbable.** *USP 34.*
Use: Lubricant.
dusting powder, surgical.
See: B-F-I.
•**dutasteride.** (doo-TASS-teer-ide) USAN.
Use: Benign prostatic hyperplasia, sex hormone, androgen hormone inhibitor.
See: Avodart.

W/Tamsulosin.
See: Jalyn.

dutch oil. Oil of turpentine, sulfurated.

•**dutogliptin.** (DOO-toe-GLIP-tin) USAN.
Use: Antidiabetc.

•**dutogliptin tartrate.** (DOO-toe-GLIP-tin) USAN.
Use: Antidiabetc.

•**duvoglustat.** (due-voe-GLUE-stat) USAN.
Use: Treatment of Pompe disease.

•**duvoglustat hydrochloride.** (due-voe-GLUE-stat) USAN.
Use: Treatment of Pompe disease.

D V Cream. (Hoechst) Dienestrol 0.01% w/lactose, propylene glycol, stearic acid, diglycol stearate, TEA, benzoic acid, butylated hydroxytoluene, disodium edetate, buffered w/lactic acid to an acid pH. Tube 3 oz, w/applicator. *Rx.*
Use: Estrogen.

Dwelle. (Dakryon Pharmaceuticals) EDTA 0.09%, sodium chloride, potassium chloride, boric acid, povidone, NPX 0.001%. Drop. Bot. 15 mL. *OTC.*
Use: Artificial tears.

DX 114 Foot Powder. (Amlab) Zinc undecylenate 1%, salicylic acid 1%, benzoic acid 1%, ammonium alum 5%, boric acid 10.5% w/zinc stearate, chlorophyll, talc, kaolin, starch, calcium silicate, oil of wormwood. Cont. 2 oz. *OTC.*
Use: Antifungal, topical.

Dyantoin Caps. (Major) Phenytoin sodium 100 mg. Cap. Bot. 100s, 1000s. *Rx.*
Use: Anticonvulsant.

Dyazide. (GlaxoSmithKline) Triamterene 37.5 mg, hydrochlorothiazide 25 mg. Cap. Bot. 1000s, UD 100s, Patient Pack 100s. *Rx.*
Use: Antihypertensive; diuretic.

Dycill. (GlaxoSmithKline) Dicloxacillin sodium 250 mg, 500 mg. Cap. Bot. 100s. *Rx.*
Use: Anti-infective; penicillin.

•**dyclonine hydrochloride.** (DIE-kloeneen) *USP 34.*
Use: Anesthetic, topical.
See: Sucrets Children's Formula.
  Sucrets Complete.
  Sucrets Maximum Strength Sore Throat.
  Sucrets Original Formula Sore Throat.
  Sucrets Throat.
W/Benzethonium Chloride.
See: Skin Shield.

Dycomene. (Hance) Hydrocodone bitartrate ⅙ g, pyrilamine maleate 1 g/fl. oz. Bot. 3 oz, gal. *c-iii.*
Use: Antitussive; sleep aid.

•**dydrogesterone.** (DIE-droe-JESS-terohn) *USP 34.*
Use: Hormone, progestin.

dyes.
See: Antiseptic, Dyes.

Dyflex-G. (Econo Med) Dyphylline 200 mg, guaifenesin 200 mg. Tab. Bot. 100s, 1000s. *Rx.*
Use: Antiasthmatic combination, xanthine combination.

Dyflex-200 Tablets. (Econo Med Pharmaceuticals) Dyphylline 200 mg. Bot. 100s, 1000s. *Rx.*
Use: Bronchodilator.

Dy-G. (Cypress) Dyphylline 100 mg, guaifenesin 100 mg/5 mL. Alcohol free. Mint flavor. Liq. Bot. 473 mL. *Rx.*
Use: Antiasthmatic combination, xanthine combination.

dylate. Clonitrate.
Use: Coronary vasodilator.

Dylix. (Lunsco) Dyphylline 100 mg per 15 mL. Alcohol 20%. Elix. 473 mL. *Rx.*
Use: Bronchodilator.

•**dymanthine hydrochloride.** (DIE-mantheen) USAN.
Use: Anthelmintic.

Dymenate. (Keene Pharmaceuticals) Dimenhydrinate 50 mg/mL. Vial 10 mL. *Rx.*
Use: Antiemetic; antivertigo.

Dynacin. (Medicis) Minocycline hydrochloride (as base). **Cap.:** 50 mg, 75 mg, 100 mg. Bot. 50s (100 mg only), 100s (except 100 mg), 500s (except 75 mg), 1000s. **Tab.:** 50 mg, 75 mg, 100 mg. Lactose. Film-coated. 50s (100 mg only), 100s (except 100 mg), 1000s. *Rx.*
Use: Anti-infective; tetracycline.

DynaCirc CR. (GlaxoSmithKline) Isradipine 5 mg, 10 mg. Film-coated. CR Tab. Bot. 30s, 100s. *Rx.*
Use: Calcium channel blocker.

Dynafed Asthma Relief. (BDI) Ephedrine hydrochloride 25 mg, guaifenesin 200 mg. Tab. Bot. 60s. *OTC.*
Use: Upper respiratory combination, decongestant, expectorant.

Dynafed Ex, Extra Strength. (BDI)
See: Extra Strength Dynafed EX.

Dynafed Jr., Children's. (BDI)
See: Children's Dynafed Jr.

Dynafed Plus, Maximum Strength.
See: Maximum Strength Dynafed Plus.

Dyna-Hex Skin Cleanser. (Western Medical) Chlorhexidine gluconate 4%,

isopropyl alcohol 4%. Liq. Bot. 120 mL,
240 mL, 480 mL, gal. *OTC.*
Use: Antimicrobial; antiseptic.
Dyna-Hex 2 Skin Cleanser. (Western
Medical) Chlorhexidine gluconate 2%,
isopropyl alcohol 4%. Liq. Bot. 120 mL,
240 mL, 480 mL, gal. *OTC.*
Use: Antimicrobial; antiseptic.
dynamine. (Mayo Foundation)
Use: Antispasmodic, Lambert-Eaton
myasthenic syndrome, hereditary
motor and sensory neuropathy type I
(Charcot-Marie-Tooth Disease).
[Orphan Drug]
Dynapen. (Apothecon) Dicloxacillin so-
dium. **Cap.:** 125 mg, 250 mg, 500 mg.
Bot. 24s (except 500 mg), 50s (500 mg
only), 100s (except 500 mg). **Pow. for
Oral Susp.:** 62.5 mg/5 mL. Bot.
100 mL, 200 mL. *Rx.*
Use: Anti-infective; penicillin.
Dynaplex. (Alton) Vitamin B complex.
Bot. 100s, 1000s. *OTC.*
Use: Vitamin supplement.
Dynatuss EX. (Breckenridge) Dextromethorphan HBr 30 mg, guaifenesin
200 mg, phenylephrine hydrochloride
10 mg per 5 mL. PEG, saccharin,
sorbitol. Syrup. 473 mL. *Rx.*
Use: Upper respiratory combination, antitussive and expectorant combination.
Dynex. (Athlon) Pseudoephedrine hydrochloride 90 mg, guaifenesin 1200 mg.
Dye free. ER Tab. Bot. 30s, 100s. *Rx.*
Use: Upper respiratory combination, decongestant, expectorant.
Dynex LA. (Athlon) Phenylephrine hydrochloride 30 mg, guaifenesin 800 mg
(400 mg extended release, 400 mg immediate release). ER Tab. 100s. *Rx.*
Use: Upper respiratory combination, decongestant and expectorant combination.
Dynex VR. (Athlon) Carbetapentane citrate (extended release) 30 mg, guaifenesin (immediate release) 400 mg.
ER Cap. 100s. *Rx.*
Use: Antitussive with expectorant.
Dy-O-Derm. (Galderma) Purified water,
isopropyl alcohol, acetone, dihydroxyacetone, FD&C yellow No. 6, FD&C
blue No. 1, FD&C red No. 33. Bot. 4 oz.
Use: Dermatologic, vitiligo stain.
Dy-Phyl-Lin. (Foy Laboratories) Dyphyl-
line 250 mg/mL with benzyl alcohol. Inj.
Vial 10 mL. *Rx.*
Use: Bronchodilator.
•**dyphylline.** (DIE-fih-lin) *USP 34.*
Use: Vasodilator; bronchodilator.
See: Dylix.

Lufyllin.
Lufyllin-400.
W/Guaifenesin.
See: Difil-G.
Difil-G Forte.
Difil-G 400.
Dilex-G.
Dilex-G 400.
Dilex-G 200.
Dyflex-G.
Dy-G Liquid.
Dyphylline and Guaifenesin.
Dyphylline-GG.
Dyphylline GG ES.
Jay-Phyl.
Lufyllin-GG.
Panfil G.
•**dyphylline and guaifenesin.** (DIE-fih-lin
and GWIE-fen-ah-sin) *USP 34.*
Use: Antiasthmatic combination, xan-
thine combination.
dyphylline and guaifenesin. (Various
Mfr.) Dyphylline 200 mg, guaifenesin
200 mg. May contain dextrose. Tab.
Bot. 100s. *Rx.*
Use: Antiasthmatic combination, xan-
thine combination.
Dyphylline GG Elixir. (Various Mfr.) Dy-
phylline 33.3 mg, guaifenesin 33.3 mg
per 5 mL. Alcohol 17%, saccharin, sucrose. Elix. Bot. 473 mL. *Rx.*
Use: Bronchodilator.
Dyphylline GG ES. (Breckenridge) Dyphylline 200 mg, guaifenesin 300 mg.
Maltodextrin, saccharin, vanilla flavoring. Tab. 100s. *Rx.*
Use: Antiasthmatic combination, xanthine combination.
Dyprotex. (Blairex) Micronized zinc ox-
ide 40%, petrolatum 37.6%, dimethi-
cone 2.5%, cod liver oil, aloe extract,
zinc stearate. Pad. Pkg. 3s (9 applications). *OTC.*
Use: Astringent.
Dyrenium. (GlaxoSmithKline) Triam-
terene 50 mg, 100 mg. Cap. Bot. 100s,
1000s (100 mg only), UD 100s. *Rx.*
Use: Diuretic.
Dyretic. (Keene Pharmaceuticals) Furo-
semide 10 mg/mL. Vial 10 mL. *Rx.*
Use: Diuretic.
Dyrexan-OD. (Trimen Laboratories, Inc.)
Phendimetrazine tartrate 105 mg. SR
Cap. Bot. 100s. *c-III.*
Use: Anorexiant.
Dyspel. (Dover Pharmaceuticals) Aceta-
minophen, ephedrine sulfate, atropine
sulfate. Sugar, lactose, salt free. Tab.
UD Box 500s. *Rx.*
Use: Analgesic.

Dysport. (Tercica) AbobotulinumtoxinA 300 units, 500 units (1 unit corresponds to the calculated median lethal intraperitoneal dose in mice). Albumin (human) 125 mg, lactose 2.5 mg. Preservative free. Inj., lyophilized powder for Soln. Single-use vial. *Rx.*
Use: Botulinum toxin.

Dytan. (Hawthorn) Diphenhydramine tannate. **Chew. Tab.:** 25 mg. Phenylalanine. Strawberry flavor. 60s. **Susp.:** 25 mg per 5 mL. Phenylalanine. Strawberry flavor. 118 mL. *Rx.*
Use: Antihistamine.

Dytan-CS. (Hawthorn) **Susp.:** Carbetapentane tannate 30 mg, diphenhydramine tannate 25 mg, phenylephrine tannate 7.5 mg per 5 mL. Aspartame, parabens, phenylalanine. Strawberry-banana flavor. 118 mL. **Tab.:** Carbetapentane tannate 30 mg, diphenhydramine tannate 25 mg, phenylephrine tannate 10 mg. 60s. *Rx.*
Use: Antitussive combination, upper respiratory combination.

Dytan-D. (Hawthorn) Phenylephrine tannate 7.5 mg, diphenhydramine tannate 25 mg per 5 mL. Phenylalanine. Bubble gum flavor. Susp. 118 mL. *Rx.*
Use: Upper respiratory combination, decongestant, antihistamine.

E

EACA. (Wyeth) Epsilon aminocaproic acid. *Rx.*
Use: Antifibrinolytic.
See: Amicar.

Ear-Dry. (Scherer) Isopropyl alcohol, boric acid 2.75%. Dropper bot. 30 mL. *OTC.*
Use: Otic preparation.

Earex Ear Drops. (Health for Life Brands) Benzocaine 0.15 g, antipyrine 0.7 g/0.5 oz. Bot. 0.5 oz. *Rx.*
Use: Otic.

Ear-Gesic. (Qualitest Pharmaceuticals) Antipyrine 5%, benzocaine 5%, phenylephrine hydrochloride 0.25%. Sodium metabisulfite. Soln., Otic. 15 mL. *Rx.*
Use: Ophthalmic and otic agent, otic preparation.

Earocol Ear Drops. (Roberts) Benzocaine 1.4%, antipyrine 5.4%, glycerin, oxyquinoline sulfate. Soln. Dropper bot. 15 mL. *Rx.*
Use: Otic preparation.

EarSol-HC. (Parnell) Hydrocortisone 1%, alcohol 44%, propylene glycol, *Derm-protective Factor* yerba santa, benzyl benzoate. Soln. 30 mL. *OTC.*
Use: Miscellaneous otic preparation.

earthnut oil. Peanut oil.

Ease. (NeuroGenesis/Matrix Tech.)
D, L-phenylalanine 500 mg, L-glutamine 15 mg, L-tyrosine 25 mg, L-carnitine 10 mg, L-arginine pyroglutamate 10 mg, L-ornithine/L-aspartate 10 mg, Cr 0.033 mg, Se 0.012 mg, B_1 0.33 mg, B_2 5 mg, B_3 3.3 mg, B_5 0.33 mg, B_6 0.33 mg, B_{12} 1 mcg, E 5 units, biotin 0.05 mg, FA 0.066 mg, Fe 1 mg, Zn 2.5 mg, Ca 35 mg, I 0.25 mg, Cu 0.33 mg, Mg 25 mg. Cap. Bot. 42s. *OTC.*
Use: Nutritional supplement.

Easprin. (Parke-Davis) Aspirin 15 g. EC Tab. Bot. 100s. *Rx.*
Use: Analgesic.

East-A. (Eastwood) Therapeutic lotion. Bot. 16 oz. *OTC.*
Use: Emollient.

Easy-Lax. (Walgreen) Docusate sodium 100 mg. Cap. Bot. 60s. *OTC.*
Use: Laxative; stool softener.

Easy-Lax Plus. (Walgreen) Docusate sodium 100 mg, casanthranol 30 mg. Cap. Bot. 60s. *OTC.*
Use: Laxative; stool softener.

Eazol. (Roberts) Fructose, dextrose, orthophosphoric acid with controlled hydrogen ion concentration. Bot. 473 mL. *OTC.*
Use: Antinauseant.

•**ebanicline tosylate.** (EE-ba-ni-kleen) USAN.
Use: Analgesic.

E-Base. (Barr) Erythromycin. **Cap.:** 333 mg. Bot. 100s, 500s, 1000s. **Tab.:** 333 mg, 500 mg. Bot. 100s, 500s. *Rx.*
Use: Anti-infective; erythromycin.

•**ebastine.** (EBB-ass-teen) USAN.
Use: Antihistamine.

EBV-VCA. (Wampole) Epstein-Barr virus, viral capsid antigen antibody test. Qualitative and semi-quantitative detection of EBV antibody in human serum. Test 100s.
Use: Diagnostic aid.

EBV-VCA Ig. (Wampole) Epstein-Barr virus, viral capsid antigen Ig antibody. Qualitative and semiqualitative detection of EBV-VCA Ig antibody in human serum. Test 50s.
Use: Diagnostic aid.

•**ecadotril.** (ee-CAD-oh-trill) USAN.
Use: Antihypertensive.

•**ecalcidene.** (ee-KAL-si-deen) USAN.
Use: Psoriasis.

•**ecallantide.** (ee-KAL-lan-tide) USAN.
Use: Hematological agent.
See: Kalbitor.

•**ecamsule.** (eh-KAM-sool) USAN.
Use: Sunscreen.
W/Avobenzone, Octocrylene.
See: Anthelios SX.
UV Protective.
W/Avobenzone, Octocrylene, Titanium Dioxide.
See: Capital Soleil 20.

Ecee Plus. (Edwards) Vitamin E 165 mg, ascorbic acid 100 mg, magnesium sulfate 70 mg, zinc sulfate 80 mg. Tab. Bot. 100s. *OTC.*
Use: Mineral, vitamin supplement.

•**echinacea angustifolia.** *NF 29.*
Use: Dietary supplement.

•**echinacea pallida.** *NF 29.*
Use: Dietary supplement.

•**echinacea purpurea.** *NF 29.*
Use: Dietary supplement.

echinocandins.
Use: Antifungal.
See: Anidulafungin.
Caspofungin Acetate.

•**echothiophate iodide.** (eck-oh-THIGH-oh-fate EYE-oh-dide) *USP 34.*
Use: Glaucoma agent.

•**eclanamine maleate.** (eh-KLAN-ah-MEEN) USAN.
Use: Antidepressant.

•**eclazolast.** (eh-CLAY-zole-AST) USAN.
Use: Antiallergic; inhibitor (mediator release).

Eclipse After Sun. (Novartis) Petrolatum, glycerin, oleth-3 phosphate, carbomer-934, imidazolidinyl urea, benzyl alcohol, cetyl esters wax. Lot. Bot. 180 mL. *OTC.*
Use: Emollient.

Eclipse Lip and Face Protectant. (Novartis) Padimate O, oxybenzone. Stick 4.5 g. *OTC.*
Use: Lip protectant.

Eclipse Original Sunscreen. (Novartis) Padimate O, glyceryl PABA. Lot. Bot. 120 mL. *OTC.*
Use: Sunscreen.

Eclipse Suntan, Partial. (Novartis) Padimate O. Lot. Bot. 120 mL. *OTC.*
Use: Sunscreen.

EC-Naprosyn. (Roche) Naproxen 375 mg, 500 mg. Enteric coated. DR Tab. Bot. 100s. *Rx.*
Use: Nonsteroidal anti-inflammatory agent.

•**econazole.** (ee-CON-uh-zole) USAN.
Use: Antifungal.

•**econazole nitrate.** (ee-CON-uh-zole) *USP 34.*
Use: Antifungal.
See: Spectazole.

econazole nitrate. (Various Mfr.) Econazole nitrate 1%. Cream. 15 g, 30 g, 85 g. *Rx.*
Use: Antifungal agent, topical anti-infective.

Econo B & C. (Vangard Labs, Inc.) Vitamins B_1 15 mg, B_2 10.2 mg, B_3 50 mg, B_5 10 mg, B_6 5 mg, C 300 mg. Cap. Bot. 100s, UD 100s. *OTC.*
Use: Vitamin supplement.

•**ecopipam hydrochloride.** (E-koe-pi-pam) USAN.
Use: Addiction disorders.

•**ecopladib.** (ek-oh-PLA-dib) USAN.
Use: Analgesic.

Ecotrin Low Strength. (GlaxoSmithKline) Aspirin 81 mg. EDTA, parabens. EC Tab. 45s. *OTC.*
Use: Analgesic.

Ecotrin Maximum Strength. (GlaxoSmithKline) Acetylsalicylic acid 500 mg. **Tab.:** Bot. 60s, 150s. **Cap.:** Bot. 60s. *OTC.*
Use: Analgesic.

Ecotrin Regular Strength. (GlaxoSmithKline) Aspirin 325 mg. EC Tab. Bot. 100s, 250s, 1000s. *OTC.*
Use: Analgesic.

•**ecraprost.** (E-kra-prost) USAN.
Use: Peripheral arterial occlusive disease.

•**ecromeximab.** (e-KROE-mek-si-mab)

USAN.
Use: Monoclonal antibody.

•**eculizumab.** (ek-yoo-LYE-zyoo-mab) USAN.
Use: Monoclonal antibody.
See: Soliris.

•**edaglitazone sodium.** (ED-a-GLI-ta-zone) USAN.
Use: Antidiabetic agent.

Ed A-Hist. (Edwards) Phenylephrine hydrochloride 10 mg, chlorpheniramine maleate 4 mg per 5 mL. Sugar free. Alcohol 5%. Grape flavor. Liq. 473 mL. *Rx.*
Use: Upper respiratory combination, decongestant and antihistamine.

Ed A-Hist DM. (Edwards) Phenylephrine hydrochloride 10 mg, chlorpheniramine maleate 4 mg, dextromethorphan 15 mg per 5 mL. Sugar free. Saccharin, sorbitol. Banana flavor. Liq. Bot. 473 mL. *Rx.*
Use: Upper respiratory combination, antitussive combination.

Ed-Apap Children's. (Edwards) Acetaminophen 160 mg/5 mL. Alcohol free. Sorbitol. Cherry flavor. Oral Soln. 236 mL. *OTC.*
Use: Analgesic.

Edarbi. (Takeda) Azilsartan medoxomil 40 mg (equiv. to azilsartan kamedoxomil 42.68 mg), 80 mg (equiv. to azilsartan kamedoxomil 85.36 mg). Mannitol. Tab. 30s, 90s. *Rx.*
Use: Renin angiotensin system antagonist, angiotensin II receptor antagonist.

edathamil. Edetate ethylenediamine tetraacetic acid.

edathamil calcium-disodium. Calcium disodium ethylenediamine tetraacetate.

edathamil disodium. Disodium salt of ethylenediamine tetraacetic acid.
See: Endrate.

•**edatrexate.** (EE-dah-TREX-ate) USAN.
Use: Antineoplastic.

Ed-Bron G. (Edwards) Theophylline 50 mg, guaifenesin 33.3 mg per 5 mL. Sugar free. Liq. 473 mL. *Rx.*
Use: Antiasthmatic combination, xanthine combination.

Ed-Bron GP. (Edwards) Guaifenesin 100 mg, phenylephrine hydrochloride 5 mg per 5 mL. Parabens, potassium citrate, potassium sorbate, propylene glycol, sorbitol, sucralose. Alcohol free, dye free, and sugar free. Orange flavor. Liq. 473 mL. *OTC.*
Use: Upper respiratory combination, decongestant and expectorant combination.

ED Chlor-Ped D. (Edwards) Phenylephrine tannate 6 mg, chlorpheniramine tannate 2 mg per 1 mL. Methylparaben, saccharin. Applesauce flavor. ER Susp. Drops. 60 mL with dropper. *Rx.*
Use: Upper respiratory combination, decongestant and antihistamine.

ED Chlorped Jr. (Edwards) Chlorpheniramine maleate 2 mg per 5 mL. Parabens, potassium sorbate, propylene glycol, sorbitol, sucralose. Alcohol free and sugar free. Cherry flavor. Syrup. 473 mL. *Rx.*
Use: Antihistamine, nonselective alkylamine.

ED Chlor-Tan. (Edwards) Chlorpheniramine tannate 8 mg. Caplets. 100s. *Rx.*
Use: Antihistamine.

Edecrin. (Aton Pharma) Ethacrynic acid 25 mg, 50 mg. Tab. Bot. 100s. *Rx.*
Use: Diuretic.

Edecrin Sodium Intravenous. (Aton Pharma) Ethacrynate sodium equivalent to 50 mg ethacrynic acid w/mannitol 62.5 mg. Inj., Pow. for Soln. Vial. 50 mL for reconstitution. *Rx.*
Use: Diuretic.

• **edetate calcium disodium.** (E-de-tate) *USP 34. Formerly Edathamil.*
Use: Chelating agent (metal).
See: Calcium Disodium Versenate.

• **edetate dipotassium.** (E-de-tate) USAN.
Use: Pharmaceutic aid (chelating agent).

• **edetate disodium.** (E-de-tate) *USP 34.*
Use: Chelating agent (metal); pharmaceutic aid (chelating agent).

• **edetate sodium.** (E-de-tate) USAN.
Use: Chelating agent.
See: Vagisec Plus.

• **edetate trisodium.** (E-de-tate) USAN.
Use: Chelating agent.

• **edetic acid.** (ED-eh-tic) *NF 29.*
Use: Pharmaceutic aid (chelating agent).

• **edetol.** (eh-deh-TOLE) USAN.
Use: Pharmaceutic aid (alkalinizing agent).

Edex. (Schwarz Pharma) Alprostadil. **Inj.:** 10 mcg, 20 mcg, 40 mcg (after reconstitution), lactose. Inj. Single-dose vial or kit containing prefilled syringe (with 1.2 mL of 0.9% sodium chloride), plunger rod, 2 one-half inch needles (one 27-gauge and one 30-gauge), 2 alcohol swabs, tape. **Pow. for Inj., lyophilized:** 10 mcg, 20 mcg, 40 mcg. Lactose. Single-dose, dual-chamber cartridges for use with reusable injection device. *Rx.*
Use: Anti-impotence agent.

Ed-Flex. (Edwards) Phenyltoloxamine citrate 20 mg, acetaminophen 300 mg, salicylamide 200 mg. Cap. Bot. 30s, 100s. *Rx.*
Use: Upper respiratory combination, antihistamine, analgesic.

• **edifoligide sodium.** (e-dif-oh-LIG-ide) USAN.
Use: Graft-vs-host disease.

• **edifolone acetate.** (EH-DIH-fah-LONE) USAN.
Use: Cardiovascular agent (antiarrhythmic).

edithamil.
See: Edathamil.

• **edivoxetine.** (E-di-VOX-e-teen) USAN.
Use: CNS agent.

• **edivoxetine hydrochloride.** (E-di-VOX-e-teen) USAN.
Use: CNS agent.

Edluar. (Meda Pharmaceuticals) Zolpidem tartrate 5 mg, 10 mg. Mannitol, saccharin. Sublingual Tab. UD 10s, UD 30s, UD 100s. *c-iv.*
Use: Sedative and hypnotic, nonbarbiturate; imidazopyridine.

• **edobacomab.** (eh-dah-BACK-ah-mab) USAN.
Use: Antiendotoxin monoclonal antibody.

• **edodekin alfa.** (e-DOE-de-kin AL-fa) USAN.
Use: Antiasthmatic.

• **edonetan.** (ed-ON-en-tan) USAN.
Use: Heart failure.

• **edotecarin.** (ed-oh-TEK-ar-in) USAN.
Use: Antineoplastic.

• **edotreotide.** (ed-oh-TREE-oh-tide) USAN.
Use: Tumor staging.

• **edoxaban.** (e-DOX-a-ban) USAN.
Use: Cardiovascular agent.

• **edoxaban tosylate.** (e-DOX-a-ban) USAN.
Use: Cardiovascular agent.

• **edoxudine.** (e-DOX-ue-deen) USAN.
Use: Antiviral.

• **edratide.** (ED-ra-tide) USAN.
Use: Lupus erythematosus.

• **edrecolomab.** (E-dre-KOL-oh-mab) USAN.
Use: Monoclonal antibody (antineoplastic adjuvant).

edrofuradene. *Name used for Nifurdazil.*

• **edrophonium chloride.** (eh-droe-FOE-nee-uhm) *USP 34.*

Use: Antidote to curare principles; diagnostic aid, myasthenia gravis.
See: Reversol.

ED-Spaz. (Edwards) Hyoscyamine sulfate 0.125 mg. Tab., dispersible. 100s. *Rx.*
Use: Anticholinergic/antispasmodic, belladonna alkaloids.

EDTA.
See: Edathamil.

E.E.S. 400. (Arbor Pharmaceuticals) Erythromycin ethylsuccinate (as base). **Tab.:** 400 mg. Sugar. Film-coated. 100s, 500s. **Susp.:** 400 mg/5 mL. Parabens, sucrose. Orange flavor. Bot. 100 mL, 473 mL. *Rx.*
Use: Anti-infective; erythromycin.

E.E.S. Granules. (Arbor Pharmaceuticals) Erythromycin ethylsuccinate (as base) 200 mg/5 mL when reconstituted. Sucrose. Cherry flavor. Pow. for Oral Susp. Bot. 100 mL, 200 mL. *Rx.*
Use: Anti-infective; erythromycin.

•**efalizumab.** (e-fa-li-ZOO-mab) USAN.
Use: Humanized anti-CD11a monoclonal antibody; immunosuppressive.

•**efaproxiral.** (ef-a-PROKS-ir-al) USAN.
Use: Investigational hemoglobin modifier.

efavirenz.
Use: Antiretroviral agent, nonnucleoside reverse transcriptase inhibitor.
See: Sustiva.
W/Emtricitabine, Tenofovir Disoproxil Fumarate.
See: Atripla.

Efedron Nasal. (Hyrex) Ephedrine hydrochloride 0.6%, chlorobutanol 0.5% w/ sodium chloride, menthol, and cinnamon oil in a water-soluble jelly base. Tube 20 g. *OTC.*
Use: Decongestant.

Efed-II. (Alto) Ephedrine sulfate 25 mg. Cap. Box 24s. *OTC.*
Use: Decongestant.

•**efegatran sulfate.** (EH-feh-GAT-ran) USAN.
Use: Antithrombotic.

E-Ferol. (Forest) **Spray:** Alpha tocopherol equivalent to 30 units vitamin E/ mL. Can 6 oz. **Vanishing Cream:** Alpha tocopherol. Jar 2 oz. *OTC.*
Use: Emollient.

E-Ferol Succinate. (Forest) d-alpha tocopherol acid succinate, equivalent to Vitamin E. **Cap. 100 units, 400 units:** Bot. 100s, 500s, 1000s. **Cap. 200 units:** Bot. 50s, 100s, 500s, 1000s. **Tab. 50 units:** Bot. 100s, 500s, 1000s. *OTC.*
Use: Vitamin supplement.

Effectin Tablets. (Sanofi-Synthelabo) Bitolterol mesylate. *Rx.*
Use: Bronchodilator.

Effective Strength Cough Formula. (Alra) Chlorpheniramine maleate 2 mg, dextromethorphan HBr 15 mg, alcohol 10%. Liq. Bot. 240 mL. *OTC.*
Use: Antihistamine, antitussive.

Effective Strength Cough w/Decongestant. (Alra) Pseudoephedrine hydrochloride 20 mg, dextromethorphan HBr 10 mg, alcohol 10%. Liq. Bot. 240 mL. *OTC.*
Use: Antitussive, decongestant.

Effer-K. (Nomax) Potassium (as bicarbonate and citrate). **10 mEq:** Sucralose (flavored only), dextrose, maltodextrin. Unflavored and cherry vanilla flavor. 30s. **20 mEq:** Sucralose (flavored only), dextrose, maltodextrin. Unflavored and orange cream flavor. 30s. **25 mEq:** Saccharin. Orange or lime flavors. 30s, 100s, 250s. Effervescent Tab. *Rx.*
Use: Electrolyte, potassium replacement product.

Effexor XR. (Wyeth Pharmaceuticals) Venlafaxine hydrochloride 37.5 mg, 75 mg, 150 mg. ER Cap. Bot. 15s, 30s, 90s, *Redipak* 100s. *Rx.*
Use: Antidepressant.

Effient. (Eli Lilly and Company) Prasugrel 5 mg, 10 mg. Film coated. Mannitol. Tab. 7s (5 mg only), 30s, UD 90s (10 mg only). *Rx.*
Use: Antiplatelet agent, aggregation inhibitor.

Efidac 24. (Hogil) Chlorpheniramine maleate 16 mg, mannitol. ER Tab. Pkg. 6s. *OTC.*
Use: Antihistamine, nonselective alkylamine.

Efidac 24 Chlorpheniramine. (Hogil) Chlorpheniramine maleate 16 mg. ER Tab. Pkg. 6s. *OTC.*
Use: Antihistamine.

•**efletirizine dihydrochloride.** (ef-le-TI-ra-zeen) USAN.
Use: Antihistaminic.

•**eflornithine hydrochloride.** (ee-FLAHR-nih-THEEN) USAN.
Use: Antineoplastic; antiprotozoal.
See: Ornidyl.
Vaniqa.

•**efungumab.** (ef-UN-gue-mab) USAN.
Use: Anti-infective.

•**egaptivon pegol.** (e-GAP-ti-von PEG-ol) USAN.
Use: Treatment of platelet dysfunction disorders.

•**eglumegad.** (e-GLUE-me-gad) USAN.

Use: Anti-anxiety agent; smoking cessation.

egraine. A protein binder from oats.

Egrifta. (EMD Serono) Tesamorelin 1 mg (equiv. to tesamorelin acetate 1.1 mg). Mannitol 50 mg. Preservative free. Inj., lyophilized Pow. for Soln. Single-use vial. *Rx.*
Use: Endocrine and metabolic agent, growth hormone–releasing factor.

•**egtazic acid.** (egg-TAY-zik) USAN.
Use: Pharmaceutic aid.

EHDP.
See: Etidronate Disodium.

8-MOP. (ICN Pharmaceuticals) Methoxsalen 10 mg. Cap. 50s. *Rx.*
Use: Pigmenting agent.

•**elacridar hydrochloride.** (eh-LACK-rih-dahr) USAN.
Use: Potentiation of chemotherapy in cancer (multidrug resistance inhibitor in cancer); antineoplastic (adjunct).

•**elacytarabine.** (EL-a-sye-TAYR-a-been) USAN.
Use: Antineoplastic.

•**elagolix.** (el-a-GOE-lix) USAN.
Use: Endometriosis.

•**elagolix sodium.** (el-a-GOE-lix) USAN.
Use: Endometriosis.

•**elantrine.** (EL-an-treen) USAN.
Use: Anticholinergic.

Elaprase. (Shire Human Genetic Therapies) Idursulfase 2 mg/mL. Sodium chloride 24 mg, sodium phosphate monobasic monohydrate 6.75 g, sodium phosphate dibasic heptahydrate 2.97 mg. Preservative free. Soln. for Inj. Singe-use vials. 5 mL. *Rx.*
Use: Hunter syndrome.

•**elarofiban.** (el-a-roe-FYE-ban) USAN.
Use: Thrombotic disorders.

•**elastofilcon A.** (ee-LASS-toe-FILL-kahn A) USAN.
Use: Contact lens material, hydrophilic.

elcatonin. (Innapharma, Inc.)
Use: Intrathecal treatment of intractable pain. [Orphan Drug]

•**eldacimibe.** (ell-DASS-ih-mibe) USAN.
Use: Antiatherosclerotic; antihyperlipidemic.

Eldec Kapseals. (Parke-Davis) Elemental iron 3.3 mg, Vitamins A 1667 units, E 10 mg, B_1 10 mg, B_2 0.9 mg, B_3 17 mg, B_5 10 mg, B_6 0.7 mg, B_{12} 2 mcg, C 67 mg, folic acid 0.3 mg, calcium iodine. Cap. Bot. 100s. *OTC.*
Use: Mineral, vitamin supplement.

Eldecort. (AstraZeneca) Hydrocortisone 2.5%, light mineral oil, propylene glycol, allantoin. Cream. Tube 15 g, 30 g.

Rx.
Use: Corticosteroid, topical.

Eldepryl. (Somerset) Selegiline hydrochloride 5 mg, lactose. Cap. Bot. 60s. *Rx.*
Use: Antiparkinsonian.

Eldercaps. (Merz) Vitamins A 4000 units, D 400 units, E 25 units, B_1 10 mg, B_2 5 mg, B_3 25 mg, B_5 10 mg, B_6 2 mg, C 200 mg, folic acid 1 mg, Zn 15.8 mg, Mg, Mn. Cap. Bot. 100s. *Rx.*
Use: Mineral, vitamin supplement.

Eldertonic. (Merz) Vitamins B_1 0.17 mg, B_2 0.19 mg, B_3 2.22 mg, B_5 1.11 mg, B_6 0.22 mg, B_{12} 0.67 mcg, alcohol 13.5%, Mg, Mn, zinc 1.7 mg/5 mL. Bot. 473 mL. *OTC.*
Use: Mineral, vitamin supplement.

Eldisine. (Eli Lilly)
See: Vindesine sulfate.

Eldo-B & C. (Canright) Vitamins C 250 mg, B_1 25 mg, B_2 10 mg, B_6 5 mg, niacinamide 150 mg, d-calcium pantothenate 20 mg. Tab. Bot. 100s, 1000s. *OTC.*
Use: Mineral, vitamin supplement.

Eldofe. (Canright) Ferrous fumarate 225 mg. Chew. Tab. Bot. 100s, 1000s. *OTC.*
Use: Mineral supplement.

Eldofe-C. (Canright) Ferrous fumarate 225 mg, ascorbic acid 50 mg. Tab. Bot. 100s. *OTC.*
Use: Mineral, vitamin supplement.

Eldopaque. (ICN) Hydroquinone 2% with sunblock. Cream. Tube. 14.2 g, 28.4 g. *OTC.*
Use: Dermatologic.

Eldopaque Forte. (ICN) Hydroquinone 4% in a sunblock base. Talc, light mineral oil, EDTA, sodium metabisulfite. Cream. Tube. 28.4 g. *Rx.*
Use: Dermatologic.

Eldoquin Forte. (ICN) Hydroquinone 4% in vanishing base. Light mineral oil, propylparaben, sodium metabisulfite. Cream. Tube. 28.4 g. *Rx.*
Use: Dermatologic.

Elecal. (Western Research) Calcium 250 mg, magnesium 15 mg. Tab. Bot. 1000s. *OTC.*
Use: Mineral supplement.

electrolyte and invert sugar solutions.
Use: Intravenous nutritional therapy, intravenous replenishment solution.
See: Invert Sugar-Electrolyte Solutions.

electrolyte concentrates, combined.
Use: Intravenous nutritional therapy, intravenous replenishment solution.
See: Hyperlyte CR.
Lypholyte.

Lypholyte-II.
Multilyte-40.
Multilyte-20.
Nutrilyte.
Nutrilyte II.
TPN Electrolytes.
TPN Electrolytes III.
TPN Electrolytes II.
electrolyte-dextrose solutions.
Use: Intravenous nutritional therapy, intravenous replenishment solution.
See: Dextrose-Electrolyte Solutions.
electrolyte No. 48 and dextrose 10%.
Use: Intravenous nutritional therapy, intravenous replenishment solution.
See: Dextrose 10% and Electrolyte No. 48.
electrolyte No. 48 injection.
Use: Intravenous nutritional therapy, intravenous replenishment solution.
See: Dextrose 5% and Electrolyte No. 48.
electrolyte No. 75 and 5% dextrose.
Use: Intravenous nutritional therapy, intravenous replenishment solution.
See: Dextrose 5% and Electrolyte No. 75.
electrolytes.
Use: Nutritional therapy.
See: Potassium Chloride.
Potassium Salts.
Sodium Chloride.
electrolyte solutions, combined.
Use: Intravenous nutritional therapy, intravenous replenishment solution.
See: Isolyte S pH 7.4.
Lactated Ringer's.
Normosol-M.
Normosol-R.
Normosol-R pH 7.4.
Plasma-Lyte A pH 7.4.
Plasma-Lyte 148.
Plasma-Lyte R.
Potassium Chloride in 0.9% Sodium Chloride.
Ringer's.
Elegen-G. (Grafton) Amitriptyline 10 mg, 25 mg, 50 mg. Tab. Bot. 100s, 1000s. *Rx.*
Use: Antidepressant, tricyclic.
elesclomol.
Use: Investigational antineoplastic agent.
Elestat. (Allergan) Epinastine hydrochloride 0.05%. Benzalkonium chloride 0.01%, EDTA. Soln., Ophthalmic. 8 mL, 15 mL. *Rx.*
Use: Ophthalmic antihistamine.
Elestrin. (Azur Pharma) Estradiol 0.06% (estradiol 0.52 mg per 0.87 g unit dose). EDTA. Top. Gel. 144 g metered-

dose pump. *Rx.*
Use: Sex hormone, estrogen.
•**eletriptan hydrobromide.** (all-eh-TRIP-tan HIGH-droe-BROE-mide)
Use: Antimigraine agent, serotonin 5-HT receptor agonist.
See: Relpax.
•**eleuthero.** *NF 29.*
Use: Dietary supplement.
Elevites. (Barth's) Vitamins A 6000 units, D 400 units, B_1 1.5 mg, B_2 3 mg, B_{12} 10 mcg, C 60 mg, niacin 1 mg, E 10 units, malt diastase 15 mg, iron 15 mg, calcium 381 mg, phosphorus 0.172 mg, citrus bioflavonoid complex 15 mg, rutin 15 mg, nucleic acid 3 mg, red bone marrow 30 mg, peppermint leaves 10 mg, wheat germ 30 mg. Tab. or Cap. Bot. 100s, 500s, 1000s. *Rx.*
Use: Mineral, vitamin supplement.
Elidel. (Novartis) Pimecrolimus 1%. Benzyl alcohol, cetyl alcohol, oleyl alcohol, stearyl alcohol. Cream. Tube. 30 g, 60 g, 100 g. *Rx.*
Use: Topical immunomodulator.
Eligard. (Sanofi-Synthelabo) Leuprolide acetate **Pow. for Inj., lyophilized:** 7.5 mg. Single-use kit w/ 2-syringe mixing system and 20-gauge, ½-inch needle. **Inj.:** 22.5 mg (3-month depot), 30 mg (4-month depot), 45 mg (6-month depot). Single-use kit with 2-syringe mixing system and 20-gauge, ½-inch needle (22.5 mg only). Single-use kit w/ 2-syringe mixing system and syringe containing *Atrigel* (30 mg, 45 mg only). *Rx.*
Use: Antineoplastic.
Eligard 22.5 mg. (Sanofi-Synthelabo) Leuprolide acetate 22.5 mg. Inj. Single-use kit w/2-syringe mixing system and 20-gauge, ½-inch needle. *Rx.*
Use: Antineoplastic.
•**eliglustat.** (EL-i-GLOO-stat) USAN.
Use: Treatment of lysosomal storage disorders.
•**eliglustat tartrate.** (EL-i-GLOO-stat) USAN.
Use: Treatment of lysosomal storage disorders.
Elimite. (Allergan) Permethrin 5%. Lanolin alcohols, coconut oil, mineral oil. Cream. Tube 60 g. *Rx.*
Use: Scabicide; pediculicide.
•**elinogrel.** (el-IN-oh-grel) USAN.
Use: Antithrombotic agent.
•**elinogrel potassium.** (el-IN-oh-grel) USAN.
Use: Antithrombotic agent.
Eliphos. (Hawthorn) Calcium acetate

667 mg. Elemental calcium 169 mg, PEG-8000. Tab. 200s. *Rx.*
Use: Mineral, calcium.

Elitek. (Sanofi-Synthelabo) Rasburicase 1.5 mg/vial (mannitol 10.6 mg), 7.5 mg (mannitol 53 mg). Pow. for Inj., lyophilized. Single-use vials with 1 mL amps of diluent (1.5 mg only). Single-use vials with 5 mL of diluent (7.5 mg only). *Rx.*
Use: Antimetabolite.

Elixicon. (Berlex) Theophylline 100 mg/5 mL with methylparabens and propylparabens. Susp. Bot. 237 mL. *Rx.*
Use: Bronchodilator.

Elixiral. (Vita Elixir) Phenobarbital 16.2 mg, hyoscyamine sulfate 0.1037 mg, atropine sulfate 0.194 mg, hyoscine HBr 0.0065 mg/5 mL. Liq. Pt, gal. *Rx.*
Use: Anticholinergic; antispasmodic; hypnotic; sedative.

Elixophyllin. (Caraco) Theophylline 80 mg/15 mL. Alcohol 20%. Saccharin. Mixed fruit flavor. Elix. 473 mL, 946 mL, 3,785 mL. *Rx.*
Use: Bronchodilator.

ElixSure Children's Congestion. (Taro Consumer) Pseudoephedrine 15 mg per 5 mL. Glycerin, propylparaben, sucralose. Bubble gum, cherry, and grape flavors. Syr. 118 mL. *OTC.*
Use: Nasal decongestant.

ElixSure Children's Cough. (Taro Consumer) Dextromethorphan hydrobromide 7.5 mg per 5 mL. Propylparaben, sorbitol, sucralose. Cherry and bubble gum flavors. Syrup. 118 mL. *OTC.*
Use: Nonnarcotic antitussive.

ElixSure Children's Fever Reducer/Pain Reliever. (Alterna) Acetaminophen 160 mg/5 mL. Butylparaben, sucralose. Cherry flavor. Oral Soln. 120 mL. *OTC.*
Use: Analgesic.

Ella. (Watson Pharma) Ulipristal acetate 30 mg. Lactose. Tab. UD 1s. *Rx.*
Use: Sex hormone, contraceptive hormone.

Ellence. (Pharmacia & Upjohn) Epirubicin hydrochloride 2 mg/mL. Preservative free. Inj. Soln. Single-use vial 25 mL, 100 mL. *Rx.*
Use: Antibiotic, anthracycline.

Ellesdine. (Janssen) Pipenperone. *Rx.*
Use: Anxiolytic.

Elliot's B Solution. (Orphan Medical)
Use: Acute lymphatic leukemias and acute lymphoblastic lymphomas. [Orphan Drug]

•**elm.** *USP 34.* Dried inner bark of *Ulmus rubra* Muhlenberg (*Ulmus fulva* Michaux).
Use: Pharmaceutic aid (suspending agent); demulcent.

Elmiron. (Janssen) Pentosan polysulfate sodium 100 mg. Cap. Bot. 100s. *Rx.*
Use: Relief of bladder pain associated with interstitial cystitis.

Elocon Cream. (Schering-Plough) **Cream:** Mometasone furoate 0.1%, hexylene glycol, phosphoric acid, propylene glycol stearate, stearyl alcohol, ceteareth-20, titanium dioxide, aluminum starch octenyl succinate, white wax, white petrolatum. Tube 15 g, 45 g. **Lot.:** Mometasone furoate 0.1%. Bot. 30 mL, 60 mL. **Oint.:** Mometasone furoate 0.1%, hexylene glycol, propylene glycol stearate, white wax, white petrolatum. Tube 15 g, 45 g. *Rx.*
Use: Corticosteroid, topical.

Elon Barrier Protectant. (Dartmouth) Paraffinum, liquidum, isopropyl palmitate, cetearyl alcohol, polyglyceryl-2, dipolyhydroxystearate, propylene glycol, cetearyl glucoside, C12-15 alkyl benzoate, stearic acid, bisabalol, petrolatum, phenoxyethanol, PEG-30 dipolyhydroxystearate, PEG-40 stearate, parabens, *Hamamelis virginiana*, denatured alcohol. Liq. 28 g. *OTC.*
Use: Protectant.

Elon Dual Defense Antifungal Formula. (Dartmouth) Undecylenic acid 25%. Alcohol. Soln. 30 mL. *OTC.*
Use: Antifungal agent.

•**elotuzumab.** (EL-oh-TOOZ-oo-mab) USAN.
Use: Antineoplastic.

Eloxatin. (Sanofi Aventis) Oxaliplatin 5 mg/mL. Preservative free. Inj.; Soln, Conc. Single-use vial. 10 mL, 20 mL, 40 mL. *Rx.*
Use: Antineoplastic agent, platinum coordination complex.

•**elpetrigine.** (EL-pe-TRI-gine) USAN.
Use: CNS agent.

Elphemet. (Canright) Phendimetrazine tartrate 35 mg. Tab. Bot. 100s, 1000s. *c-III.*
Use: Anorexiant.

Elprecal. (Canright) Vitamins A 5000 units, D 400 units, B_1 3 mg, B_2 2 mg, B_6 0.1 mg, B_{12} 1 mcg, C 50 mg, E 2 units, calcium pantothenate 2.5 mg, niacinamide 15 mg, inositol 5 mg, choline 5 mg, calcium lactate 500 mg, ferrous sulfate 50 mg, Cu 1 mg, Mn 1 mg, Mg 2 mg, K 2 mg, Zn 0.5 mg, sulfur 1 mg. Cap. Bot. 100s.

OTC.
Use: Mineral, vitamin supplement.
●**elsamitrucin.** (els-AM-ih-TRUE-sin)
USAN.
Use: Antineoplastic.
Elserpine. (Canright) Reserpine 0.25 mg.
Tab. Bot. 100s, 1000s. *Rx.*
Use: Antihypertensive.
●**elsibucol.** (el-si-BUE-kol) USAN.
Use: Immunosuppressive.
Elspar. (Merck) Asparaginase 10,000 IU.
Mannitol 80 mg. Preservative free. Pow.
for Inj., lyophilized. Vials. 10 mL. *Rx.*
Use: Antineoplastic.
Elta SilverGel. (Swiss-American) Silver
55 ppm. Gel. 30 mL, 45 mL, 236 mL,
473 mL. 2" × 2" and 4" × 4" dressings.
10s. *OTC.*
Use: Dermatological agent, wound
healing agent.
EL 10. (Elan) *Rx.*
Use: Antiviral; immunomodulator.
●**eltrombopag olamine.** (el-TROM-boe-
pag) USAN.
Use: Hematopoietic agent.
See: Promacta.
●**elucaine.** (eh-LOO-cane) USAN.
Use: Anticholinergic, gastric.
Elvanol. (DuPont) Polyvinyl alcohol. *Rx.*
Use: Pharmaceutical aid.
●**elvitegravir.** (EL-vi-TEG-ra-vir) USAN.
Use: Treatment of HIV infections.
●**elvucitabine.** (el-vue-SYE-ta-been)
USAN.
Use: Hepatitis B; HIV.
●**elzasonan citrate.** (el-za-SONE-an)
USAN.
Use: Antidepressant.
●**elzasonan hydrochloride.** (el-za-SONE-
an) USAN.
Use: Antidepressant.
Emadine. (Alcon) Emedastine difuma-
rate 0.05% (0.5 mg/mL), benzalkonium
chloride 0.01%. Ophth. Soln. Dispenser 5 mL. *Rx.*
Use: Antihistamine, ophthalmic.
embechine. Aliphatic chloroethylamine.
Use: Antineoplastic.
Embeda. (King Pharmaceuticals) Morphine sulfate/naltrexone hydrochloride
20 mg/0.8 mg, 30 mg/1.2 mg, 50 mg/
2 mg, 60 mg/2.4 mg, 80 mg/3.2 mg,
100 mg/4 mg. PEG, sugar spheres.
Gluten free. ER Cap. 100s. *c-II.*
Use: Opioid agonist-antagonist analgesic.
Embrex 600. (Andrx) Ca 240 mg, Fe (as
carbonyl iron) 90 mg, vitamin A
3500 units, D_3 400 units, E (dl-alpha
tocopherol acetate) 30 units, B_1 2 mg,

B_2 3 mg, B_6 3 mg, B_{12} 12 mg, C 60 mg,
folic acid 1 mg, Zn 20 mg, Cu, Mg, di-
octylsulfosuccinate sodium 50 mg.
Chew. Tab. Blister pack 35s, 91s. *Rx.*
Use: Vitamin, mineral supplement.
Emcodeine Tabs. (Major) Aspirin with
codeine as #2, #3, #4. Bot. 100s,
500s. *c-III.*
Use: Analgesic combination; narcotic.
Emcyt. (Pharmacia) Estramustine phosphate sodium equivalent to 140 mg
estramustine phosphate. Cap. Bot.
100s. *Rx.*
Use: Antineoplastic; hormone, alkylating agent.
Emdol. (Health for Life Brands) Salicylamide, para-aminobenzoic acid, sodium calcium succinate, vitamin D-
1250. Bot. 100s, 1000s. *OTC.*
Use: Analgesic combination.
●**emedastine difumarate.** (eh-meh-
DASS-teen die-FEW-mah-rate)
USP 34.
Use: Management of allergic conjunctivitis; antiasthmatic; antiallergic; antihistamine (H_1-receptor).
See: Emadine.
Emend. (Merck) **Cap.:** Aprepitant 40 mg,
80 mg, 125 mg. Sucrose. Bot. 30s (except 40 mg), UD 5s (40 mg only), UD
6s (except 40 mg), unit-of-use 1s
(40 mg only), unit-of-use tri-fold pack
containing one 125-mg capsule and two
80-mg capsules. **Inj., lyophilized Pow.
for Soln.:** Fosaprepitant 115 mg
(equiv. to fosaprepitant dimeglumine
188 mg), 150 mg (equiv. to fosaprepitant dimeglumine 245.3 mg). Lactose,
EDTA. Single-dose vials. 10 mL. *Rx.*
Use: Antiemetic/antivertigo agent.
●**emepepimut-S.** (EM-e-PEP-i-mut-es)
USAN.
Use: Antineoplastic.
emergency contraceptives.
See: Next Choice.
Plan B.
Plan B One.
emergency kits.
See: Cyanide Antidote Package.
Emeroid. (Delta Pharmaceutical Group)
Zinc oxide 5%, diperodon hydrochlo-
ride 0.25%, bismuth subcarbonate
0.2%, pyrilamine maleate 0.1%,
phenylephrine hydrochloride 0.25%, in
a petrolatum base containing cod liver
oil. Tube 1.25 oz. *OTC.*
Use: Anorectal preparation.
**Emerson 1% Sodium Fluoride Dental
Gel.** (Emerson) Red and plain. Bot.
2 oz. *Rx.*
Use: Dental caries agent.

emetics.
See: Ipecac.

•**emetine hydrochloride.** (EM-eh-teen)
USP 34.
Use: Antiamebic.

Emetrol. (Pharmacia) Dextrose 1.87 g,
fructose 1.87 g, phosphoric acid
21.5 mg, methylparaben, lemon, mint,
or cherry flavor. Soln. Bot. 118 mL,
236 mL, 473 mL. *OTC.*
Use: Antiemetic.

EMF. (Wesley Pharmacal) Alanine, arginine, aspartic acid, cysteine, glutamic
acid, glycine, histidine, hydroxylysine,
hydroxyproline, isoleucineline, leucine,
lysine, methionine, phenylalanine, proline, serine, threonine, tyrosine, valine,
protein 15 g, sorbitol, saccharin, cherry
flavor. Liq. Bot. Qt. *OTC.*
Use: Amino acid.

Emgel. (GlaxoSmithKline) Erythromycin
2%. Alcohol 77%. Gel. Tubes. 27 g,
50 g. *Rx.*
Use: Topical anti-infective, antibiotic.

EM-GG. (Econo Med Pharmaceuticals)
Guaifenesin 100 mg/5 mL. Bot. Pt. *OTC.*
Use: Expectorant.

•**emicerfont.** (em-eye-SER-font) USAN.
Use: CNS agent.

•**emilium tosylate.** (EE-MILL-ee-uhm
TAH-sill-ate) USAN.
Use: Cardiovascular agent (antiar-
rhythmic).

Emitrip Tabs. (Major) Amitriptyline. Tab.
10 mg, 25 mg: Bot. 100s, 250s, 1000s,
UD 100s. **50 mg:** Bot. 100s, 250s,
1000s, UD 100s. **75 mg:** Bot. 100s,
250s, UD 100s. **100 mg:** Bot. 100s,
250s, 1000s, UD 100s. **150 mg:** Bot.
100s, 250s. *Rx.*
Use: Antidepressant, tricyclic.

•**emivirine.** (e-mi-VYE-rene) USAN.
Use: HIV-1 infection.

EMLA. (Abraxis Pharm) Lidocaine 2.5%,
prilocaine 2.5%. Cream. Tube 5 g with
Tegaderm dressings, 30 g. *Rx.*
Use: Topical local anesthetic.

Emollia-Creme. (Gordon Laboratories)
Cetyl alcohol, lubricating oils in water-
soluble base. Jar 4 oz, 5 lb. *OTC.*
Use: Emollient.

Emollia-Lotion. (Gordon Laboratories)
Water-dispersable waxes, lubricating
bland oils in a water-soluble lotion base.
Bot. 1 oz, 4 oz, gal. *OTC.*
Use: Emollient.

Empirin Aspirin. (GlaxoSmithKline) Aspi-
rin 325 mg. Tab. Bot. 50s, 100s, 250s.
OTC.
Use: Analgesic.

Empirin w/Codeine. (GlaxoSmithKline)
Aspirin 325 mg with codeine phosphate
15 mg, 30 mg, 60 mg. Tab. **No. 2:** Codeine phosphate 15 mg. Bot. 100s.
No. 3: Codeine phosphate 30 mg. Bot.
100s, 500s, 1000s, *Dispenserpak* 25s.
No. 4: Codeine phosphate 60 mg. Bot.
100s, 500s, *Dispenserpak* 25s. *c-III.*
Use: Analgesic combination; narcotic.

Emsam. (Dey Labs) Selegiline hydrochloride 6 mg/24 hr (20 mg/20 cm^2),
9 mg/24 hr (30 mg/30 cm^2), 12 mg/
24 hr (40 mg/40 cm^2). Patch; transdermal system. Box. 30s. *Rx.*
Use: Antiparkinson agent.

•**emtricitabine.** (em-try-SIGH-tah-bean)
USAN.
Use: Antiviral.
See: Emtriva.
W/Efavirenz, Tenofovir Disoproxil Fumarate.
See: Atripla.
W/Tenofovir Disoproxil.
See: Truvada.

Emtriva. (Gilead) Emtricitabine. **Cap.:**
200 mg. 30s. **Oral Soln.:** 10 mg/mL.
Xylitol, parabens. Cotton-candy flavor.
170 mL with dosing cup. *Rx.*
Use: Antiviral.

Emulave. (Rydelle)
See: Aveenobar Oilated.

Emulsoil. (Paddock) Castor oil 95% w/
emulsifying agents, butylparaben.
Emulsion. Bot. 63 mL. *OTC.*
Use: Laxative.

E-Mycin. (Pharmacia) Erythromycin
250 mg, 333 mg. EC Tab. Bot. 40s
(250 mg only), 100s, 500s, UD 100s. *Rx.*
Use: Anti-infective; erythromycin.

Enablex. (Novartis) Darifenacin 7.5 mg,
15 mg. Lactose. ER Tab. 30s, 90s, UD
100s. *Rx.*
Use: Treatment of overactive bladder.

•**enadoline hydrochloride.** (en-AHD-ole-
en) USAN.
Use: Analgesic; severe head injury.
[Orphan Drug]

•**enalaprilat.** (EH-NAL-uh-prill-at) *USP 34.*
Use: Renin angiotensin system antagonist, angiotensin-converting enzyme
inhibitor.

enalaprilat. (Various Mfr.) Enalaprilat
1.25 mg/mL. Inj. Vial 1 mL, 2 mL. *Rx.*
Use: Renin angiotensin system antagonist, angiotensin-converting enzyme
inhibitor.

•**enalapril maleate.** (EH-NAL-uh-prill)
USP 34.
Use: Renin angiotensin system antagonist, angiotensin-converting enzyme
inhibitor.

See: Vasotec.
W/Diltiazem maleate.
See: Teczem.
W/Hydrochlorothiazide.
See: Enalapril Maleate/Hydrochlorothiazide.
Vaseretic.
enalapril maleate. (Various Mfr.) Enalapril maleate 2.5 mg, 5 mg, 10 mg, 20 mg. Tab. Bot. 100s, 1000s. *Rx.*
Use: Renin angiotensin system antagonist, angiotensin-converting enzyme inhibitor.
enalapril maleate/hydrochlorothiazide.
(Eon) Hydrochlorothiazide/enalapril maleate 12.5 mg/5 mg, 25 mg/10 mg. Lactose. Tab. Bot. 100s, 1000s. *Rx.*
Use: Antihypertensive.
•**enalkiren.** (en-al-KIE-ren) USAN.
Use: Antihypertensive.
•**enavatuzumab.** (EN-a-va-TOOZ-oo-mab) USAN.
Use: Antineoplastic.
•**enazadrem phosphate.** (eh-NAZZ-ah-drem) USAN.
Use: Antipsoriatic; inhibitor (5-lipoxygenase).
Enbrel. (Amgen) Etanercept. **Inj. Soln.:** 25 mg/0.5 mL, 50 mg/mL. Preservative free. Sucrose 1%, sodium chloride 100 mM, L-arginine hydrochloride 25 mM, sodium phosphate 25 mM. Single-use prefilled syringes. Single-use prefilled *Sure-Click* autoinjectors (50 mg/mL only). **Inj., Lyophilized, Pow. for Soln.:** 25 mg. Preservative free, mannitol 40 mg, sucrose 10 mg, tromethamine 1.2 mg. Multiple-use vials. Diluent contains benzyl alcohol. *Rx.*
Use: Immunologic agent, immunomodulator.
•**encaleret.** (en-KAL-er-et) USAN.
Use: Treatment of osteoporosis.
encapsulated porcine islet preparation.
Use: Type 1 diabetes. [Orphan Drug]
See: BetaRx.
Encare. (Thompson Medical) Nonoxynol 9 (2.27%). Supp. 12s. *OTC.*
Use: Vaginal contraceptive.
•**enciprazine hydrochloride.** (en-SIH-PRAH-zeen) USAN.
Use: Anxiolytic.
•**enclomiphene.** (en-KLOE-mih-FEEN) USAN. Formerly Cisclomiphene.
•**encyprate.** (en-SIGH-prate) USAN.
Use: Antidepressant.
EndaCof-AC. (Larken) Brompheniramine maleate 2 mg, codeine phosphate 10 mg per 5 mL. Alcohol free and sugar

free. Magnasweet, saccharin, sorbitol. Cotton candy flavor. Syr. 118 mL. *c-v.*
Use: Upper respiratory combination, antitussive combination.
EndaCof-C. (Larken) Codeine phosphate 10 mg, chlorpheniramine maleate 2 mg. Saccharin, sodium benzoate, sorbitol. Alcohol free, dye free, and sugar free. Cotton candy flavor. Liq. 473 mL. *c-v.*
Use: Upper respiratory combination, antitussive combination.
EndaCof-DC. (Larken) Codeine phosphate 10 mg, pseudoephedrine hydrochloride 30 mg. Saccharin, sodium benzoate, sorbitol. Alcohol free, dye free, and sugar free. Fruit gum flavor. Liq. 473 mL. *c-v.*
Use: Upper respiratory combination, antitussive combination.
Endacon. (Allegis) Dextromethorphan hydrobromide 20 mg, guaifenesin 100 mg, phenylephrine hydrochloride 10 mg. Benzoic acid, edetate disodium, glycerin, propylene glycol, sorbitol. Alcohol free and sugar free. Strawberry flavor. Liq. 473 mL. *Rx.*
Use: Upper respiratory combination, antitussive and expectorant combination.
Endafed. (Forest) Pseudoephedrine hydrochloride 120 mg, brompheniramine maleate 12 mg. SR Cap. Bot. 100s. *Rx.*
Use: Antihistamine, decongestant.
Endal CD. (Tiber Labs) Chlorpheniramine maleate 2 mg, codeine phosphate 7.5 mg, phenylephrine hydrochloride 5 mg per 5 mL. Glycerin, propylene glycol, saccharin, sorbitol. Alcohol free, dye free, and sugar free. Cherry flavor. Syr. 473 mL. *c-v.*
Use: Upper respiratory combination, antitussive combination.
EndaRoid. (Larken) Hydrocortisone acetate 1%, pramoxine hydrochloride 1%. Cream. 28 g. *Rx.*
Use: Anorectal preparation, steroid-containing product.
Endep. (Roche) Amitriptyline hydrochloride 10 mg, 25 mg, 50 mg, 75 mg, 100 mg, 150 mg. Tab. **10 mg:** Bot. 100s, *Tel-E-Dose* 100s. **25 mg:** Bot. 100s, 500s, *Tel-E-Dose* 100s. **50 mg:** Bot. 100s, 500s, *Tel-E-Dose* 100s. **75 mg:** Bot. 100s, *Tel-E-Dose* 100s. **100 mg:** Bot. 100s, *Tel-E-Dose* 100s. **150 mg:** Bot 100s. *Rx.*
Use: Antidepressant, tricyclic.
endobenziline bromide.
Use: Anticholinergic.
endocaine. Pyrrocaine.
Use: Anesthetic, local.

Endocet. (Endo) Oxycodone hydrochloride/acetaminophen 5 mg/325 mg, 7.5 mg/325 mg, 7.5 mg/500 mg, 10 mg/325 mg, 10 mg/650 mg. Tab. Bot. 100s, 500s. *c-II.*
Use: Analgesic; narcotic.

endocrine and metabolic agents.
See: Growth Hormone-Releasing Factors.
Vasopressin Receptor Antagonists.
Velaglucerase Alfa.

Endometrin. (Ferring Pharmaceuticals) Progesterone 100 mg. Vaginal Insert, Micronized. UD with 21 vaginal applicators. *Rx.*
Use: Sex hormone, progestin.

endomycin. A new antibiotic obtained from cultures of *Streptomyces endus.* Under study.

endophenolphthalein. (Roche) Diacetyl-dioxyphenylisatin-isacen-bisatin. *OTC.*
Use: Laxative.

endothelin receptor antagonists.
Use: Vasodilator.
See: Ambrisentan.
Bosentan.

•**endralazine mesylate.** (en-DRAL-ah-zeen MEH-sih-late) USAN.
Use: Antihypertensive.

•**endrysone.** (EN-drih-sone) USAN.
Use: Anti-inflammatory, topical; ophthalmic.

Enduron. (Abbott) Methyclothiazide 5 mg. Tab. Bot. 100s, 1000s, 5000s, *Abbo-Pac* 100s. *Rx.*
Use: Diuretic.

Enecat CT. (Mallinckrodt) Barium sulfate 5%. Simethicone, sorbitol. Conc. Susp. Bot. 110 mL w/480 mL bot. for dilution w/flexible tubing, clamp, enema tip. *Rx.*
Use: Radiopaque agent, GI contrast agent.

Enemark. (Lafayette) Rectal marker. 85% w/v liquid barium. Case of 12 kits.
Use: Rectal marker during radiation therapy.

enemas.
See: Fleet.
Fleet Bisacodyl.
Fleet Mineral Oil.
Therevac-SB.

Enerjets. (Chilton) Caffeine 75 mg, sugar, coffee, mocha mint, and butterscotch flavors. Loz. Pkg. 10s. *OTC.*
Use: CNS stimulant, analeptic.

Eneset 1. (Lafayette) Barium sulfate suspension 300 mL/air contrast examination kit. Unit-of-use kit. Case 12s.
Use: Radiopaque agent.

Eneset 600. (Lafayette) Barium sulfate suspension 600 mL/air contrast exami-

nation kit. Unit-of-use kit. Case 12s.
Use: Radiopaque agent.

Eneset 2. (Lafayette) Barium sulfate suspension 450 mL/contrast examination kit. Unit-of-use kit. Case 12s.
Use: Radiopaque agent.

EnfaCare. (Mead Johnson Nutritionals) Protein (nonfat milk, whey protein concentrate, taurine, L-carnitine) 2.8 g, carbohydrate (maltodextrin, lactose) 10.7 g, fat (high oleic sunflower oil, soy oil, medium chain triglycerides, coconut oil, monoglycerides and diglycerides, soy lecithin) 5.3 g/100 cal, vitamins A, B_1, B_2, B_3, B_5, B_6, B_{12}, C, D, E, K, folic acid 26 mcg/100 cal, biotin, choline, inositol, linoleic acid, Ca, chloride, Cu, Fe 1.8 mg, I, Mg, Mn, P, Se, Zn, Na 35 mg, K 105 mg/100 cal, 22 cal/oz. Liq. Pow. *Nursette* bot. 3 oz. (Liq. only). Can 14 oz (Pow. only). *OTC.*
Use: Enteral nutritional therapy.

Enfamil. (Mead Johnson Nutritionals) Vitamins A 2000 units, D 400 units, E 20 units, C 52 mg, B_1 0.5 mg, B_2 1 mg, B_6 0.4 mg, B_{12} 1.5 mcg, niacin 8 mg, Ca 440 mg, P 300 mg, folic acid 100 mcg, pantothenic acid 3 mg, inositol 30 mg, biotin 15 mcg, K-1 55 mcg, choline 100 mg, Fe 1.4 mg, K 650 mg, Cl 400 mg, Cu 0.6 mg, I 65 mcg, Na 175 mg, Mg 50 mg, Zn 5 mg, Mn 100 mg. Qt. Concentrated Liq. 13 fl oz, Instant Pow. lb. *OTC.*
Use: Nutritional supplement.

Enfamil Fer-In-Sol. (Mead Johnson Nutritionals) Iron 15 mg per mL. Alcohol, sorbitol, sugar. Drops. 50 mL. *OTC.*
Use: Trace element, iron-containing product.

Enfamil Human Milk Fortifier. (Mead Johnson Nutritionals) Whey protein, casein, corn syrup solids, lactose, protein 0.7 g, carbohydrate 2.7 g, fat 0.04 g, calories 14. Pow. Packet 0.95 g, Box 100s. *OTC.*
Use: Nutritional supplement.

Enfamil LactoFree LIPIL. (Mead Johnson Nutritionals) Protein 2.1 g, fat 5.3 g, carbohydrate 10.9 g, calories 100/serving, linoleic acid 860 mg, A 300 units, D 60 units, E 2 units, K 8 mcg, B_1 80 mcg, B_2 140 mcg, B_3 1000 mcg, B_5 500 mcg, B_6 60 mcg, B_{12} 0.3 mcg, folic acid 16 mcg, biotin 3 mcg, C 12 mg, choline 12 mg, inositol (liquid only) 17 mg, inositol (powder only) 6 mg, Ca 82 mg, P 55 mg, Mg 8 mg, Fe 1.8 mg, Zn 1 mg, Mn 15 mcg, Cu 75 mcg, I 15 mcg, Se 2.8 mcg, Na 30 mg, K 110 mg, Cl 67 mg. Liq., Liq.

Conc., Pow. Bot. 397 g (pow.), 384 mL (liq. conc.), 946 mL (liq.). *OTC.*
Use: Nutritional therapy, enteral.

Enfamil LIPIL with Iron. (Mead Johnson Nutritionals) Protein (reduced minerals, whey, nonfat milk, taurine) 2.1 g, fat (vegetable oil [palm olein, soy, coconut, and high-oleic sunflower oils], and less than 1% mortierella alpina oil, crypthecodinium cohnii oil, mono- and diglycerides, soy, lecithin) 5.3 g, carbohydrate (lactose) 10.9 g/100 cal, A, B_1, B_2, B_3, B_5, B_6, B_{12}, C, D, E, K, folic acid 16 mg/cal, biotin, chloride, choline, inositol, linoleic acid, Ca, Cu, Fe, I, Mg, Mn, P, Se, Zn, Na 27 mg and K 108 mg/100 cal. 20 cal/oz. **Liq.:** *Nursette* bottles 3 oz, 6 oz. **Liq. Conc.:** Cans 13 oz. **Pow.:** Cans. 12.9 oz, 25.7 oz. *OTC.*
Use: Nutritional therapy.

Enfamil Natalins Rx. (Mead Johnson Nutritionals) Ca 100 mg, Fe 27 mg, vitamin A 2000 units, D 200 units, E 7.5 units, B_1 0.75 mg, B_2 0.8 mg, B_3 8.5 mg, B_5 3.5 mg, B_6 2 mg, B_{12} 1.25 mcg, C 40 mg, folate 0.5 mg, biotin 15 mcg, Zn 12.5 mg, Cu, Mg. TR Tab. Bot. 200s. *Rx.*
Use: Vitamin, mineral supplement.

Enfamil Next Step. (Mead Johnson Nutritionals) Protein 17.3 g, carbohydrates 74 g, fat 33.3 g/liter, with appropriate vitamins and minerals. **Liq.:** 390 mL concentrate, 1 qt ready-to-use. **Pow.:** 360 g, 720 g. *OTC.*
Use: Nutritional supplement.

Enfamil Nursette. (Mead Johnson Nutritionals) Ready-to-feed *Enfamil* 20 kcal/fl oz, 4 fl oz, 6 fl oz and 8 fl oz. 4 bottles/sealed carton. W/Iron. Ready to use. Bot. 6 fl oz 4s, 24s. *OTC.*
Use: Nutritional supplement.

Enfamil Premature Formula. (Mead Johnson Nutritionals) Nonfat milk, whey protein concentrate, corn syrup solids, lactose, coconut oil, corn oil, medium chain triglycerides, soy lecithin. Protein 2.8 g, carbohydrate 10.7 g, fat 4.9 g, calories 96. Pow. *Nursettes* 120 mL. *OTC.*
Use: Nutritional supplement.

Enfamil Ready To Use. (Mead Johnson Nutritionals) Ready-to-use *Enfamil* infant formula 20 kcal/fl oz. Can 8 fl oz, 6-can pack; 32 fl oz, 6 cans per case. *OTC.*
Use: Nutritional supplement.

Enfamil with Iron. (Mead Johnson Nutritionals) Iron 12 mg. Qt. Pkg. Con. Liq. 13 fl oz. 24s. Pow. 1 lb. 6s. *OTC.*
Use: Nutritional supplement.

Enfamil with Iron Ready to Use. (Mead Johnson Nutritionals) Ready-to-use infant formula 20 kcal/fl oz. Can 8 fl oz, 6-can pack; 32 fl oz, 6 cans per case. *OTC.*
Use: Nutritional supplement.

•**enflurane.** (EN-flew-rane) *USP 34.*
Use: Anesthetic, inhalation.
See: Compound 347.
Ethrane.

enflurane. (Abbott) Enflurane 125 mL and 250 mL/Inhalation. *Rx.*
Use: Anesthetic, inhalation.

•**enfuvirtide.** (en-FYOO-veer-tide) USAN.
Use: Antiretroviral.
See: Fuzeon.

Engerix-B. (GlaxoSmithKline) Hepatitis B surface antigen 20 mcg/mL, thimerosal (mercury < 1 mcg), preservative free. Inj. Single-dose vial, prefilled syringe. *Rx.*
Use: Active immunization, viral vaccine.

•**englitazone sodium.** (EN-GLIH-tah-zone) USAN.
Use: Antidiabetic.

Enhancer. (Mallinckrodt) Barium sulfate 98%. Simethicone, sorbitol, sucrose, lemon-vanilla flavor. Susp. UD 312 g. *Rx.*
Use: Radiopaque agent, GI contrast agent.

•**enilconazole.** (EE-nill-KOE-nah-zole) USAN.
Use: Antifungal.

•**eniluracil.** (en-ill-YOUR-ah-sill) USAN.
Use: Potentiator of antineoplastic activity of fluorouracil (uracil reductase inhibitor); antineoplastic (adjunct).

•**enisoprost.** (en-EYE-so-prahst) USAN.
Use: Antiulcerative.

Enisyl. (Person and Covey) L-Lysine monohydrochloride 334 mg, 500 mg. Tab. Bot. 100s, 250s. *OTC.*
Use: Nutritional supplement.

Enjuvia. (Barr/Duramed) Synthetic conjugated estrogens, B, 0.3 mg, 0.45 mg, 0.625 mg, 1.25 mg. EDTA, PEG, lactose. Film-coated. Tab. 100s. *Rx.*
Use: Sex hormone, estrogen.

•**enlimomab.** (en-LIE-moe-mab) USAN.
Use: Anti-inflammatory; monoclonal antibody.

Enlive!. (Abbott) Protein (whey protein isolate) 10 g, carbohydrates (maltodextrin, sucrose) 65 g, fat 0 g, Na 65 mg, K 40 mg/L. H_2O 840 mOsm/kg, 1.25 cal/mL. Vitamin A, B_1, B_2, B_3, B_5, B_6, B_{12}, C, D, E, K, biotin, chlorine, Ca, Cl, Cu, Cr, Fe, I, Mg, Mo, P, Se, Zn. Gluten-free. Apple and peach flavors.

Liq. 240 mL. *OTC.*
Use: Enteral nutrition therapy.

•**enloplatin.** (en-LOW-PLAT-in) USAN.
Use: Antineoplastic.

Ennex Ointment. (Ennex) Aloe vera extract 37.5%. **Skin Oint.:** Zinc oxide 12.5%, coal tar 1.5%, alcohol 4.5%. Tube oz. **Hemorrhoidal Oint.:** Tube oz. *OTC.*
Use: Anti-inflammatory; astringent; antipruritic.

•**enofelast.** (EE-no-fell-ast) USAN.
Use: Antiasthmatic.

•**enokizumab.** (EN-oh-KIZ-oo-mab) USAN.
Use: Asthma.

•**enolicam sodium.** (ee-NO-lih-kam) USAN.
Use: Anti-inflammatory; antirheumatic.

Enovid-E 21. (Pharmacia) Norethynodrel 2.5 mg, mestranol 0.1 mg. Tab. Compack disp. 21s, 6 × 21. Refill 21s, 12 × 21. *Rx.*
Use: Estrogen, progestin combination.

Enovil. (Roberts) Amtriptyline hydrochloride 10 mg/mL. Vial 10 mL. *Rx.*
Use: Antidepressant.

•**enoxacin.** (en-OX-ah-SIN) USAN.
Use: Anti-infective.

•**enoxaparin sodium.** (ee-NOX-ah-PAR-in) USAN.
Use: Anticoagulant.
See: Lovenox.

enoxaparin sodium. (Sandoz) Enoxaparin sodium 30 mg per 0.3 mL, 40 mg per 0.4 mL, 60 mg per 0.6 mL, 80 mg per 0.8 mL, 100 mg/mL, 120 mg per 0.8 mL, 150 mg/mL. Preservative free. Inj., Soln. Single-dose prefilled syringe with 27-gauge × ½-inch needle. *Rx.*
Use: Anticoagulant, low molecular weight heparin.

•**enoximone.** (EN-ox-ih-MONE) USAN.
Use: Cardiovascular agent.

•**enpiroline phosphate.** (en-PIHR-oh-LEEN) USAN.
Use: Antimalarial.

Enpresse. (Barr) **Phase 1:** Levonorgestrel 0.05 mg, ethinyl estradiol 30 mcg. 6 tab. **Phase 2:** Levonorgestrel 0.075 mg, ethinyl estradiol 40 mcg. 5 tab. **Phase 3:** Levonorgestrel 0.125 mg, ethinyl estradiol 30 mcg. 10 tab. Lactose. Box. 28s with 7 inert tabs. *Rx.*
Use: Sex hormone, contraceptive hormone.

•**enprofylline.** (en-PRO-fih-lin) USAN.
Use: Bronchodilator.

•**enpromate.** (EN-pro-mate) USAN.
Use: Antineoplastic.

•**enprostil.** (en-PRAHS-till) USAN.
Use: Antisecretory; antiulcerative.

Enrich. (Ross) Liquid food with fiber providing complete, balanced nutrition as a full liquid diet, liquid supplement, or tube feeding. One serving provides 5 g dietary fiber. 1100 calories/L. 1530 calories provides 100% US RDA for vitamins and minerals. Ready-to-Use: Can 8 fl oz (vanilla, chocolate). *OTC.*
Use: Nutritional supplement, enteral.

Ensidon. (Novartis) Opipramol hydrochloride. *Rx.*
Use: Antidepressant.

•**ensituximab.** (EN-si-TUX-i-mab) USAN.
Use: Antineoplastic.

•**ensulizole.** (en-SUL-i-zole) *USP 34.* Formerly phenylbenzimidazole sulfonic acid.
Use: Sunscreen.

Ensure. (Ross) Liquid food providing 1.06 calories/mL. Can be used as a full liquid diet, liquid supplement or tube feeding. Two quarts (2000 calories) provides 100% US RDA for vitamins and minerals for adults and children over 4 yrs. **Ready-to-Use:** Bot. 8 fl oz (vanilla). Can 8 fl oz (chocolate, black walnut, coffee, strawberry, eggnog, vanilla), 32 fl oz (vanilla, chocolate). **Pow.:** Can 14 oz (400 g) (vanilla). *OTC.*
Use: Nutritional supplement.

Ensure High Protein. (Ross) Protein 50.4 g, carbohydrate 129.4 g, fat 25.2 g, < 21 mg cholesterol, Na 1218 mg, K 2100 mg, vitamin A 5250 units, D 420 units, E 47.5 units, K 84 mcg, C 125 mg, folic acid 420 mg, B_1 1.6 mg, B_2 1.8 mg, B_3 21 mg, B_5 10.5 mg, B_6 2.1 mg, B_{12} 6.3 mcg, biotin 315 mcg, Ca 1050 mg, Cl, P, Mg, I, Mn, Cu, Zn 24 mg, Fe 19 mg, Se, Cr, Mo, 945 calories per 237 mL. Liq. Bot. 237 mL. *OTC.*
Use: Nutritional supplement.

Ensure HN. (Ross) High nitrogen low residue liquid food providing complete, balanced nutrition as tube feeding or oral supplement with 1.06 calories/mL. Provides 100% US RDA for vitamins and minerals for adults and children over 4 yrs. 1400 calories (1321 mL). Ready-to-Use: Can 8 fl oz (vanilla). *OTC.*
Use: Nutritional supplement.

Ensure Osmolite. (Ross)
See: Osmolite.

Ensure Plus. (Ross) High-calorie liquid food w/caloric density of 1500 calories/L. Six servings (8 oz and 2130 calories each) provides 100% US RDA for

vitamins and minerals for adults and children. Ready-to-Use: Bot. 8 fl oz (vanilla). Can 8 fl oz (chocolate, vanilla, eggnog, coffee, strawberry). *OTC.*
Use: Nutritional supplement.

Ensure Plus HN. (Ross) High-calorie, high-nitrogen liquid food providing 1.5 calories/mL; 1420 calories provides 100% US RDA for vitamins and minerals for adults and children. Calorie/nitrogen ratio is 150:1. Can 8 fl oz (vanilla). *OTC.*
Use: Nutritional supplement.

Ensure Pudding. (Ross) Protein 6.8 g (nonfat milk), carbohydrate 34 g (sucrose, modified food starch), fat 9.7 g (partially hydrogenated soybean oil), vitamin A 850 units, D 68 units, E 7.7 units, K 12 mcg, C 15.4 mg, folic acid 68 mcg, B_1 0.25 mg, B_2 0.29 mg, B_3 3.4 mg, B_5 1.7 mg, B_6 0.34 mg, B_{12} 1.1 mcg, choline, biotin, Na 240 mg, K 330 mg, Cl 220 mg, Ca 200 mg, P, Mg, I, Mn, Cu, Zn 3.83 mg, Fe 3.06 mg, 250 calories/Can. Pudding. 150 g. *OTC.*
Use: Nutritional supplement.

Entab 650. (Merz) Aspirin 650 mg. EC tab. Bot. 100s. *OTC.*
Use: Analgesic.

•**entacapone.** (en-TACK-ah-pone) USAN.
Use: Antidyskinetic; antiparkinsonian.
See: Comtan.
W/Carbidopa and Levodopa.
See: Stalevo 50.
Stalevo 100.
Stalevo 150.
Stalevo 125.
Stalevo 75.
Stalevo 200.

•**entecavir.** (en-TE-ka-vihr) USAN.
Use: Antiviral.
See: Baraclude.

Entereg. (GlaxoSmithKline) Alvimopan 12 mg. PEG. Cap. UD 30s. *Rx.*
Use: Gastrointestinal agent.

Entero-Test. (HDC) Cap. to identify duodenal parasites; to diagnose and locate upper GI bleeding, pH disorders, achlorhydria, and esophageal reflux. Bot. 10s, 25s.
Use: Diagnostic aid.

Entero-Test Pediatric. (HDC) To identify duodenal parasites; to diagnose and locate upper GI bleeding, pH disorders, achlorhydria, and esophageal reflux. Cap. Bot. 10s, 25s.
Use: Diagnostic aid.

Enterotube. (Roche) Culture-identification method for Enterobacteriaceae ACA. Test kit 25s.
Use: Diagnostic aid.

Entero VU. (E-Z-EM) Barium sulfate 13%, 24%. Saccharin, sorbitol. Susp. 600 mL. *Rx.*
Use: GI contrast agent.

Entertainer's Secret. (KLI Corp.) Sodium carboxymethylcellulose, potassium chloride, dibasic sodium phosphate, aloe vera gel, glycerin, parabens. Soln. Bot. 60 mL spray. *OTC.*
Use: Saliva substitute.

Entex. (Andrx) Phenylephrine hydrochloride 7.5 mg, guaifenesin 100 mg per 5 mL. Alcohol, sugar, and dye free. Punch flavor. Liq. 15 mL, 473 mL. *Rx.*
Use: Upper respiratory combination, decongestant and expectorant combination.

Entex ER. (Andrx) Phenylephrine hydrochloride 10 mg, guaifenesin 300 mg. Maltodextrin, sucrose, parabens. ER Cap. 30s, 100s. *Rx.*
Use: Decongestant and expectorant.

Entex LA. (Andrx) Phenylephrine hydrochloride 30 mg, guaifenesin 800 mg (400 mg extended release/400 mg immediate release). Dye free. ER Cap. Bot. 100s. *Rx.*
Use: Upper respiratory combination, decongestant and expectorant combination.

Entex Liquid. (Andrx) Phenylephrine hydrochloride 7.5 mg, guaifenesin 100 mg/5 mL, alcohol and dye free, punch flavor. Liq. Bot. 15 mL, 473 mL. *Rx.*
Use: Upper respiratory combination, decongestant, expectorant.

Entex LQ. (WraSer) Guaifenesin 100 mg, phenylephrine hydrochloride 10 mg. Benzoic acid, edetate disodium, glycerin, propylene glycol, sorbitol. Alcohol free and sugar free. Strawberry flavor. Liq. 473 mL. *OTC.*
Use: Upper respiratory combination, decongestant and expectorant combination.

Entex PSE. (Athlon) Pseudoephedrine hydrochloride 50 mg, guaifenesin 525 mg. Dye free. ER Cap. Bot. 100s. *Rx.*
Use: Upper respiratory combination, decongestant, expectorant.

•**entinostat.** (en-tin-OH-stat) USAN.
Use: Antineoplastic agent.

Entocort EC. (Prometheus) Budesonide 3 mg (micronized), sugar spheres. Cap. Bot. 100s. *Rx.*
Use: Adrenocortical steroid, glucocorticoid.

Entolase HP. (Wyeth) Lipase 8000 units, protease 50,000 units, amylase

40,000 units. Cap. (enteric coated microbeads). Bot. 100s, 250s. *Rx.*
Use: Digestive enzyme.
Entrition Half Strength. (Biosearch Medical Products) Calcium and sodium caseinates, maltodextrin, corn oil, soy lecithin, monoglycerides and diglycerides, protein 17.5 g, carbohydrate 68 g, fat 17.5 g, Na 350 mg, K 600 mg, calories 0.5/mL, osmolarity 120 mOsm/kg, water, vitamins A, B_1, B_2, B_3, B_5, B_6, B_{12}, C, D, E, K, Ca, P, Mg, I, Fe, Zn, Mn, Cu, Cl, biotin, choline, folic acid. Pouch 1 liter. *OTC.*
Use: Nutritional supplement.
Entrition HN Entri-Pak. (Biosearch Medical Products) Sodium and calcium caseinates, soy protein isolate, maltodextrin, corn oil, soy lecithin, monoglycerides and diglycerides, vitamins A, B_1, B_2, B_3, B_5, B_6, B_{12}, C, D, E, K, folic acid, biotin, choline, Ca, Cl, Cu, Fe, I, Mg, Mn, P, Zn. Pouch 1 liter. *OTC.*
Use: Nutritional supplement.
Entrobag Set. (Lafayette) Enteroclysis set. Case 6 sets.
Use: Enteroclysis of the small intestine.
Entrobar. (Mallinckrodt) Barium sulfate 50%. Simethicone. Susp. Bot. 500 mL w/ or w/out kit. *Rx.*
Use: Radiopaque agent, GI contrast agent.
Entrokit. (Lafayette) Barium sulfate susp. (Entrobar), methylcellulose (Entrolcel). Case 4 kits.
Use: Radiopaque agent.
Entrolcel. (Lafayette) Methylcellulose 1.8% w/w concentrate for dilution at time of use. Bot. 500 mL, case 24 Bot.
Use: Diagnostic aid.
Entsol. (Kenwood Therapeutics) Sodium chloride. **Gel, intranasal:** Aloe, benzalkonium chloride, disodium EDTA, propylene glycol, glycerin, triethanolamine, vitamin E. Preservative free. 20 g. **Soln., intranasal:** Spray. 29.6 mL. *OTC.*
Use: Nasal decongestant.
•**entsufon sodium.** (ENT-sue-fahn) USAN.
Use: Detergent.
Entuss-D Junior. (Roberts) Pseudoephedrine hydrochloride 30 mg, hydrocodone bitartrate 2.5 mg, guaifenesin 100 mg w/alcohol 5%, saccharin, sorbitol, sucrose. Liq. Bot. 120 mL, pt. *c-III.*
Use: Antitussive, expectorant combination.
Entuss-D Liquid. (Roberts) Hydrocodone bitartrate 5 mg, pseudoephedrine 30 mg/5 mL. 473 mL. *c-III.*
Use: Antitussive, decongestant.

Entuss-D Tablets. (Roberts) Pseudoephedrine 30 mg, hydrocodone bitartrate 5 mg, guaifenesin 300 mg. Tab. Bot. 100s. *c-III.*
Use: Antitussive, decongestant, expectorant.
Enuclene. (Alcon) Tyloxapol 0.25%. Soln. *Drop-tainer* 15 mL. *OTC.*
Use: Artificial eye care.
Enulose. (Alra) Lactulose 10 g, (galactose < 1.6 g, lactose < 1.2 g, other sugars ≤ 1.2 g). Soln. Bot. 473 mL, 1.89 L. *Rx.*
Use: Laxative.
•**enviradene.** (en-VIE-rah-DEEN) USAN.
Use: Antiviral.
Enviro-Stress. (Vitaline) Vitamins B_1 50 mg, B_2 50 mg, B_3 100 mg, B_5 50 mg, B_6 50 mg, B_{12} 25 mcg, C 600 mg, E 30 units, folic acid 0.4 mg, zinc 30 mg, Mg, Se, PABA. SR Tab. Bot. 90s, 1000s. *OTC.*
Use: Mineral, vitamin supplement.
•**enviroxime.** (en-VIE-rox-eem) USAN.
Use: Antiviral.
Envisan Treatment Multipack. (Hoechst) Dextranomer with PEG 3000 and PEG 600. Paste 10 g packets with nylon net and semi-occlusive film. *OTC.*
Use: Dermatologic, wound therapy.
•**enzacamene.** (en-za-KAM-een) USAN.
Use: Sunscreen.
•**enzastaurin hydrochloride.** (en-za-STORE-in) USAN.
Use: Antineoplastic.
Enzest. (Barth's) Seven natural enzymes, calcium carbonate 250 mg. Tab. Bot. 100s, 250s, 500s. *OTC.*
Use: Digestive enzymes; antacid.
Enzobile Improved. (Roberts) Pancreatic enzyme concentrate 100 mg, ox bile extract 100 mg, cellulase 10 mg in inner core and pepsin 150 mg in outer layer. EC Tab. Bot. 100s. *Rx-OTC.*
Use: Digestive enzymes.
Enzone. (Forest) Hydrocortisone acetate 1%, pramoxine hydrochloride 1% in hydrophilic base w/stearic acid, aquaphor, isopropyl palmitate, polyoxyl 40, stearate, triethanolamine lauryl sulfate. Cream. Tube 30 g w/rectal applicator. *Rx.*
Use: Corticosteroid combination.
enzyme combinations, injectable.
Use: Collagenase Clostridium Histolyticum.
enzyme combinations, topical.
See: Accuzyme.
Ethezyme.
Ethezyme 830.

Gladase.
GranulDerm.
Granulex.
Panafil.
Papain.
Papain-Urea-Chlorophyllin.
Enzyme Formula #E-2. (Barth's) Amylase 30 mg, lipase 25 mg, bile salts 1 g, wilzyme 10 mg, pepsin 2 g, pancreatin 0.5 g, calcium carbonate 4 g. Tab. Bot. 100s, 250s. *Rx-OTC.*
Use: Digestive aid.
enzyme preparations.
See: Collagenase.
Enzyme Combinations, Injectable.
Enzyme Combinations, Topical.
enzymes.
See: Asparaginase.
Lactase.
Pegaspargase.
enzymes, digestive.
See: Pancreatin.
E-Oil. (Nature's Bounty) Vitamin E, corn oil, lemon oil, sesame oil, soybean oil, wheat germ oil. 74 mL. Oil, Top. *OTC.*
Use: Emollient.
E-Oil. (Nature's Bounty) Vitamin E 100 units (as d-alpha tocopheryl acetate) per 0.25 mL. Corn oil, lemon oil, sesame oil, soybean oil, wheat germ oil. 74 mL. *OTC.*
Use: Fat-soluble vitamin.
EPA. (NBTY) N-3 fat content (mg) EPA 180 mg, DHA 120 mg, vitamin E 1 units. Cap. Bot. 50s, 100s. *OTC.*
Use: Nutritional supplement.
•**eperezolid.** (eh-per-EH-zoe-lid) USAN.
Use: Anti-infective.
•**epetirimod.** (E-pe-TIR-i-mod) USAN.
Use: Antiviral; antineoplastic.
•**epetirimod esylate.** (E-pe-TIR-i-mod-ES-i-late) USAN.
Use: Antiviral, antineoplastic.
•**epetirimod esylate.** (E-pe-TIR-i-mod) USAN.
Use: Antiviral; antineoplastic.
•**ephedrine.** (eh-FED-rin) *USP 34.*
Tall Man: ePHEDrine
Use: Adrenergic (bronchodilator); vasopressor.
•**ephedrine hydrochloride.** (eh-FED-rin) *USP 34.*
Tall Man: ePHEDrine
Use: Bronchodilator.
W/Guaifenesin.
See: Broncholate.
Primatene.
ephedrine hydrochloride. (Various Mfr.)

Ephedrine hydrochloride. Cryst. Box 0.25 oz, 4 oz.
Use: Bronchodilator.
ephedrine hydrochloride nasal jelly.
See: Efedron Nasal.
•**ephedrine sulfate.** (eh-FED-rin) *USP 34.*
Tall Man: ePHEDrine
Use: Bronchodilator, sympathomimetic; vasopressor.
See: Pretz-D.
W/Guaifenesin.
See: Bronkaid Dual Action.
W/Zinc Oxide.
See: Pazo Hemorrhoid.
ephedrine sulfate. (Hospira) Ephedrine sulfate 50 mg/mL. Preservative free. Inj. Single-dose amps. 1 mL. *Rx.*
Use: Vasopressor.
ephedrine sulfate. (West-Ward) Ephedrine sulfate 25 mg. Cap. Bot. 100s. *OTC.*
Use: Bronchodilator, sympathomimetic; vasopressor.
ephedrine sulfate. (Various Mfr.) Ephedrine sulfate 50 mg/mL. Inj. Single-dose vials. *Rx.*
Use: Bronchodilator, sympathomimetic.
ephedrine sulfate and phenobarbital.
Use: Bronchodilator; hypnotic; sedative.
ephedrine tannate.
W/Carbetapentane Tannate, Chlorpheniramine Tannate, Phenylephrine Tannate.
See: Quad-Tuss Tannate Pediatric.
Rynatuss.
Rynatuss Pediatric.
Ephenyllin. (CMC) Theophylline 130 mg, ephedrine hydrochloride 24 mg, phenobarbital 8 mg. Tab. Bot. 100s, 500s, 1000s. *Rx.*
Use: Bronchodilator; decongestant; hypnotic; sedative.
Epi-C. (Mallinckrodt) Barium sulfate 150%. Simethicone, spearmint flavor. Susp. Bot. 450 mL. *Rx.*
Use: Radiopaque agent, GI contrast agent.
•**epicillin.** (EH-pih-SILL-in) USAN.
Use: Anti-infective.
EpiCream. (Promius Pharma) Disodium EDTA, glycerin, glyceryl stearate, hydroxypropyl bispalmitamide MEA (ceramide), PEG-100, petrolatum. Emulsion, Top. 90 g. *Rx.*
Use: Topical combination, miscellaneous.
epidermal growth factor (human). (Chiron Therapeutics)
Use: Accelerate corneal healing.
[Orphan Drug]
epidermal growth factor receptor inhibitors.
See: Erlotinib.

Epi-Derm Balm. (Pedinol Pharmacal) Methyl salicylate, menthol, propylene glycol, alcohol. Bot. Gal. *OTC.*
Use: Analgesic, topical.

Epidrin. (Excellium) Acetaminophen 325 mg, dichloralphenazone 100 mg, isometheptene mucate 65 mg. Cap. 100s. *c-IV.*
Use: Agent for migraine, migraine combination.

Epiduo. (Galderma) Adapalene 0.1%, benzoyl peroxide 2.5%. Edetate disodium, glycerin. Gel. 45 g. *Rx.*
Use: Acne product, combination.

Epifoam. (Alaven) Hydrocortisone acetate 1%, pramoxine hydrochloride 1% in base of propylene glycol, cetyl alcohol, PEG-100 stearate, glyceryl stearate, laureth-23, polyoxyl 40 stearate, methylparaben, propylparaben, trolamine, or hydrochloric acid to adjust pH, purified water, butane, propane inert propellant. Aerosol container 10 g. *Rx.*
Use: Corticosteroid, topical.

Epiform-HC. (Delta Pharmaceutical Group) Hydrocortisone 1%, iodohydroxyquin 3% in cream base. Tube 20 g. *Rx.*
Use: Antifungal; corticosteroid, topical.

Epilyt. (GlaxoSmithKline) Propylene glycol, glycerin, oleic acid, quaternium-26, lactic acid, BHT. Lotion. Bot. 118 mL. *OTC.*
Use: Emollient.

•**epimestrol.** (EH-pih-MESS-trole) USAN.
Use: Anterior pituitary activator.

epinastine hydrochloride. (epp-ih-NAS-teen) USAN.
Use: Ophthalmic antihistamine.
See: Elestat.

epinephran.
See: Epinephrine.

•**epinephrine.** (epp-ih-NEFF-rin) *USP 34.*
Tall Man: EPINEPHrine
Use: Bronchodilator, sympathomimetic, vasopressor.
See: Adrenalin Chloride
Epinephrine Mist.
EpiPen.
EpiPen Jr.
Nephron.
Primatene Mist.
S2.
W/Combinations.
See: Septocaine.
W/Lidocaine hydrochloride.
See: Ardecaine 1 w/epinephrine.
Ardecaine 2 w/epinephrine.
Lidocaine and Epinephrine.
Lidocaine Hydrochloride.
Lidocaine Hydrochloride and Epinephrine.

Lidosite Topical System.
Octocaine.
Xylocaine MPF.
Xylocaine w/epinephrine.

epinephrine. (Adamis Labs) Epinephrine 1:1,000 (0.3 mg per 0.3 mL) May contain sodium metabisulfite. Inj., Soln. Prefilled single-dose syringe. *Rx.*
Use: Vasopressor used in shock.

epinephrine. (Greenstone) Epinephrine 1:1,000 (0.15 mg per 0.15 mL). May contain chlorobutanol, sodium bisulfite. Inj., Soln. Single-dose injector. *Rx.*
Use: Vasopressor used in shock.

epinephrine. (Various Mfr.) Epinephrine 1:1000 (1 mg/mL as hydrochloride), 1:10,000 (0.1 mg/mL as hydrochloride). Soln. Inj. Amp. 1 mL (1:1000 only) (may contain sulfites). Prefilled syringe and vial. 10 mL (1:10,000 only) vial. 30 mL (1:1,000). *Rx.*
Use: Bronchodilator, sympathomimetic; vasopressor.

•**epinephrine bitartrate.** (epp-ih-NEFF-rin) *USP 34.*
Tall Man: EPINEPHrine
Use: Adrenergic, ophthalmic.

epinephrine borate.
Use: Adrenergic, ophthalmic.
See: Epinal.

epinephrine hydrochloride.
See: Adrenalin Cl.
EpiPen.
EpiPen Jr.
Vaponefrin.

epinephrine hydrochloride. (Ciba Vision) Epinephrine hydrochloride 0.1%. Soln. 1 mL Dropperettes (12s). *Rx.*
Use: Adrenergic, ophthalmic. Emergency kit, anaphylaxis.

Epinephrine Mist. (Various Mfr.) Epinephrine 0.22 mg/spray. May contain alcohol. Aer. 15 mL. *OTC.*
Use: Bronchodilator, sympathomimetic; vasopressor.

epinephrine, racemic.
See: AsthmaNefrin.

epinephrine-related compounds.
See: Sympathomimetic agents.

•**epinephryl borate ophthalmic solution.** (EPP-ih-NEFF-rill) *USP 34.*
Use: Adrenergic.

EpiPen. (Dey) Epinephrine 1:1,000 (0.3 mg per 0.3 mL). Latex free. Sodium metabisulfite Inj., Soln. Single-dose auto-injector. 0.3 mL (contains a total of epinephrine 2 mL). *Rx.*
Use: Emergency kit; vasopressor.

EpiPen Jr. (Dey) Epinephrine 1:2,000 (0.15 mg per 0.3 mL). Sodium meta-

bisulfite. Latex free. Inj., Soln. Single-dose autoinjector. 0.3 mL (contains a total of 2 mL of epinephrine injection solution). *Rx.*
Use: Emergency kit; vasopressor.

•**epipropidine.** (EPP-ih-PRO-pih-deen) USAN.
Use: Antineoplastic.

EpiQuin Micro. (SkinMedica) Hydroquinone 4%, vitamin A, E, and C, cetyl alcohol, benzyl alcohol, EDTA, glycerin, methylparaben, sodium metabisulfite. Cream. 30 g. *Rx.*
Use: Dermatologic, pigment agent.

epirenan.
See: Epinephrine.

•**epirizole.** (eh-PEER-IH-zole) USAN.
Use: Analgesic; anti-inflammatory.

•**epirubicin hydrochloride.** (EH-pih-ROO-bih-sin) USAN.
Use: Antineoplastic; antibiotic; anthracycline.
See: Ellence.

epirubicin hydrochloride. (Bedford) Epirubicin hydrochloride 2 mg/mL. Preservative free. Inj. Soln. Single-use vials. 25 mL, 100 mL. *Rx.*
Use: Antibiotic, anthracycline.

epirubicin hydrochloride. (Mayne) Epirubicin hydrochloride 50 mg, 200 mg. Lactose. Inj., Lyophilized, Pow. for Soln. Single-use vials. *Rx.*
Use: Antibiotic; anthracycline.

•**epitetracycline hydrochloride.** (epp-ih-TEH-trah-SIGH-kleen HIGH-droe-KLOR-ide) *USP 34.*
Use: Anti-infective.

•**epithiazide.** (EH-pih-THIGH-azz-ide) USAN.
Use: Antihypertensive; diuretic.

Epitol. (Teva) Carbamazepine 200 mg. Lactose. Tab. Bot. 100s. *Rx.*
Use: Anticonvulsant.

Epivir. (GlaxoSmithKline) Lamivudine. **Tab.:** 150 mg, 300 mg. PEG. Film-coated. Bot. 30s (300 mg only), 60s (150 mg only). **Oral Soln.:** 10 mg/mL. Parabens, sucrose 200 mg/mL, strawberry-banana flavor. Bot. 240 mL. *Rx.*
Use: Antiretroviral agent, nucleoside reverse transcriptase inhibitor.

Epivir-HBV. (GlaxoSmithKline) Lamivudine. **Tab.:** 100 mg. Film-coated. Bot. 60s. **Oral Soln.:** 5 mg/mL. Parabens, sucrose 200 mg/mL, parabens, strawberry-banana flavor. Bot. 240 mL. *Rx.*
Use: Antiretroviral agent, nucleoside reverse transcriptase inhibitor.

•**eplerenone.** (eh-PLER-en-ohn) USAN.
Use: Antihypertensive, aldosterone antagonist, renin angiotensin system antagonist.
See: Inspra.

eplerenone. (Apotex) Eplerenone 25 mg, 50 mg. Film coated. Tab. 30s, 90s, 500s (25 mg only), 1,000s, blister 100s. *Rx.*
Use: Renin angiotensin system antagonist, selective aldosterone receptor antagonist.

•**eplivanserin.** (EP-li-VAN-ser-in) USAN.
Use: Treatment of insomnia.

•**eplivanserin fumarate.** (EP-li-VAN-ser-in) USAN.
Use: Treatment of insomnia.

EPO.
See: Epogen.
Procrit.

•**epoetin alfa, recombinant.** (eh-POE-eh-tin) USAN.
Use: Antianemic; hematinic; hematopoietic.
See: Epogen.
Procrit.

•**epoetin beta.** (eh-POE-eh-tin) USAN.
Use: Hematopoietic; hematinic; antianemic. [Orphan Drug]

•**epoetin delta.** (eh-POE-eh-tin) USAN.
Use: Antianemic.

Epogen. (Amgen) Epoetin alfa (Erythropoietin; EPO) 2,000 units/mL, 3,000 units/mL, 4,000 units/mL, 10,000 units/mL, 20,000 units/mL, 40,000 units/mL. Preservative free w/2.5 mg albumin (human) per mL. Single-dose vials. 1 mL (except 20,000 units/mL and 40,000 units/mL). Multidose vials. 1 mL (20,000 units/mL, 40,000 units/mL only), 2 mL (10,000 units/mL only) (benzyl alcohol 1%). *Rx.*
Use: Hematopoietic.

•**epoprostenol.** (EH-poe-PROSTE-eh-nole) USAN. *Formerly Prostacyclin, PGI_2, Prostaglandin I_2, Prostaglandin X, PGX.*
Use: Peripheral vasodilator.

•**epoprostenol sodium.** (EH-poe-PROSTE-eh-nole) USAN.
Use: Peripheral vasodilator.
See: Flolan.

epoprostenol sodium. (Teva Parenteral Medicines) Epoprostenol sodium 0.5 mg, 1.5 mg. Sodium chloride. Inj., Pow. for Soln. Vials. 10 mL. *Rx.*
Use: Vasodilator, peripheral.

•**epostane.** (EH-poe-stain) USAN.
Use: Interceptive.

epothilones.
Use: Antimitotic agents.
See: Ixabepilone.

epoxytropine tropate methylbromide.
See: Methscopolamine Bromide.

●**epristeride.** (eh-PRISS-the-ride) USAN.
Use: Inhibitor (alpha reductase).

eprodisate.
Use: Investigational amyloid fibrinogenesis inhibitor.

Epromate. (Major) Aspirin 325 mg, meprobamate 200 mg Tab. Bot. 100s, 500s. *c-iv.*
Use: Analgesic; anxiolytic.

●**eprosartan.** (eh-pro-SAHR-tan) USAN.
Use: Antihypertensive.

eprosartan and hydrochlorothiazide.
Use: Antihypertensive.
See: Teveten HCT.

●**eprosartan mesylate.** (eh-pro-SAHR-tan) USAN.
Use: Antihypertensive.
See: Teveten.

●**eprosidate disodium.** (e-PROE-di-sate) USAN.
Use: Amyloidosis.

Epsal. (Press Chem. & Pharm Labs) Saturated soln. of Epsom salts 80% in ointment form. Jar 0.5 oz, 2 oz. *OTC.*
Use: Drawing ointment.

Epsivite Forte. (Standex) Vitamin E 1000 units. Cap. Bot. 100s. *OTC.*
Use: Vitamin supplement.

Epsivite 400. (Standex) Vitamin E 400 units. Cap. Bot. 100s. *OTC.*
Use: Vitamin supplement.

Epsivite 100. (Standex) Vitamin E 100 units. Cap. Bot. 100s. *OTC.*
Use: Vitamin supplement.

Epsivite 200. (Standex) Vitamin E 200 units. Cap. Bot. 100s. *OTC.*
Use: Vitamin supplement.

Epsom salt. (Various Mfr.) Magnesium sulfate. Gran. Bot. 120 g, 1 lb., 4 lb. *OTC.*
Use: Laxative.
See: Magnesium Sulfate.

eptifibatide.
Use: Antiplatelet agent, glycoprotein IIb/IIIa inhibitor.
See: Integrilin.

eptoin.
See: Phenytoin Sodium.

e.p.t. Stick Test. (Parke-Davis) Reagent in-home kit for urine testing. Pregnancy test. Kit 1s. *OTC.*
Use: Diagnostic aid.

Epulor. (VistaPharm) **Liq.:** Fat 31 g, carbohydrate 5 g, protein 4 g, calories 315/serving, biotin 100 mcg, B 50 mcg, Ca 333 mg, chloride 12 mg, Cr 40 mcg, Cu 200 mcg, folic acid 133 mcg, I 50 mcg, Fe 6 mg, Mg 133 mg, Mn 667 mcg, Mo 25 mcg, P 333 mg, K 35 mg, Se 23 mcg, Si 667 mcg, Na 7 mg, Sn 3 mcg, V 3 mcg, vitamin A 1667 units, B_1 500 mcg, B_2 567 mcg, B_3 7 mg, B_5 3 mg, B_6 667 mcg, B_{12} 2 mcg, Ni 2 mcg, C 20 mg, D 133 units, E 58 units, K 8 mcg, Zn 5 mg. Pkg. 24s. **Pow.:** Protein (milk protein, isoleucine, leucine, lysine, methionine/cystine, phenylalanine/tyrosine, threonine, trytophan, valine) 89 g, fat (soybean oil) 755 g/L, vitamin A, B_1, B_2, B_3, B_5, B_6, B_{12}, C, D, E, K, biotin, folate, B, Ca, chloride, Cr, Cu, Fe, I, Mg, Mn, Mo, Ni, P, Se, Si, Sn, V, Zn, lemon flavor, 7.1 cal/mL. Pouch. 1.5 oz. *OTC.*
Use: Nutritional therapy, enteral.

Epzicom. (GlaxoSmithKline) Abacavir (as sulfate) 600 mg/lamivudine 300 mg. Film-coated. Tab. 30s. *Rx.*
Use: Antiretroviral, nucleoside analog reverse transcriptase inhibitor combination.

Equagesic. (Leitner) Aspirin 325 mg, meprobamate 200 mg. Tab. 100s. *c-iv.*
Use: Nonnarcotic analgesic.

Equal. (Nutrasweet) Aspartame. **Packet:** 0.035 oz. (1 g). Box 50s, 100s, 200s. **Tab.:** Bot. 100s. *OTC.*
Use: Artificial sweetener.

Equalactin. (Numark) Calcium polycarbophil 625 mg (equivalent to 500 mg polycarbophil), citrus acid flavor. Chew. Tab. Bot. 24s, 48s. *OTC.*
Use: Antidiarrheal; laxative.

Equazine M. (Rugby) Aspirin 325 mg, meprobamate 200 mg, tartrazine. Tab. Bot. 100s, 500s. *c-iv.*
Use: Analgesic; anxiolytic.

Equetro. (Shire) Carbamazepine 100 mg, 200 mg, 300 mg. Lactose. ER Cap. 120s. *Rx.*
Use: Anticonvulsant.

Equilet. (Mission) Calcium carbonate 500 mg (elemental calcium 200 mg). Sodium up to 35 mg. Chew. Tab. 150s. *OTC.*
Use: Mineral supplement.

●**equilin.** (EK-wi-lin) *USP 34.*
Use: Estrogen.

Equipertine. (Sanofi-Synthelabo) Oxypertine. Cap. *Rx.*
Use: Anxiolytic.

Eradacil. (Sanofi-Synthelabo) Rosoxacin. Cap. *Rx.*
Use: Antigonococcal agent.

Eramycin. (Wesley) Erythromycin FC Tab. Bot. 100s, 500s. *Rx.*
Use: Anti-infective; erythromycin.

Eraxis. (Roerig) Anidulafungin 50 mg, 100 mg. Preservative free. Pow. for Inj.,

lyophilized. Single-use vial with diluent. *Rx.*
Use: Antifungal agent.

Erbitux. (Bristol-Myers Squibb) Cetuximab 2 mg/mL. Preservative-free. Sodium chloride 8.48 mg/mL, sodium phosphate dibasic heptahydrate 1.88 mg/mL, sodium phosphate monobasic monohydrate 0.41 mg/mL. Inj., Soln. Single-use vials. 50 mL, 100 mL. *Rx.*
Use: Monoclonal antibody.

•**erbulozole.** (ehr-BYOO-low-zole) USAN.
Use: Radiosensitizer; antineoplastic (adjunct).

Ergo Caff. (Rugby) Ergotamine tartrate 1 mg, caffeine 100 mg. Tab. Bot. 100s. *Rx.*
Use: Antimigraine.

•**ergocalciferol.** (ehr-go-kal-SIFF-eh-role) *USP 34. Formerly Oleovitamin D, Synthetic; Calciferol.*
Use: Treatment of refractory rickets; familial hypophosphatemia; hypoparathyroidism, vitamin (antirachitic).
See: Calciferol.
  Drisdol.
  Ergocalciferol Drops.

ergocalciferol. (Winthrop) Ergocalciferol 50,000 units. Parabens, soybean oil. Cap. 50s. *Rx.*
Use: Fat-soluble vitamin, vitamin D.

Ergocalciferol Drops. (County Line Pharmaceuticals) Ergocalciferol (D_2) 8,000 units/mL. Liq. 60 mL w/dropper in propylene glycol. *OTC.*
Use: Fat-soluble vitamin.

ergocornine. (Various Mfr.) Ergot alkaloid. *Rx.*
Use: Peripheral vascular disorders.

ergocristine. (Various Mfr.) Ergot alkaloid. *Rx.*
Use: Vascular disorders.

ergocryptine. (Various Mfr.) Ergot alkaloid. *Rx.*
Use: Peripheral vascular disorders.

•**ergoloid mesylates.** (err-GO-loyd) *USP 34. Formerly Dihydroergotoxine Mesylate; Dihydroergotoxine Methanesulfonate; Dihydrogenated Ergot Alkaloids, Hydrogenated Ergot Alkaloids.*
Use: Psychotherapeutic; cognition adjuvant.
See: Hydergine.

Ergomar. (Rosedale Therapeutics) Ergotamine tartrate 2 mg. Saccharin. Peppermint flavor. Sublingual Tab. Pkg. 20s. *Rx.*
Use: Antimigraine.

ergometrine maleate.
See: Ergonovine.

ergonovine. (Various Mfr.) Ergobasine, ergometrine, ergostetrine, ergotocine. *Rx.*
Use: Oxytocic.
See: Ergonovine Maleate.

•**ergonovine maleate.** (ehr-go-NO-veen) *USP 34.*
Use: Oxytocic.
See: Ergotrate.

ergosterol, activated, or irradiated.
See: Ergocalciferol.

ergostetrine.
See: Ergonovine.

Ergot Alkalside Dihydrogenated.
See: Ergoloid Mesylates.

ergotamine derivatives.
See: Dihydroergotamine Mesylate.
  Ergotamine Tartrate.

•**ergotamine tartrate.** (ehr-GOT-ah-mean) *USP 34.*
Use: Analgesic (specific in migraine).
See: Ergomar.
W/Bellafoline, caffeine, pentobarbital.
See: Cafergot P-B Suppositories.
W/Bellafoline, caffeine, pentobarbital sodium.
See: Cafergot P-B Tablets.
W/Caffeine.
See: Cafergot Tablets.
W/Combinations.
See: Folergot-DF.

ergotamine tartrate and caffeine. (West-Ward) Ergotamine tartrate 1 mg, caffeine 100 mg. Sugar. Tab. 30s, 100s, 500s. *Rx.*
Use: Migraine combination.

ergotamine tartrate and caffeine suppositories.
Use: Vascular headache; analgesic (specific in migraine).
See: Cafergot.

ergotamine tartrate and caffeine tablets.
Use: Vascular headache; analgesic (specific in migraine).

ergot, fluid extract. (Various Mfr.) Ergot 1 g/mL Bot. 4 oz, pt.

ergotocine.
See: Ergonovine.

Ergotrate. (HPS Rx Enterprises) Ergonovine maleate 0.2 mg. Mannitol. Tab. 100s, 500s, 1,000s. *Rx.*
Use: Oxytocic.

ergot-related products.
See: Cafergot.
  Cafergot P-B.
  D.H.E. 45.
  Ergonovine.
  Ergotamine.
  Ergotrate.
  Hydergine.

Hydro-Ergot.

• **eribulin mesylate.** (er-e-BU-lin) USAN.
Use: Halichondrin B analog.
See: Halaven.

eriodictyon. Flext., aromatic syrup.
Use: Pharmaceutic aid (flavor).

• **eritoran tetrasodium.** (ER-i-TORE-an)
USAN.
Use: Endotoxin antagonist.

• **erlotinib.** (er-LOE-tye-nib) USAN.
Use: Epidermal growth factor receptor
inhibitor.
See: Tarceva.

E•R•O Ear. (Scherer) Carbamide peroxide 6.5%, anhydrous glycerin. Drops.
15 mL. OTC.
Use: Otic preparation.

Errin. (Barr) Norethindrone 0.35 mg. Lactose. Tab. Box. 28s. Rx.
Use: Sex hormone, contraceptive hormone.

• **ersofermin.** (EER-so-FEER-min) USAN.
Use: Dermatologic, wound therapy.

Ertaczo. (OrthoNeutrogena) Sertaconazole nitrate 2%. Light mineral oil, methylparaben. Cream. Tubes. 15 g, 30 g.
Rx.
Use: Antifungal agent, topical anti-
infective.

• **ertapenem sodium.** (er-ta-PEN-em)
USAN.
Use: Antibacterial; carbapenem.
See: Invanz.

• **erteberel.** (er-TEB-er-el) USAN.
Use: Treatment of prostate diseases.

Ertine. (Health for Life Brands) Hexachlorophene, benzocaine, cod liver oil,
allantoin, boric acid, lanolin. Tube
1.5 oz. Rx.
Use: Burn and first aid remedy.

• **ertiprotafib.** (er-ti-PROE-ta-fib) USAN.
Use: Antidiabetic.

erwina L-asparaginase.
Use: Acute lymphocytic leukemia.
See: Erwinase.

Erwinase. (Porton Product Limited)
Erwinia L-asparaginase.
Use: Acute lymphocytic leukemia.
[Orphan Drug]

Erycette. (Ortho-McNeil) Erythromycin
2%. Pkg. 60 pledgets. Rx.
Use: Dermatologic, acne.

Eryderm 2%. (Abbott) Erythromycin 2%.
Alcohol 77%. Top. Soln. 60 mL with ap-
plicator. Rx.
Use: Topical anti-infective, antibiotic.

Erygel. (Merz Pharmaceuticals) Erythro-
mycin 2%. Alcohol 92%. Top. Gel. 30 g.
Rx.
Use: Topical anti-infective, antibiotic.

Erymax. (Allergan) Erythromycin 2%.
Soln. 59 mL, 118 mL. Rx.
Use: Dermatologic, acne.

Ery Pads. (Perrigo) Erythromycin 2%.
Alcohol 60.5%. Pledgets. 60s. Rx.
Use: Topical anti-infective, antibiotic.

Erypar. (Parke-Davis) Erythromycin stearate. Filmseal. **250 mg:** Bot. 100s,
500s. **500 mg:** Bot. 100s. Rx.
Use: Anti-infective; erythromycin.

EryPed Drops. (Abbott) Erythromycin
ethylsuccinate (as base) 100 mg/
2.5 mL. Sucrose, fruit flavor. Susp. Bot.
50 mL. Rx.
Use: Anti-infective; erythromycin.

EryPed 400. (Abbott) Erythromycin ethyl-
succinate (as base) 400 mg/5 mL when
reconstituted. Sucrose, banana flavor.
Pow. for Oral Susp. 100 mL, 200 mL,
UD 5 mL (100s). Rx.
Use: Anti-infective; erythromycin.

EryPed 200. (Abbott) Erythromycin ethyl-
succinate (as base) 200 mg/5 mL when
reconstituted. Sucrose, fruit flavor.
Pow. for Oral Susp. 100 mL, 200 mL.
Rx.
Use: Anti-infective; erythromycin.

Ery-Tab. (Arbor Pharmaceuticals)
Erythromycin enteric coated 250 mg,
333 mg, 500 mg. DR Tab. 100s, 500s
(except 500 mg). Rx.
Use: Anti-infective; erythromycin.

• **erythrityl tetranitrate, diluted.** (eh-
RITH-rih-till TEH-trah-NYE-trate)
USP 34. Formerly Erythrol Tetranitrate.
Use: Coronary vasodilator.
See: Cardilate.

erythrityl tetranitrate tablets. (Various
Mfr.) Erythritol, erythrol tetranitrate, ni-
troerythrite, tetranitrin, tetranitrol.
Use: Coronary vasodilator.

Erythrocin. (Abbott) Erythromycin stearate (as base) 250 mg, 500 mg. Film-
coated. Tab. Bot. 100s, 500s (250 mg
only). Rx.
Use: Anti-infective.

Erythrocin Lactobionate. (Hospira)
Erythromycin lactobionate (as base)
500 mg, 1 g. May contain benzyl alcohol. Pow. for Inj., lyophilized. Vials. Rx.
Use: Anti-infective; erythromycin.

• **erythromycin.** (eh-RITH-row-MY-sin)
USP 34.
Use: Anti-infective.
See: Akne-Mycin.
A/T/S.
Del-Mycin.
E-Base.
Emgel.
E-Mycin.
Eryderm 2%.

Erygel.
Erymax.
Ery Pads.
Erythromycin.
Erythromycin Base.
Erythromycin Ethylsuccinate.
Erythromycin Lactobionate.
Erythromycin Stearate.
Ilotycin.
Robimycin.
erythromycin. (Various Mfr.) Erythromycin base. **DR Cap.:** 250 mg. Enteric-coated pellets. 100s, 500s. **Gel:** 2%. Contains alcohol. 30 g, 60 g. **Oint.:** 0.5%. 3.5 g. **Top. Soln.:** 2%. Contains alcohol. 60 mL. *Rx.*
Use: Anti-infective.
•**erythromycin acistrate.** (eh-RITH-row-MY-sin ass-IH-strate) USAN.
Use: Anti-infective.
erythromycin base.
Use: Anti-infective.
See: Ery-Tab.
Erythromycin Filmtabs.
PCE Dispertab.
erythromycin-benzoyl peroxide. (Various Mfr.) Erythromycin 3%, benzoyl peroxide 5%. Gel. 23 g, 46 g. *Rx.*
Use: Anti-infective.
•**erythromycin estolate.** (eh-RITh-row-MY-sin ESS-toe-late) *USP 34. Formerly Erythromycin Propionate Lauryl Sulfate.*
Use: Anti-infective; erythromycin.
•**erythromycin ethylsuccinate.** (eh-RITH-row-MY-sin ETH-il-SUX-i-nate) *USP 34.*
Use: Anti-infective; erythromycin.
See: E.E.S.
EryPed.
erythromycin ethylsuccinate. (Various Mfr.) Erythromycin ethylsuccinate (as base). **Tab.:** 400 mg. Sugar. 100s, 500s. **Susp.:** 200 mg/5 mL, 400 mg/5 mL. Parabens, sucrose. 473 mL. *Rx.*
Use: Anti-infective.
•**erythromycin ethylsuccinate and sulfisoxazole acetyl for oral suspension.** (eh-RITH-row-MY-sin Eth-ill-SUCK-sih-nate and sull-fih-SOX-ah-zole ASS-eh-till) *USP 34.*
Use: Anti-infective.
erythromycin filmtabs. (Abbott) Erythromycin base 250 mg, 500 mg. Film-coated. Tab. 100s, 500s (250 mg only). *Rx.*
Use: Anti-infective; erythromycin.
erythromycin gel. (Glades) Erythromycin 2%, alcohol 95%. Gel. Tube 30 g, 60 g. *Rx.*
Use: Dermatologic, acne.

•**erythromycin gluceptate, sterile.** (eh-RITH-row-MY-sin glue-SEP-tate) *USP 34.*
Use: Anti-infective; erythromycin.
See: Ilotycin Gluceptate.
•**erythromycin lactobionate.** (eh-RITH-row-MY-sin lack-toe-BYE-oh-nate) *USP 34.*
Use: Anti-infective; erythromycin.
See: Erythrocin Lactobionate.
erythromycin ointment. (Various Mfr.) Erythromycin 0.5%. Oint. Tube 3.5 g. *Rx.*
Use: Anti-infective, topical.
erythromycin pledgets.
Use: Anti-infective; erythromycin.
Erythromycin Pledgets. (Glades) Erythromycin 2%, alcohol 68.5%. Pledgets. Bot. 60s. *Rx.*
Use: Anti-infective; erythromycin.
•**erythromycin propionate.** (eh-RITH-row-MY-sin) USAN.
Use: Anti-infective.
erythromycin propionate lauryl sulfate.
Use: Anti-infective; erythromycin.
See: Erythromycin Estolate.
Ilosone.
•**erythromycin salnacedin.** (eh-RITH-row-MY-sin sal-NAH-seh-din) USAN.
Use: Dermatologic, acne.
•**erythromycin stearate.** (eh-RITH-row-MY-sin STEE-ah-rate) *USP 34.*
Use: Anti-infective; erythromycin.
erythromycin sulfate.
Use: Anti-infective; erythromycin.
erythromycin tablets. (Various Mfr.) Erythromycin 100 mg, 250 mg. Tab. Bot. 25s (250 mg only,) 100s. *Rx.*
Use: Anti-infective.
erythromycin topical. (Various Mfr.) Erythromycin. **Gel:** 2%. Contains alcohol. Tube 30 g, 60 g. **Soln.:** 2%. Contains alcohol. Bot. 60 mL. *Rx.*
Use: Dermatologic, acne.
•**erythromycin 2-propionate dodecyl sulfate.** (e-RITH-roe-MYE-sin PROE-pee-oh-nate) *USP 34.* Erythromycin Estolate
Use: Anti-infective; erythromycin.
erythropoietin receptor activator, continuous.
Use: Investigational hematopoietic agent.
erythrosine sodium. *USP 34.*
Use: Diagnostic aid (dental disclosing agent).
•**escitalopram oxalate.** (ESS-sigh-TAL-oh-pram)
Use: Antidepressant, serotonin reuptake inhibitor.
See: Lexapro.

esclabron. Guaithylline.
Use: Antiasthmatic.

Eserdine Forte Tabs. (Major) Methyclothiazide, reserpine 0.5 mg. Bot. 100s. *Rx.*
Use: Antihypertensive; diuretic.

Eserdine Tabs. (Major) Methyclothiazide, reserpine 0.25 mg. Bot. 100s, 250s. *Rx.*
Use: Antihypertensive; diuretic.

Eserine. Physostigmine as alkaloid, salicylate or sulfate salt. *Rx.*
Use: Antiglaucoma.

Eserine Salicylate. (Alcon) Physostigmine 0.5%. Soln. 2 mL. *Rx.*
Use: Antiglaucoma.

Eserine Sulfate Sterile Ophthalmic Ointment. (Ciba Vision) Physostigmine sulfate 0.25%. Tube 3.5 g. *Rx.*
Use: Antiglaucoma.

Esgic. (Gilbert Laboratories.) Butalbital 50 mg, caffeine 40 mg, acetaminophen 325 mg. Cap. Tab. Bot. 100s. *Rx.*
Use: Analgesic; hypnotic; sedative.

Esgic-Plus. (Forest) Acetaminophen 500 mg, butalbital 50 mg, caffeine 40 mg. Tab. Bot. 100s, 500s. Cap. Bot. 20s, 100s, 500s. *Rx.*
Use: Analgesic; hypnotic; sedative.

Eskalith CR. (GlaxoSmithKline) Lithium carbonate 450 mg. CR Tab. Bot. 100s. *Rx.*
Use: Antipsychotic.

•**eslicarbazepine.** (ES-lye-kar-BAY-ze-peen) USAN.
Use: Anticonvulsant.

•**eslicarbazepine acetate.** (ES-lye-kar-BAY-ze-peen) USAN.
Use: Anticonvulsant.

•**esmirtazapine maleate.** (es-mir-TAZ-a-peen) USAN.
Use: Serotonin receptor antagonist.

•**esmolol hydrochloride.** (ESS-moe-lahl) USAN.
Use: Antiadrenergic/sympatholytic, beta-adrenergic blocking agent.
See: Brevibloc.
   Brevibloc Double Strength.

esmolol hydrochloride. (Baxter) Esmolol hydrochloride 10 mg/mL. Preservative free. Inj. Vials. 10 mL. *Rx.*
Use: Antiadrenergic/sympatholytic, beta-adrenergic blocking agent.

Esocor P. (Acella) Chlorpheniramine maleate 4 mg, dextromethorphan hydrobromide 30 mg, pseudoephedrine hydrochloride 30 mg per 5 mL. Benzoic acid, glycerin, parabens, propylene glycol, saccharin. Grape bubble gum flavor. Susp. 473 mL. *Rx.*
Use: Upper respiratory combination, antitussive combination.

•**esomeprazole magnesium.** (ES-oh-MEP-ra-zole) USAN.
Use: Proton pump inhibitor.
See: Nexium.
   Nexium I.V.

•**esomeprazole potassium.** (ES-oh-MEP-ra-zole) USAN.
Use: Gastrointestinal agent.

•**esomeprazole sodium.** (ES-oh-MEP-ra-zole) USAN.
Use: Proton pump inhibitor.

•**esorubicin hydrochloride.** (ESS-oh-ROO-bih-sin) USAN.
Use: Antineoplastic.

Esoterica Dry Skin Treatment Lotion. (GlaxoSmithKline) Bot. 13 fl oz. *OTC.*
Use: Emollient.

Esoterica Facial. (Medicis) Hydroquinone 2%, octyldimethyl PABA, benzophone, stearyl alcohol, sodium bisulfite, parabens, EDTA. Cream. Tube 90 g. *OTC.*
Use: Dermatologic.

Esoterica Regular. (Medicis) Hydroquinone 2%, light mineral oil, stearyl alcohol, parabens, sodium bisulfite, EDTA. Cream. Jar 90 g. *OTC.*
Use: Dermatologic.

Esoterica Sunscreen. (Medicis) Hydroquinone 2%, padimate O 3.3%, oxybenzone 2.5%, mineral oil, parabens, sodium bisulfite, EDTA. Cream. Jar 85 g. *OTC.*
Use: Dermatologic.

•**esoxybutynin chloride.** (es-ox-i-BUE-ti-nin) USAN.
Use: Antispasmodic, anticholinergic.

•**esproquin hydrochloride.** (ESS-pro-kwin) USAN.
Use: Adrenergic.

Essential-8. Liquid amino acid protein supplement.
Use: Protein supplement.
See: Vivonex, Standard.
   Vivonex T.E.N.

Essential ProPlus. (NutriSoy) Protein 16.3 g, fat 0.2 g, carbohydrates 6.4 g, Na 242.5 mg, K 112.5 mg, Ca 70 mg, Mg 31.3 mg, Fe 3 mg, P 187.5 mg, Cu 0.4 mg, Zn 0.5 mg, I 12.9 mcg, B_1 0.1 mg, B_3 0.2 mg, folic acid 0.1 mg/ 25 g. Pow. Cont. 2 lb. *OTC.*
Use: Nutritional supplement.

Essential Protein. (NutriSoy) Protein 16 g, fat 0.3 g, carbohydrates 5.6 g, sodium 5 mg, K 750 mg, Ca 97.5 mg, Mg 80 mg, Fe 2.5 mg, P 202.5 g, Cu 0.4 mg, Zn 0.8 mg, I 10 mcg, B_1 0.1 mg, B_3 0.2 mg, B_6 0.1 mg, folic acid

0.1 mg/25 g. Pow. Cont. 2 lb. *OTC.*
Use: Nutritional supplement.
•**estazolam.** (ess-TAZZ-OH-lam) USAN.
Use: Sedative/hypnotic, nonbarbiturate.
estazolam. (Zenith-Goldline) Estazolam
1 mg, 2 mg Tab. Bot. 30s, 100s, 500s,
1000s. *Rx.*
Use: Sedative/hypnotic, nonbarbiturate.
Ester-C Plus 500 mg Vitamin C. (Solgar) Vitamin C 500 mg, citrus bioflavonoids 25 mg, acerola 10 mg, rutin
5 mg, rose hips 10 mg, calcium 62 mg.
Sugar and sodium free. Cap. Bot.
250s. *OTC.*
Use: Water-soluble vitamin.
Ester-C Plus Multi-Mineral. (Solgar) Vitamin C 425 mg, citrus bioflavonoid
complex 50 mg, acerola 12.5 mg, rose
hips 12.5 mg, rutin 5 mg, calcium
25 mg, magnesium 13 mg, potassium
12.5 mg, zinc 2.5 mg. Sugar and sodium free. Cap. Bot. 60s, 90s. *OTC.*
Use: Water-soluble vitamin.
Ester-C Plus 1000 mg Vitamin C. (Solgar) Vitamin C 1000 mg, citrus bioflavonoid complex 200 mg, acerola 25 mg,
rutin 25 mg, rose hips 25 mg, calcium
125 mg. Sugar and sodium free. Tab.
Bot. 90s. *OTC.*
Use: Water-soluble vitamin.
esterified estrogens.
See: Estrogens, esterified.
**esterified estrogens and methyltestos-
terone.** (Various Mfr.) Esterified estro-
gens/methyltestosterone 1.25 mg/
2.5 mg. May contain lactose. Tab. 100s,
1000s. *Rx.*
Use: Sex hormone, estrogen and androgen combination.
**esterified estrogens and methyltestos-
terone H.S.** (Various Mfr.) Esterified
estrogens 0.625 mg/methyltestosterone
1.25 mg. May contain lactose. Tab.
100s, 1000s. *Rx.*
Use: Sex hormone, estrogen and androgen combination.
•**esterifilcon A.** (ess-TER-ih-FILL-kahn A)
USAN.
Use: Contact lens material, hydrophilic.
ester local anesthetics.
Use: Injectable local anesthetic, topical
local anesthetic.
See: Benzocaine.
Cocaine.
Chloroprocaine Hydrochloride.
Procaine Hydrochloride.
Tetracaine Hydrochloride.
Estilben.
See: Diethylstilbestrol Dipropionate.
Estinyl. (Schering-Plough) Ethinyl estra-
diol. **Tab., coated. 0.02 mg, 0.05 mg:**
Bot. 100s, 250s; **Tab. 0.5 mg:** Bot.
100s. *Rx.*
Use: Estrogen.
Estrace. (Warner Chilcott) Estradiol mi-
cronized 0.5 mg, 1 mg, 2 mg. Tartra-
zine (2 mg only), lactose. Tab. Bot.
100s, 500s (except 0.5 mg). *Rx.*
Use: Estrogen, sex hormone.
Estrace Vaginal. (Warner Chilcott) Estra-
diol 0.1 mg/g in a nonliquefying base.
EDTA, methylparaben, steryl alcohol.
Cream. Tube w/calibrated applicator
42.5 g. *Rx.*
Use: Estrogen, sex hormone.
Estracon. (Freeport) Conjugated estro-
gens 1.25 mg. Tab. Bot. 1000s. *Rx.*
Use: Estrogen.
Estraderm. (Novartis) Estradiol 4 mg
(0.05 mg/day), 8 mg (0.1 mg/day). Cal-
endar packs of 8 and 24 systems. *Rx.*
Use: Estrogen, sex hormone.
•**estradiol.** (ESS-truh-DIE-ole) *USP 34.*
The form now known to be physiologi-
cally active is the β form rather than
the α.
Use: Estrogen, sex hormone.
See: Alora.
Climara.
Divigel.
Elestrin.
Estrace.
Estraderm.
Estring.
EstroGel.
Evamist.
FemPatch.
Femtrace.
Gynodiol.
Vivelle.
Vivelle-Dot.
W/Drospirenone.
See: Angeliq.
W/Estrone, estriol.
See: Sanestro.
W/Levonorgestrel.
See: ClimaraPro.
W/Norethindrone acetate.
See: Activella.
CombiPatch.
Mimvey.
W/Norgestimate.
See: Prefest.
W/Testosterone and chlorobutanol in cot-
tonseed oil.
See: Depo-Testadiol.
Estraderm.
estradiol. (Various Mfr.) Micronized
estradiol 0.5 mg, 1 mg, 2 mg. May con-
tain lactose. Tab. Bot. 100s, 500s (ex-
cept 0.5 mg). *Rx.*
Use: Estrogen, sex hormone.

•**estradiol acetate.** (ESS-trah-DIE-ole)
USAN.
Use: Estrogen.

estradiol benzoate.
Use: Estrogen.

•**estradiol cypionate.** (ESS-trah-DIE-ole
SIP-ee-oh-nate) *USP 34.*
Use: Estrogen, sex hormone.
See: Depo-Estradiol.
W/Chlorobutanol, cottonseed oil
See: depGynogen.
DepoGen.
W/Testosterone cypionate.
See: Menoject, L.A.
W/Testosterone cypionate, chlorobutanol.
See: Depo-Testadiol.

estradiol cypionate. (Various Mfr.) Estradiol cypionate 5 mg/mL, cottonseed oil
w/chlorobutanol. Inj. Vial. 10 mL. *Rx.*
Use: Estrogen.

estradiol dipropionate.
Use: Estrogen.

•**estradiol enanthate.** (ESS-trah-DIE-ole
eh-NAN-thate) USAN.
Use: Estrogen.

estradiol, ethinyl.
See: Ethinyl Estradiol.

estradiol hemihydrate.
Use: Estrogen.
See: Estrasorb.
See: Vagifem.

estradiol, micronized.
Use: Estrogen.
See: Estrace.
Gynodiol.

estradiol/norethindrone acetate.
(Breckenridge) Estradiol 1 mg, norethindrone acetate 0.5 mg. May contain lactose. Tab. Blister packs. 28s. *Rx.*
Use: Sex hormone.

estradiol, oral. (Teva) Micronized estradiol 0.5 mg, 1 mg, 2 mg. Tab. Bot.
100s. *Rx.*
Use: Estrogen.

estradiol, topical emulsion.
Use: Sex hormone.

estradiol transdermal system.
Use: Estrogen, sex hormone.
See: Alora.
Climara.
Esclim.
Estraderm.
Menostar.
Vivelle.
Vivelle-Dot.
W/Levonorgestrel.
See: ClimaraPro.
W/Norethindrone Acetate.
See: CombiPatch.

estradiol transdermal system. (Mylan)
Estradiol 0.97 mg (0.025 mg/day),

1.46 mg (0.0375 mg/day), 1.94 mg
(0.05 mg/day), 2.33 mg (0.06 mg/day),
2.91 mg (0.075 mg/day), 3.88 mg
(0.1 mg/day). Patch. 4s. *Rx.*
Use: Estrogen, sex hormone.

•**estradiol undecylate.** (ESS-trah-DIE-ole
UHN-DEH-sill-ate) USAN.
See: Delestrec.

estradiol vaginal cream.
Use: Estrogen.

•**estradiol valerate.** (ESS-trah-DIE-ole
VAL-eh-rate) *USP 34.*
Use: Estrogen.
See: Ardefem 10, 20.
Delestrogen.
Duragen.
Estra-L.
Valergen.
W/Testosterone enanthate.
See: Ardiol 90/4, 180/8.
Delatestadiol.
Estra-Testrin.
Teev.
Tesogen LA.
Valertest.

estradiol valerate. (Sandoz) Estradiol
valerate 10 mg/mL, 20 mg/mL, 40 mg/
mL. Sesame oil (10 mg/mL only); benzyl alcohol, benzyl benzoate, castor oil
(20 mg, 40 mg only). Inj. Multidose vial.
5 mL. *Rx.*
Use: Estrogen, sex hormone.

estradiol valerate. (Various Mfr.) Estra-
diol valerate 20 mg/mL, 40 mg/mL. Inj.
Vial 10 mL. 40 mg/mL. Vial 10 mL. *Rx.*
Use: Estrogen.

Estra-L. (Taylor Pharmaceuticals) Estradiol valerate in oil 40 mg/mL. Vial
10 mL. *Rx.*
Use: Estrogen.

•**estramustine.** (ESS-truh-muss-TEEN)
USAN.
Use: Antineoplastic.

•**estramustine phosphate sodium.**
(ESS-truh-muss-TEEN) USAN.
Use: Antineoplastic, alkylating agent.
See: Emcyt.

Estrasorb. (Graceway) Estradiol hemihy-
drate 2.5 mg/g. Soybean oil, ethanol.
Top. Emulsion. 1.74 g pouches. *Rx.*
Use: Sex hormone; estrogen.

Estratab. (Solvay) Esterified estrogens
0.3 mg, 0.625 mg, 2.5 mg. Tab. Bot.
100s, 1000s (0.625 mg only). *Rx.*
Use: Estrogen.

Estratest. (Solvay) Esterified estrogens
1.25 mg, methyltestosterone 2.5 mg.
Lactose, sucrose, parabens. Sugar
coated. Tab. Bot. 100s, 1000s. *Rx.*
Use: Sex hormone, estrogen/androgen
combination.

Estratest H.S. (Solvay) Esterified estrogens 0.625 mg, methyltestosterone 1.25 mg. Lactose, sucrose, parabens. Sugar coated. Tab. Bot. 100s. *Rx.*
Use: Sex hormone, estrogen/androgen combination.

•**estrazinol hydrobromide.** (ESS-trazz-ih-nahl) USAN.
Use: Estrogen.

estrin.
See: Estrone.

Estrinex. (Pharmacia)
See: Toremifene.

Estring. (Pharmacia) Estradiol 2 mg. Releases estradiol 7.5 mcg/24 hours over 90 days. Vaginal ring. Single packs. *Rx.*
Use: Estrogen, sex hormone.

•**estriol.** (ESS-tree-ole) *USP 34.*
Use: Estrogen.

Estrobene DP.
See: Diethylstilbestrol Dipropionate.

Estrofem. (Taylor Pharmaceuticals) Estradiol cypionate 5 mg/mL in oil. Inj. Vial 10 mL.
Use: Estrogen.

•**estrofurate.** (ESS-troe-FYOOR-ate) USAN.
Use: Estrogen.

Estrogel. (Ascend) Estradiol 0.06% (estradiol 0.75 mg/1.25 g unit dose). Alcohol. Gel. Pump. 93 g. Tube. 80 g. *Rx.*
Use: Sex hormone, estrogen.

estrogen and androgen combinations.
Use: Sex hormone.
See: Covaryx.
Covaryx H.S.
Estratest.
Estratest H.S.

estrogen-androgen therapy.
See: Androgen-estrogen therapy.

estrogenic substance aqueous.
(Various Mfr.) Estrogenic substance or estrogens (mainly estrone) 2 mg/mL. Inj. Vial 10 mL, 30 mL. *Rx.*
Use: Estrogen.

estrogenic substances, conjugated.
(Water-soluble) A mixture containing the sodium salts of the sulfate esters of the estrogenic substances, principally estrone and equilin that are of the type excreted by pregnant mares. *Rx.*
See: Ces.
Estroquin.
Prelestrin.
Premarin.
W/Meprobamate.
See: PMB 400.
PMB 200.

estrogenic substances in aqueous suspension. (Wyeth) Sterile estrone suspension 2 mg/mL. Vial 10 mL. *Rx.*
Use: Estrogen.

estrogenic substances mixed. May be a crystalline or an amorphous mixture of the naturally occurring estrogens obtained from the urine of pregnant mares. **Aqueous Susp.:** Inj. **Cap.:** W/Androgen therapy, vitamins, iron, d-desoxyephedrine hydrochloride.

estrogen/nitrogen mustard.
Use: Alkylating agent.
See: Estramustine Phosphate Sodium.

estrogens.
Use: Sex hormones.
See: Conjugated Estrogens.
Esterified Estrogens.
Estradiol.
Estradiol Cypionate.
Estradiol Topical Emulsion.
Estradiol Transdermal System.
Estradiol Valerate in Oil.
Estropipate.
Estrogens, Miscellaneous, Vaginal.
Synthetic Conjugated Estrogens, A.
Synthetic Conjugated Estrogens, B.
Topical Estrogens, Miscellaneous.

estrogens and progestins combined.
Use: Sex hormone.
See: Activella.
Alesse.
Angeliq.
Apri.
Aviane.
Brevicon.
ClimaraPro.
CombiPatch.
Desogen.
Estrostep Fe.
Femhrt.
Jenest-28.
Levora.
Loestrin Fe 1/20.
Loestrin Fe 1.5/30.
Loestrin 21 1/20.
Loestrin 21 1.5/30.
Lo/Ovral.
Low-Ogestrel.
Microgestin Fe 1/20.
Microgestin Fe 1.5/30.
Mircette.
Modicon.
MonoNessa.
Necon 1/50.
Necon 1/35.
Necon 10/11.
Necon 0.5/35.
Nordette.
Norinyl 1 + 50.
Norinyl 1 + 35.

Nortrel 1/35.
Nortrel 0.5/35.
Ogestrel.
Ortho-Cept.
Ortho-Cyclen.
Ortho-Novum 1/50.
Ortho-Novum 1/35.
Ortho-Novum 7/7/7.
Ortho-Novum 10/11.
Ortho Tri-Cyclen.
Ovcon-50.
Ovcon-35.
Ovral-28.
Prefest.
Premphase.
Prempro.
Tri-Norinyl.
Triphasil.
Trivora-28.
Yasmin.
Yaz.
Zovia 1/50E.
Zovia 1/35E.

•**estrogens, conjugated.** (ESS-truh-janz
KAHN-juh-gay-tuhd) *USP 34.*
Use: Estrogen.
See: Conest.
Ganeake.
PMB.
Premarin.
Premarin Intravenous.
W/Meprobamate.
See: PMB.

**estrogens, conjugated and medroxy-
progesterone acetate.**
Use: Sex hormone.
See: Premphase.
Prempro.

estrogens equine.
See: Estrogen.

•**estrogens, esterified.** (ESS-troe-jenz,
ess-TER-ih-fide) *USP 34.*
Use: Estrogen.
See: Estratab.
Menest.
W/Methyltestosterone.
See: Covaryx.
Covaryx H.S.

estrogens, esterified and androgens.
Use: Estrogen, androgen supplement.
See: Covaryx.
Covaryx H.S.
Estratab.
Estratest.
Estratest H.S.
Menest.

estrogens, miscellaneous topical.
Use: Sex hormone, estrogen.
See: Divigel.
Elestrin.
Estrasorb.

Estrogel.
Evamist.

estrogens, miscellaneous, vaginal.
Use: Estrogen, sex hormone.
See: Estrace Vaginal.
Estring.
Femring.
Premarin Vaginal.
Vagifem.

estrogens, natural.
Use: Estrogen.
See: Depogen.
Estradiol.
Estrogenic Substance.
Estrone.
PMB.
Premarin.

estrogens, synthetic conjugated A.
See: Cenestin.

estrogens, synthetic conjugated B.
See: Enjuvia.

Estrogestin A. (Harvey) Estrogenic substance 1 mg, progesterone 10 mg/mL
in peanut oil. Vial 10 mL. *Rx.*
Use: Estrogen, progestin combination.

Estrogestin C. (Harvey) Estrogenic substance 1 mg, progesterone 12.5 mg/mL
in peanut oil. Vial 10 mL. *Rx.*
Use: Estrogen, progestin combination.

•**estrone.** (ESS-trone) *USP 34.*
Use: Estrogen.
See: Bestrone.
Estrogenic Substances in Aqueous
Susp.
Foygen.
Kestrone 5.
Par-Supp.
Propagon-S.
W/Estrogens.
See: Estrogenic Substances.
W/Progesterone.
See: Duovin-S.
W/Testosterone.
See: Andesterone.

estrone aqueous. (Various Mfr.) Estrone
aqueous 5 mg/mL. Inj. Vial 10 mL. *Rx.*
Use: Estrogen.

estrone sulfate, piperazine.
See: Ogen.

estrone sulfate, potassium.
See: Estrogen.

•**estropipate.** (ESS-troe-PIH-pate)
*USP 34. Formerly Piperazine Estrone
Sulfate.*
Use: Estrogen, sex hormone.

estropipate. (Various Mfr.) Estropipate
0.75 mg (sodium estrone sulfate
0.625 mg), 1.5 mg (sodium estrone sulfate 1.25 mg), 3 mg (sodium estrone
sulfate 2.5 mg), 6 mg (sodium estrone
sulfate 5 mg). Tab. Bot. 30s, 100s,

500s. *Rx.*
Use: Estrogen, sex hormone.
Estroquin. (Sheryl) Purified conjugated estrogens 1.25 mg. Tab. Bot. 100s. *Rx.*
Use: Estrogen.
Estrostep Fe. (Warner Chilcott) **Phase 1:** Norethindrone acetate 1 mg, ethinyl estradiol 20 mcg. 5 tabs. **Phase 2:** Norethindrone acetate 1 mg, ethinyl estradiol 30 mcg. 7 tabs. **Phase 3:** Norethindrone acetate 1 mg, ethinyl estradiol 35 mcg. 9 tabs. Lactose, sucrose. Box. 28s with 7 brown tabs. with ferrous fumarate 75 mg per tab. *Rx.*
Use: Sex hormone, contraceptive hormone.
●**eszopiclone.** (es-zoe-PIK-lone) USAN.
Use: Sedative and hypnotic, nonbarbiturate.
See: Lunesta.
●**etafedrine hydrochloride.** (EH-tah-FED-rin) USAN.
Use: Bronchodilator; adrenergic.
●**etafilcon A.** (EH-tah-FILL-kahn A) USAN.
Use: Contact lens material, hydrophilic.
Etalent. (Roger) Ethaverine hydrochloride 100 mg. Cap. Bot. 50s, 500s. *Rx.*
Use: Vasodilator.
●**etalocib.** (e-TAL-oh-kib) USAN.
Use: Antineoplastic.
●**etanercept.** (et-a-NER-sept) USAN.
Use: Immunologic agent, immunomodulator.
See: Enbrel.
●**etanidazole.** (ETT-ah-NIDE-ah-zole) USAN.
Use: Antineoplastic (hypoxic cell radiosensitizer).
●**etarotene.** (ett-AHR-oh-teen) USAN.
Use: Keratolytic.
●**etazolate hydrochloride.** (eh-TAY-zoe-late) USAN.
Use: Antipsychotic.
●**eteplirsen.** (e-TEP-lir-sen) USAN.
Use: Treatment of Duchenne muscular dystrophy.
Eterna 27. (Revlon) Pregnenolone acetate 0.5% in cream base. *OTC.*
Use: Emollient.
●**eterobarb.** (ee-TEER-oh-barb) USAN.
Use: Anticonvulsant.
●**ethacrynate sodium for injection.** (ETH-ah-KRIN-ate) *USP 34.*
Use: Diuretic.
See: Edecrin Sodium I.V.
●**ethacrynic acid.** (eth-uh-KRIN-ik) *USP 34.*
Use: Diuretic.
See: Edecrin.

●**ethambutol hydrochloride.** (eth-AM-byoo-tahl) *USP 34.*
Use: Anti-infective (tuberculostatic).
See: Myambutol.
ethambutol hydrochloride. (Heritage) Ethambutol hydrochloride 100 mg, 400 mg. Sorbitol, sucrose. Film-coated. Tab. 100s. *Rx.*
Use: Antituberculosis agent.
Ethamicort.
See: Hydrocortamate.
●**ethamivan.** (eth-AM-ih-van) USAN.
Use: Stimulant (central and respiratory).
Ethamolin. (Questcor) Ethanolamine oleate 5%. Inj. Amp. 2 mL. *Rx.*
Use: Sclerosing agent.
●**ethamsylate.** (ETH-AM-sill-ate) USAN.
Use: Hemostatic.
ethanol. (Various Mfr.) Alcohol, anhydrous.
ethanolamine. Olamine.
●**ethanolamine oleate.** (ETH-ah-nahl-ah-MEEN OH-lee-ate) USAN.
Use: Sclerosing agent.
See: Ethamolin.
ethanolamines, nonselective.
Use: Antihistamine.
See: Carbinoxamine Maleate.
Clemastine Fumarate.
Diphenhydramine Hydrochloride.
Doxylamine Succinate.
ethenol, homopolymer. Polyvinyl alcohol.
●**ether.** (EE-ther) *USP 34.*
Use: Anesthetic, general; inhalation.
●**ethinyl estradiol.** (ETH-in-ill ess-trah-DIE-ole) *USP 34.*
Use: Estrogen.
See: Estinyl.
Feminone.
Menolyn.
W/Desogestrel.
See: Azurette.
Caziant.
W/Drospirenone.
See: Gianvi.
Ocella.
Yaz.
W/Drospirenone, Levomefolate Calcium.
See: Beyaz.
W/Levonorgestrel.
See: LoSeasonique.
Lybrel.
W/Norethindrone.
See: Zenchent.
W/Norethindrone Acetate.
See: Femhrt.
Jinteli.
Tilia Fe.
Tri-Legest.

ETHRANE 341

W/Norgestimate.
See: Previfem.
ethinyl estradiol. (Bio-Technology General)
Use: Turner syndrome. [Orphan Drug]
ethinyl estradiol and dimethisterone tablets.
Use: Estrogen, progestin combination.
ethinyl estradiol with combinations.
See: Alesse.
   Apri.
   Aranelle.
   Aviane.
   Balziva.
   Brevicon.
   Cesia.
   Desogen.
   Estrostep Fe.
   Femcon Fe.
   GenCept.
   Jenest-28.
   Jolessa.
   Junel Fe 1/20.
   Junel Fe 1.5/30.
   Junel 21 Day 1.5/30.
   Junel 21 Day 1/20.
   Kelnor 1/35.
   Leena.
   Levora.
   Loestrin 21 1/20.
   Loestrin 21 1.5/30.
   Loestrin Fe 1/20.
   Loestrin Fe 1.5/30.
   Loestrin 24 Fe.
   Lo/Ovral.
   Low-Ogestrel.
   Lutera.
   Microgestin Fe 1/20.
   Microgestin Fe 1.5/30.
   Mircette.
   Modicon.
   MonoNessa.
   Nelulen.
   Nordette.
   Norinyl 1 + 35.
   Norlestrin.
   Norlestrin Fe.
   NuvaRing.
   Ortho-Cept.
   Ortho-Cyclen.
   Ortho-Evra.
   Ortho-Novum 1/35, 7/7/7, 10/11.
   Ortho Tri-Cyclen.
   Ovcon-50.
   Ovcon-35.
   Ovlin.
   Ovral.
   Previfem.
   Quasense.
   Reclipsen.
   Seasonale.
   Seasonique.
   Solia.
   Sronyx.
   Tri-Norinyl.
   Triphasil.
   Tri-Previfem.
   Trivora.
   Velivet.
   Yasmin.
   Zovia 1/50E.
   Zovia 1/35E.
ethinyl estrenol.
See: Lynestrenol.
•**ethiodized oil injection.** (eth-EYE-oh-dized) *USP 34.*
Use: Radiopaque agent.
•**ethiodized oil I 131.** (eth-EYE-oh-dized) USAN.
Use: Antineoplastic; radiopharmaceutical.
•**ethionamide.** (eh-THIGH-ohn-ah-mide) *USP 34.*
Use: Antituberculosis agent.
See: Trecator.
ethisterone.
See: Anhydrohydroxyprogesterone.
Ethocaine.
See: Procaine Hydrochloride.
ethodryl.
See: Diethylcarbamazine Citrate.
ethohexadiol. Used in Comp. dimethyl phthalate.
Use: Insect repellent.
•**ethonam nitrate.** (ETH-oh-nam NYE-trate) USAN.
Use: Antifungal.
•**ethosuximide.** (ETH-oh-SUX-ih-mide) *USP 34.*
Use: Anticonvulsant.
See: Zarontin.
ethosuximide. (Copley) Ethosuximide 250 mg/5 mL, saccharin, sucrose, raspberry flavor. Syr. Bot. 483 mL. *Rx.*
Use: Anticonvulsant.
ethosuximide. (Sidmark) Ethosuximide 250 mg. Cap. 100s. *Rx.*
Use: Anticonvulsant.
•**ethotoin.** (ETH-oh-toyn) *USP 34.*
Use: Anticonvulsant.
See: Peganone.
ethovan. Ethyl Vanillin.
•**ethoxazene hydrochloride.** (eth-OX-ah-zeen) USAN.
Use: Analgesic.
ethoxzolamide.
Use: Carbonic anhydrase inhibitor.
Ethrane. (Baxter Healthcare) Enflurane. Volatile Liq. Bot. 125 mL, 250 mL. *Rx.*
Use: Anesthetic, general.

•**ethybenztropine.** (ETH-ih-BENZ-troe-peen) USAN.
Use: Anticholinergic.

•**ethyl acetate.** (ETH-ill) *NF 29.*
Use: Pharmaceutic aid, flavoring; solvent.

ethyl aminobenzoate. Anesthesin, anesthrone, benzocaine, parathesin.
Use: Anesthetic, local.
See: Benzocaine.

ethyl bromide. (Various Mfr.) Bromoethane. *Rx.*
Use: Anesthetic, general.

ethyl carbamate.
See: Urethan.

•**ethylcellulose.** (eth-il-SEL-yoo-lose) *NF 29.*
Use: Tablet binder; pharmaceutic aid.

ethylcellulose aqueous dispersion.
Use: Tablet binder; pharmaceutic aid.

ethyl chaulmoograte.
Use: Hansen disease; sarcoidosis.

•**ethyl chloride.** (ETH-ill) *USP 34.*
Use: Anesthetic, topical.
W/Dichlorotetrafluoroethane.
See: Fluro-Ethyl.

ethyl chloride. (Gebauer) Chloroethane. Spray. 100 g metal tubes. *Spra-Pak.* 105 mL. Bot. 120 mL (fine, medium, and coarse spray). *Rx.*
Use: Anesthetic, local.

•**ethyl dibunate.** (ETH-ill DIE-byoo-nate) USAN.
Use: Cough suppressant; antitussive.

ethyl diiodobrassidate. Iodobrassid. Lipoiodine.

ethyldimethylammonium bromide.
See: Ambutonium Bromide.

ethylene. (Various Mfr.) Ethene. *Rx.*
Use: Anesthetic, general.

•**ethylenediamine.** (eth-ih-leen-DIE-ah-meen) *USP 34.*
Use: Component of aminophylline injection.

ethylenediamine solution. (67% w/v).
Use: Solvent (Aminophylline Inj.).

ethylenediamine tetraacetic acid disodium salt.
See: Endrate Disodium.

ethylenediaminetetraacetic acid.
See: Edathamil.
EDTA.

ethylenimines/methylmelamines.
Use: Alkylating agents.
See: Altretamine.
Mechlorethamine Derivative.
Thiotepa.

•**ethylestrenol.** (ETH-ill-ESS-tree-nahl) USAN.
Use: Anabolic.

ethylhydrocupreine hydrochloride.
Use: Antiseptic.

ethylmorphine hydrochloride.
Use: Narcotic.

ethyl nitrite spirit. Ethyl nitrite. Sweet Spirit of Niter. Spirit of Nitrous Ether.

•**ethyl oleate.** (ETH-ill) *NF 29.*
Use: Pharmaceutic aid (vehicle).

ethyl oxide; ethyl ether.
Use: Solvent.

•**ethylparaben.** (eth-ill-PAR-ah-ben) *NF 29.*
Use: Pharmaceutic aid (antifungal preservative).

ethylstibamine. Astaril, neostibosan.
Use: Antimony therapy.

•**ethyl vanillin.** (ETH-ill) *NF 29.*
Use: Pharmaceutic aid (flavor).

•**ethynerone.** (eth-EYE-ner-ohn) USAN.
Use: Hormone, progestin.

•**ethynodiol diacetate.** (eh-THIN-oh-die-ole die-ASS-eh-tate) *USP 34.*
Use: Progesterone, progestin.
W/Ethinyl estradiol.
See: Estrostep Fe.
Kelnor 1/35.
Nelulen.
Ovulen.
Zovia.
W/Mestranol.
See: Ovulen.

ethynodiol diacetate and ethinyl estradiol tablets.
Use: Contraceptive.

ethynodiol diacetate and mestranol tablets.
Use: Contraceptive.

ethynylestradiol.
See: Ethinyl Estradiol.
Mestranol.

Ethyol. (MedImmune Oncology) Amifostine 500 mg (as amifostine trihydrate). Inj., Pow. for Soln. Single-use vials. 10 mL. *Rx.*
Use: Cytoprotective agent.

•**etibendazole.** (eh-tie-BEN-dah-ZOLE) USAN.
Use: Anthelmintic.

Eticylol. (Novartis) Ethinyl estradiol. *Rx.*
Use: Estrogen.

•**etidocaine.** (eh-TIE-doe-cane) USAN.
Use: Anesthetic, local.

•**etidronate disodium.** (eh-TIH-DROE-nate) *USP 34.*
Use: Bisphosphonate.
See: Didronel.

etidronate disodium. (Genpharm) Etidronate disodium 200 mg, 400 mg. Tab. 60s. *Rx.*
Use: Bisphosphanate.

•**etidronic acid.** (eh-tih-DRAH-nik) USAN.
Use: Calcium regulator.
•**etifenin.** (EH-tih-FEN-in) USAN.
Use: Diagnostic aid.
•**etilevodopa.** (et-il-ee-voe-DOE-a) USAN.
Use: Parkinson disease.
•**etintidine hydrochloride.** (ett-IN-tih-DEEN) USAN.
Use: Antiulcerative.
etiocholanedoine. (SuperGen)
Use: Aplastic anemia; Prader-Willi syndrome. [Orphan Drug]
•**etiprednol dicloacetate.** (e-ti-PRED-nole dye-KLOE-a-se-tate) USAN.
Use: Anti-inflammatory; corticosteroid.
•**etocrylene.** (EH-toe-KRIH-leen) USAN.
Use: Ultraviolet screen.
•**etodolac.** (EE-toe-DOE-lak) *USP 34.*
Use: Analgesic; NSAID.
etodolac. (Various Mfr.) Etodolac **Tab.:** 400 mg, 500 mg. Bot. 100s, 500s, 1000s (500 mg only). **Cap.:** 200 mg, 300 mg. Bot. 100s, 500s, 1000s. **ER Tab.:** 400 mg, 500 mg, 600 mg. Bot. 100s, 500s (400 mg only). *Rx.*
Use: Analgesic; NSAID.
•**etofenamate.** (EH-toe-FEN-am-ate) USAN.
Use: Analgesic; anti-inflammatory.
•**etoformin hydrochloride.** (EH-toe-FORE-min) USAN.
Use: Antidiabetic.
•**etomidate.** (eh-TAHM-ih-date) USAN.
Use: Hypnotic; sedative.
See: Amidate.
etomidate. (Parenta) Etomidate 2 mg/mL. Inj., Soln. Single-dose vials. 10 mL, 20 mL. *Rx.*
Use: Hypnotic; sedative.
etomide hydrochloride. Bandol. Carbiphene hydrochloride.
•**etonogestrel.** (ETT-oh-no-JESS-trell) USAN.
Use: Hormone, progestin.
See: Implanon.
W/Ethinyl estradiol.
See: NuvaRing.
•**etoperidone hydrochloride.** (EH-toe-PURR-ih-dohn) USAN.
Use: Antidepressant.
Etopophos. (Bristol-Myers Squibb) Etoposide phosphate100 mg. Lyophilized Pow. for Inj. Vial. Single dose. *Rx.*
Use: Antineoplastic.
•**etoposide.** (EH-toe-POE-side) *USP 34.*
Use: Antineoplastic.
See: Etopophos.
Toposar.

Vepesid.
etoposide. (Various Mfr.) Etoposide. **Cap.:** 50 mg. Blister pack. 10s. **Inj.:** 20 mg/mL. May contain alcohol, benzyl alcohol, polysorbate 80, PEG, citric acid. Vial. 5 mL, 12.5 mL, 25 mL, 50 mL. *Rx.*
Use: Epipodophyllotoxin; antineoplastic.
etoposide. (Various Mfr.) Etoposide *Rx.*
Use: Antineoplastic.
•**etoposide phosphate.** (ee-toe-POE-side) USAN.
Use: Antineoplastic.
See: Etopophos.
•**etoprine.** (ETT-oh-preen) USAN.
Use: Antineoplastic.
etoval.
See: Butethal.
•**etoxadrol hydrochloride.** (eh-TOX-ah-drole) USAN.
Use: Anesthetic.
•**etozolin.** (EAT-oh-zoe-lin) USAN.
Use: Diuretic.
Etrafon-A (4-10). (Schering-Plough) Perphenazine 4 mg, amitriptyline hydrochloride 10 mg. Tab. Bot. 100s, UD 100s. *Rx.*
Use: Psychotherapeutic combination.
Etrafon Forte (4-25). (Schering-Plough) Perphenazine 4 mg, amitriptyline hydrochloride 25 mg. Tab. Bot. 100s, 500s, UD 100s. *Rx.*
Use: Psychotherapeutic combination.
Etrafon (2-25). (Schering-Plough) Perphenazine 2 mg, amitriptyline hydrochloride 25 mg. Tab. Bot. 100s, 500s, UD 100s. *Rx.*
Use: Psychotherapeutic combination.
•**etravirine.** (ET-ra-VIR-een) USAN.
Use: Antiretroviral, non-nucleoside reverse transcriptase inhibitor.
See: Intelence.
•**etretinate.** (eh-TRETT-ih-nate) USAN.
Use: Antipsoriatic.
•**etrolizumab.** (ET-roe-LIZ-oo-mab) USAN.
Use: Gastrointestinal agent.
etrynit. Propatyl nitrate.
Use: Cardiovascular agent.
•**etryptamine acetate.** (ee-TRIP-tah-meen) USAN.
Use: Central stimulant.
E.T.S.-2%. (Paddock) Erythromycin topical 2%. Soln. Bot. 60 mL. *Rx.*
Use: Dermatologic, acne.
ettriol trinitrate.
See: Propatyl nitrate.
etybenzatropine. Ethybenztropine.
etynodiol acetate. Ethynodiol diacetate.

eubasin.
See: Sulfapyridine.

eucaine hydrochloride. (Novartis) Menthol 8%, eucalyptus oil, SD 3A alcohol. Gel. Tube 60 g. *OTC.*
Use: Liniment.

Eucalyptamint. (Novartis) Menthol 8%, eucalyptus oil, SD 3A alcohol. Gel 60 g. *OTC.*
Use: Liniment.

Eucalyptamint Maximum Strength. (Novartis) Menthol 16%, lanolin, eucalyptus oil. Oint. Tube 60 mL. *OTC.*
Use: Liniment.

•**eucalyptol.** (yoo-ka-LIP-tol) USAN.
Use: Pharmaceutic aid (flavor); antitussive; decongestant, nasal.
See: Vicks Sinex.

eucalyptus oil.
Use: Flavor; antitussive; decongestant, nasal; expectorant; analgesic, topical.
See: Victors.
W/Combinations.
See: Mentholatum Cherry Chest Rub for Kids.
Vicks VapoRub.

•**eucatropine hydrochloride.** (you-CAT-troe-peen) USP 34.
Use: Pharmaceutical necessity for ophthalmic dosage form; anticholinergic, ophthalmic.

eucatropine hydrochloride. (Glogau) Crystal, Bot. g.
Use: Pharmaceutical necessity for ophthalmic dosage form; anticholinergic, ophthalmic.

Eucerin. (Beiersdorf) Unscented moisturizing formula. **Creme:** Jar 120 g, lb. **Lot.:** Bot. 240 mL, 480 mL. *OTC.*
Use: Emollient.

Eucerin Cleansing. (Beiersdorf) Sodium laureth sulfate, cocoamphocarboxyglycinate, cocamidopropyl betaine, cocamide MEA, PEG-7 glyceryl cocoate, PEG-5 lanolate, PEG-120 methyl glucose dioleate, lanolin alcohol, imidazolidinyl urea. Soap free. Lot. Bot. 240 mL. *OTC.*
Use: Dermatologic, cleanser.

Eucerin Dry Skin Care Daily Facial. (Beiersdorf) Ethylhexyl p-methoxycinnamate, titanium dioxide, 2-phenylbenzimidazole-5-sulfonic acid, 2-ethylhexyl salicylate, mineral oil, cetearyl alcohol, castor oil, lanolin alcohol, EDTA. SPF 20. Lot. Bot. 120 mL. *OTC.*
Use: Sunscreen.

Eucerin Itch-Relief Moisturizing. (Beiersdorf) Menthol 0.15%, glycerin, mineral oil, cetyl alcohol, *Oenothera biennis* (evening primrose oil). Spray.

200 mL. *OTC.*
Use: Emollient.

Eucerin Plus. (Beiersdorf) Mineral oil, hydrogenated castor oil, sodium lactate 5%, urea 5%, glycerin, lanolin alcohol. Lot. Bot. 177 mL. *OTC.*
Use: Emollient.

eucodal.
See: Oxycodone.

eucupin dihydrochloride. Isoamylhydrocupreine dihydrochloride.

Eudal-SR. (Forest) Pseudoephedrine 120 mg, guaifenesin 400 mg. SR Tab. Bot. 100s. *Rx.*
Use: Decongestant, expectorant.

euflavine.
See: Acriflavine.

Euflexxa. (Ferring) Sodium hyaluronate 10 mg/mL. Inj. Prefilled syringes. 2 mL. *Rx.*
Use: Physical adjunct.

•**eugenol.** (you-jeh-nole) USP 34.
Use: Dental analgesic; oral anesthetic.
See: Benzodent.

eukadol.
See: Dihydrohydroxycodeinone.

Eulcin. (Leeds) Methscopolamine bromide 2.5 mg, butabarbital sodium 10 mg, aluminum hydroxide gel, dried, 250 mg, magnesium trisilicate 250 mg. Tab. Bot. 100s. *Rx.*
Use: Antacid; anticholinergic; antispasmodic; hypnotic; sedative.

Eumydrin Drops. (Sanofi-Synthelabo) Atropine methonitrate. *Rx.*
Use: Anticholinergic; antispasmodic.

euneryl.
See: Phenobarbital.

Euphorbia Compound. (Sherwood Davis & Geck) *Euphorbia pilulifera* fluid extract 1.5 mL, lobelia tincture 2.2 mL, nitroglycerin spirit 0.29 mL, sodium iodide 1.04 g, sodium bromide 1.04 g, alcohol 24%/30 mL. Bot. Pt, gal. *Rx.*
Use: Expectorant; hypnotic; sedative.

euphorbia pilulifera.
W/Phenyl salicylate and various oils.
See: Rayderm.

Eupractone. (Baxter PPI) Dimethadione.

•**euprocin hydrochloride.** (YOU-pro-sin) USAN.
Use: Anesthetic, local.

euquinine. Quinine ethyl carbonate.
Use: Antimalarial; antipyretic.

Eurax. (Bristol-Myers Squibb) Crotamiton. **Cream:** 10% in vanishing base. Cetyl alcohol. Tube 60 g. **Lotion:** 10% in emollient base. Cetyl alcohol. Bot. 60 g, 454 g. *Rx.*
Use: Scabicide; pediculicide.

Evac. (Burgin-Arden) **Supp.:** Sodium bi-

carbonate, sodium biphosphate, dioctyl sodium sulfosuccinate 50 mg. Supp. **Tab.:** Guar gum 300 mg, danthron 50 mg, sodium 100 mg. Tab. *OTC.*
Use: Laxative.

Evactol. (Delta Pharmaceutical Group) Docusate sodium 100 mg, sodium carboxymethyl cellulose 200 mg. Cap. Pkg. 10s. Bot. 10s, 30s, 100s. *OTC.*
Use: Laxative.

Evac-U-Gen. (Lee Pharmaceuticals) Sennosides 10 mg. Sugar. Chew. Tab. 35s. *OTC.*
Use: Laxative.

Evamist. (Ther-Rx) Estradiol 1.53 mg. Alcohol, octisalate. Spray Soln. 8.1 mL (56 sprays of 90 mcL). *Rx.*
Use: Estrogen, sex hormone.

Evans Blue. *USP 34.*
Use: Diagnostic aid (blood volume determination).

Evans Blue Dye. (New World Trading Corp.) Evans blue dye 5 mL. Inj. *Rx.*
Use: Diagnostic aid.

•**evatanepag.** (EV-a-ta-NEP-ag) USAN.
Use: Treatment of fracture.

•**evatanepag sodium.** (EV-a-ta-NEP-ag) USAN.
Use: Treatment of fracture.

•**evernimicin.** (E-ver-ni-MYE-sin) USAN.
Use: Antibacterial.

•**everolimus.** (e-ver-OH-li-mus) USAN.
Use: Immunosuppressant.
See: Afinitor.

Evicyl Tablets. (Sanofi-Synthelabo) Inositol hexanicotinate. *Rx.*
Use: Hypolipidemic; peripheral vasodilator.

Eviron. (Delta Pharmaceutical Group) Ferrous fumarate 160 mg, copper 1 mg, ascorbic acid 75 mg. Tab. *OTC.*
Use: Mineral, vitamin supplement.

Evista. (Eli Lilly) Raloxifene 60 mg, lactose. Tab. Unit-of-use. 30s, 100s, 2000s. *Rx.*
Use: Osteoporosis prevention; sex hormone, selective estrogen receptor modulator.

E-Vital Creme. (Taylor Pharmaceuticals) Vitamins E 100 units, A 250 units, D 100 units, d-panthenol 0.2%, allantoin 0.1%/g. Jar 2 oz, lb. *OTC.*
Use: Emollient.

Evithrom. (J & J Wound Management) Thrombin (human origin) 800 to 1,200 units/mL. Soln., frozen; topical. Single-use vial. 2 mL, 5 mL, 20 mL. *Rx.*
Use: Topical hemostatic.

Evoclin. (Stiefel) Clindamycin 1%. Cetyl alcohol, dehydrated alcohol (ethanol

58%), stearyl alcohol. Foam. 50 g (pressurized with a hydrocarbon [propane/butane] propellant). *Rx.*
Use: Anti-infective, topical.

Evoxac. (Daiichi) Cevimeline hydrochloride 30 mg, lactose. Cap. Bot. 100s, 500s. *Rx.*
Use: Sjögran syndrome; dry mouth.

Exalgo. (Alza) Hydromorphone hydrochloride 8 mg, 12 mg, 16 mg. Lactose, PEG. ER Tab. 100s. *c-II.*
Use: Opioid analgesic.

Exall-D. (Hawthorn) Carbetapentane citrate 10 mg, guaifenesin 100 mg, pseudoephedrine hydrochloride 30 mg. Saccharin, sorbitol. Alcohol free, dye free, and sugar free. Fruit gum flavor. Liq. 473 mL. *Rx.*
Use: Upper respiratory combination, antitussive and expectorant combination.

•**exametazime.** (EX-ah-MET-ah-zeen) USAN.
Use: Diagnostic aid (regional cerebral perfusion imaging).

•**exaprolol hydrochloride.** (EX-ah-PRO-lahl) USAN.
Use: Antiadrenergic (β-receptor).

•**exatecan mesylate.** (ex-a-TE-can) USAN.
Use: Antineoplastic.

Ex-Caloric Wafers. (Eastern Research) Carboxymethylcellulose 181 mg, methylcellulose 272 mg. Bot. 100s, 500s, 5000s. *OTC.*
Use: Dietary aid.

Excedrin Back & Body Extra Strength. (Novartis Consumer Health) Acetaminophen 250 mg, buffered aspirin 250 mg. Tab. 24s. *OTC.*
Use: Nonnarcotic analgesic.

Excedrin Extra Strength. (Novartis Consumer Health) Acetaminophen 250 mg, aspirin 250 mg, caffeine 65 mg, saccharin. **Cap.:** Bot. 24s, 50s, 100s, 175s, 275s. **Tab.:** Bot. 24s, 50s, 100s, 175s, 275s. **Geltab.:** Bot. 24s, 40s, 80s. *OTC.*
Use: Analgesic combination.

Excedrin Migraine. (Novartis Consumer Health) Acetaminophen 250 mg, aspirin 250 mg, caffeine 65 mg. Tab. Bot. 50s, 100s. *OTC.*
Use: Analgesic combination.

Excedrin P.M. (Novartis Consumer Health) **Tab.:** Acetaminophen 500 mg, diphenhydramine citrate 38 mg. Parabens. Bot. 24s. **Cap.:** Acetaminophen 500 mg, diphenhydramine citrate 38 mg. Bot. 30s, 50s. **Liquigels:** Acetaminophen 500 mg, diphenhydra-

mine hydrochloride 25 mg. Bot. 20s, 40s. **Liq.:** Acetaminophen 1000 mg, diphenhydramine hydrochloride 50 mg/ 30 mL, alcohol 10%, sucrose. Bot. 180 mL. **Geltab:** Acetaminophen 500 mg, diphenhydramine citrate 38 mg, EDTA, parabens. Bot. 100s. *OTC.*
Use: Analgesic; sleep aid.

Excedrin Sinus Headache. (Novartis Consumer Health) Phenylephrine hydrochloride 5 mg, acetaminophen 325 mg. Film-coated. Tab. 24s. *OTC.*
Use: Upper respiratory combination, decongestant and analgesic.

Excedrin Tension Headache. (Novartis Consumer Health) Acetaminophen 500 mg, caffeine 65 mg. Parabens. Caplets, Geltabs. 50s, 100s. *OTC.*
Use: Nonnarcotic analgesic combination.

Excita Extra. (Durex) Nonoxynol-9 8% Ribbed Condom. Box 3s, 12s, 36s. *OTC.*
Use: Condom with spermicide.

ExeClear-C. (Larken) Codeine phosphate 10 mg, guaifenesin 200 mg per 5 mL. Magnasweet, saccharin, sorbitol. Sugar free, alcohol free, and dye free. Syr. 473 mL. *c-v.*
Use: Upper respiratory combination, antitussive with expectorant.

ExeCof. (Larken) Dextromethorphan HBr 60 mg, guaifenesin 1000 mg, phenylephrine hydrochloride 40 mg. Dye free. ER Tab. 100s. *Rx.*
Use: Upper respiratory combination, antitussive and expectorant.

ExeFen DMX. (Larken) **Tab:** Dextromethorphan hydrobromide 20 mg, guaifenesin 400 mg, pseudoephedrine hydrochloride 60 mg. Maltodextrin. 100s. **ER Tab:** Dextromethorphan hydrobromide 40 mg, guaifenesin 780 mg, pseudoephedrine hydrochloride 80 mg. Dye free. 100s. *OTC.*
Use: Upper respiratory combination, antitussive and expectorant combination.

ExeFen-PD. (Larken) Phenylephrine hydrochloride 10 mg, guaifenesin 600 mg. ER Tab. 100s. *Rx.*
Use: Upper respiratory combination, decongestant and expectorant.

Exelderm. (Ranbaxy) Sulconazole nitrate 1%. Cream: Tube. 15 g, 30 g, 60 g. Soln.: 30 mL. *Rx.*
Use: Anti-infective, antifungal agent.

Exelon. (Novartis) Rivastigmine. **Cap.:** As rivastigmine tartrate. 1.5 mg, 3 mg, 4.5 mg, 6 mg. Bot. 60s, 500s, UD 30s,

UD 100s. **Soln.:** As rivastigmine tartrate. 2 mg/mL. Bot. 120 mL. **Transdermal Patch:** 4.6 mg/24 h (rivastigmine 9 mg per transdermal system, 5 cm^2), 9.5 mg/24 h (rivastigmine 18 mg per transdermal system, 10 cm^2). 30s. *Rx.*
Use: Cholinesterase inhibitor.

•**exemestane.** (ex-e-MES-tane) USAN.
Use: Antineoplastic.
See: Aromasin.

exemestane.
Use: Hormonal therapy of metastatic breast carcinoma. [Orphan Drug]

exemestane. (Various Mfr.) Exemestane 25 mg. May contain mannitol, methylparaben, PEG, polydextrose, sucrose. Tab. 30s. *Rx.*
Use: Hormone, aromatase inhibitor.

•**exenatide.** (ex-EN-a-tide) USAN.
Use: Antidiabetic agent, incretin mimetic agent.
See: Byetta.

ExeTuss. (Larken) Phenylephrine hydrochloride 25 mg, guaifenesin 900 mg. ER Tab. 100s. *Rx.*
Use: Upper respiratory combination, decongestant and expectorant combination.

ExeTuss-DM. (Larken) Dextromethorphan hydrobromide 25 mg, guaifenesin 600 mg, phenylephrine hydrochloride 20 mg. Dye free and sugar free. ER Tab. 100s. *Rx.*
Use: Upper respiratory combination, antitussive and expectorant combination.

ExeTuss GP. (Larken) Phenylephrine hydrochloride 25 mg, guaifenesin 1200 mg. ER Tab. 100s. *Rx.*
Use: Upper respiratory combination, decongestant and expectorant combination.

Exforge. (Novartis) Amlodipine besylate/ valsartan 5 mg/160 mg, 5 mg/320 mg, 10 mg/160 mg, 10 mg/320 mg. Filmcoated. Tab. 30s, 90s, UD 100s. *Rx.*
Use: Antihypertensive combination.

Exforge HCT. (Novartis) Hydrochlorothiazide/amlodipine/valsartan. 12.5 mg/ 5 mg/160 mg, 12.5 mg/10 mg/160 mg, 25 mg/5 mg/160 mg, 25 mg/10 mg/ 160 mg, 25 mg/10 mg/320 mg. Film coated. Tab. 30s, 90s. *Rx.*
Use: Antihypertensive combination.

Exidine-4 Scrub. (Xttrium) Chlorhexidine gluconate 4%, isopropyl alcohol 4%. Soln. Bot. 120 mL, 240 mL, 480 mL, 887 mL, gal. *OTC.*
Use: Antiseptic; antimicrobial.

Exidine Skin Cleanser. (Xttrium) Chlorhexidine gluconate 4%, isopropyl alco-

hol 4%. Bot. 120 mL, 240 mL, 16 oz, 32 oz, gal. *OTC.*
Use: Antiseptic; antimicrobial.
Exidine-2 Scrub. (Baxter PPI) Chlorhexidine gluconate 2%, isopropyl alcohol 4%. Soln. Bot. 120 mL. *OTC.*
Use: Antiseptic; antimicrobial.
exisulind.
Use: Investigational apoptotic antineoplastic drug.
Exjade. (Novartis) Deferasirox 125 mg, 250 mg, 500 mg. Lactose. Tab. for Oral Susp. 30s. *Rx.*
Use: Chelating agent.
ex-lax. (Novartis Consumer Health) Sennosodes 15 mg, sucrose. Tab. Pkg. 8s, 30s, 60s. *OTC.*
Use: Laxative.
ex-lax Chocolated. (Novartis Consumer Health) Sennosides 15 mg, sugar, oil, dry milk, chocolated. Tab. Pkg. 6s, 18s, 48s. *OTC.*
Use: Laxative.
ex-lax Gentle Strength. (Novartis Consumer Health) Docusate sodium 65 mg, sennosides 10 mg, lactose, methylparaben, polydextrose. Tab. Box. 24s. *OTC.*
Use: Laxative.
ex-lax, Maximum Relief. (Novartis Consumer Health) Sennosides 25 mg, sucrose. Tab. Pkg. 24s, 48s. *OTC.*
Use: Laxative.
ex-lax Stool Softener. (Novartis Consumer Health) Docusate sodium 100 mg, methylparabens. Tab. Bot. 40s. *OTC.*
Use: Laxative.
ex-lax Ultra. (Novartis Consumer Health) Bisacodyl 5 mg. Lactose, methylparaben. Coated. Tab. 24s. *OTC.*
Use: Irritant or stimulant laxative.
Exoderm. (A.G. Marin Pharmaceuticals) Salicylic acid 3%, sulfur 10%. Soap. 91.67 mL. *OTC.*
Use: Topical anti-infective, antifungal combination.
exol. Di-isobutyl ethoxy ethyl dimethyl benzyl ammonium chloride.
exonic ot. Dioctyl sodium sulphosuccinate.
Use: Laxative.
expectorant and antitussive combinations.
Use: Upper respiratory combination.
expectorant and decongestant combinations.
Use: Upper respiratory combination.
expectorant, antihistamine, and decongestant combinations.
Use: Upper respiratory combination.

expectorant, antitussive, and decongestant combinations.
Use: Upper respiratory combination.
Expectorant DM Cough Syrup. (Weeks & Leo) Dextromethorphan HBr 15 mg, guaifenesin 100 mg/5 mL, alcohol 7.125%. Bot. 6 oz. *OTC.*
Use: Antitussive, expectorant.
expectorants.
See: Guaifenesin.
Expendable Blood Collection Unit ACD. (Baxter PPI) Citric acid 540 mg, sodium citrate 1.49 g, dextrose 1.65 g/67.5 mL. *Rx.*
Use: Anticoagulant.
Exratuss. (Midlothian) Carbetapentane tannate 30 mg, chlorpheniramine tannate 4 mg, phenylephrine tannate 12.5 mg per 5 mL. Methylparaben, saccharin, sucrose. Strawberry flavor. Susp. 118 mL. *Rx.*
Use: Antitussive.
Extavia. (Novartis) Interferon beta-1b 0.3 mg. Human albumin 15 mg, mannitol 15 mg per vial. Preservative free. Single-use 3 mL capacity vial with 1.2 mL prefilled syringe of diluents (sodium chloride 0.54%), alcohol prep pads, and vial adaptor w/attached needle for each drug vial. Blister unit 15s. *Rx.*
Use: Immunologic agent, immunomodulator.
extended-spectrum penicillins.
Use: Anti-infective.
Extendryl. (Auriga) **Chew. Tab.:** Chlorpheniramine maleate 2 mg, phenylephrine hydrochloride 10 mg, methscopolamine nitrate 1.25 mg. Mannitol, sugar. Root beer flavor. Chew. Tab. Bot. 100s. **Syrup:** Dexchlorpheniramine maleate 1 mg, phenylephrine hydrochloride 10 mg, methscopolamine nitrate 1.25 mg per 5 mL. Sorbitol, sugar. Root beer flavor. Bot. 473 mL. *Rx.*
Use: Upper respiratory combination, decongestant, antihistamine, and anticholinergic combination.
Extendryl DM. (Auriga) Dextromethorphan HBr 30 mg, chlorpheniramine maleate 8 mg, methscopolamine nitrate 2.5 mg. ER Tab. 100s. *Rx.*
Use: Upper respiratory combination, antitussive combination.
Extendryl G. (Auriga) Phenylephrine hydrochloride 30 mg, guaifenesin 1000 mg. Dye free. ER Tab. 100s. *Rx.*
Use: Upper respiratory combination, decongestant and expectorant combination.

Extendryl GCP. (Auriga) Carbetapentane citrate 15 mg, guaifenesin 100 mg, phenylephrine hydrochloride 5 mg per 5 mL. Alcohol free. Maltitol, saccharin, sorbitol. Strawberry flavor. Oral Soln. 473 mL. *Rx.*
Use: Upper respiratory combination, antitussive combination.

Extendryl PEM. (Auriga) Methscopolamine nitrate 1.25 mg, phenylephrine hydrochloride 30 mg. ER Tab. 100s. *Rx.*
Use: Upper respiratory combination, decongestant, antihistamine, and anticholinergic combination.

Exten Strone 10. (Schlicksup) Estradiol valerate 10 mg/mL. Vial 10 mL. *Rx.*
Use: Estrogen.

Extenzyme Soflens Protein Cleaner. (Allergan) Papain, sodium chloride, sodium carbonate, sodium borate, edetate disodium. Vial w/Tab. 24s. Refill 36s. *OTC.*
Use: Contact lens care.

Extina. (GlaxoSmithKline) Ketoconazole 2%. Cetyl alcohol, ethanol 58%, stearyl alcohol. Foam. 50 g, 100g. *Rx.*
Use: Topical anti-infective, antifungal agent.

Extra Action Cough. (Rugby) Dextromethorphan hydrobromide 10 mg, guaifenesin 100 mg. Cherry flavoring, corn syrup, glycerin, menthol, saccharin, sodium benzoate. Syrup. 473 mL. *OTC.*
Use: Upper respiratory combination, antitussive with expectorant.

Extraneal. (Baxter) Icodextrin 75 g, Na 132 mEq, Ca 3.5 mEq, Mg 0.5 mEq, Cl 96 mEq, lactate 40 mEq/L. Soln. *Ultrabag* and *Ambu-Flex* 1.5, 2, 2.5 L. *Rx.*
Use: Peritoneal dialysis solution.

extraocular irrigating solutions.
Use: Ophthalmic nonsurgical adjuncts.
See: AK-Rinse.
Collyrium for Fresh Eyes Wash.
Eye Stream.
Eye Irrigating Solution.
Irrigate Eye Wash.
Optigene.

Extra Strength Adprin-B. (Pfeiffer) Aspirin 500 mg, calcium carbonate, magnesium carbonate, magnesium oxide. Tab, coated. Bot. 130s. *OTC.*
Use: Analgesic.

Extra Strength Alka-Seltzer Effervescent. (Bayer Consumer Care) Sodium bicarbonate (heat-treated) 1985 mg, aspirin 500 mg, citric acid 1000 mg, sodium 588 mg. Tab. Bot. 12s and 24s. *OTC.*
Use: Antacid.

Extra Strength Aspirin Capsules. (Walgreen) Aspirin 500 mg. Bot. 80s. *OTC.*
Use: Analgesic.

Extra Strength Bayer Enteric 500 Aspirin. (Bayer) Aspirin 500 mg. Tab. Enteric coated. Bot. 60s. *OTC.*
Use: Analgesic.

Extra Strength Bayer Plus. (Bayer) Aspirin 500 mg with calcium carbonate, magnesium carbonate, magnesium oxide. Tab. Bot. 30s, 60s. *OTC.*
Use: Salicylate, aspirin, buffered.

Extra Strength Doan's PM. (Novartis Consumer Health) Magnesium salicylate 580 mg, diphenhydramine hydrochloride 25 mg. Methylparaben, PEG. Tab. 20s. *OTC.*
Use: Sleep aid.

Extra Strength Excedrin Capsules and Tablets. (Bristol-Myers Squibb) Acetaminophen 250 mg, aspirin 250 mg, caffeine 65 mg. Cap. Bot. 24s, 50s, 80s. Tab. Bot. 30s, 60s, 100s, 165s, 225s, Pkg. 12s. *OTC.*
Use: Analgesic combination.

Extra Strength 5 mg Biotin Forte. (Vitaline) Vitamins B_1 10 mg, B_2 10 mg, B_3 40 mg, B_5 10 mg, B_6 25 mg, B_{12} 10 mcg, C 100 mg, biotin 5 mg, FA 800 mcg. Tab. Bot. 60s, 1000s. *OTC.*
Use: Mineral, vitamin supplement.

Extra Strength Gas-X. (Novartis) Simethicone 125 mg. Tab. Pkg. 18s. *OTC.*
Use: Antiflatulent.

Extra Strength Pain Reliever PM. (Magno-Humphries) Diphenhydramine hydrochloride 25 mg, acetaminophen 500 mg. Tab. 100s. *OTC.*
Use: Nonprescription sleep aid.

Extreme Cold Formula. (Major) Pseudoephedrine hydrochloride 30 mg, chlorpheniramine maleate 1 mg, dextromethorphan HBr 15 mg, acetaminophen 500 mg. Cap. Bot. 10s. *OTC.*
Use: Analgesic, antihistamine, antitussive, decongestant.

Eye, Face, and Body Wash Station. (Lavoptik) Sodium chloride 0.49 g, sodium biphosphate 0.4 g, sodium phosphate 0.45 g/100 mL, benzalkonium chloride 0.005%. Bot. 32 oz. *OTC.*
Use: Emergency wash.

Eye Irrigating Solution. (Rugby) Sodium chloride, sodium phosphate mono- and dibasic, benzalkonium chloride, EDTA. Soln. Bot. 118 mL. *OTC.*
Use: Irrigant, ophthalmic.

Eye-Lube-A. (Optopics) Glycerin 0.25%, EDTA, NaCl, benzalkonium chloride. Soln. Bot. 15 mL. *OTC.*
Use: Lubricant, ophthalmic.

Eye Mo. (Sanofi-Synthelabo) Boric acid, benzalkonium chloride, phenylephrine hydrochloride, zinc sulfate. *OTC.*
Use: Astringent, ophthalmic.

Eye Scrub. (Novartis Ophthalmics) PEG-200 glyceryl monotallawate, disodium laureth sulfosuccinate, cocoamidopropylamine oxide, PEG-78 glyceryl monococoate, benzyl alcohol, EDTA. Soln. Bot. 240 mL. *OTC.*
Use: Cleanser, ophthalmic.

Eye Stream. (Alcon) Sodium chloride 0.64%, potassium chloride 0.075%, magnesium chloride hexahydrate 0.03%, calcium chloride dihydrate 0.048%, sodium acetate trihydrate 0.39%, sodium citrate dihydrate 0.17%, benzalkonium chloride 0.013%. Bot. 30 mL, 118 mL. *OTC.*
Use: Irrigant, ophthalmic.

Eye Wash. (Bausch & Lomb) Boric acid, potassium chloride, EDTA, sodium carbonate, benzalkonium chloride 0.01%. Soln. Bot. 118 mL. *OTC.*
Use: Irrigant, ophthalmic.

Eye Wash. (Goldline) Boric acid, potassium chloride, EDTA, anhydrous sodium carbonate, benzalkonium chloride 0.1%. Soln. Bot. 118 mL. *OTC.*
Use: Irrigant, ophthalmic.

Eye Wash. (Lavoptik) Sodium chloride 0.49%, sodium biphosphate 0.4%, sodium phosphate 0.45%, benzalkonium chloride 0.005%. Soln. Bot. 180 mL with eye cup. *OTC.*
Use: Irrigant, ophthalmic.

EZ Detect. (Biomerica) Occult blood screening test. Kit 3s.
Use: Diagnostic aid.

EZ Detect Strep-A Test. (Biomerica) Coated stick test for detection of group A streptococci taken directly from a throat swab.
Use: Diagnostic aid.

Eze Pain. (Halsey Drug) Acetaminophen 2.5 g, salicylamide, caffeine. Cap. Bot. 21s. *OTC.*
Use: Analgesic combination.

•**ezetimibe.** (ezz-ET-ih-mibe) USAN.
Use: Antihyperlipidemic.
See: Zetia.

ezetimibe/simvastatin.
Use: Antihyperlipidemic.
See: Vytorin.

EZFE 200. (McNeil) Iron 200 mg. Cap. 100s. *OTC.*
Use: Dietary supplement.

E-Z Gas II. (EZ EM) Citric acid 1,530 mg, simethicone 40 mg, sodium bicarbonate 2,210 mg. Saccharin. Orange flavor. Effervescent Gran. 4 g packet. 50s. *OTC.*
Use: Antacid combination.

E-Z-HD. (EZ EM) Barium sulfate 98%. Parabens, simethicone, sorbitol. Strawberry-vanilla flavor. Susp. 340 g. *Rx.*
Use: Radiopaque agent, miscellaneous gastrointestinal contrast agent.

Ezide. (Econo Med Pharmaceuticals) Hydrochlorothiazide 50 mg. Tab. Bot. 100s, 1000s. *Rx.*
Use: Diuretic.

•**ezlopitant.** (ez-LOE-pi-tant) USAN.
Use: Emesis; pain; inflammation.

•**ezogabine.** (e-ZOG-a-been) USAN.
Use: Antiepileptic.

Ezol. (Stewart-Jackson Pharmacal) Butalbital 50 mg, caffeine 40 mg, acetaminophen 325 mg. Bot. 100s. *Rx.*
Use: Analgesic; hypnotic; sedative.

Ezol #3. (Stewart-Jackson Pharmacal) Acetaminophen 650 mg, codeine 30 mg. Bot. 100s. *c-iii.*
Use: Analgesic combination; narcotic.

E-Z-Paque. (EZ EM) Barium sulfate 96%. Saccharin, simethicone, sorbitol. Strawberry-lemon flavor. Susp. 176 g, 285 g, 1,200 g. *Rx.*
Use: Radiopaque agent, miscellaneous gastrointestinal contrast agent.

E-Z-Paque Liquid. (EZ EM) Barium sulfate 60%. Saccharin, simethicone, sodium benzoate, sorbitol. Susp. 355 mL, 1,900 mL. *Rx.*
Use: Radiopaque agent, miscellaneous gastrointestinal contrast agent.

E-Z-Paste. (EZ EM) Barium sulfate 60%. Parabens, saccharin, simethicone, sorbitol. Vanilla flavor. Cream. 454 g. *Rx.*
Use: Radiopaque agent, miscellaneous gastrointestinal contrast agent.

F

Fabrase.
Use: Immunomodulator Fabry disease.
[Orphan Drug]
Fabrazyme. (Genzyme) Agalsidase beta.
5.5 mg: 5 mg/mL when reconstituted.
Mannitol 33 mg, sodium phosphate
monobasic monohydrate 3 mg, sodium
phosphate dibasic heptahydrate
8.8 mg. Preservative free. Pow. for Inj.,
lyophilized. Single-use vials. 5 mL.
37 mg (5 mg/mL when reconstituted):
Mannitol 222 mg, sodium phosphate
monobasic monohydrate 20.4 mg, sodium phosphate dibasic heptahydrate
59.2 mg/vial. Preservative free. Pow. for
Inj., lyophilized. Single-use vials.
20 mL. *Rx.*
Use: Fabry disease.
**Faces Only Moisturizing Sunblock by
Coppertone.** (Schering-Plough) Ethylhexyl p-methoxycinnamate, oxybenzone. SPF 15. Lot. Bot. 55.5 mL. *OTC.*
Use: Sunscreen.
Fact Home Pregnancy Test. (Johnson
& Johnson) Accurate test for preg-
nancy in 45 minutes, for use as early
as 3 days after a missed period. Test kit
1s.
Use: Diagnostic aid.
Factive. (Oscient) Gemifloxacin mesy-
late 320 mg, film-coated. Tab. Unit of
use 5s, 7s. *Rx.*
Use: Fluoroquinolone.
factor VIII.
See: Antihemophilic factor.
factor IX, coagulation.
See: Coagulation Factor IX.
•**factor IX complex.** (FAK-tor) *USP 34.*
Use: Hemostatic.
See: Alpha Nine SD.
Konyne 80.
Mononine.
Profilnine SD.
**factor IX complex, vapor heated Bebu-
lin VH immuno.** (Immuno U.S.) Purified, sterile, stable freeze-dried concentrate of coagulation Factor IX (Christ-
mas Factor), Factors II (prothrombin)
and X (Stuart Prower), low amounts of
Factor VII, ≤ 0.15 International Units
(units) heparin/units Factor IX. Pow. for
Inj. Single-dose vial w/Sterile Water
for Injection, double-ended needle, fil-
ter needle. *Rx.*
Use: Hemostatic.
factor IX concentrates. (FAK-tor)
Use: Antihemophilic agents.
See: AlphaNine SD.
Bebulin VH.

BeneFIX.
Mononine.
Profilnine SD.
factor XIII concentrate. (FAK-tor)
Use: Antihemophilic agent.
See: Corifact.
Fact Plus. (Johnson & Johnson) Reagent
in-home kit for urine testing. Pregnancy
test. Kit 1s, 2s.
Use: Diagnostic aid.
•**fadolmidine hydrochloride.** (fa-DOL-
mid-ine) USAN.
Use: Analgesic (spinal).
•**fadrozole hydrochloride.** (FAHD-rah-
ZOLE) USAN.
Use: Antineoplastic.
Falgos. (Sanofi-Synthelabo) Acetyl-
salicylic acid. Tab. *OTC.*
Use: Analgesic.
•**falimarev (CEA, MUC-1, fowlpox
virus).** (fa-LIM-a-rev) USAN.
Use: Antineoplastic.
Falmonox. (Sanofi-Synthelabo) Teclo-
zan. Susp., Tab. *Rx.*
Use: Amebicide.
•**famciclovir.** (fam-SIGH-kloe-veer)
USAN.
Use: Antiviral agent, antiherpes virus
agent.
See: Famvir.
famciclovir. (Teva) Famciclovir 125 mg,
250 mg, 500 mg. Polydextrose. Film-
coated. Tab. 30s. *Rx.*
Use: Antiviral agent, antiherpes virus
agent.
•**famotidine.** (fah-MOE-tih-den) *USP 34.*
Use: Histamine H$_2$ antagonist.
See: Pepcid.
Pepcid AC.
Pepcid AC Maximum Strength.
Pepcid AC Maximum Strength EZ
Chews.
Pepcid RPD.
W/Calcium Carbonate, Magnesium
Hydroxide.
See: Dual Action Complete.
Tums Dual Action.
famotidine. (Baxter) Famotidine 20 mg/
50 mL. Inj. (premixed). Single-dose
Galaxy containers. 50 mL. *Rx.*
Use: Histamine H$_2$ antagonist.
famotidine. (Ivax) Famotidine 10 mg.
Tab. Bot. 18s, 30s, 50s, 70s. *OTC.*
Use: Histamine H$_2$ antagonist.
famotidine. (Various Mfr.) Famotidine.
Tab.: 20 mg, 40 mg. May contain lac-
tose. Bot. 30s, 100s, 500s, 1000s, UD
100s; *Robot–Ready* 25s (20 mg only).
Pow. for Susp.: 40 mg per 5 mL. May-
contain parabens, sodium benzoate,

sucrose, sugar. 50 mL. **Inj.:** 10 mg/mL. May contain mannitol or benzyl alcohol. Single-dose vials. 1 mL, 2 mL. Multidose vials. 4 mL, 20 mL, 50 mL. *Rx.*
Use: Histamine H_2 antagonist.

famotidine, calcium carbonate, and magnesium hydroxide combinations.
Use: Histamine H_2 antagonist.
See: Dual Action Complete.
Pepcid Complete.

•**famotine hydrochloride.** (FAM-oh-teen) USAN.
Use: Antiviral.

•**fampridine.** (FAHM-prih-DEEN) USAN.
Use: Symptomatic treatment of multiple sclerosis.

Famvir. (Novartis) Famciclovir 125 mg, 250 mg, 500 mg. Lactose. Film-coated. Tab. Bot. 30s, UD 50s (500 mg only). *Rx.*
Use: Management of acute herpes zoster (shingles).

•**fananserin.** (fan-AN-ser-in) USAN.
Use: Antipsychotic; antischizophrenic (dual dopamine D_4 and serotonin 5-HT_2 receptor antagonist).

Fanapt. (Novartis) Iloperidone 1 mg, 2 mg, 4 mg, 6 mg, 8 mg, 10 mg, 12 mg. Lactose. Tab. 60s, titration pack (two 1 mg tablets, two 2 mg tablets, two 4 mg tablets, two 6 mg tablets) (1 mg, 2 mg, 4 mg, 6 mg). *Rx.*
Use: Antipsychotic agent, benzisoxazole derivative.

•**fandosentan potassium.** (fan-doe-SEN-tan) USAN.
Use: Pulmonary hypertension.

•**fanetizole mesylate.** (fan-EH-tih-zole) USAN.
Use: Immunoregulator.

•**fantridone hydrochloride.** (FAN-trih-dohn) USAN.
Use: Antidepressant.

Faramals. (Faraday) Vitamins A 10,000 units, D 2000 units, B_1 6 mg, B_2 4 mg, B_6 0.5 mg, folic acid 0.1 mg, C 100 mg, calcium pantothenate 5 mg, niacinamide 30 mg, E 5 units, B_{12} 3 mcg. Tab. Bot. 100s, 250s, 500s, 1000s. *OTC.*
Use: Mineral, vitamin supplement.

Faramals-M. (Faraday) Faramals plus calcium 103 mg, cobalt 0.1 mg, Cu 1 mg, I 0.15 mg, Fe 10 mg, Mg 6 mg, Mo 0.2 mg, P 80 mg, K 5 mg, Zn 1.2 mg. Tab. Bot. 100s, 250s, 500s, 1000s. *OTC.*
Use: Mineral, vitamin supplement.

Faramins. (Faraday) Vitamins B_1 20 mg, B_2 6 mg, C 40 mg, niacinamide 20 mg,

calcium pantothenate 3 mg, B_6 0.5 mg, powdered whole dried liver 125 mg, dried debittered yeast 125 mg, choline dihydrogen citrate 20 mg, inositol 20 mg, dl-methionine 20 mg, folic acid 0.1 mg, B_{12} 10 mcg, ferrous gluconate 30 mg, dicalcium phosphate 250 mg, copper sulfate 5 mg, magnesium sulfate 10 mg, manganese sulfate 5 mg, cobalt sulfate 0.2 mg, potassium Cl 2 mg, potassium iodide 0.15 mg. Tab. Bot. 100s, 250s, 500s, 1000s. *OTC.*
Use: Mineral, vitamin supplement.

Faratol. (Faraday) Vitamins A 12,500 units, D 1000 units, B_1 20 mg, B_2 6 mg, B_6 0.5 mg, B_{12} 15 mcg, folic acid 0.1 mg, niacinamide 10 mg, calcium pantothenate 3 mg, C 60 mg, E 5 units, choline dihydrogen citrate 20 mg, inositol 20 mg, dl-methionine 20 mg, whole dried liver 100 mg, dried debittered yeast 100 mg, dicalcium phosphate 200 mg, ferrous gluconate 30 mg, potassium iodide 0.2 mg, magnesium sulfate 7.2 mg, copper sulfate 5 mg, manganese sulfate 3.4 mg, cobalt sulfate 0.2 mg, potassium Cl 1.3 mg, zinc sulfate 2 mg, molybdenum 0.2 mg in a base of alfalfa. Tab. Bot. 100s, 250s, 500s, 1000s. *OTC.*
Use: Mineral, vitamin supplement.

Farbee with Vitamin C. (Major) Vitamins B_1 15 mg, B_2 10.2 mg, B_3 50 mg, B_5 10 mg, B_6 5 mg, C 300 mg. Capl. Bot. 100s, 130s, 1000s. *OTC.*
Use: Vitamin supplement.

Farbital. (Major) Butalbital. Tab. Bot. 100s. *c-III.*
Use: Hypnotic; sedative.

Farbital Compound. (Major) Butalbital, caffeine, aspirin. Cap. Bot. 100s. *c-III.*
Use: Analgesic; hypnotic; sedative.

Farbital Compound with Codeine #3. (Major) Butalbital, caffeine, aspirin, codeine 30 mg. Bot. 1000s. *c-III.*
Use: Analgesic; hypnotic; sedative.

Fareston. (Shire) Toremifene citrate 60 mg. Lactose. Tab. Bot. 30s, 100s. *Rx.*
Use: Antiestrogen, hormone.

•**farletuzumab.** (FAR-le-TOOZ-oo-mab) USAN.
Use: Antineoplastic.

•**faropenem medoxomil.** (FAR-oh-PEN-em) USAN.
Use: Anti-infective.

Faslodex. (AstraZeneca) Fulvestrant 50 mg/mL. Alcohol, benzyl alcohol, castor oil. Inj. Prefilled Syringe. 5 mL. *Rx.*
Use: Hormone, antiestrogen.

Fastlene. (BDI) Caffeine 200 mg. Cap. Bot. 100s, 500s. *OTC.*
Use: CNS stimulant, analeptic.

fat emulsion, intravenous.
See: Intralipid 30%.
Intralipid 20%.
Liposyn 10%.
Liposyn 20%.
Liposyn II 10%.
Liposyn II 20%.
Travamulsion 10%.
Travamulsion 20%.

•**fat, hard.** *NF 29.*
Use: Pharmaceutic aid (suppository base).

Father John's Medicine Plus. (Oakhurst Co.) Phenylephrine hydrochloride 1.67 mg, chlorpheniramine maleate 0.67 mg, dextromethorphan HBr 1.67 mg per 5 mL. Alcohol free. Liq. Bot. 118 mL. *OTC.*
Use: Upper respiratory combination, antitussive combination.

fat soluble vitamins.
See: Beta-carotene.
Calcifediol.
Calciferol.
Calcijex.
Calcitriol.
Cholecalciferol.
d' ALPHA E 400 Softgels.
d' ALPHA E 1000 Softgels.
Delta-D.
Doxercalciferol.
Drisdol.
Ergocalciferol.
Hectorol.
Mephyton.
Mixed E 400 Softgels.
Mixed E 1000 Softgels.
Palmitate-A 5000.
Paricalcitol.
Phytonadione.
Vita-Plus E.
Vitamin A.
Vitamin D_3.
Vitamin E.
Vitamin E with Mixed Tocopherols.
Vitamin K.
Zemplar.

Fattibase. (Paddock) Preblended fatty acid suppository base composed of triglycerides of coconut oil and palm kernel oil. Jar 1 lb, 5 lb.
Use: Pharmaceutical aid, suppository base.

•**faxeladol.** (FAX-el-a-dole) USAN.
Use: Analgesic.

FazaClo. (Azur) Clozapine 12.5 mg (phenylalanine 0.87 mg), 25 mg (phenylalanine 1.74 mg), 100 mg (phenylalanine 6.96 mg), 150 mg (phenylalanine 10.44 mg), 200 mg (phenylalanine 13.92 mg). Aspartame, mannitol. Mint flavor. Orally Disintegrating Tab. UD 48s (25 mg, 100 mg, 150 mg, 200 mg), 100s. *Rx.*
Use: Antipsychotic.

fazadinium bromide.
Use: Neuromuscular blocking agent.

•**fazarabine.** (fah-ZAY-rah-BEAN) USAN.
Use: Antineoplastic.

FE Aspartate. (Miller) Ferrous aspartate 112 mg (elemental iron 18 mg)/aspartic acid 85 mg. Tab. 90s. *OTC.*
Use: Mineral supplement.

Feberin. (Arcum) Ferrous gluconate 3 g, vitamins C 25 mg, B_1 2 mg, B_2 1 mg, B_6 1 mg, niacinamide 5 mg. Tab. Bot. 100s, 1000s. *OTC.*
Use: Mineral, vitamin supplement.

febrile antigens. (Laboratory Diagnostics) Group O antigens (somatic) are dyed blue and group H antigens (flagellars) are dyed red for clear identification for detection of bacterial agglutinins, bacterial infections. Vial 5 mL.
Use: Diagnostic aid.

Febrinol. (Eon Labs) Acetaminophen 325 mg. Tab. Bot. 100s, 1000s. *OTC.*
Use: Analgesic.

Fe-Brone. (Forest) Vitamins B_{12} 1 units, folic acid 1 mg, ferrous sulfate exsiccated (powdered) 200 mg, ferrous sulfate exsiccated (timed) 200 mg, C acid 100 mg, B_6 0.5 mg, B_1 2 mg, B_2 1 mg, copper 0.9 mg, zinc 0.5 mg, manganese 0.3 mg. Cap. Bot. 30s, 100s, 1000s. *Rx.*
Use: Mineral, vitamin supplement.

•**febuxostat.** (feb-UX-oh-stat) USAN.
Use: Hyperuricemia; xanthine oxidase/dehydrogenase inhibitor.
See: Uloric.

fecal softeners/surfactants.
See: Colace.
DC Softgels.
Diocto.
Docu.
Docusate Calcium.
Docusate Sodium.
D.O.S.
D-S-S.
ex-lax Stool Softener.
Genasoft.
Modane Soft.
Non-Habit Forming Stool Softener.
Phillips Liqui-Gels.
Regulax SS.
Silace.
Stool Softener.
Stool Softener DC.
Surfak Liquigels.

Fedahist Expectorant. (Schwarz Pharma) Guaifenesin 200 mg, pseudoephedrine hydrochloride 20 mg/5 mL, sorbitol. Alcohol free. *OTC.*
Use: Antihistamine, decongestant.

Fedahist Gyrocaps. (Schwarz Pharma) Pseudoephedrine hydrochloride 65 mg, chlorpheniramine maleate 10 mg. SR Cap. Bot. 100s. *Rx.*
Use: Antihistamine; decongestant.

Fedahist Tablets. (Schwarz Pharma) Pseudoephedrine hydrochloride 60 mg, chlorpheniramine maleate 4 mg, sorbitol (alcohol and sugar free). Tab. Bot. 100s. *Rx.*
Use: Antihistamine; decongestant.

Fedahist Timecaps. (Schwarz Pharma) Pseudoephedrine hydrochloride 120 mg, chlorpheniramine maleate 8 mg. SR Cap. Bot. 100s. *Rx.*
Use: Antihistamine; decongestant.

Feen-a-Mint. (Schering-Plough) Bisacodyl 5 mg, talc, lactose, sugar. EC Tab. Pkg. 30s. *OTC.*
Use: Laxative.

Feen-a-Mint Dual Formula. (Schering-Plough) Docusate sodium 100 mg, yellow phenolphthalein 65 mg. Tab. Box 15s, 30s, 60s. *OTC.*
Use: Laxative.

Feen-a-Mint Gum. (Schering-Plough) Yellow phenolphthalein 97.2 mg. Chewing gum. Tab. Box 5s, 16s, 40s. *OTC.*
Use: Laxative.

Feg-I. (Western Research) Ferrous gluconate 300 mg. Tab. Handicount 28s (36 bags of 28 tab.). *OTC.*
Use: Mineral supplement.

Feiba NF. (Baxter) Anti-inhibitor coagulant complex 500 units/vial, 1,000 units/vial, 2,500 units/vial. Dry natural rubber latex, sodium chloride 8 mg/mL, trisodium citrate 4 mg/mL. Nanofiltered and vapor heated. Heparin free. Inj., lyophilized Pow. for Soln. Single-dose vial w/*Baxject* needleless transfer device w/20 mL or 50 mL of diluent. *Rx.*
Use: Antihemophilic agent.

•**felbamate.** (FELL-buh-MATE) USAN.
Use: Antiepileptic; treatment of Lennox-Gastaut syndrome [Orphan Drug]
See: Felbatol.

Felbatol. (Wallace) Felbamate. **Tab.:** 400 mg, 600 mg, lactose. Bot. 100s, UD 100s. **Susp.:** 600 mg/5 mL, sorbitol, parabens, saccharin. Bot. 240 mL, 960 mL. *Rx.*
Use: Antiepileptic. It has been recommended that use of this drug be discontinued if aplastic anemia or hepatic failure occurs unless, in the judgment of the physician, continued therapy is warranted. For further information contact Wallace Labs at 609-655-6000.

•**felbinac.** (FELL-bih-nak) USAN.
Use: Anti-inflammatory.

Feldene. (Pfizer) Piroxicam 10 mg, 20 mg. Lactose. Cap. Bot. 100s. *Rx.*
Use: Nonsteroidal anti-inflammatory agent.

Fellobolic. (Forest) Methandriol dipropionate 50 mg/mL. Inj. Vial 10 mL. *Rx.*

•**felodipine.** (feh-LOW-dih-peen) *USP 34.*
Use: Vasodilator, calcium channel blocker.

felodipine. (Mutual) Felodipine 2.5 mg, 5 mg, 10 mg. Film-coated. ER Tab. 30s, 90s, 100s, 250s, 500s, 1000s. *Rx.*
Use: Vasodilator, calcium channel blocker.

felodipine and enalapril maleate.
Use: Antihypertensive.

•**felvizumab.** (fell-VYE-zoo-mab) USAN.
Use: Antiviral (systemic), monoclonal antibody.

•**felypressin.** (fell-ih-PRESS-in) USAN.
Use: Vasoconstrictor.

Femagene. (Tennessee Pharmaceutic) Boric acid, sodium borate, lactic acid, menthol, methylbenzethonium Cl, parachlorometaxylenol, lactose, surface-active agents. Pow. 6 oz. *OTC.*
Use: Feminine hygiene.

Femara. (Novartis) Letrozole 2.5 mg. Lactose. Film-coated. Tab. Bot. 30s. *Rx.*
Use: Hormone; aromatase inhibitor.

Femazole. (Major) Metronidazole 250 mg, 500 mg. Tab. **250 mg:** Bot. 100s, 250s, 500s. **500 mg:** Bot. 50s, 100s. *Rx.*
Use: Anti-infective.

Femcaps. (Buffington) Acetaminophen, caffeine, ephedrine sulfate, atropine sulfate. Tab. Sugar, lactose, and salt free. Dispens-a-Kit 500s, Aidpaks 100s. *Rx.*
Use: Analgesic; anticholinergic; antispasmodic; bronchodilator.

Femcon Fe. (Warner Chilcott) Ethinyl estradiol/norethindrone 35 mcg/0.4 mg. Lactose, maltodextrin, sucralose. Spearmint flavor. Chew. Tab. 21s with 7 brown tablets (ferrous fumarate 75 mg). *Rx.*
Use: Oral contraceptive.

Femergin.
See: Ergotamine Tartrate.

Femhrt. (Warner Chilcott) Ethinyl estradiol/norethindrone acetate 2.5 mcg/

0.5 mg, 5 mcg/1 mg. Lactose. Tab. Bot. 90s, blister card 28s. *Rx.*
Use: Sex hormone, estrogens and pro-gestins combined.

Femidyn.
See: Estrone.

Feminique Disposable Douche. (Du-rex) Sodium benzoate, sorbic acid, lac-tic acid, octoxynol-9. Twin-packs. Bot. 120 mL. *OTC.*
Use: Douche.

Feminique Disposable Douche. (Du-rex) Vinegar and water. Soln. Twin-packs. Bot. 180 mL. *OTC.*
Use: Douche.

Feminone. (Pharmacia) Ethinyl estradiol 0.05 mg. Tab. Bot. 100s. *Rx.*
Use: Estrogen.

Femiron. (Menley & James Labs, Inc.) Ferrous fumarate 63 mg (iron 20 mg). Tab. Bot. 40s, 120s. *OTC.*
Use: Mineral supplement.

Femotrone. (Bluco) Progesterone in oil 50 mg/mL. Vial 10 mL. *Rx.*
Use: Hormone, progestin.

FemPatch. (Parke-Davis) Estradiol 10.3 mg (0.025 mg/day). Patch. Box. 4s. *Rx.*
Use: Estrogen.

Fem ph. (Pharmics) Glacial acetic acid 0.9%, oxyquinoline sulfate 0.025%, gly-cerin, PEG 4500. Vaginal jelly. 50 g w/applicator. *OTC.*
Use: Vaginal preparation.

Femring. (Warner Chilcott) Estradiol ace-tate 0.05 mg/day, 0.1 mg/day. Vaginal Ring. Single packs. *Rx.*
Use: Estrogen, sex hormone.

Femtrace. (Warner Chilcott) Estradiol acetate 0.45 mg, 0.9 mg, 1.8 mg. Lac-tose. Tab. 100s. *Rx.*
Use: Sex hormone, estrogen.

•**fenalamide.** (fen-AL-am-IDE) USAN.
Use: Muscle relaxant.

fenamisal. Phenyl aminosalicylate.

•**fenamole.** (FEN-ah-mole) USAN.
Use: Anti-inflammatory.

Fenaprin. (Sanofi-Synthelabo) Aspirin, chlormezanone. Tab. *Rx.*
Use: Analgesic; anxiolytic.

Fenarol. (Sanofi-Synthelabo) Chlormeza-none 100 mg, 200 mg. Tab. Bot. 100s.
Use: Anxiolytic.

fenarsone.
See: Carbarsone.

•**fenbendazole.** (FEN-BEND-ah-zole) USAN.
Use: Anthelmintic.

•**fenbufen.** (FEN-byoo-fen) USAN.
Use: Anti-inflammatory.

•**fencibutirol.** (fen-sih-BYOO-tih-role) USAN.
Use: Choleretic.

•**fenclofenac.** (FEN-kloe-fen-ACK) USAN.
Use: Anti-inflammatory.

•**fenclonine.** (fen-KLOE-neen) USAN. Un-der study by Pfizer.
Use: Serotonin inhibitor.

•**fenclorac.** (FEN-kloe-rack) USAN.
Use: Anti-inflammatory.

Fend. (Mine Safety Appliances) **A-2:** Water-soluble cream which forms a physical barrier to water-insoluble irri-tants. Tube 3 oz, Jar lb. **E-2:** This cream combines the functions of the water-soluble Fend A-2 and water-insoluble Fend I-2 creams. Tube 3 oz, Jar lb. **I-2:** Water-insoluble cream which forms a physical barrier to water-soluble irri-tants. Tube 3 oz, Jar lb. **S-2:** A silicone cream which forms a barrier against a combination of water-soluble and water-insoluble irritants Tube 3 oz, Jar lb. **X:** Industrial cold cream which rubs well into the skin and serves as a skin con-ditioner. Tube 3 oz, Jar lb. *OTC.*
Use: Skin protectant.

Fendol. (Buffington) Salicylamide, caf-feine, acetaminophen, phenylephrine hydrochloride. Sugar, lactose and salt free. Tab. Dispens-A-Kit 500s. Bot. 100s. *OTC.*
Use: Analgesic combination.

•**fendosal.** (FEN-doe-sal) USAN.
Use: Anti-inflammatory.

Fenesin DM IR. (Pharma Medica) Dex-tromethorphan HBr 15 mg, guaifene-sin 400 mg. Tab. 100s. *OTC.*
Use: Upper respiratory combination, an-titussive with expectorant.

•**fenestrel.** (feh-NESS-trell) USAN. Under study.
Use: Estrogen.

•**fenethylline hydrochloride.** (FEN-ETH-ill-in) USAN.
Use: Stimulant (central).

•**fenfluramine hydrochloride.** (fen-FLUR-a-meen) USAN.
Use: Used as anorexic agent before withdrawal from US market.

•**fengabine.** (FEN-GAH-bean) USAN.
Use: Mood regulator.

•**fenimide.** (FEN-ih-mid) USAN.
Use: Anxiolytic; antipsychotic.

•**fenisorex.** (fen-EYE-so-rex) USAN.
Use: Anorexigenic; anorexic.

•**fenmetozole hydrochloride.** (FEN-MET-oh-zole) USAN.
Use: Antidepressant; antagonist (to nar-cotics).

•**fenmetramide.** (fen-MEH-trah-mide)
USAN.
Use: Antidepressant.
•**fennel oil.** (FEN-el) *NF 29.*
Use: Pharmaceutic aid (flavor).
•**fenobam.** (FEN-oh-bam) USAN.
Use: Hypnotic; sedative.
•**fenoctimine sulfate.** (fen-OCK-tih-
MEEN) USAN.
Use: Gastric antisecretory.
fenofibrate.
Use: Antihyperlipidemic, fibric acid de-
rivative.
See: Antara.
Fenoglide.
Fibricor.
Lipofen.
Lofibra.
TriCor.
Triglide.
Trilipix.
fenofibrate. (Global Pharmaceuticals)
Fenofibrate 160 mg. Polydextrose. Film
coated. Tab. 90s, 100s, 500s, 1,000s.
Rx.
Use: Antihyperlipidemic, fibric acid de-
rivative.
fenofibrate. (Various Mfr.) Fenofibrate.
Cap. (micronized): 67 mg, 134 mg,
200 mg. 100s. **Tab.:** 54 mg, 107 mg.
10s, 90s, 500s (54 mg only), 1000s. *Rx.*
Use: Antihyperlipidemic, fibric acid de-
rivative.
Fenoglide. (Shore Therapeutics) Fenofibrate 40 mg, 120 mg. Lactose. Tab.
90s. *Rx.*
Use: Antihyperlipidemic agent, fibric
acid derivative.
•**fenoldopam mesylate.** (feh-NAHL-doe-
pam) *USP 34.*
Use: Antihypertensive; dopamine agonist.
See: Corlopam.
fenoldopam mesylate. (Baxter)
Fenoldopam mesylate 10 mg/mL. Sodium metabisulfite. Inj. Single-dose
amps. 1 mL, 2 mL. *Rx.*
Use: Antihypertensive.
•**fenoprofen.** (FEN-oh-PRO-fen) USAN.
Use: Anti-inflammatory; analgesic.
fenoprofen. (Qualitest) Fenoprofen
200 mg, 300 mg. Cap. Bot. 100s. *Rx.*
Use: Anti-inflammatory; analgesic.
fenoprofen. (Various Mfr.) Fenoprofen
calcium. **Cap.:** 200 mg, 300 mg. Bot.
100s. **Tab.:** 600 mg. Bot. 100s, 500s,
1000s; UD 100s; unit-of-use 30s, 60s,
90s, 120s. *Rx.*
Use: Anti-inflammatory; analgesic,
NSAID.

•**fenoprofen calcium.** (FEN-oh-PRO-fen)
USP 34.
Use: Anti-inflammatory; analgesic.
See: Nalfon.
•**fenoterol hydrobromide.** (FEN-oh-TER-
ahl) USAN.
Use: Investigational bronchodilator.
•**fenpipalone.** (FEN-PIP-ah-lone) USAN.
Use: Anti-inflammatory.
•**fenprinast hydrochloride.** (fen-PRIH-
nast) USAN.
Use: Bronchodilator, antiallergic.
•**fenprostalene.** (FEN-PRAHST-ah-leen)
USAN.
Use: Luteolysin.
•**fenquizone.** (FEN-kwih-zone) USAN.
Use: Diuretic.
•**fenretinide.** (fen-RET-ih-nide) USAN.
Use: Investigational antineoplastic.
•**fenspiride hydrochloride.** (fen-SPIH-
rid) USAN.
Use: Bronchodilator; antiadrenergic (α-
receptor).
•**fentanyl.** (FEN-ta-nil) USAN.
Tall Man: fentaNYL
Use: Opioid analgesic.
See: Abstral.
Actiq.
Fentora.
•**fentanyl citrate.** (FEN-tuh-nill) *USP 34.*
Tall Man: fentaNYL
Use: Opioid analgesic.
See: Onsolis.
fentanyl citrate. (Various Mfr.) Fentanyl
citrate (as base) 50 mcg/mL. Inj. Amp.
2 mL, 5 mL, 10 mL, 20 mL. Single-
dose vials. 30 mL, 50 mL. *c-II.*
Use: Opioid analgesic.
fentanyl citrate transmucosal. (Various
Mfr.) Fentanyl citrate (as base)
200 mcg, 400 mcg, 600 mcg, 800 mcg,
1200 mcg, 1600 mcg. Sugar. Berry fla-
vor. Loz. on a Stick. 30s with carton
blister packs. *c-II.*
Use: Opioid analgesic.
fentanyl citrate transmucosal. (Various
Mfr.) Fentanyl citrate (as base)
200 mcg, 400 mcg, 600 mcg, 800 mcg,
1200 mcg, 1600 mcg. Sugar. Berry flavor. Loz. on a Stick. Blister cartons.
30s. *c-II.*
Use: Opioid analgesic.
fentanyl citrate transmucosal system.
Use: Opioid analgesic.
See: Actiq.
fentanyl transdermal system.
Use: Opioid analgesic.
See: Duragesic-12.
Duragesic-50.
Duragesic-100.

Duragesic-75.
Duragesic-25.

fentanyl transdermal system. (Sandoz) Fentanyl 1.25 mg (12.5 mcg/h). Transdermal System. Cartons containing 5 individually packaged systems. *c-II.*
Use: Opioid analgesic.

fentanyl transdermal system. (Various Mfr.) Fentanyl 2.5 to 2.55 mg (25 mcg/h); 5 to 5.1 mg (50 mcg/h); 7.5 to 7.65 mg (75 mcg/h); 10 to 10.2 mg (100 mcg/h) (for use only in opioid-tolerant patients). Transdermal system. Cartons containing 5 individually packaged systems. *c-II.*
Use: Opioid analgesic.

•**fentiazac.** (fen-TIE-azz-ACK) USAN.
Use: Anti-inflammatory.

•**fenticlor.** (FEN-tih-Klor) USAN.
Use: Antifungal; antiseptic, topical.

•**fenticonazole nitrate.** (FEN-tih-KOE-nah-zole) USAN.
Use: Antifungal.

Fenton. (Sanofi-Synthelabo) Ferrous gluconate. Elix. *OTC.*
Use: Mineral supplement.

Fentora. (Cephalon) Fentanyl citrate (as base) 100 mcg, 200 mcg, 400 mcg, 600 mcg, 800 mcg. Mannitol. Tab. Blister cards. 28s. *c-II.*
Use: Opioid analgesic.

Fenylhist. (Roberts) Diphenhydramine hydrochloride 25 mg, 50 mg. Cap. Bot. 1000s. *OTC.*
Use: Antihistamine.

fenyramidol hydrochloride. Phenyramidol hydrochloride.

•**fenyripol hydrochloride.** (FEH-nee-rih-pahl) USAN.
Use: Muscle relaxant.

Feocyte Injectable. (Oxypure) Peptonized iron 15 mg, vitamin B_{12} 200 mcg, liver injection, beef 10 units, sodium citrate 10 mg, benzyl alcohol 2%/mL. Inj. Vial 10 mL. *Rx.*
Use: Mineral, vitamin supplement.

Feocyte Tablets. (Oxypure) Iron 110 mg, vitamins C 100 mg, B_6 2 mg, B_{12} 50 mcg, copper sulfate, folic acid 0.8 mg, desiccated liver 15 mg. Prolonged Action Tab. Bot. 100s. *Rx.*
Use: Mineral, vitamin supplement.

FeoGen. (Rising) Fe 66 mg (as elemental iron), vitamin B_{12} 10 mcg, desiccated stomach substance 100 mg, C 250 mg. Cap. UD 100s. *Rx.*
Use: Vitamin, mineral supplement.

FeoGen FA. (Rising) Fe 66 mg (as elemental iron), vitamin B_{12} 10 mcg, C 250 mg, folic acid 1 mg. Cap. UD 100s.

Rx.
Use: Vitamin, mineral supplement.

FeoGen Forte. (Rising) Fe 15 mg, B_{12} 10 mcg, C 60 mg, folic acid 1 mg. Softgel Cap. 100s. *Rx.*
Use: Vitamin, mineral supplement.

Feosol. (GlaxoSmithKline) Carbonyl iron 45 mg. Tab. Bot. 30s, 60s. *OTC.*
Use: Vitamin, mineral supplement.

Feosol. (GlaxoSmithKline) Ferrous sulfate exsiccated (dried) 200 mg (iron 65 mg), 325 mg (65 mg). Glucose (200 mg only). Tab. Bot. 100s. *OTC.*
Use: Mineral supplement.

Feosol Elixir. (GlaxoSmithKline) Ferrous sulfate (44 mg iron) 220 mg/5 mL, alcohol 5%. Elix. Bot. 16 oz. *OTC.*
Use: Mineral supplement.

FE-Plus Protein. (Miller Pharmacal Group) Iron (as an iron-protein complex) 50 mg. Tab. Bot. 100s. *OTC.*
Use: Mineral supplement.

Feraheme. (AMAG Pharmaceuticals) Ferumoxytol. Elemental iron 30 mg/mL. Mannitol 44 mg. Preservative free. Single-use vial. *Rx.*
Use: Trace element.

Feratab. (Upsher-Smith) Ferrous sulfate exsiccated (dried) 300 mg (iron 60 mg. Tab. Bot. UD 100s. *OTC.*
Use: Mineral supplement.

Ferate-C. (Pal-Pak, Inc.) Ferrous fumarate 150 mg, ascorbic acid 200 mg, docusate sodium 25 mg. Tab. Bot. 100s, 1000s. *OTC.*
Use: Mineral, vitamin supplement; stool softener.

Fergon. (Bayer) Ferrous gluconate 225 mg (iron 27 mg). Tab. Bot. 100s. *OTC.*
Use: Mineral supplement.

Feridex I.V. (Bayer) Iron 11.2 mg (iron 56 mg/vial). Soln. Inj. Single-dose vials w/administration filters. 5 mL. *Rx.*
Use: Radiopaque agent, parenteral.

Fer-Iron. (Rugby) Ferrous sulfate 15 mg of iron per mL. Alcohol 0.2%, lemon flavoring, sorbitol, sucrose. Drops. 50 mL. *OTC.*
Use: Trace element, iron-containing product.

Ferocyl. (Arco) Ferrous fumarate 150 mg (iron 50 mg), docusate sodium 100 mg. TR Cap. Bot. 100s. *OTC.*
Use: Mineral supplement; stool softener.

Fero-Folic 500. (Abbott) Ferrous sulfate controlled-release (equivalent to 105 mg iron), vitamin C 500 mg, folic acid 0.8 mg. Filmtab. Bot. 100s, 500s. *Rx.*
Use: Mineral, vitamin supplement.

Fero-Grad-500. (Abbott) Sodium ascorbate 500 mg, ferrous sulfate equivalent to 105 mg iron. Castor oil. CR Tab. Blister pack 30s. *OTC.*
Use: Mineral supplement.

Ferolix. (Century) Ferrous sulfate 5 g, alcohol 5%/10 mL Elix. Bot. 8 oz, pt, gal. *OTC.*
Use: Mineral supplement.

Ferosan. (Sandia) Ferrous fumarate 91.2 mg, B_1 10 mg, B_6 3 mg, B_{12} 25 mcg/5 mL. Syr. Bot. 16 oz, gal. *OTC.*
Use: Mineral, vitamin supplement.

Ferosan Forte. (Sandia) Ferrous fumarate 300 mg, liver-stomach concentrate 150 mg, vitamin B_{12} w/intrinsic factor concentrate 7.5 mcg, intrinsic factor concentrate 150 mg, B_{12} 7.5 mcg, ascorbic acid 75 mg, folic acid 1 mg, sorbitol 50 mg. Tab. Bot. 100s. *Rx.*
Use: Mineral, vitamin supplement.

Ferospace. (Hudson Corp.) Ferrous sulfate 250 mg (iron 50 mg). TR Cap. Bot. 100s. *OTC.*
Use: Mineral supplement.

FeroSul. (Major) Ferrous sulfate 325 mg (iron 65 mg). Tab. 100s, 1,000s. *OTC.*
Use: Mineral supplement.

Ferotrinsic. (Rugby) Iron 110 mg (from ferrous fumarate), vitamins B_{12} 15 mcg, C 75 mg, intrinsic factor (as concentrate or from stomach preparations) 240 mg, folic acid 0.5 mg. Cap. 100s, 500s, 1000s. *Rx.*
Use: Mineral, vitamin supplement.

Feroweet. (Barth's) Vitamins B_1 6 mg, B_2 12 mg, niacin 4 mg, iron 30 mg, B_{12} 10 mcg, B_6 95 mcg, pantothenic acid 50 mcg. 3 Cap. Bot. 100s, 500s, 1000s. *OTC.*
Use: Mineral, vitamin supplement.

Ferracomp. (Roberts) Liver 2 mcg, vitamins B_{12} 15 mcg, B_1 10 mg, B_2 5 mg, B_6 1 mg, calcium pantothenate 1 mg, niacinamide 10 mg, iron 31.3 mg/mL. Vial 30 mL. *OTC.*
Use: Mineral, vitamin supplement.

Ferralet 90. (Mission Pharmacal) Iron 90 mg (as carbonyl iron), folic acid 1 mg, vitamin B12 12 mcg, vitamin C 120 mg, docusate sodium 50 mg. Film coated. Tab. 90s. *Rx.*
Use: Nutritional agent, trace element.

Ferralet Plus. (Mission Pharmacal) Ferrous gluconate equivalent to 46 mg iron, C 400 mg, folic acid 0.8 mg, vitamin B_{12} 25 mcg. Tab. Bot. 60s. *OTC.*
Use: Mineral, vitamin supplement.

Ferrets. (Pharmics) Ferrous fumarate 325 mg, iron 106 mg. Polydextrose.

Film-coated. Tab. Bot. 60s. *OTC.*
Use: Mineral supplement.

Ferrex 150. (Breckenridge) Iron (as polysaccharide-iron complex) 150 mg. Cap. UD 100s. *OTC.*
Use: Mineral supplement.

Ferrex 150 Forte. (Breckenridge) Iron 150 mg (as polysaccharide-iron complex), folic acid 1 mg, B_{12} 25 mcg. Cap. UD 100s. *Rx.*
Use: Vitamin, mineral supplement.

Ferrex 150 Plus. (Breckenridge) Fe (from polysaccharide iron and ferrous bisglycinate) 150 mg, ascorbic acid 50 mg. Cap. UD 100s. *OTC.*
Use: Mineral, vitamin supplement.

Ferrex PC. (Breckenridge) Iron 60 mg (as polysaccharide-iron complex), folic acid 1 mg, C 50 mg, B_{12} 3 mcg, A 4000 units, D 400 units, B_1 3 mg, B_2 3 mg, B_6 2 mg, niacinamide 10 mg, Ca 25 mg, Zn 18 mg. Tab. UD 100s. *Rx.*
Use: Vitamin, mineral supplement.

Ferrex PC Forte. (Breckenridge) Vitamins A 5000 units, C 80 mg, Ca 250 mg, iron 60 mg (as polysaccharide-iron complex), D 400 units, E (as dl–alpha–tocopheryl acetate) 30 units, B_1 3 mg, B_2 3.4 mg, niacinamide 20 mg, B_6 4 mg, folic acid 1 mg, B_{12} 12 mcg, I, Mg, Zn 25 mg, Cu. Tab. UD 100s. *Rx.*
Use: Vitamin, mineral supplement.

• **ferric ammonium citrate.** (FER-ik) *USP 34.* Ammonium iron (Fe^{+++}) citrate.
Use: Mineral supplement.

• **ferric ammonium citrate for oral solution.** (FER-ik) *USP 34.*
Use: Mineral supplement.

ferric ammonium sulfate. (Various Mfr.)
Use: Astringent.

ferric ammonium tartrate. (Various Mfr.)
Use: Mineral supplement.

ferric cacodylate. (Various Mfr.)
Use: Leukemias; hematinic.

ferric chloride. (Various Mfr.)
Use: Astringent.

• **ferric chloride Fe 59.** (FER-ik) USAN.
Use: Radiopharmaceutical.

ferric citrochloride tincture. Iron (Fe^{+++}) chloride citrate.
Use: Hematinic.

• **ferric fructose.** (FER-ik FRUKE-tose) USAN.
Use: Hematinic.

ferric glycerophosphate. Glycerol phosphate iron (Fe^{+++}) salt.
Use: Pharmaceutic necessity.

ferric hypophosphate. Iron (Fe^{+++}) phosphonate.
Use: Pharmaceutic necessity.

•**ferriclate calcium sodium.** (fer-ih-KLATE) USAN.
Use: Hematinic.

•**ferric oxide.** (FER-ik) *NF 29.*
Use: Pharmaceutic aid (color).

ferric oxide, yellow.
Use: Pharmaceutic aid (color).

ferric "peptonate". (Various Mfr.)
See: Iron Peptonized.

ferric pyrophosphate, soluble. Iron (Fe^{+++}) citrate pyrophosphate.

ferric quinine citrate, "green". (Various Mfr.)
Use: Mineral supplement.

•**ferric subsulfate solution.** (FER-ik) *USP 34.*
Use: Local use on the skin.

•**ferric sulfate.** (FER-ik) *USP 34.*
Use: Compounding agent.

•**ferristene.** (FER-ih-steen) USAN.
Use: Diagnostic aid, paramagnetic.

Ferrizyme. (Abbott Diagnostics) Enzyme immunoassay for qualitative determination of ferritin in human serum or plasma. Test kit 100s.
Use: Diagnostic aid, paramagnetic.

Ferrlecit. (Sanofi Pharmaceuticals) Sodium ferric gluconate complex 62.5 mg/5 mL (12.5 mg/mL of elemental iron), benzyl alcohol 9 mg/mL, sucrose 20%. Inj. Amp. 5 mL. *Rx.*
Use: Iron-containing product.

ferrocholate.
See: Ferrocholinate.

ferrocholinate. Ferrocholate. Ferrocholine. A chelate prepared by reacting equimolar quantities of freshly precipitated ferric hydroxide with choline dihydrogen citrate.
Use: Mineral supplement.

ferrocholine.
See: Ferrocholinate.

Ferro-Cyte. (Spanner) Iron peptonate 20 mg, liver injection (20 mg/mL) 0.25 mL, vitamins B_1 22 mg, B_2 0.5 mg, B_6 2.5 mg, B_{12} 30 mcg, niacinamide 25 mg, panthenol 1 mg/mL. Inj. Multiple-dose vial 10 mL. *Rx.*
Use: Mineral, vitamin supplement.

Ferro-Docusate TR. (Parmed Pharmaceuticals, Inc.) Ferrous fumarate 150 mg (iron 50 mg), docusate sodium 100 mg. TR Cap. Bot. 100s. *OTC.*
Use: Mineral supplement; stool softener.

Ferro-Dok TR. (Major) Ferrous fumarate 150 mg (iron 50 mg), docusate sodium 100 mg. TR Cap. Bot. 100s. *OTC.*
Use: Mineral supplement; stool softener.

Ferrodyl Chewable Tablets. (Arcum) Ferrous fumarate 320 mg, vitamin C 200 mg. Bot. 100s, 1000s. *OTC.*
Use: Mineral, vitamin supplement.

Ferromar. (Marnel) Ferrous fumarate 201.5 mg (iron 65 mg), vitamin C 200 mg. SR Capl. Bot. 100s. *OTC.*
Use: Mineral supplement.

Ferroneed. (Hanlon) Ferrous gluconate 300 mg, ascorbic acid 60 mg. Cap. Bot. 100s. *OTC.*
Use: Mineral, vitamin supplement.

Ferroneed T-Caps. (Hanlon) Ferrous fumarate 250 mg, thiamine hydrochloride 5 mg, ascorbic acid 50 mg. TD Cap. Bot. 100s. *OTC.*
Use: Mineral, vitamin supplement.

Ferronex. (Taylor Pharmaceuticals) Iron from ferrous gluconate 2.9 mg, vitamins B_{12} equivalent 1 mcg, B_2 0.75 mg, B_3 50 mg, B_5 1.25 mg, B_{12} 15 mcg, procaine 2%/mL. Inj. Vial 30 mL. *Rx.*
Use: Mineral, vitamin supplement.

Ferro-Sequels. (Can-Am/Access) Ferrous fumarate 150 mg (iron 50 mg), sodium docusate 100 mg, lactose. TR Tab. Bot. 30s, 90s. *OTC.*
Use: Mineral supplement.

Ferrospan. (Imperial Lab) Ferrous fumarate 200 mg, ascorbic acid 100 mg. Tab. Bot. 100s, 1000s. *OTC.*
Use: Mineral, vitamin supplement.

Ferrosyn Injection. (Standex) Cyanocobalamin 30 mcg, liver 2 mcg, ferrous gluconate 100 mg, riboflavin 1.5 mg, panthenol 2.5 mg, niacinamide 100 mg, procaine 2%. Inj. Vial 30 mL. *Rx.*
Use: Mineral, vitamin supplement.

Ferrosyn S.C. (Standex) Iron 60 mg, vitamin B_{12} 5 mcg, magnesium 0.6 mg, copper 0.3 mg, manganese 0.1 mg, potassium 0.5 mg, zinc 0.15 mg. Tab. Bot. 100s, 1000s. *OTC.*
Use: Mineral, vitamin supplement.

Ferrosyn See. (Standex) Iron 34 mg, ascorbic acid 60 mg. Tab. Bot. 100s, 1000s. *OTC.*
Use: Mineral, vitamin supplement.

Ferrosyn Tablets. (Standex) Fe 60 mg, vitamin B_{12} 5 mcg, Mg 0.6 mg, Cu 0.3 mg, Mn 0.1 mg, K 0.5 mg, Zn 0.15 mg. Tab. Bot. 100s. *OTC.*
Use: Mineral, vitamin supplement.

ferrous aspartate.
Use: Mineral supplement.
See: FE Aspartate.

ferrous bromide. (FER-uhs) (Various Mfr.)
Use: In chorea & tuberculous cervical adenitis.

ferrous carbonate mass. Vallet's mass.
(Various Mfr.)
Use: Mineral supplement.
ferrous carbonate, saccharated.
(Various Mfr.)
Use: Mineral supplement.
•**ferrous citrate Fe 59.** (FER-uhs) USAN.
Use: Radiopharmaceutical.
•**ferrous fumarate.** (FER-uhs) *USP 34.*
Use: Hematinic.
See: Albafort.
Ferretts.
Ferro-Sequels.
Hemocyte.
W/Ascorbic Acid.
See: Eldofe-C.
Ferrodyl.
Ferromar.
W/Ascorbic Acid and Folic Acid.
See: Fer-Regules.
Ferro-Docusate TR.
Ferro Dok TR.
Ferro-DSS SR.
Ferro-Sequels.
W/Norethindrone, Mestranol.
See: Ortho Novum Fe-28.
W/Polysaccharide Iron Complex
See: Tandem.
W/Vitamins and Minerals.
See: Stuartnatal 1 + 1.
Stuart Prenatal.
ferrous fumarate. (Mission) Ferrous
fumarate 90 mg (iron 29.5 mg). Sugar.
Tab. Bot. 100s. *OTC.*
Use: Mineral supplement.
ferrous fumarate. (Various Mfr.) Ferrous
fumarate 324 mg (iron 106 mg). Tab.
100s. *OTC.*
Use: Mineral supplement.
**ferrous fumarate and docusate so-
dium.**
Use: Mineral supplement.
•**ferrous gluconate.** (FER-uhs) *USP 34.*
Use: Hematinic.
See: Fergon.
ferrous gluconate. (Various Mfr.) Ferrous gluconate 225 mg (iron 27 mg),
324 mg (iron 38 mg), 325 mg (iron
36 mg). Tab. Bot. 100s (except
325 mg), 1,000s (325 mg only). *OTC.*
Use: Mineral supplement.
ferrous iodide. (Various Mfr.)
Use: In chronic tuberculosis.
ferrous iodide syrup. (Various Mfr.)
Use: In chronic tuberculosis.
ferrous lactate. (Various Mfr.)
Use: Mineral supplement.
•**ferrous sulfate.** (FER-uhs) *USP 34.*
Use: Hematinic.
See: Enfamil Fer-In-Sol.

Feosol.
Fer-Iron.
Ferolix.
FeroSul.
Irospan.
W/Ascorbic Acid.
See: Fero-Grad-500.
W/Ascorbic Acid, Folic Acid.
See: Fero-Folic-500.
ferrous sulfate. (Hi-Tech) Iron 15 mg/
mL. Alcohol 0.2%, sodium bisulfite,
sorbitol, sucrose. Gluten free and lactose free. Drops. 50 mL w/dropper.
OTC.
Use: Trace element, iron.
ferrous sulfate. (Magnus-Humphries
Labs) Ferrous sulfate 27 mg. PEG. Tab.
100s. *OTC.*
Use: Trace element.
ferrous sulfate. (Pharmaceutical Associates) Ferrous sulfate 300 mg per 5 mL
(60 mg iron per 5 mL). Sucrose. Cinnamon flavor. Liq. UD 100s of 5 mL
each. *OTC.*
Use: Dietary supplement.
ferrous sulfate. (Qualitest) Ferrous sulfate 75 mg per 0.6 mL (iron 15 mg per
0.6 mL). Alcohol 0.2%. Drops. 50 mL.
OTC.
Use: Trace element.
ferrous sulfate. (Rugby) Ferrous sulfate
exsiccated (dried) 160 mg (iron 50 mg).
SR Tab. Blisterpack 60s. *OTC.*
Use: Mineral supplement.
ferrous sulfate. (Various Mfr.) Ferrous
sulfate. **Tab.:** 325 mg (iron 65 mg).
100s, 1,000s, UD 100s. **Elix.:** 220 mg/
5 mL (iron 44 mg/5 mL). May contain
alcohol. Bot. 473 mL. *OTC.*
Use: Mineral supplement.
ferrous sulfate. (Ivax) Ferrous sulfate
325 mg (elemental iron 65 mg). Tab.
Bot. 100s. *OTC.*
Use: Mineral supplement.
•**ferrous sulfate, dried.** (FER-uhs)
USP 34.
Use: Antianemic.
See: Feosol.
Fer-In-Sol.
Ferrous Sulfate.
Slow Fe.
ferrous sulfate exsiccated (dried).
Use: Mineral supplement.
See: Feosol.
Feratab.
Slow FE.
Slow Release Iron.
•**ferrous sulfate Fe 59.** (FER-uhs) USAN.
Use: Radiopharmaceutical.
Fertility Tape. (Weston Labs.) Regular,
extrasensitive, less-sensitive. W/Fertil-

ity Testor, cervical glucose test. Pkg.
test 60s.
Use: Diagnostic aid.

•**ferucarbotran.** (fur-you-CAR-boe-tran)
USAN.
Use: Diagnostic aid (paramagnetic).

•**ferumoxides.** (feh-roo-MOX-ides) USAN.
Use: Radiopaque agent.
See: Feridex I.V.

•**ferumoxtran-10.** (fur-you-MOX-tran 10)
USAN.
Use: Diagnostic aid (paramagnetic).

•**ferumoxytol.** (fer-yoo-MOX-i-tole)
USAN.
Use: Diagnostic aid (MRI); iron defi-
ciency.
See: Feraheme.

Ferusal. (Eon Labs) Ferrous sulfate
325 mg. Tab. *OTC.*
Use: Mineral supplement.

•**fesoterodine fumarate.** (FES-oh-TER-
oh-deen) USAN.
Use: Treatment of overactive bladder.
See: Toviaz.

Festalan. (Hoechst) Lipase 6000 units,
amylase 30,000 units, protease
20,000 units, atropine methylnitrate
1 mg. EC Tab. Bot. 100s, 1000s. *Rx.*
Use: Digestive enzyme.

Fetinic. (Roberts) Iron 3.6 mg, vitamins
B_{12} equivalent to 2 mcg, B_1 10 mg, B_2
0.5 mg, B_3 10 mg, B_5 1 mg, B_6 1 mg,
B_{12} 15 mcg, chlorobutanol 0.5%, benzyl alcohol 2%/mL. Vial 30 mL. *Rx.*
Use: Mineral, vitamin supplement.

Fetinic-MW. (Roberts) Iron 66 mg (from
ferrous fumarate), vitamins B_{12} 5 mcg,
C 60 mg. SR Cap. Bot. 100s. *OTC.*
Use: Mineral, vitamin supplement.

Fe-Tinic 150 Forte. (Ethex) Iron 150 mg
(as polysaccharide-iron complex), folic
acid 1 mg, B_{12} 25 mcg. Cap. UD 100s. *Rx.*
Use: Vitamin, mineral supplement.

•**fetoxylate hydrochloride.** (fee-TOX-ih-
LATE) USAN.
Use: Muscle relaxant.

FeverAll. (Actavis) Acetaminophen
650 mg. Hydrogenated vegetable oil.
Supp. 50s. *OTC.*
Use: Analgesic.

FeverAll Children's. (Actavis) Acetaminophen 120 mg. Hydrogenated vegetable oil. Supp. Pkg. 6s, 50s. *OTC.*
Use: Analgesic.

FeverAll Infants. (Actavis) Acetaminophen 80 mg. Hydrogenated vegetable
oil. Supp. Pkg. 6s, 50s. *OTC.*
Use: Analgesic.

FeverAll Junior Strength. (Actavis)
Acetaminophen 325 mg. Hydrogenated

vegetable oil. Supp. Pkg. 12s, 50s.
OTC.
Use: Analgesic.

•**feverfew.** (FEE-ver-fyoo) *NF 29.*
Use: Dietary supplement.

Fexmid. (Victory) Cyclobenzaprine
hydrochloride 7.5 mg. Film-coated. Tab.
100s. *Rx.*
Use: Skeletal muscle relaxant.

•**fexofenadine hydrochloride.** (fex-oh-
FEN-ah-deen) USAN.
Use: Antihistamine, peripherally selec-
tive piperidine.

fexofenadine hydrochloride.
Use: Antihistamine, peripherally selec-
tive piperidine.
See: Allegra.
    Allegra ODT.
W/Pseudoephedrine Hydrochloride.
See: Allegra-D 12 Hour.
    Allegra-D 24 Hour.

fexofenadine hydrochloride. (Various
Mfr.) Fexofenadine hydrochloride
30 mg, 60 mg, 180 mg. May contain
lactose. Tab. 30s, 60s (60 mg only),
100s, 500s, UD 100s. *Rx.*
Use: Antihistamine, peripherally selective piperidine.

**fexofenadine hydrochloride/pseudo-
ephedrine hydrochloride.** (Various
Mfr.) Fexofenadine hydrochloride
60 mg, pseudoephedrine hydrochloride
120 mg. May contain PEG. ER Tab.
100s, 500s. *Rx.*
Use: Upper respiratory combination, decongestant and antihistamine.

•**fezakinumab.** (FEZ-a-KIN-ue-mab)
USAN.
Use: Anti-inflammatory.

•**fezolamine fumarate.** (feh-ZOLE-ah-
MEEN) USAN.
Use: Antidepressant.

fgn-1. (Cell Pathways, Inc.)
Use: Treatment of adenomatous pol-
yposis coli. [Orphan Drug]

•**fiacitabine.** (fih-AH-sit-ah-BEEN) USAN.
Use: Antiviral.

•**fialuridine.** (fie-al-YOUR-ih-deen) USAN.
Use: Antiviral.

FIAU. (Oclassen)
Use: Antiviral, hepatitis B. [Orphan Drug]

fiber.
Use: Laxative.
See: Benefiber.
    Benefiber Drink Mix.
    Benefiber for Children.
    Benefiber Plus Calcium.
    Benefiber Plus Heart Health.
    Benefiber Sticks.
    Benefiber Ultra.

Fiberall Natural Flavor. (Novartis) **Pow.:**
Psyllium hydrophilic mucilloid 3.4 g,
wheat bran, sodium < 10 mg, potassium
60 mg, calories 6/5.9 g, saccharin. Can
150 g, 300 g, 450 g. **Wafer:** Psyllium
hydrophilic mucilloid 3.4 g, wheat bran,
oats, sucrose. Box 14s. *OTC.*
Use: Laxative.

Fiberall Orange Flavor. (Heritage Consumer) Psyllium hydrophilic mucilloid
3.5 g/dose, aspartame. Pow. Can
480 g. *OTC.*
Use: Laxative.

Fiberall Tropical Fruit Flavor. (Heritage
Consumer) Psyllium hydrophilic mucilloid 3.5 g/dose, aspartame. Pow. Can.
454 g, UD 10 g packets. *OTC.*
Use: Laxative.

FiberCon. (Wyeth) Calcium polycarbophil 625 mg (equiv. to 500 mg polycarbophil). Tab. Bot. 36s, 60s, 90s.
OTC.
Use: Laxative.

Fiber Guard. (Wyeth) All natural high-
fiber supplement 530 mg. Tab. Bot.
100s, 200s. *OTC.*
Use: Fiber supplement.

Fiberlan. (Elan) Protein 50 g, fat 40 g,
carbohydrates 160 g, Na 920 mg, K
1.56 g, fiber 14 g/per L. With vitamins
A, C, B, B_2, B_3, D, E, B_5, B_6, B_{12}, K, Ca,
Fe, folic acid, P, I, Mg, Zn, Cu, biotin,
Mn, choline, Cl, Se, Cr, Mo. Liq. Bot.
237 mL. *OTC.*
Use: Nutritional supplement.

Fiber-Lax. (Rugby) Calcium polycarbophil 625 mg (equiv. to 500 mg polycarbophil). Tab. Bot. 60s, 90s, 500s.
OTC.
Use: Laxative.

Fibermed High-Fiber Snacks. (Purdue)
One serving (15 snacks) contains 5 g
dietary fiber. Box 8 oz. Packs of
24 × 1.3 oz. *OTC.*
Use: Fiber supplement.

Fibermed High-Fiber Supplement.
(Purdue) Each supplement contains 5 g
dietary fiber. Box 14s. Institutional
pack, Box 144s of two supplements.
OTC.
Use: Fiber supplement.

FiberNorm. (G & W) Polycarbophil
625 mg. Tab. Bot. 60s, 90s. *OTC.*
Use: Laxative.

•**fiboflapon.** (FYE-boe-FLAP-on) USAN.
Use: Treatment of asthma and chronic
obstructive pulmonary disease.

Fibre Trim. (Schering-Plough) Grain and
citrus fruit concentrated dietary fiber.
Tab. Bot. 100s, 250s. *OTC.*
Use: Dietary aid.

Fibre Trim w/Calcium. (Schering-
Plough) Grain and citrus fruit concentrated dietary fiber w/calcium. Tab. Bot.
90s, 225s. *OTC.*
Use: Dietary aid.

fibric acid derivatives.
Use: Antihyperlipidemic.
See: Fenofibrate.
Gemfibrozil.

Fibricor. (Mutual Pharmaceutical) Fenofibrate 35 mg, 105 mg. Tab. 30s, 60s,
90s, 100s, 250s, 500s, 1,000s. *Rx.*
Use: Antihyperlipidemic agent, fibric
acid derivative.

fibrin agents.
See: Fibrin Sealant (Human).

fibrinogen concentrate (human).
See: RiaSTAP.

fibrinogen (human). (Alpha Therapeutic) Partially purified fibrinogen prepared by fractionation from normal human plasma.
Use: Coagulant, clotting factor. [Orphan
Drug]

•**fibrinogen I 125.** (FIE-BRIN-oh-jen)
USAN.
Use: Diagnostic aid (vascular patency);
radiopharmaceutical.

fibrinogen sealant (human). (fye-BRIN-
oh-jen)
See: TachoSil.

fibrinolysis inhibitor.
See: Amicar.

fibrin sealant (human).
Use: Fibrin agent.
See: Artiss.

Fibrogammin P. (Aventis Behring)
Use: Congenital Factor XIII deficiency.
[Orphan Drug]

•**fidaxomicin.** (fye-DAX-oh-MYE-sin)
USAN.
Use: Anti-infective.

•**fidexaban.** (fye-DEX-a-ban) USAN.
Use: Anticoagulant.

•**fiduxosin hydrochloride.** (fi-DUX-oe-
sin) USAN.
Use: Benign prostatic hyperplasia.

•**figitumumab.** (FIG-i-TOOM-ue-mab)
USAN.
Use: Antineoplastic.

•**filaminast.** (fih-LAM-in-ast) USAN.
Use: Antiasthmatic (selective phosphodiesterase IV inhibitor).

Filaxis. (Amlab) Vitamins A 25,000 units,
D 1250 units, C 150 mg, E 5 units, B_1
12 mg, B_2 5 mg, B_6 0.5 mg, B_{12} 5 mcg,
calcium pantothenate 5 mg, niacin-
amide 100 mg, Fe 15 mg, I 0.15 mg,
Mg 10 mg, K 5 mg, Ca 75 mg, P 60 mg.
Tab. Bot. 30s, 100s. Available w/B_{12}.

Bot. 30s, 60s, 100s. *OTC.*
Use: Mineral, vitamin supplement.

•filgrastim. (fill-GRAH-stim) USAN.
Use: Biological response modifier; antineoplastic adjunct; antineutropenic; hematopoietic stimulant. [Orphan Drug]
See: Neupogen.

•filibuvir. (fil-i-BUE-vir) USAN.
Use: Anti-infective.

•filipin. (FIH-lih-pin) USAN.
Use: Antifungal.

Finac. (C & M Pharmacal) Salicylic acid 2%, isopropyl alcohol 22.5%, propylene glycol, acetone in lotion base. Bot. 60 mL. *OTC.*
Use: Dermatologic, acne.

Finacea. (Bayer) Azelaic acid 15%, EDTA, benzoic acid. Gel. 30 g. *Rx.*
Use: Anti-inflammatory.

•finasteride. (fih-NASS-teer-ide) *USP 34.*
Use: Benign prostatic hypertrophy therapy; antineoplastic; antineutropenic; inhibitor (alpha-reductase); androgen hormone inhibitor.
See: Propecia.
Proscar.

finasteride. (Teva Pharmaceuticals) Finasteride 5 mg. Lactose. Film-coated. Tab. 30s, 100s, 500s. *Rx.*
Use: Androgen hormone inhibitor.

Finevin. (Berlex) Azelaic acid 20%, glycerin, cetearyl alcohol. Cream. Tube. 30 g. *Rx.*
Use: Anti-infective, antibiotic, topical.

•fingolimod hydrochloride. (fin-GOLE-i-mod) USAN.
Use: Immunomodulator.
See: Gilenya.

Fioricet. (Novartis) Acetaminophen 325 mg, butalbital 50 mg, caffeine 40 mg. Tab. Bot. 100s, 500s, UD 100s. *Rx.*
Use: Analgesic; hypnotic; sedative.

Fioricet with Codeine. (Novartis) Codeine phosphate 30 mg, acetaminophen 325 mg, caffeine 40 mg, butalbital 50 mg. Cap. Bot. 100s, *ControlPak* 25s. *c-III.*
Use: Narcotic analgesic combination.

Fiorinal. (Novartis) Butalbital 50 mg, caffeine 40 mg, aspirin 325 mg, benzyl alcohol, parabens, EDTA. Cap. Bot. 100s, 500s, UD 25s. *c-III.*
Use: Analgesic; hypnotic; sedative.

Fiorinal with Codeine No. 3. (Watson) Butalbital 50 mg, caffeine 40 mg, aspirin 325 mg, codeine phosphate 30 mg. Cap. Bot. 100s. *Control Pak* 25s. *c-III.*
Use: Analgesic combination; hypnotic; sedative.

fire ant venom, allergenic extract, imported.
Use: Dermatologic aid-skin test; immunotherapy. [Orphan Drug]

Firmagon. (Ferring) Degarelix acetate 80 mg, 120 mg. Mannitol 200 mg. Inj., lyophilized Pow. for Soln. Vial. *Rx.*
Use: Sex hormone, gonadotropin-releasing hormone antagonist.

Firmdent. (Moyco Union Broach Division) *Formerly Moy.* Karaya gum 94.6%, sodium borate 5.36%. Pkg. 3 oz. *OTC.*
Use: Denture adhesive.

•firocoxib. (fir-oh-KOX-ib) USAN.
Use: Analgesic, anti-inflammatory.

First Aid Cream. (Johnson & Johnson) Cetyl alcohol, glyceryl stearate, isopropyl palmitate, stearyl alcohol, synthetic beeswax. Tube 0.8 oz, 1.5 oz, 2.5 oz. *OTC.*
Use: Antiseptic; dermatologic, protectant.

First Aid Cream. (Walgreen) Benzocaine 3%, allantoin 0.2%, benzyl alcohol 4%, phenol 0.25%. Tube 1.5 oz. *OTC.*
Use: Anesthetic; antiseptic.

First Duke's Mouthwash. (Cutis Pharma) Diphenhydramine hydrochloride 0.525 g, hydrocortisone 0.06 g, nystatin 0.6 g. Benzyl alcohol, propylene glycol, propylparabens, saccharin, sorbitol. Susp. 237 mL compounding kit. *Rx.*
Use: Mouth and throat product.

First Mary's Mouthwash. (Cutis Pharma) Diphenhydramine hydrochloride 0.45 g, hydrocortisone 0.06 g, nystatin 1.2 g, tetracycline hydrochloride 1.5 g. Benzyl alcohol, propylene glycol, propylparabens, saccharin, sorbitol. Susp. 237 mL compounding kit. *Rx.*
Use: Mouth and throat product.

First Response Ovulation Predictor. (Tambrands, Inc.) Monoclonal antibody-based enzyme immunoassay test for hLH in urine. Test kit 1s. *OTC.*
Use: Diagnostic aid.

First Response Pregnancy Test. (Tambrands, Inc.) Reagent in-home kit for urine testing. Test kit 1s. *OTC.*
Use: Diagnostic aid.

fish oil concentrate, natural. Natural fish oil concentrate containing EPA (Eicosanoic acid) and DHA (Docosahexaenoic acid).
Use: Nutritional supplement.

•fispemifene. (fis-PEM-i-feen) USAN.
Use: Selective estrogen antagonist.

FIV-ASA. (Paddock) 5-aminosalicylic acid 500 mg. Supp. Bot. 30s. *Rx.*
Use: Gastrointestinal agent.

5-FC.
See: Flucytosine
5-FU.
See: Fluorouracil.
5-HT$_{1A}$ receptor agonists.
See: Vilazodone Hydrochloride.
523. (Enzyme Process) Pancreatin
200 mg, tryspin, chymotrypsin, amylase, lipase enzymes from pancreatin,
raw beef pancreas. Tab. Bot. 100s,
250s.
Use: Digestive enzyme.
Fixodent. (Procter & Gamble) Calcium
sodium poly (vinyl methyl ether-
maleate), carboxymethylcellulose so-
dium in a petrolatum base. Tube
0.75 oz, 1.5 oz, 2.5 oz. *OTC.*
Use: Denture adhesive.
FK506.
See: Prograf.
FK-565.
Use: Immunomodulator.
Flagyl. (Pfizer) Metronidazole 250 mg,
500 mg. Bot. 50s, 100s, 500s (500 mg
only), 2500s (250 mg only). *Rx.*
Use: Anti-infective.
Flagyl ER. (Pfizer) Metronidazole
750 mg, lactose. ER Tab. Bot. 30s. *Rx.*
Use: Anti-infective.
Flagyl 375. (Pfizer) Metronidazole
375 mg. Cap. Bot. 50s, UD 100s. *Rx.*
Use: Anti-infective.
Flanders Buttocks Ointment. (Flanders)
Zinc oxide, castor oil, balsam peru, bo-
ric acid in an emollient base. Tube.
60 g. *OTC.*
Use: Dermatologic, counterirritant.
Flarex. (Alcon) Fluorometholone acetate
0.1%. Benzalkonium chloride 0.01%,
EDTA, hydroxyethylcellulose, tyloxapol,
sodium chloride, monobasic sodium
phosphate. Ophth. Susp. Bot. 2.5 mL,
5 mL, 10 mL *Drop-Tainers. Rx.*
Use: Corticosteroid, ophthalmic; anti-
inflammatory.
Flatulence. (Pal-Pak, Inc.) Nux vomica
16.2 mg, cascara sagrada extract
64.8 mg, ginger 48.6 mg, capsicum
16.2 mg, asafetida. Tab. Bot. *OTC.*
Use: Antiflatulent; laxative.
Flatulex. (Dayton) Simethicone 40 mg/
0.6 mL. Drops. 30 mL with calibrated
dropper. *OTC.*
Use: Antiflatulent.
Flatus. (Foy Laboratories) Nux vomica
extract 0.25 g, cascara extract 1 g, ginger ¾ g, capsicum g, w/asafetida qs.
Tab. Bot. 1000s. *OTC.*
Use: Antiflatulent; laxative.
Flav-A-D. (Kirkman) Vitamins A
5000 units, D 1000 units, C 100 mg.

Tab. Bot. 100s, 1000s. Also w/fluoride.
Bot. 100s, 1000s. *Rx-OTC.*
Use: Vitamin supplement.
flavine.
See: Acriflavine Hydrochloride.
Flavinoid-C. (Barth's) **Tab.:** Vitamin C
150 mg, hesperidin complex 10 mg,
citrus bioflavonoid 50 mg, rutin 20 mg.
Bot. 100s, 500s, 1000s. **Liq.:** Vitamin
C 100 mg, bioflavonoid complex
100 mg/5 mL. Bot. 4 oz. *OTC.*
Use: Vitamin supplement.
flavocoxid.
Use: Oral nutritional supplement.
See: Limbrel.
•**flavodilol maleate.** (FLAY-voe-DILL-ole)
USAN.
Use: Antihypertensive.
flavolutan.
See: Progesterone.
flavonoid compounds.
See: Bio-Flavonoid Compounds; Vitamin P.
Flavons. (Freeda) Bioflavonoids 500 mg
(also contains calcium carbonate, cal-
cium stearate). Sugar free. Tab. Bot.
100s, 250s. *OTC.*
Use: Water-soluble vitamin.
Flavons-500. (Freeda) Citrus bioflavonoids 500 mg. Sugar free. Tab. Bot.
100s, 250s. *OTC.*
Use: Water-soluble vitamin.
flavored diluent. (Roxane) Flavored vehicle for the immediate administration
of crushed tablet or capsule product.
Bot. 500 mL, UD 15 mL × 100.
Use: Flavored vehicle.
•**flavoxate hydrochloride.** (flay-VOKES-
ate) USAN.
Tall Man: flavoxATE
Use: Antispasmodic, urinary; muscle relaxant; anticholinergic.
See: Urispas.
flavoxate hydrochloride. (Global)
Flavoxate hydrochloride 100 mg. Film
coated. Tab. 100s. *Rx.*
Use: Anticholinergic.
flavurol. Merbromin.
Use: Antiseptic.
•**flazalone.** (FLAY-zah-lone) USAN.
Use: Anti-inflammatory.
Flebogamma. (Grifols) Immune globulin
(human) 5% (50 mg/mL), 10%
(100 mg/mL). Sorbitol 50 mg (5%), D-
sorbitol 5 g (10%), polyethylene glycol
≤ 6 mg/mL. Preservative free. Inj. Vials. 10 mL (except 10%), 50 mL,
100 mL, 200 mL. *Rx.*
Use: Immune globulin.

•**flecainide acetate.** (fleh-CANE-ide)
USP 34.
Use: Antiarrhythmic agent.
See: Tambocor.

flecainide acetate. (Various Mfr.)
Flecainide acetate 50 mg, 100 mg,
150 mg. Tab. 100s. *Rx.*
Use: Antiarrhythmic agent.

Fleet. (Fleet) Dibasic sodium phosphate
7 g, monobasic sodium phosphate
19 g/118 mL delivered dose (sodium
4.4 g/dose). Disp. enema. Squeeze bot.
Pediatric 66 mL, Adult 133 mL. *OTC.*
Use: Laxative, enema.

Fleet Babylax. (Fleet) Glycerin 4 mL per
applicator. Liq. Pkg. App. 6s. *OTC.*
Use: Laxative.

Fleet Bagenema. (Fleet) Castile soap or
Fleets bisacodyl prep. *OTC.*
Use: Laxative.

Fleet Bisacodyl. (Fleet) Bisacodyl
10 mg/30 mL delivered dose. Disp.
enema. Squeeze bot. 37 mL. *OTC.*
Use: Laxative, enema.

Fleet Enema. (Fleet) Sodium biphosphate 19 g, sodium phosphate 7 g/
118 mL. Bot. w/rectal tube 4.5 oz. Pediatric size 67.5 mL, 135 mL. *OTC.*
Use: Laxative.

Fleet Glycerin Suppositories. (Fleet)
Adult: Jar 12s, 24s, 50s. Child Size:
Jar 12s. *OTC.*
Use: Laxative.

Fleet Laxative. (Fleet) Bisacodyl. **EC
Tab.:** 5 mg, sucrose. Bot. 25s, 100s.
Supp.: 10 mg. Box 4s, 12s, 50s, 100s.
OTC.
Use: Laxative.

Fleet Medicated Wipes. (Fleet) Hamamelis water 50%, alcohol 7%, glycerin
10%, benzalkonium Cl, methylparaben.
Rectal pads. 100s. *OTC.*
Use: Perianal hygiene.

Fleet Mineral Oil. (Fleet) Mineral oil.
Squeeze bot. 133 mL. *OTC.*
Use: Laxative, enema.

Fleet Pain Relief. (Fleet) Pramoxine
hydrochloride 1%, glycerin 12%. Pads.
100s. *OTC.*
Use: Anorectal preparation.

Fleet Prep Kit 3. (Fleet) *Phospho-Soda*
45 mL (monobasic sodium phosphate
21.6 g, dibasic sodium phosphate
8.1 g), 4 bisacodyl tablets (5 mg each),
bisacodyl enema 30 mL (10 mg). *OTC.*
Use: Laxative, enema.

•**fleroxacin.** (fler-OX-ah-SIN) USAN.
Use: Anti-infective.

•**flestolol sulfate.** (FLESS-toe-lahl)
USAN.
Use: Antiadrenergic (β-receptor).

•**fletazepam.** (FLET-AZE-eh-pam) USAN.
Use: Muscle relaxant.

Fletcher's Castoria. (Mentholatum Co.)
Senna concentrate 33.3 mg/mL, alcohol free, sucrose, parabens. Liq. Bot.
74 mL, 150 mL. *OTC.*
Use: Laxative.

Fletcher's Castoria for Children. (Mentholatum Co.) Senna 6.5%, alcohol
3.5%. Liq. Bot. 74 mL, 150 mL. *OTC.*
Use: Laxative.

Flexall. (Chattem) Menthol 7%. Aloe leaf
juice, eucalyptus oil, glycerin, peppermint oil, methyl salicylate, SD-alcohol,
thyme oil, triethanolamine, tocopherol.
Gel. 113.3 g. *OTC.*
Use: Rub and liniment.

Flexall 454. (Chattem) Menthol 7%, alcohol, allantoin, aloe vera gel, boric acid,
carbomer 940, diazolidinyl urea, eucalyptus oil, glycerin, iodine, parabens,
methyl salicylate, peppermint oil, polysorbate 60, potassium iodide, propylene glycol, thyme oil, triethanolamine.
Gel. Tube. 240 g. *OTC.*
Use: Analgesic, topical.

Flexall 454, Maximum Strength. (Chattem) Menthol 16%, aloe vera gel, eucalyptus oil, methylsalicylate, SD alcohol 38-B, thyme oil. Gel. Tube. 90 mg.
OTC.
Use: Analgesic, topical.

Flex Anti-Dandruff Shampoo. (Revlon)
Zinc pyrithione 1% in liquid shampoo.
OTC.
Use: Antiseborrheic.

Flex Anti-Dandruff Styling Mousse.
(Revlon) Zinc pyrithione 0.1%. Aerosol
foam. *OTC.*
Use: Antiseborrheic.

Flexeril. (McNeil) Cyclobenzaprine
hydrochloride 5 mg, 10 mg. Lactose.
Film-coated. Tab. Bot. 100s. *Rx.*
Use: Muscle relaxant.

**flexible hydroactive dressings/
granules.**
See: DuoDerm.
Intra Site.
Shur-Clens.
Sorbsan.

FlexiGel Strands. (Smith-Nephew)
Single-use absorbent matrix. 6 g unit.
Absorbent wound dressing. 10s. *OTC.*
Use: Dressing.

Flexon. (Various Mfr.) Orphenadrine citrate 30 mg/mL. Inj. Vial 10 mL. *Rx.*
Use: Muscle relaxant.

Flex-Power Performance Sports. (Flex-
Power) Trolamine salicylate 10%. Cetyl
alcohol, EDTA, parabens, glycerols,
stearyl alcohol, sodium metabisulfite.

Cream. Citrus light and clean scents. 120 g. *OTC.*
Use: Rub and liniment.

Flexsol. (Alcon) Sterile, buffered, isotonic aqueous soln. of sodium Cl, sodium borate, boric acid, adsorbobase. Bot. 6 oz. *OTC.*
Use: Contact lens care.

Flextra-DS. (Poly Pharmaceuticals) Acetaminophen 500 mg, phenyltoloxamine citrate 50 mg. Tab. Bot. 100s. *OTC.*
Use: Analgesic.

•**flibanserin.** (flib-AN-ser-in) USAN.
Use: Antidepressant.

•**flindokalner.** (flin-doe-KAL-ner) USAN.
Use: Neuroprotectant.

Flintstones Children's. (Bayer Consumer Care) Vitamin A 2500 units, E 15 mg, C 60 mg, folic acid 0.3 mg, B₁ 1.05 mg, B₂ 1.2 mg, B₃ 13.5 mg, B₆ 1.05 mg, B₁₂ 4.5 mcg, D 400 units. Chew. Tab. Bot. 60s, 100s. *OTC.*
Use: Vitamin supplement.

Flintstones Complete. (Bayer Consumer Care) Elemental iron 18 mg, vitamins A 5000 units, D 400 units, E 30 mg, B₁ 1.5 mg, B₂ 1.7 mg, B₃ 20 mg, B₅ 10 mg, B₆ 2 mg, B₁₂ 6 mcg, C 60 mg, folic acid 0.4 mg, biotin 40 mcg, Ca, Cu, I, Mg, P, zinc 15 mg. Chew. Tab. Bot. 60s, 120s. *OTC.*
Use: Mineral, vitamin supplement.

Flintstones Plus Calcium. (Bayer Consumer Care) Vitamin A 2500 units, D units 400, E 15 units, C 60 mg, folic acid 0.3 mg, B₁ 1.05 mg, B₂ 1.2 mg, B₃ 13.5 mg, B₆ 1.05 mg, B₁₂ 4.5 mcg, Ca 200 mg. Chew. Tab. Bot. 60s. *OTC.*
Use: Mineral, vitamin supplement.

Flintstones Plus Extra C Children's. (Bayer Consumer Care) Vitamins A 2500 units, D 400 units, E 15 mg, C 250 mg, folic acid 0.3 mg, B₁ 1.05 mg, B₂ 1.2 mg, niacin 13.5 mg, B₆ 1.05 mg, B₁₂ 4.5 mcg. Tab. Bot. 60s, 100s. *OTC.*
Use: Vitamin supplement.

Flintstones Plus Iron Multivitamins. (Bayer Consumer Care) Vitamins A 2500 units, E 15 mg, C 60 mg, folic acid 0.3 mg, B₁ 1.05 mg, B₂ 1.2 mg, niacin 13.5 mg, B₆ 1.05 mg, B₁₂ 4.5 mcg, D 400 units, iron 15 mg. Chew. Tab. Bot. 60s, 100s. *OTC.*
Use: Mineral, vitamin supplement.

Flo-Coat. (Mallinckrodt) Barium sulfate 100%. Simethicone. Susp. Bot. 1850 mL. *Rx.*
Use: Radiopaque agent, GI contrast agent.

•**floctafenine.** (FLOCK-tah-FEN-een) USAN.
Use: Analgesic.

Flolan. (Gilead) Epoprostenol sodium 0.5 mg, 1.5 mg. Mannitol, sodium chloride. Pow. for Reconstitution. 17 mL. *Rx.*
Use: Antihypertensive; vasodilator.

Flomax. (Boehringer Ingelheim) Tamsulosin hydrochloride 0.4 mg. Cap. Bot. 100s, 1000s. *Rx.*
Use: Benign prostatic hyperplasia treatment, antiadrenergic.

Flonase. (GlaxoSmithKline) Fluticasone propionate 50 mcg/actuation. Dextrose, polysorbate 80, benzalkonium chloride 0.02% w/w, phenylethyl alcohol w/w 0.25%. Spray Susp. Intranasal. Amber glass bot. w/meterizing atomizer pump and nasal adapter. 16 g (120 actuations). *Rx.*
Use: Respiratory inhalant, intranasal steroid.

Flo-Pred. (Taro Pharmaceuticals) Prednisolone 15 mg/5 mL (equiv. to prednisolone acetate 16.7 mg). Sorbitol crystalline, sucralose, EDTA, butylparaben. Cherry flavor. Oral Susp. 120 mL. *Rx.*
Use: Adrenocortical steroid, glucocorticoid.

Floranex. (Rising) Mixed culture of *Lactobacillus acidophilus* and *L. bulgaricus* 1 million CFU. Lactose, non-fat dried milk, sucrose. Chew. Tab. 50s. *OTC.*
Use: Nutritional supplement.

Florastor. (Biocodex) *Saccharomyces boulardii lyo* 250 mg. Lactose. Cap. 10s, 50s. *OTC.*
Use: Oral nutritional supplement.

Florastor Kids. (Biocodex) *Saccharomyces boulardii lyo* 250 mg. Tutti-frutti flavor. Oral Pow. 10s. *OTC.*
Use: Oral nutritional supplement.

•**florbenazine F 18.** (flor-BEN-a-zeen) USAN.
Use: Diagnostic imaging agent.

•**florbetapir F 18.** (flor-BAY-ta-pir) USAN.
Use: Diagnostic imaging agent.

Flor-D Chewable Tab. (Derm Pharm.) Fluoride 1 mg, vitamins A 4000 units, D 400 units, C 75 mg, B₁ 1.5 mg, B₂ 1.8 mg, niacinamide 15 mg, B₆ 1 mg, B₁₂ 3 mcg, calcium pantothenate 10 mg. Chew. Tab. Bot. 100s. *Rx.*
Use: Mineral, vitamin supplement.

Flor-D Drops. (Derm Pharm.) Fluoride 0.5 mg, vitamins A 3000 units, D 400 units, C 60 mg, B₁ 1 mg, B₂ 1.2 mg, niacinamide 8 mg/0.6 mL. Drops. Bot. 60 mL. *Rx.*
Use: Mineral, vitamin supplement.

•**flordipine.** (FLORE-dih-peen) USAN.
Use: Antihypertensive.

Florical. (Mericon) Ca 145 mg (calcium content expressed in mg elemental calcium), fluoride 3.75 mg (fluoride content expressed in mg elemental fluoride. Cap. 100s. *OTC.*
Use: Nutritional supplement, multimineral.

Florical. (Mericon) Sodium fluoride 8.3 mg, calcium carbonate 364 mg (elemental calcium 145.6 mg). Cap. and Tab. 100s, 500s. *OTC.*
Use: Mineral supplement, calcium.

Florida Foam. (Hill Dermaceuticals) Benzalkonium Cl, aluminum subacetate, boric acid 2%. Bot. 8 oz. *OTC.*
Use: Soap substitute; antiseborrheic; antifungal; dermatologic-acne.

Florida Sunburn Relief. (Pharmacel Laboratory, Inc.) Benzyl alcohol 3%, phenol 0.4%, camphor 0.2%, menthol 0.15%. Lot. Bot. 60 mL. *OTC.*
Use: Sunburn relief.

Florinef Acetate. (Monarch) Fludrocortisone acetate, 0.1 mg, lactose. Tab. Bot. 100s. *Rx.*
Use: Corticosteroid.

Florone Cream. (Dermik) Diflorasone diacetate 0.5 mg/g (0.05%) w/stearic acid, sorbitan mono-oleate, polysorbate 60, sorbic acid, citric acid, propylene glycol, purified water. Cream. Tube 15 g, 30 g, 60 g. *Rx.*
Use: Corticosteroid, topical.

Florone E. (Dermik) Diflorasone diacetate 0.5 mg. Tube 15 g, 30 g, 60 g. *Rx.*
Use: Corticosteroid, topical.

Florone Ointment. (Dermik) Diflorasone diacetate 0.5 mg/g (0.05%), polyoxypropylene 15-stearyl ether, stearic acid, lanolin alcohol, white petrolatum. Oint. Tube 15 g, 30 g, 60 g. *Rx.*
Use: Corticosteroid, topical.

Floropryl. (Merck & Co.) Isoflurophate 0.025% in sterile ophthalmic ointment in polyethylene-mineral oil gel. Tube 3.5 g. *Rx.*
Use: Agent for glaucoma.

Florvite Drops. (Everett) Fluoride 0.25 mg, 0.5 mg, A 1500 units, D 400 units, E 5 units, B_1 0.5 mg, B_2 0.6 mg, B_3 8 mg, B_6 0.4 mg, B_{12} 2 mcg, C 35 mg. Bot. 50 mL. *Rx.*
Use: Mineral, vitamin supplement; dental caries agent.

Florvite Half Strength. (Everett) Elemental fluoride 0.5 mg, vitamins A 2500 units, D 400 units, E 15 mg, B_1 1.05 mg, B_2 1.2 mg, B_3 13.5 mg, B_6 1.05 mg, B_{12} 4.5 mcg, C 60 mg, folic acid 0.3 mg. Chew. Tab. Bot. 100s. *Rx.*
Use: Mineral, vitamin supplement; dental caries agent.

Florvite Pediatric Drops. (Everett) Elemental fluorine, 0.25 mg/mL, 0.5 mg/mL, Vitamins A 1500 units, D 400 units, E 5 mg, B_1 0.5 mg, B_2 0.6 mg, B_3 8 mg, B_6 0.4 mg, B_{12} 2 mcg, C 35 mg/mL. Bot. 50 mL *Rx.*
Use: Mineral, vitamin supplement; dental caries agent.

Florvite + Iron Chewable. (Everett) Fluoride 1 mg, iron 12 mg, vitamins A 2500 units, D 400 units, E 15 mg, B_1 1.05 mg, B_2 1.2 mg, B_3 13.5 mg, B_6 1.05 mg, B_{12} 4.5 mcg, C 60 mg, folic acid 0.3 mg, Cu, Zn 10 mg, sucrose. Chew. Tab. Bot. 100s. *Rx.*
Use: Mineral, vitamin supplement; dental caries agent.

Florvite + Iron Drops. (Everett) Elemental fluorine 0.25 mg, 0.5 mg, Vitamins A 1500 units, D 400 units, E 5 mg, B_1 0.5 mg, B_2 0.6 mg, B_3 8 mg, B_6 0.4 mg, C 35 mg, iron 10 mg/mL. Liq. Bot. 50 mL. *Rx.*
Use: Mineral, vitamin supplement; dental caries agent.

Florvite Tablets. (Everett) Fluoride 1 mg, vitamins A 2500 units, D 400 units, E 15 mg, B_1 1.05 mg, B_2 1.2 mg, B_3 13.5 mg, B_6 1.05 mg, B_{12} 4.5 mcg, C 60 mg, folic acid 0.3 mg. Chew. Tab. Bot. 100s, 1000s. *Rx.*
Use: Mineral, vitamin supplement; dental caries agent.

•**flosequinan.** (flow-SEH-kwih-NAHN) USAN.
Use: Antihypertensive (vasodilator).

Flovent Diskus. (GlaxoSmithKline) Fluticasone propionate 50 mcg/actuation, 100 mcg/actuation, 250 mcg/actuation. Lactose. Pow., Inhal. Inhalation device containing 60 blisters. *Rx.*
Use: Respiratory inhalant, corticosteroid.

Flovent HFA. (GlaxoSmithKline) Fluticasone propionate/actuation 44 mcg, 110 mcg, 220 mcg. Aerosol. Susp. Inh. Canister with actuator. 10.6 g (120 metered inhalations) (44 mcg only), 12 g (120 metered inhalations) (110 mcg and 220 mcg only). *Rx.*
Use: Respiratory inhalant, corticosteroid.

•**floxacillin.** (FLOX-ah-SILL-in) USAN.
Use: Anti-infective.

Floxin. (Ortho-McNeil) Ofloxacin, 200 mg, 300 mg, 400 mg. Lactose. Tab. Bot. 50s (except 400 mg), 100s (400 mg only); UD 6s (200 mg only),

100s. *Rx.*
Use: Anti-infective, fluoroquinolone.
Floxin Otic. (Daiichi) Ofloxacin 3 mg/mL. Benzalkonium chloride 0.0025%. Otic Soln. Dropper Bot. 5 mL, 10 mL. *Rx.*
Use: Otic antibiotic.
•**floxuridine.** (flox-YOUR-ih-deen) *USP 34.*
Use: Antiviral; antineoplastic.
See: FUDR.
floxuridine. (Bedford) Floxuridine 500 mg. Pow. for Inj., lyophilized. Vial 5 mL. *Rx.*
Use: Antiviral; antineoplastic.
Fluarix. (GlaxoSmithKline) Hemagglutinin 15 mcg each of A/California/7/2009 NYMC X-181 (H1N1), A/Victoria/210/2009 NYMC X-187 (H3N2) (an A/Perth/16/2009-like virus), and B/Brisbane/60/2008 per 0.5 mL. Dry natural latex rubber. Each 0.5 mL dose also contains octoxynol-10 ≤ 0.085 mg, alpha-tocopheryl hydrogen succinate ≤ 0.1 mg, and ≤ 0.415 mg of polysorbate 80. Each dose also may contain residual amounts of hydrocortisone ≤ 0.0016 mcg, gentamicin sulfate ≤ 0.15 mcg, ovalbumin ≤ 0.05 mcg, formaldehyde ≤ 5 mcg, and sodium deoxycholate ≤ 50 mcg. Inj., Susp. (purified split virus). Preservative free 0.5 mL prefilled, single-dose syringe. *Rx.*
Use: Viral vaccine.
•**fluazacort.** (flew-AZE-ah-kort) USAN.
Use: Anti-inflammatory.
•**flubanilate hydrochloride.** (flew-BAN-ill-ate) USAN.
Use: Antidepressant; CNS stimulant.
•**flubendazole.** (FLEW-BEN-dah-zole) USAN.
Use: Antiprotozoal.
Flucaine. (Altaire) Proparacaine hydrochloride 0.5%, fluorescein sodium 0.25%. Soln. 5 mL. *Rx.*
Use: Ophthalmic local anesthetic.
flucarbril.
Use: Muscle relaxant; analgesic.
•**fluciclatide F 18.** (floo-SIK-la-tide) USAN.
Use: Radiopharmaceutical.
•**flucindole.** (flew-SIN-dole) USAN.
Use: Antipsychotic.
•**flucloronide.** (flew-KLOR-oh-nide) USAN.
Use: Corticosteroid, topical.
Flu, Cold & Cough Medicine. (Major) Pseudoephedrine hydrochloride 60 mg, chlorpheniramine 4 mg, dextromethorphan HBr 20 mg, acetaminophen

500 mg. Pow. Pck. 6s. *OTC.*
Use: Analgesic; antihistamine; antitussive; decongestant.
•**fluconazole.** (flew-KOE-nuh-sole) *USP 34.*
Use: Antifungal.
See: Diflucan.
fluconazole. (Hospira) Fluconazole 2 mg/mL. Sodium chloride 9 mg/mL or dextrose 56 mg/mL. Inj. 100 mL, 200 mL. *Rx.*
Use: Antifungal agent.
fluconazole. (Mayne) Fluconazole 2 mg/mL. Inj. 100 mL, 200 mL. *Rx.*
Use: Antifungal.
fluconazole. (Various Mfr.) Fluconazole 50 mg, 100 mg, 150 mg, 200 mg. May contain lactose. Tab. 30s, 100s, UD 100s (except 150 mg); unit-of-use cards (150 mg only). *Rx.*
Use: Antifungal agent.
fluconazole. (West-Ward Pharmaceutical Corp.) Fluconazole 2 mg/mL. Inj. Glass Bot. 100 mL. *Rx.*
Use: Antifungal agent.
•**flucrylate.** (FLEW-krih-late) USAN.
Use: Surgical aid (tissue adhesive).
•**flucytosine.** (flew-SITE-oh-seen) *USP 34.*
Use: Antifungal.
See: Ancobon.
•**fludalanine.** (flew-DAL-AH-neen) USAN.
Use: Anti-infective.
Fludara. (Bayer) Fludarabine 50 mg. Mannitol 50 mg. Inj., lyophilized, cake. Single-dose vial. *Rx.*
Use: Antineoplastic.
•**fludarabine phosphate.** (flew-DAR-uh-BEAN) USAN.
Use: Antineoplastic. [Orphan Drug]
See: Fludara.
  Oforta.
fludarabine phosphate. (Various Mfr.) Fludarabine phosphate. **Inj., Lyophilized, Cake:** 50 mg. Preservative free. Single-dose vials. **Inj.:** 25 mg/mL. Preservative free. Mannitol 25 mg/mL, sodium hydroxide. Single-dose vial. 2 mL. *Rx.*
Use: Antimetabolite.
•**fludazonium chloride.** (FLEW-dazz-OH-nee-uhm) USAN.
Use: Anti-infective, topical.
•**fludeoxyglucose F 18 injection.** (FLEW-dee-OX-ee-GLUE-kose) *USP 34.*
Use: Diagnostic aid (brain disorders, thyroid disorders, liver disorders, cardiac disease, and neoplastic disease); radiopharmaceutical.

•**fludorex.** (FLEW-doe-rex) USAN.
Use: Anorexic; antiemetic.

•**fludrocortisone acetate.** (flew-droe-CORE-tih-sone) *USP 34.*
Use: Adrenocortical steroid (salt-regulating).
See: Florinef Acetate.

fludrocortisone acetate. (Various Mfr.)
Fludrocortisone acetate 0.1 mg. Tab.
Bot. 100s. *Rx.*
Use: Adrenocortical steroid.

•**flufenamic acid.** (FLEW-fen-AM-ik)
USAN.
Use: Anti-inflammatory.

•**flufenisal.** (flew-FEN-ih-sal) USAN.
Use: Analgesic.

Fluidex. (Columbia) Natural botanical ingredients. Tab. Bot. 36s, 72s.
Use: Diuretic.

Flu-Imune. (Wyeth) Influenza virus vaccine. Vial 5 mL (10 doses). (Purified surface antigen.) *Rx.*
Use: Immunization.

fluitran. Trichlormethiazide.

FluLaval. (GlaxoSmithKline) Hemagglutinin 15 mcg each of A/California/7/2009 NYMC X-179A (H1N1), A/Victoria/210/2009 NYMC X-187 (H3N2) (an A/Perth/16/2009-like virus), and B/Brisbane/60/2008 per 0.5 mL. Thimerosal, mercury 25 mcg/dose. Each dose may also contain residual amounts of egg protein (ovalbumin ≤ 1 mcg), formaldehyde ≤ 25 mcg, and sodium deoxycholate ≤ 50 mcg. Inj., Susp. (purified split virus). Multidose vial. 5 mL. *Rx.*
Use: Viral vaccine.

Flumadine. (Caraco) Rimantadine hydrochloride 100 mg. Film-coated. Tab. 100s. *Rx.*
Use: Antiviral.

•**flumazenil.** (flew-MAZ-ah-nil) USAN.
Use: Antagonist (to benzodiazepine), antidote.
See: Romazicon.

flumazenil. (Various Mfr.) Flumazenil 0.1 mg/mL. May contain EDTA, parabens, sodium chloride. Inj. Multidose vials. 5 mL, 10 mL. *Rx.*
Use: Antidote.

•**flumequine.** (FLEW-meh-kwin) USAN.
Use: Anti-infective.

•**flumeridone.** (FLEW-MER-ih-dohn)
USAN.
Use: Antiemetic.

•**flumethasone.** (FLEW-meth-ah-zone)
USAN.
Use: Corticosteroid, topical.

•**flumethasone pivalate.** (FLEW-meth-ah-zone PIH-vah-late) *USP 34.*
Use: Corticosteroid, topical.

flumethiazide.
Use: Diuretic.

•**flumetramide.** (flew-MEH-trah-mide)
USAN.
Use: Muscle relaxant.

•**flumezapine.** (FLEW-MEZZ-ah-peen)
USAN.
Use: Antipsychotic; neuroleptic.

•**fluminorex.** (flew-MEE-no-rex) USAN.
Use: Anorexic.

FluMist. (MedImmune Vaccines) Fluorescent focus units $10^{6.5-7.5}$ of A/California/7/2009 (H1N1), A/Perth/16/2009 (H3N2), and B/Brisbane/60/2008 per 0.2 mL actuation. Each 0.2 mL dose also contains monosodium glutamate 0.1888 mg, hydrolyzed porcine gelatin 2 mg, arginine 2.42 mg, sucrose 13.68 mg, dibasic potassium phosphate 2.26 mg, monobasic potassium phosphate 0.96 mg, and gentamicin sulfate < 0.015 mcg/mL. Preservative free. Spray, Soln.; intranasal. Prefilled, single-use sprayer. 0.2 mL. *Rx.*
Use: Viral vaccine.

•**flumizole.** (FLEW-mih-zole) USAN.
Use: Anti-inflammatory.

•**flumoxonide.** (flew-MOX-OH-nide)
USAN.
Use: Adrenocortical steroid.

flunarizine.
Use: Alternating hemiplegia. [Orphan Drug]
See: Sibelium.

•**flunarizine hydrochloride.** (flew-NAR-ih-zeen) USAN.
Use: Vasodilator.

•**flunidazole.** (FLEW-nih-dah-ZOLE)
USAN.
Use: Antiprotozoal.

•**flunisolide.** (flew-NIH-sole-ide) *USP 34.*
Use: Corticosteroid, topical, respiratory inhalant.
See: Aerospan.

flunisolide. (Bausch & Lomb) Flunisolide 0.025% (25 mcg/actuation), propylene glycol, polyethylene glycol 3350, EDTA, benzalkonium chloride. Soln. Bot. 25 mL nasal pump dispenser (200 sprays/bot). *Rx.*
Use: Corticosteroid, topical; intranasal steroid.

•**flunisolide acetate.** (flew-NIH-sole-ide)
USAN.
Use: Anti-inflammatory.

•**flunitrazepam.** (flew-NYE-TRAY-zeh-pam) USAN.
Use: Hypnotic; sedative.

•**flunixin.** (flew-NIX-in) USAN.
Use: Analgesic; anti-inflammatory.

•**flunixin meglumine.** (flew-NIX-in meh-GLUE-meen) *USP 34.*
Use: Analgesic; anti-inflammatory.

Fluocet. (Alra) Fluocinolone acetonide 0.025%, 0.01%. Cream. Tube 15 g, 60 g. *Rx.*
Use: Corticosteroid, topical.

fluocinolide. (flew-oh-SIN-oh-lide)
See: Fluocinonide.

•**fluocinolone acetonide.** (flew-oh-SIN-oh-lone ah-SEE-toe-nide) *USP 34.*
Use: Corticosteroid, topical; corticosteroid, ophthalmic.
See: Fluonid.
Retisert.
W/Combinations.
See: Tri-Luma.

•**fluocinonide.** (FLEW-oh-SIN-oh-nide) *USP 34. Formerly Fluocinolide.*
Use: Corticosteroid, topical.
See: Lidex.
Lidex-E.
Vanos.

fluocinonide. (E. Fougera) Fluocinonide 0.05%. Tube 15 g, 60 g.
Use: Corticosteroid, topical.

fluocinonide topical solution. (E. Fougera) Fluocinonide 0.05%. Soln. Bot. 60 mL.
Use: Corticosteroid, topical.

•**fluocortin butyl.** (FLEW-oh-CORE-tin BYOO-tuhl) USAN.
Use: Anti-inflammatory.

•**fluocortolone.** (FLEW-oh-CORE-toe-lone) USAN.
Use: Corticosteroid, topical.

•**fluocortolone caproate.** (FLEW-oh-CORE-toe-lone) USAN.
Use: Corticosteroid, topical.

Fluonex. (AstraZeneca) Fluocinonide 0.05%. Cream. Tube. 15 g, 30 g. *Rx.*
Use: Corticosteroid, topical.

Fluonid. (Allergan) Fluocinolone acetonide 0.01%. Soln. Bot. 20 mL, 60 mL. *Rx.*
Use: Corticosteroid, topical.

Fluoracaine. (Akorn) Proparacaine hydrochloride 0.5%, fluorescein sodium 0.25%. Glycerin, povidone, polysorbate 80, thimerosal 0.01%, boric acid, sodium hydroxide and/or hydrochloric acid. Soln. 5 mL. *Rx.*
Use: Anesthetic, local; ophthalmic.

Fluor-A-Day. (Arbor Pharmaceuticals) Fluoride 0.25 mg (from 0.55 mg of sodium fluoride), 0.5 mg (from 1.1 mg of sodium fluoride), 1 mg (from 2.2 mg of sodium fluoride). Maltodextrin, sorbitol, xylitol. Sugar free. Raspberry flavor. Chew. Tab. 120s. *Rx.*
Use: Trace element, fluoride.

•**fluorescein.** (FLURE-eh-seen) *USP 34.*
Use: Diagnostic aid (corneal trauma indicator).
See: Fluorescite.

Fluorescein Injection Lite. (HUB) Fluorescein sodium 10%. Inj., Soln. Single-dose vials. 5 mL. *Rx.*
Use: Ophthalmic diagnostic product.

•**fluorescein sodium.** (FLURE-eh-seen) *USP 34. Formerly Fluorescein, soluble.*
Use: Diagnostic aid, corneal trauma indicator.
See: AK-Fluor.
Fluorescein Injection Lite.
Fluorescite.
Fluorets.
Fluor-I-Strips.
Ful-Glo.
Funduscein.
Ophthifluor.
W/Benoxinate Hydrochloride.
See: Fluress.
Flurox.
W/Proparacaine Hydrochloride.
See: Flucaine.
Fluoracaine.

fluorescein sodium/benoxinate hydrochloride. (Bausch & Lomb) Benoxinate hydrochloride 0.4%, fluorescein sodium 0.25%. Povidone, boric acid, chlorobutanol 1%. Soln., Ophth. 5 mL w/dropper. *Rx.*
Use: Ophthalmic local anesthetic.

fluorescein sodium intravenous.
See: Fluorescite.

fluorescein sodium/sodium hyaluronate.
See: Sodium Hyaluronate and Fluorescein Sodium Healon Yellow.

fluorescein sodium 2%. (Ciba Vision) Sterile aqueous solution containing fluorescein sodium 2%. *Dropperette* 1 mL, Box 12s.
Use: Diagnostic aid, ophthalmic.

fluorescein sodium 2% solution. (Alcon) *Drop-Tainer* 15 mL, *Steri-Unit* 2 mL 12s.
Use: Diagnostic aid, ophthalmic.

fluorescein sodium with proparacaine hydrochloride. (Various Mfr.) Proparacaine hydrochloride 0.5%, fluorescein sodium 0.25%. Povidone, glycerin, EDTA, thimerosal 0.01%. Soln. Bot. 5 mL with dropper. *Rx.*
Use: Anesthetic, local; diagnostic aid, ophthalmic.

Fluorescite. (Alcon) Fluorescein sodium 10%. Inj. Amp. 5 mL with syringes. *Rx.*
Use: Diagnostic aid, ophthalmic.

Fluoresoft 0.35%. (Various Mfr.) Fluorexon 0.35%. Preservative free. Soln. 0.35 mL ampules. 20s. *OTC.*
Use: Diagnostic aid, ophthalmic.

Fluorets. (Bausch & Lomb) Fluorescein sodium 1 mg. Strip. Box 100s. *OTC.*
Use: Diagnostic aid, ophthalmic.

fluorexon.
Use: Ophthalmic diagnostic product.
See: Fluoresoft 0.35%.

fluoride. (Kirkman) Fluoride 1 mg (sodium fluoride 2.21 mg). Tab. Bot. 1000s. *Rx.*
Use: Dental caries agent.

Fluoride Loz. (Kirkman) Fluoride 1 mg (sodium fluoride 2.21 mg). Bot. 1000s. *Rx.*
Use: Dental caries agent.

fluoride sodium.
See: Ludent.
ReNaf.
Sodium Fluoride.

fluoride therapy.
See: Cari-Tab.
ControlRx.
Coral.
Fluor-A-Day.
Fluorineed.
Fluorinse.
Monocal.
Mulvidren-F.
OrthoWash.
PerioMed.
Point Two.
SF 5000 Plus.
SF 1.1%.
SodiPhluor.
Soluvite-F.
Tri-Vi-Flor.

Fluoridex Daily Defense Sensitivity Relief. (Discus Dental) Sodium fluoride 1.1%, potassium nitrate 5%. Saccharin, sorbitol. Mint flavor. Dental paste. 112 g. *Rx.*
Use: Mouth and throat product, preparation for sensitive teeth.

Fluorigard. (Colgate Oral) Fluoride 0.02% (from sodium fluoride 0.05%), alcohol 6%, tartrazine. Bot. 180 mL, 300 mL, 480 mL. *Rx.*
Use: Dental caries agent.

Fluorineed. (Hanlon) Fluoride 1 mg. Chew. Tab. Bot. 100s, 1000s. *Rx.*
Use: Dental caries agent.

Fluorinse. (Oral-B) Fluoride 0.09% from sodium fluoride 0.2%. Bot. 480 mL. *Rx.*
Use: Dental caries agent.

Fluorinse. (Pacemaker) Fluoride mouthwash. Pack. Fluoride ion level 0.05%, 0.2%. UD Bot. 32 oz. Concentrate 1 oz, 4 oz, gal. *Rx.*
Use: Dental caries agent.

Fluoritab. (Fluoritab) Sodium fluoride 2.2 mg equivalent to 1 mg of fluorine (as fluoride ion) w/inert organic filler 75.8 mg. Tab. 100s; Liq. Dropper Bot. Fluoride 0.125 mg from sodium fluoride 0.275 mg. Drop 30 mL. *Rx.*
Use: Dental caries agent.

5-fluorocytosine.
See: Ancobon.

•**fluorodopa F 18 injection.** (FLEW-roe-DOE-pah) *USP 34.*
Use: Diagnostic aid (brain imaging); radiopharmaceutical.

fluorogestone acetate.
Use: Hormone, progestin.

fluorohydrocortisone acetate. 9-α-Fluorohydrocortisone.

•**fluorometholone.** (flure-oh-METH-oh-lone) *USP 34.*
Use: Corticosteroid, ophthalmic.
See: Flarex.
FML.

fluorometholone. (Various Mfr.) Fluorometholone 0.1%. Benzalkonium chloride 0.004%, EDTA, polysorbate 80, polyvinyl alcohol 1.4%. Ophth. Susp. Bot. 5 mL, 10 mL, 15 mL. *Rx.*
Use: Corticosteroid, ophthalmic; anti-inflammatory.

•**fluorometholone acetate.** (flure-oh-METH-oh-LONE) USAN.
Use: Corticosteroid, ophthalmic; anti-inflammatory.

fluorophene.
Use: Antiseptic.

Fluoroplex. (Allergan) Fluorouracil 1%. Benzyl alcohol, emulsifying wax, mineral oil. Cream. Tube 30 g. *Rx.*
Use: Pyrimidine antagonist, topical.

fluoroquinolones.
Use: Anti-infective.
See: Ciprofloxacin.
Enoxacin.
Gemifloxacin Mesylate.
Levofloxacin.
Lomefloxacin Hydrochloride.
Moxifloxacin Hydrochloride.
Norfloxacin.

•**fluorosalan.** (FLEW-oh-row-SAH-lan) USAN.
Use: Antiseptic; disinfectant.

fluorothyl.
See: Flurothyl.

•**fluorouracil.** (FLURE-oh-YOUR-uh-sill) *USP 34.*

Use: Antimetabolite; antineoplastic; pyrimidine antagonist, topical.
See: Adrucil.
Carac.
Fluoroplex.
fluorouracil. (Oceanside Pharmaceuticals) Fluorouracil 5%. Parabens, stearyl alcohol, white petrolatum. Cream. 40 g. *Rx.*
Use: Pyrimidine antagonist, topical.
fluorouracil. (Taro) Fluorouracil 2%, 5%. Soln. Dropper bot. 10 mL. *Rx.*
Use: Pyrimidine antagonist, topical.
fluorouracil. (Various Mfr.) Fluorouracil 50 mg/mL. Vial 10 mL, 20 mL, 100 mL. Amp. 10 mL. *Rx.*
Use: Antineoplastic; antimetabolite.
•**fluotracen hydrochloride.** (FLEW-oh-TRAY-sen) USAN.
Use: Antipsychotic; antidepressant.
•**fluoxetine hydrochloride.** (flew-OX-eh-teen) *USP 34.*
Tall Man: FLUoxetine
Use: Antidepressant, selective serotonin reuptake inhibitor.
See: Prozac.
Prozac Weekly.
Sarafem.
Selfemra.
W/Olanzapine.
See: Symbyax.
fluoxetine hydrochloride. (Various Mfr.) Fluoxetine hydrochloride. **Cap.:** 10 mg, 20 mg, 40 mg. May contain parabens, EDTA, lactose (except 40 mg). Bot. 30s (except 10 mg), 60s (except 10 mg), 100s; 1000s, 2000s, unit-of-use 30s (except 40 mg); UD 100s (10 mg only). **Cap., delayed release:** 90 mg. May contain isopropyl alcohol, PEG, sugar. UD 4s. **Tab.:** 10 mg, 20 mg. Bot. 30s, 60s, 90s, 100s, 500s (10 mg only), 1000s, 5000s (10 mg only), UD 100s (10 mg only). **Oral Soln.:** 20 mg/5 mL. May contain alcohol, sucrose. Bot. 120 mL, 473 mL. *Rx.*
Use: Antidepressant, selective serotonin reuptake inhibitor.
•**fluoxymesterone.** (flew-ox-ee-MESS-teh-rone) *USP 34.*
Use: Sex hormone, androgen.
See: Androxy.
fluoxymesterone. (Various Mfr.) Fluoxymesterone 10 mg. Tab. Bot. 100s. *c-III.*
Use: Sex hormone, androgen.
•**fluparoxan hydrochloride.** (flew-pah-ROX-an) USAN.
Use: Antidepressant.
•**fluperamide.** (flew-purr-ah-mide) USAN.

Use: Antiperistaltic.
•**fluperolone acetate.** (FLEW-per-oh-lone) USAN.
Use: Corticosteroid, topical.
•**fluphenazine decanoate.** (flew-FEN-uh-zeen) *USP 34.*
Tall Man: fluPHENAZine
Use: Antipsychotic.
fluphenazine decanoate. (Various Mfr.) Fluphenazine decanoate 25 mg/mL, may contain sesame oil and benzyl alcohol. Inj. Multidose vials 5 mL. *Rx.*
Use: Antipsychotic.
•**fluphenazine enanthate.** (flew-FEN-uh-zeen) *USP 34.*
Tall Man: fluPHENAZine
Use: Antipsychotic; anxiolytic.
•**fluphenazine hydrochloride.** (flew-FEN-uh-zeen) *USP 34.*
Tall Man: fluPHENAZine
Use: Antipsychotic; anxiolytic.
fluphenazine hydrochloride. (American Pharmaceutical Partners) Fluphenazine hydrochloride. **Elix.:** 2.5 mg/mL. May contain alcohol 14% and sucrose. 60 mL, 473 mL. **Inj.:** 2.5 mg/mL. Parabens. Vial. 10 mL. *Rx.*
Use: Antipsychotic.
fluphenazine hydrochloride. (Pharmaceutical Associates) Fluphenazine hydrochloride 5 mg/mL. Alcohol 14%. Oral Soln., concentrated. 120 mL with safety-cap dropper calibrated at 0.1 mL and in 0.2 mL increments. *Rx.*
Use: Antipsychotic agent.
fluphenazine hydrochloride. (Various Mfr.) Fluphenazine hydrochloride. **Tab.:** 1 mg, 2.5 mg, 5 mg, 10 mg. Bot. 50s, 100s, 500s, 1000s, UD 100s. **Elixir:** 2.5 mg/mL. May contain alcohol 14% and sucrose. 60 mL, 473 mL. *Rx.*
Use: Antipsychotic.
•**flupirtine maleate.** (flew-PIHR-teen) USAN.
Use: Investigational analgesic.
•**fluprednisolone.** (FLEW-pred-NIH-so-lone) USAN.
Use: Corticosteroid, topical.
•**fluprednisolone valerate.** (FLEW-pred-NIH-so-lone VAL-eh-rate) USAN.
Use: Corticosteroid, topical.
•**fluproquazone.** (FLEW-PRO-kwah-zone) USAN.
Use: Analgesic.
•**fluprostenol sodium.** (flew-PROSTE-een-ole) USAN.
Use: Prostaglandin.
•**fluquazone.** (FLEW-kwah-zone) USAN.
Use: Anti-inflammatory.

• **fluradoline hydrochloride.** (FLURE-ade-OLE-een) USAN.
Use: Analgesic.

Flura-Drops. (Kirkman) Fluoride. **Drops:** 0.25 mg (from 0.55 mg sodium fluoride). Bot. 30 mL. **Rinse:** 0.02% (from 0.05% sodium fluoride). Bot. 480 mL. *Rx.*
Use: Dental caries agent.

Flura-Loz. (Kirkman) Sodium fluoride 2.2 mg providing 1 mg fluoride. Loz. Bot. 100s, 1000s. *Rx.*
Use: Dental caries agent.

• **flurandrenolide.** (FLURE-an-DREEN-oh-lide) *USP 34.* Cream; Ointment, USP. *Formerly Flurandrenolone.*
Use: Corticosteroid, topical.
See: Cordran.

flurandrenolone. (FLURE-an-DREE-nahl-ohn)
Use: Corticosteroid, topical.

Flura-Tablets. (Kirkman) Sodium fluoride 2.21 mg, equivalent to 1 mg fluoride ion. Tab. Bot. 100s, 1000s. *Rx.*
Use: Dental caries agent.

• **flurazepam hydrochloride.** (flure-AZE-uh-pam) *USP 34.*
Use: Anticonvulsant; hypnotic; muscle relaxant; sedative/hypnotic, nonbarbiturate.

flurazepam hydrochloride. (Various Mfr.) Flurazepam hydrochloride 15 mg, 30 mg. Cap. 100s. *c-iv.*
Use: Sedative/hypnotic, nonbarbiturate.

• **flurbiprofen.** (FLURE-bih-PRO-fen) *USP 34.*
Use: Analgesic; anti-inflammatory.

flurbiprofen. (Various Mfr.) Flurbiprofen 50 mg, 100 mg. Tab. 100s, 500s (100 mg only). *Rx.*
Use: Analgesic, NSAID.

• **flurbiprofen sodium.** (FLURE-bih-PRO-fen) *USP 34.*
Use: Analgesic, NSAID; prostaglandin synthesis inhibitor.
See: Ocufen.

flurbiprofen sodium. (Various Mfr.) Flurbiprofen sodium 0.03%. Polyvinyl alcohol 1.4%, thimerosal 0.005%, EDTA. Ophth. Soln. Bot. 2.5 mL. *Rx.*
Use: Analgesic, NSAID.

Fluress. (Akorn) Fluorescein sodium 0.25%, benoxinate hydrochloride 0.4%. Povidone, boric acid, chlorobutanol 1%, sodium hydroxide and/or hydrochloric acid. Bot. 5 mL. *Rx.*
Use: Local anesthetic, ophthalmic.

• **fluretofen.** (flure-EH-TOE-fen) USAN.
Use: Anti-inflammatory; antithrombotic.

flurfamide. (FLURE-fah-MIDE)
See: Flurofamide.

• **flurocitabine.** (FLEW-row-SIGH-tah-bean) USAN.
Use: Antineoplastic.

Fluro-Ethyl. (Gebauer) Ethyl chloride 25%, dichlorotetrafluoroethane 75%. Aer. Spray. 270 mL. *Rx.*
Use: Anesthetic, topical.

• **flurofamide.** (FLEW-row-fah-MIDE) USAN. *Formerly Flurfamide.*
Use: Enzyme inhibitor (urease).

• **flurogestone acetate.** (FLEW-row-JEST-ohn) USAN.
Use: Hormone, progestin.

• **flurothyl.** (FLURE-oh-thill) USAN.
Use: Stimulant (central).

Flurox. (Ocusoft) Benoxinate hydrochloride 0.4%, fluorescein sodium 0.25%. Soln. 5 mL. *Rx.*
Use: Ophthalmic local anesthetic.

• **fluroxene.** (flure-OX-een) USAN.
Use: General inhalation anesthetic.

• **flurpiridaz F 18.** (flur-PIR-i-daz) USAN.
Use: Diagnostic imaging agent.

• **fluspiperone.** (FLEW-spih-per-OHN) USAN.
Use: Antipsychotic.

• **fluspirilene.** (flew-SPIRE-ih-leen) USAN.
Use: Antipsychotic; anxiolytic.

Flutabs. (Breckenridge) Dextromethorphan HBr 20 mg, guaifenesin 200 mg, pseudoephedrine hydrochloride 60 mg, acetaminophen 500 mg. Dye free. Tab. 100s. *Rx.*
Use: Upper respiratory combination, antitussive and expectorant combination.

• **flutamide.** (FLEW-tuh-mide) *USP 34.*
Use: Hormone, antiandrogen.

flutamide. (Various Mfr.) Flutamide 125 mg, may contain lactose. Cap. Bot. 100s, 180s, 500s, UD 100s. *Rx.*
Use: Hormone, antiandrogen.

• **fluticasone furoate.** (floo-TICK-a-sone FUR-oh-ate) USAN.
Use: Anti-inflammatory, intranasal steroid, corticosteroid, respiratory inhalant.
See: Veramyst.

• **fluticasone propionate.** (flew-TICK-ah-SONE) USAN.
Use: Anti-inflammatory, respiratory inhalant, intranasal steroid, corticosteroid.
See: Cutivate.
Flonase.
Flovent Diskus.
Flovent HFA.
Veramyst.
W/Salmeterol
See: Advair Diskus.
Advair HFA.

fluticasone propionate. (Fougera) Fluticasone propionate 0.005%. Oint. Tubes. 15 g, 30 g, 60 g. *Rx.*
Use: Anti-inflammatory agent.

fluticasone propionate. (Par) Fluticasone propionate 50 mcg/actuation. Dextrose, polysorbate 80, 0.02% w/w benzalkonium chloride, 0.25% w/w phenylethyl alcohol. Spray. Susp. Intranasal. Amber glass bot. 16 g (120 actuations) with metering atomizing pump and nasal adapter. *Rx.*
Use: Intranasal steroid, respiratory inhalant.

fluticasone propionate. (Sandoz) Fluticasone propionate 0.05%. Cetostearyl alcohol, mineral oil. Cream. Tubes. 15 g, 30 g, 60 g. *Rx.*
Use: Anti-inflammatory agent.

fluticasone propionate. (Various Mfr.) Fluticasone propionate 0.05%. Cetostearyl alcohol, mineral oil. Cream. 15 g, 30 g, 60 g. *Rx.*
Use: Anti-inflammatory agent.

Flutra. Trichlormethiazide.
Use: Diuretic.

•**flutroline.** (FLEW-troe-LEEN) USAN.
Use: Antipsychotic.

•**fluvastatin sodium.** (FLEW-vah-STAT-in) USAN.
Use: Antihyperlipidemic inhibitor, HMG-CoA reductase inhibitor.
See: Lescol.
Lescol XL.

Fluvirin. (Novartis Vaccines) Hemagglutinin 15 mcg each of A/California/7/2009 NYMC X-181 (H1N1), A/Victoria/210/2009 NYMC X-187 (H3N2) (an A/Perth/16/2009-like strain), and B/Brisbane/60/2008 per 0.5 mL. Inj., Susp. (purified split virus). Preservative-free 0.5 mL prefilled, single-dose syringe (formulated without preservative; however, thimerosal is used during manufacturing and is removed by subsequent purification steps to a trace amount [mercury ≤ 1 mcg per 0.5 mL dose]); 5 mL multidose vial with preservative (thimerosal) (with mercury 25 mcg/dose). Each dose from the multidose vial or prefilled syringe may also contain residual amounts of ovalbumin (≤ 1 mcg), polymyxin (≤ 3.75 mcg), neomycin (≤ 2.5 mcg), betapropiolactone (≤ 0.5 mcg), and nonylphenol ethoxylate (≤ 0.015%). *Rx.*
Use: Viral vaccine.

•**fluvoxamine maleate.** (flew-VOX-ah-meen) USAN.
Tall Man: fluvoxaMINE
Use: Antidepressant; selective serotonin reuptake inhibitor.
See: Luvox.
Luvox CR.

fluvoxamine maleate. (Various Mfr.) Fluvoxamine maleate 25 mg, 50 mg, 100 mg. Tab. 100s, 500s. *Rx.*
Use: Antidepressant, selective serotonin reuptake inhibitor.

•**fluzinamide.** (flew-ZIN-ah-mide) USAN.
Use: Anticonvulsant.

Fluzone. (Sanofi Pasteur) Hemagglutinin 15 mcg each of A/California/7/2009 NYMC X-179A (H1N1), A/Victoria/210/2009 NYMC X-187 (H3N2) (an A/Perth/16/2009-like virus), and B/Brisbane/60/2008 per 0.5 mL. Mercury 25 mcg/dose. Each 0.5 mL dose may contain residual amounts of formaldehyde (≤ 100 mcg), octylphenol ethoxylate (≤ 100 mcg), and gelatin (0.05%). Inj., Susp. (purified split virus). Preservative-free 0.25 mL and 0.5 mL prefilled syringes; preservative-free 0.5 mL single-dose vial; 5 mL multiple-dose vial with preservative (thimerosal). *Rx.*
Use: Viral vaccine.

Fluzone High-Dose. (Sanofi Pasteur) Hemagglutinin 60 mcg each of A/California/7/2009 NYMC X-179A (H1N1), A/Victoria/210/2009 NYMC X-187 (H3N2) (an A/Perth/16/2009-like virus), and B/Brisbane/60/2008 per 0.5 mL. Each 0.5 mL dose may contain residual amounts of formaldehyde (≤ 100 mcg) and octylphenol ethoxylate (≤ 250 mcg). Preservative free. Inj., Susp. (purified split virus). Prefilled, single-dose syringe. 0.5 mL. *Rx.*
Use: Viral vaccine.

FML. (Allergan) Fluorometholone 0.1%. Benzalkonium chloride 0.004%, EDTA, polysorbate 80, polyvinyl alcohol 1.4%, sodium chloride, sodium phosphate. Ophth. Susp. Bot. 5 mL, 10 mL, 15 mL. *Rx.*
Use: Corticosteroid, ophthalmic; anti-inflammatory.

FML Forte. (Allergan) Fluorometholone 0.25%. Benzalkonium chloride 0.005%, EDTA, polysorbate 80, polyvinyl alcohol 1.4%, sodium chloride, sodium phosphate. Ophth. Susp. Bot. 5 mL, 10 mL, 15 mL. *Rx.*
Use: Corticosteroid, ophthalmic; anti-inflammatory.

FML S.O.P. (Allergan) Fluorometholone 0.1%. Phenylmercuric acetate 0.0008%, white petrolatum, mineral oil, lanolin alcohol. Ophth. Oint. Tube 3.5 g. *Rx.*

Use: Corticosteroid, ophthalmic; anti-inflammatory.

Focalin. (Novartis) Dexmethylphenidate hydrochloride 2.5 mg, 5 mg, 10 mg. Lactose. Tab. Bot. 100s. *c-II.*
Use: Central nervous system stimulant.

Focalin XR. (Novartis) Dexmethylphenidate hydrochloride 5 mg, 10 mg, 15 mg, 20 mg, 30 mg, 40 mg. Sugar spheres. ER Cap. 100s. *c-II.*
Use: Central nervous system stimulant.

•**focofilcon A.** (FOE-koe-FILL-kahn) USAN.
Use: Contact lens material (hydrophilic).

•**fodipir.** (FO-di-pir) USAN.
Use: Excipient.

Foillecort. (Blairex) Hydrocortisone acetate 0.5%. Cream. Tube 3.5 g. *OTC.*
Use: Corticosteroid, topical.

Foille Medicated First Aid. (Blistex) **Oint.:** Benzocaine 5% with chloroxylenol 0.1%, benzyl alcohol, EDTA in a corn oil base. 3.5 g, 28 g. **Aerosol:** Benzocaine 5% with chloroxylenol 0.6%, benzyl alcohol in corn oil. 92 mL. *OTC.*
Use: Topical local anesthetic, ester local anesthetic.

Folacin.
See: Folic acid.

folate.
Use: Water-soluble vitamin.
See: DuLeek-DP 7.5.
DuLeek-DP 15.

Folgard. (Upsher-Smith) B_6 10 mg, B_{12} 115 mcg, folic acid 0.8 mg. Tab. Bot. 60s. *OTC.*
Use: Vitamin, mineral supplement.

Folgard Rx. (Upsher-Smith) B_6 25 mg, B_{12} 500 mcg, folic acid 2.2 mg. Tab. Bot. 100s. *Rx.*
Use: Vitamin, mineral supplement.

•**folic acid.** (FOLE-ik) *USP 34.*
Use: Anemia; vitamin (hematopoietic).
See: Deplin.
W/Iron.
See: Tandem F.

folic acid. (Fujisawa Healthcare) Folic acid 5 mg/mL w/benzyl alcohol 1.5%, EDTA. Inj. Vials 10 mL. *Rx.*
Use: Vitamin supplement.

folic acid. (Various Mfr.) Folic acid. Tab. **0.4 mg, 0.8 mg:** Bot. 100s. **1 mg:** Bot. 30s, 100s, 1000s, UD 100s. *Rx.*
Use: Vitamin supplement.

folic acid antagonists.
See: Daraprim.
Methotrexate.
Pemetrexed.
Pralatrexate.
Pyrimethamine.

folinic acid. Leucovorin Calcium, USP.
Fol-Li-Bee. (Foy Laboratories) Liver inj. equivalent to cyanocobalamin 10 mcg, folic acid 1 mg, cyanocobalamin 100 mcg/mL, phenol 0.5% pH adjusted w/sodium hydroxide and/or hydrochloride. Vial 10 mL multi-dose, Monovials. *Rx.*
Use: Anemia.

follicle-stimulating hormone, human. Menotropins.

Follicormon.
See: Estradoil Benzoate.

follicular hormones.
See: Estrone.

Follistim AQ. (Organon) Follicle-stimulating hormone 75 units per 0.5 mL, 150 units per 0.5 mL. Sucrose 25 mg, sodium 7.35 mg. Inj. Single-use vials. *Rx.*
Use: Ovulation stimulant.

Follistim AQ Cartridge. (Organon) Follicle-stimulating hormone activity 150 units (175 units per 0.2 mL), 300 units (350 units per 0.42 mL), 600 units (650 units per 0.78 mL), 900 units (975 units per 1.17 mL). Benzyl alcohol 10 mg/mL, sucrose 50 mg/mL. Inj. Cartridges with *BD* micro-fine pen needles. *Rx.*
Use: Ovulation stimulants.

follitropin alfa.
Use: Sex hormone, ovulation stimulant.
See: Gonal-F.
Gonal-f RFF Pen.

follitropin beta.
Use: Sex hormone, ovulation stimulant.
See: Follistim AQ.

Folotyn. (Allos Therapeutics Inc) Pralatrexate 20 mg/mL. Preservative free. Inj., Soln. Single-use vial. 1 mL, 2 mL. *Rx.*
Use: Antimetabolite, folic acid antagonist.

Folpace. (Alaven) Vitamin B_6 25 mg, vitamin B_{12} 425 mcg, FA 2.05 mg, E 100 units, Mg 100 mg. Tab. 90s. *Rx.*
Use: Nutritional product.

Foltrin. (Eon Labs) Liver and stomach concentrate 240 mg, B_{12} 15 mcg, iron 110 mg, C 75 mg, folic acid 0.5 mg. Cap. Bot. 100s, 1000s. *Rx.*
Use: Mineral, vitamin supplement.

FOLTX. (PAMLAB) B_{12} 2,000 mcg, B_6 25 mg, folic acid 2.5 mg, sugar free, dye free. Tab. Bot. 90s. *Rx.*
Use: Vitamin, mineral supplement.

•**fomepizole.** (foe-MEH-pih-ZOLE) USAN.
Use: Antidote (alcohol dehydrogenase inhibitor).
See: Antizol.

fomepizole. (X-Gen) Fomepizole 1 g/mL. Preservative free. Inj., Soln. Vials. 1.5 mL. *Rx.*
Use: Antidote.

Fonatol.
See: Diethylstilbestrol.

•**fonazine mesylate.** (FAH-nazz-een) USAN.
Use: Serotonin inhibitor.

•**fondaparinux sodium.** (fon-da-PAR-in-ux) USAN.
Use: Anticoagulant, selective factor Xa inhibitor.
See: Arixtra.

fontarsol.
See: Dichlorophenarsine Hydrochloride.

•**fontolizumab.** (fon-toe-LIZ-oo-mab) USAN.
Use: Immunoregulator.

Foradil Aerolizer. (Schering) Formoterol fumarate 12 mcg. Lactose. Inh. Pow. in Cap. Blister Pack 12s, 60s w/*Aerolizer Inhaler. Rx.*
Use: Bronchodilator, sympathomimetic.

Foralicon Plus. (Forbes) Vitamins B_{12} 16.7 mcg, B_6 4 mg, iron 200 mg (equivalent to elemental iron 24 mg), niacinamide 40 mg, folic acid 0.8 mg, sorbitol soln. q.s./15 mL. Elix. Bot. 8 oz, 16 oz. *Rx.*
Use: Mineral, vitamin supplement.

Forane. (Baxter Healthcare) Isoflurane. Gas. Volume 100 mL. *Rx.*
Use: Anesthetic, general.

•**forasartan.** (far-ah-SAHR-tan) USAN.
Use: Antihypertensive.

Fordustin. (Sween) Cornstarch based powder with deodorizing action. Bot. 3 oz, 8 oz. *OTC.*
Use: Powder, topical.

•**foretinib.** (for-e-TIN-ib) USAN.
Use: Antineoplastic.

•**forigerimod.** (FOR-eye-JIR-i-mod) USAN.
Use: Treatment of systemic lupus erythematosus.

•**forigerimod acetate.** (FOR-eye-JIR-i-mod) USAN.
Use: Treatment of systemic lupus erythematosus.

Formadon. (Gordon Laboratories) Formalin 3.7% to 4% (10% of USP strength) in an aqueous perfumed base. Soln. Bot. 1 oz, 4 oz, 0.5 gal, 1 gal. *Rx.*
Use: Bromhidrosis, hyperhidrosis agent.

Formalaz. (River's Edge) Formaldehyde 10%. Liq. Roll-on plastic bot. 85.05 g. *Rx.*
Use: Drying agent.

•**formaldehyde.** (for-MAL-deh-hide) *USP 34.*
Use: Drying agent.
See: Formalyde 10.
Lazer Formalyde.

Formalin.
See: Formaldehyde.

Formalyde-10. (Pedinol) Formaldehyde 10%, SD-40 alcohol. Spray. Bot. 60 mL. *Rx.*
Use: Drying agent.

Forma-Ray. (Gordon Laboratories) Formalin 7.4% to 8% (20% of USP strength) in aqueous, scented, tinted solution. Soln. Bot. 1.5 oz, 4 oz. *OTC.*
Use: Drying.

•**formocortal.** (FORE-moe-CORE-tal) USAN.
Use: Corticosteroid, topical.

•**formoterol fumarate.** (fore-MOE-ter-ole) USAN.
Use: Bronchodilator, sympathomimetic.
See: Foradil Aerolizer.
Perforomist.
W/Budesonide.
See: Symbicort.
W/Mometasone Furoate.
See: Dulera.

Formula B. (Major) Vitamins B_1 15 mg, B_2 15 mg, B_3 100 mg, B_5 18 mg, B_6 4 mg, B_{12} 5 mcg, C 500 mg, folic acid 0.5 mg. Tab. Bot 250 g. *Rx.*
Use: Vitamin supplement.

Formula B Plus. (Major) Iron 27 mg, A 5000 units, E 30 units, B_1 20 mg, B_2 20 mg, B_3 100 mg, B_5 25 mg, B_6 25 mg, B_{12} 50 mcg, C 500 mg, folic acid 0.8 mg, biotin 0.15 mg, Cr, Cu, Mg, Mn, Zn. Tab. Bot 100s, 500s. *Rx.*
Use: Mineral, vitamin supplement.

Formula EM. (Major) Dextrose 1.87 g, fructose 1.87 g, phosphoric acid 21.5 mg/5 mL, methylparaben, cherry-flavor. Soln. Bot. 118 mL. *OTC.*
Use: Antiemetic, antivertigo agent.

Formula 44 Cough Mixture. (Procter & Gamble) Chlorpheniramine maleate 2 mg, dextromethorphan HBr 15 mg, alcohol 10%/5 mL. Liq. Bot. 120 mL, 240 mL. *OTC.*
Use: Antihistamine; antitussive.

Formula 44D Decongestant Cough Mixture. (Procter & Gamble) Pseudoephedrine hydrochloride 20 mg, dextromethorphan HBr 10 mg, guaifenesin 67 mg, alcohol 10%/5 mL. Liq. Bot. 120 mL, 240 mL. *OTC.*
Use: Antitussive; decongestant; expectorant.

Formula 44M Cough and Cold. (Procter & Gamble) Pseudoephedrine hydro-

chloride 15 mg, dextromethorphan HBr 7.5 mg, chlorpheniramine maleate 1 mg, acetaminophen 125 mg/5 mL, alcohol 20%, saccharin, sucrose. Liq. Bot. 120 mL, 240 mL. *OTC.*
Use: Analgesic; antihistamine; antitussive; decongestant.

Formula 405. (Doak Dermatologics) **Bar:** Sodium tallowate, sodium cocoate, Doak Additive A, PPF-20 methyl glucose ether, titanium dioxide, trochlorocarbanilide, pentasodium pentatate, EDTA. 100 g. **Cream:** Coconut oil, beeswax, PEG-40, petrolatum, mineral oil, lanolin alcohol, isopropyl palmitate, sweet almond oil, ceresin, stearyl alcohol, lanolin, vitamin E, urea parabens. 56.7 g. *OTC.*
Use: Dermatologic, cleanser.

Formula No. 81. (Fellows) Liver (beef) 1 mcg, ferrous gluconate 100 mg, niacinamide 100 mg, B_2 1.5 mg, panthenol 2.5 mg, B_{12} 3 mcg, procaine hydrochloride 25 mg/2 mL. Inj. Vial 30 mL. *OTC.*
Use: Mineral, vitamin supplement.

Formula 1207. (Thurston) Iodine, liver fraction No. 2, caseinates. Tab. Bot. 100s, 250s. *OTC.*
Use: Mineral supplement.

Formulation R. (G & W Labs) **Cream:** Glycerin 12%, petrolatum 18%, phenylephrine hydrochloride 0.025%. Tube. 52 g. **Oint.:** Petrolatum 71.9%, mineral oil 14%, phenylephrine hydrochloride 0.25%, parabens. Tube. 28.4 g, 56.8 g. *OTC.*
Use: Anorectal preparation.

Formula VM-2000. (Solgar) Iron 5 mg, A 12,500 units, D 200 units, E 100 units, B_1 50 mg, B_2 50 mg, B_3 50 mg, B_5 50 mg, B_6 50 mg, B_{12} 50 mcg, C 150 mg, folic acid 0.2 mg, B, Ca, Cr, Cu, I, K, Mg, Mn, Mo, Se, Zn 7.5 mg, betaine, biotin 50 mcg, choline, bioflavonoids, amino acids, hesperidin, inositol, l-glutethione, PABA, rutin. Tab. Bot. 30s, 60s, 90s, 180s. *OTC.*
Use: Mineral, vitamin supplement.

formyl tetrahydropteroylglutamic acid. Leucovorin Calcium.

•**forodesine.** (FORE-oh-de-seen) USAN.
Use: Antineoplastic.

•**forodesine hydrochloride.** (fore-OH-de-seen) USAN.
Use: Antineoplastic.

Forta Drink. (Ross) Whey protein concentrate, sucrose, vitamins A, B_1, B_2, B_3, B_5, B_6, B_{12}, C, D, E, folic acid, biotin, Ca, Cu, Fe, I, Mg, Mn, P, Zn. Pow. Can. 482 g. *OTC.*
Use: Nutritional supplement.

Forta-Flora. (Barth's) Whey-lactose 90%, pectin. Pow. Jar lb. Wafer. Bot. 100s. *OTC.*

Forta Instant Cereal. (Ross) Lactose-free oat or bran cereal provides 6.25 g dietary fiber/serving. Can 1 lb 1 oz. *OTC.*
Use: Nutritional supplement.

Forta Instant Pudding. (Ross) Lactose-free in pudding base. Can 1 lb 12 oz. Vanilla, chocolate, butterscotch flavors. *OTC.*
Use: Nutritional supplement.

Fortamet. (First Horizon) Metformin hydrochloride 500 mg, 1000 mg. Film-coated. ER Tab. 60s. *Rx.*
Use: Antidiabetic agent, biguanide.

Forta Pudding Mix. (Ross) Milk protein isolate, sucrose, hydrolyzed cornstarch, modified tapioca starch, partially hydrogenated soybean oil, vitamins A, B_1, B_2, B_3, B_5, B_6, B_{12}, C, D, E, folic acid, biotin, Ca, Fe, P, I, Mg, Zn, Cu, Mn, tartrazine. Can 794 g. *OTC.*
Use: Nutritional supplement.

Forta Shake Powder. (Ross) Nonfat dry milk, sucrose, vitamins A, B_1, B_2, B_3, B_5, B_6, B_{12}, C, D, E, folic acid, biotin, Ca, Cu, Fe, I, Mg, Mn, P, Zn, tartrazine. Can lb, pkt. 1.4 oz. Can 1 lb 2.7 oz, pkt. 1.6 oz. *OTC.*
Use: Nutritional supplement.

Forta Soup Mix. (Ross) Milk protein isolate, sodium and calcium caseinate, hydrolyzed cornstarch, modified tapioca starch, powdered shortening (partially hydrogenated coconut oil), vitamins A, B_1, B_2, B_3, B_5, B_6, B_{12}, C, D, E, folic acid, biotin, Ca, Cu, Fe, I, Mg, Mn, P, Zn. Chicken flavor. Can. 454 g. *OTC.*
Use: Nutritional supplement.

Fortaz. (GlaxoWellcome) Ceftazidime Pow. for Inj. Sodium 2.3 mEq/g.
500 mg: Vial. **1 g:** Vial, *ADD-Vantage* vial, Infusion Pack. **2 g:** Vial, *ADD-Vantage* vial, Infusion Pack. **6 g:** Bulk Pkg. **Inj.:** 1 g (dextrose hydrous 2.2 g), 2 g (dextrose hydrous 1.6 g). Vial 50 mL, premixed, frozen. *Rx.*
Use: Anti-infective, cephalosporin.

Forte L.I.V. (Foy Laboratories) Cyanocobalamin 15 mcg liver injection equivalent to vitamin B_{12} activity 1 mcg, ferrous gluconate 50 mg, B_2 0.75 mg, panthenol 1.25 mg, niacinamide 50 mg, citric acid 8.2 mg, sodium citrate 118 mg/mL, procaine hydrochloride 2%. Bot. 30 mL. *OTC.*
Use: Mineral, vitamin supplement.

Fortel Midstream. (Biomerica) Reagent

in-home urine test for pregnancy. 1 test stick per kit.
Use: Diagnostic aid, pregnancy.

Fortel Ovulation. (Biomerica) Monoclonal antibody-based home test to predict ovulation. Kit 1s.
Use: Diagnostic aid.

Fortel Plus. (Biomerica) Reagent in-home urine pregnancy test. Kit contains urine collection cup, dropper, test device.
Use: Diagnostic aid, pregnancy.

Forteo. (Lilly) Teriparatide 250 mcg/mL, mannitol 45.4 mg. Inj. Prefilled pen delivery device 2.4 mL (20 mcg of teriparatide per dose). *Rx.*
Use: Parathyroid hormone.

Fortesta. (Endo Pharmaceuticals Inc) Testosterone 10 mg per 0.5 g. Ethanol, propylene glycol. Gel. 60 g metered-dose pumps (each metered-dose pump delivers 120 metered 10 mg doses). *c-III.*
Use: Sex hormone, androgen.

Fortical. (Upsher-Smith) Calcitonin-salmon 200 units per activation (0.09 mL/dose). Sodium chloride, benzyl alcohol, phenylethyl alcohol. Nasal spray. Metered-dose, glass bot. with pump. 3.7 mL. *Rx.*
Use: Antihypercalcemic.

Fortral. (Sanofi-Synthelabo) Pentazocine as solution and tablets. *c-IV.*
Use: Analgesic, narcotic.

Fortramin. (Thurston) Vitamins E 200 units, A 6000 units, D 600 units, B_1 4.5 mg, B_2 4.5 mg, B_6 4.5 mg, B_{12} 5 mcg, C 2.75 mg, rutin 8 mg, hesperidin complex 10 mg, lemon bioflavonoids 15 mg, d-calcium pantothenate 50 mg, para-aminobenzoic acid 7.5 mg, biotin 10 mg, folic acid 24 mcg, niacinamide 20 mg, desiccated liver 25 mg, iron 3 mg, calcium 75 mg, phosphorus 34 mg, manganese 10 mg, copper 0.5 mg, zinc 0.5 mg, iodine 0.375 mg, potassium 500 mg, magnesium 5 mg. Tab. Bot. 100s, 250s. *OTC.*
Use: Mineral, vitamin supplement.

.44 Magnum. (BDI) Caffeine 200 mg. Cap. Bot. 100s, 500s. *OTC.*
Use: CNS stimulant, analeptic.

40 Winks. (Roberts) Diphenhydramine hydrochloride 50 mg. Cap. Bot. 30s. *OTC.*
Use: Sleep aid.

Fosamax. (Merck) Alendronate sodium (as base). **Oral Soln.:** 70 mg. Parabens, saccharin. Raspberry flavor. 75 mL. **Tab.:** 5 mg, 10 mg, 35 mg, 40 mg, 70 mg. Lactose. Unit-of-use 30s (5 mg, 10 mg, 40 mg), 100s (5 mg, 10 mg); unit-of-use 4s and UD 20s (35 mg, 70 mg); Bot. 1000s, *Uniblister* cards of 31, UD 100s (10 mg). *Rx.*
Use: Bone resorption inhibitor; bisphosphonate.

Fosamax Plus D. (Merck) Alendronate/ vitamin D_3 70 mg/70 mcg (equiv. to vitamin D 2800 units), 70 mg/140 mcg (equiv. to vitamin D 5600 units). Lactose, sucrose. Tab. Unit-of-use blisters of 4, UD 20s. *Rx.*
Use: Bisphosphonate.

•**fosamprenavir calcium.** (FOSS-am-PREN-ah-veer) USAN.
Use: Antiretroviral agents.
See: Lexiva.

•**fosamprenavir sodium.** (FOSS-am-PREN-ah-veer) USAN.
Use: Antiviral.

•**fosaprepitant dimeglumine.** (FOS-ap-RE-pi-tant)
Use: Antiemetic/antivertigo agent.
See: Emend.

•**fosarilate.** (FOSS-ah-RILL-ate) USAN.
Use: Antiviral.

•**fosazepam.** (foss-AZZ-eh-pam) USAN.
Use: Hypnotic; sedative.

•**fosbretabulin disodium.** (fos-BRE-ta-BUE-lin) USAN.
Use: Antineoplastic.

•**fosbretabulin tromethamine.** (fos-BRE-ta-BUE-lin troe-METH-a- meen) USAN.
Use: Antineoplastic.

•**foscarnet sodium.** (foss-CAR-net) USAN.
Use: Antiviral.

foscarnet sodium. (Hospira) Foscarnet sodium 24 mg per mL. Inj. 250 mL, 500 mL. *Rx.*
Use: Antiviral agent.

•**fosdevirine.** (FOS-de-VIR-een) USAN.
Use: Antiviral.

•**fosfomycin.** (foss-foe-MY-sin) USAN.
Use: Anti-infective.
See: Monurol.

•**fosfomycin tromethamine.** (foss-foe-MY-sin troe-METH-ah-meen) USAN.
Use: Anti-infective.
See: Monurol.

•**fosfonet sodium.** (FOSS-foe-net) USAN.
Use: Antiviral.

Fosfree. (Mission Pharmacal) Iron 14.5 mg, A 1500 units, D_3 150 units, B_1 4.5 mg, B_2 2 mg, B_3 10.5 mg, B_5 1 mg, B_6 2.5 mg, B_{12} 2 mcg, C 50 mg, Ca 175.5 mg, sugar. Tab. Bot. 120s. *OTC.*
Use: Mineral, vitamin supplement.

fosinopril. (FAH-sen-oh-PRIL)

Use: Angiotensin-converting enzyme inhibitor; antihypertensive.
See: Monopril.

●**fosinoprilat.** (fah-SIN-oh-prill-at) USAN.
Use: Antihypertensive.

●**fosinopril sodium.** (FAH-sen-oh-PRIL) USAN.
Use: Renin angiotensin system antagonist, angiotensin-converting enzyme inhibitor.
See: Monopril.
W/Hydrochlorothiazide.
See: Monopril-HCT.

fosinopril sodium. (Teva) Fosinopril sodium 10 mg, 20 mg, 40 mg. Isopropyl alcohol, lactose. Tab. 90s, 1,000s. *Rx.*
Use: Renin angiotensin system antagonist, angiotensin-converting enzyme inhibitor.

fosinopril sodium and hydrochlorothiazide. (Ranbaxy) Hydrochlorothiazide/fosinopril sodium 12.5 mg/10 mg, 12.5 mg/20 mg. Lactose. Tab. 30s, 100s, 1,000s. *Rx.*
Use: Antihypertensive combination.

●**fosphenytoin sodium.** (FOSS-FEN-ih-toe-in) USAN.
Use: Anticonvulsant.
See: Cerebyx.

fosphenytoin sodium. (Various Mfr.) Fosphenytoin sodium 75 mg/mL (equiv. to phenytoin sodium 50 mg/mL). Inj., Soln.; concentrate. Vial. 2 mL, 10 mL. *Rx.*
Use: Anticonvulsant, hydantoin.

●**fospropofol disodium.** (fos-proe-POE-fol) USAN.
Use: Sedative/hypnotic agent.
See: Lusedra.

●**fosquidone.** (FOSS-kwih-dohn) USAN.
Use: Antineoplastic.

Fosrenol. (Shire) Lanthanum carbonate 500 mg, 750 mg, 1000 mg. Chew. Tab. 90s. *Rx.*
Use: Phosphate binder.

●**fostamatinib.** (FOS-tam-A-ti-nib) USAN.
Use: Immunomodulator.

●**fostamatinib disodium.** (FOS-tam-A-ti-nib) USAN.
Use: Immunomodulator.

●**fostedil.** (FOSS-teh-dill) USAN.
Use: Vasodilator, calcium channel blocker.

Fostex. (Bristol-Myers Squibb) Benzoyl peroxide 10%, EDTA, urea. Bar. 106 g. *OTC.*
Use: Dermatologic, acne.

Fostex Acne Cleansing Cream. (Bristol-Myers Squibb) Salicylic acid 2%, EDTA, stearyl alcohol. Cream. Bot. 118 g.

OTC.
Use: Dermatologic, acne.

Fostex Acne Medication Cleansing Bar. (Bristol-Myers Squibb) Salicylic acid 2%, EDTA. Bar. 106 g. *OTC.*
Use: Dermatologic, acne.

●**fostriecin sodium.** (FOSS-try-eh-SIN) USAN.
Use: Antineoplastic.

●**fosveset.** (FOS-ve-set) USAN.
Use: Ligant excipient.

Fototar. (ICN Pharm) Coal tar extract (equiv. to 2% coal tar) in emollient moisturizing cream base. Cream. Tube 85 g, 454 g. *OTC.*
Use: Dermatologic.

4 Hair Softgel. (Marlyn Nutraceuticals) Iron 2.5 mg, A 1250 units, E 10 units, B_3 5 mg, B_5 2.5 mg, B_6 1.5 mg, B_{12} 44 mcg, C 25 mg, folic acid 33.3 mg, biotin 250 mcg, I, Mg, Cu, Zn 7.5 mg, choline bitartrate, inositol, Mn, methionine, PABA, B_1, L-cysteine, tyrosine, Si. Cap. Bot 60s. *OTC.*
Use: Mineral, vitamin supplement.

4 Nails Softgel. (Marlyn Nutraceuticals) Ca 167 mg, iron 3 mg, A 833 units, D 67, E 10 mg, B_1 3.3 mg, B_2 1.7 mg, B_3 8.3 mg, B_5 8.3 mg, B_6 8.3 mg, B_{12} 8.3 mcg, C 10 mg, folic acid 33.3 mg, biotin 8.3 mcg, P, I, Mg, Cu, Zn 3.3 mg, Cr, Mn, methionine, inositol, choline bitartrate, Se, PABA, protein isolate, gelatin, lecithin, unsaturated fatty acid, predigested protein L-cysteine, B mucopolysaccharides, silicon amino acid chelate, Si. Cap. Bot. 60s. *OTC.*
Use: Mineral, vitamin supplement.

4-N-1. (DermaRite) Dimethicone 1%, alcohols, parabens, PEG. Latex free. Cream. 114 g. *OTC.*
Use: Miscellaneous protectant.

4 Trace Elements. (Hospira) Chromium (as chloride) 6 mcg, copper (as chloride) 0.42 mg, manganese (as chloride) 0.37 mg, zinc (as chloride) 1.67 mg. Vial. 5 mL. *Rx.*
Use: Intravenous nutritional therapy.

4-Way Fast Acting Nasal Spray. (Novartis Consumer Health) Phenylephrine hydrochloride 1%, benzalkonium chloride, boric acid, sodium borate. Soln. Spray Bot. 30 mL. *OTC.*
Use: Nasal decongestant, arylalkylamine.

4-Way Menthol. (Novartis Consumer Health) Phenylephrine hydrochloride 1%. Menthol. Nasal Spray. 14.8 mL. *OTC.*
Use: Nasal decongestant, arylalkylamine.

4-Way Moisturizing Relief. (Novartis Consumer Health) Xylometazoline hydrochloride 0.1%. Benzalkonium chloride, edetate disodium. Spray, Soln. Intranasal. 14.8 mL. *c-v.*
Use: Nasal decongestant, imidazoline.

Fowler's Solution. Potassium Arsenite Solution.

Foxalin. (Standex) Digitoxin 0.1 mg, sodium carboxymethylcellulose. Cap. Bot. 100s. *Rx.*
Use: Cardiovascular agent.

foxglove.
See: Digitalis.

Foygen Aqueous. (Foy Laboratories) Estrogenic substance or estrogens 2 mg/mL with sodium carboxymethylcellulose, povidone, benzyl alcohol, methyl and propyl parabens. Inj. Vial 10 mL. *Rx.*
Use: Estrogen.

Foyplex. (Foy Laboratories) Sterile injectable soln. of nine water-soluble vitamins. Packaged as 2 separate solutions for extemporaneous combination. Inj. *Rx.*
Use: Nutritional supplement, parenteral.

Fragmin. (Eisai) Dalteparin sodium 2,500 units/0.2 mL (16 mg/0.2 mL), 5,000 units/0.2 mL (32 mg/0.2 mL), 7,500 units/0.3 mL (48 mg/0.3 mL), 10,000 units/mL (64 mg/mL), 10,000 units/0.4 mL (64 mg/0.4 mL), 12,500 units/0.5 mL (80 mg/0.5 mL), 15,000 units/0.6 mL (96 mg/0.6 mL), 18,000 units/0.72 mL (115.2 mg/0.72 mL), 95,000 units/3.8 mL (160 mg/mL), 95,000 units/9.5 mL (64 mg/mL). Preservative free (except 95,000 units/3.8 mL, 95,000 units/9.5 mL). Anti-Factor Xa International Units. Inj. Soln. Single-dose prefilled syringe 0.2 mL with 27-gauge × ½-inch needle (2,500 units/0.2 mL, 5,000 units/0.2 mL only), single-dose prefilled syringe 0.3 mL with 27-gauge × ½-inch needle (7,500 units/0.3 mL only), single-dose prefilled syringe 0.4 mL with 27-gauge × ½-inch needle (10,000 units/0.4 mL only), single-dose graduated syringes 1 mL with 27-gauge × ½-inch needle (10,000 units/mL only), single-dose prefilled syringes 0.5 mL with 27-gauge × ½-inch needle (12,500 units/0.5 mL only), single-dose prefilled syringes 0.6 mL with 27-gauge × ½-inch needle (15,000 units/0.6 mL only), single-dose prefilled syringes 0.72 mL with 27-gauge × ½-inch needle (18,000 units/0.72 mL only), multidose vials 9.5 mL with benzyl alcohol 14 mg/mL (95,000 units/9.5mL only), multidose vials 3.8 mL with benzyl alcohol 14 mg/mL (95,000 units/3.8 mL only). *Rx.*
Use: Anticoagulant.

FreAmine HBC 6.9%. (B. Braun) High branched 6.9% amino acid formulation for hypercatabolic patients. Bot. 1000 mL. *Rx.*
Use: Nutritional supplement, parenteral.

FreAmine III. (B. Braun) Amino acid 8.5%, 10%. Bot. 500 mL, 1000 mL. *Rx.*
Use: Nutritional supplement, parenteral.

FreAmine III 3% w/Electrolytes. (B. Braun) Amino acid 3% with electrolytes. Bot. 1000 mL. *Rx.*
Use: Nutritional supplement, parenteral.

Free & Clear. (Pharmaceutical Specialties) Ammonium laureth sulfate, disodium cocamide MEA sulfosuccinate, cocamidopropyl hydroxysultaine, cocamide DEA, PEG-120 methyl glucose dioleate, EDTA, potassium sorbate, citric acid. Shampoo. Bot. 240 mL. *OTC.*
Use: Dermatologic, cleanser.

Freedavite. (Freeda) Iron 10 mg (from ferrous fumarate), vitamins A 5000 units, D 400 units, E 3 units, B_1 5 mg, B_2 3 mg, B_3 25 mg, B_5 5 mg, B_6 2 mg, B_{12} 2 mcg, C 60 mg, choline, inositol, potassium iodide, Ca, Cu, K, Mg, Mn, Se, Zn 0.2 mg. Bot. 100s, 250s. *OTC.*
Use: Mineral, vitamin supplement.

Freedox. (Pharmacia) Tirilazad.
Use: A 21 aminosteroid antioxidant.

•**frentizole.** (FREN-tih-zole) USAN.
Use: Immunoregulator.

Fresenius Propoven. (APP Pharmaceutical) Propofol 10 mg/mL. Glycerol, oleic acid, purified egg phosphatides, soybean oil, medium chain triglycerides. Inj., Emuls. Single-use ampule, 20 mL. Single-use vial, 20 mL, 50 mL, 100 mL. *Rx.*
Use: General anesthetic.

FreshBurst Listerine. (Warner Lambert) Thymol 0.064%, eucalyptol 0.092%, methyl salicylate 0.06%, menthol 0.042%, alcohol 21.6%. Rinse. Bot. 250 mL. *OTC.*
Use: Mouthwash.

FreshKote. (Focus Labs) Polyvinyl alcohol 2.7%, polyvinyl pyrrolidone 2%, boric acid, disodium EDTA, polixetonium, potassium chloride, sodium chloride. Soln., Ophth. 15 mL. *OTC.*
Use: Artificial tear solution.

Fresh n' Feminine. (Walgreen) Benzethonium Cl 0.2% Bot. 8 oz. *OTC.*
Use: Vaginal agent.

•**fresolimumab.** (FRE-soe-LIM-ue-mab) USAN.
Use: Monoclonal antibody.

Frova. (Elan) Frovatriptan succinate 2.5 mg, lactose. Tab. Blister card 9s. *Rx.*
Use: Agent for migraine, serotonin 5-HT$_1$ receptor agonist.

•**frovatriptan succinate.** (froe-va-TRIP-tan) USAN.
Use: Antimigraine, serotonin 5-HT$_1$ receptor agonist.
See: Frova.

•**fructose.** (FRUK-tose) *USP 34.*
Use: Nutritional supplement.
See: Frutabs.
W/Dextrose, Phosphoric Acid.
See: Emetrol.
  Nausatrol.
  Nausea Relief.
  Nausetrol.

fructose. (Various Mfr.) Fructose 10%. Soln. Bot. 1000 mL.
Use: Nutritional supplement.

fructose and sodium chloride injection.
Use: Electrolyte, fluid, nutrient replacement.

Fruit C 500. (Freeda) Vitamin C 500 mg (as calcium ascorbate and ascorbic acid). Rose hips. Sugar free. Chew. Tab. Bot. 100s, 250s. *OTC.*
Use: Water-soluble vitamin.

Fruit C 100. (Freeda) Vitamin C 100 mg (as calcium ascorbate and ascorbic acid). Sugar free. Chew. Tab. Bot. 250s. *OTC.*
Use: Water-soluble vitamin.

Fruit C 200. (Freeda) Vitamin C 200 mg (as calcium ascorbate and ascorbic acid). Rose hips. Sugar free. Chew. Tab. Bot. 100s, 250s. *OTC.*
Use: Water-soluble vitamin.

Fruity Chews. (Ivax) Vitamins A 2500 units, D 400 units, E 15 mg, B$_1$ 1.05 mg, B$_2$ 1.2 mg, B$_3$ 13.5 mg, B$_6$ 1.05 mg, B$_{12}$ 4.5 mcg, C (as sodium ascorbate and ascorbic acid) 60 mg, folic acid 0.3 mg. Chew. Tab. Bot. 100s. *OTC.*
Use: Mineral, vitamin supplement.

Fruity Chews w/Iron. (Ivax) Elemental iron 12 mg, vitamins A 2500 units, D 400 units, E 15 mg, B$_1$ 1.05 mg, B$_2$ 1.2 mg, B$_3$ 13.5 mg, B$_6$ 1.05 mg, B$_{12}$ 4.5 mcg, C (as sodium ascorbate and ascorbic acid) 60 mg, folic acid 0.3 mg, zinc 8 mg. Chew. Tab. Bot. 100s. *OTC.*
Use: Mineral, vitamin supplement.

Frutabs. (Pfanstiehl) Fructose 2 g. Tab. Bot. 100s. *OTC.*
Use: Carbohydrate supplement.

FS Shampoo. (Hill Dermaceuticals) *OTC.*
See: Capex.

FTA-ABS. (Wampole) Fluorescent treponemal antibody-absorbed test in vitro for confirming a positive reagent test for syphilis. Test 100s.
Use: Diagnostic aid.

FTA-ABS/DS. (Wampole) Fluorescent treponemal antibody-absorbed test in vitro for confirming a positive reagent test for syphilis. Test 100s.
Use: Diagnostic aid.

•**fuchsin, basic.** (FYOO-sin) *USP 34.*
Use: Anti-infective, topical.

FUDR. (Roche) Floxuridine 500 mg. Pow. for Inj., lyophilized. Vial 5 mL. *Rx.*
Use: Antineoplastic; antimetabolite.

Ful-Glo. (Akorn) Fluorescein sodium 0.6 mg. Strip. Box 300s. *OTC.*
Use: Diagnostic aid, ophthalmic.

Fuller. (Birchwood) Pkg. 1 shield.
Use: Anorectal preparation.

Full Spectrum B. (National Vitamin) Vitamin B$_1$ 1.5 mg, B$_2$ 1.7 mg, B$_3$ 20 mg, B$_5$ 10 mg, B$_6$ 10 mg, B$_{12}$ 6 mcg, C 60 mg, FA 800 mcg, biotin 3 mg. Preservative-free. Tab. 100s. *OTC.*
Use: Nutrition combination product.

•**fulranumab.** (ful-RAN-ue-mab) USAN.
Use: Treatment of pain.

•**fulvestrant.** (ful-VES-trant)
Use: Hormone, antiestrogen.
See: Faslodex.

•**fumaric acid.** (fyoo-MAR-ik) *NF 29.*
Use: Acidifier.

Fumatinic. (Laser) Iron 90 mg (from ferrous fumarate equivalent to elemental iron 66 mg), vitamins C 60 mg, B$_{12}$ 5 mcg. ER Cap. Bot. 100s. *Rx.*
Use: Mineral, vitamin supplement.

•**fumoxicillin.** (fyoo-MOX-ih-SILL-in) USAN.
Use: Antibacterial.

Fungacetin. (Blair) Triacetin (glyceryl triacetate) 25% in a water-miscible ointment base. Tube 30 g. *Rx.*
Use: Antifungal, topical.

Fungatin. (Major) Tolnaftate 1%. Cream. Tube 15 g. *OTC.*
Use: Antifungal, topical.

fungicides.
See: Amphotericin B.
  Ancobon.
  Asterol.
  Desenex.
  Diflucan.
  Fluconazole.
  Griseofulvin Ultramicrosize.
  Gris-PEG.
  Itraconazole.

Miconazole Nitrate.
Mycostatin.
Nifuroxime.
Nilstat.
Nizoral.
Nystatin.
Sporanox.
Undecylenic Acid.
Fungi Cure Intensive. (Alva-Amco) Clotrimazole 1%. Alcohol. Spray, Soln. Pump spray. 60 mL. *OTC.*
Use: Topical anti-infective, antifungal agent.
Fungi Cure Maximum Strength. (Alva-Amco) Undecylenic acid 25%. Aloe vera, isopropyl alcohol 70%. Liq., topical. 30 mL. *OTC.*
Use: Topical anti-infective.
•**fungimycin.** (FUN-jih-MY-sin) USAN.
Use: Antifungal.
Fungi-Nail. (Kramer) Resorcinol 1%, salicylic acid 2%, parachlorometaxylenol 2%, benzocaine 0.5%, acetic acid 2.5%, propylene glycol, hydroxypropyl methylcellulose, alcohol 0.5%. Bot. 30 mL. *OTC.*
Use: Antifungal, topical.
Fungizone for Laboratory Use in Tissue Culture. (Bristol-Myers Squibb) Amphotericin B 50 mg, sodium desoxycholate 41 mg. Vial 20 mL.
Use: Diagnostic aid.
Fungoid-HC Creme. (Pedinol Pharmacal) Miconazole nitrate 2%, hydrocortisone 1%. Cream. In 56.7 g, 1 g dual packets. *Rx.*
Use: Antifungal, topical.
Fungoid Tincture. (Pedinol) Miconazole nitrate 2%. Alcohol. Soln. Bot. with brush applicator 7.39 mL, 29.57 mL. *Rx.*
Use: Antifungal agent, topical antiinfective.
Furadantin. (Sciele) Nitrofurantoin 25 mg per 5 mL. Glycerin, parabens, saccharin, sorbitol. Oral Susp. Bot. 60 mL, 470 mL. *Rx.*
Use: Anti-infective, urinary.
furalazine hydrochloride.
Use: Antimicrobial compound.
Furanite. (Major) Nitrofurantoin 50 mg, 100 mg. Tab. Bot. 100s. *Rx.*
Use: Anti-infective, urinary.
•**furaprofen.** (FYOOR-ah-PRO-fen) USAN. *Formerly Enprofen.*
Use: Anti-inflammatory.
•**furazolidone.** (fyoor-ah-ZOE-lih-dohn) *USP 34.*
Use: Antiprotozoal.
•**furazolium chloride.** (FYOOR-ah-zoe-lee-uhm) USAN.

Use: Anti-infective.
•**furazolium tartrate.** (FYOOR-ah-ZOE-lee-uhm) USAN.
Use: Anti-infective.
•**furazosin hydrochloride.** (FYOOR-ah-zoe-sin) Under study.
Use: Antihypertensive.
•**furegrelate sodium.** (fyoor-eh-GRELL-ate) USAN.
Use: Inhibitor (thromboxane synthetase).
•**furobufen.** (FER-oh-BYOO-fen) USAN.
Use: Anti-inflammatory.
•**furodazole.** (fyoor-OH-dah-zole) USAN.
Use: Anthelmintic.
Furonatal FA. (Lexis Laboratories) Vitamins A 8000 units, D 400 units, E 30 units, C 60 mg, folic acid 1 mg, B_1 2 mg, B_2 2.8 mg, B_6 2.5 mg, B_{12} 8 mcg, niacinamide 20 mg, iron 65 mg, calcium 125 mg. Tab. Bot. 100s, 1000s. *Rx.*
Use: Mineral, vitamin supplement.
•**furosemide.** (fyu-ROH-se-mide) *USP 34.* Oral Solution, USP.
Use: Diuretic.
furosemide. (Roxane) Furosemide.
10 mg/mL: Soln. Dropper bot. 60 mL.
40 mg/5 mL: Soln. Bot. 5 mL, 10 mL, 500 mL. *Rx.*
Use: Diuretic.
furosemide. (Various Mfr.) **Tab.:** 20 mg, 40 mg, 80 mg. Bot. 60s (40 mg only), 100s, 500s, 1000s, UD 100s. **Oral Soln.:** 10 mg/mL Bot. 60 mL, 120 mL.
Inj.: 10 mg/mL Vial 10 mL; single-dose vial 2 mL, 10 mL; partial fill single-dose vial 4 mL. *Rx.*
Use: Diuretic.
•**fursalan.** (FYOOR-sal-an) USAN. Under study.
Use: Disinfectant.
•**fusidate sodium.** (FEW-sih-DATE) USAN.
Use: Anti-infective.
•**fusidic acid.** (few-SIH-dik) USAN.
Use: Anti-infective.
Fusilev. (Spectrum Pharmaceuticals) *Formerly levoleucovorin.* Levoleucovorin 50 mg (equiv. to levoleucovorin calcium 64 mg). Contains mannitol 50 mg. Inj., Lyophilized, Pow. for Soln. Single-use vials. *Rx.*
Use: Water-soluble vitamin.
Fuzeon. (Hoffman-LaRoche) Enfuvirtide 108 mg. Pow. for Inj., lyophilized. Convenience Kit with single-use vials, syringes, diluent, alcohol wipes. *Rx.*
Use: Anti-infective, tetracycline.

G

•**gabapentin.** (GAB-uh-PEN-tin) USAN.
Use: Anticonvulsant; amyotrophic lateral sclerosis agent.
See: Gabarone.
Gralise.
Neurontin.

gabapentin. (Ivax) Gabapentin 100 mg, 300 mg, 400 mg. Tab. 100s, 200s, 500s, 1000s (400 mg only), 2000s (300 mg only), 5000s (100 mg only), UD 100s. *Rx.*
Use: Anticonvulsant.

gabapentin. (Various Mfr.) Gabapentin 100 mg, 300 mg, 400 mg. Cap. 100s, 500s. *Rx.*
Use: Anticonvulsant.

•**gabapentin enacarbil.** (GAB-uh-PEN-tin EN-a-KAR-bil) USAN.
Use: Treatment of neuropathic pain and restless legs syndrome.

Gabarone. (Ivax) Gabapentin 100 mg, 300 mg, 400 mg. Lactose. Tab. 100s, 500s, 1000s (400 mg only), 2,000s (300 mg only), 5,000s (100 mg only), UD 100s. *Rx.*
Use: Anticonvulsant.

Gabbromicina. Aminosidine.
Use: Anti-infective. [Orphan Drug]

Gabitril Filmtabs. (Cephalon) Tiagabine hydrochloride 2 mg, 4 mg, 12 mg, 16 mg. Lactose. Tab. 30s. *Rx.*
Use: Anticonvulsant.

Gablofen. (CNS Therapeutics) Baclofen 0.05 mg/mL, 10 mg/20 mL, 10 mg/5 mL. Preservative free. Inj., Soln.; intrathecal. Single-use syringe. *Rx.*
Use: Skeletal muscle relaxant, centrally acting.

•**gaboxadol.** (gab-OX-a-dol) USAN.
Use: Insomnia.

Gacid. (Arcum) Magnesium trisilicate 500 mg, aluminum hydroxide 250 mg. Tab. Bot. 100s, 1000s. *OTC.*
Use: Antacid.

Gadavist. (Bayer Health Care) Gadobutrol 1 mmol/mL (equiv. to gadobutrol 604.72 mg/mL). Preservative free. Inj., Soln. Single-dose vial and pre-filled syringe. 7.5 mL, 10 mL, 15 mL. *Rx.*
Use: Miscellaneous radiopaque agent.

•**gadobenate dimeglumine.** (gad-oh-BEN-ate die-meh-GLUE-meen) USAN.
Use: Radiopaque agent.
See: MultiHance.

•**gadobutrol.** (GAD-oh-BUE-trol) USAN.
Use: Miscellaneous radiopaque agent.
See: Gadavist.

•**gadodiamide.** (GAD-oh-DIE-ah-mide) *USP 34.*
Use: Radiopaque agent, parenteral.
W/Caldiamide.
See: Omniscan.

•**gadofosveset trisodium.** (gad-oh-FOS-ve-set) USAN.
Use: Diagnostic contrast agent.
See: Ablavar.

•**gadopentetate dimeglumine.** (GAD-oh-PEN-teh-tate die-meh-GLUE-meen) *USP 34.*
Use: Radiopaque agent, parenteral.
See: Magnevist.

•**gadoteridol.** (GAD-oh-TER-ih-dahl) *USP 34.*
Use: Radiopaque agent, parenteral.
See: ProHance.

•**gadoversetamide.** (gad-oh-ver-SET-ah-mide) *USP 34.*
Use: Radiopaque agent, parenteral.
See: OptiMARK.

•**gadoxanum.** (gad-oh-ZAN-uhm) USAN.
Use: Diagnostic aid.

•**gadoxetate disodium.** (gad-OX-e-tate) USAN.
Use: Contrast agent.

•**gadozelite.** (gad-oh-ZEH-lite) USAN.
Use: Diagnostic aid.

•**galantamine.** (ga-LAN-ta-meen) USAN.
Use: Alzheimer disease; cholinesterase inhibitor.

galantamine hydrobromide.
Use: Cholinesterase inhibitor; Alzheimer disease.
See: Razadyne.
Razadyne ER.

galantamine hydrobromide. (Various Mfr.) Galantamine hydrobromide. **Tab.:** 4 mg, 8 mg, 12 mg. May contain lactose. 60s, 1000s. **ER Cap.:** 8 mg, 16 mg, 24 mg. May contain sugar spheres. 30s, 500s, unit-use 30s. *Rx.*
Use: CNS agent, cholinesterase inhibitor.

Galardin. (Glycomed, Inc.) Matrix metalloproteinase inhibitor.
Use: Corneal ulcers. [Orphan Drug]

•**galasomite.** (GAL-ah-som-ite) USAN.
Use: Verocytotoxogenic *E. coli* infections.

•**galdansetron hydrochloride.** (gahl-DAN-seh-trahn) USAN.
Use: Antiemetic.

•**galiximab.** (gal-IX-i-mab) USAN.
Use: Psoriasis.

•**gallamine triethiodide.** (GAL-ah-meen try-eth-EYE-oh-dide) *USP 34.*
Use: Neuromuscular blocker.

•**gallium citrate Ga 67 injection.** (GAL-ee-uhm SIH-trate) *USP 34.*
Use: Diagnostic aid (radiopaque medium); radiopharmaceutical.

•**gallium nitrate.** (GAL-ee-uhm NYE-trate) USAN.
Use: Calcium regulator; antihypercalcemic.
See: Ganite.

gallochrome.
See: Merbromin.

gallotannic acid.
See: Tannic Acid.

gallstone solubilizing agents.
See: Chenodiol.
Ursodiol.

•**galsulfase.** (gal-SUL-fase) USAN.
Use: Mucopolysaccharidosis VI.
See: Naglazyme.

Galzin. (Gate Pharmaceuticals) Zinc 25 mg, 50 mg. Cap. 250s. *Rx.*
Use: Trace element.

Galzin. (Lemmon) Zinc acetate.
Use: Wilson disease. [Orphan Drug]

GamaSTAN S/D. (Talecris Biotherapeutics) Immune globulin (human) 15% to 18% protein, glycine 0.21 to 0.32 M, solvent/detergent treated, preservative free. Soln. for Inj. Single-dose vial 2 mL, 10 mL; single-dose syringe 2 mL. *Rx.*
Use: Immune globulin.

Gamazole Tabs. (Major) Sulfamethoxazole 500 mg. Tab. Bot. 100s, 500s, 1000s. *Rx.*
Use: Anti-infective; sulfonamide.

•**gamfexine.** (gam-FEX-ine) USAN.
Use: Antidepressant.

gamma benzene hexachloride.
See: Lindane.

Gammagard. (Baxter) Immune globulin (human) 10%. Preservative free. Inj. Single-use bot. 1 g, 2.5 g, 5 g, 10 g, 20 g. *Rx.*
Use: Immune globulin.

Gammagard S/D. (Baxter Healthcare) Immune globulin (human) 0.5 g. Glycine 22.5 mg/mL, glucose 20 mg/mL, PEG 2 mg/mL, 100 mcg/mL of polysorbate 80 in a 5% solution. Inj., freeze-dried Pow. for Soln. Single-use bottle. *Rx.*
Use: Immune globulin.

gamma globulin.
See: Immune Globulin Intramuscular.
Immune Globulin Intravenous.
Immune Globulin Subcutaneous.

gamma-hydroxybutyrate. (Biocraft)
Use: Narcolepsy. [Orphan Drug]

gamma-hydroxybutyric acid. Under study.

Use: Anesthetic adjuvant, sleep disorders. [Orphan Drug]

gamma interferon.
See: Actimmune.

gammalinolenic acid.
Use: Juvenile rheumatoid arthritis. [Orphan Drug]

Gamunex. (Talecris Biotherapeutics) Immune globulin (human) 10%. Glycine 0.16 to 0.24 M. Caprylate/chromatography purified. Inj. 10 mL, 25 mL, 50 mL, 100 mL, 200 mL. *Rx.*
Use: Immune globulin.

Gamunex-C. (Talecris Biotherapeutics) Immune globulin (human) 10% (100 mg/mL) (each vial consists of 9% to 11% protein in 0.16 to 0.24 M of glycine). Preservative free. Inj., Soln. Single-use vial. 10 mL, 25 mL, 50 mL, 100 mL, 200 mL. *Rx.*
Use: Immune globulin.

ganaxolone. (Cocensys, Inc.)
Use: Infantile spasms; epilepsy; migraine. [Orphan Drug]

•**ganciclovir.** (gan-SIGH-kloe-VIHR) *USP 34.*
Use: Antiviral.
See: Cytovene.
Zirgan.

ganciclovir. (APP) Ganciclovir sodium 500 mg. Sodium 46 mg. Inj., lyophilized Pow. for Soln. Vial. 10 mL. *Rx.*
Use: Anti-infective, antiviral agent.

ganciclovir. (Ranbaxy) Ganciclovir 250 mg, 500 mg. Cap. 100s. *Rx.*
Use: Antiviral.

ganciclovir intravitreal implant.
Use: Cytomegalovirus retinitis. [Orphan Drug]
See: Vitrasert.

•**ganciclovir sodium.** (gah-SIGH-kloe-VIHR) USAN.
Use: Antiviral.
See: Cytovene.

Ganeake. (Geneva) Conjugated Estrogens, 0.625 mg, 1.25 mg, 2.5 mg. Tab. Bot. 100s, 1000s. *Rx.*
Use: Estrogen.

ganeden BC30.
See: Ganeden Sustenex.

Ganeden Sustenex. (Ganeden) Ganeden BC30 2 billion cells. Lactose free. Cap. 30s. *OTC.*
Use: Oral nutritional supplement, probiotic.

ganglionic blocking agents.
See: Dibenzyline Hydrochloride.
Hexamethonium Chloride and Bromide.
Hydergine.
Priscoline Hydrochloride.
Regitine.

Ganidin NR. (Cypress) Guaifenesin 100 mg/5 mL. Liq. 473 mL. *Rx.*
Use: Expectorant.

•**ganirelix acetate.** (ga-ni-REL-ix) USAN.
Use: Sex hormone.

ganirelix acetate. (Organon) Ganirelix acetate 250 mcg/0.5 mL. Inj. Prefilled disp. syr. 1 mL. Box 1s, 5s, 50s. *Rx.*
Use: Sex hormone.

Ganite. (Genta) Gallium nitrate 25 mg/mL. Preservative free. Inj. Single-dose vials. 20 mL. *Rx.*
Use: Calcium regulator; antihypercalcemic.

•**ganitumab.** (ga-NIT-ue-mab) USAN.
Use: Antineoplastic.

Gani-Tuss-DM NR. (Cypress) Dextromethorphan HBr 10 mg, guaifenesin 100 mg per 5 mL. Raspberry flavor. Alcohol and sugar free. Liq. Bot. 473 mL. *Rx.*
Use: Upper respiratory combination, antitussive with expectorant.

Gani-Tuss NR. (Cypress) Codeine phosphate 10 mg, guaifenesin 100 mg per 5 mL. Raspberry flavor, alcohol free, sugar free. Liq. Bot. 120 mL, 473 mL. *c-v.*
Use: Upper respiratory combination, antitussive with expectorant.

•**gantenerumab.** (GAN-te-NER-ue-mab) USAN.
Use: Alzheimer disease.

Gardasil. (Merck) Approximately 20 mcg of human papillomavirus (HPV) 6 L1 protein, 40 mcg of HPV 11 L1 protein, 40 mcg of HPV 16 L1 protein, 20 mcg of HPV 18 L1 protein per 0.5 mL. Preservative free. Soln. for Inj. Single-dose vials. 0.5 mL. *Rx.*
Use: Active immunization; viral vaccine.

gardinol type detergents. Aurinol, cyclopon, dreft, drene, duponol, lissapol, maprofix, modinal, orvus, sandopan, sadipan.
Use: Detergent.

gardol. Sodium lauryl sarcosinate.

•**garenoxacin mesylate.** (gar-en-OX-a-sin) USAN.
Use: Antibacterial.

Garfield's Tea. (Last) Senna leaf powder 68.3%. Bot. 2 oz. *OTC.*
Use: Laxative.

Garitabs. (Halsey Drug) Iron 50 mg, vitamins B_1 5 mg, B_2 5 mg, B_5 2 mg, B_6 0.5 mg, B_{12} 3 mcg, C 75 mg, niacinamide 30 mg. Bot. 1000s. *OTC.*
Use: Mineral, vitamin supplement.

Gari-Tonic Hematinic. (Halsey Drug) Vitamins B_1 5 mg, B_2 5 mg, B_6 1 mg,

B_{12} 6 mcg, pantothenic acid 4 mg, niacinamide 100 mg, choline bitartrate 100 mg, iron 100 mg/30 mL Bot. 16 oz. *OTC.*
Use: Mineral, vitamin supplement.

•**garlic.** (GAR-lik) *NF 29.* Allium.
Use: Antispasmodic.

garlic capsules. (Miller Pharmacal Group) Garlic 166 mg. Cap. Bot. 100s. *OTC.*
Use: Antispasmodic.

garlic oil.
See: Natural Garlic Oil.

garlic oil capsules. (Kirkman) Bot. 100s. *OTC.*

•**garnocestim.** (gar-no-SES-tim) USAN.
Use: Chemotherapeutic aid.

Gas Ban. (Roberts) Calcium carbonate 300 mg, simethicone 40 mg. Tab. Bot. UD 8s, 1000s. *OTC.*
Use: Antacid.

Gas Ban DS. (Roberts) Aluminum hydroxide 400 mg, magnesium hydroxide 400 mg, simethicone 40 mg/5 mL. Liq. Bot. 150 mL. *OTC.*
Use: Antacid.

Gas Permeable Lens Starter System. (PBH Wesley Jessen) **Daily cleanser:** Bot. 3 mL **Wetting and soaking soln.:** Bot. 60 mL *Hydra-Mat II* spin cleansing unit. Kit. *OTC.*
Use: Contact lens care.

Gas Permeable Wetting & Soaking Solution. (PBH Wesley Jessen) Sterile aqueous, isotonic soln. of low viscosity, buffered to physiological pH. Bot. 60 mL, 120 mL. *OTC.*
Use: Contact lens care.

Gas Relief. (Rugby) Simethicone 80 mg, 125 mg. Chew. Tab. Bot. 60s (125 mg only), 100s (80 mg only). *OTC.*
Use: Antiflatulant.

gastric acidifiers.
See: Glutamic Acid Hydrochloride.

Gastroccult. (SmithKline Diagnostics) Occult blood screening test. In 40s.
Use: Diagnostic aid.

Gastrocrom. (Celltech) Cromolyn sodium 100 mg/5 mL. Oral Conc. 8 UD Amps/foil pouch. *Rx.*
Use: Antiasthmatic.

Gastrografin. (Bracco Diagnostics) Diatrizoate meglumine 660 mg, diatrizoate sodium 100 mg, iodine 367 mg/mL. EDTA, polysorbate 80, saccharin, simethicone, lemon flavor. Soln. Bot. 120 mL. *Rx.*
Use: Radiopaque agent, GI contrast agent.

gastrointestinal agents.
See: Antidiarrheals.

Antiflatulents.
Mesalamine.

gastrointestinal anticholinergics/anti-spasmodics.
See: Belladonna Alkaloids.
Quaternary Anticholinergics.

gastrointestinal contrast agents (iodinated).
Use: Radiopaque agent.
See: Diatrizoate Meglumine and Diatrizoate Sodium.
Diatrizoate Sodium.

gastrointestinal contrast agents (miscellaneous).
Use: Radiopaque agent.
See: Barium Sulfate.
Radiopaque Polyvinyl Chloride.
Sodium Bicarbonate and Tartaric Acid.

gastrointestinal function tests.
See: Secretin.
Simethicone-coated Cellulose Suspension.
Sincalide.

gastrointestinal stimulants.
See: Maxolon.
Metoclopramide.
Metoclopramide Hydrochloride.
Octamide.
Reclomide.
Reglan.

gastrointestinal tests.
See: Entero-Test.
Gastro-Test.

Gastrosed. (Roberts) Hyoscyamine sulfate. **Soln.:** 0.125 mg/mL. Dropper Bot. 5 mL. Alcohol free. **Tab.:** 0.125 mg. Bot. 100s. *Rx.*
Use: Anticholinergic; antispasmodic.

Gastro-Test. (HDC) To determine stomach pH and to diagnose and locate gastric bleeding. Test 25s.
Use: Diagnostic aid.

Gas-X. (Novartis) Simethicone 80 mg. Softgel Cap. Pkg. 12s, 30s. *OTC.*
Use: Antiflatulent.

Gas-X, Extra Strength. (Novartis) Simethicone 125 mg, sorbitol. Softgel Cap. Box 30s, 100s. *OTC.*
Use: Antiflatulent.

Gas-X Thin Strips. (Novartis) Simethicone 62.5 mg. Maltodextrin, menthol, sorbitol, sucralose. Orally Disintegrating Strips. 18s. *OTC.*
Use: Antiflatulent.

Gas-X with Maalox Extra Strength. (Novartis) Calcium carbonate 500 mg, simethicone 125 mg. Dextrose, mannitol. Orange and wild berry flavors. Chew. Tab. 8s, 24s. *OTC.*
Use: Antacid.

• **gataparsen.** (GAT-a-PAR-sen) USAN.
Use: Antineoplastic.

• **gataparsen sodium.** (GAT-a-PAR-sen) USAN.
Use: Antineoplastic.

• **gatifloxacin.** (gat-ih-FLOX-ah-sin) USAN.
Use: Fluoroquinolone, antibiotic.
See: Zymar.

• **gauze, absorbent.** (gawz) *USP 34.*
Use: Surgical aid.

• **gauze, petrolatum.** (gawz PET-roe-LAY-tum) *USP 34.*
Use: Surgical aid.

• **gavestinel.** (ga-VE-sti-nel) USAN.
Use: Stroke.

GaviLAX. (Gavis) 17 g of PEG 3350. Pow. for oral Soln. 238 g, 510 g. *OTC.*
Use: Laxative, bowel evacuant.

GaviLyte-C. (Gavis Pharmaceuticals) 240 g of PEG 3350, sodium bicarbonate 6.72 g, sodium chloride 5.84 g, sodium sulfate 22.72 g, potassium chloride 2.98 g. Pow. for Soln. 4 L w/lemon flavor pack. *Rx.*
Use: Laxative, bowel evacuant.

GaviLyte-G. (Gavis Pharmaceuticals) 236 g of PEG 3350, sodium bicarbonate 6.74 g, sodium chloride 5.86 g, sodium sulfate 22.74 g, potassium chloride 2.97 g. Pow. for Soln. 4 L w/lemon flavor pack. *Rx.*
Use: Laxative, bowel evacuant.

Gaviscon. (GlaxoSmithKline) Aluminum hydroxide 80 mg. Magnesium 5 mg, magnesium trisilicate 14.2 mg, alginic acid, sodium bicarbonate, sucrose. Chew. Tab. 100s. *OTC.*
Use: Antacid.

Gaviscon Extra Strength Antacid. (GlaxoSmithKline) Aluminum hydroxide 160 mg, magnesium carbonate 105 mg. Acesulfame K, alginic acid, corn syr., mannitol, sodium bicarbonate, sucrose, calcium stearate, sodium 19 mg. Cherry flavor. Chew. Tab. 30s, 100s. *OTC.*
Use: Antacid.

Gaviscon Extra Strength Relief Formula. (GlaxoSmithKline) Aluminum hydroxide 254 mg, magnesium carbonate 237.5 mg. Parabens, EDTA, saccharin, sorbitol, simethicone, sodium alginate/5 mL. Liq. Bot. 355 mL. *OTC.*
Use: Antacid.

Gaviscon Liquid. (GlaxoSmithKline) Aluminum hydroxide 31.7 mg, magnesium carbonate 119.3 mg/5 mL. Bot. 177 mL, 355 mL. *OTC.*
Use: Antacid.

Gaviscon-2, Double Strength Tablets.
(GlaxoSmithKline) Aluminum hydroxide 160 mg, magnesium trisilicate 40 mg, alginic acid, sodium bicarbonate, sucrose. Chew. Tab. Bot. 48s. *OTC.*
Use: Antacid.

GBA.
See: Gamma Hydroxybutyrate.

G-BID DM TR. (Boca Pharmacal) Dextromethorphan HBr 60 mg, guaifenesin 1200 mg. ER Tab. 100s. *Rx.*
Use: Antitussive with expectorant.

G.B.S. (Forest) Dehydrocholic acid 125 mg, phenobarbital 8 mg, homatropine methylbromide 2.5 mg. Tab. 100s, 1000s. *Rx.*
Use: Hydrocholeretic.

G-CSF. Granulocyte Colony-Stimulating Factor.
See: Neupogen.

Gebauer's 114. (Gebauer) Dichlorotetrafluoroethane 100%. Can 8 oz.
Use: Anesthetic, local.

Gebauer's Spray and Stretch. (Gebauer) Tetrafluoroethane and pentafluoropropane. Spray. 103.5 mL. *Rx.*
Use: Local anesthetic, topical.

•**gefitinib.** (ge-FI-tye-nib) USAN.
Use: Antineoplastic.
See: Iressa.

Geladine. (Barth's) Gelatin, protein, vitamin D. Cap. Bot. 100s, 500s. *OTC.*

Gelamal. (Halsey Drug) Magnesium-aluminum hydroxide gel. Bot. 12 oz. *OTC.*
Use: Antacid.

•**gelatin.** (JEL-a-tin) *NF 29.*
Use: Pharmaceutic aid (encapsulating, suspending agent, tablet binder, tablet coating agent).

•**gelatin film, absorbable.** (JEL-a-tin) *USP 34.*
Use: Local hemostatic.
See: Gelfilm.

gelatin film, sterile.
See: Neupogen.

gelatin powder, sterile.
See: Gelfoam.

gelatin sponge.
See: Gelfilm.

•**gelatin sponge, absorbable.** (JEL-a-tin) *USP 34.*
Use: Hemostatic, local.
See: Gelfoam.

gelatin, zinc.
See: Zinc Gelatin.

Gelclair. (EKR Therapeutics) Water, maltodextrin, propylene glycol, PVP, sodium hyaluronate, potassium sorbate, sodium benzoate, hydroxyethylcellulose, PEG-40 hydrogenated castor oil, EDTA, benzalkonium chloride, flavoring, saccharin sodium, glycyrrhetinic acid. Gel. Single-use packets. 15 mL. *Rx.*
Use: Mouth and throat preparation.

Gel-Clean. (PBH Wesley Jessen) Gel formulated with nonionic surfactant. Tube 30 g. *OTC.*
Use: Contact lens care.

G-11. (Givaudan) Hexachlorophene Pow. for Mfg.
See: Hexachlorophene.

Gelfilm. (Pharmacia) Sterile, absorbable gelatin film. Envelope 1s. 100 mm × 125 mm. Also available as Ophth. Sterile 25 × 50 mm. Box 6s. *Rx.*
Use: Hemostatic, topical.

Gelfoam Dental Pack. (Pharmacia) Size 4, 20 mm × 20 mm × 7 mm. Jar 15 sponges. *Rx.*
Use: Hemostatic, topical.

Gelfoam Powder. (Pharmacia) Sterile Jar 1 g. *Rx.*
Use: Hemostatic, topical.

Gelfoam Prostatectomy Cones. (Pharmacia) Prostatectomy cones (for use with Foley catheter) 13 cm, 18 cm in diameter. Box 6s. *Rx.*
Use: Hemostatic.

Gelhist Pediatric Suspension. (Econolab) Phenylephrine tannate 5 mg, chlorpheniramine tannate 2 mg, pyrilamine tannate 12.5 mg/5 mL, methylparaben, saccharin, sucrose. Susp. Bot. 118 mL, 473 mL. *Rx.*
Use: Antihistamine, decongestant.

Gel Jet Gelatin Capsules. (Kirkman) Bot. 100s, 250s.

Gel-Kam. (Colgate Oral) **Gel:** Fluoride 0.1% (stannous fluoride 0.4%). Mint, fruit, berry, bubble gum, cinnamon flavors. Bot. w/applicator tip. 4.3 oz, 7 oz. **Rinse:** Sodium fluoride 0.04%. Mint, fruit and berry, bubblegum, and cinnamon flavors. 4.3 oz, 7 oz. **Rinse Concen.:** Stannous fluoride 0.63%. Glycerin. Cinnamon and mint flavors. 283 g. *Rx-OTC.*
Use: Dental caries agent.

Gelnique. (Watson) Oxybutynin chloride 10%. Alcohol, glycerin. Gel. Sachet. 1 g. Carton. 30s. *Rx.*
Use: Renal and genitourinary agent, anticholinergic.

Gelocast. (Beiersdorf) Unna's Boot medicated bandage: Unna's semi-rigid cast impregnated with zinc oxide mixtures. Box 4 inches × 10 yd, 3 inches × 10 yd.
Use: Unna's cast dressing.

gelsemium. (Various Mfr.) Pkg. oz.

Use: Neuralgia.
W/A.P.C.
See: APC Combinations.
W/Combinations
See: UB.
Urisan-P.
gelsolin, recombinant human. (Biogen)
Use: Cystic fibrosis. [Orphan Drug]
Gel-Tin. (Young Dental) Fluoride 0.1%
(from stannous fluoride 0.4%). Gel Bot.
57 g, 623 g. *Rx.*
Use: Dental caries agent.
•**gemcabene calcium.** (JEM-ka-been)
USAN.
Use: Atherosclerosis.
•**gemcadiol.** (JEM-kah-DIE-ole) USAN.
Use: Antihyperlipoproteinemic.
•**gemcitabine.** (JEM-sit-ah-BEAN) USAN.
Use: Antineoplastic.
gemcitabine. (Various Mfr.) Gemcitabine
hydrochloride 200 mg, 1 g, 2 g. Mannitol. Inj., lyophilized Pow. for Soln.
Single-use vial. 10 mL (200 mg), 50 mL
(1 g), 100 mL (2 g). *Rx.*
Use: Antimetabolite, pyrimidine analog.
•**gemcitabine hydrochloride.** (JEM-sit-
ah-BEAN) *USP 34.*
Use: Antineoplastic; antimetabolite.
See: Gemzar.
•**gemeprost.** (JEH-meh-PRAHST) USAN.
Use: Prostaglandin.
•**gemfibrozil.** (gem-FIE-broe-ZILL)
USP 34.
Use: Antihyperlipidemic.
See: Lopid.
gemfibrozil. (Various Mfr.) Gemfibrozil
600 mg. Tab., Bot. 60s, 500s; blister-
pack 25s; UD 100s. *Rx.*
Use: Antihyperlipidemic.
•**gemifloxacin mesylate.** (jeh-mih-
FLOKS-ah-sin MEH-sih-LATE) USAN.
Use: Fluoroquinolone.
See: Factive.
•**gemopatrilat.** (ge-moe-PA-tril-at) USAN.
Use: Hypertension; congestive heart
failure.
•**gemtuzumab ozogamicin.** (jem-TOOZ-
ue-mab OH-zoe-ga-MYE-sin) USAN.
Use: Monoclonal antibody.
Gemzar. (Eli Lilly) Gemcitabine hydrochloride 200 mg, 1 g. Mannitol. Pow. for Inj.,
lyophilized. Single-use vials. 10 mL
(200 mg only), 50 mL (1 g only). *Rx.*
Use: Antineoplastic.
Genac. (Ivax) Triprolidine hydrochloride
2.5 mg, pseudoephedrine hydrochloride 60 mg. Lactose. Tab. Bot. 24s, 48s.
OTC.
Use: Upper respiratory combination, antihistamine, and decongestant.

Genacol. (Ivax) Pseudoephedrine hydrochloride 30 mg, chlorpheniramine
maleate 2 mg, dextromethorphan HBr
10 mg, acetaminophen 325 mg. Tab.
Bot. 50s. *OTC.*
Use: Analgesic, antihistamine, antitussive, decongestant.
**Genacol Maximum Strength Cold & Flu
Relief.** (Ivax) Dextromethorphan HBr
15 mg, chlorpheniramine maleate 2 mg,
pseudoephedrine hydrochloride 30 mg,
acetaminophen 500 mg. Tab. Bot. 50s.
OTC.
Use: Upper respiratory combination, antitussive, antihistamine, decongestant, analgesic.
Genagesic. (Ivax) Propoxyphene hydro-
chloride 165 mg, acetaminophen
650 mg. Tab. Bot. 100s, 500s. *c-iv.*
Use: Analgesic combination, narcotic.
Genahist. (Goldline) Diphenhydramine
hydrochloride. **Liq.:** 12.5 mg/5 mL,
cherry flavor. Bot. 118 mL. **Tab.:** 25 mg.
24s. **Cap.:** 25 mg, lactose, parabens.
100s. *OTC.*
Use: Antihistamine.
Genallerate. (Ivax) Chlorpheniramine
maleate 4 mg, lactose. Tab. Bot. 24s.
OTC.
Use: Antihistamine.
Genapap. (Ivax) Acetaminophen 325 mg.
Tab. Bot. 100s. *OTC.*
Use: Analgesic.
Genapap Children's. (Ivax) Acetamino-
phen 80 mg. Grape flavor. Chew. Tab.
Bot. 30s. *OTC.*
Use: Analgesic.
Genapap Extra Strength. (Ivax) Aceta-
minophen 500 mg. Tab., Rapid Re-
lease. 100s. *OTC.*
Use: Analgesic.
Genapax. (Key) Gentian violet 5 mg.
Tampon. Box 12s.
Use: Antifungal, vaginal.
Genaphed. (Ivax) Pseudoephedrine
hydrochloride 30 mg, lactose. Tab. Bot.
24s. *OTC.*
Use: Nasal decongestant, arylalkyl-
amine.
Genaphed Plus. (Ivax) Pseudoephed-
rine hydrochloride 60 mg, chlorphenir-
amine maleate 4 mg. Lactose. Tab. 24s.
OTC.
Use: Upper respiratory combination, de-
congestant and antihistamine.
Genasal. (Goldline) Oxymetazoline
hydrochloride 0.05%, benzalkonium
chloride, edetate disodium, PEG 1450.
Soln. Spray Bot. 15 mL, 30 mL. *OTC.*
Use: Nasal decongestant, arylalkylamine.

Genaspor Antifungal. (Ivax) Tolnaftate 1%. Cream. Bot. 15 g. *OTC.*
Use: Antifungal, topical.

Genasyme. (Ivax) Simethicone 80 mg. Tab. Bot. 100s. *OTC.*
Use: Antiflatulent.

Genaton. (Ivax) Aluminum hydroxide 80 mg, magnesium trisilicate 20 mg, alginic acid, sodium bicarbonate, sodium 18.4 mg, sucrose, sugar. Chew. Tab. Bot. 100s. *OTC.*
Use: Antacid.

Genaton, Extra Strength. (Ivax) Aluminum hydroxide 160 mg, magnesium carbonate 105 mg, alginic acid, sodium bicarbonate, sodium 29.9 mg, sucrose, calcium stearate. Chew. Tab. Bot. 100s. *OTC.*
Use: Antacid.

Genaton Liquid. (Ivax) Aluminum hydroxide 31.7 mg, magnesium carbonate 137.3 mg, sodium alginate, sodium 13 mg, EDTA, saccharin, sorbitol/ 5 mL. Bot. 355 mL. *OTC.*
Use: Antacid.

genatropine hydrochloride. (jen-AT-row-peen) Atropine-N-oxide hydrochloride. Aminoxytropine tropate hydrochloride.
See: X-tro.

Genatuss DM. (Ivax) Dextromethorphan HBr 10 mg, guaifenesin 100 mg per 5 mL. Corn syr., menthol, saccharin, sodium 3 mg/mL. Alcohol free. Syr. Bot. 118 mL. *OTC.*
Use: Upper respiratory combination, antitussive with expectorant.

Gen-bee with C. (Ivax) Vitamins B_1 15 mg, B_2 10.2 mg, B_3 50 mg, B_5 10 mg, B_6 5 mg, C 300 mg. Cap. Bot. 130s, 1000s. *OTC.*
Use: Vitamin supplement.

Gencept. (Gencon) **0.5/35:** Norethindrone 0.5 mg, ethinyl estradiol, 35 mcg. Tab (with 7 inert tabs). Pkgs 21s and 28s. **1/35:** Norethindrone 1 mg, ethinyl estradiol 35 mcg. Tab (with 7 inert tabs). Pkgs 21s and 28s. **10/11:** Norethindrone 0.5 mg and 1 mg, ethinyl estradiol 35 mcg. Tab (with 7 inert tabs). Pkg 21s and 28s. *Rx.*
Use: Contraceptive.

Gendecon. (Ivax) Phenylephrine hydrochloride 5 mg, chlorpheniramine maleate 2 mg, acetaminophen 325 mg. Tab. Bot. 50s. *OTC.*
Use: Analgesic, antihistamine, decongestant.

Genebrom-DM. (PGD) Dextromethorphan HBr 10 mg, brompheniramine maleate 2 mg, pseudoephedrine hydrochloride 30 mg per 5 mL. Alcohol free. Parabens, sugar, saccharin. Cherry flavor. Liq. 473 mL. *Rx.*
Use: Antitussive combination.

Genelan-NF. (PGD) Dextromethorphan HBr 15 mg, guaifenesin 100 mg, phenylephrine hydrochloride 10 mg, chlorpheniramine maleate 2 mg per 5 mL. Sugar, alcohol, and dye free. Parabens, aspartame, phenylalanine. Liq. 473 mL. *Rx.*
Use: Antitussive and expectorant combination.

general anesthetics.
Use: Anesthetics, general.
See: Barbiturates.
Fospropofol Disodium.

Generet-500. (Ivax) Iron 105 mg, Vitamins B_1 6 mg, B_2 6 mg, B_3 30 mg, B_5 10 mg, B_6 5 mg, B_{12} 25 mcg, C (as sodium ascorbate) 500 mg. TR Tab. Bot. 60s. *OTC.*
Use: Mineral, vitamin supplement.

Generix-T. (Ivax) Iron 15 mg, vitamins A 10,000 units, D 400 units, E 5.5 mg, B_1 15 mg, B_2 10 mg, B_3 100 mg, B_5 10 mg, B_6 2 mg, B_{12} 7.5 mcg, C 150 mg, Cu, I, Mg, Mn, zinc 1.5 mg. Tab. Bot. 100s. *OTC.*
Use: Mineral, vitamin supplement.

Generlac. (Morton Grove Pharmaceuticals) Lactulose 10 g per 15 mL. Soln., Oral and Rectal. 473 mL, 1,892 mL. *Rx.*
Use: Laxative, hyperosmotic agent.

Gene-T-Press. (PGD) Dextromethorphan HBr 15 mg, guaifenesin 200 mg, phenylephrine hydrochloride 5 mg per 5 mL. Sugar and alcohol free. Parabens, aspartame, phenylalanine. Cherry flavor. Liq. 473 mL. *Rx.*
Use: Antitussive and expectorant combination.

Genfiber. (Goldline Consumer) Psyllium hydrophilic mucilloid fiber 3.4 g, 14 cal/ dose, dextrose. Pow. Can 595 g. *OTC.*
Use: Laxative.

Genfiber, Orange Flavor. (Goldline Consumer) Psyllium hydrophilic mucilloid fiber 3.4 g/dose, sucrose, orange flavor. Pow. Can 397 g. *OTC.*
Use: Laxative.

Gengraf. (Abbott) Cyclosporine. **Cap.:** 25 mg, 100 mg, alcohol 12.8%, castor oil. UD 30s. **Oral Soln.:** 100 mg/mL. Castor oil. 50 mL. *Rx.*
Use: Immunosuppressant.

genital herpes treatment.
See: Acyclovir.
Zovirax.

Genite. (Ivax) Pseudoephedrine hydrochloride 10 mg, doxylamine succinate

1.25 mg, dextromethorphan HBr 5 mg, acetaminophen 167 mg, alcohol 25%/ 5 mL. Bot. 177 mL. *OTC.*
Use: Analgesic, antihistamine, antitussive, decongestant.

genitourinary irrigants.
See: Acetic Acid for Irrigation.
   Glycine (Aminoacetic Acid) for Irrigation.
   Hexitol Irrigants.
   Neosporin G.U. Irrigant.
   Renacidin.
   Sodium Chloride for Irrigation.
   Sorbitol.
   Sorbitol-Mannitol.
   Sterile Water for Irrigation.
   Suby's Solution G.

Gen-K. (Ivax) **Pow.:** Potassium chloride. Bot. 20 mEq. Pkt. Box 30s. **Tab.:** Effervescent potassium. Bot. 30s. *Rx.*
Use: Electrolyte supplement.

Genna Tablets. (Ivax) Senna concentrate 217 mg. Bot. 100s, 1000s. *OTC.*
Use: Laxative.

Gennin. (Ivax) Buffered aspirin 5 g. Tab. Bot. 100s. *OTC.*
Use: Analgesic.

genophyllin.
See: Aminophylline.

Genotropin. (Pfizer) Somatropin 5.8 mg (≈ 17.4 units)/cartridge. Glycine 2.2 mg, mannitol 46.8 mg, metacresol 0.3%. Pow. for Inj., lyophilized. 1s, 5s. Somatropin 13.8 mg (≈ 41.4 units)/cartridge. Glycine 2.3 mg, mannitol 46 mg, metacresol 0.3%. Pow. for Inj., lyophilized. 1s, 5s. *Rx.*
Use: Growth hormone.

Genotropin MiniQuick. (Pfizer) Somatropin 0.2 mg (≈ 0.6 units), 0.4 mg (≈ 1.2 units), 0.6 mg (≈ 1.8 units), 0.8 mg (≈ 2.4 units), 1 mg (≈ 3 units), 1.2 mg (≈ 3.6 units), 1.4 mg (≈ 4.2 units), 1.6 mg (≈ 4.8 units), 1.8 mg (≈ 5.4 units), 2 mg (≈ 6 units) per cartridge. Glycine 0.23 mg, mannitol 13.74 mg, preservative free. Pow. for Inj., lyophilized. Single-use syringe w/2-chamber cartridge. Box 7s. *Rx.*
Use: Growth hormone.

Genprep Ointment. (Ivax) Live yeast cell derivative supplying 2000 units skin respiratory factor/oz of ointment w/shark liver oil 3%, phenylmercuric nitrate 1:10,000. Tube 2 oz. *OTC.*
Use: Anorectal preparation.

Genprin. (Ivax) Aspirin 325 mg. Tab. 100s. *OTC.*
Use: Analgesic.

gensalate sodium.
Use: Analgesic.

Gentafair. (Bausch & Lomb) **Oint.:** Gentamicin 3 mg/g with liquid lanolin, white petrolatum, mineral oil, parabens. Tube 3.75 g, 15 g. **Soln.:** Gentamicin 3 mg/mL, polyoxyl 40 stearate, polyethylene glycol. Dropper bot. 5 mL, 15 mL. *Rx.*
Use: Anti-infective, ophthalmic.

Gentak. (Akorn) Gentamicin sulfate 3 mg/g. White petrolatum, parabens. Oint. 3.5 g. *Rx.*
Use: Anti-infective, ophthalmic.

gentamicin. (Various Mfr.) Gentamicin sulfate. **Oint.:** 0.1% (as base), may contain white petrolatum, parabens. 15 g. **Cream:** 0.1% (as base), may contain propylene glycol, parabens. 15 g. *Rx.*
Use: Anti-infective, topical.

gentamicin and prednisolone acetate ophthalmic suspension.
Use: Anti-infective; anti-inflammatory.

gentamicin impregnated PMMA beads on surgical wire.
Use: Chronic osteomyelitis. [Orphan Drug]

gentamicin liposome injection.
Use: Mycobacterium avium-intracellulare infection. [Orphan Drug]

gentamicin ophthalmic. (Various Mfr.) Gentamicin sulfate 3 mg/mL. Soln. 5 mL, 15 mL. *Rx.*
Use: Antibiotic.

•**gentamicin sulfate.** (JEN-tuh-MY-sin) *USP 34.*
Use: Anti-infective.
See: Gentak.
   W/Combinations.
   See: Pred-G.
   Pred-G Ophthalmic Suspension.

gentamicin sulfate. (Hospira) Gentamicin (as sulfate) 10 mg/mL. Inj. Vials. 60 mg, 80 mg, 100 mg. *Rx.*
Use: Aminoglycoside.

gentamicin sulfate. (Various Mfr.) Gentamicin (as sulfate) 40 mg/mL. Inj. Vial 2 mL, 20 mL. Cartridge-needle units 1.5 mL, 2 mL. *Rx.*
Use: Anti-infective.

gentamicin sulfate in 0.9% sodium chloride. (Hospira) Gentamicin sulfate (as gentamicin base) 0.8 mg, 0.9 mg, 1 mg, 1.2 mg, 1.4 mg, 1.6 mg. Sodium chloride 0.9% per mL. Inj. Single-dose flexible containers. 50 mL (1.2 mg, 1.4 mg, 1.6 mg only), 100 mL (0.8 mg, 0.9 mg, 1 mg only). *Rx.*
Use: Aminoglycoside.

gentamicin sulfate ophthalmic. (E. Fougera) Gentamicin sulfate 3 mg/g. In a base of white petrolatum and

mineral oil. Oint. 3.5 g. *Rx.*
Use: Antibiotic.

gentamicin sulfate, pediatric.
(Fujisawa) Gentamicin (as sulfate)
10 mg/mL. Inj. Vial. 2 mL. *Rx.*
Use: Anti-infective.

GenTeal. (Novartis Ophthalmics) **Drops:**
Hydroxypropyl methylcellulose 0.3%,
boric acid, phosphone acid, sodium
chloride, sodium perborate. 15 mL,
25 mL. **Gel:** Carboxymethylcellulose
sodium 0.25%, hypromellose 0.3%, boric acid, calcium chloride dihydrate, citric acid monohydrate, sodium perborate, magnesium chloride hexahydrate,
phosphoric acid, potassium chloride,
sodium chloride. 25 mL. *OTC.*
Use: Lubricant, ophthalmic.

GenTeal Mild. (Novartis) Hypromellose
0.2%, boric acid, phosphonic acid, potassium chloride, sodium chloride, sodium perborate. Preservative free.
Soln., Ophth. 25 mL. *OTC.*
Use: Artificial tear solution.

GenTeal Mild to Moderate. (Novartis)
Hypromellose 0.3%, boric acid, phosphonic acid, potassium chloride, sodium
chloride, sodium perborate. Preservative free. Soln., Ophth. 25 mL. *OTC.*
Use: Artificial tear solution.

GenTeal Moderate to Severe. (Novartis)
Carboxymethylcellulose sodium 0.25%,
hypromellose 0.3%, boric acid, sodium
perborate, magnesium chloride, phosphonic acid, potassium chloride, sodium
chloride. Preservative free. Soln., gel
forming; Ophth. 25 mL. *OTC.*
Use: Artificial tear solution.

Gentex LA. (Gentex) Phenylephrine
hydrochloride 23.75 mg, guaifenesin
650 mg. ER Tab. 100s. *Rx.*
Use: Upper respiratory combination, decongestant, and expectorant combination.

Gentex 30. (Gentex) Carbetapentane citrate 30 mg, guaifenesin 200 mg,
phenylephrine hydrochloride 8 mg per
5 mL. EDTA, parabens, saccharin.
Cherry flavor. Liq. 118 mL. *Rx.*
Use: Upper respiratory combination, antitussive, and expectorant combination.

•**gentian violet.** (JEN-shun) *USP 34.*
Formerly Methylrosaniline Chloride.
Use: Topical anti-infective, antifungal
agent.

gentian violet. (Various Mfr.) Gentian violet 1%, 2%. Top. Soln. Bot. 30 mL. *OTC.*
Use: Anti-infective; antifungal, topical.

gentisic acid ethanolamide.
Use: Pharmaceutic aid, complexing
agent.

Gentle Cream. (Geritrex) Mineral oil, cetearyl alcohol, petrolatum, castor oil,
lanolin, triethanolamine, propylene glycol, EDTA, zinc oxide, vitamins A, D,
& E, aloe vera oil. Cream. 120 g. *OTC.*
Use: Emollient.

Gentle Iron. (Nature's Bounty) Fe 28 mg
(as ferrous bisglycinate), vitamin B_{12}
8 mcg, C 60 mg, FA 0.4 mg. Cap. 90s.
OTC.
Use: Vitamin.

**Gentle Nature Natural Vegetable Laxa-
tive.** (Novartis) Sennosides A and B as
calcium salts. 20 mg. Tab. Box 16s,
32s. *OTC.*
Use: Laxative.

Gentle Shampoo. (Ulmer Pharmacal)
Bot. 4 oz, gal. *OTC.*
Use: Dermatologic, hair.

Gentran 40. (Baxter PPI) Dextran 40
10% w/sodium chloride 0.9% or Dextran
40 10% w/dextrose 5%. Inj. Plastic
Bot. 500 mL. *Rx.*
Use: Plasma expander.

Gentran 70. (Baxter PPI) Dextran 70 6%
w/sodium chloride 0.9%. Inj. Plastic Bot.
500 mL. *Rx.*
Use: Plasma expander.

Gentran 75. (Baxter PPI) Dextran 75 6%
in sodium chloride 0.9%. Inj. Bot.
500 mL. *Rx.*
Use: Plasma expander.

Gentrasul. (Bausch & Lomb) Gentamicin. **Oint.:** 3 mg. **Soln.:** 3.5 g. Dropper bot. 5 mL. *Rx.*
Use: Anti-infective, ophthalmic.

Genuine Bayer Aspirin. (Bayer Con-
sumer Care) Aspirin 325 mg. FC Tab.
Bot. 12s, 24s, 50s, 200s, 300s. *OTC.*
Use: Analgesic.

Geodon. (Pfizer) **Cap.:** Ziprasidone
hydrochloride 20 mg, 40 mg, 60 mg,
80 mg. Lactose. Bot. 60s, UD 80s. **Pow.
for Inj.:** Ziprasidone mesylate 20 mg.
Vials. Single use. *Rx.*
Use: Antipsychotic; benzisoxazole derivative.

Geopen. (Roerig) Carbenicillin disodium.
Inj. **Vial:** 1 g, 2 g, 5 g. Pkg. 10s. **Piggyback Vial:** 2 g, 5 g, 10 g. **Bulk Pharmacy Pack:** 30 g. *Rx.*
Use: Anti-infective, penicillin.

•**gepirone hydrochloride.** (jeh-PIE-rone)
USAN.
Use: Anxiolytic; antidepressant.

Gera Plus. (Towne) Iron 50 mg, vitamins
B_1 5 mg, B_2 5 mg, B_6 0.5 mg, B_{12}
3 mcg, C 75 mg, niacinamide 30 mg,
calcium pantothenate 2 mg. Tab. Bot.
100s. *OTC.*
Use: Mineral, vitamin supplement.

Geravim. (Major) Vitamins B$_1$ 0.83 mg, B$_2$ 0.42 mg, B$_3$ 8.3 mg, B$_5$ 1.67 mg, B$_6$ 0.17 mg, B$_{12}$ 0.17 mg, I, Fe 2.5 mg, Zn 0.3 mg, choline, Mn, alcohol 18%. Liq. Bot. Pt, gal. *OTC.*
Use: Mineral, vitamin supplement.

Geravite. (Roberts) Vitamins B$_1$ 0.3 mg, B$_2$ 0.4 mg, B$_3$ 33.3 mg, B$_{12}$ 3.3 mcg, L-lysine, alcohol 15%, parabens, sorbitol, sucrose. Elix. Bot. 480 mL. *OTC.*
Use: Mineral, vitamin supplement.

Gerber Baby Formula Low Iron Formula. (Bristol-Myers Squibb) Protein (from non-fat milk) 14.7 g, carbohydrate (from lactose) 71.3 g, fat (from palm olein, soy, coconut, and high oleic sunflower oils) 36 g, linoleic acid 5.9 g, vitamins A, D, E, K, C, B$_1$, B$_2$, B$_3$, B$_5$, B$_6$, B$_{12}$, folic acid, biotin, choline, inositol, Ca, P, Mg, Fe 3.4 mg, Zn, Mn, Cu, I, Na 220 mg, K 720 mg, Cl, taurine, calories per L 666.7. **Ready to use liq.:** Bot. 943 mL. **Concentrated liq.:** Bot. 433 mL. **Pow.:** Can 457 g and 914 g. *OTC.*
Use: Nutritional supplement.

Geri-All-D. (Barth's) Vitamins A 10,000 units, D 400 units, B$_1$ 7 mg, B$_2$ 14 mg, B$_6$ 0.35 mg, B$_{12}$ 25 mcg, C 200 mg, niacin 4.17 mg, E 50 units, pantothenic acid 0.63 mg, trace minerals, and other factors. 2 Cap. Bot. 1 mo., 3 mo., and 6 mo. supply of Geri-All. regular and Geri-All-D. *OTC.*
Use: Mineral, vitamin supplement.

geriatric supplements with multivitamins/minerals.
See: Geravite.
Gerimed.
Geriot.
Geri-Plus.
Geritol Complete.
Gerivite.
Gerix.
Hep-Forte.
Mega VM-80.
Optivite P.M.T.
Strovite Plus.
Ultra Freeda.
Ultra Freeda Iron Free.
Vigortol.
Viminate.
Vita-Plus G.

Geriatroplex. (Morton Grove) Cyanocobalamin 30 mcg, liver inj. 0.1 mL, vitamins B$_2$ 1.5 mg, B$_{12}$ activity 2 mcg, ferrous gluconate 50 mg, calcium pantothenate 2.5 mg, niacinamide 100 mg, citric acid 16.4 mg, sodium citrate 23.6 mg/2 mL. Vial 30 mL. *OTC.*
Use: Mineral, vitamin supplement.

Geri-Derm. (Barth's) Vitamins A 400,000 units, D 40,000 units, E 200 units, panthenol 800 mg/4 oz. Jar 4 oz. *OTC.*
Use: Skin supplement.

Geridium. (Goldline) Phenazopyridine hydrochloride 100 mg, 200 mg. Sugar coated. Tab. Bot. 100s, 1000s (100 mg only). *Rx.*
Use: Analgesic; anti-infective, urinary.

Geri-Hydrolac. (Geritrex) **Cream:** Ammonium lactate (equiv. to 12% lactic acid), light mineral oil, petrolatum, propylene glycol, glycerin, cetyl alcohol, parabens. Cream. 140 g. **Lot.:** Lactic acid buffered 5%, ammonium hydroxide, cetyl alcohol, dimethicone, EDTA, glycerin, parabens, petrolatum. 237 mL. *OTC.*
Use: Emollient.

Geri-Hydrolac 12. (Geritrex Corp) Ammonium lactate 12%, cetyl alcohol, glycerin, mineral oil, parabens, PEG-100, propylene glycol. Lot. 225 g, 400 g. *OTC.*
Use: Emollient.

Gerilets. (Abbott) Vitamins A 5000 units, D 400 units, E 45 units, C 90 mg (from sodium ascorbate), folic acid 0.4 mg, B$_1$ 2.25 mg, B$_2$ 2.6 mg, niacin 30 mg, B$_6$ 3 mg, B$_{12}$ 9 mcg, biotin 0.45 mg, pantothenic acid 15 mg, iron 27 mg (from ferrous sulfate). Tab. Bot. 100s. *OTC.*
Use: Mineral, vitamin supplement.

Gerimal. (Rugby) Ergoloid mesylates. **Sublingual Tab.:** 0.5 mg, 1 mg. Bot. 100s, 500s, 1000s. **Oral Tab.:** 1 mg. Bot. 100s, 500s, 1000s. *Rx.*
Use: Psychotherapeutic agent.

Gerimed. (Fielding) Vitamins A 5000 units, D 400 units, E 30 mg, B$_1$ 3 mg, B$_2$ 3 mg, B$_3$ 25 mg, B$_6$ 2 mg, B$_{12}$ 6 mcg, C 120 mg, calcium 370 mg, zinc 15 mg, Mg, Fe. Tab. Bot. 60s. *OTC.*
Use: Mineral, vitamin supplement.

Geri-Mucil. (Geri-Care) Psyllium husk 3.4 g. Sodium 10 mg, 14 calories/dose, dextrose. Pow. 368 g. *OTC.*
Use: Laxative, bulk-producing laxative.

Geriot. (Ivax) Vitamins A 6000 units, D 400 units, E 30 units, B$_1$ 1.5 mg, B$_2$ 1.7 mg, B$_3$ 20 mg, B$_5$ 10 mg, B$_6$ 2 mg, B$_{12}$ 6 mcg, C 60 mg, folic acid 0.4 mg, iron 50 mg (from ferrous sulfate), biotin 45 mcg, Ca, Cl, Cr, Cu, I, K, Mg, Mn, Mo, Ni, P, Se, Si, Sn, V, Zn, vitamin K. Tab. Bot. 100s. *OTC.*
Use: Mineral, vitamin supplement.

Geri-Plus. (Health for Life Brands) **Cap.:** Vitamins A 12,500 units, D 1200 units,

B_1 15 mg, B_2 10 mg, B_6 0.5 mg, B_{12} 15 mcg, C 75 mg, niacinamide 30 mg, calcium pantothenate 2 mg, E 5 units, Brewer's yeast 10 mg, iron 11.58 mg, desiccated liver 15 mg, choline bitartrate 30 mg, inositol 30 mg, Ca 59 mg, P 45 mg, Zn 0.68 mg, francium dicalcium phosphate 200 mg, Mn, enzymatic factors, amino acids. Cap. Bot. 50s, 100s, 1000s. **Elix.:** Vitamins B_1 25 mg, B_2 10 mg, B_6 1 mg, B_{12} 20 mcg, niacinamide 100 mg, calcium pantothenate 5 mg, iron ammonium citrate 100 mg, choline 200 mg, inositol 100 mg, magnesium chloride 2 mg, manganese citrate 2 mg, zinc acetate 2 mg, amino acids/fl oz. Bot. Pt. *OTC.*
Use: Mineral, vitamin supplement.

Geri-Silk Bath Oil. (Geritrex) Mineral oil, PEG-4 dilaurate, lanolin oil. Oil. 237 mL. *OTC.*
Use: Emollient.

Geri-Soft. (Geritrex) Mineral oil, propylene glycol, cetearyl alcohol, sorbitol, petrolatum, dimethicone, lanolin, castor oil, stearic acid, parabens, stearyl alcohol, EDTA, lemon oil. Lot. 240 g. *OTC.*
Use: Emollient.

Geri SS. (Geritrex) Mineral oil, propylene glycol, cetearyl alcohol, petrolatum, glycerin, dimethicone, colloidal oatmeal, hydrogenated castor oil, parabens, stearyl alcohol, EDTA, lemon oil, tocopheryl acetate. Lot. 240 g. *OTC.*
Use: Emollient.

Geritol Complete. (GlaxoSmithKline) **Complete:** Vitamins A 6000 units, E 30 units, C 60 mg, folic acid 400 mcg, B_1 1.5 mg, B_2 1.7 mg, B_3 20 mg, B_5 10 mg, B_6 2 mg, B_{12} 6 mcg, D 400 units, K, biotin 45 mcg, iron 18 mg, Ca, Cl, Cr, Cu, I, K, Mg, Mn, Mo, Ni, P, Se, Si, Sn, V, Zn, vitamin K. Tab. Bot. 14s, 40s, 100s, 180s. **Extended:** Iron 10 mg, vitamins A 3333 units, D 200 units, E 15 units, B_1 1.2 mg, B_2 1.4 mg, B_3 15 mg, B_6 2 mg, B_{12} 2 mg, C 60 mg, folic acid 0.2 mg, vitamin K, Ca, I, Mg, Se, Zn 15 mg. Capl. Bot. 40s, 100s. **Tonic Liq.:** Iron 18 mg, vitamins B_1 2.5 mg, B_2 2.5 mg, B_3 50 mg, B_5 2 mg, B_6 0.5 mg, methionine 25 mg, choline bitartrate 50 mg/15 mL, alcohol 12%. Bot. 120 mL, 360 mL. *OTC.*
Use: Mineral, vitamin supplement.

Geri-Tussin DM. (Geri-Care) Dextromethorphan hydrobromide 10 mg, guaifenesin 100 mg. Fructose, glucose, saccharin. Alcohol free. Liq. 473 mL. *OTC.*

Use: Upper respiratory combination, antitussive with expectorant.

Gerivite. (Ivax) Vitamins B_1 0.8 mg, B_2 0.4 mg, B_3 8.3 mg, B_5 1.7 mg, B_6 0.2 mg, B_{12} 0.2 mcg, iron 0.3 mg, Zn 0.3 mg, choline, I Mg, Mn, alcohol 18%, methylparaben, sorbitol. Liq. Bot. 473 mL. *OTC.*
Use: Mineral, vitamin supplement.

Gerix. (Abbott) Vitamins B_1 6 mg, B_2 6 mg, B_6 1.6 mg, niacin 100 mg, iron 15 mg, cyanocobalamin 6 mcg, alcohol 20%/30 mL. Elix. Bot. 480 mL. *OTC.*
Use: Mineral, vitamin supplement.

germanin. (Centers for Disease Control & Prevention) *Rx.*
Use: Anti-infective.
See: Suramin Sodium (Naphuride Sodium).

Germicin. (CMC) Benzalkonium chloride 50%. Bot. Pt, gal. *OTC.*
Use: Antiseptic; antimicrobial.

Ger-O-Foam. (Roberts) Methyl salicylate 30%, benzocaine 3%, volatile oils. Aerosol Can 4 oz. *OTC.*
Use: Analgesic; anesthetic.

Geroton Forte. (Kenwood) Vitamin B_1 1.7 mg, B_2 1.9 mg, B_3 2.22 mg, B_5 1.11 mg, B_6 0.22 mg, B_{12} 0.67 mcg, Zn 1.7 mg, Mg, Mn, alcohol 13%. Liq. Bot. 473 mL. *OTC.*
Use: Mineral, vitamin supplement.

Gerterol Depo. (Fellows) Medroxyprogesterone acetate 50 mg, 100 mg/mL. Vial 5 mL. *Rx.*
Use: Hormone, progestin.

Gesic. (Lexalabs) Aspirin 226.8 mg, caffeine 32.4 mg, codeine 32.4 mg. Tab. Bot. 100s. *c-III.*
Use: Analgesic combination, narcotic.

•**gestaclone.** (JEST-ah-klone) USAN.
Use: Hormone, progestin.

•**gestodene.** (JEST-oh-deen) USAN.
Use: Hormone, progestin.

Gestoneed. (Hanlon) Calcium lactate 1069 mg, vitamins C 100 mg, nicotinic acid 18 mg, B_1 1.8 mg, B_2 2.4 mg, B_6 9 mg, D 500 units, A 6000 units. Cap. Bot. 100s. *OTC.*
Use: Mineral, vitamin supplement.

•**gestonorone caproate.** (jess-TOE-noreohn CAP-row-ate) USAN.
Use: Hormone, progestin.

•**gestrinone.** (JESS-trih-nohn) USAN.
Use: Hormone, progestin.

Get Better Bear Sore Throat Pops. (Whitehall-Robins) Pectin 19 mg, corn syr., sucrose, parabens. Loz. on a stick. Pkg. 10s. *OTC.*
Use: Mouth and throat product.

Gets-It. (Oakhurst) Salicylic acid, zinc chloride, collodion in ether ≈ 35%, alcohol ≈ 28%. Liq. Bot. 12 mL. *OTC.*
Use: Keratolytic.

• **gevokizumab.** (JEV-oh-KIZ-oo-mab) USAN.
Use: Treatment of diabetes, inflammatory disorders.

• **gevotroline hydrochloride.** (jeh-VOE-troe-LEEN) USAN.
Use: Antipsychotic.

Gevrabon. (Wyeth) Vitamins B_1 0.83 mg, B_2 0.42 mg, B_3 8.3 mg, B_5 1.67 mg, B_6 0.17 mg, B_{12} 0.17 mcg, Fe 2.5 mg, choline, I, Mg, Mn, Zn 0.3 mg, alcohol 18%. Liq. Bot. 480 mL. *OTC.*
Use: Mineral, vitamin supplement.

Gevral. (Wyeth) Vitamins A 5000 units, B_1 1.5 mg, B_2 1.7 mg, B_3 20 mg, B_6 2 mg, B_{12} 6 mcg, folic acid 0.4 mg, C 60 mg, E 30 mg, Ca, P, iron 18 mg, Mg, I, lactose, parabens, sucrose. Tab. Bot. 100s. *OTC.*
Use: Mineral, vitamin supplement.

GFN 1000/DM 50. (Cypress) Dextromethorphan HBr 50 mg, guaifenesin 1000 mg. ER Tab. 100s. *Rx.*
Use: Antitussive, expectorant.

GFN 1000/DM 60. (Cypress) Dextromethorphan HBr 60 mg, guaifenesin 1000 mg. Dye free. ER Tab. Bot. 100s. *Rx.*
Use: Upper respiratory combination, antitussive with expectorant.

GFN 1200/DM 60. (Cypress) Dextromethorphan HBr 60 mg, guaifenesin 1200 mg. Dye free. ER Tab. Bot. 100s. *Rx.*
Use: Upper respiratory combination, antitussive with expectorant.

GFN 1200/DM 60/PSE 120. (Cypress) Dextromethorphan HBr 60 mg, guaifenesin 1200 mg, pseudoephedrine hydrochloride 120 mg, dye free. SR Tab. Bot. 100s. *Rx.*
Use: Upper respiratory combination, antitussive, expectorant, decongestant.

GFN 1200/DM 20/PE 40. (Cypress) Dextromethorphan HBr 20 mg, guaifenesin 1200 mg, phenylephrine hydrochloride 40 mg. Dye free. ER Tab. 100s. *Rx.*
Use: Upper respiratory combination, antitussive and expectorant combination.

GFN/PSE. (Cypress) Pseudoephedrine hydrochloride 120 mg, guaifenesin 1200 mg. ER Tab. Bot. 100s. *Rx.*
Use: Upper respiratory combination, decongestant with expectorant.

GFN 600/Phenylephrine 20. (Cypress) Phenylephrine hydrochloride 20 mg, guaifenesin 600 mg. Dye free. ER Tab. Bot. 100s. *Rx.*
Use: Upper respiratory combination, decongestant, and expectorant combination.

GFN 600/PSE 60/DM 30. (Cypress) Dextromethorphan HBr 30 mg, guaifenesin 600 mg, pseudoephedrine hydrochloride 60 mg. Dye free. ER Tab. 100s. *Rx.*
Use: Upper respiratory combination, antitussive and expectorant combination.

G-4.
See: Dichlorophene.

Gianvi. (Teva) Ethinyl estradiol 20 mcg, drospirenone 3 mg. Film coated. Lactose, PEG, polysorbate 80. Tab. 24s w/ 4 white, round, inert tablets. Blister pack. 28s. *Rx.*
Use: Oral contraceptive.

Gilenya. (Novartis) Fingolimod 0.5 mg (equiv. to fingolimod hydrochloride 0.56 mg). Mannitol. Cap. UD 7s, 28s. *Rx.*
Use: Immunologic agent, immunomodulator.

Gilphex TR. (GIL) Guaifenesin 388 mg, phenylephrine hydrochloride 10 mg. Maltodextrin. Film-coated. Tab. 100s, 500s, 1000s. *Rx.*
Use: Decongestant and expectorant combination, upper respiratory combination.

Giltuss. (GIL) Dextromethorphan HBr 15 mg, guaifenesin 300 mg, phenylephrine hydrochloride 10 mg per 5 mL. Alcohol and sugar free. Phenylalanine 3.75 mg/5 mL. Grape flavor. Liq. 473 mL. *Rx.*
Use: Upper respiratory combination, antitussive and expectorant combination.

Giltuss Ped-C. (GIL) Codeine phosphate 3 mg, guaifenesin 50 mg, phenylephrine hydrochloride 25 mg per 5 mL. Alcohol and sugar free. Phenylalanine 0.6 mg/mL. Strawberry-banana flavor. Liq. 60 mL. *Rx.*
Use: Upper respiratory combination, antitussive and expectorant combination.

Giltuss Pediatric. (GIL) Dextromethorphan HBr 5 mg, guaifenesin 50 mg, phenylephrine hydrochloride 2.5 mg per 5 mL. Alcohol and sugar free. Grape flavor. Liq. 60 mL. *Rx.*
Use: Upper respiratory combination, antitussive and expectorant combination.

Giltuss TR. (GIL) **Cap.:** Dextromethorphan HBr 14 mg, guaifenesin 288 mg, phenylephrine hydrochloride 7 mg.

Maltodextrin. Sugar free. 100s, 500s, 1000s. **Tab.**: Dextromethorphan HBr 30 mg, guaifenesin 600 mg, phenylephrine hydrochloride 20 mg. Dye, sugar, and preservative free. 100s, 1000s. *Rx.*
Use: Upper respiratory combination, antitussive and expectorant combination.

•**ginger.** *NF 29.*
Use: Dietary supplement.

•**ginseng, American.** *NF 29.*
Use: Dietary supplement.

•**ginseng, Asian.** *NF 29.*
Use: Dietary supplement.

•**ginseng extract.** *NF 29.*
Use: Dietary supplement.

•**girentuximab.** (JIR-en-TUK-see-mab) USAN.
Use: Antineoplastic.

•**giripladib.** (jir-IP-la-dib) USAN.
Use: Analgesic.

•**gisadenafil.** (JEES-a-DEN-a-fil) USAN.
Use: Genitourinary agent.

•**gisadenafil besylate.** (JEES-a-DEN-a-fil) USAN.
Use: Genitourinary agent.

glandubolin.
See: Estrone.

•**glatiramer acetate.** (glah-TEER-ah-mer ASS-eh-tate) USAN.
Use: Multiple sclerosis; immunosuppressant.
See: Copaxone.

glauber's salt.
See: Sodium Sulfate.

glaucoma, agents for.
See: Brimonidine Tartrate/Timolol.
Brinzolamide.
Carbonic Anhydrase Inhibitors.
Dorzolamide Hydrochloride.
Dorzolamide Hydrochloride/Timolol Maleate.
Echothiophate Iodide.
Latanoprost.
Miotics, Cholinesterase Inhibitors.
Prostaglandin Agonists.

•**glaze, pharmaceutical.** *NF 29.*
Use: Pharmaceutic aid (tablet coating agent).

Gleevec. (Novartis) Imatinib mesylate 100 mg, 400 mg. Film-coated. Tab. Bot. 30s (400 mg only), 100s (100 mg only). *Rx.*
Use: Protein-tyrosine kinase inhibitor.

•**glemanserin.** (gleh-MAN-ser-in) USAN.
Use: Anxiolytic.

•**glembatumumab.** (GLEM-ba-TOOM-oo-mab) USAN.
Use: Antineoplastic.

•**glembatumumab vedotin.** (GLEM-ba-TOOM-oo-mab ve-DOE-tin) USAN.
Use: Antineoplastic.

Gliadel. (Guilford Pharm) Carmustine (BCNU) 7.7 mg, preservative free. Wafer. Single-dose treatment box with 8 individually pouched wafers. *Rx.*
Use: Alkylating agent.

•**gliamilide.** (glie-AM-ih-lide) USAN.
Use: Antidiabetic.

glibenclamide.
See: Glyburide.

•**glibornuride.** (glie-BORN-you-ride) USAN.
Use: Oral hypoglycemic agent; antidiabetic.

•**glicetanile sodium.** (glie-SET-AH-nile) USAN. *Formerly Glydanile Sodium.*
Use: Antidiabetic.

•**gliflumide.** (GLIH-flew-mide) USAN.
Use: Antidiabetic.

glim.
See: Gardinol Type Detergents.

•**glimepiride.** (GLIE-meh-pie-ride) USAN.
Use: Hypoglycemic; antidiabetic.
See: Amaryl.
W/Pioglitazone Hydrochloride.
See: Duetact.
W/Rosiglitazone Maleate.
See: Avandaryl.

glimepiride. (Various Mfr.) Glimepiride 1 mg, 2 mg, 4 mg. May contain lactose. Tab. 30s, 100s, 250s, (4 mg only), 500s, 1000s, UD 100s (except 1 mg). *Rx.*
Use: Antidiabetic agent.

•**glipizide.** (GLIP-ih-zide) *USP 34.*
Tall Man: glipiZIDE
Use: Antidiabetic.
See: Glucotrol.
Glucotrol XL.
W/Metformin Hydrochloride.
See: Metaglip.

glipizide. (Various Mfr.) Glipizide 5 mg, 10 mg. Tab. 100s, 500s, 1000s, UD 100s. *Rx.*
Use: Antidiabetic.

glipizide ER. (Watson) Glipizide 5 mg, 10 mg. Film-coated. ER Tab. 100s. *Rx.*
Use: Antidiabetic.

glipizide extended-release. (Andrx) Glipizide 2.5 mg. ER Tab. 30s. *Rx.*
Use: Antidiabetic.

glipizide extended-release. (Various Mfr.) Glipizide 5 mg, 10 mg. ER Tab. 100s, 500s. *Rx.*
Use: Antidiabetic.

glipizide/metformin hydrochloride. (Various Mfr.) Glipizide/metformin hydrochloride 2.5 mg/250 mg, 2.5 mg/

500 mg, 5 mg/500 mg. Tab. 100s. *Rx.*
Use: Antidiabetic combination.

globulin, cytomegalovirus immune.
See: CytoGam.

globulin, gamma.
See: Immune Globulin Intramuscular.
Immune Globulin Intravenous.

globulin, hepatitis B immune.
See: BayHep B.
H-BIG.

•**globulin, immune.** (GLAH-byoo-lin)
USP 34. Formerly Globulin, Immune Human Serum.
Use: IM, measles prophylactic and polio; immunization.

globulin, immune, intravenous.
Use: Immunodeficiency; immune thrombocytopenia purpura; Kawasaki syndrome.
See: Gamimune N.
Gammagard S/D.
Iveegam.
Polygam S/D.
Sandoglobulin.
Venoglobulin-I.
Venoglobulin-S.

globulin, rabies immune.
Use: Immunization.
See: Imogam Rabies.

globulin, Rh$_o$(D) immune.
Use: Prevention of Rh isoimmunization; immune thrombocytopenic purpura.
See: BayRho D.
Gamulin Rh.
MICRhoGAM.
Mini-Gamulin Rh.
RhoGAM.
WinRho SD.

•**globulin serum, anti-human.** (GLOB-ue-lin) *USP 34.*
Use: Immunization.

globulin, tetanus immune.
Use: Immunization.
See: Baytet.

globulin, vaccinia immune.
Use: Immunization.

globulin, varicella-zoster immune.
Use: Immunization.
See: Varicella-zoster Immune Globulin.

•**gloximonam.** (GLOX-ih-MOE-nam)
USAN.
Use: Anti-infective.

GL-7 Skin Adherent. (Gordon Laboratories) Plastic material which may be used full strength or diluted with 3 to 10 parts 99% isopropyl alcohol, acetone or naphtha. Pkg. Pt, qt, gal. *OTC.*

GL-2 Skin Adherent. (Gordon Laboratories) Ready-to-use. Bot. Pt, qt, gal. *OTC.*

GlucaGen. (Bedford Laboratories) Glucagon 1 mg (1 unit), lactose 107 mg. Pow. for Inj. Vials with 1 mL diluent. *Rx.*
Use: Glucose-elevating agent, diagnostic aid, emergency kit.

GlucaGen HypoKit. (Novo Nordisk) Glucagon 1 mg (1 unit). Lactose 107 mg. Pow. for Inj. Disposable syringe w/1 mL diluent. *Rx.*
Use: Glucose-elevating agent.

•**glucagon.** (GLUE-kuh-gahn) *USP 34.*
Use: Emergency treatment of hypoglycemia; antidiabetic.
See: GlucaGen.
Glucagon Diagnostic Kit.
Glucagon Emergency Kit.

glucagon. (Eli Lilly) 1 unit/mL w/diluent. 10 units w/10 mL diluent. Glucagon hydrochloride 1 mg, 10 mg w/diluent; soln. contains lactose, glycerin 1.6% w/ phenol 0.2% as a preservative. Vial. *Rx.*
Use: Hypoglycemic shock; antidiabetic.

Glucagon Diagnostic Kit. (Bedford) Glucagon 1 mg (1 unit), lactose 107 mg. Pow. for Inj. Vial w/1 mL syringe diluent. *Rx.*
Use: Glucose-elevating agent.

Glucagon Emergency Kit. (Eli Lilly) Glucagon 1 mg (1 unit), lactose 49 mg, glycerin 12 mg/mL. Pow. for Inj. Vial w/ 1 mL syr. diluent. *Rx.*
Use: Glucose-elevating agent.

glucagon-like peptide 1 receptor agonists.
See: Liraglutide.

Glucamide. (Teva) Chlorpropamide 100 mg, 250 mg. Tab. Bot. 100s, 250s, 500s, 1000s, UD 100s. *Rx.*
Use: Antidiabetic.

•**gluceptate sodium.** (GLUE-sep-tate)
USAN.
Use: Pharmaceutic aid.

Glucerna. (Ross) Protein 41 g (amino acids), carbohydrate 93 g (hydrolyzed cornstarch, fructose, soy fiber), fat 55 g (high oleic safflower oil, soy oil, soy lecithin), sodium 917 mg (40 mEq), potassium 1542 mg (40 mEq), vitamins A, B$_1$, B$_2$, B$_3$, B$_5$, B$_6$, B$_{12}$, C, D, E, K, folic acid, Cl, Ca, P, Mg, I, Mn, Cu, Zn, Fe, Se, Cr, Mo, biotin, choline. Liq. Can 240 mL, Cont. 1 L. Ready-to-use. *OTC.*
Use: Nutritional supplement.

Glucerna Select. (Abbott) Protein (sodium and calcium caseinates, soy protein isolate) 50 g, carbohydrates (fructose, fructooligosaccharides, maltodextrin, soy fiber, sugar alcohols) 95.7 g, fat (canola oil, high oleic safflower oil, soy lecithin) 54.4 g, Na 940 mg,

1810 mg K/L. H_2O 470 mOsm/kg, 1 cal/mL. Vitamin A, B_1, B_2, B_3, B_5, B_6, B_7, B_9, B_{12}, C, D, E, K, choline, Ca, Cl, Cu, Cr, Fe, I, Mg, Mn, Mo, P, Se, Zn. Gluten-free. Vanilla flavor. Liq. 240 mL, 1000 mL, 1500 mL. *OTC.*
Use: Enteral nutrition therapy.

Glucerna Weight Loss Shake. (Abbott) Protein (sodium and calcium caseinates, soy protein isolate) 54.6 g, carbohydrates (fructose, fructooligosaccharides, maltodextrin, soy fiber, sugar alcohols) 163.8 g, fat (canola oil, high oleic safflower oil, soy lecithin) 46.2 g, Na 1176 mg, K 2100 mg. 0.89 cal/mL. Vitamin A, B_1, B_2, B_3, B_5, B_6, B_{12}, FA, C, D, E, K, biotin, choline, Ca, Cl, Cu, Cr, Fe, I, Mg, Mn, Mo, P, Se, Zn. Gluten-free. Vanilla, chocolate, banana, peach, dulce de leche flavors. Liq. 325 mL. *OTC.*
Use: Enteral nutrition therapy.

glucocerebrosidase-beta-glucosidase.
Use: Treatment of Gaucher disease.
See: Ceredase.

glucocerebrosidase (PEG).
See: PEG-glucocerebrosidase.

glucocerebrosidase, recombinant retroviral vector. (Genetic Therapy)
Use: Treatment for Gaucher disease.
[Orphan Drug]

glucocorticoids.
See: Betamethasone.
Betamethasone Sodium Phosphate and Betamethasone Acetate.
Budesonide.
Cortical Hormone Products.
Cortisone.
Dexamethasone.
Dexamethasone Acetate.
Dexamethasone Sodium Phosphate.
Dexamethasone Sodium Phosphate with Lidocaine Hydrochloride.
Hydrocortisone.
Hydrocortisone Acetate.
Hydrocortisone Cypionate.
Hydrocortisone Sodium Phosphate.
Hydrocortisone Sodium Succinate.
Methylprednisolone.
Methylprednisolone Acetate.
Methylprednisolone Sodium Succinate.
Prednisolone.
Prednisolone Acetate.
Prednisolone Sodium Phosphate.
Prednisolone Tebutate.
Prednisone.
Triamcinolone.
Triamcinolone Acetonide.
Triamcinolone Hexacetonide.

Glucolet Automatic Lancing Device. (Bayer Consumer Care) To obtain sample for blood glucose testing. Automatic spring-loaded lancing device.
Use: Diagnostic aid.

Glucolet Endcaps. (Bayer Consumer Care) To obtain sample for blood glucose testing. Controls depth of lancet penetration. Regular or super puncture.
Use: Diagnostic aid.

Glucometer II Blood Glucose Meter. (Bayer Consumer Care) Electronic meter for blood glucose testing. *OTC.*
Use: Diagnostic aid.

d-gluconic acid, calcium salt. Calcium gluconate.

gluconic acid salts.
See: Calcium Gluconate.
Ferrous Gluconate.
Magnesium Gluconate.
Potassium Gluconate.

•**gluconolactone.** (glue-koe-no-LACK-tone) *USP 34.*
Use: Chelating agent.

Glucophage. (Bristol-Myers Squibb) Metformin hydrochloride 500 mg, 850 mg, 1000 mg. Film-coated. Tab. Bot. 100s, 500s (500 mg only). *Rx.*
Use: Antidiabetic, biguanide.

Glucophage XR. (Bristol-Myers Squibb) Metformin hydrochloride 500 mg, 750 mg. ER Tab. Bot. 100s. *Rx.*
Use: Antidiabetic, biguanide.

•**glucosamine.** (glue-KOSE-ah-meen) USAN.
Use: Pharmaceutic aid.
W/Tetracycline.
See: Tetracyn.

glucose.
See: Glutose.
Insta-Glucose.

glucose-elevating agents.
See: B-D Glucose.
Glucagon.
Glutose.
Insta-Glucose.
Insulin Reaction.
Proglycem.

glucose and ketone urine test. (Major) Reagent test for glucose and ketones in urine. Bot. 100s.
Use: Diagnostic aid.

glucose enzymatic test strip.
Use: Diagnostic aid (in vitro, reducing sugars in urine).

glucose (HK) reagent strips. Reagent strip test for detection of glucose in serum or plasma. Bot. 50s.
Use: Diagnostic aid.

•**glucose, liquid.** (GLUE-kose) *NF 29.*
Use: As a 5% to 50% solution as nutrient; for acute hepatitis and dehydra-

tion; to increase blood volume; pharmaceutic aid (tablet binder, tablet-coating agent).

d-glucose, monohydrate. Dextrose.

•**glucose oxidase.** (GLOO-kose OX-i-dase) USAN.
Use: Anti-infective.

glucose polymers.
See: Polycose.

glucose reagent strips. (Bayer Consumer Care) A quantitative strip test for glucose in serum or plasma. Seralyzer reagent strips. Bot. 50s.
Use: Diagnostic aid.

glucose test.
See: Combistix.
First Choice.
Glucose Reagent.

Glucostix Reagent Strips. (Bayer Consumer Care) Cellulose strip containing glucose oxidase and indicator system. Bot. 50s, 100s, UD 25s. *OTC.*
Use: Diagnostic aid.

glucosulfone sodium, injection.
See: Sodium Glucosulfone.

Gluco System Lancets. (Bayer Consumer Care) Disposable lancets for use in Miles diagnostic autolet or glucolet.
Use: Diagnostic aid.

Glucotrol. (Pfizer) Glipizide 5 mg, 10 mg. Lactose. Tab. Bot. 100s, 500s, UD 100s. *Rx.*
Use: Antidiabetic.

Glucotrol XL. (Pfizer) Glipizide 2.5 mg, 5 mg, 10 mg. ER Tab. Bot. 30s (2.5 mg only); 100s, 500s (except 2.5 mg). *Rx.*
Use: Antidiabetic.

Glucovance. (Bristol-Myers Squibb) Glyburide/metformin hydrochloride 1.25 mg/250 mg, 2.5 mg/500 mg, 5 mg/500 mg. Film-coated. Tab. Bot. 100s. *Rx.*
Use: Antidiabetic combination.

Glucovite. (Pal-Pak, Inc.) Ferrous gluconate 260 mg, vitamins B_1 1 mg, B_2 0.5 mg, C 10 mg. Tab. Bot. 1000s, 5000s. *OTC.*
Use: Mineral, vitamin supplement.

glucurolactone. Gamma lactone of glucofuranuronic acid.

glufanide disodium. (GLOO-fa-nide)
See: Oglufanide Disodium.

Glu-K. (Western Research) Potassium gluconate 486 mg. Tab. Bot. 1000s. *OTC.*
Use: Electrolyte supplement.

Glumetza. (Depomed) Metformin hydrochloride 500 mg, 1000 mg. Film-coated. ER Tab. 90s (1000 mg), 100s (500 mg). *Rx.*
Use: Antidiabetic agent.

gluside.
See: Saccharin.

•**glutamic acid.** (gloo-TAM-ik AS-id) USP 34.
Use: Nutritional supplement.
See: Glutamic Acid.

glutamic acid. (J. R. Carlson Laboratories) Glutamic acid. Pow. Bot. 100 g. *OTC.*
Use: Nutritional supplement.

glutamic acid. (Various Mfr.) Glutamic acid 500 mg. Tab. Bot. 100s, 500s. *OTC.*
Use: Nutritional supplement.

glutamic acid hydrochloride. Acidogen, aciglumin, glutasin. *OTC.*
Use: Gastric acidifier.

glutamic acid salts.
See: Calcium Glutamate.

•**glutamine.** (GLOO-ta-meen) USP 34.
Use: Dietary supplement; treatment of short bowel syndrome. [Orphan Drug]

•**glutaral concentrate.** (GLUE-tah-ral) USP 34.
Use: Disinfectant.
See: Cidex.

glutaraldehyde.
Use: Sterilizing, disinfecting agent.
See: Cidex.
Cidex Plus.
Cidex-7.

Glutarex-1. (Ross) Protein 15 g, fat 23.9 g, carbohydrates 46.3 g, linoleic acid 1800 mg, Fe 9 mg, Na 190 mg, K 675 mg, Ca, vitamins A, B_1, B_2, B_3, B_5, B_6, B_{12}, C, D, E, K, biotin, choline, folic acid, inositol, Cl, Cu, I, Mg, Mn, P, Se, Zn, and 480 Cal per 100 g, lysine and tryptophan free. Pow. Can 350 g. *OTC.*
Use: Nutritional supplement.

Glutarex-2. (Ross) Protein 30 g, fat 15.5 g, carbohydrates 30 g, Fe 13 mg, Na 880 mg, K 1370 mg, Ca, vitamins A, B_1, B_2, B_3, B_5, B_6, B_{12}, C, D, E, K, biotin, choline, folic acid, inositol, Cl, Cu, I, Mg, Mn, P, Se, Zn, and 410 Cal per 100 g, lysine and tryptophan free. Pow. Can 325 g. *OTC.*
Use: Nutritional supplement.

l-glutathione, reduced.
Use: Treatment of AIDS-associated cachexia. [Orphan Drug]
See: Cachexon.

Glutofac. (Kenwood) Vitamins A 500 units, E 30 units, B_1 15 mg, B_2 10 mg, B_3 50 mg, B_5 20 mg, B_6 50 mg, C 300 mg, Zn 5 mg, Ca, Cr, Cu, Fe, K, Mg, Mn, P, Se. Capl. Bot. 90s. *OTC.*
Use: Mineral, vitamin supplement.

Glutofac-ZX. (Kenwood) Vitamin A 5000 units, D 400 units, E (succinate) 50 units, B 20 mg, B_2 20 mg, B_3 100 mg, B_5 25 mg, B_6 25 mg, B_{12} 50 mcg, C 500 mg, folic acid 1 mg, Zn, Ca, Cr, Cu, Mg, Mn, Se 20 mg, biotin 200 mg. Parabens, sorbitol. Capl. 60s. *Rx.*
Use: Mineral, vitamin supplement.
Glutol. (Paddock) Dextrose 100 g/ 180 mL. Bot. 180 mL.
Use: Diagnostic aid.
Glutose. (Paddock) Liquid glucose (40% dextrose). Concentrated glucose for insulin reactions. Gel. Bot. 60 g. *OTC.*
Use: Hyperglycemic.
•**glyburide.** (glie-BYOO-ride) *USP 34.*
Tall Man: glyBURIDE
Use: Antidiabetic.
See: DiaBeta.
Glynase PresTab.
W/Metformin Hydrochloride.
See: Glucovance.
glyburide. (Various Mfr.) Glyburide. Tab. **1.25 mg:** Bot. 50s, 100s, 500s. **1.5 mg (micronized):** Bot. 100s, 500s, 1000s, UD 100s. **2.5 mg & 5 mg:** Bot. 90s, 100s, 500s, 1000s, UD 100s; Blister pack 25s, 100s, 600s. **3 mg (micronized):** Bot. 100s, 500s, 1000s, UD 100s. **4.5 mg (micronized):** Bot. 100s, 500s, 1000s. **6 mg (micronized):** 100s, 500s, 1000s. *Rx.*
Use: Antidiabetic.
glyburide/metformin hydrochloride.
(PAR) Glyburide/metformin hydrochloride 1.25 mg/250 mg, 2.5 mg/500 mg, 5 mg/500 mg. Film-coated. Tab. 100s. *Rx.*
Use: Antidiabetic combination.
glyburide, micronized. (Various Mfr.) Micronized glyburide 1.5 mg, 3 mg, 4.5 mg, 6 mg. Tab. Bot. 100s, 500s (except 4.5 mg), 1000s, UD 100s (1.5 mg and 3 mg only). *Rx.*
Use: Antidiabetic.
Glycate Chewables. (Forest) Glycine 150 mg, calcium carbonate 300 mg. Chew. Tab. Bot. 1000s. *OTC.*
Use: Antacid.
•**glycerin.** (GLIH-suh-rin) *USP 34.*
Use: Pharmaceutic aid (humectant, solvent).
See: Colace.
Corn Huskers.
Fleet Babylax.
Sani-Supp.
W/Antipyrine, Benzocaine, Zinc Acetate Dihydrate.
See: Neotic.
W/Benzocaine.
See: Cēpacol Dual Relief Sore Throat + Coating Spray.

W/Carboxymethylcellulose Sodium.
See: Optive.
W/Chloroxylenol, Pramoxine Hydrochloride, Zinc Acetate Dihydrate Acetate Dihydrate.
See: Zinotic.
Zinotic ES.
W/Combinations.
See: Clear Eyes for Dry Eyes.
Dermasil.
W/Polysorbate 80.
See: Refresh Dry Eye Therapy.
glycerin suppositories. (Various Mfr.) Glycerin. **Adults:** Box 10s, 12s, 25s, 50s, 100s. **Pediatric:** 10s, 12s, 25s. *OTC.*
Use: Rectal evacuant, cathartic.
glycerol.
See: Glycerin.
•**glycerol, iodinated.** (GLIH-ser-ole EYE-oh-dih-nay-tehd) *USAN.*
Use: Expectorant.
•**glyceryl behenate.** (GLIS-er-il be-HEN-ate) *NF 29.*
Use: Pharmaceutic aid (tablet/capsule lubricant).
glyceryl guaiacolate.
Use: Expectorant.
See: Guaifenesin.
glyceryl guaiacolate carbamate. Methocarbamol.
See: Robaxin.
Robaxin 750.
glyceryl guaiacolether.
See: Guaifenesin.
•**glyceryl monostearate.** (GLIS-ir-il mon-oh-STEER-ate) *NF 29.*
Use: Pharmaceutic aid (emulsifying agent).
glyceryl triacetate.
See: Triacetin.
glyceryl triacetin. (Various Mfr.) Triacetin.
See: Fungacetin.
glyceryl trierucate.
Use: Adrenoleukodystrophy. [Orphan Drug]
glyceryl trinitrate ointment.
See: Nitrol.
glyceryl trinitrate tablets.
See: Nitroglycerin.
Nitroglyn.
glyceryl trioleate.
Use: Adrenoleukodystrophy. [Orphan Drug]
Glycets-Antacid Tablets. (Weeks & Leo) Calcium carbonate 350 mg, simethicone 25 mg. Chew. Tab. Bot. 100s. *OTC.*
Use: Antacid; antiflatulent.

glycinato dihydroxyaluminum hydrate.
See: Dihydroxyaluminum Aminoacetate.

•**glycine.** (GLIE-seen) *USP 34. Formerly Aminoacetic Acid.*
Use: Myasthenia gravis treatment, irrigating solution.
W/Aluminum Hydroxide-Magnesium Carbonate Coprecipitated Gel.
See: Glycogel.
W/Calcium Carbonate.
See: Antacid No. 6.
   Glycate Chewables.
   Titralac.
W/Glutamic Acid, Alanine.
See: Prostall.

glycine, aluminum salt.
See: Dihydroxyaluminum Aminoacetate.

glycine hydrochloride. (Various Mfr.)
Use: Gastric acidifier.

glycobiarsol.
Use: Amebiasis, *Trichomonas vaginalis, Monilia albicans*.

glycocoll. Glycine.
See: Aminoacetic Acid.

glycocyamine. Guanidoacetic acid.

Glycofed. (Pal-Pak, Inc.) Pseudoephedrine 30 mg, guaifenesin 100 mg. Tab. Bot. 1000s. *OTC.*
Use: Decongestant, expectorant.

GlycoLax. (Kremers Urban) PEG 3350 17 g in 14 single-dose packets, 255 g in 16 oz with dosing cup. Pow. for Oral Soln. *Rx.*
Use: Laxative.

•**glycol distearate.** (GLIE-kole dih-STEE-ah-rate) USAN.
Use: Pharmaceutic aid (thickening agent).

glycol monosalicylate.
W/Oil of Mustard, Camphor, Menthol, Methyl Salicylate.
See: Musterole.

glycophenylate bromide.
See: Mepenzolate Methylbromide.

glycoprotein.
Use: Antiplatelet agent.
See: Kogenate FS.

glycoprotein IIb/IIIa inhibitors.
Use: Antiplatelet agent.
See: Abciximab.
   Eptifibatide.
   Tirofiban Hydrochloride.

•**glycopyrrolate.** (glie-koe-PIE-row-late) *USP 34.*
Use: Anticholinergic.
See: Cuvposa.
   Robinul.
   Robinul Forte.

glycopyrrolate. (Rising) Glycopyrrolate 1 mg, 2 mg. Lactose. Tab. 100s, 1000s. *Rx.*
Use: Gastrointestinal anticholinergic/antispasmodic.

glycopyrrolate. (Various Mfr.) Glycopyrrolate 0.2 mg/mL. Inj. Vials. 1 mL, 2 mL, 5 mL, 20 mL. *Rx.*
Use: Anticholinergic.

Glycotuss. (Pal-Pak, Inc.) Guaifenesin 100 mg. Tab. Bot. 100s, 1000s. *OTC.*
Use: Expectorant.

Glycotuss-DM. (Pal-Pak, Inc.) Guaifenesin 100 mg, dextromethorphan HBr 10 mg. Tab. Bot. 100s, 1000s. *OTC.*
Use: Antitussive, expectorant.

glycylclines.
See: Tigecycline.

glycyrrhiza. Pure extract, fluid extract. Licorice root.
Use: Flavoring agent.

glycyrrhiza extract, pure.
Use: Flavoring agent.

glycyrrhiza fluid extract.
Use: Flavoring agent.

glydanile sodium. (GLIE-dah-neel SO-dee-uhm)
See: Glicetanile Sodium.

•**glyhexamide.** (glie-HEX-ah-mid) USAN.
Use: Antidiabetic.

Glylorin. (Cellegy) Monolaurin.
Use: Congenital primary ichthyosis.
[Orphan Drug]

•**glymidine sodium.** (GLIE-mih-deen) USAN.
Use: Oral hypoglycemic agent; antidiabetic.

glymol.
See: Petrolatum Liquid.

Glynase PresTab. (Pharmacia & Upjohn) Glyburide. Tab., micronized. Lactose.
1.5 mg: Tab. Bot. 100s, UD 100s. **3 mg:** Tab. Bot. 100s, 500s, 1000s, UD 100s.
6 mg: Tab. Bot. 100s, 500s. *Rx.*
Use: Antidiabetic.

•**glyoctamide.** (glie-OCKT-am-id) USAN.
Use: Hypoglycemic agent; antidiabetic.

Gly-Oxide Liquid. (GlaxoSmithKline) Carbamide peroxide 10%. Soln. Bot. 15 mL, 60 mL. *OTC.*
Use: Mouth and throat product.

glyoxyldiureide.
See: Allantoin.

•**glyparamide.** (glie-PAR-am-ide) USAN.
Use: Oral hypoglycemic agent; antidiabetic.

Glypressin. (Ferring) Terlipressin.
Use: Bleeding esophageal varicies.
[Orphan Drug]

Glyquin. (ICN) Hydroquinone 4%, padimate O, oxybenzone, octyl methoxycinnamate, methylparaben. SPF 15. In a vanishing base. Cream. Tube. 28 g. *Rx.*
Use: Pigment agent.

Glyquin-XM. (ICN) Hydroquinone 4%. Octocrylene, oxybenzone, avobenzone, vitamin E, methylparaben, EDTA, SPF 15. In a vanishing base. Cream. 28 g. *Rx.*
Use: Pigment agent.

Glyset. (Bayer Consumer Care) Miglitol 25 mg, 50 mg, 100 mg. Tab. Bot. 100s, 1000s (except 25 mg), UD 100. *Rx.*
Use: Antidiabetic.

GM-CSF. Granulocyte macrophage colony-stimulating factor.
See: Leukine.

gododiamide.
Use: Diagnostic aid.

Golacol. (Arcum) Codeine sulfate 30 mg, papaverine hydrochloride 30 mg, emetine hydrochloride 2 mg, ephedrine hydrochloride 15 mg, q.s./30 mL, alcohol 6.25%. Syr. Bot. 4 oz, 16 oz, gal. Orange flavor. *c-III.*
Use: Antitussive; bronchodilator.

Gold Alka-Seltzer Effervescent. (Bayer Consumer Care) Sodium bicarbonate (heat treated) 958 mg, citric acid 832 mg, potassium bicarbonate 312 mg. Tab. Bot. 20s, 36s. *OTC.*
Use: Antacid.

Gold Bond Antiseptic First Aid Quick Spray. (Chattem) Benzethonium chloride 0.13%, menthol 1%. Glycerin, parabens, SD alcohol 40, urea. Spray. 60 mL. *OTC.*
Use: Anti-infective, topical; antiseptic and germicide.

Gold Bond Foot Pain Relieving. (Chattem) Menthol 16%, aloe, benzyl alcohol, capsaicin, cetyl alcohol, cetearyl alcohol, disodium EDTA, SD alcohol, stearyl alcohol, urea. Cream. 113 g. *OTC.*
Use: Emollient.

Gold Bond Intensive Healing. (Chattem) Dimethicone 6%, pramoxine hydrochloride 1%. Aloe, cetearyl alcohol, cetyl alcohol, EDTA, glycerin, glyceryl stearate, parabens, petrolatum, propylene glycol, stearyl alcohol, urea. Cream. 28 g. *OTC.*
Use: Topical local anesthetic.

Gold Bond Medicated Triple Action Relief. (Chattem) Dimethicone 5%, menthol 0.15%, aloe, alcohols, EDTA, glycerin, parabens, petrolatum. Lot. 236 mL. *OTC.*
Use: Emollient.

Gold Bond Pain Relieving Foot Roll-On. (Chattem) Menthol 16%. Capsaicin, glycerin, propylene glycol, SD alcohol, triethanolamine. Liq., topical. 73 mL. *OTC.*
Use: Rub and liniment.

gold compounds.
See: Gold Sodium Thiosulfate.
Ridaura.
Solganal.

•**goldenseal.** (GOLD-n-seal) *NF 29.*
Use: Dietary supplement.

Golden-West Compound. (Golden-West) Gentian root, licorice root, cascara sagrada, damiana leaves, senna leaves, psyllium seed, buchu leaves, crude pepsin. Box 1.5 oz. *OTC.*
Use: Laxative.

Goldicide Concentrate. (Pedinol Pharmacal) Bot. oz. Ctn. 10s.
Use: Disinfectant.

Gold Seal Calcium 600. (Walgreen) Calcium 1200 mg. Tab. Bot. 60s. *OTC.*
Use: Mineral supplement.

Gold Seal Calcium 600 with Vitamin D. (Walgreen) Calcium 1200 mg, vitamin D. Tab. Bot. 60s. *OTC.*
Use: Mineral supplement.

Gold Seal Chewable Vitamin C. (Walgreen) Ascorbic acid 250 mg, 500 mg. Tab. Bot. 100s. *OTC.*
Use: Vitamin supplement.

Gold Seal Ferrous Gluconate. (Walgreen) Iron 37 mg. Tab. Bot. 100s. *OTC.*
Use: Mineral supplement.

Gold Seal Ferrous Sulfate. (Walgreen) Ferrous sulfate 325 mg. Tab. Bot. 100s, 1000s. *OTC.*
Use: Mineral supplement.

Gold Seal Time Release Ferrous Sulfate. (Walgreen) Iron 50 mg. Tab. Bot. 100s. *OTC.*
Use: Mineral supplement.

•**gold sodium thiomalate.** (gold SO-dee-uhm thigh-oh-MAL-ate) *USP 34.*
Use: Antirheumatic.
See: Aurolate.
Myochrisine.

gold sodium thiomalate. (Parenta) Gold sodium thiomalate 50 mg/mL. Benzyl alcohol 0.5%. Inj. 1 mL single-dose and 10 mL multidose vials. *Rx.*
Use: Antirheumatic agent.

gold sodium thiosulfate. Sterile, auricidine, aurocidin, aurolin, auropin, aurosan, novacrysin, solfocrisol, thiochrysine.
Use: Antirheumatic.

gold thioglucose.
See: Aurothioglucose.

- **golimumab.** (goe-li-MUE-mab) USAN.
  Use: Monoclonal antibody.
  See: Simponi.
- **golnerminogene pradenovec.** (GOL-ner-MIN-oh-jeen PRA-den-oh-vek) USAN.
  Use: Antineoplastic.
- **golotimod.** (goe-LOE-ti-mod) USAN.
  Use: Anti-infective agent.
  GoLYTELY. (Braintree) **Disp. Jug:** PEG 3350 236 g, sodium sulfate 22.74 g, sodium bicarbonate 6.74 g, sodium chloride 5.86 g, potassium chloride 2.97 g. Pow. for Oral Soln. **Packet:** PEG 3350 227.1 g, sodium sulfate 21.5 g, sodium bicarbonate 6.36 g, sodium chloride 5.53 g, potassium chloride 2.82 g. *Rx.*
  Use: Bowel evacuant.
- **gomiliximab.** (goe-mi-LIX-i-mab) USAN.
  Use: Allergic asthma.
  gonacrine.
  See: Acriflavine.
- **gonadorelin hydrochloride.** (go-NAD-oh-RELL-in) USAN. *Formerly Luteinizing Hormone-releasing Factor Dihydrochloride.*
  Use: In vivo diagnostic aid.
  gonadotropic substance.
  See: Gonadotropin Chorionic.
- **gonadotropin, chorionic.** (go-NAD-oh-TROE-pin, core-ee-AHN-ik) *USP 34.*
  Use: Gonad-stimulating principle. In women: Chronic cystic mastitis, functional sterility, dysmenorrhea, premenstrual tension, threatened abortion. In men: Cryptorchidism, hypogenitalism, dwarfism, impotency, enuresis.
  See: A.P.L.
  Chorex-10.
  Choron 10.
  Gonic.
  Pregnyl.
  Profasi.
  gonadotropin, pituitary anterior lobe.
  Extracted from anterior lobe of equine pituitaries (not pregnant mare urine) (rat unit = 1 Fevold-Hisaw unit).
  gonadotropin-releasing hormone analog.
  See: Goserelin Acetate.
  Histrelin Acetate.
  Leuprolide Acetate.
  Triptorelin Pamoate.
  gonadotropin-releasing hormone antagonists.
  Use: Sex hormone.
  See: Abarelix.
  Cetrorelix Acetate.
  Degarelix.

Ganirelix Acetate.
gonadotropin-releasing hormones.
Use: Sex hormone.
See: Gonadorelin Acetate.
Histrelin Acetate.
Nafarelin Acetate.
gonadotropins.
Use: Ovulation stimulant.
See: Lutropin Alfa.
Menotropins.
Pergonal.
gonadotropins, follitropin alfa.
Use: Sex hormone, ovulation stimulant.
See: Gonal-f.
Gonal-f RFF Pen.
gonadotropins, follitropin beta.
Use: Sex hormone, ovulation stimulant.
See: Follistim.
gonadotropins, menotropins.
Use: Sex hormone, ovulation stimulant.
See: Pergonal.
Repronex.
gonadotropins, urofollitropin.
Use: Sex hormone, ovulation stimulant.
See: Bravelle.
Gonak. (Akorn) Hydroxypropyl methylcellulose 2.5%. Soln. Bot. 15 mL. *OTC.*
Use: Ophthalmic.
Gonal-f. (Serono) Follitropin alfa 82 units (to deliver 75 units), 600 units (to deliver 450 units), 1200 units (to deliver 1050 units) FSH activity, sucrose 30 mg. Pow. for Inj., lyophilized. Single-dose vials with sterile water for injection as diluent. 1, 10 (82 units only). Multi-dose vials with prefilled syringes of bacteriostatic water (with 0.9% benzyl alcohol) for injection as diluent. 1 (600 units and 1200 units only), 5, 10 (1200 units only). *Rx.*
Use: Sex hormone, ovulation stimulant.
Gonal-f RFF Pen. (Serono) Follitropin alfa 415 units (to deliver ≥ 300 units/0.5 mL), 568 units (to deliver ≥ 450 units/ 0.75 mL), 1026 units (to deliver ≥ 900 units/1.5 mL) FSH activity. Inj. Prefilled pens with needles with benzyl alcohol 0.9%. *Rx.*
Use: Ovulation stimulant.
gonioscopic hydroxypropyl methylcellulose.
See: Goniosol.
Goniosoft. (Ocusoft) Hydroxypropyl methylcellulose 2.5%. Benzalkonium chloride 0.01%, EDTA. Ophth. Soln. 15 mL. *OTC.*
Use: Ophthalmic and otic agent, ophthalmic surgical adjunct.
Goniosol. (Novartis Ophthalmics) Gonioscopic hydroxypropyl methylcellulose 2.5%. Bot. 15 mL. *OTC.*
Use: Ophthalmic.

Gonodecten Test Kit. (United States Packaging) Tube test for urethral discharge from males, for detection of *Neisseria gonorrhoeae.* Test kit 10s, 25s.
Use: Diagnostic aid.
gonorrhea tests.
See: Biocult-GC.
Gonodecten Test Kit.
Gonozyme.
Isocult for *Neisseria gonorrhoeae.*
MicroTrak *Neisseria gonorrhoeae* Culture Test.
Gonozyme. (Abbott Diagnostics) Enzyme immunoassay for detection of *Neisseria gonorrhoeae* in urogenital swab specimens. Test kit 100s.
Use: Diagnostic aid.
Good Samaritan Ointment. (Good Samaritan) Tube 1.25 oz. *OTC.*
Use: Counterirritant.
Good Sense Maximum Strength Dose Sinus. (Perrigo) Pseudoephedrine hydrochloride 30 mg, chlorpheniramine maleate 2 mg, acetaminophen 500 mg. Tab. Pkg. 24s. *OTC.*
Use: Upper respiratory combination, decongestant, antihistamine, analgesic.
Good Sense Maximum Strength Pain Relief Allergy Sinus. (Perrigo) Pseudoephedrine hydrochloride 30 mg, chlorpheniramine maleate 2 mg, acetaminophen 500 mg. Gelcap. Pkg. 24s. *OTC.*
Use: Upper respiratory combination, decongestant, antihistamine, analgesic.
Goody's Body Pain Powder. (Glaxo Consumer) Acetaminophen 325 mg, aspirin 500 mg, lactose. Pow. Pkg. 6s, 24s. *OTC.*
Use: Analgesic.
Goody's Extra Strength. (Glaxo Consumer) Acetaminophen 260 mg, aspirin 520 mg, caffeine 32.5 mg. Potassium 51.1 mg. Pow., Oral. 2s, 6s, 24s, 50s. *OTC.*
Use: Nonnarcotic analgesic.
Goody's PM. (GlaxoSmithKline) Diphenhydramine citrate 38 mg, acetaminophen 500 mg. Lactose. Pow. Packets. 6s. *OTC.*
Use: Nonprescription sleep aid.
Gordobalm. (Gordon Laboratories) Chloroxylenol, methyl salicylate, menthol, camphor, thymol, eucalyptus oil, isopropyl alcohol 16%, fast-drying gum base. Bot. 4 oz, gal. *OTC.*
Use: Analgesic, topical.
Gordochom. (Gordon Laboratories) Undecylenic acid 25%, chloroxylenol in an oily base. Soln. Bot. 30 mL. *OTC.*
Use: Antifungal, topical.

Gordofilm. (Gordon Laboratories) Salicylic acid 16.7%, lactic acid 16.7% in flexible colloidan. Bot. 15 mL. *OTC.*
Use: Keratolytic.
Gordogesic Cream. (Gordon Laboratories) Methyl salicylate 10% in absorption base. Jar 2.5 oz, 1 lb. *OTC.*
Use: Analgesic, topical.
Gordomatic. (Gordon Laboratories) **Crystals:** Sodium borate, sodium bicarbonate, sodium chloride, thymol, menthol, eucalyptus oil. Jar 8 oz, 7 lb. **Lot.:** Menthol, camphor, propylene glycol, isopropyl alcohol. Bot. 1 oz, 4 oz, gal. **Pow.:** Menthol, thymol camphor, eucalyptus oil, salicylic acid, alum bentonite, talc. Shaker can 3.5 oz. Can 1 lb, 5 lb. *OTC.*
Use: Counterirritant.
Gordon's Urea. (Gordon Laboratories) Urea 40% in petrolatum base. Jar oz. *Rx.*
Use: Emollient.
Gordophene. (Gordon Laboratories) Neutral coconut oil soap 15%, glycerin with Septi-Chlor (trichlorohydroxy diphenyl ether) broad-spectrum antimicrobial and bacteriostatic agent. Bot. 4 oz, gal.
Use: Dermatologic, cleanser.
Gordo-Vite A. (Gordon Laboratories) **Creme:** Vitamin A 100,000 units/oz. in water-soluble base. Jar 0.5 oz, 2.5 oz, 4 oz, lb, 5 lb. **Lot.:** Vitamin A 100,000 units/oz. Plastic bot. 4 oz, gal. *OTC.*
Use: Emollient.
Gordo-Vite E Creme. (Gordon Laboratories) Vitamin E 1500 units/oz in water-soluble base. Jar 2.5 oz, lb. *OTC.*
Use: Emollient.
Gormel Cream. (Gordon Laboratories) Urea 20% in emollient base. Jar 0.5 oz, 2.5 oz, 4 oz, 1 lb, 5 lb. *OTC.*
Use: Emollient.
•**goserelin.** (GO-suh-REH-lin) USAN.
Use: LHRH agonist.
See: Zoladex.
goserelin acetate.
Use: Gonadotropin-releasing hormone analog.
See: Zoladex.
•**gosogliptin.** (goe-soe-GLIP-tin) USAN.
Use: Antidiabetic.
gossypol.
Use: Antineoplastic. [Orphan Drug]
gotamine. (Vita Elixir) Ergotamine tartrate 1 mg, caffeine 100 mg. Tab. *Rx.*
Use: Antimigraine.
gout, agents for.
See: Allopurinol.

Colchicine.
Lesinurad.
Lesinurad Sodium.
Pegloticase.
Probenecid.
Probenecid with Colchicine.
Sulfinpyrazone.
•**govafilcon A.** (GO-vaff-ILL-kahn A)
USAN.
Use: Contact lens material, hydrophilic.
•**goxalapladib.** (gox-a-LAP-la-dib) USAN.
Use: Atherosclerosis.
G Phen. (Boca Pharmacal) Dextromethorphan HBr 60 mg, guaifenesin
600 mg, phenylephrine hydrochloride
40 mg. Film-coated. ER Tab. 100s. *Rx.*
Use: Antitussive and expectorant combination.
gp100 adenoviral gene therapy. (Genzyme)
Use: Antineoplastic. [Orphan Drug]
G/P 1200/60. (Cypress) Pseudoephedrine hydrochloride 60 mg, guaifenesin
1200 mg. SR Tab. Bot. 100s. *Rx.*
Use: Upper respiratory combination, decongestant, expectorant.
Grafco. (Graham-Field) Potassium nitrate 25%, silver nitrate 75%. Swab,
topical. 100s. *Rx.*
Use: Topical antiseptic, antiseptic and
germicide.
Gralise. (Abbott Laboratories) Gabapentin 300 mg, 600 mg. Tab. 30s (300 mg
only), 90s, 300s, UD 10s, 30-day
starter packs (contains 78 tablets:
9 × 300 mg and 69 × 600 mg tablets).
Rx.
Use: Anticonvulsant.
•**gramicidin.** (gram-ih-SIH-din) *USP 34.*
Use: Anti-infective.
W/Neomycin.
See: Spectrocin.
W/Benzocaine, Neomycin Sulfate, Polymyxin B Sulfate.
See: Mycolog Cream.
W/Hydrocortisone Acetate, Neomycin
Sulfate, Polymyxin B Sulfate.
See: Cortisporin.
W/Neomycin Sulfate, Polymyxin B Sulfate.
See: AK-Spore.
Neosporin.
Neosporin-G.
Ocutricin.
W/Neomycin Sulfate, Polymyxin B Sulfate, Thimerosal.
See: AK-Spore Ophthalmic Solution.
Neo-Polycin.
Neosporin Ophthalmic Solution.
Grandpa's Wonder Pin Tar Conditioner. (Grandpa Brands) Pin tar oil.

Cetearyl alcohol, glyceryl, sunflower
seed oil. Liq. 237 mL. *OTC.*
Use: Miscellaneous tar-containing
product.
•**granisetron.** (gran-IH-SEH-trahn) USAN.
Use: Antiemetic.
See: Granisol.
Kytril.
Sancuso.
granisetron. (Bedford Laboratories)
Granisetron 0.1 mg/mL. Preservative
free. May contain sodium chloride. Inj.,
Soln. Single-dose vial. *Rx.*
Use: Antiemetic/antivertigo agent,
$5-HT_3$ receptor antagonist.
•**granisetron hydrochloride.** (gran-IH-SEH-trahn) USAN.
Use: Antiemetic.
See: Kytril.
granisetron hydrochloride. (Various
Mfr.) Granisetron. **Inj., Soln.:** 0.1 mg/
mL (may contain sodium chloride),
1 mg/mL (may contain benzyl alcohol,
parabens, sodium chloride). Single-use
vials. 1 mL. Multiple-use vials (1 mg/
mL only). 4 mL. **Tab.:** 1 mg. May contain lactose. 20s, 100s, blister 2s, blister 20s. *Rx.*
Use: Antiemetic/antivertigo agent,
$5-HT_3$ receptor antagonist.
Granisol. (PediatRx) Granisetron 1 mg
per 5 mL. Sorbitol. Orange flavor. Oral
Soln. 30 mL. *Rx.*
Use: Antiemetic/antivertigo agent,
$5-HT_3$ receptor antagonist.
Granulex. (Bertek) Trypsin 0.12 mg, balsam Peru 87 mg, castor oil 788 mg/g.
Aerosol. 113.4 g. *Rx.*
Use: Enzyme preparation, topical.
granulocyte colony-stimulating factor.
See: Neupogen.
granulocyte macrophage colony-stimulating factor.
See: Leukine.
gratus strophanthin. Ouabain.
Gravineed. (Hanlon) Vitamins C 100 mg,
E 10 units, B_1 3 mg, B_2 2 mg, B_6 10 mg,
B_{12} 5 mcg, A 4000 units, D 400 units,
niacin 10 mg, folic acid 0.1 mg, iron
fumarate 40 mg, calcium 67 mg. Cap.
Bot. 100s. *OTC.*
Use: Mineral, vitamin supplement.
Green Glo. (Hub Pharmaceuticals) Lissamine green 1.5 mg. Strip, Ophth. 100s.
Rx.
Use: Ophthalmic diagnostic product.
Green Mint. (Block Drug) Urea, glycine,
polysorbate 60, sorbitol, alcohol 12.2%,
peppermint oil, menthol, chlorophyllin-
copper complex. Bot. 7 oz, 12 oz. *OTC.*
Use: Mouth and throat preparation.

green soap.
Use: Detergent.
Green Throat Spray. (Clay-Park Labs) Phenol 1.4%. Glycerin, saccharin. Alcohol-free. Throat spray. 473 mL. *OTC.*
Use: Mouth and throat product.
•**grepafloxacin hydrochloride.** (grep-ah-FLOX-ah-sin) USAN.
Use: Antibacterial.
Grifulvin V. (Ortho) Griseofulvin microsize 500 mg. Tab. 100s, 500s. *Rx.*
Use: Antifungal.
•**griseofulvin.** (griss-ee-oh-FULL-vin) *USP 34.*
Use: Antifungal.
See: Fulvicin P/G.
Fulvicin U/F.
Grifulvin V.
Griseofulvin Ultramicrosize.
Gris-PEG.
griseofulvin. (Various Mfr.) Griseofulvin 165 mg, 330 mg. Tab. Bot. 100s. *Rx.*
Use: Antifungal.
griseofulvin microsize.
Use: Antifungal.
See: Grifulvin V.
griseofulvin microsize. (Glades) Griseofulvin microsize 125 mL per 5 mL. Alcohol 0.2%, menthol, parabens, saccharin, sucrose. Orange-cream flavor. Susp. 120 mL. *Rx.*
Use: Antifungal.
griseofulvin ultramicrosize.
Use: Antifungal.
See: Gris-PEG.
Gris-PEG. (Pedinol) Griseofulvin ultramicrosize 125 mg, 250 mg. Lactose (125 mg only), parabens. Tab. 100s, 500s (250 mg only). *Rx.*
Use: Antifungal.
growth hormone. Extract of human pituitaries containing predominantly growth hormone.
See: Crescormon.
Somatropin.
growth hormone-releasing factor. (ICN)
Use: Long-term treatment of growth failure. [Orphan Drug]
See: Tesamorelin.
g-strophanthin. Ouabain.
guaiacol carbonate. (Various Mfr.) Duotal.
Use: Expectorant.
guaiacol glyceryl ether.
See: Guaifenesin.
guaiacol potassium sulfonate.
See: Bronchial.
W/Ammonium Chloride, Sodium Citrate, Benzyl Alcohol, Carbinoxamine Maleate.
See: Clistin Expectorant.

W/Dextromethorphan Hydrobromide.
See: Bronchial DM.
W/Pheniramine Maleate, Pyrilamine Maleate, Codeine Phosphate.
See: Tritussin.
guaianesin.
Use: Expectorant.
See: Guaifenesin.
•**guaiapate.** (GWIE-ah-pate) USAN.
Use: Antitussive.
GUAI 800 mg/DM 30 mg. (Brighton) Dextromethorphan HBr 30 mg, guaifenesin 800 mg. Dye and sugar free. ER Tab. 100s.
Use: Antitussive with expectorant, upper respiratory combination.
Guaifed. (Victory) Guaifenesin 400 mg, phenylephrine 15 mg. Sucrose, parabens. ER Cap. Bot. 30s, 100s. *Rx.*
Use: Upper respiratory combination, decongestant and expectorant combination.
Guaifed-PD. (Victory) Guaifenesin 200 mg, phenylephrine hydrochloride 7.5 mg. Parabens, sucrose. ER. Cap. Bot. 30s, 100s. *Rx.*
Use: Upper respiratory combination, decongestant, and expectorant combination.
Guaifed Syrup. (Muro) Pseudoephedrine hydrochloride 30 mg, guaifenesin 200 mg/5 mL, EDTA, menthol, saccharin, sorbitol, sucrose, cherry flavor, alcohol free. Syr. Bot. 473 mL. *OTC.*
Use: Upper respiratory combination, decongestant, expectorant.
Guaifen DM. (Breckenridge) Dextromethorphan HBr 20 mg, guaifenesin 1200 mg, phenylephrine hydrochloride 40 mg. Dye free. ER Tab. 100s. *Rx.*
Use: Upper respiratory combination, antitussive and expectorant combination.
•**guaifenesin.** (GWIE-fen-ah-sin) *USP 34.*
Formerly Glyceryl Guaiacolate. Synonyms: Glyceryl guaiacolate, glyceryl guaiacol ether, guaianesin, guaifylline, guayanesin.
Tall Man: guaiFENesin
Use: Expectorant.
See: AMBI.
Buckley's Chest Congestion.
Consin-GG.
Diabetic Tussin.
Diabetic Tussin EX.
Duratuss-G.
GG-Cen.
Glycotuss.
G-100.
G-Tussin.
Guiatuss.
Humibid Maximum Strength.

Liquibid.
Monafed.
Mucinex.
Mucinex Children's.
Mucinex Mini-Melts Children's.
Mucinex Mini-Melts Junior Strength.
Muco-Fen-LA.
Mucus Relief.
Organ-I NR.
Pheunomist.
Robitussin.
Scot-Tussin Expectorant.
Siltussin.
Tusibron.
2/G.
Vicks DayQuil Mucus Control.
W/Acetaminophen.
  See: Comtrex Multi-Symptom Deep
    Chest Cold.
  Theraflu Chest Congestion.
  Tylenol Chest Congestion.
W/Acetaminophen, Dextromethorphan
  Hydrobromide, Phenylephrine Hydro-
  chloride.
  See: Phenflu G.
  Sine-Off Cough/Cold.
  Sudafed PE Multi-Symptom Cold and
    Cough.
W/Acetaminophen, Dextromethorphan
  Hydrobromide, Pseudoephedrine
  Hydrochloride.
  See: Duraflu.
  Flutabs.
  Maxiflu DM.
  Maxiflu G.
  Tylenol Cold Severe Congestion.
W/Acetaminophen, Phenylephrine Hydro-
  chloride.
  See: Coldonyl.
  Duratuss A.
  Tylenol Sinus Severe Congestion &
    Pain Severe Daytime.
W/Acetaminophen, Pseudoephedrine
  Hydrochloride.
  See: Poly-Vent Plus.
  Tylenol Sinus Severe Congestion.
W/Brompheniramine Maleate, Dextro-
  methorphan Hydrobromide, Phenyl-
  ephrine Hydrochloride.
  See: AccuHist PDX.
  Bromhist-PDX.
W/Brompheniramine Maleate, Dextro-
  methorphan Hydrobromide, Pseudo-
  ephedrine Hydrochloride.
  See: Bromhist DM Pediatric.
  Histacol DM Pediatric.
  Pediahist DM.
W/Carbetapentane Citrate.
  See: Allfen C.
  AMBI 1000/5.
  BetaVent.

Duratuss CS.
Dynex VR.
Tusso-ZMR.
Tusso-ZR.
XPect-AT.
W/Carbetapentane Citrate, Phenyl-
  ephrine Hydrochloride.
  See: Albatussin.
  Carbatab-12.
  Carbatuss.
  Extendryl GCP.
  Gentex 30.
  Levall.
  Phencarb GG.
  Zinx GCP.
W/Carbetapentane Citrate, Pseudo-
  ephedrine Hydrochloride.
  See: Exall-D.
W/Chlophedianol Hydrochloride, Pseudo-
  ephedrine Hydrochloride.
  See: Vanacof DX.
W/Chlorpheniramine Maleate, Dextro-
  methorphan Hydrobromide, Phenyl-
  ephrine Hydrochloride.
  See: Chlordex GP.
  DM/CPM/PE/GG.
  Donatussin.
  Genelan-NF.
  Qual-Tussin.
W/Chlorpheniramine Maleate, Hydro-
  codone Bitartrate, Pseudoephedrine
  Hydrochloride.
  See: Tussend.
  ZTuss Expectorant.
W/Chlorpheniramine Maleate, Phenyl-
  ephrine Hydrochloride.
  See: P Chlor C.
W/Codeine Phosphate.
  See: Allfen CDX.
  Brontex.
  CGU WC.
  Cheracol Cough.
  Cheratussin AC Expectorant Cough
    Suppressant.
  ExeClear-C.
  Gani-Tuss NR.
  Guiatuss AC.
  Iophen C-NR.
  Iophen DM-NR.
  Mar-Cof-CG.
  M-Clear.
  M-Clear WC.
  Myci-GC.
  Mytussin AC Cough.
  Pro-Clear.
  Romilar AC.
  Tussi-Organidin NR.
  Tussi-Organidin-S NR.
  Tusso-C.

W/Codeine Phosphate, Phenylephrine
Hydrochloride.
See: Giltuss Ped-C.
Tridal.
W/Codeine Phosphate, Pseudoephed-
rine Hydrochloride.
See: Cheratussin DAC.
Guiatuss DAC.
Lortuss EX.
Mytussin DAC.
Novagest Expectorant with Codeine.
Sudatuss-2 DF.
Tusnel C.
Zodryl DEC 80.
Zodryl DEC 50.
Zodryl DEC 40.
Zodryl DEC 60.
Zodryl DEC 30.
Zodryl DEC 35.
Zodryl DEC 25.
W/Dexbrompheniramine Maleate, Dextro-
methorphan Hydrobromide, Pseudo-
ephedrine Hydrochloride.
See: DEKA.
DEKA Pediatric.
W/Dextromethorphan Hydrobromide.
See: Alka-Seltzer Plus Mucus & Con-
gestion.
Allfen DM.
AMBI 1000/55.
Atuss-12 DX.
Bidex-A.
Biospec DMX.
Cheracol D Cough Formula.
Cheracol Plus.
Congesta DM.
Coricidin HBP Chest Congestion &
Cough.
Dex-Tuss DM.
Diabetic Tussin DM.
Diabetic Tussin Maximum Strength
DM.
Extra Action Cough.
Fenesin DM IR.
Gan-Tuss DM NR.
Genatuss DM.
Geri-Tussin DM.
GFN 1000/DM 60.
GFN 1200/DM 60.
GUAI 800 mg/DM 30 mg.
Guaifenesin DM.
Guaifenesin DM 1000/60.
Guaifenex DM.
Iobid DM.
Kolephrin GG/DM.
Mucinex Cough for Kids.
Mucinex Cough Mini-Melts for Kids.
Mucinex DM.
Mucinex DM Maximum Strength.
MucusRelief DM.
NeoTuss.

Phanatuss DM.
Pulexn DM.
Respa-DM.
Robafen DM Max.
Robitussin Cough & Congestion.
Robitussin Cough DM.
Robitussin Cough Sugar-Free DM.
Robitussin DM.
Safe Tussin DM.
Scot-Tussin Senior Clear.
Siltussin DM.
Touro DM.
TUSSI-bid.
Tussi-Organidine DM-S NR.
Vicks Formula 44E Cough & Chest
Congestion Relief.
Vicks Formula 44e Pediatric Cough &
Chest Congestion Relief.
Zotex-EX.
W/Dextromethorphan Hydrobromide,
Phenylephrine Hydrochloride.
See: AMBI 10PEH/400GFN/20DM.
Biobron SF.
Biogil.
BioGtuss.
Bio T Pres.
Bio T Pres Pediatric.
Biotuss.
Bio-Tussi.
Broncotron-D.
Brontuss DX.
Dacex PE.
Deconex DM.
Deconex DMX.
Despec DM.
Despec NR.
Dynatuss EX.
Endacon.
ExeCof.
ExeTuss-DM.
Gene-T-Pres.
GFN 1200/DM 20/PE 40.
Giltuss.
Giltuss Pediatric.
Giltuss TR.
Guaifen.
Maxiphen DM.
NeoTuss-D.
Phlemex Forte.
Phlemex-PE.
Phenydex Pediatric.
Robitussin Children's Cough & Cold CF.
Robitussin Pediatric Cough/Cold CF.
SINUtuss DM.
TriTuss.
TriTuss ER.
Tussi-Pres.
Tussi-Pres Pediatric.
Tusso DMR.
Tusso XR.
Z-Dex.

Z-Dex Pediatric.
Zotex.
Zotex-D.
Zotex Pediatric.
W/Dextromethorphan Hydrobromide,
  Phenylephrine Hydrochloride, Pyril-
  amine Maleate.
  See: Phenydex.
W/Dextromethorphan Hydrobromide,
  Potassium Citrate.
  See: Sorbutuss NR.
W/Dextromethorphan Hydrobromide,
  Pseudoephedrine Hydrochloride.
  See: Aldex GS DM.
    Ambifed-G DM.
    AMBI 40PSE/400GFN/20DM.
    AMBI 60/580/30.
    AMBI 60PSE/400GFN/20DM.
    Bionel.
    Bionel Pediatric.
    Capmist DM.
    Despec.
    Donatussin DM.
    ExeFen DMX.
    GFN 600/PSE 60/DM 30.
    Iophen NR.
    Liquicough DM.
    Maxifed DM.
    Maxifed DMX.
    Medent DMI.
    PanMist-DM.
    Poly-Vent DM.
    Pseudo Cough.
    Q-Tussin CF.
    Relacon DM NR.
    Relasin DM.
    Robaben CF.
    Robitussin Cough & Cold D.
    Sudafed Multi-Symptom Cold &
      Cough.
    TGQ 30PSE/150GFN/15DM.
    Tidafen DM.
    TL-DEX DM.
    Touro CC-LD.
    Tusnel.
    Tusnel-DM Pediatric.
    Tusnel Pediatric.
    Z-Cof DMX.
    Z-Cof 8 DM.
    Z-Cof I.
W/Dihydrocodeine Bitartrate.
  See: J-Max DHC.
W/Dihydrocodeine Bitartrate, Phenyl-
  ephrine Hydrochloride.
  See: Donatuss DC.
    Poly-Tussin EX.
W/Dihydrocodeine Bitartrate, Pseudo-
  ephedrine Hydrochloride.
  See: Despec-EXP.
W/Dyphylline.
  See: Difil-G.

Difil-G Forte.
Difil-G 400.
Dilex-G.
Dilex-G 400.
Dilex-G 200.
Dyflex-G.
Dy-G.
Dyphylline-GG.
Dyphylline GG ES.
Ed-Bron G.
Jay-Phyl.
Lufyllin-GG.
W/Ephedrine Hydrochloride.
  See: Primatene.
W/Ephedrine Sulfate.
  See: Broncholate.
    Bronkaid Dual Action.
W/Hydrocodone Bitartrate.
  See: ZTuss ZT.
W/Phenylephrine Hydrochloride.
  See: AMBI 1PEH/400GFN.
    Crantex.
    Deconex.
    Deconsal II.
    Despec.
    Donatussin.
    D-Phen 1000.
    D-Tab.
    Duratuss GP.
    Dynex LA.
    ED Bron GP.
    Entex.
    Entex LA.
    Entex LQ.
    Exefen-PD.
    ExeTuss.
    ExeTuss GP.
    Extendryl G.
    Gentex LA.
    GFN 600/Phenylephrine 20.
    Gilphex TR.
    Guaifed.
    Guaifed-PD.
    Guaifen PE.
    Guaphenyl LA.
    J-Max.
    Liquibid-D.
    Liquibid-PD.
    Liquibid PD-R.
    Medent-PE.
    Mucinex Cold for Kids.
    MucusRelief Sinus.
    MyDex.
    Nariz.
    Nasex.
    Nasex-G.
    Norel EX.
    PE/GG.
    PhenaVent D.
    PhenaVent LA.
    Reluri.

Rescon GG.
Robitussin PE Head and Chest Congestion.
Sil-Tex.
Simuc-GP.
Sinutab Non-Drying.
SINUtab PE.
Sitrex.
Sitrex PD.
Sudafed PE Non-Drying Sinus.
SymPak.
Triaminic Chest & Nasal Congestion.
Tussbid.
Tussbid PD.
Visonex.
Zinx GP.
Zotex GPX.
W/Phenylephrine Tannate.
See: Sina-12X.
W/Phenylephrine Tannate, Pyrilamine Tannate.
See: Ryna-12X.
W/Pseudoephedrine Hydrochloride.
See: Altarussin-PE.
Ambifed.
Ambifed-G.
AMBI 40PSE/400GFN.
AMBI 60/580.
AMBI 60PSE/400GFN.
Coldmist JR.
Coldmist LA.
Congestac.
Despec-Tab.
Dynex.
Entex PSE.
GFN-PSE.
Guaifenex GP.
Guaifenex PSE.
Guaifenex PSE 85.
Guaifenex PSE 60.
GuaiMAX-D.
Iosal II.
LEV/PSE/GG.
Maxifed.
Maxifed-G.
Mucinex D.
Mucinex D Maximum Strength.
Nasatab LA.
Nomuc-PE.
Respa-1st.
Respaire-120 SR.
Respaire-60 SR.
Severe Congestion Tussin.
Stamoist E.
Sudafed Maximum Strength Non-Drowsy Non-Drying Sinus.
SudaTex G.
Tenar PSE.
Touro LA.
Triacting.
Zephrex.

guaifenesin. (URL) Guaifenesin 400 mg. Dye-free. Tab. 50s, 100s. *OTC.*
Use: Expectorant.
guaifenesin. (Various Mfr.) Guaifenesin.
ER Tab.: 600 mg. Bot. 100s, **SR Tab.:** 1000 mg. Bot. 100s. **Syr.:** 100 mg/ 5 mL. Bot. 473 mL. **Tab.:** 200 mg. 100s. *Rx-OTC.*
Use: Expectorant.
•**guaifenesin and codeine phosphate oral solution.** (GWIE-fen-ah-sin and KOE-deen) *USP 34.*
Use: Antitussive, expectorant.
guaifenesin and phenylephrine hydrochloride. (River's Edge) Phenylephrine hydrochloride 30 mg, guaifenesin 900 mg. Dye free. SR Tab. 100s. *Rx.*
Use: Decongestant and expectorant.
Guaifenesin DAC. (Cypress) Codeine phosphate 10 mg, pseudoephedrine hydrochloride 30 mg, guaifenesin 100 mg/5 mL, alcohol 1.9%, saccharin, sorbitol. Liq. Bot. 480 mL. *OTC.*
Use: Antitussive, decongestant, expectorant.
Guaifenesin DM. (UDL) Dextromethorphan HBr 10 mg, guaifenesin 100 mg per 5 mL. Saccharin, sorbitol, alcohol free. Syr. UD 5 mL, 10 mL. *OTC.*
Use: Upper respiratory combination, antitussive with expectorant.
Guaifenesin-DM NR. (Silarx) Dextromethorphan HBr 10 mg, guaifenesin 100 mg per 5 mL. Methylparaben, saccharin, sorbitol, raspberry flavor, alcohol free, sugar free. Liq. Bot. 118 mL, 473 mL, 3785 mL. *Rx.*
Use: Upper respiratory combination, antitussive with expectorant.
Guaifenesin DM 1000/60. (Prasco) Dextromethorphan HBr 60 mg, guaifenesin 1000 mg. Dye free. ER Tab. 100s. *Rx.*
Use: Upper respiratory combination, antitussive with expectorant.
guaifenesin 900 mg/phenylephrine hydrochloride 25 mg. (Brighton) Phenylephrine hydrochloride 25 mg, guaifenesin 900 mg. Dye free. ER Tab. 100s. *Rx.*
Use: Upper respiratory combination, decongestant and expectorant combination.
Guaifenesin NR. (Silarx) Guaifenesin 100 mg/5 mL. Raspberry flavor. Liq. 473 mL. *Rx.*
Use: Expectorant.
guaifenesin 1000 mg and dextromethorphan HBr 60 mg. (URL Laboratories) Dextromethorphan HBr 60 mg, guaifenesin 1000 mg. LA Tab. Bot.

100s. *Rx.*
Use: Upper respiratory combination, antitussive, expectorant.

guaifenesin/phenylephrine hydrochloride. (Various Mfr.) Phenylephrine hydrochloride 30 mg, guaifenesin 900 mg. ER Tab. 100s. *Rx.*
Use: Upper respiratory combination, decongestant and expectorant combination.

guaifenesin/pseudoephedrine hydrochloride. (Major) Pseudoephedrine hydrochloride 60 mg, guaifenesin 600 mg. SR Tab. Bot. 100s. *Rx.*
Use: Upper respiratory combination, decongestant, expectorant.

guaifenesin/pseudoephedrine hydrochloride/codeine phosphate syrup. (Schein) Pseudoephedrine hydrochloride 30 mg, codeine phosphate 10 mg, guaifenesin 100 mg, alcohol 1.4%/ 5 mL. Bot. 473 mL. *c-v.*
Use: Antitussive, decongestant, expectorant.
See: Guaifenesin DAC.

guaifenesin/pseudoephedrine hydrochloride/dextromethorphan HBr 800/90/60. (Medicosa) Dextromethorphan HBr 60 mg, guaifenesin 800 mg, pseudoephedrine hydrochloride 90 mg. ER Tab. 100s. *Rx.*
Use: Antitussive and expectorant combination.

Guaifenex DM. (Ethex) Guaifenesin 600 mg, dextromethorphan HBr 30 mg. ER Tab. Bot. 100s. *Rx.*
Use: Upper respiratory combination, antitussive with expectorant.

Guaifenex GP. (Ethex) Pseudoephedrine hydrochloride 120 mg, guaifenesin 1200 mg. Lactose, dye free. Film-coated. ER Tab. Bot. 100s. *Rx.*
Use: Upper respiratory combination, decongestant, expectorant.

Guaifenex PSE 85. (Ethex) Pseudoephedrine hydrochloride 85 mg, guaifenesin 795 mg. Lactose. ER Tab. 100s. *Rx.*
Use: Upper respiratory combination, decongestant and expectorant combination.

Guaifenex PSE 120. (Ethex) Guaifenesin 600 mg, pseudoephedrine hydrochloride 120 mg. Dye free. ER Tab. Bot. 100s. *Rx.*
Use: Upper respiratory combination, decongestant, expectorant.

Guaifenex PSE 60. (Ethex) Guaifenesin 600 mg, pseudoephedrine hydrochloride 60 mg. Lactose. ER Tab. Bot. 100s. *Rx.*
Use: Upper respiratory combination, decongestant, expectorant.

Guaifen PE. (Breckenridge) Phenylephrine hydrochloride 25 mg, guaifenesin 800 mg. Dye free. ER Tab. 100s. *Rx.*
Use: Upper respiratory combination, decongestant and expectorant combination.

GuaiMAX-D. (Schwarz Pharma) Pseudoephedrine hydrochloride 120 mg, guaifenesin 600 mg. ER Tab. Bot. 100s. *Rx.*
Use: Upper respiratory combination, decongestant, expectorant.

GuaiMist DM. (Scientific Laboratories) Dextromethorphan hydrobromide 15 mg, guaifenesin 100 mg, pseudoephedrine hydrochloride 40 mg per 5 mL. Sugar, alcohol, and dye free. Syr. 473 mL. *Rx.*
Use: Antitussive and expectorant combination.

Guaipax PSE. (Eon) Pseudoephedrine hydrochloride 120 mg, guaifenesin 600 mg. SR Tab. Bot. 100s, 250s, 500s. *Rx.*
Use: Upper respiratory combination, decongestant, expectorant.

Guaiphotol. (Foy Laboratories) Iodine 1/30 g, calcium creosote 4 g. Tab. Bot. 1000s. *Rx.*
Use: Expectorant.

Guaitab. (Muro) Pseudoephedrine hydrochloride 60 mg, guaifenesin 400 mg, lactose. Tab. Bot. 100s. *OTC.*
Use: Decongestant; expectorant.

Guaitex PSE. (Rugby) Pseudoephedrine hydrochloride 120 mg, guaifenesin 500 mg. Tab. Bot. 100s. *Rx.*
Use: Decongestant, expectorant.

•**guaithylline.** (GWIE-thill-in) USAN.
Use: Bronchodilator; expectorant.

Guaivent. (Ethex) Guaifenesin 250 mg, pseudoephedrine hydrochloride 120 mg, parabens, EDTA, sucrose. Cap. Bot. 100s, 500s. *Rx.*
Use: Decongestant, expectorant.

Guaivent PD. (Ethex) **300:** Guaifenesin 300 mg, pseudoephedrine hydrochloride 60 mg, parabens, sucrose. Cap. Bot. 100s, 500s. **600:** Guaifenesin 600 mg, pseudoephedrine hydrochloride 60 mg, parabens, EDTA, sucrose. Cap. Bot. 100s, 500s. *Rx.*
Use: Decongestant, expectorant.

guamide.
See: Sulfaguanidine.

•**guanabenz.** (GWAHN-uh-benz) USAN.
Use: Antihypertensive.
See: Wytensin.

•**guanabenz acetate.** (GWAHN-uh-benz) USP 34.
Use: Antihypertensive.

guanabenz acetate. (Various Mfr.)
Guanabenz acetate 4 mg, 8 mg. Tab.
Bot. 30s, 100s, 500s.
Use: Antihypertensive.

•**guanacline sulfate.** (GWAHN-ah-kleen)
USAN.
Use: Antihypertensive.

•**guanadrel sulfate.** (GWAHN-uh-drell)
USP 34.
Use: Antihypertensive.

•**guancydine.** (GWAHN-sigh-deen)
USAN.
Use: Antihypertensive.

•**guanethidine sulfate.** (gwahn-ETH-ih-
deen) USAN.
Use: Antihypertensive.
See: Ismelin.
W/Hydrochlorothiazide.
See: Esimil.

•**guanfacine hydrochloride.** (GWAHN-
fay-seen) *USP 34.*
Tall Man: guanFACINE
Use: Antihypertensive.
See: Intuniv.
Tenex.

guanfacine hydrochloride. (Various
Mfr.) Guanfacine 1 mg, 2 mg. May contain lactose. Tab. 100s, 500s . *Rx.*
Use: Antiadrenergic/sympatholytic; antiadrenergic agent, centrally acting.

guanidine hydrochloride. (Key) Guani-
dine hydrochloride 125 mg. Mannitol.
Tab. Bot. 100s. *Rx.*
Use: Muscle stimulant.

•**guanisoquin sulfate.** (GWAHN-eye-so-
kwin) USAN.
Use: Antihypertensive.

•**guanoclor sulfate.** (GWAHN-oh-klahr)
USAN.
Use: Antihypertensive.

•**guanoctine hydrochloride.** (GWAHN-
ock-teen) USAN.
Use: Antihypertensive.

•**guanoxabenz.** (gwahn-OX-ah-benz)
USAN.
Use: Antihypertensive.

•**guanoxan sulfate.** (GWAHN-ox-an)
USAN.
Use: Antihypertensive.

•**guanoxyfen sulfate.** (GWAHN-OX-eh-
fen) USAN.
Use: Antihypertensive; antidepressant.

Guaphenyl LA. (River's Edge) Phenylephrine hydrochloride 30 mg (extended
release), guaifenesin 40 mg (immediate release). Sucrose. ER Cap. 100s.
Rx.
Use: Upper respiratory combination, decongestant and expectorant combination.

Guaphenyl II. (River's Edge) Phenylephrine hydrochloride 20 mg, guaifenesin 375 mg. Maltodextrin, sucrose.
Cap. 100s. *Rx.*
Use: Decongestant and expectorant
combination.

Guardal. (Morton Grove) Vitamins A
10,000 units, B_1 20 mg, B_2 8 mg, B_6
0.5 mg, B_{12} 8 mcg, C 50 mg, niacinamide 10 mg, calcium d-pantothenate
5 mg, iron 10 mg, dried whole liver
100 mg, yeast 100 mg, choline bitartrate 30 mg, mixed tocopherols 5 mg,
dicalcium phosphate anhydrous
150 mg, magnesium sulfate dried
7.2 mg, sodium 1 mg, potassium chloride 1.3 mg. Tab. Bot. 100s. *OTC.*
Use: Mineral, vitamin supplement.

Guardex. (Archer-Taylor) Tube 4 oz, 1 lb,
4.5 lb. *OTC.*
Use: Emollient.

•**guar gum.** *NF 29.*
Use: Pharmaceutic aid (tablet binder;
tablet disintegrant).
See: Benefiber.
W/Danthron, Docusate Sodium.
See: Guarsol.
W/Standardized Senna Concentrate.
See: Gentlax B.

guayanesin.
Use: Expectorant.
See: Guaifenesin.

Guiadrine DM. (Breckenridge Pharmaceutical) Dextromethorphan HBr
30 mg, guaifenesin 600 mg. SR Tab.
Bot. 100s, 250s. *Rx.*
Use: Upper respiratory combination, antitussive, expectorant.

Guiamid Expectorant. (Vangard Labs,
Inc.) Guaifenesin 100 mg/5 mL, alco-
hol 3.5%. Bot. Pt, gal. *OTC.*
Use: Expectorant.

Guiaphed. (Various Mfr.) Theophylline
45 mg, ephedrine sulfate 36 mg, guaifenesin 150 mg, phenobarbital 12 mg,
alcohol 19%/15 mL. Elix. Bot. 480 mL.
Rx.
Use: Antiasthmatic combination.

Guiatex PSE. (Rugby) Pseudoephedrine
hydrochloride, guaifenesin 500 mg. Tab.
Bot. 100s. *Rx.*
Use: Decongestant, expectorant.

Guiatuss. (Various Mfr.) Guaifenesin
100 mg/5 mL, may contain saccharin,
menthol, corn syr. Syr. Bot. 118 mL.
OTC.
Use: Expectorant.

Guiatuss AC. (Ivax) Codeine phosphate
10 mg, guaifenesin 100 mg per 5 mL.
Sugar free, alcohol 3.5%. Saccharin,
sorbitol, sodium 4 mg/5 mL. Syr. Bot.

118 mL, 473 mL. *c-v.*
Use: Upper respiratory combination, antitussive, expectorant.
Guiatuss DAC. (Various Mfr.) Pseudoephedrine hydrochloride 30 mg, codeine phosphate 10 mg, guaifenesin 100 mg per 5 mL. Alcohol 1.9%, menthol, saccharin, sodium 4 mg/5 mL, sorbitol. Syr. Bot. 473 mL. *c-v.*
Use: Upper respiratory combination, antitussive and expectorant combination.
Guiatuss-DM. (Ivax) Dextromethorphan HBr 10 mg, guaifenesin 100 mg per 5 mL. Alcohol free. Corn syr., menthol, saccharin. Syr. 473 mL, 3785 mL. *OTC.*
Use: Antitussive with expectorant, upper respiratory combination.
Guiatussin/Codeine Expectorant. (Rugby) Codeine phosphate 10 mg, guaifenesin 100 mg/5 mL, alcohol 3.5%. Syr. Bot. 120 mL, pt, gal. *c-v.*
Use: Antitussive, expectorant.
Guiatussin/Dextromethorphan. (Rugby) Dextromethorphan HBr 15 mg, guaifenesin 100 mg, alcohol 1.4%/5 mL. Liq. Bot. 480 mL. *OTC.*
Use: Antitussive, expectorant.
Guiatuss Syrup. (Various Mfr.) Guaifenesin 100 mg/5 mL. Syr. Bot. 120 mL, 240 mL, pt, gal. *OTC.*
Use: Expectorant.
Guistrey Fortis. (Jones Pharma) Guaifenesin 100 mg, phenylephrine hydrochloride 10 mg, chlorpheniramine maleate 1 mg. Tab. Bot. 1000s. *OTC.*
Use: Antihistamine, decongestant, expectorant.
Gulfasin. (Major) Sulfisoxazole 500 mg. Tab. Bot. 100s, 250s, 1000s.
Use: Anti-infective, sulfonamide.
guncotton, soluble. Pyroxylin.
gusperimus.
Use: Acute renal graft-rejection episodes.
•**gusperimus trihydrochloride.** (guss-PURR-ih-muss try-HIGH-droe-KLOR-ide) USAN.
Use: Immunosuppressant.
Gustalac. (Roberts) Calcium carbonate 300 mg, defatted skim milk pow. 200 mg. Tab. Bot. 100s, 250s, 1000s. *OTC.*
Use: Antacid; calcium supplement.
•**gutta percha.** (GUT-a-PER-cha) *USP 34.*
Use: Dental restoration agent.

G-vitamin.
See: Riboflavin.
Gynazole-1. (Ther-Rx) Butoconazole nitrate 2%, EDTA, parabens, mineral oil. Vag. Cream. Prefilled, single-dose applicator 5 g (1s). *Rx.*
Use: Antifungal, vaginal.
Gynecort 10, Extra Strength. (Combe) Hydrocortisone acetate 1%, parabens, zinc pyrithione. Cream. Tube 15 g. *OTC.*
Use: Corticosteroid, topical.
Gyne-Lotrimin 3. (Schering-Plough) Clotrimazole. **Vag. Supp.:** 200 mg. Pkg. 3s w/applicator. **Vag. Cream:** 2%, benzyl alcohol. Tube 21 g w/3 disp. applicators. *OTC.*
Use: Antifungal, vaginal.
Gyne-Lotrimin 3 Combination Pack. (Schering-Plough) **Vaginal Supp.:** Clotrimazole 200 mg, lactose. Pkg. 3s w/ applicator. **Topical Cream:** Clotrimazole 1%, benzyl alcohol, cetyl stearyl alcohol. Tube 7 g. *OTC.*
Use: Antifungal, vaginal.
gynergon.
See: Estradiol.
Gynodiol. (Fielding) Estradiol, micronized 0.5 mg, 1 mg, 1.5 mg, 2 mg, lactose. Tab. Bot. 30s, 100s. *Rx.*
Use: Estrogen, sex hormone.
Gynogen L.A. (Forest) **10:** Estradiol valerate in sesame oil 10 mg/mL. Vial 10 mL. **20:** Estradiol valerate in castor oil 20 mg/mL. Inj. Multi-dose Vial 10 mL. **40:** Estradiol valerate in castor oil 40 mg/mL. Inj. Vial 10 mL. *Rx.*
Use: Estrogen.
Gynol II Extra Strength Contraceptive. (Johnson & Johnson) Nonoxynol-9 3%. Jelly. 75 g, 114 g. *OTC.*
Use: Contraceptive, spermicide.
Gyno-Petraryl. (Janssen) Econazole nitrate. *Rx.*
Use: Antifungal, vaginal.
Gynovite Plus. (Optimox) Vitamins A 833 units, D 67 units, E 67 mg (as d-alpha tocopheryl acid succinate), B_1 1.7 mg, B_2 1.7 mg, B_3 3.3 mg, B_5 1.7 mg, B_6 3.3 mg, B_{12} 21 mcg, C 30 mg, calcium 83 mg, iron 3 mg, folic acid 0.07 mg, boron, betaine, biotin, Cr, Cu, hesperidin, I, inositol, Mg, Mn, PABA, pancreatin, rutin, Se, Zn 2.5 mg. Tab. Bot. 100s. *OTC.*
Use: Mineral, vitamin supplement.

H

Habitrol. (Basel Pharm.) Nicotine transdermal system. Dose absorbed in 24 hours. Patch 21 mg, 14 mg, 7 mg. Box 30 systems. *OTC.*
Use: Smoking deterrent, nicotine.

Haemophilus b conjugate vaccine.
Use: Agent for active immunization, bacterial vaccine.
See: ActHIB.
Hiberix.
Liquid PedvaxHIB.
W/DTP vaccine.
See: ActHIB/DTP.

Haemophilus b conjugate vaccine with hepatitis B vaccine.
Use: Agent for active immunization, bacterial vaccine.
See: Comvax.

Haemophilus influenzae type b conjugate vaccine (DTaP-HIB).
Use: Active immunization, toxoid.

Hair Booster Vitamin. (NBTY) Vitamin B_3 35 mg, B_5 100 mg, B_{12} 6 mcg, folic acid 0.4 mg, zinc 15 mg, Cu, iron 18 mg, I, Mn, choline bitartrate, inositol, PABA, protein. Tab. Bot. 60s. *OTC.*
Use: Mineral, vitamin supplement.

Halac Kit. (Acella) Halobetasol propionate 0.05%. Beeswax, petrolatum, propylene glycol. Kit. 50 g w/225 g of ammonium lactate lotion 12%. *Rx.*
Use: Anti-inflammatory agent, topical corticosteroid.

Halaven. (Eisai) Eribulin mesylate 0.5 mg/mL. Ethanol. Inj., Soln. Single-use vial. 2 mL. *Rx.*
Use: Antimitotic agent, halichondrin B analog.

•**halazone.** (HAL-ah-zone) *USP 34.*
Use: Disinfectant.

•**halcinonide.** (hal-SIN-oh-nide) *USP 34.*
Use: Corticosteroid, topical; anti-inflammatory.
See: Halog.

Halcion. (Upjohn) Triazolam 0.25 mg. Tab. 500s. *c-iv.*
Use: Sedative/hypnotic, nonbarbiturate.

Haldol. (McNeil) Haloperidol 5 mg (as lactate)/mL. Inj. Amp. 1 mL. *Rx.*
Use: Antipsychotic, phenylbutylpiperadine derivative.

Haldol Decanoate 100. (McNeil) Haloperidol 100 mg/mL (141.04 mg decanoate), sesame oil, benzyl alcohol 1.2%. Amp. 1 mL. *Rx.*
Use: Antipsychotic.

Haldrone. (Eli Lilly) Paramethasone acetate 1 mg, 2 mg. Tab. Bot. 100s. *Rx.*
Use: Corticosteroid.

Halercol. (Roberts) Vitamins A 5000 units, D 400 units, E 1.36 mg, B_1 1.5 mg, B_2 2 mg, B_3 20 mg, B_5 1 mg, B_6 0.1 mg, B_{12} 1 mcg, C 37.5 mg. Cap. Bot. 100s. *OTC.*
Use: Vitamin supplement.

Haley's M-O. (Bayer Consumer Care) Magnesium hydroxide ≈ 900 mg, mineral oil 3.75 mL/15 mL, saccharin (vanilla creme only). Regular or vanilla creme. Liq. Bot. 360 mL, 780 mL (vanilla creme only). *OTC.*
Use: Laxative.

HalfLytely. (Braintree) **DR Tab.:** Bisacodyl 5 mg. Lactose, sucrose, sugar. Enteric-coated. 4s. Kit. **Pow. for Oral Soln.:** PEG 3350 210 g, sodium chloride 5.6 g, sodium bicarbonate 2.86 g, potassium chloride 0.74 g. Lemon-lime flavor. Bot. 2 L. *Rx.*
Use: Bowel evacuant.

Halfort-T. (Halsey Drug) Vitamins C 300 mg, B_1 15 mg, B_2 10 mg, niacin 100 mg, B_6 5 mg, B_{12} 4 mcg, pantothenic acid 20 mg. Tab. Bot. 100s. *OTC.*
Use: Vitamin supplement.

Halfprin 81. (Kramer) Aspirin 81 mg. EC Tab. Bot. 90s. *OTC.*
Use: Analgesic.

Half Strength Entrition Entri-Pak. (Biosearch Medical Products) Protein 17.5 g (Na and Ca caseinates), carbohydrate 68 g (maltodextrin), fat 17.5 g (corn oil, soy lecithin, monoglycerides and diglycerides), sodium 350 mg, potassium 600 mg, mOsm/120 kg H_2O, calories 0.5/mL, vitamins A, B_1, B_2, B_3, B_5, B_6, B_{12}, C, D, E, K, P, Ca, Mg, I, Fe, Zn, Mn, Cu, Cl, biotin, choline, folic acid. Liq. Pouch 1 L. *OTC.*
Use: Nutritional supplement.

Half Strength Florvite with Iron. (Everett) Fluoride 0.5 mg, Vitamins A 2500 units, D 400 units, E 15 units, B_1 1.05 mg, B_2 1.2 mg, B_3 13.5 mg, B_6 1.05 mg, B_{12} 4.5 mcg, C 60 mg, folic acid 0.3 mg, Cu, iron 12 mg, Zn 10 mg, sucrose. Tab. Bot. 100s. *Rx.*
Use: Mineral, vitamin supplement; dental caries agent.

Half Strength Introlan. (Elan) Protein 22.5 g, fat 18 g, carbohydrates 70 g, Na 345 mg, K 585 mg/L. Vitamins A, C, B_1, B_2, B_3, B_5, B_6, B_{12}, D, E, K, Ca, Fe, folic acid, P, I, Mg, Zn, Cu, biotin, Mn, choline, Cl, Se, Cr, Mo. Liq. In 1,000 mL *New Pak* closed systems with and without color check. *OTC.*
Use: Nutritional supplement.

Half-Strength Lactated Ringer's in 2.5% Dextrose. (Various Mfr.) Dextrose

25 g/L, calories 85 to 89/L, Na$^+$
$\approx$ 65.5 mEq, K$^+$ 2 mEq, Ca^{++}
$\approx$ 1.5 mEq, Cl$^-$ $\approx$ 55 mEq, lactate
14 mEq/L, osmolarity $\approx$ 264 mOsm/L.
Soln. Bot. 250 mL, 500 mL, 1,000 mL.
Rx.
Use: Intravenous nutritional therapy,
intravenous replenishment solution.

Hali-Best. (Barth's) Vitamins A
10,000 units, D 400 units. Cap. Bot.
100s, 500s. *OTC.*
Use: Vitamin supplement.

halibut liver oil.
Use: Vitamin supplement.

halichondrin B analogs.
See: Eribulin Mesylate.

haliver oil.
See: Halibut Liver Oil.

**Hall's Mentho-Lyptus Cough Loz-
enges.** (Warner Lambert) Menthol and
eucalyptus oil in varying amounts and
flavors. *Stick-Pack* 9s. Bag 30s. *OTC.*
Use: Mouth and throat preparation.

Hall's Mentho-Lyptus Sugar Free.
(Warner Lambert) Menthol 5 mg, 6 mg,
eucalyptus oil 2.8 mg. Tab. Pkg. 25s.
OTC.
Use: Mouth and throat preparation.

Hall's-Plus Maximum Strength. (Warner
Lambert) Menthol 10 mg, corn syrup,
sugar. Cherry, honey-lemon, and regular flavors. Tab. Pkg. 10s, 25s. *OTC.*
Use: Mouth and throat preparation.

Hall's Zinc Defense. (Warner Lambert)
Zinc acetate 5 mg, sugar, cherry, or
peppermint flavor. Loz. 24s. *OTC.*
Use: Mineral supplement.

• **halobetasol propionate.** (hal-oh-BEH-
tah-sahl) USAN.
Use: Anti-inflammatory; corticosteroid,
topical.
See: Halac Kit.
Ultravate.
Ultravate PAC.

halobetasol propionate. (Various Mfr.)
Halobetasol propionate. **Cream:**
0.05%. May contain cetyl alcohol, glycerin, diazolidinyl urea. 15 g, 50 g.
Oint.: 0.05%. May contain petrolatum.
15 g, 50 g. *Rx.*
Use: Anti-inflammatory.

Halofed. (Halsey Drug) **Tab.:** Pseudoephedrine hydrochloride 30 mg, 60 mg.
Bot. 100s, 1000s. **Syr.:** Pseudoephedrine hydrochloride 30 mg/5 mL. Bot.
120 mL, 240 mL, pt, gal. *OTC.*
Use: Decongestant.

• **halofenate.** (HAY-low-FEN-ate) USAN.
Use: Antihyperlipoproteinemic; uricosuric.

• **halofuginone hydrobromide.** (HAY-low-
FOO-jin-ohn) USAN.
Use: Antiprotozoal.

Halog. (Ranbaxy) Halcinonide. **Cream:**
0.1%, in specially formulated cream
base consisting of glyceryl monostearate, cetyl alcohol, myristyl stearate, isopropyl palmitate, polysorbate 60, propylene glycol, purified water. Tube 15 g,
30 g, 60 g. Jar 240 g. **Oint.:** Halcinonide 0.1%, in *Plastibase* (plasicized hydrocarbon gel), PEG 400, PEG 6000
distearate, PEG 300, PEG 1540, butylated hydroxy toluene. Tube 15 g, 30 g,
60 g. Jar 240 g. **Sol.:** 0.1%, EDTA,
PEG 300, purified water, butylated hydroxy toluene as preservative. Bot.
20 mL, 60 mL. *Rx.*
Use: Corticosteroid, topical.

• **halopemide.** (hal-OH-pe-mide) USAN.
Use: Antipsychotic.

• **haloperidol.** (HAY-low-PURR-ih-dahl)
USP 34.
Use: Antipsychotic; tranquilizer; antidys-
kinetic (in Gilles de la Tourette dis-
ease).
See: Haldol.

haloperidol. (Various Mfr.) Haloperidol.
Tab.: 0.5 mg, 1 mg, 2 mg, 5 mg,
10 mg, 20 mg. Tab. Bot. 100s, 1000s
(except 0.5 mg and 20 mg), UD 100s
(except 20 mg). **Conc.:** 2 mg/mL. Bot.
15 mL, 120 mL, and 5 mL, UD 100s.
Inj.: 5 mg/mL. May contain parabens.
Vial 1 mL, 2 mL, 10 mL. *Rx.*
Use: Antipsychotic.

• **haloperidol decanoate.** (HAY-low-
PURR-ih-dahl deh-KAN-oh-ate) USAN.
Use: Antipsychotic.
See: Haldol Decanoate.

haloperidol decanoate. (Various Mfr.)
Haloperidol 50 mg/mL (70.5 mg decanoate), 100 mg/mL (141.04 mg decanoate), may contain sesame oil, benzyl alcohol 1.2%. Inj. Single-dose vial.
1 mL. Multidose vial. 5 mL. *Rx.*
Use: Antipsychotic.

• **halopredone acetate.** (HAY-low-PREH-
dohn) USAN.
Use: Anti-inflammatory, topical.

• **haloprogesterone.** (HAL-oh-pro-jeh-
STEE-rone) USAN.
Use: Hormone, progestin.

• **halothane.** (HAL-oh-thane) *USP 34.*
Use: General anesthetic, inhalation.

Halotussin. (Halsey Drug) Guaifenesin
100 mg/5 mL. Bot. 4 oz, 8 oz, pt, gal.
OTC.
Use: Expectorant.

• **halquinols.** (HAL-kwin-oles) USAN.
Use: Anti-infective, topical; antimicrobial.
HAMA. Hydroxyaluminum magnesium aminoacetate.
hamamelis water.
See: Witch Hazel.
Tucks.
• **hamycin.** (HAY-MY-sin) USAN.
Use: Antifungal.
Hang-Over-Cure. (Silvers) Calcium carbonate, glycine, thiamine hydrochloride, pyridoxine hydrochloride, aspirin. Cont. Tab. 6 g. *OTC.*
Use: Antacid; analgesic combination.
Haniform. (Hanlon) Vitamins A 25,000 units, D 1000 units, B_1 10 mg, B_2 5 mg, C 150 mg, niacinamide 150 mg. Cap. Bot. 100s. *OTC.*
Use: Vitamin supplement.
Haniplex. (Hanlon) Vitamins B_1 20 mg, B_2 10 mg, B_6 1 mg, B_{12} 5 mcg, calcium pantothenate 10 mg, niacin 20 mg, liver concentrate 50 mg, C 150 mg. Cap. Bot. 100s. *OTC.*
Use: Mineral, vitamin supplement.
Harbolin. (Arcum) Hydralazine hydrochloride 25 mg, hydrochlorothiazide 15 mg, reserpine 0.1 mg. Tab. Bot. 100s, 1000s. *Rx.*
Use: Antihypertensive combination.
hard fat.
Use: Pharmaceutic necessity.
hartshorn. Ammonium carbonate.
Haugase. (Madland) Trypsin, chymotrypsin. Bot. 50s, 250s.
Use: Enzyme preparation.
Havab. (Abbott Diagnostics) Radioimmunoassay or enzyme immunoassay for detection of antibody to hepatitis A virus. Test kit 100s.
Use: Diagnostic aid.
Havab EIA. (Abbott Diagnostics) Enzyme immunoassay for the detection of antibody to hepatitis A virus.
Use: Diagnostic aid.
Havab-M. (Abbott Diagnostics) Radioimmunoassay for the detection of specific Ig antibody to hepatitis A virus. Test kit 100s.
Use: Diagnostic aid.
Havab-M EIA. (Abbott Diagnostics) Enzyme immunoassay for the detection of Ig antibody to hepatitis A virus.
Use: Diagnostic aid.
Havrix. (GlaxoSmithKline) Hepatitis A vaccine, inactivated. **Adult:** 1440 ELU (ELISA [enzyme-linked immunosorbent assay] units) of viral antigen per mL. Inj. Single-dose vial; prefilled syringe.
Pediatric: 720 ELU of viral antigen per

0.5 mL. Inj. Single-dose vial; prefilled syringe. *Rx.*
Use: Immunization, viral vaccine.
Hawaiian Tropic Aloe Paba Sunscreen. (Tanning Research Labs) Padimate O, oxybenzone. Cream. Bot. 120 g. *OTC.*
Use: Sunscreen.
Hawaiian Tropic Baby Faces. (Tanning Research Labs) SPF 20. Octyl methoxycinnamate, octocrylene, benzophenone-3, menthyl anthranilate, PABA free, waterproof. Gel. Tube 120 g. *OTC.*
Use: Sunscreen.
Hawaiian Tropic Baby Faces Sunblock. (Tanning Research Labs) Octyl methoxycinnamate, benzophenone-3, octyl salicylate, titanium dioxide, octocrylene, PABA free, waterproof. **SPF 35:** Lot. Bot. 60 mL, 120 mL, 300 mL. **SPF 50:** Lot. Bot. 120 mL. *OTC.*
Use: Sunscreen.
Hawaiian Tropic Cool Aloe with I.C.E. (Tanning Research Labs) Lidocaine, menthol, aloe, SD alcohol 40, diazolidinyl urea, EDTA, vitamins A and E, tartrazine. Gel. Jar 360 g. *OTC.*
Use: Emollient.
Hawaiian Tropic Dark Tanning. (Tanning Research Labs) **Gel:** Phenylbenzimidazole sulfonic acid. SPF 2. Bot. 240 mL. **Oil:** 2-ethylhexyl methoxycinnamate, octyl dimethyl, PABA, waterproof. Bot. 240 mL. *OTC.*
Use: Sunscreen.
Hawaiian Tropic Dark Tanning with Sunscreen. (Tanning Research Labs) **Oil:** Ethylhexyl p-methoxycinnamate, octyl dimethyl, PABA, waterproof. SPF 4. Bot. 240 mL. **Gel:** Phenylbenzimidazole, sulfonic acid. PABA free. SPF 4. Tube 240 g. *OTC.*
Use: Sunscreen.
Hawaiian Tropic 8 Plus. (Tanning Research Labs) Octyl methoxycinnamate, benzophenone-3, menthyl anthranilate, PABA free, waterproof. SPF 8+. Gel. Tube 120 g. *OTC.*
Use: Sunscreen.
Hawaiian Tropic 15 Plus. (Tanning Research Labs) Octyl methoxycinnamate, octocrylene, benzophenone-3, menthyl anthranilate, PABA free, waterproof. Gel. Tube 120 g. *OTC.*
Use: Sunscreen.
Hawaiian Tropic 15 Plus Sunblock. (Tanning Research Labs) Menthyl anthranilate, octyl methoxycinnamate, benzophenone-3, PABA free, waterproof. Lot. Bot. 7.5 mL, 15 mL, 60 mL, 120 mL, 240 mL, 300 mL. *OTC.*
Use: Sunscreen.

Hawaiian Tropic 15 Plus Sunblock Lip Balm. (Tanning Research Labs) Padimate O, oxybenzone. SPF 15, waterproof. Stick 4.2 g. *OTC.*
Use: Sunscreen.

Hawaiian Tropic 45 Plus Sunblock Lip Balm. (Tanning Research Labs) Octyl methoxycinnamate, benzophenone-3, octyl salicylate, titanium dioxide, menthyl anthranilate, PABA free, waterproof. SPF 45+. Lip balm 4.2 g. *OTC.*
Use: Sunscreen.

Hawaiian Tropic Just for Kids Sunblock. (Tanning Research Labs) **SPF 30:** Homosalate, octyl methoxycinnamate, benzophenone-3, menthyl anthranilate, octyl salicylate, PABA free, waterproof. Lot. Bot. 88.7 mL. **SPF 45:** Octyl methoxycinnamate, benzophenone-3, octyl salicylate, octocrylene, titanium dioxide, PABA free, waterproof. Lot. Bot. 88.7 mL. *OTC.*
Use: Sunscreen.

Hawaiian Tropic Lip Balm Sunblock. (Tanning Research Labs) Padimate O, oxybenzone. Stick 4 g. *OTC.*
Use: Sunscreen.

Hawaiian Tropic Protective Tanning. (Tanning Research Labs) Titanium dioxide, PABA free, waterproof. SPF 6. Lot. Bot. 240 mL. *OTC.*
Use: Sunscreen.

Hawaiian Tropic Protective Tanning Dry. (Tanning Research Labs) SPF 6. **Oil:** 2-ethylhexyl p-methoxycinnamate, homosalate, menthyl anthranilate, waterproof. Bot. 180 mL. **Gel:** Phenylbenzimidazole, sulfonic acid, benzophenone-4. Tube 180 g. *OTC.*
Use: Sunscreen.

Hawaiian Tropic Self Tanning Sunblock. (Tanning Research Labs) Octyl methoxycinnamate, benzophenone-3, aloe, cetyl alcohol, stearyl alcohol, cocoa butter, parabens, vitamin E, PABA free. SPF 15. Cream. Tube 93.75 mL. *OTC.*
Use: Sunscreen.

Hawaiian Tropic Sport Sunblock. (Tanning Research Labs) SPF 15, SPF 30. Methoxycinnamate, octocrylene, benzophenone-3, octyl salicylate, titanium dioxide, PABA free, waterproof. Lot. Bot. 88.7 mL. *OTC.*
Use: Sunscreen.

Hawaiian Tropic Sunblock. (Tanning Research Labs) Titanium dioxide, octyl methoxycinnamate, benzophenone-3, octyl salicylate, octocrylene, PABA free, waterproof. **SPF 30+:** Lot. Bot. 120 mL. **SPF 45+:** Lot. Bot. 120 mL, 300 mL. *OTC.*
Use: Sunscreen.

Hawaiian Tropic Swim 'n' Sun. (Tanning Research Labs) Padimate O, oxybenzone. Lot. Bot. 120 mL. *OTC.*
Use: Sunscreen.

Hawaiian Tropic 10 Plus. (Tanning Research Labs) Octyl methoxycinnamate, benzophenone-3, menthyl anthranilate, PABA free, waterproof. SPF 10+. Gel. Tube 120 g. *OTC.*
Use: Sunscreen.

•**hawthorne leaf with flower.** (HAWthorn) *NF 29.*
Use: Dietary supplement.

Hayfebrol Liquid. (Scot-Tussin) Pseudoephedrine hydrochloride 30 mg, chlorpheniramine 2 mg. Syr. Bot. 118 mL. *OTC.*
Use: Antihistamine; decongestant.

1% HC. (C & M Pharmacal) Hydrocortisone 1%, petrolatum base. Oint. Tube 15, 20, 30, 60, 120, 240 g, lb. *OTC.*
Use: Corticosteroid, topical.

HC Derma-Pax. (Recsei) Hydrocortisone 0.5% in liquid base. Dropper Bot. 2 oz. *OTC.*
Use: Corticosteroid, topical.

HCG.
See: Chorionic Gonadotropin.

HCG-Nostick. (Organon Teknika) Sol Particle Immunoassay (SPIA) for detection of hCG in urine. Stick 30s.
Use: Diagnostic aid, pregnancy.

HC Pram 1%. (River's Edge) Hydrocortisone acetate 1%, pramoxine hydrochloride 1%. Cetearyl alcohol, glycerin, phenoxyethanol, safflower seed oil, stearyl alcohol, tetrasodium EDTA. Cream. 30 g. *Rx.*
Use: Anti-inflammatory agent, topical corticosteroid.

HC Pram 2.5%. (River's Edge) Hydrocortisone acetate 2.5%, pramoxine hydrochloride 1%. Cetearyl alcohol, glycerin, phenoxyethanol, safflower seed oil, stearyl alcohol, tetrasodium EDTA. Cream. 4 g (UD 12s and UD 30s), 30 g. *Rx.*
Use: Anti-inflammatory agent, topical corticosteroid.

HC Pramoxine. (Veracity) Hydrocortisone acetate 2.5%, pramoxine hydrochloride 1%. Cetyl alcohol. Cream. 28 g. *Rx.*
Use: Anorectal preparations.

HD 85. (Mallinckrodt) Barium sulfate 85%. Simethicone, saccharin, Raspberry flavor. Susp. Kits. 150 mL, 450 mL. Bot. 1900 mL. *Rx.*
Use: Radiopaque agent, GI contrast agent.

HD 200 Plus. (Mallinckrodt) Barium sulfate 98%. Simethicone, sorbitol, sucrose. Strawberry flavor. Pow. for Susp. UD 312 g. *Rx.*
Use: Radiopaque agent, GI contrast agent.

Head & Shoulders. (Procter & Gamble) Pyrithione zinc 1%. **Cream:** Tube 51 g, 75 g, 120 g, 210 g. **Lot.:** Bot. 120 mL, 210 mL, 330 mL, 450 mL. **Shampoo:** Cetyl and benzyl alcohol. Normal to oily and normal to dry formulas. 200 mL, 400 mL, 750 mL. *OTC.*
Use: Dermatologic agent.

Head & Shoulders Conditioner. (Procter & Gamble) Pyrithione zinc 0.3%. Bot. 4 oz, 11 oz. *OTC.*
Use: Antiseborrheic.

Head & Shoulders Dry Scalp. (Procter & Gamble) Pyrithione zinc 1%. Cetyl and benzyl alcohol, regular and conditioning formulas. Shampoo. Bot. 200 mL, 400 mL, 750 mL, 1000 mL. *OTC.*
Use: Dermatologic agent.

Head & Shoulders Intensive Treatment. (Procter & Gamble) Selenium sulfide 1%. Lotion/Shampoo. Bot. 400 mL. *OTC.*
Use: Antiseborrheic.

Healon. (Abbott) Sodium hyaluronate 10 mg/mL. Inj. Syringe 0.4 mL, 0.55 mL, 0.85 mL, 2 mL. *Rx.*
Use: Surgical aid, ophthalmic.

Healon5. (Advanced Medical Optics) Sodium hyaluronate 23 mg/mL. Sodium chloride 8.5 mg/mL. Inj. Disposable syringe. 0.6 mL. *Rx.*
Use: Ophthalmic surgical adjunct.

Healon GV. (Abbott) Sodium hyaluronate 14 mg/mL. Inj. Syringe 0.55 mL, 0.85 mL. *Rx.*
Use: Surgical aid, ophthalmic.

Healthbreak. (Lemar Labs) Silver acetate 6 mg. Chewing gum. Pack 24s. *OTC.*
Use: Smoking deterrent.

Heartburn Antacid. (Walgreen) Aluminum hydroxide dried gel 80 mg, magnesium trisilicate 60 mg. Tab. Bot. 100s. *OTC.*
Use: Antacid.

Heartline. (BDI) Aspirin 81 mg. EC Tab. Bot. 36s. *OTC.*
Use: Anti-inflammatory.

Heather. (Glenmark Generics) Norethindrone 0.35 mg. Lactose. Tab. 28s. *Rx.*
Use: Oral contraceptive, progestin.

heavy metal poisoning, antidote.
See: BAL.
Calcium Disodium Versenate.

Hectorol. (Genzyme) Doxercalciferol. **Cap.:** 0.5 mcg, 1 mcg, 2.5 mcg. Ethanol (1 mcg and 2.5 mcg only). Peach flavor (1 mcg). Bot. 50s. **Inj.:** 2 mcg/mL. 100% ethanol 0.05 mL, disodium edetate 1.1 mg, sodium chloride 1.5 mg, sodium phosphate dibasic, sodium phosphate monobasic. Amps. 2 mL. *Rx.*
Use: Hyperparathyroidism.

Heet Liniment. (Whitehall-Robins Laboratories) Methyl salicylate 15%, camphor 3.6%, oleoresin capsicum 0.025%, alcohol 70%. Bot. 2⅓ oz, 5 oz. *OTC.*
Use: Analgesic-topical.

•**hefilcon A.** (heh-FILL-kahn A) USAN.
Use: Contact lens material (hydrophilic).

•**hefilcon B.** (heh-FILL-kahn B) USAN.
Use: Contact lens material (hydrophilic).

•**hefilcon C.** (heh-FILL-kahn C) USAN.
Use: Contact lens material (hydrophilic).

Helidac. (Promethus) **Chew Tab.:** Bismuth subsalicylate 262.4 mg. **Tab.:** Metronidazole 250 mg. **Cap.:** Tetracycline 500 mg.14 blister cards of 4s (Cap. and Tab. only), 8s (Chew. Tab. only). *Rx.*
Use: Antiulcerative.

Helistat. (Hoechst) Absorbable collagen hemostatic sponge. 1" × 2" and 3" × 4" in 10s, 9" × 10" in 5s. *Rx.*
Use: Hemostatic.

•**helium.** (HEE-lee-uhm) *USP 34.*
Use: Diluent for gases.

Helixate. (Aventis) Concentrated recombinant hemophilic factor. After reconstitution, also contains glycine 10 to 30 mg, imidazole ≤ 500 mcg/ 1000 units, polysorbate 80 H 600 mcg/ 1000 units, Calcium Cl 2 to 5 mM, sodium 100 to 130 mEq/L, chloride 100 to 130 mEq/L, albumin (human) 4 to 10 mg/mL. units 250, 500, 1000. *Rx.*
Use: Antihemophilic.

Helixate FS. (CSL Behring) Recombinant antihemophilic factor 250 units, 500 units, 1,000 units, 2,000 units. Glycine, histidine, sodium, sucrose. Preservative free and albumin free. Solvent/detergent treated. Inj., lyophilized Pow. for Soln. Single-dose Bot. and diluent (2.5 mL sterile water for injection). *Rx.*
Use: Antihemophilic agent.

Hemabate. (Pharmacia) Carboprost tromethamine equivalent to 250 mcg carboprost, tromethamine 83 mcg/mL. Inj. Amp. 1 mL. *Rx.*
Use: Abortifacient.

Hema-Chek Slides. (Bayer Consumer Care) Fecal occult blood test containing slide tests, developer, and applicators. Pkg. 100s, 300s, 1000s.
Use: Diagnostic aid.

Hema-Combistix Reagent Strips. (Seimans Medical) Four-way strip test for urinary pH, glucose, protein, and occult blood. Strip. Bot. 100s.
Use: Diagnostic aid.

Hemaferrin. (Western Research) Ferrous fumarate 150 mg, desiccated liver 50 mg, docusate sodium 25 mg, betaine hydrochloride 100 mg, folic acid 0.4 mg, vitamins C 50 mg, B_6 2 mg, B_{12} 5 mcg, Mn 2 mg, Cu 1 mg, Zn 2 mg, Mo 0.4 mg. Tab. 28s. Pack 1000s. *OTC.*
Use: Mineral, vitamin supplement; stool softener.

Hemafolate. (Canright) Ferrous gluconate 293 mg, liver fraction II 250 mg, gastric substance 100 mg, vitamins C 50 mg, B_{12} 10 mcg. Tab. Bot. 100s, 1000s. *OTC.*
Use: Mineral, vitamin supplement.

Hemalive. (Barth's) **Liq.:** Vitamins B_1 3.15 mg, B_2 3.33 mg, B_6 0.81 mg, B_{12} 6 mcg, biotin 3.6 mcg, iron 60 mg, choline, inositol, liver fraction No. 1, niacin 22.5 mg, pantothenic acid/15 mL. Bot. 8 oz, 24 oz. **Tab.:** Vitamins B_1 2.5 mg, B_2 5 mg, B_6, B_{12} 25 mcg, iron 75 mg, niacin 1.4 mg, C 30 mg, liver 240 mg, pantothenic acid, aminobenzoic acid, choline, inositol, biotin, Mg, Mn, Cu. Tab. Bot. 100s, 500s, 1000s. *OTC.*
Use: Mineral, vitamin supplement.

Hemaneed. (Hanlon) Hematinic B_{12}, intrinsic factor, Fe. Cap. Bot. 100s. *OTC.*
Use: Mineral, vitamin supplement.

Hemastix Reagent Strips. (Bayer Consumer Care) Cellulose strip, impregnated with a peroxide and orthotolidine for detection of hematuria and hemoglobinuria. Strip Bot. 50s.
Use: Diagnostic aid.

Hematest Reagent Tablets. (Bayer Consumer Care) Reagent Tab. for blood in the feces. Bot. 100s.
Use: Diagnostic aid.

hematin.
Use: Porphyria.
See: Panhematin.

Hematinic. (Cypress) Ferrous fumarate 106 mg, folic acid 1 mg. Tab. Bot. 100s. *Rx.*
Use: Mineral, vitamin supplement.

Hematinic Plus. (Cypress) Ferrous fumarate 106 mg, vitamin B_1 10 mg, B_2 6 mg, B_3 30 mg, B_6 5 mg, B_{12} 15 mcg, C 200 mg, folic acid 1 mg, pantothenic acid, Cu, Mg, Mn, Zn 18.2 mg. Tab. 100s. *Rx.*
Use: Mineral, vitamin supplement.

hematinics.
See: Iron Products.
  Ferric Compounds.
  Ferrous Compounds.
  Liver Products.
  Vitamin B_{12}.
  Vitamin Products.

hematological agents.
See: Antihemophilic Combinations.
  Hemostatics, Systemic.
  Hemostatics, Topical.
  Kallikrein Inhibitors.
  Protein C1 Inhibitors.

hematopoietic agents.
See: Colony Stimulating Factors.
  Interleukins.
  Methoxy Polyethylene Glycol-Epoetin Beta.
  Recombinant Human Erythropoietin.
  Stem Cell Mobilizers.
  Thrombopoietin Receptor Agonists.

Hematrin. (Towne) Iron 50 mg, vitamins B_1 10 mg, B_2 10 mg, B_6 2 mg, B_{12} 10 mcg, C 150 mg, copper 2 mg, niacinamide 50 mg, calcium pantothenate 5 mg, desiccated liver 200 mg. Captab. Bot. 60s, 100s. *OTC.*
Use: Mineral, vitamin supplement.

heme arginate.
Use: Acute porphyria; myelodysplastic syndromes. [Orphan Drug]

HemeSelect. (SmithKline Diagnostics) Occult blood screening test. Box 40 test kits.
Use: Diagnostic aid, fecal.

Hemex. Hemin and zinc mesoporphyrin.
Use: Acute porphyric syndromes. [Orphan Drug]

Hemex. (Vogarell) Oint. Tube 1.25 oz. Supp. Box 12s.
Use: Anorectal preparation.

Hemiacidrin. Citric acid, glucono-delta-lactone, magnesium carbonate.
Use: Genitourinary irrigant.
See: Renacidin.

hemin.
Use: Acute intermittent porphyria. [Orphan Drug]
See: Panhematin.

hemin and zinc mesoporphyrin.
Use: Acute porphyric syndromes. [Orphan Drug]
See: Hemex.

hemisine.
See: Epinephrine.

Hemoccult SENSA. (SmithKline Diagnostics) Occult blood screening tests.
Use: Diagnostic aid, fecal.

Hemoccult Slides. (SmithKline Diagnostics) Occult blood detection (fecal). In 100s, 1000s, and tape dispensers (test 100s).
Use: Diagnostic aid.

Hemoccult II. (SmithKline Diagnostics) Occult blood detection (fecal). In 102s, kit 100s.
Use: Diagnostic aid.

Hemocitrate. (Hemotec Medical Products) Trisodium citrate concentrate.
Use: Leukapheresis procedures.
   [Orphan Drug]

Hemocyte. (US Pharmaceutical Corp.) Ferrous fumarate 324 mg (iron 106 mg). Tab. Bot. 30s, 100s. *OTC.*
Use: Mineral supplement.

Hemocyte-F. (US Pharmaceutical Corp.) **Elix.:** Fe (as polysaccharide-iron complex) 100 mg, B_{12} 25 mcg, folic acid 1 mg/5 mL, alcohol 10%, parabens, saccharin, sorbitol, sherry wine flavor. 473 mL. **Tab.:** Iron 106 mg (from ferrous fumarate), folic acid 1 mg. 100s. *Rx.*
Use: Mineral supplement.

Hemocyte Plus. (US Pharmaceutical Corp.) Iron 106 mg (from ferrous fumarate), sodium ascorbate 200 mg, vitamins B_1 10 mg, B_2 6 mg, B_3 30 mg, B_5 10 mg, B_6 5 mg, B_{12} 15 mcg, folic acid 1 mg, zinc 18.2 mg, Mg, Mn sulfate, Cu. Tab. Bot. 100s. *Rx.*
Use: Mineral, vitamin supplement.

Hemocyte Plus Elixir. (US Pharmaceutical Corp.) Polysaccharide iron complex 12 mg, vitamin B_3 13.3 mg, B_5 3.3 mg, B_6 1.3 mg, B_{12} 4 mcg, folic acid 0.33 mg, zinc 5 mg, Mn 1.3 mg/15 mL. Bot. 473 mL. *Rx.*
Use: Mineral, vitamin supplement.

Hemofil M. (Baxter) Preparation of human antihemophilic factor in concentrated form. When reconstituted, contains human albumin ≤ 12.5 mg/mL, PEG 3350 0.07 mg/mL, histidine 0.39 mg, glycine 0.1 mg, mouse protein ≤ 1 ng. Tri-n-butyl-phosphate 18 ng. Solvent/detergent-treated. Monoclonal purified. Inj. Single-dose bot. w/diluent, double-ended needle, filter needle. Actual number of antihemophilic factor units indicated on vials. *Rx.*
Use: Antihemophilic agent.

Hemofil T. (Baxter PPI) Antihemophilic factor (human), method four, dried, heat-treated 225 to 375 units/10 mL; 450 to 650 units/20 mL; 675 to 999 units/30 mL; 1000 to 1600 units/30 mL. *Rx.*
Use: Antihemophilic.

• **hemoglobin crosfumaril.** (HEE-moe-GLOBE-in CROSS-FEW-mah-ril) USAN.
Use: Red cell substitute; treatment of prefusion deficit disorders.

• **hemoglobin raffimer.** (HEE-moe-GLOBE-in RAF-fi-mer) USAN.
Use: Blood substitute.

Hemoglobin Reagent Strips. (Bayer Consumer Care) Seralyzer reagent strips. Bot. 50s. Quantitive strip test for hemoglobin in whole blood.
Use: Diagnostic aid.

Hemopad. (AstraZeneca) Fibrous absorbable collagen hemostat. 2.5 cm × 5 cm, 5 cm × 8 cm, 8 cm × 10 cm. *Rx.*
Use: Hemostatic.

Hemorid for Women. (Thompson Medical) **Lotion:** Mineral oil, petrolatum, diazolidinyl urea, cetyl alcohol, glycerin, parabens. Bot. 118 mL. **Cream:** White petrolatum 30%, mineral oil 20%, pramoxine hydrochloride 1%, phenylephrine hydrochloride 0.25%, aloe vera gel, parabens, cetyl and stearyl alcohols. Tube 28.3 g. **Supp.:** Zinc oxide 11%, phenylephrine hydrochloride 0.25%, hard fat 88.25%, aloe vera. Box 12s. *OTC.*
Use: Perianal hygiene.

hemorrheologic agent.
See: Pentoxifylline.

Hemorrhoidal HC. (Various Mfr.) Hydrocortisone acetate 25 mg. Supp. Box 12s, 24s, 50s, 100s, UD 12s. *Rx.*
Use: Anorectal preparation.

Hemorrhoidal Ointment. (Ivax) Live yeast cell derivative supplying skin respiratory factor 2000 units/oz of ointment w/shark liver oil 3%, phenyl mercuric nitrate 1:10,000. *OTC.*
Use: Anorectal preparation.

Hemorrhoidal Suppositories. (Ivax) Bismuth subgallate 2.25%, bismuth resorcin compound 1.75%, benzyl benzoate 1.2%, balsam Peru 1.8%, zinc oxide 11%. Supp. Box 12s. *OTC.*
Use: Anorectal preparation.

Hemorrhoidal Uniserts. (Upsher-Smith) Bismuth subgallate 2.25%, bismuth resorcin compound 1.75%, benzyl benzoate 1.2%, balsam Peru 1.8%, zinc oxide 11%. Supp. Carton 12s, 50s. *OTC.*
Use: Anorectal preparation.

hemostatics, local.
See: Absorbable Gelatin Sponge.
   Gelfilm.
   Helistat.
   Oxidized Cellulose.
   Thrombin.

hemostatics, systemic.
See: Amicar.
Aminocaproic Acid.
Fibrinogen Concentrate (Human).
Tranexamic Acid.
hemostatics, topical. Thrombin.
See: Fibrinogen Sealant (Human).
Thrombin.
Thrombinar.
Thrombostat.
hemostatin.
See: Epinephrine.
Hemovit. (Dayton) Vitamin B₁ 1.5 mg, B₂
1.7 mg, B₃ 20 mg, B₅ 10 mg, B₆ 10 mg,
B₁₂ 6 mcg, C 60 mg, folic acid 1 mg, d-
biotin 300 mcg, dye free. Tab. Blister
100s. *Rx.*
Use: Nutritional product.
Hemozyme Elixir. (Barrows) Vitamins B₁
5 mg, B₂ 5 mg, B₆ 1 mg, panthenol
4 mg, niacinamide 100 mg, B₁₂ 3 mcg,
iron 100 mg, choline bitartrate 100 mg,
dl-methionine 100 mg, yeast extract,
alcohol 12%/fl oz. Bot. 12 oz. *OTC.*
Use: Mineral, vitamin supplement.
Hem-Prep. (G & W) Phenylephrine
hydrochloride 0.25%, zinc oxide 11%.
Supp. Bot. 12s. *OTC.*
Use: Anorectal preparation.
Hem-Prep Ointment. (G & W) Phenylephrine hydrochloride 0.025%, zinc oxide 11%, white petrolatum. Oint.
42.5 g. *OTC.*
Use: Anorectal preparation.
Hemril-HC Uniserts. (Upsher-Smith)
Hydrocortisone acetate 25 mg. Supp.
12s. *Rx.*
Use: Anorectal preparation.
Hemril Uniserts. (Upsher-Smith) Bis-
muth subgallate 2.25%, bismuth resor-
cin compound 1.75%, benzyl benzo-
ate 1.2%, balsam Peru 1.8%, zinc ox-
ide 11%. Supp. Box 12s, 50s. *OTC.*
Use: Anorectal preparation.
henbane.
See: Hyoscyamus.
Henydin-M. (Arcum) Thyroid desiccated
pow. 0.5 g, vitamins B₁ 1 mg, B₂
0.5 mg, B₆ 0.5 mg, niacinamide 2.5 mg.
Tab. Bot. 100s, 1000s. *Rx.*
Use: Vitamin supplement.
Henydin-R. (Arcum) Thyroid desiccated
pow. 1 g, vitamins B₁ 2 mg, B₂ 1 mg,
B₆ 1 mg, niacinamide 5 mg. Tab. Bot.
100s, 1000s. *Rx.*
Use: Vitamin supplement.
HepaGam B. (Cangene Biopharma)
Hepatitis B immune globulin. Protein
5% (50 mg/mL). Solvent/detergent
treated. Maltose 10%, polysorbate 80
0.03%. Preservative free. Soln. for Inj.

Single-dose vials. 1 mL, 5 mL. *Rx.*
Use: Immune globulin.
heparin.
Use: Anticoagulant.
See: Heparin Sodium and Sodium
Chloride.
Heparin Sodium Injection.
Heparin Sodium Lock Flush Solution.
heparin antagonist.
Use: Coagulant.
See: Protamine Sulfate.
•**heparin calcium.** (HEP-uh-rin) *USP 34.*
Use: Anticoagulant.
heparin I.V. flush syringe. (Medefil)
Heparin sodium 1 unit/mL. Inj. Syringe
1 mL, 2 mL, 2.5 mL, 5 mL, 10 mL. *Rx.*
Use: Anticoagulant.
heparin lock flush solution. (Sanofi-
Synthelabo) **10 USP units/1 mL:** Cartridge 2 mL *HEP-PAK* containing 1 cartridge heparin lock flush soln. (1 mL)
and 2 cartridges sodium Cl Inj. *HEP-
PAK-2* containing 1 cartridge heparin
lock flush soln. (1 mL) and 1 cartridge
sodium Cl Inj. **10 USP units/2 mL:**
Cartridge 2 mL. **100 USP units/1 mL:**
Cartridge 2 mL *HEP-PAK* containing
1 cartridge heparin lock flush soln.
(1 mL) and 2 cartridges sodium Cl Inj.
HEP-PAK-2 containing 1 cartridge of
heparin lock flush soln. (1 mL) and
1 cartridge sodium Cl Inj. **100 USP
units/2 mL:** Cartridge 2 mL. *Rx.*
Use: Catheter patency agent.
heparin lock flush solution. (Wyeth)
Heparin sodium 10 units/mL, 100 units/
mL vial. Pkg. 50 *Tubex* 1 mL, 2 mL.
Rx.
Use: Infusion set patency agent.
•**heparin sodium.** (HEP-uh-rin) *USP 34.*
Use: Anticoagulant. Note: Protamine
sulfate is antidote.
See: Hepathrom.
Hepflush-10.
Heprinar.
Lipo-Hepin.
Lipo-Hepin/BL.
Liquaemin.
heparin sodium. (Hospira) Heparin sodium 2000 units/mL, 2500 units/mL. Inj.
Vials. 5 mL, 10 mL. *Rx.*
Use: Anticoagulant.
heparin sodium. (Pharmacia) Heparin
sodium 1000 units/mL. Vial 10 mL,
30 mL. 5000 units/mL. Vial 1 mL,
10 mL. 10,000 units/mL. Vial 1 mL,
4 mL. (Sanofi Winthrop Pharmaceuticals) 5000 USP units/1 mL. *Carpuject*
1 mL fill in 2 mL cartridge.
Use: Anticoagulant. Note: Protamine
sulfate is antidote.

HERPECIN-L 421

heparin sodium and 0.45% sodium chloride. (Abbott) Heparin sodium 12,500, 25,000 units in 250 mL Inj. *Rx.*
Use: Anticoagulant.

heparin sodium and 0.9% sodium chloride. (Baxter PPI) Heparin sodium 1000 units in 500 mL *Viaflex.* 2000 units in 1000 mL *Viaflex.* Inj. *Rx.*
Use: Anticoagulant.

heparin sodium in 5% dextrose injection. (Hospira) Heparin sodium 40 units in 5% dextrose injection per mL, 50 units in 5% dextrose injection per mL. Sodium 17 mEq. Inj. Single-dose containers. 500 mL. *Rx.*
Use: Anticoagulants.

heparin sodium lock flush solution. *Rx.*
Use: Anticoagulant.
See: Heparin Lock Flush.
Hepflush-10.
Hep-Lock.
Hep-Lock U/P.

heparin, 2-0-desulfated.
Use: Cystic fibrosis. [Orphan Drug]
See: Aeropin.

HepatAmine. (McGaw) Amino acid 8%. Inj. Bot. 500 mL. *Rx.*
Use: Nutritional supplement, parenteral.

hepatitis A, inactivated and hepatitis B, recombinant vaccine.
Use: Active immunization, viral vaccine.
See: Twinrix.

hepatitis A vaccine, inactivated. *Rx.*
Use: Immunization, active.
See: Havrix.
Vaqta.

hepatitis B and Haemophilus type b vaccine, combined.
See: Comvax.

•**hepatitis B immune globulin.** (hep-uh-TIGHT-iss B ih-myoon GLAH-byoo-lin)
USP 34.
Use: Immunization.
See: H-BIG.
HepaGam B.
HyperHEP B S/D.
Nabi-HB.

hepatitis B immune globulin intravenous (human).
Use: Prophylaxis against hepatitis B virus reinfection in liver transplant patients. [Orphan Drug]
See: H-BIGIV.

hepatitis B vaccine, recombinant.
Use: Immunization.
See: Engerix-B.
Recombivax HB.

hepatitis B vaccine (recombinant) and inactivated poliovirus vaccine combined, diphtheria and tetanus tox-

oids and acellular pertussis adsorbed.
Use: Active immunization, toxoid.
See: Diphtheria and tetanus toxoids and acellular vaccine adsorbed and hepatitis B vaccine (recombinant) and inactivated poliovirus vaccine combined.

•**hepatitis B virus vaccine inactivated.** (hep-uh-TIGHT-iss B vak-SEEN)
USP 34.
Use: Immunization.

Hepflush-10. (American Pharmaceutical Partners) Heparin sodium 10 units/mL, preservative free. Inj. Single-dose vial 10 mL. *Rx.*
Use: Catheter patency agent.

Hepfomin R Injection. (Keene Pharmaceuticals) Liver inj. equivalent to cyanocobalamin 10 mcg, folic acid 0.4 mg, cyanocobalamin 100 mcg. Vial 10 mL. *Rx.*
Use: Nutritional supplement, parenteral.

Hep-Forte. (Marlyn Nutraceuticals) Vitamins A 1200 units, E 10 mg, B₁ 1 mg, B₂ 1 mg, B₃ 10 mg, B₅ 2 mg, B₆ 0.5 mg, B₁₂ 1 mcg, C 10 mg, folic acid 0.06 mg, zinc 0.5 mg, choline, inositol, biotin, dl-methionine, desiccated liver, liver concentrate, liver fraction No. 2. Cap. Bot. 100s, 300s, 500s. *OTC.*
Use: Vitamin, liver supplement.

Hep-Lock. (Various Mfr.) Sterile heparin sodium soln. in saline 10 units/mL. *Dosette* vial. 1 mL, 2 mL. Vial. 10 mL, 30 mL. *Dosette* cartridge 1 mL, 2.5 mL. *Rx.*
Use: Catheter patency agent.

Hep-Lock PF. (Wyeth) Preservative-free heparin flush soln. 10 units/mL, 100 units/mL. Vial 1 mL. *Rx.*
Use: Catheter patency agent.

Hepsera. (Gilead Sciences) Adefovir dipivoxil 10 mg. Lactose. Tab. Bot. 30s. *Rx.*
Use: Antiviral.

Herbal Cellulex. (NBTY) Vitamin C 83 mg, K 33 mg, iron 9 mg. Tab. Bot. 90s. *OTC.*
Use: Vitamin supplement.

Herceptin. (Genentech) Trastuzumab 440 mg. Pow. for Inj., lyophilized. Preservative free. Vials. Diluent 20 mL vial of Bacteriostatic Water for Inj. w/1.1% benzyl alcohol. *Rx.*
Use: Monoclonal antibody.

Hermal Bath Oil. (Healthpoint Medical) Soybean oil-based bath oil. Bot. 8 oz, 32 oz. *OTC.*
Use: Emollient.

Herpecin-L. (Chattem Consumer Products) Dimethicone 1%, meradimate

5%, octinoxate 7.5%, octisalate 5%, oxybenzone 6%. *Helianthus annuus* (hybrid sunflower) oil, petrolatum mineral oil, talc, titanium dioxide. Lip balm stick. 1 tube per package. *OTC.*
Use: Cold sores.

herpes simplex virus gene. (Genetic Therapy)
Use: Antineoplastic. [Orphan Drug]

Herrick Lacrimal Plug. (Lacrimedics) Silicone plug 0.3 mm, 0.5 mm Pkg. 2 plugs. *Rx.*
Use: Punctal plug.

HES. Hetastarch.
Use: Plasma expander.
See: Hespan.

Hespan. (B. Braun Medical) Hetastarch 6 g, sodium Cl 0.9%/100 mL. Inj. Bot. 500 mL. *Rx.*
Use: Plasma volume expander.

hesperidin.
Use: Capillary fragility and permeability; hemorrhage.
See: Vitamin P; also Rutin.
W/Combinations.
See: A.C.N.
  Hesper Bitabs.
  Nialex.
  Vita Cebus.

hesperidin methyl chalcone.
Use: Vitamin P supplement.

hesperidin w/C. (Various Mfr.)
Use: Vitamin supplement.

•**hetacillin.** (HET-ah-SILL-in) USAN.
Use: Anti-infective.

•**hetacillin potassium.** (HET-ah-SILL-in) *USP 34.*
Use: Anti-infective.

•**hetaflur.** (HEH-tah-flure) USAN.
Use: Dental caries prophylactic.

•**hetastarch.** (HET-uh-starch) USAN.
Use: Plasma volume expander.
See: Hespan.

hetastarch, 6%. (Hospira) Hetastarch 6 g/100 mL in sodium chloride 0.9%. Inj. 500 single-dose containers. *Rx.*
Use: Plasma volume expander.

•**heteronium bromide.** (HET-er-oh-nee-uhm) USAN.
Use: Anticholinergic.

Hexabamate #1. (Rugby) Tridihexethyl Cl 25 mg, meprobamate 200 mg. Tab. Bot. 100s, 500s. *Rx.*
Use: Anticholinergic combination.

Hexabamate #2. (Rugby) Tridihexethyl Cl 25 mg, meprobamate 400 mg. Tab. Bot. 100s, 500s. *Rx.*
Use: Anticholinergic combination.

Hexa-Betalin. (Eli Lilly) Pyridoxine hydrochloride. Inj. Vial 100 mg/mL. Ctn. 10s,

vial 10 mL. *Rx.*
Use: Vitamin supplement.

Hexabrix. (Mallinckrodt) Ioxaglate meglumine 393 mg, ioxaglate sodium 196 mg, iodine 320 mg/mL, EDTA. Inj. Vials. 20 mL, 30 mL, 50 mL. Bot. 150 mL, 75 mL fill in 150 mL, 100 mL fill in 150 mL, 200 mL fill in 250 mL. Power injector syringes. 125 mL, 50 mL fill in 125 mL, 100 mL fill in 125 mL. *Rx.*
Use: Radiopaque agent, parenteral.

•**hexachlorophene.** (hex-ah-KLOR-oh-feen) *USP 34.*
Use: Anti-infective, topical; antiseptic; detergent.
See: Deri.
  Gamophen, Leaves.
  pHisoHex.

hexachlorophene cleansing emulsion.
Use: Anti-infective, topical detergent.

hexachlorophene liquid soap, detergent liquid.
Use: Anti-infective, topical detergent.
See: pHisoHex.

hexacose. Mixture of C-6 alcohols derived from oxidation of tetracosane $C_{24}H_{50}$.

hexadecadrol.
See: Dexamethasone.

hexadienol. Hexacose.

Hexafed. (Alaven Pharmaceuticals) Pseudoephedrine hydrochloride 60 mg, dexchlorpheniramine maleate 4 mg. Sugar free. Film-coated. ER Tab. 100s. *Rx.*
Use: Decongestant and antihistamine.

•**hexafluorenium bromide.** (HEK-sah-flure-EE-nee-uhm) USAN.
Use: Muscle relaxant, synergist (succinylcholine).

hexafluorodiethyl ether. *Name used for Flurothyl.*

hexahydroxycyclohexane.
See: Inositol.

hexakose. Mixture of tetracosanes and oxidation products.

Hexalen. (EISAI) Altretamine 50 mg. Lactose. Cap. 100s. *Rx.*
Use: Antineoplastic.

hexamethonium chloride. (Various Mfr.) Hexamethylene (bistrimethylammonium) chloride.

hexamethylamine.
Use: Hypotensive.
See: Hexastat.

hexamethylenamine.
See: Methenamine.

hexamethylenetetramine.
See: Methenamine.

hexamethylmelamine. Altretamine.
Use: Antineoplastic.
See: Hexalen.

hexamethylpararosaniline chloride.
See: Bismuth Violet.
hexamethylrosaniline chloride.
See: Gentian Violet.
hexamine.
See: Methenamine.
•**hexaminolevulinate hydrochloride.**
(hex-a-MIN-oh-le-VUE-lin-ate) USAN.
Use: Diagnostic agent, bladder cancer.
See: Cysview.
hexapradol hydrochloride.
Use: CNS stimulant.
Hexate. (Davis & Sly) Atropine sulfate
$\frac{1}{2000}$ g, extract of hyoscyamus 0.25 g,
methylene blue g, methenamine 0.5 g,
benzoic acid 0.5 g, salol 0.5 g. Tab. Bot.
1000s. *Rx.*
Use: Anti-infective, urinary.
Hexavitamin SC. (Halsey Drug)
Use: Vitamin supplement.
Hexavitamin Tablets. (Various Mfr.) Vita-
mins A 5000 units, B_1 2 mg, B_2 3 mg,
B_3 20 mg, C 75 mg, D 400 units. Bot.
100s, 1000s, UD 100s. *OTC.*
Use: Vitamin supplement.
•**hexedine.** (HEX-eh-deen) USAN.
Use: Anti-infective.
hexene-ol. Hexacose.
hexenol. Hexacose.
hexitol irrigants.
Use: Irrigant, genitourinary.
See: Sorbitol.
Sorbitol-mannitol.
hexobarbital. *Name previously used*
Hexobarbitone.
•**hexobendine.** (HEX-oh-BEN-deen)
USAN.
Use: Vasodilator.
Hexopal. (Bayer Consumer Care) Inositol hexanicotinate. *Rx.*
Use: Hypolipidemic; peripheral vasodi-
lator.
•**hexoprenaline sulfate.** (hex-oh-PREN-
ah-leen) USAN.
Use: Tocolytic.
•**hexylene glycol.** (HEX-il-een-GLYE-kol)
NF 29.
Use: Pharmaceutic aid (humectant, sol-
vent).
•**hexylresorcinol.** (hex-ill-reh-SORE-sih-
nole) *USP 34.*
Use: Anthelmintic (intestinal round-
worms and trematodes); throat
preparation.
See: Sucrets Original Formula Sore
Throat.
H-F Gel. (Paddock) Calcium gluconate
gel 2.5%.
Use: Emergency burn treatment.
[Orphan Drug]

H5N1 influenza vaccine. (Sanofi Pasteur) A/Vietnam/1203/2004 (H5N1,
clade 1) 90 mcg HA/mL. Thimerosal
(not more than 98.2 mcg/mL [$\approx$ 50 mcg
mercury per dose]), formaldehyde (not
more than 200 mcg), polyethylene glycol p-isooctylphenyl ether (not more
than 0.05%), sucrose (not more than
2%). Inj. Susp. (purified split-virus). Multidose vials. 5 mL. *Rx.*
Use: Active immunization; viral vaccine.
H.H.R. (Geneva) Hydralazine hydrochloride 25 mg, hydrochlorothiazide 15 mg,
reserpine 0.1 mg. Tab. Bot. 100s,
1000s. *Rx.*
Use: Antihypertensive.
Hiberix. (GlaxoSmithKline) Purified haemophilus B capsular polysaccharide
10 mcg, tetanus toxoid 25 mcg per
0.5 mL. Lactose. Preservative free.
Single-dose vial w/*Tip-Lok* syringe containing 0.7 mL of saline diluent. *Rx.*
Use: Agent for active immunization,
bacterial vaccine.
Hibistat. (J & J Merck Consumer Pharm.)
Chlorhexidine gluconate 0.5%. **Liq.:**
Isopropyl alcohol 70%, emollients. Bot.
4 oz, 8 oz. **Towelettes:** Unit-of-use
pocket-size towelette impregnated with
5 mL. *OTC.*
Use: Antimicrobial; antiseptic.
Hibplex. (Standex) Vitamins B_1 100 mg,
B_2 2 mg, B_3 100 mg, panthenol 2 mg/
mL. Vial 30 mL. *Rx.*
Use: Vitamin supplement.
Hi B with C. (Towne) Vitamin C 300 mg,
B_1 15 mg, B_2 10.2 mg, B_6 5 mg, niacin
50 mg, pantothenic acid 10 mg. Cap.
Bot. 100s. *Rx.*
Use: Vitamin supplement.
Hicon. (DRAXIMAGE) Sodium iodide I-
131 1000 mCi/mL. Disodium edetate
dihydrate < 2 mg. Oral Soln. In 0.25 mL,
0.5 mL, 1 mL kits with 10 capsules of
dibasic sodium phosphate 300 mg and
10 empty large hard gelatin capsules.
Rx.
Use: Radiopharmaceutical.
Hi-Cor 1.0. (C & M Pharmacal) Hydrocortisone 1%% in a nonionic, ester-
free, salt-free, paraben-free washable
base. Tube 30 g. Jar 60 g, lb. *Rx.*
Use: Corticosteroid, topical.
Hi-Cor 2.5. (C & M Pharmacal) Hydrocortisone 2.5% in a nonionic, ester-
free, salt-free, paraben-free washable
base. Tube 30 g. Jar 60 g. *Rx.*
Use: Corticosteroid, topical.
hiestrone.
See: Estrone.
High B12. (Barth's) Vitamin B_{12}, desic-

cated liver. Cap. Bot. 100s, 500s. *OTC.*
Use: Vitamin supplement.
High Potency Cold Cap. (Weeks & Leo)
Salicylamide 325 mg, chlorpheniramine
maleate 4 mg, dextromethorphan HBr
15 mg, caffeine 16.2 mg. Tab. Bot. 18s.
OTC.
Use: Analgesic; antihistamine; antitus-
sive.
High Potency D-1000. (Nature's Bounty)
Cholecalciferol 1,000 units. Glycerin,
soybean oil. Cap., softgel. 200s. *OTC.*
Use: Fat-soluble vitamin.
high potency insulin.
Use: Antidiabetic.
See: Humulin R Regular U-500 (Con-
centrated).
Insulin Injection Concentrated.
High Potency N-Vites. (Nion Corp.) Vita-
mins B_1 15 mg, B_2 10 mg, B_3 100 mg,
B_5 20 mg, B_{12} 10 mcg, C 500 mg. Tab.
Bot. 100s. *OTC.*
Use: Vitamin supplement.
High Potency Pain Relievers. (Weeks
& Leo) Acetaminophen 300 mg, sali-
cylamide 300 mg. Cap. Bot. 20s, 40s.
OTC.
Use: Analgesic.
High Potency Vitamins and Minerals.
(Burgin-Arden) Vitamins A 25,000 units,
D 400 units, B_1 10 mg, B_2 5 mg, B_6
1 mg, B_{12} 5 mcg, C 150 mg, niacin-
amide 100 mg, calcium 103 mg, phos-
phorus 80 mg, iron 10 mg, magnesium
5.5 mg, manganese 1 mg, potassium
5 mg, zinc 1.4 mg. Tab. Bot. 100s. *OTC.*
Use: Mineral, vitamin supplement.
•**hilafilcon A.** (high-lah-FILL-kahn A)
USAN.
Use: Contact lens material (hydrophilic).
•**hilafilcon B.** (high-lah-FILL-kahn B)
USAN.
Use: Contact lens material (hydrophilic).
Hill-Shade Lotion. (Hill Dermaceuticals)
Para-aminobenzoic acid, alcohol 65%.
SPF 22. *OTC.*
Use: Sunscreen.
•**hioxifilcon A.** (high-ock-sih-FILL-kahn A)
USAN.
Use: Contact lens material (hydrophilic).
Hipotest. (Marlop) Ca 53.5 mg, iron
50 mg, vitamins A 10,000 units, D
400 units, E 2.5 mg, B_1 25 mg, B_2
25 mg, B_3 50 mg, B_5 13 mg, B_6 15 mg,
B_{12} 50 mcg, C 150 mg, choline, beta-
ine, PABA, rutin, bioflavonoids, biotin
1 mg, desiccated liver, bone meal, Cu,
Mg, Mn, Zn 2.2 mg, I, P, lecithin. Tab.
Bot. 100s. *OTC.*
Use: Mineral, vitamin supplement.

Hi-Po-Vites Tablets. (Hudson Corp.) Iron
6 mg, vitamins A 10,000 units, D
400 units, E 13 mg, B_1 25 mg, B_2
25 mg, B_3 50 mg, B_5 12.5 mg, B_6
15 mg, B_{12} 50 mcg, C 150 mg, folic acid
0.4 mg, Ca, Cr, Cu, I, K, Mg, Mn, Mo,
P, Se, Zn 5 mg, biotin 1 mg, bioflavonoids, bone meal, PABA, choline bitartrate, betaine, inositol, lecithin, desiccated liver, rutin. Tab. Bot. 100s. *OTC.*
Use: Mineral, vitamin supplement.
hippramine.
See: Methenamine Hippurate.
hipputope. (Bristol-Myers Squibb) Radio-
iodinated sodium iodohippurate (^{131}I)
Inj. Bot. 1 m Ci, 2 m Ci.
Use: Diagnostic aid.
Hiprex. (Hoechst) Methenamine hippurate 1 g. Tab. Bot. 100s. *Rx.*
Use: Anti-infective, urinary.
Histacol DM Pediatric. (Breckenridge)
Pseudoephedrine hydrochloride 15 mg,
brompheniramine maleate 1 mg, dextromethorphan HBr 4 mg per 1 mL.
Sugar and alcohol free. Sorbitol. Grape
flavor. Drops 30 mL with 1 mL dropper. *Rx.*
Use: Upper respiratory combination, antitussive and expectorant combination.
Histade. (Breckenridge) Pseudoephedrine hydrochloride 120 mg, chlorpheniramine maleate 12 mg, sucrose. SR
Cap. Bot. 100s. *Rx.*
Use: Upper respiratory combination, antihistamine, decongestant.
Histagesic Modified Tablets. (Jones
Pharma) Phenylephrine hydrochloride
10 mg, chlorpheniramine maleate 4 mg,
acetaminophen 324 mg. Tab. Bot.
1000s. *OTC.*
Use: Analgesic, antihistamine, decongestant.
Histalet. (Solvay) Pseudoephedrine
hydrochloride 45 mg, chlorpheniramine
maleate 3 mg/5 mL. Syr. Bot. 473 mL.
Rx.
Use: Antihistamine, decongestant.
Histalet X. (Solvay) **Syr.:** Pseudoephedrine hydrochloride 45 mg, guaifenesin
200 mg/5 mL, alcohol 15%. Bot.
480 mL. **Tab.:** Pseudoephedrine hydrochloride 120 mg, guaifenesin 400 mg.
Tab. Bot. 100s. *Rx.*
Use: Decongestant, expectorant.
Histamax D. (Laser) Phenylephrine
hydrochloride 1.5 mg, carbinoxamine
maleate 1.5 mg per 1 mL. Cotton candy
flavor. Drops. 30 mL with dropper. *Rx.*
Use: Upper respiratory combination, decongestant and antihistamine.

•**histamine dihydrochloride.** (HISS-tah-meen die-HIGH-droe-KLOR-ide) *USP 34.*
Use: Analgesic, topical.

histamine H₂ antagonists.
See: Cimetidine.
Famotidine.
Nizatidine.
Ranitidine Hydrochloride.

Histatab D. (Breckenridge) Dexchlorpheniramine maleate 3.5 mg, methscopolamine nitrate 1 mg, pseudoephedrine hydrochloride 45 mg. Tab. 100s. *Rx.*
Use: Upper respiratory combination, decongestant, antihistamine, and anticholinergic combination.

Histatab Plus. (Century) Phenylephrine hydrochloride 5 mg, chlorpheniramine maleate 2 mg. Tab. Bot. 30s, 100s, 1000s. *OTC.*
Use: Upper respiratory combination, decongestant, antihistamine.

Histatrol. (Center) 2.75 mg/mL histamine phosphate, equivalent to 1 mg/mL histamine base, in 50% glycerin w/v, 5 mL vial; available in a Multitest dosage form or dropper bottle; 0.275 mg/mL histamine phosphate, equivalent to 0.1 mg/mL histamine base, 5 mL vial.
Use: Diagnostic aid, skin test control.

Histenol-Forte. (Zee Medical) Acetaminophen 325 mg, pseudoephedrine hydrochloride 30 mg, dextromethorphan HBr 10 mg. Tab. 24s. *OTC.*
Use: Antitussive combination.

Histex. (Tiber) Pseudoephedrine hydrochloride 30 mg, chlorpheniramine maleate 2 mg per 5 mL. Peach flavor. Liq. 15 mL, 29.6 mL, 473 mL. *Rx.*
Use: Upper respiratory combination, decongestant and antihistamine.

Histex CT. (Teamm) Carbinoxamine maleate 8 mg. Film-coated. TR Tab. Bot. 30s, 100s. *Rx.*
Use: Antihistamine, nonselective ethanolamine.

Histex I/E. (Teamm) Carbinoxamine maleate 10 mg. ER Cap. 60s. *Rx.*
Use: Antihistamine.

Histex Pd. (Teamm) Carbinoxamine maleate 4 mg/5 mL. Dye, alcohol, and sugar free. Saccharin, sorbitol, gum fruit flavor. Liq. Bot. 473 mL. *Rx.*
Use: Antihistamine.

Histex SR. (Tiber) Pseudoephedrine hydrochloride 120 mg, brompheniramine maleate 10 mg. **ER Cap.:** Sucrose. 100s. **ER Tab.:** Lactose. 100s. *Rx.*

Use: Upper respiratory combination, antihistamine, decongestant.

•**histidine.** (HISS-tih-deen) *USP 34.*
Use: Amino acid.
W/Combinations.
See: Monarc-M.

histidine monohydrochloride.
Use: I.M., peptic and jejunal ulcers.

Histine-8. (Freeport) Chlorpheniramine maleate 8 mg. TR Tab. Bot. 1000s. *OTC.*
Use: Antihistamine.

Histine-50. (Freeport) Diphenhydramine hydrochloride 50 mg. Cap. Bot. 1000s. *OTC.*
Use: Antihistamine, antitussive; anticholinergic; antiemetic; sedative.

Histine-4. (Freeport) Chlorpheniramine maleate 4 mg. Tab. Bot. 1000s. *OTC.*
Use: Antihistamine.

Histine-1. (Freeport) Diphenhydramine hydrochloride 10 mg, alcohol 12% to 14%/4 mL. Bot. 4 oz. *OTC.*
Use: Antihistamine, antitussive; anticholinergic; antiemetic; sedative.

Histine-12. (Freeport) Chlorpheniramine maleate 12 mg. TR Tab. Bot. 1000s. *OTC.*
Use: Antihistamine.

Histine-25. (Freeport) Diphenhydramine hydrochloride 25 mg. Cap. Bot. 1000s. *OTC.*
Use: Antihistamine, antitussive; anticholinergic; antiemetic; sedative.

Histine-2. (Freeport) Diphenhydramine hydrochloride 12.5 mg/5 mL w/alcohol 5%. Bot. 4 oz. *OTC.*
Use: Antihistamine, antitussive; anticholinergic; antiemetic; sedative.

Histinex HC. (Ethex) Hydrocodone bitartrate 2.5 mg, phenylephrine hydrochloride 5 mg, chlorpheniramine maleate 2 mg per 5 mL. Sorbitol, saccharin. Alcohol free, sugar free. Syrup. Bot. 473 mL, 946 mL. *c-III.*
Use: Upper respiratory combination, antitussive combination.

histone deacetylase inhibitors.
Use: Antineoplastic agents.
See: Vorinostat.

•**histoplasmin.** (hiss-toe-PLAZZ-min) *USP 34.* (Parke-Davis) An aqueous solution containing standardized sterile culture filtrate of *Histoplasma capsulatum* grown on liquid synthetic medium.
Use: Diagnostic aid (dermal reactivity indicator).
See: Histoplasmin, Diluted.

histoplasmin, diluted. (Parke-Davis) 1:100 w/v. Standardized sterile filtrate from cultures of *Histoplasma capsula-*

tum, 0.5% phenol, polysorbate 80.
1 mL. Inj. *Rx.*
Use: Diagnostic aid.
•**histrelin.** (hiss-TRELL-in) USAN.
Use: LHRH agonist; treatment of por-
phyria. [Orphan Drug]
See: Supprelin.
histrelin acetate.
Use: Hormone, gonadotropin-releasing
hormone analog.
See: Supprelin LA.
Vantas.
Hitone. (Lafayette) Barium sulfate suspension 125% w/v. Bot. 2000 mL.
Case 4s.
Use: Radiopaque agent.
Hi-Tor. (Barth's) B₁ 6 mg, B₂ 12 mg, B₆
54 mcg, Vitamins B₁₂ 15 mcg, niacin
1.5 mg, pantothenic acid 150 mcg, cho-
line 3.75 mg, inositol 5.25 mg. Tab.
Bot. 100s, 500s, 1000s. *OTC.*
Use: Vitamin supplement.
Hi-Tor 900. (Barth's) Vitamins B₁
13.5 mg, B₂ 5.2 mg, B₆ 0.6 mg, B₁₂
2.5 mcg, niacin 15 mg, pantothenic acid
1.2 mg, biotin, iron 0.9 mg, protein
7.5 g, inositol 50 mg, choline 40 mg,
aminobenzoic acid 0.15 to 2.4 mg/15 g.
Bot. 1 lb, 3 lb. *OTC.*
Use: Mineral, vitamin supplement.
HIVAG HIV-1/HIV-2 (rDNA) EIA. (Abbott)
Enzyme immunoassay for qualitative
detection of antibodies to human
immunodeficiency virus type 1 or type
2 in human serum or plasma. Test kits
100s, 1000s, 5000s.
Use: Diagnostic aid.
Hi-Vegi-Lip Tablets. (Freeda) Pancreatin
2400 mg, lipase 12,000 units, protease
60,000 units, amylase 60,000 units.
Tab. Bot. 100s, 250s. *OTC.*
Use: Digestive aid.
Hivig. (NABI) Human immunodeficiency
virus immune globulin.
Use: Antiviral, HIV. [Orphan Drug]
Hiwolfia. (Jones Pharma) Rauwolfia
25 mg, 50 mg, 100 mg. Tab. Bot. 100s,
1000s.
Use: Antihypertensive.
HMG-CoA reductase inhibitors.
Use: Antihyperlipidemic agents.
See: Atorvastatin.
Fluvastatin.
Lovastatin.
Pitavastatin.
Pravastatin Sodium.
Rosuvastatin Calcium.
Simvastatin.
HMM.
See: Hexamethylmelamine.
HN₂. Mechlorethamine hydrochloride.

Use: Antineoplastic.
See: Mustargen.
H 9600. (Cypress) Pseudoephedrine
hydrochloride 90 mg, guaifenesin
600 mg, dye free. SR Tab. Bot. 100s.
Rx.
Use: Upper respiratory combination, de-
congestant, expectorant.
•**hofocon A.** (hoe-FOE-kon) USAN.
Use: Hydrophobic.
H₂ OEX. (Fellows) Benzthiazide 50 mg.
Tab. Bot. 100s, 1000s. *Rx.*
Use: Diuretic.
Hold. (GlaxoSmithKline) Dextromethor-
phan HBr 5 mg. Loz. Plastic tube
10 oz. *OTC.*
Use: Antitussive.
Hold DM. (B.F. Ascher) Dextromethor-
phan HBr 5 mg. Corn syrup, sucrose.
Original and cherry flavor. Loz. Pkg.
10s. *OTC.*
Use: Nonnarcotic antitussive.
holocaine hydrochloride. (Various Mfr.)
Phenacaine hydrochloride.
Use: Anesthetic, local.
homarylamine hydrochloride. N-
Methyl-3,4-methylenedioxyphenethyl-
amine hydrochloride.
•**homatropine hydrobromide.** (hoe-MA-
troe-peen) *USP 34.*
Use: Anticholinergic, ophthalmic; mydri-
atic, cycloplegic.
See: Isopto Homatropine.
Murocoll.
W/Hydrocodone Bitartrate.
See: Tussigon.
homatropine hydrobromide. (Various
Mfr.) Homatropine HBr 5%. Soln. Bot.
1 mL, 2 mL, 5 mL. *Rx.*
Use: Mydriatic, cycloplegic.
homatropine hydrochloride.
Use: Anticholinergic, topical; mydriatic,
cycloplegic.
•**homatropine methylbromide.** (hoe-MA-
troe-peen) *USP 34.*
Use: Anticholinergic.
W/Combinations.
See: Hydromide.
Hydropane.
Panitol H.M.B.
Spasmatol.
Tapuline.
W/Hydrocodone Bitartrate.
See: Hydromet.
**homatropine methylbromide and
phenobarbital combinations.**
Use: Anticholinergic.
See: Gustase Plus.
Hominex-1. (Ross) Protein 15 g, fat
23.9 g, carbohydrate 46.3 g, linoleic

acid 1800 mg, Fe 9 mg, Na 190 mg, K 675 mg, Ca, vitamins A, B_1, B_2, B_3, B_5, B_6, B_{12}, C, D, E, K, biotin, choline, folic acid, inositol, Cl, Cu, I, Mg, Mn, P, Se, Zn and 480 Cal per 100 g. Methionine free. Pow. Can 350 g. *OTC.*
Use: Nutritional supplement.

Hominex-2. (Ross) Protein 30 g, fat 15.5 g, carbohydrate 30 g, Fe 13 mg, Na 880 mg, K 1370 mg, Ca, vitamins A, B_1, B_2, B_3, B_5, B_6, B_{12}, C, D, E, K, biotin, choline, folic acid, inositol, Cl, Cu, I, Mg, Mn, P, Se, Zn and 410 Cal per 100 g. Methionine free. Pow. Can 325 g. *OTC.*
Use: Nutritional supplement.

Homogene-S. (Spanner) Testosterone 25 mg/mL, 50 mg/mL, 100 mg/mL. Vial 10 mL. *c-III.*
Use: Androgen.

•**homosalate.** (hoe-moe-SAL-ate) USAN. Formerly Homomenthyl Salicylate.
Use: Ultraviolet screen.
W/Avobenzone, Octisalate, Octocrylene, Oxybenzone.
See: Neutrogena Ultra Sheer Dry-Touch Sunblock.
W/Combinations.
See: Coppertone.

honey bee venom.
See: Albay.
Pharmalgen.
Venomil.

•**hoquizil hydrochloride.** (HOE-kwih-zill) USAN.
Use: Bronchodilator.

hormofollin.
See: Estrone.

hormones.
See: Androgens.
Antiandrogens.
Antiestrogens.
Aromatase Inhibitors.
Cetrorelix Acetate.
Choriogonadotropin Alfa.
Clomiphene Citrate.
Estrogen/Nitrogen Mustard.
Estrogens.
Ganirelix Acetate.
Gonadotropin-Releasing Hormone Analog.
Intrauterine Progesterone Contraceptive System.
Levonorgestrel-Releasing Intrauterine System.
Medroxyprogesterone Acetate/Estradiol Cypionate.
Medroxyprogesterone Contraceptive Injection.
Progestins.
Raloxifene.

hormones, contraceptive.
Use: Contraceptive hormones.

hormones, growth.
Use: Growth hormones.

hormones, posterior pituitary.
Use: Posterior pituitary hormones.

hormones, sex.
Use: Sex hormones.

hornet venom.
See: Albay.
Pharmalgen.
Venomil.

•**horse chestnut.** *NF 29.*
Use: Anti-inflammatory.

Hospital Foam Cleaner. (Health & Medical Techniques) 0-phenylphenol 0.1%, 4-chloro-2-cyclopentyl-phenol 0.08%, lauric diethanolamide 0.2%, triethanolamine dodecylbenzenesulfonate 0.3%. Aerosol spray 19 oz.
Use: Antimicrobial; disinfectant.

Hospital Lotion. (Paddock) Diisobutyl-cresoxyethoxy-ethyl dimethyl benzyl ammonium chloride, menthol, lanolin, mineral and vegetable oils. Bot. 4 oz, 8 oz, gal. *OTC.*
Use: Emollient.

H.P. Acthar. (Questcor) Repository corticotropin injection 80 units/mL, gelatin 16%. Multidose vial 5 mL. *Rx.*
Use: Corticosteroid.

HRC-Tylaprin. (Cenci, H.R. Labs, Inc.) Acetaminophen 120 mg, alcohol 7%/5 mL. Elix. Bot. 2 oz, 4 oz. *OTC.*
Use: Analgesic.

H-R Lubricating Jelly. (Wallace) Hydroxypropyl methycellulose, parabens. Jelly 150 g. *OTC.*
Use: Lubricant.

H.S. Need. (Hanlon) Chloral hydrate 3¾ g, 7.5 g. Cap. Bot. 100s. *Rx.*
Use: Sedative.

HSV-1. (Wampole) Herpes simplex virus type 1 test system. For the qualitative and semi-quantitative detection of HSV-1 antibody in human serum. Test 100s.
Use: Diagnostic aid.

HSV-2. (Wampole) Herpes simplex virus type 2 antibody test. For the qualitative and semi-quantitative detection of HSV-2 antibody in human serum. Test 100s.
Use: Diagnostic aid.

H.T. Factorate. (Centeon) Antihemophilic factor (human) dried, heat treated for IV administration only. Single-dose vial w/diluent and needles. *Rx.*
Use: Antihemophilic.

H.T. Factorate Generation II. (Centeon) Antihemophilic factor (human) dried, heat treated for IV administration only.

Single-dose vial w/diluent and needles. *Rx.*
Use: Antihemophilic.

HTSH EIA. (Abbott Diagnostics) Enzyme immunoassay for the quantitative determination of human thyroid-stimulating hormone (TSH) in human serum or plasma.
Use: Diagnostic aid.

HTSH RIAbead. (Abbott Diagnostics) Immunoradiometric assay for the quantitative measurement of human thyroid-stimulating hormone (TSH) in serum.
Use: Diagnostic aid.

5-HT₃ receptor antagonists.
See: Alosetron Hydrochloride.
  Dolasetron Mesylate.
  Granisetron Hydrochloride.
  Ondansetron Hydrochloride.
  Palonosetron Hydrochloride.

H-Tuss-D. (Cypress) Hydrocodone bitartrate 5 mg, pseudoephedrine hydrochloride 60 mg/5 mL, Liq. Bot. 473 mL. *Rx.*
Use: Expectorant.

Hulk Hogan Multi-Vitamins Plus Extra C. (S.G. Labs, Inc.) Vitamins A 2500 units, E 15 units, D_3 400 units, B_1 1.05 mg, B_2 1.2 mg, B_3 13.5 mg, B_6 1.05 mg, B_{12} 4.5 mcg, C 300 mg, folic acid 300 mcg, sucrose. Chew. Tab. Bot. 60s. *OTC.*
Use: Mineral, vitamin supplement.

Humalog. (Lilly) Human insulin lispro 100 units/mL. Inj. Vials. 10 mL. Cartridges. 5 × 1.5 mL, 5 × 3 mL. Disp. pen insulin delivery devices. 5 × 3 mL. *Rx.*
Tall Man: HumaLOG
Use: Antidiabetic, insulin.

Humalog Mix 50/50. (Lilly) Insulin lispro (human) 100 units/mL. Metacresol 2.2 mg/mL, protamine sulfate 0.19 mg/mL. Contains 50% insulin lispro protamine (rDNA origin) suspension and 50% insulin lispro (rDNA origin) injection. Inj., Susp. Vial. 10 mL. Disposable pen and *KwikPen* insulin delivery device. 5 × 3 mL. *Rx.*
Tall Man: HumaLOG
Use: Antidiabetic agent, insulin.

Humalog Mix 75/25. (Lilly) Human insulin lispro 100 units/mL. Protamine sulfate 0.28 mg. Contains 75% insulin lispro protamine suspension and 25% insulin lispro injection (rDNA). Inj. Disp. pen insulin delivery devices. 5 × 3 mL. Vials. 10 mL. *Rx.*
Tall Man: HumaLOG
Use: Antidiabetic, insulin.

human albumin grifols. (Grifols) Human albumin 25%. Inj. 50 mL, 100 mL.

Rx.
Use: Plasma expander.

human antihemophilic factor.
See: Antihemophilic.

human B-type natriuretic peptide.
Use: Vasodilator.
See: Nesiritide.

human growth hormone function test.
See: R-Gene 10.

•**human insulin.** *USP 34.* Insulin human.
Use: Hypoglycemic.
See: Humulin.

humanized anti-tac.
Use: Immunosuppressant. [Orphan Drug]
See: Zenapax.

•**human papillomaviros recombinant vaccine, bivalent.**
Use: Cervarix.

human papillomavirus recombinant vaccine, quadrivalent.
Use: Active immunization; viral vaccine.
See: Gardasil.

human protein C.
Use: Thrombolytic agent.
See: Drotrecogin Alfa (Activated).
  Protein C Concentrate (Human).

human serum albumin.
See: Albumotope.

human T-lymphotropic virus type III Gp 160 antigens.
Use: AIDS. [Orphan Drug]
See: Vaxsyn HIV-1.

Humate-P. (CSL Behring) Antihemophilic factor and von Willebrand factor: Ristocetin cofactor (vWF/RCo) 250 units/600 units per vial, 500 units/1200 units per vial, 1,000 units/2400 units per vial. When reconstituted, each milliliter contains Factor VIII activity 40 to 80 units, vWF/RCo activity 72 to 224 units, glycine 15 to 33 mg, sodium citrate 3.5 to 9.3 mg, sodium chloride 2 to 5.3 mg, albumin (human) 8 to 16 mg, other proteins 2 to 14 mg, total proteins 10 to 30 mg. Contains anti-A and anti-B blood group isoagglutinins. Heat-treated. Pow. for Inj., Soln. Lyophilized. Single-dose vials with 5 mL (250 units/600 units), 10 mL (500 units/1200 units), 15 mL (1000 units/2400 units) diluent, filter transfer set for reconstitution, and a vented filter spike for withdrawal. *Rx.*
Use: Antihemophilic agent.

Humatin. (Parke-Davis) Paromomycin sulfate 250 mg. Cap. Bot. 16s. *Rx.*
Use: Amebicide.

Humatrope. (Eli Lilly) Somatropin. 5 mg (≈ 15 units)/vial. Mannitol 25 mg, glycine 5 mg. Pow. for Inj., lyophilized. Vial with 5 mL diluent (water for injection

with metacresol 0.3%, glycerin 1.7%). *Rx.*
Use: Hormone, growth.

HumatroPen. (Eli Lilly) Somatropin. **6 mg (18 units)/cartridge:** Mannitol 18 mg, glycine 6 mg. **12 mg (36 units)/cartridge:** Mannitol 36 mg, glycine 12 mg. **24 mg (72 units)/cartridge:** Mannitol 72 mg, glycine 24 mg. Inj., lyophilized Pow. for Soln. Cartridges w/prefilled syringe of diluents (metacresol 0.3% as preservative, glycerin 1.7% (6 mg only) and 0.29% (12 mg and 24 mg). *Rx.*
Use: Growth hormone.

Humibid CS. (Cornerstone Biopharma) Dextromethorphan HBr 20 mg, guaifenesin 400 mg. Saccharin. Tab. 24s. *OTC.*
Use: Antitussive with expectorant.

Humibid DM. (Carolina Pharmaceuticals) Dextromethorphan HBr 50 mg, guaifenesin 400 mg, potassium guaiacolsulfonate 200 mg. Sucrose. ER Cap. Bot. 30s, 100s. *Rx.*
Use: Upper respiratory combination, antitussive and expectorant combination.

Humibid Maximum Strength. (Adams) Guaifenesin 1200 mg. ER Tab. 100s. *OTC.*
Use: Expectorant.

Humira. (Abbott) Adalimumab 20 mg/0.4 mL, 40 mg/0.8 mL. Preservative free. Inj. Soln. Single-use prefilled syringes. Single-use prefilled pens (40 mg/0.8 mL only). Each dose tray consists of a single-use syringe or pen with a fixed 27-gauge ½-inch needle. *Rx.*
Use: Immunomodulator.

HuMist. (Scherer) Sodium Cl 0.65%, chlorobutanol. Soln. Bot. 45 mL. *OTC.*
Use: Nasal decongestant.

Humulin 50/50. (Lilly) Human insulin (rDNA) 100 units/mL. Inj. Vials. 10 mL. *OTC.*
Tall Man: HumuLIN
Use: Antidiabetic, insulin.

Humulin N. (Lilly) Human insulin (rDNA) 100 units/mL. Inj. Disp. pen insulin delivery device 5 × 3 mL, Vials. 10 mL. *OTC.*
Tall Man: HumuLIN
Use: Antidiabetic, insulin.

Humulin R. (Lilly) Regular insulin (rDNA) 100 units/mL. Inj. Vials. 10 mL. *OTC.*
Tall Man: HumuLIN
Use: Antidiabetic, insulin.

Humulin R Regular U-500 (Concentrated). (Lilly) Insulin concentrate regular 500 units/mL. M-cresol 2.5 mg, gly-

cerin 16 mg/mL. Inj. Vials. 20 mL. *Rx.*
Tall Man: HumuLIN

Humulin 70/30. (Lilly) Human insulin (rDNA) 100 units/mL. Inj. Disp. pen insulin delivery devices. 5 × 3 mL. Vials. 10 mL. *OTC.*
Tall Man: HumuLIN
Use: Antidiabetic, insulin.

Hurricaine. (Beutlich) Benzocaine 20%. **Gel:** Alcohol 60%, saccharin. 7 g. **Spray:** Cherry flavor. 60 mL. **Swab:** Polyethylene glycol, saccharin. 72s. *OTC.*
Use: Topical local anesthetic, ester local anesthetic.

Hurricaine Topical Anesthetic Spray Kit. (Beutlich) Benzocaine 20%. Kit: Aerosol 60 g plus 200 disposable extension tubes. *OTC.*
Use: Anesthetic, topical.

HVS 1 & 2. (Chemi-Tech Laboratories) Benzalkonium Cl in a specially formulated base. Soln. Bot. 15 mL. *OTC.*
Use: Cold sores, fever blisters, herpes virus.

Hyacide. (Niltig) Benzethonium chloride 0.1%, sodium nitrite 0.55%. Soln. Bot. oz. *OTC.*
Use: Antiseptic.

Hyalex. (Miller Pharmacal Group) Magnesium salicylate 260 mg, magnesium p-aminobenzoate 163 mg, vitamins A 1500 units, C 30 mg, D 100 units, E 3 units, B_{12} 2 mcg, pantothenic acid 5 mg, zinc 0.7 mg. Tab. Bot. 100s. *OTC.*
Use: Mineral, vitamin supplement.

Hyalgan. (Sanofi-Synthelabo) Sodium hyaluronate 10 mg/mL. Prefilled syringes and vials. 2 mL. Prefilled Syringe. *Rx.*
Use: Antiarthritic.

hyalidase.
See: Hyaluronidase.

hyaluronan.
See: Orthovisc.

hyaluronic acid derivatives.
Use: Physical adjunct, correction of facial wrinkles and folds.
See: Bionect.
   Euflexxa.
   Hyalgan.
   Hylaform.
   Hylira.
   Juvederm 30.
   Juvederm 30HV.
   Juvederm 24HV.
   Juvederm Ultra.
   Juvederm Ultra Plus.
   Juvederm Ultra Plus XC.
   Juvederm Ultra XC.

Orthovisc.
Perlane.
Perlane-L.
Restylane.
Restylane-L.
Sodium Hyaluronate.
Supartz.
Synvisc.
Synvisc-One.
•hyaluronidase. (hye-al-ur-ON-i-dase)
USP 34.
Use: Physical adjunct.
See: Amphadase.
Hylenex.
Vitrase.
•hyaluronidase (human recombinant).
(hye-al-ur-ON-i-dase) USAN.
Use: Spreading agent.
•hyaluronidase injection. (high-uhl-yur-
AHN-ih-dase) USP 34. Hyalidase, Hy-
dase Enzymes which depolymerize hy-
aluronic acid. Hyalase, Rondase.
Use: Hypodermoclyses, promotion of
diffusion, spreading agent.
See: Wydase.
•hyaluronidase ovine. (hye-al-ur-ON-i-
dase) USAN.
Use: Spreading agent.
hyamagnate. Hydroxy-Aluminum-
Magnesium-Aminoacetate, Sodium-free.
Hybec Forte. (Amlab) Vitamins B₁
100 mg, B₂ 20 mg, B₆ 2.5 mg, B₁₂
10 mcg, niacinamide 25 mg, C 200 mg,
calcium pantothenate 5 mg, iron
10 mg, choline bitartrate 24 mg, inositol
10 mg, biotin 5 mcg, liver 50 mg, yeast
100 mg. Tab. Bot. 30s, 100s. OTC.
Use: Mineral, vitamin supplement.
Hycamtin. (GlaxoSmithKline) Topotecan
(as topotecan hydrochloride). Cap.:
0.25 mg, 1 mg. Hydrogenated vegetable oil. 10s. Inj., Lyophilized. Pow.
for Soln.: 4 mg. Preservative free.
Single-dose vials. Rx.
Use: Antineoplastic; DNA topoisomerase inhibitor.
•hycanthone. (HIGH-kan-thone) USAN.
Use: Antischistosomal.
Hycet. (Xanodyne) Hydrocodone bitartrate 2.5 mg/acetaminophen 108 mg
per 5 mL. Alcohol 7%, glycerin, parabens, saccharin, sorbitol, sucrose. Oral
Soln. 473 mL. c-III.
Use: Analgesic, narcotic.
Hyclorite. USP 34. Sodium hypochlorite
soln.
HycoClear Tuss. (Ethex) Hydrocodone
bitartrate 5 mg, guaifenesin 100 mg/
5 mL. Alcohol, dye, sugar free. Syrup.

Bot. 118 mL, 473 mL. c-III.
Use: Antitussive, expectorant.
Hycort. (Everett) Cream: Hydrocortisone
1% in a cream base. Tube oz. Oint.:
Hydrocortisone 1% in ointment base.
Tube oz. Rx.
Use: Corticosteroid, topical.
Hycortole. (Teva) Hydrocortisone.
Cream: 0.5%: 5 g, 20 g; 1%: 5 g, 20 g,
4 oz; 2.5%: Tube 5 g, 20 g. Oint.: 1%,
2.5%. Tube 5 g, 20 g.
Use: Corticosteroid, topical.
Hycosin Expectorant. (Alpharma)
Hydrocodone bitartrate 5 mg, guaifenesin
100 mg per 5 mL. Alcohol 10%, para-
bens, saccharin, sorbitol, sucrose, butter-
scotch flavor. Syr. Bot. 473 mL. c-III.
Use: Upper respiratory combination, an-
titussive, expectorant.
hydantoin derivatives.
Use: Anticonvulsant.
See: Dilantin.
Diphenylhydantoin Sodium.
Mesantoin.
Phenantoin.
hydantoins.
See: Ethotoin.
Fosphenytoin Sodium.
Phenytoin.
Hydergine. (Novartis) Liq.: Equal parts
of dihydroergocornine, dihydroergocristine, dihydroergocryptine (Ergoloid
Mesylates). 1 mg/mL. Bot. 100 mL w/
dropper. Oral: Equal parts of dihydroergocornine, dihydroergocristine, dihydroergocryptine (Ergoloid Mesylates).
1 mg. Tab. Bot. 100s, 500s. SandoPak
(UD) 100s, 500s. Sublingual: Equal
parts of dihydroergocornine, dihydroergocristine, dihydroergocryptine (Ergoloid Mesylates). 0.5 mg, 1 mg. Tab. Bot.
100s, 1000s, SandoPak (UD) 100s. Rx.
Use: Psychotherapeutic agent.
Hydoril. (Cenci, H.R. Labs, Inc.) Hydrochlorothiazide 25 mg, 50 mg. Tab. Bot.
100s, 1000s. Rx.
Use: Diuretic.
hydrabamine phenoxymethyl penicillin.
See: Penicillin V Hydrabamine.
hydracrylic acid beta lactone.
See: Propiolactone.
hydralazine. (Solopak Pharmaceuticals,
Inc.) Hydralazine hydrochloride 20 mg/
mL Inj. Vial 1 mL. Rx.
Use: Antihypertensive.
•hydralazine hydrochloride. (high-
DRAL-uh-zeen) USP 34.
Tall Man: hydrALAZINE
Use: Antihypertensive.
See: Apresoline.

W/Hydrochlorothiazide.
See: Apresoline-Esidrix.
Hydralazide.
Hydroserpine Plus.
W/Isosorbide Dinitrate.
See: BiDil.
W/Reserpine.
See: Dralserp.
Serpasil-Apresoline.
W/Reserpine, hydrochlorothiazide.
See: Harbolin.
hydralazine hydrochloride. (Various Mfr.) Hydralazine hydrochloride 10 mg, 25 mg, 50, mg 100 mg. Tab. Bot. 100s, 1000s, UD 100s (except 100 mg).
Use: Antihypertensive.
•**hydralazine polistirex.** (high-DRAL-ah-zeen pahl-ee-STIE-rex) USAN.
Tall Man: hydrALAZINE
Use: Antihypertensive.
Hydra Mag Tablets. (Pal-Pak, Inc.) Aluminum hydroxide gel, dried, 195 mg, magnesium trisilicate 195 mg, kaolin 162 mg. Tab. Bot. 1000s. *OTC.*
Use: Antacid.
Hydramine Cough. (Various Mfr.) Diphenhydramine hydrochloride 12.5 mg/mL, may contain alcohol. Syr. Bot. 473 mL. *Rx-OTC.*
Use: Antitussive.
Hydraserp. (Geneva) Hydrochlorothiazide 25 mg, 50 mg, reserpine 0.1 mg. Tab. Bot. 100s, 1000s. *Rx.*
Use: Antihypertensive combination.
hydrastine hydrochloride. (Penick) Pow. Bot. oz.
Use: Hemostatic.
Hydrazide. (Ivax) **25/25:** Hydrochlorothiazide 25 mg, hydralazine 25 mg. Cap. **50/50:** Hydrochlorothiazide 50 mg, hydralazine 50 mg. Cap. Bot. 100s. *Rx.*
Use: Antihypertensive.
Hydra-Zide. (Par Pharmaceuticals) Hydralazine hydrochloride 50 mg, hydrochlorothiazide 50 mg. Cap. Bot. 100s, 500s, 1000s. *Rx.*
Use: Antihypertensive.
hydrazone.
Use: Pulmonary tuberculosis.
See: Rimactane.
Hydrea. (Bristol-Myers Squibb) Hydroxyurea 500 mg, lactose. Cap. Bot. 100s. *Rx.*
Use: Antineoplastic.
hydriodic acid. (Various Mfr.)
Use: Expectorant.
hydriodic acid therapy.
See: Aminoacetic Acid Hydrochloride.
Hydrisalic. (Pedinol) Salicylic acid 6%. Alcohol. Gel. 28.35 g. *OTC.*
Use: Keratolytic agent.

Hydrisinol. (Pedinol Pharmacal) Sulfonated hydrogenated castor oil. **Cream:** Spout Cap Jar 4 oz, lb. **Lot.:** Bot. 8 oz. *OTC.*
Use: Emollient.
Hydro-Ban. (Whiteworth Towne) Juniper oil 10 mg, uva ursi 50 mg, buchu extract 50 mg, parsley piert extract 50 mg, iron 6 mg. Cap. Bot. 42s. *OTC.*
Use: Diuretic.
Hydrocare Cleaning and Disinfecting. (Allergan) Buffered, isotonic. Tris (2-hydroxyethyl) tallow ammonium Cl, thimerosal 0.002%, bis (2-hydroxyethyl) tallow ammonium Cl, sodium bicarbonate, sodium phosphates, hydrochloric acid, propylene glycol, polysorbate 80, polyhema. Soln. Bot. 240 mL, 360 mL. *OTC.*
Use: Contact lens care, disinfective.
Hydrocare Preserved Saline. (Allergan) Isotonic, buffered, NaCl, sodium hexametaphosphate, boric acid, sodium borate, EDTA 0.01%, thimerosal 0.001%. Soln. Bot. 240 mL, 360 mL. *OTC.*
Use: Contact lens care, rinsing/storage solution.
Hydrocerin. (Geritrex) **Cream:** Petrolatum, mineral oil, mineral wax, ceresin, lanolin alcohol, parabens. 480 g. **Lotion:** EDTA, lanolin alcohol, parabens, PEG-40 sorbitan, peroleate, propylene glycol, sorbitol, water. 240 g. *OTC.*
Use: Emollient.
hydrochlorate. Same as Hydrochloride.
•**hydrochloric acid.** (HYE-droe-KLOR-ik) *NF 29.*
Use: Well diluted, achlorhydria; pharmaceutic aid (acidifying agent).
hydrochloric acid. (Various Mfr.) Muriatic acid, Absolute 38%. Diluted 10%.
hydrochloric acid therapy.
Use: Well diluted, achlorhydria; pharmaceutic aid (acidifying agent); gastric acidifier.
See: Betaine Hydrochloride.
Glutamic Acid Hydrochloride.
Glycine Hydrochloride.
Hydrochloroserpine. (Freeport) Hydralazine hydrochloride 25 mg, hydrochlorothiazide 15 mg, reserpine 0.1 mg. Tab. Bot. 1000s.
Use: Antihypertensive combination.
•**hydrochlorothiazide.** (high-droe-klor-oh-THIGH-uh-zide) *USP 34.*
Use: Diuretic.
See: Ezide.
HydroDiuril.
Hydro-Par.
Microzide.

W/Aliskirin.
  See: Tekturna HCT.
W/Amlodipine/Valsartan.
  See: Exforge HCT.
W/Combinations.
  See: Accuretic.
  Apresoline-Esidrix.
  Atacand HCT.
  Avalide.
  Benicar HCT.
  Capozide.
  Diovan HCT.
  Dyazide.
  Hydralazide.
  Hyzaar.
  Lopressor HCT.
  Lotensin HCT.
  Micardis HCT.
  Monopril-HCT.
  Oreticyl.
  Prinzide.
  Quinaretic.
  Teveten HCT.
  Uniretic.
  Vaseretic.
  Zestoretic.
  Ziac.
hydrochlorothiazide. (Various Mfr.)
  Hydrochlorothiazide. **Cap.:** 12.5 mg.
  Bot. 100s, 500s. **Tab.:** 12.5 mg (100s,
  1000s), 25 mg (30s, 100s, 500s,
  1000s, 5000s, UD 32s, UD 100s),
  50 mg (30s, 100s, 500s, 1000s, 5000s,
  UD 100s), 100 mg (30s, 100s, 250s,
  500s, 1000s, UD 100s). *Rx.*
  Use: Diuretic.
hydrochlorothiazide/amiloride.
  See: Amiloride Hydrochloride and
    Hydrochlorothiazide.
**hydrochlorothiazide and benazepril
  hydrochloride.**
  See: Benazepril Hydrochloride/Hydro-
    chlorothiazide.
hydrochlorothiazide/hydralazine.
  (Various Mfr.) Hydrochlorothiazide/hy-
  dralazine hydrochloride 25 mg/25 mg,
  50 mg/50 mg. Cap. Bot. 100s, 500s,
  1000s. *Rx.*
  Use: Antihypertensive.
**hydrochlorothiazide/metoprolol tar-
  trate.**
  See: Metoprolol Tartrate/Hydrochloro-
    thiazide.
hydrocholeretic combinations.
  See: G.B.S.
hydrocholeretics.
  See: Bile Salts.
    Dehydrocholic Acid.
    Ox Bile Extract.
Hydrocil Instant. (Numark) Psyllium hydrophilic mucilloid 3.5 g/dose. Pow. Jar

250 g. *OTC.*
  Use: Laxative.
•**hydrocodone bitartrate.** (HIGH-droe-
  KOE-dohn by-TAR-TRATE) *USP 34.*
  Dihydrocodeinone bitartrate.
  Tall Man: HYDROcodone
  Use: Antitussive, analgesic, narcotic.
  W/Acetaminophen.
    See: Anexsia 7.5/650.
    Anexsia 10/660.
    Co-Gesic.
    Hycet.
    Hydrogesic.
    Liquicet.
    Lorcet Plus.
    Lorcet 10/650.
    Lortab.
    Lortab 5/500.
    Lortab 7.5/500.
    Lortab 10/500.
    Margesic H.
    Maxidone.
    Norco.
    Norco 5/325.
    Stagesic.
    T-Gesic.
    Vicodin.
    Vicodin ES.
    Vicodin HP.
    Xodol.
    Zamicet.
    Zydone.
  W/Aspirin.
    See: Lortab ASA.
  W/Chlorpheniramine Maleate.
    See: TussiCaps Full Strength.
    TussiCaps Half Strength.
  W/Chlorpheniramine Maleate, Guaifene-
  sin, Pseudoephedrine Hydrochloride.
    See: ZTuss Expectorant.
  W/Chlorpheniramine Maleate, Phenyl-
  ephrine Hydrochloride.
    See: Histinex HC.
    Neo HC.
    Notuss-Forte.
    Relacon-HC.
    Vanex-HD.
  W/Chlorpheniramine Maleate, Phenyl-
  ephrine Hydrochloride, Pseudoephed-
  rine Hydrochloride, Pyrilamine Maleate.
    See: Statuss Green.
  W/Chlorpheniramine Maleate, Pseudo-
  ephedrine Hydrochloride.
    See: Notuss-Forte.
  W/Chlorpheniramine Polistirex.
    See: Tussionex Pennkinetic.
  W/Guaifenesin.
    See: ZTuss ZT.
  W/Homatropine Hydrobromide.
    See: Tussigon.

W/Ibuprofen.
 See: Ibudone.
 Reprexain.
 Vicoprofen.
W/Methylbromide.
 See: Hydromet.
W/Phenylephrine Hydrochloride, Pyrilamine Maleate.
 See: Tussplex.
**hydrocodone bitartrate/acetamino-
phen.** (Boca Pharmacal) Hydrocodone
 bitartrate 5 mg, acetaminophen
 300 mg. Tab. 100s. *c-III.*
 Use: Opioid analgesic combination.
**hydrocodone bitartrate and aceta-
minophen.** (Qualitest) Hydrocodone bitartrate 2.5 mg, acetaminophen
 500 mg. Sucrose. Tab. 100s, 500s,
 1,000s. *c-III.*
 Use: Narcotic analgesic.
**hydrocodone bitartrate and aceta-
minophen.** (Various Mfr.) **Caplets:**
 Hydrocodone bitartrate 7.5 mg, acetaminophen 650 mg. Cap. Bot. 100s,
 500s. **Capsules:** Hydrocodone bitartrate 5 mg, acetaminophen 500 mg.
 Cap. Bot. 100s, 500s. **Elixir:** Hydrocodone bitartrate 2.5 mg, acetaminophen 167 mg/5 mL, alcohol 7%. Bot.
 473 mL. **Tab.:** Hydrocodone bitartrate
 5 mg, 7.5 mg, 10 mg, acetaminophen
 325 mg, 500 mg, 650 mg, 660 mg,
 750 mg. Tab. Bot. 30s, 60s, 90s, 120s
 (10 mg/500 mg only); 100s; 500s;
 1,000s (except 10 mg/500 mg and
 10 mg/750 mg); UD 100s. *c-III.*
 Use: Analgesic combination, narcotic.
**hydrocodone bitartrate and homatro-
pine methylbromide.** (Alpharma)
 Hydrocodone bitartrate 5 mg, homatropine methylbromide 1.5 mg per 5 mL.
 Methylparaben, saccharin, sucrose.
 Cherry flavor. Syrup. 473 mL, 3785 mL.
 c-III.
 Use: Antitussive combination.
hydrocodone bitartrate and ibuprofen.
 (Qualitest) Hydrocodone bitartrate/ibu-
 profen 7.5 mg/200 mg, 10 mg/200 mg.
 Film-coated. Tab. 10, 100s, 500s
 (7.5 mg/200 mg only), 1000s. *c-III.*
 Use: Narcotic analgesic.
hydrocodone bitartrate and ibuprofen.
 (Breckenridge) Hydrocodone bitartrate
 7.5 mg, ibuprofen 200 mg. PEG, polydextrose. Aqueous film coated. Tab.
 100s. *c-III.*
 Use: Narcotic analgesic.
hydrocodone bitartrate and ibuprofen.
 (Teva) Hydrocodone bitartrate 7.5 mg, ibuprofen 200 mg, lactose. Tab. 100s. *c-III.*
 Use: Narcotic analgesic.

**hydrocodone bitartrate 5 mg/pseudo-
ephedrine hydrochloride 30 mg/
carbinoxamine maleate 2 mg.** (URL)
 Hydrocodone bitartrate 5 mg, carbinoxamine maleate 2 mg, pseudoephedrine hydrochloride 30 mg per 5 mL. Alcohol free. Liq. Bot. 473 mL. *c-III.*
 Use: Upper respiratory combination, antitussive, antihistamine, decongestant.
**hydrocodone bitartrate/homatropine
methylbromide.** (Pharmaceutical Associates) Hydrocodone bitartrate 5 mg,
 homatropine methylbromide 1.5 mg.
 Alcohol < 0.1%, glycerin, parabens,
 sorbitol, sugar. Cherry flavor. Syr. UD
 5 mL. *c-III.*
 Use: Upper respiratory combination, antitussive combination.
**hydrocodone bitartrate, phenylephrine
hydrochloride, chlorpheniramine
maleate.** (Cypress) Hydrocodone bitartrate 1.67 mg, phenylephrine hydrochloride 5 mg, chlorpheniramine
 maleate 2 mg/5 mL. Syr. Bot. Pt, gal.
 c-III.
 Use: Decongestant, antihistamine, antitussive.
•**hydrocodone bitartrate tablets.** (hye-
 droe-KOE-done) *USP 34.*
 Tall Man: HYDROcodone
 Use: Analgesic, narcotic.
hydrocodone comp. syrup. (Various
 Mfr.) Hydrocodone bitartrate 5 mg, homatropine methylbromide 1.5 mg. Bot.
 473 mL, gal. *c-III.*
 Use: Antitussive.
Hydrocodone CP. (Morton Grove)
 Hydrocodone bitartrate 2.5 mg, phenylephrine hydrochloride 5 mg, chlorpheniramine maleate 2 mg per 5 mL.
 Saccharin, sorbitol, fruit flavor, alcohol
 free. Syr. Bot. 237 mL, 473 mL. *c-III.*
 Use: Upper respiratory combination, antitussive, antihistamine, decongestant.
Hydrocodone GF. (Morton Grove Pharmaceuticals) Hydrocodone bitartrate
 5 mg, guaifenesin 100 mg per 5 mL.
 Saccharin, sorbitol, fruit flavor. Alcohol,
 sugar, and dye free. Syrup. Bot.
 237 mL, 473 mL. *c-III.*
 Use: Upper respiratory combination, antitussive, expectorant.
Hydrocodone HD. (Morton Grove)
 Hydrocodone bitartrate 1.67 mg,
 phenylephrine hydrochloride 5 mg,
 chlorpheniramine maleate 2 mg per
 5 mL. Sugar, menthol, parabens, cherry
 flavor, alcohol free. Liq. Bot. 236 mL,
 473 mL. *c-III.*
 Use: Upper respiratory combination, antihistamine, decongestant, antitussive.

•**hydrocodone polistirex.** (high-droe-KOE-dohn pahl-ee-STIE-rex) USAN.
Tall Man: HYDROcodone
Use: Antitussive.
W/Chlorpheniramine Maleate.
See: Tussionex Pennkinetic.
hydrocodone resin complex.
Use: Antitussive.
W/Phenyltoloxamine Resin Complex.
See: Tussionex.
hydrocodone w/acetaminophen.
Use: Analgesic combination, narcotic.
See: Alor 5/500.
  Anexsia 10/660.
  Lortab.
  Vicodin.
hydrocodone w/acetaminophen. (Pharmics) Hydrocodone bitartrate 7.5 mg, acetaminophen 500 mg. Tab. Bot. 100s, 500s. *c-III.*
Use: Analgesic combination, narcotic.
Hydrocof-HC. (Morton Grove) Hydrocodone bitartrate 3 mg, chlorpheniramine maleate 2 mg, pseudoephedrine hydrochloride 15 mg per 5 mL. Sugar, alcohol, and dye free. Saccharin, sorbitol. Grape flavor. Liq. 473 mL. *c-III.*
Use: Antitussive combination.
hydrocortamate hydrochloride. 17-Hydroxycorticosterone-21-diethylaminoacetate hydrochloride.
Use: Anti-inflammatory, topical.
•**hydrocortisone.** (HIGH-droe-CORE-tih-sone) *USP 34.*
Use: Anti-inflammatory, topical; corticosteroid, topical.
See: Acticort Lotion 100.
  Alphaderm.
  Balneol For Her.
  Caldecort.
  Cetacort.
  Colocort.
  Cort-Dome.
  Cortef.
  Cortizone for Kids.
  Cortizone-10.
  Cortizone-10 External Anal Itch.
  Cortizone-10 Plus.
  Cortizone-10 Quickshot.
  Cortril.
  Delacort.
  Dermacort.
  Dermolate.
  Dermol HC.
  Eldecort.
  HC Derma-Pax.
  Hi-Cor 1.0.
  Hi-Cor 2.5.
  Hycort.
  Hycortole.
  Hydrocortone.

  Hydroskin.
  Hytone.
  Ivy Soothe.
  Ivy Stat.
  My Cort.
  Proctocort.
  proctoCream•HC 2.5%.
  Scalacort.
  Scalpicin.
  Signef.
  Synacort.
  Texacort.
  T/Scalp.
  Xolegel CorePak.
W/Acyclovir.
  See: Xerese.
W/Benzalkonium Chloride, Chloroxylenol, Pramoxine Hydrochloride.
  See: Cortic-ND.
  Mediotic-HC.
W/Benzoyl Peroxide.
  See: Bencort.
  Vanoxide HC.
W/Chloroxylenol, Pramoxine Hydrochloride.
  See: Oto-End 10.
  Zoto-HC.
W/Clioquinol, Pramoxine Hydrochloride.
  See: 1 + 1-F Creme.
W/Combinations.
  See: AnaMantle HC.
  Carmol HC.
  Cipro HC.
  Cortane-B.
  Cortef.
  Cortisporin.
  Cortisporin-TC.
  Doak Oil Forte.
  Fostril HC.
  Hysone.
  Kleer.
  Neo-Cort Dome.
  Neo Cort Top.
  Nutracort.
  1 + 1.
  Oti-Med.
  Oto.
  Otomar-HC.
  Pyocidin-Otic.
  Rectal Medicone-HC.
  Terra-Cortril.
  Vanoxide-HC.
  Vytone.
W/Diphenhydramine Hydrochloride, Nystatin.
  See: First Duke's Mouthwash.
W/Diphenhydramine Hydrochloride, Nystatin, Tetracycline Hydrochloride.
  See: First Mary's Mouthwash.
hydrocortisone. (Pharmacia) Micronized nonsterile powder for prescription compounding.

Use: Anti-inflammatory, topical; corticosteroid, topical.

hydrocortisone. (Various Mfr.) Hydrocortisone 2.5%, may contain stearyl
alcohol, cetyl alcohol, light mineral oil.
Lot. Bot. 59 mL. *Rx.*
Use: Anti-inflammatory, corticosteroid,
topical.

hydrocortisone. (Various Mfr.) Hydrocortisone 5 mg. May contain lactose.
Tab. 10s, 50s, 100s, 1000s. *Rx.*
Use: Adrenocortical steroid, glucocorticoid.

•**hydrocortisone acetate.** (HYE-droe-
KOR-ti-sone) *USP 34.*
Use: Glucocorticoid.
See: AlcortinA.
Anucort-HC.
Anuprep HC.
Anusol-HC.
Caldecort.
Caldecort Light.
Cortifoam.
Cortril Acetate.
Gynecort.
Hemril-HC Uniserts.
Hydrocort.
Hydrocortone Acetate.
Hydrosone.
Keratol HC.
Maximum Strength Corticaine.
Maximum Strength Dermarest Dri-
cort.
Novacort.
NuCort.
Pramosone Cream.
Proctocort.
Tucks Ointment.
U-cort.
W/Benzocaine, Chloroxylenol.
See: TriOxin.
W/Combinations.
See: AnaMantle HC 2.5%.
Anusol-HC.
Carmol HC.
Coly-Mycin S Otic Drops w/Neomycin
and Hydrocortisone.
Cortaid.
Cortisporin-TC.
Derma Medicone-HC.
Epifoam.
Furacin HC.
Neo-Cortef.
Otomar-HC.
Rectal Medicone-HC.
Wyanoids HC.
W/Iodoquinol.
See: Hydro-Iodoquinol 2-1.
W/Lidocaine.
See: Lida-Mantle HC.
Lida-Mantle HC Relief.

LidoCort.
Xyralid.
Xyralid RC.
W/Pramoxine Hydrochloride.
See: Analpram-E.
EndaRoid.
HC Pram 1%
HC Pramoxine.
HC Pram 2.5%.
Pramosone E.
Proctofoam-HC.
Zypram.

hydrocortisone acetate. (Pharmacia)
Micronized nonsterile powder for prescription compounding.
Use: Anti-inflammatory, topical; corticosteroid, topical.

hydrocortisone acetate. (Various Mfr.)
Hydrocortisone acetate 25 mg. Supp.
12s, 24s. *Rx.*
Use: Anorectal preparation.

**hydrocortisone acetate maximum
strength.** (Clay-Park) Hydrocortisone
acetate 1% (equiv. to hydrocortisone
10 mg/g), aloe extract, white petrolatum. Oint. Tube 28 g. *OTC.*
Use: Anti-inflammatory, corticosteroid,
topical.

**hydrocortisone acetate 2.5% with
pramoxine hydrochloride 1%.** (Brookstone) Hydrocortisone acetate 2.5%,
pramoxine hydrochloride 1%. Cetostearyl alcohol, lanolin alcohol, mineral
oil, parabens, PEG-40, white petrolatum. Cream. 4 g. *Rx.*
Use: Topical corticosteroid, corticosteroid combination.

hydrocortisone acetate with aloe. (Riv-
er's Edge) Hydrocortisone acetate 2%.
Aloe, benzyl alcohol, camphor, cetyl
alcohol, dimethicone, glycerin, menthol,
PEG-7, triethanolamine. Lot. 59.14 mL.
Rx.
Use: Anti-inflammatory agent, topical
corticosteroid.

hydrocortisone and acetic acid. (Taro)
Hydrocortisone 1%, acetic acid 2%,
propylene glycol diacetate 3%, sodium
acetate 0.015%, benzethonium chloride 0.02%. Citric acid 0.2%. Otic Soln.
10 mL dropper tip bottle. *Rx.*
Use: Otic preparation.

**hydrocortisone and acetic acid otic so-
lution.**
Use: Anti-inflammatory, otic.

hydrocortisone and iodoquinol 1%.
(Various Mfr.) Hydrocortisone 1%, iodoquinol 1%, may contain cetearyl alcohol, EDTA. Cream. Tube 30 g. *Rx.*
Use: Anti-inflammatory, corticosteroid,
topical.

• **hydrocortisone butyrate.** (HIGH-droe-CORE-tih-sone) *USP 34.*
Use: Corticosteroid, topical.
See: Locoid.

hydrocortisone butyrate. (Taro) Hydrocortisone butyrate. **Cream:** 0.1%. 5 g, 10 g, 15 g, 30 g, 45 g. **Oint.:** 0.1%. 5 g, 10 g, 15 g, 30 g, 45 g. **Soln.:** 0.1%. Isopropyl alcohol 50%, glycerin. 20 mL, 60 mL. *Rx.*
Use: Anti-inflammatory agent.

• **hydrocortisone cypionate.** (HIGH-droe-CORE-tih-sone) *USP 34.* Oral Susp.
Use: Corticosteroid, topical.

hydrocortisone diethylaminoacetate hydrochloride.
See: Hydrocortamate.

• **hydrocortisone hemisuccinate.** (HIGH-droe-CORE-tih-sone hem-ih-SUCK-sih-nate) *USP 34.*
Use: Adrenocortical steroid.

hydrocortisone intravenous.
See: A-Hydro Cort.
Solu-Cortef.

hydrocortisone/iodochlorhydroxyquin. (Various Mfr.) **Cream:** Hydrocortisone 0.5%, 3%, iodochlorhydroxyquin 3%. 15 g, 30 g, 480 g. **Oint.:** Hydrocortisone 1%, iodochlorhydroxyquin 3%. 20 g, 30 g. *Rx-OTC.*
Use: Corticosteroid, topical.

hydrocortisone-neomycin. (Various Mfr.) Hydrocortisone 1%, neomycin sulfate 0.5%. Oint. 20 g. *Rx-OTC.*
Use: Corticosteroid, topical.

hydrocortisone phosphate.
See: Hydrocortone Phosphate.

• **hydrocortisone probutate.** (HYE-droe-KOR-ti-sone proe-BUE-tate) USAN.
Use: Atopic dermatitis (glucocorticoid).
See: Pandel.

• **hydrocortisone sodium phosphate.** (HIGH-droe-CORE-tih-sone) *USP 34.*
Use: Adrenocortical steroid (anti-inflammatory); corticosteroid, topical.

• **hydrocortisone sodium succinate.** (HIGH-droe-CORE-tih-sone) *USP 34.*
Use: Adrenocortical steroid (anti-inflammatory); corticosteroid, topical.
See: A-hydroCort.
Solu-Cortef.

• **hydrocortisone valerate.** (HIGH-droe-CORE-tih-sone VAL-eh-rate) *USP 34.*
Use: Corticosteroid, topical.
See: Westcort.

hydrocortisone valerate. (Copley) Hydrocortisone valerate 0.2% in hydrophilic base, white petrolatum, alcohol. Cream. Tube 15 g, 45 g, 60 g. *Rx.*
Use: Corticosteroid, topical.

hydrocortisone valerate. (Taro) Hydrocortisone valerate 0.2% in hydrophilic base, white petrolatum, alcohol, mineral oil. Oint. Tube 15 g, 45 g, 60 g. *Rx.*
Use: Corticosteroid, topical.

hydrocortisone with aloe. (G & W Labs) Hydrocortisone 1%. Aloe, mineral oil, white petrolatum, parabens. Oint. 28.4 g. *OTC.*
Use: Anti-inflammatory agent.

Hydrocortone Acetate Saline Suspension. (Merck & Co.) Hydrocortisone acetate 25 mg, 50 mg/mL, sodium Cl 9 mg, polysorbate 80 4 mg, sodium carboxymethylcellulose 5 mg/mL, benzyl alcohol 9 mg q.s. water for injection to 1 mL. Vial 5 mL. *Rx.*
Use: Corticosteroid.

Hydrocortone Tablets. (Merck & Co.) Hydrocortisone 10 mg, 20 mg. Bot. 100s. *Rx.*
Use: Corticosteroid.

Hydrocream Base. (Paddock) Petrolatum, mineral oil, woolwax alcohol, imidazolidinyl urea, methyl- and propylparabens. Cream. Jar lb.
Use: Emollient.

HydroDIURIL. (Merck) Hydrochlorothiazide 25 mg. Lactose. Tab. Bot. 100s, 1000s. *Rx.*
Use: Diuretic.

Hydro-D Tablets. (Halsey Drug) Hydrochlorothiazide. 25 mg, 50 mg. Tab. Bot. 1000s. *Rx.*
Use: Diuretic.

Hydro-Ergot. (Henry Schein) Hydrogenated ergot alkaloids 0.5 mg, 1 mg. Tab. Bot. 100s. *Rx.*
Use: Psychotherapeutic agent.

• **hydrofilcon A.** (HIGH-droe-FILL-kahn A) USAN.
Use: Contact lens material (hydrophilic).

• **hydroflumethiazide.** (HIGH-droe-flew-meth-EYE-ah-zide) *USP 34.*
Use: Antihypertensive; diuretic.

Hydro 40. (Quinnova) Urea 40%. Glycerin, parabens. Aerosol Foam. 70 g. *Rx.*
Use: Emollient.

hydrogen dioxide.
See: Hydrogen Peroxide.

hydrogen iodide.
Use: Expectorant.
See: Hydriodic Acid.

• **hydrogen peroxide concentrate.** (HIGH-droe-jen per-OX-ide) *USP 34.*
Use: Anti-infective, topical.

hydrogen peroxide solution 30%. Perhydrol, hydrogen peroxide. Bot. 0.25 lb, 0.5 lb, 1 lb.

Use: Dentistry, preparing the 3% solution.

hydrogen peroxide topical solution. (Various Mfr.) Hydrogen peroxide (3%). Bot. 4 oz, 8 oz, pt.
Use: Anti-infective, topical.

Hydrogesic. (Edwards) Hydrocodone bitartrate 5 mg, acetaminophen 500 mg. Cap. Bot. 100s. *c-III.*
Use: Analgesic combination, narcotic.

Hydro-Iodoquinol 2-1. (Seton Pharmaceuticals) Hydrocortisone acetate 2%, iodoquinol 1%. Aloe polysaccharide 1%, amino methylpropanol 95%, benzyl alcohol, glycerin, glyceryl, propylene glycol, SD alcohol. Gel. Packettes. 2 g. *Rx.*
Use: Anti-inflammatory agent, topical corticosteroid.

Hydroloid-G Sublingual. (Major) Ergoloid mesylates 0.5 mg, 1 mg. Tab. Bot. 100s, 250s, 500s (0.5 mg only), 1000s (1 mg only), UD 100s. *Rx.*
Use: Psychotherapeutic agent.

Hydroloid-G Tabs. (Major) Ergoloid mesylates 1 mg. Tab. Bot. 100s, 250s, 1000s, UD 100s. *Rx.*
Use: Psychotherapeutic agent.

Hydromet. (Alpharma) Hydrocodone bitartrate 5 mg, homatropine methylbromide 1.5 mg per 5 mL. Saccharin, sucrose, methylparaben, cherry flavor. Syr. Bot. 473 mL, 3.8 L. *c-III.*
Use: Upper respiratory combination, antitussive combination.

Hydromide. (Major) Hydrocodone bitartrate 5 mg, homatropine methylbromide 1.5 mg per 5 mL. Alcohol < 0.1%, cherry flavor. Syrup. Bot. 473 mL. *c-III.*
Use: Upper respiratory combination, antitussive combination.

hydromorphone. *c-II.*
Tall Man: HYDROmorphone
Use: Analgesic, narcotic.

•**hydromorphone hydrochloride.** (HIGH-droe-MORE-phone) *USP 34. Formerly Dihydromorphinone Hydrochloride.*
Tall Man: HYDROmorphone
Use: Opioid analgesic.
See: Dilaudid.
  Dilaudid-HP.

hydromorphone hydrochloride. (Paddock) Hydromorphone hydrochloride 3 mg. Supp. Box 6s. *c-II.*
Use: Opioid analgesic.

hydromorphone hydrochloride. (Various Mfr.) Hydromorphone hydrochloride. **Tab.:** 2 mg, 4 mg, 8 mg. Bot. 100s, UD 25s (except 8 mg), UD 100s. **Inj., Soln.:** 1 mg/mL, 2 mg/mL, 4 mg/mL. Prefilled syringes. 1 mL. Vials

(2 mg/mL only). 1 mL, 20 mL. **Inj., Soln., Conc.:** 10 mg/mL. Single-dose vials. 1 mL, 5 mL, 50 mL. **Liq.:** 1 mg/ 1 mL. UD patient cups. 4 mL, 8 mL. Bot. 250 mL. *c-II.*
Use: Opioid analgesic.

hydromorphone sulfate.
Use: Analgesic, narcotic.

Hydropane. (Watson) Hydrocodone bitartrate 5 mg, homatropine methylbromide 1.5 mg per 5 mL. Parabens, sucrose, cherry flavor. Syrup. Bot. 473 mL, 3.8 L. *c-III.*
Use: Upper respiratory combination, antitussive combination.

Hydro-Par. (Parmed) Hydrochlorothiazide 25 mg, 50 mg. Tab. 1000s, 5000s (50 mg only). *Rx.*
Use: Diuretic.

Hydropel. (C & M Pharmacal) Silicone 30%, hydrophobic starch derivative 10%, petrolatum. Jar 2 oz, lb. *OTC.*
Use: Emollient.

Hydrophed. (Rugby) Theophylline 130 mg, ephedrine sulfate 25 mg, hydroxyzine hydrochloride 10 mg. Tab. Bot. 100s, 1000s. *Rx.*
Use: Antiasthmatic combination.

hydrophilic ointment. (E. Fougera) Stearyl alcohol, white petrolatum, propylene glycol, sodium lauryl sulfate, water. Jar lb.
Use: Pharmaceutic aid, ointment base.

hydrophilic ointment base. (Emerson) Oil in water emulsion bases. 1 lb.
Use: Pharmaceutic aid, ointment base.
See: Aquaphilic.
  Cetaphil.
  Dermovan.
  Lanaphilic.
  Polysorb.
  Unibase.

Hydropine. (Rugby) Hydroflumethiazide 25 mg, reserpine 0.125 mg. Tab. Bot. 100s. *Rx.*
Use: Antihypertensive combination.

Hydropine H.P. Tablets. (Rugby) Hydroflumethiazide 50 mg, reserpine 0.125 mg. Bot. 100s, 500s, 1000s. *Rx.*
Use: Antihypertensive combination.

•**hydroquinone.** (high-DROE-KWIN-ohn) *USP 34.*
Use: Depigmentor.
See: Aclaro PD.
  Artra Skin Tone, Cream.
  Black and White Bleaching.
  Eldopaque.
  Eldopaque Forte.
  Eldoquin Forte.
  EpiQuin Micro.
  Esoterica.

Glyquin.
Lustra.
Lustra-AF.
Melpaque HP.
Melquin HP.
Nuquin HP.
Solaquin.
W/Combinations.
See: Tri-Luma.
hydroquinone. (Glades) Hydroquinone.
Gel: 3%, 4%. Padimate O, dioxybenzone, EDTA, sodium metabisulfite, alcohol (4% only), hydroalcoholic base. 30 g (3% only), 28.35 g (4% only).
Soln.: 3%, SD Alcohol 40-B, isopropyl alcohol. 29 mL with applicator. *Rx.*
Use: Depigmentor.
hydroquinone. (River's Edge) Hydroquinone 4%. Benzyl alcohol, cetyl alcohol, EDTA. Emulsion, Top. 48 g. *Rx.*
Use: Depigmentor.
hydroquinone. (Various Mfr.) Hydroquinone 4%. May contain EDTA, parabens, mineral oil, sodium metabisulfite. Cream 28.35 g. *Rx.*
Use: Depigmentor.
hydroquinone monobenzyl ether.
See: Benoquin.
hydroquinone with sunscreen. (Various Mfr.) Hydroquinone 4%. May contain padimate O, dioxybenzone, oxybenzone, octyl methoxycinnamate, octyl dimethyl-p-aminobenzoate, cetearyl alcohol, vitamin E, parabens, mineral oil, stearyl alcohol, lactic acid, EDTA, sodium metabisulfite. Cream 28.35 g. *Rx.*
Use: Depigmentor.
Hydrosal. (Hydrosal Co.) Aluminum acetate 5%. **Susp.:** Bot. 16 oz, gal. **Oint.:** 54 g, 113.4 g, Jar 54 g, 454 g. *OTC.*
Use: Astringent.
Hydrosine 50. (Major) Hydrochlorothiazide 50 mg, reserpine 0.125 mg. Tab. Bot. 100s. *Rx.*
Use: Antihypertensive combination.
Hydrosine 25. (Major) Hydrochlorothiazide 25 mg, reserpine 0.125 mg. Tab. Bot. 100s. Tartrazine. *Rx.*
Use: Antihypertensive combination.
HydroSKIN. (Rugby) Hydrocortisone 1%.
Cream: Mineral oil, lanolin alcohol, cetyl alcohol, parabens. Tube 113.4 g.
Lot.: Cetyl alcohol, parabens. Bot. 118 mL. *OTC.*
Use: Anti-inflammatory, corticosteroid, topical.
Hydrosone. (Sigma-Tau) Hydrocortisone acetate 25 mg, 50 mg, lactose/mL. Vial 5 mL. *Rx.*
Use: Corticosteroid.

Hydro-T. (Major) Hydrochlorothiazide 25 mg, 50 mg, 100 mg. Tab. Bot. 100s, 250s (100 mg only), 1000s, UD 100s. *Rx.*
Use: Diuretic.
Hydrotensin. (Merz) Hydrochlorothiazide 50 mg, reserpine 0.125 mg. Tab. Bot. 100s, 1000s. *Rx.*
Use: Antihypertensive combination.
Hydro 35. (Quinnova) Urea 35%. Dimethicone, glycerin, lactic acid, parabens. Aer. Foam. 150 g. *Rx.*
Use: Emollient.
Hydro-12. (Table Rock) Crystalline hydroxocobalamin 1000 mcg/mL. Pkg. 10 mL. *Rx.*
Use: Vitamin supplement.
• **hydroxocobalamin.** (high-DROX-oh-koe-BAL-ah-meen) *USP 34.*
Use: Treatment of megaloblastic anemia; vitamin (hematopoietic); detoxification agent, antidote.
See: Cyanokit.
• **hydroxyamphetamine hydrobromide.** (high-DROX-ee-am-FET-uh-meen) *USP 34.*
Use: Adrenergic (ophthalmic); mydriatic.
2-hydroxybenzamide.
See: Salicylamide.
hydroxy bis (acetato-O) aluminum.
Aluminum Subacetate.
hydroxy bis (salicylato) aluminum diacetate.
See: Aluminum Aspirin.
hydroxybutyrate, sodium/gamma.
See: Sodium Gamma-Hydroxybutyrate Acid.
• **hydroxychloroquine sulfate.** (high-drox-ee-KLOR-oh-kwin) *USP 34.*
Use: Antimalarial; lupus erythematosus suppressant; antirheumatic agent.
hydroxycholecalciferol. (D_3).
Use: Antihypocalcemia.
See: Calcifediol.
• **hydroxyethyl cellulose.** (high-drox-ee-ETH-ill SELL-you-lohs) *NF 29.*
Use: Pharmaceutic aid (suspending, viscosity-increasing agent).
hydroxyethyl starch. (hye-DROX-ee-ETH-il stahrch) USAN. (HES).
Use: Plasma volume expander; prevention of hypervolemia.
See: Hespan.
Voluven.
hydroxyisoindolin. Under study.
Use: Antihypertensive.
hydroxymagnesium aluminate.
Use: Antacid.
See: Magaldrate.

hydroxymycin. An antibiotic substance obtained from cultures of *Streptomyces paucisporogenes.*
●**hydroxyphenamate.** (high-DROX-ee-FEN-ah-mate) USAN.
Use: Anxiolytic.
4-hydroxyphenylpyruvate dioxygenase inhibitor.
Use: Tyrosinemia.
See: Nitisinone.
●**hydroxyprogesterone caproate.** (hye-DROX-ee-proe-JES-ter-one KAP-roe-ate) USP 34.
Use: Sex hormone, progestin.
See: Makena.
●**hydroxypropyl cellulose.** (high-drox-ee-PRO-pill SELL-you-lohs) NF 29.
Use: Topical protectant; pharmaceutic aid, emulsifying tablet-coating agent.
hydroxypropyl methylcellulose.
See: Goniosoft.
Hypromellose.
●**hydroxypropyl methylcellulose phthalate.** (high-drox-ee-PRO-pill) NF 29.
Use: Pharmaceutic aid (coating agent).
See: Hypromellose Phthalate.
hydroxypropyl methylcellulose phthalate 200731.
Use: Pharmaceutic aid (coating agent).
hydroxypropyl methylcellulose phthalate 220824.
Use: Pharmaceutic aid (coating agent).
hydroxystearin sulfate. Sulfonate hydrogenated castor oil.
L-5-hydroxytryptophan. (Circa) L-5HTP.
Use: Postanoxic intention myoclonus. [Orphan Drug]
●**hydroxyurea.** (high-DROX-ee-you-REE-uh) USP 34.
Use: Antineoplastic; sickle cell disease.
See: Droxia.
Hydrea.
hydroxyurea. (Various Mfr.) Hydroxyurea 500 mg. Cap. Bot. 100s, UD 100s. Rx.
Use: Antineoplastic.
●**hydroxyzine.** (high-DROX-ih-zeen) USP 34.
Tall Man: hydrOXYzine
Use: Anxiolytic; antihistamine, nonselective piperazine.
See: Vistaril.
W/Ephedrine Sulfate, Theophylline.
See: Marax.
Marax DF.
Theo-Drox.
hydroxyzine. (Various Mfr.) Hydroxyzine. **Tab.:** 10 mg, 25 mg, 50 mg. Bot. 100s, 500s, 1000s. **Syrup:** 10 mg/5 mL. May contain alcohol. 118 mL,

473 mL. Rx.
Use: Antihistamine, nonselective piperazine; anxiolytic.
hydroxyzine hydrochloride. (Various Mfr.) Hydroxyzine hydrochloride 25 mg/mL, 50 mg/mL. May contain benzyl alcohol. Vials. 1 mL, 2 mL, 10 mL (50 mg/mL only). Rx.
Use: Antihistamine.
●**hydroxyzine pamoate.** (hye-DROX-i-zeen PAM-oh-ate) USP 34.
Tall Man: hydrOXYzine
Use: Tranquilizer (minor); antihistamine.
See: Vistaril.
hydroxyzine pamoate. (Various Mfr.) Hydroxyzine pamoate 25 mg, 50 mg, 100 mg (equivalent to hydrochloride). Cap. 100s, 500s, 1000s, UD 100s (except 100 mg). Rx.
Use: Antihistamine, nonselective piperazine; anxiolytic.
Hydro-Z-50. (Merz) Hydrochlorothiazide 50 mg. Tab. Bot. 100s, 1000s. Rx.
Use: Diuretic.
Hy-Flow Solution. (Ciba Vision) Polyvinyl alcohol with hydroxyethylcellulose, benzalkonium Cl, EDTA. Bot. 60 mL. OTC.
Use: Contact lens care.
HyGel. (Aletheia) Sodium hyaluronate 0.2%. Parabens. Gel. 340 mL. Rx.
Use: Physical adjunct; hyaluronic acid derivative, dermal.
Hygienic Cleansing. (Rugby) Witch hazel 50%, glycerin, benzalkonium Cl, methylparaben. Pads 100s. OTC.
Use: Anorectal preparation.
hylan polymers.
See: Synvisc.
Synvisc-One.
Hylatopic. (Onset Therapeutics) Cetearyl alcohol, disodium EDTA, glycerin, petrolatum, parabens, theobroma gradiflorum seed butter. Foam. 100 g. Rx.
Use: Emollient.
Hylenex. (Baxter Anesthesia) Hyaluronidase (recombinant human) 150 units/mL. Sodium chloride 8.5 mg, sodium phosphate dibasic dihydrate 1.8 mg, sodium hydroxide 4.2 mg, human serum albumin 1 mg, EDTA 1 mg, calcium chloride dihydrate 0.4 mg. Soln. for Inj. Single-dose vials. 1 mL. Rx.
Use: Physical adjunct.
Hylidone. (Major) Chlorthalidone. Tab. **25 mg, 50 mg:** Bot. 100s, 250s, 1000s, UD 100s. **100 mg:** Bot. 100s, 250s, 500s, 1000s. Rx.
Use: Diuretic.
Hylira. (Hawthorn) Hyaluronic acid 0.2%. Parabens. Top. Gel. 113 g, 340 g. Rx.
Use: Physical adjunct.

Hyliver Plus. (Hyrex) Folic acid 0.4 mg, liver 10 mcg, vitamin B_{12} 100 mcg/mL. Vial 10 mL with phenol. *Rx.*
Use: Vitamin supplement.
•**hymecromone.** (HIGH-meh-KROE-mone) USAN.
Use: Choleretic.
hymenoptera venom/venom protein. Purified venoms of honeybee, wasp, white faced hornet, yellow hornet, yellow jacket, and mixed vespids (both hornets and yellow jackets). *Rx.*
Use: Allergenic extract.
See: Albay.
Venomil.
HY-N.B.P. Ointment. (Jones Pharma) Bacitracin zinc 400 units, neomycin sulfate 5 mg, polymyxin B sulfate 10,000 units/g. Tube ⅛ oz. *Rx.*
Use: Anti-infective, topical.
HyoMax. (Aristos) Hyoscyamine sulfate 0.125 mg. Lactose, mannitol. Tab. 100s. *Rx.*
Use: Gastrointestinal anticholinergic/ antispasmodic, belladonna alkaloid.
HyoMax-FT. (Aristos) Hyoscyamine sulfate 125 mg. Lactose, mannitol. Mint flavor. Tab. 100s. *Rx.*
Use: Gastrointestinal anticholinergic/ antispasmodic, belladonna alkaloid.
hyoscine hydrobromide. Scopolamine HBr.
Use: Antispasmodic.
W/Combinations.
See: Phenazopyridine Plus.
Pyridium Plus.
W/Butalbital, Phenazopyridine Hydrochloride.
See: PhenazoForte Plus.
•**hyoscyamine.** (high-oh-SIGH-ah-meen) *USP 34.*
Use: Anticholinergic.
See: Cystospaz.
hyoscyamine-atropine-hyoscine.
Use: Anticholinergic.
See: Atropine w/hyoscyamine w/hyoscine.
•**hyoscyamine hydrobromide.** (HYE-oh-SYE-a-meen) *USP 34.*
Use: Anticholinergic.
W/Atropine Sulfate, Phenobarbital, Scopolamine Hydrobromide.
See: PB-Hyos.
W/Combinations.
See: Phenazopyridine Plus.
hyoscyamine hydrochloride. (Various Mfr.)
hyoscyamine salts.
Use: Anticholinergic.
W/Atropine salts.
See: Atropine w/hyoscyamine.

•**hyoscyamine sulfate.** (HYE-oh-SYE-a-meen) *USP 34.*
Use: Anticholinergic.
See: Cystospaz.
ED-Spaz.
HyoMax.
HyoMax-FT.
IB-Stat.
Levbid.
Levsin.
Levsinex Timecaps.
Levsin/SL.
Mar-Spas.
Neosol.
NuLev.
Symax Duotab.
Symax FasTab.
Symax-SL.
Symax-SR.
W/Amylase, Cellulase, Lipase, Phenytoloxamine Citrate, Protease.
See: Digex.
W/Atropine Sulfate, Benzoic Acid, Methenamine, Methylene Blue, Phenyl Salicylate.
See: Uritact DS.
W/Atropine Sulfate, Chlorpheniramine Maleate, Phenylephrine Hydrochloride, Scopolamine Hydrobromide.
See: Bellahist-D LA.
W/Atropine Sulfate, Chlorpheniramine Maleate, Pseudoephedrine Hydrochloride, Scopolamine Hydrobromide.
See: Stahist.
W/Atropine Sulfate, Phenobarbital, Scopolamine Hydrobromide.
See: Antispasmodic.
Donnatal.
Donnatal Extentabs.
PB-Hyos.
Quadrapax.
W/Methenamine, Methylene Blue, Phenyl Salicylate, Sodium Biphosphate.
See: Urimax.
W/Methenamine, Methylene Blue, Phenyl Salicylate, Sodium Phosphate Monobasic.
See: Uticap.
Ultrona-C.
W/Phenyltoloxamine Citrate.
See: Digex NF.
hyoscyamine sulfate. (Ethex) Hyoscyamine sulfate 0.375 mg. ER Cap. Bot. 100s. *Rx.*
Use: Anticholinergic.
hyoscyamine sulfate. (Franklin Pharmaceuticals) Hyoscyamine sulfate 0.125 mg. Lactose, mannitol. Tab. 100s. *Rx.*
Use: Gastrointestinal anticholinergic/ antispasmodic, belladonna alkaloid.

hyoscyamine sulfate. (Goldline) Hyoscyamine sulfate 0.125 mg/mL, alcohol 5%. Soln. Bot. with dropper. 15 mL. *Rx.*
Use: Anticholinergic.

hyoscyamine sulfate. (River's Edge Pharmaceuticals) Hyoscyamine sulfate 0.125 mg (immediate release), hyoscyamine 0.25 mg (controlled release). Tab. 90s. *Rx.*
Use: Gastrointestinal anticholinergic/ antispasmodic, belladonna alkaloid.

hyoscyamine sulfate. (Various Mfr.) Hyoscyamine sulfate. **ER Tab.:** 0.375 mg. Bot. 100s, 1,000s. **Sublingual Tab.:** 0.125 mg. 100s. **TR Cap.:** 0.375 mg. Bot. 100s. *Rx.*
Use: Anticholinergic.

hyoscyamine sulfate. (Vision Pharma) Hyoscyamine sulfate 0.125 mg. Aspartame, mannitol, phenylalanine 2.2 mg. Mint flavor. Tab. 90s, 100s. *Rx.*
Use: Gastrointestinal anticholinergic/ antispasmodic, belladonna alkaloid.

hyoscyamus extract.
W/A.P.C.
See: Valacet Junior.
W/A.P.C., gelsemium extract.
See: Valacet.

hyoscyamus products and phenobarbital combinations.
Use: Anticholinergic, sedative.
See: Anaspaz PB.
Donnatal.
Elixiral.

Hyosophen Elixir. (Rugby) Atropine sulfate 0.0194 mg, scopolamine HBr 0.0065 mg, hyoscyamine HBr or sulfate 0.1037 mg, phenobarbital 16.2 mg, alcohol 23%, sugar, sorbitol. Bot. 120 mL, pt, gal. *Rx.*
Use: Gastrointestinal, anticholinergic.

Hyosophen Tablets. (Rugby) Atropine sulfate 0.0194 mg, scopolamine HBr 0.0065 mg, hyoscyamine HBr or SO$_4$ 0.1037 mg, phenobarbital 16.2 mg. Bot. 1000s. *Rx.*
Use: Anticholinergic combination.

Hypaque-M 90%. (Sanofi-Synthelabo) Diatrizoate meglumine 60%, diatrizoate sodium 30%, EDTA. Vial 50 mL.
Use: Radiopaque agent.

Hypaque-M 75%. (Sanofi-Synthelabo) Diatrizoate meglumine 50%, diatrizoate sodium 25%, iodine 38.5%, EDTA. Vial 20 mL, 50 mL.
Use: Radiopaque agent.

Hypaque Oral. (Sanofi-Synthelabo)
Pow.: Diatrizoate sodium oral pow. containing iodine 600 mg/g. Can 250 g,

Bot. 10 g. **Liq.:** Soln. 41.66%. Bot. 120 mL.
Use: Radiopaque agent.

Hypaque-76. (Nycomed) Diatrizoate meglumine 660 mg, diatrizoate sodium 100 mg, iodine 370 mg/mL. EDTA. Inj. Vials. 50 mL. Bot. 200 mL. 100 mL and 150 mL in 200 mL dilution bot. *Rx.*
Use: Radiopaque agent, parenteral.

HyperHEP B S/D. (Talecris Biotherapeutics) Hepatitis B immune globulin (human) 15% to 18% protein. 0.21 to 0.32 M glycine, solvent/detergent treated, preservative free. Soln. for Inj. Single-dose vials. 1 mL, 5 mL. Neonatal single-dose syringes. 0.5 mL. Single-dose syringes. 1 mL. *Rx.*
Use: Immune globulin.

hypericin. (VIMRxyn Pharm/NIH) *Rx.*
Use: Antiviral.

hyperlipidemia, agents for.
See: Atromid-S.
Choloxin.
Clofibrate.
Colestid.
Lescol.
Lopid.
Lorelco.
Mevacor.
Pravachol.
Questran.
Questran Light.
Zocor.

Hyperlyte. (B. Braun) Sodium 25 mEq, potassium 40.5 mEq, calcium 5 mEq, magnesium 8 mEq, chloride 33.5 mEq, acetate 40.6 mEq, gluconate 5 mEq, 6050 mOsm/L. Inj. Vial 25 mL fill in 50 mL. *Rx.*
Use: Nutritional supplement, parenteral.

Hyperlyte CR. (B. Braun) Sodium 25 mEq, potassium 20 mEq, calcium 5 mEq, magnesium 5 mEq, chloride 30 mEq, acetate 30 mEq, 5500 mOsm/ L. Inj. Pharmacy bulk packaging. *Super-vial* 250 mL. *Rx.*
Use: Intravenous nutritional therapy, intravenous replenishment solution.

Hyperlyte R. (B. Braun) Sodium 25 mEq, potassium 20 mEq, calcium 5 mEq, magnesium 5 mEq, chloride 30 mEq, acetate 25 mEq, 4200 mOsm/L. Inj. Vial 25 mL fill in 50 mL. *Rx.*
Use: Nutritional supplement, parenteral.

Hypermune RSV. (MedImmune) Respiratory syncytial virus immune globulin, human.
Use: Respiratory syncytial virus treatment. [Orphan Drug]

Hyperopto 5%. (Professional Pharmacal) Sodium Cl 5%. Oint. Tube 3.5 g.

OTC.
Use: Ophthalmic.
Hyperopto Ointment. (Professional Pharmacal) Sodium hydrochloride 50 mg, D.I. water 150 mg, anhydrous lanolin 150 mg, liquid petrolatum 50 mg, white petrolatum 599 mg, methylparaben 7 mg, propylparaben 3 mg/g. Tube 3.5 g. *OTC.*
Use: Ophthalmic.
hyperosmotic agents.
Use: Laxative.
See: Cephulac.
 Cholac.
 Chronulac.
 Colace.
 Constulose.
 Duphalac.
 Enulose.
 Fleet Babylax.
 Glycerin.
 Lactulose.
 Sani-Supp.
HyperRab S/D. (Talecris Biotherapeutics) Rabies immune globulin, human, 150 units/mL. Preservative free. Glycine 0.21 to 0.32 M. Solvent/detergent treated. Inj. Single-dose vials. 2 mL, 10 mL. *Rx.*
Use: Immune globulin.
HyperRHO S/D Full Dose. (Talecris Biotherapeutics) $Rh_o(D)$ immune globulin 15% to 18% protein ($\geq$ 1,500 units). Glycine 0.21 to 0.32 M. Solvent/detergent treated. Preservative free. Inj., Soln. Single-dose syringe w/attached needle. 1s. *Rx.*
Use: Biologic and immunological agent, immune globulin.
HyperRHO S/D Mini-Dose. (Talecris Biotherapeutics) $Rh_o(D)$ immune globulin micro-dose 15% to 18% protein ($\geq$ 250 units). Glycine 0.21 to 0.32 M. Solvent/detergent treated. Preservative free. Inj., Soln. Single-dose syringe. 10s. *Rx.*
Use: Immune globulin.
hypertension diagnosis.
See: Regitine.
hypertensive emergency agents.
See: Diazoxide.
 Fenoldopam Mesylate.
 Nitroprusside Sodium.
Hyphylline. Dyphylline. *Rx.*
See: Neothylline.
hypnogene.
See: Barbital.
Hypnomidate. (Janssen) Etomidate. *Rx.*
Use: Anesthetic, general.
hypnotics.
See: Sedative/Hypnotic Agents.

"hypo".
See: Sodium thiosulfate.
Hypo-Bee. (Towne) Vitamins B_1 50 mg, B_2 20 mg, B_6 5 mg, B_{12} 15 mcg, niacinamide 25 mg, calcium pantothenate 5 mg, C 300 mg, E 200 units, iron 10 mg. Tab. Bot. 30s, 100s. *OTC.*
Use: Mineral, vitamin supplement.
hypochlorite preps.
See: Antiformin.
 Dakin's.
 Hyclorite.
Hypoclear. (Bausch & Lomb) Isotonic soln. with sodium Cl 0.9%. Aerosol soln. 240 mL, 300 mL. *OTC.*
Use: Contact lens care.
hypoglycemic agents.
See: Chlorpropamide.
 Diabeta.
 Diabinese.
 Dymelor.
 Glucotrol.
 Glynase.
 Micronase.
 Orinase.
 Phenformin Hydrochloride.
 Tolbutamide.
 Tolinase.
α-hypophamine. Oxytocin.
•**hypophosphorous acid.** (high-poe-FOSS-for-uhs) *NF 29.*
Use: Pharmaceutic aid (antioxidant).
HypoTears Ophthalmic Liquid. (Novartis Ophthalmics) Polyvinyl alcohol 1%, PEG-400, dextrose 1%, benzalkonium Cl 0.01%, EDTA. Bot. 15 mL, 30 mL. *OTC.*
Use: Lubricant, ophthalmic.
HypoTears Ophthalmic Ointment. (Novartis Ophthalmics) White petrolatum, light mineral oil. Tube 3.5 g. *OTC.*
Use: Lubricant, ophthalmic.
hypotensive agents.
See: Antihypertensives.
•**hypromellose.** (hye-PROE-me-lose) *USP 34.* Formerly hydroxypropyl methylcellulose.
Use: Pharmaceutical aid (suspending agent), tablet excipient, viscosity-increasing agent.
See: Bion Tears.
 GenTeal.
 Goniosol.
 Gonak.
 OcuCoat.
 Tears Naturale Free.
 Tears Naturale II.
 Tears Renewed.
 W/Combinations.
See: Clear Eyes Plus Redness Relief.
 Isopto Plain.

Isopto Tears.
Lacril.
Tearisol.
Tears Naturale.
Ultra Tears.
Hyrexin-50. (Hyrex) Diphenhydramine hydrochloride 50 mg/mL, benzethonium chloride. Vial 10 mL. Amp. 1 mL. *Rx.*
Use: Antihistamine.
Hyscorbic Plus Tablets. (Sanofi-Synthelabo) Vitamins E 45 units, C 600 mg, folic acid 400 mcg, B_1 20 mg, B_2 10 mg, niacinamide 100 mg, B_6 10 mg, B_{12} 25 mcg, pantothenic acid 25 mg, copper 3 mg, zinc 23.9 mg. Tab. Bot. 60s. *OTC.*
Use: Mineral, vitamin supplement.
Hyserp. (Freeport) Reserpine alkaloid 0.25 mg. Tab. Bot. 1000s. *Rx.*
Use: Antihypertensive.
Hyskon. (Pharmacia) Dextran 70 32% in 10% w/v dextrose. Bot. 100 mL, 250 mL. *Rx.*
Use: Diagnostic aid. For distending the uterine cavity and irrigating and visualizing its surfaces.
Hysone. (Roberts) Clioquinol 30 mg, hydrocortisone 10 mg/g. Cream. Tube 20 g. *OTC.*
Use: Antifungal; corticosteroid, topical.
hysteroscopy fluid.
Use: Diagnostic aid.
See: Hyskon.

Hytone Cream. (Dermik) Hydrocortisone in cream base. **1%:** 1 oz. Jar 4 oz. **2.5%:** Tube 1 oz, 2 oz. *Rx-OTC.*
Use: Corticosteroid, topical.
Hytone Lotion. (Dermik) Hydrocortisone 2.5% (25 mg/mL) in lotion base. Bot. 60 mL. *Rx.*
Use: Corticosteroid, topical.
Hytone Ointment. (Dermik) Hydrocortisone in ointment base, mineral oil, white petrolatum. **1%:** Tube 28.3 g, 113.4 g. **2.5%:** Tube 28.3 g. *Rx.*
Use: Corticosteroid, topical.
Hytone Spray. (Dermik) Hydrocortisone 1%. 45 mL. *Rx.*
Use: Corticosteroid, topical.
Hytrin. (Abbott) Terazosin hydrochloride 1 mg, 2 mg, 5 mg, 10 mg, parabens. Cap. Bot. 100s, UD 100s. *Rx.*
Use: Antihypertensive, antiadrenergic.
Hyzaar. (Merck) Losartan potassium/hydrochlorothiazide 50 mg/12.5 mg (potassium 4.24 mg), 100 mg/12.5 mg (potassium 8.48 mg), 100 mg/25 mg (potassium 8.48 mg). Lactose. Tab. Bot. 30s, 90s, 1000, 5000s (except 100 mg/25 mg), 4000s (100 mg/25 mg only), UD 100s. *Rx.*
Use: Antihypertensive.
Hyzine-50. (Hyrex) Hydroxyzine hydrochloride 50 mg as hydrochloride/mL. Vial 10 mL. *Rx.*
Use: Anxiolytic.

I

•**ibafloxacin.** (ih-BAH-FLOX-ah-sin) USAN.
Use: Anti-infective.

•**ibalizumab.** (I-ba-LIZ-oo-mab) USAN.
Use: Treatment of HIV/AIDS.

•**ibandronate sodium.** (ih-BAN-droe-nate) USAN.
Use: Bone resorption inhibitor; antihypercalcemic; bisphosphonate.
See: Boniva.

ibenzmethyzin. *Name used for Procarbazine Hydrochloride.*

•**iboctadekin.** (ib-OK-ta-DE-kin) USAN.
Use: Immunologic mediator.

•**ibopamine.** (EYE-BOE-pah-meen) USAN.
Use: Dopaminergic (peripheral).

•**ibritumomab tiuxetan.** (ib-ri-TYOO-mo-mab tye-UX-e-tan) USAN.
Use: Monoclonal antibody.
See: Zevalin.

•**ibrolipim.** (ib-ROE-li-pim) USAN.
Use: Antiatherogenic; anti-obesity; antidyslipidemia; anticachexia; antidiabetes agent.

IB-Stat. (InKine) L-hyoscyamine sulfate 0.125 mg/mL. Alcohol 5.3%, liquid sugar, methylparaben, sorbitol. Oral Spray. 30 mL. *Rx.*
Use: Anticholinergic/antispasmodic, belladonna alkaloid.

Ibudone. (ProEthic Pharmaceuticals) Hydrocodone bitartrate/ibuprofen 5 mg/200 mg, 10 mg/200 mg. PEG. Film-coated. Tab. 100s. *c-III.*
Use: Narcotic analgesic.

•**ibufenac.** (eye-BYOO-feh-nak) USAN.
Use: Antirheumatic; anti-inflammatory; analgesic; antipyretic.

•**ibuprofen.** (eye-BYOO-pro-fen) *USP 34.*
Use: Anti-inflammatory; analgesic.
See: Advil.
 Advil Migraine.
 Caldolor.
 Children's Advil.
 Children's Motrin.
 Dynafed IB.
 Ibuprin.
 Ibutab.
 Infants' Motrin.
 Junior Strength Motrin.
 Menadol.
 Midol Cramp & Body Aches
 Midol Maximum Strength Cramp Formula.
 Motrin IB.
 Motrin, Junior Strength.
 Motrin Migraine Pain.
 Pediatric Advil.
 Saleto.
W/Diphenhydramine Hydrochloride
See: Advil PM.
W/Hydrocodone Bitartrate.
See: Ibudone.
 Reprexain.
 Vicoprofen.
W/Pseudoephedrine Hydrochloride.
See: Advil Cold & Sinus.
 Children's Ibuprofen Cold.
 Children's Motrin Cold.
W/Pseudoephedrine Hydrochloride, Chlorpheniramine Maleate.
See: Advil Allergy Sinus.

ibuprofen. (Perrigo) Ibuprofen 40 mg/mL. Oral Drops. Bot. 15 mL. *OTC.*
Use: Analgesic; NSAID.

ibuprofen. (Various Mfr.) Ibuprofen. **Tab.:** 200 mg, 400 mg, 600 mg, 800 mg. Bot. **200 mg:** 24s, 50s, 100s, 250s, 1000s, UD 100s. **400 mg, 600 mg, 800 mg:** 100s, 270s (600 mg, 800 mg only), 360s (400 mg only), 500s, UD 100s, UD 300s, unit-of-use 100s, *Robot* ready 25s, *Emergi-script* 60s. **Susp.:** 100 mg/5 mL. Bot. 118 mL. *Rx-OTC.*
Use: Analgesic; NSAID.

•**ibuprofen aluminum.** (eye-BYOO-profen ah-LOO-min-uhm) USAN.
Use: Anti-inflammatory.

•**ibuprofen lysine.** (EYE-bue-PROE-fen LYE-seen) USAN.
Use: Anti-inflammatory.
See: NeoProfen.

•**ibuprofen piconol.** (eye-BYOO-pro-fen PIK-oh-nahl) USAN.
Use: Anti-inflammatory, topical.

•**ibuprofen sodium.** (EYE-bue-PROE-fen) USAN.
Use: Treatment of pain, fever, and rheumatic disorders.

ibuprofen suspension. (Various Mfr.) Ibuprofen 100 mg/5 mL. UD 50s. *Rx.*
Use: Analgesic; NSAID.

Ibutab. (Zee Medical) Ibuprofen 200 mg. Tab. 24s. *OTC.*
Use: Analgesic; NSAID.

•**ibutilide fumarate.** (ih-BYOO-tih-lide) USAN.
Use: Cardiac depressant (antiarrhythmic).
See: Corvert.

ibutilide fumarate. (Bioniche Pharma Group) Ibutilide fumarate 0.1 mg/mL (equiv. to ibutilide 0.087 mg). Inj., Soln. Single-dose vial. 10 mL. *Rx.*
Use: Antiarrhythmic agent.

ICAPS Plus. (Ciba Vision) Vitamin A 6000 units, C 200 mg, E 60 units,

B_2 20 mg, Zn 14.25 mg, Cu, Se, Mn. Sugar free. Tab. Bot. 60s, 120s. *OTC.*
Use: Mineral, vitamin supplement.

ICAPS Time Release. (Ciba Vision) Vitamin A 7000 units, C 200 mg, E 100 units, B_2 20 mg, Zn 14.25 mg, Cu, Se. Sugar free. Tab. Bot. 60s, 120s. *OTC.*
Use: Mineral, vitamin supplement.

Icar. (Hawthorn) Carbonyl iron. **Chew. Tab.:** 15 mg. Sorbitol, grape flavor. 60s. **Susp.:** 15 mg/1.25 mL. Fructose, parabens, grape and lemon flavors. Bot. 118 mL. *OTC.*
Use: Mineral supplement.

● **icatibant acetate.** (eye-CAT-ih-bant) USAN.
Use: Investigational bradykinin antagonist.

Ice Mint. (Bristol-Myers Squibb) Stearic acid, synthetic cocoa butter, lanolin oil, camphor, menthol, beeswax, mineral oil, sodium borate, aromatic oils, emulsifiers. Jar 4 oz. *OTC.*
Use: Emollient; counterirritant.

IC-Green. (Akorn) Indocyanine green 25 mg. Pow. for Inj. Vials with 10 mL amps of aqueous solvent. 6s. *Rx.*
Use: Ophthalmic diagnostic product.

I-Chlor 0.5%. (Akorn) Chloramphenicol 5 mg/mL. Bot. 7.5 mL, 15 mL. *Rx.*
Use: Anti-infective, ophthalmic.

● **ichthammol.** (ICK-thah-mole) *USP 34.*
Use: Anti-infective, topical.
W/Aluminum Hydroxide, Phenol, Zinc Oxide, Camphor, Eucalyptol.
See: Boil-Ease Anesthetic Drawing Salve.
W/Hydrocortisone Acetate, Benzocaine, Oxyquinoline Sulfate, Ephedrine Hydrochloride.
See: Derma Medicone-HC.
W/Naftalan, Calamine, Amber Pet.
See: Naftalan.

ichthammol. (Allan Pharmaceutical) Ichthammol 20%. Lanolin, mineral oil, petrolatum. Oint. 30 g. *OTC.*
Use: Dermatological agent, miscellaneous topical combination.

ichthammol. (Alra) Ichthammol 10%, 20% in a lanolin-petrolatum base. Oint. Tube 28.4 g. *OTC.*
Use: Antiseptic.

ichthammol. (Eli Lilly) Ichthammol 10%, 20% Oint. *OTC.*
Use: Antiseptic.

ichthynate.
See: Ichthammol.

● **iclaprim.** (EYE-kla-prim) USAN.
Use: Anti-infective agent.

● **iclaprim mesylate.** (EYE-kla-prim) USAN.
Use: Anti-infective agent.

● **icodextrin.** (eye-koe-DEX-trin) USAN.
Use: Osmotic.

● **icopezil maleate.** (eye-KOE-peh-zill) USAN.
Use: Alzheimer disease treatment (cognition enhancer); cognition adjuvant; acetylcholinesterase inhibitor.

● **icotidine.** (eye-KOE-tih-DEEN) USAN.
Use: Antagonist (to histamine H_2 and H_1 receptors).

● **icrucumab.** (ey-KROO-kue-mab) USAN.
Use: Antineoplastic.

● **ictasol.** (IK-tah-sahl) USAN.
Use: Disinfectant.

Ictotest Reagent Tablets. (Bayer Consumer Care) Reagent Tab. for urinary bilirubin. Bot. 100s.
Use: Diagnostic aid.

Icy Hot Back Pain Relief. (Chattem) Menthol 5%, glycerin. Patch. 5s. *OTC.*
Use: Rub and liniment.

Icy Hot Balm. (Chattem) Methyl salicylate 29%, menthol 7.6%. Jar 3.5 oz, 7 oz. *OTC.*
Use: Analgesic, topical.

Icy Hot Chill Stick. (Chattem) Methyl salicylate 30%, menthol 10%, hydrogenated castor oil, stearyl alcohol. Stick. 49 g. *OTC.*
Use: Rub and liniment.

Icy Hot Cream. (Chattem) Methyl salicylate 30%, menthol 10%. Tube 0.25 oz, 1.25 oz, 3 oz. *OTC.*
Use: Analgesic, topical.

Icy Hot, Extra Strength. (Chattem) Methyl salicylate 30%, menthol 10%, ceresin, cyclomethicone, hydrogenated castor oil, PEG-150 distearate, propylene glycol, stearic acid, stearyl alcohol. Stick 52.5 g. *OTC.*
Use: Liniment.

Icy Hot Pain Relieving Gel. (Chattem) Menthol 2.5%. Alcohol 15%, aloe, parabens, triethanolamine. Gel. 70.8 g. *OTC.*
Use: Rub and liniment, gel.

Icy Hot PM. (Chattem) Capsaicin 0.025%. Menthol 5%, benzyl alcohol, disodium EDTA. Patch. 6s. *OTC.*
Use: Dermatological agent, counterirritant.

Icy Hot PM Medicated. (Chattem) Menthol 7.5%. Aloe, benzyl alcohol, capsaicin, cetearyl alcohol, cetyl alcohol, disodium EDTA, ethanol, PEG-2, stearyl alcohol. Lot. 113 g. *OTC.*
Use: Rub and liniment, lotion and liniment.

Icy Hot Pop & Peel. (Chattem) Menthol 5%, glycerin. Patch. 5s. *OTC.*
Use: Rub and liniment.

Icy Hot Pro-Therapy. (Chattem) Menthol 5%. Diazolidinyl urea, parabens. Top. Pad. 4s. *OTC.*
Use: Rubs and liniments.

Icy Hot Roll. (Chattem) Menthol 7.5%. Mineral oil. Patch. 3s. *OTC.*
Use: Rub and liniment.

I.D.A. Capsules. (Ivax) Isometheptene mucate 65 mg, dichloralphenazone 100 mg, acetaminophen 324 mg. Bot. 100s. *Rx.*
Use: Analgesic.

Idamycin PFS. (Pfizer) Idarubicin hydrochloride 1 mg/mL. Preservative free. Inj. Single-use vials. 5 mL, 10 mL, 20 mL. *Rx.*
Use: Antibiotic, anthracycline.

•**idarubicin hydrochloride.** (eye-DUH-RUE-bih-sin) *USAN.*
Tall Man: IDArubicin
Use: Antineoplastic; antibiotic, anthracycline.
See: Idamycin PFS.

idarubicin hydrochloride. (GensiaSicor) Idarubicin hydrochloride 1 mg/mL. Preservative free. Inj. Single-use vials. 5 mL, 10 mL, 20 mL. *Rx.*
Use: Antibiotic, anthracycline.

•**idoxifene.** (ih-dox-ih-feen) *USAN.*
Use: Antineoplastic; hormone replacement therapy (estrogen receptor antagonist); osteoporosis treatment and prevention.

•**idronoxil.** (id-roe-NOX-il) *USAN.*
Use: Antineoplastic agent.

I-Drops. (Akorn) Tetrahydrozoline hydrochloride 0.5%. Ophthalmic Soln. Bot. 0.5 oz. *Rx.*
Use: Mydriatic, vasoconstrictor.

•**idursulfase.** (eye-dur-SUL-fase) *USAN.*
Use: Hunter syndrome.
See: Elaprase.

iFerex 150. (Nnodum Pharmaceuticals) Iron 150 mg. Cap. 100s. *OTC.*
Use: Trace element, iron.

•**ifetroban.** (ih-FEH-troe-ban) *USAN.*
Use: Antithrombotic.

•**ifetroban sodium.** (ih-FEH-troe-ban) *USAN.*
Use: Antithrombotic.

Ifex. (Baxter) Ifosfamide 1 g, 3 g. Pow. for Inj. Vial single dose. *Rx.*
Use: Antineoplastic.

•**ifosfamide.** (eye-FOSS-fuh-MIDE) *USP 34.*
Use: Antineoplastic.
See: Ifex.

ifosfamide. (American Pharmaceutical Partners) Ifosfamide 1 g, 3 g. Pow. for Inj., lyophilized. Vials. Single-dose. *Rx.*
Use: Antineoplastic.

I-Gent. (Akorn) Gentamicin sulfate 3 mg/mL. Ophthalmic soln. Bot. 5 mL. *Rx.*
Use: Anti-infective, ophthalmic.

Igepal Co-880. (General Aniline & Film) Nonoxynol-30. *OTC.*
Use: Contraceptive, spermicide.

Igepal Co-430. (General Aniline & Film) Nonoxynol-4. *OTC.*
Use: Contraceptive, spermicide.

Igepal Co-730. (General Aniline & Film) Nonoxynol-15. *OTC.*
Use: Contraceptive, spermicide.

IgG monoclonal anti-CD4.
See: Chimeric m-t412 (Human-Murine) IgG Monoclonal Anti-CD4.

IGIV. (Various Mfr.) Immune globulin intravenous. *Rx.*
Use: Immunomodulator (Phase II/III pediatric HIV), immunization.
See: Immune Globulin Intravenous

•**igmesine hydrochloride.** (IGG-meh-seen) *USAN.*
Use: Antidepressant.

I-Homatrine 5%. (Akorn) Homatropine hydrobromide 5%. Ophth. Soln. Bot. 5 mL. *Rx.*
Use: Cycloplegic; mydriatic.

Ilaris. (Novartis) Canakinumab 180 mg. Preservative free. Inj., lyophilized Pow. for Soln. Single-use vial. 6 mL. *Rx.*
Use: Immunologic agent, immunomodulator.

•**ilepcimide.** (eye-LEPP-sih-mide) *USAN.*
Formerly antiepileptsirine.
Use: Anticonvulsant.

Iletin I. (Eli Lilly) Regular and modified insulin products from beef and pork.
Regular: 100 units/mL. Bot. 10 mL.
Lente: 100 units/mL. Bot. 10 mL. **NPH:** 100 units/mL. Bot. 10 mL. *OTC.*
Use: Antidiabetic.

Iletin II Concentrated. (Eli Lilly) Purified pork regular insulin 500 units/mL. Vial 20 mL. *Rx.*
Use: Antidiabetic.

Iletin II Regular. (Eli Lilly) Insulin 100 units/mL purified pork. Inj. Vial 10 mL. *OTC.*
Use: Antidiabetic.

•**ilmofosine.** (ill-MOE-fose-een) *USAN.*
Use: Antineoplastic.

•**ilomastat.** (eye-LOW-mah-stat) *USAN.*
Use: Corneal ulcers; inflammatory conditions; cancers.

•**ilonidap.** (ile-OHN-ih-dap) *USAN.*
Use: Anti-inflammatory.

Ilopan. (Pharmacia) Dexpanthenol
250 mg/mL. Disp. syringe 2 mL. *Rx.*
Use: Gastrointestinal stimulant.

• **iloperidone.** (ill-oh-PURR-ih-dohn)
USAN.
Use: Antipsychotic.
See: Fanapt.

• **iloprost.** (EYE-loe-prost) USAN.
Use: Treatment of pulmonary arterial
hypertension.
See: Ventavis.

Ilosone. (Eli Lilly) Erythromycin estolate.
Tab.: 500 mg, Bot. 50s. **Susp.:** 125 mg,
250 mg/5 mL. Bot. 100 mL (250 mg
only), 480 mL. *Rx.*
Use: Anti-infective, erythromycin.

Ilosone Pulvules. (Eli Lilly) Erythromycin
estolate 250 mg. Cap. Bot. 100s. *Rx.*
Use: Anti-infective, erythromycin.

Ilotycin. (Fera Pharmaceuticals) Erythromycin 0.5%. Mineral oil, white petrolatum. Oint., Ophth. 1 g. *Rx.*
Use: Ophthalmic and otic agent, ophthalmic antibiotic.

Ilotycin Gluceptate. (Eli Lilly) Erythro-
mycin gluceptate 1 g. Inj. Vial 30 mL.
Rx.
Use: Anti-infective, erythromycin.

Ilozyme. (Pharmacia) Pancrelipase
equivalent to lipase 11,000 units,
protease 30,000 units, amylase
30,000 units. Tab. Bot. 250s. *Rx.*
Use: Digestive enzymes.

IL-2. (Various Mfr.) Interleukin-2. *Rx.*
Use: Immunomodulator.
See: Proleukin.

I.L.X. B12 Elixir. (Kenwood) Liver fraction 98 mg, iron 102 mg, vitamins B_1
5 mg, B_2 2 mg, B_3 10 mg, B_{12} 10 mcg/
15 mL. Bot. 240 mL. *OTC.*
Use: Mineral, vitamin supplement.

I.L.X. B12 Tablets and Caplets. (Kenwood) Iron 37.5 mg, vitamins C
120 mg, desiccated liver 130 mg, B_1
2 mg, B_2 2 mg, B_3 20 mg, B_{12} 12 mcg.
Tab. Bot. 100s. *OTC.*
Use: Mineral, vitamin supplement.

I.L.X. Elixir. (Kenwood) Iron 70 mg, liver
concentrate 98 mg, vitamins B_1 5 mg,
B_2 2 mg, B_3 10 mg/15 mL. Bot. 240 mL.
OTC.
Use: Mineral, vitamin supplement.

• **imafen hydrochloride.** (IH-mah-fen)
USAN.
Use: Antidepressant.

• **imagabalin.** (IM-a-GAB-a-lin) USAN.
Use: CNS agent.

• **imagabalin hydrochloride.** (IM-a-GAB-
a-lin) USAN.
Use: CNS agent.

Imager ac. (Mallinckrodt) Barium sulfate
100%. Simethicone, sorbitol, sodium
benzoate. Susp. Bot. 650 mL w/enema
tip-tubing assemblies w/kit, 1900 mL
bot. *Rx.*
Use: Radiopaque agent, gastrointestinal contrast agent.

imatinib.
Use: Protein-tyrosine kinase inhibitor.
See: Gleevec.

• **imazodan hydrochloride.** (ih-MAY-zoe-
DAN) USAN.
Use: Cardiovascular agent.

• **imciromab pentetate.** (im-SIHR-ah-
mab) USAN.
Use: Monoclonal antibody (antimyosin).
[Orphan Drug]
See: Myoscint.

Imdur. (Key) Isosorbide mononitrate
30 mg, 60 mg, 120 mg. ER Tab. Bot.
100s, UD 100s. *Rx.*
Use: Vasodilator.

Imenol. (Sigma-Tau) Guaiacol 0.1 g, eucalyptol 0.08 g, iodoform 0.02 g, camphor 0.05 g/mL. Vial 30 mL. *Rx.*
Use: Expectorant.

• **imetelstat.** (im-e-TEL-stat) USAN.
Use: Antineoplastic.

• **imetelstat sodium.** (im-e-TEL-stat)
USAN.
Use: Antineoplastic.

l-methorphinan levorphanol.
See: Levo-Dromoran.

• **imexon.** (eye-MEX-on) USAN.
Use: Antineoplastic.

Imexon. (Amplimed) DM 06.002.
Use: Multiple myeloma. [Orphan Drug]

Imferon. (Medeva) An iron-dextran complex containing iron 50 mg/mL. Amp.
2 mL. Box 10s. Vial (w/phenol 0.5%)
10 mL. Box 2s. *Rx.*
Use: Mineral supplement.

imidazole antifungal.
Use: Antifungal agent.
See: Ketoconazole.
Miconazole.

imidazole carboxamide.
Use: Antineoplastic.
See: Dacarbazine.
DTIC-Dome.

imidazolines.
Use: Nasal decongestant.
See: Afrin No-Drip Sinus with Vapor-
nase.
Afrin Sinus with Valpornase.
Benzedrex.
Dristan Fast Acting Formula.
Dristan 12-Hr Nasal.
Duramist Plus 12-Hr Decongestant.
Duration.

Genasal.
Naphazoline Hydrochloride.
Nasal Decongestant Combinations.
Nasal Decongestant Inhalers.
Nasal Decongestant, Maximum
  Strength.
Nasal Relief.
Neo-Synephrine 12-Hour.
Neo-Synephrine 12-Hour Extra Mois-
  turizing.
Nōstrilla 12-Hour.
Otrivin.
Otrivin Pediatric Nasal.
Oxymetazoline Hydrochloride.
Privine.
Tetrahydrozoline Hydrochloride.
12 Hour Nasal.
Twice-A-Day 12-Hour Nasal.
Tyzine.
Tyzine Pediatric.
Xylometazoline Hydrochloride.

imidazopyridines.
Use: Sedative/hypnotic nonbarbiturate.
See: Zolpidem Tartrate.

imidazotetrazine derivatives.
Use: Antineoplastic agents.
See: Temozolomide.

•**imidecyl iodine.** (IH-mih-DEH-sill EYE-
uh-dine) USAN.
Use: Anti-infective, topical.

•**imidocarb hydrochloride.** (ih-MIH-doe-
KARB) USAN.
Use: Antiprotozoal (Babesia).

•**imidoline hydrochloride.** (im-ID-oh-
leen) USAN.
Use: Anxiolytic; antipsychotic.

•**imidurea.** (ih-mid-your-EE-ah) *NF 29.*
Use: Antimicrobial.

•**imiglucerase.** (ih-mih-GLUE-ser-ACE)
USAN.
Use: Enzyme replenisher; treatment for
Gaucher disease (glucocerebrosi-
dase). [Orphan Drug]
See: Cerezyme.

•**imiloxan hydrochloride.** (ih-mill-OX-
ahn) USAN.
Use: Antidepressant.

imipemide.
Use: Anti-infective.
See: Imipenem.

•**imipenem.** (ih-mih-PEN-em) *USP 34.*
Formerly imipemide.
Use: Anti-infective.
W/Cilastatin for Injection.
See: Primaxin.

•**imipramine hydrochloride.** (im-IPP-ruh-
meen) *USP 34.*
Use: Antidepressant.
See: Tofranil.

imipramine hydrochloride. (Various
Mfr.) Imipramine hydrochloride 10 mg,
25 mg, 50 mg. Tab. Bot. 50s (50 mg
only), 100s, 250s, 500s, 1000s, UD 20s
(50 mg only). *Rx.*
Use: Antidepressant.

imipramine pamoate.
Use: Antidepressant.
See: Tofranil-PM.

imipramine pamoate. (Mallinckrodt)
Imipramine pamoate 75 mg, 100 mg,
125 mg, 150 mg. Parabens. Cap. 30s.
Rx.
Use: Antidepressant.

•**imiquimod.** (ih-mih-KWIH-mahd) USAN.
Use: Immunomodulator.
See: Aldara.
  Zyclara.

imiquimod. (Fougera) Imiquimod 5%.
May contain benzyl alcohol, cetyl alcohol, parabens, stearyl alcohol, white
petrolatum. Cream. Single-use packet.
24s. *Rx.*
Use: Topical immunomodulator.

Imitrex. (GlaxoSmithKline) Sumatriptan.
Inj. Soln.: As sumatriptan succinate.
4 mg/0.5 mL (sodium chloride 3.8 mg/
mL), 6 mg/0.5 mL (sodium chloride
3.5 mg/mL). **4 mg/0.5 mL:** 4 mg *STAT-
dose System* (2 prefilled single-dose
syringe cartridges, 1 *STATdose Pen*,
and instructions for use), injection cartridge pack. Contains 2 prefilled syringe cartridges for refill of *STATdose
System* only. **6 mg/0.5 mL:** 6 mg single-
dose vials and *STATdose System*
(2 prefilled single-dose syringes,
1 *STATdose Pen* and instructions for
use) injection cartridge pack. Contains
2 prefilled syringe cartridges for refill
of *STATdose System* only. **Soln. Intranasal:** 5 mg, 20 mg. Unit-dose spray
device. 100 mcL. Box 6s. **Tab.:** 25 mg
(equiv. to sumatriptan succinate
35 mg), 50 mg (equiv. to sumatriptan
succinate 70 mg), 100 mg (equiv. to
sumatriptan succinate 140 mg). Blister
pack 9s. *Rx.*
Use: Antimigraine, serotonin 5-HT$_1$ receptor agonist.

ImmTher. (Immuno Therapeutics) Disaccharide tripeptide glycerol dipalmitoyl.
Use: Antineoplastic. [Orphan Drug]

Immun-Aid. (McGaw) A custard flavored
liquid containing 18.5 g protein, 60 g
carbohydrate, 11 g fat, sodium 290 mg,
potassium 530 mg per liter. 1 calorie/
mL. With appropriate vitamins and minerals. Pow. Packets 123 g. 24s. *OTC.*
Use: Nutritional supplement, enteral.

immune globulin. (ih-MYOON GLAH-byoo-lin) Immune Serum Globulin Human. Gamma-globulin fraction of normal human plasma. Vial 10 mL. Tubex 1 mL, 2 mL w/thimerosal 1:10,000. *Rx.*
Use: Modification of active measles; prophylaxis of hepatitis A; treatment of immune deficiencies; prevention of infection associated with bone marrow transplantation (BMT); decrease frequency of certain pediatric HIV-related infections and conjunctive therapy for Kawasaki syndrome.

immune globulin, antithymocyte (rabbit).
Use: Immunization.
See: Thymoglobulin.

immune globulin, cytomegalovirus.
See: CytoGam.

immune globulin, hepatitis B.
See: BayHep B.
H-BIG.
Nabi-HB.

immune globulin (human).
See: GamaSTAN S/D.
Gammagard S/D.
Privigen.

immune globulin intramuscular.
Use: Immunization.

immune globulin intravenous.
Use: Immunization.
See: BayGam.
Carimune NF.
Flebogamma 5%.
GamaSTAN S/D.
Gammagard.
Gamunex.
Privigen.
Rho₀(D) Immune Globulin IV (Human).
Sandoglobulin.
Venoglobulin-I.
WinRho SDF.

immune globulin intravenous, botulism.
Use: Infant botulism.
See: BabyBIG.

•**immune globulin intravenous pentetate.** (ih-MYOON GLAH-byoo-lin in-trah-VEE-nuhs) USAN.
Use: Diagnostic aid.

immune globulin intravenous/subcutaneous.
See: Gamunex-C.

immune globulin intravenous, vaccinia.
Use: Immunization.

immune globulin, lymphocyte, antithymocyte (equine).
Use: Immunization.
See: Atgam.

immune globulin, rabies.
Use: Immunization.
See: Imogam Rabies-HT.

immune globulin, Rh₀(D).
See: BayRho D Full Dose.
BayRho D Mini Dose.
MICRhoGAM.
RhoGAM.
WinRho SDF.

immune globulins.
See: Antithymocyte Globulin (Rabbit).
Botulism Immune Globulin IV.
Cytomegalovirus Immune Globulin Intravenous, Human.
Hepatitis B Immune Globulin (Human).
Immune Globulin (Human).
Immune Globulin Intravenous.
Immune Globulin Subcutaneous (Human).
Lymphocyte Immune Globulin, Antithymocyte Globulin (Equine).
Rabies Immune Globulin, Human.
Rho₀(D) Immune Globulin.
Rho₀(D) Immune Globulin IV Human.
Rho₀(D) Immune Globulin Micro-Dose.
Respiratory Syncytial Virus Immune Globulin Intravenous (Human).
Tetanus Immune Globulin (Human).
Vaccinia Immune Globulin IV.

immune globulin subcutaneous (human).
Use: Immune globulin.
See: Vivaglobin.

immune globulin, tetanus.
Use: Immunization.
See: BayTet.

immune globulin, varicella-zoster.
Use: Immunization.
See: Varicella-Zoster Immune Globulin (Human).

immune serum (animal).
See: Botulism Antitoxin.
Diphtheria Antitoxin.

immune serums.
See: Cytomegalovirus Immune Globulin Intravenous (Human).
Hepatitis B Immune Globulin.
Immune Globulin Intramuscular.
Immune Globulin Intravenous.
Immune Serum Globulin (Human).
Rabies Immune Globulin.
Rho₀(D) Immune Globulin.
Tetanus Immune Globulin.
Vaccinia Immune Globulin.
Varicella-Zoster Immune Globulin.

Immunex C-RP. (Wampole) Two-minute latex agglutination slide test for the qualitative detection of C-Reactive protein in serum. Kit 100s.
Use: Diagnostic aid.

immunization, active.
See: Toxoids.
Vaccines, Bacterial.
Vaccines, Viral.
Immuno-C. (Biomune Systems, Inc.)
Bovine Whey Protein Concentrate.
Use: Cryptosporidiosis treatment.
[Orphan Drug]
Immunocal. (Immunotech Research)
Protein (from milk protein isolate) 9 g/
10 g, vitamin A, Ca, chloride, Fe, MG, P,
Na 25 mg, K 30 mg/10 g, 37 cal/10 g.
Pow. Pouch. 10 g. OTC.
Use: Enteral nutritional therapy.
Immunocal. (Immunotech Research)
Protein (from milk protein isolate) 9 g/
10 g, sodium 25 mg, potassium 30 mg,
calcium 60 mg, magnesium 9 mg, P
21 mg, calories 37/pkt. Pow. Pkt. 10 g
(30s). OTC.
Use: Nutritional supplement.
immunologic agents.
See: Immunomodulators.
Immunostimulants.
Immunosuppressives.
immunomodulators.
See: Abatacept.
Adalimumab.
Anakinra.
Canakinumab.
Certolizumab Pegol.
Etanercept.
Fingolimod.
Golimumab.
Imiquimod.
Infliximab.
Interferon alfacon-1.
Interferon alfa-n3 (Human Leukocyte
Derived).
Interferon alfa-2b, Recombinant.
Interferon beta-1a.
Interferon beta-1b.
Interferon gamma-1b.
Lenalidomide.
Mitoxantrone Hydrochloride.
Natalizumab.
Peginterferon alfa-2a.
Peginterferon alfa-2b.
Pimecrolimus.
Rilonacept.
Thalidomide.
Tocilizumab.
Ustekinumab.
immunomodulators, topical.
See: Imiquimod.
Pimecrolimus.
Tacrolimus.
Immunorex. (Antigen Laboratories) Aller-
genic extracts, various. Vial. Rx.
Use: Allergen desensitization.

immunostimulants.
See: Pegademase Bovine.
immunosuppressives.
See: Alefacept.
Azathioprine.
Basiliximab.
Cylcosporine.
Daclizumab.
Efalizumab.
Glatiramer Acetate.
Muromonab-CD3.
Mycophenolate Mofetil.
Mycophenolate Sodium.
Sirolimus.
Tacrolimus.
ImmuRAID. (Immunomedics) Techne-
tium Tc-99M murine monoclonal anti-
body to hCG and human AFP.
Use: Diagnostic aid. [Orphan Drug]
ImmuRAIT. (Immunomedics) Iodine I^{131}
murine monoclonal antibody IgG2a to
B cell.
Use: Antineoplastic, investigational.
Imodium A-D. (Ortho-McNeil) Loper-
amide 1 mg/5 mL, 1 mg/7.5 mL. Alcohol
5.25%. Cherry/licorice flavor (except
1 mg/7.5 mL), mint flavor (1 mg/7.5 mL
only). Liq. Bot. 60 mL, 90 mL (except
1 mg/7.5 mL); 120 mL. OTC.
Use: Antidiarrheal.
Imodium Capsules. (Janssen) Loper-
amide 2 mg. Cap. Bot. 100s, 500s,
UD 100s. Rx.
Use: Antidiarrheal.
Imodium Multi-Symptom Relief. (Mc-
Neil Consumer) Loperamide hydrochlo-
ride 2 mg, simethicone 125 mg. **Tab.**
Chew.: Calcium 50 mg, saccharin,
sorbitol, sugar. Mint flavor. 18s, 42s.
Tab.: Acesulfame K, calcium 165 mg,
sodium 4 mg. 12s, 18s, 30s, 42s. OTC.
Use: Antidiarrheal combination product.
Imogam Rabies-HT. (Sanofi Pasteur)
Rabies immune globulin (human) (RIG)
150 units/mL. Preservative free, glycine 0.3 M, heat treated. Vials. 2 mL,
10 mL. Rx.
Use: Immunization, rabies.
**Imovax Rabies Vaccine (Human Dip-
loid Cell).** (Aventis Pasteur) Rabies
antigen ≥ 2.5 IU/mL. Freeze-dried suspension of Wistar rabies virus strain
PM-1503-3M grown in human diploid
cell cultures (inactivated whole virus).
Human albumin < 100 mg, neomycin
sulfate < 150 mcg, phenol red indicator
20 mcg. Inj., Lyophilized Pow. for Reconstitution. In single-dose vial with disposable needle and syringe containing diluent and disposable needle for

administration. *Rx.*
Use: Active immunization, viral vaccine.

Impact Advanced Recovery. (Nestle Nutrition) Protein 18.1 g (caseinate, L-arginine), carbohydrate 44.7 g (sucrose), fat 9.2 g (corn oil, medium chain triglycerides), sodium 350 mg, potassium 450 mg. Fiber 3.3 g, vitamins A, B_1, B_2, B_3, B_5, B_6, B_{12}, C, D, E, K, Ca, Cl, Cr, Cu, Fe, I, Mg, Mn, Mo, P, Se, Zn, biotin, choline, folic acid. Lactose free. Chocolate and vanilla flavors. Liq. 273 mL. *OTC.*
Use: Defined formula diet, lactose-free product.

Implanon. (Organon) Etonogestrel 68 mg. Implant. Preloaded needle with disposable applicator. *Rx.*
Use: Contraceptive hormone.

imported fire ant venom, allergenic extract. (ALK)
Use: Allergy testing. [Orphan Drug]

impotence agents.
See: Alprostadil.
Phosphodiesterase Type 5 Inhibitors.
Sildenafil Citrate.
Tadalafil.
Vardenafil Hydrochloride.
Yohimbine Hydrochloride.

Impromen. (Janssen) Bromperidol decanoate. *Rx.*
Use: Antipsychotic.

Impromen Decanoate. (Janssen) Bromperidol decanoate. *Rx.*
Use: Antipsychotic.

•**impromidine hydrochloride.** (im-PRAH-mid-deen) USAN.
Use: Diagnostic aid (gastric secretion indicator).

Improved Congestant Tablets. (Rugby) Chlorpheniramine maleate 2 mg, acetaminophen 325 mg. Tab. Bot. 100s, 1000s. *OTC.*
Use: Antihistamine, analgesic.

Impruv Deep Moisturizing. (GlaxoSmithKline) Cetyl alcohol, glyceryl, lactic acid, mineral oil, myristyl alcohol, parabens, PEG-100, stearyl alcohol. Lot. 200 mL. *OTC.*
Use: Emollient.

Impruv Natural Repair. (Stiefel) Caprylic/capric triglyceride, glycerin, *butyrispermum parkii*, cocos nucifera, squalane. Cream. 156 g. *OTC.*
Use: Emollient.

Imreg-1. (Imreg) *Rx.*
Use: Immunomodulator.

Imreg-2. (Imreg) *Rx.*
Use: Immunomodulator.

Imuran. (Prometheus) Azathioprine 50 mg. Tab. Bot. 100s, UD 100s. *Rx.*
Use: Immunosuppressant.

Imuthiol. (Aventis Pasteur) Diethyldithiocarbamate. *Rx.*
Use: Immunomodulator.

Imuvert. (Celltech) *Serratia marcescens* extract (polyribosomes).
Use: Primary brain malignancies. [Orphan Drug]

•**inalimarev (CEA, MUC-1, vaccinia virus).** (in-a-LIM-a-rev) USAN.
Use: Antineoplastic.

•**inamrinone.** (eye-NAM-ri-none) *USP 34.* Formerly Amrinone.
Use: Cardiovascular agent.

•**inamrinone lactate.** (eye-NAM-ri-none) *USP 34. Formerly Amrinone Lactate.*
Use: Cardiovascular agent.

inamrinone lactate. (Abbott Hospital Products) Inamrinone lactate 5 mg/mL, sodium metabisulfate 0.25 mg/mL. Inj. Amp. 20 mL. *Rx.*
Use: Inotropic agent.

•**incobotulinumtoxinA.** (IN-koe-BOT-ue-LYE-num-TOX-in-AY) USAN.
Use: Botulinum toxin.
See: Xeomin.

Increlex. (Tercica) Mecasermin (rDNA origin) 10 mg/mL. Benzyl alcohol 9 mg/mL, sodium chloride 5.84 mg/mL, polysorbate 20 2 mg/mL, acetate 0.5 M. Inj. Multiple-dose vials. 40 mL. *Rx.*
Use: Insulin-like growth factor.

incretin mimetic agents.
Use: Antidiabetic agent.
See: Exenatide.

•**incyclinide.** (in-SYE-kli-nide) USAN.
Use: Anti-inflammatory.

•**indacaterol.** (in-da-KAT-er-ol) USAN.
Use: Treatment of COPD.

•**indacaterol maleate.** (in-da-KAT-er-ol) USAN.
Use: iTreatment of COPD.

•**indacrinone.** (IN-dah-KRIH-nohn) USAN.
Use: Antihypertensive, diuretic.

indalone.
See: Butopyronoxyl.

Indamix DM. (Centurion Labs) Dexchlorpheniramine tannate 3 mg, dextromethorphan tannate 27.5 mg, pseudoephedrine tannate 50 mg per 5 mL. Grape flavor. Oral Susp. 473 mL. *Rx.*
Use: Upper respiratory combination, antitussive combination.

indandione derivative.
Use: Anticoagulant.
See: Anisindione.

•**indapamide.** (IN-DAP-uh-mide) *USP 34.*
Use: Diuretic.

indapamide. (Mylan) Indapamide 2.5 mg. Lactose. Film-coated. Tab. 100s, 1000s. *Rx.*
Use: Diuretic.

indapamide. (Various Mfr.) Indapamide 1.25 mg. Tab. Bot. 100s, 500s, 1000s. *Rx.*
Use: Diuretic.

•indeglitazar. (IN-de-GLIT-a-zar) USAN.
Use: Antidiabetic agent.

•indeloxazine hydrochloride. (in-DELL-OX-ah-zeen) USAN.
Use: Antidepressant.

Inderal LA. (Akrimax) Propranolol hydrochloride 60 mg, 80 mg, 120 mg, 160 mg. ER Cap. 100s. *Rx.*
Use: Antiadrenergic/sympatholytic; beta-adrenergic blocker.

indian gum.
See: Karaya Gum.

indigo carmine. (Akorn) Sodium indigotindisulfonate 8 mg/mL. Amp. 5 mL. Box. 10s, 100s.
Use: Diagnostic aid.
See: Sodium Indigotindisulfonate.

indigo carmine solution. (Becton Dickinson & Co.) Indigotindisulfonate sodium (0.8% aqueous soln. sodium salt of indigotindisulfonic acid) 40 mg/5 mL. Inj. Amp. 5 mL, 10s.
Use: Diagnostic aid.

•indigotindisulfonate sodium. (IN-dih-go-tin-die-SULL-foe-nate) *USP 34.* Indigo Carmine.
Use: Diagnostic aid (cystoscopy).
See: Sodium Indigotindisulfonate.

•indinavir. (in-DIN-ah-veer) USAN.
Use: Antiviral (HIV-protease inhibitor).

•indinavir sulfate. (in-DIN-ah-veer) USAN.
Use: Antiretroviral, protease inhibitor.
See: Crixivan.

•indiplon. (IN-di-plon) USAN.
Use: Sedative, hypnotic.

•indisulam. (IN-di-SOO-lam) USAN.
Use: Antineoplastic.

•indium chlorides In 113m. (IN-dee-uhm) USAN.
Use: Radiopharmaceutical.

Indium DTPA In 111. (GE Healthcare) Pentetate indium disodium In 111 37 MBq (1 mCi) per mL at calibration. Inj. Single-dose vials. 1.5 mL. *Rx.*
Use: In vivo diagnostic aid.

•indium In 111 chloride solution. (IN-dee-uhm) *USP 34.*
Use: Radiopharmaceutical.

•indium In 111 ibritumomab tiuxetan injection. (IN-dee-uhm) *USP 34.*
Use: Radiopharmaceutical.

indium In 111 murine monoclonal antibody fab to myosin.
Use: Diagnostic aid in myocarditis. [Orphan Drug]
See: Myoscint.

•indium In 111 oxyquinoline solution. (IN-dee-uhm OX-ee-KWIN-oh-lin) *USP 34.*
Use: Radiopharmaceutical, diagnostic aid.

•indium In 111 pentetate injection. (IN-dee-uhm) *USP 34.*
Use: Diagnostic aid (radionuclide cisternography), radiopharmaceutical.

•indium In 111 pentetreotide. (IN-dee-uhm In 111 pen-teh-TREE-oh-tide) *USP 34.*
Use: Diagnostic aid, radiopharmaceutical.

•indium In 111 satumomab pendetide. (IN-dee-uhm sat-YOU-mah-mab PEN-deh-TIDE) USAN.
Use: Radiodiagnostic monoclonal antibody (ovarian and colorectal carcinoma), radiopharmaceutical.

Indocin. (Iroko) Indomethacin. Oral Susp.: 25 mg/5 mL. Alcohol 1%. Sorbitol. Pineapple, coconut, and mint flavor. Bot. 237 mL. Supp.: 50 mg. 30s. *Rx.*
Use: Analgesic; nonsteroidal anti-inflammatory drug.

Indocin I.V. (Lundbeck) Indomethacin sodium trihydrate equivalent to 1 mg indomethacin/Vial. Vial single-dose. *Rx.*
Use: Arterial patency agent.

•indocyanine green. (in-doe-SIGH-ah-neen) *USP 34.*
Use: Diagnostic aid (cardiac output determination, hepatic function determination); ophthalmic diagnostic product.
See: Cardio-Green.
IC-Green.

Indogesic. (Century) Acetaminophen 32.5 mg, butalbital 50 mg. Tab. Bot. 100s, 1000s. *Rx.*
Use: Analgesic; hypnotic, sedative.

Indoklon. Hexafluorodiethyl ether. Fluorothyl. Bis-(2,2,2-trifluoroethyl) ether. *Rx.*
Use: Shock-inducing agent (convulsant).

•indolapril hydrochloride. (in-DAHL-ah-PRILL) USAN.
Use: Antihypertensive.

•indolidan. (in-DOE-lih-DAN) USAN.
Use: Cardiovascular agent.

Indometh. (Major) Indomethacin. Cap. 25 mg: Bot. 100s, 1000s. 50 mg: Bot. 100s, 500s. *Rx.*
Use: Nonsteroidal anti-inflammatory agent.

• **indomethacin.** (in-doe-METH-ah-sin)
USP 34.
Use: Nonsteroidal anti-inflammatory
agent.
See: Indocin.

indomethacin. (Bedford Labs) Indo-
methacin sodium 1 mg. Inj., lyophilized
Pow. for Soln. Single-dose vial. Rx.
Use: Agent for patent ductus arteriosus.

indomethacin. (G & W Laboratories) Indomethacin 50 mg. Rectal Supp. 30s. *Rx.*
Use: Nonsteroidal anti-inflammatory
agent.

indomethacin. (Various Mfr.) Indomethacin sodium 1 mg. Inj., lyophilized Pow.
for Soln. Single-dose vial. *Rx.*
Use: Agent for patent ductus arteriosus.

indomethacin. (Various Mfr.) Indomethacin 25 mg, 50 mg. Cap. Bot. 50s (25 mg
only), 100s, 500s, 1000s, UD 100s,
Robot ready 25s. *Rx.*
Use: Nonsteroidal anti-inflammatory
agent.

indomethacin extended-release. (Inwood) Indomethacin 75 mg. Sucrose,
parabens. SR Cap. Bot. 60s, 100s. *Rx.*
Use: Nonsteroidal anti-inflammatory
agent.

• **indomethacin sodium.** (in-doe-METH-
ah-sin) *USP 34.*
Use: Nonsteroidal anti-inflammatory
agent.

indomethacin sodium trihydrate. *Rx.*
Use: Arterial patency agent.
See: Indocin I.V.

indomethacin SR. (Various Mfr.) Indomethacin 75 mg. SR Cap. Bot. 60s,
100s, 500s. *Rx.*
Use: Nonsteroidal anti-inflammatory
agent.

• **indoprofen.** (in-doe-PRO-fen) USAN.
Use: Analgesic; anti-inflammatory.

• **indoramin.** (in-DAHR-ah-min) USAN.
Use: Antihypertensive.

• **indoramin hydrochloride.** (in-DAHR-ah-
min) USAN.
Use: Antihypertensive.

• **indorenate hydrochloride.** (in-DAHR-
en-ATE) USAN.
Use: Antihypertensive.

• **indoxole.** (IN-dox-OLE) USAN.
Use: Antipyretic; anti-inflammatory.

• **indriline hydrochloride.** (IN-drih-leen)
USAN.
Use: Stimulant, central.

I-Neocort. (American Pharmaceutical)
Neomycin sulfate 5 mg, hydrocortisone
acetate 15 mg/5 mL. Ophth. Susp. Bot.
5 mL. *Rx.*
Use: Anti-infective; corticosteroid.

I-Neospor. (American Pharmaceutical)
Polymyxin B sulfate, gramicidin, neo-
mycin sulfate. Ophth. Soln. Bot. 10 mL.
Rx.
Use: Anti-infective, ophthalmic.

Infalyte Oral Solution. (Bristol-Myers
Squibb) Electrolyte mixture with 30 g/L
rice syrup solids containing 4.2 calo-
ries/fl. oz. In 1 liter. *OTC.*
Use: Nutritional supplement.

Infanrix. (GlaxoSmithKline) Diphtheria
toxoid 25 Lf units, tetanus toxoid 10 Lf
units, inactivated pertussis toxin
25 mcg, filamentous hemagglutinin
25 mcg, pertactin 8 mcg/0.5 mL. Formaldehyde, sodium chloride, phenoxyethanol. Inj. Single-dose Vials and disposable *Tip-Lok* syringes. *Rx.*
Use: Immunization, active toxoid.

Infantaire. (Altaire) Acetaminophen
100 mg/mL. Soln., Conc., Oral. 15 mL,
30 mL with 0.8 mL dropper. *OTC.*
Use: Analgesic.

infant foods.
Use: Nutritional supplement.
See: Enfamil.
Enfamil Human Milk Fortifier.
Enfamil Premature 20 Formula.
RCF.
Similac.
Similac PM 60/40.

infant foods, hypoallergenic.
Use: Nutritional supplement.
See: Isomil.
Isomil SF.
I-Soyalac.
Nutramigen.
Pregestimil.
ProSobee.
Soyalac.

Infants' Motrin. (McNeil) Ibuprofen
40 mg/mL. Sorbitol, sucrose, berry flavor. Oral drops. Bot. 15 mL w/dropper.
OTC.
Use: Anti-inflammatory; analgesic.

Infants' No-Aspirin Drops. (Walgreen)
Acetaminophen 80 mg/0.8 mL. Nonal-
coholic. Bot. 15 mL. *OTC.*
Use: Analgesic.

Infants' Silapap. (Silarx) Acetaminophen
80 mg/0.8 mL. Drops. Bot. 15 mL. Alcohol free. *OTC.*
Use: Analgesic; antipyretic.

Infarub Cream. (Whitehall-Robins Laboratories) Methyl salicylate 35%, menthol 10% in vanishing cream base. Tube
1.25 oz, 3.5 oz. *OTC.*
Use: Analgesic, topical.

Infasurf. (Forest) Phospholipids 35 mg/
mL suspended in 0.9% sodium chloride solution, 0.65 mg proteins. Intratra-

cheal Susp. Single-use vial 6 mL. *Rx.*
Use: Lung surfactant.

Infectrol Ointment. (Bausch & Lomb) Dexamethasone 0.1%, neomycin sulfate equivalent to 0.35% neomycin base, 10,000 units polymyxin B sulfate/g. White petrolatum, lanolin, mineral oil, parabens. Tube 3.5, 3.75 g. *Rx.*
Use: Anti-infective, corticosteroid, topical.

Infectrol Suspension. (Bausch & Lomb) Dexamethasone 0.1%, neomycin sulfate equivalent to 0.35% neomycin base, 10,000 units polymyxin B sulfate/mL. Hydroxypropyl methylcellulose, polysorbate 20, benzalkonium chloride. Drop. Bot. 5 mL. *Rx.*
Use: Anti-infective; corticosteroid, ophthalmic.

INFeD. (Schein) Iron 50 mg/mL (as dextran), sodium chloride approximately 0.9%. Inj. Single-dose Vial 2 mL. *Rx.*
Use: Mineral supplement.

Infergen. (Three Rivers) Interferon alfacon-1 9 mcg, 15 mcg, preservative free. Inj. Single-dose vial. 0.3 mL (9 mcg), 0.5 mL (15 mcg). *Rx.*
Use: Immunologic, immunomodulator.

• **infliximab.** (in-FLIX-i-mab) USAN.
Tall Man: inFLIXimab
Use: Immunologic agent; immunomodulator.
See: Remicade.

• **influenza virus vaccine.** (in-flew-EN-zuh) *USP 34.*
Use: Immunization.
See: Afluria.
  Agriflu.
  Fluarix.
  FluLaval.
  FluMist.
  Fluvirin.
  Fluzone.
  Fluzone High-Dose.

Infumorph 500. (Baxter) Morphine sulfate 25 mg/mL. Soln. for Inj. Amp. 20 mL (500 mg). *c-II.*
Use: Opioid analgesic.

Infumorph 200. (Baxter) Morphine sulfate 10 mg/mL. Inj. Amp. 20 mL (200 mg). *c-II.*
Use: Opioid analgesic.

Infuvite Adult. (Baxter) Vitamin A 2300 units, D_3 200 units, E (dl-alpha tocopheryl acetate) 10 units, B_1 6 mg, B_2 3.6 mg, B_3 40 mg, B_5 15 mg, B_6 6 mg, B_{12} 5 mcg, C 200 mg, K 150 mcg, biotin 60 mcg, folic acid 600 mcg/10 mL (after combining vials), polysorbate 80. Inj. Vials. 2.5 mL. *Rx.*
Use: Nutritional supplement.

Infuvite Pediatric. (Baxter) Vitamin A

2300 units, D_3 400 units, E (dl-alpha tocopheryl acetate) 7 units, B_1 1.2 mg, B_2 14 mg, B_3 17 mg, B_5 15 mg, B_6 1 mg, B_{12} 1 mcg, C 80 mg, K 0.2 mg, biotin 20 mcg, folic acid 140 mcg/5 mL (after combining vials), polysorbate 80. Inj. 2 vials (4 mL and 1 mL). *Rx.*
Use: Nutritional supplement.

Ingadine Tabs. (Major) Guanethidine sulfate 10 mg, 25 mg. Bot. 100s, 1000s. *Rx.*
Use: Antihypertensive.

• **ingenol mebutate.** (IN-jen-ol me-BUE-tate) USAN.
Use: Antineoplastic agent.

• **ingliforib.** (in-gli-FOE-rib) USAN.
Use: Antidiabetic.

INH. (Novartis) Isoniazid 300 mg. Tab. *Rx.*
Use: Antituberculosis agent.

Inhal-Aid. (Key)
Use: Respiratory drug delivery system.

Inhibace. (Roche) Cilazapril. *Rx.*
Use: Antihypertensive.

• **iniparib.** (in-i-PAR-ib) USAN.
Use: Antineoplastic.

injectable local anesthetics.
See: Anesthetics, Injectable Local.

Innerclean Herbal Laxative. (Last) Senna leaf powder, psyllium seed, buckthorne, anise seed, fennel seed. Bot. 1 oz, 2 oz. *OTC.*
Use: Laxative.

Innertabs. (Last) Senna leaf powder and psyllium seed tablets. Bot. 80s, 200s. *OTC.*
Use: Laxative.

Innohep. (Leo Pharma) Tinzaparin sodium 20,000 units/mL (Anti-Factor Xa International Units). Sodium metabisulfite 3.1 mg/mL, benzyl alcohol 10 mg/mL. Inj. Multidose vial 2 mL. *Rx.*
Use: Anticoagulant; low molecular weight heparin.

InnoPran XL. (GlaxoSmithKline) Propranolol hydrochloride 80 mg, 120 mg, sugar spheres. ER Cap. 30s, 100s. *Rx.*
Use: Antiadrenergic/sympatholytic, beta-adrenergic blocking agent.

Inocor Lactate. (Sanofi-Synthelabo) Amrinone lactate (base equivalent) 5 mg/mL, sodium metabisulfite 0.25 mg. Inj. Amp. 20 mL. Box 5s. *Rx.*
Use: Inotropic.

• **inocoterone acetate.** (ih-NO-koe-ter-ohn) USAN.
Use: Dermatologic, acne.

INOmax. (INO Therapeutics) Nitric oxide 100 ppm, 800 ppm. Gas. 353 L (delivered volume 344 L), 1963 L (delivered

volume 1918 L). *Rx.*
Use: Respiratory inhalant.
inophylline.
See: Aminophylline.
inosine pranobex. Isoprinosine.
Use: Antiviral. [Orphan Drug]
See: Isoprinosine.
Inosiplex. (Newport Pharmaceuticals)
Isoprinosine. *Rx.*
Use: Antiviral.
inosit.
See: Inositol.
Inositech. (Bio-tech) Inositol 324 mg.
Cap. 100s. *OTC.*
Use: Lipotropic product.
inositol.
Use: Lipotropic.
See: Inositech.
•**inositol niacinate.** (in-OH-sih-tole NIE-ah-sin-ate) USAN.
Use: Vasodilator.
inositol nicotinate.
See: Inositol Niacinate.
inotropic agents.
See: Digitek.
Digoxin.
Digoxin Injection, Pediatric.
Inamrinone Lactate.
Lanoxin.
Milrinone Lactate.
Primacor.
Inova Easy Pad. (JSJ Pharmaceuticals)
Benzoyl peroxide 4%, 8%. Disodium
EDTA, glycerin, methylparaben. Pad.
Kit w/30 pads and 28 tocopherol 5%
topical capsules. *Rx.*
Use: Anti-infective, topical; antibiotic
agent.
Inova 8/2 Acne Control Therapy. (JSJ
Pharmaceuticals) Benzoyl peroxide
8%, salicylic acid 2%, tocopherol 5%.
Disodium EDTA, glycerin, methylpara-
ben. Pad. Kit w/30 benzoyl peroxide
pads, 30 salicylic acid pads, and 28 to-
copherol 5% topical capsules. *Rx.*
Use: Acne product combination
Inova 4/1 Acne Control Therapy. (JSJ
Pharmaceuticals) Benzoyl peroxide
4%, salicylic acid 1%, tocopherol 5%.
Disodium EDTA, glycerin, methylpara-
ben. Pad. Kit w/30 benzoyl peroxide
pads, 30 salicylic acid pads, and 28 tocopherol 5% topical capsules. *Rx.*
Use: Acne product combination.
InspirEase. (Key) *Rx.*
Use: Respiratory drug delivery system.
Inspra. (Searle) Eplerenone 25 mg,
50 mg, lactose. Tab. Bot. 30s, 90s, unit
doses (25 mg only). *Rx.*
Use: Renin angiotensin system antagonist.

Insta-Char. (Kerr Drug) **Regular:** Aqueous suspension activated charcoal
50 g/8 oz. **Pediatric:** Aqueous suspen-
sion activated charcoal 15 g/4 oz. *OTC.*
Use: Antidote.
Insta-Glucose. (ICN) Undiluted USP glu-
cose. UD tube containing liquid glu-
cose 31 g. *OTC.*
Use: Hyperglycemic.
Inst-E-Vite. (Barth's) Vitamin E 100 units,
200 units. Cap. **100 units:** Bot 100s,
500s, 1000s. **200 units:** Bot. 100s,
250s, 500s. *OTC.*
Use: Vitamin supplement.
•**insulin.** (IN-suh-lin) *USP 34.*
Use: Antidiabetic.
See: Insulin Analog.
Insulin Detemir.
Insulin Glargine.
Insulin Glulisine.
Insulin Human (Inhalation).
Insulin Injection Concentrated.
Insulin Injection (Regular).
Insulin Regular Concentrate.
Insulin Zinc Suspension, Extended
(Ultralente).
Insulin Zinc Suspension (Lente).
Isophane Insulin Suspension (NPH).
Isophane Insulin Suspension (NPH)
and Insulin Injection (Regular).
insulin analog.
Use: Antidiabetic.
See: Humalog.
Humalog Mix 75/25.
NovoLog.
•**insulin aspart.** (IN-suh-lin ASS-part)
USAN.
Use: Antidiabetic.
•**insulin, dalanated.** (IN-suh-lin dah-
LAHN-ate-ed) USAN.
Use: Antidiabetic.
•**insulin degludec.** (IN-su-lin de-GLOO-
dek) USAN.
Use: Antidiabetic.
•**insulin detemir.** (IN-suh-lin DEHT-ih-
meer) USAN.
Use: Antidiabetic.
See: Levemir.
•**insulin glargine.** (IN-suh-lin GLAHR-
gine) USAN.
Use: Antidiabetic.
See: Lantus.
•**insulin glulisine.** (IN-suh-lin gloo-LIS-
een) USAN.
Use: Antidiabetic.
See: Apidra.
•**insulin human.** (IN-suh-lin) *USP 34.*
Use: Antidiabetic.
See: Humulin.

•**insulin human, isophane, suspension.** (IN-suh-lin hue-man EYE-so-fane) *USP 34.*
Use: Antidiabetic.

•**insulin human zinc, extended, suspension.** (IN-suh-lin) *USP 34.*
Use: Antidiabetic.

•**insulin human zinc suspension.** (IN-suh-lin) *USP 34.*
Use: Antidiabetic.

insulin inhaled.
Use: Investigational antidiabetic agent.

insulin injection, concentrated.
Use: Antidiabetic.
See: Humulin R Regular U-500 (Concentrated).

insulin injection (regular).
Use: Antidiabetic.
See: Humulin R.
  Novolin R.
  Novolin R PenFill.
  Novolin R Prefilled.

•**insulin, isophane, suspension.** (IN-suh-lin EYE-so-fane) *USP 34.*
Use: Antidiabetic.
See: NPH.

•**insulin I 131.** (IN-suh-lin) USAN.
Use: Radiopharmaceutical.

•**insulin I 125.** (IN-suh-lin) USAN.
Use: Radiopharmaceutical.

insulin-like growth factor.
See: Mesermin.
  Mecasermin Rinfabate.

insulin-like growth factor-1, recombinant.
Use: Amyotrophic lateral sclerosis. [Orphan Drug]

•**insulin lispro.** (IN-suh-lin LICE-pro) *USP 34.*
Use: Antidiabetic.
See: Humalog.
  Humalog Mix 50/50.
  Humalog Mix 75/25.

•**insulin, neutral.** (IN-suh-lin) USAN.
Use: Antidiabetic.

insulin Novo rapitard. Biphasic Insulin.

•**insulin, protamine zinc suspension.** (IN-suh-lin PRO-tah-meen zingk) *USP 34.* 40 units, 100 units/mL. Vials 10 mL.
Use: Antidiabetic.

insulin, regular.
Use: Antidiabetic.
See: Humulin BR.
  Humulin R.
  Novolin R.
  Novolin R PenFill.
  Velosulin.
  Velosulin (Pork).

insulin, regular concentrate.
Use: Antidiabetic.
See: Humulin R.
  Regular U-500 (Concentrated).

insulin suspension, isophane.
Use: Antidiabetic.
See: Humulin 50/50.
  Humulin 70/30.
  Novolin 70/30.
  Novolin 70/30 PenFill.

insulin suspension, lente.
Use: Antidiabetic.
See: Lente Insulin.
  Lente Insulin (Beef).
  Lente L.
  Lente Iletin II (Beef).
  Lente Purified Pork Insulin.
  Novolin L.

insulin suspension, NPH.
Use: Antidiabetic.
See: Beef NPH Iletin II.
  Humulin N.
  Novolin N.
  Novolin N PenFill.
  NPH Iletin I (Beef and Pork).
  NPH Insulin (Beef).
  NPH-N Purified (Pork).

insulin suspension, PZI. *OTC.*
Use: Antidiabetic.

insulin suspension semilente. *OTC.*
Use: Antidiabetic.

insulin suspension, ultralente. *OTC.*
Use: Antidiabetic.
See: Ultralente Insulin (Beef).

•**insulin zinc, prompt, suspension.** (IN-suh-lin) *USP 34.*
Use: Antidiabetic.

•**insulin zinc, suspension, extended (ultralente).** (IN-suh-lin) *USP 34.*
Use: Antidiabetic.

•**insulin zinc suspension (lente).** (IN-suh-lin) *USP 34.*
Use: Antidiabetic.

Intal. (King) Cromolyn sodium 800 mcg/actuation. Aerosol. 8.1 g (≥ 112 metered sprays), 14.2 g (≥ 200 metered sprays). *Rx.*
Use: Antiasthmatic.

integrase inhibitors.
Use: Antiretroviral agents.
See: Raltegravir.

Integrilin. (Schering) Eptifibatide 0.75 mg/mL, 2 mg/mL. Inj. for Soln. Vial 10 mL (2 mg/mL only), 100 mL. *Rx.*
Use: Antiplatelet, glycoprotein IIb/IIIa inhibitor.

Integrin Caps. (Sanofi-Synthelabo) Oxypertine. *Rx.*
Use: Anxiolytic.

Intelence. (Centocor Ortho Biotech) Etravirine 100 mg, 200 mg. Lactose. Tab.

60s (200 mg), 120s (100 mg). *Rx.*
Use: Antiretroviral agent, non-nucleoside reverse transcriptase inhibitors.
Intensol. (Roxane) A system of concentrated solutions of drugs w/calibrated dropper: Chlorpromazine hydrochloride 30 mg/mL, 100 mg/mL; dexamethasone 1 mg/mL; dihydrotachysterol 0.2 mg/mL; hydrochlorothiazide 100 mg/mL; prednisone 5 mg/mL; thioridazine hydrochloride 30 mg/mL, 100 mg/mL.
interferon. A family of naturally occurring, small protein molecules with molecular weights of approximately 15,000 to 21,000 daltons. They are formed by the interaction of animal cells with viruses capable of conferring on animal cells' resistance to virus infection. Three major classes of interferons have been identified: alpha, beta, and gamma. Interferon was first derived from human white blood cells and originally used in Finland.
Use: Antineoplastic, antiviral; treatment of breast cancer lymphoma, multiple melanoma, and malignant melanoma.
See: Actimmune.
Avonex.
Betaseron.
Intron A.
interferon alfacon-1.
Use: Immunologic, immunomodulator.
See: Infergen.
•**interferon alfa-n1.** (IN-ter-FEER-ahn AL-fuh) USAN.
Use: Antineoplastic, antiviral; biological response modifier. [Orphan Drug]
interferon alfa-n3 (human leukocyte derived).
Use: Immunologic agent, immunomodulator.
See: Alferon N.
•**interferon alfa-2a, recombinant.** (IN-ter-FEER-ahn AL-fuh-2a ree-KAHM-bih-nent) USAN.
Use: Antineoplastic, antiviral; biological response modifier; immunomodulator. [Orphan Drug]
•**interferon alfa-2b, recombinant.** (IN-ter-FEER-ahn AL-fuh-2b) USAN.
Use: Antineoplastic, antiviral; biological response modifier; immunomodulator.
See: Intron A.
interferon, beta.
Use: Immunomodulator; treatment of multiple sclerosis.
See: Avonex.
Betaseron.

•**interferon beta-1a.** (in-ter-FEER-ohn BAY-tuh-1a) USAN.
Use: Biological response modifier; immunologic agent, immunomodulator.
See: Avonex.
Rebif.
•**interferon beta-1b.** (IN-ter-FEER-ahn BAY-tuh-1b) USAN.
Use: Immunologic agent, immunomodulator.
See: Betaseron.
Extavia.
•**interferon gamma-1b.** (IN-ter-FEER-ahn GAM-uh-1b) USAN.
Use: Antineoplastic, antiviral; immunoregulator, biological response modifier; immunomodulator.
See: Actimmune.
interleukin-1 receptor antagonist, human recombinant.
Use: Juvenile rheumatoid arthritis; graft-vs-host disease in transplant patients. [Orphan Drug]
See: Antril.
interleukins.
Use: Hematopoietic.
See: Oprelvekin.
interleukin-3, human recombinant. (Novartis) *Rx.*
Use: Immunomodulator. [Orphan Drug]
interleukin-2.
Use: Immunomodulator; antineoplastic. [Orphan Drug]
See: Proleukin.
Teceleukin.
interleukin-2 PEG. (Cetus) *Rx.*
Use: Immunomodulator.
interleukin-2, recombinant liposome encapsulated.
Use: Antineoplastic. [Orphan Drug]
interstitial cystitis agents.
See: Dimethyl Sulfoxide.
Interstitial Cystitis Combinations.
Pentosan Polysulfate Sodium.
Phenazopyridine Hydrochloride.
interstitial cystitis combinations.
See: Phenazopyridine Hydrochloride, Hyoscyamine Hydrobromide, Butabarbital.
Intestinex. (A.G. Marin) *Lactobacillus acidophilus* 100 million units. Cap. 24s. *OTC.*
Use: Nutritional supplement.
•**intetumumab.** (IN-te-TUM-ue-mab) USAN.
Use: Antineoplastic.
Intralipid 30%. (Baxter) Soybean oil 30%, egg yolk phospholipids 1.2%, glycerin 1.7%. 200 mOsmol/L. 3 kcal/mL. Inj., Emulsion. Pharmacy bulk pack-

ages. 500 mL. *Rx.*
Use: Intravenous fat emulsion, lipid, intravenous nutritional therapy.
Intralipid 20% I.V. Fat Emulsion. (Baxter) IV fat emulsion containing soybean oil 20%, egg yolk phospholipids 1.2%, glycerin 2.25%, water for injection. I.V. Flask 50 mL, 100 mL, 250 mL, 500 mL. *Rx.*
Use: Nutritional supplement, parenteral.
intranasal steroids.
See: Beclomethasone Dipropionate.
Budesonide.
Ciclesonide.
Flunisolide.
Fluticasone.
Mometasone Furoate Monohydrate.
Triamcinolone Acetonide.
IntraSite. (Smith & Nephew) Graft T starch copolymer 2%, water 8%, propylene glycol 20%. Sterile amorphous interactive hydrogel dressing. 25 g. *Rx.*
Use: Dermatologic, wound therapy.
intraval sodium.
See: Pentothal Sodium.
intravenous nutritional therapy.
See: Combined Electrolyte Concentrates.
Combined Electrolyte Solutions.
Dextrose 2.5% with 0.45% Sodium Chloride.
Dextrose 3.3% and 0.3% Sodium Chloride.
Dextrose 5% and Electrolyte No. 48.
Dextrose 5% and Electrolyte No. 75.
Dextrose 5% with 0.2% Sodium Chloride.
Dextrose 5% and 0.225% Sodium Chloride.
Dextrose 5% with 0.3% Sodium Chloride.
Dextrose 5% with 0.33% Sodium Chloride.
Dextrose 5% with 0.45% Sodium Chloride.
Dextrose 5% with 0.9% Sodium Chloride.
Dextrose 10% and Electrolyte No. 48.
Dextrose 10% with 0.2% Sodium Chloride.
Dextrose 10% with 0.225% Sodium Chloride.
Dextrose 10% with 0.45% Sodium Chloride.
Dextrose 10% and 0.9% Sodium Chloride.
Electrolytes.
Half-Strength Lactated Ringer's in 2.5% Dextrose.
Hyperlyte CR.
Invert Sugar-Electrolyte Solutions.
Isolyte H in 5% Dextrose.
Isolyte M in 5% Dextrose.
Isolyte P in 5% Dextrose.
Isolyte R in 5% Dextrose.
Isolyte S pH 7.4.
Isolyte S with 5% Dextrose.
Lactated Ringer's.
Lactated Ringer's in 5% Dextrose.
Lypholyte.
Lypholyte-II.
Magnesium.
Minerals.
Multilyte-20.
Multilyte-40.
Multiple Electrolytes and 5% Travert.
Multiple Electrolytes and 10% Travert.
Normosol-M.
Normosol-M and 5% Dextrose.
Normosol-R.
Normosol-R and 5% Dextrose.
Normosol-R pH 7.4.
Nutrilyte.
Nutrilyte II.
Phosphate.
Plasma-Lyte A pH 7.4.
Plasma-Lyte 56 and 5% Dextrose.
Plasma-Lyte 148.
Plasma-Lyte 148 and 5% Dextrose.
Plasma-Lyte R.
Plasma-Lyte R and 5% Dextrose.
Potassium Chloride in 0.9% Sodium Chloride.
Potassium Chloride in 3.3% Dextrose and 0.3% Sodium Chloride.
Potassium Chloride in 5% Dextrose.
Potassium Chloride in 5% Dextrose and Lactated Ringer's.
Potassium Chloride in 5% Dextrose and 0.2% Sodium Chloride.
Potassium Chloride in 5% Dextrose and 0.33% Sodium Chloride.
Potassium Chloride in 5% Dextrose and 0.45% Sodium Chloride.
Potassium Chloride in 5% Dextrose and 0.9% Sodium Chloride.
Potassium Chloride in 10% Dextrose and 0.2% Sodium Chloride.
Potassium Salts.
Ringer's.
Ringer's in 5% Dextrose.
Sodium Chloride.
TPN Electrolytes.
TPN Electrolytes II.
TPN Electrolytes III.
intravenous replenishment solutions.
Use: Intravenous nutritional therapy.
See: Intravenous Nutritional Therapy.
•**intrazole.** (IN-trah-zole) USAN.
Use: Anti-inflammatory.

•**intriptyline hydrochloride.** (in-TRIP-tih-leen) USAN.
Use: Antidepressant.

Introlite. (Ross) Protein 22.2 g, carbohydrate 70.5 g, fat 18.4 g, Na 930 mg, K 1570 mg/L with 200 mOsm/kg water, with appropriate vitamins and minerals, 0.53 Cal/mL. Liq. *OTC.*
Use: Nutritional supplement.

Intron A. (Schering) Interferon alfa-2b, recombinant. **Inj., Pow. for Soln.:** 10 million, 18 million, 50 million units/vial. Each mL contains human albumin 1 mg, glycine 20 mg, sodium phosphate dibasic 2.3 mg, sodium phosphate monobasic 0.55 mg. Vials w/1 mL diluent vial. Diluent is sterile water for injection. **Inj. Soln.:** 3 million, 5 million, 10 million, 18 million, 25 million units/vial. Each mL contains sodium chloride 7.5 mg, sodium phosphate dibasic 1.8 mg, sodium phosphate monobasic 1.3 mg, EDTA 0.1 mg, polysorbate 80 0.1 mg, m-cresol 1.5 mg as preservative. Vials. Pak-10 (6 vials, 6 B-D Safety-Lok syringes) (10 million). Multidose vials. 22.8 million units/3.8 mL (18 million units). Multidose vials. 32 million units/3.2 mL (25 million units). Multidose pens (6 doses) with needles. 22.5 million units/1.5 mL/pen (3 million units), 37.5 million units/1.5 mL/pen (5 million units), 75 million units/1.5 mL/pen (10 million units). *Rx.*
Use: Immunologic agent, immunomodulator.

Intropaque Liquid. (Lafayette) Barium sulfate 60% w/v suspension. Bot. Gal. Case 4s.
Use: Radiopaque agent.

Intropaste. (Mallinckrodt) Barium sulfate 70%. Simethicone, sorbitol, saccharin, parabens. Paste. Tube 454 g. *Rx.*
Use: Radiopaque agent, GI contrast agent.

Intuniv. (Shire) Guanfacine 1 mg, 2 mg, 3 mg, 4 mg. Lactose. ER Tab. 100s. *Rx.*
Use: Antiadrenergic/sympatholytic; antiadrenergic agent, centrally acting.

•**inulin.** (IN-you-lin) *USP 34.*
Use: Diagnostic aid (renal function determination).

inulin. (DuPont) Purified inulin 5 g/50 mL sodium Cl 0.9%, sodium hydroxide to adjust pH. Amp. 50 mL.
Use: Diagnostic aid.

Invanz. (Merck) Ertapenem sodium 1.046 g (equivalent to ertapenem 1 g). Sodium bicarbonate 175 mg, sodium 6 mEq. Pow., for Inj., lyophilized. Single-dose vials. *Rx.*
Tall Man: INVanz
Use: Anti-infective.

Invega. (Janssen) Paliperidone 3 mg (lactose), 6 mg, 9 mg. ER Tab. 30s, 350s, UD 100s. *Rx.*
Use: Antipsychotic agent.

Invega Sustenna. (Janssen) Paliperidone 39 mg, 78 mg, 117 mg, 156 mg, 234 mg. PEG 4000. Kit w/prefilled syringe and 2 safety needles. *Rx.*
Use: Antipsychotic agent, benzisoxazole derivative.

invert sugar. (Abbott) 10%. Soln. Bot. 1000 mL. *Rx-OTC.*
Use: Nutritional supplement, parenteral.
See: Travert.

invert sugar-electrolyte solutions. *Rx.*
Use: Nutritional supplement, parenteral.
See: 5% Travert and Electrolyte No. 2.
10% Travert and Electrolyte No. 2.
Multiple Electrolytes and 5% Travert.
Multiple Electrolytes and 10% Travert.
Multiple Electrolyte 2 w/5% Invert Sugar.
Multiple Electrolyte 2 w/10% Invert Sugar.

invert sugar injection.
Use: Fluid, nutrient replacement.

Invirase. (Roche) Saquinavir mesylate. **Cap.:** 200 mg. Lactose. Bot. 270s. **Tab.:** 500 mg. Lactose. 120s. *Rx.*
Use: Antiviral.

Invites Rx. (Breckenridge Pharmaceuticals) Vitamin C 60 mg, B_1 1.5 mg, B_2 1.7 mg, B_3 20 mg, B_6 10 mg, B_{12} 6 mcg, folic acid 1 mcg, biotin 300 mcg, Zn. Film-coated. Tab. 100s. *Rx.*
Use: Multivitamin with minerals.

in vivo diagnostic aids.
See: Benzypenicilloyl Polylysine.
Capromab Pendetide.
Gadofosveset Trisodium.
Gastrointestinal Function Tests.
Gonadorelin Hydrochloride.
Hexaminolevulinate Hydrochloride.
Ioflupane I 123.
Methacholine Chloride.
Metyrapone.
Pentetate Indium Disodium In 111.
Regadenoson.
Tolbutamide Sodium.
Thyroid Function Tests.
Tuberculin Purified Protein Derivative.

•**iobenguane I 131.** (EYE-oh-BEN-gwane) USAN.
Use: Diagnostic aid; radiopharmaceutical.

• **iobenguane I 123 injection.** (EYE-oh-BEN-gwane) *USP 34.*
Use: Radiopharmaceutical.
See: AdreView.

• **iobenguane sulfate I 131.** (EYE-oh-BEN-gwane) USAN.
Use: Diagnostic aid; radiopharmaceutical.

• **iobenguane sulfate I 123.** (EYE-oh-BEN-gwane) USAN.
Use: Diagnostic aid, radioactive, adrenomedullary disorders, and neuroendocrine tumors; radiopharmaceutical.

• **iobenzamic acid.** (EYE-oh-ben-ZAM-ik) USAN.
Use: Diagnostic aid (radiopaque medium, cholecystographic).

Iobid DM. (Iopharm) Dextromethorphan HBr 30 mg, guaifenesin 600 mg. ER Tab. Bot. 100s. *Rx.*
Use: Upper respiratory combination, antitussive, expectorant.

• **iocanlidic acid I 123.** (eye-oh-kan-LIH-dik) USAN.
Use: Diagnostic aid (radioactive, cardiac disease) for assessment of viable myocardium.

Iocare Balanced Salt Solution. (Novartis Ophthalmic) Sodium Cl 0.64%, potassium Cl 0.075%, magnesium Cl 0.03%, calcium Cl 0.048%, sodium acetate 0.39%, sodium citrate 0.17%, sodium hydroxide or hydrochloric acid. Soln. Bot. 15 mL. *Rx.*
Use: Irrigant, ophthalmic.

• **iocarmate meglumine.** (EYE-oh-KAR-mate meh-GLUE-meen) USAN.
Use: Diagnostic aid (radiopaque medium).

• **iocarmic acid.** (EYE-oh-KAR-mik) USAN.
Use: Diagnostic aid (radiopaque medium).

• **iocetamic acid.** (eye-oh-seh-TAM-ik) *USP 34.*
Use: Diagnostic aid (radiopaque medium).

i-octadecanol. *NF 29.*
See: Stearyl Alcohol.

• **iodamide.** (EYE-oh-dah-MIDE) USAN.
Use: Diagnostic aid (radiopaque medium).

• **iodamide meglumine.** (EYE-oh-dah-MIDE meh-GLUE-meen) USAN.
Use: Diagnostic aid (radiopaque medium).
W/Combinations.
See: Renovue-Dip.
Renovue-65.

Iodex. (Lee) Iodine 4.7% in petrolatum ointment base. 28.35 g. *OTC.*
Use: Antimicrobial; antiseptic.

Iodex with Methyl Salicylate. (Lee) Iodine 4.7%, methyl salicylate 4.8%. Oleic acid, paraffin, petrolatum. Oint. 28 g. *OTC.*
Use: Antiseptic; analgesic, topical.

iodide, sodium, I-131 capsules.
Use: Antineoplastic; diagnostic aid (thyroid function determination); radiopharmaceutical.
See: Iodotope.

iodide, sodium, I-131 solution.
Use: Antineoplastic; diagnostic aid (thyroid function determination); radiopharmaceutical.
See: Iodotope.

iodide, sodium, I-125 capsules.
Use: Diagnostic aid (thyroid function determination); radiopharmaceutical.

iodide, sodium, I-125 solution.
Use: Diagnostic aid (thyroid function determination), radiopharmaceutical.

iodide, sodium, I-123 capsules.
Use: Diagnostic aid (thyroid function determination).

iodide, sodium, I-123 tablets.
Use: Diagnostic aid (thyroid function determination).

iodinated glycerol and codeine phosphate liquid. (Various Mfr.) Codeine phosphate 10 mg, iodinated glycerol 30 mg. Liq. Bot. Pt, gal. *c-v.*
Use: Antitussive, expectorant, narcotic.

iodinated human serum albumin.
See: Albumotope.

iodinated I-131 albumin aggregated injection.
Use: Radiopharmaceutical.
See: Albumin, Aggregated Iodinated I-131 serum.

iodinated I-131 albumin injection.
Use: Diagnostic aid (blood volume determination and intrathecal imaging); radiopharmaceutical.
See: Albumin, Iodinated I-131.

iodinated I-125 albumin injection.
Use: Diagnostic aid (blood volume determination); radiopharmaceutical.
See: Albumin, Iodinated I-125.

• **iodine.** (EYE-uh-dine) *USP 34.*
Use: Anti-infective, topical; source of iodine.
See: Curity Sponge Sticks.
Curity Wet Skin Scrub Pack.
Iodex.
Kelp.
W/Methyl Salicylate
See: Iodex with Methyl Salicylate.
W/Potassium Iodide.
See: Strong Iodine Solution (Lugol's Solution).

iodine cacodylate, colloidal. Cacodyne Iodine.

iodine combination.
See: Calcidrine.

iodine-iodophor.
See: Betadine.

iodine I 131 murine monoclonal antibody IgG2a to B cell.
Use: Antineoplastic. [Orphan Drug]
See: Immurait.

iodine I 131 murine monoclonal antibody to alpha-fetoprotein. (Immunomedics)
Use: Antineoplastic. [Orphan Drug]

iodine I 131 murine monoclonal antibody to hCG. (Immunomedics)
Use: Antineoplastic. [Orphan Drug]

iodine I 131 6b-iodomethyl-19-norcholesterol.
Use: Diagnostic aid. [Orphan Drug]

iodine I 131 tositumomab and tositumomab.
Use: Antineoplastic.
See: Bexxar.

• **iodine I 124 girentuximab.** (JIR-en-TUX-i-mab) USAN.
Use: Diagnostic agent.

iodine I 123 murine monoclonal antibody to alpha-fetoprotein. (Immunomedics)
Use: Diagnostic aid. [Orphan Drug]

iodine I 123 murine monoclonal antibody to hCG. (Immunomedics)
Use: Diagnostic aid. [Orphan Drug]

iodine 131: capsules diagnostic-capsules therapeutic-solution therapeutic oral.
See: Iodotope.

• **iodine povacrylex.** (poe-va-KREYE-lex) USAN.
Use: Topical antiseptic.

iodine povidone.
See: Iodophor.
Mallisol.

iodine products, anti-infective.
See: Anayodin.
Betadine.
Chiniofon.
Diiodohydroxyquinoline.
Prepodyne.
Quinoxyl.
Surgidine.
Vioform.

iodine products, diagnostic.
See: Chloriodized Oil.
Ethyl Iodophenylundecylate.
Iodoalphionic Acid.
Iodobrassid.
Iodohippurate Sodium.
Iodopanoic Acid.
Iodophthalein Sodium.
Iodopyracet.

Methiodal Sodium.
Optiray 350.
Pantopaque.
Sodium Acetrizoate.
Sodium Iodomethamate.
Telepaque.

iodine products, nutritional.
See: Calcium Iodobehenate.
Entodon.
Hydriodic Acid.
Iodobrassid.
Potassium Iodide.

iodine ration. (Barth's) Iodine (from kelp) 0.15 mg, trace minerals. Tab. Bot. 90s, 180s, 360s. *OTC.*
Use: Mineral supplement.

iodine ration. (Nion Corp.) Iodine (from kelp) 0.15 mg. 3 Tab. Bot. 175s, 500s. *OTC.*
Use: Mineral supplement.

iodine surface active complex.
See: Ioprep.

iodine tincture, strong.
Use: Anti-infective, topical.

• **iodipamide.** (eye-oh-DIH-pah-mide) *USP 34.*
Use: Pharmaceutic necessity for Iodipamide Meglumine Injection.

• **iodipamide meglumine 52%.** (eye-oh-DIH-pah-mide meh-GLUE-meen) *USP 34.*
Use: Radiopaque agent, parenteral.
See: Cholografin Meglumine.

iodipamide methylglucamine. Also sodium salt injection.
W/Diatrizoate Methylglucamine.
See: Sinografin.

iodipamide sodium injection.
See: Cholografin Sodium.

• **iodipamide sodium I 131.** (eye-oh-DIH-pah-mide) USAN.
Use: Radiopharmaceutical.

iodipamide 26.8% and diatrizoate meglumine 52.7%.
Use: Radiopaque agent.
See: Diatrizoate Meglumine 52.7% and Iodipamide Meglumine 26.8% (38% Iodine).

• **iodixanol.** (EYE-oh-DIX-an-ole) *USP 34.*
Use: Radiopaque agent, parenteral.
See: Visipaque 270.
Visipaque 320.

iodoalphionic acid. Biliselectan dikol, pheniodol.

• **iodoantipyrine I 131.** (EYE-oh-doe-ANN-tee-PI-reen) USAN.
Use: Radiopharmaceutical.

iodobehenate calcium. Calcium iododocosanoate.
Use: Antigoitrogenic.

iodobrassid. Ethyl Diiodobrassidate.
Lipoiodine.
•**iodocetylic acid I 123.** (eye-OH-doe-SEE-till-ik) USAN.
Use: Diagnostic aid; radiopharmaceutical.
iodochlorhydroxyquin.
Use: Antiamebic; anti-infective, topical.
See: Clioquinol.
•**iodocholesterol I 131.** (EYE-oh-DOE-koe-LESS-teh-role) USAN.
Use: Radiopharmaceutical.
Iodo Cream. (Day-Baldwin) Clioquinol 3%. Tube 1 oz, Jar 1 lb. *OTC.*
Use: Antifungal, topical.
•**iodofiltic acid I 123.** (eye-oh-doe-FIL-tic) USAN.
Use: Metabolic imaging agent.
•**iodoform.** (EYE-oh-doe-form) *USP 34.*
Iodo H-C. (Day-Baldwin) Clioquinol 3%, hydrocortisone 1%. **Oint.:** Tube 20 g, Jar 1 lb. **Cream:** Tube 20 g, Jar 1 lb. *Rx.*
Use: Antifungal; corticosteroid.
•**iodohippurate, sodium I 131 injection.** (EYE-oh-doe-HIP-you-rate) *USP 34.*
Use: Diagnostic aid (renal function determination); radiopharmaceutical.
See: Hipputope.
•**iodohippurate sodium I 125.** (EYE-oh-doe-HIP-you-rate) USAN.
Use: Radiopharmaceutical.
See: Hipputope I 125.
•**iodohippurate sodium I 123 injection.** (EYE-oh-doe-HIP-you-rate) *USP 34.*
Use: Radiopharmaceutical; diagnostic aid (renal function determination).
iodohippuric acid.
See: Hipputope.
Iodo Ointment. (Day-Baldwin) Clioquinol 3%. Tube 1 oz, Jar 1 lb. *Rx.*
Use: Antifungal, topical.
Iodo-Pak. (SoloPak Pharmaceuticals, Inc.) Iodine 100 mcg/mL. Inj. Vial 10 mL. *Rx.*
Use: Nutritional supplement, parenteral.
iodopanoic acid.
Use: Diagnostic aid (radiopaque medium).
Iodopen. (American Pharmaceutical Partners) Sodium iodide 118 mcg/mL. Inj. 10 mL. *Rx.*
Use: Nutritional supplement, parenteral.
iodophene. Iodophthalein.
iodophene sodium.
See: Iodophthalein Sodium.
iodophor.
See: Betadine.
iodophthalein sodium. Tetraiodophenolphthalein Sodium, Tetraiodophthalein Sodium, Tetiothalein Sodium (Antinosin,

Cholepulvis, Cholumbrin, Foriod, Iodophene, Iodorayoral, Nosophene Sodium, Opacin, Photobiline, Piliophen, Radiotetrane).
Use: Radiopaque agent.
iodopropylidene glycerol.
See: Organidin.
iodopyracet compound. Diodrast.
iodopyracet concentrated. Diodrast.
iodopyracet injection. Diatrast, Diodone, Iopyracil, Neo-Methiodal, NeoSkiodan.
Use: Radiopaque medium.
•**iodopyracet I 131.** (EYE-oh-doe-peer-ah-set) USAN.
Use: Radiopharmaceutical.
•**iodopyracet I 125.** (EYE-oh-doe-peer-ah-set) USAN.
Use: Radiopharmaceutical.
iodopyrine. Antipyrine iodide.
Use: Iodides, analgesic.
•**iodoquinol.** (EYE-oh-doe-KWIH-nole) *USP 34. Formerly Diiodohydroxyquin.*
Use: Antiamebic.
See: Floraquin.
Sebaquin.
Yodoxin.
W/9-Aminoacridine Hydrochloride.
See: Vagitric.
Yodoxin.
W/Hydrocortisone Acetate.
See: Hydro-Iodoquinol 2-1.
Vytone.
W/Hydrocortisone, Coal Tar Solution.
See: Gynben.
Gynben Insufflate.
W/Surfactants.
See: Lycinate.
W/Sulfanilamide, Diethylstilbestrol.
See: Amide V/S.
D.I.T.I.
•**iodoxamate meglumine.** (EYE-oh-DOX-ah-mate meh-GLUE-meen) USAN.
Use: Diagnostic aid (radiopaque medium).
•**iodoxamic acid.** (EYE-oh-dox-AM-ik) USAN.
Use: Diagnostic aid (radiopaque medium).
iodoxyl.
See: Sodium Iodomethamate.
Iofed. (Iomed) Brompheniramine maleate 12 mg, pseudoephedrine hydrochloride 120 mg. ER Cap. Bot. 100s. *Rx.*
Use: Antihistamine, decongestant.
Iofed PD. (Iomed) Brompheniramine maleate 6 mg, pseudoephedrine hydrochloride 60 mg. ER Cap. Bot. 100s. *Rx.*
Use: Antihistamine, decongestant.

•**iofetamine hydrochloride I 123.** (EYE-oh-FET-ah-meen) USAN.
Use: Diagnostic aid; radiopharmaceutical.

•**ioflubenzamide I 131.** (EYE-oh-floo-BEN-za-mide) USAN.
Use: Radiotherapeutic agent.

•**ioflupane I 123.** (EYE-oh-FLOO-pane) USAN.
Use: Imaging agent.
See: DaTscan.

•**iofolastat I 123.** (EYE-oh-FOL-a-stat)
Use: Diagnostic agent.

•**ioglicic acid.** (eye-oh-GLIH-sick) USAN.
Use: Diagnostic aid (radiopaque medium).

•**ioglucol.** (EYE-oh-GLUE-kahl) USAN.
Use: Diagnostic aid (radiopaque medium).

•**ioglucomide.** (EYE-oh-GLUE-koe-mide) USAN.
Use: Diagnostic aid (radiopaque medium).

•**ioglycamic acid.** (EYE-oh-glie-KAM-ik) USAN.
Use: Diagnostic aid (radiopaque medium, cholecystographic).

•**iogulamide.** (EYE-oh-GULL-ah-mide) USAN.
Use: Diagnostic aid (radiopaque medium).

•**iohexol.** (EYE-oh-HEX-ole) *USP 34.*
Use: Radiopaque agent, parenteral.
See: Omnipaque 140.
   Omnipaque 300.
   Omnipaque 350.
   Omnipaque 240.

•**iomeprol.** (EYE-oh-MEH-prole) USAN.
Use: Diagnostic aid (radiopaque medium).

•**iomethin I 131.** (EYE-oh-METH-in) USAN.
Use: Diagnostic aid (neoplasm); radiopharmaceutical.

•**iomethin I 125.** (EYE-oh-METH-in) USAN.
Use: Diagnostic aid (neoplasm); radiopharmaceutical.

•**iometopane I 123.** (eye-oh-meh-TOE-pane) USAN.
Use: Diagnostic aid.

Ionamin. (Celltech) Phentermine resin 15 mg, 30 mg, lactose. Cap. Bot. 100s, 400s. *c-iv.*
Use: CNS stimulant, anorexiant.

Ionax Astringent Cleanser. (Galderma) Isopropyl alcohol 48%, acetone, salicylic acid. Bot. 240 mL. *OTC.*
Use: Dermatologic, acne.

Ionax Foam. (Galderma) Benzalkonium Cl, propylene glycol. Aerosol Can 150 mL. *OTC.*
Use: Dermatologic, acne.

Ionax Scrub. (Galderma) SD alcohol 40, benzalkonium Cl. Tube 60 g, 120 g. *OTC.*
Use: Dermatologic, acne.

ion-exchange resins.
See: Polyamine Methylene Resin.
   Resins, Sodium-Removing.

Ionil Plus Shampoo. (Galderma) Salicylic acid 2%, sodium laureth sulfate, lauramide DEA, quaternium-22, talloweth-60 myristyl glycol, laureth-23, TEA lauryl sulfate, glycol disterate, laureth-4, TEA-abietoyl hydrolyzed collagen, DMDM hydantoin, tetrasodium EDTA, sodium hydroxide, FD&C blue No. 1. Bot. 4 oz, 8 oz. *OTC.*
Use: Antiseborrheic.

Ionil Rinse. (Galderma) Conditioners with benzalkonium Cl in water base. Bot. 16 oz. *OTC.*
Use: Dermatologic, hair.

Ionil Shampoo. (Galderma) Salicylic acid, benzalkonium Cl, alcohol 12%, polyoxyethylene ethers. Plastic bot. w/ dispenser cap 4 oz, 8 oz, 16 oz, 32 oz. *OTC.*
Use: Antiseborrheic.

Ionil T. (Valeant) Coal tar solution 1%. Alcohols, benzalkonium chloride, EDTA. Shampoo. 237 mL, 473 mL. *OTC.*
Use: Antiseborrheic.

Ionosol B and 5% Dextrose. (Hospira) Dextrose 50 g, Na^+ 57 mEq, K^+ 25 mEq, Mg^{++} 5 mEq, Cl^- 49 mEq, phosphate 7 millimoles, lactate 25 mEq, 426 mOsm per L. Inj. Single-dose containers. 500 mL, 1000 mL. *Rx.*
Use: Intravenous nutritional therapy.

Ionosol D-CM. (Abbott Hospital Products) Sodium Cl 516 mg, potassium Cl 89.4 mg, calcium Cl anhydrous 27.8 mg, magnesium Cl anhydrous 14.2 mg, sodium lactate 560 mg/100 mL. Bot. 1000 mL. *Rx.*
Use: Nutritional supplement, parenteral.

Ionosol-T and 5% Dextrose. (Hospira) Dextrose 50 g, sodium 40 mEq, potassium 35 mEq, chloride 40 mEq, phosphate 15 mM, lactate 20 mEq, 432 mOsm per L. Inj., Soln. 500 mL, 1000 mL. *Rx.*
Use: Intravenous nutritional therapy, intravenous replenishment solutions.

•**iopamidol.** (EYE-oh-PAM-ih-dahl) *USP 34.*
Use: Radiopaque agent, parenteral.
See: Isovue-M 300.
   Isovue-M 200.

Isovue 300.
Isovue 370.
Isovue-200.
Isovue-250.

•**iopentol.** (EYE-oh-PEN-tole) USAN.
Use: Diagnostic aid (radiopaque medium).

Iophen-C. (Various Mfr.) Codeine phosphate 10 mg, iodinated glycerol 30 mg/5 mL. Liq. Bot. Pt, gal. *c-v.*
Use: Antitussive, expectorant.

Iophen C-NR. (Qualitest) Codeine phosphate 10 mg, guaifenesin 100 mg per 5 mL. Glycerin, propylene glycol, raspberry flavoring, saccharin, sodium benzoate, sorbitol. Liq. 473 mL. *c-v.*
Use: Upper respiratory combination, antitussive with expectorant.

Iophen-DM. (Various Mfr.) Dextromethorphan HBr, iodinated glycerol 30 mg/5 mL. Liq. Bot. 120 mL, pt, gal. *Rx.*
Use: Antitussive, expectorant.

Iophen DM-NR. (Qualitest) Dextromethorphan hydrobromide 10 mg, guaifenesin 100 mg. Glycerin, propylene glycol, raspberry flavoring, saccharin, sodium benzoate, sorbitol. Liq. 473 mL. *OTC.*
Use: Upper respiratory combination, antitussive with expectorant.

Iophendylate injection. Ethiodan, Myodil. Ethyl Iodophenylundecylate.
Use: Diagnostic aid (radiopaque medium).
See: Pantopaque.

Iophen NR. (Qualitest) Guaifenesin 100 mg per 5 mL. Glycerin, propylene glycol, raspberry flavoring, saccharin, sodium 2 mg, sodium benzoate, sorbitol. Liq. 473 mL. *OTC.*
Use: Expectorant.

Iopidine. (Alcon) Apraclonidine 0.5%, 1%, benzalkonium Cl 0.01%. Dispenser Bot. 0.25 mL (1%), *Drop-Tainer* 5 mL (0.5%). *Rx.*
Use: Antiglaucoma agent.

Iopodate sodium.
See: Ipodate Sodium.

Ioprep. (Johnson & Johnson) Nonylphenoxypolyethyleneoxy (4) ethanol and nonylphenoxypolyethyleneoxy (15) ethanol iodine complex 5.5%, nonylphenoxypolyethyleneoxy (30) ethanol 10%. Solution provides 1% available iodine. Plastic bot. Gal.
Use: Antiseptic.

•**ioprocemic acid.** (EYE-oh-pro-SEH-mik acid) USAN.
Use: Diagnostic aid (radiopaque medium).

•**iopromide.** (eye-oh-PRO-mide) *USP 34.*
Use: Radiopaque agent, parenteral.
See: Ultravist 150.
Ultravist 300.
Ultravist 370.
Ultravist 240.

•**iopronic acid.** (eye-oh-PRO-nik acid) USAN.
Use: Diagnostic aid (radiopaque medium, cholecystographic).

•**iopydol.** (eye-oh-PIE-dahl) USAN.
Use: Diagnostic aid (radiopaque medium, bronchographic).

•**iopydone.** (eye-oh-PIE-dohn) USAN.
Use: Diagnostic aid (radiopaque medium, bronchographic).

Iosal II. (Iopharm) Pseudoephedrine hydrochloride 60 mg, guaifenesin 600 mg. ER Tab. Bot. 100s. *Rx.*
Use: Upper respiratory combination, decongestant, expectorant.

Iosat. (Anbex) Potassium iodide 130 mg. Tab. 14s. *OTC.*
Use: Thyroid drug.

•**iosefamic acid.** (EYE-oh-seh-FAM-ik) USAN.
Use: Diagnostic aid; radiopaque medium.

•**ioseric acid.** (eye-oh-SEH-rik) USAN.
Use: Diagnostic aid (radiopaque medium).

•**iosimenol.** (EYE-oh-SIM-e-nol) USAN.
Use: Iodinated x-ray contrast agent.

Iosopan. (Ivax) Magaldrate 540 mg/5 mL. Liq. Bot. 355 mL. *OTC.*
Use: Antacid.

Iosopan Plus. (Ivax) Magaldrate 540 mg, simethicone 40 mg/5 mL. Liq. Bot. 355 mL. *OTC.*
Use: Antacid.

•**iosulamide meglumine.** (eye-oh-SULL-ah-mide meh-GLUE-meen) USAN.
Use: Diagnostic aid (radiopaque medium).

•**iosumetic acid.** (eye-oh-sue-MEH-tick) USAN.
Use: Diagnostic aid (radiopaque medium).

•**iotasul.** (EYE-oh-tah-sull) USAN.
Use: Diagnostic aid (radiopaque medium).

•**iotetric acid.** (eye-oh-TEH-trick) USAN.
Use: Diagnostic aid (radiopaque medium).

iothalamate meglumide and iothalmate sodium injection.
Use: Diagnostic aid (radiopaque medium).

iothalamate meglumine.
Use: Radiopaque agent.
See: Conray.

Conray 43.
Conray 30.

• **iothalamate sodium injection.** (eye-oh-THAL-am-ate) *USP 34.*
Use: Diagnostic aid (radiopaque medium).
See: Conray.

• **iothalamate sodium I 131.** (eye-oh-THAL-am-ate) USAN.
Use: Radiopharmaceutical.

• **iothalamate sodium I 125 injection.** (eye-oh-THAL-am-ate) *USP 34.*
Use: Radiopharmaceutical.

• **iothalamic acid.** (eye-oh-THAL-am-ik) *USP 34.*
Use: Diagnostic aid (radiopaque medium).

iothiouracil sodium. Sodium salt of 5-iodo-2-thiouracil.

• **iotrolan.** (EYE-oh-TRAHL-an) USAN.
Formerly Iotrol.
Use: Diagnostic aid (radiopaque medium).

• **iotroxic acid.** (EYE-oh-TRAHK-sick) USAN.
Use: Diagnostic aid (radiopaque medium).

• **iotyrosine I 131.** (eye-oh-TYE-roe-seen) USAN.
Use: Radiopharmaceutical.

• **ioversol.** (EYE-oh-ver-sole) *USP 34.*
Use: Radiopaque agent, parenteral.
See: Optiray 160.
 Optiray 300.
 Optiray 350.
 Optiray 320.
 Optiray 240.

 ioversol 74%.
Use: Radiopaque agent, parenteral.
See: Optiray 350.

 ioversol 68%.
Use: Radiopaque agent, parenteral.
See: Optiray 320.

 ioversol 64%.
Use: Radiopaque agent, parenteral.
See: Optiray 300.

 ioversol 34%.
Use: Radiopaque agent, parenteral.
See: Optiray 160.

• **ioxaglate meglumine.** (eye-ox-AGG-late meh-GLUE-meen) USAN.
Use: Diagnostic aid (radiopaque medium).
See: Hexabrix.

 ioxaglate meglumine 39.3% and ioxaglate sodium 19.6%.
Use: Radiopaque agent, parenteral.
See: Hexabrix.

• **ioxaglate sodium.** (eye-ox-AGG-late) USAN.

Use: Diagnostic aid (radiopaque medium).

• **ioxaglic acid.** (eye-ox-AGG-lick) *USP 34.*
Use: Diagnostic aid (radiopaque medium).

• **ioxilan.** (eye-OX-ee-lan) USAN.
Use: Diagnostic aid.

• **ioxotrizoic acid.** (eye-OX-oh-TRY-zoe-ik) USAN.
Use: Diagnostic aid (radiopaque medium).

• **ipazilide fumarate.** (ih-PAZZ-ih-LIDE) USAN.
Use: Cardiovascular agent.

• **ipecac.** (IPP-uh-kak) *USP 34.*
Use: Emetic.
W/Combinations.
See: Ipsatol.
 Mallergan.

 ipecac. (Various Mfr.) Ipecac alcohol 1.5% to 1.75%, 2%. Syrup. Bot. 15 mL, 30 mL. *OTC.*
Use: Antidote.

• **ipexidine mesylate.** (eye-PEX-ih-DEEN) USAN.
Use: Dental caries agent.

• **ipilimumab.** (i-pi-LIM-ue-mab) USAN.
Use: Antineoplastic.
See: Yervoy.

 I-Pilopine. (Akorn) Pilocarpine hydrochloride 1%. Ophthalmic soln. Bot. 15 mL. *Rx.*
Use: Antiglaucoma agent.

• **ipodate calcium.** (EYE-poe-date) *USP 34.*
Use: Diagnostic aid (radiopaque medium).
See: Oragrafin Calcium.

• **ipodate sodium.** (EYE-poe-date) *USP 34.*
Use: Diagnostic aid (radiopaque medium).

 IPOL. (Connaught) Suspension of 3 types of poliovirus (Types 1, 2, and 3) grown in monkey kidney cell cultures. Each dose contains 2-phenoxyethanol 0.5%, formaldehyde 0.02% (maximum), streptomycin ≤ 200 ng, polymyxin B 25 ng, neomycin 5 ng. Inj. Single-dose syringe with integrated needle. 0.5 mL. *Rx.*
Use: Immunization.

 Ipran. (Major) Propranolol hydrochloride 10 mg, 20 mg, 40 mg, 60 mg, 80 mg, 90 mg. Tab. **10 mg, 20 mg, 40 mg:** Bot. 100s, 250s, 1000s, UD 100s. **60 mg:** Bot. 100s, 500s. **80 mg:** Bot. 100s, 500s, 1000s, UD 100s. **90 mg:** Bot. 100s, 500s. *Rx.*
Use: Beta-adrenergic blocker.

• **ipratropium bromide.** (IH-pruh-TROE-pee-uhm) USAN.
Use: Bronchodilator.
See: Atrovent.
Atrovent HFA.

ipratropium bromide. (Dey) Ipratropium bromide 0.02% (500 mcg/vial). Preservative free. Soln. for Inh. Vial 2.5 mL each. 25, 60 unit-dose. *Rx.*
Use: Anticholinergic.

ipratropium bromide. (Various Mfr.) Ipratropium bromide 0.03% (21 mcg/spray), 0.06% (42 mcg/spray). Nasal Spray. 30 mL with spray pump (345 sprays) (0.03% only), 15 mL with spray pump (165 sprays) (0.06% only). *Rx.*
Use: Anticholinergic.

ipratropium bromide/albuterol sulfate.
Use: Bronchodilator, anticholinergic.
See: Combivent.
DuoNeb.

ipratropium bromide and albuterol sulfate. (Sandoz) Albuterol sulfate 3 mg (equiv. to 2.5 mg base), ipratropium bromide 0.5 mg/3 mL. Inh. Soln. 3 mL unit-dose vials. 30s, 60s. *Rx.*
Use: Bronchodilator, anticholinergic.

I-Pred. (Akorn) Prednisolone sodium phosphate 0.5%, 1%. Ophth. Soln. Bot. 5 mL. *Rx.*
Use: Corticosteroid, ophthalmic.

• **iprindole.** (IH-prin-dole) USAN.
Use: Antidepressant.

Iprivask. (Aventis) Desirudin 15 mg, preservative free. Pow. for Inj., lyophilized. Single-use vials with diluent (mannitol 0.6 mL [3%] in water for injection). *Rx.*
Use: Anticoagulant, antithrombin agent.

• **iprofenin.** (IH-pro-FEN-in) USAN.
Use: Diagnostic aid (hepatic function determination).

• **ipronidazole.** (ih-pro-NIH-dah-zole) USAN.
Use: Antiprotozoal *Histomonas.*

• **iproplatin.** (IH-pro-PLAT-in) USAN.
Use: Antineoplastic.

iproveratril. *Name used for Verapamil.*

• **iproxamine hydrochloride.** (IH-PROX-ah-meen) USAN.
Use: Vasodilator.

• **ipsapirone hydrochloride.** (ipp-sah-PIE-rone) USAN.
Use: Anxiolytic.

IPV.
Use: Immunization.
See: IPOL.
Polio Virus Vaccine, Inactivated.

Iquix. (Vistakon) Levofloxacin 1.5%. Gly-cerin. Ophth. Soln. 5 mL. *Rx.*
Use: Antibiotic.

• **iratumumab.** (IR-a-TOOM-ue-mab) USAN.
Use: Antineoplastic.

• **irbesartan.** (ihr-beh-SAHR-tan) *USP 34.*
Use: Renin angiotensin system antagonist, angiotensin II receptor antagonist.
See: Avapro.
W/Hydrochlorothiazide.
See: Avalide.

Ircon. (Kenwood) Iron (as carbonyl iron) 66 mg. Tab. Blister Pack 100s. *OTC.*
Use: Mineral supplement.

Iressa. (AstraZeneca) Gefitinib 250 mg. Lactose. Film-coated Tab. 30s. *Rx.*
Use: Antineoplastic.

Irgasan CF3. Cloflucarban.
Use: Antiseptic, topical.

• **iridium Ir 192.** (ih-RID-ee-uhm) USAN.
Use: Radioactive agent.

• **irinotecan hydrochloride.** (eye-rih-no-TEE-can) USAN.
Use: DNA topoisomerase inhibitor.
See: Camptosar.

irinotecan hydrochloride. (Various Mfr.) Irinotecan 20 mg. May contain sorbitol. IV Inj. Vials. 2 mL, 5 mL. *Rx.*
Use: DNA topoisomerase inhibitor.

irisin. A polysaccharide found in several species of iris.

irocaine.
See: Procaine Hydrochloride.

Irodex. (Keene Pharmaceuticals) Iron dextran complex 50 mg/mL. Vial 10 mL. *Rx.*
Use: Mineral supplement.

Iromin-G. (Mission Pharmacal) Ferrous gluconate 260 mg (iron 30 mg), vitamins B_{12} (crystalline on resin) 2 mcg, C 100 mg, A acetate 4000 units, D 400 units, B_1 5 mg, B_2 2 mg, B_3 10 mg, B_5 1 mg, B_6 20.6 mg, folic acid 0.8 mg, Ca. Tab. Bot. 100s. *OTC.*
Use: Mineral, vitamin supplement.

iron.
See: Carbonyl Iron.
Ferrous Fumarate.
Ferrous Gluconate.
Ferrous Sulfate.
Ferrous Sulfate Exsiccated (Dried).
Iron Dextran.
Iron Sucrose.
Iron with Vitamin C.
Polysaccharide-Iron Complex.
Sodium Ferric Gluconate Complex.

iron carbonate complex.
See: Polyferose.

Iron Chews. (Midlothian) Carbonyl iron 15 mg. Sorbitol, grape flavor. Chew.

Tab. 60s. *OTC.*
Use: Nutritional supplement.
Ironco-B. (Pal-Pak, Inc.) Ferrous sulfate
120.4 mg, manganese sulfate 21.6 mg,
dicalcium phosphate 129.6 mg, vitamins
B_1 1 mg, B_2 1 mg, niacin 6 mg,
D 100 units. Tab. Bot. 100s, 1000s. *OTC.*
Use: Mineral, vitamin supplement.
• **iron dextran.** (iron DEX-tran) *USP 34.*
Use: Hematinic.
See: DexFerrum.
Ferumoxytol.
INFeD.
Iron-Folic 500. (Major) Ferrous sulfate
105 mg, B_1 6 mg, B_2 6 mg, B_3 30 mg,
B_5 10 mg, B_{12} 25 mcg, C 500 mg, folic
acid 0.8 mg. Tab. Bot. 100s, 500s. *OTC.*
Use: Mineral, vitamin supplement.
iron/liver combinations, injection.
See: Hemocyte.
Liver-Iron B Complex w/Vitamin B_{12}.
iron/liver combination, oral.
See: Feocyte.
I-L-X.
I-L-X B_{12}.
Liquid Geritonic.
iron oxide mixture with zinc oxide.
Calamine, USP.
iron, parenteral.
See: DexFerrum.
Ferumoxytol.
INFeD.
iron products, injection.
See: INFeD.
• **iron sorbitex injection.** (SORE-bih-tex)
USP 34.
Use: Hematinic.
• **iron sucrose.** (EYE-urn-SOO-krose)
USP 34.
Use: Trace element.
See: Venofer.
iron (2+) fumarate. Ferrous Fumarate,
USP.
iron (2+) gluconate.
See: Ferrous Gluconate, USP.
iron with vitamin B_{12} and IFC.
See: Albafort.
Contrin.
Chromagen.
Fergon Plus.
Ferotrinsic.
Livitrinsic-f.
Multigen.
Pronemia Hematinic.
TriHEMIC 600.
Trinsicon.
Vitagen Advance.
iron with vitamin C.
See: Fero-Grad-500.
Ferrex 150 Plus.

Niferex-150.
Vitelle Irospan.
Vitron-C.
iron with vitamins.
See: Gentle Iron.
Tandem F.
Irospan. (Fielding) Ferrous sulfate
65 mg, vitamin C 150 mg. Cap. Bot.
60s. Tab. Bot. 100s. *OTC.*
Use: Mineral, vitamin supplement.
• **irosustat.** (IR-oh-SOO-stat) USAN.
Use: Antineoplastic.
irradiated ergosterol.
See: Calciferol.
Irrigate Eye Wash. (Optopics) Sodium
chloride, monobasic and dibasic so-
dium phosphate, benzalkonium chlor-
ide, EDTA. Soln. Bot. 118 mL. *OTC.*
Use: Irrigant, ophthalmic.
irrigating solutions, physiological.
Use: Irrigant.
See: Lactated Ringer's Irrigation.
Physiolyte.
PhysioSol.
Tis-U-Sol.
irrigating solutions, urinary.
Use: Irrigant.
See: Acetic Acid.
Glycine (Aminoacetic acid).
Neosporin G.U. Irrigant.
Renacidin.
Resectisol.
Sodium Chloride.
Sorbitol-Mannitol.
Sterile Water.
irritant or stimulant laxatives.
See: Agoral.
Aromatic Cascara Fluid Extract.
Bisac-Evac.
Bisacodyl.
Bisacodyl Uniserts.
Black-Draught.
Caroid.
Cascara Aromatic.
Cascara Sagrada.
Correctol.
Dulcolax.
ex-lax.
ex-lax chocolated.
Feen-a-mint.
Fleet Laxative.
Fletcher's Castoria.
Maximum Relief ex-lax.
Modane.
Reliable Gentle Laxative.
Senexon.
Senna-Gen.
Sennosides.
Senokot.
Senokot XTRA.
Women's Gentle Laxative.

•**irtemazole.** (ihr-TEH-mah-zole) USAN.
Use: Uricosuric.

isacen.
See: Oxyphenisatin.

•**isamoxole.** (eye-SAH-MOX-ole) USAN.
Use: Antiasthmatic.

•**isatoribine.** (eye-sah-TORE-ih-been)
USAN.
Use: Immunomodulator.

Iscador. (Weleda) Mistletoe.
Use: Cancer (not FDA-approved).

•**iscotrizinol.** (IS-koe-TRIZ-i-nol) USAN.
Use: Sunscreen.

•**iseganan hydrochloride.** (eye-se-GAN-
an) USAN.
Use: Antimicrobial.

Isentress. (Merck) Raltegravir 400 mg
(equiv. to raltegravir potassium
434.4 mg). Lactose. Film-coated. Tab.
60s. *Rx.*
Use: Antiretroviral agent, integrase inhibitor.

•**isepamicin.** (eye-SEP-ah-MY-sin) USAN.
Use: Antibacterial (aminoglycoside).

ISG. Immune globulin intramuscular. *Rx.*
Use: Immunization.

Ismo. (Reddy Pharmaceuticals) Isosor-
bide mononitrate 20 mg. Lactose. Tab.
Bot. 100s, UD 100s. *Rx.*
Use: Vasodilator.

•**ismomultin alpha.** (IZ-moe-MUL-tin)
USAN.
Use: Rheumatoid arthritis.

iso-alcoholic elixir.
Use: Vehicle.

isoamylhydrocupreine dihydrochloride.
See: Eucupin Dihydrochloride.

isoamyl methoxycinnamate.
See: Amiloxate.

isoamyl nitrate.
See: Amyl Nitrite.

isoamyne.
See: Amphetamine.

Iso-B. (Tyson) Vitamins B_1 25 mg, B_2
25 mg, B_3 75 mg, B_5 125 mg, B_6 50 mg,
B_{12} 100 mcg, FA 0.2 mg, pyridoxal 5
phosphate 2.5 mg, PABA 50 mg, inositol 50 mg, choline bitartrate 125 mg,
biotin 100 mcg. Cap. Bot. 120s. *OTC.*
Use: Mineral, vitamin supplement.

isobornyl thiocyanoacetate, technical.
Use: Pediculicide.
See: Barc.
W/Docusate Sodium and Related
Terpenes.
See: Barc.

•**isobucaine hydrochloride.** (eye-so-
BYOO-kane) *USP 34.*
Use: Anesthetic, local.

•**isobucaine hydrochloride and epinephrine injection.** (eye-so-BYOO-
kane HIGH-droe-KLOR-ide & epp-ih-
NEFF-rin) *USP 34.*
Use: Anesthetic, local.

•**isobutamben.** (EYE-so-BYOO-tam-ben)
USAN.
Use: Anesthetic, local.

•**isobutane.** (eye-so-BYOO-tane) *NF 29.*
Use: Aerosol propellant.

isobutylallylbarbituric acid.
W/Aspirin, Phenacetin, Caffeine.
See: Buff-A-Comp.
Fiorinal.
Palgesic.
Tenstan.
W/Codeine Phosphate.
See: Fiorinal w/Codeine.

isobutyl p-aminobenzoate.
See: Isobutamben, USAN.

isobutyramide. (Vertex)
Use: Sickle cell disease; beta-
thalassemia. [Orphan Drug]

isobutyramide oral solution. (Alpha
Therapeutic)
Use: Sickle call disease; beta-
thalassemia. [Orphan Drug]

isocaine. Isobutamben, USP.

Isocal. (Bristol-Myers Squibb) Lactose-
free isotonic liquid containing as a per-
centage of the calories protein 13% as
caseinate and soy protein; fat 37% as
soy oil and medium chain triglycerides;
carbohydrate 50% as corn syrup solids
w/vitamins and minerals for the tube-
fed patient. Bot. 8 fl oz, 12 fl oz, 32 fl oz.
OTC.
Use: Nutritional supplement.

Isocal HCN. (Bristol-Myers Squibb) High
calorie nitrogen nutritionally complete
food. Protein 15%, fat 45%, carbohydrate 40%. Can 8 fl oz. *OTC.*
Use: Nutritional supplement.

Isocal HN. (Bristol-Myers Squibb)
≈ 1 Kcal/mL with protein 44 g, fat 45 g,
carbohydrates 124 g/L. In 237 mL.
OTC.
Use: Nutritional supplement.

•**isocarboxazid.** (eye-so-car-BOX-ah-zid)
USP 34.
Use: Antidepressant.
See: Marplan.

Isochron. (Forest) Isosorbide dinitrate
40 mg. Lactose. ER Tab. 100s. *Rx.*
Use: Vasodilator.

Isoclor Expectorant. (Medeva) Codeine
phosphate 10 mg, pseudoephedrine
hydrochloride 30 mg, guaifenesin
100 mg/5 mL, alcohol 5%. Bot. Pt. *c-v.*
Use: Antitussive, decongestant, expectorant.

isococaine. Pseudococaine.

Isocom. (Nutripharm Laboratories, Inc.) Isometheptene mucate 65 mg, dichloralphenazone 100 mg, acetaminophen 325 mg. Cap. Bot. 50s, 100s, 250s. Rx.
Use: Antimigraine.

•isoconazole. (EYE-so-CONE-ah-zole) USAN.
Use: Anti-infective; antifungal.

isoephedrine hydrochloride.
d-Isoephedrine hydrochloride.
See: Pseudoephedrine Hydrochloride.

d-isoephedrine sulfate.
See: Pseudoephedrine Sulfate.

•isoetharine. (EYE-so-ETH-uh-reen) USAN.
Use: Bronchodilator.

•isoetharine hydrochloride. (EYE-so-ETH-uh-reen) USP 34.
Use: Bronchodilator, sympathomimetic.

•isoetharine mesylate. (EYE-so-ETH-uh-reen) USP 34.
Use: Bronchodilator.
See: Bronkometer.

•isoflupredone acetate. (eye-so-FLEW-PREH-dohn) USAN.
Use: Anti-inflammatory.

•isoflurane. (EYE-so-FLEW-rane) USP 34.
Use: Anesthetic, general.
See: Terrell.

•isoflurophate. (eye-so-FLURE-oh-fate) USP 34.
Use: Cholinergic, ophthalmic.
See: Floropryl.

iso-iodeikon.
See: Phentetiothalein Sodium.

Isoject. (Roerig) A purified, sterile, disposable injection system.
Use: Injection system.
See: Permapen (Benzathine Penicillin G) Aqueous Soln. 1,200,000 units/ 2 mL. 10s.

Isolan. (Elan) Protein 40 g, fat 36 g, carbohydrates 144 g, Na 690 g, K 1.17 g/ L, with appropriate vitamins and minerals. Lactose free. Liq. In 237 mL Tetra Pak containers and 1000 mL New Pak closed systems with and without Color Check. OTC.
Use: Nutritional supplement.

Isolate Compound Elixir. (Various Mfr.) Theophylline 45 mg, ephedrine sulfate 12 mg, isoproterenol hydrochloride 2.5 mg, potassium iodide 150 mg, phenobarbital 6 mg/15 mL, alcohol 19%. Elix. Bot. Pt, gal. Rx.
Use: Antiasthmatic combination.

•isoleucine. (EYE-so-LOO-seen) USP 34.
Use: Amino acid.

isoleucine. (Pfaltz & Bauer) Pow. 10 g.
Use: Amino acid.

Isolyte G with Dextrose. (McGaw) Sodium 65 mEq, potassium 17 mEq, chloride 150 mEq, NH_4 70 mEq, dextrose 50 g, 170 Cal, 555 mOsm/L. Bot. 1000 mL. Rx.
Use: Nutritional supplement, parenteral.

Isolyte H in 5% Dextrose. (B. Braun) Dextrose 50 g/L, calories 170 Cal/L, Na^+ 39 mEq, K^+ 13 mEq, Mg^{++} 3 mEq, Cl^- 44 mEq, acetate 16 mEq/L, osmolarity 360 mOsm/L. Inj. Soln. 1000 mL. Rx.
Use: Intravenous nutritional therapy, intravenous replenishment solution.

Isolyte M in 5% Dextrose. (B. Braun) Dextrose 50 g/L, calories 170 cal/L, Na^+ 36 mEq, K^+ 35 mEq, Cl^- 49 mEq, phosphate 15 mEq, acetate 20 mEq/L, osmolarity 390 mOsm/L. Inj. Soln. 500 mL, 1000 mL. Rx.
Use: Intravenous nutritional therapy, intravenous replenishment solution.

Isolyte P in 5% Dextrose. (B. Braun) Dextrose 50 g/L, calories 170 Cal/L, Na^+ 23 mEq, K^+ 20 mEq, Mg^{++} 3 mEq, Cl^- 29 mEq, phosphate 3 mEq, acetate 23 mEq/L, osmolarity 340 mOsm/L. Inj. Soln. 250 mL, 500 mL, 1000 mL. Rx.
Use: Intravenous nutritional therapy, intravenous replenishment solution.

Isolyte R in 5% Dextrose. (B. Braun) Sodium 39 mEq, potassium 16 mEq, calcium 5 mEq, magnesium 3 mEq, chloride 46 mEq, acetate 24 mEq, dextrose 50 g, 170 Cal, 375 mOsm/L. Inj. Soln. 1000 mL. Rx.
Use: Intravenous nutritional therapy, intravenous replenishment solution.

Isolyte S pH 7.4. (B. Braun) Sodium 141 mEq, potassium 5 mEq, magnesium 3 mEq, chloride 98 mEq, acetate 27 mEq, gluconate 23 mEq, phosphate 1 mEq, 295 mOsm/L, preservative free. Inj. Bot. Soln. 500 mL, 1000 mL. Rx.
Use: Intravenous nutritional therapy, intravenous replenishment solution.

Isolyte S with 5% Dextrose. (B. Braun) Sodium 140 mEq, potassium 5 mEq, magnesium 3 mEq, chloride 106 mEq, acetate 27 mEq, gluconate 23 mEq, dextrose 50 g, Cal 170, 550 mOsm/L. Inj. Soln. 1000 mL. Rx.
Use: Intravenous nutritional therapy, intravenous replenishment solution.

•isomazole hydrochloride. (eye-SO-mah-ZOLE) USAN.
Use: Cardiovascular agent.

isomeprobamate.
See: Carisoprodol.
•**isomerol.** (EYE-so-MER-ole) USAN. *Formerly Parahydrecin.*
Use: Antiseptic.
•**isometheptene/dichloralphenazone/ acetaminophen.** (eye-so-meth-EPP-teen/die-klor-uhl-FEN-uh-zone/ASS-et-ah-MEE-noe-fen) *USP 34.*
Use: Antimigraine.
See: Epidrin.
  Midrin.
  Migrazone.
isometheptene/dichloralphenazone/ acetaminophen. (Various Mfr.) Isometheptene 65 mg, dichloralphenazone 100 mg, acetaminophen 325 mg. Cap. 50s, 100s, 250s, 500s. *c-iv.*
Use: Antimigraine.
•**isometheptene mucate.** (eye-so-meth-EPP-teen MYOO-kate) *USP 34.*
See: Midrin.
W/Acetaminophen, Caffeine.
See: MigraTen.
  Prodrin.
W/Acetaminophen, Dichloralphenazone.
See: Migragesic IDA.
  Nodolor.
Isomil. (Ross) Soy protein isolate infant formula containing 20 calories/fl oz. **Pow.:** Can 14 oz. **Concentrated Liq.:** Can 13 fl oz. **Ready-to-feed:** Can 32 fl oz. **Nursing Bottles:** Hospital use. Bot. 8 fl oz. *OTC.*
Use: Nutritional supplement.
Isomil DF. (Ross) Protein 17.9 g, carbohydrates 67.3 g, fat 36.7 g, Fe 12 mg, Na 293 mg, K 720 mg, with appropriate vitamins and minerals. 676 cal/L. Lactose free. Liq. 960 mL prediluted, ready-to-use cans. *OTC.*
Use: Nutritional supplement.
Isomil SF. (Ross) Low osmolar sucrose-free soy protein isolate infant formula containing 20 calories/fl oz. **Concentrated Liq.:** Can 13 fl oz. **Ready-to-feed:** Can 32 fl oz. **Nursing Bottles:** Hospital use. Bot. 8 fl oz. *OTC.*
Use: Nutritional supplement, enteral.
Isomune-CK. (Roche) Rapid immunochemical separation method of the heart specific CK-MB isoenzyme for quantitating when used with an appropriate CK substrate reagent. Test kit 100s, 250s.
Use: Diagnostic aid.
Isomune-LD. (Roche) Rapid immunochemical separation method of the heart specific LD-1 isoenzyme for quantitating when used with an appro-

priate LD substrate reagent. Test kit 40s, 100s.
Use: Diagnostic aid.
•**isomylamine hydrochloride.** (EYE-so-MILL-ah-meen) USAN.
Use: Muscle relaxant.
isomyn.
See: Amphetamine.
IsonaRif. (VersaPharm) Rifampin 300 mg, isoniazid 150 mg. Lactose. Cap. 60s. *Rx.*
Use: Antituberculosis agent.
Isonate Sublingual. (Major) Isosorbide 2.5 mg, 5 mg. Sublingual Tab. Bot. 100s, 1000s, UD 100s. *Rx.*
Use: Antianginal.
Isonate Tablets. (Major) Isosorbide. **5 mg, 10 mg:** Bot. 100s, 1000s, UD 100s. **20 mg, 30 mg:** Bot. 100s, 1000s. *Rx.*
Use: Antianginal.
Isonate TD-Caps. (Major) Isosorbide 40 mg. Bot. 100s, 1000s. *Rx.*
Use: Antianginal.
Isonate T.R. Tabs. (Major) Isosorbide 40 mg. Bot. 100s, 1000s. *Rx.*
Use: Antianginal.
•**isoniazid.** (eye-so-NYE-uh-zid) *USP 34.*
Use: Antituberculosis agent.
See: Calpas-INH.
  Dow-Isoniazid.
  INH.
  Laniazid.
  Nydrazid.
W/Calcium P-Aminosalicylate, Vitamin B$_6$.
See: Calpas-INAH-6.
  Calpas Isoxine.
W/Pyridoxine Hydrochloride (Vitamin B$_6$).
See: Niadox.
  Pasna, Tri-Pack 300.
  Teebaconin w/B$_6$.
W/Rifampin.
See: IsonaRif.
  Rifater.
isoniazid. (Carolina Medical Products) Isoniazid 50 mg/5 mL, sorbitol, orange flavor. Syr. Bot. Pt. *Rx.*
Use: Antituberculosis agent.
isoniazid. (Sandoz) Isoniazid 100 mg/mL. Inj., Soln. Vials. 10 mL. *Rx.*
Use: Antituberculosis agent.
isoniazid. (Various Mfr.) Isoniazid 100 mg, 300 mg. Tab. Bot. 30s, 60s (300 mg only), 100s, 200s (300 mg only), 1000s. *Rx.*
Use: Antituberculosis agent.
isoniazid combinations.
Use: Antituberculous agent.
See: Rifamate.
  Rifater.

isonicotinic acid hydrazide.
See: Isoniazid.
isonicotinyl hydrazide.
See: Isoniazid.
isonipecaine hydrochloride.
See: Meperidine Hydrochloride.
isopentaquine.
Use: Antimalarial.
isophane insulin suspension (NPH).
Use: Antidiabetic.
See: Humulin N.
    Novolin N.
    Novolin N PenFill.
    Novolin N Prefilled.
**isophane insulin suspension (NPH)/
insulin injection (regular).**
Use: Antidiabetic.
See: Humulin 50/50.
    Humulin 70/30.
    Novolin 70/30.
    Novolin 70/30 Penfill.
    Novolin 70/30 Prefilled.
isopregnenone.
See: Dydrogesterone.
Isoprinosine. (Newport Pharmaceuticals) Inosine pranobex.
Use: Antiviral; immunomodulator.
isopropanol.
Use: Antiseptic.
W/Combinations.
See: Ivy-Dry.
    Ivy-Dry Super.
isoprophenamine hydrochloride. Name used for Clorprenaline Hydrochloride.
isopropicillin potassium.
Use: Anti-infective.
•**isopropyl alcohol.** (eye-so-PRO-pill ALkoe-hahl) USP 34.
Use: Topical anti-infective; pharmaceutic aid (solvent).
isopropyl alcohol spray. (Morton Grove) Isopropyl alcohol w/propellant. Aer. Can 6 oz. OTC.
Use: Anti-infective.
isopropylarterenol hydrochloride.
Use: Asthma; vasoconstrictor, allergic states.
isopropylarterenol sulfate.
See: Isoproterenol Sulfate.
•**isopropyl myristate.** (eye-so-PRO-pill mih-RIST-ate) NF 29.
Use: Pharmaceutic aid (emollient).
isonoradrenaline.
See: Isoproterenol.
isopropyl-noradrenaline hydrochloride.
See: Isoproterenol Hydrochloride.
•**isopropyl palmitate.** (eye-so-PRO-pill pal-mih-tate) NF 29.
Use: Pharmaceutic aid (oleaginous vehicle).
See: Versa PLO20.

isopropyl phenazone. 4-Isopropyl antipyrine. Larodon.
isopropyl rubbing alcohol.
Use: Rubefacient, solvent.
isoproterenol.
See: Norisodrine.
isoproterenol. (Various Mfr.) Isoproterenol 1:5000 solution (0.2 mg/mL with sodium metabisulfite). Inj. Vials. 5 mL, 10 mL. Rx.
Use: Vasopressor.
•**isoproterenol hydrochloride.** (eye-sopro-TER-uh-nahl) USP 34.
Use: Bronchodilator; vasoconstrictor.
See: Isuprel.
isoproterenol hydrochloride. (Abbott) Isoproterenol hydrochloride 0.02 mg/mL (1:50,000), sodium metabisulfite. Inj. Prefilled syr. 10 mL. Rx.
Use: Bronchodilator, sympathomimetic.
isoproterenol hydrochloride. (ESI Lederle) Isoproterenol hydrochloride 0.2 mg/mL (1:5000 solution), sodium bisulfite. Inj. Amp. 5 mL. Rx.
Use: Bronchodilator, sympathomimetic.
•**isoproterenol sulfate.** (eye-so-pro-TERuh-nahl) USP 34.
Use: Bronchodilator.
See: Medihaler-Iso.
W/Calcium Iodide (Anhydrous), Alcohol.
See: Norisodrine.
Isoptin SR. (FSC Laboratories) Verapamil hydrochloride 120 mg, 180 mg, 240 mg. Film-coated. ER Tab. Bot. 100s, 500s (240 mg only). Rx.
Use: Calcium channel blocker.
Isopto Alkaline. (Alcon) Hydroxypropyl methylcellulose 1%, benzalkonium Cl 0.01%. Sterile ophthalmic soln. Dropper bot. 15 mL. OTC.
Use: Artificial tears.
Isopto Carbachol. (Alcon) Carbachol 1.5%, 3%. Benzalkonium chloride 0.005%, hydroxypropyl methylcellulose 1%, sodium chloride, boric acid, sodium borate. Soln. Drop-Tainer 15 mL, 30 mL. Rx.
Use: Antiglaucoma agent.
Isopto Carpine. (Alcon) Pilocarpine hydrochloride 1%, 2%, 4%, 6%. Soln. Bot. 15 mL, 30 mL. Rx.
Use: Antiglaucoma agent.
Isopto Cetamide. (Alcon) Sodium sulfacetamide 15%. Soln. Drop-Tainer 5 mL, 15 mL. Rx.
Use: Anti-infective, ophthalmic.
Isopto Frin. (Alcon) Phenylephrine hydrochloride 0.12% in a methylcellulose Soln. Drop-Tainer 15 mL. Rx.
Use: Mydriatic; vasoconstrictor.

Isopto Homatropine. (Alcon) Homatropine HBr 2%, 5%. Soln. *Drop-Tainer* 5 mL, 15 mL. *Rx.*
Use: Cycloplegic; mydriatic.

Isopto Hyoscine. (Alcon) Hyoscine HBr 0.25%. Soln. *Drop-Tainer* 5 mL, 15 mL. *Rx.*
Use: Cycloplegic; mydriatic.

Isopto Plain. (Alcon) Hydroxypropyl methylcellulose 2910 0.5%, benzalkonium Cl 0.01%, sodium Cl, sodium phosphate, sodium citrate. *Drop-Tainer* 15 mL. *OTC.*
Use: Artificial tears.

Isopto Tears. (Alcon) Hydroxypropyl methylcellulose 0.5%, benzalkonium Cl 0.01%, sodium Cl, sodium phosphate, sodium citrate. Bot. *Drop-Tainer* 15 mL, 30 mL. *OTC.*
Use: Artificial tears.

Isordil Sublingual. (Wyeth) Isosorbide dinitrate. Tab. **2.5 mg, 5 mg:** Bot. 100s, 500s, *Redi-pak* 100s. **10 mg:** Bot. 100s. *Rx.*
Use: Antianginal.

Isordil Titradose. (Wyeth) Isosorbide dinitrate 5 mg, 10 mg, 20 mg, 30 mg, 40 mg. Lactose. Tab. Bot. 100s, 500s (20 mg only), 1000s (5 mg, 10 mg only). *Rx.*
Use: Vasodilator.

Isorgen-G. (Grafton) Isosorbide 5 mg, 10 mg. Tab. Bot. 1000s. *Rx.*
Use: Antianginal.

• **isosorbide concentrate.** (EYE-sos-ORE-bide) *USP 34.*
Use: Diuretic.

• **isosorbide dinitrate.** (EYE-sos-ORE-bide die-NYE-trate dye-LOOT-ed) *USP 34.*
Use: Vasodilator, nitrate.
See: Dilatrate-SR.
  Isochron.
  Isordil.
W/Hydralazine Hydrochloride.
See: BiDil.

isosorbide dinitrate. (Rising Pharmaceuticals) Isosorbide dinitrate 40 mg. Lactose. ER Tab. 100s. *Rx.*
Use: Vasodilator, nitrate.

isosorbide dinitrate. (Various Mfr.) Isosorbide dinitrate. **Sublingual Tab.:** 2.5 mg, 5 mg. May contain lactose. Bot. 100s, 1000s, UD 100s. **Tab.:** 5 mg, 10 mg, 20 mg, 30 mg. 100s, 500s (except 20 mg), 1000s, UD 100s. *Rx.*
Use: Vasodilator, nitrate.

• **isosorbide mononitrate.** (EYE-sos-ORE-bide MAH-no-NYE-trate) USAN.
Use: Coronary vasodilator.

See: Imdur.
  ISMO.
  Monoket.

isosorbide mononitrate. (Teva) Isosorbide mononitrate 20 mg, lactose. Tab. Bot. 100s, 500s. *Rx.*
Use: Coronary vasodilator.

isosorbide mononitrate. (Various Mfr.) Isosorbide mononitrate. **ER Tab.:** 30 mg, 60 mg, 120 mg. May contain lactose. ER Tab. Bot. 100s, 1000s. **Tab.:** 10 mg, 20 mg. May contain lactose. 100s, 500s (20 mg only). *Rx.*
Use: Coronary vasodilator.

isosorbide oral solution.
Use: Diuretic.

Isosource. (Novartis) Protein (Ca and Na caseinate, soy protein isolate) 43.2 g, carbohydrate (maltodextrin) 1755 g, fat (MCT, canola oil, lecithin) 443.9 g, Na 760 mg, K 1182 mg, mOsm/kg H_2O 390, Cal/mL 1.2, vitamins A, B_1, B_2, B_3, B_5, B_6, B_{12}, C, D, E, K, FA, biotin, choline, Ca, Cl, Cu, Fe, I, Mg, Mn, P, Zn, Se, Cr, Mo. Liq. Bot. 250 mL, 1000 mL. *OTC.*
Use: Nutritional supplement.

Isosource HN. (Novartis) Protein (Ca and Na caseinate, soy protein isolate) 56.1 g, carbohydrate (maltodextrin) 165 g, fat (MCT, canola oil, lecithin) 43.9 g, Na 760 mg, K 1772 mg, mOsm/kg H_2O 390, Cal/mL 1.2, vitamins A, B_1, B_2, B_3, B_5, B_6, B_{12}, C, D, E, K, FA, biotin, choline, Ca, P, I, Fe, Mg, Cu, Zn, Cl, Mn, Se, Cr, Mo. Liq. Bot. 250 mL, 1000 mL. *OTC.*
Use: Nutritional supplement.

Isosource 1.5 Cal. (Nestle Nutrition) Protein 68 g (L-carnitine, sodium caseinate, taurine), carbohydrate 170 g (maltodextrin), fat 65 g (canola oil, medium chain triglycerides), sodium 1,290 mg, potassium 2,250 mg. Fiber 8 g, vitamins A, B_1, B_2, B_3, B_5, B_6, B_{12}, C, D, E, K, Ca, Cl, Cr, Cu, Fe, I, Mg, Mn, Mo, P, Se, Zn, biotin, choline, folic acid. Lactose free. Liq. 250 mL, 1,000 mL, 1,500 mL. *OTC.*
Use: Defined formula diet, lactose-free product.

Isosource VHN. (Nestle Nutrition) Protein 62.7 g (Ca caseinate, Na caseinate, L-carnitine, soy fiber, taurine), carbohydrate 126.7 g (maltodextrin), fat 28.7 g (canola oil, medium chain triglycerides, soy lecithin), Na 1,346.7 mg, K 1,800 mg, vitamin A, B_1, B_2, B_3, B_5, B_6, B_{12}, C, D, E, K, Ca, Cl, Cu, Fe, I, Mg, Mn, P, Se, Zn, folic acid, biotin, choline, folic acid, biotin, choline. Methyl-

paraben. Lactose free. Vanilla flavor. Liq. 250 mL, 1 L, 1.5 L. *OTC.*
Use: Defined formula diet, supplemental nutritional formula.

•**isostearyl alcohol.** (EYE-so-STEE-rill AL-koe-hahl) USAN.
Use: Pharmaceutic aid (emollient, solvent).

•**isosulfan blue.** (EYE-so-SULL-fan) USAN.
Use: Radiopaque agent, parenteral.
See: Lymphazurin 1%.

isosulfan blue 1%. (Bioniche Pharma) Isosulfan blue 10 mg/mL. Preservative free. Inj., Soln. Single-use vial. 5 mL. *Rx.*
Use: Radiopaque agent.

Isotein HN. (Novartis) Vanilla Flavor. Maltodextrin, delactosed lactalbumin, partially hydrogenated soy oil with BHA, fructose, medium chain triglycerides, artificial flavor, sodium caseinate, monoglycerides and diglycerides, sodium Cl, vitamins, minerals. Pow. Packet 2.75 oz. *OTC.*
Use: Nutritional supplement.

•**isotiquimide.** (eye-so-TIH-kwih-MIDE) USAN.
Use: Antiulcerative.

Isotrate ER. (Apothecon) Isosorbide mononitrate 60 mg, lactose. ER Tab. Bot. 100s, 500s. *Rx.*
Use: Coronary vasodilator.

•**isotretinoin.** (EYE-so-TREH-tin-NO-in) *USP 34.*
Tall Man: ISOtretinoin
Use: Retinoid, first generation.
See: Amnesteem.
   Claravis.
   Sotret.

•**isovaleramide.** (EYE-soe-val-ER-a-mide) USAN.
Use: Agent for migraine.

•**isotretinoin anisatil.** (eye-so-TRETT-ih-noyn ah-NIH-sah-till) USAN.
Use: Dermatologic, acne.

Isovorin. (Wyeth) L-leucovorin.
Use: Antineoplastic. [Orphan Drug]

Isovue-M 300. (Bracco Diagnostics) Iopamidol 612 mg, iodine 300 mg/mL. EDTA. Inj. Vials. 15 mL. For intrathecal use *Rx.*
Use: Radiopaque agent, parenteral.

Isovue-M 200. (Bracco Diagnostics) Iopamidol 408 mg, iodine 200 mg/mL. EDTA. Inj. Vials. 10 mL, 20 mL. For intrathecal use. *Rx.*
Use: Radiopaque agent, parenteral.

Isovue-300. (Bracco Diagnostics) Iopamidol 612 mg, iodine 300 mg/mL.

EDTA. Inj. Vials. 30 mL, 50 mL. Bot. 75 mL, 100 mL, 150 mL w/wo administration sets. Power injector syringes. 100 mL, 150 mL. *Rx.*
Use: Radiopaque agent, parenteral.

Isovue-370. (Bracco Diagnostics) Iopamidol 755 mg, iodine 370 mg/mL. EDTA. Inj. Vials. 20 mL, 30 mL, 50 mL. Bot. 50 mL, 75 mL, 100 mL, 125 mL, 150 mL, 175 mL, 200 mL. Power injector syringes. 75 mL, 100 mL. *Rx.*
Use: Radiopaque agent, parenteral.

Isovue-200. (Bracco Diagnostics) Iopamidol 408 mg, iodine 200 mg/mL. EDTA. Inj. Vials. 50 mL. Bot. 100 mL, 200 mL w/infusion set. *Rx.*
Use: Radiopaque agent, parenteral.

Isovue-250. (Bracco Diagnostics) Iopamidol 510 mg, iodine 250 mg/mL. EDTA. Inj. Vials. 50 mL. Bot. 100 mL, 150 mL, 200 mL. Power injector syringes. 150 mL. *Rx.*
Use: Radiopaque agent, parenteral.

•**isoxepac.** (EYE-SOX-eh-pack) USAN.
Use: Anti-inflammatory.

•**isoxicam.** (eye-SOX-ih-kam) USAN.
Use: Anti-inflammatory.

•**isoxsuprine hydrochloride.** (eye-SOX-you-preen) *USP 34.*
Use: Vasodilator.
See: Vasodilan.
   Voxsuprine.

isoxsuprine hydrochloride. (Various Mfr.) Isoxsuprine hydrochloride 10 mg, 20 mg. Tab. 60s, 100s, 500s, 1000s, UD 100s. *Rx.*
Use: Vasodilator.

I-Soyalac. (Mt. Vernon Foods, Inc.) P-soy protein isolate, l-methionine, CHO-sucrose, tapioca dextrin. F-soy oil, soy lecithin. Corn free. Protein 20.2 g, carbohydrate 63.4 g, fat 35.5 g, iron 12 mg, 640 Cal/serving (1 qt). Concentrate 390 mL, ready-to-use 1 qt. *OTC.*
Use: Nutritional supplement.

•**ispinesib mesylate.** (is-PIN-es-ib) USAN.
Use: Antineoplastic.

•**ispronicline.** (eyes-PRON-i-kleen) USAN.
Use: CNS agent, Alzheimer disease.

•**isradipine.** (iss-RAHD-ih-peen) *USP 34.*
Use: Calcium channel blocker; antagonist (calcium channel).
See: DynaCirc CR.

isradipine. (Various Mfr.) Isradipine 2.5 mg, 5 mg. May contain lactose. Cap. 60s, 100s, 500s. *Rx.*
Use: Calcium channel blocker.

Istodax. (Celgene) Romidepsin 10 mg. Povidone 20 mg. Inj. Kit w/single-use vial and diluent. *Rx.*
Use: Cutaneous T-cell lymphoma.

Istalol. (Ista Pharmaceuticals) Timolol maleate 0.5%, benzalkonium chloride 0.005%, monobasic sodium phosphate monohydrate, potassium sorbate 0.47%, sodium hydroxide. Soln. 5 mL. *Rx.*
Use: Agents for glaucoma.

• **istradefylline.** (iz-TRA-de-fye-leen) USAN.
Use: Parkinson disease.

I-Sulfacet. (American Pharmaceutical) Sulfacetamide sodium 10%, 15%, 30% ophthalmic soln. Bot. 2 mL, 5 mL, 15 mL. *Rx.*
Use: Anti-infective, ophthalmic.

Isuprel Inhalation Solution. (Sanofi-Synthelabo) Isoproterenol hydrochloride 0.5% (1:200), 1% (1:100). Soln. for Inh. Bot. 10 mL. *Rx.*
Use: Bronchodilator; sympathomimetic.

Isuprel Mistometer. (Sanofi-Synthelabo) Isoproterenol hydrochloride 103 mcg/dose. Aer. Bot. 15 mL. Refill 15 mL. *Rx.*
Use: Bronchodilator; sympathomimetic.

Isuprel Sterile Injection. (Abbott) Isoproterenol hydrochloride 0.2 mg/mL (1:5000), sodium metabisulfite. Inj. Amp. 1 mL, 5 mL. *Rx.*
Use: Bronchodilator; sympathomimetic.

isuprene.
See: Isoproterenol.

• **itasetron.** (eye-tah-SEH-trahn) USAN.
Use: Antidepressant; antiemetic; anxiolytic.

• **itazigrel.** (ih-TAY-zih-GRELL) USAN.
Use: Platelet aggregation inhibitor.

Itchaway. (Moyco Union Broach Division) Zinc undecylenate 20%, undecylenic acid 2%. Pow. Can 1.5 oz. *OTC.*
Use: Antifungal, topical.

Itch Relief Gel Spritz. (Band-Aid) Camphor 0.5%, benzyl alcohol, glycerin SD alcohol 40 B (43%). Spray. 56 g. *OTC.*
Use: Poison ivy treatment.

Itch-X. (Ascher & Co.) Pramoxine hydrochloride 1%. **Gel:** Benzyl alcohol 10%, aloe vera gel, diazolidinyl urea, SD alcohol 40, parabens. 35.4 g. **Foam:** Hydrocortisone 1%. Cetyl alcohol, mineral oil, parabens, white petrolatum. 88.7 mL. **Spray:** Benzyl alcohol 10%, aloe vera gel, SD alcohol 40. In 60 mL. *OTC.*
Use: Topical local anesthetic.

Itchy Eye Drops. (Major) Ketotifen 0.025% (as ketotifen fumarate). Benz-

alkonium chloride 0.01%, glycerin, sodium hydroxide, and/or hydrochloric acid. Soln., Ophth. 5 mL. *OTC.*
Use: Ophthalmic and otic agent, ophthalmic antihistamine.

itobarbital.
W/Acetaminophen.
See: Panitol.

• **itraconazole.** (ih-truh-KAHN-uh-zole) USAN.
Use: Antifungal, triazole.
See: Sporanox.

itraconazole. (Various Mfr.) Itraconazole 100 mg. Cap. 28s, 30s, 100s, 500s, UD 28s, UD 30s. *Rx.*
Use: Antifungal agent.

• **ivacaftor.** (EYE-va-KAF-tor) USAN.
Use: Treatment of cystic fibrosis.

I-Valex-1. (Ross) Protein 15 g, fat 23.9 g, carbohydrates 46.3 g, linoleic acid 1800 mg, Fe 9 mg, Na 190 mg, K 675 mg, with appropriate vitamins and minerals. 480 Cal/100 g. Leucine free. Pow. Can 350 g. *OTC.*
Use: Nutritional supplement.

I-Valex-2. (Ross) Protein 30 g, fat 15.5 g, carbohydrates 30 g, Na 880 mg, K 1370 mg, with appropriate vitamins and minerals. 410 Cal/100 g. Leucine free. Pow. Can 325 g. *OTC.*
Use: Nutritional supplement.

Ivarest Maximum Strength. (Blistex) Calamine 14%, diphenhydramine hydrochloride 2%, lanolin oil, petrolatum, propylene glycol. Cream. Tube. 56 g. *OTC.*
Use: Poison ivy product, topical.

• **ivermectin.** (eye-VER-MEK-tin) *USP 34.*
Use: Anthelmintic.
See: Stromectol.

Ivocort. (Roberts) Micronized hydrocortisone alcohol 0.5%, 1%. Bot. 4 oz. *OTC.*
Use: Corticosteroid, topical.

Ivy Block. (EnviroDerm) Bentoquatam 5%, benzyl alcohol, methylparaben, SDA 40 denatured alcohol. Lot. 118 mL. *OTC.*
Use: Poison ivy treatment.

Ivy Cleanse. (EnviroDerm) Isopropyl alcohol, cetyl alcohol. Wipes. Packets of 12 individually wrapped towelettes. *OTC.*
Use: Poison ivy treatment.

Ivy-Dry. (Ivy Corp.) Zinc acetate 2%, isopropanol 12.5%. Glycerin, methylparaben. Lot. Bot. 118 mL. *OTC.*
Use: Poison ivy product, topical.

Ivy-Dry Super. (Ivy Corp.) Zinc acetate 2%, benzyl alcohol 10%, isopropanol 35%, menthol, camphor. Glycerin, para-

bens. Lot. Bot. 177 mL. *OTC.*
Use: Poison ivy product, topical.

Ivy Soothe. (Enviroderm) Hydrocortisone 1%, parabens, cetyl alcohol, glycerin, white petrolatum. Cream. 28 g. *OTC.*
Use: Poison ivy treatment.

Ivy Stat. (Tec Labs) Hydrocortisone 1%, propylene glycol, menthol, SD alcohol 40–B. Gel. 89 mL. *OTC.*
Use: Poison ivy treatment.

I-Wash. (Akorn) Phosphate buffered saline soln. Bot. 4 oz, 8 oz. *OTC.*
Use: Irrigant, ophthalmic.

I-White. (Akorn) Phenylephrine 0.12%, polyvinyl alcohol, hydroxyethyl cellulose. Soln. Bot. 15 mL. *OTC.*
Use: Mydriatic; vasoconstrictor.

• **ixabepilone.** (ix-ab-EP-i-lone) USAN.
Use: Antimitotic, epothilone.
See: Ixempra.

• **ixekizumab.** (IX-e-KIZ-ue-mab) USAN.
Use: Treatment of autoimmune diseases.

Ixempra. (Bristol-Myers Squibb) Ixabepilone 15 mg, 45 mg. Inj., Lyophilized Pow. for Soln., Conc. Single-use kits. Kit contains 1 vial of ixabepilone and 1 vial of diluent. Diluent contains purified polyoxyethylated castor oil 52.8%, dehydrated alcohol 39.8%. *Rx.*
Use: Antimitotic agent, epothilone.

Ixiaro. (Novartis) Japanese encephalitis virus vaccine 6 mcg per 0.5 mL (contains ≈ 6 mcg of purified inactivated Japanese encephalitis virus proteins and aluminum hydroxide 250 mcg). Each 0.5 mL dose contains formaldehyde ≤ 200 ppm, bovine serum albumin ≤ 100 ng/mL, host cell DNA ≤ 200 pg/mL, sodium metabisulfite ≤ 200 ppm, host cell proteins ≤ 300 ng/mL, protamine sulfate ≤ 1 mcg/mL. Preservative free. Single-dose prefilled syringes. 0.5 mL. *Rx.*
Use: Agent for active immunization, viral vaccine.

Izonid. (Major) Isoniazid 300 mg. Tab. Bot. 100s. *Rx.*
Use: Antituberculosis agent.

J

Jalovis.
See: Hyaluronidase.

Jalyn. (GlaxoSmithKline) Dutasteride 0.5 mg/tamsulosin hydrochloride 0.4 mg. Glycerin. Cap. 30s, 90s. *Rx.*
Use: Androgen hormone inhibitor, benign prostatic hyperplasia combination.

Jantoven. (Upsher-Smith) Warfarin sodium 1 mg, 2 mg, 2.5 mg, 3 mg, 4 mg, 5 mg, 6 mg, 7.5 mg, 10 mg. Lactose. Dye free (10 mg only). Tab. 100s, 500s (7.5 mg, 10 mg only), 1000s (except 7.5 mg, 10 mg), UD 100s. *Rx.*
Use: Anticoagulant.

Janumet. (Merck) Sitagliptin (as sitagliptin phosphate)/metformin hydrochloride 50 mg/500 mg, 50 mg/1000 mg. Film-coated. Tab. 60s, 180s, 1000s, UD 50s. *Rx.*
Use: Antidiabetic combination.

Januvia. (Merck) Sitagliptin phosphate 25 mg, 50 mg, 100 mg. Film-coated. Tab. 30s, 90s, 500s (100 mg only), 1000s (100 mg only), UD blister pack 100s. *Rx.*
Use: Antidiabetic agent.

Japan agar.
See: Agar.

Japanese encephalitis virus vaccine.
Use: Agent for active immunization, viral vaccine.
See: Ixiaro.
JE-VAX.

Japan gelatin.
See: Agar.

Japan isinglass.
See: Agar.

Jay-Phyl. (Jaymac) Dyphilline 100 mg, guaifenesin 50 mg per 5 mL. Alcohol and sugar free. Vanilla flavor. Syr. 473 mL. *Rx.*
Use: Antiasthmatic combination, xanthine combination.

J-COF DHC. (JayMac Pharmaceuticals) Brompheniramine maleate 3 mg, dihydrocodeine bitartrate 7.5 mg, pseudoephedrine hydrochloride 15 mg per 5 mL. Alcohol free, dye free, and sugar free. Saccharin, sorbitol. Grape flavor. Liq. 473 mL. *c-III.*
Use: Upper respiratory combination, antitussive combination.

Jenest-28. (Organon) 7 white tablets norethindrone 0.5 mg, ethinyl estradiol 35 mcg; 14 peach tablets norethindrone 1 mg, ethinyl estradiol 35 mcg; 7 inert tablets. Lactose. *Cyclic Tablet dispenser* 28s. *Rx.*

Use: Sex hormone, contraceptive hormone.

Jenloga. (UPM Inc) Clonidine hydrochloride 0.1 mg (equiv. to 0.087 mg of clonidine base). Lactose. Tab., Modified release. 60s, 180s. *Rx.*
Use: Antiadrenergic/sympatholytic; antiadrenergic agent, centrally acting.

Jeri-Bath. (Dermik) Concentrated moisturizing bath oil. Plastic Bot. 8 oz. *OTC.*
Use: Dermatologic.

Jets. (Freeda) L-lysine 300 mg, vitamins C 25 mg, B_{12} 25 mcg, B_6 5 mg, B_1 10 mg. Chew. Tab. Bot. 100s. *OTC.*
Use: Vitamin supplement; amino acid.

JE-VAX. (Sanofi Pasteur) Japanese encephalitis virus vaccine. Thimerosal 0.007%. Gelatin ≈ 500 mcg, formaldehyde < 100 mcg, mouse serum protein < 50 ng per each 1 mL dose. Pow. for Inj., lyophilized. Single-dose vial with 1.3 mL diluent (sterile water for injection); 10-dose vial with 11 mL diluent (sterile water for injection). *Rx.*
Use: Agent for active immunization, viral vaccine.

Jevity. (Ross) Calcium and sodium caseinates, soy fiber, hydrolyzed cornstarch, MCT (fractionated coconut oil), soy oil, corn oil, soy lecithin, vitamins A, B_1, B_2, B_3, B_5, B_6, B_{12}, C, D, E, K, folic acid, biotin, choline, Ca, P, Mg, Fe, Mn, Cu, Zn, I, Cl. Liq. Bot. 240 mL. *OTC.*
Use: Nutritional supplement.

Jevity 1.5 Cal. (Ross) Protein 63.4 g, carbohydrate 214.2 g, fat 49.6 g/L. Na 1386 mg/L, K 1848 mg/L, cal 1.5/mL. Vitamins A, B_1, B_2, B_3, B_5, B_6, B_{12}, C, D, E, K, Ca, Cu, Fe, I, Mg, Mn, Mo, P, Se, Zn, biotin, chloride, choline, folic acid. Liq. Can. 237 mL. Ready-to-hang containers 1 L, 1.5 L. *OTC.*
Use: Enteral nutrition therapy.

Jevtana. (Sanofi-Aventis) Cabazitaxel 40 mg/mL. Polysorbate 80. Inj., Soln. Single-use vial w/diluents. *Rx.*
Use: Antimitotic agent, taxoid.

Jiffy. (Block Drug) Benzocaine, menthol, eugenol in glycerin-water base with SD alcohol 38-B 76%. Bot. 0.125 oz. *OTC.*
Use: Anesthetic, local.

Jinteli. (Teva) Ethinyl estradiol 5 mcg/norethindrone acetate 1 mg. Lactose. Tab. 90s, blister card 28s. *Rx.*
Use: Sex hormone, estrogen/progestin combination.

J-Liberty. (J Pharmacal) Chlordiazepoxide hydrochloride 5 mg, 10 mg, 25 mg. Cap. *c-IV.*
Use: Anxiolytic.

J-Max. (Jaymac) **ER Tab.**: Phenylephrine hydrochloride 35 mg, guaifenesin 1200 mg. 100s. **Syr.**: Phenylephrine hydrochloride 5 mg, guaifenesin 200 mg per 5 mL. Dye and gluten free. Aspartame, parabens. Strawberry cream flavor. 473 mL. *Rx.*
Use: Decongestant and expectorant combination, upper respiratory combination.

J-Max DHC. (JayMac Pharmaceuticals) Dihydrocodeine bitartrate 7.5 mg, guaifenesin 100 mg per 5 mL. Menthol, saccharin, sorbitol. Alcohol free. Grape flavor. Liq. 473 mL. *c-III.*
Use: Upper respiratory combination

Johnson's Baby. (Johnson & Johnson) Dimethicone 2%. Cream. Jar 4 oz, 6 oz; Tube 2 oz. *OTC.*
Use: Dermatologic protectant.

Johnson's Baby Sunblock Extra Protection. (Johnson & Johnson) Octyl methoxycinnamate, octyl salicylate, titanium dioxide, oxybenzone, C12-15 alcohols benzoate, cetyl alcohol, EDTA, vitamin E. Lot. Bot. 120 mL. *OTC.*
Use: Sunscreen.

Johnson's Baby Sunblock SPF 15. (Johnson & Johnson) Octyl methoxycinnamate, octyl salicylate, oxybenzone, titanium dioxide, benzyl alcohol, cetyl alcohol. PABA free. Waterproof. **Cream:** Tube. 60 g. **Lot.**: Bot. 60 g. *OTC.*
Use: Sunscreen.

Johnson's Baby Sunblock SPF 30. (Johnson & Johnson) Benzophenone-3, octyl methoxycinnamate, octyl salicylate, titanium dioxide. PABA free. Waterproof. Lot. Bot. 120 mL.
Use: Sunscreen.

Johnson's Medicated. (Johnson & Johnson) Bentonite, kaolin, talc, zinc oxide. Pow. Bot. Small, Medium, Large. *OTC.*
Use: Diaper rash preparation.

Johnson's Shea & Cocoa Butter Baby Lotion. (J & J Consumer) Butyrospermum parkii (shea butter), glycerin, mineral oil, parabens, stearyl alcohol, theobroma cacao. Lot. 798 mL. *OTC.*
Use: Emollient.

Jolessa. (Barr) Ethinyl estradiol 30 mcg, levonorgestrel 0.15 mg. Lactose. Film-coated. Tab. 91s with 7 inert tablets (lactose). *Rx.*
Use: Contraceptive hormone, sex hormone.

Jolivette. (Watson) Norethindrone 0.35 mg. Lactose. Tab. 28s. *Rx.*
Use: Contraceptive hormone, sex hormone.

• **josamycin.** (JOE-sah-MYsin) USAN.
Use: Anti-infective.

J-Tan. (Jaymac) Brompheniramine tannate 4 mg. Strawberry cream flavor. Oral Susp. 473 mL. *Rx.*
Use: Antihistamine.

J-Tan D. (Jaymac) Brompheniramine tannate 2.2 mg, phenylephrine tannate 1.58 mg per 5 mL. Phenylalanine 5 mg. Strawberry cream flavor. Susp. 473 mL. *Rx.*
Use: Upper respiratory combination, decongestant and antihistamine.

J-Tan D PD. (Jaymac) Pseudoephedrine hydrochloride 7.5 mg, brompheniramine maleate 1 mg per 1 mL. Alcohol, sugar, and dye free. Saccharin, sorbitol. Strawberry-banana flavor. Drops. 30 mL with dropper. *Rx.*
Use: Upper respiratory combination, decongestant and antihistamine.

Junel Fe 1/20. (Barr) Norethindrone acetate 1 mg, ethinyl estradiol 20 mcg. Tab. 28s with 7 brown tablets (ferrous fumarate 75 mg/tab). *Rx.*
Use: Contraceptive hormone, sex hormone.

Junel Fe 1.5/30. (Barr) Norethindrone acetate 1.5 mg, ethinyl estradiol 30 mcg. Tab. 28s with 7 brown tablets (ferrous fumarate 75 mg/tab). *Rx.*
Use: Contraceptive hormone, sex hormone.

Junel 21 Day 1.5/30. (Barr) Ethinyl estradiol 30 mcg, norethindrone acetate 1.5 mg. Lactose, sugar. Tab. 21s. *Rx.*
Use: Contraceptive hormone, sex hormone.

Junel 21 Day 1/20. (Barr) Ethinyl estradiol 20 mcg, norethindrone acetate 1 mg. Lactose, sugar. Tab. 21s. *Rx.*
Use: Contraceptive hormone, sex hormone.

Junior Strength Motrin. (McNeil) Ibuprofen. **Chew. Tab.**: 100 mg. Aspartame, phenylalanine 6 mg. Orange flavor. 24s. **Tab.**: 100 mg. Bot. 24s. *OTC.*
Use: Analgesic, NSAID.

Junior Strength Panadol. (Bayer Consumer Care) Acetaminophen 160 mg. Capl. Bot. 30s. *OTC.*
Use: Analgesic.

• **juniper tar.** (JOO-nih-per tar) *USP 34.*
Use: Local antieczematic, pharmaceutic necessity.

Junyer-All. (Barth's) Vitamins A 6000 units, D 400 units, B_1 3 mg, B_2 6 mg, C 120 mg, niacin 1 mg, E 12 units, B_{12} 10 mcg, calcium 217 mg, phosphorus 97.5 mg, red bone mar-

row 10 mg, organic iron 15 mg, iodine 0.1 mg, beef peptone 20 mg/2 Cap. Bot. 10 month, 3 month, 6 month supply. OTC.
Use: Vitamin, mineral supplement.
Just For Kids. (3M ESPE) Stannous fluoride 0.4%. Bubble gum flavor. Dental gel. 121.9 g. OTC.
Use: Nutritional agent, trace element.
Just Tears. (Blairex) Benzalkonium chloride, EDTA, NaCl, polyvinyl alcohol 1.4%. Soln. Bot. 15 mL. OTC.
Use: Lubricant, ophthalmic.
Juvederm 30. (Inamed) Hyaluronic acid 24 mg/mL. Gel for Inj. Single-use prefilled syringes with 27-gauge needle. Rx.
Use: Physical adjunct.
Juvederm 30HV. (Inamed) Hyaluronic acid 24 mg/mL. Gel for Inj. Single-use prefilled syringes with 27-gauge needle. Rx.
Use: Physical adjunct.
Juvederm 24HV. (Inamed) Hyaluronic acid 24 mg/mL. Gel for Inj. Single-use prefilled syringes with 30-gauge needles. Rx.
Use: Physical adjunct.

Juvederm Ultra. (Allergan) Hyaluronic acid 24 mg/mL. Gel; intradermal. Single-use, prefilled syringe w/30-gauge needle. Rx.
Use: Physical adjunct, dermal hyaluronic acid derivative.
Juvederm Ultra Plus. (Allergan) Hyaluronic acid 24 mg/mL. Gel; intradermal. Single-use, prefilled syringe w/27-gauge needle. Rx.
Use: Physical adjunct, dermal hyaluronic acid derivative.
Juvederm Ultra Plus XC. (Allergan) Hyaluronic acid 24 mg/mL, lidocaine 0.3%. Gel; intradermal. Single-use syringe. Rx.
Use: Physical adjunct, dermal hyaluronic acid derivative.
Juvederm Ultra XC. (Allergan) Hyaluronic acid 24 mg/mL, lidocaine 0.3%. Gel; intradermal. Single-use, prefilled syringe w/30-gauge needle. Rx.
Use: Physical adjunct, dermal hyaluronic acid derivative.
Juvocaine.
See: Procaine Hydrochloride.

K

Kadian. (Actavis) Morphine sulfate 10 mg, 20 mg, 30 mg, 50 mg, 60 mg, 80 mg; 100 mg, 200 mg (for use only in opioid-tolerant patients). Sucrose. ER Pellet Cap. Bot. 100s. *c-II*.
Use: Opioid analgesic.

Kaergona.
See: Menadione.

Kala. (Freeda) Soy-based acidophilus 2 million units. Tab. Bot. 100s, 250s, 500s. *OTC*.
Use: Nutritional supplement.

•**kalafungin.** (kal-ah-FUN-jin) USAN.
Use: Antifungal.

Kalbitor. (Dyax Corp) Ecallantide 10 mg/ mL (produced in Pichia pastoris yeast cells by recombinant DNA technology). Disodium hydrogen orthophosphate (dihydrate) 0.76 mg, monopotassium phosphate 0.2 mg, potassium chloride 0.2 mg, sodium chloride 8 mg. Preservative free. Inj., Soln. Single-use vial. *Rx*.
Use: Hematological agent, kallikrein inhibitor.

Kaletra. (Abbott) **Oral Soln.:** Lopinavir 80 mg, ritonavir 20 mg/mL. Alcohol 42.4%, menthol, acesulafme K, corn syrup, saccharin, peppermint and castor oils, cotton candy or vanilla flavor. Bot. with dosing cup. 160 mL. **Tab.:** Lopinavir/ritonavir. 100 mg/25 mg, 200 mg/50 mg. Film-coated. 60s (100 mg/25 mg only), 120s (200 mg/ 50 mg only). *Rx*.
Use: Antiretroviral, protease inhibitor combination.

Kallikrein inhibitors.
See: Ecallantide.

Kaltostat. (GlaxoSmithKline) Calcium-sodium alginate fiber, 3" × 4¾" sterile dressing. In 1s. *OTC*.
Use: Dressing, hydroactive.

Kaltostat Forte. (GlaxoSmithKline) Calcium-sodium alginate fiber, 4" × 4" sterile dressing. In 1s. *OTC*.
Use: Dressing, hydroactive.

Kamfolene. (Wade) Camphor, menthol, methyl salicylate, turpentine and eucalyptus oils, carbolic acid 2%, calamine, zinc oxide in lanolin base. Jar 2 oz, lb. *OTC*.
Use: Antiseptic.

•**kanamycin sulfate.** (kan-uh-MY-sin) USP 34.
Use: Anti-infective.
See: Kantrex.

Kank-A. (Blairex) Benzocaine 5%, cetylpyridinium chloride, castor oil, benzoin

compound. Liq. Bot. 3.75 mL. *OTC*.
Use: Anesthetic, local.

Kantrex. (Bristol-Myers Squibb) Kanamycin sulfate. **Vial:** 0.5 g/2 mL or 1 g/ 3 mL. **Pediatric Inj.:** 75 mg/2 mL. **Disposable Syringe:** 500 mg/2 mL. *Rx*.
Use: Anti-infective aminoglycoside.

Kaochlor-Eff. (Pharmacia) Elemental potassium 20 mEq, chloride 20 mEq. Tab. Supplied by: Potassium Cl 0.6 g, potassium citrate 0.22 g, potassium bicarbonate 1 g, betaine hydrochloride 1.84 g, saccharin 20 mg, artificial fruit flavor, tartrazine (color). Tab. Sugar free. Carton 60s. *Rx*.
Use: Electrolyte supplement.

Kaodene Non-Narcotic. (Pfeiffer) Kaolin 3.9 g, pectin 194.4 mg/30 mL, bismuth subsalicylate. Alcohol free. Liq. Bot. 120 mL. *OTC*.
Use: Antidiarrheal.

Kaodene with Codeine. (Pfeiffer) Codeine phosphate 32.4 mg, kaolin 3.9 g, pectin 194.4 mg, sodium carboxymethylcellulose, bismuth subsalicylate/ 30 mL. Susp. Bot. 120 mL. *OTC*.
Use: Antidiarrheal.

•**kaolin.** (KAY-oh-lin) *USP 34*.
Use: Adsorbent.
W/Cornstarch, camphor, zinc oxide, eucalyptus oil.
See: Mexsana Medicated Powder.
W/Furazolidone, pectin.
See: Furoxone.
W/Pectin.
See: Kapectin.
W/Pectin, paregoric (equivalent).
See: Kapectin.

kaolin with pectin. (Various Mfr.) Kaolin 90 g, pectin 2 g/30 mL. Susp. Bot. 180 mL, pt, UD 30 mL. *OTC*.
Use: Antidiarrheal combination.

Kaon Cl. (Savage) Potassium Cl 500 mg, FD&C Yellow No. 5. CR Tab. Bot. 100s, 250s, 1000s. *Rx*.
Use: Electrolyte supplement.

Kaon Cl-10. (Savage) Potassium Cl 750 mg. CR Tab. Bot. 100s, 500s, 1000s. *Stat-Pak* 100s. *Rx*.
Use: Electrolyte supplement.

Kaon Cl 20%. (Savage) Potassium and chloride 40 mEq (to potassium Cl 3 g)/ 15 mL, saccharin, flavoring, alcohol 5%. Bot. Pt. *Rx*.
Use: Electrolyte supplement.

Kaon Elixir. (Savage) Elemental potassium 20 mEq (as potassium gluconate 4.68 g)/15 mL, aromatics, grape and lemon-lime flavors, alcohol 5%, saccharin. Elix. Unit pkg. Pt, gal. *Rx*.
Use: Electrolyte supplement.

Kaon Tablets. (Savage) Elemental potassium 5 mEq obtained from potassium gluconate 1.17 g. SC Tab. Bot. 100s, 500s. *Rx.*
Use: Electrolyte supplement.

Kaopectate. (Chattem) Bismuth subsalicylate 262 mg. Tab. 12s, 20s. *OTC.*
Use: Antidiarrheal.

Kaopectate, Children's. (Chattem) Bismuth subsalicylate 87 mg/5 mL, sucrose, cherry flavor. Liq. 177 mL. *OTC.*
Use: Antidiarrheal combination.

Kaopectate Extra Strength. (Chattem) Bismuth subsalicylate 175 mg/5 mL, sucrose, peppermint flavor. Liq. 236 mL. *OTC.*
Use: Antidiarrheal.

Kaopectate, Maximum Strength. (Chattem) Attapulgite 750 mg, Capl. Pkg. 12s, 20s. *OTC.*
Use: Antidiarrheal combination.

Kaopectate Tablet Formula. (Chattem) Attapulgite 750 mg. Tab. Blister pak 12s, 20s. *OTC.*
Use: Antidiarrheal.

Kaophen. (Pal-Pak, Inc.) Phenobarbital 6.5 mg, belladonna extract 0.1 mg, kaolin 388.8 mg. Tab. Bot. 100s, 1000s. *OTC.*
Use: Antidiarrheal.

Kao-Spen. (Century) Kaolin 5.2 g, pectin 260 mg/30 mL. Susp. Bot. 120 mL, pt, gal. *OTC.*
Use: Antidiarrheal.

Kao-Tin. (Major) Bismuth subsalicylate 262 mg per 15 mL. Saccharin, sorbitol. Liq. 236 mL, 473 mL. *OTC.*
Use: Antidiarrheal.

Kapectin. (Health for Life Brands) Kaolin 90 g, pectin 2 g/oz. Bot. Gal. *OTC.*
Use: Antidiarrheal.

Ka-Pek. (A.P.C.) Kaolin 90 g, pectin 4.5 g/fl oz. Bot. 6 oz, gal. *OTC.*
Use: Antidiarrheal.

kapilin.
See: Menadione.

Kapvay. (Shionogi Pharma) Clonidine hydrochloride 0.1 mg (equiv. to clonidine base 0.087 mg), 0.2 mg (equiv. to clonidine base 0.174 mg). Lactose. ER Tab. 60s, 180s. *Rx.*
Use: Antiadrenergic/sympatholytic; antiadrenergic agent, centrally acting.

karaya gum. (Penick) Indian Gum. Sterculia Gum.

karaya powder. (Sween) Bot. 3 oz.
Use: Deodorant, ostomy.

Kareon.
See: Menadione.

Karidium. (Young Dental) **Tab.:** Sodium fluoride 2.21 mg, sodium Cl 94.49 mg,

disintegrant 0.5 mg. Bot. 180s, 1000s.
Liq.: Sodium fluoride 2.21 mg, sodium Cl 10 mg, purified water q.s./8 drops. Bot. 30 mL, 60 mL. *Rx.*
Use: Dental caries agent.

Karigel. (Young Dental) Fluoride ion 0.5%, pH 5.6. Gel. Bot. 30 mL, 130 mL, 250 mL. *Rx.*
Use: Dental caries agent.

Karigel-N. (Young Dental) Fluoride ion 0.5% in neutral pH gel. Bot. 24 mL, 125 mL. *Rx.*
Use: Dental caries agent.

Kariva. (Barr) **Phase 1:** Desogestrel 0.15 mg, ethinyl estradiol 20 mcg. 21 tabs. **Phase 2:** Ethinyl estradiol 10 mcg. 5 tabs. Lactose. Tab. Blister card. 28s with 2 inert tabs. *Rx.*
Use: Sex hormone, contraceptive update.

•**kasal.** (KAY-sal) USAN. Approximately Na_8Al_2 $(OH)_2$ $(PO_4)_4$ with ≈ 30% of dibasic sodium phosphate; sodium aluminum phosphate, basic.
Use: Food additive.

kasugamycin. Under study.
Use: Anti-infective.

Kaviton.
See: Menadione, USP.

Kayexalate. (Sanofi-Synthelabo) Sodium polystyrene sulfonate (sodium content ≈ 100 mg/g). Jar 1 lb. *Rx.*
Use: Potassium-removing resin.

K-C. (Century) **Susp.:** Kaolin 5.2 g, pectin 260 mg, bismuth subcarbonate 260 mg/30 mL. Bot. 120 mL, pt, gal.
Liq.: Kaolin 5.2 g, pectin 260 mg, bismuth subcarbonate 260 mg/oz. Bot. 4 oz, pt, gal. *OTC.*
Use: Antidiarrheal.

KCl-20. (Western Research) Potassium Cl 1.5 g (potassium 20 mEq, chloride 20 mEq) Packet. Box 30s. *Rx.*
Use: Electrolyte supplement.

K-Dur 10 & 20. (Key) **10:** Potassium Cl 750 mg (10 mEq). SR Tab. **20:** Potassium Cl 1500 mg (20 mEq). SR Tab. Bot. 100s. *Rx.*
Use: Electrolyte supplement.

KE.
See: Cortisone Acetate.

Keelamin. (Mericon Industries) Zinc 20 mg, manganese 5 mg, copper 3 mg. Tab. Bot. 100s. *OTC.*
Use: Mineral supplement.

Keep Alert. (Magno-Humphries Labs) Caffeine 200 mg. Tab. Bot. 60s. *OTC.*
Use: CNS stimulant, analeptic.

Keep Going. (Block Drug) Caffeine 200 mg. Tab. Pkg. 4s. *OTC.*
Use: CNS stimulant, analeptic.

Keflex. (Victory Pharma) **Cap.:** Cephalexin 250 mg, 333 mg, 500 mg, 750 mg. Bot. 20s, 100s (250, 500 mg only); 50s (333 mg, 750 mg only). **Pow. for Oral Susp.:** Cephalexin 125 mg/ 5 mL, 250 mg/5 mL. Sucrose. Bot. 100 mL, 200 mL. *Rx.*
Use: Anti-infective, cephalosporin.
Kell E. (Canright) dl-α Tocopheryl 100 units, 200 units, 400 units. Tab. Bot. 100s. *OTC.*
Use: Vitamin supplement.
Kellogg's Tasteless Castor Oil. (GlaxoSmithKline) Castor oil 100%. Bot. 2 oz. *OTC.*
Use: Laxative.
Kelnor 1/35. (Barr) Ethinyl estradiol 35 mcg, ethynodiol diacetate 1 mg. Tab. 28s with 7 inert tablets. *Rx.*
Use: Contraceptive hormone, sex hormone.
Kelp. (Arcum) Tab. Bot. 100s, 1000s. *OTC.*
Use: Supplement.
Kelp. (Faraday) Iodine from kelp 0.15 mg. Tab. Bot. 100s. *OTC.*
Use: Supplement.
Kelp Plus. (Barth's) Iodine from kelp plus 16 trace minerals. Tab. Bot. 100s, 500s, 1000s. *OTC.*
Use: Supplement.
Kemstro. (Schwarz) Baclofen 10 mg (with phenylalanine 3.7 mg), 20 mg (phenylalanine 7.9 mg). Mannitol, aspartame. Orally Disintegrating Tab. 100s. *Rx.*
Use: Skeletal muscle relaxant.
Kenac. (Alra) Triamcinolone acetonide. **Cream:** 0.025%, 0.1%. Tube 15 g, 60 g, 80 g; Jar 240 g. **Oint.:** 0.1%. Tube 15 g, 80 g. *Rx.*
Use: Corticosteroid, topical.
Kenakion. (Harriett Lane Home of Johns Hopkins Hospital) Vitamin K-1 oxide. *Rx.*
Use: Vitamin K-induced kernicterus.
Kenalog. (Bristol-Myers Squibb) Triamcinolone acetonide. 0.1% (w/base of polyethylene, mineral oil). Oint. Tubes. 15 g, 60 g, 80 g. Jars. 240 g. *Rx.*
Use: Corticosteroid, topical.
Kenalog. (Ranbaxy) Aer. 6.6 mg/100 g, alcohol 10.3%. Cans. 23 g, 63 g.
Kenalog-40. (Bristol-Myers Squibb) Triamcinolone acetonide 40 mg/mL. Benzyl alcohol 0.9%, carboxymethylcellulose, polysorbate 80. Inj., Susp. Vials. 1 mL, 5 mL, 10 mL. *Rx.*
Use: Adrenocortical steroid, glucocorticoid.
Kenalog-10. (Bristol-Myers Squibb) Triamcinolone acetonide 10 mg/mL. Ben-

zyl alcohol 0.9%, carboxymethylcellulose, polysorbate 80. Inj., Susp. Vials. 5 mL. *Rx.*
Use: Adrenocortical steroid, glucocorticoid.
Kenalog 0.025%. (Bristol-Myers Squibb) Triamcinolone acetonide. **Cream:** Tube 15 g, 80 g; Jar 240 g. **Oint.:** Plastibase (w/base of polyethylene and mineral oil gel). Tube 15 g, 80 g, 240 g. *Rx.*
Use: Corticosteroid, topical.
Kendall's "Compound E".
See: Cortisone Acetate.
Kendall's "Desoxy Compound B".
See: Desoxycorticosterone Acetate.
Kenwood Therapeutic. (Kenwood) Vitamins A 3333 units, D 133 units, E 1.5 units, C 50 mg, B_1 2 mg, B_2 1 mg, B_3 20 mg, B_5 2 mg, B_6 0.33 mg, Ca, K, Mg, Mn, P per 5 mL. Liq. Bot. 240 mL. *OTC.*
Use: Mineral, vitamin supplement.
Kepivance. (Biovitrum AB) Palifermin 6.25 mg. Sucrose. Preservative free. Pow. for Inj. Single-use vials. *Rx.*
Use: Keratinocyte growth factor.
Keppra. (UCB) Levetiracetam. **Inj. Concentrate:** 100 mg/mL. 5 mL single-use vials. **Oral Soln.:** 100 mg/mL. Dyefree. Acesulfame K, ammonium glycyrrhizinate, parabens, maltitol. Grape flavor. 480 mL. **Tab.:** 250 mg, 500 mg, 750 mg, 1000 mg. Film-coated. PEG, polyvinyl alcohol. Lactose free and gluten free. 60s (1000 mg only); 120s (except 1000 mg). *Rx.*
Use: Anticonvulsant.
Keppra XR. (UCB) Levetriacetam 500 mg, 750 mg. Film-coated. PEG 6000, polyvinyl alcohol. ER Tab. 60s. *Rx.*
Use: Anticonvulsant.
Kerafoam. (Onset Therapeutics) Urea 30%. Cetyl alcohol, parabens. Foam. 60 g. *Rx.*
Use: Emollient.
Kerafoam 42. (Onset Therapeutics) Urea 42%. Cetearyl alcohol, edetate disodium, parabens. Aer. Foam. 60 g. *Rx.*
Use: Emollient.
Keralac. (Pharmaderm) Urea. **Cream:** 50%. EDTA. 18 mL. **Lot.:** 35%. Cetyl alcohol, EDTA. 207 mL, 325 mL. **Oint.:** Urea 50%. Vitamin E, lactic acid, zinc pyrithione, glycerin, EDTA, cetyl alcohol. 45 g. *Rx.*
Use: Emollient.
Keralac Nail Gel. (Pharmaderm) Urea 50%. EDTA. Gel. 18 mL. *Rx.*
Use: Emollient.
Keralac Nailstik. (Pharmaderm) Urea 50%. EDTA. Soln., Top. Cartons of

6 nailsticks containing 2.4 mL. *Rx.*
Use: Emollient.

Keralyt. (Summers) Salicylic acid 3%, 6%. Alcohol 21%, propylene glycol. Gel. 28.4 g. *OTC.*
Use: Keratolytic agent.

Kerasal AL. (Taro Consumer) Ammonium lactate, light mineral oil, glycerin, propylene glycol, cetyl alcohol, glyceryl monostearate, polyoxyethylene 100 stearate, magnesium aluminum silicate, methylcellulose, polyoxyl 40 stearate, laureth-4, parabens. May contain ammonium hydroxide and lactic acid. Cream. 42 g. *OTC.*
Use: Emollient.

Kerasal Ultra 20. (Alterna) Ammonium lactate 5%, urea 20%, cetyl alcohol, disodium EDTA, glycerin, glyceryl, mineral oil, parabens, PEG-100, petrolatum, propylene glycol. Cream. 56.8 g. *OTC.*
Use: Emollient.

keratinocyte growth factors.
See: Palifermin.

Keratol HC. (Breckenridge) Hydrocortisone acetate 1%. Cetyl alcohol, disodium edetate, urea 10%. Cream. 28.3 g, 95 g. *Rx.*
Use: Anti-inflammatory agent; corticosteroid, topical.

keratolytic agents.
See: Acne Products, Combinations.
Masoprocol.
Salicylic Acid.
Sulfur Preparations.

Keri. (Novartis Consumer Health) Mineral oil, lanolin oil, water, propylene glycol, glyceryl stearate, PEG-100 stearate, PEG 40 stearate, PEG-4 dilaurate, laureth-4, parabens, docusate sodium, triethanolamine, quaternium 15, carbomer 934. Lot. Bot. 6.5 oz, 13 oz, 20 oz. *OTC.*
Use: Emollient.

Keri Advanced. (Novartis Consumer Health) Glycerin, petrolatum, cetyl alcohol, aloe, tocopheryl acetate, dimethicone, PEG-100 stearate, parabens, EDTA, diazolidinyl urea. Oil free. Lot. 241 g. *OTC.*
Use: Emollient.

Keri Age Defy & Protect. (Novartis Consumer Health) Octinoxate 7.5%, oxybenzone 2%, cetearyl alcohol, glycerin, ammonium lactate, dimethicone, tocopheryl, EDTA. SPF +15. Lot. 425 g. *OTC.*
Use: Emollient.

Keri Deep Conditioning Overnight. (Novartis Consumer Health) Castor oil, cetyl alcohol, cetearyl alcohol, disodium EDTA, glycerin, glyceryl, parabens, PEG-8, shea butter, vitamins A, C, and E. Lt. 425 g. *OTC.*
Use: Emollient, miscellaneous.

Keri Facial Soap. (Novartis Consumer Health) Sodium tallowate, sodium cocoate, mineral oil, octyl hydroxystearate, fragrance, glycerin, titanium dioxide, PEG-75, lanolin oil, docusate sodium, PEG-4 dilaurate, propylparaben, PEG-40 stearate, glyceryl monostearate, PEG-100 stearate, sodium Cl, BHT, EDTA. Bar 3.25 oz. *OTC.*
Use: Dermatologic cleanser.

Keri Long Lasting. (Novartis Consumer Health) Cetearyl alcohol, polysorbate 60, mineral oil, cetyl alcohol, caprylic/carpic triglycerides, propylene glycol, dimethicone, parabens, tocopheryl acetate, disodium EDTA. Cream, Top. 113 g. *OTC.*
Use: Emollient, miscellaneous.

Keri Nourishing Shea Butter. (Novartis Consumer Health) Mineral oil, glycerin, shea butter, vitamin E acetate, parabens, sunflower seed oil, EDTA, aloe. Lot. 425 g. *OTC.*
Use: Emollient.

Keri Original. (Novartis Consumer Health) Mineral oil, glycerin, PEG-40 stearate, glyceryl stearate, PEG-100 stearate, PEG-4 dilaurate, laureth-4, aloe, sunflower seed oil, tocopheryl acetate, parabens, EDTA. Scented and unscented. Lot. 241 g. *OTC.*
Use: Emollient.

Keri Renewal Milk Body. (Novartis Consumer Health) Caprylic/carpic triglyceride, sunflower oil, glycerin, PEG-20, methyl glucose sesquistearate, laureth-7, C-13-14 isoparaffin, polyacrylamide, parabens, phenoxyethanol, dimethicone, cera alba, sodium pyruvate, tocopheryl acetate, borage oil, lactic acid, propylene glycol, hydrolyzed fibronectin, bifida fermen lysate, carbomer, sodium hydroxide, acrylates/C10-30 alkyl acrylate, crosspolymer, allantoin, disodium EDTA, citric acid, glyceryl oleate, glyceryl stearate, ascorbyl palmitate, BHT, glycosphingolipids, phospholipids, cholesterol, whey protein. Top. Lot. 241 g. *OTC.*
Use: Emollient, miscellaneous.

Keri Renewal Skin Firming. (Novartis Consumer Health) Cetyl alcohol, ceteareth-20, isostearyl isostearate, hydrolyzed fibronectin, propylene glycol, glyceryl stearate, steareth-20, PEG-6 stearate, dimethicone, tocopheryl ace-

tate, sodium pyruvate, collagen, hydrolyzed elastin, methyl silanol, sodium mannuronate, parabens, phenoxyethanol, carbomer, sodium hydroxide, madecassicoside. Top. Lot. 119 g. *OTC.*
Use: Emollient, miscellaneous.

Keri Sensitive Skin. (Novartis Consumer Health) Glycerin, hydrogenated polyisobutane, petrolatum, cetyl alcohol, aloe, barbadensis gel, vitamin E acetate, EDTA, parabens. Lot. 241 g. *OTC.*
Use: Emollient.

Keri Shave Minimizing. (Novartis Consumer Health) Glycerin, cetearyl alcohol, mineral oil, petrolatum, SD alcohol 40-B, glyceryl dilaurate, dimethicone, parabens, hydrolyzed soy protein. Lot. 425 g. *OTC.*
Use: Emollient.

Kerlone. (Sanofi) Betaxolol hydrochloride 10 mg, 20 mg. Lactose. Film-coated. Tab. Bot. 100s. *Rx.*
Use: Antiadrenergic/sympatholytic, beta-adrenergic blocker.

Kerocaine.
See: Procaine hydrochloride.

Kerodex. (Wyeth) **No. 51:** Water-miscible. Tube 4 oz, Jar lb. **No. 71:** Water-repellent Tube 4 oz, Jar lb. *OTC.*
Use: Emollient.

kerohydric. A de-waxed, oil-soluble fraction of lanolin.
Use: Emollient, cleanser.
See: Alpha-Keri.
Keri.
W/Docusate Sodium, Sodium Alkyl Polyether Sulfonate, Sodium Sulfoacetate, Sulfur, Salicylic Acid, Hexachlorophene.
See: Sebulex with Conditioners.

Kerol. (Doak) Urea 50%. Cetyl alcohol, EDTA, glycerin, PEG-6. Top. Susp. 284 g. *Rx.*
Use: Emollient.

Kerol. (PharmaDerm) Urea 50%. Cetyl alcohol, disodium EDTA, glycerin, lactic acid, PEG-6, vitamin E. Top. Emulsion. 284 g. *Rx.*
Use: Emollient.

Kerol AD. (Pharmaderm) Urea 45%. Cetyl alcohol, EDTA disodium, glycerin, lactic acid, PEG, titanium dioxide. Emuls. 240 mL. *Rx.*
Use: Emollient.

Kerol ZX. (PharmaDerm) Urea 50%. Disodium EDTA, lactic acid, PEG-6, vitamin E. Top. Soln. 12 mL prefilled applicator. *Rx.*
Use: Emollient.

Kerr Insta-Char. (Kerr Drug) **Regular:** Aqueous suspension activated charcoal 50 g/8 oz. **Pediatric:** Aqueous suspension activated charcoal 15 g/4 oz. *OTC.*
Use: Antidote.

Kerr Triple Dye. (Kerr Drug) Gentian violet, proflavine hemisulfate, brilliant green in water. Dispensing bot. 15 mL. Single Use *Dispos-A-Swab* 0.65 mL, Box 10s, Case 10 × 50 Box. *OTC.*
Use: Antiseptic.

Kestrone 5. (Hyrex) Estrone 5 mg/mL, sodium carboxymethylcellulose, povidone, benzyl alcohol, propylparabens Inj. Multi-dose vial 10 mL. *Rx.*
Use: Estrogen.

Ketalar. (JHP Pharmaceuticals) Ketamine hydrochloride 10 mg, 50 mg, 100 mg/mL. Inj. Vial 20 mL (10 mg), 10 mL (50 mg), 5 mL (100 mg). Ctn. 10s. *c-III.*
Use: Anesthetic.

•**ketamine hydrochloride.** (KEET-uh-MEEN) *USP 34.*
Use: Anesthetic.
See: Ketalar.

•**ketanserin.** (KEET-AN-ser-in) USAN.
Use: Serotonin antagonist.

•**ketazocine.** (key-TAY-zoe-seen) USAN.
Use: Analgesic.

•**ketazolam.** (keet-AZE-oh-lam) USAN.
Use: Anxiolytic.

Ketek. (Sanofi-Aventis) Telithromycin 300 mg, 400 mg. Cornstarch (400 mg only), lactose. Film-coated. Tab. 20s (300 mg only); 60s, *Ketek Pak*, blister pack 10s (400 mg only). *Rx.*
Use: Anti-infective.

•**kethoxal.** (KEY-thox-al) USAN.
Use: Antiviral.

•**ketipramine fumarate.** (key-TIH-prah-MEEN) USAN.
Use: Antidepressant.

KetoCare. (Home Diagnostics) Reagent strips for urine tests. 50s. *OTC.*
Use: Diagnostic aid.

•**ketoconazole.** (KEY-toe-KOE-nuh-zole) *USP 34.*
Use: Antifungal agent, topical anti-infective.
See: Extina.
Nizoral A-D.
Xolegel.
Xolegel CorePak.
W/Pyrithione Zinc.
See: Xolegel Duo Convenience Pack.

ketoconazole. (Various Mfr.) Ketoconazole. **Cream:** 2%. Cetyl alcohol, stearyl alcohol, sodium sulfite. Cream. Tube. 15 g, 30 g, 60 g. **Shampoo:** 2%. 120 mL. *Rx.*

Use: Antifungal agent, topical anti-infective.

ketoconazole. (Various Mfr.) Ketoconazole 200 mg. Tab. Bot. 30s, 50s, 100s, 250s, 500s, 1000s; blister pack 10s, 30s, 50s, 100s. *Rx.*
Use: Antifungal.

Ketodestrin.
See: Estrone.

ketohexazine. (Wyeth)
Use: Hypnotic.

ketohydroxyestratriene.
See: Estrone.

ketohydroxyestrin.
See: Estrone.

ketolides.
Use: Anti-infectives.
See: Telithromycin.

ketone tests.
Use: Diagnostic aid.
See: Acetest Reagent.
  Chemstrip K.

Ketonex-1. (Ross) Protein 15 g, fat 23.9 g, carbohydrates 46.3 g, linoleic acid 1800 mg, Fe 9 mg, Na 190 mg, K 675 mg. With appropriate vitamins and minerals. 480 Cal/100 g. Isoleucine, leucine, and valine free. Pow. Can 350 g. *OTC.*
Use: Nutritional supplement.

Ketonex-2. (Ross) Protein 30 g, fat 15.5 g, carbohydrates 30 g, Fe 13 mg, Na 880 mg, K 1370 mg. With appropriate vitamins and minerals. 410 Cal/100 g. Isoleucine, leucine and valine free. Pow. Can 325 g. *OTC.*
Use: Nutritional supplement.

•**ketoprofen.** (KEY-to-pro-fen) *USP 34.*
Use: Nonsteroidal anti-inflammatory agent.

ketoprofen. (Andrx) Ketoprofen 100 mg, 150 mg, 200 mg. ER Cap. Bot. 100s, 1000s. *Rx.*
Use: Nonsteroidal anti-inflammatory agent.

ketoprofen. (Various Mfr.) Ketoprofen 50 mg, 75 mg. Cap. Bot. 100s, 500s (75 mg only). *Rx.*
Use: Nonsteroidal anti-inflammatory agent.

•**ketorfanol.** (key-TAR-fan-AHL) USAN.
Use: Analgesic.

•**ketorolac tromethamine.** (KEY-TOR-oh-lak tro-METH-uh-meen) *USP 34.*
Use: Analgesic, NSAID, ophthalmic.
See: Acular.
  Acular LS.
  Acuvail.
  Sprix.

ketorolac tromethamine. (Apotex) Ketorolac tromethamine. **0.4%:** EDTA

0.015%, benzalkonium chloride 0.006%, sodium chloride, hydrochloric acid, and/or sodium hydroxide. **0.5%:** Benzalkonium chloride 0.01%, EDTA disodium 0.1%, octoxynol 40, sodium chloride, hydrochloric acid, and/or sodium hydroxide. Soln., Ophth. 5 mL, 10 mL. *Rx.*
Use: Ophthalmic and otic agent, nonsteroidal anti-inflammatory agent.

ketorolac tromethamine. (Bedford) Ketorolac tromethamine 15 mg/mL, 30 mg/mL. Inj. Vial 1 mL (15 mg/mL only). Single dose vial 1 mL, 2 mL; multiple-dose vial 10 mL (30 mg/mL only). *Rx.*
Use: Nonsteroidal anti-inflammatory agent.

ketorolac tromethamine. (Various Mfr.) Ketorolac tromethamine 10 mg. Tab. Bot. 100s, 500s. *Rx.*
Use: Nonsteroidal anti-inflammatory agent.

•**ketotifen fumarate.** (KEY-toe-TIE-fen) USAN.
Use: Antiasthmatic.
See: Alaway.
  Claritin Eye.
  Itchy Eye Drops.
  Visine All Day Eye Itch.
  Zaditor.
  Zyrtec Itchy Eye.

ketotifen fumarate. (Various Mfr.) Ketotifin fumarate 0.025%. Benzalkonium chloride 0.01%, glycerol, sodium hydroxide and/or hydrochloric acid. Soln., Ophth. 5 mL. *Rx.*
Use: Ophthalmic decongestant agent.

K-4. Menadiol sodium diphosphate.
Use: Vitamin K.

K-G Elixir. (Geneva) Potassium (as potassium gluconate) 20 mEq/15 mL, alcohol 5%. Elix. Bot. Pt. *Rx.*
Use: Electrolyte supplement.

khellin.
Use: Coronary vasodilator.

Kiddie Powder. (Gordon Laboratories) Pure fine Italian talc. Can. 3.5 oz. *OTC.*
Use: Antifungal.

Kiddi-Vites, Improved. (Geneva) Vitamins A 5000 units, D 500 units, B_1 1 mg, B_2 1.5 mg, B_{12} 2 mcg, C 50 mg, B_6 1 mg, pantothenate 2 mg, niacinamide 10 mg. Tab. Bot. 100s, 1000s. *OTC.*
Use: Vitamin supplement.

Kid Kare. (Rugby) Pseudoephedrine hydrochloride 7.5 mg/0.8 mL, sorbitol, sugar, cherry flavor, alcohol free. Drops. Bot. 30 mL w/dropper. *OTC.*
Use: Nasal decongestant, arylalkylamine.

Kid Kare Children's Cough/Cold.
(Rugby) Pseudoephedrine hydrochloride 15 mg, chlorpheniramine maleate 1 mg, dextromethorphan HBr 5 mg per 5 mL. Sorbitol, corn syrup, cherry flavor, alcohol free. Liq. Bot. 118 mL. *OTC.*
Use: Upper respiratory combination, antitussive combination.

kidney function agents.
See: Indigo Carmine.
Inulin.
Iodohippurate Sodium.
Methylene Blue.

KIE. (Laser) Potassium iodide 150 mg, ephedrine hydrochloride 8 mg/5 mL, saccharin, sorbitol, sucrose, cherry flavor. Syr. Bot. 473 mL. *Rx.*
Use: Upper respiratory combination, decongestant, expectorant.

kinase inhibitors.
See: MTOR Inhibitors.
Tyrosine Kinase Inhibitors.

kinate. Hexahydrotetra hydroxybenzoate salt, quinic acid salt.

Kindercal. (Mead Johnson Nutritionals) Protein 13%, carbohydrate 50%, fat 37%, 30 cal/oz, sucrose, vanilla flavor, lactose free, 30 cal/oz. Liq. Can. 8 oz. *OTC.*
Use: Nutritional supplement.

Kinerase Intensive Eye Cream.
(Valeant) Kinetin 0.125%, safflower seed oil, cetyl alcohol, urea, parabens. Cream. 20 g. *OTC.*
Use: Emollient.

Kineret. (Amgen) Anakinra 100 mg/ 0.67 mL. Sodium chloride, EDTA, preservative free. Inj. Single-use Prefilled syringe 1 mL w/27-gauge needle. *Rx.*
Use: Immunologic, immunomodulator.

Kinevac. (Bracco Diagnostics) Sincalide 5 mcg/vial. Pow. for Inj., lyophilized. Vials. *Rx.*
Use: Diagnostic aid, gastrointestinal function test.

Kinrix. (GlaxoSmithKline) Diphtheria toxoid 25 Lf, tetanus toxoid 10 Lf, inactivated pertussis toxin 25 mcg, filamentous hemaglutinin 25 mcg, pertactin 8 mcg, type 1 poliovirus (Mahoney) 40 D-antigen units, type 2 poliovirus (MEF-1) 8 D-antigen units, type 3 poliovirus (Saukett) 32 D-antigen units per 0.5 mL. Sodium chloride 4.5 mg, alumin adjuvant (≤ 0.6 mg aluminum by assay), residual formaldehyde ≤ 100 mcg, polysorbate 80 (*Tween 80*) ≤ 100 mcg, neomycin ≤ 0.05 ng, polymyxin B ≤ 0.01 ng per dose. Preservative free. Inj., Susp. 0.5 mL single-dose vial, prefilled *Tip-Lok* syringe. *Rx.*

Use: Vaccine combination, diphtheria toxoid/tetanus toxoid/acellular pertussis, adsorbed/inactivated poliovirus combination vaccine.

Kin White. (Whiteworth Towne) Triamcinolone acetonide. **Cream:** 0.025%, 1%. Tube 15 g, 80 g. **Oint.:** 1%. Tube 15 g, 80 g. *OTC.*
Use: Corticosteroid, topical.

Kionex. (Paddock) **Pow. for Susp.:** Finely ground sodium polystyrene sulfonate (4 level tsp ≈ 15 g), sodium content ≈ 100 mg (4.1 mEq)/g. 454 g. **Susp.:** Sodium polystyrene sulfonate 15 g per 60 mL. Alcohol 0.2%, parabens, propylene glycol, saccharin, sodium 1.5 g (65 mEq) per 60 mL, sorbitol 19.3 g per 60 mL. Raspberry flavor. 480 mL, UD 60 mL. *Rx.*
Use: Potassium-removing resin.

• **kitasamycin.** (kit-ah-sah-MY-sin) USAN. An antibiotic substance obtained from cultures of *Streptomyces kitasatoensis.* Under study.
Use: Anti-infective.

Klaron. (Dermik) Sodium sulfacetamide 10%, propylene glycol, polyethylene glycol 400, methylparaben, EDTA. Lot. Bot. 59 mL. *Rx.*
Use: Dermatologic.

Klaron 10%. (Dermik) Sulfacetamide sodium 100 mg/mL. Methylparaben, EDTA. Lot. 59 mL, 118 mL. *Rx.*
Use: Dermatologic agent.

Klavikordal. (US Ethicals) Nitroglycerin 2.6 mg. SR Tab. Bot. 100s, 1000s. *Rx.*
Use: Antianginal.

KLB6. (NBTY) Vitamin B$_6$ 3.5 mg, soya lecithin 100 mg, kelp 25 mg, cider vinegar 80 mg Softgels. Bot. 100s. *OTC.*
Use: Vitamin supplement.

KLB6 Complete. (NBTY) Vitamins A 833.3 units, E 5 mg (as units), B$_3$ 3.3 mg, C 10 mg, soya lecithin 200 mg, kelp 25 mg, cider vinegar 40 mg, wheat bran 83.3 mg, D 66.7 units, FA 0.067 mg, B$_1$ 0.25 mg, B$_2$ 0.28 mg, B$_6$ 8.3 mg, B$_{12}$ 1 mcg, biotin 0.05 mg. Tab. Bot. 100s. *OTC.*
Use: Vitamin supplement.

Kleer Improved. (Scrip) Atropine sulfate 0.2 mg, chlorpheniramine maleate 5 mg/mL. *Rx.*
Use: Anticholinergic; antihistamine.

Klerist-D. (Nutripharm Laboratories, Inc.) **Cap. SR:** Pseudoephedrine hydrochloride 120 mg, chlorpheniramine maleate 8 mg. Bot. 100s, 500s. **Tab.:** Pseudoephedrine hydrochloride 60 mg, chlorpheniramine maleate 4 mg. Bot. 24s,

100s. *Rx.*
Use: Antihistamine; decongestant.

Kler-Ro. (Ulmer Pharmacal) Surgical cleanser and laboratory detergent. **Liq.:** Bot. Gal. **Pow.:** Can 2 lb, Bot. 6 lb. *Rx.*
Use: Antiseptic.

Klonopin. (Roche) Clonazepam. **Orally Disintegrating Tab.:** 0.125 mg, 0.25 mg, 0.5 mg, 1 mg, 2 mg. Mannitol, parabens. Blister pack 60s. **Tab.:** 0.5 mg, 1 mg, 2 mg. Lactose. 100s.
c-IV.
Tall Man: KlonoPIN
Use: Anticonvulsant; antianxiety agent.

K-Lor. (Abbott) Potassium Cl equivalent to potassium 20 mEq and Cl 20 mEq/ 2.6 g for oral soln. w/saccharin. Pkg. 30s, 100s. 15 mEq/2 g Pkg. 100s. *Rx.*
Use: Electrolyte supplement.

Klor-Con 8. (Upsher-Smith) Potassium Cl 8 mEq. ER Tab. Bot. 100s, 500s. *Rx.*
Use: Electrolyte supplement.

Klor-Con M15. (Upsher-Smith) Potassium 15 mEq (from potassium chloride 1125 mg). ER Tab. Bot. 100s, 1000s, UD 100s. *Rx.*
Use: Electrolyte supplement.

Klor-Con M10. (Upsher-Smith) Potassium 10 mEq (from potassium chloride 750 mg). ER Tab. Bot. 90s, 100s, 1000s, UD 100s. *Rx.*
Use: Electrolyte supplement.

Klor-Con M20. (Upsher-Smith) Potassium 20 mEq (from potassium chloride 1500 mg). ER Tab. Bot. 90s, 100s, 500s, 1000s, UD 100s. *Rx.*
Use: Electrolyte supplement.

Klor-Con 10. (Upsher-Smith) Potassium Cl 10 mEq. ER Tab. Bot. 100s, 500s. *Rx.*
Use: Electrolyte supplement.

Klorvess. (Novartis) **Liq.:** Potassium Cl 1.5 g (20 mEq)/15 mL, alcohol 0.75%. Bot. pt. **Effervescent Granules:** Potassium 20 mEq, Cl 20 mEq supplied by potassium Cl 1.125 g, potassium bicarbonate 0.5 g, L-lysine monohydrochloride 0.913 g. Pkt. w/saccharin. Box 30s. **Effervescent Tablets:** Potassium Cl 1.125 g, potassium bicarbonate 0.5 g, L-lysine hydrochloride 0.913 g. Sodium and sugar free, saccharin. Pkg. 60s, 1000s. *Rx.*
Use: Electrolyte supplement.

Klotrix. (Bristol-Myers Squibb) Potassium Cl 10 mEq. SR Tab. Bot. 100s, 1000s, UD 100s. *Rx.*
Use: Electrolyte supplement.

Klout. (PediaMed) Acetic acid, isopropanol, sodium laureth sulfate. Parabens.

Shampoo. 118.3 mL with comb. *OTC.*
Use: Scabicide/pediculicide.

K-Lyte. (Bristol-Myers Squibb) Potassium bicarbonate and citrate 25 mEq, saccharin. Lime and orange flavors. Effervescent Tab. Pkg. 30s, 100s, 250s. *Rx.*
Use: Electrolyte supplement.

K-Lyte/Cl. (Bristol-Myers Squibb) Potassium Cl 25 mEq, saccharin. Citrus and fruit punch flavor. Bulk powder 225 g Can. *Rx.*
Use: Electrolyte supplement.

K-Lyte/Cl 50. (Bristol-Myers Squibb) Potassium Cl 50 mEq, saccharin. Citrus and fruit punch flavors. Pkg. 30s, 100s. *Rx.*
Use: Electrolyte supplement.

K-Lyte DS. (Bristol-Myers Squibb) Potassium bicarbonate and citrate 50 mEq, saccharin. Lime and orange flavor. Effervescent Tab. Pkg. 30s, 100s. *Rx.*
Use: Electrolyte supplement.

Koate-DVI. (Talecris) Human antihemophilic factor 250 units, 500 units, 1000 units. Albumin (human) ≤ 10 mg/ mL, aluminum ≤ 1 mcg/mL, glycine, histidine, PEG. Solvent/detergent treated, heat treated. Inj., lyophilized Pow. for Soln. Single-dose Bot. and sterile water for injection. *Rx.*
Use: Antihemophilic agent.

Kodonyl Expectorant. (Halsey Drug) Bromodiphenhydramine hydrochloride 3.75 mg, diphenhydramine hydrochloride 8.75 mg, ammonium Cl 80 mg, potassium guaiacolsulfonate 80 mg, menthol 0.5 mg/5 mL. Bot. 16 oz. *OTC.*
Use: Antihistamine; expectorant.

Kof-Eze. (Roberts) Menthol 6 mg. Loz. Pkg. 4s, Bot. 500s. *OTC.*
Use: Mouth and throat preparation.

Kogenate. (Bayer) Concentrate of AHF (recombinant). When reconstituted, contains glycine 10 to 30 mg/mL, imidazole ≤ 500 mcg/1000 units, CaCl 2 to 5 mM, chloride 100 to 130 mEq/L, human albumin 4 to 10 mg/mL, monoclonal purified, Na 100 to 130 mEq/ L. Preservative free. Inj., lyophilized. Single-dose bottles (actual number of AHF units indicated on bottles) with diluent, double-ended needle, filter needle, administration set. *Rx.*
Use: Antihemophilic.

Kogenate FS. (Bayer) Recombinant antihemophilic factor 250 units, 500 units, 1,000 units, 2,000 units, 3,000 units. Glycine, histidine, polysorbate 80, sodium, sucrose. Preservative free and albumin free. Solvent/detergent treated, monoclonal antibody purified. Inj., ly-

ophilized Pow. for Soln. Kit w/single-use vial and diluent (2.5 mL sterile water for injection [250 unit, 500 unit, 1,000 unit], 5 mL sterile water for injection [2,000 unit, 3,000 unit]). *Rx.*
Use: Antihemophilic agent.

Kolephrin GG/DM. (Pfeiffer) Dextromethorphan HBr 10 mg, guaifenesin 150 mg per 5 mL. Glucose, saccharin, sucrose, cherry flavor, alcohol free, sodium 0.9 mg/5 mL. Liq. Bot. 118 mL. *OTC.*
Use: Upper respiratory combination, antitussive and expectorant combination.

•**kolfocon A.** (KAHL-FOE-kahn A) USAN.
Use: Contact lens material (hydrophobic).

•**kolfocon B.** (KAHL-FOE-kahn B) USAN.
Use: Contact lens material (hydrophobic).

•**kolfocon C.** (KAHL-FOE-kahn C) USAN.
Use: Contact lens material (hydrophobic).

•**kolfocon D.** (KAHL-FOE-kahn D) USAN.
Use: Contact lens material (hydrophobic).

Kombiglyze XR. (Bristol-Myers Squibb) Saxagliptin/metformin hydrochloride 5 mg/500 mg (equiv. to saxagliptin hydrochloride 5.58 mg), 5 mg/1,000 mg (equiv. to saxagliptin hydrochloride 5.58 mg), 2.5 mg/1,000 mg (equiv. to saxagliptin hydrochloride 2.79 mg). Film coated. ER Tab. 30s (5 mg/500 mg); 30s, 90s, 500s (5 mg/1,000 mg); 60s, 500s (2.5 mg/1,000 mg). *Rx.*
Use: Antidiabetic combination product.

Kondon's Nasal Jelly. (Kondon) Tube 20 g w/ephedrine alkaloid. *OTC.*
Use: Decongestant.

Kondremul Plain. (Heritage Consumer) Mineral oil, Irish moss, acacia, glycerin. Emulsion Bot. 480 mL. **W/Cascara:** 0.66 g/15 mL. Bot. 14 oz. *OTC.*
Use: Laxative.

K-1. Phytonadione.
Use: Vitamin K.
See: Aqua MEPHYTON.
Mephyton.

Konsto. (Freeport) Docusate sodium 100 mg. Cap. Bot. 1000s. *OTC.*
Use: Laxative.

Konsyl. (Konsyl) Psyllium 6 g. Pow. Canister 300 g, 450 g, UD Packet 6 g. *OTC.*
Use: Laxative.

Konsyl-D. (Konsyl) Psyllium 3.4 g, 14 cal/tsp, dextrose. Pow. Canister 325 g, 500 g, UD 6.5 g. *OTC.*
Use: Laxative.

Konsyl Easy Mix Formula. (Konsyl) Psyllium 6 g, Na 4.4 mg, Ca 48 mg, P 4 mg, Zn 0.06 mg, K 42 mg, carbohydrates 0.35 g, 4 cal/5 mL. Pow. Can.

200 g, Packets. *OTC.*
Use: Laxative

Konsyl Fiber. (Konsyl) Polycarbophil 500 mg Tab. Bot. 90s. *OTC.*
Use: Laxative.

Konsyl-Orange. (Konsyl) Psyllium fiber 3.4 g/tbsp., sucrose, orange flavor. Pow. Can. 538 g and Packets. *OTC.*
Use: Laxative.

Konsyl Orange Sugar Free. (Konsyl) Psyllium 3.5 g/tsp. Aspartame, calcium 6 mg, maltodextrin, phenylalanine 21 mg, potassium 32 mg, sodium 3 mg. Sugar free. Orange flavor. Pow. 450 g. *OTC.*
Use: Laxative, bulk-producing laxative.

Koro-Flex. (Holland-Rantos) Improved contouring-spring, natural latex diaphragm 60 mm to 95 mm. *OTC.*
Use: Contraceptive.

Korum. (Geneva) Acetaminophen 5 g. Tab. Bot. 1000s. *OTC.*
Use: Analgesic.

Kotabarb. (Wesley) Phenobarbital ¼ g. Tab. Bot. 1000s. *Rx.*
Use: Hypnotic, sedative.

Kovitonic. (Freeda) Iron 42 mg, vitamins B_1 5 mg, B_6 10 mg, B_{12} 30 mcg, folic acid 0.1 mg, l-lysine 10 mg/15 mL. Liq. Bot. 120 mL, 240 mL. *OTC.*
Use: Mineral, vitamin supplement.

K-P. (Century) Kaolin 5.2 g, pectin 260 mg/oz. Susp. Bot. Gal. *OTC.*
Use: Antidiarrheal.

K-PAX Immune Support. (K-PAX) Fe 1.125 mg, Ca 50 mg, vitamin A 1,250 units, D_3 25 units, E 25 units, B_1 3.75 mg, B_2 3.75 mg, B_3 3.75 mg, B_5 3.75 mg, B_6 12.5 mg, B_{12} 0.16 mcg, C 125 mg, folate 0.05 mg, B, Cr, Cu, I, K, Mg, Mn, Mo, Se, Z. N-acetyl-L-cysteine, acetyl-L-carnitine HCl, alpha lipoic acid, betaine HCl, biotin, choline, citrus bioflavonoid complex, inositol (from soy), L-glutamic acid, mixed tocopherol blend. Cap. 240s (60 packets of 8 capsules). *OTC.*
Use: Multivitamin with minerals.

K-PAX Immune Support Protein Blend Powder. (K-PAX) Protein 20 g (from brown rice protein, N-acetyl-cysteine, L-glutamine), carbohydrate 7 g (as sugar), fat < 1 g, vitamin K 50 mg, A, B_1, B_2, B_3, B_5, B_6, B_{12}, C, D, E, alpha lipoic acid, betaine HCl, biotin, choline, citrus bioflavonoid complex, folic acid, inositol, mixed tocopherols, B, Ca, Cr, Cu, I, Mg, Mn, Mo, Se, Zn. Vegetarian formula. Pow. 505 g. *OTC.*
Use: Enteral nutritional therapy, defined formula diet.

K-PAX Protein Blend Powder. (K-PAX) Protein 10 g (from acetyl-L-carnitine HCl, N-acetyl-L-cysteine, L-glutamic acid), carbohydrate 16 g (as sugar), fat < 1 g, vitamin K 25 mg, A, B_1, B_2, B_3, B_5, B_6, B_{12}, C, D, E, alpha lipoic acid, betaine HCl, biotin, choline, citrus bioflavonoid complex, folic acid, inositol, mixed tocopherol blend, B, Ca, Cr, Cu, I, Mg, Mn, Mo, Se, Zn. Pow. 908 g. *OTC.*
Use: Enteral nutritional therapy, defined formula diet.

K-Pek II. (Rugby) Loperamide hydrochloride 2 mg, lactose. Tab, Pkg. 12s. *OTC.*
Use: Antidiarrheal.

K-Phos M.F. (Beach) Potassium acid phosphate 155 mg, sodium acid phosphate 350 mg Tab. Bot. 100s, 500s. *Rx.*
Use: Acidifier, urinary.

K-Phos Neutral. (Beach) Phosphorus 250 mg, potassium 45 mg, sodium 298 mg. Film-coated. Tab. 100s, 500s. *Rx.*
Use: Mineral supplement.

K-Phos No. 2. (Beach) Potassium acid phosphate 305 mg, sodium acid phosphate, anhydrous 700 mg. Tab. Bot. 100s, 500s. *Rx.*
Use: Acidifier, urinary.

K-Phos Original. (Beach) Potassium acid phosphate 500 mg. Tab. Bot. 100s, 500s. *Rx.*
Use: Urinary acidifier; electrolyte supplement.

K + 10. (Edwards) Potassium Cl 10 mEq. Tab. Bot. 100s, 500s, 1000s. *Rx.*
Use: Electrolyte supplement.

K.P.N. (Freeda) Vitamins C 333 mg, Fe 11 mg, A 2667 units, D 133 units, E 10 mg, B_1 2 mg, B_2 2 mg, B_3 10 mg, B_5 3.3 mg, B_6 0.83 mg, B_{12} 2 mcg, C 33 mg, FA 0.27 mg, I, Cu, Mn, K, Mg, Zn 6.7 mg, bioflavonoids. Tab. Bot. 100s, 250s, 500s. *OTC.*
Use: Mineral, vitamin supplement.

Kristalose. (Bertek) Lactulose (galactose and lactose < 0.3 g/10 g). Crystals for reconstitution. Pack 10 g, 20 g. Box. 30s. *Rx.*
Use: Laxative, hyperosmotic agent.

Kronofed-A. (Ferndale) Pseudoephedrine hydrochloride 120 mg, chlorpheniramine maleate 8 mg. SR Cap. Bot. 100s, 500s. *Rx.*
Use: Upper respiratory combination, antihistamine, decongestant.

Kronofed-A Jr. (Ferndale) Pseudoephedrine hydrochloride 60 mg, chlorpheniramine maleate 4 mg. SR Cap.

Bot. 100s, 500s. *Rx.*
Use: Upper respiratory combination, antihistamine, decongestant.

• **krypton clathrate Kr 85.** (KRIPP-tahn KLATH-rate) USAN.
Use: Radiopharmaceutical.

• **krypton Kr 81m.** (KRIP-tahn Kr 81 m) *USP 34.*
Use: Radiopharmaceutical.

Krystexxa. (Savient Pharmaceuticals) Pegloticase 8 mg/mL (as uricase protein [recombinant]). Inj., Soln., Conc. Single-use vial. 2 mL. *Rx.*
Use: Agent for gout.

K-Tab. (Abbott) Potassium Cl (10 mEq) 750 mg. ER Tab. Bot. 100s, 1000s, UD 100s. *Rx.*
Use: Electrolyte supplement.

K 34. Hexachlorophene.

K.T.V. (Knight) Vitamin B_{12}, minerals. Tab. Bot. 50s. *OTC.*
Use: Mineral, vitamin supplement.

kunecatechins. (koo-ne-KAT-e-kins)
Use: Treatment of external genital and perianal warts.
See: Veregen.

Kuvan. (BioMarin Pharmaceuticals) Sapropterin dihydrochloride 100 mg (equiv. to sapropterin base 76.8 mg). D-mannitol. Tab. 120s. *Rx.*
Use: Phenylketonuria agent.

K-Vescent Potassium Chloride. (Major) Potassium and chloride 20 mEq from potassium chloride 1.5 g, saccharin. Pow. Pkt. 30s, 100s. *Rx.*
Use: Potassium replacement product.

Kwikderm. (Alra) Tolnaftate 1%. **Cream:** Tube. 15 g. **Soln.:** Bot. 10 mL. *OTC.*
Use: Antifungal, topical.

Kwildane. (Major) Gamma benzene hexachloride 1%. Shampoo. Bot. 60 mL, pt, gal. *OTC.*
Use: Pediculicide.

K-Y. (Johnson & Johnson) Glycerin, methylparaben, hydroxyethylcellulose. Sterile or regular. Jelly. Tube. 12 g, 60 g, 120 g. *OTC.*
Use: Lubricant.

Kyodex Reagent Strips. (Kyoto) A disposable plastic reagent strip for determination of glucose in whole blood. Vial 25s.
Use: Diagnostic aid.

Kyotest UGK Reagent Strip. (Kyoto) Disposable reagent strip for measurement of glucose and ketones in the urine. Vial 50s, 100s.
Use: Diagnostic aid.

Kyotest UG Reagent Strips. (Kyoto) Reagent strips for glucose and ketones in urine.
Use: Diagnostic aid.

Kyotest UK Reagent Strips. (Kyoto) Reagent strip for ketones in urine. Vial 50s.
Use: Diagnostic aid.

KY Plus. (Johnson & Johnson) Nonoxynol-9 2%, methylparaben. Nongreasy. 113 g. *OTC.*
Use: Lubricant.

Kytril. (Roche) Granisetron hydrochloride. **Inj.:** 0.1 mg/mL (0.112 mg/mL as hydrochloride), 1 mg/mL (1.12 mg/mL as hydrochloride) (benzyl alcohol 10 mg, sodium chloride 9 mg/mL). Preservative free. Single-use vials. 1 mL (0.1 mg/mL). Multidose vials. 4 mL (1 mg/mL). **Oral Soln.:** 1 mg/mL (1.12 mg/5 mL as hydrochloride). Sorbitol, orange flavor. Bot. 30 mL. *Rx.*
Use: Antiemetic (cancer therapy).

L

• **labetalol hydrochloride.** (la-BET-ul-lahl) *USP 34.*
Use: Alpha/beta-adrenergic blocking agent; antiadrenergic/sympatholytic.
See: Trandate.

labetalol hydrochloride. (Various Mfr.) Labetalol hydrochloride. **Inj.:** 5 mg/mL, EDTA 0.1 mg, methylparaben 0.8 mg, propylparaben 0.1 mg, dextrose. Multidose vial 20 mL, 40 mL. **Tab.:** 100 mg, 200 mg, 300 mg. Bot. 30s, 100s, 250s, 500s, 1000s. *Rx.*
Use: Antiadrenergic/sympatholytic; alpha/beta-adrenergic blocker.

• **labetuzumab.** (la-be-too-zoo-mab) USAN.
Use: Monoclonal antibody.

• **labradimil.** (la-BRAY-da-mil) USAN.
Use: Adjuvant.

Labstix Reagent Strips. (Siemans Medical) Urine screening test. Bot. 100s.
Use: Diagnostic aid.

Lac-Dose. (Rugby) Lactase 3,000 FCC units. Dextrose, mannitol, sodium 4 mg. Tab. 50s. *OTC.*
Use: Enzyme.

Lac-Hydrin Cream. (Bristol-Myers Squibb) Ammonium lactate 12%. Cetyl alcohol, glycerin, glyceryl stearate, light mineral oil, parabens. Cream. 280 g, 385 g. *Rx.*
Use: Emollient.

Lac-Hydrin Five. (Ranbaxy) Lactic acid, glycerin, petrolatum, squalane, steareth-2, PCE-21-stearyl ether, propylene glycol dioctanoate, dimethicone, cetyl palmitate, diazolidinyl urea. Unscented. Lot. 120 mL, 240 mL. *OTC.*
Use: Emollient.

Lac-Hydrin Lotion. (Ranbaxy) Lactic acid 12% neutralized w/ammonium hydroxide, light mineral oil, cetyl alcohol, parabens. Tube 150 mL, 360 mL. *Rx.*
Use: Emollient.

• **lacidipine.** (lah-SIH-dih-PEEN) USAN.
Use: Antihypertensive.

Laclede Cleaner. (Laclede) Container. 2 lb. *OTC.*
Use: Detergent.

Laclede Disclosing Swab. (Laclede) Swabs 6". 100s, 500s, 1000s. *OTC.*
Use: Dentifrice.

Laclede Topi-Fluor A.P.F. Topical Cream. (Laclede) Fluoride ion 1.23% (from sodium fluoride) in orthophosphoric acid 0.98%. Jar 50 mL, 500 mL, 1000 mL, 2000 mL. *Rx.*
Use: Dental caries agent.

LAC-Lotion. (Paddock) Ammonium lactate 12% (12% lactic acid neutralized with ammonium hydroxide), mineral oil, cetyl alcohol, parabens, glycerin. Lotion. 225 g, 400 g. *Rx.*
Use: Emollient.

lacosamide.
Use: Investigational anticonvulsant.
See: Vimpat.

Lacotein. (Christina) Protein digest 5% w/preservatives. Vial 30 mL (w/iodochin), vial 30 mL. *Rx.*
Use: Protein supplement.

Lacril. (Allergan) Hydroxypropyl methylcellulose 0.5%, gelatin A 0.01%, chlorobutanol 0.5%, polysorbate 80, dextrose, magnesium Cl, sodium borate, sodium chloride. Soln. Dropper bot. 15 mL. *OTC.*
Use: Lubricant; ophthalmic.

Lacri-Lube NP. (Allergan) White petrolatum 55.5%, mineral oil 42.5%, petrolatum/lanolin alcohol 2%. Oint. 0.7 g. *OTC.*
Use: Lubricant; ophthalmic.

Lacri-Lube S.O.P. (Allergan) White petrolatum 56.8%, mineral oil 41.5%, lanolin alcohols, chlorobutanol. Tube 3.5 g, 7 g. *OTC.*
Use: Lubricant; ophthalmic.

Lacrisert. (Aton Pharma) Hydroxypropyl cellulose 5 mg/insert. Pkg. 60s w/applicators. *Rx.*
Use: Artificial tears.

Lactaid. (Ortho-McNeil) **Liq.:** Beta-D-galactosidase derived from Kluyveromyces lactis yeast (1000 Neutral Lactase units/5 drop dosage) in carrier of glycerol 50%, water 30%, inert yeast dry matter 20%. Units of 4, 12, 30, 75 one-quart dosages at 5 drops/dose. **Tab.:** Beta-D-galactosidase from Aspergillus oryzae (3300 FCC lactase units/Tab.) In 12s, 100s. *OTC.*
Use: Digestive aid.

lactalbumin hydrolysate.
See: Aminonat.

• **lactase.** (LAK-tase) USAN.
Use: Digestive aid.
See: Dairy Ease.
Lac-Dose.
. Lactaid.
Lactase Fast Acting.
Lactrase.
SureLac.

Lactase Fast Acting. (Major) Lactase 9,000 FCC units. Dextrose, fructose, sugar. Tab. 32s. *OTC.*
Use: Nutritional agent, lactase enzyme.

lactated Ringer's. (Various Mfr.) Na$^+$ 130 mEq, K$^+$ 4 mEq, Ca^{++} ≈ 3 mEq, Cl$^-$

≈ 109 mEq, lactate 28 mEq, osmolarity ≈ 274 mOsm/L. Soln. Inj. Bot. 250 mL, 500 mL, 1000 mL. *Rx.*
Use: Intravenous nutritional therapy, intravenous replenishment solution.

lactated Ringer's in 5% dextrose. (Various Mfr.) Dextrose 50 g, calories 170, Na+ 130 mEq, K+ 4 mEq, Ca++ ≈ 3 mEq, Cl- 109–112 mEq, lactate 28 mEq, osmolarity 525–530 mOsm/L. Soln. Bot. 250 mL, 500 mL, 1000 mL. *Rx.*
Use: Intravenous nutritional therapy, intravenous replenishment solution.

lactated Ringer's irrigation. (Hospira) Sodium chloride 600 mg, anhydrous sodium lactate 310 mg, potassium chloride 30 mg, calcium chloride dihydrate 20 mg per 100 mL. Soln. 300 mL. *Rx.*
Use: Irrigating solution.

•**lactic acid.** (LACK-tick) *USP 34.*
Use: Pharmaceutic necessity for sodium lactate injection.
See: Lactic Acid E.
  Lactrex 12%.
  Penecare.
W/Sodium Pyrrolidone Carboxylate.
See: LactiCare.
  Lactinol.

Lactic acid E. (Stratus Pharmaceutical) Lactic acid 10%, vitamin E, cetyl alcohol, disodium EDTA, glycerin, glyceryl, PEG-40, PEG-100, parabens. Cream. 113.4 g. *Rx.*
Use: Emollient.

lactic acid, lyophilized.
See: VSL#3 The Living Shield.
  VSL#3 DS Double Strength.

lactic acid 10% E. (Sonar Products) Lactic acid 10%, vitamin E 3500 units per 30 g. Cetyl alcohol, EDTA, glycerin, parabens. Cream. 113.4 g, 226.8 g. *Rx.*
Use: Emollient.

LactiCare. (GlaxoSmithKline) Lactic acid 5%, sodium pyrrolidone carboxylate 2.5% in an emollient lotion base. Lot. Bot. 8 oz, 12 oz, w/pump dispenser. *OTC.*
Use: Emollient.

Lactinex. (Becton Dickinson & Co.) *Lactobacillus acidophilus* & *Lactobacillus bulgaricus* mixed culture. **Tab.:** 250 mg, Bot. 50s. **Gran.:** 1 g pkt. Box 12s. *OTC.*
Use: Antidiarrheal; nutritional supplement.

Lactinol. (Pedinol Pharmacal) Lactic acid 10%. Lot. Bot. 237 mL. *Rx.*
Use: Emollient.

Lactobacillin Acidophilus. (Nature's Blend) *Lactobacillus acidophilus* 25 million units. Lactose. Cap. 100s. *OTC.*
Use: Nutritional supplement, probiotic.

Lactobacillus acidophilus. Preparation made from acid-producing bacterium.
Use: Antidiarrheal; nutritional supplement.
See: Acidophilus.
  Bacid.
  Dofus.
  Intestinex.
  Lactobacillin Acidophilus.
  Lacto-Key-100.
  Lacto-Key-600.
  More Dophilus.
  Pro-Bionate.
  Superdophilus.
W/Lactobacillus Bifidus.
See: Acidophilus with Bifidus.

Lactobacillus acidophilus and bulgaricus mixed culture.
See: Floranex.
  Lactinex.

Lactobacillus acidophilus, viable culture.
See: Dofus.

Lactobacillus and Bifidobacterium.
See: ReZyst IM.

Lactobacillus bifidus.
Use: Nutritional supplement.
W/Lactobacillus Acidophilus.
See: Acidophilus with Bifidus.

Lactobacillus bulgaricus.
Use: Antidiarrheal.
See: Bacid.
  More Dophilus.

Lactobacillus GG.
See: Culturelle For Kids.
  Culturelle with Lactobacillus GG.

Lactobacillus reuteri Protectis.
Use: Nutritional supplement.
See: BioGaia.

Lactocal-F. (Laser) Vitamin A 4000 units, D 400 units, E 30 units, C 100 mg, folic acid 1 mg, B_1 3 mg, B_2 3.4 mg, B_3 20 mg, B_6 5 mg, B_{12} 12 mcg, calcium 200 mg, I, Fe 65 mg, Mg, Cu, Zn 15 mg. Tab. Bot. 100s, 1000s. *Rx.*
Use: Mineral; vitamin supplement.

lactoflavin.
See: Riboflavin.

Lacto-Key-100. (Key) *Lactobacillus acidophilus* ≥ 1 billion CFU. Cap. 60s, 120s, 500s. *OTC.*
Use: Nutritional supplement.

Lacto-Key-600. (Key) *Lactobacillus acidophilus* ≥ 6 billion CFU. Cap. 60s, 120s. *OTC.*
Use: Nutritional supplement.

lactose. Milk sugar.
Use: Pharmaceutic aid (tablet and capsule diluent).
See: Natur-Aid.

• **lactose anhydrous.** (LAK-tose an-HIGH-druss) *NF 29.*
Use: Pharmaceutic aid (tablet and capsule diluent).

• **lactose monohydrate.** (LAK-tose) *NF 29.*
Use: Pharmaceutic aid (tablet and capsule diluent).

Lactrase. (Aventis) Standardized enzyme lactase (β-D-galactosidase) 125 mg dispersed in maltodextrins. Cap. Bot. 100s. *OTC.*
Use: Nutritional supplement.

Lactrodectus Mactans Antivenin. (Merck & Co.) Antivenin 6000 units per vial (with 1:10,000 thimerosal), supplied with a 2.5 mL vial of Sterile Water for Injection and a 1 mg vial (with 1:10,000 thimerosal) of normal horse serum (1:10 dilution) for sensitivity testing. *Rx.*
Use: Antivenin (Black Widow spider).
See: Antivenin (Lactrodectus Mactans).

lactulose.
Use: Laxative.
See: Cephulac.
　Chronulac.
　Constilac.
　Constulose.
　Duphalac.
　Enulose.
　Generlac.
　Kristalose.

lactulose. (Various Mfr.) Lactulose 10 g/15 mL (galactose < 1.6 g, lactose 1.2 g, other sugars 1.2 g). Soln. Bot. 237 mL, 473 mL, 960 mL, 1873 mL. *Rx.*
Use: Laxative.

• **lactulose concentrate.** (LAK-tyoo-lohs) *USP 34.*
Use: Laxative, treatment of hepatic coma and chronic constipation.
See: Cephulac.
　Chronulac.

ladakamycin.
Use: Refractory acute myelogenous leukemia (AML) agent.
See: Azacitidine.

Ladogal. (Sanofi-Synthelabo) Danazol. *Rx.*
Use: Androgen.

Ladogar. (Sanofi-Synthelabo) Danazol. *Rx.*
Use: Androgen.

• **ladostigil.** (LAD-oh-STIJ-il) USAN.
Use: Alzheimer disease.

Lady Esther. (Menley & James Labs, Inc.) Mineral oil. Cream. 120 g. *OTC.*
Use: Emollient.

L.A.E. 40. (Seatrace) Estradiol valerate 40 mg/mL. Inj. Vial 10 mL. *Rx.*
Use: Estrogen.

L.A.E. 20. (Seatrace) Estradiol valerate 20 mg/mL. Inj. Vial 10 mL. *Rx.*
Use: Estrogen.

Lagesic. (Laser) Phenyltoloxamine citrate 66 mg, acetaminophen 600 mg. Lactose. ER Tab. 100s. *Rx.*
Use: Nonnarcotic analgesic.

Lamictal. (GlaxoSmithKline) Lamotrigine. **Chew. Dispersible Tab.:** 2 mg, 5 mg, 25 mg. Saccharin. Black currant flavor. 30s (2 mg only), 100s (except 2 mg). **Tab.:** 25 mg, 100 mg, 150 mg, 200 mg. Lactose. 60s (150 mg, 200 mg), 100s (25 mg, 100 mg). **Orally disintegrating Tab.:** 25 mg, 50 mg, 100 mg, 200 mg. Mannitol, sucralose. Cherry flavor. 30s. *Rx.*
Tall Man: LaMICtal
Use: Anticonvulsant.

Lamictal ODT Patient Titration Kit. (GlaxoSmithKline) Lamotrigine. Tab., orally disintegrating. **Blue ODT kit:** 25 mg, 50 mg. Mannitol, sucralose. Cherry flavor. (Titration kits contain 21 of the 25 mg tablets and 7 of the 50 mg tablets.) **Green ODT kit:** 50 mg, 100 mg. Mannitol, sucralose. Cherry flavor. (Titration kits contain 42 of the 50 mg tablets and 14 of the 100 mg tablets.) **Orange ODT kit:** 25 mg, 50 mg, 100 mg. Mannitol, sucralose. Cherry flavor. (Titration kits contain 14 of the 25 mg tablets, 14 of the 50 mg tablets, and 7 of the 100 mg tablets.) *Rx.*
Tall Man: LaMICtal
Use: Anticonvulsant.

Lamictal Starter Kit. (GlaxoSmithKline) Lamotrigine 25 mg, 100 mg. Lactose. Tab. Blue kit (contains 35 of the 25 mg tablets), green kit (contains 84 of the 25 mg tablets and 14 of the 100 mg tablets), orange kit (contains 42 of the 25 mg tablets and 7 of the 100 mg tablets). *Rx.*
Tall Man: LaMICtal
Use: Anticonvulsant.

Lamictal XR. (GlaxoSmithKline) Lamotrigine 25 mg, 50 mg, 100 mg, 200 mg. Film coated. Lactose. ER Tab. 30s. *Rx.*
Tall Man: LaMICtal
Use: Anticonvulsant.

Lamictal XR Patient Titration Kit. (GlaxoSmithKline) Lamotrigine. ER Tab. **Blue XR kit:** 25 mg, 50 mg. Film coated. Lactose. (Titration kits contain 21 of the 25 mg ER tablets and 7 of the 50 mg ER tablets.) **Orange XR kit:** 25 mg, 50 mg, 100 mg. Film coated.

Lactose. (Titration kits contain 14 of the 25 mg ER tablets, 14 of the 50 mg ER tablets, and 7 of the 100 mg ER tablets.) **Green XR kit:** 50 mg, 100 mg, 200 mg. Film coated. Lactose. (Titration kits contain 14 of the 50 mg ER tablets, 14 of the 100 mg ER tablets, and 7 of the 200 mg ER tablets.) *Rx.*
Tall Man: LaMICtal
Use: Anticonvulsant.

• **lamifiban.** (la-mih-FIE-ban) USAN.
Use: Antithrombotic; platelet aggregation inhibitor; fibrinogen receptor antagonist.

Lamisil. (Novartis) Terbinafine hydrochloride. **Gran.:** 125 mg/packet, 187.5 mg/packet. Film-coated. Cartons. 14s, 42s. **Tab.:** 250 mg. Tab. Bot. 30s, 100s. *Rx.*
Tall Man: LamISIL
Use: Antifungal, allyamine.

Lamisil AF. (Novartis) Tolnaftate 1%. Talc. Top. Pow. 113 g. *OTC.*
Tall Man: LamISIL
Use: Topical anti-infective, antifungal agent.

Lamisil AT. (Novartis) Terbinafine hydrochloride. **Gel:** 1%. Benzyl alcohol. 6 g, 12 g. **Spray:** 1%, ethanol, propylene glycol. Bot. 30 mL. *OTC.*
Tall Man: LamISIL
Use: Antifungal.

Lamisil Cream. (Novartis) Terbinafine 1%, benzyl alcohol, cetyl alcohol, stearyl alcohol. Cream. Tube. 15 g, 30 g. *OTC.*
Tall Man: LamISIL
Use: Antifungal.

• **lamivudine.** (la-MIH-view-deen) USAN.
Tall Man: lamiVUDine
Use: Antiretroviral, nucleoside reverse transcriptase inhibitor.
See: Epivir.
   Epivir-HBV.
W/Abacavir.
See: Epzicom.
W/Zidovudine.
See: Combivir.

lamivudine and zidovudine.
Use: Antiretroviral; AIDS.
See: Combivir.

• **lamotrigine.** (lah-MOE-trih-JEEN) USAN.
Tall Man: lamoTRIgine
Use: Anticonvulsant; Lennox-Gastaut syndrome. [Orphan Drug]
See: Lamictal.
   Lamictal ODT Patient Titration Kit.
   Lamictal Starter Kit.
   Lamictal XR.
   Lamictal XR Patient Titration Kit.

lamotrigine. (Various Mfr.) Lamotrigine. **Tab.:** 25 mg, 100 mg, 150 mg, 200 mg. May contain lactose. 25s (25 mg only), 30s, 60s, 90s, 100s, 500s, 1,000s, 1,500s (200 mg only), 2,000 (150 mg only), 3,000 (100 mg only), UD 100s. **Chew. Dispersible Tab.:** 5 mg, 25 mg. May contain mannitol, saccharin, and/or sucralose. 30s, 90s, 100s, 500s, 1,000s, UD 100s. *Rx.*
Use: Anticonvulsant.

lamotrigine. (ZyGenerics) Lamotrigine 50 mg, 250 mg. May contain lactose. Tab. 60s (250 mg), 90s, 100s (50 mg), 500s, 1,000s (50 mg). *Rx.*
Use: Anticonvulsant.

lamotrigine starter kit. (Various Mfr.) Lamotrigine 25 mg, 100 mg. May contain lactose. Tab. Blue kit (contains 35 of the 25 mg tablets), green kit (contains 84 of the 25 mg tablets and 14 of the 100 mg tablets), orange kit (contains 42 of the 25 mg tablets and 7 of the 100 mg tablets). *Rx.*
Use: Anticonvulsant.

Lampit. (Bayer) Nifurtimox.
Use: Anti-infective.

Lanabiotic. (Combe) Polymyxin B sulfate 10,000 units, neomycin (as sulfate) 3.5 mg, bacitracin zinc 500 units, lidocaine 40 mg. Aloe, lanolin, mineral oil, petrolatum. Oint. Tubes. 28 g. *OTC.*
Use: Anti-infective; antibiotic, topical; anesthetic, local.

Lanacane. (Combe) **Spray:** Benzocaine 20%. Benzethonium chloride 0.1%, ethanol 36%, aloe extract. 113 mL. **Cream:** Benzocaine 6%. Benzethonium chloride 0.1%, aloe, parabens, castor oil, glycerin, isopropyl alcohol. 28 g, 56 g. *OTC.*
Use: Anesthetic, local.

Lanacort. (Combe) Hydrocortisone acetate 0.5%. Cream. Tube 0.5 oz, 1 oz. *OTC.*
Use: Corticosteroid, topical.

Lanacort 10. (Combe) Hydrocortisone acetate 1%. **Cream:** Tube 15, 30 g. **Oint.:** Tube 15 g. *OTC.*
Use: Corticosteroid, topical.

Lanaphilic. (Medco Lab) Sorbitol, isopropyl palmitate, stearyl alcohol, white petrolatum, lanolin oil, sodium lauryl sulfate, propylene glycol, methylparaben, propylparaben. Oint. Jar 16 oz. Also available w/urea 10% or 20%. *OTC.*
Use: Emollient.

Lanaphilic w/Urea 10%. (Medco Lab) Urea, stearyl alcohol, white petrolatum, isopropyl palmitate, propylene gly-

col, sorbitol, sodium lauryl sulfate, lactic acid, parabens. Oint. Jar 1 lb. *OTC.*
Use: Emollient.
•**lanimostim.** (LAN-i-MOE-stim) USAN.
Use: Antineoplastic agent.
•**lanolin.** (LAN-oh-lin) *USP 34.* Formerly *Anhydrous lanolin.*
Use: Pharmaceutic aid (ointment base, absorbent).
See: Kerohydric.
Lan-O-Soothe.
Lansinoh.
Lantiseptic Therapeutic.
W/Diiosbutylcresoxyethoxyethyl, Dimethyl Benzyl Ammonium Chloride, Menthol.
See: Hospital Lotion.
•**lanolin alcohols.** (LAN-oh-lin) *NF 29.*
Use: Pharmaceutic aid (emulsifying agent).
Lanoline. (GlaxoSmithKline) Perfumed emollient. Oint. Tube 1.75 oz. *OTC.*
Use: Pharmaceutic aid; ointment base; absorbent; emollient.
•**lanolin, modified.** (LAN-oh-lin) *USP 34.*
Use: Pharmaceutic aid (ointment base, absorbent).
Lano-Lo Bath Oil. (Whorton Pharmaceuticals, Inc.) 8 oz. *OTC.*
Lanolor. (Numark) Lanolin oil, glyceryl stearates, propylene glycol, sodium lauryl sulfate, simethicone, polyoxyl 40 stearate, cetyl esters wax, methylparaben. Cream Jar 60 g, 240 g. *OTC.*
Use: Emollient.
Lan-O-Smooth. (Geritrex) Lanolin 100%. Oint. 56 g. *OTC.*
Use: Emollient.
•**lanoteplase.** (lan-OH-teh-place) USAN.
Use: Thrombolytic; plasminogen activator.
Lanoxin. (GlaxoSmithKline) Digoxin.
Tab.: 0.125 mg, 0.25 mg, lactose. Bot. 30s, 100s, 1000s, 5000s, UD 100s.
Inj.: (w/propylene glycol 40%, alcohol 10%). Amp. 2 mL. **Pediatric Inj.:** 0.1 mg/mL (w/propylene glycol 40%, alcohol 10%). Amp. 1 mL. *Rx.*
Use: Inotropic agent; cardiac glycoside.
•**lanreotide acetate.** (lan-REE-oh-tide) USAN.
Use: Antineoplastic.
See: Somatuline Depot.
Lansinoh. (Lansinoh) Lanolin 100%. Oint. 59 g. *OTC.*
Use: Emollient.
Lansinoh Diaper Rash. (Lansinoh) Lanolin 15.5%, zinc oxide 5.5%, dimethicone 5%. Beeswax, petrolatum. Oint. 90 g. *OTC.*

Use: Diaper rash product.
•**lansoprazole.** (lan-SO-pruh-zole) *USP 34.*
Use: Proton pump inhibitor.
See: Prevacid.
Prevacid 24 Hour.
W/Amoxicillin and clarithromycin.
See: Prevpac.
lansoprazole. (Various Mfr.) Lansoprazole 15 mg, 30 mg (contain enteric-coated granules). May contain PEG, sugar spheres, sucrose. Cap., delayed release. 30s (15 mg only), 90s (30 mg only), 100s, 500s (30 mg only), 1,000s. *Rx.*
Use: Proton pump inhibitor.
•**lanthanum carbonate.** (LAN-tha-num KAR-bo-nate)
Use: Phosphate binder.
See: Fosrenal.
Lantiseptic Therapeutic. (Summit) Lanolin 37%. Beeswax, HEEDTA, lanolin alcohol, mineral oil, petrolatum. Cream. 113 g. *OTC.*
Use: Emollient.
Lanturil. (Sanofi-Synthelabo) Oxypertine. *Rx.*
Use: Anxiolytic.
Lantus. (Aventis) Insulin glargine 100 units/mL. Inj. Vials. 10 mL. Cartridge system for use with *OptiClik.* 3 mL. *Rx.*
Use: Antidiabetic, insulin.
Ianum. (Various Mfr.) Lanolin. *OTC.*
Use: Pharmaceutic aid.
lapatinib.
Use: Antineoplastic, tyrosine kinase inhibitor.
See: Tykerb.
•**lapatinib ditosylate.** (la-PA-tin-ib) USAN.
Use: Antineoplastic; tyrosine kinase inhibitor.
•**lapuleucel-T.** (LA-pul-OO-sel) USAN.
Use: Antineoplastic.
•**lapyrium chloride.** (LAH-pihr-ee-uhm KLOR-ide) USAN.
Use: Pharmaceutic aid (surfactant).
•**larazotide.** (lar-a-ZOE-tide) USAN.
Use: Immunomodulator.
Lariam. (Roche) Mefloquine hydrochloride 250 mg, lactose. Tab. UD 25s. *Rx.*
Use: Antimalarial.
•**laronidase.** (lare-AHN-ih-dase) USAN.
Use: Enzyme replacement in Mucopolysaccharidosis.
See: Aldurazyme.
Larotid. (GlaxoSmithKline) Amoxicillin.
Cap.: 250 mg: Bot. 100s, 500s, UD 100s, unit-of-use 18s. **500 mg:** Bot. 50s, 500s. **Oral Susp.:** 125 mg, 250 mg

(as trihydrate)/5 mL. Bot. 80 mL,
100 mL, 150 mL. **Pediatric drops:**
50 mg (as trihydrate)/mL. Bot. 15 mL.
Rx.
Use: Anti-infective, penicillin.

Larynex. (Dover Pharmaceuticals)
Benzocaine. Sugar, lactose and salt
free. Loz. UD Box 500s. *OTC.*
Use: Anesthetic, local.

Lasix. (Aventis) Furosemide. **Tab.:**
20 mg, 40 mg. Tab. Bot. 100s, 500s,
1000s, UD 100s; 80 mg. Tab. Bot. 50s,
500s, UD 100s. **Inj.:** 10 mg/mL. 2 mL
Amp. Box 5s, 50s, 4 mL Amp. Box 5s,
25s; 10 mL Amp. Box 5s, 25s; Syringe
2 mL, 4 mL, 10 mL. Box 5s. Single-use
Vial 2 mL, 4 mL, 10 mL. *Rx.*
Use: Diuretic.

•**lasofoxifene tartrate.** (la-soe-FOX-i-
feen) USAN.
Use: Osteoporosis; breast cancer.

lassar's paste.
See: Zinc Oxide Paste.

Lastacaft. (Vistakon Pharmaceuticals)
Alcaftadine 0.25%. Benzalkonium
chloride 0.005%, edetate disodium.
Soln., Ophth. 3 mL. *Rx.*
Use: Ophthalmic and otic agent, oph-
thalmic antihistamine.

•**latanoprost.** (lah-TAN-oh-prahst) USAN.
Use: Antiglaucoma agent.
See: Xalatan.

latanoprost. (Various Mfr.) Latanoprost
0.005%. May contain benzalkonium
chloride 0.02%, sodium chloride. Soln.,
Ophth. 2.5 mL. *Rx.*
Use: Agent for glaucoma, prostaglandin
agonist.

Latest-CRP Kit. (Fischer) Measures C-
reactive protein in serum. Kit 1s.
Use: Diagnostic aid.

Latisse. (Allergan) Bimatoprost 0.03%.
Benzalkonium chloride. Soln., Ophth.
60 disposable applicators. 3 mL. *Rx.*
Use: Agent for glaucoma, prostaglandin
agonist.

•**latrepirdine.** (la-TRE-pir-deen) USAN.
Use: CNS agent.

•**latrepirdine dihydrochloride.** (la-TRE-
pir-deen) USAN.
Use: CNS agent.

Latrix XM. (Stratus) Urea 45%. Caprylic/
capric triglycerides, cetyl alcohol, EDTA
disodium, glycerin, lactic acid, linoleic
acid, PEG 300, titanium dioxide. Emuls.
240 mL. *Rx.*
Use: Emollient.

Latuda. (Sunovion) Lurasidone hydrochloride 40 mg, 80 mg. Mannitol. Tab.
30s, 90s, 500s, UD 70s, UD 100s. *Rx.*

Use: Antipsychotic agent, benzoisothiazol derivative.

•**laureth 4.** (LAH-reth 4) USAN.
Use: Pharmaceutic aid (surfactant).

•**laureth 9.** (LAH-reth 9) USAN.
Use: Pharmaceutical aid (surfactant);
emulsifier; spermicide.

•**laureth 10.** (LAH-reth 10) USAN.
Use: Spermaticide.

•**laurocapram.** (LAHR-oh-KAH-pram)
USAN.
Use: Pharmaceutic aid (excipient).

lauromacrogol 400. Laureth 9.

•**lauryl isoquinolinium bromide.** (LAH-
rill EYE-so-KWIN-oh-lih-nee-uhm)
USAN.
Use: Anti-infective.

lauryl sulfoacetate.
See: Lowila Cake.

Lavacol. (Parke-Davis) Ethyl alcohol
70%. Bot. Pt.
Use: Anti-infective, topical.

Lavatar. (Doak Dermatologics) Coal tar
distillate 25.5% in a bath oil base. Liq.
Bot. 4 oz, pt. *OTC.*
Use: Antipsoriatic; antipruritic.

•**lavoltidine succinate.** (lahv-OLE-tih-
DEEN) USAN. *Formerly Loxotidine.*
Use: Antiulcerative (histamine H_2-
receptor blocker).

Lavoptik Emergency Wash. (Lavoptik)
Eye, face, body wash. 32 oz/emer-
gency station. *OTC.*
Use: Emergency wash.

Lavoptik Eye Wash. (Lavoptik) Sodium
Cl 0.49%, sodium biphosphate 0.4%,
sodium phosphate 0.45%/100 mL w/
benzalkonium Cl 0.005%. Bot. 6 oz.
OTC.
Use: Irrigant; ophthalmic.

Lavoris. (Procter & Gamble) Zinc Cl, glycerin, poloxamer 407, saccharin, polysorbate 80, flavors, clove oil, alcohol,
citric acid, water. Bot. 6 oz, 12 oz,
18 oz, 24 oz. *OTC.*
Use: Mouthwash.

Laxative & Stool Softener. (Rugby)
Docusate sodium 100 mg, casanthranol
30 mg, parabens, sorbitol. Softgel.
Cap. Bot. 100s. *OTC.*
Use: Laxative.

Laxative Caps. (Weeks & Leo) Docusate sodium 100 mg, casanthranol
30 mg. Cap. Bot. 30s, 60s. *OTC.*
Use: Laxative.

laxatives.
See: Aloe.
   Aloin.
   Bile Salts.
   Bisacodyl.

Bisacodyl Tannex.
Bowel Evacuants.
Bulk-Producing Laxatives.
Carboxymethylcellulose Sodium.
Casanthranol.
Cascara.
Cascara Sagrada.
Castor Oil.
Citrucel.
Correctol.
Docusate Sodium.
Emulsoil.
Enemas.
ex-lax.
Fecal Softeners/Surfactants.
Feen-a-Mint.
Fleet Prep Kit 1.
Fleet Prep Kit 2.
Fleet Prep Kit 3.
Hyperosmotic Agents.
Irritant or Stimulant Laxatives.
Karaya Gum.
Liquid Petrolatum Emulsion.
Magnesia Magma.
Maltsupex.
Methylcellulose.
Mucilloid of Psyllium Seed W/Dex-
   trose.
Nature's Remedy.
Neoloid.
Oxyphenisatin Acetate.
Petrolatum.
Phenolphthalein.
Plantago Ovata, Coating.
Poloxalkol.
Senna Conc., Standardized.
Senna Fruit Extract, Standardized.
Sodium Biphosphate.
Sodium Phosphate.
Tridrate Bowel Cleansing System.
Unifiber.
X-Prep.
X-Prep Bowel Evacuant Kit-1.
W/Choline Base, Cephalin, Lipositol.
   See: Alcolec.
W/CO$_2$-Releasing Suppositories.
   See: Ceo-Two.
W/Polycarbophil.
   See: Bulk Forming Fiber Laxative.
   Cephulac.
   Cholac.
   Chronulac.
   Citrucel Sugar Free.
   Colace.
   Constulose.
   DC Softgels.
   Diocto.
   Docu.
   Docusate Calcium.
   D.O.S.
   D-S-S.

Duphalac.
Enulose.
Equalactin.
ex-lax Stool Softener.
FiberCon.
Fiber-Lax.
FiberNorm.
Fleet.
Fleet Babylax.
Fleet Bisacodyl.
Fleet Mineral Oil.
Genasoft.
Glycerin.
Kondremul Plain.
Konsyl Fiber.
Mineral Oil.
Non-Habit Forming Stool Softener.
Phillips' Liqui-Gels.
Regulax SS.
Sani-Supp.
Silace.
Stool Softener.
Stool Softener DC.
Surfak.
Therevac-Plus.
Therevac-SB.
W/Polyethylene Glycol-Electrolyte.
   See: CoLyte.
   Concentrated Milk of Magnesia-
      Cascara.
   DOK-Plus.
   Emulsoil.
   Evac-Q-Kwik.
   Fleet Prep Kit 1.
   Fleet Prep Kit 2.
   Fleet Prep Kit 3.
   GoLYTELY.
   Haley's M-O.
   Liqui-Doss.
   MiraLax.
   Neoloid.
   NuLYTELY.
   OCL.
   Perdiem Overnight Relief.
   Tridrate Bowel Cleansing System.
   X-Prep.
   X-Prep Bowel Evacuant Kit-1.
   X-Prep Bowel Kit-2.
W/Psyllium.
   See: Fiberall Orange Flavor.
   Fiberall Tropical Fruit Flavor.
   Genfiber.
   Genfiber, Orange Flavor.
   Hydrocil Instant.
   Konsyl.
   Konsyl-D.
   Konsyl Easy Mix Formula.
   Konsyl-Orange.
   Konsyl Orange Sugar Free.
   Metamucil.
   Metamucil, Orange Flavor, Original
      Texture.

Metamucil Orange Flavor, Smooth Texture.
Metamucil, Original Texture.
Metamucil, Sugar Free, Orange Flavor, Smooth Texture.
Metamucil, Sugar Free, Smooth Texture.
Natural Fiber Laxative.
Perdiem Fiber Therapy.
Reguloid.
Reguloid, Orange.
Reguloid, Sugar Free Orange.
Reguloid, Sugar Free Regular.
Serutan.
Syllact.
W/Saline Laxatives.
See: Aromatic Cascara Fluid Extract.
Cascara Aromatic.
Epsom Salt.
Fleet Phospho-soda.
Magnesium Citrate.
Milk of Magnesia.
Milk of Magnesia-Concentrated.
Phillips' Milk of Magnesia.
Phillips' Milk of Magnesia, Concentrated.
W/Sennosides.
See: Agoral.
Bisac-Evac.
Bisacodyl Uniserts.
Black Draught.
Caroid.
Doxidan.
Dulcolax.
ex-lax Chocolated.
Fleet Laxative.
Fletcher's Castoria.
Maximum Relief ex•lax.
Modane.
Nature's Remedy.
Peri-Colace.
Reliable Gentle Laxative.
Senexon.
Senna-Gen.
Senokot.
Senokot-S.
SenokotxTRA.
Women's Gentle Laxative.
W/Vitamins.
See: Lec-E-Plex.
Laxinate 100. (Roberts) Dioctyl sodium sulfosuccinate 100 mg. Cap. Bot. 100s, 1000s.
Use: Laxative.
Lax Pills. (G & W Labs) Sennosides 15 mg, 25 mg, EDTA, parabens, sucrose. Tab. Blister pack 24s, 48s (25 mg only); 30s, 60s (15 mg only). *OTC.*
Use: Laxative.
layor carang.
See: Agar.

• **Iazabemide.** (Iazz-AH-bem-ide) USAN.
Use: Antiparkinsonian.
• **Iazabemide hydrochloride.** (Iazz-AH-bem-ide) USAN.
Use: Antiparkinsonian.
Lazer Creme. (Pedinol) Vitamins E 3500 units, A 100,000 units/oz. Cream. Jar 2 oz. *OTC.*
Use: Emollient.
Lazer Formalyde. (Pedinol) Formaldehyde 10%. Soln. Bot. 90 mL. *Rx.*
Use: Drying agent.
LazerSporin-C. (Pedinol) Neomycin sulfate 5 mg, polymyxin B sulfate 10,000 units, hydrocortisone 1%. Soln. Bot. 10 mL with dropper. *Rx.*
Use: Anti-infective combination, topical.
L-baclofen.
Use: Antispasmodic. [Orphan Drug]
L-Caine E. (Century) Lidocaine hydrochloride 1%, 2%, epinephrine 1:100,000/mL. Inj. 20 mL, 50 mL. *Rx.*
Use: Anesthetic, local.
L-Caine Viscous. (Century) Lidocaine hydrochloride 2% with sodium carboxymethylcellulose. Soln. Bot. 100 mL. *Rx.*
Use: Anesthetic, local.
l-carnitine. (Freeda Vitamins) Levocarnitine 500 mg. Tab. Bot. 50s, 100s. *OTC.*
Use: Amino acid.
l-carnitine. (Various Mfr.) Amino acid derivative 250 mg. Cap. Bot. 30s, 60s, 100s. *OTC.*
Use: Amino acid.
L.C.D. (Almay) Alcohol extractions of crude coal tar. Cream, soln. Bot. 4 oz, pt. *OTC.*
Use: Antipsoriatic; antipruritic; topical.
See: Coal Tar Topical Solution.
LCR. *Rx.*
Use: Antineoplastic.
See: Vincristine sulfate.
LCx Neisseria gonorrhoeae Assay. (Abbott) Reagent kit for the detection of *Neisseria gonorrhoeae* in female endocervical, male urethral, and urine swab specimens. Kit. 96s. *Rx.*
Use: Diagnostic aid.
L-cycloserine.
Use: Gaucher disease. [Orphan Drug]
L-cysteine. (Tyson)
Use: Erythropoietic protoporphyria. [Orphan Drug]
L-deprenyl.
See: Selegiline hydrochloride.
LDH Reagent Strip. (Bayer Consumer Care) A quantitative strip test for LDH in serum or plasma. *Seralyzer* reagent strip. Bot. 25s. *Rx.*
Use: Diagnostic aid.
Leber Tabulae. (Paddock) Aloe 0.09 g,

extract of rhei 0.03 g, myrrh 0.01 g, frangula 5 mg, galbanum 2 mg, olibanum 3 mg. Tab. Bot. 100s, 500s, 1000s. *OTC.*

•**lebrikizumab.** (LEB-ri-KIZ-ue-mab) USAN.
Use: Respiratory agent.

Lec-E-Plex. (Barth's) Vitamin E 100 units, 200 units, 400 units. Cap. w/ lecithin. Bot. 100s, 500s, 1000s. *OTC.*
Use: Vitamin E supplement.

•**lecimibide.** (leh-SIM-ih-bide) USAN.
Use: Antihyperlipidemic.

•**lecithin.** (LESS-ih-thin) *NF 29.*
Use: Pharmaceutic aid (emulsifying agent).

lecithin. (Arcum) Lecithin 1200 mg. Cap. Bot. 100s, 1000s; Gran. Bot. 8 oz; Pow. Bot. 4 oz. (Barth's) 8 gr. Cap. Bot. 100s, 500s, 1000s; Gran. Can 8 oz, 16 oz; Pow. Can 10 oz. (Cavendish) Tab. (0.5 g) Bot. 500s. (Quality Formulations, Inc.) 1200 mg, Cap. 100s. (De Pree) Cap. Bot 100s. (Pfanstiehl) 25 g, 100 g, 500 g Pkg.
Use: Pharmaceutic aid (emulsifying agent).

lecithin. (Various Mfr.) Lecithin. **Cap.:** 520 mg. Bot. 100s, 250s, 1000s; 650 mg. Bot. 90s, 100s, 250s, 500s. **Pow.:** 120 g, kg, lb. *OTC.*
Use: Nutritional supplement.

•**lecozotan hydrochloride.** (le-KOE-zoe-tan) USAN.
Use: 5-HT$_{1A}$ receptor antagonist; Alzheimer disease.

•**ledoxantrone trihydrochloride.** (led-OX-an-trone try-HIGH-droe-KLOR-ide) USAN.
Use: Antineoplastic.

Leena. (Watson) **Phase 1:** Norethindrone 0.5 mg, ethinyl estradiol 35 mcg. 7 tabs. **Phase 2:** Norethindrone 1 mg, ethinyl estradiol 35 mcg. 9 tabs. **Phase 3:** Norethindrone 0.5 mg, ethinyl estradiol 35 mcg. 5 tabs. Lactose. Tab. 28s with 7 inert tabs. *Rx.*
Use: Contraceptive hormone, sex hormone.

•**leflunomide.** (le-FLOO-noe-mide) USAN.
Use: Antirheumatic agent.
See: Arava.

leflunomide. (Various Mfr.) Leflunomide 10 mg, 20 mg. May contain lactose. Tab. 30s. *Rx.*
Use: Antirheumatic agent.

Legatrin PM. (Columbia) Acetaminophen 500 mg, diphenhydramine hydrochloride 50 mg. Capl. Bot. 30s, 50s. *OTC.*

Use: Sleep aid.

•**lemon oil.** *NF 29.*
Use: Pharmaceutic aid (flavor).

•**lemon tincture.** *NF 29.*
Use: Pharmaceutic aid (flavor).

Lemotussin-DM. (Seneca) Dextromethorphan HBr 7.5 mg, guaifenesin 50 mg, potassium guaiacolsulfonate 50 mg, pseudoephedrine hydrochloride 10 mg, chlorpheniramine maleate 2 mg per 5 mL. Parabens, saccharin, sorbitol, alcohol free. Liq. 473 mL. *Rx.*
Use: Antitussive and expectorant combination.

•**lenalidomide.** (le-na-LID-oh-mide) USAN.
Use: Immunomodulator.
See: Revlimid.

•**lenefilcon A.** (len-e-FIL-kon A) USAN.
Use: Hydrophilic.

•**lenercept.** (LEH-ner-sept) USAN.
Use: Treatment of septic shock, multiple sclerosis, inflammatory bowel disease, rheumatoid arthritis.

lenetran. Mephenoxalone.
Use: Anxiolytic.

•**leniquinsin.** (LEN-ih-KWIN-sin) USAN. Under study.
Use: Antihypertensive.

Lenium Medicated Shampoo. (Sanofi-Synthelabo) Selenium sulfide. *OTC.*
Use: Antiseborrheic.

•**lenograstim.** (leh-no-GRAH-stim) USAN.
Use: Antineutropenic; hematopoietic stimulant; immunomodulator (granulocyte colony-stimulating factor).

•**lenperone.** (LEN-per-OHN) USAN.
Use: Antipsychotic.

Lens Clear. (Allergan) Sterile, isotonic solution surfactant cleaner w/sorbic acid 0.1%, edetate disodium 0.2%. Bot. 15 mL. *OTC.*
Use: Contact lens care.

Lensept Disinfecting Solution. (Ciba Vision) Micro-filtered hydrogen peroxide with sodium stannate 3%, sodium nitrate, phosphate buffers. Soln. Bot. 237, 355 mL. *OTC.*
Use: Disinfecting solution.

Lensept Rinse and Neutralizer. (Ciba Vision) Sodium chloride, sodium borate decahydrate, boric acid, bovine catalase, sorbic acid, EDTA. Soln. Bot. 237 mL. System includes lens cup and holder. *OTC.*
Use: Contact lens care, rinsing, neutralizing.

Lens Fresh. (Allergan) Sterile, buffered, isotonic aqueous soln., hydroxyethyl cellulose, sodium Cl, boric acid, sodium

borate, sorbic acid 0.1%, edetate disodium 0.2%. Bot. 0.5 oz. *OTC.*
Use: Contact lens care.

Lensine Extra Strength. (Ciba Vision) Cleaning agent with benzalkonium Cl 0.01%, EDTA 0.1%. Soln. Bot. 45 mL. *OTC.*
Use: Contact lens care.

Lens Plus. (Allergan) Isotonic soln. w/ sodium Cl 0.9%. Aerosol 3 oz, 8 oz, 12 oz. Preservative free. *OTC.*
Use: Contact lens care.

Lens Plus Oxysept Disinfecting Solution. (Allergan) Hydrogen peroxide with sodium stannate 3%, sodium nitrate, phosphate buffer. Soln. Bot. 240 mL. *OTC.*
Use: Contact lens care.

Lens Plus Oxysept Rinse and Neutralizer. (Allergan) Isotonic with sodium chloride, mono- and dibasic sodium phosphates, catalytic neutralizing agent, EDTA. Soln. Bot. 15 mL. *OTC.*
Use: Contact lens care.

Lens Plus Oxysept 2 Neutralizing. (Allergan) Catalase with buffering agents used to neutralize the Lens Plus Oxysept 1 disinfecting solution in a chemical lens care system. For soft contact lens. Tabs. Box 12s. Bot. 36s. *OTC.*
Use: Contact lens care.

Lens Plus Preservative Free. (Allergan) Isotonic sodium chloride 9%. Soln. Bot. 90 mL, 240 mL, 360 mL. *OTC.*
Use: Contact lens care.

Lens Plus Sterile Saline. (Allergan) Sodium Cl, boric acid, nitrogen. Soln. Bot. 90 mL, 240 mL, 360 mL. Aerosol. *OTC.*
Use: Contact lens care.

Lensrins. (Allergan) Sterile preserved saline for heat disinfection, rinsing and storage of soft (hydrophilic) contact lenses, rinsing solution for chemical disinfection. Soln. Bot. 8 oz. *OTC.*
Use: Contact lens care.

Lens-Wet. (Allergan) Isotonic, buffered soln. of polyvinyl alcohol, thimerosal 0.002%, EDTA 0.01%. Bot. 0.5 fl oz. *OTC.*
Use: Contact lens care.

lente insulin. Susp. of zinc insulin crystals.
See: Lente lletin II.

lente insulin. (Novo/Nordisk) Insulin zinc susp. 100 units/mL Beef. Inj. Vial 10 mL. *OTC.*
Use: Antidiabetic.

lentinan. (Lenti-Chemico Pharmaceuticals)
Use: Immunomodulator.

• **lenvatinib.** (len-VA-ti-nib) USAN.
Use: Antineoplastic.

• **lenvatinib mesylate.** (len-VA-ti-nib) USAN.
Use: Antineoplastic.

lepirudin. (LEP-ih-ru-din)
Use: Thrombin inhibitor. [Orphan Drug]
See: Refludan.

lepromin. (Louisiana State University) Lepromin, 30 to 40 million acid-fast bacilli/mL. Vial 5 mL, 10 mL, 20 mL, 50 mL.

leprostatics.
Use: Bactericidal.
See: Dapsone.

• **lercanidipine hydrochloride.** (ler-can-i-DIP-een) USAN.
Use: Antihypertensive; calcium channel blocker.

• **lergotrile.** (LER-go-trill) USAN.
Use: Enzyme inhibitor (prolactin).

• **lergotrile mesylate.** (LER-go-trill) USAN.
Use: Enzyme inhibitor (prolactin).

• **lersivirine.** (ler-si-VIR-een) USAN.
Use: Antiretroviral.

Lerton Ovules. (Vita Elixir) Caffeine 250 mg. Cap. *OTC.*
Use: CNS stimulant.

Lescol. (Novartis) Fluvastatin 20 mg, 40 mg. May contain benzyl alcohol, parabens, EDTA. Cap. Bot. 30s, 100s. *Rx.*
Use: Antihyperlipidemic, HMG-CoA reductase inhibitor.

Lescol XL. (Novartis) Fluvastatin 80 mg. Film-coated. ER Tab. Bot. 30s, 100s. *Rx.*
Use: Antihyperlipidemic, HMG-CoA reductase inhibitor.

• **lesinurad.** (le-SIN-ure-ad) USAN.
Use: Treatment of gout.

• **lesinurad sodium.** (le-SIN-ure-ad) USAN.
Use: Treatment of gout.

Lessina. (Barr) Levonorgestrel 0.1 mg, ethinyl estradiol 20 mcg. Lactose. Film-coated. Tab. Packs. 21s, 28s with 7 inert tabs. *Rx.*
Use: Sex hormone, contraceptive hormone.

• **lestaurtinib.** (le-STOR-tin-ib) USAN.
Use: Antineoplastic agent.

Lesterol. (Dram) Nicotinic acid 500 mg. Tab. Bot. 250s. *OTC.*
Use: Antihyperlipidemic.

Letairis. (Gilead) Ambrisentan 5 mg, 10 mg. Lactose (10 mg only). Film-coated. Tab. UD 30s. *Rx.*
Use: Vasodilator, endothelin receptor antagonist.

•**letaxaban.** (le-TAX-a-ban) USAN.
Use: Anticoagulant.

•**leteprinim potassium.** (leh-TEPP-rin-nim) USAN.
Use: Central neurodegenerative disease; Alzheimer disease; spinal cord injury; stroke.

•**letimide hydrochloride.** (LET-ih-mide) USAN.
Use: Analgesic.

•**letrozole.** (let-ROW-zahl) *USP 34.*
Use: Antineoplastic, hormone, aromatase inhibitor.
See: Femara.

letrozole. (Mylan) Letrozole 2.5 mg. Film coated. Lactose, PEG, polydextrose. Tab. 30s, 500s. *Rx.*
Use: Hormone, aromatase inhibitor.

•**leucine.** (LOO-SEEN) *USP 34.*
Use: Amino acid.

•**leucovorin calcium.** (loo-koe-VORE-in) *USP 34.*
Use: Antianemic; folate-deficiency; antidote to folic acid antagonists.

leucovorin calcium. (American Regent) Leucovorin calcium 10 mg/mL. Inj. Single-dose vial 5 mg. 25s (10 mg/mL only). *Rx.*
Use: Antianemic; folate-deficiency; antidote to folic acid antagonists.

leucovorin calcium. (Various Mfr.) Leucovorin calcium. **Tab.:** 5 mg, 15 mg, 25 mg (as calcium). 30s, 100s, UD 50s (5 mg); 12s, 24s, UD 50s (15 mg); 25s (25 mg). **Inj., Soln.; lyophilized:** 50 mg/vial, 100 mg/vial, 200 mg/vial, 350 mg/vial. Preservative free. *Rx.*
Use: Antineoplastic agent, cytoprotective agent.

Leukeran. (GlaxoSmithKline) Chlorambucil 2 mg. Film-coated. Tab. Bot. 50s. *Rx.*
Use: Antineoplastic; alkylating agent.

Leukine. (Genzyme) Sargramostim. Mannitol 40 mg, sucrose 10 mg, tromethamine 1.2 mg/mL. **Liq.:** 500 mcg/mL. Benzyl alcohol 1.1%. Multiple-dose vial. **Pow. for Inj., lyophilized:** 250 mcg. Preservative free. Vial. *Rx.*
Use: Hematopoietic, colony stimulating factor.

leukocyte protease inhibitor, secretory.
Use: Bronchopulmonary dysplasia. [Orphan Drug]

leukocyte typing serum. (LOO-koe-site)
Use: Diagnostic aid, blood, in vitro.

leukotriene formation inhibitor.
Use: Antiasthmatic.
See: Zileuton.

leukotriene receptor antagonists.
Use: Antiasthmatic.
See: Montelukast Sodium.
Zafirlukast.

leupeptin. (Neuromuscular Agents)
Use: Adjunct to nerve repair. [Orphan Drug]

•**leuprolide acetate.** (loo-PRO-lide) USAN.
Use: Antineoplastic; LHRH agonist; central precocious puberty. [Orphan Drug]
See: Eligard.
Lupron Depot.
Lupron Depot-4 Month.
Lupron Depot-Ped.
Lupron Depot-3 Month.
Lupron for Pediatric Use.

leuprolide acetate. (Various Mfr.) Leuprolide acetate 5 mg/mL. Benzyl alcohol 9 mg/mL, sodium chloride. Inj. Multiple-dose vial. 2.8 mL. *Rx.*
Use: Antineoplastic; hormone; gonadotropin-releasing hormone analog.

leurocristine.
See: Vincristine Sulfate.

leurocristine sulfate (1:1) (salt). Vincristine Sulfate, USP.
Use: Antineoplastic.

Leustatin. (Ortho Biotech) Cladribine. Soln. 1 mg/mL. Vial. 20 mL single-use. *Rx.*
Use: Antineoplastic.

Levacet. (Pharmakon) Phenyltoloxamine citrate 50 mg, acetaminophen 400 mg, salicylamide 150 mg, aspirin 400 mg, caffeine 40 mg. Tab. 50s. *Rx.*
Use: Narcotic analgesic.

levalbuterol. (Mylan) Levalbuterol hydrochloride 1.25 mg per 0.5 mL. Preservative free. Soln.; Conc., Inhal. Vial. UD 0.5 mL. *Rx.*
Use: Bronchodilator, sympathomimetic.

•**levalbuterol hydrochloride.** (lev-al-BYOO-ter-ole) USAN.
Use: Bronchodilator, sympathomimetic.
See: Xopenex.

•**levalbuterol sulfate.** (lev-al-BYOO-ter-ole) USAN.
Use: Bronchodilator, antiasthmatic.

•**levalbuterol tartrate.** (lev-al-BYOO-ter-ole) USAN.
Use: Bronchodilator.
See: Xopenex HFA.

Levall. (Auriga) Carbetapentane citrate 15 mg, guaifenesin 100 mg, phenylephrine hydrochloride 5 mg per 5 mL. Maltitol, saccharin, sorbitol. Strawberry flavor, alcohol free. Liq. Bot. 473 mL. *Rx.*

Use: Upper respiratory combination, antitussive and expectorant combination.

Levall 12. (Auriga) Carbetapentane tannate 30 mg, phenylephrine tannate 30 mg per 5 mL. Parabens, aspartame, phenylalanine 7 mg/5 mL. Strawberry flavor. Susp. 118 mL. *Rx.*
Use: Antitussive combination, upper respiratory combination.

• **levamfetamine succinate.** (LEV-am-FET-ah-meen) USAN.
Use: Anorexic.

Levaquin. (Ortho-McNeil) Levofloxacin. **Tab.:** 250 mg, 500 mg, 750 mg. Film-coated. Bot. 20s (750 mg only), 50s (except 750 mg), UD 100s, *Leva-Pak* 5s (750 mg only). **Inj., Soln., Conc.:** 500 mg (25 mg/mL), preservative free, single-use vial 20 mL; 750 mg (25 mg/mL), preservative free, single-use vial 20 mL, 30 mL. **Inj., Soln.:** 250 mg (5 mg/mL), 500 mg (5 mg/mL), 750 mg (5 mg/mL). Preservative free. Flex. Cont 50 mL (250 mg only), 100 mL (500 mg only), 150 mL (750 mg only) w/dextrose solution 5%. **Oral Soln.:** 25 mg/mL. Benzyl alcohol, sucralose, sucrose. 480 mL. *Rx.*
Use: Fluoroquinolone.

levarterenol.
See: Norepinephrine Bitartrate.

Levatol. (Schwarz Pharma) Penbutolol sulfate 20 mg. Tab. Bot. 100s. *Rx.*
Use: Antiadrenergic/sympatholytic, beta-adrenergic blocker.

Levbid. (Alaven Pharmaceuticals) L-hyoscyamine sulfate 0.375 mg. ER Tab. Bot. 100s. *Rx.*
Use: Anticholinergic; antispasmodic.

• **levcromakalim.** (lev-KROE-mah-KAY-lim) USAN.
Use: Antihypertensive; antiasthmatic.

• **levcycloserine.** (LEV-sigh-kloe-SER-een) USAN.
Use: Enzyme inhibitor (Gaucher disease).

• **levdobutamine lactobionate.** (LEV-dah-BYOOT-ah-meen LACK-toe-BYE-oh-nate) USAN.
Use: Cardiovascular agent.

Levemir. (Novo Nordisk) Insulin detemir 100 units/mL. Inj. Vials. 10 mL. *PenFill* cartridges. 3 mL. Prefilled syringes (use with *FlexPen*). 3 mL. *Rx.*
Use: Antidiabetic, insulin.

• **levetiracetam.** (lee-ve-tye-RA-se-tam) USAN.
Tall Man: levETIRAcetam
Use: Antiepileptic.

See: Keppra.
Keppra XR.

levetiracetam. (Mylan) Levetiracetam 250 mg, 500 mg, 750 mg. Film-coated. Polydextrose. Tab. 120s, 500s. *Rx.*
Use: Anticonvulsant.

levetiracetam. (Sun Pharmaceuticals) Levetiracetam 100 mg/mL. Inj., Soln. Single-use vial. 5 mL. *Rx.*
Use: Anticonvulsant.

Leviron. (Health for Life Brands) Desiccated liver 7 gr, iron and ammonium citrate 3 gr, vitamins B$_1$ 1 mg, B$_2$ 0.5 mg, B$_6$ 0.5 mg, calcium pantothenate 0.3 mg, niacinamide 2.5 mg, B$_{12}$ 1 mcg. Cap. Bot. 100s, 1000s. *OTC.*
Use: Mineral, vitamin supplement.

Levitra. (Schering-Plough) Vardenafil hydrochloride 2.5 mg, 5 mg, 10 mg, 20 mg. Film-coated. Tab. 30s. *Rx.*
Use: Impotence agents.

levmetamfetamine.
Use: Nasal decongestant.
See: Vicks Vapor Inhaler.

• **levoamphetamine.** (lee-voe-am-FET-uh-meen) *USP 34.*
Use: Nasal decongestant.

levo-amphetamine. Alginate (l-isomer) alpha-2-phenylaminopropane succinate.

• **levobetaxolol hydrochloride.** (LEE-voe-beh-TAX-oh-lahl) USAN.
Use: Antiadrenergic, β-receptor.

• **levobunolol hydrochloride.** (LEE-voe-BYOO-no-lahl) *USP 34.*
Use: Antiadrenergic, β-receptor.
See: AK-Beta.
Betagan Liquifilm.

levobunolol hydrochloride. (Various Mfr.) Levobunolol hydrochloride 0.25%, 0.5% Ophth. Soln. Bot. 5 mL, 10 mL, 15 mL (0.5% only). *Rx.*
Use: Antiglaucoma agent; beta-adrenergic blocker.

• **levocarnitine.** (LEE-voe-KAR-nih-teen) *USP 34.*
Tall Man: levOCARNitine
Use: Amino acid.
See: Carnitor.
L-Carnitine.
Vitacarn.

levocarnitine. (Rising) Levocarnitine. **Soln.:** 100 mg/mL. Sucrose, parabens. Cherry flavor. 118 mL. **Tab.:** 330 mg. Blisters of 90. *Rx.*
Use: Amino acid.

levocarnitine. (Various Mfr.) Levocarnitine 200 mg/mL. Inj. Single-dose vial. *Rx.*
Use: Amino acid.

- **levocarnitine propionate hydrochloride.** (lee-voe-KAR-ni-teen) USAN.
  Use: Peripheral arterial disease.
- **levocetirizine.** (LEE-vo-se-TIR-a-zeen) USAN.
  Use: Antihistamine.
- **levocetirizine.** (Winthrop US) Levocetirizine dihydrochloride 0.5 mg/mL. May contain glycerin, maltitol, parabens, saccharin. Soln. 150 mL. *Rx.*
  Use: Antihistamine; piperazine, peripherally selective.
- **levocetirizine.** (Various Mfr.) Levocetirizine dihydrochloride 5 mg. May contain lactose. Tab. 30s, 90s. *Rx.*
  Use: Antihistamine; piperazine, peripherally selective.
- **levocetirizine dihydrochloride.** (LEE-vo-se-TIR-a-zeen) USAN.
  Use: Antihistamine.
  See: Xyzal.
- **levodopa.** (LEE-voe-DOE-puh) *USP 34.*
  Use: Antiparkinsonian.
  W/Carbidopa.
  See: Parcopa.
  Sinemet CR.
  Sinemet 10/100.
  Sinemet 25/100.
  Sinemet 25/250.
  W/Carbidopa, Entacapone.
  See: Stalevo 50.
  Stalevo 100.
  Stalevo 150.
  Stalevo 125.
  Stalevo 75.
  Stalevo 200.
- **levofloxacin.** (lee-voe-FLOX-ah-sin) USAN.
  Use: Anti-infective, fluoroquinolone.
  See: Iquix.
  Levaquin.
  Quixin.
- **levofloxacin.** (Pack Pharmaceuticals) Levofloxacin 0.5%. Benzalkonium chloride 0.005%. Soln., Ophth. 5 mL. *Rx.*
  Use: Ophthalmic and otic agent, ophthalmic antibiotic.
- **levofuraltadone.** (LEE-voe-fer-AL-tah-dohn) USAN.
  Use: Anti-infective; antiprotozoal.
- **levoglucose.** (LEE-voe-GLOO-kose) USAN.
  Use: Colon cleansing before colonoscopy.
- **levoleucovorin calcium.** (LEE-voe-loo-koe-VORE-in) USAN.
  Use: Antidote to folic acid antagonist; water-soluble vitamin.
  See: Fusilev.
  Isovorin.

- **levomefolate calcium.** (LEE-voe-FOE-late) USAN.
  Use: Nutritional agent.
  W/Drospirenone, Ethinyl Estradiol.
  See: Beyaz.
- **levomefolic acid.** (LEE-voe-me-FOE-lik) USAN.
  Use: Nutritional agent.
- **levomepromazine.** (LEE-voe-me-PROE-ma-zeen) USAN.
  Use: Analgesic.
- **levomepromazine hydrochloride.** (LEE-voe-me-PROE-ma-zeen) USAN.
  Use: Analgesic.
- **levomepromazine maleate.** (LEE-voe-me-PROE-ma-zeen) USAN.
  Use: Analgesic.
- **levomethadyl acetate hydrochloride.** (LEE-voe-METH-uh-dill) USAN.
  Use: Analgesic; narcotic. [Orphan Drug]
- **levomilnacipran.** (LEE-voe-mil-NA-si-pran) USAN.
  Use: Antidepressant.
- **levonantradol hydrochloride.** (LEE-voe-NAN-trah-DAHL) USAN.
  Use: Analgesic.
- **levonordefrin.** (lee-voe-nore-DEFF-rin) *USP 34.*
  Use: Adrenergic, vasoconstrictor.
  W/Mepivacaine Hydrochloride.
  See: Scandonest L.
- **levonorgestrel.** (LEE-voe-nor-JESS-truhl) *USP 34.*
  Use: Hormone, progestin.
  See: Alesse.
  Levora.
  Plan B.
  Plan B One-Step.
  W/Estradiol.
  See: ClimaraPro.
  W/Ethinyl Estradiol.
  See: Alesse.
  Aviane.
  Jolessa.
  Levora.
  LoSeasonique.
  Lutera.
  Lybrel.
  Nordette.
  Plan B.
  Quasense.
  Seasonale.
  Seasonique.
  Sronyx.
  Triphasil.
  Trivora.
- **levonorgestrel.** (Perrigo Pharmaceuticals) Levonorgestrel 0.75 mg. Lactose. Tab. UD 2s. *OTC.*
  Use: Emergency contraceptive.

levonorgestrel-releasing intrauterine system.
Use: Sex hormone, contraceptive system.
See: Mirena.

Levophed. (Hospira) Norepinephrine bitartrate (as base) 1 mg/mL. Metabisulfite ≤ 2 mg. Inj. Amp. 4 mL. *Rx.*
Use: Vasoconstrictor.

•**levopropoxyphene napsylate.** (lee-voe-pro-POX-ee-feen NAP-sih-late) *USP 34.*
Use: Antitussive.

•**levopropylcillin potassium.** (lee-voe-pro-pihl-SILL-in) USAN.
Use: Anti-infective.

Levora. (Watson) Ethinyl estradiol 30 mcg, levonorgestrel 0.15 mg. Lactose. Tab. Pkt. 28s with 7 inert tabs. *Rx.*
Use: Sex hormone, contraceptive hormone.

levorenine.
See: Epinephrine.

Levoroxine. (Bariatric) Sodium levothyroxine 0.05 mg, 0.1 mg, 0.2 mg, 0.3 mg. Tab. Bot. 100s, 500s. *Rx.*
Use: Hormone, thyroid.

•**levorphanol tartrate.** (lee-VORE-fah-nole) *USP 34.*
Use: Opioid analgesic.

levorphanol tartrate. (Roxane) Levorphanol tartrate 2 mg. Lactose. Tab. Bot. 100s. *c-II.*
Use: Opioid analgesic.

•**levosimendan.** (lee-voe-sih-MEN-dan) USAN.
Use: Investigational for congestive heart failure.

Levo-T. (Wyeth) Levothyroxine sodium 0.025 mg, 0.05 mg, 0.075 mg, 0.1 mg, 0.125 mg, 0.15 mg, 0.2 mg, 0.3 mg. Tab. Bot. 100s (all strengths), 1000s (0.05, 0.1, 0.15, 0.2 mg only). *Rx.*
Use: Hormone, thyroid.

Levothroid. (Forest) Levothyroxine sodium. **Tab.:** 0.025 mg, 0.05 mg, 0.075 mg, 0.088 mg, 0.1 mg, 0.112 mg, 0.125 mg, 0.150 mg, 0.175 mg, 0.2 mg, 0.3 mg. Bot. 100s, 1000s. *Rx.*
Use: Hormone, thyroid.

•**levothyroxine sodium.** (lee-voe-thigh-ROX-een) *USP 34.*
Use: Hormone, thyroid.
See: Levothroid.
  Levoxyl.
  Synthroid.
  Unithroid.
W/Mannitol.
See: Synthroid.

W/Sodium liothyronine.
See: Thyrolar.

levothyroxine sodium. (Sandoz) Levothyroxine sodium (T_4, L-thyroxine) 0.137 mg. Tab. 100s. *Rx.*
Use: Hormone, thyroid.

levothyroxine sodium. (Various Mfr.) Levothyroxine sodium. **Pow. for Inj.:** 200 mcg, 500 mcg. Vial. 10 mL. **Tab.:** 0.025 mg, 0.05 mg, 0.075 mg, 0.088 mg, 0.1 mg, 0.112 mg, 0.125 mg, 0.15 mg, 0.175 mg, 0.2 mg, 0.3 mg. Bot. 100s. *Rx.*
Use: Hormone, thyroid.

•**levotofisopam.** (LEV-oh-toe-FIS-oh-pam) USAN.
Use: Anxiolytic agent.

•**levoxadrol hydrochloride.** (lev-OX-ah-drole) USAN.
Use: Anesthetic, local; muscle relaxant.

Levoxyl. (Jones Pharma) Levothyroxine sodium 0.025 mg, 0.05 mg, 0.075 mg, 0.088 mg, 0.1 mg, 0.112 mg, 0.125 mg, 0.137 mg, 0.15 mg, 0.175 mg, 0.2 mg, 0.3 mg. Tab. Bot. 100s, 1000s, UD 100s. *Rx.*
Use: Hormone, thyroid.

LEV/PSE/GG. (Varsity) Pseudoephedrine hydrochloride 90 mg, guaifenesin 400 mg. ER Cap. 100s. *Rx.*
Use: Upper respiratory combination, decongestant and expectorant combination.

Levsin. (Alaven) L-hyoscyamine sulfate. **Tab.:** 0.125 mg. Bot. 100s, 500s. **Inj.:** 0.5 mg/mL. Amp. 1 mL, Vial 10 mL with benzyl alcohol 1.5%, sodium metabisulfite 0.1%. *Rx.*
Use: Anticholinergic; antispasmodic.

Levsin Drops. (Alaven) L-hyoscyamine sulfate 0.125 mg/mL, alcohol 5%, sorbitol, orange flavor. Soln. Bot. 15 mL. *Rx.*
Use: Anticholinergic; antispasmodic.

Levsinex Timecaps. (Alaven) L-hyoscyamine sulfate 0.375 mg. TR Cap. Bot. 100s, 500s. *Rx.*
Use: Anticholinergic; antispasmodic.

Levsin/SL. (Alaven) L-hyoscyamine sulfate 0.125 mg. Peppermint flavor. Tab. Sublingual. Bot. 100s, 500s. *Rx.*
Use: Anticholinergic; antispasmodic.

Levulan Kerastick. (DUSA) Aminolevulinic acid hydrochloride 20% (354 mg), ethanol v/v 48%, isopropyl alcohol. Top. Soln. Applicator (2 glass Amp, applicator tip. One amp 1.5 mL soln. vehicle, other amp aminolevulinic acid hydrochloride 354 mg). Box 4s, 6s, 12s. *Rx.*
Use: Photochemotherapy.

levulose. Fructose.
levulose-dextrose.
See: Invert Sugar.
Lexapro. (Forest) Escitalopram oxalate.
Tab.: 5 mg, 10 mg, 20 mg. Film-coated. Bot. 100s, UD 100s (except 5 mg). **Oral Soln.:** 1 mg/mL. Sorbitol, parabens, peppermint flavor. Bot. 240 mL. Rx.
Use: Antidepressant, selective serotonin reuptake inhibitor.
•**lexatumumab.** (LEX-a-TOO-moo-mab) USAN.
Use: Antineoplastic.
•**lexibulin.** (LEX-i-BUE-lin) USAN.
Use: Antineoplastic.
•**lexipafant.** (lex-IH-pah-fant) USAN.
Use: Platelet-activating factor (PAP) antagonist.
Lexiscan. (Astellas Pharma) Regadenoson 0.4 mg/5 mL. Preservative free. Edetate disodium dihydrate. Inj., Soln. 5-mL single-use vials and single-use prefilled syringes. Rx.
Use: In vivo diagnostic aid.
•**lexithromycin.** (lex-ith-row-MY-sin) USAN.
Use: Anti-infective.
Lexiva. (GlaxoSmithKline) Fosamprenavir calcium. **Susp.:** 50 mg/mL (equiv. to amprenavir 43 mg/mL). Parabens, sucralose. Grape-bubblegum-peppermint flavor. 225 mL. **Tab.:** 700 mg (equiv. to amprenavir 600 mg). Film-coated. 60s. Rx.
Use: Antiretroviral agent, protease inhibitor.
Lextron. (Eli Lilly) Liver-stomach concentrate 50 mg, iron 30 mg, vitamins B_1 1 mg, B_2 0.25 mg, B_{12} (activity equivalent) 2 mcg, other factors of vitamin B complex present in the liver-stomach concentrate. Pulv. Bot. 84s. OTC.
Use: Mineral; vitamin supplement.
Lexuss 210. (Centurion) Codeine phosphate 10 mg, chlorpheniramine maleate 2 mg. Alcohol 0.1%, parabens, potassium citrate, potassium sorbate, sucralose, sorbitol. Sugar free. Vanilla cream flavor. Liq. 473 mL. c-v.
Use: Upper respiratory combination, antitussive combination.
L-5-hydroxytryptophan. (Circa)
Use: Postanoxic intention myoclonus. [Orphan Drug]
L'Homme. (Armenpharm Ltd.) Vitamins A 4000 units, D 400 units, B_1 1 mg, B_2 1.2 mg, B_3 10 mg, B_{12} 2 mcg, calcium pantothenate 5 mg, C 30 mg, Ca 100 mg, P 76 mg, Fe 10 mg, Mn 1 mg,

Mg 1 mg, Zn 1 mg. Bot. 100s. OTC.
Use: Mineral, vitamin supplement.
Lialda. (Shire US) Mesalamine 1.2 g. Film-coated. DR Tab. 120s. Rx.
Use: Treatment of chronic inflammatory bowel disease.
•**liarozole fumarate.** (lie-AHR-oh-zole) USAN.
Use: Antipsoriatic.
•**liarozole hydrochloride.** (lie-AHR-oh-zole) USAN.
Use: Antineoplastic.
Li Ban. (Pfizer) Synthetic pyrethroid 0.5%, related compounds 0.065%, aromatic petroleum hydrocarbons 0.664%. Spray. Bot. 5 oz, Box 6s. OTC.
Use: Pediculicide, inanimate objects. (Not to be used on humans or animals).
•**libenzapril.** (lie-BENZ-ah-prill) USAN.
Use: ACE inhibitor.
Librax. (Valeant) Clidinium bromide 2.5 mg, chlordiazepoxide hydrochloride 5 mg. Lactose, parabens. Cap. Bot. 100s. Rx.
Use: Gastrointestinal anticholinergic combination.
Lice Treatment. (Goldline) Pyrethrins 0.33%, piperonyl butoxide. Benzyl alcohol. Shampoo. 59 mL, 118 mL with comb. OTC.
Use: Pediculicide.
Licide Complete Lice Treatment Kit. (Reese Chemical) Piperonyl butoxide 4%, pyrethrins 0.33%. Castor oil, PEG-25, SD alcohol. Shampoo. Kit w/gel, comb, and lice control spray. 118 mL. OTC.
Use: Scabicide/pediculicide.
•**licorice.** (LIK-o-ris) NF 29.
Use: Pharmaceutic aid (flavor).
•**licostinel.** (li-KOS-ti-nel) USAN.
Use: Treatment of stroke (NMDA receptor antagonist, glycine site).
•**licryfilcon A.** (lih-krih-FILL-kahn A) USAN.
Use: Contact lens material (hydrophilic).
•**licryfilcon B.** (lih-krih-FILL-kahn B) USAN.
Use: Contact lens material, hydrophilic.
LidaMantle. (Doak Dermatologics) Lidocaine hydrochloride 3%. Cetyl alcohol, stearyl alcohol, glycerin, petrolatum, parabens, light mineral oil. Cream. 28 g, 85 g. Rx.
Use: Topical local anesthetic, amide local anesthetic.
LidaMantle HC. (Doak Dermatologics) Lidocaine hydrochloride 3%, hydrocortisone acetate 0.5%. Cetyl alcohol,

mineral oil, methylparaben, petrolatum. Lot. 177 mL. *Rx.*
Use: Corticosteroid, topical.

LidaMantle HC Cream. (Doak Dermatologics) Lidocaine 3%, hydrocortisone acetate 0.5% in cream base. Tube 1 oz. *Rx.*
Use: Corticosteroid; anesthetic, local.

LidaMantle HC Relief. (Doak Dermatologics) Hydrocortisone acetate 2%, lidocaine hydrochloride 2%. Mineral oil, parabens, urea. Pad. 60s. *Rx.*
Use: Anorectal preparation, steroid-containing product.

•**lidamidine hydrochloride.** (LIE-DAM-ih-deen) USAN.
Use: Antiperistaltic.

Lidex. (Roche) Fluocinonide 0.05%.
Cream: Tube 15 g, 30 g, 60 g, 120 g.
Oint.: Tube 15 g, 30 g, 60 g, 120 g.
Soln.: Bot. 20 mL, 60 mL. *Rx.*
Use: Corticosteroid, topical.

Lidex-E. (Roche) Fluocinonide 0.05% in aqueous emollient base. Tube 15 g, 30 g, 60 g, 120 g. *Rx.*
Use: Corticosteroid, topical.

•**lidocaine.** (LIE-doe-cane) USP 34.
Use: Anesthetic, local.
See: Anestafoam.
W/Benzalkonium Chloride.
See: Bactine Pain Relieving Cleansing.
W/Benzethonium Chloride.
See: Dr. Scholl's Cracked Heel Relief.
W/Hyaluronic Acid.
See: Juvederm Ultra Plus XC.
Juvederm Ultra XC.
W/Phenol.
See: Skeeter Stik.
W/Polymyxin B Sulfate, Neomycin Sulfate, Bacitracin Zinc.
See: Lanabiotic.
W/Prilocaine.
See: EMLA.
EMLA Anesthetic.
Oraqix.
W/Tetracaine.
See: Pliaglis.
Synera.

lidocaine and epinephrine. (Abbott) Lidocaine 0.5%, epinephrine 1:200,000, methylparaben, sodium metabisulfite. Inj. Multidose vial 50 mL. Lidocaine 1%, epinephrine 1:100,000, methylparaben, sodium metabisulfite. Inj. Multidose vial 20 mL, 30 mL, 50 mL. Lidocaine 1%, epinephrine 1:200,000, sodium metabisulfite. Inj. Single-dose amp. 30 mL. Lidocaine 1.5%, epinephrine 1:200,000. Inj. Single-dose amp. 5 mL, 30 mL. Single-dose vial 30 mL (sodium metabisulfite). Lidocaine 2%, epinephrine 1:200,000, sodium metabisulfite. Inj. Single-dose vial 20 mL. *Rx.*
Use: Injectable local anesthetic, amide.

lidocaine and epinephrine. (Various Mfr.) Lidocaine 2%, epinephrine 1:100,000. Inj. Cart. 1.8 mL. Multidose vial 20 mL, 30 mL, 50 mL (may contain sodium metabisulfite and methylparaben) *Rx.*
Use: Injectable local anesthetic, amide.

•**lidocaine hydrochloride.** (LIE-doe-cane) USP 34.
Use: Cardiovascular agent; antiarrhythmic agent; anesthetic, local.
See: AneCream.
Anestacon.
Ardecaine 1%, 2%.
Burn-o-Jel.
L-Caine.
LidaMantle.
Lidoderm.
LidoPen Auto-Injector.
L-M-X4.
LTA 360 Kit.
Numby Stuff.
Octocaine.
Regenecare HA.
Regenecare Wound.
Solarcaine Aloe Extra Burn Relief.
Topicaine.
Topicaine 5.
Xylocaine.
Xylocaine MPF.
W/Benzalkonium Chloride.
See: Bactine Antiseptic Anesthetic.
Medi-Quik.
W/Benzethonium Hydrochloride.
See: StaphAseptic.
W/Camphor.
See: TheraPatch Cold Sore.
W/Capsaicin, Menthol, Methyl Salicylate.
See: Terocin.
W/Epinephrine.
See: Lidocaine and Epinephrine.
Lidocaine Hydrochloride.
Lidosite Topical System.
Xylocaine.
Xylocaine MPF.
W/Epinephrine, Methyl Parasept.
See: L-Caine-E.
W/Hydrocortisone.
See: AnaMantle HC.
LidaMantle HC.
LidaMantle HC Relief.
LidoCort.
W/Hydrocortisone Acetate.
See: AnaMantle HC 2.5%.
Xyralid.
Xyralid RC.
W/Methyl Parasept.
See: L-Caine.

W/Povidone Iodine.
See: ProTech First-Aid Stik.
lidocaine hydrochloride. (Abbott) Lidocaine hydrochloride. Inj. **1.5%:** With 1:200,000 epinephrine. Amp. 5 mL, 30 mL. Single-dose vial 30 mL (with sodium metabisulfite). With 7.5% dextrose. Amp. 2 mL **4%:** Single-dose amp. 5 mL. **5%:** With 7.5% dextrose. Single-dose amp. *Rx.*
Use: Injectable local anesthetic, amide.
lidocaine hydrochloride. (IMS) Lidocaine hydrochloride 2%. Preservative free. Jelly. UD 5, 10, and 20 mL single-use vials. 25s. *Rx.*
Use: Anesthetic, local.
lidocaine hydrochloride. (Moore) Lidocaine hydrochloride 5%. Oint. 50 g. *Rx.*
Use: Topical local anesthetic.
lidocaine hydrochloride. (River's Edge) Lidocaine hydrochloride. **Cream:** 3%. Alcohols, aluminum sulfate, glycerin, light mineral oil, parabens, petrolatum. 28.35 g, 85 g. **Lot.:** 3%. Alcohols, aluminum sulfate, glycerin, light mineral oil, parabens, petrolatum. Lot. 177 mL. *Rx.*
Use: Local anesthetic, topical.
lidocaine hydrochloride. (Various Mfr.) Lidocaine hydrochloride. Inj. **0.5%:** May contain methylparaben. Single-dose vial 50 mL; multidose vial 50 mL. **1%:** Amp. 2 mL, 5 mL. Vial 5 mL (preservative free). Single-dose vial 30 mL. Multidose vial 20 mL, 30 mL, 50 mL (may contain methylparaben). Syr. 5 mL. Cartridge. **1.5%:** Amp. 20 mL. **2%:** Amp. 2 mL, 10 mL. Vial 5 mL (preservative free). Single-dose vial 10 mL. Multidose vial 20 mL, 50 mL (may contain methylparaben). Syr. 5 mL *Rx.*
Use: Injectable local anesthetic, amide.)
lidocaine hydrochloride. (Various Mfr.) Lidocaine hydrochloride 4%. May contain parabens. Top. Soln. 50 mL. *Rx.*
Use: Topical local anesthetic.
lidocaine hydrochloride and epinephrine. (Eastman Kodak) Lidocaine 2%, epinephrine 1:50,000, sodium metabisulfite. Dental cart. 1.8 mL *Rx.*
Use: Injectable local anesthetic, amide.
lidocaine hydrochloride cream. (River's Edge) Lidocaine hydrochloride 3%. Alcohols, aluminum sulfate, glycerin, light mineral oil, parabens, petrolatum. Cream. 28.35 g, 85 g. *Rx.*
Use: Local anesthetic, topical.
lidocaine hydrochloride for cardiac arrhythmias. (Abbott) Lidocaine hydrochloride. **1%:** 10 mg/mL. Inj. (for direct IV administration). Amps. 5 mL. Vi-

als. 20 mL, 30 mL, 50 mL. *Abboject* syringes. 5 mL. **10%:** 100 mg/mL. Inj. (for IV admixture). Additive vials. 10 mL. **20%:** 200 mg/mL. Inj. (for IV admixture). Syringes. 5 mL, 10 mL. Vials. 10 mL. *Rx.*
Use: Antiarrhythmic agent.
lidocaine hydrochloride for cardiac arrhythmias. (Various Mfr.) Lidocaine hydrochloride. **2%:** 20 mg/mL. Inj. (for direct IV administration). Vials. 5 mL, 10 mL. 20 mL, 30 mL, 50 mL. Syringes. 5 mL. **4%:** 40 mg/mL. Inj. (for IV admixtures). Amps. 5 mL. Vials. 25 mL, 50 mL. *Rx.*
Use: Antiarrhythmic agent.
lidocaine hydrochloride/hydrocortisone acetate. (River's Edge) Hydrocortisone acetate 0.55%, lidocaine hydrochloride 2.8%. Aloe, parabens, PEG-4. Gel. 100 g w/single-use applicators. *Rx.*
Use: Anorectal preparation, steroid-containing product.
lidocaine hydrochloride in 5% dextrose. (Various Mfr.) Lidocaine hydrochloride 0.2% (2 mg/mL), 0.4% (4 mg/mL), 0.8% (8 mg/mL). Inj. (for IV infusion). 250 mL (except 0.2%), 500 mL, 1,000 mL (0.2% only). *Rx.*
Use: Antiarrhythmic agent.
lidocaine hydrochloride monohydrate.
Use: Topical local anesthetic, amide local anesthetic.
See: Zingo.
lidocaine hydrochloride 3%-hydrocortisone acetate 2.5%. (River's Edge) Hydrocortisone acetate 25 mg, lidocaine hydrochloride 30 mg per g. Cetyl alcohol, mineral oil, parabens, petrolatum, stearyl alcohol, urea. Rectal Gel. 20 single-use 7 g tubes with applicators and cleansing wipes. *Rx.*
Use: Anorectal preparation.
lidocaine/hydrocortisone cream. (River's Edge) Hydrocortisone acetate 0.5%, lidocaine hydrochloride 3%. Aluminum sulfate, alcohols, glycerin, light mieral oil, parabens, petrolatum. Cream. 28.5 g, 85 g. *Rx.*
Use: Topical corticosteroid.
lidocaine/hydrocortisone rectal. (River's Edge) Hydrocortisone acetate 0.5%, lidocaine hydrochloride 3%. Aluminum sulfate, alcohols, glycerin, light mineral oil, parabens, petrolatum. Cream. Single-use units with applicator. 7 g. *Rx.*
Use: Anorectal preparation.
lidocaine patch 5%.
Use: Anesthetic, local topical.

See: Lidoderm.
TheraPatch Cold Sore.
lidocaine/prilocaine. (Various Mfr.) Lidocaine 2.5%, prilocaine 2.5%. Cream. 5 g, 15 g, 30 g. *Rx.*
Use: Local anesthetic, topical.
lidocaine 2% viscous. (Various Mfr.) Lidocaine hydrochloride 2%. May contain parabens, sodium carboxymethylcelluose, saccharin. Soln. 50 mL, 100 mL, UD 20 mL. *Rx.*
Use: Anesthetic, local.
LidoCort. (Aristos) Hydrocortisone acetate 2.5%, lidocaine 3%. Mineral oils, parabens, petrolatum. Gel, Rectal. 20 single-use 7 g tube w/applicators and cleansing wipes. *Rx.*
Use: Anorectal preparation, steroid-containing product.
Lidoderm. (Endo) Lidocaine 5%. EDTA, glycerin, parabens, polyvinyl alcohol. Patch. 10 × 14 cm. Box 5s. *Rx.*
Use: Anesthetic, local topical.
•**lidofenin.** (LIE-doe-FEN-in) USAN.
Use: Diagnostic aid (hepatic function determination).
•**lidofilcon A.** (lih-DAH-FILL-kahn A) USAN.
Use: Contact lens material (hydrophilic).
•**lidofilcon B.** (lih-DAH-FILL-kahn B) USAN.
Use: Contact lens material (hydrophilic).
•**lidoflazine.** (LIE-dah-FLAY-zeen) USAN.
Use: Coronary vasodilator.
Lidopen Auto-Injector. (Survival Technical) Lidocaine hydrochloride 300 mg/3 mL. EDTA, methylparaben. Inj. (for IM administration). Automatic-injection device. *Rx.*
Use: Antiarrhythmic.
•**lidorestat.** (lye-DOE-res-tat) USAN.
Use: Selective aldose reductase inhibitor.
Lidox Caps. (Major) Chlordiazepoxide hydrochloride 10 mg, clidinium bromide 2.5 mg. Cap. Bot. 100s, 500s, 1000s, UD 100s. *Rx.*
Use: Anticholinergic combination.
Lidoxide. (Henry Schein) Chlordiazepoxide hydrochloride 5 mg, clidinium bromide 2.5 mg. Tab. Bot. 100s, 500s. *Rx.*
Use: Anticholinergic combination.
lid scrubs.
Use: Cleanser, ophthalmic.
See: Eye Scrub.
OCuSOFT.
•**lifarizine.** (lih-FAR-ih-ZEEN) USAN.
Use: Cerebral anti-ischemic; platelet aggregation inhibitor.

Lifer-B. (Burgin-Arden) Cyanocobalamin 30 mcg, liver inj. 0.1 mL, ferrous gluconate 100 mg, riboflavin 1.5 mg, panthenol 2.5 mg, niacinamide 100 mg, citric acid 16.4 mg, sodium citrate 23.6 mg/mL. Vial 30 mL. *Rx.*
Use: Mineral; vitamin supplement.
Life Saver Kit. (Whiteworth Towne) Ipecac syr. two 1 oz bottles, activated charcoal pow. 1 oz, poison treatment instruction booklet. *OTC.*
Use: Antidote; poisons.
Life Spanner. (Spanner) Vitamins A 12,500 units, D 400 units, E 5 units, B$_1$ 10 mg, B$_2$ 5 mg, B$_6$ 2 mg, B$_{12}$ 5 mcg, niacinamide 50 mg, calcium pantothenate 10 mg, biotin 10 mcg, C 100 mg, hesperidin complex 10 mg, rutin 20 mg, choline bitartrate 40 mg, inositol 30 mg, betaine anhydrous 15 mg, l-lysine monohydrochloride 25 mg, Fe 30 mg, Cu 1 mg, Mn 1 mg, K 5 mg, Ca 105 mg, P 82 mg, Mg 5.56 mg, Zn 1 mg. Cap. Bot. 100s. *OTC.*
Use: Mineral; vitamin supplement.
•**lifibrate.** (lih-FIE-brate) USAN.
Use: Antihyperlipoproteinemic.
•**lifibrol.** (lie-FIB-rahl) USAN.
Use: Hypercholesterolemic.
Lifol-B. (Burgin-Arden) Liver inj. 10 mcg, folic acid 1 mg, cyanocobalamin 100 mcg, phenol 0.5%/mL. Inj. Vial 10 mL. *Rx.*
Use: Nutritional supplement.
Lifolex. (Taylor Pharmaceuticals) Liver 10 mcg, cyanocobalamin 100 mcg, folic acid 5 mg/mL. Inj. Vial 10 mL. *Rx.*
Use: Nutritional supplement.
Lilly Bulk Products. (Eli Lilly) The following products are supplied by Eli Lilly under the USP, NF, or chemical name as a service to the health professions:
See: Amyl Nitrite.
Analgesic Balm.
Apomorphine Hydrochloride.
Aromatic Elix.
Atropine Sulfate.
Bacitracin.
Belladonna Tincture.
Benzoin.
Boric Acid.
Caffeine Citrated.
Calcium Gluconate.
Calcium Hydroxide.
Calcium Lactate.
Carbarsone.
Cascara Fluid Extract, Aromatic.
Cascara Sagrada Fluid Extract.
Cocaine Hydrochloride.
Codeine Phosphate.
Codeine Sulfate.

Colchicine.
Diethylstilbestrol Dipropionate.
Ephedrine Sulfate.
Ferrous Gluconate.
Ferrous Sulfate.
Folic Acid.
Glucagon.
Green Soap.
Heparin Sodium.
Ipecac.
Isoniazid.
Isopropyl Alcohol.
Liver.
Magnesium Sulfate.
Mercuric Oxide Ophthalmic Ointment,
    Yellow.
Methadone Hydrochloride.
Methyltestosterone.
Milk of Bismuth.
Morphine Sulfate.
Neomycin Sulfate.
Niacin.
Niacinamide.
Nitroglycerin.
Opium Tincture, Deodorized.
Ox Bile Extract.
Pancreatin.
Papaverine Hydrochloride.
Paregoric.
Penicillin G Potassium.
Phenobarbital.
Phenobarbital Sodium.
Potassium Chloride.
Potassium Iodide.
Progesterone.
Propylthiouracil.
Protamine Sulfate.
Pyridoxine Hydrochloride.
Quinidine Gluconate.
Quinidine Sulfate.
Quinine Sulfate.
Riboflavin.
Silver Nitrate.
Sodium Bicarbonate.
Sodium Chloride.
Sodium Salicylate.
Streptomycin Sulfate.
Sulfadiazine.
Sulfapyridine.
Sulfur.
Terpin Hydrate Oral Solution.
Terpin Hydrate and Codeine Oral
    Solution.
Testosterone Propionate.
Thiamine Hydrochloride.
Thyroid.
Tylosterone.
Whitfield's Ointment.
Wild Cherry Syrup.
Zinc Oxide.
Limbitrol. (Valeant) Chlordiazepoxide

5 mg, amitriptyline hydrochloride
12.5 mg. Film-coated. Tab. 100s. *c-IV.*
Use: Psychotherapeutic agent.
Limbitrol DS. (Valeant Pharmaceuticals,
Inc.) Chlordiazepoxide 10 mg, amitriptyline hydrochloride 25 mg. Film-
coated. Tab. Bot. 100s. *c-IV.*
Use: Psychotherapeutic agent.
Limbrel. (Primus) Flavocoxid 250 mg,
500 mg. Maltodextrin. Cap. 60s. *Rx.*
Use: Nutrition supplement.
•**lime.** *USP 34.*
Use: Pharmaceutical necessity.
•**lime solution, sulfurated.** *USP 34.*
Use: Scabicide.
lime sulfur solution. Calcium poly-
sulfide, calcium thiosulfate.
Use: Wet dressing.
•**linaclotide.** (LIN-a-KLOE-tide) USAN.
Use: Gastrointestinal agent.
•**linaclotide acetate.** (LIN-a-KLOE-tide)
USAN.
Use: Gastrointestinal agent.
•**linagliptin.** (LIN-a-GLIP-tin) USAN.
Use: Antidiabetic agent.
See: Tradjenta.
•**linarotene.** (lin-AHR-oh-teen) USAN.
Use: Antikeratolytic.
Lincocin. (Pfizer) Lincomycin hydrochlo-
ride 300 mg/mL. Benzyl alcohol
9.45 mg/mL. Inj. Vial 2 mL, 10 mL. *Rx.*
Use: Anti-infective.
•**lincomycin.** (LIN-koe-MY-sin) *USP 34.*
Antibiotic produced by *Streptomyces
lincolnensis* variant.
Use: Anti-infective; infections due to
gram-positive organisms.
•**lincomycin hydrochloride.** (LIN-koe-
MY-sin) *USP 34.*
Use: Anti-infective.
See: Lincocin.
Lincorex.
Lincorex. (Hyrex) Lincomycin hydrochlo-
ride 300 mg/mL. Benzyl alcohol
9.45 mg/mL. Inj. Vial 10 mL. *Rx.*
Use: Anti-infective.
lincosamides.
Use: Anti-infective.
See: Clindamycin.
Lincomycin.
•**lindane.** (LIN-dane) *USP 34.* Gamma-
benzene-hexachloride; hexachlorocy-
clohexane.
Use: Pediculicide, scabicide.
lindane. (Various Mfr.) Lindane. **Lot.:** 1%.
30 mL, 59 mL, pharmacy-size only pint.
Shampoo: 1%. 30 mL, 59 mL, pharmacy-
size only pint. *Rx.*
Use: Pediculicide, scabicide.
Lindora. (Bristol-Myers Squibb) Sodium

laureth sulfate, cocamide DEA, sodium Cl, lactic acid, tetra sodium EDTA, benzophenone-4, FD&C Blue No. 1. Bot. 8 oz. *OTC.*
Use: Dermatologic, cleanser.

•**linezolid.** (lin-EH-zoe-lid) USAN.
Use: Anti-infective, oxalodinone.
See: Zyvox.

•**linifanib.** (lin-i-FAN-ib) USAN.
Use: Antineoplastic.

Linodil. (Sanofi-Synthelabo) Inositol hexanicotinate. Cap. *Rx.*
Use: Hyperlipidemic; peripheral vasodilator.

•**linogliride.** (LIN-oh-GLYE-ride) USAN.
Use: Antidiabetic.

•**linogliride fumarate.** (LIN-oh-GLYE-ride) USAN.
Use: Antidiabetic.

•**linopirdine.** (lih-no-PIHR-deen) USAN.
Use: Treatment of Alzheimer disease (cognition enhancer).

•**linsitinib.** (lin-SYE-ti-nib) USAN.
Use: Antineoplastic.

Lioresal. (Novartis) Baclofen 10 mg, 20 mg. Tab. Bot. 100s, UD 100s. *Rx.*
Use: Muscle relaxant.

Lioresal Intrathecal. (Medtronic) Baclofen 0.05 mg/mL (50 mcg/mL), 10 mg/20 mL (500 mcg/mL), 10 mg/5 mL (2000 mcg/mL), preservative free. Single-use amps. 1 amp refill kit (10 mg/20 mL only), 2 and 4 amp refill kits (10 mg/5 mL only). *Rx.*
Use: Muscle relaxant.

•**liothyronine I 131.** (lie-oh-THIGH-row-neen) USAN.
Use: Radiopharmaceutical.

•**liothyronine I 125.** (lie-oh-THIGH-row-neen) USAN.
Use: Radiopharmaceutical.

•**liothyronine sodium.** (lie-oh-THIGH-row-neen) *USP 34.*
Use: Hormone, thyroid.
See: Cytomel.
Triostat.

liothyronine sodium. (Various Mfr.) Liothyronine sodium 5 mcg, 25 mcg, 50 mcg. May contain sucrose. Tab. 100s, 1000s. *Rx.*
Use: Thyroid hormone.

liothyronine sodium. (X-Gen) Liothyronine sodium 10 mcg. Alcohol 6.8%, ammonia 2.19 mg. Inj. Vials. 1 mL. *Rx.*
Use: Thyroid hormone.

liothyronine sodium injection.
Use: Myxedema coma/precoma. [Orphan Drug]

•**liotrix.** (LIE-oh-trix) *USP 34.*
Use: Hormone, thyroid.

See: Thyrolar.

lipase.
Use: Digestive enzyme.
W/Alpha-Amylase W-100, Proteinase W-300, Cellase W-100, Estrone, Testosterone, Vitamins, Minerals.
See: Kutrase.
Ku-Zyme.
W/Amylase, Bile Salts, Pepsin, Pancreatin, Calcium.
See: Enzymes.
W/Amylase, Cellulase, Hyoscyamine Sulfate, Phenyltoloxamine Citrate, Protease.
See: Digex.
W/Amylase, Protease.
See: Creon.
Palcaps 10.
Pancrelipase.
Tri-Pase 8.
Tri-Pase 16.
Zenpep.
W/Amylolytic, Proteolytic, Cellulolytic Enzymes.
See: Arco-Lase.

lipase inhibitors.
See: Orlistat.

lipid/DNA human cystic fibrosis gene. (Genzyme)
Use: Cystic fibrosis. [Orphan Drug]

lipids.
Use: Intravenous nutritional therapy.
See: Intralipid 30%.
Intralipid 20%.
Liposyn II.
Liposyn III.

Lipisorb. (Bristol-Myers Squibb) Protein 35 g/L, fat 48 g/L, carbohydrates 115 g/L, Na 733.3 mg/L, K 1250 mg/L, H_2O 320 mOsm/kg. With appropriate vitamins and minerals. 1 calorie/mL. Vanilla flavored. Pow. Can 1 lb. *OTC.*
Use: Nutritional supplement.

Lipitor. (Pfizer) Atorvastatin 10 mg, 20 mg, 40 mg, 80 mg. Lactose. Film-coated. Tab. Bot. 90s, 500s (40 mg, 80 mg only), 5000s (10 mg, 20 mg only), UD 100s (10 mg, 20 mg only). *Rx.*
Use: Antihyperlipidemic; HMG-CoA reductase inhibitor.

Lipkote by Coppertone. (Schering-Plough) Padimate O, oxybenzone. SPF 15. Lip balm 4.2 g. *OTC.*
Use: Sunscreen.

Lipkote SPF 15 Ultra Sunscreen Lipbalm. (Schering-Plough) Tube 0.15 oz. *OTC.*
Use: Sunscreen.

Lip Medex. (Blairex) Petrolatum, camphor 1%, phenol 0.54%, cocoa but-

ter, lanolin. Oint. 210 g. *OTC.*
Use: Fever blisters; lip protectant.

lipocholine.
See: Choline dihydrogen citrate.

Lipofen. (Kowa Pharmaceuticals) Fenofibrate 50 mg, 150 mg. Cap. 90s. *Rx.*
Use: Antihyperlipidemic agent, fibric acid derivative.

Lipoflavonoid. (Numark) Vitamins C 100 mg, B_1 0.33 mg, B_2 0.33 mg, B_3 3.33 mg, B_5 1.66 mg, B_6 0.33 mg, B_{12} 1.66 mcg, choline 111 mg, bioflavonoids 100 mg, inositol 111 mg. Capl. Bot. 100s, 500s. *OTC.*
Use: Vitamin supplement.

Lipogen. (Ivax) Choline 111 mg, inositol 111 mg, vitamins B_1 0.33 mg, B_2 0.33 mg, B_3 3.33 mg, B_5 1.7 mg, B_6 0.33 mg, B_{12} 1.7 mcg, C 20 mg, A 1667 units, E 10 units, Zn 30 mg, Cu, Se. Capl. Bot. 60s. *OTC.*
Use: Mineral, vitamin supplement.

Lipogen. (Various Mfr.) Choline 111 mg, inositol, vitamins B_1 0.33 mg, B_2 0.33 mg, B_3 3.33 mg, B_5 1.7 mg, B_6 0.33 mg, B_{12} 1.7 mcg, C 100 mg. Cap. Bot. 60s. *OTC.*
Use: Vitamin supplement.

lipoglycopeptides.
Use: Anti-infective.
See: Telavancin.

•**lipoic acid, alpha.** (li-POE-ik) *NF 29.*
Use: Dietary supplement.

Lipo-Nicin/100 mg. (ICN Pharm) Niacin 100 mg, niacinamide 75 mg, vitamins C 150 mg, B_1 25 mg, B_2 2 mg, B_6 10 mg. Tab. Bot. 100s. *Rx.*
Use: Vasodilator combination.

Lipo-Nicin/300 mg. (ICN Pharm) Niacin 300 mg, vitamin C 150 mg, B_1 25 mg, B_2 2 mg, B_6 10 mg. TR Cap. 100s. *Rx.*
Use: Vasodilator.

Liponol. (Rugby) Choline, inositol 83 mg, methionine 110 mg, vitamins B_1 3 mg, B_2 3 mg, B_3 10 mg, B_5 2 mg, B_6 2 mg, B_{12} 2 mcg, desiccated liver 56 mg, liver concentrate 30 mg, sorbitol, lecithin. Cap. Bot. 60s. *OTC.*
Use: Nutritional supplement.

lipopeptides.
Use: Anti-infectives.
See: Daptomycin.

liposomal amphotericin B.
Use: Antifungal. [Orphan Drug]
See: AmBisome.

liposomal doxorubicin.
See: Doxorubicin Hydrochloride.

liposome encapsulated recombinant interleukin-2. (Biomerica)
Use: Antineoplastic. [Orphan Drug]

Liposyn. (Abbott Hospital Products) Intravenous fat emulsion containing safflower oil 10%, egg phosphatides 1.2%, glycerin 2.5% in water for inj. **10%:** Single-dose container 50 mL, 100 mL, 200 mL, 500 mL; Syringe Pump Unit 50 mL single-dose. **20%:** Single-dose container 200 mL, 500 mL Syringe Pump Unit 25 mL, 50 mL single-dose. *Rx.*
Use: Nutritional supplement, parenteral.

Liposyn II. (Hospira) Intravenous fat emulsion: **10%:** Safflower oil 5%, soybean oil 5%. Bot. 100 mL, 200 mL, 500 mL. **20%:** Safflower oil 10%, soybean oil 10%, egg phosphatides 1.2%, glycerin 2.5%. 200 mL, 500 mL. Bot. Syringe pump unit 25 mL, 50 mL. *Rx.*
Use: Nutritional supplement, parenteral.

Liposyn III. (Hospira) **10%:** Soybean oil 10%, linoleic acid 54.5%, oleic acid 22.4%, palmitic acid 10.5%, linolenic acid 8.3%, stearic acid 4.2%, egg phosphatides 1.2%, glycerin 2.5%, 1.1 kcal/mL, 284 mOsmol/L. 100, 200, 500 mL. **20%:** Soybean oil 10%, linoleic acid 54.5%, oleic acid 22.4%, palmitic acid 10.5%, linolenic acid 8.3%, stearic acid 4.2%, egg phosphatides 1.2%, glycerin 2.5%, 2 kcal/mL, 292 mOsmol/L. 200, 500 mL. **30%:** Soybean oil 10%, linoleic acid 54.5%, oleic acid 22.4%, palmitic acid 10.5%, linolenic acid 8.3%, stearic acid 4.2%, egg phosphatides 1.8%, glycerin 2.5%, 2.9 kcal/mL, 293 mOsmol/L. 500 mL. *Rx.*
Use: Nutritional supplement, parenteral.

Lipo-Tears. (Spectra Pharmaceuticals) Mineral oil, petrolatum, preservative free. Drops. Bot. 1 mL. 30s. *OTC.*
Use: Lubricant, ophthalmic.

Lipotriad. (Numark) Zn 30 mg, vitamin A 5000 units, C 60 mg, E 30 units, Cu, Se, B_3 20 mg, B_1 1.5 mg, B_2 1.7 mg, B_6 2 mg, B_{12} 6 mcg, B_5 10 mg, choline bitartrate, inositol. Capl. Bot. 60s. *OTC.*
Use: Mineral, vitamin supplement.

lipotropics with vitamins.
Use: Nutritional supplement.
See: Cholidase.
  Cholinoid.
  Lipoflavonoid.
  Lipogen.
  Liponol.
  Lipotriad.
  Methatropic.

Lipoxide. (Major) Chlordiazepoxide hydrochloride 5 mg, 10 mg, 25 mg. Cap. Bot. 100s, 500s, 1000s. *c-IV.*
Use: Anxiolytic.

• **liprotamase.** (li-PROE-tam-ase) USAN.
Use: Treatment of malabsorption.

Liqua-Gel. (Paddock) Boric acid, glycerine, propylene glycol, methylparaben, propylparaben, Irish moss extract, methylcellulose. Bot. 4 oz, 16 oz. *OTC.*
Use: Lubricant.

Liquibid. (Capellon) Guaifenesin 400 mg. Tab. 100s. *Rx.*
Use: Expectorant.

Liquibid-D. (Capellon) Guaifenesin 650 mg (250 mg immediate release/400 mg extended release), phenylephrine hydrochloride 40 mg (extended release). Lactose. ER Tab. Bot. 90s. *Rx.*
Use: Upper respiratory combination, decongestant and expectorant combination.

Liquibid-PD. (Capellon) Phenylephrine hydrochloride 5 mg, guaifenesin 120 mg (immediate-release layer). Phenylephrine hydrochloride 15 mg, guaifenesin 195 mg (extended-release layer). ER Tab. 90s. *Rx.*
Use: Upper respiratory combination, decongestant and expectorant combination.

Liquibid PD-R. (Capellon) Guaifenesin 200 mg, phenylephrine hydrochloride 5 mg. Tab. 90s. *OTC.*
Use: Upper respiratory combination, expectorant, decongestant.

Liquicet. (Mallinckrodt) Hydrocodone bitartrate 10 mg, acetaminophen 500 mg per 15 mL. Saccharin, sorbitol, sucrose. Raspberry flavor. Soln. 473 mL. *c-III.*
Use: Narcotic analgesic.

Liqui-Char. (Jones Pharma) Activated charcoal. **Liq. Bot.:** 12.5 g/60 mL, 15 g/75 mL. **Squeeze container:** 25 g/120 mL, 50 g/240 mL, 30 g/120 mL. *OTC.*
Use: Antidote.

Liqui-Coat HD. (Mallinckrodt) Barium sulfate 210%. Simethicone, sorbitol, saccharin, sodium benzoate, vanilla-raspberry flavor. Susp. UD Bot. 150 mL. *Rx.*
Use: Radiopaque agent, GI contrast agent.

Liquicough DM. (Breckenridge) Dextromethorphan hydrobromide 15 mg, guaifenesin 175 mg, pseudoephedrine hydrochloride 32 mg per 5 mL. Alcohol free. Saccharin, sorbitol, acesulfame K. Grape flavor. Sugar free. Liq. 473 mL. *Rx.*
Use: Upper respiratory combination, antitussive and expectorant combination.

Liquid Barosperse. (Mallinckrodt) Barium sulfate 60%. Simethicone, vanilla flavor. Susp. Bot. 355 mL, 1900 mL. *Rx.*
Use: Radiopaque agent, GI contrast agent.

Liquid Geritonic. (Roberts) Fe 105 mg, liver fraction 1 375 mg, B_1 3 mg, B_2 3 mg, B_3 30 mg, B_6 0.3 mg, B_{12} 9 mcg, inositol 60 mg, glycine 180 mg, yeast concentrate 375 mg, Ca, I, K, Mg, Mn, P, alcohol 20%. Liq. Bot. 240 mL, gal. *OTC.*
Use: Nutritional supplement.

Liquid Lather. (Ulmer Pharmacal) Gentle wash for hands, body, face, hair. Bot. 8 oz, gal. *OTC.*
Use: Cleanser.

Liqui-Doss. (Ferndale) Mineral oil in emulsifying base, alcohol free. Emulsion. Bot. 60 mL, 480 mL. *OTC.*
Use: Laxative.

Liquid PedvaxHIB. (Merck) *Haemophilus* b PRP 7.5 mcg, *Neisseria meningitidis* OMPC 125 mcg, aluminum hydroxide 225 mcg/0.5 mL. Inj. Single-dose vials. *Rx.*
Use: Agent for active immunization, bacterial vaccine.

liquid petrolatum emulsion.
See: Mineral Oil.

Liquid Polibar. (E-Z-EM) Barium sulfate 100%. Potassium sorbate, saccharin, simethicone, sodium benzoate, sorbitol. Orange flavoring. Susp. (oral and rectal). 1,900 mL. *Rx.*
Use: Radiopaque agent, miscellaneous gastrointestinal contrast agent.

Liquid Polibar Plus. (EZ EM) Barium sulfate 105%. PEG, saccharin, sorbitol. Susp. 1,900 mL. *Rx.*
Use: Radiopaque agent, miscellaneous gastrointestinal contrast agent.

Liquifilm Forte. (Allergan) Polyvinyl alcohol 3%, thimerosal 0.002%, EDTA, sodium Cl. Soln. Bot. 15 mL, 30 mL. *OTC.*
Use: Artificial tears.

Liquimat. (Galderma) Sulfur 5%, SD alcohol 40 22%, cetyl alcohol in drying makeup base. Plastic Bot. 45 mL. *OTC.*
Use: Dermatologic, acne.

Liquipake. (Lafayette) Barium sulfate suspension 100% w/v for dilution. Bot. 1850 mL, Case 4s.
Use: Radiopaque agent.

liquor carbonis detergens.
See: Coal Tar Topical Solution.

• **liraglutide.** (lir-A-gloo-tide) USAN.
Use: Antidiabetic agent.
See: Victoza.

•**lisadimate.** (liss-AD-ih-mate) USAN.
Use: Sunscreen.

•**lisdexamfetamine dimesylate.** (lis-DEX-am-FET-a-meen) USAN.
Use: CNS stimulant, amphetamine.
See: Vyvanse.

•**lisinopril.** (lie-SIN-oh-pril) *USP 34.*
Use: Renin angiotensin system antagonist, angiotensin-converting enzyme inhibitor.
See: Prinivil.
Zestril.
W/Hydrochlorothiazide.
See: Prinzide.
Zestoretic.

lisinopril. (Various Mfr.) Lisinopril 2.5 mg, 5 mg, 10 mg, 20 mg, 30 mg, 40 mg. Tab. 30s, 100s, 500s (except 20 mg), 1000s, UD 25s (10 mg, 40 mg only), UD 100s (except 20 mg, 30 mg), UD 300s (5 mg, 10 mg only). *Rx.*
Use: Renin angiotensin system antagonist, angiotensin-converting enzyme inhibitor.

lisinopril/hydrochlorothiazide. (Various Mfr.) Lisinopril/hydrochlorothiazide 10 mg/12.5 mg, 20 mg/12.5 mg, 20 mg/25 mg. Tab. 100s, 500s, 1000s, UD 100s. *Rx.*
Use: Antihypertensive combination.

•**lisofylline.** (lie-SO-fih-lin) USAN.
Use: Immunomodulator.

lissamine green. (Rose Stone Enterprises) Lissamine green 1.5 mg. Strip, Ophth. 100s. *Rx.*
Use: Ophthalmic diagnostic product.
See: Green Glo.

Listerine Antiseptic. (Johnson & Johnson) Thymol 0.06%, eucalyptol 0.09%, methyl salicylate 0.06%, menthol 0.04%. Alcohol 26.9% (regular flavor), 21.6% (cool mint flavor), sorbitol, saccharin. Bot. 90 mL, 180 mL, 360 mL, 540 mL, 720 mL, 960 mL, 1440 mL. *OTC.*
Use: Mouthwash, antiseptic.

Listerine, Natural Citrus. (Johnson & Johnson) Thymol 0.064%, eucalyptol 0.092%, methyl salicylate 0.06%, menthol 0.042%. Alcohol 21.6%, sorbitol, sucralose. Mouthwash. 250 mL, 500 mL, 1 L, 1.5 L. *OTC.*
Use: Mouth and throat product.

Listerine, Tartar Control. (Johnson & Johnson) Thymol 0.064%, eucalyptol 0.092%, methyl salicylate 0.06%, menthol 0.042%. Alcohol 21.6%, sorbitol, sucralose. Wintermint flavor. Mouthwash. 250 mL, 500 mL, 1 L, 1.5 L. *OTC.*
Use: Mouth and throat product.

Listerine Tooth Defense. (Johnson and Johnson) Sodium fluoride 0.0221% (fluoride 0.01%). Alcohol 21.6%, sorbitol, sucralose. Mint flavor. Dental Liq. Rinse. 500 mL. *OTC.*
Use: Fluoride.

Listermint Arctic Mint Mouthwash. (Warner Lambert) Glycerin, poloxamer 335, PEG 600, sodium lauryl sulfate, sodium benzoate, benzoic acid, zinc chloride, saccharin. Liq. 946 mL. *OTC.*
Use: Antiseptic, mouthwash.

Lite Pred. (Horizon) Prednisolone sodium phosphate 0.125%. Soln. Bot. 5 mL. *Rx.*
Use: Corticosteroid, ophthalmic.

lithium. (Roxane) Lithium 8 mEq (equiv. to lithium carbonate 300 mg) per 5 mL. Alcohol, sorbitol. Soln., Oral. Patient cups. 5 mL. Bot. 500 mL. *Rx.*
Use: Antipsychotic agent.

lithium. (Various Mfr.) Lithium carbonate 300 mg (lithium 8.12 mEq). May contain sorbitol. ER Tab. 100s, 500s. *Rx.*
Use: Antipsychotic agent.

•**lithium carbonate.** (LITH-ee-uhm CAR-boe-nate) *USP 34.*
Use: Antipsychotic, manic-depressive state; antidepressant.
See: Eskalith CR.
Lithonate.
Lithotabs.

lithium carbonate. (Roxane) Lithium carbonate. **ER Tab.:** 450 mg. 100s. **Tab.:** 300 mg. Bot. 100s, 1000s, UD 100s. **Cap.:** 150 mg, 300 mg, 600 mg. Bot. 100s, 1000s, UD 100s. *Rx.*
Use: Antipsychotic, manic-depressive state; antidepressant.

•**lithium citrate.** (LITH-ee-uhm) *USP 34.*
Use: Antimanic.

lithium citrate. (Various Mfr.) Lithium citrate 8 mEq (equivalent to 300 mg lithium carbonate)/5 mL. Syr. Bot. 480 mL, 500 mL, UD 5 mL, 10 mL. *Rx.*
Use: Antipsychotic.

•**lithium hydroxide.** (LITH-ee-uhm high-DROX-ide) *USP 34.*
Use: Antipsychotic, manic-depressive state; antidepressant.

Lithonate. (Solvay) Lithium carbonate 300 mg. Cap. Bot. 100s, 1000s, UD 100s. *Rx.*
Use: Antipsychotic.

Lithostat. (Mission Pharmacal) Aceto-hydroxamic acid 250 mg. Tab. Bot. 100s. *Rx.*
Use: Anti-infective; urinary.

Lithotabs. (Solvay) Lithium carbonate 300 mg. Tab. Bot. 100s, 1000s, UD

100s. *Rx.*
Use: Antipsychotic.
•**litronesib.** (lit-ron-NES-ib) USAN.
Use: Antineoplastic.
Little Colds Cough Formula. (Vetco)
Dextromethorphan hydrobromide
7.5 mg per mL. Glycerin, corn syr.
Natural grape flavor. Soln., Conc., Oral.
30 mL. *OTC.*
Use: Nonnarcotic antitussive.
Little Colds Decongestant Plus Cough.
(Medtech) Dextromethorphan hydrobro-
mide 5 mg, phenylephrine hydrochlo-
ride 2.5 mg. Corn syrup, glycerin, sodium benzoate, sucralose. Gluten free.
Grape flavor. Soln., concentrate. 30 mL
w/dropper. *OTC.*
Use: Upper respiratory combination, antitussive combination.
Little Colds for Infants and Children.
(Vetco) Phenylephrine hydrochloride
0.25%, sorbitol, sucralose, grape flavor,
alcohol free. Soln. Oral Drops. Bot.
30 mL w/dropper. *OTC.*
Use: Nasal decongestant, arylalkylamine.
Little Fevers. (Little Remedies) Acetaminophen 80 mg/mL. Corn syrup, sucralose. Alcohol free. Soln., concentrate. 30 mL. *OTC.*
Use: Analgesic.
**Little Noses Gentle Formula, Infants &
Children.** (Vetco) Phenylephrine hydrochloride 0.125%, EDTA, benzalkonuim
chloride, alcohol free. Soln. Drops. Bot.
15 mL w/dropper. *OTC.*
Use: Nasal decongestant, arylalkylamine.
Little Tummys Laxative. (Vetco) Sennosides 8.8 mg/mL. Alcohol free. Methylparaben, sorbitol. Drops, Oral. 30 mL
with dropper. *OTC.*
Use: Laxative.
Livalo. (Lilly) Pitavastatin 1 mg, 2 mg,
4 mg. Film-coated. Tab. 90s. *Rx.*
Use: Antihyperlipidemic agent, HMG-
COA reductase inhibitor.
Livec. (Enzyme Process) Vitamins A
5000 units, B₁ 1.5 mg, B₂ 1.7 mg, niacin
20 mg, C 60 mg, B₆ 2 mg, pantothenic
acid 10 mg, E 30 units, B₁₂ 6 mcg, Ca
250 mg, Fe 5 mg, D 400 units, folacin
0.075 mg/3 Tab. Bot. 100s, 300s. *OTC.*
Use: Mineral, vitamin supplement.
Liverbex. (Spanner) Liver 2 mcg, vitamins B₁, B₂, B₆, B₁₂, niacinamide,
pantothenate/mL. Vial 30 mL. *OTC.*
Use: Nutritional supplement.
liver desiccated. Desiccated liver substance.
liver extract. Dry liver extract w/Vitamin
B₁₂, folic acid.

liver function agents.
See: Sulfobromophthalein Sodium.
Livergran. (Rawl) Desiccated whole liver
9 g, vitamins B₁ 18 mg, B₂ 36 mg, niacinamide 90 mg, choline bitartrate
216 mg, B₆ 3.6 mg, calcium pantothenate 3.6 mg, inositol 90 mg, biotin
6 mcg, vitamins B₁₂ 5.4 mcg, methionine 198 mg, arginine 242 mg, cysteine
72 mg, glutamic acid 675 mg, histidine
99 mg, isoleucine 333 mg, leucine
495 mg, lysine 297 mg, phenylalanine
189 mg, threonine 333 mg, tryptophan
45 mg, tyrosine 180 mg, valine
306 mg/3 Tsp. Bot. 15 oz. *OTC.*
Use: Nutritional supplement.
liver injection. (Various Mfr.) Liver extract for parenteral use. *Rx.*
Use: Parenteral liver supplement.
liver injection. (Arcum; Lederle Laboratories) Vitamin B₁₂ 20 mcg/mL. Vial
10 mL. *Rx.*
Use: Nutritional supplement.
liver injection, crude. (Eli Lilly and Co.)
2 mcg/mL. Vial 30 mL; (Medwick)
2 mcg/mL. Vial 30 mL. *Rx.*
Use: Liver supplement.
Liver Iron Vitamins. (Arcum) Liver inj.
(10 mcg B₁₂ activity/mL) 0.1 mL, crude
liver inj. (2 mcg B₁₂ activity/mL)
0.125 mL, green ferric ammonium citrate 20 mg, niacinamide 50 mg, vitamin
B₆ 0.3 mg, B₂ 0.3 mg, procaine hydrochloride 0.5%, phenol 0.5%/2 mL. Inj.
Vial 30 mL. *Rx.*
Use: Nutritional supplement.
•**liver, refined.** (Medwick) 20 mcg/mL. Vial
10 mL, 30 mL. *Rx.*
Use: Nutritional supplement.
Livifol. (Oxypure) Vitamin B₁₂ activity from
liver inj. equivalent to cyanocobalamin
10 mcg, folic acid 1 mg, cyanocobalamin
100 mcg/mL. Vial 10 mL. *Rx.*
Use: Vitamin supplement.
•**lixazinone sulfate.** (lix-AZE-ih-NOHN)
USAN.
Use: Cardiotonic (phosphodiesterase
inhibitor).
•**lixivaptan.** (lix-i-VAP-tan) USAN.
Use: Nonhypovolemic hyponatremia.
Lixoil. (Lixoil Labs.) Sulfonated fatty oils
and one or more esters of higher fatty
acids. Bot. 16 oz. *OTC.*
Use: Dermatologic.
LKV-Drops. (Freeda) Vitamins A
5000 units, D 400 units, E 2 mg, B₁
1.5 mg, B₂ 1.5 mg, B₃ 10 mg, B₅ 2 mg,
B₆ 2 mg, B₁₂ 6 mcg, C 50 mg, biotin
50 mcg/0.6 mL. Bot. 60 mL. *OTC.*
Use: Vitamin supplement.

LKV Infant Drops. (Freeda) Vitamins A 2500 units, D 400 units, E 5 units, B$_1$ 1 mg, B$_2$ 1 mg, B$_3$ 10 mg, B$_5$ 3 mg, B$_6$ 1 mg/0.5 mL. Bot. 60 mL. OTC.
Use: Vitamin supplement.

lld factor.
See: Vitamin B$_{12}$.

L-leucovorin.
Use: Antineoplastic.
See: Isovorin.

L-Lysine. (Various Mfr.) L-lysine 312 mg, 500 mg. Tab. Bot. 100s. 1000 mg. Tab. Bot. 60s. 500 mg. Cap. Bot. 100s, 250s. OTC.
Use: Dietary supplement; amino acid.

LMD. (Hospira) Dextran 40 10%. 500 mL. With 0.9% sodium chloride or in 5% dextrose. Rx.
Use: Plasma volume expander.

L-methylfolate.
Use: Water-soluble vitamin.
See: ViloFane-Dp.

LM-427. Ribabutin.
Use: CDC anti-infective agent.

LMWD-Dextran 40. (Pharmachemie USA, Inc.) Normal saline 0.9%, dextrose 10%. Rx.
Use: Plasma volume expander.

L-M-X4. (Ferndale) Lidocaine hydrochloride 4% (40 mg/g), benzyl alcohol. Cream. 5 g, 30 g. OTC.
Use: Topical local anesthetic, amide local anesthetic.

Lobak. (Sanofi-Synthelabo) Chlormezanone 250 mg, acetaminophen 300 mg. Tab. 40s, 100s, 1000s. Rx.
Use: Anxiolytic; analgesic.

Lobana Body. (Ulmer Pharmacal) Mineral oil, triethanolamine stearate, stearic acid, lanolin, cetyl alcohol, potassium stearate, propylene glycol, parabens. Lot. Bot. 120, 240 mL, gal. OTC.
Use: Emollient.

Lobana Body Shampoo. (Ulmer Pharmacal) Chloroxylenol. Bot. 240 mL, gal. OTC.
Use: Dermatologic, hair and skin.

Lobana Conditioning Shampoo. (Ulmer Pharmacal) Bot. 8 oz, gal. OTC.
Use: Dermatologic, hair and scalp.

Lobana Derm-Ade. (Ulmer Pharmacal) Vitamin A, D, E. Cream Jar 2 oz, 8 oz. OTC.
Use: Dermatologic; counterirritant.

Lobana Liquid Lather. (Ulmer Pharmacal) Sodium laureth sulfate, sodium lauroyl sarcosinate, sodium myristyl sarcosonate, lauramide DEA, linoleamide DEA, octyl hydroxystearate, polyquaternium 7, tetrasodium EDTA, quaternium 15, sodium chloride, citric acid. Liq. Bot. 240 mL, gal. OTC.
Use: Cleanser.

Lobana Peri-Gard. (Ulmer Pharmacal) Water-resistant ointment containing vitamins A & D. Oint. Jar 2 oz, 8 oz. OTC.
Use: Dermatologic, protectant.

Lobana Perineal Cleanser. (Ulmer Pharmacal) Sprayer 4 oz, 8 oz. Bot. Gal. OTC.
Use: Urine and fecal cleanser.

•**lobenzarit sodium.** (low-BENZ-ah-RIT) USAN.
Use: Antirheumatic.

Lobidram. (Dram) Lobeline sulfate 2 mg. Tab. Pkg. 15s, 30s. OTC.
Use: Smoking cessation aid.

•**lobucavir.** (lah-BYOO-kah-vihr) USAN.
Use: Antiviral.

Locoid. (Triax) **Cream:** Hydrocortisone butyrate 0.1%. Tube 15 g, 45 g. **Lot.:** Hydrocortisone butyrate 0.1%. Cetostearyl alcohol, light mineral oil, parabens, safflower oil, white petrolatum. 60 mL, 120 mL. **Oint.:** Hydrocortisone butyrate 0.1%. Tube 15 g, 45 g. **Soln.:** Hydrocortisone butyrate 0.1%, isopropyl alcohol 50%, glycerin, povidone. Bot. 20 mL, 60 mL. Rx.
Use: Corticosteroid, topical.

Locoid Lipocream. (Triax) Hydrocortisone butyrate 0.1%. Alcohol, mineral oil, parabens, white petrolatum. Cream. 15 g, 45 g. Rx.
Use: Anti-inflammatory agent.

•**lodelaben.** (low-DELL-ah-ben) USAN.
Formerly Declaben.
Use: Antiarthritic; emphysema therapy adjunct.

•**lodenosine.** (loh-DEN-oh-seen) USAN.
Use: Antiviral (HIV reverse transcriptase inhibitor).

Lodosyn. (Valeant) Carbidopa 25 mg. Tab. Bot. 100s. Rx.
Use: Antiparkinsonian.

•**lodoxamide ethyl.** (low-DOX-ah-mide ETH-uhl) USAN.
Use: Antiasthmatic, antiallergic, bronchodilator.

•**lodoxamide tromethamine.** (low-DOX-ah-mide troe-METH-ah-meen) USAN.
Use: Antiasthmatic, antiallergic, bronchodilator; vernal keratoconjunctivitis.
See: Alomide.

Lodrane. (ECR) Pseudoephedrine hydrochloride 60 mg, brompheniramine maleate 4 mg/5 mL. Cherry flavor, alcohol, sugar, and dye free. Liq. Bot. 473 mL Rx.

Use: Upper respiratory combination, decongestant, antihistamine.

Lodrane D. (ECR) Pseudoephedrine tannate 90 mg, brompheniramine tannate 8 mg per 5 mL. Alcohol free, sugar free. Strawberry flavor. Susp. 473 mL. *Rx.*
Use: Upper respiratory combination, decongestant and antihistamine.

Lodrane LD. (ECR) Brompheniramine maleate 6 mg, pseudoephedrine hydrochloride 60 mg, dye free. Cap. Bot. 100s. *Rx.*
Use: Upper respiratory combination, antihistamine, decongestant.

Lodrane 12 D. (ECR) Pseudoephedrine hydrochloride 45 mg, brompheniramine maleate 6 mg. Dye free. ER Tab. 100s. *Rx.*
Use: Upper respiratory combination, decongestant and antihistamine.

Lodrane 12 Hour. (ECR Pharmaceuticals) Brompheniramine maleate 6 mg. Dye free. ER Tab. 100s. *Rx.*
Use: Antihistamine.

Lodrane 24. (ECR Pharmaceuticals) Brompheniramine maleate 12 mg. ER Cap. 100s. *Rx.*
Use: Antihistamine.

Lodrane 24 D. (ECR) Pseudoephedrine hydrochloride 90 mg, brompheniramine maleate 12 mg. ER Cap. 60s. *Rx.*
Use: Upper respiratory combination, decongestant and antihistamine.

Lodrane XR. (ECR Pharmaceuticals) Brompheniramine tannate 8 mg/5 mL. Alcohol free, sugar free. Strawberry flavor. Oral Susp. Pints, 10 mL. *Rx.*
Use: Antihistamine.

Loestrin Fe 1/20. (Teva) Norethindrone acetate 1 mg, ethinyl estradiol 20 mcg. Lactose, sugar (active tablets), sucrose (inert tablets), ferrous fumarate 75 mg per tab. (brown tab. only). Tab. Pack 28s. *Rx.*
Use: Sex hormone, contraceptive hormone.

Loestrin Fe 1.5/30. (Teva) Norethindrone acetate 1.5 mg, ethinyl estradiol 30 mcg. Lactose, sugar (active tablets), sucrose (inert tablets), ferrous fumarate 75 mg per tab. (brown tab. only). Tab. Pack 28s. *Rx.*
Use: Sex hormone, contraceptive hormone.

Loestrin 24 Fe. (Warner Chilcott) Ethinyl estradiol 20 mcg, norethindrone acetate 1 mg. Sugar, lactose, ferrous fumarate 75 mg per tab. (brown tab. only). Tab. 28s. *Rx.*
Use: Contraceptive hormone, sex hormone.

Loestrin 21 1/20. (Teva) Norethindrone acetate 1 mg, ethinyl estradiol 20 mcg. Lactose, sugar. Tab. Packs 21s. *Rx.*
Use: Sex hormone, contraceptive hormone.

Loestrin 21 1.5/30. (Teva) Norethindrone acetate 1.5 mg, ethinyl estradiol 30 mcg. Lactose, sugar. Tab. Packs 21s. *Rx.*
Use: Sex hormone, contraceptive hormone.

•**lofemizole hydrochloride.** (low-FEM-ih-ZOLE) USAN.
Use: Anti-inflammatory; analgesic; antipyretic.

•**lofentanil oxalate.** (low-FEN-tah-NILL OX-ah-late) USAN.
Use: Analgesic, narcotic.

•**lofepramine hydrochloride.** (low-FEH-prah-MEEN) USAN.
Use: Antidepressant.

•**lofexidine hydrochloride.** (low-FEX-ih-DEEN) USAN.
Use: Treatment of opioid withdrawal symptoms.

Lofibra. (Gate) **Cap.:** Fenofibrate (micronized) 67 mg, 134 mg, 200 mg. Lactose. 100s. **Tab.:** Fenofibrate 54 mg, 160 mg. Lactose. Film-coated. 90s. *Rx.*
Use: Antihyperlipidemic agent, fibric acid derivative.

Logen. (Ivax) Diphenoxylate hydrochloride, atropine sulfate. **Liq.:** Bot. 2 oz. **Tab.:** Bot. 100s, 500s, 1000s. *c-v.*
Use: Antidiarrheal.

LoHist-D. (Larken Laboratories) Chlorpheniramine maleate 2 mg, pseudoephedrine hydrochloride 30 mg. Saccharin, sorbitol. Alcohol free and dye free. Peach flavor. Liq. 473 mL. *Rx.*
Use: Upper respiratory combinations, decongestant and antihistamine.

LoHist-DM. (Larken) Brompheniramine maleate 2 mg, dextromethorphan hydrobromide 10 mg, phenylephrine hydrochloride 5 mg per 5 mL. Parabens, saccharin, sorbitol. Strawberry flavor. Syr. 473 mL. *Rx.*
Use: Upper respiratory combination, antitussive combination.

LoHist-LQ. (Larken) Pseudoephedrine hydrochloride 60 mg, brompheniramine maleate 4 mg per 5 mL. Alcohol, sugar, and dye free. Saccharin, sorbitol. Cherry flavor. Liq. 473 mL. *Rx.*
Use: Upper respiratory combination, decongestant and antihistamine.

LoHist PEB. (Larken Labs) Brompheniramine maleate 4 mg, phenylephrine hydrochloride 10 mg. Benzoic acid,

edetate disodium, glycerin, propylene glycol, saccharin, sorbitol. Alcohol free, dye free, and sugar free. Bubble gum flavor. Liq. 118 mL. *OTC.*
Use: Upper respiratory combination, decongestant and antihistamine.

LoHist PSB. (Larken Labs) Brompheniramine maleate 4 mg, pseudoephedrine hydrochloride 20 mg. Benzoic acid, glycerin, PEG, saccharin, sorbitol. Alcohol free, dye free, and sugar free. Cherry flavor. Liq. 473 mL. *OTC.*
Use: Upper respiratory combination, decongestant and antihistamine.

LoHist 12D. (Larken) Pseudoephedrine hydrochloride 45 mg, brompheniramine maleate 6 mg. Dye free. ER Tab. 100s. *Rx.*
Use: Upper respiratory combination, decongestant and antihistamine.

LoHist 12 Hour. (Larken) Brompheniramine tannate 6 mg. ER Tab. 100s. *Rx.*
Use: Antihistamine.

LoKara. (PharmaDerm) Desonide 0.05%. Light mineral oil, cetyl alcohol, stearyl alcohol, parabens, EDTA. Lot. 59 mL, 118 mL. *Rx.*
Use: Topical corticosteroid.

Lomanate. (Various Mfr.) Diphenoxylate hydrochloride 2.5 mg, atropine sulfate 0.025 mg/5 mL. Bot. 60 mL. *c-v.*
Use: Antidiarrheal.

•**lomefloxacin.** (low-MEH-FLOX-ah-sin) USAN.
Use: Anti-infective, fluoroquinolone.

•**lomefloxacin hydrochloride.** (low-MEH-FLOX-ah-sin) USAN.
Use: Anti-infective, fluoroquinolone.

•**lomefloxacin mesylate.** (low-MEH-FLOX-ah-sin) USAN.
Use: Anti-infective.

•**lometraline hydrochloride.** (low-MET-rah-LEEN) USAN.
Use: Antipsychotic; antiparkinsonian.

•**lometrexol sodium.** (LOW-meh-TREX-ole) USAN.
Use: Antineoplastic.

•**lomitapide.** (lom-i-TA-pide) USAN.
Use: Treatment of hypercholesterolemia and hypertriglyceridemia.

•**lomitapide mesylate.** (lom-i-TA-pide) USAN.
Use: Treatment of hypercholesterolemia and hypertriglyceridemia.

•**lomofungin.** (low-moe-FUN-jin) USAN.
Use: Antifungal.

Lomotil. (Pfizer) Diphenoxylate hydrochloride 2.5 mg, atropine sulfate 0.025 mg. Tab. or 5 mL. **Tab.:** Bot.

100s, 500s, 1000s, 2500s, UD 100s.
Liq.: Bot. w/dropper 2 oz. *c-v.*
Use: Antidiarrheal.

•**lomustine.** (LOW-muss-teen) USAN.
Use: Antineoplastic, alkylating agent.
See: CeeNu.

•**lonafarnib.** (loe-na-FAR-nib) USAN.
Use: Chemotherapeutic.

Lonalac. (Bristol-Myers Squibb) Protein as casein 21%, fat as coconut oil 49%, carbohydrate as lactose 30%, vitamins A 1440 units, B_1 0.6 mg, B_2 2.6 mg, niacin 1.2 mg, Ca 1.69 g, P 1.5 g, Cl 750 mg, K 1.88 g, Na 38 mg, Mg 135 mg/qt. Pow. Can 16 oz. *OTC.*
Use: Nutritional supplement.

•**lonapalene.** (loe-NA-pa-leen) USAN.
Use: Antipsoriatic.

•**lonaprisan.** (loe-na-PRIS-an) USAN.
Use: Progesterone receptor antagonist; antineoplastic.

Long Acting Nasal Spray. (Weeks & Leo) Oxymetazoline hydrochloride 0.05%. Soln. Bot. 0.75 oz. *OTC.*
Use: Decongestant.

Lonox. (Sandoz) Diphenoxylate hydrochloride 2.5 mg, atropine sulfate 0.025 mg. Tab. Bot. 100s, 500s, 1000s, UD 100s. *c-v.*
Use: Antidiarrheal.

•**lontucirev.** (lon-TOO-si-rev) USAN.
Use: Antineoplastic agent.

Lo/Ovral. (Akrimax Pharmaceuticals) Norgestrel 0.3 mg, ethinyl estradiol 30 mcg. Lactose. Tab. *Pilpak* 21s, 28s (with 7 inert tabs.). *Rx.*
Use: Sex hormone, contraceptive hormone.

loperamide. (Geri-Care) Loperamide hydrochloride 2 mg. Tab. 24s. *OTC.*
Use: Antidiarrheal.

•**loperamide hydrochloride.** (low-PURR-ah-mide) *USP 34.*
Use: Antiperistaltic.
See: Imodium.
     K-Pek II.
     Neo-Diaral.
W/Simethicone.
See: Imodium Multi-Symptom Relief.

Lopid. (Parke-Davis) Gemfibrozil 600 mg, parabens. Tab. Bot. 60s, 500s, UD 100s. *Rx.*
Use: Antihyperlipidemic; fibric acid derivative.

lopinavir and ritonavir.
Use: Antiretroviral; protease inhibitor combination.
See: Kaletra.

Lopressor. (Novartis) Metoprolol 50 mg, 100 mg. Lactose. Tab. 100s, 1000s, UD

100s (50 mg only). *Rx.*
Use: Antiadrenergic/sympatholytic, beta-adrenergic blocking agent.
Lopressor HCT. (Novartis) Metoprolol tartrate/hydrochlorothiazide. 50/25 mg, 100/25 mg, 100/50 mg. Lactose, sucrose. Tab. Bot. 100s. *Rx.*
Use: Antihypertensive combination.
Loprox. (Medicis) Ciclopirox. **Gel:** 0.77%. Isopropyl alcohol. 30 g, 45 g, 100 g. **Shampoo:** 1%. 120 mL. *Rx.*
Use: Topical antifungal, anti-infective.
Lopurin. (Knoll) Allopurinol 100 mg, 300 mg. Tab. Bot. 100s, 1000s, UD 100s. *Rx.*
Use: Antigout agent.
•**loracarbef.** (LOW-ra-CAR-beff) *USP 34.*
Use: Anti-infective.
•**lorajmine hydrochloride.** (lahr-AZH-meen) USAN.
Use: Cardiovascular agent.
•**loratadine.** (lor-AT-uh-DEEN) *USP 34.*
Use: Antihistamine, peripherally-selective piperidine.
See: Alavert.
Alavert Children's.
Children's Loratadine.
Claritin.
Claritin Children's Allergy.
Claritin Hives Relief.
Claritin Non-Drowsy Liqui-Gels.
Claritin RediTabs.
Claritin 24-Hour Allergy.
Clear-Atadine.
Clear-Atadine Children's.
Dimetapp Children's ND Non-Drowsy Allergy.
Loratadine Hives Relief.
Non-Drowsy Allergy Relief.
Non-Drowsy Allergy Relief for Kids.
Triaminic AllerChews.
W/Pseudoephedrine Sulfate.
See: Alavert Allergy & Sinus D-12 Hour.
Allergy Relief & Nasal Decongestant.
Claritin-D 12 Hour.
Claritin-D 24 Hour.
Clear-Atadine D.
Loratadine D.
loratadine. (Ranbaxy) Loratadine 5 mg per 5 mL. Sucrose. Fruit flavor. Syr. 480 mL. *OTC.*
Use: Antihistamine, peripherally selective piperidine.
loratadine. (Various Mfr.) Loratadine 10 mg. Tab. 100s. *OTC.*
Use: Antihistamine, peripherally selective piperidine.
Loratadine D. (Major) Loratadine 10 mg, pseudoephedrine sulfate 240 mg. Lactose, PEG, sodium 10 mg. ER Tab.

10s, 15s. *OTC.*
Use: Upper respiratory combination, decongestant and antihistamine.
Loratadine Hives Relief. (Silarx) Loratadine 5 mg per 5 mL. Glycerin, propylene glycol, sodium benzoate, sucralose. Alcohol free, dye free, and sugar free. Grape flavor. Syrup. 120 mL. *OTC.*
Use: Antihistamine; piperidine, peripherally selective.
•**lorazepam.** (lor-AZ-e-pam) *USP 34.*
Tall Man: LORazepam
Use: Anxiolytic; anticonvulsant.
See: Alzapam.
Ativan.
lorazepam. (Hospira) Lorazepam 2 mg/mL, 4 mg/mL. PEG 400, propylene glycol, benzyl alcohol 2%. Inj. Prefilled syringe. 1 mL. Single-dose vials. 1 mL. Multidose vials. 10 mL. *c-IV.*
Use: Anxiolytic; hypnotic; sedative.
lorazepam. (Pharmaceutical Associates) Lorazepam 2 mg/mL. PEG, propylene glycol. Soln., concentrate. 30 mL w/dropper. *c-IV.*
Use: Antianxiety agent, benzodiazepine.
lorazepam. (Various Mfr) Lorazepam 0.5 mg, 1 mg, 2 mg. Tab. Bot. 100s, 500s, 1000s. *c-IV.*
Use: Anxiolytic; hypnotic; sedative.
Lorazepam Intensol. (Roxane) Lorazepam 2 mg/mL. Alcohol and dye free. Concentrated oral soln. Dropper Bot. 10 mL, 30 mL. *c-IV.*
Use: Anxiolytic; hypnotic; sedative.
•**lorbamate.** (lore-BAM-ate) USAN.
Use: Muscle relaxant.
•**lorcainide hydrochloride.** (lahr-CANE-ide) USAN.
Use: Cardiovascular agent; antiarrhythmic.
•**lorcaserin hydrochloride.** (lor-ca-SER-in) USAN.
Use: Anorexiant; obesity.
Lorcet Plus. (Forest) Hydrocodone bitartrate 7.5 mg, acetaminophen 650 mg. Tab. Bot. 100s, 500s, UD 100s. *c-III.*
Use: Analgesic combination, narcotic.
Lorcet 10/650. (Forest) Hydrocodone bitartrate 10 mg, acetaminophen 650 mg. Tab. Bot. 20s, 100s, UD 100s. *c-III.*
Use: Analgesic combination, narcotic.
•**lorcinadol.** (LORE-sin-ah-dole) USAN.
Use: Analgesic.
•**loreclezole.** (lahr-EH-kleh-zole) USAN.
Use: Antiepileptic.
Lorelco. (Hoechst) Probucol 250 mg. Tab. Bot. 120s. *Rx.*
Use: Antihyperlipidemic.

- **lormetazepam.** (lor-me-TAZ-e-pam) USAN.
  Use: Hypnotic, sedative.
- **lornoxicam.** (lore-NOX-ih-kam) USAN.
  Use: Anti-inflammatory; analgesic.

Lortab. (UCB) Hydrocodone bitartrate 2.5 mg, acetaminophen 167 mg/5 mL, alcohol 7%, parabens, saccharin, sorbitol, sucrose. Elix. Bot. pt. *c-III*.
  Use: Analgesic combination, narcotic.

Lortab 5/500. (UCB) Hydrocodone 5 mg, acetaminophen 500 mg. Tab. Bot. 100s, 500s, UD 100s. *c-III*.
  Use: Analgesic combination, narcotic.

Lortab 7.5/500. (UCB) Hydrocodone 7.5 mg, acetaminophen 500 mg. Tab. Bot. 100s, 500s, UD 100s. *c-III*.
  Use: Analgesic combination, narcotic.

Lortab 10/500. (UCB) Hydrocodone bitartrate 10 mg, acetaminophen 500 mg. Tab. Bot. 100s, 500s. *c-III*.
  Use: Analgesic combination, narcotic.

- **lortalamine.** (lahr-TAHL-ah-MEEN) USAN.
  Use: Antidepressant.

Lortuss EX. (Poly Pharmaceuticals) Codeine phosphate 10 mg, guaifenesin 100 mg, pseudoephedrine hydrochloride 22.5 mg per 5 mL. Glycerin, propylene glycol, saccharin, sorbitol. Alcohol free, dye free, and sugar free. Cotton candy flavor. Susp. 473 mL. *c-v.*
  Use: Upper respiratory combination, antitussive and expectorant combination.

Lortuss DM. (Poly Pharmaceuticals) Dextromethorphan hydrobromide 15 mg, doxylamine succinate 6.25 mg, pseudoephedrine hydrochloride 30 mg per 5 mL. Glycerin, propylene glycol, saccharin, sorbitol. Alcohol free, dye free, and sugar free. Candy apple flavor. Liq. 473 mL. *Rx.*
  Use: Upper respiratory combination, antitussive combination.

Lortuss LQ. (Poly Pharmaceuticals) Doxylamine succinate 6.25 mg, pseudoephedrine hydrochloride 30 mg. Glycerin, propylene glycol, saccharin, sorbitol. Alcohol free, dye free, and sugar free. Grape flavor. Liq. 473 mL. *OTC.*
  Use: Upper respiratory combination, decongestant and antihistamine.

- **lorvotuzumab mertansine.** (LOR-voe-TOOZ-oo-mab) USAN.
  Use: Antineoplastic.
- **lorzafone.** (LAHR-zah-FONE) USAN.
  Use: Anxiolytic.
- **losartan potassium.** (low-SAHR-tan) USP 34.
  Use: Renin angiotensin system antagonist, angiotensin II receptor antagonist.
  See: Cozaar.
  W/Hydrochlorothiazide and Potassium.
  See: Hyzaar.

losartan potassium. (Various Mfr.) Losartan potassium 25 mg, 50 mg, 100 mg. May contain lactose; PEG; potassium 2.12 mg (25 mg), 4.24 mg (50 mg), 8.48 mg (100 mg). Tab. 30s (except 25 mg), 90s, 1000s. *Rx.*
  Use: Renin angiotensin system antagonist, angiotensin II receptor antagonist.

losartan potassium. (ZyGenerics) Losartan potassium 25 mg, 50 mg, 100 mg. May contain lactose; PEG; potassium 2.12 mg (25 mg), 4.24 mg (50 mg), 8.48 mg (100 mg). Tab. 30s, 90s, 100s, 1000s, 5000s (except 50 mg), 10,000s (except 100 mg). *Rx.*
  Use: Renin angiotensin system antagonist, angiotensin II receptor antagonist.

losartan potassium/hydrochlorothiazide. (Various Mfr.) Losartan potassium/hydrochlorothiazide 50 mg/12.5 mg, 100 mg/12.5 mg, 100 mg/25 mg. May contain lactose; PEG; potassium 4.24 mg (50 mg/12.5 mg), 8.48 mg (100 mg/12.5 mg and 100 mg/25 mg). Tab. 20s, 90s, 500s, 1000s. *Rx.*
  Use: Antihypertensive combination.

losartan potassium/hydrochlorothiazide. (ZyGenerics) Losartan potassium/hydrochlorothiazide 50 mg/12.5 mg, 100 mg/12.5 mg, 100 mg/25 mg. May contain lactose; potassium 4.24 mg (50 mg/12.5 mg), 8.48 mg (100 mg/12.5 mg and 100 mg/25 mg). Tab. 30s, 90s, 1000s, 5000s. *Rx.*
  Use: Antihypertensive combination.

LoSeasonique. (Teva) **Phase 1:** Ethinyl estradiol 0.02 mg, levonorgestrel 0.1 mg. Lactose. Tab. 84s. **Phase 2:** Ethinyl estradiol 0.01 mg. Lactose, PEG. Tab. 7s. *Rx.*
  Use: Oral contraceptive, biphasic contraceptive.

Losec.
  See: Prilosec.
- **losmapimod.** (los-MAP-i-mod) USAN.
  Use: CNS agent.

Losopan. (Ivax) Magaldrate 540 mg/5 mL. Liq. Bot. 12 oz. *OTC.*
  Use: Antacid.

Losopan Plus. (Ivax) Magaldrate 540 mg, simethicone 20 mg/5 mL. Liq. Bot. 12 oz. *OTC.*
  Use: Antacid; antiflatulent.

Losotron Plus. (Various Mfr.) Magaldrate 540 mg, simethicone 20 mg/5 mL. Liq. Bot. 360 mL. *OTC.*
Use: Antacid; antiflatulent.

• **losoxantrone hydrochloride.** (low-SOX-an-trone) USAN.
Use: Antineoplastic.

• **losulazine hydrochloride.** (low-SULL-ah-zeen) USAN.
Use: Antihypertensive.

Lotawin. (Sanofi-Synthelabo) Oxypertine. Cap. *Rx.*
Use: Anxiolytic.

Lotemax. (Bausch & Lomb) Loteprednol etabonate 0.5%. **Ophth. Susp.:** EDTA, benzalkonium chloride 0.01%, glycerin, povidone. 2.5 mL, 5 mL, 10 mL, 15 mL. **Oint., Ophth.:** Mineral oil, white petrolatum. 3.5 g. *Rx.*
Use: Ophthalmic corticosteroid.

Lotensin. (Novartis) Benazepril hydrochloride 10 mg, 20 mg, 40 mg. Castor oil (except 40 mg), lactose. Tab. 100s. *Rx.*
Use: Renin angiotensin system antagonist, angiotensin-converting enzyme inhibitor.

Lotensin HCT. (Novartis) Hydrochlorothiazide/benazepril 12.5 mg/10 mg, 12.5 mg/20 mg, 25 mg/20 mg. Lactose. Tab. 100s. *Rx.*
Use: Antihypertensive.

• **loteprednol etabonate.** (low-TEH-PRED-nole ET-a-BOE-nate) USAN.
Use: Ophthalmic corticosteroid.
See: Alrex.
  Lotemax.

lotio alba. White lotion. *OTC.*
Use: Antiseborrheic; dermatologic, acne.

lotio alsulfa. (Doak Dermatologics) Colloidal sulfur 5%. Bot. 4 oz. *OTC.*
Use: Antiseborrheic; dermatologic, acne.

Lotion-Jel. (C.S. Dent & Co.) Benzocaine in gel base. Tube 0.2 oz. *OTC.*
Use: Anesthetic, local.

• **lotrafiban hydrochloride.** (low-TRAFF-ih-ban) USAN.
Use: Antiplatelet.

• **lotrafilcon A.** (lo-tra-FIL-kon A) USAN.
Use: Contact lens material.

• **lotrafilcon B.** (lo-tra-FIL-kon B) USAN.
Use: Contact lens material.

Lotrel. (Novartis) Amlodipine/benazepril hydrochloride 2.5 mg/10 mg, 5 mg/10 mg, 5 mg/20 mg, 5 mg/40 mg, 10 mg/20 mg, 10 mg, 40 mg. Lactose (5 mg/40 mg, 10 mg/20 mg, 10 mg/40 mg only). Cap. Bot. 100s. *Rx.*

Use: Antihypertensive combination.

Lotrimin AF. (Schering-Plough) Clotrimazole 1%. **Cream:** Benzyl alcohol, cetearyl alcohol. Tube. 12 g, 24 g. **Top. Soln.:** PEG. Bot. 10 mL. **Lot.:** Benzyl alcohol, cetearyl alcohol. Bot. 20 mL. *OTC.*
Use: Antifungal, topical.

Lotrimin AF. (Schering-Plough) Miconazole nitrate. **Pow.:** 2%. Talc. 90 g. **Spray Liq.:** 2%. SD alcohol 40 17%. 113 mL. **Spray Pow.:** 2%. SD alcohol 40 10%. 100 g. *OTC.*
Use: Topical anti-infective, antifungal agent.

Lotrimin Ultra. (Schering-Plough) Butenafine hydrochloride 1%. Benzyl alcohol, cetyl alcohol, glycerin, white petrolatum. Cream. 12 g, 24 g. *OTC.*
Use: Antifungal, topical anti-infective.

Lotrisone. (Schering) Betamethasone (as dipropionate) 0.05%, clotrimazole 1%. Alcohols, hydrophilic, mineral oil, white petrolatum. Lot. 30 mL. *Rx.*
Use: Antifungal, topical.

Lotronex. (Promethus) Alosetron hydrochloride (as base) 0.5 mg, 1 mg. Lactose. Film-coated. Tab. Bot. 30s. *Rx.*
Use: Antiemetic; antivertigo.

Lo-Trop. (Vangard Labs, Inc.) Diphenoxylate hydrochloride 2.5 mg, atropine sulfate 0.025 mg. Tab. Bot. 100s, 1000s. *c-v.*
Use: Antidiarrheal.

• **lovastatin.** (LOW-vuh-STAT-in) *USP 34.* Formerly Mevinolin.
Use: Antihypercholesterolemic; antihyperlipidemic, HMG-CoA reductase inhibitor.
See: Altoprev.
  Mevacor.

lovastatin. (Various Mfr.) Lovastatin 10 mg, 20 mg, 40 mg. May contain lactose. Tab. Bot. 30s, 60s, 90s (except 10 mg), 100s, 500s, 1000s. *Rx.*
Use: Antihypercholesterolemic; antihyperlipidemic; HMG-CoA reductase inhibitor.

lovastatin/niacin.
Use: Antihyperlipidemic.
See: Advicor.

Lovaza. (GlaxoSmithKline) Omega-3 fatty acids 900 mg (EPA 465 mg and DHA 375 mg). Soybean oil, partially hydrogenated vegetable oils. Cap. 60s, 120s. *Rx.*
Use: Fish oil.

Love Longer. (Durex) Benzocaine 7.5% in water-soluble lubricant base. Tube 0.5 oz. *OTC.*
Use: Anesthetic, local.

Lovenox. (Sanofi-Aventis) Enoxaparin sodium. 30 mg/0.3 mL, 40 mg/0.4 mL, 60 mg/0.6 mL, 80 mg/0.8 mL, 100 mg/ 1 mL, 120 mg/0.8 mL, 150 mg/1 mL, 300 mg/3 mL. Benzyl alcohol 15 mg/ 15 mL (300 mg/3 mL only). Preservative free (except 300 mg/3 mL). Approximate anti-factor Xa activity of 1000 units (30 mg/0.3 mL, 40 mg/0.4 mL, 60 mg/ 0.6 mL, 80 mg/0.8 mL, 100 mg/mL, 300 mg/3 mL), 1500 units (120 mg/ 0.8 mL, 150 mg/1 mL) (with reference to the WHO First International Low Molecular Weight Heparin Reference Standard). Inj. **30 mg/0.3 mL:** Single-dose prefilled syringes w/27-gauge ×½-inch needle. **40 mg/0.4 mL:** Single-dose prefilled syringes with a 27-gauge ×½-inch needle. **60 mg/ 0.6 mL, 80 mg/0.8 mL, 100 mg/1 mL, 120 mg/0.8 mL, 150 mg/mL:** Graduated single-dose prefilled syringes with a 27-gauge ×½-inch needle. **300 mg/ 3 mL:** 3 mL multidose vial. *Rx.*
Use: Anticoagulant, low molecular weight heparin (LMWH).

•**loviride.** (LOW-vihr-ide) USAN.
Use: Antiviral for chronic oral treatment of HIV-seropositive patients (non-nucleoside reverse transcriptase inhibitor).

Lowila Cake. (Bristol-Myers Squibb) Sodium lauryl sulfoacetate, dextrin, boric acid, urea, sorbitol, mineral oil, PEG 14 M, lactic acid, cellulose gum, docusate sodium. Cake 112.5 g. *OTC.*
Use: Dermatologic, cleanser.

low molecular weight heparins. LMWH.
Use: Anticoagulant.
See: Dalteparin Sodium.
Enoxaparin Sodium.
Tinzaparin Sodium.

Low-Ogestrel. (Watson) Ethinyl estradiol 30 mcg, norgestrel 0.3 mg. Lactose. Tab. Pack 28s (with 7 inert tabs.). *Rx.*
Use: Sex hormone, contraceptive hormone.

Low-Quel. (Halsey Drug) Diphenoxylate hydrochloride 2.5 mg, atropine sulfate 0.025 mg. Tab. Bot. 100s. *c-v.*
Use: Antidiarrheal.

Lowsium. (Rugby) Magaldrate 540 mg/ 5 mL. Susp. Bot. 360 mL. *OTC.*
Use: Antacid.

Lowsium Plus. (Rugby) **Tab.:** Magaldrate 480 mg, simethicone 20 mg. Bot. 60s. **Susp.:** Magaldrate 540 mg, simethicone 40 mg/5 mL. Bot. 360 mL. *OTC.*
Use: Antacid; antiflatulent.

•**loxapine.** (LOX-ah-peen) USAN.
Use: Anxiolytic; antipsychotic, dibenzapine derivative.
See: Loxapine Succinate.
Loxitane.

loxapine hydrochloride.
Use: Anxiolytic.
See: Loxitane.

•**loxapine succinate.** (LOX-ah-peen) *USP 34.*
Use: Anxiolytic; antipsychotic, dibenzapine derivative.
See: Loxitane.

loxapine succinate. (Various Mfr.) Loxapine 5 mg (loxapine succinate 6.8 mg), 10 mg (loxapine succinate 13.6 mg), 25 mg (loxapine succinate 34 mg), 50 mg (loxapine succinate 68.1 mg). Cap. Bot. 100s, 1000s (5 mg only). *Rx.*
Use: Antipsychotic, dibenzapine derivative.

Loxitane. (Watson) Loxapine 5 mg (loxapine succinate 6.8 mg), 10 mg (loxapine succinate 13.6 mg), 25 mg (loxapine succinate 34 mg), 50 mg (loxapine succinate 68.1 mg). Lactose. Cap. Bot. 100s, 1000s. *Rx.*
Use: Antipsychotic, dibenzapine derivative.

•**loxoribine.** (LOX-ore-ih-BEAN) USAN.
Use: Immunostimulant; vaccine adjuvant.

L-2-oxothiazolidine-4-carboxylic acid.
Use: Treatment of adult respiratory distress syndrome. [Orphan Drug]
See: Procysteine.

L-PAM.
See: Melphalan.

LTA 360 Kit. (Hospira) Lidocaine hydrochloride 4%. Preservative free. Soln., Top. Single-use 4 mL prefilled vial. *Rx.*
Use: Topical local anesthetic.

Lubafax. (GlaxoSmithKline) Surgical lubricant, sterile, water-soluble, nonstaining. Foil wrapper 2.7 g, 5 g. Box 144s.
Use: Lubricant.

Lubath. (Warner Lambert) Mineral oil, PPG-15, stearyl ether, oleth-2, nonoxynol 5, fragrance, FD&C Green No. 6. Bot. 4 oz, 8 oz, 16 oz. *OTC.*
Use: Emollient.

•**lubazodone hydrochloride.** (LOO-ba-zoe-done) USAN.
Use: Antidepressant; SSRI.

•**lubeluzole.** (loo-BELL-you-zole) USAN.
Use: Stroke treatment.

Lubinol. (Purepac) Light, heavy, and extra heavy mineral oil. Bot. Pt, qt, gal. (Extra heavy Bot.) 8 oz, pt, qt, gal. *OTC.*
Use: Emollient.

•**lubiprostone.** (loo-bi-PROS-tone) USAN.
Use: Treatment of chronic constipation.
See: Amitiza.

Lubraseptic Jelly. (Guardian Laboratories) Water-soluble amyl phenyl phenol complex 0.12%, phenylmercuric nitrate, 0.007%. Bellows-type tube 10 g, 24s.
Use: Genitourinary aid.

Lubricating Jelly. (Taro) Glycerin, propylene glycol. Tube. 60 g, 125 g. *OTC.*
Use: Vaginal agent.

Lubriderm. (Johnson & Johnson) Mineral oil, petrolatum, sorbitol, lanolin, lanolin alcohol, stearic acid, TEA, cetyl alcohol, fragrance (if scented), butylparaben, methylparaben, propylparaben, sodium Cl. Lot. Bot. (scented), 4 oz, 8 oz, 16 oz; (unscented) 8 oz, 16 oz. *OTC.*
Use: Emollient.

Lubriderm Daily Moisture with SPF 15. (Johnson & Johnson) Octinoxate 7.5%, octisalate 4%, oxybenzone 3%. Lot. 100 mL, 177 mL, 296 mL, 473 mL. *OTC.*
Use: Emollient.

Lubriderm Intense Skin Repair. (Johnson & Johnson) Avena sativa (oat), kernel flour, benzaldehyde (shea butter), benzalkonium chloride, C12-15 alkyl benzoate, carbomer, ceteareth-6, cetyl alcohol, citric acid, dimethicone, glycerin, glyceryl stearate, glycine soja (soybean) sterols, hydrolyzed milk protein, hydrolyzed soy protein, mineral oil, parabens, petrolatum, stearyl alcohol, tetrasodium EDTA. Cream. 141.7 g. *OTC.*
Use: Dermatological agent.

Lubriderm Skin Nourishing with Sea Kelp Extract. (Johnson & Johnson) Glycerin, glyceryl stearate SE, cetyl alcohol, emulsifying wax, petrolatum, caprylic/capric triglyceride, castor oil, octyldodecanol, dimethicone, diazolidinyl urea, propylene glycol, xanthan gum, disodium EDTA, fragrance, giant kelp leaf extract, iodopropynyl butylcarbamate. Lot. 100 mL, 177 mL, 473 mL. *OTC.*
Use: Emollient.

LubriFresh P.M. (Major) White petrolatum 83%, mineral oil 15%, lanolin oil. Preservative free. Oint. 3.5 g. *OTC.*
Use: Ocular lubricant.

Lubrin. (Kenwood) Glycerin, caprylic/capric triglyceride. Inserts. Pkg. 5s, 12s. *OTC.*
Use: Lubricant.

Lubriskin. (Geritrex) Mineral oil, petrolatum, lanolin, lanolin alcohol, cetearyl alcohol, castor oil, triethanolamine, stearyl alcohol, propylene glycol, parabens, EDTA. Lot. 240 g. *OTC.*
Use: Emollient.

LubriTears. (Bausch & Lomb) White petrolatum, mineral oil, lanolin, chlorobutanol 0.5%. Oint. Tube 3.5 g. *OTC.*
Use: Lubricant, ophthalmic.

LubriTears Solution. (Bausch & Lomb) Hydroxypropyl methylcellulose 2906 0.3%, dextran 70 0.1%, EDTA, KCl, NaCl, benzalkonium chloride 0.01%. Bot. 15 mL. *OTC.*
Use: Artificial tears.

•**lucanthone hydrochloride.** (LOO-kanthone) USAN.
Use: Antischistosomal.

•**lucatumumab.** (LOO-ka-TOOM-oo-mab) USAN.
Use: Treatment of cancer.

Lucentis. (Genentech) Ranibizumab 10 mg/mL (delivers 0.05 mL). Polysorbate 20 0.01%. Preservative free. Inj., Ophth. Single-use glass vial. Carton contains 2 mL single-use vial, one 5-micron 19-gauge × 1½-filter needle, and one 30-gauge × ½-injection needle. *Rx.*
Use: Macular degeneration.

•**lucinactant.** (loo-sin-AK-tant) USAN.
Use: Respiratory distress syndrome.

Ludent. (Sancilio) Fluoride 0.25 mg (from sodium fluoride 0.55 mg), 0.5 mg (from sodium fluoride 1.1 mg), 1 mg (from sodium fluoride 2.2 mg). Sucralose, xylitol. Dye free and sugar free. Orange flavor. Chew. Tab. 30s, 90s, blister pack 30s. *Rx.*
Use: Trace element, fluoride.

•**lufironil.** (loo-FIHR-ah-nill) USAN.
Use: Collagen inhibitor.

Lufyllin. (Medpointe) Dyphylline 200 mg. Tab. 100s. *Rx.*
Use: Bronchodilator.

Lufyllin-400. (Medpointe) Dyphylline 400 mg. Tab. 100s. *Rx.*
Use: Bronchodilator.

Lufyllin-GG. (Medpointe) Dyphylline 33.3 mg, guaifenesin 33.3 mg per 5 mL. Alcohol 17%, saccharin, sucrose. Wine flavor. Elix. Bot. 473 mL, 3785 mL. *Rx.*
Use: Antiasthmatic combination, xanthine combination.

Lugol's Solution. (Lyne) Iodine 5 g, potassium iodide 10 g, in purified water to make 100 mL. Soln. Bot. 15 mL. (Wisconsin Pharmacal Co.) Bot. Pt. *Rx-OTC.*
Use: Antithyroid; antiseptic, topical.

•**luliconazole.** (LOO-li-KON-a-zole) USAN.
Use: Antifungal agent.

•**lumefantrine.** (lue-mee-FAN-treen) USAN.
Use: Antimalarial.

Lumigan. (Allergan) Bimatoprost 0.03%, benzalkonium chloride 0.05 mg/mL. Soln. 2.5 mL, 5 mL, 7.5 mL. *Rx.*
Use: Antiglaucoma; prostaglandin agonist.

•**lumiliximab.** (loo-mil-IX-i-mab) USAN.
Use: Monoclonal antibody.

Luminal Sodium. (Hospira) Phenobarbital 60 mg, 130 mg. Alcohol 10%, propylene glycol 67.8%. Inj. 1 mL *Carpuject* with *Luer Lock. c-IV.*
Use: Hypnotic, sedative.

•**lumiracoxib.** (lue-mye-ra-KOX-ib) USAN.
Use: Rheumatoid arthritis; osteoarthritis.

Lumitene. (Tishcon Corp) Beta-carotene 30 mg. Glucose. Cap. 100s. *OTC.*
Use: Vitamin, fat-soluble vitamin.

Lumizyme. (Genzyme Corp) Alglucosidase alfa 50 mg. Mannitol 210 mg, 0.5 mg of polysorbate 80. Preservative free. Inj., lyophilized Pow. for Soln. Single-use vial. 20 mL. *Rx.*
Use: Endocrine and metabolic agent.

Lumopaque Capsules. (Sanofi-Synthelabo) Tyropanoate sodium.
Use: Radiopaque agent.

•**lunacalcipol.** (LOO-na-KAL-si-pol) USAN.
Use: Treatment of secondary hyperparathyroidism.

Lunesta. (Sepracor) Eszopiclone 1 mg, 2 mg, 3 mg. Lactose. Film-coated. Tab. 100s, cartons of 90s (except 1 mg). *c-IV.*
Use: Sedative/hypnotic, nonbarbiturate.

lung surfactants.
Use: Surfactant replacement therapy in neonatal respiratory distress syndrome.
See: Beractant.
 Calfactant.
 Poractant Alfa.

Lupron Depot. (Abbott) Leuprolide acetate 3.75, 7.5 mg. Mannitol, preservative free. Lyophilized microspheres for injection. Single kits, multi-packs, prefilled dual-chamber syringe. *Rx.*
Use: Hormone, gonadotropin-releasing hormone analog.

Lupron Depot-4 Month. (TAP Pharm) Leuprolide acetate 30 mg. Mannitol, preservative free. Microspheres for injection, lyophilized. Single-use kit w/ diluent 1.5 mL and in prefilled dual-chamber syringe. *Rx.*
Use: Hormone, gonadotropin-releasing hormone analog.

Lupron Depot-Ped. (Abbott) Leuprolide acetate 7.5 mg, 11.25 mg, 15 mg. Mannitol. Preservative free. Microspheres for Inj., lyophilized. Single-dose kit, prefilled dual-chamber syringe. *Rx.*
Use: Hormone, gonadotropin-releasing hormone analog.

Lupron Depot-3 Month. (TAP Pharm) Leuprolide acetate 11.25 mg, 22.5 mg. Mannitol, preservative free. Microspheres for Inj., lyophilized. Single-use Kit, w/diluent 1.5 mL and in prefilled dual-chamber syringe. *Rx.*
Use: Hormone, gonadotropin-releasing hormone analog.

Lupron for Pediatric Use. (TAP Pharm) Leuprolide acetate 5 mg/mL. Benzyl alcohol 9 mg/mL, sodium chloride. Inj. Multiple-dose vial 2.8 mL. *Rx.*
Use: Hormone, gonadotropin-releasing hormone analog.

Lupron Injection. (TAP) Leuprolide acetate 1 mg/0.2 mL. Vial 2.8 mL. *Rx.*
Use: Antineoplastic.

Luramide. (Major) Furosemide 20 mg, 40 mg, 80 mg. Tab. Bot. 100s, 1000s. *Rx.*
Use: Diuretic.

•**lurasidone hydrochloride.** (loo-RAS-i-done) USAN.
Use: Antipsychotic.
See: Latuda.

Luride Drops. (Colgate Oral) Sodium fluoride equivalent to 0.5 mg of fluoride. Plastic dropper bot. 50 mL. *Rx.*
Use: Dental caries agent.

Luride-F Lozi Tablets. (Colgate Oral) Sodium fluoride in Lozi base tab. available as fluoride. **0.25 mg:** Bot. 120s; **0.5 mg:** Bot. 120s, 1200s; **1 mg:** Bot. 120s, 1000s, 5000s. *Rx.*
Use: Dental caries agent.

Luride Gel. (Colgate Oral) Fluoride (from sodium fluoride and hydrogen fluoride) 1.2%. Tube 7 g. *Rx.*
Use: Dental caries agent.

Luride Lozi-Tabs. (Colgate Oral Pharmaceuticals) Sodium fluoride 0.25 mg Chew. Tab. Sugar free. Bot. 120s. *Rx.*
Use: Dental caries agent.

Luride Prophylaxis Paste. (Colgate Oral Pharmaceuticals) Acidulated phosphate sodium fluoride containing 0.4% fluoride ion w/silicon dioxide abrasive. UD 3 g, Jar 50 g. *OTC.*
Use: Dentrifice.

Luride-SF Lozi Tablets. (Colgate Oral Pharmaceuticals) Sodium fluoride equivalent to 1 mg. Bot. 120s. *Rx.*
Use: Dental caries agent.

Luride Topical Gel. (Colgate Oral Pharmaceuticals) Fluoride 1.2%. Tube 7 g. *Rx.*
Use: Dental caries agent.

Luride Topical Solution. (Colgate Oral Pharmaceuticals) Acidulated phosphate sodium fluoride w/pH 3.2. Bot. 250 mL. *OTC.*
Use: Dental caries agent.

Lurline PMS. (Fielding) Acetaminophen 500 mg, pamabrom 25 mg, pyridoxine 50 mg. Tab. Bot. 24s, 50s. *OTC.*
Use: Analgesic combination.

•**lurosetron mesylate.** (loo-ROW-set-rahn) USAN.
Use: Antiemetic.

Lurotin Caps. (BASF) Beta-carotene 25 mg. Cap. Bot. 100s. *OTC.*
Use: Nutritional supplement.

•**lurtotecan dihydrochloride.** (lure-toe-TEE-kan die-HIGH-droe-KLOR-ide) USAN.
Use: Antineoplastic (DNA topoisomerase I inhibitor).

Lusedra. (Eisai) Fospropofol disodium 35 mg/mL. Preservative free. Inj., Soln. Single-use vial. 30 mL. *Rx.*
Use: General anesthetic.

Lusonal. (Wraser) Pseudoephedrine hydrochloride 7.5 mg per 5 mL. Aspartame, parabens, phenylalanine. Liq. 473 mL. *Rx.*
Use: Decongestant.

Lustra. (Medicis) Hydroquinone 4%, glycerin, alcohol, cetyl alcohol, cetearyl alcohol, benzyl alcohol, sodium metabisulfite, EDTA. Cream. Tube. 28.4 g. *Rx.*
Use: Depigmentor.

Lustra-AF. (Medicis) Hydroquinone 4%, glycerin, alcohol, cetyl alcohol, cetearyl alcohol, benzyl alcohol, sodium metabisulfite, EDTA, octyl methoxycinnamate, arobenzone. Cream. Tube. 28.4 g. *Rx.*
Use: Depigmentor.

luteogan.
See: Progesterone.

luteosan.
See: Progesterone.

Lutera. (Watson) Ethinyl estradiol 20 mcg, levonorgestrel 0.1 mg. Lactose. Tab. 28s. 7 inert tablets. *Rx.*
Use: Contraceptive hormone, sex hormone.

lutocylol. (Novartis) Ethisterone.

Lutolin-F. (Spanner) Progesterone 25 mg, 50 mg/mL. Vial 10 mL. *Rx.*
Use: Hormone, progestin.

Lutolin-S. (Spanner) Progesterone 25 mg/mL. Vial 10 mL. *Rx.*
Use: Hormone, progestin.

•**lutrelin acetate.** (loo-TRELL-in) USAN.
Use: LHRH agonist.

lutren.
See: Progesterone.

•**lutropin alfa.** (LOO-troe-pin alfa) USAN.
Use: Ovulation stimulant.
See: Luveris.

Luveris. (Serono) Lutropin alfa 82.5 units/vial. Sucrose 48 mg. Pow. for Inj., lyophilized. Single-dose vials. Delivers 75 units lutropin alfa after reconstitution. *Rx.*
Use: Ovulation stimulant.

Luvox. (Jazz Pharmaceuticals) Fluvoxamine maleate 25 mg, 50 mg, 100 mg. Mannitol, PEG. Film-coated. Tab. 100s. *Rx.*
Use: Antidepressant, selective serotonin reuptake inhibitor.

Luvox CR. (Jazz Pharmaceuticals) Fluvoxamine maleate 100 mg, 150 mg. Sugar spheres. Gluten free. ER Cap. 30s. *Rx.*
Use: Antidepressant, selective serotonin reuptake inhibitor.

Luxiq. (GlaxoSmithKline) Betamethasone valerate 1.2 mg/g, cetyl alcohol, stearyl alcohol. Foam. Can. 100 g. *Rx.*
Use: Anti-inflammatory.

•**lyapolate sodium.** (lie-APP-oh-late) USAN.
Use: Anticoagulant.
See: Peson.

Lybrel. (Wyeth) Levonorgestrel 0.09 mg, ethinyl estradiol 20 mcg. Lactose. Film-coated. Tab. 28s. *Rx.*
Use: Sex hormone, contraceptive hormone.

•**lycetamine.** (lie-SEET-ah-meen) USAN.
Use: Antimicrobial, topical.

lycine hydrochloride.
See: Betaine hydrochloride.

Lydia E. Pinkham Herbal Compound. (Numark) Vitamin C, iron. Liq. Bot. 8 fl oz, 16 fl oz.

Lydia E. Pinkham Tablets. (Numark) Vitamin C, iron, calcium. Bot. 72s, 150s. *OTC.*

•**lydimycin.** (lie-dih-MY-sin) USAN.
Use: Antifungal.

Lymphazurin 1%. (United States Surgical Corp.) Isosulfan blue 10 mg/mL. Preservative free. Inj. Vials. 5 mL. *Rx.*
Use: Radiopaque agent, parenteral.

lymphocyte immune globulin antithymocyte globulin (equine).
Use: Immune globulin.
See: Atgam.

LymphoScan. (Immunomedics) Technetium TC-99M murine monoclonal antibody (IgG2a) to B-cell.
Use: Diagnostic aid. [Orphan Drug]

•**lynestrenol.** (lin-ESS-tree-nahl)
USP 34.
Use: Hormone, progestin.

lynoestrenol. Lynestrenol.

lyophilized vitamin B complex and vitamin C with B$_{12}$. (McGuff) B$_1$ 50 mg, B$_2$ 5 mg, B$_3$ 125 mg, B$_5$ 6 mg, B$_6$ 5 mg, B$_{12}$ 1000 mcg, C 50 mg/mL. Inj. Vial 10 mL. *Rx.*
Use: Vitamin supplement; parenteral.

Lyphocin P. (Fujisawa Healthcare) Vancomycin hydrochloride 500 mg. Vial 10 mL. *Rx.*
Use: Anti-infective.

Lypholyte. (American Pharmaceutical Partners) Na$^+$ 25 mEq, K$^+$ ≈ 40 mEq, Ca^{++} 5 mEq, Mg^{++} 8 mEq, Cl$^-$ ≈ 33 mEq, acetate ≈ 41 mEq, gluconate 5 mEq, osmolarity ≈ 7562/20 mL or 25 mL after dilution. Conc. Single-dose vial 20 mL, 40 mL, *Maxivial* (pharmacy bulk packaging) 100 mL, 200 mL. *Rx.*
Use: Intravenous nutritional therapy, intravenous replenishment solution.

Lypholyte II. (American Pharmaceutical Partners) Na$^+$ 35 mEq, K$^+$ 20 mEq, Ca^{++} 4.5 mEq, Mg^{++} 5 mEq, Cl 35 mEq, acetate 29.5 mEq, osmolarity ≈ 6200/ 20 mL or 25 mL after dilution. Single-dose vial 20 mL, 40 mL; *Maxivial* (pharmacy bulk packaging) 100 mL, 200 mL. *Rx.*
Use: Intravenous nutritional therapy, intravenous replenishment solution.

•**lypressin nasal solution.** (LIE-PRESS-in) *USP 34.*
Use: Antidiuretic; vasoconstrictor.

Lyrica. (Pfizer) **Cap.:** Pregabalin 25 mg, 50 mg, 75 mg, 100 mg, 150 mg, 200 mg, 225 mg, 300 mg. Lactose. 90s, UD 100s (50 mg, 75 mg, 100 mg, 150 mg only). **Soln.:** Pregabalin 20 mg/mL. Parabens, sucralose. Strawberry flavor. 473 mL. *c-v.*
Use: Anticonvulsant.

lysidin. Methyl glyoxalidin.

•**lysine.** (LIE-SEEN) USAN.
Use: Nutrient; rapid weight gain; amino acid.

•**lysine acetate.** (LIE-SEEN) *USP 34.*
Use: Amino acid.

•**lysine hydrochloride.** (LIE-SEEN) *USP 34.*
Use: Amino acid.
See: Enisyl.

Lysodase. (Enzon) PEG-glucocerebrosidase.
Use: Gaucher disease. [Orphan Drug]

Lysodren. (Bristol-Myers Squibb Oncology) Mitotane 500 mg. Tab. Bot. 100s. *Rx.*
Use: Antineoplastic.

•**lysostaphin.** (LIE-so-STAFF-in) USAN. Enzyme produced by *Staphylococcus staphylolyticus.*
Use: Antibiotic; antibacterial enzyme.

Lysteda. (Ferring) Tranexamic acid 650 mg. Tab. 30s, 100s, 500s, UD 30s. *Rx.*
Use: Hematological agent; hemostatic, systemic.

Lytren. (Bristol-Myers Squibb) Dextrose, sodium citrate, citric acid, sodium Cl, potassium citrate. Ready-to-use Bot. 8 fl. oz. *OTC.*
Use: Electrolyte, fluid replacement.

M

Maagel. (Health for Life Brands) Aluminum and magnesium hydroxide. Bot. 12 oz, gal. *OTC.*
Use: Antacid.

Maalox Advanced Maximum Strength. (Novartis Consumer Health) **Chew. Tab.:** Calcium carbonate 1,000 mg, simethicone 60 mg. Dextrose, maltodextrin, mannitol. Assorted fruit flavor. 35s. **Liq.:** Aluminum hydroxide 400 mg, magnesium hydroxide 400 mg, simethicone 40 mg per 5 mL. Potassium 5 mg, parabens, saccharin, sorbitol. Mint flavor. 355 mL. *OTC.*
Use: Mineral supplement; antacid.

Maalox Advanced Regular Strength. (Novartis Consumer Health) Aluminum hydroxide 200 mg, magnesium hydroxide 200 mg, simethicone 20 mg. Potassium 5 mg, parabens, saccharin sodium, sorbitol. Mint flavor. Liq. 140 mL, 355 mL, 473 mL. *OTC.*
Use: Antacid.

Maalox Children's. (Novartis Consumer Health) Calcium carbonate 400 mg (elemental calcium 160 mg). Aspartame, dextrose, maltodextrin, mannitol, phenylalanine 0.3 mg. Wild berry flavor. Chew. Tab. 32s. *OTC.*
Use: Mineral supplement.

Maalox Junior. (Novartis Consumer Health) Calcium carbonate 400 mg (elemental calcium 160 mg), simethicone 24 mg. Dextrose, maltodextrin, mannitol. Wild berry flavor. Chew. Tab. 24s. *OTC.*
Use: Antacid.

Maalox Regular Strength. (Novartis Consumer Health) Calcium carbonate 600 mg (elemental calcium 240 mg). Aspartame, dextrose, maltodextrin, mannitol. Wild berry flavor. Chew. Tab. 150s. *OTC.*
Use: Mineral supplement; antacid.

Maalox Total Relief. (Novartis Consumer Health) Bismuth subsalicylate 525 mg per 15 mL. Sodium 6 mg, parabens, sorbitol, sucralose, xanthan gum, ethyl alcohol. Strawberry flavor. Liq. 140 mL, 355 mL, 473 mL. *OTC.*
Use: Antidiarrheal.

MacPac. (Procter & Gamble) Nitrofurantoin macrocrystals 50 mg, 100 mg. Cap. UD 28s. *Rx.*
Use: Anti-infective, urinary.

macroaggregated albumin. (Bristol-Myers Squibb) Albumotope I-131.

Macrobid. (Procter & Gamble) Nitrofurantoin (as monohydrate/macrocrystals) 100 mg. Lactose, talc. Cap. Bot. 100s. *Rx.*
Use: Anti-infective, urinary.

Macrodantin. (Procter & Gamble) Nitrofurantoin macrocrystals 25 mg, 50 mg, 100 mg. Lactose, talc. Cap. Bot. 100s, 1000s. *Rx.*
Use: Anti-infective, urinary.

Macrodex. (Pharmacia) Dextran 6% w/v in normal saline, 6% w/v in Dextrose 5% in water. Bot. 500 mL. *Rx.*
Use: Plasma volume expander.

macrogol stearate 2000. Polyoxyl 40 Stearate.

macrolides.
Use: Anti-infective.
See: Azithromycin.
  Clarithromycin.
  Erythromycin.

Macrotec. (Bristol-Myers Squibb) Technetium Tc 99m Medronate kit. Vial Kit 10s.
Use: Radiopaque agent.

Macugen. (Eyetech) Pegaptanib sodium 0.3 mg (equiv. to 1.6 mg or 3.2 mg when expressed as the sodium salt form). Inj. Glass syringes. 1 mL with 27-gauge needle and shield. *Rx.*
Use: Treatment of age-related macular degeneration.

MacuTrition. (Advanced Vision Research) **Cap., softgels.:** Fish oil 0.8 g (DHA 149 mg, EPA 283.5 mg), mixed tocopherol 8.5 mg, tocotrienols 6 mg, phytosterol 0.45 mg, plant squaiane 1.25 mg, vitamin D3 1,332.5 units, vitamin E 76.5 units. 60s. **Tab.:** Cu 0.25 mg, green tea leaf extract 171 mg, lutein 8 mg, vitamin C 500 mg, zeaxanthin 2 mg, Zn 9 mg. Dextrose, maltodextrose, polydextrose. 30s. *OTC.*
Use: Nutritional supplement.

• **maduramicin.** (mad-UHR-ah-MY-sin) USAN.
Use: Anticoccidal.

• **mafenide.** (MAY-feh-NIDE) USAN.
Use: Anti-infective.

• **mafenide acetate.** (MAY-feh-NIDE) *USP 34.*
Use: Anti-infective, topical.
See: Sulfamylon.

mafenide acetate solution.
Use: Prevent graft loss on burn wounds. [Orphan Drug]

• **mafilcon A.** (MAY-fill-kahn) USAN.
Use: Contact lens material (hydrophilic).

Mafylon Cream. (Sanofi-Synthelabo) Mafenide acetate.
Use: Burn therapy.

• **magaldrate.** (MAG-al-drate) *USP 34.*

Monalium Hydrate. Aluminum Magnesium Hydroxide.
Use: Antacid.
See: Iosopan.
Lowsium.
Monalium Hydrate.
W/Simethicone.
See: Lowsium Plus.
Riopan Plus.

magaldrate plus suspension. (Various Mfr.) Magaldrate 540 mg, simethicone 40 mg/5 mL. Susp. Bot. 360 mL. *OTC.*
Use: Antacid; antiflatulent.

Magan. (Pharmacia) Magnesium salicylate (anhydrous) 545 mg. Tab. Bot. 100s, 500s. *Rx.*
Use: Analgesic.

Mag-Cal Mega. (Freeda) Mg 800 mg, Ca 400 mg, kosher, sugar free. Tab. Bot. 100s, 250s. *OTC.*
Use: Mineral, vitamin supplement.

Mag-Caps. (Genesis) Magnesium oxide ≈ 140 mg (elemental magnesium 85 mg). Cap. 100s. *OTC.*
Use: Dietary supplement.

Magdrox. (Vita Elixir) Magnesium hydroxide, aluminum hydroxide. *OTC.*
Use: Antacid.

Mag-G. (Cypress) Magnesium gluconate dihydrate 500 mg (elemental magnesium 27 mg). Tab. Bot. 100s. *OTC.*
Use: Mineral supplement.

Magmalin. (Pal-Pak, Inc.) Magnesium hydroxide 0.2 g, aluminum hydroxide gel, dried 0.2 g/Loz. Bot. 1000s. *OTC.*
Use: Antacid.

Magnacal Liquid. (Biosearch Medical Products) Protein (from calcium, sodium caseinate), carbohydrate (from maltodextrin, sucrose), fat (partially hydrogenated from soy oil, lecithin, mono- and diglycerides). 1.5 Cal/mL, 590 mOsm/kg H_2O. Protein 70 g, CHO 250 g, fat 80 g, Na 1000 mg, K 1250 mg/L. Can 120 mL, 240 mL. *OTC.*
Use: Nutritional supplement.

Magnacet. (Victory Pharma) Oxycodone hydrochloride/acetaminophen, 5 mg/400 mg, 7.5 mg/400 mg, 10 mg/400 mg. Tab. 100s. *c-II.*
Use: Narcotic analgesic.

Magnalum. (Global Source) Magnesium hydroxide 3.75 g, aluminum hydroxide 2 g. Tab. Bot. 1000s. *OTC.*
Use: Antacid.

MagneBind 400 Rx. (Nephro-Tech) Magnesium carbonate 400 mg, calcium carbonate 200 mg, folic acid 1 mg. Tab. Bot. 150s. *Rx.*
Use: Mineral supplement.

MagneBind 300. (Nephro-Tech) Magnesium carbonate 300 mg, calcium carbonate 250 mg. Tab. Bot. 150s. *OTC.*
Use: Mineral supplement.

MagneBind 200. (Nephro-Tech) Magnesium carbonate 200 mg, calcium carbonate 400 mg. Tab. Bot. 150s. *OTC.*
Use: Mineral supplement.

magnesia tablets.
Use: Antacid.

magnesia and alumina oral suspension. (Roxane) Oral Susp. 6 fl oz. 25s.
Use: Antacid.

•**magnesia, milk of.** (mag-NEE-zee-uh) *USP 34.*
Use: Antacid; laxative.

magnesium.
Use: Mineral.
See: Magnesium Citrate.
Magnesium Gluconate.
Magonate Natal.
Mag-Tab SR.
Mag-200.
Slow-Mag.

magnesium. (21st Century) Magnesium oxide 250 mg. Calcium 47 mg. Gluten free and preservative free. Tab. 110s. *OTC.*
Use: Antacid.

magnesium. (Various Mfr.) Elemental magnesium 30 mg. Tab. Bot. 100s. *OTC.*
Use: Mineral.

magnesium acetylsalicylate. Apyron, Magnespirin, Magisal, Novacetyl.
Use: Analgesic.

magnesium aluminate hydrated.
Use: Antacid.
See: Riopan.

•**magnesium aluminometasilicate.** (mag-NEE-zee-uhm ah-LOO-mihn-oh-met-uh-sill-ih-CATE) *NF 29.*

•**magnesium aluminosilicate.** (mag-NEE-zee-uhm ah-LOO-mihn-oh-sill-ih-CATE) *NF 29.*

magnesium aluminum hydroxide.
Use: Antacid.
See: Medalox Gel.

•**magnesium aluminum silicate.** (mag-NEE-zee-uhm ah-LOO-mihn-num sill-ih-CATE) *NF 29.*
Use: Pharmaceutic aid; suspending agent.

magnesium aspartate/potassium aspartate. (The Key Co.) Magnesium 90 mg (magnesium content expressed in mg elemental magnesium), potassium 90 mg. Sugar free. Cap. 100s. *OTC.*
Use: Nutritional supplement, multimineral.

- **magnesium carbonate.** (mag-NEE-zee-uhm kar-BAHN-ate) *USP 34.*
  Use: Antacid.
  W/Aluminum Hydroxide.
  See: Acid Gone.
  Gaviscon Extra Strength Antacid.
  W/Aspirin, Calcium Carbonate, Magnesium Oxide.
  See: Bayer Plus, Extra Strength.
  Bufferin.
  Bufferin Extra Strength.
  W/Combinations.
  See: Antacid #2.
  MagneBind 400 Rx.
  MagneBind 300.
  MagneBind 200.
  Marblen.
- **magnesium chloride.** (mag-NEE-zee-uhm) *USP 34.*
  Use: Electrolyte replacement; pharmaceutical necessity for hemodialysis and peritoneal dialysis.
  See: Chloromag.
- **magnesium citrate.** (mag-NEE-zee-uhm) *USP 34.*
  Use: Cathartic; laxative.
  magnesium citrate. (Various Mfr.) Elemental magnesium 100 mg. Tab. Bot. 100s, 250s. *OTC.*
  Use: Mineral.
  magnesium citrate solution. (Humco Holding Group) Magnesium citrate 1.75 g/30 mL, saccharine, cherry, lemon flavors. Soln. Bot. 2% mL. *OTC.*
  Use: Laxative.
- **magnesium gluconate.** (mag-NEE-zee-um glu-ca-nate) *USP 34.*
  Use: Vitamin supplement, replacement.
  See: Mag-G.
  Magonate.
  Magtrate.
  magnesium gluconate. (Various Mfr.) Elemental magnesium 27.5 mg. Tab. Bot. 100s, 500s. *OTC.*
  Use: Mineral.
  magnesium hydroxide. (mag-NEE-zee-uhm) *USP 34.*
  Use: Antacid; cathartic; laxative.
  See: Dulcolax.
  Magnesia Magma.
  Milk of Magnesia.
  Pedia-Lax.
  Phillips' Chewable.
  Phillips' Milk of Magnesia.
  W/Aluminum Hydroxide, Simethicone.
  See: Maalox Advanced Maximum Strength.
  Maalox Advanced Regular Strength.
  Mi-Acid Maximum Strength.

W/Aspirin, Aluminum Hydroxide, Calcium Carbonate.
See: Ascriptin Maximum Strength.
W/Calcium Carbonate, Famotidine.
See: Dual Action Complete.
Tums Dual Action.
W/Combinations.
See: Aludrox.
Ascriptin.
Delcid.
Gas Ban DS.
Maagel.
Mylanta Gelcaps.
Mylanta Supreme.
Mylanta Ultra.
Pepcid Complete.
Rolaids.
Rolaids Extra Strength.
Rolaids Multi-Symptom.
Trial AG.
magnesium-L-aspartate.
Use: Mineral.
- **magnesium oxide.** (mag-NEE-zee-uhm) *USP 34.*
  Use: Pharmaceutic aid (sorbent).
  See: Mag-Caps.
  Mag-Ox 400.
  Niko-Mag.
  Phillips'.
  Uro-Mag.
  W/Aspirin, Calcium Carbonate, Magnesium Carbonate.
  See: Bufferin.
  Bufferin Extra Strength.
  Bayer Plus, Extra Strength.
  magnesium oxide. (Manne) Magnesium oxide 420 mg. Tab. Bot. 250s, 1000s. *OTC.*
  Use: Mineral.
  magnesium oxide. (Stanlabs) Magnesium oxide 10 g. Tab. Bot. 100s, 1000s. *OTC.*
  Use: Mineral.
  magnesium oxide. (Various Mfr.) Magnesium oxide 400 mg (elemental magnesium 241.3 mg). Tab. 120s, 400s. *OTC.*
  Use: Dietary supplement.
- **magnesium phosphate.** (mag-NEE-zee-uhm) *USP 34.*
  Use: Antacid.
- **magnesium salicylate.** (mag-NEE-zee-uhm suh-LIH-sih-late) *USP 34.*
  Use: Analgesic; antipyretic; antirheumatic.
  See: Doan's.
  Magan.
  W/Combinations.
  See: Durabac Forte.
  W/Diphenhydramine Hydrochloride.
  See: Extra Strength Doan's PM.

magnesium salicylate tetrahydrate.
Use: Nonnarcotic analgesic.
See: Backache Maximum Strength
Relief.
Bayer Select Maximum Strength
Backache.
Momentum Muscular Backache
Formula.
Painaid BRF Back Relief Formula.

•**magnesium silicate.** (mag-NEE-zee-uhm sill-IH-cate) *NF 29.*
Use: Pharmaceutic aid (tablet excipient).

•**magnesium stearate.** (mag-NEE-zee-uhm STEER-ate) *NF 29.*
Use: Pharmaceutic aid (tablet and capsule lubricant).

•**magnesium sulfate.** (mag-NEE-zee-uhm) *USP 34.*
Use: Anticonvulsant; electrolyte replacement; laxative.
W/Potassium Sulfate, Sodium Sulfate.
See: Suprep Bowel Prep.

magnesium sulfate. (Abbott) Magnesium sulfate (as heptahydrate) 4%
(0.325 mEq/mL), 8% (0.65 mEq/mL).
Inj. Single-dose flexible containers.
50 mL (8% only); 100 mL, 500 mL,
1000 mL (except 8%). *Rx.*
Use: Anticonvulsant.

magnesium sulfate. (Various Mfr.) Magnesium sulfate (as heptahydrate). Inj.
12.5%: (1 mEq/mL). Preservative-free.
Single-dose vials. 8 mL. **50%:** (4 mEq/
mL). Preservative-free. Single-dose
amps. 2 mL, 10 mL. Single-dose vials.
2 mL, 10 mL, 20 mL. Multidose vials.
50 mL. Syringes. 5 mL, 10 mL. *Rx.*
Use: Anticonvulsant; electrolyte replacement; laxative.

•**magnesium trisilicate.** (mag-NEE-zee-uhm try-SILL-ih-cate) *USP 34.*
Use: Antacid.
See: Banacid.
W/Aluminum hydroxide gel.
See: Gacid.
Gaviscon.
Maracid 2.

Magnevist. (Bayer Healthcare Pharma)
Gadopentetate dimeglumine
469.01 mg/mL. Preservative free. Inj.
Pharmacy bulk pkg. 100 mL. *Rx.*
Use: Radiopaque agent, parenteral.

Magonate. (Fleming) **Tab.:** Magnesium
gluconate dihydrate 500 mg (elemental magnesium 27 mg), Ca 87.5 mg,
P 66 mg (dibasic calcium phosphate dihydrate 376 mg). Bot. 1000s. **Liq.:**
Magnesium gluconate dihydrate
1000 mg/5 mL (elemental magnesium
54 mg/5 mL), sorbitol, magnesium
carbonate, melon flavored. Bot. 473 mL.
OTC.
Use: Mineral supplement.

Magonate Natal. (Fleming) Elemental
magnesium 3.52 mg (as gluconate)/mL.
Liq. Bot. 480 mL. *OTC.*
Use: Mineral.

Mag-Ox 400. (Blaine) Magnesium oxide
400 mg (elemental magnesium
241.3 mg). Tab. Bot. 120s, 1000s, UD
100s. *OTC.*
Use: Antacid; vitamin, mineral supplement.

Mag-Tab SR. (Niche) Elemental magnesium (as L-lactate dihydrate) 84 mg.
SR Tab. 60s, 100s, 1000s. *OTC.*
Use: Mineral supplement.

Magtrate. (Mission) Magnesium gluconate 500 mg (elemental magnesium
29 mg). Tab. Bot. 100s. *OTC.*
Use: Mineral supplement.

Mag-200. (Optimox) Elemental magnesium (as oxide) 200 mg, PABA 300 mg.
Tab. Bot. 120s. *OTC.*
Use: Mineral supplement.

Maintenance Vitamin Formula w/Minerals. (Towne) Vitamins A palmitate
10,000 units, D 400 units, B_1 5 mg, B_2
2.5 mg, C 75 mg, niacinamide 40 mg,
B_6 1 mg, calcium pantothenate 4 mg,
B_{12} 2 mcg, E 2 units, choline bitartrate
31.4 mg, inositol 15 mg, Ca 75 mg, P
58 mg, Fe 30 mg, Mg 3 mg, Mn 0.5 mg,
K 2 mg, Zn 0.5 mg. Cap. Bot. 100s.
OTC.
Use: Mineral, vitamin supplement.

majeptil. Thioproperazine. Psychopharmacologic agent; pending release.

Major-gesic. (Major) Phenyltoloxamine
citrate 30 mg, acetaminophen 325 mg.
Tab. Bot. 100s, 1000s. *OTC.*
Use: Upper respiratory combination, antihistamine, analgesic.

Makena. (Ther-Rx) Hydroxyprogesterone
caproate 250 mg/mL. Benzyl alcohol,
benzyl benzoate, castor oil. Inj., Soln.
Multidose vial. 5 mL. *Rx.*
Use: Sex hormone, progestin.

Malaraquin. (Sanofi-Synthelabo) Chloroquine phosphate. *Rx.*
Use: Antimalarial.

Malarone. (GlaxoSmithKline) Atovaquone 250 mg, proguanil hydrochloride
100 mg. Film-coated. Tab. Bot. 100s,
UD 24s. *Rx.*
Use: Antimalarial.

Malarone Pediatric. (GlaxoSmithKline)
Atovaquone 62.5 mg, proguanil hydrochloride 25 mg. Film-coated. Tab. Bot.
100s. *Rx.*
Use: Antimalarial.

•**malathion.** (mal-ah-THIGH-ahn) *USP 34.*
Use: Pediculicide.

malathion. (Various Mfr) Malathion 0.5%
(in a vehicle of isopropyl alcohol 78%,
terpineol, dipentene, and pine needle
oil). Lot. 59 mL. *Rx.*
Use: Dermatological agent, scabicide/
pediculicide.

•**malic acid.** (MAL-ik) *NF 29.*
Use: Pharmaceutic aid (acidifying
agent).

Mallergan-VC w/Codeine Syrup. (Roberts) Phenylephrine hydrochloride
5 mg, promethazine hydrochloride
6.25 mg, codeine phosphate 10 mg/
5 mL, alcohol 7%. Syrup. Bot. 120 mL.
c-v.
Use: Antihistamine, antitussive, decongestant.

Malogen Cyp. (Forest) Testosterone
cypionate in oil 100 mg, 200 mg/mL. Inj.
Vial 10 mL. *c-III.*
Use: Androgen.

Malogen Injection Aqueous. (Forest)
Testosterone. **25 mg/mL:** 10 mL,
30 mL. **50 mg/mL:** 10 mL. **100 mg/mL:**
10 mL. *c-III.*
Use: Androgen.

Malogen 100 L.A. in Oil. (Forest) Testosterone enanthate 100 mg/mL. Inj.
10 mL. *c-III.*
Use: Androgen.

Malogen 200 L.A. in Oil. (Forest) Testosterone enanthate 200 mg/mL. Inj.
10 mL. *c-III.*
Use: Androgen.

malonal. (Various Mfr.) Barbital.

•**malotilate.** (mal-OH-tih-LATE) USAN.
Use: Liver disorder treatment.

Malotrone Aqueous Injection. (Bluco)
Testosterone, USP 25 mg, 50 mg/mL
in aqueous susp. Vial 10 mL. *c-III.*
Use: Androgen.

•**maltitol solution.** (MAL-tih-tahl) *NF 29.*
Use: Sweetener.

•**maltodextrin.** (MAWL-toe-DEX-trin)
NF 29.
Use: Pharmaceutic aid (coating agent,
tablet binder, tablet and capsule diluent, viscosity-increasing agent).

•**maltose.** (MAWL-toes) *NF 29.*
Use: Pharmaceutic aid.

Maltsupex. (Wallace) Malt soup extract
8 g/level scoop. Pow. Can. 227 g,
454 g. *OTC.*
Use: Laxative.

Mammol Ointment. (Abbott) Bismuth
subnitrate 40%, castor oil 30%, anhydrous lanolin 22%, ceresin wax 7%,
balsam Peru 1%. Tube ⅞ oz. Ctn. 12s.

OTC.
Use: Dermatologic; protectant; emollient.

mandameth. (Major) Methenamine mandelate 0.5 g. EC Tab. Bot. 1000s. *Rx.*
Use: Anti-infective, urinary.

mandelic acid.
Use: Anti-infective, urinary.

mandelic acid salts. (Various Mfr.) Calcium mandelate.

mandelyltropeine. (Various Mfr.) Homatropine Salts.

•**mangafodipir trisodium.** (man-gah-
FOE-dih-pihr try-SO-dee-uhm) *USP 34.*
Use: Radiopaque agent, parenteral.

manganese.
Use: Dietary supplement.
See: Chelated Manganese.
Mangimin.

•**manganese chloride.** (MANG-ah-neese)
USP 34. For Oral Solution.
Use: Manganese deficiency treatment;
trace mineral supplement.

•**manganese gluconate.** (MANG-ah-
neese GLOO-kahn-ate) *USP 34.*
Use: Manganese deficiency; trace mineral supplement.

manganese glycerophosphate. Glycerol phosphate manganese salt.
Use: Pharmaceutical necessity.

manganese hypophosphite. Manga-
nese⁺⁺ phosphinate.
Use: Pharmaceutical necessity.

•**manganese sulfate.** (MANG-ah-neese)
USP 34.
Use: Trace mineral supplement.

Manga-Pak. (SoloPak Pharmaceuticals,
Inc.) Manganese 0.1 mg/mL. Inj. Vial
10 mL, 30 mL. *Rx.*
Use: Nutritional supplement, parenteral.

Mangimin. (The Key Company) Manganese 10 mg. Tab. 100s. *OTC.*
Use: Nutrient and nutritional agent,
trace element.

Maniron. (Jones Pharma) Ferrous fumarate 3 mg. Tab. Bot. 100s, 1000s,
5000s. *OTC.*
Use: Mineral supplement.

Mannan. (Rugby) Purified glucomannan
500 mg. Cap. Bot. 90s. *OTC.*
Use: Nutritional supplement.

**Mann Astringent Mouth Wash Concen-
trate.** (Manne) Bot. 4 oz, qt, 0.5 gal, gal.
Mint flavored. Bot. 4 oz, qt, 0.5 gal, gal.
OTC.
Use: Mouthwash.

manna sugar. (Various Mfr.) Mannitol.

Mann Body Deodorant. (Manne) Bot.
4 oz, 8 oz, pt, qt. *OTC.*
Use: Deodorant.

Mann Breath Deodorant. (Manne) Bot. 1 oz, 4 oz, 8 oz, pt, qt, 0.5 gal. *OTC.*
Use: Mouthwash.
Mann Emollient. (Manne) Jar. 100 g. *OTC.*
Use: Emollient.
Mannest. (Manne) Conjugated estrogens 0.625 mg, 1.25 mg, or 2.5 mg. Tab. Bot. 100s, 200s. *Rx.*
Use: Estrogen.
Mann Eugenol U.S.P. Extra. (Manne) 0.06 lb, 0.13 lb, 0.25 lb, 0.5 lb, 1 lb. *OTC.*
Use: Dermatologic, protectant.
Mann Germicidal Solution. (Manne) **Regular:** Bot. Gal, 4 gal. **Conc.:** 12.8%. Bot. Pt, qt, 0.5 gal, gal. *OTC.*
Use: Antimicrobial.
Mann Hand Lotion. (Manne) Twin pack, gal. *OTC.*
Use: Emollient.
Mann Hemostatic. (Manne) Bot. 1 oz, 4 oz, 8 oz, pt, qt. *OTC.*
Use: Hemostatic.
mannite.
See: Mannitol.
•**mannitol.** (MAN-ih-tole) *USP 34.*
Use: Diagnostic aid.
See: Osmitrol.
mannitol and sorbitol.
See: Sorbitol-Mannitol.
mannitol hexanitrate.
Use: Coronary vasodilator.
See: Vascunitol.
W/Phenobarbital.
See: Manotensin.
  Vascused.
mannitol hexanitrate and phenobarbital tablets. (Jones Pharma) Mannitol hexanitrate 0.5 g, phenobarbital 0.25 g. Tab. Bot. 1000s. *c-IV.*
Use: Vasodilator.
mannitol injection. (Abbott) Mannitol 15%, 20%. *Abbo-Vac* single-dose container 500 mL.
Use: Diagnostic aid (renal function determination); diuretic.
mannitol in sodium chloride injection.
Use: Diuretic.
Mann Liquid Soap. (Manne) Concentrated cococastile. Bot. Qt, 0.5 gal, gal. *OTC.*
Use: Emollient.
Mann Lubricant and Cleanser. (Manne) Bot. Pt, qt. *OTC.*
Use: Emollient.
Mann Superfatted Bar Soap. (Manne) Rich in lanolin. Cake. 12s. *OTC.*
Use: Emollient.
Mann Talbot's Iodine. (Manne) Glycerin

base. Bot. 1 oz, 4 oz, 8 oz, pt, qt. *OTC.*
Use: Antiseptic.
Mann Topical Anesthetic. (Manne) Bot. 1 oz, 4 oz, 8 oz, pt. W/stain to indicate area treated. Bot. 1 oz, 4 oz, 8 oz. *OTC.*
Use: Anesthetic, local.
Manotensin. (Oxypure) Mannitol hexanitrate 32 mg, phenobarbital 16 mg. Tab. Bot. 100s, 1000s. *c-IV.*
Use: Vasodilator.
Mantoux Test.
Use: Tuberculin test.
manvene.
Use: Antineoplastic.
MAOI.
See: Monoamine Oxidase Inhibitors.
Maox 420. (Manne) Magnesium oxide 420 mg. Tab. Bot. 250s, 1000s. *OTC.*
Use: Antacid.
Mapap. (Major) Acetaminophen. **Cap.:** 500 mg. 24s, 50s, 100s, 175s, 500s, 1000s. **Tab.:** 500 mg. Tab. Bot. 24s, 50s, 100s, 175s, 500s, 1000s. **Tab., Rapid Release:** 500 mg. 24s, 50s, 100s, 175s, 500s, 1000s. *OTC.*
Use: Analgesic.
Mapap Arthritis Pain. (Major) Acetaminophen 650 mg. ER Tab. 100s. *OTC.*
Use: Analgesic.
Mapap Children's. (Major) **Chew. Tab.:** Acetaminophen 80 mg. Aspartame, mannitol, phenylalanine 3 mg, sucrose. Grape, fruit, and bubble gum flavors. 30s. **Elix.:** Acetaminophen 160 mg/5 mL. Alcohol free. Sorbitol, sucrose. Cherry flavor. Bot. 118 mL. *OTC.*
Use: Analgesic.
Mapap Cold Formula Multi-Symptom. (Major) Acetaminophen 325 mg, phenylephrine hydrochloride 5 mg, dextromethorphan HBr 10 mg. Polyvinyl alcohol, sucralose. Tab. Pkg. 24s. *OTC.*
Use: Upper respiratory combination, antitussive combination.
Mapap Infant. (Major) Acetaminophen 100 mg/mL. Alcohol free. Cherry flavor. Soln., Conc., Oral. Bot. 15 mL, 30 mL. *OTC.*
Use: Analgesic.
Mapap Junior Strength. (Major) Acetaminophen 160 mg. Grape flavor. Chew. Tab. 24s. *OTC.*
Use: Analgesic.
Mapap Regular Strength. (Major) Acetaminophen 325 mg. Tab. Bot. 100s, 1000s, UD 100s. *OTC.*
Use: Analgesic.
Mapap Sinus Congestion and Pain Maximum Strength. (Major) Phenylephrine hydrochloride 5 mg, aceta-

minophen 325 mg. Acesulfame K. Tab. 24s. *OTC.*
Use: Upper respiratory combination, decongestant and analgesic combination.

Mapap Sinus Maximum Strength. (Major) Pseudoephedrine hydrochloride 30 mg, acetaminophen 500 mg. PEG. Tab. Pkg. 24s. *OTC.*
Use: Upper respiratory combination, decongestant, analgesic.

• **mapatumumab.** (MAP-a-TOOM-ue-mab) USAN.
Use: Antineoplastic.

Maprofix.
See: Gardinol Type Detergents.

• **maprotiline.** (map-ROW-tih-leen) USAN.
Use: Antidepressant.

• **maprotiline hydrochloride.** (map-ROW-tih-leen) *USP 34.*
Use: Antidepressant, tetracyclic compound.

maprotiline hydrochloride. (Mylan) Maprotiline hydrochloride 25 mg, 50 mg, 75 mg. PEG, polydextrose. Film coated. Tab. 100s. *Rx.*
Use: Antidepressant, tetracyclic compound.

• **maraciclatide.** (MAR-a-SIK-la-tide) USAN.
Use: Diagnostic agent.

Maracid 2. (Marlin Industries) Magnesium trisilicate 150 mg, aluminum hydroxide dried gel 90 mg, aminoacetic acid 75 mg. Tab. Bot. *OTC.*
Use: Antacid; adsorbent.

maraviroc. (mah-RAV-er-rock)
Use: Antiretroviral, cellular chemokine receptor antagonist.
See: Selzentry.

Marbaxin 750. (Vortech Pharmaceuticals) Methocarbamol 750 mg. Tab. Bot. 500s. *Rx.*
Use: Muscle relaxant.

Marblen Liquid. (Fleming & Co.) Magnesium carbonate 400 mg, calcium carbonate 520 mg/5 mL. Bot. 473 mL. *OTC.*
Use: Antacid.

Marblen Tablets. (Fleming & Co.) Calcium carbonate 520 mg, magnesium carbonate 400 mg. Tab. Bot. 100s, 1000s. *OTC.*
Use: Antacid.

Marcaine. (Eastman-Kodak) Bupivacaine 0.5%, epinephrine 1:200,000, sodium metabisulfite, EDTA 0.1 mg/mL. Inj. Dental Cart. 1.8 mL. *Rx.*
Use: Anesthetic, local amide.

Marcaine. (Hospira) Bupivacaine hydrochloride. Multiple-dose vial also contains methylparaben 1 mg/mL as preservative. **0.25%:** Single-dose amp. 50 mL. Single-dose vial 10 mL, 30 mL. Multiple-dose vial 50 mL. **0.5%:** Single-dose amp. 30 mL. Single-dose vial 10 mL, 30 mL. Multiple-dose vial 50 mL. **0.75%:** Single-dose amp. 30 mL. Single-dose vial 10 mL, 30 mL. **0.25% with epinephrine 1:200,000:** Sodium metabisulfite 0.5 mg, edetate calcium disodium 0.1 mg. Amp. 50 mL, 5s. Vial 10 mL, 30 mL, 50 mL (methylparaben 1 mg/mL). **0.5% with epinephrine 1:200,000:** Sodium metabisulfite 0.5 mg, edetate calcium disodium 0.1 mg. Single-dose amp. 3 mL, 30 mL. Single-dose vial 10 mL, 30 mL. **0.75% with epinephrine 1:200,000:** Sodium metabisulfite 0.5 mg, edetate calcium disodium 0.1 mg. Amp. 30 mL. Inj. *Rx.*
Use: Anesthetic, local amide.

Marcillin. (Marnel) Ampicillin trihydrate 500 mg. Cap. Bot. 100s. *Rx.*
Use: Anti-infective; penicillin.

Mar-Cof BP. (Marnel Pharmaceutical) Brompheniramine maleate 2 mg, codeine phosphate 7.5 mg, pseudoephedrine hydrochloride 30 mg. Magnasweet, saccharin, sorbitol. Alcohol free and sugar free. Liq. 473 mL. *c-v.*
Use: Upper respiratory combination, antitussive combination.

Mar-Cof-CG. (Marnel) Codeine phosphate 7.5 mg, guaifenesin 225 mg per 5 mL. PEG, saccharin, sorbitol. Alcohol free and sugar free. Liq. 473 mL. *c-v.*
Use: Upper respiratory combination, antitussive with expectorant.

Mardon. (Armenpharm Ltd.) Propoxyphene hydrochloride. **Cap.:** 32 mg Bot. 100s, 1000s. **65 mg:** Bot. 100s, 500s, 1000s. *c-iv.*
Use: Analgesic; narcotic.

Mardon Compound. (Armenpharm Ltd.) Propoxyphene compound 65 mg, aspirin 3.5 g, phenacetin 2.5 g, caffeine 0.5 g. Cap. Bot. 100s, 500s, 1000s. *c-iv.*
Use: Analgesic combination; narcotic.

Marezine. (Himmel) Cyclizine hydrochloride 50 mg. Tab. Bot. 100s. Box 12s. *OTC.*
Use: Anticholinergic.

Margesic. (Marnel) Butalbital 50 mg, acetaminophen 325 mg, caffeine 40 mg. Cap. Bot. 100s. *Rx.*
Use: Analgesic; hypnotic; sedative.

Margesic H. (Marnel) Hydrocodone bitartrate 5 mg, acetaminophen 500 mg. Cap. Bot. 100s. *c-iii.*
Use: Analgesic combination; narcotic.

Margesic No. 3. (Marnel) Codeine phosphate 30 mg, acetaminophen 300 mg. Tab. Bot. 100s. *c-III.*
Use: Analgesic combination; narcotic.
•**marimastat.** (mah-RIH-mah-stat) USAN.
Use: Antineoplastic (matrix metalloproteinase inhibitor).
Marine Lipid Concentrate. (Vitaline) Omega-3 1200 mg, EPA 360 mg, DHA 240 mg, E 5 units/Cap., sodium free. Bot. 90s. *OTC.*
Use: Nutritional supplement.
Marinol. (Unimed) Dronabinol 2.5 mg, 5 mg, 10 mg, in sesame oil. Parabens. Gelatin Cap. Bot. 25s, 60s (except 5 mg), 100s (except 10 mg). *c-III.*
Use: Antiemetic, antivertigo agent.
•**maritime pine.** (mair-ih-time) *NF 29.*
Use: Pharmaceutic aid.
•**marizomib.** (MAR-i-ZOE-mib) USAN.
Use: Antineoplastic.
Marlyn Formula 50. (Marlyn Nutraceuticals) Vitamin B$_6$ with 18 amino acids. Cap. Bot. 100s, 250s, 1000s. *OTC.*
Use: Nutritional supplement.
Marnatal-F. (Marnel) Ca 250 mg, Fe 60 mg, vitamins A 4000 units, D 400 units, E 30 mg, B$_1$ 3 mg, B$_2$ 3.4 mg, B$_3$ 20 mg, B$_6$ 5 mg, B$_{12}$ 12 mcg, C 100 mg, folic acid 1 mg, Mg, Zn 25 mg, Cu, I. Tab. Bot. 30s, 100s. *Rx.*
Use: Mineral, vitamin supplement; dental caries agent.
•**maropitant citrate.** (mar-oh-PIT-ant) USAN.
Use: Antiemetic.
Marplan. (Validus) Isocarboxazid 10 mg. Lactose. Tab. Bot. 100s. *Rx.*
Use: Antidepressant.
Mar-Spas. (Marnel) L-hyoscyamine sulfate 0.25 mg. Aspartame, phenylalanine 3.5 mg. Spearmint flavor. Orally Disintegrating Tab. 100s. *Rx.*
Use: Gastrointestinal anticholinergic/antispasmodic.
Marten-Tab. (Marnel) Butalbital 50 mg, acetaminophen 325 mg. Tab. Bot. 100s. *Rx.*
Use: Analgesic.
Marthritic. (Marnel) Salsalate 750 mg. Tab. Bot. 100s. *Rx.*
Use: Analgesic.
Masophen. (Mason) Acetaminophen 325 mg, 500 mg. Tab. 100s. *OTC.*
Use: Analgesic.
Masophen Extra Strength. (Mason) Acetaminophen 500 mg. Cap. 100s. *OTC.*
Use: Analgesic.

Masse Breast Cream. (Johnson & Johnson) Glyceryl monostearate, glycerin, cetyl alcohol, lanolin, peanut oil, Span-60, stearic acid, Tween-60, sodium benzoate, propylparaben, methylparaben, potassium hydroxide. Tube 2 oz. *OTC.*
Use: Emollient.
Massengill Baking Soda Freshness. (GlaxoSmithKline) Sanitized water, sodium bicarbonate. Soln. Bot. 180 mL. *OTC.*
Use: Vaginal agent.
Massengill Disposable Douche. (GlaxoSmithKline) Water, SD alcohol 40, lactic acid, sodium lactate, octoxynol-9, cetylpyridinium chloride, propylene glycol, diazolidinyl urea, EDTA, parabens, fragrance, color. Bot. 180 mL. *OTC.*
Use: Vaginal agent.
Massengill Extra Cleansing w/Puraclean. (GlaxoSmithKline) Vinegar, water, cetylpyridinium chloride, diazolidinyl urea, EDTA. Soln. Bot. 180 mL. *OTC.*
Use: Vaginal agent.
Massengill Feminine Cleansing Wash. (GlaxoSmithKline) Sodium laureth sulfate, magnesium oleth sulfate, sodium oleth sulfate, magnesium oleth sulfate, PEG-120 methyl glucose dioleate, parabens. Liq. Bot. 240 mL. *OTC.*
Use: Vaginal agent.
Massengill Feminine Deodorant Spray. (GlaxoSmithKline) Aerosol Bot. 3 oz. *OTC.*
Use: Vaginal agent.
Massengill Liquid. (GlaxoSmithKline) Lactic acid, SD alcohol 40, octoxynol-9, water, sodium bicarbonate. Bot. 120 mL. *OTC.*
Use: Vaginal agent.
Massengill Medicated. (GlaxoSmithKline) Povidone-iodine 0.3% when added to sanitized fluid. Bot. 6 oz. *OTC.*
Use: Vaginal agent.
Massengill Medicated Disposable Douche w/Cepticin. (GlaxoSmithKline) Povidone-iodine 10%. Liq. Vial 5 mL w/180 mL bot. of sanitized water. *OTC.*
Use: Vaginal agent.
Massengill Medicated Douche w/Cepticin. (GlaxoSmithKline) Povidone-iodine 12%. Liq. concentrate. Bot. 120 mL, 240 mL. *OTC.*
Use: Vaginal agent.
Massengill Powder. (GlaxoSmithKline) Ammonium alum, PEG-8, methyl salicylate, eucalyptus oil, menthol, thymol, phenol. Jar 120 g, 240 g, 480 g, 660 g. UD Packette 10s, 12s. *OTC.*
Use: Vaginal agent.

Massengill Soft Cloth. (GlaxoSmith-Kline) Hydrocortisone 0.5%, diazolidinyl urea, DMDM hydantoin, isopropyl myristate, methylparaben, polysorbate 60, propylene glycol, propylparaben, sorbitan stearate, steareth-2, steareth-21. Towelettes 10s. *OTC.*
Use: Vaginal agent.

Massengill Unscented. (GlaxoSmith-Kline) Water, SD alcohol 40, lactic acid, sodium lactate, octoxynol-9, cetylpyridinium chloride, propylene glycol, diazolidinyl urea, parabens, EDTA. Soln. Bot. 180 mL. *OTC.*
Use: Vaginal agent.

Massengill Vinegar & Water Extra Cleansing with Puraclean. (Glaxo-SmithKline) Vinegar, water, cetylpyridinium chloride, diazolidinyl urea, EDTA. Soln. Bot. 180 mL. *OTC.*
Use: Vaginal agent.

Massengill Vinegar & Water Extra Mild. (GlaxoSmithKline) Vinegar, water, preservative free. Soln. Bot. 180 mL. *OTC.*
Use: Vaginal agent.

Massengill Vinegar-Water Disposable Douche. (GlaxoSmithKline) Water and vinegar solution. Bot. 180 mL. *OTC.*
Use: Vaginal agent.

mast cell stabilizer.
Use: Ophthalmic agent.
See: Bepotastine Besilate.
    Cromolyn Sodium.
    Pemirolast Potassium.

Master Formula. (Barth's) Vitamins A 10,000 units, D 400 units, C 180 mg, B_1 7 mg, B_2 14 mg, niacin 4.6 mg, B_6 292 mcg, pantothenic acid 210 mcg, B_{12} 25 mcg, biotin 2.9 mcg, E 50 units, Ca 800 mg, P 387 mg, Fe 10 mg, I 0.1 mg, Cl 7.78 mg, inositol 11.6 mg, aminobenzoic acid 35 mcg, rutin 30 mg, citrus bioflavonoid complex 30 mg/4 Tab. Bot. 120s, 600s, 1200s. *OTC.*
Use: Mineral, vitamin supplement.

Mastisol. (Ferndale) Nonirritating medical adhesive. Bot. 4 oz.
Use: Adhesive.

matrix metalloproteinase inhibitor.
Use: Corneal ulcers. [Orphan Drug]

Matulane. (Sigma-Tau) Procarbazine hydrochloride 50 mg. Talc, mannitol, parabens. Cap. Bot. 100s. *Rx.*
Use: Antineoplastic.

Matzim LA. (Watson Pharma) Diltiazem hydrochloride 180 mg, 240 mg, 300 mg, 360 mg, and 420 mg. Lactose, sucrose. ER Tab. 30s, 90s, 1,000s. *Rx.*
Use: Calcium channel blocking agent.

• **mavacoxib.** (MAY-va-KOX-ib) USAN.
Use: Anti-inflammatory; analgesic.

Mavik. (Abbott) Trandolapril 1 mg, 2 mg, 4 mg, lactose. Tab. Bot. 100s, UD 100s. *Rx.*
Use: Antihypertensive; renin angiotensin system antagonist; angiotensin-converting enzyme inhibitor.

• **mavrilimumab.** (MAV-ri-LIM-ue-mab) USAN.
Use: Antirheumatic agent.

Maxair Autohaler. (Graceway) Pirbuterol acetate 0.2 mg/actuation. Aer. Autohaler 2.8 g (80 inhalations), 14 g (400 inhalations). *Rx.*
Use: Bronchodilator, sympathomimetic.

Maxalt. (Merck) Rizatriptan benzoate 5 mg, 10 mg, lactose. Tab. Unit-of-use carrying case 6s. *Rx.*
Use: Antimigraine, serotonin 5-HT$_1$ receptor agonist.

Maxalt-MLT. (Merck) Rizatriptan benzoate 5 mg, 10 mg, lyophilized, mannitol, aspartame, phenylalanine 1.05 mg (5 mg only), 2.1 mg (10 mg only). Orally disintegrating Tab. 2 unit-of-use carrying cases of 3 tabs (6 tabs total). *Rx.*
Use: Antimigraine, serotonin, 5-HT$_1$ receptor agonist.

Max EPA. (Various Mfr.) Omega-3 polyunsaturated fatty acids 1000 mg. Cap. containing EPA 180 mg, DHA 60 mg. Cap. Bot. 50s, 60s, 100s. *OTC.*
Use: Nutritional supplement.

Maxichlor PEH DM. (MCR American) Chlorpheniramine maleate 4 mg, dextromethorphan hydrobromide 20 mg, phenylephrine hydrochloride 10 mg. Tab. 100s. *Rx.*
Use: Upper respiratory combination, antitussive combination.

Maxidex. (Alcon) Dexamethasone 0.1%. Benzalkonium chloride 0.01%, EDTA, hypromellose 0.5%, polysorbate 80, sodium chloride, dibasic sodium phosphate. Ophth. Susp. *Drop-Tainers* 5 mL, 15 mL. *Rx.*
Use: Corticosteroid, ophthalmic.

Maxidone. (Watson) Hydrocodone bitartrate 10 mg, acetaminophen 750 mg, lactose. Tab. Bot. 100s, 500s. *c-III.*
Use: Narcotic analgesic combination.

Maxifed. (MCR American) Guaifenesin 400 mg, pseudoephedrine hydrochloride 60 mg. ER Tab. Bot. 100s. *Rx.*
Use: Upper respiratory combination, decongestant, expectorant.

Maxifed DM. (MCR American) **Liq.:** Dextromethorphan hydrobromide 10 mg, guaifenesin 200 mg, pseudoephedrine hydrochloride 20 mg per 5 mL. Alcohol 0.1%, parabens, sorbitol, sucralose.

Sugar free. Orange cream flavor. 473 mL. **Tab.:** Dextromethorphan hydrobromide 20 mg, guaifenesin 400 mg, pseudoephedrine hydrochloride 40 mg. 100s. *Rx.*
Use: Upper respiratory combination, antitussive and expectorant.

Maxifed DMX. (MCR American) Dextromethorphan HBr 20 mg, guaifenesin 400 mg, pseudoephedrine hydrochloride 60 mg. Tab. 100s. *Rx.*
Use: Upper respiratory combination, antitussive and expectorant combination.

Maxifed-G. (MCR American) Guaifenesin 580 mg, pseudoephedrine hydrochloride 60 mg. ER Tab. Bot. 100s. *Rx.*
Use: Upper respiratory combination, decongestant, expectorant.

Maxiflor. (Allergan) Diflorasone diacetate 0.05%. Cream, Oint. Tubes 15 g, 30 g, 60 g. *Rx.*
Use: Corticosteroid, topical.

Maxiflu DM. (MCR American) Acetaminophen 500 mg, dextromethorphan hydrobromide 20 mg, guaifenesin 400 mg, pseudoephedrine hydrochloride 60 mg. Tab. 100s. *Rx.*
Use: Upper respiratory combination, antitussive and expectorant combination.

Maxilube. (Mission Pharmacal) Water, silicone oil, glycerin, carbomer 934, triethanolamine, sodium lauryl sulfate, parabens. Jelly 90 g, 150 g. *OTC.*
Use: Vaginal agent.

Maximum Bayer Aspirin. (Bayer Consumer Care) Aspirin (Acetylsalicylic Acid; ASA) 500 mg. **Tab.:** 10s, 30s, 60s, 100s. **Capl.:** 60s. *OTC.*
Use: Analgesic.

Maximum Blue Label. (Vitaline) Vitamins A 2500 units, D 16.7 units, E 66.7 mg, B_1 16.7 mg, B_2 8.3 mg, B_3 31.7 mg, B_5 66.7 mg, B_6 16.7 mg, B_{12} 16.7 mcg, C 200 mg, folic acid 0.13 mg, Zn 5 mg, Ca, Cr, Cu, I, K, Mg, Mn, Mo, Se, Si, V, biotin 50 mcg, SOD, l-lysine. Tab. Bot. 180s. *OTC.*
Use: Mineral, vitamin supplement.

Maximum D3. (Pro-Pharma) Cholecalciferol 10,000 IU. Cap. 5s. *OTC.*
Use: Vitamin supplement.

Maximum Green Label. (Vitaline) Vitamins A 2500 units, D 16.7 units, E 66.7 mg, B_1 16.7 mg, B_2 8.3 mg, B_3 31.7 mg, B_5 66.7 mg, B_6 16.7 mg, B_{12} 16.7 mcg, C 200 mg, folic acid 0.13 mg, Zn 5 mg, Ca, Cr, I, K, Mg, Mn, Mo, Se, Si, V, biotin 50 mcg, SOD, l-lysine. Tab. Bot. 180s. *OTC.*
Use: Mineral, vitamin supplement.

Maximum Pain Relief Pamprin. (Chattem) Acetaminophen 250 mg, magnesium salicylate 250 mg, pamabrom 25 mg. Capl. Bot. 16s, 32s. *OTC.*
Use: Analgesic combination.

Maximum Red Label. (Vitaline) Iron 3.3 mg, vitamins A 2500 units, D 67 units, E 66.7 mg, B_1 16.7 mg, B_2 8.3 mg, B_3 31.7 mg, B_5 66.7 mg, B_6 16.7 mg, B_{12} 16.7 mcg, C 200 mg, folic acid 0.13 mg, Zn 5 mg, Ca, Cr, Su, I, K, Mg, Mo, Se, Si, V, biotin 50 mcg, choline, inositol, bioflavonoids, l-lysine, PABA. Tab. Bot. 180s. *OTC.*
Use: Mineral, vitamin supplement.

Maximum Relief ex•lax. (Novartis) Sennosides 25 mg, sucrose. Tab. Bot. 24s, 48s. *OTC.*
Use: Laxative.

Maximum Strength Anbesol. (Whitehall) Benzocaine 20%. Alcohol 50%, saccharin. Liq. Bot. 9 mL. *OTC.*
Use: Topical local anesthetic.

Maximum Strength Aqua-Ban. (Thompson Medical) Pamabrom 50 mg, lactose. Tab. Bot. 30s. *OTC.*
Use: Diuretic.

Maximum Strength Benadryl. (Parke-Davis) **Cream:** Diphenhydramine hydrochloride 2%, parabens in a greaseless base. Jar 15 g. **Spray, non-aerosol:** Diphenhydramine hydrochloride 2%, alcohol 85%. Bot. 60 mL. *OTC.*
Use: Antihistamine, topical.

Maximum Strength Benadryl Itch Relief. (Warner Lambert) Diphenhydramine hydrochloride. **Cream:** 2%, zinc acetate 1%, parabens, aloe vera. 14.2 g. **Stick:** 2%, zinc acetate 1%. Alcohol 73.5%, aloe vera. 14 mL. *OTC.*
Use: Antihistamine.

Maximum Strength Clearasil Clearstick.
See: Clearasil.

Maximum Strength Clearasil Clearstick for Sensitive Skin.
See: Clearasil.

Maximum Strength Cortaid. (Pharmacia) Hydrocortisone 1% in parabens, mineral oil, white petrolatum. Oint. Tube 15 g, 30 g. *OTC.*
Use: Corticosteroid, topical.

Maximum Strength Cortaid Faststick. (Pharmacia) Hydrocortisone 1%, alcohol 55%, methylparaben. Stick, roll-on. 14 g. *OTC.*
Use: Corticosteroid, topical.

Maximum Strength Corticaine. (UCB) Hydrocortisone acetate 1%, glycerin, menthol, EDTA, parabens. Cream Tube

30 g. *OTC.*
Use: Corticosteroid, topical.
Maximum Strength Dermarest Dricort Creme. (Del) Hydrocortisone (as acetate) 1%, white petrolatum. Cream Tube 14 g. *OTC.*
Use: Corticosteroid, topical.
Maximum Strength Dristan. (Whitehall-Robins) Pseudoephedrine hydrochloride 30 mg, acetaminophen 500 mg. Cap. Bot. 24s, 48s, 100s. *OTC.*
Use: Decongestant, analgesic.
Maximum Strength Dristan Cold. (Whitehall-Robins) Pseudoephedrine hydrochloride 30 mg, brompheniramine maleate 2 mg, acetaminophen 500 mg. Capl. Pkg. 16s, Bot. 36s. *OTC.*
Use: Decongestant, analgesic, antihistamine.
Maximum Strength D-2000. (21st Century) Cholecalciferol 2,000 units. Calcium 180 mg. Gluten free. Tab. 110s. *OTC.*
Use: Fat-soluble vitamin.
Maximum Strength Dynafed Plus. (BDI) Acetaminophen 500 mg, pseudoephedrine 30 mg. Tab. Bot. 30s. *OTC.*
Use: Analgesic, decongestant.
Maximum Strength Flexall 454. (Chattem) Menthol 16%, aloe vera gel, eucalyptus oil, methyl salicylate, SD alcohol 38-B, thyme oil. Gel Tube 90 g. *OTC.*
Use: Liniment.
Maximum Strength Halls-Plus. (Warner Lambert) Menthol 10 mg, corn syrup, sucrose. Loz. Pkg. 10s, 20s. *OTC.*
Use: Anesthetic.
Maximum Strength Ivarest. (Blistex) Calamine 14%, diphenhydramine hydrochloride 2%. Lanolin oil, petrolatum, propylene glycol. Cream. 56 g. *OTC.*
Use: Poison ivy treatment.
Maximum Strength KeriCort-10. (Bristol-Myers Squibb) Hydrocortisone 1%, parabens, cetyl alcohol, stearyl alcohol. Cream Tube 56.7 g. *OTC.*
Use: Corticosteroid, topical.
Maximum Strength Meted. (Sirius Labs) Sulfur 5%, salicylic acid 3%. Shampoo. Bot. 118 mL. *OTC.*
Use: Antiseborrheic combination.
Maximum Strength Nasal Decongestant. (Taro) Oxymetazoline hydrochloride 0.05%, 0.002% phenylmercuric acetate, benzalkonium chloride. Spray Bot. 15 mL, 30 mL. *OTC.*
Use: Decongestant.
Maximum Strength No-Aspirin Sinus Medication. (Walgreen) Acetamino-

phen 500 mg, pseudoephedrine hydrochloride 30 mg. Tab. Bot. 50s. *OTC.*
Use: Analgesic, decongestant.
Maximum Strength NoDoz. (Novartis Consumer Health) Caffeine 200 mg, sucrose. Tab. Pkg. 36s. *OTC.*
Use: CNS stimulant, analeptic.
Maximum Strength Nytol. (Block Drug) Diphenhydramine hydrochloride 50 mg. Tab., lactose. Pkg. 8s, 16s. *OTC.*
Use: Sleep aid.
Maximum Strength Orajel Gel. (Del) Benzocaine 20%, saccharin. Tube 9.45 mL. *OTC.*
Use: Anesthetic, local.
Maximum Strength Orajel Liquid. (Del) Benzocaine 20%, ethyl alcohol 44.2%, phenol, tartrazine, saccharin. Liq. Bot. 13.3 mL. *OTC.*
Use: Anesthetic, local.
Maximum Strength Ornex. (Menley & James Labs, Inc.) Pseudoephedrine hydrochloride 30 mg, acetaminophen 500 mg. Cap. Bot. 24s, 48s. *OTC.*
Use: Analgesic, decongestant.
Maximum Strength Sine-Aid. (McNeil Consumer) Pseudoephedrine hydrochloride 30 mg, acetaminophen 500 mg. Cap., Tab., or Gelcap. **Cap. & Tab.:** Bot. 50s. **Gelcaps:** Bot. 40s. *OTC.*
Use: Analgesic, decongestant.
Maximum Strength Sinutab Nighttime. (Warner Lambert) Pseudoephedrine hydrochloride 10 mg, diphenhydramine hydrochloride 8.33 mg, acetaminophen 167 mg/5 mL. Liq. Alcohol free. 120 mL. *OTC.*
Use: Analgesic, antihistamine, decongestant.
Maximum Strength Sinutab Without Drowsiness. (Warner Lambert) Pseudoephedrine hydrochloride 30 mg, acetaminophen 500 mg. Tab. or Capl. Bot. 24s, 48s (tab. only). *OTC.*
Use: Analgesic, decongestant.
Maximum Strength Sleepinal. (Thompson Medical) **Cap.:** Diphenhydramine hydrochloride 50 mg, lactose. Pkg. 16s. **Soft gel:** Diphenhydramine hydrochloride 50 mg, sorbitol. Pkg. 16s. *OTC.*
Use: Sleep aid.
Maximum Strength Sudafed Severe Cold Formula. (McNeil-PPC) Dextromethorphan HBr 15 mg, pseudoephedrine hydrochloride 30 mg, acetaminophen 500 mg. Tab. 10s. *OTC.*
Use: Analgesic, antitussive, decongestant.
Maximum Strength Sudafed Sinus. (McNeil-PPC) Pseudoephedrine hydro-

chloride 30 mg, acetaminophen 500 mg. Tab. or Capl. Bot. 24s, 48s. *OTC.*
Use: Analgesic, decongestant.

Maximum Strength Unisom SleepGels. (Pfizer) Diphenhydramine hydrochloride 50 mg, sorbitol. Cap. Pkg. 8s. *OTC.*
Use: Sleep aid.

Maximum Strength Wart Remover. (Stiefel) Salicylic acid 17%, alcohol 29%, castor oil, flexible collodion. Liq. 13.3 mL. *OTC.*
Use: Keratolytic.

Maxiphen DM. (MCR American) Dextromethorphan HBr 20 mg, guaifenesin 400 mg, phenylephrine hydrochloride 10 mg. Tab. 100s. *Rx.*
Use: Upper respiratory combination, antitussive and expectorant.

Maxiphen-G DM. (AMBI) Dextromethorphan HBr 30 mg, phenylephrine hydrochloride 20 mg, guaifenesin 1000 mg. ER Tab. 100s. *Rx.*
Use: Upper respiratory combination, antitussive and expectorant combination.

Maxitrol Ointment. (Alcon) Dexamethasone 0.1%, neomycin 0.35%, polymyxin B sulfate 10,000 units/g. Tube 3.5 g. *Rx.*
Use: Anti-infective, ophthalmic.

Maxitrol Ophthalmic Suspension. (Alcon) Dexamethasone 0.1%, neomycin (as sulfate) 0.35%, polymyxin B sulfate 10,000 units/mL, benzalkonium chloride 0.004%, hydroxypropyl methylcellulose 0.5%, hydrochloric acid, sodium chloride, polysorbate 20, sodium hydroxide. *Drop-Tainer* 5 mL. *Rx.*
Use: Anti-infective, ophthalmic; steroid antibiotic combination.

Maxi-Tuss DM. (MCR American Pharmaceuticals) Dextromethorphan HBr 20 mg, guaifenesin 200 mg per 5 mL. Glucose, menthol, parabens, saccharin, black cherry flavor. Liq. Bot. 473 mL. *Rx.*
Use: Upper respiratory combination, antitussive, expectorant.

Maxi-Tuss HC. (MCR American) Hydrocodone bitartrate 2.5 mg, chlorpheniramine maleate 4 mg, phenylephrine hydrochloride 10 mg per 5 mL. Liq. Bot. 473 mL. *c-III.*
Use: Upper respiratory combination, antitussive, antihistamine, decongestant.

Maxivate. (Bristol-Myers Squibb) Betamethasone dipropionate 0.05%. Cream. Oint. Tube 15 g. 45 g. *Rx.*
Use: Corticosteroid, topical.

Maxi-Vite. (Ivax) Vitamins A 10,000 units, D 400 units, E 15 mg, B_1 10 mg, B_2 10 mg, B_3 100 mg, B_5 20 mg, B_6 5 mg, B_{12} 5 mcg, C 200 mg, Ca 53.5 mg, Fe 1.5 mg, folic acid 0.4 mg, biotin 1 mcg, I, P, Cu, Mg, Mn, Zn 1.5 mg, PABA, rutin, glutamic acid, inositol, choline bitartrate, bioflavonoids, l-lysine, betaine, lecithin. Tab. Bot. 60s. *OTC.*
Use: Mineral, vitamin supplement.

Maxovite. (Tyson) Vitamins A 2083 units, D 16.7 units, E 16.7 mg, B_1 5 mg, B_2 4.2 mg, B_3 4.2 mg, B_5 4.2 mg, B_6 54.2 mg, B_{12} 10.8 mcg, C 250 mg, folic acid 0.33 mg, Zn 5 mg, Ca, Cr, Cu, Fe, I, K, Mg, Mn, Se, biotin 11.7 mcg. Tab. Bot. 120s, 240s. *OTC.*
Use: Mineral, vitamin supplement.

Maxzide. (Bertek) Hydrochlorothiazide 50 mg, triamterene 75 mg. Tab. Bot. 100s, 500s, UD 100s. *Rx.*
Use: Antihypertensive; diuretic.

Maxzide-25MG. (Bertek) Triamterene 37.5 mg, hydrochlorothiazide 25 mg. Tab. Bot. 100s, UD 100s. *Rx.*
Use: Diuretic combination.

Mayotic. (Merz) Hydrocortisone 1%, neomycin sulfate 5 mg, polymyxin B sulfate 10,000 units/mL, thimerosal 0.01%. Susp. Bot. 10 mL w/dropper. *Rx.*
Use: Otic.

•**maytansine.** (MAY-tan-SEEN) USAN.
Use: Antineoplastic.

•**mazapertine succinate.** (mazz-ah-PURR-teen) USAN.
Use: Antipsychotic.

Mazicon. (Roche) Flumazenil 0.1 mg/mL. Inj. Vial 5 mL, 10 mL. *Rx.*
Use: Antidote.

•**mazindol.** (MAZE-in-dole) *USP 34.*
Use: Anorexic; appetite suppressant; Duchenne muscular dystrophy. [Orphan Drug]

M-Caps. (Mill-Mark) Methionine 200 mg. Cap. Bot. 50s, 1000s. *Rx.*
Use: Diaper rash preparation.

M-Clear. (R.A. McNeil) Codeine phosphate 9 mg, guaifenesin 200 mg. Maltodextrin, tartrazine. Cap. 100s. *c-v.*
Use: Upper respiratory combination, antitussive with expectorant.

M-Clear Jr. (R.A. McNeil) Hydrocodone bitartrate 2.5 mg, potassium guaiacolsulfonate 175 mg per 5 mL. Sugar, alcohol, and dye free. Saccharin, sorbitol. Syrup. 473 mL. *c-III.*
Use: Antitussive with expectorant.

M-Clear WC. (R.A. McNeil) Codeine phosphate 6.3 mg, guaifenesin 100 mg per 5 mL. Alcohol and sugar free.

PEG, saccharin, sorbitol. Liq. 473 mL.
c-v.
Use: Upper respiratory combination, antitussive with expectorant.

MCT Oil. (Bristol-Myers Squibb) Triglycerides of medium chain fatty acids. Lipid fraction of coconut oil; fatty acid shorter than $C_8 < 6\%$, C_8 (octanoic) 67%, C_{10} (decanoic) 23%, longer than C_{10} 4%. Bot. Qt. *OTC.*
Use: Nutritional supplement, enteral.

MDP-Squibb. (Bristol-Myers Squibb) Technetium Tc 99 medronate. Reaction vial pkg. 10s.
Use: Radiopaque agent.

MD-76 R. (Mallinckrodt) Diatrizoate meglumine 660 mg, diatrizoate sodium 100 mg, iodine 370 mg/mL. Inj. Vials. 50 mL. Bot. 100 mL, 150 mL, 200 mL. Power injector syringe. 125 mL. *Rx.*
Use: Radiopaque agent, parenteral.

MD-60. (Mallinckrodt) Diatrizoate meglumine 52%, diatrizoate sodium 8% (29.2% iodine). Inj. Vial 30 mL, 50 mL.
Use: Radiopaque agent.

meadinin. Mixture of Amoidin & Amidin alk. of Ammi Majus Linn.

measles, mumps, and rubella virus vaccine live. (MEE-zuhls, mumps, and ru-BELL-uh)
Use: Immunization.
See: M-M-R II.

measles, mumps, rubella, and varicella virus vaccine, live, attenuated.
Use: Immunization.
See: ProQuad.

measles prophylactic serum.
See: Immune Globulin (Intramuscular).

•**measles virus vaccine, live.** (MEE-zuhls) *USP 34.* Modified live-virus measles vaccine.
Use: Immunization.
See: Attenuvax.
W/Mumps virus vaccine, rubella virus vaccine.
See: M-M-R II.

measles virus vaccine, live attenuated. Moratenline derived from Enders' attenuated Edmonston strain grown in cell cultures of chick embryos.
See: Attenuvax.
W/Mumps virus vaccine, rubella virus vaccine.
See: M-M-R II.

Mebaral. (Ovation) Mephobarbital 0.5 gr, 0.75 gr, 1.5 gr. Tab. Bot. 250s. *c-iv.*
Use: Anticonvulsant; sedative.

•**mebendazole.** (meh-BEND-uh-zole) *USP 34.*
Use: Anthelmintic.
See: Vermox.

mebendazole. (Copley) Mebendazole 100 mg. Chew. Tab. Pkg. 12s, 36s. *Rx.*
Use: Anthelmintic.

•**mebeverine hydrochloride.** (MEH-BEH-ver-een) USAN.
Use: Spasmolytic agent; muscle relaxant.

•**mebrofenin.** (MEH-broe-FEN-in) *USP 34.*
Use: Diagnostic aid (hepatobiliary function determination).

•**mebutamate.** (meh-BYOO-ta-mate) USAN.
Use: Antihypertensive.

•**mecamylamine hydrochloride.** (mek-ah-MILL-ah-meen) *USP 34.*
Use: Antihypertensive, antiadrenergic.

•**mecasermin.** (mek-a-SER-min) USAN.
Use: Insulin-like growth factor.
See: Increlex.

•**mecetronium ethylsulfate.** (MEH-seh-TROE-nee-uhm ETH-ill-SULL-fate) USAN.
Use: Antiseptic.

mechlorethamine derivative.
Use: Alkylating agent; ethylenimine/methylmelamine.
See: Bendamustine Hydrochloride.

•**mechlorethamine hydrochloride.** (meh-klor-ETH-ah-meen) *USP 34.*
Use: Antineoplastic, alkylating agent.
See: Mustargen.

mecholin hydrochloride.
See: Methacholine Chloride.

Mecholyl Ointment. (Gordon Laboratories) Methacholine chloride 0.25%, methyl salicylate 10% in ointment base. Jar 4 oz, 1 lb, 5 lb. *OTC.*
Use: Analgesic, topical.

meclastine. Clemastine.

•**meclizine hydrochloride.** (MEK-lih-zeen) *USP 34.*
Use: Antinauseant; antiemetic.
See: Antivert.
Antivert/50.
Antivert/25.
Antrizine.
Bonine.
Dizmiss.
Dramamine II.
Dramamine Less Drowsy Formula.

meclizine hydrochloride. (Various Mfr.) Meclizine hydrochloride. **Tab.: 12.5 mg:** Bot. 30s, 60s, 100s, 500s, 1000s, UD 100s. **25 mg:** Bot. 12s, 20s, 30s, 60s, 100s, 500s, 1000s, UD 32s, 100s. **50 mg:** Bot. 100s. **Chew Tab.: 25 mg:** Bot. 20s, 30s, 60s, 100s, 1000s, UD 100s. *Rx-OTC.*
Use: Antiemetic/antivertigo agent.

• **meclocycline.** (meh-kloe-SIGH-kleen) USAN.
Use: Anti-infective.

• **meclofenamate sodium.** (mek-loe-FEN-uh-mate) *USP 34.*
Use: Nonsteroidal anti-inflammatory agent.

meclofenamate sodium. (Various Mfr.) Meclofenamate sodium 50 mg, 100 mg. Cap. Bot. 100s, 500s, 1000s. *Rx.*
Use: Nonsteroidal anti-inflammatory agent.

• **meclofenamic acid.** (MEH-kloe-fen-AM-ik) USAN.
Use: Anti-inflammatory.

• **mecloqualone.** (MEH-kloe-KWAH-lone) USAN.
Use: Sedative; hypnotic.

• **meclorisone dibutyrate.** (MEH-KLAHR-ih-sone die-BYOO-tih-rate) USAN.
Use: Anti-inflammatory, topical.

• **mecobalamin.** (MEH-koe-BAHL-ah-min) USAN.
Use: Vitamin (hematopoietic).

Mecodrin.
See: Amphetamine.

• **mecrylate.** (MEH-krih-late) USAN.
Use: Surgical aid (tissue adhesive).

mecysteine. Methyl Cysteine.

Medadyne. (Dal-Med Pharmaceuticals)
Liq.: Methyl benzethonium chloride, benzocaine, tannic acid, camphor, chlorothymol, menthol, benzyl alcohol, alcohol 61%. Bot. 15 mL, 30 mL. **Throat Spray:** Lidocaine, cetyl dimethyl ammonium chloride, ethyl alcohol. Bot. 30 mL. *OTC.*
Use: Mouth and throat preparation.

Meda-Hist Expectorant. (Medwick) Bot. 4 oz, pt, gal.
Use: Decongestant, antitussive.

Medalox Gel. (Davol) Magnesium aluminum hydroxide gel. Bot. 12 oz, pt, gal. *OTC.*
Use: Antacid.

Medamint. (Dal-Med Pharmaceuticals) Benzocaine 10 mg/Loz. Pkg. 12s, 24s. *OTC.*
Use: Mouth and throat preparation.

Medatussin Pediatric. (Dal-Med Pharmaceuticals) Dextromethorphan HBr 5 mg, guaifenesin 50 mg, potassium citrate, citric acid, sorbitol, saccharin. Syr. Bot. 120 mL. *OTC.*
Use: Antitussive, expectorant.

• **medazepam hydrochloride.** (med-AZE-eh-pam) USAN. Under study.
Use: Anxiolytic.

Medebar Plus. (Mallinckrodt) Barium sulfate 100%. Simethicone. Susp. Bot. 1900 mL. 650 mL w/enema tip-tubing assemblies. *Rx.*
Use: Radiopaque agent; GI contrast agent.

Medent. (SJ Pharmaceuticals) Pseudoephedrine hydrochloride 120 mg, guaifenesin 500 mg. Tab. Bot. 100s.
Use: Decongestant, expectorant.

Medent-DMI. (SJ Pharmaceuticals) Dextromethorphan hydrobromide 20 mg, guaifenesin 400 mg, pseudoephedrine hydrochloride 60 mg. Tab. 100s. *OTC.*
Use: Upper respiratory combination, antitussive and expectorant combination.

Medent-PE. (SJ Pharmaceuticals) Phenylephrine hydrochloride 12.5 mg, guaifenesin 600 mg. Dye free. ER Tab. 100s. *Rx.*
Use: Decongestant and expectorant, upper respiratory combination.

Mederma. (Merz) PEG-4, onion (allium cepa) extract, xanthan gum, allantoin, fragrance, methylparaben. Gel. Tube. 50 g. *OTC.*
Use: Helps scars appear softer and smoother.

Medescan. (Mallinckrodt) Barium sulfate 2.3%. Sorbitol, saccharin, sodium benzoate. Susp. Bot. 250 mL, 450 mL, 1900 mL. *Rx.*
Use: Radiopaque agent; GI contrast agent.

Medicaine Cream. (Walgreen) Benzocaine 3%, resorcinol 2%. Tube 1.25 oz. *OTC.*
Use: Antipruritic.

Medicated Acne Cleanser. (C & M Pharmacal) Sulfur 4%, resorcinol 2%, SD alcohol 40 11.65%, methylparaben. Lot. Bot. 120 mL. *OTC.*
Use: Dermatologic, acne.

Medicated Healer. (Walgreen) Strong ammonia soln. 10%, camphor 2.6%. Bot. 6 oz. *OTC.*
Use: Emollient.

Medicated Powder. (Johnson & Johnson) Zinc oxide, talc, fragrance, menthol. Plastic container 3 oz, 6 oz, 11 oz. *OTC.*
Use: Antipruritic.

Medicidin-D. (Medique) Phenylephrine hydrochloride 5 mg, chlorpheniramine maleate 2 mg, acetaminophen 325 mg. Sucrose. Tab. 100s, 200s, 500s. *OTC.*
Use: Upper respiratory combination, decongestant, antihistamine, and analgesic.

Medi-Derm. (Two Hip) Capsaicin 0.035%, menthol 5%, methyl salicylate

20%. Alcohols, cypress oil, glyceryl, propylene glycol, polysorbate 80. Cream 120 g. *OTC.*
Use: Rub and liniment.

Medi-First Extra Strength Pain Relief. (Medique Products) Acetaminophen 110 mg, aspirin 162 mg, caffeine 32.4 mg, salicylamide 152 mg. Tab. 100s, 250s, 500s. *OTC.*
Use: Nonnarcotic analgesic combination.

Medihaler-Iso. (3M) Isoproterenol sulfate 80 mcg/actuation. Aer. Inhaler 15 mL ($\geq$ 300 doses) with adapter and 15 mL refill. *Rx.*
Use: Sympathomimetic bronchodilator.

Mediotic-HC. (Dayton) Hydrocortisone 1%, pramoxine hydrochloride 1%, chloroxylenol 0.1%, benzalkonium chloride 0.01%. Drops. Vial. 15 mL with dropper. *Rx.*
Use: Miscellaneous otic preparation.

Medipak. (Armenpharm Ltd.) First-aid kit.

Medi-Phite. (Davol) Vitamins B_1 and B_{12}. Syr. Bot. 4 oz, pt, gal. *OTC.*
Use: Vitamin supplement.

Mediplast. (Beiersdorf) Salicylic acid plaster 40%. Box 25s. *OTC.*
Use: Keratolytic.

Mediplex Plus. (US Pharm) Vitamins E (dl-alpha tocopheryl) 50 units, B_1 25 mg, B_2 10 mg, B_3 100 mg, B_5 25 mg, B_6 10 mg, B_{12} 25 mcg, C 300 mg, folic acid 0.4 mg, Zn 18 mg, Cu, Mg, Mn. Bot. Tab. 100s. *OTC.*
Use: Multivitamin.

Mediplex Tabules. (US Pharm) Vitamins E 60 units, B_1 25 mg, B_2 10 mg, B_3 100 mg, B_5 25 mg, B_6 10 mg, B_{12} 25 mcg, C 300 mg, Zn 4 mg, Cu, Mg, Mn. Bot. 100s. *OTC.*
Use: Mineral, vitamin supplement.

Medi-Quik. (Mentholatum) **Aerosol:** Lidocaine hydrochloride, benzalkonium chloride. 90 mL. **Spray:** Lidocaine 2%, benzalkonium chloride 0.13%, camphor 0.2%, benzyl alcohol. 85 mL. *OTC.*
Use: Antiseptic; anesthetic, local.

•**medorinone.** (MEH-doe-RIH-nohn) USAN.
Use: Cardiovascular agent.

Medotar. (Medco) Coal tar 1%, octoxynol-5, zinc oxide, white petrolatum. Oint. 454 g. *OTC.*
Use: Antipsoriatic; antipruritic.

•**medrogestone.** (MEH-droe-JEST-ohn) USAN.
Use: Hormone, progestin.

Medrol. (Upjohn) Methylprednisolone. Lactose, sucrose. Tab. **2 mg:** 100s. **4 mg:** Bot. 30s, 100s, UD 100s. Dosep-ack 21s. **8 mg:** 25s. **16 mg:** 50s. ADT Pak 14s. **24 mg:** 25s. **32 mg:** 25s. *Rx.*
Use: Corticosteroid.

•**medronate disodium.** (MEH-droe-nate) USAN. *Formerly Disodium Methylene Diphosphonate; MDP.*
Use: Pharmaceutic aid.

•**medronic acid.** (meh-DRAH-nik) USAN.
Use: Pharmaceutic aid.

Medrosphol Hg-197. Merprane.

Medrox. (Pharmaceutica North America) Capsaicin 0.0375%, menthol 5%, methyl salicylate 20%. Cetyl alcohol, glycerin, parabens, PEG-150. Oint. 60 g. *OTC.*
Use: Rub and liniment.

•**medroxalol.** (meh-DROX-ah-LAHL) USAN.
Use: Antihypertensive.

•**medroxalol hydrochloride.** (meh-DROX-ah-LAHL) USAN.
Use: Antihypertensive.

•**medroxyprogesterone acetate.** (meh-DROX-ee-pro-JESS-tuh-rone) *USP 34. Tall Man:* medroxyPROGESTERone
Use: Hormone, progestin.
See: Depo-Provera.
  Depo-Sub Q Provera 104.
  Provera.
W/Conjugated Estrogens.
See: Premphase.
  Prempro.

medroxyprogesterone acetate. (CMC) Medroxyprogesterone acetate 50 mg, 100 mg/mL. Vial 5 mL.
Use: Hormone, progestin.

medroxyprogesterone acetate. (Sicor) Medroxyprogesterone acetate 150 mg/mL. PEG 28.9 mg, polysorbate 80 2.41 mg, sodium chloride 8.68 mg, methylparaben 1.37 mg, propylparaben 0.15 mg. Inj. Vials. 1 mL. *Rx.*
Use: Contraceptive.

medroxyprogesterone acetate. (Wyeth) Medroxyprogesterone acetate 10 mg. Tab. Bot. 50s, 250s. *Rx.*
Use: Sex hormone, progestin.

medroxyprogesterone acetate. (Various Mfr.) Medroxyprogesterone acetate 2.5 mg, 5 mg, 10 mg. Tab. Bot. 30s, 40s (10 mg only), 50s (10 mg only), 90s (2.5 mg only), 100s, 250s (10 mg only), 500s, 1000s (2.5 and 5 mg only). *Rx.*
Use: Sex hormone, progestin.

MED-Rx. (Iopharm) Pseudoephedrine hydrochloride 60 mg, guaifenesin 600 mg. CR Tab. Box 28s. Guaifenesin 600 mg. CR Tab. Box 28s. *Rx.*
Use: Decongestant, expectorant.

•**medrysone.** (MEH-drih-sone) USAN.

Use: Ophthalmic, corticosteroid, topical.

• **mefenamic acid.** (MEH-fen-AM-ik)
USP 34.
Use: Nonsteroidal anti-inflammatory
agent.
See: Ponstel.

mefenamic acid. (Paddock) Mefenamic
acid 250 mg. Lactose. Cap. 100s. *Rx.*
Use: Nonsteroidal anti-inflammatory
agent.

• **mefenidil.** (meh-FEN-ih-dill) USAN.
Use: Cerebral vasodilator.

• **mefenidil fumarate.** (meh-FEN-ih-dill)
USAN.
Use: Cerebral vasodilator.

• **mefenorex hydrochloride.** (meh-FEN-
oh-rex) USAN. Under study.
Use: Anorexic.

• **mefexamide.** (meh-FEX-am-IDE) USAN.
Use: Stimulant (central).

• **mefloquine hydrochloride.** (MEH-flow-
kwin) USAN.
Use: Antimalarial.
See: Lariam.

mefloquine hydrochloride. (Geneva)
Mefloquine hydrochloride 250 mg. Tab.
Bot. 25s. *Rx.*
Use: Antimalarial.

• **mefruside.** (MEFF-ruh-side) USAN.
Use: Diuretic.

Mega B. (Arco) Vitamins B_1 100 mg,
B_2 100 mg, B_3 100 mg, B_5 100 mg,
B_6 100 mg, B_{12} 100 mcg, folic acid
100 mcg, d-biotin 100 mcg, PABA
100 mg. Tab. Bot. 100s. *OTC.*
Use: Vitamin supplement.

Megace. (Bristol-Myers Oncology) Megestrol acetate. **Tab.:** 40 mg. Lactose.
Bot. 250s, 500s. **Susp.:** 40 mg/mL. Alcohol ≤ 0.06%, sucrose, lemon-lime
flavor. Bot. 240 mL. *Rx.*
Use: Sex hormone, progestin.

Megace ES. (Par Pharmaceutical, Inc.)
Megestrol acetate 125 mg/mL. Alcohol ≤ 0.06%, sucrose. Lemon-lime flavor. Susp. 150 mL. *Rx.*
Use: Sex hormone, progestin.

• **megalomicin potassium phosphate.**
(meh-GAL-OH-my-sin) USAN.
Use: Anti-infective.

Mega VM-80. (NBTY) Vitamins A
10,000 units, D 1000 units, E 100 mg,
B_1 80 mg, B_2 80 mg, B_3 80 mg, B_5
80 mg, B_6 80 mg, B_{12} 80 mcg, C
250 mg, Fe 1.2 mg, folic acid 0.4 mg,
Ca 4.5 mg, Zn 3.58 mg, choline, inositol, biotin 80 mcg, PABA, bioflavonoids, betaine, hesperidin, Cu, I, K, Mg,
Mn. Tab. Bot. 60s, 100s. *OTC.*
Use: Mineral, vitamin supplement.

• **megestrol acetate.** (meh-JESS-trole)
USP 34.
Use: Sex hormone, progestin.
See: Megace.
Megace ES.

megestrol acetate. (Various Mfr.) Megestrol acetate. **Susp.:** 40 mg/mL. Alcohol, sorbitol, sucrose. 240 mL. **Tab.:**
20 mg, 40 mg. Bot. 100s, 500s (40 mg
only), UD 100s. Blister pkg. 25s
(40 mg only). *Rx.*
Use: Sex hormone, progestin.

meglitinides.
Use: Antidiabetic.
See: Nateglinide.
Repaglinide.

• **meglumine.** (meh-GLUE-meen) *USP 34.*
Use: Diagnostic aid (radiopaque medium).

meglumine, diatrizoate injection.
Use: Diagnostic aid (radiopaque me-
dium).
See: Cystografin.
Gastrografin.
Hypaque-M 90%.
Hypaque-M 75%.
Hypaque-76.
Reno-M-Dip.
W/Meglumine iodipamide.
See: Sinografin.
W/Sodium diatrizoate.
See: Gastrografin.
Renografin-60.
Renovist II.

meglumine, iodipamide injection.
Use: Diagnostic aid; radiopaque me-
dium.
See: Cholografin Meglumine.
W/Meglumine diatrizoate.
See: Sinografin.

meglumine, iothalamate injection.
Use: Diagnostic aid; radiopaque medium.

• **meglutol.** (MEH-glue-tahl) USAN.
Use: Antihyperlipoproteinemic.

• **melafocon A.** (MEH-lah-FOE-kahn)
USAN.
Use: Contact lens material (hydro-
phobic).

melanoma cell vaccine.
Use: Invasive melanoma. [Orphan
Drug]

melanoma vaccine.
Use: Stage III to IV melanoma. [Orphan
Drug]

melarsoprol. (Mel B)
Use: Anti-infective.
See: Arsobal.

melatonin.
Use: Treatment of circadian rhythm sleep disorders in blind patients. [Orphan Drug]

melatonin receptor agonists.
Use: Sedative and hypnotic, nonbarbiturate.
See: Ramelteon.

Mel B.
See: Melarsoprol.

•**melengestrol acetate.** (meh-len-JESS-trole) USAN.
Use: Antineoplastic; hormone, progestin.

Melfiat-105 Unicelles. (Numark) Phendimetrazine tartrate 105 mg, sucrose. SR Cap. Bot. 100s. *c-III.*
Use: CNS stimulant, anorexiant.

Melhoral Child Tablet. (Sanofi-Synthelabo) Acetylsalicylic acid. *OTC.*
Use: Analgesic.

melitoxin.
See: Dicumarol.

•**melitracen hydrochloride.** (meh-lih-TRAY-sen) USAN.
Use: Antidepressant.

•**melizame.** (MEH-lih-zame) USAN.
Use: Sweetener.

mellose. Methylcellulose.

Melonex. Metahexamide.
Use: Oral antidiabetic.

•**meloxicam.** (mell-OX-ih-kam) USAN.
Use: Nonsteroidal anti-inflammatory agent.
See: Mobic.

meloxicam. (Roxane) Meloxicam 7.5 mg/5 mL. Oral Susp. 100 mL. *Rx.*
Use: Nonsteroidal anti-inflammatory agent.

meloxicam. (Various Mfr.) Meloxicam 7.5 mg, 15 mg. Tab. 30s, 60s, 100s, 250s, 500s, 1000s. *Rx.*
Use: Nonsteroidal anti-inflammatory agent.

Melpaque HP. (Stratus) Hydroquinone 4% in a sunblocking base of mineral oil, parabens, talc, EDTA, sodium metabisulfite. Cream. Tinted. Tube 14.2 g, 28.4 g. *Rx.*
Use: Dermatologic.

•**melphalan.** (MELL-fuh-lan) *USP 34.*
Use: Alkylating agent, nitrogen mustard.
See: Alkeran.

melphalan. (Bioniche Pharma Group) Melphalan hydrochloride 50 mg. Inj., lyophilized Pow. For Soln. Single-use vial (with povidone 20 mg) with 10 mL vial of sterile diluents (with sodium citrate 0.2 g, propylene glycol 6 mL, ethanol (96%) 0.52 mL. *Rx.*

Use: Alkylating agent, nitrogen mustard.

Melquin HP. (Stratus) Hydroquinone 4%, mineral oil, petrolatum, cetostearyl alcohol, glycerin, sodium metabisulfite. Vanishing base. Cream. Tube 14.2 g, 28.4 g. *Rx.*
Use: Dermatologic.

•**memantine hydrochloride.** (me-MAN-teen) USAN.
Use: Alzheimer disease.
See: Namenda.
Namenda XR.

MembraneBlue. (Dutch Ophthalmic) Trypan blue 0.15%. Ophth. Soln. 0.5 mL single-use *Luer Lok* with glass syringe. *Rx.*
Use: Ophthalmic surgical adjunct.

•**memotine hydrochloride.** (MEH-moe-teen) USAN.
Use: Antiviral.

•**menabitan hydrochloride.** (meh-NAB-ih-tan) USAN.
Use: Analgesic.

Menactra A/C/Y/W-135. (Sanofi Pasteur) Each 0.5 mL contains 4 mcg each of groups A, C, Y, and W-135. Inj. Soln. Single-dose syringes and vials (conjugated to approximately 48 mcg of diphtheria toxoid protein carrier). Stopper to the vial contains dry, natural latex rubber. *Rx.*
Use: Agent for active immunization, bacterial vaccine.

•**menadiol sodium diphosphate.** (men-ah-DIE-ole) *USP 34.*
Use: Vitamin (prothrombogenic).

•**menadione.** (men-ah-DIE-ohn) *USP 34.*
Use: Oral & IM; Vitamin K therapy; vitamin (prothrombogenic).

menadione diphosphate sodium.
See: Menadiol sodium diphosphate.

menaphthene.
See: Menadione.

menaphthone.
See: Menadione.

menaquinone.
See: Menadione.

M-End PE. (R.A. McNeil) Brompheniramine maleate 1.33 mg, codeine phosphate 6.33 mg, phenylephrine hydrochloride 3.33 mg per 5 mL. Saccharin, sorbitol. Cotton candy flavor. Liq. 354 mL. *c-v.*
Use: Upper respiratory combination, antitussive combination.

M-End WC. (R.A. McNeil) Brompheniramine maleate 1.3 mg, codeine phosphate 6.3 mg, pseudoephedrine hydrochloride 10 mg per 5 mL. Saccharin,

sorbitol. Cherry flavor. Liq. 473 mL. *c-v.*
Use: Upper respiratory combination, antitussive combination.

Menest. (Monarch) Esterified estrogens. 0.3 mg, 0.625 mg, 1.25 mg, 2.5 mg. Lactose. Film-coated. Tab. Bot. 50s. (2.5 mg only), 100s (except 2.5 mg). *Rx.*
Use: Estrogen, hormone.

meningococcal vaccine.
Use: Agent for active immunization, bacterial vaccine.
See: Menactra A/C/Y/W-135.
Menomune A/C/Y/W-135.

•**menoctone.** (meh-NOCK-tone) USAN. Under study.
Use: Antimalarial.

•**menogaril.** (MEN-oh-gar-ILL) USAN.
Use: Antineoplastic.

Menoject L.A. (Merz) Testosterone cypionate, estradiol cypionate. Vial 10 mL. *Rx.*
Use: Androgen; estrogen combination.

Menolyn. (Arcum) Ethinyl estradiol 0.05 mg. Tab. Bot. 100s, 1000s. *Rx.*
Use: Estrogen.

Menomune A/C/Y/W-135. (Sanofi Pasteur) When reconstituted, each 0.5 mL contains 50 mcg isolated product from each of groups A, C, Y, and W-135. Freeze-dried. Lactose 2.5 to 5 mg per dose. Inj. Lyophilized Pow. for Soln. Single-dose vial w/preservative-free distilled water diluent 0.78 mL. 10-dose vial w/diluent 6 mL w/thimerosal 1:10,000 (stopper to vial contains dry, natural latex rubber). *Rx.*
Use: Immunization.

Menopur. (Ferring) Follicle-stimulating hormone activity 75 units, luteinizing hormone activity 75 units. Pow. or Pellets for Inj., lyophilized. In vials with diluent. *Rx.*
Use: Ovulation stimulant.

Menostar. (Berlex) Estradiol 1 mg (0.014 mg/day). Transdermal system. 4s. *Rx.*
Use: Sex hormone, estrogen.

•**menotropins.** (MEN-oh-trope-inz) USAN. *Formerly Human Follicle-Stimulating Hormone.*
Use: Sex hormone; ovulation stimulant; gonadotropin; gonad-stimulating principle.
See: Follistim AQ.
Menopur.
Pergonal.
Repronex.

Men-Phor. (Geritrex) Camphor 0.5%, menthol 0.5%, carbopol, cetearyl alco-

hol, cetyl alcohol, hydantoin, castor oil, petrolatum. Lot. 222 mL. *OTC.*
Use: Topical combination.

Mentane. (Hoechst) Velnacrine.
Use: Cholinesterase inhibitor for Alzheimer disease.

Mentax. (Mylan) Butenafine hydrochloride 1%. Benzyl and cetyl alcohol, glycerin, white petrolatum. Cream. Tubes. 15 g, 30 g. *Rx.*
Use: Anti-infective, antifungal, topical.

Menthoderm. (Pharmaceutica North America) Methyl salicylate 15%, menthol 10%. Glycerin, parabens, polysorbate 20, propylene glycol, tartrazine, triethanolamine, SD-alcohol, urea. Oint. 60 g, 120 g. *OTC.*
Use: Rub and liniment.

•**menthol.** (MEN-thole) *USP 34.*
Use: Topical antipruritic; local analgesic; nasal decongestant; antitussive.
See: Absorbine Jr Back Patch.
Bengay Patch.
Blue Gel Muscular Pain Reliever.
Blue Ice.
Breathe Right Children's Colds.
Breathe Right Colds.
Cēpacol Menthol Regular Strength.
Cold & Hot Pain Relief Therapy Patch.
Flexall.
Gold Bond Pain Relieving Foot Roll-On.
Icy Hot Back Pain Relief.
Icy Hot Pain Relieving Gel.
Icy Hot PM Medicated.
Icy Hot Pop & Peel.
Icy Hot Pro-Therapy.
Icy Hot Roll.
Menthol Cough Drops.
Mineral Freez.
Therapy Ice.
Vicks Sinex.
Vicks VapoRub.
Vicks VapoSteam.
Victors.
W/Benzethonium Chloride.
See: Gold Bond Antiseptic First Aid Quick Spray.
W/Benzocaine.
See: Cēpacol Maximum Numbing Sore Throat.
Cēpacol Sore Throat Pain Relief Maximum Numbing.
Sting-Kill.
W/Benzocaine, Camphor.
See: Chiggerex.
W/Benzocaine, Methyl Salicylate.
See: Dendracin Neurodendtraxcin.
W/Camphor
See: Tiger Balm.
W/Capsaicin.
See: Capzasin Quick Relief.

W/Capsaicin, Lidocaine, Methyl Salicylate.
See: Terocin.
W/Capsaicin, Methyl Salicylate.
See: Medi-Derm.
Medrox.
W/Combinations.
See: Cēpacol Sore Throat.
Cēpacol Sore Throat From Post Nasal Drip.
Chloraseptic Kids Sore Throat.
Chloraseptic Sore Throat.
Chloraseptic Sore Throat Relief.
Eucalyptamint.
Eucalyptamint Maximum Strength.
Hall's Mentho-Lyptus Sugar Free.
Icy Hot Chill Stick.
Listerine Antiseptic.
Mentholatum Cherry Chest Rub for Kids.
Nose Better.
Sōltice Quick-Rub.
TheraPatch Vapor Patch for Kids Cough Suppressant.
Tom's of Maine Natural Cough & Cold Rub Cough Suppressant.
Vicks VapoRub.
W/Methyl Salicylate.
See: Analgesic Balm-GRX.
Menthoderm.
Pain Relieving Rub.
W/Zinc Oxide.
See: Calmoseptine.
Mentholatum. (Mentholatum Co.) Menthol 1.3%, camphor 9%. Petrolatum. Oint. Tube 28 g, 84 g. *OTC.*
Use: Upper respiratory combination, topical.
Mentholatum Cherry Chest Rub for Kids. (Mentholatum Co.) Camphor 4.7%, menthol 2.6%, eucalyptus oil 1.2%. Petrolatum. Oint. Tube 28 g. *OTC.*
Use: Upper respiratory combination, topical.
Mentholatum Deep Heating Lotion. (Mentholatum Co.) Menthol 6%, methyl salicylate 20%, lanolin derivative in lotion base. Bot. 2 oz, 4 oz. *OTC.*
Use: Analgesic, topical.
Mentholatum Deep Heating Rub. (Mentholatum Co.) Menthol 5.8%, methyl salicylate 12.7%, eucalyptus oil, turpentine oil, anhydrous lanolin, vehicle and fragrance. Tube 1.25 oz, 3.33 oz, 5 oz. *OTC.*
Use: Analgesic, topical.
Menthol Cough Drops. (Major) Menthol 6.5 mg. Eucalyptus oil, glucose syrup, sucrose. Lozenges. 30s. *OTC.*
Use: Mouth and throat product.

Mentholin. (Apco) Methyl salicylate 30%, chloroform 20%, hard soap 3%, camphor gum 2.2%, menthol 0.8%, alcohol 35%. Bot. 2 oz. *OTC.*
Use: Analgesic, topical.
menthyl anthranilate.
See: Meradimate
Menveo. (Novartis) Serogroups A 10 mcg, C 5 mcg, Y 5 mcg, W-135 5 mcg per 0.5 mL. Preservative free. Inj., Soln. Single-dose vial (supplied as a vial containing group A meningococcal (MenA) lyophilized conjugate component and a vial containing Men-CYW-135 liquid. *Rx.*
Use: Agent for active immunization, bacterial vaccine.
•**meobentine sulfate.** (meh-OH-BEN-teen) USAN.
Use: Cardiovascular agent (antiarrhythmic).
mepacrine hydrochloride.
Use: Anthelmintic; antimalarial.
•**mepartricin.** (meh-PAR-trih-sin) USAN.
Use: Antifungal; antiprotozoal.
mepavlon. Meprobamate.
•**mepenzolate bromide.** (meh-PEN-zoe-late) *USP 34.*
Use: Anticholinergic.
See: Cantil.
mepenzolate methyl bromide. Mepenzolate bromide.
Use: Anticholinergic.
•**meperidine hydrochloride.** (meh-PEHR-ih-deen) *USP 34.*
Use: Opioid analgesic.
See: Demerol.
W/Promethazine Hydrochloride.
See: Meprozine.
meperidine hydrochloride. (Hospira) Meperidine hydrochloride 10 mg/mL. Inj. Single-dose container (this vial only for use with a compatible Hospira *PCA* pump set with injector and a compatible Hospira infusion device). 30 mL. *c-II.*
Use: Opioid analgesic.
meperidine hydrochloride. (Roxane) Meperidine hydrochloride 50 mg/5 mL. Sorbitol. Oral Soln. 500 mL. *c-II.*
Use: Opioid analgesic.
meperidine hydrochloride. (Various Mfr.) Meperidine hydrochloride **Tab.:** 50 mg, 100 mg. Bot. 100s, 500s, 1000s, UD 25s. **Inj.:** 25 mg/mL, 50 mg/mL, 75 mg/mL, 100 mg/mL. Vials. 1 mL. Amps. 1 mL. *c-II.*
Use: Opioid analgesic.
meperidine hydrochloride and promethazine hydrochloride. (Various Mfr.) Meperidine hydrochloride 50 mg,

promethazine hydrochloride 25 mg.
Cap. 100s. *c-II.*
Use: Narcotic analgesic combination.
mephenesin.
Use: Muscle relaxant.
See: Myanesin.
mephenesin carbamate. Methoxydone.
•**mephobarbital.** (meh-foe-BAR-bih-tahl)
USP 34.
Use: Anticonvulsant; hypnotic; sedative.
See: Mebaral.
mephone. Mephentermine.
Mephyton. (Aton Pharma) Phytonadione (vitamin K) 5 mg. Lactose. Tab. Bot. 100s. *Rx.*
Use: Fat-soluble vitamin.
Mepiben. (Schein) Methylpiperidyl benzhydryl ether.
Use: Antihistamine.
mepiperphenidol bromide.
Use: Anticholinergic.
•**mepivacaine hydrochloride.** (meh-PIHV-ah-cane) *USP 34.*
Use: Anesthetic, local amide.
See: Carbocaine.
  Polocaine.
  Polocaine MPF.
  Scandonest.
W/Levonordefrin.
See: Carbocaine with Neo-Cobefrin.
  Scandonest L.
mepivacaine hydrochloride. (Septodont) Mepivacaine hydrochloride 3%. Inj. Dental Cart. 1.8 mL. *Rx.*
Use: Anesthetic, local amide.
mepivacaine hydrochloride and levonordefrin. (Septodont) Mepivacaine hydrochloride 2%, levonordefrin 1:20,000, sodium bisulfite. Inj. Dental Cart. 1.8 mL. *Rx.*
Use: Anesthetic, local amide.
•**meprednisone.** (meh-PRED-nih-sone) *USP 34.*
Use: Corticosteroid, topical.
•**meprobamate.** (meh-pro-BAM-ate) *USP 34.*
Use: Anxiolytic; hypnotic; sedative; antianxiety agent.
See: Arcoban.
W/Conjugated Estrogens.
See: PMB 400.
  PMB 200.
meprobamate. (Various Mfr.) Meprobamate 200 mg, 400 mg. Tab. Bot. 20s, 100s, 500s (400 mg only), 1000s, UD 100s (400 mg only). *c-IV.*
Use: Antianxiety agent.
meprobamate/aspirin. (Various Mfr.) Aspirin 325 mg, meprobamate 200 mg.

Tab. Bot. 100s, 500s. *Rx.*
Use: Analgesic combination.
meprobamate/benactyzine.
Use: Miscellaneous psychotherapeutic agent.
meprobamate, n-isopropyl.
See: Carisoprodol.
Meprogesic Q. (Various Mfr.) Aspirin 325 mg, meprobamate 200 mg. Tab. Bot. 100s, 500s. *Rx.*
Use: Analgesic combination.
Meprolone Tabs. (Major) Methylprednisolone 4 mg. Bot. 25s, 100s. *Rx.*
Use: Corticosteroid.
Mepron. (GlaxoSmithKline) Atovaquone 750 mg/5 mL. Susp. Bot. 210 mL. *Rx.*
Use: Anti-infective.
Meprozine. (Qualitest) Meperidine hydrochloride 50 mg, promethazine hydrochloride 25 mg. Lactose. Cap. 100s. *c-II.*
Use: Opioid analgesic combination.
meprylcaine hydrochloride.
Use: Anesthetic, local.
•**meptazinol hydrochloride.** (mep-TAZE-ih-nahl) USAN.
Use: Analgesic.
mepyrapone.
See: Metopirone.
•**mequidox.** (MEH-kwih-dox) USAN. Under study.
Use: Anti-infective.
•**mequinol.** (MEH-kwih-noll) USAN.
Use: Hyperpigmentation.
mequinolate. Name used for Proquinolate.
•**meradimate.** (mer-ADD-ih-mate) USAN.
Formerly menthyl anthranilate.
Use: Sunscreen.
•**meralein sodium.** (MER-ah-leen) USAN.
Use: Anti-infective, topical.
merbromin. *OTC.*
Use: Antiseptic, topical.
•**mercaptopurine.** (mer-cap-toe-PURE-een) *USP 34.*
Use: Antineoplastic.
See: Purinethol.
mercaptopurine. (PAR) Mercaptopurine 50 mg. Lactose. Tab. 60s. *Rx.*
Use: Antineoplastic.
mercazole.
See: Methimazole.
•**mercufenol chloride.** (MER-cue-FEEN-ole) USAN.
Use: Anti-infective, topical.
mercuranine.
See: Merbromin.
mercurial, antisyphilitics. Mercuric oleate, mercuric salicylate.
mercuric oleate. Oleate of mercury.
Use: Parasitic and fungal skin diseases.

mercuric oxide ophthalmic ointment, yellow.
Use: Local anti-infective, ophthalmic.
mercuric salicylate. Mercury subsalicylate.
Use: Parasitic and fungal skin diseases.
mercuric succinimide. Bis-Succinimidato-mercury.
mercurochrome.
See: Merbromin.
•mercury, ammoniated. (mer-cue-REE, ah-MOHN-ee-ated) *USP 34.*
Use: Anti-infective, topical.
mercury compounds.
See: Antiseptic, Mercurials.
mercury oleate. Mercury++ oleate.
Use: Pharmaceutic aid.
mercury-197-203.
See: Chlormerodrin.
Merdex. (Faraday) Docusate sodium 100 mg. Tab. Vial 60 mL. *Rx-OTC.*
Use: Laxative.
Meridia. (Abbott) Sibutramine 5 mg, 10 mg, 15 mg, lactose. Cap. Bot. 100s. *c-IV.*
Use: CNS stimulant; anorexiant.
•merimepodib. (me-ri-ME-poe-dib) USAN.
Use: Inosine monophosphate dehydrogenase inhibitor.
•merisoprol acetate Hg 197. (mer-EYE-so-prole) USAN.
Use: Radiopharmaceutical.
•merisoprol acetate Hg 203. (mer-EYE-so-prole) USAN.
Use: Radiopharmaceutical.
Meritene Powder. (Novartis) Vanilla flavor: Specially processed nonfat dry milk, corn syrup solids, sucrose, fructose, calcium caseinate, sodium chloride, natural and artificial flavors, lecithin, vitamins and minerals. Can 1 lb, 4.5 lb, 25 lb. Packet 1.14 oz. Vanilla, chocolate, eggnog, milk chocolate, plain flavors. *OTC.*
Use: Nutritional supplement.
merodicein. Sodium meralein.
•meropenem. (meh-row-PEN-em) USAN.
Use: Anti-infective.
See: Merrem I.V
meropenem. (Hospira) Meropenem 500 mg, 1 g. Sodium 45.1 mg (500 mg), 90.2 mg (1 g). Inj., Pow. for Soln. Vial. 20 mL, 30 mL. *Rx.*
Use: Anti-infective agent, carbapenem.
meroxapol 105.
Use: Irrigating solution.
See: Saf-Clens.
merprane.
Use: Diagnostic aid.

Merrem I.V. (AstraZeneca) Meropenem 500 mg, 1 g. Pow. for Inj. Vial 20 mL, 30 mL. *Rx.*
Use: Anti-infective.
Mervan. (Continental Pharma, Belgium) Alclofenac.
Use: Anti-inflammatory.
•mesalamine. (me-SAL-uh-MEEN) *USP 34.*
Use: Anti-inflammatory.
See: Apriso.
Asacol.
Canasa.
Lialda.
Pentasa.
Rowasa.
sfRowasa.
mesalamine. (Various Mfr.) Mesalamine 4 g/60 mL. May contain EDTA, potassium metabisulfite. Enemas. 7s in disposable bot. *Rx.*
Use: Treatment of inflammatory bowel disease.
mescomine.
See: Methscopolamine Bromide.
•meseclazone. (meh-SAK-lah-zone) USAN.
Use: Anti-inflammatory.
Mesehist DM. (Trigen Laboratories) Chlorpheniramine maleate 2 mg, dextromethorphan hydrobromide 15 mg, pseudoephedrine hydrochloride 15 mg per 5 mL. Parabens, potassium citrate, potassium sorbate, propylene glycol, sorbitol, sucralose. Orange flavor. Liq. 473 mL. *Rx.*
Use: Upper respiratory combination, antitussive combination.
Mesehist WC. (Trigen Laboratories) Brompheniramine maleate 1.3 mg, codeine phosphate 6.3 mg, pseudoephedrine hydrochloride 10 mg. Cherry flavoring, parabens, potassium citrate, potassium sorbate, propylene glycol, sorbitol, sucralose. Alcohol free and sugar free. Liq. 473 mL. *c-v.*
Use: Upper respiratory combination, antitussive combination.
•mesifilcon A. (MEH-sih-FILL-kahn A) USAN.
Use: Contact lens material; hydrophilic.
•mesna. (MESS-nah) USAN.
Use: Cytoprotective agent.
See: Mesnex.
mesna. (Baxter) Mesna 400 mg. Lactose. Film-coated. Tab. 10 blisters. *Rx.*
Use: Cytoprotective agent.
mesna. (Various Mfr.) Mesna 100 mg/mL. Benzyl alcohol 10.4 mg, EDTA

0.25 mg/mL. Inj. Multidose vials. 10 mL.
Rx.
Use: Cytoprotective agent.
Mesnex. (Bristol-Myers Squibb) Mesna.
Inj.: 100 mg/mL. EDTA 0.25 mg/mL, ben-
zyl alcohol 10.4 mg. Multidose vials.
10 mL. **Tab.:** 400 mg. Lactose, simethi-
cone. Film-coated. Blisters. 10. *Rx.*
Use: Antidote; cytoprotective agent.
• **mespiperone C 11.** (meh-SPIH-peh-rone
c 11) USAN.
Use: Radiopharmaceutical.
• **mesterolone.** (MESS-TER-oh-lone)
USAN.
Use: Androgen.
mestibol. Monomestrol.
Mestinon. (ICN) Pyridostigmine bromide.
ER Tab.: 180 mg. 30s. **Syrup:** 60 mg/
5 mL. Sucrose, sorbitol, alcohol 5%,
raspberry flavor. 480 mL. **Tab.:** 60 mg.
Lactose. 100s, 500s. *Rx.*
Use: Muscle stimulant.
• **mestranol.** (MESS-trah-nole) *USP 34.*
Use: Contraceptive; estrogen.
W/Ethynodiol Diacetate.
See: Ovulen-28.
Ovulen-21.
W/Norethindrone.
See: Necon 1/50.
Norinyl.
Norinyl 1 + 50.
Ortho-Novum 1/50.
W/Norethynodrel.
See: Enovid-E 21.
• **mesuprine hydrochloride.** (MEH-suh-
PREEN) USAN.
Use: Vasodilator; muscle relaxant.
Metabolin. (Thurston) Vitamins A
833 units, D 66 units, B_1 833 mcg, B_2
500 mcg, B_6 0.083 mcg, calcium panto-
thenate 833 mcg, niacinamide 5 mg,
folic acid 0.066 mcg, p-aminobenzoic
acid 0.416 mcg, inositol 833 mcg, B_{12}
500 mcg, C 5 mg, Ca 33.1 mg, P
14.6 mg, Fe 2.5 mg, I 0.15 mg. Tab.
Bot. 100s, 500s, 1000s. *OTC.*
Use: Mineral, vitamin supplement.
• **metabromsalan.** (MET-ah-BROME-sah-
lan) USAN.
Use: Antimicrobial; disinfectant.
metabutethamine hydrochloride.
Use: Anesthetic, local.
metabutoxycaine hydrochloride.
Use: Anesthetic, local.
metacaraphen hydrochloride.
See: Netrin.
metacortandracin.
See: Prednisone.
metacortandralone.
See: Prednisolone.

metacortin.
See: Meticorten.
• **metacresol.** (met-ah-KREE-sole)
USP 34.
Use: Antiseptic, topical; antifungal.
Metadate CD. (UCB) Methylphenidate
hydrochloride 10 mg, 20 mg, 30 mg,
40 mg, 50 mg, 60 mg. Sugar spheres.
ER Cap. 100s, UD 100s (except 40 mg,
50 mg, 60 mg), dosepack 30s (20 mg
only). *c-II.*
Use: Central nervous system stimulant.
Metadate ER. (Celltech) Methylphenidate
hydrochloride 10 mg, 20 mg. Cetyl alco-
hol, lactose, color-additive free. ER
Tab. Bot. 100s. *c-II.*
Use: Central nervous system stimulant.
meta-delphene. Diethyltoluamide.
Metaglip. (Bristol-Myers Squibb) Glipi-
zide/metformin hydrochloride 2.5 mg/
250 mg. Film-coated. Tab. 100s. *Rx.*
Use: Antidiabetic combination.
metaglycodol.
Use: Central nervous system depressant.
• **metalol hydrochloride.** (MEH-ta-lahl)
USAN. Under study.
Use: Antiadrenergic beta-receptor.
Metamucil. (Procter & Gamble) **Cap.:**
Psyllium husk 0.52 g. 100s, 160s. **Pow.:**
Psyllium hydrophilic mucilloid, sodium
1 mg, potassium 31 mg/Dose. **Regular
Flavor:** w/dextrose. Jar 7 oz, 14 oz,
21 oz. Packette 5.4 g. Box 100s.
Orange and Strawberry Flavors:
w/flavoring, sucrose and coloring. Jar
7 oz, 14 oz, 21 oz. **Wafer:** Psyllium husk
3.4 g, carbohydrates 17 g, sodium
20 mg, fat 5 g, 120 cal/dose, sugar,
fructose, molasses, sucrose, cinnamon
spice, apple crisp flavors. Ctn. 24s. *OTC.*
Use: Laxative.
Metamucil Instant Mix. (Procter &
Gamble) Psyllium hydrophilic mucilloid
with citric acid, sucrose, potassium bicarbonate, sodium bicarbonate. Powder when combined with water forms an
effervescent, flavored liquid. **Lemon
Lime Flavor:** w/calcium carbonate.
Cartons of 16, 30, or 100 packets of
3.4 g. **Orange Flavor:** w/flavoring and
coloring. Ctn. 16 or 30 packets of
3.4 g. *OTC.*
Use: Laxative.
**Metamucil Orange Flavor, Original Tex-
ture.** (Procter & Gamble) Approximately
psyllium husk 3.4 g, carbohydrates
10 g, sodium 5 mg, 40 cal/dose, sucrose. Pow. Can. 210 g, 420 g, 538 g,
630 g. *OTC.*
Use: Laxative.

Metamucil Orange Flavor, Smooth Texture. (Procter & Gamble) Approximately psyllium husk 3.4 g, sodium 5 mg, carbohydrates 12 g, 45 cal/dose, sucrose. Pow. Can. 420 g, 630 g, 1368 g, 100 UD single-dose packs (100s). *OTC.*
Use: Laxative.

Metamucil Original Texture. (Procter & Gamble) Approximately psyllium husk 3.4 g, carbohydrates 6 g, sodium 3 mg, 25 cal/dose, sucrose. Pow. Can. 822 g, Pack. 30. *OTC.*
Use: Laxative.

Metamucil, Sugar Free. (Procter & Gamble) Psyllium hydrophilic mucilloidin sugar-free formula. **Regular Flavor:** Jar 3.7 oz, 7.4 oz, 11.1 oz. Packet 3.4 g. Box 100s. **Orange Flavor:** Jar 3.7 oz, 7.4 oz, 11.1 oz. *OTC.*
Use: Laxative.

Metamucil Sugar Free, Orange Flavor, Smooth Texture. (Procter & Gamble) Approximately psyllium husk 3.4 g, carbohydrates 5 g, sodium 5 mg, 20 cal/dose, aspartame, phenylalanine 25 mg. Pow. Can. 210 g, 420 g, 630 g, 660 g. *OTC.*
Use: Laxative.

Metamucil, Sugar Free, Smooth Texture. (Procter & Gamble) Approximately psyllium husk 3.4 g, carbohydrates 5 g, sodium 4 mg, 20 cal/dose. Pow. Can. 425 g, Pack. 30s, 100s. *OTC.*
Use: Laxative.

Metandren. (Novartis) Methyltestosterone. **Linguet:** 5 mg, 10 mg Bot. 100s. **Tab.:** 10 mg, 25 mg Bot. 100s. *Rx.*
Use: Androgen.

Metanx. (Pamlab) Vitamins B$_6$ 35 mg (as pyridoxal-5' phosphate), B$_{12}$ 2,000 mcg (as methylcobalamin), folate 3 mg (as L-methylfolate calcium). Tab. 90s, 500s. *OTC.*
Use: Nutritional supplement, multivitamin.

metaphenylbarbituric acid.
See: Mephobarbital.

metaphyllin.
See: Aminophylline.

Metaprel Syrup. (Novartis) Metaproterenol sulfate 10 mg/5 mL. Bot. Pt. *Rx.*
Use: Bronchodilator.

•**metaproterenol polistirex.** (MEH-tuh-pro-TEHR-uh-nahl pahl-ee-STIE-rex) USAN.
Use: Bronchodilator.

•**metaproterenol sulfate.** (MEH-tuh-pro-TEHR-uh-nahl) *USP 34.*
Use: Bronchodilator, sympathomimetic.

metaproterenol sulfate. (Silarx) Meta-

proterenol sulfate 10 mg per 5 mL. EDTA, saccharin, sorbitol. Black cherry flavor. Syrup. 473 mL. *Rx.*
Use: Bronchodilator, sympathomimetic.

metaproterenol sulfate. (Various Mfr.) Metaproterenol sulfate 10 mg, 20 mg. Tab. 100s, 1000s. *Rx.*
Use: Bronchodilator, sympathomimetic.

•**metaraminol bitartrate.** (met-uh-RAM-in-ole) *USP 34.*
Use: Adrenergic; vasopressor.

Metastron. (Medi-Physics, Amersham Healthcare) Strontium-89 chloride 10.9 to 22.6 mg/mL. Preservative free. Inj. Vial 10 mL.
Use: Radiopharmaceutical.

•**metaxalone.** (meh-TAX-ah-lone) USAN.
Use: Muscle relaxant.
See: Skelaxin.

metaxalone. (Various Mfr.) Metaxalone 800 mg. Tab. 100s, 500s, 1,000s. *Rx.*
Use: Skeletal muscle relaxant, centrally acting.

Meted, Maximum Strength. (Medicis) Sulfur 5%, salicylic acid 3%. Shampoo. Bot. 118 mL. *OTC.*
Use: Antiseborrheic combination.

•**meteneprost.** (meh-TEN-eh-PRAHST) USAN.
Use: Oxytocic; prostaglandin.

•**metesind glucuronate.** (MEH-teh-sind glue-CURE-oh-nate) USAN.
Use: Antineoplastic (specific thymidylate synthase inhibitor).

metethoheptazine.
Use: Analgesic.

•**metformin.** (MET-fore-min) USAN.
Tall Man: metFORMIN
Use: Oral hypoglycemic; antidiabetic.
See: Riomet.

•**metformin hydrochloride.** (MET-fore-min) *USP 34.*
Tall Man: metFORMIN
Use: Antidiabetic agent, biguanide.
See: Fortamet.
Glucophage.
Glucophage XR.
Glumetza.
Riomet.
W/Glipizide.
See: Metaglip.
W/Glyburide.
See: Glucovance.
W/Pioglitazone Hydrochloride.
See: ActoPlus Met.
ActoPlus Met XR.
W/Rosiglitazone Maleate.
See: Avandamet.
W/Saxagliptin.
See: Kombiglyze XR.

W/Sitagliptin.
See: Janumet.
metformin hydrochloride. (Various Mfr.)
Metformin hydrochloride. **ER Tab.:**
500 mg, 750 mg. 100s. **Tab.:** 500 mg,
850 mg, 1,000 mg. Bot. 100s, 500s,
1,000s, 2,000s (500 mg only), UD 100s.
Rx.
Use: Antidiabetic agent, biguanide.
methacholine bromide. Mecholin bro-
mide.
Use: Cholinergic.
• **methacholine chloride.** (METH-uh-
KOH-leen) *USP 34.*
Use: Cholinergic.
See: Mecholyl Ointment.
Provocholine.
• **methacrylic acid copolymer.** (meth-ah-
KRILL-ik ASS-id koe-PAHL-ih-mer)
NF 29.
Use: Pharmaceutic aid (tablet coating
agent).
• **methacycline.** (meth-ah-SIGH-kleen)
USAN.
Use: Anti-infective.
• **methadone hydrochloride.** (METH-uh-
dohn) *USP 34.*
Use: Opioid analgesic; narcotic absti-
nence syndrome suppressant.
See: Diskets.
Dolophine Hydrochloride.
Methadose.
methadone hydrochloride. (AAI
Pharma) Methadone hydrochloride
10 mg/mL. Chlorobutanol 0.5%. Inj.
Multidose vial 20 mL. *c-II.*
Use: Opioid analgesic.
methadone hydrochloride. (Roxane)
Methadone hydrochloride 5 mg/mL,
10 mg/5 mL. May contain alcohol,
sorbitol. Citrus flavor. Oral Soln.
500 mL. *c-II.*
Use: Opioid analgesic.
methadone hydrochloride. (Various
Mfr.) Methadone hydrochloride. **Dispersible Tab. for Susp.:** 40 mg. Bot.
100s. **Oral Conc.:** 10 mg/mL. 946 mL,
1 L. **Tab.:** 5 mg, 10 mg. 100s, UD
100s. *c-II.*
Use: Opioid analgesic.
methadone hydrochloride diskets.
(Various Mfr.) Methadone hydrochloride
40 mg. Dispersible Tab. Bot. 100s. *c-II.*
Use: Opioid analgesic.
methadone hydrochloride intensol.
(Roxane) Methadone hydrochloride
10 mg/mL. Oral Conc. Bot. 30 mg with
calibrated dropper. *c-II.*
Use: Opioid analgesic.

Methadose. (Mallinckrodt) Methadone
hydrochloride. **Tab.:** 5 mg, 10 mg. Bot.
100s. **Disp. Tab.:** 40 mg. Bot. 100s.
Oral Conc.: 10 mg/mL. Sucrose, cherry
flavor. Also available sugar free, dye
free, unflavored. Bot. 1 L. *c-II.*
Use: Opioid analgesic.
• **methadyl acetate.** (METH-ah-dill) USAN.
Use: Analgesic, narcotic.
• **methafilcon B.** (METH-ah-FILL-kahn B)
USAN.
Use: Contact lens material (hydrophilic).
Methagual. (Gordon Laboratories)
Guaiacol 2%, methyl salicylate 8% in
petrolatum. Oint. 2 oz, lb. *OTC.*
Use: Analgesic, topical.
methalamic acid. Name used for lotha-
lamic acid.
• **methalthiazide.** (METH-al-THIGH-ah-
zide) USAN.
Use: Antihypertensive; diuretic.
methaminodiazepoxide.
See: Librium.
methamoctol.
Use: Adrenergic.
methamphetamine-dl hydrochloride.
See: dl-Methamphetamine Hydrochloride.
• **methamphetamine hydrochloride.**
(meth-am-FET-uh-meen) *USP 34.*
Use: CNS stimulant, amphetamine.
See: Desoxyn.
methamphetamine hydrochloride.
(Mylan) Methamphetamine hydrochloride 5 mg. Lactose. Tab. 100s. *c-II.*
Use: CNS stimulant, amphetamine.
methampyrone.
See: Dipyrone.
methandriol. (Various Mfr.) Methylandrostenediol.
methandriol dipropionate.
See: Arbolic.
Methaphor. (Borden) Protein hydrolysate
(l-leucine, l-isoleucine, l-methionine, l-
phenylalanine, l-tyrosine); methionine,
camphor, benzethonium chloride, in
Dermabase vehicle. Oint. Tube 1.5 oz.
OTC.
Use: Dermatologic, amino acid supplement.
• **methaqualone.** (METH-ah-kwan-lone)
USAN.
Use: Hypnotic, sedative.
Methatropic Capsules. (Ivax) Choline
115 mg, inositol 83 mg, methionine
110 mg, vitamins B_1 3 mg, B_2 3 mg,
B_3 10 mg, B_5 2 mg, B_6 2 mg, B_{12} 2 mcg,
desiccated liver 86 mg. Bot. 100s. *OTC.*
Use: Vitamin supplement.

• **methazolamide.** (meth-ah-ZOLE-ah-mide) *USP 34.*
Use: Carbonic anhydrase inhibitor.
methazolamide. (Various Mfr.) Methazolamide 25 mg or 50 mg. Tab. Bot. 100s. *Rx.*
Use: Carbonic anhydrase inhibitor.
Methblue 65. (Manne) Methylene blue 65 mg. Tab. Bot. 100s, 1000s. *Rx.*
Use: Antidote, cyanide.
Meth-Choline. (Schein) Choline 115 mg, inositol 83 mg, methionine 110 mg, vitamins B_1 3 mg, B_2 3 mg, B_3 10 mg, B_5 2 mg, B_6 2 mg, B_{12} 2 mcg, desiccated liver 56 mg, liver concentrate 30 mg. Cap. Bot. 100s, 250s, 1000s. *OTC.*
Use: Vitamin supplement.
Meth-Dia-Mer Sulfa. Trisulfapyrimidines. Tab.
Use: Triple sulfonamide therapy.
See: Chemozine.
Triple Sulfa.
Meth-Dia-Mer Sulfonamides Suspension. Trisulfapyrimidines Oral Suspension.
Use: Triple sulfonamide therapy.
See: Chemozine.
Triple Sulfa.
• **methdilazine hydrochloride.** (METH-dill-ah-ZEEN) *USP 34.*
Use: Antipruritic.
• **methenamine.** (meh-THEN-uh-meen) *USP 34. Formerly Hexamethylenamine.*
Use: Anti-infective, urinary.
W/Atropine Sulfate, Benzoic Acid, Hyoscyamine Sulfate, Methylene Blue, Phenyl Salicylate.
See: Uritact DS
W/Combinations.
See: Cystamine.
Cystex.
Cysto.
MHP-A.
Prosed/DS.
Urelle.
Uretron D/S.
Urimar-T.
Urisan-P.
Uriseptic.
Uro Blue.
Urogesic Blue.
Uro Phosphate.
W/Hyoscyamine Sulfate, Methylene Blue, Phenyl Salicylate, Sodium Biphosphate.
See: Urimax.
W/Hyoscyamine Sulfate, Methylene Blue, Phenyl Salicylate, Sodium Phosphate Monobasic.
See: Uticap.
Utrona-C.

methenamine and monobasic sodium phosphate tablets.
Use: Anti-infective, urinary.
methenamine anhydromethylene citrate. Formanol, uropurgol, urotropin.
• **methenamine hippurate.** (meth-EE-nah-meen HIP-you-rate) *USP 34.*
Use: Anti-infective, urinary.
See: Hiprex.
Urex.
methenamine hippurate. (CorePharma) Methenamine hippurate 1 g. Saccharin. Tab. 100s. *Rx.*
Use: Anti-infective, methenamine.
methenamine hippurate. (Mylan) Methenamine hippurate 1 g. Saccharin. Tabs. 100s. Rx. Anti-effective, methenamine.
• **methenamine mandelate.** (meth-EE-nah-meen MAN-deh-late) *USP 34.*
Use: Anti-infective, urinary.
W/Hyoscyamine.
See: Urisedamine.
W/Sodium Acid Phosphate Monobasic Monohydrate.
See: Utac.
methenamine mandelate. (Various Mfr.)
Tab.: 0.5 g, 1 g. Tab. 100s, 1000s.
Susp.: 0.5 g/5 mL. Susp. Bot. 480 mL.
Use: Anti-infective, urinary.
• **methenolone acetate.** (meth-EEN-oh-lone) USAN.
Use: Anabolic.
• **methenolone enanthate.** (meth-EEN-oh-lone eh-NAN-thate) USAN.
Use: Anabolic.
Metheponex. (Rawl) Choline 0.54 g, dl-methionine 1.80 g, inositol 0.27 g, whole desiccated liver 8.10 g, vitamins B_1 18 mg, B_2 36 mg, niacinamide 90 mg, B_6 3.6 mg, calcium pantothenate 3.6 mg, biotin 10.8 mcg, B_{12} 5.4 mcg and amino acid/daily therapeutic dose. Cap. Bot. 100s, 500s. *Rx.*
Use: Antidiabetic; nutritional supplement.
metheptazine.
Use: Analgesic.
Methergine. (Sandoz) Methylergonovine maleate. **Inj.:** 0.2 mg/mL. Ampuls. 1 mL. **Tab.:** 0.2 mg. Lactose, FD&C Blue No. 1, parabens, sucrose, coated. Bot. 100s. *Rx.*
Use: Oxytocic.
methestrol.
See: Promethestrol Dipropionate.
methetharimide bemegride. USAN.
Use: Anticonvulsant.
Methibon. (Barrows) Choline dihydrogen citrate 278 mg, dl-methionine 111 mg,

inositol 83.3 mg, vitamin B_{12} 2 mcg, liver concentrate, desiccated liver 86.6 mg. Cap. Bot. 100s. *Rx.*
Use: Antidiabetic; nutritional supplement.

•**methicillin sodium.** (meth-ih-SILL-in) USAN.
Use: Anti-infective.

•**methimazole.** (meth-IMM-uh-zole) *USP 34.*
Use: Antithyroid agent.
See: Northyx.
Tapazole.

methimazole. (Par Pharm) Methimazole 5 mg, 10 mg. Lactose. Tab. Bot. 100s. *Rx.*
Use: Antithyroid agent.

Methiokaps. (Pal-Pak, Inc.) dl-methionine 200 mg. Cap. Bot. 1000s. *Rx.*
Use: Diaper rash product.

methiomeprazine hydrochloride. (GlaxoSmithKline)
Use: Antiemetic.

•**methionine.** (meh-THIGH-oh-NEEN) *USP 34.*
Note: Also see Racemethionine.
Use: Amino acid.
See: M-Caps.

•**methionine C 11 injection.** (meh-THIGH-oh-NEEN) *USP 34.*
Use: Radiopharmaceutical.

methionyl brain-derived neurotrophic factor, recombinant.
Use: Amyotrophic lateral sclerosis agent. [Orphan Drug]

Methioplex. (Lincoln Diagnostics) Methionine 25 mg, vitamins B_1 50 mg, niacinamide 100 mg, B_2 2 mg, choline 50 mg, B_6 2 mg, panthenol 2 mg, benzyl alcohol 1%, distilled water q.s./mL. Vial 30 mL. *Rx.*
Use: Nutritional supplement.

•**methisazone.** (METH-eye-SAH-zone) USAN.
Use: Antiviral.

Methitest. (Global) Methyltestosterone 10 mg. Lactose, sugar. Tab. Bot. 100s. *c-III.*
Use: Sex hormone, androgen.

methitural sodium.
Use: Hypnotic, sedative.

•**methixene hydrochloride.** (meh-THIX-een) USAN.
Use: Muscle relaxant.

•**methocarbamol.** (meth-oh-CAR-buh-mahl) *USP 34.*
Use: Muscle relaxant.
See: Robaxin.
Robaxin-750.

methocarbamol. (Various Mfr.) Methocarbamol. **Tab.:** 500 mg, 750 mg. Bot. 60s (750 mg only), 100s, 500s, UD 100s.
Use: Muscle relaxant.

methocel. Methylcellulose.

•**methohexital.** (meth-oh-HEX-ih-tahl) *USP 34.*
Use: Pharmaceutic necessity for methohexital sodium for injection.

•**methohexital sodium for injection.** (METH-oh-HEX-ih-tahl) *USP 34.*
Use: Anesthetic, general; anesthetic (intravenous).
See: Brevital Sodium.

•**methoin.** (METH-eh-toe-in) USAN.
Use: Anticonvulsant.

•**methopholine.** (METH-oh-foe-leen) USAN.
Use: Analgesic.
See: Versidyne.

Methopto Forte 1%. (Professional Pharmacal) Methylcellulose pow. 10 mg (1% soln.), boric acid 12 mg, potassium chloride 7.3 mg, benzalkonium chloride 0.04 mg, glycerin 12 mg/mL w/sodium carbonate to adjust pH and purified water. Bot. 15 mL. *OTC.*
Use: Artificial tears.

Methopto Forte 0.5%. (Professional Pharmacal) Methylcellulose pow. 5 mg (0.5% soln.), boric acid 12 mg, potassium chloride 7.3 mg, benzalkonium chloride 0.4 mg, glycerin 12 mg/mL w/ sodium carbonate to adjust pH and purified water. Bot. 15 mL. *OTC.*
Use: Artificial tears.

Methopto 0.25%. (Professional Pharmacal) Methylcellulose pow. 2.5 mg (0.25% soln.), boric acid 12 mg, potassium chloride 7.3 mg, benzalkonium chloride 0.04 mg, glycerin 12 mg/mL w/sodium carbonate to adjust pH and purified water. Bot. 15 mL, 30 mL. *OTC.*
Use: Artificial tears.

methopyraphone.
See: Metopirone.

methorate.
See: Dextromethorphan Hydrobromide.

Methorbate S.C. (Standex) Methenamine 40.8 mg, atropine sulfate 0.03 mg, hyoscyamine sulfate 0.03 mg, salol 18.1 mg, benzoic acid 4.5 mg, methylene blue 5.4 mg. Tab. Bot. 100s. *Rx.*
Use: Anti-infective, urinary.

d-methorphan hydrobromide.
See: Dextromethorphan Hydrobromide.

methorphinan. Racemorphan hydrobromide. Dromoran.

•**methotrexate.** (meth-oh-TREK-sate) *USP 34. Formerly Amethopterin.*

Use: Leukemia in children; antineoplastic; antipsoriatic; juvenile rheumatoid arthritis; folic acid antagonist.
See: Mexate-AQ.
Rheumatrex Dose Pack.
Trexall.
methotrexate. (Immunex) **Inj.:** 25 mg/mL as sodium, benzyl alcohol 0.9%, sodium chloride 0.26% and water for inj. Vials 2 mL, 10 mL. **Pow. for Inj.:** 20 mg or 1 g/vial as sodium. Single-use vials. *Rx.*
Use: Antipsoriatic.
methotrexate. (Various Mfr.) Methotrexate 2.5 mg (as sodium). Tab. Bot. 36s, 100s. *Rx.*
Use: Antineoplastic; antirheumatic.
methotrexate LPF sodium. (Xanodyne) Methotrexate sodium 25 mg/mL (as base). Preservative free. Single-use vials. 2 mL (sodium 0.43 mEq/vial), 4 mL (sodium 0.86 mEq/vial), 10 mL (sodium 2.15 mEq/vial). *Rx.*
Use: Antimetabolite.
methotrexate sodium. (Various Mfr.) Methotrexate sodium. **Inj.:** 25 mg/mL (as base). Preservative free. Single-use vials. 2 mL, 4 mL, 8 mL, 10 mL, 20 mL, 40 mL. **Pow. for Inj., lyophilized:** 20 mg (as base) (sodium 0.14 mEq/vial), 1 g (as base) (sodium 7 mEq/vial). Preservative free. Single-use vials. *Rx.*
Use: Antimetabolite.
methotrexate sodium. (Various Mfr.) Methotrexate sodium 25 mg/mL (as base). Benzyl alcohol 0.9%. Must not be used for intrathecal or high-dose therapy. Vials. 2 mL, 10 mL. *Rx.*
Use: Antimetabolite.
methotrexate sodium. (Wyeth) Methotrexate sodium 2.5 mg/mL Vial 2 mL; 25 mg/mL. Vial 2 mL w/preservatives; 20 mg, 50 mg, 100 mg Vial cryodesiccated, preservative free; 50 mg, 100 mg, 200 mg Vial; 25 mg/mL solution preservative free.
Use: Leukemia therapy; psoriasis; osteogenic sarcoma. [Orphan Drug]
methotrexate with laurocapram.
Use: Topical treatment of *Mycosis fungoides.* [Orphan Drug]
•**methoxsalen.** (meth-OX-ah-len) *USP 34.*
Use: Pigmenting agent.
See: 8-MOP.
Oxsoralen.
Oxsoralen Ultra.
Uvadex.
8-methoxsalen.
Use: Treatment of diffuse systemic sclerosis, rejection of cardiac allografts. [Orphan Drug]

See: Uvadex.
methoxyphenamine hydrochloride.
USP 34.
Use: Adrenergic (bronchodilator).
W/Dextromethorphan hydrochloride, orthoxine, sodium citrate.
See: Orthoxicol.
methoxy polyethylene glycol-epoetin beta. (meth-ox-ee POL-ee-eth-i-leen GLYE-kol e-POE-e-tin BAY-ta)
Use: Hematopoietic agent.
See: Mircera.
methoxypromazine maleate.
Use: CNS depressant.
methoxypsoralen, oral.
Use: Psoralen.
See: Oxsoralen.
Oxsoralen Ultra.
•**methscopolamine bromide.** (METH-skoe-POL-a-meen) *USP 34.*
Use: Anticholinergic.
See: Pamine.
Pamine Forte.
Pamine FQ Kit.
W/Butabarbital Sodium, Dried Aluminum Hydroxide Gel and Magnesium Trisilicate.
See: Eulcin.
methscopolamine bromide. (Boca Pharmacal) Methscopolamine bromide 2.5 mg, 5 mg. Tab. 60s (5 mg only), 100s (2.5 mg only), 5 blisters of 12 tablets (5 mg only). *Rx.*
Use: Anticholinergic/antispasmodic.
methscopolamine nitrate. Scopolamine methyl nitrate, preps. Mescomine.
W/Chlorpheniramine Maleate.
See: AeroHist.
AllePak Dose Pack.
Allergy DN.
AlleRx DF Dose Pack.
AlleRx Dose Pack.
NoHist EXT.
RelCof CPM.
SymPak PDX.
W/Chlorpheniramine Maleate, Phenylephrine Hydrochloride.
See: AeroHist Plus.
AeroKid.
CPM 8/PE 20/MSC 1.25.
Dallergy.
Dallergy PE.
Dehistine.
Denaze.
DriHist SR.
Drysec.
Duradryl.
Extendryl.
NoHist-Plus.
OMNIhist II LA.
PCM.

PE-CPM-MSN 8-2-0.75.
PE-HCL-CPM-MSN 10-2-0.75.
Phenylephrine CM.
QV Allergy.
Ralix.
Rescon.
Rescon-MX.
SymPak.
SymPak PDX.
Zinx PCM.
W/Chlorpheniramine Maleate, Pseudo-
ephedrine Hydrochloride.
See: CPM 8/PSE 90/MSC 2.5.
DryMax.
Relcof PSE.
Time-Hist QD.
W/Chlorpheniramine Tannate.
See: Dexodryl.
W/Chlorpheniramine Tannate, Phenyl-
ephrine Tannate.
See: AH-chew.
AH-chew Ultra.
Redur-PCM.
W/Dexchlorpheniramine Maleate, Phenyl-
ephrine Hydrochloride.
See: Dexphen M.
Extendryl.
W/Dexchlorpheniramine Maleate,
Pseudoephedrine Hydrochloride.
See: D-Hist D.
Histatab D.
W/Dextromethorphan Hydrobromide,
Chlorpheniramine Maleate.
See: Extendryl DM.
W/Phenylephrine Hydrochloride.
See: Extendryl PEM.
W/Pseudoephedrine Hydrochloride.
See: AllePak Dose Pack.
Allergy DN.
AlleRx-D.
AlleRx Dose Pack.
Amdry-D.
PSE 120/MSC 2.5.
• **methsuximide.** (meth-SUCK-sih-mide)
USP 34.
Use: Anticonvulsant.
See: Celontin.
• **methyclothiazide.** (METH-ee-kloe-
THIGH-ah-zide) *USP 34.*
Use: Antihypertensive; diuretic.
See: Enduron.
W/Deserpidine.
See: Enduronyl.
methyclothiazide. (Various Mfr.) Methy-
clothiazide 2.5 mg, 5 mg. Tab. 100s
(2.5 mg only), 100s. *Rx.*
Use: Diuretic.
methylacetylcholine.
See: Methacholine.
• **methyl alcohol.** (METH-ill) *NF 29.*
Use: Pharmaceutic acid (solvent).

methyl aminolevulinate.
Use: Photochemotherapy.
See: Metvixia.
• **methyl aminolevulinate hydrochloride.**
(METH-il a-MEE-noe-LEV-ue-LIN-ate)
USAN.
Use: Antineoplastic.
**methylamphetamine hydrochloride
and sulfate.**
See: Desoxyephedrine Hydrochloride.
methylandrostenediol. Methandriol.
• **methylatropine nitrate.** (METH-ill-AT-
row-peen) USAN.
Use: Anticholinergic.
• **methylbenzethonium chloride.** (meth-
ill-benz-eth-OH-nee-uhm) *USP 34.*
Use: Bactericide, local anti-infective
(topical).
See: Diaparene.
methylbenztropine.
See: Ethybenztropine.
methylbromtropin mandelate. Homatropine Methylbromide, USP.
• **methylcellulose.** (METH-ill-SELL-you-
lohs) *USP 34.*
Use: Pharmaceutic aid (suspending
agent).
See: Cellothyl.
Citrucel Fiber Shake.
Cologel.
W/Carboxymethylcellulose.
See: Ex-Caloric.
methyl cysteine hydrochloride. Cys-
teine methyl ester hydrochloride.
Use: Mucolytic agent.
• **methyldopa.** (meth-ill-DOE-puh)
USP 34. Formerly Alpha-Methyldopa.
Use: Antihypertensive.
W/Chlorothiazide.
See: Aldoclor.
methyldopa. (Various Mfr.) Methyldopa
250 mg, 500 mg. Tab. Bot. 100s, 500s,
1000s (250 mg only), UD 100s. *Rx.*
Use: Antihypertensive.
methyldopa/hydrochlorothiazide.
(Various Mfr.) Methyldopa/hydrochloro-
thiazide 250 mg/15 mg, 250 mg/25 mg.
Tab. Bot. 100s, 500s, 1000s, UD 100s.
Rx.
Use: Antihypertensive combination.
methyldopa/hydrochlorothiazide.
(Various Mfr.) Methyldopa/hydrochloro-
thiazide 500 mg/30 mg, 500 mg/50 mg.
Tab. Bot. 100s, 250s, 500s. *Rx.*
Use: Antihypertensive combination.
• **methyldopate hydrochloride.** (meth-ill-
DOE-pate) *USP 34.*
Use: Antihypertensive.
• **methylene blue.** (METH-ih-leen)
USP 34.

Use: Antidote; cyanide.
See: Methblue 65.
W/Atropine Sulfate, Benzoic Acid, Hyoscyamine Sulfate, Methenamine, Phenyl Salicylate.
See: Uritact DS.
W/Hyoscyamine Sulfate, Methenamine, Phenyl Salicylate, Sodium Biphosphate.
See: Urimax.
W/Hyoscyamine Sulfate, Methenamine, Phenyl Sailcylate, Sodium Phosphate Monobasic.
See: Uticap.
Utrona-C.
methylene blue. (Various Mfr.) Methylene blue 10 mg/mL. Inj. Vial 1 mL, 10 mL. *Rx.*
Use: GU antiseptic; antidote; cyanide.
• **methylene chloride.** (METH-ih-leen) *NF 29.*
Use: Pharmaceutic aid (solvent).
• **methylergonovine maleate.** (METH-ill-err-go-NO-veen) *USP 34.*
Use: Oxytocic.
See: Methergine.
methylergonovine maleate. (PharmaForce) Methylergonovine maleate 0.2 mg/mL. Inj., Soln. Vial. 1 mL. *Rx.*
Use: Uterine-active agent.
methylglucamine diatrizoate, injection. A water-soluble radiopaque iodine cpd. N-methylglucamine salt of Diatrizoate.
See: Diatrizoate Meglumine.
methylglucamine iodipamide, injection.
See: Meglumine Iodipamide, Injection.
W/Diatrizoate methylglucamine.
See: Sinografin.
methylglyoxal-bis-guanylhydrazone. Methyl GAG.
Methylin. (Shionogi Pharm) Methylphenidate hydrochloride. **Chew. Tab.:** 2.5 mg, phenylalanine 0.42 mg; 5 mg, phenylalanine 0.84 mg; 10 mg, phenylalanine 1.68 mg. Aspartame, grape flavor. 100s. **Oral Soln.:** 5 mg per 5 mL, 10 mg per 5 mL. Glycerin. Grape flavor. 500 mL. *c-II.*
Use: Central nervous system stimulant.
Methylin. (Shionogi Pharm) Methylphenidate hydrochloride 5 mg, 10 mg, 20 mg. Lactose, talc. Tab. Bot. 100s, 1,000s. *c-II.*
Use: Central nervous system stimulant.
Methylin ER. (Mallinckrodt) Methylphenidate hydrochloride 10 mg, 20 mg. Talc, color-additive free. ER Tab. Bot. 100s. *c-II.*
Use: Central nervous system stimulant.

• **methyl isobutyl ketone.** (METH-ill eye-so-BYOO-till KEE-tone) *NF 29.*
Use: Pharmaceutic aid (alcohol denaturant).
methylmelamines/ethylenimines.
See: Ethylenimines/Methylmelamines.
methylmercadone. Name used for Nifuratel.
• **methylnaltrexone bromide.** (METH-il-nal-TREX-one BROE-mide)
Use: Detoxification agent, antidote.
See: Relistor.
• **methyl nicotinate.** (METH-ill NIK-oh-TIN-ate) *USAN.*
W/Methyl salicylate, menthol.
See: Musterole Deep Strength.
Methylone. (Paddock) Methylprednisolone acetate 40 mg/mL. Vial 5 mL. *Rx.*
Use: Corticosteroid.
• **methyl palmoxirate.** (METH-ill pal-MOX-ihr-ate) *USAN.*
Use: Antidiabetic.
• **methylparaben.** (meth-ill-PAR-ah-ben) *NF 29.*
Use: Pharmaceutic aid (antifungal agent).
• **methylparaben sodium.** (meth-ill-PAR-ah-ben) *NF 29.*
Use: Pharmaceutic aid (antimicrobial preservative).
methylphenethylamine.
See: Amphetamine Hydrochloride.
• **methylphenidate.** (meth-ill-FEN-ih-date) *USAN.*
Use: Central nervous system stimulant.
methylphenidate. (Breckenridge) Methylphenidate hydrochloride 5 mg per 5 mL. Glycerin, PEG. Grape flavor. Soln. 500 mL. *c-II.*
Use: CNS stimulant.
• **methylphenidate hydrochloride.** (meth-ill-FEN-ih-date) *USP 34.*
Use: Central nervous system stimulant.
See: Concerta.
Daytrana.
Metadate CD.
Metadate ER.
Methylin.
Methylin ER.
Ritalin.
Ritalin LA.
Ritalin-SR.
methylphenidate hydrochloride. (Various Mfr.) Methylphenidate hydrochloride. **Tab.:** 5 mg, 10 mg, 20 mg. Bot. 100s, 1000s. **ER Tab.:** 20 mg, Bot. 30s, 100s. *c-II.*
Use: Central nervous system stimulant.
methylphenidylacetate hydrochloride.
See: Methylphenidate Hydrochloride.

methylphenobarbital.
See: Mephobarbital.
d-methylphenylamine sulfate.
See: Dextroamphetamine Sulfate.
methylphytyl naphthoquinone.
Use: Vitamin supplement.
See: Phytonadione.
methyl polysiloxane.
See: Mylicon.
Simethicone.
methylpred-40. (Seatrace) Methylpred-
nisolone acetate 40 mg/mL. Vial 5 mL,
10 mL. *Rx.*
Use: Corticosteroid.
•**methylprednisolone.** (METH-ill-pred-
NIH-suh-lone) *USP 34.*
Tall Man: methylPREDNISolone
Use: Adrenocortical steroid, glucocorti-
coid.
See: Medrol.
methylprednisolone. (Cadista) Methyl-
prednisolone 32 mg. Lactose. Tab. 25s.
Rx.
Use: Adrenocortical steroid, glucocorti-
coid.
methylprednisolone. (Various Mfr.)
Methylprednisolone 4 mg, 8 mg, 16 mg.
May contain lactose (except 4 mg).
Tab. **4 mg:** 21s, 100s, unit-of-use 21s.
8 mg: 25s. **16 mg:** 50s. *Rx.*
Use: Adrenocortical steroid, glucocorti-
coid.
•**methylprednisolone acetate.** (METH-ill-
pred-NIH-suh-lone) *USP 34.*
Tall Man: methylPREDNISolone
Use: Adrenocortical steroid, glucocorti-
coid.
See: Depo-Medrol.
methylprednisolone acetate. (Various
Mfr.) Methylprednisolone acetate
20 mg/mL, 40 mg/mL, 80 mg/mL. Susp.
Inj. Vials. 5 ml, 10 mL (except 80 mg).
Rx.
Use: Adrenocortical steroids, glucocorti-
coids.
•**methylprednisolone hemisuccinate.**
(METH-ill-pred-NIH-suh-lone hem-ih-
SUCK-sih-nate) *USP 34.*
Tall Man: methylPREDNISolone
Use: Adrenocortical steroid.
•**methylprednisolone sodium phos-
phate.** (METH-ill-pred-NIH-suh-lone)
USAN.
Tall Man: methylPREDNISolone
Use: Corticosteroid, topical.
•**methylprednisolone sodium succinate.**
(METH-ill-pred-NIH-suh-lone) *USP 34.*
Tall Man: methylPREDNISolone
Use: Adrenocorticoid steroid; corticoste-
roid, topical; glucocorticoid.

See: A-Methapred.
Solu-Medrol.
methylprednisolone sodium succinate.
(Various Mfr.) Methylprednisolone sodium succinate 40 mg/vial, 125 mg/vial,
500 mg/vial, 1 g/vial. Inj., Pow. for
Soln. Vials. 1 mL (except 125 mg), 2 mL
(125 mg only), 3 mL (40 mg only),
4 mL (500 mg only), 5 mL (125 mg
only), 8 mL (1 g only), 20 mL (500 mg
only), 50 mL (1 g only). *Rx.*
Use: Adrenocortical steroid, glucocorticoid.
•**methylprednisolone suleptanate.**
(METH-ill-pred-NIH-suh-lone sull-EPP-
tah-NATE) USAN.
Tall Man: methylPREDNISolone
Use: Adrenocortical steroid; anti-inflam-
matory.
methylpyrimal.
See: Sulfamerazine.
methylrosaniline chloride.
Use: Anthelmintic; anti-infective.
See: Gentian Violet.
•**methyl salicylate.** (METH-ill sal-ISS-ih-
late) *NF 29.*
Use: Rubefacient rub (topical).
W/Benzocaine, Menthol.
See: Dendracin Neurodendtraxcin.
W/Capsaicin, Lidocaine, Menthol.
See: Terocin.
W/Capsaicin, Menthol.
See: Medi-Derm.
Medrox.
W/Combinations.
See: Analbalm.
Analgesic Balm.
Bayer Muscle Joint Cream.
Cydonol.
Gordobalm.
Icy Hot Chill Stick.
Listerine Antiseptic.
Musterole.
Pain Bust-R II.
Sloan's Liniment.
Ziks.
W/Iodine.
See: Iodex With Methyl Salicylate.
W/Menthol.
See: Analgesic Balm-GRX.
Menthoderm.
Pain Relieving Rub.
methyl sulfanil amidoisoxazole. Sulfa-
methoxazole.
•**methyltestosterone.** (METH-ill-tess-
TAHS-ter-ohn) *USP 34.*
Tall Man: methylTESTOSTERone
Use: Sex hormone, androgen.
See: Methitest.
Testred.

Virilon.
W/Esterified Estrogens.
See: Covaryx.
  Covaryx HS.
  Estratest.
  Estratest H.S.
methyltestosterone. (Various Mfr.)
Methyltestosterone. **Tab.:** 10 mg,
25 mg. Bot. 100s. **Tab., buccal:** 10 mg.
Bot. 100s. *c-III.*
Use: Sex hormone, androgen.
**methyltestosterone and esterified
estrogens.** (Lannett) Esterified estrogens 1.25 mg, methyltestosterone
2.5 mg. Tartrazine. Film-coated. Tab.
100s, 1000s. *Rx.*
Use: Sex hormone.
**methyltestosterone and esterified
estrogens H.S.** (Lannett) Esterified
estrogens 0.625 mg, methyltestosterone 1.25 mg. Lactose. Film-coated.
Tab. 100s, 1000s. *Rx.*
Use: Sex hormone.
methylthionine chloride. *Name used
for Methylene Blue.*
methylthionine hydrochloride. *Name
used for Methylene Blue.*
methylthiouracil. *USP 34.*
Use: Antithyroid agent.
methyl violet.
See: Gentian Violet, Crystal Violet,
  Methylrosaniline Chloride.
methyndamine. *Name used for Tetrydamine.*
●**metiamide.** (meh-TIE-aim-ide) USAN.
Histamine H₂ antagonist.
Use: Treatment for peptic ulcer; antiulcerative.
●**metiapine.** (meh-TIE-ah-PEEN) USAN.
Use: Antipsychotic.
meticlopindol. *Name used for Clopidol.*
Metimyd Ophthalmic Oint. Sterile.
(Schering-Plough) Prednisolone acetate
0.5% (5 mg), sulfacetamide sodium
10%. Tube 3.5 g. *Rx.*
Use: Corticosteroid; sulfonamide,
topical.
●**metioprim.** (meh-TIE-oh-PRIM) USAN.
Use: Anti-infective.
●**metipranolol.** (meh-tih-PRAN-oh-lahl)
USAN.
Use: Antihypertensive (beta-blocker,
ophthalmic).
metipranolol. (Falcon Ophthalmics)
Metipranolol 0.3%, povidone, hydrochloric acid, NaCl, EDTA, benzalkonium
chloride 0.004%. Ophth. Soln. Bot.
5 mL, 10 mL. *Rx.*
Use: Antihypertensive, beta-blocker,
ophthalmic.

metipranolol hydrochloride.
Use: Antihypertensive (beta-blocker,
ophthalmic).
See: OptiPranolol.
metizoline.
Use: Decongestant.
●**metizoline hydrochloride.** (meh-TIH-
zoe-leen) USAN.
Use: Adrenergic vasoconstrictor.
●**metkephamid acetate.** (MET-KEFF-am-
id) USAN.
Use: Analgesic.
●**metoclopramide hydrochloride.** (MET-
oh-kloe-PRA-mide) *USP 34.*
Use: Antiemetic; gastrointestinal stimulant.
See: Metozolv.
metoclopramide hydrochloride.
(Various Mfr.) Metoclopramide hydrochloride (as monohydrochloride monohydrate). **Inj.:** 5 mg/mL. Vials. 2 mL,
10 mL, 30 mL. Amps. 2 mL. **Syrup:**
5 mg/mL. 480 mL, UD 10 mL. **Tab.:**
5 mg, 10 mg. 100s; 500s; 1000s;
2500s, UD 100s (10 mg only). *Rx.*
Use: Gastrointestinal stimulant.
metofurone. Name used for Nifurmerone.
●**metogest.** (MET-oh-JEST) USAN.
Use: Hormone.
●**metolazone.** (meh-TOLE-uh-ZONE)
USP 34.
Use: Antihypertensive; diuretic.
See: Zaroxolyn.
metolazone. (Various Mfr.) Metolazone
2.5 mg, 5 mg, 10 mg. Tab. 100s, 1000s
(2.5 mg only). *Rx.*
Use: Diuretic.
●**metopimazine.** (meh-toe-PIH-mazz-
EEN) USAN.
Use: Antiemetic.
Metopirone. (Novartis) Metyrapone
250 mg. Softgel Cap. Pkg. 18s. *Rx.*
Use: In vivo diagnostic aid.
●**metoprine.** (MET-oh-preen) USAN.
Use: Antineoplastic.
●**metoprolol.** (meh-TOE-pro-lahl) USAN.
Use: Antiadrenergic/sympatholytic,
beta-adrenergic blocker.
●**metoprolol fumarate.** (meh-TOE-pro-
lahl) *USP 34.*
Use: Antihypertensive.
●**metoprolol succinate.** (meh-TOE-pro-
lahl) USAN.
Use: Antihypertensive; antianginal;
treatment of myocardial infarction.
See: Toprol XL.
metoprolol succinate. (Various Mfr.)
Metoprolol 25 mg (metoprolol succinate
23.75 mg equiv. to metoprolol tartrate

25 mg), 50 mg (metoprolol succinate 47.5 mg equiv. to metoprolol tartrate 50 mg), 100 mg (metoprolol succinate 95 mg equiv. to metoprolol tartrate 100 mg), 200 mg (metoprolol succinate 190 mg equiv. to metoprolol tartrate 200 mg). May contain maltodextrin, polydextrose (100 mg, 200 mg only). Film-coated. ER Tab. 100s, 1000s (except 50 mg), UD 100s (100 mg, 200 mg only). *Rx.*
Use: Antiadrenergic/sympatholytic.

● **metoprolol tartrate.** (meh-TOE-pro-lahl) *USP 34.*
Use: Antiadrenergic (beta-receptor).
W/Hydrochlorothiazide
See: Lopressor.
Lopressor HCT.

metoprolol tartrate. (Hospira) Metoprolol tartrate 1 mg/mL. Inj. Amp. *Carpuject* sterile cartridge units with Interlink System Cannula, *Carpuject* sterile cartridge units with *Luer-Lock.* *Rx.*
Use: Antiadrenergic/sympatholytic, beta-adrenergic blocker.

metoprolol tartrate. (Purepac) Metoprolol tartrate. **Tab.:** 50 mg, 100 mg, lactose. Bot. 100s, 1000s, UD 100s. **Inj.:** 1 mg/mL. Amp. 5 mL. *Rx.*
Use: Antiadrenergic/sympatholytic; beta-adrenergic blocker.

metoprolol tartrate. (Various Mfr.) Metoprolol tartrate 25 mg, 50 mg, 100 mg. Tab. 30s, 90s, 100s, 1000s. *Rx.*
Use: Antiadrenergic, sympatholytic, beta-adrenergic blocker.

metoprolol tartrate/hydrochlorothiazide. (Mylan) Hydrochlorothiazide/metoprolol tartrate 25 mg/50 mg, 25 mg/100 mg, 50 mg/100 mg. Lactose. Tab. 100s, 500s. *Rx.*
Use: Antihypertensive.

metoquine.
Use: Antimalarial.

● **metoquizine.** (MET-oh-kwih-zeen) USAN.
Use: Anticholinergic; antiulcerative.

Metozolv ODT. (Salix) Metoclopramide 5 mg (equiv. to metoclopramide hydrochloride 5.91 mg), 10 mg (equiv. to metoclopramide hydrochloride 11.82 mg). Acesulfate K, mannitol. Mint flavor. Tab., orally disintegrating. UD 100s. *Rx.*
Use: GI stimulant.

● **metreleptin.** (MET-re-LEP-tin) USAN.
Use: Obesity and related disorders.

Metric 21. (Fielding) Metronidazole 250 mg. Tab. Bot. 100s. *Rx.*
Use: Anti-infective.

● **metrifonate.** (meh-TRIH-foe-nate) *USP 34. Formerly trichlorfon.*
Use: Cholinesterase inhibitor.

● **metrizamide.** (meh-TRIH-zam-ide) USAN.
Use: Myelography; diagnostic aid (radiopaque medium).
See: Amipaque.

● **metrizoate sodium.** (meh-trih-ZOE-ate) USAN.
Use: Diagnostic aid (radiopaque medium).

MetroCream. (Galderma) Metronidazole 0.75%. Glycerin, benzyl alcohol. Cream. Tube. 45 g. *Rx.*
Use: Topical anti-infective, antibiotic.

MetroGel. (Galderma) Metronidazole 1%. Parabens, EDTA. Gel. Tubes. 45 g. *Rx.*
Use: Dermatologic, acne.

MetroGel-Vaginal. (Graceway Pharmaceuticals) Metronidazole 0.75%, EDTA, parabens. Gel Tube (with 5 applicators) 70 g. *Rx.*
Use: Anti-infective, vaginal.

Metrogesic. (Lexis Laboratories) Salicylamide 325 mg, acetaminophen 162 mg, phenacetin 65 mg. Tab. Bot. 100s.
Use: Analgesic.

metrogestone.
Use: Hormone, progestin.

MetroLotion. (Galderma) Metronidazole 0.75%. Benzyl alcohol, stearyl alcohol, glycerin, mineral oil. Lot. Bot. 59 mL. *Rx.*
Use: Topical anti-infective, antibiotic.

● **metronidazole.** (meh-troe-NID-uh-zole) *USP 34.*
Tall Man: metroNIDAZOLE
Use: Antiprotozoal (trichomonas); antitrichomonal.
See: Flagyl.
Flagyl ER.
Flagyl 375.
MetroCream.
MetroGel.
MetroGel-Vaginal.
MetroLotion.
Metryl.
Noritate.
Rozex.
Vandazole.
Vitazol.
W/Bismuth Subcitrate Potassium, Tetracycline Hydrochloride.
See: Pylera.

metronidazole. (Able) Metronidazole 375 mg. Cap. 30s, 50s, 100s, 500s, 1000s. *Rx.*
Use: Anti-infective.

metronidazole. (B. Braun) Metronidazole 5 mg/mL. Inj. Vial 100 mL. *Rx.*
Use: Anti-infective.

metronidazole. (Fougera) Metronidazole. **Cream:** 0.75%. Benzyl alcohol, glycerin, lactic acid. 45 g. **Gel:** 0.75%. EDTA, parabens. 45 g. *Rx.*
Use: Topical anti-infective, antibiotic.

metronidazole. (Prasco) Metronidazole 0.75%. EDTA, parabens. Vaginal Gel. Tubes with vaginal applicators. 70 g. *Rx.*
Use: Vaginal preparation; anti-infective.

metronidazole. (Various Mfr.) Metronidazole. **Lot.:** 0.75%. May contain benzyl alcohol. 59 mL. **Tab.:** 250 mg, 500 mg. Bot. 25s, 50s (500 mg only), 100s, 250s, (250 mg only), 500s. *Rx.*
Use: Anti-infective.

• **metronidazole benzoate.** (meh-troe-NIH-dah-zole BEN-zoe-ate) *USP 34.*
Tall Man: metroNIDAZOLE
Use: Anti-infective.

• **metronidazole hydrochloride.** (meh-troe-NIH-dah-zole) USAN.
Tall Man: metroNIDAZOLE
Use: Anti-infective.

metronidazole in sodium chloride. (Claris Lifesciences) Metronidazole 5 mg/mL. Sodium chloride 7.9 mg/mL. Inj., Soln. Single-dose container. 100 mL. *Rx.*
Use: Anti-infective agent.

• **metronidazole phosphate.** (meh-troe-NIH-dah-zole) USAN.
Tall Man: metroNIDAZOLE
Use: Antibacterial; anti-infective; antiprotozoal.

Metrozole. (Lexis Laboratories) Metronidazole 250 mg, 500 mg. Tab. **250 mg:** Bot. 100s, 250s. **500 mg:** Bot. 100s. *Rx.*
Use: Amebicide; anti-infective.

MET-RX. (Met-Rx USA) **Pow. for Drink:** Fat 2 g, Na 37 mg, K 900 mg, carbohydrate 22 g, protein, < 1 g dietary fiber, sugar, vitamins A, D, C, E, B_1, B_5, B_6, B_{12}, biotin, Mg, Zn, Ca, folate, P, Cu, Fe, riboflavin, iodine. 72 g. **Food Bar:** Fat 4 g, Na 110 mg, K 700 mg, carbohydrate 50 g, protein 27 g, sugar, Ca, vitamins A, D, B_1, B_2, B_3, B_5, B_6, B_{12}, C, E, folate, biotin, P, Mg, Cu, Fe, I, Zn. 100 g. *OTC.*
Use: Nutritional therapy.

Metryl. (Teva) Metronidazole 250 mg. Tab. Bot. 100s, 250s, 500s, UD 100s. *Rx.*
Use: Amebicide, anti-infective.

Metryl 500. (Teva) Metronidazole 500 mg. Tab. Bot. 100s, 500s. *Rx.*
Use: Amebicide; anti-infective.

• **meturedepa.** (meh-TOO-ree-DEH-pah) USAN.
Use: Antineoplastic.

Metussin. (Faraday) Dextromethorphan. Bot. 4 oz. *OTC.*
Use: Antitussive.

Metussin Jr. (Faraday) Dextromethorphan. Bot. 4 oz. *OTC.*
Use: Antitussive.

Metvixia. (PhotoCure ASA) Methyl aminolevulinate 16.8%. Almond oil, EDTA, glycerin, parabens, peanut oil, white petrolatum. Cream. 2 g. *Rx.*
Use: Photochemotherapy.

• **metyrapone.** (meh-TEER-ah-pone) *USP 34.*
Use: In vivo diagnostic aid (pituitary function determination); adrenocortical enzyme inhibitor.
See: Metopirone.

• **metyrapone tartrate.** (meh-TEER-ah-pone) USAN.
Use: Diagnostic aid (pituitary function determination).

metyrapone tartrate injection.
Use: Diagnostic aid.

• **metyrosine.** (meh-TIE-roe-seen) *USP 34.*
Use: Antihypertensive.
See: Demser.

Mevacor. (Merck) Lovastatin 20 mg, 40 mg. Lactose. Tab. Bot. 1000s, 10,000s; UD 100s (20 mg only); unit-of-use 60s; unit-of-use 90s. *Rx.*
Use: Antihyperlipidemic; HMG-CoA reductase inhibitor.

mevinolin.
See: Lovastatin.

Mexate-AQ. (Bristol-Myers Squibb Oncology/Virology) Methotrexate 50 mg, 100 mg, 250 mg/preservative-free liquid vial. *Rx.*
Use: Antineoplastic.

• **mexiletine hydrochloride.** (MEX-ih-leh-teen) *USP 34.*
Use: Antiarrhythmic agent.
See: Mexitil.

mexiletine hydrochloride. (Various Mfr.) Mexiletine hydrochloride 150 mg, 200 mg, 250 mg. Cap. 30s, 60s, 90s (150 mg only); 100s; 120s, 240s (150 mg only). *Rx.*
Use: Antiarrhythmic agent.

Mexitil. (Boehringer Ingelheim) Mexiletine hydrochloride 150 mg, 200 mg, 250 mg. Cap. Bot. 100s, UD 100s. *Rx.*
Use: Antiarrhythmic.

• **mexrenoate potassium.** (mex-REN-oh-ate) USAN.
Use: Aldosterone antagonist.

Mexsana Medicated Powder. (Schering-Plough) Corn starch, kaolin, triclosan, zinc oxide. Can 3 oz, 6.25 oz, 11 oz. *OTC.*
Use: Diaper rash preparation.

Meyenberg Goat Milk. (Jackson-Mitchell) Evaporated and powdered cans of goat milk. Foil pack 4 oz. (makes 1 quart). *OTC.*
Use: Cows' milk allergies.

MG Cold Sore Formula. (Outdoor Recreation) Menthol 1%, lidocaine, propylene glycol in alcohol base. Soln. Bot. 7.5 mL. *OTC.*
Use: Cold sores; fever blisters.

MG400. (Triton) Colloidal sulfur in Guy-Base II 5%, salicylic acid 3%. Shampoo. Bot. 240 mL, pt. *OTC.*
Use: Antiseborrheic.

MG-Oroate. (Miller Pharmacal Group) Magnesium (as magnesium orotate) 33 mg. Tab. Bot. 100s. *OTC.*
Use: Vitamin supplement.

MG-Plus Protein. (Miller Pharmacal Group) Magnesium-protein complex made with specially isolated soy protein 133 mg. Tab. Bot. 100s. *OTC.*
Use: Vitamin supplement.

MG217 Medicated Tar. (Triton) **Shampoo:** Coal tar solution 15%. Bot. 120 mL, 240 mL. **Oint.:** Coal tar solution 10%, petrolatum, cetyl alcohol. 107 g. **Lot.:** Coal tar solution 5%, moisturizing base, cetyl alcohol, mineral oil. 120 mL. *OTC.*
Use: Antipruritic; antieczematic; keratolytic.

MG217 Medicated Tar-Free. (Triton) Colloidal sulfur 5%, salicylic acid 3%. Shampoo. Bot. 120 mL, 240 mL. *OTC.*
Use: Antiseborrheic; antipruritic.

MG217 Sal-Acid. (Triton) Salicylic acid 3%, vitamin E. Oint. Tube. 60 g. *OTC.*
Use: Keratolytic.

MHP-A. (Cypress) Methenamine 40.8 mg, phenyl salicylate 18.1 mg, atropine sulfate 0.03, hyoscyamine sulfate 0.03 mg, benzoic acid 4.5 mg, methylene blue 5.4 mg. Tab. 100s. *Rx.*
Use: Anti-infective, urinary.

Miacalcin. (Novartis) Calcitonin-salmon. **Inj.:** 200 units/mL. Phenol. Vial 2 mL. **Nasal Spray:** 200 units/activation (0.09 mL/dose). Sodium chloride 8.5 mg. Metered dose glass bot. with pump. 2 mL. *Rx.*
Use: Paget disease; antihypercalcemic; postmenopausal osteoporosis.

Mi-Acid Gelcaps. (Major) Calcium carbonate 311 mg, magnesium carbonate 232 mg, parabens, EDTA. Bot. 50s.
OTC.
Use: Antacid.

Mi-Acid Liquid. (Major) Aluminum hydroxide 200 mg, magnesium hydroxide 200 mg, simethicone 20 mg/5 mL. Bot. 355 mL, 780 mL. *OTC.*
Use: Antacid; antiflatulent.

Mi-Acid II Liquid. (Major) Aluminum hydroxide 400 mg, magnesium hydroxide 400 mg, simethicone 40 mg/5 mL. Bot. 355 mL. *OTC.*
Use: Antacid; antiflatulent.

Mi-Acid Maximum Strength. (Major) Aluminum hydroxide 400 mg, magnesium hydroxide 400 mg, simethicone 40 mg per 5 mL. Parabens, saccharin, sorbitol. Lemon/mint flavor. Liq. 360 mL.
Use: Antacid combination.

miadone.
See: Methadone Hydrochloride.

•**mianserin hydrochloride.** (my-AN-ser-in) USAN. Under study.
Use: Serotonin inhibitor; antihistamine.

•**mibampator.** (mye-BAM-pa-tor) USAN.
Use: CNS agent.

•**mibolerone.** (my-BOLE-ehr-ohn) USAN.
Use: Anabolic; androgen.

•**micafungin sodium.** (mi-ka-FUN-gin) USAN.
Use: Antifungal.
See: Mycamine.

Micardis. (Boehringer Ingelheim) Telmisartan 20 mg, 40 mg, 80 mg. Sorbitol. Tab. Blister Pack. 28s. *Rx.*
Use: Antihypertensive.

Micardis HCT. (Boehringer Ingelheim) Telmisartan/hydrochlorothiazide 40 mg/12.5 mg, 80 mg/12.5 mg, 80 mg/25 mg. Sorbitol, lactose. Tab. Blister pack 30s. *Rx.*
Use: Antihypertensive.

Micatin. (Ortho) Miconazole nitrate 2%. **Cream:** Mineral oil. 15 g, 30 g. **Pow.:** 90 g. **Spray powder:** Alcohol. Available with and without deodorant. 90 g. **Spray Liquid:** Alcohol. 105 mL. *OTC.*
Use: Antifungal, topical.

Mi-Cebrin. (Eli Lilly) Vitamins B_1 10 mg, B_2 5 mg, B_6 1.7 mg, pantothenic acid 10 mg, niacinamide 30 mg, B_{12} (activity equivalent) 3 mcg, C 100 mg, E 5.5 units, A 10,000 units, D 400 units, Fe 15 mg, Cu 1 mg, I 0.15 mg, Mn 1 mg, Mg 5 mg, Zn 1.5 mg. Tab. Pkg. 60s, 100s, 1000s, Blister pkg. 10 × 10s. *OTC.*
Use: Mineral, vitamin supplement.

Mi-Cebrin T. (Eli Lilly) Vitamins B_1 15 mg, B_2 10 mg, B_6 2 mg, pantothenic acid

10 mg, niacinamide 100 mg, B_{12} 7.5 mcg, C 150 mg, E 5.5 units, A 10,000 units, D 400 units, Fe 15 mg, Cu 1 mg, I 0.15 mg, Mn 1 mg, Mg 5 mg, Zn 1.5 mg. Tab. Bot. 30s, 100s, 1000s, Blister pkg. 10 × 10s. *OTC.*
Use: Mineral, vitamin supplement.

micofur.
Use: Antifungal; anti-infective, topical.

• **miconazole.** (my-KAHN-uh-zole) *USP 34.*
Use: Antifungal.
See: Oravig.

• **miconazole nitrate.** (my-CONE-ah-zole) *USP 34.*
Use: Antifungal agent, topical anti-infective.
See: Aloe Vesta.
  Cruex.
  Desenex.
  Desenex Liquid Spray.
  Fungoid Tincture.
  Lotrimin AF.
  Micatin.
  Monistat.
  Monistat 7.
  Monistat 7 Combination Pack.
  Monistat 3.
  Monistat 3 Combination Pack.
  Neosporin AF.
  Prescription Strength Desenex.
  Tetterine.
  Ting.
  Triple Paste AF.
  Vagistat-3 Combination Pack.
  Zeasorb-AF.

miconazole nitrate. (Taro) Miconazole nitrate 2%. Benzoic acid, mineral oil, apricot kernel oil. Cream. Tube 15 g, 30 g. *OTC.*
Use: Antifungal agent, topical anti-infective.

miconazole nitrate. (Various Mfr.) Miconazole nitrate 2%. Vag. Cream. Tube 15 g, 30 g, 45 g. *OTC.*
Use: Antifungal, vaginal.

micoren. (Novartis) A respiratory stimulant; pending release.

MICRhoGAM. (Ortho-Clinical Diagnostics) Rh_0 (D) immune globulin microdose ≈ 5% ± 1% gamma globulin, sodium chloride 2.9 mg/mL, polysorbate 80 0.01%, glycine 15 mg/mL, preservative free. Soln. for Inj. Pkg. containing single-dose prefilled syringes, injection control form, patient ID card 5s, 25s. *Rx.*
Use: Immune globulin.

MICRhoGAM Ultra-Filtered Plus.
(Ortho-Clinical Diagnostics) Rh_0(D) immune globulin microdose 50 mcg

(250 units/dose). Glycine 15 mg/mL, polysorbate 80 0.01%, sodium chloride 2.9 mg/mL. Preservative free. Inj., Soln. Package w/single-dose syringe, control form, and patient ID card. 1s, 5s, 25s. *Rx.*
Use: Biologic and immunologic agent, immune globulin.

microbubble contrast agent.
Use: Aid in ID of intracranial tumors. [Orphan Drug]

Microcult-GC Test. (Bayer Consumer Care) Miniaturized culture test for the detection of *Neisseria gonorrhoeae.* Test Kit 25s.
Use: Diagnostic aid.

microfibrillar collagen hemostat.
Use: Hemostatic, topical.
See: Hemopad.

Microgestin Fe 1/20. (Watson) Ethinyl estradiol 20 mcg, norethindrone acetate 1 mg. Lactose. Tab. Pack 28s with 7 tabs. with ferrous fumarate 75 mg per tab. *Rx.*
Use: Sex hormone, contraceptive hormone.

Microgestin Fe 1.5/30. (Watson) Ethinyl estradiol 30 mcg, norethindrone acetate 1.5 mg. Lactose. Tab. Pack 28s with 7 tabs with ferrous fumarate 75 mg per tab. *Rx.*
Use: Sex hormone, contraceptive hormone.

Micro-Guard. (Sween) Antimicrobial skin cream. Tube 0.5 oz, Jar 2 oz. *OTC.*
Use: Antifungal, topical.

Micro-K Extencaps. (Wyeth) Potassium chloride (8 mEq) 600 mg. Cap. Bot. 100s, 500s, *Dis-Co* pack 100s. *Rx.*
Use: Electrolyte supplement.

Micro-K 10 Extencaps. (Wyeth) Potassium chloride 750 mg (10 mEq). Cap. Bot. 100s, 500s, *Dis-co* UD 100s. *Rx.*
Use: Electrolyte supplement.

Microlipid. (Nestle Healthcare Nutrition) Fat emulsion 50%, safflower oil, polyglycerol esters of fatty acids, soy lecithin, xanthan gum, ascorbic acid. Cal 4500, fat 500 g/L, 80 mOsm/Kg. H_2O. 120 mL. *Rx.*
Use: Nutritional supplement.

Micronor.
See: Ortho Micronor.

Microsol. (Star) Sulfamethizole 0.5 g, 1 g. Tab. Bot. 100s, 1000s. *Rx.*
Use: Anti-infective; urinary.

Microsol-A. (Star) Phenazopyridine 50 mg, sulfamethizole 0.5 g. Tab. Bot. 100s, 1000s. *Rx.*
Use: Anti-infective; urinary.

Microstix Candida. (Bayer Consumer Care) Test for *Candida* species in vaginal specimens. Box 25s.
Use: Diagnostic aid.

Microstix-3 Reagent Strips. (Bayer Consumer Care) For recognition of nitrite in urine and for semiquantitation of bacterial growth. Bot. 25s with 25 incubation pouches.
Use: Diagnostic aid.

MicroTrak Chlamydia Trachomatis Direct Specimen Test. (Syva) To detect and identify chlamydia trachomatis. Slide test 60s.
Use: Diagnostic aid.

MicroTrak HSV 1/HSV 2 Culture Confirmation/Typing Test. (Syva) For identification and typing of herpes simplex in tissue culture. Test kit 1s.
Use: Diagnostic aid.

MicroTrak Neisseria Gonorrhea Culture Test. (Syva) For endocervical, urethral, rectal, and pharyngeal cultures. Test kit 85s.
Use: Diagnostic aid.

Microzide. (Watson) Hydrochlorothiazide 12.5 mg. Lactose. Cap. Bot. 100s. *Rx.*
Use: Diuretic.

Micrurus fulvius antivenin. (Wyeth) Inj. Combination package: One vial antivenin, one vial diluent (Bacteriostatic Water for Injection 10 mL).
Use: Antivenin.

Mictrin Plus. (Johnson & Johnson) Water, SD alcohol 38-B, glycerin, poloxamer 407, flavor, sodium saccharin, glutamic acid buffer, cetylpyridinium chloride, FD & C Yellow #5, Blue #1. Bot. 12 oz, 24 oz. *OTC.*
Use: Mouth preparation.

• **midaflur.** (MY-dah-flure) USAN.
Use: Hypnotic; sedative.

midamaline hydrochloride.
Use: Anesthetic, local.

Midamor. (Merck & Co.) Amiloride 5 mg. Tab. Bot. 100s. *Rx.*
Use: Diuretic; antihypertensive.

Midaneed. (Hanlon) Vitamins A 5000 units, D 500 units, B_1 5 mg, B_2 3 mg, B_6 0.5 mcg, B_{12} 5 mcg, C 100 mg, niacinamide 10 mg, calcium pantothenate 5 mg. Cap. Bot. 100s. *OTC.*
Use: Mineral, vitamin supplement.

• **midazolam hydrochloride.** (meh-DAZE-oh-lam) USAN.
Use: Anesthetic (injectable).

midazolam hydrochloride. (Roxane) Midazolam hydrochloride 2 mg/mL. EDTA, saccharin, sorbitol, cherry flavor. Syrup. 118 mL. *c-iv.*
Use: General anesthetic.

midazolam hydrochloride. (Various Mfr.) Midazolam hydrochloride 1 mg/mL, 5 mg/mL. Inj. Vial 1 mL (5 mg only), 2 mL, 5 mL. *Carpuject* Vial 10 mL. Syr. 2 mL (5 mg only). *c-iv.*
Use: Anesthetic.

• **midazolam maleate.** (meh-DAZE-oh-lam) USAN.
Use: Anesthetic, intravenous.

• **midodrine hydrochloride.** (MIH-doe-DREEN) USAN.
Use: Antihypotensive; vasoconstrictor.
See: ProAmatine.

midodrine hydrochloride. (Avkare) Midodrine hydrochloride 10 mg. Tab. 90s. *Rx.*
Use: Vasopressor used in shock.

midodrine hydrochloride. (Global) Midodrine hydrochloride 2.5 mg, 5 mg. Tab. 100s, 500s, 1,000s. *Rx.*
Use: Vasopressor used in shock.

midodrine hydrochloride. (Mylan) Midodrine hydrochloride 10 mg. Tab. 100s. *Rx.*
Use: Vasopressor used in shock.

midodrine hydrochloride. (Various Mfr.) Midodrine hydrochloride 2.5 mg, 5 mg. Tab. 100s, 500s (except 2.5 mg). *Rx.*
Use: Vasopressor used in shock.

Midol Cramp & Body Aches. (Bayer Consumer Care) Ibuprofen 200 mg. Tab. Bot. 24s. *OTC.*
Use: Analgesic; NSAID.

Midol Extended Relief. (Bayer Consumer Care) Naproxen 200 mg (naproxen sodium 220 mg). Sodium 20 mg. Tab. 24s. *OTC.*
Use: Nonsteroidal anti-inflammatory agent.

Midol Maximum Strength Cramp Formula. (Bayer Consumer Care) Ibuprofen 200 mg. Tab. 24s. *OTC.*
Use: Nonsteroidal anti-inflammatory agent.

Midol Menstrual Complete. (Bayer Consumer Care) Acetaminophen 500 mg, caffeine 60 mg, pyrilamine maleate 15 mg. Capl. Pkg. 8s, 16s, 32s. Gelcaps. Pkg. 12s, 24s. *OTC.*
Use: Analgesic combination.

Midol Pre-Menstrual Syndrome. (Bayer Consumer Care) Acetaminophen 500 mg, pamabrom 25 mg, pyrilamine maleate 15 mg. Capl. Bot. 24s. Gelcap: EDTA. Bot. 24s. *OTC.*
Use: Analgesic.

Midol Teen Formula. (Bayer Consumer Care) Acetaminophen 500 mg, pamabrom 25 mg. Capl. Bot. 24s. *OTC.*
Use: Analgesic.

- **midostaurin.** (mi-doe-STOR-in) USAN.
  Use: Antineoplastic.

Midrin. (Caraco) Isometheptene mucate 65 mg, acetaminophen 325 mg, dichloralphenazone 100 mg. Cap. 100s. *c-iv.*
  Use: Antimigraine.

Midstream Pregnancy Test Kit. (Ivax) Stick for urine test. Kit 1s. *OTC.*
  Use: Pregnancy test.

- **mifamurtide.** (mif-AM-ure-tide) USAN.
  Use: Investigational treatment for osteosarcoma.

Mifeprex. (Danco Labs) Mifepristone 200 mg. Tab. Single-dose blister pack containing 3 tabs. *Rx.*
  Use: Uterine-active agent; abortifacient.

mifepristone.
  Use: Uterine-active agent; abortifacient.
  See: Mifeprex.

- **mifobate.** (mih-FOE-bate) USAN.
  Use: Antiatherosclerotic.

- **migalastat hydrochloride.** (mi-GAL-a-stat) USAN.
  Use: Treatment of Fabry disease.

Migergot. (G & W) Caffeine 100 mg, ergotamine tartrate 2 mg. Supp. 12s. *Rx.*
  Use: Agent for migraine, migraine combination.

- **miglitol.** (mih-GLIH-tole) USAN.
  Use: Antidiabetic.
  See: Glyset.

- **miglustat.** (MIG-loo-stat)
  Use: Gaucher disease.
  See: Zavesca.

Migragesic IDA. (Acella) Acetaminophen 325 mg, dichloralphenazone 100 mg, isometheptene mucate 65 mg. Cap. 100s. *c-iv.*
  Use: Agent for migraine, migraine combination.

migraine agents.
  See: Ergotamine Derivatives.
    Serotonin 5-HT$_1$ Receptor Antagonist.

migraine combinations.
  See: Isometheptene/Dichloralphenazone/Acetaminophen.

Migranal. (Valeant) Dihydroergotamine mesylate 4 mg/mL, caffeine 10 mg, dextrose 50 mg. Nasal spray. Vial w/ nasal sprayer. 3.5 mL. *Rx.*
  Use: Antimigraine.

MigraTen. (Pharmelle) Isometheptene mucate 65 mg, caffeine 100 mg, acetaminophen 325 mg. Cap. 100s. *Rx.*
  Use: Migraine combination.

Migrazone. (Breckenridge) Acetaminophen 325 mg, dichloralphenazone

100 mg, isometheptene mucate 65 mg. Cap. 100s. *c-iv.*
  Use: Agent for migraine, migraine combination.

MIH.
  Use: Antineoplastic.
  See: Matulane.

- **milacemide hydrochloride.** (mill-ASS-eh-mide) USAN.
  Use: Anticonvulsant; antidepressant.

- **milameline hydrochloride.** (mill-AM-eh-leen) USAN.
  Use: Antidementia (partial muscarinic agonist).

mild silver protein.
  See: Silver Protein, Mild.

- **milenperone.** (mih-LEN-per-OHN) USAN.
  Use: Antipsychotic.

Miles Nervine. (Bayer Consumer Care) Diphenhydramine hydrochloride 25 mg. Tab. Pkg. 12s, Bot. 30s.
  Use: Nonprescription sleep aid.

- **milipertine.** (MIH-lih-PURR-teen) USAN.
  Use: Antipsychotic.

milk of bismuth. (Various Mfr.) Bismuth hydroxide, bismuth subcarbonate.
  Use: Orally; intestinal disturbances.

- **milk of magnesia.** (mag-NEE-zhuh) USP 34. Formerly Magnesia Magma.
  Use: Antacid; laxative.
  See: Magnesium hydroxide.

Milk of Magnesia. (Various Mfr.). Magnesium hydroxide 325 mg, 390 mg. **Tab.:** 250s, 1000s. **Liq.:** 120 mL, 360 mL, 720 mL, pt, qt, gal, UD 10 mL, 15 mL, 20 mL, 30 mL, 100 mL, 180 mL, 400 mL. **Susp.:** 400 mg/5 mL. Bot. 180 mL, 360 mL, 480 mL, UD 30 mL, gal. *OTC.*
  Use: Antacid; laxative.

Milk of Magnesia-Concentrated. (Roxane) Equivalent to milk of magnesia 30 mL susp. Bot. 100 mL, 400 mL, UD 10 mL. *OTC.*
  Use: Antacid; laxative.

- **milk thistle extract.** *NF 29.*
  Use: Anti-inflammatory.

Millazine. (Major) Thioridazine. **10 mg, 15 mg/Tab.:** Bot. 100s. **25 mg/Tab.:** Bot. 100s, 1000s. **100 mg, 150 mg, 200 mg/Tab.:** Bot. 100s, 500s. *Rx.*
  Use: Antipsychotic.

Millipred. (Laser Pharmaceutical) Prednisolone. **Oral Soln.:** 10 mg/5 mL. Dye free. Corn syrup, edetate disodium, methylparaben, saccharin. Grape flavor. 237 mL. **Tab.:** 5 mg. Lactose. 100s, 1,000s. *Rx.*
  Use: Adrenocortical steroid, glucocorticoid.

•**milnacipran hydrochloride.** (mil-NA-si-pran) USAN.
Use: Treatment of fibromyalgia.
See: Savella.

•**milodistim.** (my-low-DIH-stim) USAN.
Use: Immunomodulator (antineutropenic).

Milophene. (Milex) Clomiphene citrate 50 mg. Tab. Bot. 30s. *Rx.*
Use: Sex hormone; ovulation stimulant.

Milpar. (Sanofi-Synthelabo) Magnesium hydroxide, mineral oil. *OTC.*
Use: Antacid; laxative.

•**milrinone lactate.** (MILL-rih-nohn) *USP 34.*
Use: Cardiovascular agent, congestive heart failure.

milrinone lactate. (Bedford) Milrinone lactate (as base) 1 mg/mL, dextrose 47 mg/mL, lactic acid 0.282 mg/mL. Single-dose vials. 10 mL, 20 mL, 50 mL. *Rx.*
Use: Cardiovascular agent, congestive heart failure.

Milroy Artificial Tears. (Milton Roy) Bot. 22 mL.
Use: Artificial tears.

Miltown. (Wallace) Meprobamate 200 mg, 400 mg. Tab. Bot. 100s; 500s, 1000s (400 mg only). *c-iv.*
Use: Anxiolytic; antianxiety agent.

Miltown 600. (Wallace) Meprobamate 600 mg. Tab. Bot. 100s. *c-iv.*
Use: Anxiolytic.

•**mimbane hydrochloride.** (MIM-bane) USAN.
Use: Analgesic.

Mimvey. (Teva) Estradiol 1 mg/norethindrone acetate 0.5 mg. Film coated. Lactose, PEG. Tab. Blister pack. 28s. *Rx.*
Use: Sex hormone, estrogen/progestin combination.

Mimyx. (GlaxoSmithKline) Betaine, olive oil, glycerin, pentylene glycol, palm glycerides, vegetable oil, squalene, hydroxyethyl cellulose, carbomer, xanthan gum. Preservative free. Cream. 70 g. *Rx.*
Use: Miscellaneous topical combination.

•**minalrestat.** (min-AL-reh-stat) USAN.
Use: Aldose reductase inhibitor.

•**minaprine.** (MIN-ah-preen) USAN.
Use: Psychotherapeutic agent.

•**minaprine hydrochloride.** (MIN-ah-preen) USAN.
Use: Antidepressant.

•**minaxolone.** (min-AX-oh-lone) USAN.
Use: Anesthetic.

mincard.
Use: Diuretic.

Mineral Freez. (Geritrex) Menthol 2%. Alcohol. Gel. 226.8 g. *OTC.*
Use: Rub and liniment.

Mineral Ice, Therapeutic. (Bristol-Myers Squibb) Menthol 2%, ammonium hydroxide, carbomer 934, cupric sulfate, isopropyl alcohol, magnesium sulfate, thymol. Gel Tube 105 g, 240 g, 480 g. *OTC.*
Use: Liniment.

mineralocorticoids.
Use: Adrenalocortical steroids.
See: Fludrocortisone Acetate.

•**mineral oil.** (MIN-er-al) *USP 34.*
Use: Laxative; pharmaceutic aid (solvent, oleaginous vehicle).
See: Kondremul Plain.
Liqui-Doss.
Min-O-Ear.
Petrolatum.
Soothe XP.

mineral oil. (Various Mfr.) Mineral oil. Liq. Bot. 180 mL, 473 mL. *OTC.*
Use: Laxative.

•**mineral oil, light.** (MIN-er-al) *NF 29.*
Use: Pharmaceutic aid (tablet and capsule lubricant, vehicle).
See: Soothe XP.

minerals.
See: Calcium.
Calcium Acetate.
Calcium Carbonate.
Calcium Citrate.
Calcium Glubionate.
Calcium Gluconate.
Calcium Lactate.
Calcium Microcrystalline Hydroxyapatite.
Magnesium.
Magnesium Citrate.
Magnesium Gluconate.
Magnesium Oxide.
Phosphate.
Sodium Phosphates.
Tricalcium Phosphate.

Mineral Zinc. (Mason) Ca 122 mg (calcium content expressed in mg elemental calcium), zinc 10 mg. Gluten free, preservative free, and sugar free. Tab. 100s. *OTC.*
Use: Nutritional supplement, multimineral.

Minibex. (Faraday) Vitamins B₁ 6 mg, B₂ 3 mg, B₆ 0.5 mg, C 50 mg, niacinamide 10 mg, calcium pantothenate 3 mg, B₁₂ 2 mcg, folic acid 0.1 mg. Cap. Bot. 100s, 250s, 1000s. *OTC.*
Use: Mineral, vitamin supplement.

Minidyne 10%. (Pedinol Pharmacal) Povidone-iodine 10%, citric acid, sodium

phosphate dibasic. Soln. Bot. 15 mL. OTC.
Use: Antimicrobial; antiseptic.

Minipress. (Pfizer) Prazosin hydrochloride 1 mg, 2 mg, 5 mg. Cap. Bot. 250s. Rx.
Use: Antihypertensive, antiadrenergic.

Miniprin Low Dose. (Time-Cap Labs) Aspirin 81 mg. Lactose. Tab., enteric coated. 120s. OTC.
Use: Salicylate.

Minirin. (Ferring) Desmopressin acetate 0.1 mg, chlorobutanol 5 mg/mL. Nasal spray. 5 mL (50 doses of 10 mcg). Rx.
Use: Posterior pituitary hormones.

Minitec. (Bristol-Myers Squibb) Sodium pertechnetate Tc 99 m generator.
Use: Radiopaque agent.

Minitec Generator (Complete with Components). (Bristol-Myers Squibb) Medotopes Kit.
Use: Diagnostic aid.

Minitran. (3M) Nitroglycerin 0.1 mg/h (9 mg), 0.2 mg/h (18 mg), 0.4 mg/h (36 mg), 0.6 mg/h (54 mg). Transdermal Patch. 30s. Rx.
Use: Antianginal.

Minit-Rub. (Bristol-Myers Squibb) Methyl salicylate 15%, menthol 3.5%, camphor 2.3% in anhydrous base. Tube 1.5 oz, 3 oz. OTC.
Use: Analgesic, topical.

Minocin. (Lederle) Minocycline hydrochloride (as base). **Cap., Pellet-filled:** 50 mg, 100 mg. Bot. 50s (100 mg only), 100s (50 mg only). **Oral Susp.:** 50 mg/5 mL. Alcohol 5%, parabens, EDTA, saccharin, custard flavor. Bot. 60 mL. Rx.
Use: Anti-infective, tetracycline.

•**minocromil.** (MIH-no-KROE-mill) USAN.
Use: Antiallergic (prophylactic).

•**minocycline.** (mihn-oh-SIGH-kleen) USAN.
Use: Anti-infective.
See: Cleeravue-M.
Vectrin.

•**minocycline hydrochloride.** (mihn-oh-SIGH-kleen) USP 34.
Use: Anti-infective, mouth and throat product.
See: Arestin.
Dynacin.
Minocin.
Myrac.
Solodyn.

minocycline hydrochloride. (Par) Minocycline hydrochloride (as base) 50 mg, 75 mg, 100 mg. Lactose. Film-coated. Tab. 50s (100 mg only), 100s (except

100 mg), 1000s. Rx.
Use: Tetracycline.

minocycline hydrochloride. (Teva) Minocycline hydrochloride 45 mg, 90 mg, 135 mg. Lactose. Film coated. ER Tab. 30s, 100s, 1,000s. Rx.
Use: Anti-infective agent, tetracycline.

minocycline hydrochloride. (Various Mfr.) Minocycline hydrochloride (as base) 50 mg, 75 mg, 100 mg. Cap. Bot. 50s (100 mg only), 100s (except 100 mg). Rx.
Use: Anti-infective, tetracycline.

Min-O-Ear. (Geritrex) Mineral oil. Otic Soln. 22 mL. Rx.
Use: Otic preparation.

•**minoxidil.** (min-OX-ih-dill) USP 34.
Use: Antihypertensive; vasodilator; antialopecia agent.
See: Rogaine.
Rogaine Extra Strength for Men.
Rogaine Men's Extra Strength.

minoxidil. (Rugby) Minoxidil 10 mg. Tab. Bot. 500s. Rx.
Use: Antihypertensive.

minoxidil. (Schein) Minoxidil 2.5 mg. Tab. Bot. 100s, 500s, 1000s. Rx.
Use: Antihypertensive.

minoxidil extra strength for men. (Apotex USA) Minoxidil 5%. Alcohol 30%. Top. Soln. Bot. 60 mL (1s and 2s). OTC.
Use: Alopecia.

Minoxidil for Men. (Actavis Mid Atlantic) Minoxidil 2%. Alcohol 60%, propylene glycol. Soln., Top. 60 mL. OTC.
Use: Dermatological agent.

Minto-Chlor Syrup. (Pal-Pak, Inc.) Codeine sulfate 10 mg, potassium citrate 219 mg/5 mL, alcohol 2%. Gal. c-v.
Use: Antitussive, expectorant.

Mintox. (Major) **Susp.:** Aluminum hydroxide 200 mg, magnesium hydroxide 200 mg, simethicone 20 mg. Benzyl alcohol, parabens, saccharin, sorbitol, sodium 1 mg per 5 mL. Mint creme flavor. 355 mL. **Chew. Tab.:** Aluminum hydroxide/magnesium hydroxide. **200 mg/200 mg:** Saccharin. Mint flavor. 100s. **300 mg/150 mg:** Aspartame, phenylalanine, sorbitol. 24s. OTC.
Use: Antacid.

Mintox Plus Extra Strength Liquid. (Major) Aluminum hydroxide 500 mg, magnesium hydroxide 450 mg, simethicone 40 mg/5 mL. Bot. 355 mL. OTC.
Use: Antacid, antiflatulent.

Mintox Plus Tablets. (Major) Aluminum hydroxide 200 mg, magnesium hydroxide 200 mg, simethicone 25 mg. Chew. Tab. 100s. OTC.
Use: Antacid; antiflatulent.

Mint Sensodyne. (Block Drug) Potassium nitrate 5%, saccharin, sorbitol. Toothpaste. Tube 28.3 g. *OTC.*
Use: Toothpaste for sensitive teeth.

Mintuss MR. (Breckenridge) Hydrocodone bitartrate 5 mg, pyrilamine maleate 5 mg, phenylephrine hydrochloride 5 mg per 5 mL. Sugar and alcohol free. Menthol, sucrose. Pineapple-orange flavor. Syrup. 473 mL. *c-III.*
Use: Antitussive combination.

Minute-Gel. (Oral-B) Acidulated phosphate fluoride 1.23%. Gel. Bot. 16 oz. *Rx.*
Use: Dental caries agent.

Miochol-E. (Novartis Ophthalmic) Acetylcholine chloride 1:100, mannitol 2.8% when reconstituted. Soln. In 2 mL Univials. *Rx.*
Use: Antiglaucoma agent.

•**mioflazine hydrochloride.** (MY-ah-FLAY-zeen) USAN.
Use: Vasodilator (coronary).

Miostat Intraocular Solution. (Alcon) Carbachol 0.01%. Vial 1.5 mL. Pkg. 12s.
Use: Antiglaucoma agent.

miotics, cholinesterase inhibitors.
Use: Glaucoma agents.
See: Echothiophate Iodide.
 Eserine Salicylate.
 Eserine Sulfate.
 Floropryl.

•**mipafilcon A.** (mih-paff-ILL-kahn A) USAN.
Use: Contact lens material (hydrophilic).

•**mirabegron.** (mye-ra-BE-ron) USAN.
Use: Genitourinary agent.

MiraFlow Extra Strength. (Ciba Vision) Isopropyl alcohol 15.7%, poloxamer 407, amphoteric 10. Thimerosal free. Soln. Bot. 12 mL. *OTC.*
Use: Contact lens care.

Miral. (Armenpharm Ltd.) Dexamethasone 0.75 mg. Tab. Bot. 100s, 1000s.
Use: Corticosteroid.

MiraLax. (Schering-Plough) Polyethylene glycol 3350 17 g, 119 g, 238 g, 510 g. Pow. for oral soln. Single-dose packet (17 g only). 12s. 119 g (119 g), 239 g (238 g), 510 g (510 g). *OTC.*
Use: Laxative; bowel evacuant.

Mirapex. (Boehringer Ingelheim) Pramipexole dihydrochloride 0.125 mg, 0.25 mg, 0.5 mg, 0.75 mg, 1 mg, 1.5 mg. Mannitol. Tab. Bot. 90s, UD 100s (except 0.125 mg, 0.75 mg). *Rx.*
Use: Antiparkinson agent.

Mirapex XR. (Boehringer Ingelheim) Pramipexole dihydrochloride 0.375 mg,

0.75 mg, 1.5 mg, 3 mg, 4.5 mg. ER Tab. 30s. *Rx.*
Use: Dopaminergic, dopamine receptor agonist, nonergot.

Miraphen PSE. (Major) Pseudoephedrine hydrochloride 120 mg, guaifenesin 600 mg. ER Tab. Bot. 500s. *Rx.*
Use: Upper respiratory combination, decongestant, expectorant.

Mircette. (Duramed) **Phase 1:** Desogestrel 0.15 mg, ethinyl estradiol 20 mcg. 21 tabs. **Phase 2:** Ethinyl estradiol 10 mcg. 5 tabs. Latose. Tab. Blister Cards. 28s with 2 inert tabs. *Rx.*
Use: Sex hormone, contraceptive hormone.

Mircera. (Hoffman-LaRoche) Methoxy polyethylene glycol-epoetin beta 50 mcg/0.3 mL, 50 mcg/mL, 75 mcg/ 0.3 mL, 100 mcg/0.3 mL, 100 mcg/mL, 150 mcg/0.3 mL, 200 mcg/0.3 mL, 200 mcg/mL, 250 mg/0.3 mL, 300 mcg/ mL, 400 mcg/0.6 mL, 400 mcg/mL, 600 mcg/0.6 mL, 600 mcg/mL, 800 mcg/0.6 mL, 1000 mcg/mL. Preservative free. Inj., Soln. Single-use prefilled syringes. 1s (50 mcg/0.3 mL, 75 mcg/0.3 mL, 100 mcg/0.3 mL, 150 mcg/0.3 mL, 200 mcg/0.3 mL, 250 mcg/0.3 mL, 400 mcg/0.6 mL, 600 mcg/0.6 mL, 800 mcg/0.6 mL). Single-use vials. 1s, 12s (50 mcg/mL, 100 mcg/mL, 200 mcg/mL, 300 mcg/ mL, 400 mcg/mL, 600 mcg/mL, 1000 mcg/mL). *Rx.*
Use: Hematopoietic agent.

Mirena. (Bayer) T-shaped unit containing a reservoir of levonorgestrel 52 mg covered by a silicone membrane. Intrauterine system. Pkg. 1s w/inserter. *Rx.*
Use: Sex hormone; contraceptive.

•**mirfentanil hydrochloride.** (MIHR-FEN-tan-ill) USAN.
Use: Analgesic.

•**mirincamycin hydrochloride.** (mihr-IN-kah-MY-sin) USAN.
Use: Anti-infective; antimalarial.

•**mirisetron maleate.** (my-RIH-seh-trahn) USAN.
Use: Antianxiety.

•**mirtazapine.** (mihr-TAZZ-ah-PEEN) USAN.
Use: Antidepressant, tetracyclic compound.
See: Remeron.
 Remeron SolTab.

mirtazapine. (Various Mfr.) Mirtazapine. **Orally Disintegrating Tab.:** 15 mg, 30 mg, 45 mg. May contain aspartame, corn syrup, mannitol, phenylalanine,

xylitol. UD 30s. **Tab.:** 7.5 mg, 15 mg, 30 mg, 45 mg. May contain lactose. 30s, 90s (15 mg, 30 mg, 45 mg), 100s (15 mg, 30 mg, 45 mg), 500s, 1000s. Rx.
Use: Antidepressant, tetracyclic compound.

● **misonidazole.** (MY-so-NIH-dah-zole) USAN.
Use: Antiprotozoal (trichomonas).

● **misoprostol.** (MY-so-PRAHST-ole) USAN.
Use: Antiulcerative.
See: Cytotec.
W/Diclofenac sodium.
See: Arthrotec.

misoprostol. (Various Mfr.) Misoprostol 100 mcg, 200 mcg. Tab. Unit-of-use 60s, 100s (200 mcg only), 120s (120 mcg only). *Rx.*
Use: Antiulcerative.

Mission Prenatal. (Mission Pharmacal) Ferrous gluconate 260 mg (iron 30 mg), vitamins C 100 mg, B₁ 5 mg, B₆ 3 mg, B₂ 2 mg, B₃ 10 mg, B₅ 1 mg, B₁₂ 2 mcg, A 4000 units, D 400 units, Ca, zinc 15 mg. Tab. Bot. 100s. *OTC.*
Use: Mineral, vitamin supplement.

Mission Prenatal F.A. (Mission Pharmacal) Ferrous gluconate 260 mg (iron 30 mg), vitamins C 100 mg, B₁ 5 mg, B₆ 10 mg, B₂ 2 mg, B₃ 10 mg, B₁₂ 2 mcg, folic acid 0.8 mg, A acetate 4000 units, D 400 units, Ca, B₅ 1 mg. Tab. Bot. 100s. *OTC.*
Use: Mineral, vitamin supplement.

Mission Prenatal H.P. (Mission Pharmacal) Ferrous gluconate 260 mg (iron 30 mg), vitamins C 100 mg, B₁ 5 mg, B₆ 25 mg, B₂ 2 mg, B₃ 10 mg, B₅ 1 mg, B₁₂ 2 mcg, folic acid 0.8 mg, A 4000 units, D 400 units, Ca. Tab. Bot. 100s. *OTC.*
Use: Mineral, vitamin supplement.

Mission Prenatal Rx. (Mission Pharmacal) Vitamins A 8000 units, D 400 units, C 240 mg, B₁ 4 mg, B₂ 2 mg, B₃ 20 mg, B₅ 10 mg, B₆ 20 mg, B₁₂ 8 mcg, folic acid 1 mg, Fe 60 mg, Ca 175 mg, I, Zn 15 mg, Cu. Tab. Bot. 100s. *Rx.*
Use: Mineral, vitamin supplement.

Mission Surgical Supplement. (Mission Pharmacal) Vitamins C 500 mg, B₁ 2.5 mg, B₂ 2.6 mg, B₃ 30 mg, B₅ 16.3 mg, B₆ 3.6 mg, B₁₂ 9 mcg, A 5000 units, D 400 units, E 45 units, Fe 27 mg, Zn 22.5 mg. Tab. Bot. 100s. *OTC.*
Use: Mineral, vitamin supplement.

● **mitemcinal fumarate.** (mye-TEM-cin-al)

USAN.
Use: GERD.

● **mitindomide.** (my-TIN-doe-MIDE) USAN.
Use: Antineoplastic.

● **mitocarcin.** (MY-toe-CAR-sin) USAN. Antibiotic derived from *Streptomyces* species.
Use: Antineoplastic.

● **mitocromin.** (MY-toe-KROE-min) USAN. Produced by *Streptomyces virdochromogenes.*
Use: Antineoplastic.

● **mitogillin.** (MY-toe-GIH-lin) USAN. An antibiotic obtained from a "unique strain" of *Aspergillus restrictus.*
Use: Antitumorigenic antibiotic; antineoplastic.

mitoguazone. (CTRC Research Foundation)
Use: Treatment of diffuse non-Hodgkin lymphoma. [Orphan Drug]

mitolactol.
Use: Adjuvant therapy in the treatment of primary brain tumors. [Orphan Drug]

● **mitomalcin.** (MY-toe-MAL-sin) USAN. Produced by *Streptomyces malayensis.* Under study.
Use: Antineoplastic.

● **mitomycin.** (MY-toe-MY-sin) *USP 34.* In literature as Mitomycin C. Antibiotic isolated from *Streptomyces caespitosis.*
Tall Man: mitoMYcin
Use: Anti-infective, antibiotic; antineoplastic.

mitomycin. (Various Mfr.) Mitomycin 5 mg (mannitol 10 mg), 20 mg (mannitol 40 mg), 40 mg (mannitol 80 mg). Pow. for Inj. Vials. *Rx.*
Use: Antibiotic.

mitomycin C.
See: Mitomycin.

● **mitosper.** (MY-toe-sper) USAN. Substance derived from *Aspergillus* of the glaucus group.
Use: Antineoplastic.

● **mitotane.** (MY-toe-TANE) *USP 34.* Formerly o,p'-DDD.
Use: Antineoplastic.
See: Lysodren.

● **mitoxantrone hydrochloride.** (MY-toe-ZAN-trone) *USP 34.*
Tall Man: mitoXANtrone
Use: Antineoplastic; immunologic agent; anthracenedione.
See: Novantrone.

mitoxantrone hydrochloride. (Various Mfr.) Mitoxantrone free base 2 mg/mL. Preservative free. Inj. Multi-dose vi-

als. 10 mL, 12.5 mL, 15 mL. *Rx.*
Use: Anthracenedione; antineoplastic.

• **mitumomab.** (mih-TOO-moe-mab) USAN.
Use: Antitumor monoclonal antibody.

• **mitumprotimut-T.** (MYE-tum-PROE-ti-mut T) USAN.
Use: Treatment of B-cell non-Hodgkin lymphoma.

• **mivacurium chloride.** (MYE-va-KUE-ree-um) *Rx.*
Use: Muscle relaxant–adjunct to anesthesia, nondepolarizing neuromuscular blockers.

• **mivobulin isethionate.** (mih-VOE-byoo-lin eye-seh-THIGH-oh-nate) USAN.
Use: Antineoplastic (microtubule inhibitor).

Mixed E 400 Softgels. (Naturally) Vitamin E 400 IU. Cap. Bot. 60s, 90s, 180s. *OTC.*
Use: Vitamin supplement.

Mixed E 1000 Softgels. (Naturally) Vitamin E 1000 IU. Cap. Bot. 30s, 60s *OTC.*
Use: Vitamin supplement.

Mixed Respiratory Vaccine. Each mL contains *Staphylococcus aureus* 1,200 million organisms, *Streptococcus* (both *viridans* and nonhemolytic) 200 million organisms, *Streptococcus (Diplococcus) pneumoniae* 150 million organisms, *Moraxella (Branhamella, Neisseria) catarrhalis* 150 million organisms, *Klebsiella pneumoniae* 150 million organisms, and *Haemophilus influenzae* types a and b 150 million organisms. Vial. 20 mL.
Use: Bacterial vaccine.
See: MRV.

mixed vespid Hymenoptera venom. *Rx.*
Use: Agent for immunization.
See: Albay.
Pharmalgen.
Venomil.

• **mixidine.** (MIX-ih-deen) USAN.
Use: Vasodilator (coronary).

mixture 612. Dimethyl phthalate solution, compound.

M-M-R II. (Merck) Mixture of 3 viruses: ≥ 1000 measles $TCID_{50}$ (tissue culture infectious doses), ≥ 20,000 mumps $TCID_{50}$, and ≥ 1000 rubella $TCID_{50}$ per 0.5 mL dose. Neomycin 25 mcg. Pow. for Inj. Single dose vial w/diluent. *Rx.*
Use: Agent for immunization.

Mobic. (Boehringer Ingelheim/Abbott) Meloxicam. **Oral Susp.:** 7.5 mg/5 mL. Saccharin, sorbitol. Raspberry flavor. 100 mL. **Tab.:** 7.5 mg, 15 mg. Lactose. Bot. 100s. *Rx.*

Use: Nonsteroidal anti-inflammatory agent.

Mobidin. (B.F. Ascher) Magnesium salicylate, anhydrous 600 mg. Tab. Bot. 100s, 500s. *Rx.*
Use: Antiarthritic.

Mobisyl Creme. (B.F. Ascher) Trolamine salicylate in vanishing creme base. Tube 100 g. *OTC.*
Use: Analgesic, topical.

• **mocetinostat.** (MOE-se-TIN-oh-stat) USAN.
Use: Antineoplastic.

• **mocetinostat dihydrobromide.** (MOE-se-TIN-oh-stat dye-HYE-droe-BROE-mide) USAN.
Use: Antineoplastic.

• **moclobemide.** (moe-KLOE-beh-mide) USAN.
Use: Antidepressant.

• **modafinil.** (moe-DAFF-ih-nill) USAN.
Use: CNS stimulant, analeptic.
See: Provigil.

• **modaline sulfate.** (MODE-al-een) USAN.
Use: Antidepressant.

Modane. (Savage) Bisacodyl 5 mg, lactose. EC Tab. Bot. 10s, 30s, 100s. *OTC.*
Use: Laxative.

Modane Mild. (Pharmacia) Phenolphthalein 60 mg. Tab. Bot. 10s, 30s, 100s. *OTC.*
Use: Laxative.

Modane Versabran. (Pharmacia) Psyllium hydrophilic mucilloid in wheat bran base. Dose 3.4 g, Bot. 10 oz. *OTC.*
Use: Laxative.

• **modecainide.** (moe-deh-CANE-ide) USAN.
Use: Cardiovascular (antiarrhythmic).

Modicon. (Ortho-McNeil) Norethindrone 0.5 mg, ethinyl estradiol 35 mcg. Lactose. Tab. *Dialpak* and *Veridate* 28s with 7 inert tabs. *Rx.*
Use: Sex hormone, contraceptive hormone.

modinal.
See: Gardinol Type Detergents.

• **modithromycin.** (moe-IDTH-roe-MYE-sin) USAN.
Use: Antibiotic.

Moducal. (Bristol-Myers Squibb) Maltodextrin. Pow. Can 13 oz. *OTC.*
Use: Nutritional supplement.

Moduretic. (Merck & Co.) Hydrochlorothiazide 50 mg, amiloride 5 mg. Tab. Bot. 100s, UD 100s. *Rx.*
Use: Antihypertensive; diuretic.

moenomycin. Phosphorus-containing glycolipide antibiotic. Active against gram-positive organisms. Under study.

• **moexipril hydrochloride.** (moe-EX-ah-prill) USAN.
Use: Renin angiotensin system antagonist, angiotensin-converting enzyme inhibitor.
See: Univasc.
W/Hydrochlorothiazide.
See: Uniretic.

moexipril hydrochloride. (Various Mfr.) Moexipril hydrochloride 7.5 mg, 15 mg. Lactose. Film-coated. Tab. Unit-of-use 90s, 100s, 500s. *Rx.*
Use: Renin angiotensin system antagonist, angiotensin-converting enzyme inhibitor.

moexipril hydrochloride/hydrochlorothiazide. (Teva) Moexipril hydrochloride/hydrochlorothiazide 7.5 mg/12.5 mg, 15 mg/12.5 mg, 15 mg/25 mg. Tartrazine (except 15 mg/12.5 mg). Film-coated. Tab. 100s. *Rx.*
Use: Antihypertensive combination.

• **mofegiline hydrochloride.** (moe-FEH-jih-leen) USAN.
Use: Antiparkinsonian.

• **mogamulizumab.** (moe-GAM-ue-LIZ-oo-mab) USAN.
Use: Antineoplastic.

Moist Again. (Lake Consumer) Aloe vera, EDTA, methylparaben, glycerin. Gel. Tube 70.8 g. *OTC.*
Use: Vaginal agent.

Moi-Stir. (Kingswood) Dibasic sodium phosphate, calcium chloride, sodium chloride, potassium chloride, Mg, sorbitol, sodium carboxymethylcellulose, parabens. Soln. Bot. 120 mL spray. *OTC.*
Use: Saliva substitute.

Moi-Stir Swabsticks. (Kingswood) Dibasic sodium phosphate, Mg, calcium chloride, sodium chloride, potassium chloride, sorbitol, sodium carboxymethylcellulose, parabens. Swabsticks. Pkt. 3s. *OTC.*
Use: Saliva substitute.

Moisture Drops. (Bausch & Lomb) Hydroxypropyl methylcellulose 0.5%, povidone 0.1%, glycerin 0.2%, benzalkonium chloride 0.01%, EDTA, NaCl, boric acid, KCl, sodium borate. Soln. Bot. 0.5 oz, 1 oz. *OTC.*
Use: Artificial tears.

molar phosphate.
W/Fluoride ion.
See: Coral.

• **molgramostim.** (mahl-GRAH-moe-STIM) USAN.
Use: Hematopoietic stimulant; antineutropenic.

• **molinazone.** (moe-LEEN-ah-zone) USAN.
Use: Analgesic.

• **molindone hydrochloride.** (moe-LIN-dohn) *USP 34.*
Use: Antipsychotic.

Mollifene Ear Drops. (Pfeiffer) Glycerin, camphor, cajaput oil, eucalyptus oil, thyme oil. Soln. Bot. 24 mL. *OTC.*
Use: Otic.

Mollifene Ear Wax Removing Formula. (Pfeiffer) Carbamide peroxide 6.5%, anhydrous glycerin. Propylene glycol, sodium stannate. Drops. 15 mL with dropper. *OTC.*
Use: Otic preparation.

• **molsidomine.** (mole-SIH-doe-meen) USAN.
Use: Antianginal; vasodilator (coronary).

molybdenum solution. (American Quinine) Molybdenum 25 mcg/mL (as 46 mcg/mL ammonium molybdate tetrahydrate). Inj. Vial 10 mL. *Rx.*
Use: Nutritional supplement, parenteral.

Molycu. (Burns) Meprobamate 400 mg, copper 60 mg/mL. *Rx.*
Use: Antidote.

Moly-Pak. (SoloPak Pharmaceuticals, Inc.) Molybdenum 25 mcg. Inj. Vial 10 mL. *Rx.*
Use: Nutritional supplement, parenteral.

Momentum. (Whitehall-Robins) Aspirin 500 mg, phenyltoloxamine citrate 15 mg. Capl. Bot. 24s, 48s. *OTC.*
Use: Analgesic.

Momentum Muscular Backache Formula. (Whitehall-Robins) Magnesium salicylate tetrahydrate 580 mg (equivalent to 467 mg magnesium salicylate anhydrous). Capl. Box. 48s. *OTC.*
Use: Analgesic compound.

• **mometasone furoate.** (moe-MET-uh-SONE FEW-roh-ate) *USP 34.*
Use: Corticosteroid, topical; intranasal steroid; oral inhalation.
See: Asmanex Twisthaler.
Elocon.
Momexin.
W/Formoterol Fumarate.
See: Dulera.

mometasone furoate. (Clay Park) Mometasone furoate. **Cream:** 0.1%. White petrolatum, stearyl alcohol. 15 g, 45 g. **Top. Soln.:** 0.1%. Isopropyl alcohol 40%, glycerin. 30 mL, 60 mL. *Rx.*
Use: Topical corticosteroid.

mometasone furoate. (Taro) Mometasone furoate 0.1%. Isopropyl alcohol. Lot. Bot. 30 mL, 60 mL. *Rx.*

Use: Anti-inflammatory agent; topical corticosteroid.

mometasone furoate. (Various Mfr.) Mometasone furoate 0.1%. Oint. 15 g, 45 g. *Rx.*
Use: Topical corticosteroid.

mometasone furoate monohydrate.
Use: Respiratory inhalant, intranasal steroid.
See: Nasonex.

Momexin. (JSJ Pharmaceuticals) Mometasone furoate 0.1%. Stearyl alcohol, titanium dioxide, white petrolatum, white wax. Cream. 45 g. *Rx.*
Use: Anti-inflammatory agent, topical corticosteroid.

monacetyl pyrogallol. Eugallol. Pyrogallol monoacetate.
Use: Keratolytic.

Monafed. (Monarch) Guaifenesin 600 mg, lactose. SR Tab. Bot. 100s. *Rx.*
Use: Expectorant.

monalium hydrate. Hydrated magnesium aluminate. Magaldrate.
See: Riopan.

•**monatepil maleate.** (moe-NAT-eh-pill) USAN.
Use: Antianginal; antihypertensive.

•**monensin.** (mah-NEN-sin) *USP 34.*
Use: Antifungal; anti-infective; antiprotozoal.

•**monensin sodium.** (mah-NEN-sin) *USP 34.*
Use: Antifungal; anti-infective; antiprotozoal.

Monistat. (Personal Products) Miconazole nitrate 2%. Top. Cream. Tube 9 g. *OTC.*
Use: Antifungal, vaginal.

Monistat 1. (Personal Products) Tioconazole 6.5%. Vag. Oint. Prefilled single-dose applicator 4.6 g. *OTC.*
Use: Antifungal, vaginal.

Monistat 1 Combination Pack. (Personal Products) Miconazole nitrate. **Supp.:** 1200 mg, petrolatum w/parafin. Pkg. 1s w/applicator. **Cream:** 2%, stearyl and cetyl alcohol. Tube 9 g. *Rx.*
Use: Antifungal, vaginal.

Monistat 7. (Personal Products) Miconazole nitrate. **Vag. Supp.:** 100 mg. Box 7s w/applicator. **Vag. Cream:** 2%. Tube 35 g, 45 g w/1 applicator or 7 *Ultraslim* disp. applicators, or 7 prefilled applicators w/5 g cream. *OTC.*
Use: Antifungal, vaginal.

Monistat 7 Combination Pack. (Personal Products) **Vaginal Supp.:** Miconazole nitrate 100 mg. In 7s with

applicator. **Topical Cream:** Miconazole nitrate 2%. Tube. *OTC.*
Use: Antifungal, vaginal.

Monistat 3. (Personal Products) Miconazole nitrate 2%. Vag. Cream. Pkg. Pre-filled applicator (3). *OTC.*
Use: Antifungal, vaginal.

Monistat 3 Combination Pack. (Personal Products) Miconazole nitrate. **Vag. Supp.:** 200 mg. 3s w/1 reusable applicator or 3 disp. applicators. **Top. Cream:** 2%. Tube. *OTC.*
Use: Antifungal, vaginal.

monoamine oxidase inhibitors.
Use: Antidepressant.
See: Isocarboxazid.
Phenelzine Sulfate.
Tranylcypromine Sulfate.

•**mono- and di-acetylated monoglycerides.** (mahn-OH and di-ah-SEE-till-ated mahn-OH-GLIH-sir-ides) *NF 29.* A mixture of glycerin esterified mono- and diesters of edible fatty acids followed by direct acetylation.
Use: Pharmaceutic aid (plasticizer).

•**mono- and di-glycerides.** (mahn-OH and di-GLIH-sir-ides) *NF 29.* A mixture of mono- and diesters of fatty acids from edible oils.
Use: Fatty acids; pharmaceutic aid (emulsifying agent).

monobactams.
See: Aztreonam.

•**monobenzone.** (MON-oh-BEN-zone) *USP 34.*
Use: Pigment agent.

Monocal. (Mericon) Fluoride 3 mg, Ca 250 mg. Tab. Bot. 100s. *OTC.*
Use: Mineral supplement.

Monocaps Tablets. (Freeda) Iron 14 mg, vitamins A 10,000 units, D 400 units, E 15 units, B_1 15 mg, B_2 15 mg, B_3 41 mg, B_5 15 mg, B_6 15 mcg, B_{12} 15 mcg, C 125 mg, folic acid 0.1 mg, biotin 15 mg, PABA, L-lysine, Ca, Cu, I, K, Mg, Mn, Se, Zn 12 mg, lecithin. Tab. Bot. 100s, 250s, 500s. *OTC.*
Use: Mineral, vitamin supplement.

Monocete EZ Swabs. (Pedinol) Monochloroacetic acid 80%. PEG 200. Swab. 15s. *Rx.*
Use: Destructive agent, chloroacetic acid.

monochloroacetic acid.
Use: Cauterizing agent.
See: Monocete EZ Swabs.

monochlorophenol-para.
See: Camphorated Para-chlorophenol.

Monoclate-P. (CSL Behring) Human anti-hemophilic factor 250 units, 500 units,

1,000 units, 1,500 units. Albumin (human) ≈ 1% to 2%, histidine, mannitol 0.8%, ≤ 50 ng murine monoclonal antibody per 100 AHF units, sodium. Heat treated, monoclonal antibody purified. Inj., lyophilized Pow. for Soln. Single-dose vial and diluent. *Rx.*
Use: Antihemophilic agent.

monoclonal antibodies.
See: Alemtuzumab.
Belimumab.
Bevacizumab.
Cetuximab.
Denosumab.
Eculizumab.
Gemtuzumab Ozogamicin.
Ibritumomab Tiuxetan.
Ipilimumab.
Ofatumumab.
Omalizumab.
Palivizumab.
Panitumumab.
Rituximab.
Tositumomab and Iodine I 131 Tositumomab.
Trastuzumab.

monoclonal antibodies (murine) anti-idiotype melanoma associated antigen.
Use: Invasive cutaneous melanoma. [Orphan Drug]

monoclonal antibody for immunization against lupus nephritis. (Medclone, Inc.)
Use: Immunization. [Orphan Drug]

monoclonal antibody (human) against hepatitis B virus.
Use: Prophylaxis in hepatitis B reinfection in liver transplants. [Orphan Drug]

monoclonal antibody to CD4, 5a8. (Biogen)
Use: Postexposure prophylaxis for HIV. [Orphan Drug]

• **monoctanoin.** (MAHN-ahk-tuh-NO-in) USAN.

monocycline hydrochloride.
See: Minocin IV.

Mono-Diff Test. (Wampole)
Use: Diagnostic aid; mononucleosis.

Monodox. (Oclassen) Doxycycline monohydrate 50 mg, 100 mg. Cap. Bot. 50s (100 mg only), 100s (50 mg only), 250s, (100 mg only) *Rx.*
Use: Anti-infective; tetracycline.

• **monoethanolamine.** (mahn-oh-eth-an-OLE-ah-meen) *NF 29.*
Use: Pharmaceutic aid (surfactant).

Monojel. (Sherwood Davis & Geck) Glucose 40%. UD 25 g. *OTC.*
Use: Hyperglycemic.

Monoket. (Schwarz Pharma) Isosorbide

mononitrate 10 mg, 20 mg. Lactose. Tab. Bot. 100s; 180s, UD 100s (20 mg only). *Rx.*
Use: Vasodilator.

Mono-Latex. (Wampole) Two-minute latex agglutination slide test for the qualitative or semiquantitative detection of infectious mononucleosis heterophile antibodies in serum or plasma. Test kit 20s, 50s, 1000s.
Use: Diagnostic aid.

monolaurin.
Use: Treatment of congenital primary ichthyosis. [Orphan Drug]
See: Glylorin.

MonoNessa. (Watson) Norgestimate 0.25 mg, ethinyl estradiol 35 mcg. Tab. Pkg. 28s. *Rx.*
Use: Sex hormone, contraceptive hormone.

Mononine. (CSL Behring) Factor IX (human) ≈ 500 units, ≈ 1,000 units (monoclonal antibody purified). Actual number of units shown on each bottle. Histidine, mannitol, polysorbate 80, ≤ 50 ng of mouse protein per 100 factor IX activity units. Inj., lyophilized Pow. for Soln. Kit w/single-dose vial and sterile water for injection. *Rx.*
Use: Antihemophilic agent.

mononucleosis tests.
Use: Diagnostic aid.
See: Mono-Diff Test.
Mono-Latex.
Mono-Plus.
Monospot.
Monosticon Dri-Dot.
Mono-Sure Test.

Monopar. Stilbazium Iodide.
Use: Anthelmintic.

monophen.
Use: Cholecystography.

Mono-Plus. (Wampole) To diagnose infectious mononucleosis from serum, plasma, or fingertip blood. Test kits 24s.
Use: Diagnostic aid.

Monopril. (Bristol-Myers Squibb) Fosinopril sodium 10 mg, 20 mg, 40 mg. Lactose. Tab. Bot. 90s, 1000s (except 40 mg), UD 100s (20 mg only). *Rx.*
Use: Renin angiotensin system antagonist, angiotensin-converting enzyme inhibitor.

Monopril-HCT. (Bristol-Myers Squibb) Fosinopril sodium/hydrochlorothiazide 10 mg/12.5 mg, 20 mg/12.5 mg. Lactose. Tab. Bot. 100s. *Rx.*
Use: Antihypertensive.

• **monosodium glutamate.** (mahn-oh-SO-dee-uhm GLUE-tah-mate) *NF 29.*
Use: Pharmaceutic aid (flavor, perfume).

monosodium phosphate.
See: Sodium Biphosphate.
Monospot. (Ortho-Clinical Diagnostics) Diagnosis of infectious mononucleosis. Test kit 20s.
Use: Diagnostic aid.
monostearin. (Various Mfr.) Glyceryl monostearate.
Monosticon Dri-Dot. (Organon Teknika) Diagnosis of infectious mononucleosis. Test kit 40s, 100s.
Use: Diagnostic aid.
Mono-Sure Test. (Wampole) One-minute hemagglutination slide test for the differential qualitative detection and quantitative determination of infectious mononucleosis heterophile antibodies in serum or plasma. Kit 20s.
Use: Diagnostic aid.
Monosyl. (Arcum) Secobarbital sodium 1 gr, butabarbital 0.5 gr. Tab. Bot. 100s, 1000s. *c-II.*
Use: Hypnotic; sedative.
Monotard Human Insulin. (Bristol-Myers Squibb; Novo/Nordisk) Human insulin zinc 100 units/mL. Susp. Vial 10 mL. *OTC.*
Use: Antidiabetic.
•**monothioglycerol.** (mahn-oh-thigh-oh-GLIS-er-ole) *NF 29.*
Use: Pharmaceutic aid (preservative).
Mono-Vacc Test O.T. (Aventis Pasteur) 5 tuberculin units by the Mantoux method. Multiple puncture disposable device. Box 25s (tamper-proof). *Rx.*
Use: Diagnostic aid, tuberculosis.
monoxychlorosene. A stabilized, buffered, organichypochlorous acid derivative.
See: Oxychlorosene.
Monsel Solution. (Wade) Bot. 2 oz, 4 oz.
Use: Styptic solution.
•**montelukast sodium.** (mahn-teh-LOO-kast) USAN.
Use: Antiasthmatic, leukotriene receptor antagonist.
See: Singulair.
Monurol. (Forest) Fosfomycin tromethamine 3 g/Gran. Single-dose packet. *Rx.*
Use: Anti-infective, urinary.
•**morantel tartrate.** (moe-RAN-tell) USAN.
Use: Anthelmintic.
Moranyl. Suramin.
Morco. (Archer-Taylor) Cod liver oil ointment, zinc oxide, benzethonium chloride, benzocaine 1%. 1.5 oz, lb. *OTC.*
Use: Antiseptic; antipruritic, topical.
More Dophilus. (Freeda) Acidophilus-carrot derivative 4 billion units/g. Pow.

Bot. 120 g. *OTC.*
Use: Antidiarrheal; nutritional supplement.
•**moricizine hydrochloride.** (MAHR-IH-sizz-een) USAN.
Use: Cardiovascular agent (antiarrhythmic).
•**morniflumate.** (MAR-nih-FLEW-mate) USAN.
Use: Anti-inflammatory.
Moroline. (Schering-Plough) Petrolatum. Jar 1.75 oz, 3.75 oz, 15 oz. *OTC.*
Use: Dermatologic; lubricant; protectant.
Morpen. (Major) Ibuprofen 400 mg, 600 mg. Tab. Bot. 500s. *Rx.*
Use: Analgesic; NSAID.
morphine hydrochloride. (Various Mfr.) Pow. Bot. 1 oz, 5 oz. *c-II.*
Use: Analgesic.
•**morphine sulfate.** (MORE-feen) *USP 34.*
Use: Opioid analgesic; sedative.
See: Astramorph PF.
Avinza.
DepoDur.
Duramorph.
Infumorph 500.
Infumorph 200.
Kadian.
MS Contin.
MSIR.
Oramorph SR.
RMS.
Roxanol.
Roxanol 100.
Roxanol T.
morphine sulfate. (Abbott, Baxter) Morphine sulfate 0.5 mg/mL. Inj. Amps and vials 10 mL. *c-II.*
Use: Analgesic, narcotic agonist.
morphine sulfate. (Eli Lilly) Morphine sulfate 10 mg, 15 mg, 30 mg, Soln. Tab. Bot. 100s. *c-II.*
Use: Analgesic, narcotic.
morphine sulfate. (Endo) Morphine sulfate 15 mg, 30 mg, 60 mg, 100 mg, lactose. ER Tab. Bot. 100s, 500s. *c-II.*
Use: Analgesic, narcotic agonist.
morphine sulfate. (Ethex) Morphine sulfate 20 mg/mL, alcohol free. Soln. Bot 30 mL, 120 mL, 240 mL. *c-II.*
Use: Analgesic, narcotic agonist.
morphine sulfate. (Paddock) Morphine sulfate. Compounding Pow. Bot. 25 g. *c-II.*
Use: Analgesic, narcotic agonist.
morphine sulfate. (Ranbaxy) Morphine sulfate 10 mg, 15 mg, 30 mg. Lactose, sucrose. Soluble Tab. for Inj. Bot.

100s. *c-II.*
Use: Opioid analgesic.
morphine sulfate. (Roxane) Morphine
sulfate 10 mg/5 mL, 20 mg/5 mL. Oral
Soln. Bot. 100 mL, 500 mL. UD 5 mL
(10 mg only), 10 mL (10 mg only). *c-II.*
Use: Opioid analgesic.
morphine sulfate. (Various Mfr.) Morphine sulfate. **ER Tab.:** 15 mg, 30 mg,
60 mg, 100 mg, 200 mg (for use only
in opioid-tolerant patients). 50s (30 mg
only), 100s, 500s (except 200 mg),
UD 100s (except 200 mg). 150 punch
cards (15 mg, 30 mg, 60 mg only). **Inj.:**
1 mg/mL (Vial 10 mL, 30 mL. Amp.
10 mL), 2 mg/mL (Vial 30 mL, syringe,
Carpuject, Tubex 1 mL); 4 mg/mL (Disp.
Syringe 1 mL, 2 mL. *Tubex* and *Carpuject* 1 mL), 5 mg/mL (Vial 1 mL), 8 mg/
mL (Vial, Amp., *Carpuject,* 1 mL),
10 mg/mL (1 mL *Carpuject,* Vial, Amp.;
Multidose vial 10 mL), 15 mg/mL
(Amp., *Carpuject,* Vial 1 mL, Multidose
vial 20 mL). **Oral Soln. (concentrate):**
20 mg/mL. Alcohol free. 15 mL, 30 mL,
120 mL, 240 mL with calibrated dropper or spoon. **Rec. Supp.:** 5 mg, 10 mg,
20 mg, 30 mg. Box 12s. **Soln. for Inj.:**
25 mg/mL (Syringe 4 mL, 10 mL, 20 mL,
40 mL; Single-use vials [may contain sul-
fites]); 50 mg/mL (Syringe 10 mL, 20 mL,
40 mL, 50 mL; Single-use vials [may contain sulfites]). **Tab.:** 15 mg, 30 mg. Bot.
100s, UD 100s. *c-II.*
Use: Opioid analgesic.
morphine sulfate. (Watson) Morphine
sulfate 15 mg; 30 mg; 60 mg; 100 mg,
200 mg (for use in opioid-tolerant patients only). Lactose (except 100 mg,
200 mg). Film-coated. CR Tab. 100s.
c-II.
Use: Opioid analgesic.
morphine sulfate in 5% dextrose.
(Hospira) Morphine sulfate 1 mg/mL.
Inj. 100 mL, 250 mL. *c-II.*
Use: Opioid analgesic.
•**morrhuate sodium.** (MORE-you-ate)
USP 34.
Use: Sclerosing agent.
See: Scleromate.
morrhuate sodium. (Various Mfr.) Morrhuate sodium 50 mg/mL. Inj. Multiple-
use vials. 30 mL. *Rx.*
Use: Sclerosing agent.
Morton Salt Substitute. (Morton Grove)
Potassium chloride, fumaric acid, tri-
calcium phosphate, monocalcium phos-
phate. Na < 0.5 mg/5 g (0.02 mEq/5 g),
K 2800 mg/5 g (72 mEq/5 g) 88.6 g.
OTC.
Use: Salt substitute.

Morton Seasoned Salt Substitute.
(Morton Grove) Potassium chloride,
spices, sugar, fumaric acid, tricalcium
phosphate, monocalcium phosphate.
Na < 1 mg/5 g (< 0.04 mEq/5 g), K
2165 mg/5 g (56 mEq/5 g). Bot. 85.1 g.
OTC.
Use: Salt substitute.
Mosco. (Medtech) Salicylic acid 17.6%.
Jar. 10 mL. *OTC.*
Use: Keratolytic.
•**motavizumab.** (moe-ta-VIZ-ue-mab)
USAN.
Use: Prevention of respiratory syncytial
virus.
•**motesanib.** (moe-TES-a-nib) USAN.
Use: Antiangiogenesis agent.
•**motexafin gadolinium.** (moe-TEX-a-fin
gad-OH-lihn-ee-uhm) USAN.
Use: Investigational antineoplastic.
•**motexafin lutetium.** (moe-TEX-a-fin)
USAN.
Use: Photoantineoplastic.
Motilium. (Janssen) Domperidone
maleate. *Rx.*
Use: Antiemetic.
Motion Aid. (Vangard Labs, Inc.) Dimen-
hydrinate 50 mg. Tab. Bot. 100s, 1000s,
UD 10 × 10s.
Use: Antiemetic; antivertigo.
Motion Cure. (Wisconsin Pharmacal Co.)
Meclizine 25 mg. Chew. Tab. 12s.
Use: Antiemetic; antivertigo.
motion sickness agents.
See: Antinauseants.
Bucladin.
Dramamine.
Emetrol.
Marezine.
Scopolamine Hydrobromide.
Motofen. (Valeant) Difenoxin hydrochlo-
ride 1 mg, atropine sulfate 0.025 mg.
Tab. Bot. 50s, 100s. *c-IV.*
Use: Antidiarrheal.
•**motretinide.** (MOE-TREH-tih-nide)
USAN.
Use: Keratolytic.
Motrin, Children's. (McNeil Consumer
Healthcare) Ibuprofen 100 mg/5 mL,
sucrose. Susp. Bot. 120 mL, 480 mL.
Rx-OTC.
Use: Analgesic, nonsteroidal anti-
inflammatory agent.
Motrin Children's Cold. (McNeil Con-
sumer Healthcare) Pseudoephedrine
hydrochloride 15 mg, ibuprofen 100 mg/
5 mL. Acesulfame K, sucrose, sucra-
lose. Tropical punch, berry, or grape fla-
vors. Dye free. Susp. Bot. 118 mL.
OTC.

Use: Upper respiratory combination, decongestant, analgesic.

Motrin, Infant's. (McNeil Consumer Healthcare) Ibuprofen 40 mg/mL. Sorbitol, sucrose. Berry flavor. Oral Drops. 30 mL with dropper. *OTC.*
Use: Nonsteroidal anti-inflammatory agent.

Motrin, Junior Strength. (McNeil Consumer Healthcare) Ibuprofen. **Chew. Tab.:** 100 mg. Aspartame, phenylalanine 6 mg, orange flavor. Pkg. 24s **Tab.:** 100 mg. 24s. *OTC.*
Use: Analgesic, nonsteroidal anti-inflammatory agent.

Motrin IB. (McNeil Consumer Healthcare) Ibuprofen. **Tab.:** 200 mg. Bot. 100s. **Gelcap.:** 200 mg. Pkg. 8s. *OTC.*
Use: Analgesic; nonsteroidal anti-inflammatory agent.

Motrin Migraine Pain. (McNeil Consumer Healthcare) Ibuprofen 200 mg. Capl. Bot. 24s, 50s, 100s. *OTC.*
Use: Analgesic, nonsteroidal anti-inflammatory agent.

mouth and throat products.
See: Amlexanox.
Benzocaine.
Benzyl Alcohol.
Carbamide Peroxide.
Doxycycline.
Menthol.
Minocycline Hydrochloride.
Pilocarpine Hydrochloride.
Saliva Substitutes.
Sulfuric Acid/Sulfonated Phenolics.
Tetracycline Hydrochloride.

MouthKote. (Parnell) Xylitol, sorbitol, yerba santa, citric acid, ascorbic acid, sodium benzoate, saccharin, lemonlime flavor. Soln. Spray Bot. 60 mL, 240 mL. *OTC.*
Use: Saliva substitute.

MoviPrep. (Salix) PEG 3350 100 g, sodium sulfate 7.5 g, sodium chloride 2.691 g, potassium chloride 1.015 g. Ascorbic acid 4.7 g, sodium ascorbate 5.9 g, phenylalanine 2.33 mg. Lemon flavor. Pow. for Reconstitution. Cartons with disposable container and 4 pouches. *Rx.*
Use: Laxative.

Moxatag. (Middlebrook) Amoxicillin 775 mg. Film-coated. ER Tab. 30s, UD 10s. *Rx.*
Use: Penicillin, aminopenicillin.

•**moxalactam disodium for injection.** (MOX-ah-LACK-tam) *USP 34.*
Use: Anti-infective.
See: Moxam.

Moxam. (Eli Lilly) Moxalactam disodium.

Vial 1 g/10 mL Traypak 10s; Vial 2 g/ 20 mL Traypak 10s; Vial 10 g/100 mL Traypak 6s. *Rx.*
Use: Anti-infective; cephalosporin.

•**moxazocine.** (MOX-AZE-oh-seen) USAN.
Use: Analgesic; antitussive.

•**moxetumomab pasudotox.** (MOX-e-TOOM-oh-mab pa-SOO-doe-tox) USAN.
Use: Antineoplastic.

Moxeza. (Alcon Vision) Moxifloxacin hydrochloride 0.5%. Boric acid, sodium chloride. Soln., Ophth. 3 mL *DropTainer. Rx.*
Use: Ophthalmic and otic agent, ophthalmic antibiotic.

•**moxifloxacin hydrochloride.** (mox-ih-FLOX-ah-sin) USAN.
Use: Anti-infective; fluoroquinolone; antibiotic, ophthalmic.
See: Avelox.
Avelox IV.
Moxeza.
Vigamox.

•**moxilubant maleate.** (MOX-ill-yoo-bahnt) USAN.
Use: Treatment of rheumatoid arthritis and psoriasis (leukotriene B_4 receptor antagonist).

•**moxnidazole.** (MOX-NIH-dazz-ole) USAN.
Use: Antiprotozoal (trichomonas).

M-Oxy. (Mallinckrodt) Oxycodone hydrochloride 5 mg. Tab. Bot. 100s. *c-II.*
Use: Opioid analgesic.

Moxy Compound. (Major) Theophylline 130 mg, ephedrine 25 mg, hydroxyzine hydrochloride 10 mg. Tab. Bot. 100s. *Rx.*
Use: Antiasthmatic compound.

Moyco Fluoride Rinse. (Moyco Union Broach Division) Fluoride 2%. Flavor. Bot. 128 oz. with pump. *Rx-OTC.*
Use: Dental caries agent.

Mozobil. (Genzyme) Plerixafor 20 mg/ mL. Sodium chloride 5.9 mg. Preservative free. Inj., Soln. Single-use vial. *Rx.*
Use: Hematopoietic agent, stem cell mobilizer.

6-MP.
Use: Antimetabolite.
See: Purinethol.

MRV. (Bayer Consumer Care) 2000 million organisms/mL from *Staphylococcus aureus* (1200 million), *Streptococcus,* viridans and nonhemolytic (200 million), *Streptococcus pneumoniae* (150 million), *Branhamella*

catarrhalis (150 million), *Klebsiella pneumoniae* (150 million), *Haemophilus influenzae* (150 million). Inj. Vial 20 mL. *Rx.*
Use: Immunization.

MS Contin. (Purdue Frederick) Morphine sulfate 15 mg; 30 mg; 60 mg; 100 mg, 200 mg (for use only in opioid-tolerant patients). Lactose (except 100 mg, 200 mg). CR Tab. Bot. 100s, 500s (except 200 mg), UD 25s (except 200 mg). *c-II.*
Use: Opioid analgesic.

MSIR. (Purdue Frederick) Morphine sulfate. **Oral Soln.:** 10 mg/5 mL, 20 mg/5 mL. Sugar, sucrose. EDTA. Bot. 120 mL. **Oral Soln. (concentrate):** 20 mg/mL. EDTA. 30 mL with calibrated dropper. *c-II.*
Use: Opioid analgesic.

MS/L-Concentrate. (Richwood Pharmaceuticals) Morphine sulfate 100 mg/5 mL. Oral Soln. Bot. 120 mL w/calibrated dropper. *c-II.*
Use: Analgesic; narcotic.

MS/S. (Richwood Pharmaceuticals) Morphine sulfate 5 mg, 10 mg, 20 mg, 30 mg. Supp. 12s. *c-II.*
Use: Analgesic; narcotic.

MTC. Mitomycin. *Rx.*
Use: Anti-infective.
See: Mutamycin.

mTOR inhibitor.
Use: Protein-tyrosine kinase inhibitor.
See: Everolimus.
Temsirolimus.

MTP-PE. (Novartis) Muramyl-tripeptide.
Use: Immunomodulator.

MTX. *Rx.*
Use: Antineoplastic; antipsoriatic.
See: Methotrexate.

• **mubritinib.** (mue-bri-TYE-nib) USAN.
Use: Antineoplastic agent.

mucilloid of psyllium seed.
W/Dextrose.
See: Metamucil.

mucin.
See: Gastric Mucin.

Mucinex. (Reckitt Benckiser) Guaifenesin 600 mg (100 mg immediate-release, 500 mg extended-release). ER Tab. Bot. 20s, 40s, 500s. *OTC.*
Use: Expectorant.

Mucinex Children's. (Reckitt Benckiser) Guaifenesin 100 mg per 5 mL. Alcohol free. Parabens, saccharin. Grape flavor. Liq. 118 mL. *OTC.*
Use: Expectorant.

Mucinex Cold for Kids. (Reckitt Benckiser) Guaifenesin 100 mg, phenylephrine hydrochloride 2.5 mg. Dextrose, parabens, saccharin, sorbitol, sucralose. Alcohol free. Mixed berry flavor. Liq. 118 mL. *OTC.*
Use: Upper respiratory combination, decongestant and expectorant combination.

Mucinex Cough for Kids. (Reckitt Benckiser) Dextromethorphan hydrobromide 5 mg, guaifenesin 100 mg. Dextrose, parabens, saccharin, sucralose. Alcohol free. Cherry flavor. Liq. 118 mL. *OTC.*
Use: Upper respiratory combination, antitussive with expectorant.

Mucinex Cough Mini-Melts for Kids. (Reckitt Benckiser) Dextromethorphan hydrobromide 5 mg, guaifenesin 100 mg. Aspartame, phenylalanine 2 mg, sorbitol. Orange cream flavor. Gran. 12s. *OTC.*
Use: Upper respiratory combination, antitussive with expectorant.

Mucinex D. (Reckitt Benckiser) Pseudoephedrine hydrochloride 60 mg, guaifenesin 600 mg. ER Tab. 18s. *OTC.*
Use: Upper respiratory combination, decongestant and expectorant combination.

Mucinex DM. (Reckitt Benckiser) Dextromethorphan HBr 30 mg, guaifenesin 600 mg. ER Tab. 20s, 40s. *OTC.*
Use: Antitussive with expectorant, upper respiratory combination.

Mucinex D Maximum Strength. (Reckitt Benckiser) Guaifenesin 1,200 mg, pseudoephedrine hydrochloride 120 mg. ER Tab. 24s. *OTC.*
Use: Upper respiratory combination, decongestant/expectorant combination.

Mucinex DM Maximum Strength. (Reckitt Benckiser) Dextromethorphan hydrobromide 60 mg, guaifenesin 1,200 mg. ER Tab. 14s. *OTC.*
Use: Upper respiratory combination, antitussive with expectorant.

Mucinex Maximum Strength. (Reckitt Benckiser) Guaifenesin 1,200 mg. ER Tab. 28s. *OTC.*
Use: Expectorant.

Mucinex Mini-Melts for Kids. (Reckitt Benckiser) Guaifenesin 50 mg, 100 mg per packet. Aspartame, phenylalanine 0.6 mg, 1 mg, sorbitol. Grape, bubble gum flavor. Gran. 12s. *OTC.*
Use: Expectorant.

MUC 9 + 4 Pediatric. (Fujisawa Healthcare) Vitamin A 2300 units, D 400 units, E 7 mg, B_1 1.2 mg, B_2 1.4 mg, B_3 17 mg, B_5 5 mg, B_6 1 mg, B_{12} 1 mcg, C 80 mg, biotin 20 mcg, folic acid 0.14 mg, K 200 mcg/5 mL, mannitol 375 mg. Pow.

Vial. 10 mL. *Rx.*
Use: Nutritional supplement, parenteral.

Muco-Fen DM. (Ivax) Guaifenesin 1000 mg, dextromethorphan HBr 60 mg. Dye free. Long-acting Tab. Bot. 100s. *Rx.*
Use: Upper respiratory combination, antitussive, expectorant.

Muco-Fen LA. (Ivax) Guaifenesin 600 mg, dye free. TR Tab. Bot. 100s. *Rx.*
Use: Expectorant.

mucolytics.
Use: Respiratory.

Mucus Relief. (Major) Guaifenesin 400 mg. Maltodextrin. Dye free. Tab. 60s. *OTC.*
Use: Respiratory agent, expectorant.

Mucus Relief DM. (Major) Dextromethorphan hydrobromide 20 mg, guaifenesin 400 mg. Maltodextrin. Tab. 60s. *OTC.*
Use: Upper respiratory combination, antitussive with expectorant.

MucusRelief Sinus. (Major) Phenylephrine hydrochloride 10 mg, guaifenesin 400 mg. Tab. 60s. *OTC.*
Use: Upper respiratory combination, decongestant and expectorant combination.

Mudd. (Chattem) Natural hydrated magnesium aluminum silicate. Topical preparation. *OTC.*
Use: Cleanser.

Mudrane GG Elixir. (ECR) Theophylline 20 mg, ephedrine hydrochloride 4 mg, guaifenesin 26 mg, phenobarbital 2.5 mg/5 mL, alcohol 20%. Bot. pt, 0.5 gal. *Rx.*
Use: Antiasthmatic combination.

Mudrane-2. (ECR) Potassium iodide 195 mg, aminophylline (anhydrous) 130 mg. Tab. Bot. 100s. *Rx.*
Use: Antiasthmatic combination.

MuGard. (Access Pharmaceuticals) Benzyl alcohol, carbomer homopolymer A, citric acid, glycerin, potassium hydroxide, saccharin. Oral Rinse. 237 mL. *Rx.*
Use: Mouth and throat product.

Multa-Gen 12 + E. (Jones Pharma) Vitamin A 5000 units, D 400 units, B_1 2 mg, B_2 2 mg, B_6 0.5 mg, B_{12} 3 mcg, C 37.5 mg, E 15 units, folic acid 0.2 mg, nicotinamide 20 mg. Cap. Bot. 60s, 500s, 1000s. *OTC.*
Use: Vitamin supplement.

Multaq. (Sanofi-Aventis) Dronedarone 400 mg. Film coated. Tab. Lactose. 60s, 180s, 500s, UD 100s. *Rx.*
Use: Cardiovascular agent, antiarrhythmic agent.

Multi-B-Plex. (Forest) Vitamins B_1 100 mg, B_2 1 mg, nicotinamide 100 mg, pantothenic acid 10 mg, B_6 10 mg/mL. Inj. Vial 10 mL, 30 mL. *Rx.*
Use: Mineral, vitamin supplement.

Multi-B-Plex Capsules. (Forest) Vitamins B_1 50 mg, B_2 5 mg, niacinamide 50 mg, calcium pantothenate 5.4 mg, B_6 0.2 mg, C 150 mg, B_{12} 1 mcg. Cap. Bot. 100s, 1000s. *OTC.*
Use: Mineral, vitamin supplement.

Multi-Day. (NBTY) Vitamins A 5000 units, D 400 units, E 30 mg, B_1 1.5 mg, B_2 1.7 mg, B_3 20 mg, B_5 10 mg, B_6 2 mg, B_{12} 6 mcg, C 60 mg, FA 0.4 mL. Tab. Bot. 100s. *OTC.*
Use: Vitamin supplement.

Multi-Day Plus Iron. (NBTY) Fe 18 mg, A 5000 units, D 400 units, E 15 mg, B_1 1.5 mg, B_2 1.7 mg, B_3 20 mg, B_6 2 mg, B_{12} 6 mcg, C 60 mg, FA 0.4 mg. Tab. Bot. 100s. *OTC.*
Use: Vitamin supplement.

Multi-Day Plus Minerals. (NBTY) Fe 18 mg, A 6500 units, D 400 units, E 30 mg, B_1 1.5 mg, B_2 1.7 mg, B_3 20 mg, B_5 10 mg, B_6 2 mg, B_{12} 6 mcg, C 60 mg, FA 0.4 mg, Ca, Cl, Cr, Cu, I, K, Mg, Mn, Mo, P, Se, Zn 15 mg, biotin 30 mcg. Tab. Bot. 100s. *OTC.*
Use: Vitamin supplement.

Multi-Day with Calcium and Extra Iron Tablets. (NBTY) Fe 27 mg, A 5000 units, D 400 units, E 30 mg, B_1 1.5 mg, B_2 1.7 mg, B_3 20 mg, B_5 10 mg, B_6 2 mg, B_{12} 6 mcg, C 60 mg, FA 0.4 mg, Ca, Zn 15 mg, tartrazine. Tab. Bot. 100s. *OTC.*
Use: Mineral, vitamin supplement.

Multifol. (Breckenridge) Ca 125 mg, iron (as ferrous fumarate) 65 mg, vitamin A 6000 units, D 400 units, E 30 units, B_1 1.1 mg, B_2 1.8 mg, B_3 15 mg, B_6 2.5 mg, B_{12} 5 mcg, C 60 mg, FA 1 mg. Tab. UD 100s. *Rx.*
Use: Multivitamin.

Multigen. (Breckenridge Pharmaceutical) Vitamin B_{12} 10 mcg, desiccated stomach substance 50 mg, Fe 70 mg (from ferrous asparto glycinate), succinic acid 75 mg, vitamin C 152 mg (as calcium ascorbate and calcium threonate). Film coated. Tab. 90s. *Rx.*
Use: Trace element, iron.

Multi-Germ Oil. (Viobin) Corn, sunflower and wheat germ oils. Bot. 4 oz, 8 oz, pt, qt. *OTC.*
Use: Nutritional supplement.

MultiHance. (Bracco Diagnostics) Gadobenate dimeglumine 529 mg/mL. Preservative free. Single-dose vials. 5 mL, 10 mL, 15 mL, 20 mL. *Rx.*
Use: Radiopaque agent.

Multi-Jets. (Kirkman) Vitamins A 10,000 units, D_2 400 units, B_1 20 mg, B_2 8 mg, C 120 mg, niacinamide 10 mg, calcium pantothenate 5 mg, B_6 0.5 mg, E 50 units, desiccated liver 100 mg, dried debittered yeast 100 mg, choline bitartrate 62 mg, inositol 30 mg, dl-methionine 30 mg, B_{12} 7 mcg, Fe 2.6 mg, Ca (dical phosphate) 58 mg, P (dical phosphate) 45 mg, I (potassium iodide) 0.114 mg, Mg sulfate 1 mg, Cu sulfate 1.99 mg, Mn sulfate 1.11 mg, KCl iodide 79 mg. Tab. Bot. 100s. *OTC.*
Use: Mineral, vitamin supplement.

multikinase inhibitor.
Use: Treatment of advanced renal cell carcinoma.
See: Sorafenib.

Multilex. (Rugby) Fe 15 mg, vitamins A 10,000 units, D 400 units, E 5.5 mg, B_1 10 mg, B_2 5 mg, B_3 30 mg, B_5 10 mg, B_6 1.7 mg, B_{12} 3 mcg, C 100 mg, Zn 1.5 mg, Cu, I, Mg, Mn. Film coated. Mannitol, PEG, sodium benzoate. Tab. 100s. *OTC.*
Use: Mineral, vitamin supplement.

Multilex T & M Tablets. (Rugby) Fe 15 mg, vitamins A 10,000 units, D 400 units, E 5.5 mg, B_1 15 mg, B_2 10 mg, B_3 100 mg, B_5 10 mg, B_6 2 mg, B_{12} 7.5 mcg, C 150 mg, Cu, I, Mg, Mn, Zn 1.5 mg, sugar. Tab. Bot. 100s. *OTC.*
Use: Mineral, vitamin supplement.

Multilyte. (Fujisawa Healthcare) Vitamins A 5000 units, D 400 units, E 15 mg, B_1 3 mg, B_2 3.4 mg, B_3 36 mg, B_5 14 mg, B_6 4.4 mg, B_{12} 6 mcg, C 120 mg, FA 0.4 mg, Zn 10.5 mg, biotin 100 mcg, Ca, K, Mg, Mn, phenylalanine. Tab. Pkg. 12s. *OTC.*
Use: Mineral, vitamin supplement.

Multilyte-40. (American Pharmaceutical Partners) Na 25 mEq, K $\approx$ 40 mEq, Ca 5 mEq, Mg 8 mEq, Cl $\approx$ 33 mEq, acetate $\approx$ 40 mEq, gluconate 5 mEq/25 mL, osmolarity $\approx$ 6015 mOsm/L. Single-dose vial 25 mL. *Rx.*
Use: Intravenous nutritional therapy, intravenous replenishment solution.

Multilyte-20. (American Pharmaceutical Partners) Na 25 mEq, K 20 mEq, Ca 5 mEq, Mg 5 mEq, Cl 30 mEq, acetate 25 mEq/25 mL, osmolarity $\approx$ 4205 mOsm/L. Single-dose vial 25 mL. *Rx.*
Use: Intravenous nutritional therapy, intravenous replenishment solution.

Multi-Mineral Tablets. (NBTY) Ca 166.7 mg, P 75.7 mg, I 25 mcg, Fe 3 mg, Mg 66.7 mg, Cu 0.33 mg, Zn 2.5 mg, K 12.5 mg, Mn 8.3 mg. Tab.

Bot. 100s. *OTC.*
Use: Mineral, vitamin supplement.

Multinatal Plus. (Brookstone Pharmaceuticals) Vitamin C 60 mg, E 30 units, B1 3 mg, B2 3.4 mg, B3 20 mg, B6 50 mg, B12 12 mcg. Folic acid 1 mg, Ca 200 mg, Fe 30 mg, Mg 100 mg, Zn 15 mg, Cu 2 mg. Film coated. Tab. 30s. *Rx.*
Use: Vitamin supplement.

Multipals. (Faraday) Vitamins A 5000 units, D 400 units, C 50 mg, B_1 3 mg, B_6 0.5 mg, B_2 3 mg, calcium pantothenate 5 mg, niacinamide 20 mg, B_{12} 2 mcg. Tab. Bot. 100s, 250s, 1000s. *OTC.*
Use: Mineral, vitamin supplement.

Multipals-M. (Faraday) Vitamins A 6000 units, D 400 units, B_1 3 mg, B_2 3 mg, B_6 0.5 mg, B_{12} 5 mcg, C 60 mg, E 2 units, niacinamide 20 mg, calcium pantothenate 5 mg, Fe 10 mg, I 0.15 mg, Cu 1 mg, Mg 6 mg, Mn 1 mg, K 5 mg. Tab. Bot. 100s, 250s, 1000s. *OTC.*
Use: Mineral, vitamin supplement.

Multiple Electrolytes and 5% Travert. (Baxter Healthcare) Invert sugar 50 g/L, calories 196 cal/L, Na^+ 56 mEq, K^+ 25 mEq, Mg^{++} 6 mEq, Cl^- 56 mEq, phosphate 12.5 mEq, lactate 25 mEq/L, osmolarity 449 mOsm/L, sodium 5 mEq/L sodium bisulfite. Soln. Bot. 1000 mL. *Rx.*
Use: Intravenous nutritional therapy, intravenous replenishment solution.

Multiple Electrolytes and 10% Travert. (Baxter Healthcare) Invert sugar 100 g/L, calories 384 cal/L, Na^+ 56 mEq, K^+ 25 mEq, Mg^{++} 6 mEq, Cl^- 56 mEq, phosphate 12.5 mEq, lactate 25 mEq/L, osmolarity 726 mOsm/L, sodium 5 mEq/L, sodium bisulfite. Soln. Bot. 1000 mL. *Rx.*
Use: Intravenous nutritional therapy, intravenous replenishment solution.

Multiple Vitamin Mineral Formula. (Kirkman) Vitamins A 5000 units, D_2 400 units, C 50 mg, B_1 2.5 mg, B_2 2.5 mg, B_6 0.5 mg, B_{12} 1 mcg, niacinamide 15 mg, calcium pantothenate 5 mg, E 0.1 units, Ca 100 mg, Fe 7.5 mg, Mg 2.5 mg, K 2.5 mg, Zn 0.15 mg, Mn 0.5 mg, I 0.07 mg. Tab. Bot. 100s. *OTC.*
Use: Mineral, vitamin supplement.

Multiple Vitamins Chewable. (Kirkman) Vitamins A 5000 units, D 400 units, C 50 mg, B_1 3 mg, B_2 2.5 mg, B_6 1 mg, B_{12} 1 mcg, niacinamide 20 mg. Tab. Bot. 100s. *OTC.*
Use: Vitamin supplement.

Multiple Vitamins w/Iron. (Kirkman) Vitamins A 5000 units, D 400 units, C 50 mg, B$_1$ 3 mg, B$_2$ 2.5 mg, B$_6$ 1 mg, B$_{12}$ 1 mcg, niacinamide 20 mg, Fe 10 mg. Tab. Bot. 100s. *OTC.*
Use: Mineral, vitamin supplement.

Multi 75. (Fibertone) Vitamins A 25,000 units, D 500 units, E 150 units, B$_1$ 75 mg, B$_2$ 75 mg, B$_3$ 75 mg, B$_5$ 75 mg, B$_6$ 75 mg, B$_{12}$ 75 mcg, C 250 mg, FA 0.4 mg, Ca 50 mg, Fe 10 mg, biotin, I, Mg, Zn 15 mg, Cu, PABA, K, Mn, Cr, Se, Mo, B, Si, choline bitartrate, inositol, rutin, lemon bioflavonoid complex, hesperidin, betaine, hydrochloride. TR Tab. Bot. 60s, 90s. *OTC.*
Use: Mineral, vitamin supplement.

Multistix 8 Reagent Strips. (Siemans Medical) Urinalysis reagent strip test for detecting glucose, ketone, blood, pH, protein, nitrite, bilirubin, leukocytes. Strip Box. 100s.
Use: Diagnostic aid.

Multistix 8 SG Reagent Strips. (Siemans Medical) Urinalysis reagent strip test for glucose, ketone, specific gravity, blood, pH, protein nitrite, leukocytes. Strip Box 100s.
Use: Diagnostic aid.

Multistix-N. (Bayer Consumer Care) Glucose, protein, pH, blood, ketones, bilirubin, urobilinogen, nitrate, leukocytes. Kit. 100s.
Use: Diagnostic aid.

Multistix 9 Reagent Strips. (Siemans Medical) Urinalysis reagent strip test for glucose, bilirubin, ketone, blood, pH, protein, urobilinogen, nitrite, leukocytes. Strip Box 100s.
Use: Diagnostic aid.

Multistix 9 SG Reagent Strips. (Siemans Medical) Urinalysis reagent strip test for glucose, bilirubin, ketone, specific gravity, blood, pH, protein, nitrite, leukocytes. Strip Box 100s.
Use: Diagnostic aid.

Multistix-N S.G. Reagent Strips. (Bayer Consumer Care) Urinalysis reagent strip test for pH, protein, glucose, ketones, bilirubin, blood nitrite, urobilinogen, specific gravity. Strip Bot. 100s.
Use: Diagnostic aid.

Multistix Reagent Strips. (Siemans Medical) Urinalysis reagent strip test for pH, protein, glucose, ketone, bilirubin, blood. Strip Box 100s.
Use: Diagnostic aid.

Multistix 7. (Siemans Medical) Urinalysis reagent strip test for glucose ketone, blood, pH, protein, nitrite, leuko-

cytes. Strip Box 100s.
Use: Diagnostic aid.

Multistix 10 SG Reagent Strips. (Siemans Medical) Reagent strip test for glucose, bilirubin, ketone, specific gravity, blood, pH, protein, urobilinogen, nitrite, leukocytes in urine. Strip Box 100s.
Use: Diagnostic aid.

Multistix 2 Reagent Strips. (Siemans Medical) Urinalysis reagent strip test for nitrite and leukocytes. Strip Bot. 100s.
Use: Diagnostic aid.

Multi-Symptom Tylenol Cold. (McNeil Consumer) Pseudoephedrine hydrochloride 30 mg, chlorpheniramine maleate 2 mg, dextromethorphan HBr 15 mg, acetaminophen 325 mg. Capl. or Tab. Bot. 24s, 50s. *OTC.*
Use: Analgesic, antihistamine, antitussive, decongestant.

Multi-Thera-M. (NBTY) Iron 27 mg, vitamins A 5500 units, D 400 units, E 30 mg, B$_1$ 3 mg, B$_2$ 3.4 mg, B$_3$ 30 mg, B$_5$ 10 mg, B$_6$ 3 mg, B$_{12}$ 9 mcg, C 120 mg, folic acid 0.4 mg, biotin 15 mcg, Zn 15 mg, Ca, Cl, Cr, Cu, I, K, Mg, Mn, Mo, Se. Tab. Bot. 130s. *OTC.*
Use: Mineral, vitamin supplement.

Multi-Thera Tablets. (NBTY) Vitamins A 5500 units, D 400 units, E 30 mg, B$_1$ 3 mg, B$_2$ 3.4 mg, B$_3$ 30 mg, B$_5$ 10 mg, B$_6$ 3 mg, B$_{12}$ 9 mcg, C 120 mg, folic acid 0.4 mg, biotin 15 mcg. Tab. Bot. 100s. *OTC.*
Use: Vitamin supplement.

Multitrace-5. (American Regent) Chromium (as chloride) 4 mcg, copper (as sulfate) 0.4 mg, manganese (as sulfate) 0.1 mg, selenium (as selenious acid) 20 mcg, zinc (as sulfate) 1 mg. Benzyl alcohol 0.9%. Inj. Multidose vial. 10 mL. *Rx.*
Use: Trace metal combination.

Multitrace-5 Concentrate. (American Regent) Zinc sulfate 5 mg, copper sulfate 1 mg, manganese sulfate 0.5 mg, chromium chloride 10 mcg, selenium 60 mcg, benzyl alcohol 0.9%. Inj. Soln. Vial 1 mL, 10 mL. *Rx.*
Use: Mineral supplement.

Multitrace-4. (American Regent) Chromium (as chloride) 4 mcg, copper (as sulfate) 0.4 mg, manganese (as sulfate) 0.1 mg, zinc (as sulfate) 1 mg. Benzyl alcohol 0.9%. Inj. Multidose vial. 10 mL. *Rx.*
Use: Trace metal combination.

Multitrace-4 Concentrate. (American Regent) Chromium (as chloride) 10 mcg, copper (as sulfate) 1 mg,

manganese (as sulfate) 0.5 mg, zinc (as sulfate) 5 mg. Benzyl alcohol 0.9%. Inj. 1 mL single-dose vial, 10 mL multidose vial. *Rx.*
Use: Trace metal combination.

Multitrace-4 Neonatal. (American Regent) Chromium (as chloride) 0.85 mcg, copper (as sulfate) 0.1 mg, manganese (as sulfate) 0.025 mg, zinc (as sulfate) 1.5 mg. Inj. Single-dose vial. 2 mL. *Rx.*
Use: Trace metal combination.

Multitrace-4 Pediatric. (American Regent) Chromium (as chloride) 1 mcg, copper (as sulfate) 0.1 mg, manganese (as sulfate) 0.025 mg, zinc (as sulfate) 1 mg. Preservative free. Inj. Single-dose vial. 3 mL. *Rx.*
Use: Trace metal combination.

Multi-Vita. (Rosemont) Vitamins A 1500 units, D 400 units, E 5 mg, B_1 0.5 mg, B_2 0.6 mg, B_3 8 mg, B_6 0.4 mg, B_{12} 2 mcg, C 35 mg/mL. Alcohol free. Drop. Bot. 50 mL. *OTC.*
Use: Vitamin supplement.

Multi-Vita Drops. (Rosemont) Vitamins A 1500 units, D 400 units, E 5 mg, B_1 0.5 mg, B_2 0.6 mg, B_3 8 mg, B_6 0.4 mg, B_{12} 2 mcg, C 35 mg/mL. Alcohol free. Drop. Bot. 50 mL. *OTC.*
Use: Mineral, vitamin supplement.

Multi-Vita Drops w/Fluoride. (Rosemont) Fluoride 0.5 mg, vitamins A 1500 units, D 400 units, E 5 mg, B_1 0.5 mg, B_2 0.6 mg, B_3 8 mg, B_6 0.4 mg, B_{12} 2 mcg, C 35 mg/mL. Alcohol free. Drop. Bot. 50 mL. *Rx.*
Use: Vitamin supplement; dental caries agent.

Multi-Vita Drops w/Iron. (Rosemont) Iron 10 mg, vitamins A 1500 units, D 400 units, E 5 mg, B_1 0.5 mg, B_2 0.6 mg, B_3 8 mg, B_6 0.4 mg, C 35 mg/mL. Alcohol free. Drop. Bot. 50 mL. *OTC.*
Use: Mineral, vitamin supplement.

multivitamin concentrate injection. (Fujisawa Healthcare) Vitamins A 10,000 units, D 1000 units, E 5 units, B_1 50 mg, B_2 10 mg, B_3 100 mg, B_5 25 mg, B_6 15 mg, C 500 mg/Inj. Vial 5 mL. *Rx.*
Use: Vitamin supplement.

multivitamin infusion (neonatal formula).
Use: Nutritional supplement for low birth weight infants. [Orphan Drug]

Multi-Vitamin Mineral w/Beta Carotene. (Mission Pharmacal) Iron 27 mg, A 5000 units, D 400 units, E 30 units, B_1 2.25 mg, B_2 2.6 mg, B_3 20 mg, B_5

10 mg, B_6 3 mg, B_{12} 9 mcg, C 90 mg, folic acid 0.4 mg, biotin 0.45 mg, Ca, Cl, Cr, Cu, I, K, Mg, Mn, Mo, P, Se, Zn 15 mg, Vitamin K. Tab. Bot. 130s. *OTC.*
Use: Mineral, vitamin supplement.

Multi-Vitamins Capsules. (Forest) Vitamins A 5000 units, D 400 units, B_1 1.5 mg, B_2 2 mg, B_6 0.1 mg, C 37.5 mg, calcium pantothenate 1 mg, niacinamide 20 mg. Cap. Bot. 100s, 1000s, 5000s. *OTC.*
Use: Mineral, vitamin supplement.

Multivitamins Capsules. (Solvay) Vitamins A 5000 units, D 400 units, B_1 2.5 mg, B_2 2.5 mg, C 50 mg, B_3 20 mg, B_5 5 mg, B_6 0.5 mg, B_{12} 2 mcg, E 10 units. Cap. Bot. 100s, UD 100s. *OTC.*
Use: Mineral, vitamin supplement.

Multivitamins with A, B, D, E and K Plus Zinc. (SourceCF) **Tab., Chew.:** Vitamins A 16,000 units, D 1,000 units, E 200 units, B_1 1.5 mg, B_2 1.7 mg, B_3 10 mg, B_5 12 mg, B_6 1.9 mg, B_{12} 6 mcg, C 100 mg, K 800 mcg, folic acid 200 mcg, Zn, biotin 100 mcg. Sucralose, sucrose. Bubble gum flavor. 90s.
Cap. softgels: Vitamins A 16,000 units, D 1,000 units, E 200 units, B_1 1.5 mg, B_2 1.7 mg, B_3 20 mg, B_5 12 mg, B_6 1.9 mg, B_{12} 6 mcg, C 100 mg, K 800 mcg, folic acid 200 mcg, Zn, biotin 100 mcg. Hydrogenated vegetable oil, soybean oil, sucralose. 60s.
Pediatric Drops: Vitamins A 4,627 units, D 500 units, E 50 units, B_1 0.5 mg, B_2 0.6 mg, B_3 6 mg, B_5 3 mg, B_6 0.6 mg, B_{12} 4 mcg, C 45 mg, K 400 mcg, Zn, biotin 15 mcg per mL. EDTA, sucralose, sucrose. 60 mL w/ dropper.
Use: Nutritional supplement, multivitamin.

multivitamins with iron.
Use: Nutritional combination products.
See: BiferaRx.
Tandem DHA.

multivitamins with iron and other minerals.
Use: Nutritional combination products.
See: Biotect Plus.
Tandem OB.
Tandem Plus.
TotalDay.

multivitamins with minerals.
Use: Nutritional combination products.
See: Advanced Ear Health Formula.
Calcium-Folic Acid Plus D.
Corvite Free.
Daily Betic.
D1000 Plus.

Invites Rx.
K-PAX Immune Support.
Multivitamin with A, B, D, E, and K
  Plus Zinc.
Nutravance.
One-Daily.
PreserVision Lutein.
Prosteon.
Strovite One.
Udamin.
Udamin SP.
UpCal D.

Multivitamin with Fluoride Drops. (Major) Fluoride 0.5 mg, vitamins A 1500 units, D 400 units, E 4.1 units, B_1 0.5 mg, B_2 0.6 mg, B_3 8 mg, B_6 0.4 mg, B_{12} 2 mg, C 35 mg. Drop. Bot. 50 mL. *OTC.*
Use: Vitamin supplement; dental caries agent.

Multivitamin with Fluoride Drops. (Major) Fluoride 0.5 mg, vitamins A 1500 units, D 400 units, E 5 units, B_1 0.5 mg, B_2 0.6 mg, B_3 8 mg, B_6 0.4 mg, B_{12} 2 mcg, C 35 mg, F 0.25 mg. Drop. Bot. 50 mL. *Rx.*
Use: Vitamin supplement; dental caries agent.

Multi-Vit Drops. (Alra) Vitamins A 500 units, D 400 units, E 5 mg, B_1 0.5 mg, B_2 0.6 mg, B_3 8 mg, B_6 0.4 mg, B_{12} 2 mcg, C 35 mg/mL. Bot. 50 mL. *OTC.*
Use: Vitamin supplement.

Multi-Vit Drops w/Iron. (Alra) Iron 10 mg, vitamins A 1500 units, D 400 units, E 5 units, B_1 0.5 mg, B_2 0.6 mg, B_3 8 mg, B_6 0.4 mg, C 35 mg/mL. Methylparaben. Drop. Bot. 50 mL. *OTC.*
Use: Mineral, vitamin supplement.

Multi-Vit with Fluoride. (Qualitest) Fluoride 0.25 mg, vitamins A 1,500 units (as vitamin A palmitate), D_3 400 units (as cholecalciferol), E 5 units (as d-alpha-tocopheryl acid succinate), B_1 0.5 mg, B_2 0.6 mg, B_3 8 mg, B_6 0.4 mg, B_{12} 2 mcg, C 35 mg. Glycerin. Drops. 50 mL. *Rx.*
Use: Multivitamin.

Multorex. (Health for Life Brands) Vitamins A 6000 units, D 1250 units, C 50 mg, E 5 units, B_1 3 mg, B_2 3 mg, B_6 0.5 mg, niacinamide 20 mg, calcium pantothenate 5 mg, B_{12} 5 mcg, Ca 59 mg, P 45 mg. Cap. Bot. 100s, 250s, 1000s.
Use: Mineral, vitamin supplement.

Mulvidren-F Softabs. (Wyeth) Fluoride 1 mg, vitamins A 4000 units, D 400 units, B_1 1.6 mg, B_2 2 mg, B_3 10 mg, B_5 2.8 mg, B_6 1 mg, B_{12} 3 mcg, C 75 mg, saccharin. Tab. Bot. 100s. *Rx.*
Use: Mineral, vitamin supplement; dental caries agent.

• **mumps skin test antigen.** *USP 34.*
Use: Diagnostic aid (dermal reactivity indicator).

• **mumps virus vaccine live.** *USP 34.*
Use: Immunization.

mumps virus vaccine, live attenuated. Jeryl Lynn (B level) strain.
W/Measles virus vaccine, rubella virus vaccine.
See: M-M-R.

• **mupirocin.** (myoo-PIHR-oh-sin) *USP 34.*
Use: Anti-infective (topical and nasal).
See: Bactroban.
  Centany.

mupirocin. (Various Mfr.) Mupirocin 2%. Polyethylene glycol base. Oint. 15 g, 22 g, 30 g. *Rx.*
Use: Topical anti-infective, antibiotic.

• **mupirocin calcium.** (myoo-PIHR-oh-sin) USAN.
Use: Anti-infective, topical.
See: Bactroban.

• **muplestim.** (myoo-PLEH-stim) USAN.
Use: Hematopoietic stimulant; antineutropenic.

• **muraglitazar.** (myoo-ra-GLI-ta-zar) USAN.
Use: Investigational antidiabetic.

muriatic acid.
See: Hydrochloric Acid.

Muri-Lube. (Fujisawa Healthcare) Mineral Oil "Light." Vial 2 mL, 10 mL. *Rx.*
Use: Lubricant.

Murine Ear Drops. (Ross) Carbamide peroxide 6.5%, alcohol 6.3%, glycerin, polysorbate 20. Drops. 15 mL. *OTC.*
Use: Otic preparation.

Murine Ear Wax Removal System. (Ross) Carbamide peroxide 6.5% in anhydrous glycerin w/ear washing syringe. Bot. 0.5 oz. and ear washer 1 oz. *OTC.*
Use: Otic.

Murine Regular Formula. (Ross) Sodium chloride, potassium chloride, sodium phosphate, glycerin, benzalkonium chloride 0.01%, EDTA 0.05%. Drop. Bot. 15, 30 mL. *OTC.*
Use: Artificial tears.

Murine Plus. (MedTech) Tetrahydrozoline hydrochloride 0.05%. Polyvinyl alcohol 0.5%, povidone 0.6%, benzalkonium chloride, dextrose, EDTA, sodium bicarbonate, sodium chloride, sodium citrate, sodium phosphate mono- and dibasic. Ophth. Soln. Bot. 15 mL. *OTC.*

Use: Vasoconstrictor; ophthalmic decongestant.

Murocel Solution. (Bausch & Lomb) Methylcellulose 1%, propylene glycol, sodium chloride, methylparaben 0.046%, propylparaben 0.02%, boric acid, sodium borate. Soln. Bot. 15 mL. *OTC.*
Use: Artificial tears.

• **muromonab-CD3.** (MYOO-row-MOE-nab) USAN.
Use: Monoclonal antibody (immunosuppressant).
See: Orthoclone OKT3.

Muro 128 Ointment. (Bausch & Lomb) Sodium chloride 5% in sterile ointment base. Tube 3.5 g. *OTC.*
Use: Hyperosmolar.

Muro 128 Solution. (Bausch & Lomb) Sodium chloride 2%, 5%. Soln. Bot. 15 mL, 30 mL (5% only). *OTC.*
Use: Hyperosmolar.

Muroptic-5. (Optopics) Sodium chloride, hypertonic 5%. Soln. Bot. 15 mL. *OTC.*
Use: Hyperosmolar.

Muro's Opcon A Solution. (Bausch & Lomb) Naphazoline hydrochloride 0.025%, pheniramine maleate 0.3%. Bot. 15 mL. *OTC.*
Use: Antihistamine (ophthalmic), decongestant.

Muro's Opcon Solution. (Bausch & Lomb) Naphazoline hydrochloride 0.1%. Bot. 15 mL. *OTC.*
Use: Decongestant; ophthalmic.

Muro Tears Solution. (Bausch & Lomb) Hydroxypropyl methylcellulose, dextran 40. Soln. Bot. 15 mL. *OTC.*
Use: Artificial tears.

muscle adenylic acid. (Various Mfr.) Active form of adenosine 5-monophosphate.

muscle relaxants.
See: Curare.
  Flexeril.
  Lioresal.
  Mephenesin.
  Meprobamate.
  Neuromuscular Blockers, Nondepolarizing.
  Norflex.
  Pancuronium Bromide.
  Parafon Forte DSC.
  Robaxin.
  Rocuronium Bromide.
  Soma.
  Succinylcholine Chloride.

Muse. (Meda Pharmaceuticals) Alprostadil 125 mcg, 250 mcg, 500 mcg, 1000 mcg. Pellet. Individual foil pouches. *Rx.*
Use: Anti-impotence agent.

mustaral oil.
See: Allyl Isothiocyanate.

Mustargen. (Lundbeck) Mechlorethamine hydrochloride 10 mg. Pow. for Inj. Vial. Set of 4s. *Rx.*
Use: Antineoplastic, alkylating agent.

Musterole. (Schering-Plough) **Regular:** Camphor 4%, menthol 2%. Jar 0.9 oz.
Extra Strength: Camphor 5%, menthol 3%. Jar 0.9 oz., Tube 1 oz, 2.25 oz. *OTC.*
Use: Analgesic, topical.

Musterole Deep Strength. (Schering-Plough) Methyl salicylate 30%, menthol 3%, methyl nicotinate 0.5%. Jar 1.25 oz, Tube 3 oz. *OTC.*
Use: Analgesic, topical.

Musterole Extra Strength. (Schering-Plough) Camphor 5%, menthol 3%, methyl salicylate, lanolin, oil of mustard, petrolatum. 27 g, 30 g, 67.5 g. *OTC.*
Use: Liniment.

mustin.
See: Mechlorethamine Hydrochloride.

mutalin. (Spanner) Protein and iodine. Vial 30 mL.

• **muzolimine.** (MYOO-ZOLE-ih-meen) USAN.
Use: Antihypertensive; diuretic.

M.V.I. Pediatric. (Hospira) Vitamin A 2300 units, D 400 units, E 7 units, B_1 1.2 mg, B_2 1.4 mg, B_3 17 mg, B_5 5 mg, B_6 1 mg, B_{12} 1 mcg, C 80 mg, biotin 20 mcg, FA 0.14 mg, vitamin K 200 mcg, mannitol 375 mg. Inj. Vial. *Rx.*
Use: Nutritional supplement, parenteral.

M.V.I.-12. (Mayne) Vitamins A 3300 units, D 200 units, E 10 units, B_1 3 mg, B_2 3.6 mg, B_3 40 mg, B_5 15 mg, B_6 4 mg, B_{12} 5 mcg, C 100 mg, biotin 60 mcg, FA 0.4 mg. Inj. Vials. 5 mL single-dose, 50 mL multiple-dose; Unit vial: 10 mL two-chambered vials. *Rx.*
Use: Nutritional supplement, parenteral.

M.V.M. (Tyson) Iron 3.6 mg, vitamins A 400 units, E 60 units, B_1 20 mg, B_2 10 mg, B_3 10 mg, B_5 100 mg, B_6 31 mg, B_{12} 160 mcg, C 50 mg, folic acid 0.08 mg, Ca, Cr, Cu, I, K, Mg, Mo, Zn 6 mg, biotin 160 mcg, PABA, Mn, Se, tryptophan. Cap. Bot. 150s. *OTC.*
Use: Mineral, vitamin supplement.

Myadec. (Parke-Davis) Iron 18 mg, A 5000 units, D 400 units, E 30 units, B_1 1.7 mg, B_2 2 mg, B_3 20 mg, B_5 10 mg, B_6 3 mg, B_{12} 6 mcg, C 60 mg, folic acid 0.4 mg, biotin 30 mcg, vitamin K, Ca, P, I, Mg, Cu, Zn 15 mg, Mn, K, Cl, Cr, Mo, Se, Ni, Si, V, B, Sn. Tab. Bot. 130s. *OTC.*
Use: Mineral, vitamin supplement.

myagen. Bolasterone.
Use: Anabolic agent.

Myambutol. (X-Gen) Ethambutol hydrochloride. Tab. **100 mg:** Bot. 100s.
400 mg: Bot. 100s, 1000s, UD 10s. *Rx.*
Use: Antituberculous.

myanesin.
See: Mephenesin.

Myapap Drops. (Rosemont) Acetaminophen 80 mg/0.8 mL. Bot. 15 mL w/dropper. *OTC.*
Use: Analgesic.

Myapap Elixir. (Rosemont) Acetaminophen 160 mg/5 mL. Bot. 4 oz, pt, gal. *OTC.*
Use: Analgesic.

Myapap with Codeine Elixir. (Rosemont) Acetaminophen 120 mg, codeine phosphate 12 mg/5 mL. Bot. 4 oz, pt, gal. *c-v.*
Use: Analgesic, antitussive.

Mybanil. (Rosemont) Codeine phosphate 10 mg, bromodiphenhydramine hydrochloride 12.5 mg/5 mL, alcohol 5%. Bot. 4 oz, pt, gal. *c-v.*
Use: Antihistamine, antitussive.

Mycadec DM Drops. (Rosemont) Pseudoephedrine 25 mg, carbinoxamine maleate 2 mg, dextromethorphan HBr 4 mg/mL. Bot. 30 mL. *Rx.*
Use: Antihistamine, antitussive, decongestant.

Mycadec DM Syrup. (Rosemont) Carbinoxamine maleate 4 mg, pseudoephedrine hydrochloride 60 mg, dextromethorphan HBr 15 mg/5 mL, alcohol 0.6%. Bot. 4 oz, pt, gal. *Rx.*
Use: Antihistamine, antitussive, decongestant.

Mycadec Drops. (Rosemont) Pseudoephedrine hydrochloride 25 mg, dextromethorphan HBr 4 mg, carbinoxamine maleate 2 mg/mL. Bot. 30 mL. *Rx.*
Use: Antihistamine, antitussive, decongestant.

Mycamine. (Astellas Pharma, Inc.) Micafungin sodium 50 mg, 100 mg. Lactose. Pow. for Inj., lyophilized. Single-use vials. *Rx.*
Use: Antifungal agent.

Mycartal. (Sanofi-Synthelabo) Pentaerythritol tetranitrate. *Rx.*
Use: Coronary vasodilator.

Mycelex. (Ortho McNeil) Clotrimazole.
Cream: 1%. Tube 15 g, 30 g, 90 g (2 × 45 g). **Topical Soln.:** 1%. Bot. 10 mL, 30 mL. *Rx-OTC.*
Use: Antifungal, topical.

Mycelex-7. (Ortho-McNeil) Clotrimazole 1%, benzyl alcohol, cetostearyl alcohol. Vag. Cream. Tube 45 g w/1 applicator or 7 disp. applicators. *OTC.*
Use: Antifungal, vaginal.

Mycelex-7 Combination Pack. (Ortho-McNeil) Clotrimazole. **Cream:** 1%, benzyl alcohol, cetostearyl alcohol, polysorbate 80. Tube 7 g. **Supp.:** 100 mg, lactose, povidone. Pkg. 7s w/applicator. *OTC.*
Use: Antifungal, vaginal.

Mycelex-3. (Ortho-McNeil) Butoconazole nitrate 2%, cetyl and stearyl alcohol, parabens, mineral oil. Vag. Cream. Prefilled single-dose applicators (3s), 3 disp. applicators 20 g. *OTC.*
Use: Antifungal, vaginal.

Mycelex Troches. (Bayer Consumer Care) Clotrimazole 10 mg. Troche 70s, 140s. *Rx.*
Use: Antifungal.

Mychel-S. (Houba) Sterile chloramphenicol sodium succinate. Vial 1 g/15 mL. Box 5s. *Rx.*
Use: Anti-infective.

Mycifradin. (Pharmacia) Neomycin sulfate 125 mg/5 mL (equivalent to 87.5 mg neomycin). Oral soln. Bot. Pt. *Rx.*
Use: Anti-infective.

Myci-GC. (Misemer Pharmaceuticals) Codeine phosphate 10 mg, guaifenesin 100 mg per 5 mL. Saccharin, sorbitol. Alcohol free and sugar free. Liq. 236 mL. *c-v.*
Use: Upper respiratory combination, antitussive with expectorant.

Mycinaire Saline Mist. (Pfeiffer) Sodium chloride 0.65%, benzalkonium chloride. Soln. Spray Bot. 45 mL. *OTC.*
Use: Nasal decongestant.

Mycinette. (Pfeiffer) Benzocaine 15 mg, sorbitol, saccharin, menthol. Loz. 12s. *OTC.*
Use: Anesthetic, local; antiseptic; expectorant.

Mycinette Sore Throat. (Pfeiffer) Phenol 1.4%, alum 0.3%, alcohol free, sugar free. Spray 180 mL. *OTC.*
Use: Mouth and throat preparation.

Myci-Spray. (Edwards) Phenylephrine hydrochloride 0.25%, pyrilamine maleate 0.15%/mL. Bot. 20 mL. *OTC.*
Use: Antihistamine, decongestant.

Mycitracin. (Pharmacia) Bacitracin 500 units, neomycin sulfate 5 mg, polymyxin B sulfate 5000 units/g. Oint. Tube 0.5 oz. Box 36s; 1 oz; UD ¹⁄₃₂ oz. Box 144s. *OTC.*
Use: Anti-infective, topical.

Mycitracin Triple Antibiotic, Maximum Strength. (Pharmacia) Polymyxin B

sulfate 5000 units/g, neomycin 3.5 mg/
g, bacitracin 500 units/g, parabens,
mineral oil, white petrolatum. Oint. Tube
30 g, UD 0.94 g. *OTC.*
Use: Anti-infective, topical.

Mycobutin. (Pharmacia) Rifabutin
150 mg. Cap. Bot. 100s. *Rx.*
Use: Antituberculosal.

Mycocide NS. (Woodward) Benzalkonium chloride, propylene glycol,
methylparaben. Soln. Bot. 30 mL. *OTC.*
Use: Antimicrobial; antiseptic.

Mycodone Syrup. (Rosemont) Hydrocodone bitartrate 5 mg, homatropine
HBr 1.5 mg/5 mL. Bot. 4 oz, pt, gal.
c-III.
Use: Antitussive.

Mycogen-II Cream. (Ivax) Nystatin
100,000 units, triamcinolone acetonide
1 mg/g. Cream Tube 15 g, 30 g, 60 g,
120 g, lb. *Rx.*
Use: Antifungal; corticosteroid, topical.

Mycogen-II Ointment. (Ivax) Nystatin
100,000 units, triamcinolone acetonide
1 mg/g. Oint. Tube 15 g, 30 g, 60 g.
Rx.
Use: Antifungal; corticosteroid, topical.

Mycolog-II Cream and Ointment.
(Bristol-Myers Squibb) Triamcinolone
acetonide 1 mg, nystatin 100,000 units/
g. Ointment base w/Plastibase (polyethylene, mineral oil). Tube 15 g, 30 g,
60 g, Jar 120 g. *Rx.*
Use: Antifungal; corticosteroid, topical.

Mycomist. (Gordon Laboratories)
Chlorophyll, formalin, benzalkonium
chloride. Bot. 4 oz, plastic bot. 1 oz.
OTC.
Use: Antifungal for clothing.

mycophenolate. (Various Mfr.) Mycophenolate mofetil 250 mg. Cap. 30s, 100s,
120s, 500s, 1,000s, 3,500s. *Rx.*
Use: Immunologic agent, immunosuppressive.

• **mycophenolate mofetil.** (my-koe-FEN-
oh-late MOE-fe-till) USAN.
Use: Transplantation (immunosuppressant).
See: CellCept.

• **mycophenolate sodium.** (mye-koe-
FEN-oh-late) USAN.
Use: Immunosuppressant (transplanta-
tion).
See: Myfortic.

• **mycophenolic acid.** (MY-koe-fen-AHL-
ik) USAN.
Use: Antineoplastic.
See: Myfortic.

Mycoplasma Pneumonia IFA IgM Test.
(Wampole) Indirect fluorescent assay

for IgM antibodies to *Mycoplasma pneumoniae.* Box test 100s.
Use: Diagnostic aid.

Mycoplasma Pneumonia IFA Test.
(Wampole) Indirect fluorescent assay
for antibodies to *Mycoplasma pneumoniae* Box test 100s.
Use: Diagnostic aid.

Mycostatin. (Bristol-Myers Squibb) Nystatin. **Tab.:** 500,000 units, lactose.
Bot. 100s. **Cream:** 100,000 units/g in
aqueous base. Tube 15 g, 30 g. **Oint.:**
100,000 units/g in Plastibase (polyethylene and mineral oil). Tube 15 g,
30 g. **Troche:** 200,000 units. 30s. **Vaginal Tab:** 100,000 units, lactose 0.95 g,
ethyl cellulose, stearic acid, starch.
Pkg. 15s, 30s. **Pow.:** (topical)
100,000 units/g in talc. Shaker bot.
15 g. *Rx.*
Use: Antifungal.

Mycostatin Pastilles. (Bristol-Myers
Squibb Oncology/Virology) Nystatin,
200,000 units. Troche. 30s. *Rx.*
Use: Antifungal.

Myco-Triacet. (Various Mfr.) Triamcinolone acetonide 0.1%, neomycin sulfate 0.25%, gramicidin 0.25 mg, nystatin
100,000 units/g. **Cream:** 15 g, 30 g,
60 g, 480 g. **Oint.:** 15 g, 30 g, 60 g. *Rx.*
Use: Antifungal; corticosteroid, topical.

Myco-Triacet II. (Teva) Nystatin
100,000 units, triamcinolone acetonide
1 mg/g. **Cream:** White petrolatum and
mineral oil. Tube 15 g, 30 g, 60g. **Oint.:**
Tube 15 g, 30 g, 60 g. *Rx.*
Use: Antifungal; corticosteroid, topical.

Mycotussin Expectorant. (Rosemont)
Pseudoephedrine hydrochloride 60 mg,
hydrocodone bitartrate 5 mg, guaifenesin 200 mg/5 mL, alcohol 12.5%. Liq.
Bot. 4 oz, pt, gal. *c-III.*
Use: Antitussive, decongestant, expectorant.

Mycotussin Liquid. (Rosemont)
Pseudoephedrine hydrochloride 60 mg,
hydrocodone bitartrate 5 mg/5 mL, alcohol 5%. Bot. 4 oz, pt, gal. *c-III.*
Use: Antitussive, decongestant.

Mydacol. (Rosemont) Vitamins B_1 5 mg,
B_2 2.5 mg, niacinamide 50 mg, B_6
1 mg, B_{12} 1 mcg, pantothenic acid
10 mg, I 100 mcg, Fe 15 mg, Mg 2 mg,
Zn 2 mg, choline 100 mg, Mn 2 mg/
30 mL. Liq. Bot. Pt, gal. *OTC.*
Use: Mineral, vitamin supplement.

MyDex. (Larken) Phenylephrine hydrochloride 30 mg, guaifenesin 900 mg.
ER Tab. 100s. *Rx.*
Use: Upper respiratory combination, decongestant and expectorant combination.

Mydfrin 2.5%. (Alcon) Phenylephrine hydrochloride 2.5%. Benzalkonium chloride 0.01%, EDTA, sodium bisulfite, boric acid. Ophth. Soln. *Drop-Tainers.* 3 mL, 5 mL. *Rx.*
Use: Mydriatic; ophthalmic decongestant.

Mydral. (OcuSoft) Tropicamide 0.5%, 1%. Benzalkonium chloride 0.01%, EDTA. Soln. 2 mL (1% only), 15 mL. *Rx.*
Use: Ophthalmic and otic agent, cycloplegic mydriatic.

Mydriacyl. (Alcon) Tropicamide 1%. Soln. 3 mL, 15 mL *Drop-Tainer. Rx.*
Use: Cycloplegic; mydriatic.

mydriatics, parasympatholytic types.
See: Homatropine Hydrobromide.
Scopolamine Salts.

mydriatics, sympathomimetic types.
See: Amphetamine Sulfate.
Ephedrine Sulfate.
Epinephrine Hydrochloride.
Neo-Synephrine Hydrochloride.
Phenylephrine Hydrochloride.

Myelo-Kit. (Sanofi-Synthelabo) Omnipaque 180, 240 in various sizes and one sterile myelogram tray.
Use: Radiopaque agent.

•**myeloperoxidase.** (MY-el-oh-per OX-i-dase) USAN.
Use: Anti-infective.

Myfed. (Rosemont) Triprolidine hydrochloride 1.25 mg, pseudoephedrine hydrochloride 30 mg/5 mL. Syr. Bot. 4 oz, pt, gal. *OTC.*
Use: Antihistamine, decongestant.

Myfedrine. (Rosemont) Pseudoephedrine 30 mg/5 mL. Liq. Bot. 473 mL. *OTC.*
Use: Decongestant.

Myfedrine Plus. (Rosemont) Pseudoephedrine hydrochloride 30 mg, chlorpheniramine maleate 2 mg/5 mL. Syr. Bot. 4 oz, pt, gal. *OTC.*
Use: Antitussive, decongestant.

Myferon 150. (M.E. Pharmaceuticals) Polysaccharide iron complex 150 mg. Cap. UD 100s. *OTC.*
Use: Trace element.

Myfortic. (Novartis) Mycophenolate (as sodium) 180 mg, 360 mg. Lactose. Film-coated. DR Tab. 120s. *Rx.*
Use: Immunosuppressant.

Mygel Liquid. (Geneva) Aluminum hydroxide 200 mg, magnesium hydroxide 200 mg, simethicone 20 mg, Na 1.38 mg/5 mL. Liq. Bot. 360 mL. *OTC.*
Use: Antacid; antiflatulent.

Mygel Suspension. (Geneva) Aluminum hydroxide 200 mg, magnesium hydroxide 200 mg, simethicone 20 mg/5 mL. Bot. 360 mL. *OTC.*
Use: Antacid; antiflatulent.

Mygel II Suspension. (Geneva) Aluminum hydroxide 400 mg, magnesium hydroxide 400 mg, simethicone 40 mg/5 mL. Bot. 360 mL. *OTC.*
Use: Antacid; antiflatulent.

MyHist-DM. (Larken) Dextromethorphan HBr 15 mg, pyrilamine maleate 12.5 mg, phenylephrine hydrochloride 7.5 mg per 5 mL. Alcohol, dye, and sugar free. EDTA, parabens, saccharin, sorbitol. Grape flavor. Liq. 473 mL. *Rx.*
Use: Upper respiratory combination, antitussive combination.

Myhistine DH. (Rosemont) Codeine phosphate 10 mg, chlorpheniramine maleate 2 mg, pseudoephedrine hydrochloride 30 mg/5 mL. Liq. Bot. 4 oz, pt, gal. *c-v.*
Use: Antihistamine, antitussive, decongestant.

Myhistine Elixir. (Rosemont) Chlorpheniramine maleate 2 mg, phenylephrine hydrochloride 5 mg/5 mL, alcohol 5%. Liq. Bot. 4 oz, pt, gal. *OTC.*
Use: Antihistamine, decongestant.

Myhistine Expectorant. (Rosemont) Codeine phosphate 10 mg, guaifenesin 100 mg, pseudoephedrine hydrochloride 30 mg/5 mL, alcohol 7.5%. Liq. Bot. 4 oz, pt, gal. *c-v.*
Use: Antitussive, decongestant, expectorant.

MyHist-PD. (Larken) Phenylephrine hydrochloride 7.5 mg, chlorpheniramine maleate 2 mg, pyrilamine maleate 12.5 mg per 5 mL. Alcohol, dye, and sugar free. Parabens, sorbitol, saccharin. Bubble gum flavor. Liq. 473 mL. *Rx.*
Use: Upper respiratory combination, decongestant and antihistamine.

Myidone Tabs. (Major) Primidone 250 mg. Tab. Bot. 100s, 1000s. *Rx.*
Use: Anticonvulsant.

Mykacet Cream. (Alra) Nystatin 100,000 units, triamcinolone acetonide 0.1%/g. Tube 15 g, 30 g, 60 g. *Rx.*
Use: Antifungal; corticosteroid, topical.

My-K Elixir. (Rosemont) Potassium 20 mEq/15 mL, alcohol 5%, saccharin. Bot. Pt, gal. *Rx.*
Use: Electrolyte supplement.

My-K Formula 77 Liquid. (Rosemont) Doxylamine succinate 3.75 mg, dextromethorphan HBr 7.5 mg/5 mL, alcohol 10%. Liq. Bot. 180 mL. *OTC.*
Use: Antihistamine, antitussive.

Mykinac. (Alra) Nystatin 100,000 units/g in cream base. Cream Tube 15 g, 30 g. *OTC.*
Use: Antifungal, topical.

My-K Nasal Spray. (Rosemont) Oxymetazoline hydrochloride 0.05%. Soln. Bot. 0.5 oz. *OTC.*
Use: Decongestant.

Mykrox. (Medeva) Metolazone 0.5 mg. Tab. Bot. 100s. *OTC.*
Use: Diuretic.

Mylagen Gelcaps. (Ivax) Calcium carbonate 311 mg, magnesium carbonate 232 mg. Pkg. 24s. *OTC.*
Use: Antacid.

Mylagen Liquid. (Ivax) Magnesium hydroxide 200 mg, aluminum hydroxide 200 mg, simethicone 20 mg/5 mL. Bot. 355 mL. *OTC.*
Use: Antacid; antiflatulent.

Mylagen II Liquid. (Ivax) Aluminum hydroxide 400 mg, magnesium hydroxide 400 mg, simethicone 40 mg/5 mL. Bot. 355 mL. *OTC.*
Use: Antacid; antiflatulent.

Mylanta, Children's. (J & J/Merck Consumer) Calcium carbonate 400 mg (elemental calcium 160 mg). Sorbitol. Bubble gum flavor. Chew. Tab. 24s. *OTC.*
Use: Mineral supplement; antacid.

Mylanta Gas. (J & J/Merck Consumer) Simethicone 80 mg. Mint flavor. Chew. Tab. Pkg. 100s. *OTC.*
Use: Antiflatulent.

Mylanta Gas Maximum Strength. (J & J/ Merck Consumer) Simethicone. **Softgels:** 125 mg. Peppermint oil. 24s, 48s. **Chew. Tab.:** 125 mg. Mint and cherry flavors. 12s, 24s, 60s. *OTC.*
Use: Antiflatulent.

Mylanta Gelcaps. (J & J/Merck Consumer) Calcium carbonate 550 mg, magnesium hydroxide 125 mg. Bot. 24s, 50s, 100s. *OTC.*
Use: Antacid.

Mylanta Maximum Strength. (J & J/ Merck Consumer) Aluminum hydroxide 400 mg, magnesium hydroxide 400 mg, simethicone 40 mg/5 mL, parabens, saccharin, sorbitol. Original, cherry, mint, and orange flavors. Liq. 360 mL, 720 mL (original only). *OTC.*
Use: Antacid.

Mylanta Regular Strength. (J & J/Merck Consumer) Aluminum hydroxide 200 mg, magnesium hydroxide 200 mg, simethicone 20 mg/5 mL, parabens, sorbitol, saccharin. Original, mint, cherry flavors. Liq. Bot. 150 mL (original), 360 mL (all flavors), 720 mL (original, cherry). *OTC.*
Use: Antacid.

Mylanta Supreme. (J & J/Merck Consumer) Calcium carbonate 400 mg, magnesium hydroxide 135 mg/5 mL. Saccharin, sorbitol. Cherry flavor. Liq. Bot. 355 mL. *OTC.*
Use: Antacid.

Mylanta Ultra Tabs. (J & J/Merck Consumer) Magnesium hydroxide 300 mg, calcium carbonate 700 mg. Sugar, sorbitol. Cool mint and cherry creme flavors. Chew. Tab. 35s, 70s, 3 roll packs. *OTC.*
Use: Antacid.

Mylase 100. Alpha-amylase.
See: Diastase.

Myleran. (GlaxoSmithKline) Busulfan 2 mg. Lactose. Film-coated. Tab. Bot. 25s. *Rx.*
Use: Alkylating agent.

Mylicon. (AstraZeneca) Simethicone 40 mg. **Chew. Tab.:** Bot. 100s, 500s, UD 100s. **Drops:** 40 mg/0.6 mL. Bot. 30 mL. *OTC.*
Use: Antiflatulent.

Mylicon-80. (AstraZeneca) Simethicone 80 mg. Chew. Tab. Bot. 100s, Box 12s, 48s, UD 100s. *OTC.*
Use: Antiflatulent.

Mylicon-125. (AstraZeneca) Simethicone 125 mg. Chew. Tab. In 12s, 50s. *OTC.*
Use: Antiflatulent.

Mylocaine 4% Solution. (Rosemont) Lidocaine hydrochloride 4%. Bot. 50 mL, 100 mL. *Rx.*
Use: Anesthetic, local.

Mylocaine 2% Viscous Solution. (Rosemont) Lidocaine hydrochloride 2%. Bot. 100 mL. *Rx.*
Use: Anesthetic, local.

Mymethasone. (Rosemont) Dexamethasone 0.5 mg/5 mL, alcohol 5%. Elix. Bot. 100 mL, 240 mL. *Rx.*
Use: Corticosteroid.

Mynatal. (ME Pharmaceuticals) Ca 300 mg, Fe 65 mg, vitamins A 5000 units, D 400 units, E 30 mg, B_1 3 mg, B_2 3.4 mg, B_3 20 mg, B_5 10 mg, B_6 10 mg, B_{12} 12 mcg, C 120 mg, folic acid 1 mg, biotin 30 mcg, Cr, Cu, I, Mg, Mn, Mo, Zn 25 mg. Cap. Bot. 100s, 500s. *Rx.*
Use: Mineral, vitamin supplement.

Mynatal FC. (ME Pharmaceuticals) Ca 250 mg, Fe 60 mg, vitamin A 5000 units, D 400 units, E 30 units, B_1 3 mg, B_2 3.4 mg, B_3 20 mg, B_5 10 mg, B_6 10 mg, B_{12} 12 mcg, C 100 mg, folic acid 1 mg, biotin 30 mcg, Zn 25 mg, I,

Mg, Cr, Cu, Mo, Mn. Capl. Bot. 100s. *Rx.*
Use: Mineral, vitamin supplement.

Mynatal P.N. Captabs. (ME Pharmaceuticals) Ca 125 mg, Fe 60 mg, vitamins A 4000 units, D 400 units, B_1 3 mg, B_2 3 mg, B_3 10 mg, B_6 2 mg, B_{12} 3 mcg, C 50 mg, folic acid 1 mg, Zn 18 mg. Tab. Bot. 100s. *Rx.*
Use: Mineral, vitamin supplement.

Mynatal P.N. Forte. (ME Pharmaceuticals) Fe 60 mg, vitamin A 5000 units, D 400 units, E 30 units, C 80 mg, B_1 3 mg, B_2 3.4 mg, B_3 20 mg, B_6 4 mg, B_{12} 12 mcg, folic acid 1 mg, Ca 250 mg, Zn 25 mg, I, Mg, Cu. Capl. Bot. 100s. *Rx.*
Use: Mineral, vitamin supplement.

Mynatal Rx. (ME Pharmaceuticals) Ca 200 mg, Fe 60 mg, vitamin A 4000 units, D 400 units, E 15 mg, B_1 1.5 mg, B_2 1.6 mg, B_3 17 mg, B_5 7 mg, B_6 4 mg, B_{12} 2.5 mcg, C 80 mg, folic acid 1 mg, biotin 0.03 mg, Zn 25 mg, Mg, Cu. Capl. Bot. 100s. *Rx.*
Use: Mineral, vitamin supplement.

Mynate 90 Plus. (ME Pharmaceuticals) Ca 250 mg, Fe 90 mg, vitamin A 4000 units, D 400 units, E 30 units, B_1 3 mg, B_2 3.4 mg, B_3 20 mg, B_6 20 mg, B_{12} 12 mcg, C 120 mg, folic acid 1 mg, Zn 25 mg, DSS, I, Cu. Capl. Bot. 100s. *Rx.*
Use: Mineral, vitamin supplement.

Myo-B. (Sigma-Tau) Adenosine-5-monophosphoric acid, vitamin B_{12}. Inj. Vial 10 mL. *Rx.*

Myobloc. (Solstice Neurosciences) RimabotulinumtoxinB 5,000 units/mL, human serum albumin 0.05%, sodium succinate 0.01 M, sodium chloride 0.1 M. Preservative free. (One unit corresponds to the calculated median lethal intraperitoneal dose (LD_{50}) in mice.) Inj. Soln. Single-use vial. 0.5 mL, 1 mL, 2 mL. *Rx.*
Use: Botulinum toxin.

Myochrysine. (Akorn) Gold sodium thiomalate 50 mg/mL. Benzyl alcohol 0.5%. Inj. Vials. 2 mL, 10 mL. *Rx.*
Use: Antirheumatic agent.

Myocide NS. (Woodward) Benzalkonium chloride, propylene glycol, methylparaben. Soln. 30 mL. *OTC.*
Use: Antiseptic.

Myodil.
See: Iophendylate Injection.

Myoflex Creme. (Novartis Consumer) Trolamine salicylate 10% in a vanishing cream base. Tube 2 oz, 4 oz, Jar 8 oz, lb, Pump dispenser 3 oz. *OTC.*
Use: Analgesic, topical.

Myolin. (Roberts) Orphenadrine citrate 30 mg/mL. Inj. Vial 10 mL. *Rx.*
Use: Muscle relaxant.

Myorgal. (Mysuran) Ambenonium Chloride.
Use: Cholinergic.

Myoscint. (Centocor) Imciromab pentetate 0.5 mg for conjugation with indium-111. Kit.
Use: Radioimmunoscintigraphy agent. [Orphan Drug]

Myotalis. (Vita Elixir) Digitalis 1.5 gr. EC Tab. *Rx.*
Use: Cardiovascular agent.

Myotonachol. (Glenwood) Bethanechol chloride 10 mg, 25 mg. Tab. Bot. 100s. *Rx.*
Use: Urinary tract product.

Myotoxin. (Vita Elixir) **#1:** Digitoxin 0.1 mg. Tab. **#2:** Digitoxin 0.2 mg. Tab. *Rx.*
Use: Cardiovascular agent.

Myozyme. (Genzyme Corporation) Alglucosidase alfa 50 mg. Preservative free. Pow. for Inj., lyophilized. Single-use vials. 20 mL. *Rx.*
Use: Enzyme replacement therapy.

Myphentol Elixir. (Rosemont) Phenobarbital 16.2 mg, hyoscyamine SO_4 or HBr 0.1037 mg, atropine sulfate 0.0194 mg, scopolamine HBr 0.0065 mg/5 mL, alcohol 23%. Bot. 4 oz, pt, gal. *Rx.*
Use: Anticholinergic; antispasmodic; hypnotic; sedative.

Myphetane DX Cough. (Morton Grove) Brompheniramine maleate 2 mg, pseudoephedrine hydrochloride 30 mg, dextromethorphan HBr 10 mg/5 mL. Alcohol 0.95%, methylparaben, sugar. Butterscotch flavor. Syrup. 473 mL. *Rx.*
Use: Upper respiratory combination, antitussive combination.

Myproic Acid. (Rosemont) Valproic acid 250 mg (as sodium valproate)/5 mL. Syrup. Bot. Pt. *Rx.*
Use: Anticonvulsant.

Myrac. (Glades) Minocycline hydrochloride (as base) 50 mg, 75 mg, 100 mg. Lactose. Film-coated. Tab. 50s (100 mg only), 100s (except 100 mg). *Rx.*
Use: Anti-infective.

Myriatin Drops. (Sanofi-Synthelabo) Atropine methonitrate BP. *Rx.*
Use: Antispasmodic.

myristica oil.
Use: Flavor.

•**myristyl alcohol.** (mih-RIST-ill) *NF 29.*
Use: Pharmaceutic aid (stiffening agent).

Myrj 53. (AstraZeneca) Polyoxyl 50 stearate.
Use: Surface active agent.

Myrj 52 and M2s. (AstraZeneca) Polyoxyethylene 40 stearate. Mixture of free polyoxyethylene glycol and its mono- and di-stearates.
Use: Surface active agent.

Myrj 45. (AstraZeneca) Mixture of free polyoxyethylene glycol and its mono- and di-stearates. Polyoxyl 8 stearate.
Use: Surface active agent.

Mysoline. (Valeant) Primidone 50 mg, 250 mg. Lactose. Tab. 100s, 500s (50 mg only); 1000s, UD 100s (250 mg only). *Rx.*
Use: Anticonvulsant.

Mysuran. Ambenonium Chloride.
Use: Muscle stimulant.
See: Mytelase.

Mytelase. (Sanofi-Synthelabo) Ambenonium chloride 10 mg. Cap. Bot. 100s. *Rx.*
Use: Muscle stimulant.

Mytussin. (Morton Grove Pharmaceuticals) Guaifenesin 100 mg/5 mL, alcohol 3.5%. Syrup. Bot. 4 oz, pt, gal. *OTC.*
Use: Expectorant.

Mytussin AC Cough. (Morton Grove Pharmaceuticals) Codeine phosphate 10 mg, guaifenesin 100 mg per 5 mL. Alcohol 3.5%, menthol, saccharin, sorbitol. Sugar free. Syr. 473 mL. *c-v.*
Use: Upper respiratory combination, antitussive with expectorant.

Mytussin DAC. (Morton Grove Pharmaceuticals) Guaifenesin 100 mg, pseudoephedrine hydrochloride 30 mg, codeine phosphate 10 mg per 5 mL. Sugar free. Menthol, saccharin, sorbitol. Liq. Bot. 118 mL. *c-v.*
Use: Upper respiratory combination, antitussive and expectorant combination.

Mytussin DM. (Morton Grove Pharmaceuticals) Guaifenesin 100 mg, dextromethorphan HBr 10 mg per 5 mL. Alcohol free, sugar, menthol, saccharin, cherry flavor. Syrup. Bot. 118 mL, 3.8 L. *OTC.*
Use: Upper respiratory combination, antitussive, expectorant.

Myverol. (Eastman Kodak) Glyceryl monostearate.

My-Vitalife. (ME Pharmaceuticals) Ca 130 mg, Fe 27 mg, vitamins A 6500 units, D 400 units, E 30 mg, B_1 1.5 mg, B_2 1.7 mg, B_3 20 mg, B_5 10 mg, B_6 2 mg, B_{12} 6 mcg, C 60 mg, folic acid 0.4 mg, Cr, Cu, K, I, Mg, Mn, Mo, P, Se, Zn 15 mg, vitamin K, biotin 30 mcg. Cap. Bot. 60s. *OTC.*
Use: Mineral, vitamin supplement.

N

Na-Ana-Tal. (Churchill) Phenobarbital 0.25 g, phenacetin 2 g, aspirin 3 g, nicotinic acid 50 mg. Tab. Bot. 100s, Liq. Bot. 16 oz. *c-IV.*
Use: Analgesic; hypnotic; sedative.

•**nabazenil.** (nab-AZE-eh-nill) USAN.
Use: Anticonvulsant.

Nabi-HB. (Nabi Biopharmaceuticals) Hepatitis B immune globulin (human) 5% ± 1% protein. Glycine 0.15 M, solvent/detergent treated. Preservative free. Soln. for Inj. Single-dose vial 1 mL, 5 mL. *Rx.*
Use: Immune globulin.

•**nabilone.** (NAB-ih-lone) USAN.
Use: Anxiolytic; antiemetic/antivertigo agent.
See: Cesamet.

•**nabitan hydrochloride.** (NAB-ih-tan) USAN. *Formerly Nabutan Hydrochloride.*
Use: Analgesic.

•**nabiximols.** (nab-IX-i-mols) USAN.
Use: Analgesic.

•**naboctate hydrochloride.** (NAB-ocktate) USAN.
Use: Antiglaucoma agent; antinauseant.

•**nabumetone.** (nab-YOU-meh-TONE) *USP 34.*
Use: Nonsteroidal anti-inflammatory agent.

nabumetone. (Various Mfr.) Nabumetone 500 mg, 750 mg. Tab. 100s, 500s, 1000s. *Rx.*
Use: Nonsteroidal anti-inflammatory agent.

n-acetylcysteine.
See: Acetylcysteine.

n-acetyl-p-aminophenol. Acetaminophen.

•**nadide.** (NAD-ide) USAN. *Formerly Diphosphopyridine Nucleotide, Nicotinamide Adenine Dinucleotide.*
Use: Antagonist to alcohol and narcotics.

Nadinola (Deluxe) for Oily Skin. (Strickland) Hydroquinone 2%. Bot. 1.25 oz, 2.25 oz. *Rx.*
Use: Dermatologic.

Nadinola for Dry Skin. (Strickland) Hydroquinone 2%. Bot. 1.25 oz, 2.25 oz. *Rx.*
Use: Dermatologic.

Nadinola (Ultra) for Normal Skin. (Strickland) Hydroquinone 2%. Bot. 1.25 oz, 3.75 oz, Tube 1.85 oz. *Rx.*
Use: Dermatologic.

•**nadolol.** (nay-DOE-lahl) *USP 34.*
Use: Antihypertensive; antianginal; beta-adrenergic blocker.
See: Corgard.

nadolol. (Various Mfr.) Nadolol 20 mg, 40 mg, 80 mg, 120 mg, 160 mg. Tab. Bot. 30s (80 mg only), 100s; 500s (80 mg, 120 mg, 160 mg only); 1000s (except 20 mg); UD 100s (20 mg, 40 mg, 80 mg only). *Rx.*
Use: Antiadrenergic/sympatholytic, beta-adrenergic blocker.

nadolol and bendroflumethiazide.
Use: Antihypertensive; antianginal beta blocker.
See: Corzide.

nadolol/bendroflumethiazide. (IMPAX Laboratories) Nadolol/bendroflumethiazide 40 mg/5 mg, 80 mg/5 mg. Lactose, mannitol. Tab. 100s, 500s. *Rx.*
Use: Antihypertensive combination.

naepaine hydrochloride.
Use: Anesthetic, local.

•**nafamostat mesylate.** (naff-AM-oh-stat) USAN.
Use: Anticoagulant; antifibrinolytic.

•**nafarelin acetate.** (NAFF-uh-RELL-in) USAN.
Use: LHRH agonist; agonist; hormone. [Orphan Drug]
See: Synarel.

Nafazair A. (Bausch & Lomb) Naphazoline hydrochloride 0.025%, pheniramine maleate 0.3%, benzalkonium chloride 0.01%, EDTA, boric acid, sodium borate. Bot. 15 mL. *Rx.*
Use: Decongestant combination, ophthalmic.

nafcillin. (Baxter) Inj., Soln. Nafcillin. **1 g:** Dextrose 1.8 g. Premixed, frozen 50 mL single-dose *Galaxy* container. **2 g:** Dextrose 3.6 g. Premixed, frozen 100 mL single-dose *Galaxy* container. *Rx.*
Use: Penicillin, penicillin-resistant penicillin.

Nafcillin Injection. (Baxter) Nafcillin sodium 1 g, 2 g (as base). Premixed, frozen, single-dose *Galaxy* containers. 50 mL (1 g only), 100 mL (2 g only). *Rx.*
Use: Anti-infective, penicillin.

•**nafcillin sodium.** (naff-SILL-in) *USP 34.*
Use: Anti-infective.
See: Nafcillin Injection.

nafcillin sodium. (Sandoz) Nafcillin sodium (as base) 1 g, 2 g. Pow. for Inj. *Add-Vantage* vials. *Rx.*
Use: Penicillin, anti-infective.

Na-Feen. (Pacemaker) Fluoride 1 mg/Dose. Tab. Bot. 100s, 500s, 1000s; Liq.

2 oz. *Rx.*
Use: Dental caries agent.

•**nafenopin.** (naff-EN-oh-pin) USAN.
Use: Antihyperlipoproteinemic.

•**nafimidone hydrochloride.** (naff-IH-mih-DOHN) USAN.
Use: Anticonvulsant.

•**naflocort.** (NAFF-lah-cort) USAN.
Use: Adrenocortical steroid (topical).

•**nafoxidine hydrochloride.** (naff-OX-ih-deen) USAN.
Use: Antiestrogen.

•**nafronyl oxalate.** (NAFF-row-NILL OX-ah-late) USAN.
Use: Vasodilator.

•**naftifine hydrochloride.** (NAFF-tih-FEEN) USAN.
Use: Antifungal agent, topical anti-infective.
See: Naftin.

Naftin. (Merz Pharmaceutical) Naftifine hydrochloride. **Cream:** 1%. 15 g, 30 g, 60 g. **Gel:** 1%. 20 g, 40 g, 60 g. *Rx.*
Use: Antifungal agent, topical anti-infective.

Naganol.
See: Suramin.
Naphuride Sodium.

Naglazyme. (BioMarin) Galsulfase 1 mg/mL (expressed as protein content). Preservative free. Soln. for Inj. Single-use vial (contains sodium chloride 43.8 mg, sodium phosphate monobasic monohydrate 6.2 mg, sodium phosphate dibasic heptahydrate 1.34 mg, polysorbate 80 0.25 mg) 5 mL. *Rx.*
Use: Mucopolysaccharidosis VI.

•**nagrestipen.** (na-GRES-ti-pen) USAN.
Use: Stem cell inhibitory protein.

Nailicure. (Purepac) Denatonium benzoate in a clear nail polish base. Liq. Bot. 0.33 oz. *OTC.*
Use: Nail-biting deterrent.

Nail Plus. (Faraday) Gelatin Cap. Bot. 100s, 200s.

•**nalbuphine hydrochloride.** (NAL-byoo-FEEN) USAN.
Use: Narcotic agonist-antagonist analgesic.
See: Nubain.

nalbuphine hydrochloride. (Various Mfr.) Nalbuphine hydrochloride 10 mg/mL, 20 mg/mL. Inj. Vials. 1 mL, 10 mL. *Rx.*
Use: Narcotic agonist-antagonist analgesic.

Naldecon Senior EX. (Sandoz) Guaifenesin 200 mg/5 mL, saccharin, sorbitol. Alcohol free. Liq. Bot. 120 mL. *OTC.*
Use: Expectorant.

NalDex. (Blansett Pharmacal) Dexchlorpheniramine maleate 3.5 mg, phenylephrine hydrochloride 18.5 mg. Cap. 100s. *Rx.*
Use: Upper respiratory combination, decongestant and antihistamine.

Nalex-A. (Blansett Pharmacal) **Liq.:** Phenylephrine hydrochloride 5 mg, chlorpheniramine maleate 2.5 mg, phenyltoloxamine citrate 7.5 mg per 5 mL. Alcohol free, sugar free. Cotton-candy flavor. 473 mL. **Tab.:** Phenylephrine hydrochloride 20 mg, chlorpheniramine maleate 4 mg, phenyltoloxamine 40 mg. Lactose. 100s. *Rx.*
Use: Upper respiratory combination, decongestant and antihistamine.

Nalex AC. (Blansett Pharmacal) Brompheniramine maleate 2 mg, codeine phosphate 10 mg per 5 mL. Alcohol free. Saccharin, sorbitol. Blueberry flavor. Syrup. 118 mL. *c-v.*
Use: Upper respiratory combination, antitussive combination.

Nalex-A 12. (Blansett Pharmacal) Phenylephrine tannate 5 mg, chlorpheniramine tannate 2 mg, pyrilamine tannate 12.5 mg per 5 mL. Methylparaben, saccharin, sucrose. Raspberry flavor. Susp. 120 mL. *Rx.*
Use: Upper respiratory combination, decongestant and antihistamine.

Nalfon. (Pedinol) Fenoprofen calcium 200 mg, 400 mg. Cap. 90s (400 mg only), 100s (200 mg only), 500s (400 mg only). *Rx.*
Use: Analgesic; NSAID.

Nalfrx. (Blansett Pharmacal) Dexchlorpheniramine tannate 2.5 mg, pseudoephedrine tannate 75 mg, pyrilamine tannate 12.5 mg per 5 mL. Methylparaben, saccharin, sucrose. Orange-pineapple flavor. Susp. 118 mL. *Rx.*
Use: Upper respiratory combination, decongestant and antihistamine.

•**nalidixate sodium.** (nal-ih-DIK-sate) USAN. Under study.
Use: Anti-infective.

•**nalidixic acid.** (nal-ih-DIK-sik) *USP 34.*
Use: Anti-infective.

•**nalmefene hydrochloride.** (NAL-meh-FEEN) USAN. *Formerly Naletrene.*
Use: Antagonist to narcotics.

nalmetrene.
Use: Antagonist to narcotics.

•**nalmexone hydrochloride.** (NAL-mex-ohn) USAN.
Use: Analgesic; narcotic.

•**nalorphine hydrochloride.** (nal-OR-feen) *USP 34.*

• **naloxone hydrochloride.** (nal-OX-one) *USP 34.*
Use: Detoxification agent, antidote.
See: Narcan.

naloxone hydrochloride. (Various Mfr.) Naloxone hydrochloride 0.4 mg/mL. Amps. 1 mL. Syringes. 1 mL. Vials. 1 mL, 2 mL, 10 mL. *Rx.*
Use: Detoxification agent, antidote.

• **naltrexone hydrochloride.** (nal-TREX-ohn) USAN.
Use: Antidote, antagonist to narcotics.
See: ReVia.
Vivitrol.

naltrexone hydrochloride. (Various Mfr.) Naltrexone hydrochloride 50 mg. Tab. Bot. 30s, 100s, 500s. *Rx.*
Use: Narcotic antagonist; antidote.

• **naluzotan.** (na-lue-ZOE-tan) USAN.
Use: CNS agent.

• **naluzotan hydrochloride.** (na-lue-ZOE-tan) USAN.
Use: CNS agent.

Namenda. (Forest Laboratories) Memantine hydrochloride. **Oral Soln.:** 2 mg/mL. Sorbitol, parabens. Alcohol free. Peppermint flavor. 360 mL. **Tab.:** 5 mg, 10 mg. Lactose. Film-coated. 60s, 200s, 2000s, UD 100s, titration paks (blister pack containing 49 tabs [28 × 5 mg and 21 × 10 mg]). *Rx.*
Use: Alzheimer disease.

Namenda XR. (Forest Laboratories) Memantine hydrochloride 7 mg, 14 mg, 21 mg, 28 mg. PEG, sugar. ER Cap. 30s, 90s (14 mg, 28 mg), UD 100s (14 mg, 28 mg), titration pack (contains 28 capsules [7 × 7 mg, 7 × 14 mg, 7 × 21 mg, 7 × 28 mg]). *Rx.*
Use: NMDA receptor antagonist.

• **naminidil.** (nam-IN-i-dil) USAN.
Use: Alopecia.

namol xenyrate.
See: Namoxyrate.

• **namoxyrate.** (nam-OX-ee-rate) USAN.
Use: Analgesic.
See: Namol Xenyrate.

namuron.
See: Cyclobarbital Calcium.

• **nandrolone cyclotate.** (NAN-drole-ohn SIH-kloe-tate) USAN.
Use: Anabolic.

• **nandrolone decanoate.** (NAN-drole-ohn deh-KAN-oh-ate) *USP 34.*
Use: Anabolic steroid.

• **nandrolone phenpropionate.** (NAN-drole-ohn PROE-pee-oh-nate) *USP 34.*
Use: Androgen.

• **nantradol hydrochloride.** (NAN-trah-DAHL) USAN.
Use: Analgesic.

Naotin. (Drug Products) Sodium nicotinate. Amp. (equivalent to 10 mg nicotinic acid/mL) 10 mL, Box 25s, 100s. *Rx.*
Use: Vitamin B_3 supplement.

NAPA. (Medco Research; Parke-Davis) Acecainide hydrochloride.
Use: Cardiovascular agent.

• **napactadine hydrochloride.** (nap-ACK-tah-deen) USAN.
Use: Antidepressant.

• **napamezole hydrochloride.** (nap-am-EH-zole) USAN.
Use: Antidepressant.

NAPAmide Caps. (Major) Disopyramide phosphate 100 mg or 150 mg. Bot. 100s, 500s, UD 100s. *Rx.*
Use: Antiarrhythmic.

naphazoline. (Various Mfr.) Naphazoline hydrochloride. 0.1%. Ophth. Soln. Bot. 15 mL. *Rx.*
Use: Adrenergic, vasoconstrictor; ophthalmic decongestant.

• **naphazoline hydrochloride.** (naff-AZZ-oh-leen) *USP 34.*
Use: Adrenergic, vasoconstrictor; nasal decongestant, arylalkylamine; ophthalmic decongestant.
See: Advanced Eye Relief, Redness Instant Relief.
Advanced Eye Relief, Redness Maximum Relief.
AK-Con.
Clear Eyes ACR Seasonal Relief.
Clear Eyes for Redness Relief.
Clear Eyes Tears Plus Redness Relief.
Muro's Opcon.
Naphcon.
Privine.
20/20 Eye Drops.
W/Pheniramine Maleate.
See: Naphcon-A.
Opcon-A.
Visine-A.

naphazoline hydrochloride and antazoline phosphate. (Various Mfr.) Naphazoline hydrochloride 0.05%, antazoline phosphate 0.5%. Soln. 5 mL, 15 mL. *OTC.*
Use: Antihistamine; decongestant, ophthalmic.

naphazoline hydrochloride and pheniramine maleate. (Various Mfr.) Naphazoline hydrochloride 0.025%, pheniramine maleate 0.3%. Soln. Bot. 15 mL. *OTC.*
Use: Antihistamine; decongestant, ophthalmic.

Naphcon. (Alcon) Naphazoline hydrochloride 0.012%. Benzalkonium chloride 0.01%, EDTA. Ophth. Soln. Bot. 15 mL. *OTC.*
Use: Mydriatic; vasoconstrictor; ophthalmic decongestant.

Naphcon-A. (Alcon) Naphazoline hydrochloride 0.025%, pheniramine maleate 0.3%. Soln. Bot. 15 mL. *OTC.*
Use: Decongestant combination, ophthalmic.

Napholine. (Horizon) Naphazoline hydrochloride 0.1%. Soln. Bot. 15 mL. *Rx.*
Use: Mydriatic; vasoconstrictor.

Naphthyl-B Salicylate. Betol, Naphthosalol, Salinaphthol.
Use: GI & GU, antiseptic.

naphuride sodium. Suramin Sodium.

• **napitane mesylate.** (NAP-ih-tane) USAN.
Use: Antidepressant.

Naprelan. (Victory Pharma) Naproxen 375 mg (naproxen sodium 412.5 mg), 500 mg (naproxen sodium 550 mg), 750 mg (naproxen sodium 825 mg). CR Tab. 30s (750 mg), 100s (375 mg), 60s (750 mg), 75s (500 mg). *Rx.*
Use: Nonsteroidal anti-inflammatory agent.

Naprosyn. (Roche) Naproxen. **Tab.:** 250 mg, 375 mg, 500 mg. Bot. 100s, 500s. **Susp.:** 125 mg/5 mL. Sorbitol, sucrose, parabens, orange-pineapple flavor. Bot. 473 mL. *Rx.*
Use: Analgesic; nonsteroidal anti-inflammatory agent.

• **naproxcinod.** (na-PROKS-sin-od) USAN.
Use: Osteoarthritis.

• **naproxen.** (nah-PROX-ehn) *USP 34.*
Use: Analgesic; nonsteroidal anti-inflammatory agent; antipyretic.
See: EC-Naprosyn.
Naprosyn.

naproxen. (Various Mfr.) Naproxen. **Tab.:** 250 mg, 375 mg, 500 mg. Bot. 30s, 100s, 500s, 1000s, UD 100s, UD 300s (500 mg only); unit-of-use 30s, 60s, 90s, 120s; *Robot ready* 25s (except 375 mg). **DR Tab.:** 375 mg, 500 mg. Bot. 100s, 500s. **Susp.:** 125 mg/5 mL. Methylparaben, sorbitol, sucrose, pineapple-orange flavor. Bot. 15 mL, 20 mL, 500 mL. *Rx.*
Use: Analgesic; nonsteroidal anti-inflammatory agent; antipyretic.

• **naproxen etemesil.** (na-PROX-en et-e-ME-sil) USAN.
Use: CNS agent.

• **naproxen sodium.** (nah-PROX-ehn) *USP 34.*
Use: Analgesic; nonsteroidal anti-inflammatory agent; antipyretic.
See: Aleve.
Anaprox.
Anaprox DS.
Midol Extended Relief.
Naprelan.
W/Pseudoephedrine Hydrochloride.
See: Aleve-D Sinus & Cold.

naproxen sodium. (Ivax) Naproxen sodium 200 mg (220 mg naproxen sodium). Tab. Bot. 24s. *OTC.*
Use: Anti-inflammatory.

naproxen sodium. (Various Mfr.) Naproxen 200 mg (naproxen sodium 220 mg), 250 mg (naproxen sodium 275 mg), 500 mg (naproxen sodium 550 mg). Tab. Bot. 24s, 50s (200 mg only); 100s, 500s, 1000s, UD 100s (except 200 mg). *Rx-OTC.*
Use: Analgesic; nonsteroidal anti-inflammatory agent.

naproxen sodium and pseudoephedrine hydrochloride.
Use: Upper respiratory combination, decongestant, analgesic.
See: Aleve Cold & Sinus.
Aleve Sinus & Headache.

• **naproxol.** (nay-PROX-ole) USAN.
Use: Analgesic; anti-inflammatory; antipyretic.

• **napsagatran.** (nap-sah-GAT-ran) USAN.
Use: Antithrombotic.

• **narafilcon B.** (NAR-a-FIL-kon) USAN.
Use: Contact lens material (hydrophilic).

• **naranol hydrochloride.** (NARE-ah-nahl) USAN.
Use: Antipsychotic.

• **naratriptan hydrochloride.** (NAHR-ah-trip-tan) *USP 34.*
Use: Antimigraine, serotonin 5-HT$_1$ receptor antagonist.
See: Amerge.

naratriptan hydrochloride. (Various Mfr.) Naratriptan hydrochloride 1 mg, 2.5 mg. Film coated. May contain lactose, PEG, polyvinyl alcohol. Tab. Blister pack. 9s. *Rx.*
Use: Agent for migraine, serotonin 5-HT$_1$ receptor agonist.

Narcan. (DuPont Pharm) Naloxone hydrochloride 0.4 mg/mL. Inj. Amps. 1 mL. Vials (available with or without parabens). 10 mL. *Rx.*
Use: Detoxification agent, antidote.

narcotic agonist-antagonist analgesics.
See: Buprenorphine Hydrochloride.

Butorphanol Tartrate.
Nalbuphine Hydrochloride.
Pentazocine.
narcotic antitussive.
See: Codeine Sulfate.
Nardil. (Parke-Davis) Phenelzine sulfate 15 mg. Mannitol. Film-coated. Tab. Bot. 60s. *Rx.*
Use: Antidepressant, monoamine oxidase inhibitor.
Nariz. (Hawthorn) Phenylephrine hydrochloride 7.5 mg, guaifenesin 200 mg per 5 mL. Saccharin, sorbitol. Bubble gum flavor. Liq. 473 mL. *Rx.*
Use: Upper respiratory combination, decongestant and expectorant combination.
•**narlaprevir.** (nar-la-PRE-vir) USAN.
Use: Antiviral.
•**narnatumab.** (nar-NAT-ue-mab) USAN.
Use: Antineoplastic.
•**naronapride.** (nar-ON-a-pride) USAN.
Use: Gastrointestinal agent.
•**naronapride dihydrochloride.** (nar-ON-a-pride) USAN.
Use: Gastrointestinal agent.
Naropin. (AAP Pharmaceuticals) Ropivacaine hydrochloride 0.2%, 0.5%, 0.75%, 1%, preservative free. Inj. *PolyAmp DuoFit Sterile Paks* 10 mL (0.2%, 1% only), 20 mL. Single-dose vial 30 mL (0.5% only). Single-dose infusion bot. 100 mL, 200 mL (0.2% only). *Rx.*
Use: Anesthetic, local injectable.
Nasabid. (Jones Pharma) Pseudoephedrine hydrochloride 90 mg, guaifenesin 250 mg, sucrose. Cap., prolonged-action. Bot. 100s. *Rx.*
Use: Decongestant; expectorant.
Nasabid SR. (Jones Medical) Pseudoephedrine hydrochloride 90 mg, guaifenesin 600 mg. SR Tab. Bot. 100s. *Rx.*
Use: Decongestant; expectorant.
Nasacort AQ. (Sanofi Aventis) Triamcinolone acetonide 55 mcg per actuation. Polysorbate 80, edetate disodium. Spray Susp., Intranasal. Bot. 16.5 g (120 actuations) w/metered dose pump unit w/nasal adapter. *Rx.*
Use: Respiratory inhalant, intranasal steroid.
Nasadent. (Scherer) Sodium metaphosphate, glycerin, dicalcium phosphate dihydrate, sodium carboxymethylcellulose, oil of spearmint, sodium benzoate, saccharin. *OTC.*
Use: Ingestible dentifrice.
NaSal. (Bayer Consumer Care) Sodium chloride 0.65%, benzalkonium chloride. Alcohol free. Soln. Drop bot. 15 mL.

Spray bot. 30 mL. *OTC.*
Use: Nasal decongestant.
NasalCrom. (Pharmacia) Cromolyn sodium 40 mg/mL, benzalkonium Cl, EDTA. Nasal Soln. Delivers 5.2 mg/spray. Metered spray device 13 mL or 26 mL. *OTC.*
Use: Antiasthmatic.
Nasal Decongestant, Children's Non-Drowsy. (Various Mfr.) Pseudoephedrine hydrochloride 15 mg/5 mL. Liq. Bot. 118 mL. *OTC.*
Use: Nasal decongestant, arylalkylamine.
Nasal Decongestant, Maximum Strength. (Taro) Oxymetazoline hydrochloride 0.05%. Soln. Spray bot. 15 mL, 30 mL. *OTC.*
Use: Nasal decongestant, imidazoline.
Nasal Decongestant Oral. (Various Mfr.) Pseudoephedrine hydrochloride 7.5 mg/0.8 mL. Drops. Bot. 15 mL, 30 mL w/dropper. *OTC.*
Use: Nasal decongestant, arylalkylamine.
nasal decongestants.
See: Adrenalin Chloride.
Afrin No-Drip Sinus with Vapornase.
Afrin Saline, Extra Moisturizing.
Afrin Sinus with Vapornase.
AH-Chew D.
Arylalkylamines.
Ayr Saline.
Benzedrex.
Breathe Free.
Cenafed.
Decofed.
Dimetapp Decongestant Pediatric.
Dimetapp, Maximum Strength, Non-Drowsy.
Dimetapp, Maximum Strength 12-Hour Non-Drowsy.
Dristan Fast Acting Formula.
Dristan 12-Hour Nasal.
Drixoral 12-Hour Non-Drowsy Formula.
Duramist Plus 12-Hour Decongestant.
Duration.
Efidac 24.
Ephedrine Sulfate.
Epinephrine Hydrochloride.
4-Way Fast Acting.
Genaphed.
Genasal.
HuMist.
Imidazolines.
Kid Kare.
Little Colds for Infants & Children.
Little Noses Gentle Formula, Infants & Children.

Medi-First Sinus Decongestant.
Mycinaire Saline Mist.
Naphazoline hydrochloride.
NaSal.
Nasal Decongestant, Children's Non-Drowsy.
Nasal Decongestant, Maximum Strength.
Nasal Decongestant Oral.
Nasal•Ease with Zinc.
Nasal•Ease with Zinc Gluconate.
Nasal Moist.
Nasal Relief.
Nasal Spray.
Neo-Synephrine 4-Hour Extra Strength.
Neo-Synephrine 4-Hour Mild Formula.
Neo-Synephrine 4-Hour Regular Strength.
Neo-Synephrine 12-Hour.
Neo-Synephrine 12-Hour Extra Moisturizing.
Nōstrilla 12-Hour.
Ocean.
Otrivin.
Otrivin Pediatric Nasal.
Oxymetazoline Hydrochloride.
Phenylephrine Hydrochloride.
Pretz-D.
Pretz Irrigation.
Pretz Moisturizing.
Privine.
Pseudoephedrine Hydrochloride.
Pseudoephedrine Sulfate.
Rhinall.
Rhinaris Lubricating Mist.
Salinex.
Silfedrine, Children's.
Simply Saline.
Simply Stuffy.
Sinustop.
Sodium Chloride.
Sudafed, Children's Non-Drowsy.
Sudafed Non-Drowsy, Maximum Strength.
Sudafed Non-Drowsy 12 Hour Long-Acting.
Sudafed Non-Drowsy 24 Hour Long-Acting.
Sudodrin.
Tetrahydrozoline Hydrochloride.
Triaminic Allergy Congestion.
12–Hour Nasal.
Twice-A-Day 12-Hour Nasal.
Tyzine.
Tyzine Pediatric.
Vicks Sinex.
Vicks Sinex 12 Hour.
Vicks Sinex 12 Hour UltraFine Mist for Sinus Relief.
Vicks Sinex UltraFine Mist.

Vicks Vapor Inhaler.
Xylometazoline Hydrochloride.
Nasal Decongestant Sinus Non-Drowsy. (Topco) Pseudoephedrine hydrochloride 30 mg, acetaminophen 500 mg. Tab. Pkg. 24s. *OTC.*
Use: Upper respiratory combination, decongestant, analgesic.
Nasal•Ease with Zinc. (Health Care Products) Zinc acetate, aloe vera, calendula extract, parabens, tocopherol acetate, EDTA, glycerin. Soln. Gel. Tube 14.1 g. *OTC.*
Use: Nasal decongestant.
Nasal•Ease with Zinc Gluconate. (Health Care Products) Zinc gluconate, sodium chloride, benzalkonium chloride, glycerin. Soln. Spray. Bot. 30 mL. *OTC.*
Use: Nasal decongestant.
Nasal Jelly. (Kondon) Phenol, camphor, menthol, eucalyptus oil, lavender oil. Oint. Tube. 20 g. *OTC.*
Use: Decongestant.
Nasal Moist. (Blairex) Sodium chloride 0.65%, alcohol and dye free. Soln. Spray bot. 45 mL. Mist pump bot. 15 mL. Gel bot. 28.5 g, unit-of-use 2 mL, aloe vera. *OTC.*
Use: Nasal decongestant.
Nasal Relief. (Rugby) Oxymetazoline hydrochloride 0.05%, EDTA, phenylmercuric acetate, sodium chloride. Soln. Spray bot. 15 mL. *OTC.*
Use: Nasal decongestant, imidazoline.
Nasal Saline. (Sanofi-Synthelabo) Nasal spray and drops. Sodium Cl 0.65% buffered w/phosphates, preservatives. Bot. 15 mL. Spray Bot. 15 mL. *OTC.*
Use: Moisturizer, nasal.
NaSal Saline Nasal. (Sanofi-Synthelabo) Sodium Cl 0.65%. Drops, Spray. Bot. 15 mL. *OTC.*
Use: Moisturizer, nasal.
Nasal Spray. (Various Mfr.) Sodium chloride. Soln. Spray bot. 45 mL. *OTC.*
Use: Nasal decongestant.
•**nasaruplase beta.** (na-SA-rue-plase) USAN.
Use: Ischemic stroke, acute.
Nasatab LA. (ECR) Guaifenesin 500 mg, pseudoephedrine hydrochloride 120 mg. ER Tab. Bot. 100s. *Rx.*
Use: Upper respiratory combination, decongestant, expectorant.
Nascobal. (Par Pharmaceuticals) Cyanocobalamin 500 mcg per 0.1 mL (500 mcg/actuation). Benzalkonium chloride. Intranasal spray. 2.3 mL (≈ 8 doses/bottle). *Rx.*
Use: Water-soluble vitamin.

Nasex. (Cypress) Phenylephrine hydrochloride 25 mg, guaifenesin 650 mg. ER Tab. 100s. *Rx.*
Use: Upper respiratory combination, decongestant and expectorant combination.

Nasex-G. (Cypress) Phenylephrine hydrochloride 25 mg, guaifenesin 835 mg. Dye free. ER Tab. 100s. *Rx.*
Use: Upper respiratory combination, decongestant and expectorant combination.

Nashville Rabbit Antithymocyte. (Applied Medical Research) Antithymocyte serum. *Rx.*
Use: Immunosuppressant.

Nasohist. (Hawthorn) Chlorpheniramine maleate 1 mg, phenylephrine hydrochloride 2 mg per mL. Saccharin, sorbitol. Orange-vanilla flavor. Soln., Conc. 30 mL. *Rx.*
Use: Upper respiratory combination, decongestant and antihistamine.

Nasohist DM. (Hawthorn) Chlorpheniramine maleate 1 mg, phenylephrine hydrochloride 2 mg, dextromethorphan HBr 3 mg per mL. Saccharin, sorbitol. Orange-vanilla flavor. Soln., Conc. 30 mL. *Rx.*
Use: Upper respiratory combination, antitussive combination.

Nasonex. (Schering) Mometasone furoate monohydrate 0.05% (50 mcg/actuation). Glycerin, 0.25% w/w phenylethyl alcohol, citric acid, benzalkonium chloride, polysorbate 80. Spray Susp. Intranasal. Bot. 17 g (120 sprays) w/ metered-dose manual pump spray unit. *Rx.*
Use: Respiratory inhalant, intranasal steroid.

Nasophen. (Premo) Phenylephrine hydrochloride 0.25%, 1%. Bot. Pt. *OTC.*
Use: Decongestant.

Nasotuss. (Hawthorn Pharmaceuticals) Chlorcyclizine hydrochloride 25 mg, codeine phosphate 10 mg, phenylephrine hydrochloride 10 mg. Glycerin, propylene glycol, sorbitol, sucralose. Alcohol free, dye free, and sugar free. Raspberry flavor. Liq. 473 mL. *c-v.*
Use: Upper respiratory combination, antitussive combination.

Natabec. (Parke-Davis) Vitamins A 4000 units, D 400 units, B_1 3 mg, B_2 2 mg, B_6 3 mg, C 50 mg, B_{12} 5 mcg, B_3 10 mg, elemental calcium 240 mg, elemental iron 30 mg. Kapseal. Bot. 100s. *OTC.*
Use: Mineral, vitamin supplement.

Natabec-F.A. (Parke-Davis) Vitamins A 4000 units, D 400 units, B_1 3 mg, B_2 2 mg, B_6 3 mg, C 50 mg, B_{12} 5 mcg, B_3 10 mg, elemental calcium 240 mg, elemental iron 30 mg, folic acid 0.1 mg. Kapseal, magnesium, bisulfites. Bot. 100s. *OTC.*
Use: Mineral, vitamin supplement.

Natabec with Fluoride. (Parke-Davis) Vitamins A 4000 units, D 400 units, B_1 3 mg, B_2 2 mg, B_6 3 mg, C 50 mg, B_{12} 5 mcg, B_3 10 mg, elemental calcium 240 mg, elemental iron 30 mg, elemental fluoride 1 mg. Kapseal. Bot. 100s. *Rx.*
Use: Vitamin supplement, dental caries agent.

NataChew. (Warner Chilcott) Vitamin A 1000 units, D_3 400 units, E (as dl-alpha tocopheryl acetate) 11 units, C 120 mg, folic acid 1 mg, B_1 2 mg, B_2 3 mg, niacinamide 20 mg, B_6 10 mg, B_{12} 12 mcg, Fe (as ferrous fumarate) 29 mg, wildberry flavor. Chew. Tab. Bot. 90s. *Rx.*
Use: Vitamin, mineral supplement.

Natacyn. (Alcon) Natamycin 5%. Bot. 15 mL. *Rx.*
Use: Antifungal agent, ophthalmic.

NataFort. (Warner Chilcott) Vitamin A (as acetate and beta carotene) 1000 units, D_3 400 units, E (as dl-alpha tocopheryl acetate) 11 units, C 120 mg, folic acid 1 mg, B_1 2 mg, B_2 3 mg, niacinamide 20 mg, B_6 10 mg, B_{12} 12 mcg, Fe (as carbonyl iron and ferrous sulfate) 60 mg, lactose. Tab. UD 90s. *Rx.*
Use: Vitamin, mineral supplement.

NatalCare Plus. (Ethex) Vitamin A 4000 units, C 120 mg, calcium sulfate 200 mg, Fe 27 mg, D 400 units, E 22 units, B_1 1.84 mg, B_2 3 mg, niacinamide 20 mg, B_6 10 mg, folic acid 1 mg, B_{12} 12 mcg, Zn 25 mg, Cu 2 mg. Tab. Bot. 100s. *Rx.*
Use: Mineral, vitamin supplement.

NatalCare Three. (Ethex) Ca 200 mg, Fe (as ferrous fumarate) 27 mg, vitamin A (as beta carotene) 3000 units, D 400 units, E (as dl-alpha tocopheryl acetate) 30 units, B_1 1.8 mg, B_2 4 mg, B_3 20 mg, B_6 25 mg, B_{12} 12 mcg, C 120 mg, folic acid 1 mg, Zn 25 mg, Cu, Mg. Tab. Bot. 100s. *Rx.*
Use: Vitamin, mineral supplement.

Natalins. (Bristol-Myers Squibb) Ca 200 mg, Fe 30 mg, vitamins A 4000 units, D 400 units, E 15 units, B_1 1.5 mg, B_2 1.6 mg, B_3 17 mg, B_6 2.6 mg, B_{12} 2.5 mcg, C 70 mg, folic acid 0.5 mg, Mg, Cu, Zn 15 mg. Tab. Bot. 100s. *OTC.*
Use: Mineral, vitamin supplement.

•**natalizumab.** (nay-tal-IZ-oo-mab) USAN.
Use: Immunomodulator, immunologic
agent.
See: Tysabri.

•**natamycin.** (NAT-uh-MY-sin) *USP 34.*
Use: Anti-infective, ophthalmic.
See: Natacyn.

Natarex Prenatal. (Major) Ca 200 mg,
iron 60 mg, vitamins A 4000 units, D
400 units, E 15 mg, B_1 1.5 mg, B_2
1.6 mg, B_3 17 mg, B_5 7 mg, B_6 4 mg,
B_{12} 2.5 mcg, C 80 mg, folic acid 1 mg,
Cu, Mg, Zn 25 mg, biotin 30 mcg. Tab.
Bot 100s. *Rx.*
Use: Mineral, vitamin supplement.

Nata-San. (Sandia) Vitamins A
4000 units, D 400 units, B_1 5 mg, B_2
4 mg, B_6 10 mg, nicotinic acid 10 mg,
C 100 mg, B_{12} activity 5 mcg, ferrous
fumarate 200 mg (elemental iron
65 mg), calcium carbonate 500 mg
(Ca 196 mg), Cu (sulfate) 0.5 mg, Mg
(sulfate) 0.1 mg, Mn (sulfate) 0.1 mg,
K (sulfate) 0.1 mg, Zn (sulfate) 0.5 mg.
Tab. Bot. 100s, 1000s. *OTC.*
Use: Mineral, vitamin supplement.

Nata-San F.A. (Sandia) Vitamins A
4000 units, D 400 units, B_1 5 mg, B_2
4 mg, B_6 10 mg, nicotinic acid 10 mg,
C 100 mg, B_{12} activity 5 mcg, folic acid
1 mg, Fe 65 mg, Ca 200 mg, Cu (sulfate) 0.5 mg, Mg (sulfate) 0.1 mg, Mn
(sulfate) 0.1 mg, K (sulfate) 0.1 mg,
Zn (sulfate) 0.5 mg. Tab. Bot. 100s,
1000s. *Rx.*
Use: Mineral, vitamin supplement.

NataTab FA. (Ethex) Vitamin A
4000 units, C 120 mg, Ca 200 mg,
Fe 29 mg, D 400 units, E 30 units, B_1
3 mg, B_2 3 mg, niacin 20 mg, B_6 3 mg,
folic acid 1 mg, B_{12} 8 mcg, iodine, zinc
15 mg, lactose. Tab. Bot. 100s. *Rx.*
Use: Vitamin, mineral supplement.

•**nateglinide.** (na-te-GLYE-nide) USAN.
Use: Antidiabetic; meglitinide.
See: Starlix.

nateglinide. (Dr Reddy's Labs) Nateglinide 60 mg, 120 mg. Mannitol. Tab. 30s,
90s, 100s, 500s, UD 100s. *Rx.*
Use: Antidiabetic agent, meglitinide.

nateglinide. (Par Pharmaceutical) Nateglinide 60 mg, 120 mg. Lactose. Tab. UD
30s. *Rx.*
Use: Antidiabetic agent, meglitinide.

Natelle-EZ. (Tiber Labs) Ca 100 mg, Fe
25 mg, vitamin A 2700 units, D_3
400 units, E 20 units, B_1 3 mg, B_2
3.5 mg, B_3 20 mg, B_5 8 mg, B_6 30 mg,
B_{12} 12 mcg, C 120 mg, folic acid
800 mcg, biotin 30 mcg, Cu, Mg, Se,
Zn, choline bitartrate. PEG, polyvinyl al-

cohol. Tab. 30s. *Rx.*
Use: Multivitamin with calcium and iron.

Natodine. (Faraday) Iodine in organic
form as found in kelp 1 mg. Tab. Bot.
100s, 250s. *OTC.*

Natrapel. (Tender) Citronella 10% in 15%
Aloe vera base. *OTC.*
Use: Insect repellent.

Natrecor. (Scios Nova) Nesiritide
1.58 mg, mannitol. Pow. for Inj., lyophilized. Single-use vial 1.5 mg. *Rx.*
Use: Vasodilator, human B-type natriuretic peptide.

Natrico. (Drug Products) Potassium nitrate 2 g, sodium nitrite 1 g, nitroglycerin 0.25 g, crataegus oxycantha
0.25 g. Pulvoid. Bot. 100s, 1000s. *Rx.*
Use: Antihypertensive.

Natroba. (ParaPRO/Pernix Therapeutics) Spinosad 0.9%. Alcohols, butylated
hydroxytoluene, propylene glycol.
Susp. 120 mL. *Rx.*
Use: Scabicide/Pediculicide.

Naturacil. (Bristol-Myers Squibb) Psyllium seed husks 3.4 g, carbohydrate
9.6 g, Na 11 mg, 54 cal/2 pieces. Ctn.
24s, 40s. *OTC.*
Use: Laxative.

Natur-Aid. (Scot-Tussin) Lactose, pectin,
and carob-lemon juice. Pow. 90%. Bot.
8 oz. *OTC.*
Use: Increase in normal intestinal flora.

Natural Diuretic Water Tablet. (AmLab)
Buchu leaves 1 g, uva ursi 1 g, trilicum
1 g, parsley 1 g, juniper berries 1 g,
asparagus 1 g, alfalfa powder 1 gr. Tab.
Bot. 100s. *OTC.*
Use: Diuretic.

Natural E 200. (Mason) Vitamin E
200 units. Preservative free and sugar
free. Cap., softgels. 100s. *OTC.*
Use: Fat-soluble vitamin.

Natural Fiber Laxative. (Apothecary
Prods.) Approx. psyllium hydrophilic
mucilloid 3.4 g/7 g dose, 14 cal/dose,
sodium free. Pow. Can. 390 g. *OTC.*
Use: Laxative.

natural lung surfactant.
See: Survanta.

natural penicillins.
Use: Anti-infective.
See: Penicillin G (Aqueous).
Penicillin G Potassium.
Pfizerpen.

Natural Psyllium Fiber. (Plus Pharma)
Psyllium hydrophilic mucilloid fiber
3.4 g, sodium 3 mg, 25 calories per
dose. Dextrose. Pow. 368 g. *OTC.*
Use: Laxative.

Natural Psyllium Fiber, Orange. (Plus
Pharma) Psyllium hydrophilic mucil-

loid fiber 3.4 g, sodium 3 mg, 25 calories per dose. Sucrose. Orange flavor. Pow. 368 g. *OTC.*
Use: Laxative.

natural vitamin A in oil.
See: Oleovitamin A.

Natural Vitamin E. (Freeda Vitamins) Vitamin E 1,150 units (as d-alpha tocopherol) per 1.25 mL. Gluten, lactose, and sugar free. Liq. 114 mL. *OTC.*
Use: Fat-soluble vitamin.

Naturalyte. (Unico Holdings) Na 45 mEq, K 20 mEq, Cl 35 mEq, citrate 48 mEq, dextrose 25 g/L. Soln. Bot. 240 mL, 1 liter. *OTC.*
Use: Electrolyte, mineral supplement.

Naturalyte Oral Electrolyte Solution. (Unico Holdings) Dextrose 20 g, K 20 mEq, fructose 5 g, Cl 35 mEq, Na 45 mEq, citrate 30 mEq. Soln. Bot. 1 liter. *OTC.*
Use: Mineral, electrolyte supplement.

Nature's Aid Laxative Tabs. (Walgreen) Docusate sodium 100 mg, yellow phenolphthalein 65 mg. Tab. Bot. 60s. *OTC.*
Use: Laxative.

Nature's Remedy. (Block Drug) Aloe 100 mg, cascara sagrada 150 mg, lactose. Tab. Bot. 15s, 30s, 60s. *OTC.*
Use: Laxative.

Nature's Tears. (Rugby) Hydroxypropyl methylcellulose 2906 0.4%, KCl, NaCl, sodium phosphate, benzalkonium Cl 0.01%, EDTA. Soln. Bot. 15 mL. *OTC.*
Use: Artificial tears.

Nature's Wash Plus. (Geritrex) Aloe vera, parabens, propylene glycol, urea, vitamin E, wheat germ oil. Soap. 3,785 mL. *OTC.*
Use: Emollient bath preparation.

Nature-Throid. (RLC Labs) Thyroid desiccated 16.25 mg (¼ gr) (lactose, PEG 400), 32.4 mg (½ gr), 48.75 mg (¾ gr) (lactose), 64.8 mg (1 gr), 81.25 mg (1 ¼ gr) (lactose), 97.5 mg (1 ½ gr) (lactose), 113.75 mg (1 ¾ gr) (lactose), 129.6 mg (2 gr), 146.25 mg (2 ¼ gr) (lactose), 162.5 mg (2 ½ gr) (lactose), 194.4 mg (3 gr), 260 mg (4 gr) (lactose), 325 mg (5 gr) (lactose). Note: 1 grain (gr) = 64.8 mg. Tab. 100s; 30s, 60s, 90s, 990s, 1,000s, 1,008s (48.75 mg, 81.25 mg, 97.5 mg, 113.75 mg, 146.25 mg, 162.5 mg, 260 mg, 325 mg). *Rx.*
Use: Thyroid hormone.

Natur-Lax Tablets. (Faraday) Rhubarb root, cape aloes, cascara sagrada extract, mandrake root, parsley, carrot.

Protein-coated tab. Bot. 100s. *OTC.*
Use: Laxative.

Naus-A-Tories. (Table Rock) Pyrilamine maleate 25 mg, secobarbital 30 mg. Supp. Box 12s. *c-II.*
Use: Antiemetic.

Nausatrol. (Medique Products) Dextrose 1.87 g, fructose 1.87 g, phosphoric acid 21.5 mg per 5 mL. Cherry flavoring, glycerin, methylparaben, potassium sorbate. Soln. 15 mL packet (20s). *OTC.*
Use: Miscellaneous antiemetic, phosphorated carbohydrate solution.

Nausea Relief. (Ivax) Dextrose 1.87 g, fructose 1.87 g, phosphoric acid 21.5 mg, methylparaben. Soln. Bot. 118 mL. *OTC.*
Use: Antiemetic; antivertigo.

Nausetrol. (Walsh Dohmen) Dextrose 1.87 g, fructose 1.87 g, phosphoric acid 21.5 mg per 5 mL. Glycerin, methylparaben. Cherry flavor. Soln. Bot. 118 mL. *OTC.*
Use: Antiemetic; antivertigo.

Navane. (Roerig) Thiothixene 1 mg, 2 mg, 5 mg, 10 mg, 20 mg. Lactose. Cap. 100s, 1,000s (1 mg only). *Rx.*
Use: Antipsychotic.

•**navarixin.** (NAV-a-RIX-in) USAN.
Use: Treatment of asthma and chronic obstructive pulmonary disease.

•**naveglitazar.** (nav-e-GLI-ta-zar) USAN.
Use: Diabetes.

Navelbine. (Pierre Fabre Pharmaceuticals) Vinorelbine tartrate 10 mg/mL, preservative free. Inj. Single-use Vial 1 mL, 5 mL. *Rx.*
Use: Antineoplastic; vinca alkaloid.

•**navitoclax.** (na-VIT-oh-klax) USAN.
Use: Antineoplastic.

•**navitoclax dihydrochloride.** (na-VIT-oh-klax) USAN.
Use: Antineoplastic.

•**naxagolide hydrochloride.** (nax-A-go-LIDE) USAN.
Use: Antiparkinsonian; dopamine agonist.

•**naxifylline.** (na-xee-FYE-leen) USAN.
Use: Edema.

Nazafair. (Various Mfr.) Naphazoline hydrochloride 0.1%. Soln. Bot. 15 mL. *Rx.*
Use: Mydriatic; vasoconstrictor.

ND-Gesic. (Hyrex) Acetaminophen 300 mg, pyrilamine maleate 12.5 mg, chlorpheniramine maleate 2 mg, phenylephrine hydrochloride 5 mg. Tab. Bot. 100s, 1000s. *OTC.*
Use: Analgesic; antihistamine; decongestant.

n-diethylvanillamide.
See: Ethamivan.

NDNA. (Wampole) Anti-native DNA test
by IFA. Confirmatory test for active
SLE. Test 48s. *Rx.*
Use: Diagnostic aid.

•**nebacumab.** (neh-BACK-you-mab)
USAN. *Formerly Septomonab.*
Use: Monoclonal antibody, antiendo-
toxin.

•**nebivolol.** (neh-BIV-oh-lole) USAN.
Use: Antiadrenergic/sympatholytic,
beta-adrenergic blocking agents.
See: Bystolic.

•**nebivolol hydrochloride.** (neh-BIV-oh-
lole) USAN.
Use: Antihypertensive, beta blocker.

•**nebramycin.** (neh-brah-MY-sin) USAN.
A complex of antibiotic substances pro-
duced by *Streptomyces tenebrarius.*
Use: Anti-infective.

NebuPent. (American Pharmaceutical
Partners) Pentamidine isethionate
300 mg. Aer. single-dose vial. *Rx.*
Use: Anti-infective.

Nebu-Prel. (Mahon) Isoproterenol sulfate
0.4%, phenylephrine hydrochloride 2%,
propylene glycol 10%. Liq. Vial 10 mL.
Rx.
Use: Bronchodilator.

•**necitumumab.** (NE-si-TOOM-oo-mab)
USAN.
Use: Antineoplastic.

Necon 1/50. (Watson) Mestranol 50 mcg,
norethindrone 1 mg. Lactose. Tab. Pkt.
21s, 28s (7 inert tabs.). *Rx.*
Use: Sex hormone, contraceptive hormone.

Necon 1/35. (Watson) Ethinyl estradiol
35 mcg, norethindrone 1 mg. Lactose.
Tab. Pkt. 21s, 28s (7 inert tabs.). *Rx.*
Use: Sex hormone, contraceptive hormone.

Necon 7/7/7. (Watson) **Phase 1:** Norethindrone 0.5 mg, ethinyl estradiol
35 mcg. 7 tabs. **Phase 2:** Norethindrone 0.75 mg, ethinyl estradiol 35 mcg.
7 tabs. **Phase 3:** Norethindrone 1 mg,
ethinyl estradiol 35 mcg. 7 tabs. Tab.
28s (7 inert tabs.). *Rx.*
Use: Sex hormone, contraceptive hormone.

Necon 10/11. (Watson) **Phase 1:** Norethindrone 0.5 mg, ethinyl estradiol
35 mcg. 10 tabs. **Phase 2:** Norethindrone 1 mg, ethinyl estradiol 35 mcg.
11 tabs. Lactose. Tab. Pkt. 28s (7 inert
tabs.). *Rx.*
Use: Sex hormone, contraceptive hormone.

Necon 0.5/35. (Watson) Ethinyl estradiol
35 mcg, norethindrone 0.5 mg. Lactose. Tab. Pkt. 21s, 28s (7 inert tabs).
Rx.
Use: Sex hormone, contraceptive hormone.

•**nedocromil.** (NEH-doe-KROE-mill)
USAN.
Use: Antiallergic, prophylactic.

•**nedocromil calcium.** (NEH-doe-KROE-
mill) USAN.
Use: Antiallergic, prophylactic.

•**nedocromil sodium.** (NEH-doe-KROE-
mill) USAN.
Use: Mast cell stabilizer, ophthalmic
agent.
See: Alocril.

N.E.E. (Lexis Laboratories) Ethinyl estradiol 35 mcg, norethindrone 1 mg. Tab.
6 pcks. 21s, 28s. *Rx.*
Use: Contraceptive.

•**nefazodone hydrochloride.** (neff-AZE-
oh-dohn) USAN.
Use: Antidepressant.

nefazodone hydrochloride. (Various
Mfr.) Nefazodone hydrochloride 50 mg,
100 mg, 150 mg, 200 mg, 250 mg. Tab.
60s, 100s (50 mg only). *Rx.*
Use: Antidepressant.

•**neflumozide hydrochloride.** (neh-
FLEW-moe-ZIDE) USAN.
Use: Antipsychotic.

•**nefocon A.** (NEE-FOE-kahn A) USAN.
Use: Contact lens material, hydrophilic.

•**nefopam hydrochloride.** (NEFF-oh-
pam) USAN.
Use: Muscle relaxant; analgesic.

Negacide. (Sanofi-Synthelabo) Nalidixic
acid. *Rx.*
Use: Anti-infective, urinary.

•**nelarabine.** (neh-LAY-rah-bean) USAN.
Use: Antineoplastic; DNA demethyl-
ation agent.
See: Arranon.

•**nelezaprine maleate.** (neh-LEH-zah-
PREEN) USAN.
Use: Muscle relaxant.

•**nelfilcon A.** (nell-FILL-kahn A) USAN.
Use: Contact lens material, hydrophilic.

•**nelfinavir mesylate.** (nell-FIN-ah-veer)
USAN.
Use: Antiviral.
See: Viracept.

•**nelotanserin.** (NEL-oh-tan-SER-in)
USAN.
Use: CNS agent.

Nelulen. (Watson) **1/35 E:** Ethynodiol diacetate 1 mg, ethinyl estradiol 35 mcg.
Tab. Pack 21s, 28s. **1/50 E:** Ethyno-

diol diacetate 1 mg, ethinyl estradiol 50 mcg. Tab. Pack 21s, 28s. *Rx.*
Use: Contraceptive.

•**nelzarabine.** (nell-ZARE-ah-bean) USAN.
Use: Antineoplastic.

nemazine. Under study.
Use: Anti-inflammatory.

•**nemazoline hydrochloride.** (neh-MAZZ-oh-leen) USAN.
Use: Decongestant, nasal.

Nembutal Sodium. (Ovation) Pentobarbital sodium. **Inj.:** 50 mg/mL. Amp 2 mL; Vial 20 mL, 50 mL. Box 5s. **Cap.:** 50 mg. Bot. 100s; 100 mg. Bot. 100s, 500s. Display pack 100s. **Supp.:** 30 mg, 60 mg, 120 mg, 200 mg. Box 12s. *c-II.*
Use: Hypnotic; sedative.

•**nemifitide ditriflutate.** (ne-MI-fi-tide dye-trye-FLOO-tate) USAN.
Use: Antidepressant.

Neoasma. (Tarmac Products) Theophylline 125 mg, guaifenesin 100 mg. Tab. UD 30s. *Rx.*
Use: Antiasthmatic combination.

Neo-Benz-All. (Xttrium) Benzalkonium Cl 20.1%. Packet 25 mL 15s. To make gal of 1:750 soln. Also Aqueous Neo-Benz-All 1:750 soln. Packet 20 mL, 50s. *OTC.*
Use: Antiseptic; antimicrobial.

NeoBenz Micro. (SkinMedica) Benzoyl peroxide 3.5%, 5.5%, 8.5%. Cetyl alcohol, stearyl alcohol, parabens. Cream. 45 g. *Rx.*
Use: Topical anti-infective, antibiotic.

NeoBenz Micro SD. (SkinMedica) Benzoyl peroxide 3.5%, 5.5%, 8.5%. Cetyl alcohol, stearyl alcohol, parabens. Cream. 0.5 g applicators. 30s. *Rx.*
Use: Topical anti-infective.

NeoBenz Micro Wash. (SkinMedical) Benzoyl peroxide 7%. Castor oil, edetate disodium, methylparaben, PEG-6, PEG-15, PEG-40. Top. Wash. 180 g. *Rx.*
Use: Anti-infective, topical; antibiotic agent.

Neo Beserol. (Sanofi-Synthelabo) Aspirin, methocarbamol. *Rx.*
Use: Analgesic; muscle relaxant.

Neocalamine. (Various Mfr.) Red ferric oxide 30 g, yellow ferric oxide 40 g, zinc oxide 930 g. *OTC.*
Use: Astringent; antiseptic.

Neocate One +. (Scientific Hospital Supplies, Inc.) Protein 2.5 g (amino acids 3 g), carbohydrates 14.6 g, fat 3.5 g, vitamins A, D, E, K, B_1, B_2, B_3, B_5, B_6,

B_{12}, folic acid, biotin, C, choline, inositol, Ca, P, Mg, Fe, Zn, Mn, Cu, I, Mo, Cr, Se, Cl, Na 20 mg (0.9 mEq), K 93 mg (2.4 mEq) per 100 mL, 100 cal/mL. Liq. Bot. 237 mL. *OTC.*
Use: Nutritional supplement, enteral.

Neo-Cholex. (Lafayette) Fat emulsion containing 40% w/v pure vegetable oil. Bot. 60 mL. *Rx.*
Use: Cholecystokinetic.

Neocidin. (Major) Polymyxin B sulfate 10,000 units, neomycin sulfate 1.75 mg, gramicidin 0.025 mg/mL. Soln. Bot. 10 mL. *Rx.*
Use: Anti-infective, ophthalmic.

Neo-Cobefrin.
Use: Vasoconstrictor.

Neocurb. (Taylor Pharmaceuticals) Phendimetrazine tartrate 35 mg. Tab. Bot. 100s, 1000s. *c-III.*
Use: Anorexiant.

Neocylate. (Schwarz Pharma) Potassium salicylate 280 mg, aminobenzoic acid 250 mg. Tab. Bot. 100s, 1000s. *OTC.*
Use: Analgesic.

Neocyten. (Schwarz Pharma) Orphenadrine citrate 30 mg/mL. Vial 10 mL. *Rx.*
Use: Muscle relaxant.

Neo-Dexair. (Bausch & Lomb) Dexamethasone sodium phosphate 0.1%, neomycin sulfate 0.35%, polysorbate 80, EDTA, benzalkonium Cl 0.02%, sodium bisulfite 0.1%. Soln. Bot. 5 mL. *Rx.*
Use: Anti-infective; corticosteroid, ophthalmic.

Neo-Diaral. (Roberts) Loperamide 2 mg. Cap. Bot. UD 8s, 250s. *OTC.*
Use: Antidiarrheal.

Neo DM. (Laser) **Drops:** Dextromethorphan HBr 2.75 mg, chlorpheniramine maleate 0.75 mg, phenylephrine hydrochloride 1.75 mg per 1 mL. Alcohol and sugar free. Saccharin, sorbitol. Black cherry flavor. 30 mL with dropper. **Syrup:** Dextromethorphan HBr 30 mg, pseudoephedrine hydrochloride 50 mg, brompheniramine maleate 3 mg per 5 mL. Saccharin, sorbitol. Berry vanilla flavor. 30 mL, 470 mL. **Susp.:** Dextromethorphan tannate 30 mg, brompheniramine tannate 10 mg, phenylephrine tannate 25 mg per 5 mL. Alcohol and sugar free. Aspartame, parabens, phenylalanine 7 mg/5 mL. Cherry flavor. 473 mL. **Elix:** Brompheniramine maleate 3 mg, dextromethorphan hydrobromide 30 mg, pseudoephedrine hydrochloride 15 mg per 5 mL saccharin, sorbitol. Berry vanilla flavor. 473 mL. *Rx.*

Use: Upper respiratory combination, antitussive combination.

neodrenal.
See: Isoproterenol.

Neo-Durabolic. (Roberts) Nandrolone decanoate injection. **50 mg/mL, 100 mg/mL:** Vial 2 mL. **200 mg/mL:** Vial 1 mL. *c-III.*
Use: Anabolic steroid.

Neo-fradin. (Pharma-Tek) Neomycin sulfate 125 mg/5 mL, parabens. Oral Soln. Bot. 480 mL. *Rx.*
Use: Amebicide.

Neofrin. (Ocusoft) Phenylephrine hydrochloride 2.5% (benzalkonium chloride 0.01%, boric acid, EDTA, sodium borate, sodium bisulfite), 10% (benzalkonium chloride, sodium phosphate mono- and dibasic). Ophth. Soln. 15 mL. *Rx.*
Use: Ophthalmic decongestant.

Neogesic. (Pal-Pak, Inc.) Aspirin 194.4 mg, acetaminophen 129.6 mg, caffeine 32.4 mg. Tab. Bot. 1000s. *OTC.*
Use: Analgesic combination.

Neo HC. (Laser) Chlorpheniramine maleate 3 mg, hydrocodone bitartrate 5 mg, phenylephrine hydrochloride 7.5 mg. Glycerin, saccharin, sorbitol. Alcohol free and sugar free. Orange cream flavor. Syr. 473 mL. *c-III.*
Use: Upper respiratory combination, antitussive combination.

Neo-Mist Nasal Spray. (A.P.C.) Phenylephrine hydrochloride 0.5%, cetalkonium Cl 0.02%. Spray Bot. 20 mL. *OTC.*
Use: Antiseptic; decongestant.

Neo-Mist Pediatric 0.25% Nasal Spray. (A.P.C.) Phenylephrine hydrochloride 0.25%, cetalkonium Cl 0.02%. Squeeze Bot. 20 mL. *OTC.*
Use: Antiseptic; decongestant.

neomycin.
W/Polymyxin B Sulfate, Bacitracin Zinc.
See: Neosporin Original.
Triple Antibiotic.
W/Polymyxin B Sulfate, Bacitracin Zinc, Lidocaine.
See: Lanabiotic.
W/Polymyxin B Sulfate, Bacitracin Zinc, Pramoxine Hydrochloride.
See: Neosporin Plus Pain Relief.
Tri-Biozene.
W/Pramoxine Hydrochloride, Polymyxin B Sulfate.
See: Neosporin Plus Pain Relief.

neomycin and polymyxin B sulfate. (Watson Pharma) Neomycin 40 mg, polymyxin B sulfate 200,000 units/mL. Soln., intravesical. Amp. 1 mL. *Rx.*
Use: Anti-infective.

• **neomycin and polymyxin B sulfates and bacitracin ointment.** *USP 34.*
Use: Anti-infective, antibiotic, topical.
See: Bacitracin/Neomycin/Polymyxin B Ointment.

• **neomycin and polymyxin B sulfates and bacitracin ophthalmic ointment.** *USP 34.*
Use: Anti-infective, topical.

• **neomycin and polymyxin B sulfates and bacitracin zinc ointment.** *USP 34.*
Use: Anti-infective, topical.

• **neomycin and polymyxin B sulfates and bacitracin zinc ophthalmic ointment.** *USP 34.*
Use: Anti-infective, ophthalmic.

neomycin and polymyxin B sulfates and bacitracin zinc ophthalmic ointment. (Various Mfr.) Polymyxin B sulfate 10,000 units, neomycin 3.5 mg, bacitracin zinc 400 units/g, white petrolatum, mineral oil. Tube. 3.5 g. *Rx.*

neomycin and polymyxin B sulfates and dexamethasone ophthalmic ointment. (Various Mfr.) Dexamethasone 0.1%, neomycin sulfate 0.35%, polymyxin B sulfate 10,000 units. Tube 3.5 g.

• **neomycin and polymyxin B sulfates and dexamethasone ophthalmic suspension.** *USP 34.*
Use: Anti-infective; corticosteroid, ophthalmic.

neomycin and polymyxin B sulfates and dexamethasone ophthalmic suspension. (Various Mfr.) Dexamethasone 0.1%, neomycin sulfate 0.35%, polymyxin B sulfate 10,000 units/mL, benzalkonium chloride 0.004%, hydroxypropyl methylcellulose 0.5%, hydrochloric acid, sodium chloride, polysorbate 20, sodium hydroxide. Bot. 5 mL. *Rx.*

• **neomycin and polymyxin B sulfates and gramicidin cream.** *USP 34.*
Use: Anti-infective, topical.

• **neomycin and polymyxin B sulfates and gramicidin ophthalmic solution.** *USP 34.*
Use: Anti-infective, ophthalmic.

neomycin and polymyxin B sulfates and hydrocortisone. (Falcon) Hydrocortisone 1%, neomycin sulfate equiv. to 0.35% neomycin as base, polymyxin B sulfate 10,000 units/mL. Thimerosal 0.001%, cetyl alcohol, glyceryl monostearate, mineral oil, propylene glycol. Susp. 7.5 mL *Drop-Tainers. Rx.*
Use: Otic preparations.

• **neomycin and polymyxin B sulfates and hydrocortisone acetate cream.** *USP 34.*
Use: Anti-infective; corticosteroid, topical.

• **neomycin and polymyxin B sulfates and hydrocortisone acetate ophthalmic suspension.** *USP 34.*
Use: Anti-infective; corticosteroid, ophthalmic.

neomycin and polymyxin B sulfates and hydrocortisone acetate ophthalmic suspension. (Various Mfr.) Hydrocortisone 1%, neomycin sulfate 0.35%, polymyxin B sulfate 10,000 units. Bot. 7.5 mL, 10 mL.
Use: Anti-infective; corticosteroid, ophthalmic.

• **neomycin and polymyxin B sulfates and hydrocortisone otic suspension.** *USP 34.*
Use: Anti-infective; corticosteroid, otic.

neomycin and polymyxin B sulfates and hydrocortisone otic suspension. (Steris) Polymyxin B sulfate equiv. to 10,000 polymyxin B units, neomycin sulfate equiv. to 3.5 mg neomycin base/mL. Hydrocortisone 1%, thimerosal 0.01%, cetyl alcohol, propylene glycol, polysorbate 80. Susp. Bot. 10 mL.

• **neomycin and polymyxin B sulfates and pramoxine hydrochloride cream.** *USP 34.*
Use: Anti-infective, topical anesthetic.

• **neomycin and polymyxin B sulfates and prednisolone acetate ophthalmic suspension.** *USP 34.*
Use: Anti-infective; corticosteroid, ophthalmic.

• **neomycin and polymyxin B sulfates, bacitracin, and hydrocortisone acetate ointment.** *USP 34.*
Use: Anti-infective; corticosteroid, topical.

• **neomycin and polymyxin B sulfates, bacitracin, and hydrocortisone acetate ophthalmic ointment.** *USP 34.*
Use: Anti-infective; corticosteroid, topical.

• **neomycin and polymyxin B sulfates, bacitracin, and hydrocortisone ointment.** *USP 34.*
Use: Anti-infective; corticosteroid.

• **neomycin and polymyxin B sulfates, bacitracin, and lidocaine ointment.** *USP 34.*
Use: Anti-infective; anesthetic, topical.

• **neomycin and polymyxin B sulfates, bacitracin zinc, and hydrocortisone acetate ophthalmic ointment.** *USP 34.*
Use: Anti-infective; antifungal; anti-inflammatory, topical.

• **neomycin and polymyxin B sulfates, bacitracin zinc, and hydrocortisone ophthalmic ointment.** *USP 34.*
Use: Anti-infective, corticosteroid.

neomycin and polymyxin B sulfates cream.
Use: Anti-infective, topical.

• **neomycin and polymyxin B sulfates, gramicidin, and hydrocortisone acetate cream.** *USP 34.*
Use: Anti-infective; corticosteroid.

neomycin and polymyxin B sulfates, gramicidin, and hydrocortisone acetate cream.
Use: Anti-infective; corticosteroid, topical.

neomycin and polymyxin B sulfates ophthalmic ointment.
Use: Anti-infective, ophthalmic.

neomycin and polymyxin B sulfates ophthalmic solution.
Use: Anti-infective, ophthalmic.

neomycin and polymyxin B sulfates solution for irrigation.
Use: Irrigant, ophthalmic; anti-infective, topical.
See: Neosporin G.U. Irrigant.

neomycin base.
Use: Anti-infective.
W/Combinations.
See: Maxitrol.
Neosporin Plus.
Neotal.

• **neomycin boluses.** *USP 34.*
Use: Anti-infective.

• **neomycin palmitate.** (NEE-oh-MY-sin PAL-mih-tate) USAN.
Use: Anti-infective.

neomycin/polymyxin B sulfates/hydrocortisone otic. (Steris) Hydrocortisone 1%, neomycin sulfate 5 mg, polymyxin B 10,000 units. Cetyl alcohol, propylene glycol, polysorbate 80, thimerosal. Susp. 10 mL with dropper. *Rx.*
Use: Steroid and antibiotic combination.

• **neomycin sulfate.** (NEE-oh-MY-sin) *USP 34.* Cream; Ointment; Ophthalmic Ointment, Oral Solution; Tablets.
Use: Anti-infective.
See: Mycifradin.
Neo-fradin.
Neo-Tabs.
W/Combinations.
See: Bacitracin Neomycin.

Coracin.
Cortisporin.
Maxitrol.
Mycitracin.
Neosporin.
Neotal.
Neo-Thrycex.
Ocutricin.
Tigo.
Trimixin.

neomycin sulfate. (Pharmacia) Neomycin sulfate. Pow. micronized for compounding. Bot. 100 g.
Use: Anti-infective.

•**neomycin sulfate and bacitracin ointment.** *USP 34.*
Use: Anti-infective, topical.

•**neomycin sulfate and bacitracin zinc ointment.** *USP 34.*
Use: Anti-infective, topical.

•**neomycin sulfate and dexamethasone sodium phosphate cream.** *USP 34.*
Use: Anti-infective; corticosteroid, topical.

•**neomycin sulfate and dexamethasone sodium phosphate ophthalmic ointment.** *USP 34.*
Use: Anti-infective; corticosteroid, ophthalmic.

•**neomycin sulfate and dexamethasone sodium phosphate ophthalmic solution.** *USP 34.* (Various Mfr.) Dexamethasone sodium phosphate 0.1%, neomycin sulfate 0.35%. Bot. 5 mL.
Use: Anti-infective; corticosteroid, ophthalmic.

•**neomycin sulfate and fluocinolone acetonide cream.** *USP 34.*
Use: Anti-infective; corticosteroid, topical.

•**neomycin sulfate and fluorometholone ointment.** *USP 34.*
Use: Anti-infective; corticosteroid, topical.

•**neomycin sulfate and flurandrenolide cream.** *USP 34.*
Use: Anti-infective; corticosteroid, topical.

•**neomycin sulfate and gramicidin ointment.** *USP 34.*
Use: Anti-infective, topical.

•**neomycin sulfate and hydrocortisone.** *USP 34.* Cream; Ointment; Otic Suspension, USP.
Use: Anti-infective; corticosteroid, topical.

•**neomycin sulfate and hydrocortisone acetate.** *USP 34.* Cream; Lotion; Ointment; Ophthalmic Ointment; Ophthalmic Suspension, USP.
Use: Anti-infective; corticosteroid.

•**neomycin sulfate and methylprednisolone acetate cream.** *USP 34.*
Use: Anti-infective; corticosteroid, topical.

•**neomycin sulfate and prednisolone acetate ointment.** *USP 34.*
Use: Anti-infective; corticosteroid, topical.

•**neomycin sulfate and prednisolone acetate ophthalmic ointment.** *USP 34.*
Use: Anti-infective; corticosteroid, topical.

•**neomycin sulfate and prednisolone acetate ophthalmic suspension.** *USP 34.*
Use: Anti-infective; corticosteroid, topical.

•**neomycin sulfate and prednisolone sodium phosphate ophthalmic ointment.** *USP 34.*
Use: Anti-infective; corticosteroid, topical.

•**neomycin sulfate and triamcinolone acetonide cream.** *USP 34.*
Use: Anti-infective; corticosteroid, topical.

•**neomycin sulfate and triamcinolone acetonide ophthalmic ointment.** *USP 34.*
Use: Anti-infective; corticosteroid, ophthalmic.

neomycin sulfate, polymyxin B sulfate, and gramicidin solution. (Various Mfr.) Polymyxin B sulfate 10,000 units/mL, neomycin sulfate 1.75 mg/mL, gramicidin 0.025 mg/mL, sodium chloride, alcohol 0.5%, propylene glycol, hydrochloric acid, thimerosal 0.001%, poloxamer 188, ammonium hydroxide. Bot. 10 mL. *Rx.*
Use: Anti-infective, ophthalmic.

neomycin sulfate, polymyxin B sulfate, and lidocaine.
Use: Anti-infective; anesthetic, local.

•**neomycin sulfate, sulfacetamide sodium, and prednisolone acetate ophthalmic ointment.** *USP 34.*
Use: Anti-infective; corticosteroid, topical.

•**neomycin undecylenate.** (NEE-oh-MY-sin UHN-de-sih-LEN-ate) USAN.
Use: Anti-infective; antifungal.

Neopham 6.4%. (Pharmacia) Essential and nonessential amino acids 6.4%. Inj. 250 mL, 500 mL. *Rx.*
Use: Nutritional supplement, parenteral.

Neo Picatyl. (Sanofi-Synthelabo) Gly-

cobiarsoln. *Rx.*
Use: Amebicide.

NeoProfen. (Ovation) Ibuprofen lysine 17.1 mg (equiv. to ibuprofen 10 mg/mL [±]). Preservative free. Soln. for Inj. Single-use vials. *Rx.*
Use: Agent for patent ductus arteriousus.

Neo Quipenyl. (Sanofi-Synthelabo) Primaquine phosphate. *Rx.*
Use: Antimalarial.

Neoral. (Novartis) Cyclosporine. **Soft Gelatin Cap.:** 25 mg, 100 mg, dehydrated alcohol 11.9%. UD 30s. **Oral Soln.:** 100 mg/mL, dehydrated alcohol 11.9%. Bot. 50 mL. *Rx.*
Use: Immunosuppressant.

Neosalus. (Quinnova) **Aer., Foam.:** Dimethicone, glycerin, parabens. 70 g, 200 g. **Cream:** Dimethicone, glycerin, parabens, trolamine. 60 g, 100 g. *Rx.*
Use: Emollient.

neo-skiodan. Iodopyracet, Diodrast.

Neosol. (Breckenridge) L-hyoscyamine sulfate 0.125 mg, mint flavor. Orally Disintegrating Tab. 100s. *Rx.*
Use: Gastrointestinal anticholinergic/antispasmodic.

Neosporin AF. (Johnson & Johnson) Miconazole nitrate 2%. Mineral oil. Cream. 14 g. *OTC.*
Use: Anti-infective, topical; antifungal agent.

Neosporin AF. (Johnson & Johnson) Miconazole nitrate 2%. Alcohol. Spray Liq. 105 g. *OTC.*
Use: Anti-infective, topical; antifungal agent.

Neosporin G.U. Irrigant. (Monarch) Neomycin sulfate 40 mg, polymyxin B sulfate 200,000 units/mL. Amp. 1 mL. Box 10s, 50s, Multiple-dose vial 20 mL. *Rx.*
Use: Irrigant, genitourinary.

Neosporin Maximum Strength. (Johnson & Johnson) Polymyxin B sulfate 10,000 units, neomycin 3.5 mg, bacitracin 500 units/g, white petrolatum. Oint. Tube 15 g. *OTC.*
Use: Anti-infective, topical.

Neosporin Ophthalmic Solution. (Monarch) Polymyxin B sulfate 10,000 units, neomycin 1.75 mg, gramicidin 0.025 mg/mL, alcohol 0.5%, thimerosal 0.001%, propylene glycol, sodium chloride. Bot. 10 mL. *Drop-dose. Rx.*
Use: Anti-infective, ophthalmic.

Neosporin Original. (Johnson & Johnson) Polymyxin B sulfate 5000 units, neomycin 3.5 mg, bacitracin zinc 400 units per g. Cocoa butter, cottonseed oil, olive oil, white petrolatum. Oint. Tubes. 14 g, 28 g, UD 0.9 g (10s). *OTC.*
Use: Anti-infective, antibiotic, topical.

Neosporin Plus Pain Relief. (Johnson & Johnson) **Oint.:** Polymyxin B sulfate 10,000 units, neomycin 3.5 mg, bacitracin zinc 500 units, pramoxine hydrochloride 10 mg per g. White petrolatum. Tubes. 15 g, 30 g. **Cream:** Polymyxin B sulfate 10,000 units, neomycin 3.5 mg, pramoxine hydrochloride 10 mg per g. Methylparaben, mineral oil, white petrolatum. Tubes. 15 g. *OTC.*
Use: Anti-infective, antibiotic, topical.

neostibosan. Ethylstibamine.

neostigmine.
Use: Cholinergic.
See: Neostigmine Bromide.
Neostigmine Methylsulfate.
Prostigmin.

neostigmine and atropine sulfate.
Use: Muscle stimulant.
See: Neostigmine Min-I-Mix.

•**neostigmine bromide.** (nee-oh-STIGG-meen) *USP 34.*
Use: Cholinergic.
See: Prostigmin Bromide.

neostigmine bromide. (Lannett) Neostigmine bromide. 15 mg. Tab. 100s and 1000s.
Use: Cholinergic.

•**neostigmine methylsulfate.** (nee-oh-STIGG-meen METH-ill-SULL-fate) *USP 34.*
Use: Cholinergic.
See: Prostigmin.

neostigmine methylsulfate. (Various Mfr.) Neostigmine methylsulfate 1:2000 (0.5 mg/mL), 1:1000 (1 mg/mL). Inj. Vials. 1 mL, 2 mL, 10 mL (1:2000 only). Multidose vials. 10 mL. *Rx.*
Use: Cholinergic; urinary cholinergic.

Neostigmine Min-I-Mix. (I.M.S., Ltd.) Atropine sulfate 1.2 mg, neostigmine methylsulfate 2.5 mg. Inj. Vial. *Rx.*
Use: Cholinergic muscle stimulant.

Neo-Strepsan.
See: Sulfathiazole.

Neo-Synephrine. (Hospira) Phenylephrine hydrochloride 1% (10 mg/mL). Sodium bisulfite. Inj. Uni-Nest amps. 1 mL. *Rx.*
Use: Mydriatic; vasopressor.

Neo-Synephrine Extra Strength. (Bayer Consumer Care) Phenylephrine hydrochloride 1%, benzalkonium chloride. Drop. bot., Spray bot. 15 mL. *Formerly Neo-Synephrine 4-Hour Extra Strength. OTC.*
Use: Nasal decongestant, arylalkylamine.

Neo-Synephrine Mild Strength. (Bayer Consumer Care) Phenylephrine hydrochloride 0.25%, benzalkonium chloride. Soln. Spray bot. 15 mL. *Formerly Neo-Synephrine 4-Hour Mild Formula. OTC.*
Use: Nasal decongestant, arylalkylamine.

Neo-Synephrine Regular Strength. (Bayer Consumer Care) Phenylephrine hydrochloride 0.5%, benzalkonium chloride. Soln. Spray bot., Drop. bot. 15 mL. *Formerly Neo-Synephrine 4-Hour Regular Formula. OTC.*
Use: Nasal decongestant, arylalkylamine.

Neo-Synephrine Hydrochloride. (Sanofi-Synthelabo) Phenylephrine hydrochloride. **Spray:** 0.25% children and adult, 0.5% adult. **Regular:** Squeeze bot. 0.5 oz. **0.5% mentholated:** Squeeze bot. 0.5 oz. **Drops:** 0.125% infant; 0.25% children and adult; 0.5% adult; 1% adult extra strength. Bot. 1 oz; 0.25% and 1%, also bot. 16 oz. **Jelly:** 0.5%. Tube. 18.75 g. *OTC.*
Use: Decongestant.

Neo-Synephrine 12-Hour Extra Moisturizing. (Bayer Consumer Care) Oxymetazoline hydrochloride 0.05%, benzalkonium chloride, edetate sodium, sodium chloride. Soln. Spray Bot. 15 mL. *OTC.*
Use: Nasal decongestant, imidazoline.

Neo-Tabs. (Pharma-Tek) Neomycin sulfate 500 mg (equivalent to 350 mg neomycin base). Tab. Bot. 100s. *Rx.*
Use: Amebicide.

Neotal. (Roberts) Zinc bacitracin 400 units, polymyxin B sulfate 5000 units, neomycin sulfate 5 mg, petrolatum and mineral oil base/g. Tube 3.5 g. *Rx.*
Use: Anti-infective, ophthalmic.

Neo-Thrycex. (Del) Bacitracin, neomycin sulfate, polymyxin B sulfate. Oint. Tube 0.5 oz. *Rx.*
Use: Anti-infective, topical.

Neotic. (Arbor) Benzocaine 1%, antipyrine 5.4%, glycerin 2%, zinc acetate dehydrate 1%. Drops; otic. 10 mL w/ dropper. *Rx.*
Use: Miscellaneous otic preparation.

Neotricin HC. (Bausch & Lomb) Hydrocortisone acetate 1%, neomycin sulfate 0.35%, bacitracin zinc 400 units, polymyxin B sulfate 10,000 units. Oint. Tube 3.5 g. *Rx.*
Use: Anti-infective; corticosteroid, ophthalmic.

Neotricin Ophthalmic Ointment. (Bausch & Lomb) Polymyxin B sulfate 10,000 units, neomycin sulfate 3.5 mg, bacitracin 400 units/g. In 3.5 g. *Rx.*
Use: Anti-infective, ophthalmic.

Neotricin Ophthalmic Solution. (Bausch & Lomb) Polymyxin B sulfate 10,000 units, neomycin sulfate 1.75 mg, gramicidin 0.025 mg/mL. Dropper bot. 10 mL. *Rx.*
Use: Anti-infective, ophthalmic.

Neo-Trobex Injection. (Forest) Vitamins B_1 150 mg, B_6 10 mg, riboflavin 5-phosphate sodium 2 mg, niacinamide 150 mg, panthenol 10 mg, choline Cl 20 mg, inositol 20 mg/mL. Vial 30 mL. *Rx.*
Use: Vitamin supplement.

Neotrol. (Horizon) Phenylephrine hydrochloride 0.25%, pyrilamine maleate 0.2%, cetalkonium Cl 0.05%, tyrothricin 0.03%, phenylmercuric acetate 1:50,000. Soln. Squeeze Bot. 20 mL. *OTC.*
Use: Antihistamine; decongestant.

NeoTuss. (A.G. Marin Pharmaceuticals) Dextromethorphan hydrobromide 30 mg, guaifenesin 200 mg. Glycerin, menthol, parabens, propylene glycol, sorbitol, sucralose. Alcohol free, dye free, and sugar free. Grape menthol flavor. Liq. 473 mL. *OTC.*
Use: Upper respiratory combination, antitussive with expectorant.

NeoTuss-D. (A.G. Marin Pharmaceuticals) Dextromethorphan hydrobromide 30 mg, guaifenesin 200 mg, phenylephrine hydrochloride 7.5 mg. Glycerin, parabens, propylene glycol, sucralose. Alcohol free, dye free, and sugar free. Raspberry flavor. Liq. 474 mL. *Rx.*
Use: Upper respiratory combination, antitussive and expectorant combination.

Neoval. (Halsey Drug) Vitamins A 10,000 units, D 400 units, B_1 10 mg, B_2 5 mg, B_6 2 mg, B_{12} 3 mcg, C 100 mg, E 5 mg, pantothenic acid 10 mg, niacinamide 30 mg, Fe 15 mg, Cu 1 mg, Mg 5 mg, Mn 1 mg, Zn 1.5 mg, I 0.15 mg. Tab. Bot. 100s. *OTC.*
Use: Mineral, vitamin supplement.

Neoval T. (Halsey Drug) Vitamins A 10,000 units, D 400 units, B_1 15 mg, B_2 10 mg, B_6 2 mg, C 150 mg, B_{12} 7.5 mcg, E 5 mg, pantothenic acid 10 mg, E 5 mg, niacinamide 100 mg, Fe 15 mg, Mg 5 mg, Mn 1 mg, Zn 1.5 mg, Cu 1 mg. Tab. Bot. 1000s. *OTC.*
Use: Mineral, vitamin supplement.

•**nepafenac.** (neh-pah-FEN-ack) USAN.
Use: Ophthalmic nonsteroidal anti-
inflammatory agent.
See: Nevanac.

NephPlex Rx. (Nephro-Tech) B_1 1.5 mg,
B_2 1.7 mg, B_3 20 mg, B_5 10 mg, B_6
10 mg, B_{12} 6 mcg, C 60 mg, folic acid
1 mg, biotin 300 mcg, Zn 12.5 mg. Tab.
Bot. 100s. *Rx.*
Use: Mineral, vitamin supplement.

5.4% NephrAmine. (McGaw) Amino acid
concentration 5.4%, nitrogen 0.65 g/
100 mL. **Essential amino acids:** Isoleucine 560 mg, leucine 880 mg, lysine
640 mg, methionine 880 mg, phenylalanine 880 mg, threonine 400 mg, tryptophan 200 mg, valine 640 mg, histidine 250 mg/100 mL. **Nonessential
amino acids:** Cysteine < 20 mg/
100 mL, sodium 5 mEq, acetate
44 mEq, chloride 3 mEq/L, sodium bisulfite. Inj. 250 mL. *Rx.*
Use: Nutritional supplement, parenteral.

nephridine.
See: Epinephrine.

Nephro-Calci. (Watson) Calcium carbonate 1500 mg (elemental calcium
600 mg). Tab. Bot. 100s. *OTC.*
Use: Mineral supplement, calcium.

Nephrocaps. (Fleming & Co.) Vitamins
B_1 1.5 mg, B_2 1.7 mg, B_3 20 mg, B_5
5 mg, B_6 10 mg, B_{12} 6 mcg, C 100 mg,
folic acid 1 mg, biotin 150 mcg. Cap.
Bot. 100s. *Rx.*
Use: Vitamin supplement.

Nephronex. (Llorens) Biotin 300 mcg, folic acid 0.9 mg, vitamins B_1 1.5 mg, B_2
1.7 mg, B_3 20 mg, B_5 10 mg, B_6
10 mg, B_{12} 10 mcg, C 60 mg per 5 mL.
Aspartame, parabens, phenylalanine.
Alcohol free, dye free, and sugar free.
Liq. 236.5 mL. *OTC.*
Use: Nutritional supplement, multivitamin.

Nephron FA. (Nephro-Tech) Fe 66.6 mg,
C 40 mg, B_1 1.5 mg, B_2 1.7 mg, B_3
20 mg, B_5 10 mg, B_6 10 mg, B_{12} 6 mcg,
biotin 300 mcg, FA 1 mg, docusate sodium 75 mg. Tab. Bot. 100s. *Rx.*
Use: Mineral, vitamin supplement.

Nephro-Vite Rx. (R & D Laboratories,
Inc.) Vitamins B_1 1.5 mg, B_2 1.7 mg,
B_3 20 mg, B_5 10 mg, B_6 10 mg, B_{12}
6 mcg, C 60 mg, folic acid 1 mg, d-
biotin 300 mcg. Tab. Bot. 100s. *Rx.*
Use: Mineral, vitamin supplement.

**Nephro-Vite Vitamin B Complex & C
Supplement.** (R & D Laboratories,
Inc.) Vitamins B_1 1.5 mg, B_2 1.7 mg,
B_3 20 mg, B_5 10 mg, B_6 10 mg, B_{12}
6 mcg, C 60 mg, folic acid 800 mcg,

biotin 300 mcg. Tab. Bot. 100s. *OTC.*
Use: Mineral, vitamin supplement.

Nephrox. (Fleming & Co.) Aluminum
hydroxide 320 mg, mineral oil 10%/
5 mL. Bot. Pt. *OTC.*
Use: Antacid.

Nepro. (Ross) Protein 6.6 g (as Ca, Mg,
and Na caseinates), fat 22.7 g (as 90%
high-oleic safflower oil, 10% soy oil),
carbohydrate 51.1 g (as sucrose, hydrolyzed corn starch), vitamins A, D, E, K,
C, B_1, B_2, B_5, B_6, B_{12}, biotin, FA, Na,
K, Cl, Ca, P, Mg, I, Mn, Cu, Zn, Fe, Se/
240 mL. 59.4 calories. Liq. Can.
240 mL. *OTC.*
Use: Nutritional supplement, enteral.

•**neramexane mesylate.** (ner-a-MEX-ane)
USAN.
Use: Depression; Alzheimer disease;
pain.

neraval.
Use: Anesthetic, general.

•**nerelimomab.** (neh-reh-LI-moe-mab)
USAN.
Use: Monoclonal antibody.

Nervine Nighttime Sleep-Aid. (Bayer
Consumer Care) Diphenhydramine
hydrochloride 25 mg. Tab. Bot. 12s,
30s, 50s. *OTC.*
Use: Sleep aid.

Nesacaine. (AAP Pharmaceuticals)
Chloroprocaine hydrochloride 1%, 2%,
methylparaben, EDTA. Inj. Multidose
vial. 30 mL. *Rx.*
Use: Anesthetic, local injectable.

Nesacaine-MPF. (AAP Pharmaceuticals)
Chloroprocaine hydrochloride 2%, 3%,
preservative free. Inj. Single-dose vials. 20 mL. *Rx.*
Use: Anesthetic, local injectable.

Nesa Nine Cap. (Standex) Vitamins A
5000 units, D 400 units, C 37.5 mg,
B_1 1.5 mg, B_2 2 mg, niacinamide 20 mg,
B_6 0.1 mg, calcium pantothenate 1 mg,
E 2 units. Cap. Bot. 100s. *OTC.*
Use: Mineral, vitamin supplement.

nesdonal sodium.
See: Pentothal.
Thiopental Sodium.

•**nesiritide.** (ni-SIR-i-tide) USAN.
Use: Vasodilator, human B-type natri-
uretic peptide.
See: Natrecor.

•**nesiritide citrate.** (ni-SIR-i-tide) USAN.
Use: Treatment of congestive heart
failure.

Nestabs. (Fielding) See Vitelle Nestabs.

Nestabs CBF. (Fielding) Vitamins A
4000 units, D 400 units, E 30 units, C
120 mg, folic acid 1 mg, B_1 3 mg, B_2

3 mg, niacinamide 20 mg, B_6 3 mg, B_{12} 8 mcg, Ca 200 mg, I, Zn 15 mg, Fe 50 mg. Tab. Bot. 100s. *Rx.*
Use: Mineral, vitamin supplement.

Nestabs FA. (Fielding) Vitamins A 4000 units, D 400 units, E 30 units, C 120 mg, B_1 3 mg, B_2 3 mg, B_3 20 mg, B_6 3 mg, B_{12} 8 mcg, Ca 200 mg, Fe 29 mg, folic acid 1 mg, Zn 15 mg, I. Tab. Bot. 100s. *Rx.*
Use: Mineral, vitamin supplement.

Nestle VHC 2.25. (Nestle Clinical Nutrition) Protein 90 g, carbohydrate 196 g, fat 120 g, vitamins A, B_1, B_2, B_3, B_5, B_6, B_{12}, C, D, E, K, folic acid, biotin, chloride, choline, Ca, Cr, Cu, Fe, I, Mg, Mn, Mo, P, Se, Zn, Na 1200 mg, K 1732 mg/L. Liq. Can. 250 mL. *OTC.*
Use: Enteral nutrition.

•**netilmicin sulfate.** (ne-til-MYE-sin) USAN.

•**netoglitazone.** (net-oh-GLIT-a-zone) USAN.
Use: Antidiabetic.

•**netrafilcon a.** (NET-rah-FILL-kahn A) USAN.
Use: Contact lens material, hydrophilic.
netrin. Under Study.
Use: Anticholinergic.
See: Metacaraphen Hydrochloride.

•**netupitant.** (net-UE-pi-tant) USAN.
Use: Antiemetic.

Neulasta. (Amgen) Pegfilgrastim 10 mg/mL, preservative free. Soln. for Inj. Dispensing pack containing single-dose syr. w/needle. *Rx.*
Use: Hematopoietic, colony stimulating factor.

Neumega. (Wyeth) Oprelvekin 5 mg. Dibasic sodium phosphate heptahydrate 1.6 mg, monobasic sodium phosphate monohydrate 0.55 mg. Preservative free. Pow. for Inj. Soln., lyophilized. Single-dose vial with diluent. *Rx.*
Use: Hematopoietic, interleukin.

Neupogen. (Amgen) Filgrastim (G-CSF). Inj. **300 mcg/0.5 mL:** Acetate 0.295 mg, sorbitol 25 mg, 0.004% Tween 80, 0.0175 mg Na/0.5 mL. Preservative free. Inj. Prefilled syringe. 0.5 mL, 0.8 mL. **300 mcg/mL:** Acetate 0.59 mg, sorbitol 50 mg, 0.004% Tween 80, 0.035 mg Na/mL. Preservative free. Single-dose vial. 1 mL, 1.6 mL. *Rx.*
Use: Immunomodulator.

NeuRecover-DA. (NeuroGenesis) DL-phenylalanine 460 mg, L-glutamine 25 mg, vitamin A 333.3 units, B_1 1.65 mg, B_2 0.85 mg, B_3 33 mg, B_5 15 mg, B_6 3 mg, B_{12} 5 mcg, FA

0.065 mg, C 100 mg, E 5 units, biotin 0.05 mg, Ca 25 mg, Cr 0.01 mg, Fe 1.5 mg, Mg 25 mg, Zn 2.5 mg. Cap. Bot. 180s. *OTC.*
Use: Amino acid.

NeuRecover-SA. (NeuroGenesis) DL-phenylalanine 250 mg, L-tyrosine 150 mg, L-glutamine 50 mg, vitamins B_1 1.65 mg, B_2 2.5 mg, B_3 16.6 mg, B_5 15 mg, B_6 3.36 mg, B_{12} 5 mcg, FA 0.067 mg, C 100 mg, Ca 25 mg, Fe 1.5 mg, Mg 25 mg, Zn 5 mg. Cap. Bot. 180s. *OTC.*
Use: Amino acid.

Neurodep-Caps. (Medical Products Panamericana) Vitamins B_1 125 mg, B_6 125 mg, B_{12} 1000 mcg. Cap. Bot. 50s. *OTC.*
Use: Vitamin supplement.

Neurodep Injection. (Medical Products Panamericana) Vitamins B_1 50 mg, B_2 5 mg, B_3 125 mg, B_5 6 mg, B_6 5 mg, B_{12} 1000 mcg, C 50 mg/mL. Inj. Vial 10 mL. *Rx.*
Use: Vitamin supplement, parenteral.

neuromuscular blockers, nondepolarizing.
Use: Muscle relaxants; adjuncts to anesthesia.
See: Mivacurium Chloride.
Pancuronium Bromide.
Rocuronium Bromide.

Neurontin. (Pfizer) Gabapentin. **Cap.:** 100 mg, 300 mg, 400 mg, lactose, talc. Bot. 100s, UD 50s. **Tab.:** 600 mg, 800 mg, talc. Bot. 100s, 500s, UD 50s. **Oral Soln.:** 250 mg/5 mL, xylitol, cool strawberry anise flavor. Bot. 480 mL. *Rx.*
Use: Anticonvulsant.

neurosin.
See: Calcium Glycerophosphate.

NeuroSlim. (NeuroGenesis) DL-phenylalanine 500 mg, L-glutamine 15 mg, L-tyrosine 25 mg, L-carnitine 10 mg, L-arginine pyroglutamate 10 mg, ornithine aspartate 10 mg, Cr 0.033 mg, Se 0.012 mg, vitamins B_1 0.33 mg, B_2 0.5 mg, B_3 3.3 mg, B_5 0.012 mg, B_6 0.333 mg, B_{12} 1 mcg, E 5 units, biotin 0.05 mg, FA 0.066 mg, Fe 1 mg, Zn 2.5 mg, Ca 35 mg, I 0.025 mg, Cu 0.33 mg, Mg 25 mg. Cap. Bot. 180s. *OTC.*
Use: Amino acid.

neurotrophin-1.
Use: Motor neuron disease/amyotrophic lateral sclerosis. [Orphan Drug]

Neut. (Abbott) Sodium bicarbonate 4%. Vial (2.4 mEq each of sodium and bicarbonate), disodium edetate anhy-

drous 0.05% as stabilizer. Pintop Vial 5 mL, 10 mL. Box 25s, 100s. *Rx.*
Use: Nutritional supplement, parenteral.

NeutraGuard Advanced. (Pascal) Fluoride sodium 1.1%, wintermint flavor. Dental Gel. 60 g. *Rx.*
Use: Prevention of dental caries.

Neutrahist. (Cypress Pharmaceuticals) Chlorpheniramine maleate 0.8 mg, pseudoephedrine hydrochloride 9 mg per 5 mL. Saccharin, sorbitol. Cherry flavor. Drops. 30 mL w/dropper. *Rx.*
Use: Upper respiratory combination, decongestant and antihistamine.

Neutrahist PDX. (Cypress) Dextromethorphan hydrobromide 3 mg, chlorpheniramine maleate 0.8 mg, pseudoephedrine hydrochloride 9 mg. Glycerin, propylene glycol, saccharin, sorbitol. Alcohol free and sugar free. Grape flavor. Drops. 30 mL w/dropper. *OTC.*
Use: Upper respiratory combination, antitussive combination.

neutral acriflavine.
See: Acriflavine.

Neutralin. (Dover Pharmaceuticals) Calcium carbonate, magnesium oxide. Tab. Sugar, lactose, and salt free. UD Box 500s. *OTC.*
Use: Antacid.

neutral protamine hagedorn-insulin.
See: Insulin.
N.P.H. Iletin II.

•**neutramycin.** (NEW-trah-MY-sin) USAN. A neutral macrolide antibiotic produced by a variant strain of *Streptomyces rimosus.*
Use: Anti-infective.

NeutraSal. (Invado Pharmaceuticals) Calcium chloride 50 mg, dibasic sodium phosphate 10 mg, monobasic sodium phosphate 10 mg, silicon dioxide 2 mg, sodium chloride 450 mg, sodium bicarbonate 16 mg. Pow. 30s, 120s. *OTC.*
Use: Saliva substitute.

neutroflavin.
See: Acriflavine.

Neutrogena Antiseptic Cleanser for Acne-Prone Skin. (Neutrogena) Benzethonium Cl, butylene glycol, methylparaben, menthol, peppermint oil, eucalyptus, mint, rosemary oils, witch hazel extract, camphor. Liq. Bot. 135 mL. *OTC.*
Use: Dermatologic, acne.

Neutrogena Body Lotion. (Neutrogena) Glyceryl stearate, isopropyl myristate, PEG-100 stearate, butylene glycol, imidazolidinyl urea, carbomer 934, parabens, sodium lauryl sulfate, triethanolamine, cetyl alcohol. Lot. Bot. 240 mL.

OTC.
Use: Emollient.

Neutrogena Body Oil. (Neutrogena) Isopropyl myristate, sesame oil, PEG-40 sorbitan peroleate, parabens. Bot. 240 mL. *OTC.*
Use: Emollient.

Neutrogena Chemical-Free Sunblocker. (Neutrogena) Titanium dioxide, parabens, diazolidinyl urea, shea butter. SPF 17. Lot. Bot. 120 mL. *OTC.*
Use: Sunscreen.

Neutrogena Cleansing for Acne-Prone Skin. (Neutrogena) TEA-stearate, triethanolamine, glycerin, sodium tallowate, sodium cocoate, TEA-oleate, sodium ricinoleate, acetylated lanolin alcohol, cocamide DEA, TEA lauryl sulfate, tocopherol. Bar 105 g. *OTC.*
Use: Dermatologic, cleanser.

Neutrogena Clear Pore. (Neutrogena) Benzoyl peroxide 3.5%, glycerin, titanium dioxide, EDTA, menthol. Cleanser/mask. 125 mL. *OTC.*
Use: Dermatologic, acne.

Neutrogena Drying. (Neutrogena) Witch hazel, isopropyl alcohol, EDTA, parabens, tartrazine. Gel. Tube 22.5 mL. *OTC.*
Use: Dermatologic, acne.

Neutrogena Dry Skin Soap. (Neutrogena) Triethanolamine, stearic acid, tallow, glycerin, coconut oil, castor oil, sodium hydroxide, oleic acid, laneth-10 acetate, cocamide DEA, nonoxynol-14, PEG-14 octoate, BHT, O-tolyl biguanide. Bar 105 g, 165 g. Scented or unscented. *OTC.*
Use: Dermatologic, cleanser.

Neutrogena Glow Sunless Tanning. (Neutrogena) Octyl methoxycinnamate, cetyl alcohol, diazolidinyl urea, parabens, EDTA. SPF 8. Lot. Bot. 120 mL. *OTC.*
Use: Sunscreen.

Neutrogena Intensified Day Moisture. (Neutrogena) Octyl methoxycinnamate, 2-phenylbenzimidazole sulfonic acid, titanium dioxide, cetyl alcohol, diazolidinyl urea, parabens, EDTA. SPF 15. Cream 67.5 g. *OTC.*
Use: Dermatologic, moisturizer.

Neutrogena Lip Moisturizer. (Neutrogena) Octyl methoxycinnamate, benzophenone-3, corn oil, castor oil, mineral oil, lanolin oil, petrolatum, lanolin, stearyl alcohol. SPF 15. Lip balm 4.5 g. *OTC.*
Use: Lip protectant.

Neutrogena Moisture SPF 15. (Neutrogena) Octyl methoxycinnamate, benzo-

phenone-3, glycerin, PEG-100 stearate, dimethicone, PEG-6000 monostearate, triethanolamine, parabens, imidazolidinyl urea, carbomer 954, PABA free. Lot. Bot. 120 mL. *OTC.*
Use: Sunscreen.

Neutrogena Moisture SPF 5. (Neutrogena) Octyl methoxycinnamate, petrolatum, cetyl alcohol, parabens, diazolidinyl urea, EDTA, cetyl alcohol. Lot. Bot 60 mL, 120 mL. *OTC.*
Use: Dermatologic, moisturizer.

Neutrogena Non-Drying Cleansing. (Neutrogena) Glycerin, caprylic/capric triglyceride, PEG-20 almond glycerides, cetyl ricinoleate, isohexadecane, TEA-cocoyl glutamate, PEG-20 methyl glucose sesquistearate, stearyl alcohol, cetyl alcohol, EDTA, dipotassium glycyrrhizate, stearyl glycyrrhetinate, bisabolol, parabens, acrylates/C 10-30 alkyl acrylate crosspolymer, triethanolamine, diazolidinyl urea. Lot. Bot. 165 mL. *OTC.*
Use: Dermatologic, cleanser.

Neutrogena Norwegian Formula Emulsion. (Neutrogena) Glycerin base 2%. Pump dispenser 5.25 oz. *OTC.*
Use: Emollient.

Neutrogena Norwegian Formula Hand Cream. (Neutrogena) Glycerin base 41%. Tube 2 oz. *OTC.*
Use: Emollient.

Neutrogena No-Stick Sunscreen. (Neutrogena) SPF 30. Homosalate 15%, octyl methoxycinnamate 7.5%, benzophenone-36%, octyl salicylate 5%, EDTA, parabens, diazolidinyl urea/ Cream. Waterproof 118 g. *OTC.*
Use: Sunscreen.

Neutrogena Oil-Free Acne Wash. (Neutrogena) Salicylic acid 2%, EDTA, propylene glycol, tartrazine, aloe extract. Liq. Bot. 180 mL. *OTC.*
Use: Dermatologic, acne.

Neutrogena Oily Skin Formula Soap. (Neutrogena) Triethanolamine, glycerin, fatty acids. Bar 3.5 oz. *OTC.*
Use: Dermatologic, cleanser.

Neutrogena Original Formula Soap. (Neutrogena) Triethanolamine, glycerin, fatty acids. Bar 3.5 oz, 5.5 oz. *OTC.*
Use: Dermatologic, cleanser.

Neutrogena Soap. (Neutrogena) TEA-stearate, triethanolamine, glycerin, sodium tallowate, sodium cocoate, sodium ricinoleate, TEA-oleate, cocamide DEA, tocopherol. Bar 105 g, 165 g. *OTC.*
Use: Dermatologic, cleanser.

Neutrogena Sunblock. (Neutrogena)

SPF 8: Octyl methoxycinnamate, menthyl anthranilate, titanium dioxide, mineral oil. Cream 67.5 g. **SPF 15:** Octyl methoxycinnamate, octyl salicylate, menthyl anthranilate, mineral oil, titanium dioxide, propylparaben. Cream 67.5 g. **SPF 25:** Octyl methoxycinnamate, benzophenone-3, octyl salicylate, castor oil, cetearyl alcohol, propylparaben, shea butter. Stick 12.6 g. **SPF 30:** Octocrylene, octyl methoxycinnamate, menthyl anthranilate, zinc oxide, mineral oil, vitamin E. Cream 67.5 g. *OTC.*
Use: Sunscreen.

Neutrogena Sunscreen. (Neutrogena) Ethylhexyl p-methoxycinnamate 7%, oxybenzone 4%, titanium dioxide 2%. Tube 3 oz. *OTC.*
Use: Sunscreen.

Neutrogena T/Gel Original. (Neutrogena Corp) Coal tar extract 2%. Shampoo. Bot. 132 mL, 255 mL, 480 mL. *OTC.*
Use: Dermatologic.

Neutrogena T/Sal. (Neutrogena) Salicylic acid 2%, solubilized coal tar extract 2%. Shampoo. Bot. 135 mL. *OTC.*
Use: Antiseborrheic.

Neutrogena Ultra Sheer Dry-Touch Sunblock. (Neutrogena) Avobenzone 3%, homosalate 15%, octisalate 5%, octocrylene 2.8%, oxybenzone 6%. EDTA, glyceryl, PEG 100. SPF 70. Lot. 88 mL. *OTC.*
Use: Sunscreen.

Nevanac. (Alcon) Nepafenac 0.1%. Benzalkonium chloride 0.005%, EDTA, sodium chloride, tyloxapol, sodium hydroxide, hydrochloric acid. Ophth. Susp. Bot. 3 mL with dropper. *Rx.*
Use: Ophthalmic nonsteroidal anti-inflammatory drug.

•**nevirapine.** (neh-VIE-rah-peen) *USP 34.*
Use: Antiviral.
See: Viramune.

Nexavar. (Bayer) Sorafenib 200 mg (equiv. to sorafenib tosylate 274 mg). Polyethylene glycol. Film-coated. Tab. 120s. *Rx.*
Tall Man: NexAVAR
Use: Multikinase inhibitor.

•**nexeridine hydrochloride.** (NEX-eh-RIH-deen) *USAN.*
Use: Analgesic.

Nexiclon XR. (Nextwave Pharmaceuticals) Clonidine hydrochloride 0.09 mg/mL. Corn syrup, glycerin, parabens, polysorbate 80, sucrose. ER Susp. 118 mL. *Rx.*
Use: Antiadrenergic/sympatholytic; antiadrenergic agent, centrally acting.

Nexium. (AstraZeneca) Esomeprazole.

DR Cap.: 20 mg, 40 mg. Sugar spheres. Enteric-coated Gran. Bot. 90s, 1000s, unit-of-use 30s, UD 100s.
DR Pow. for Susp.: 10 mg, 20 mg, 40 mg. Dextrose. Contains enteric-coated granules. Unit-dose packets. 30s. *Rx.*
Tall Man: NexIUM
Use: Proton pump inhibitor.
Nexium I.V. (AstraZeneca) Esomeprazole 20 mg, 40 mg. EDTA. Inj., Pow. or Cake for Soln. Single-use vials. 10s. *Rx.*
Tall Man: NexIUM
Use: Proton pump inhibitor.
Next Choice. (Watson Laboratories) Levonorgestrel 0.75 mg. Lactose. Tab. UD 2s. *OTC.*
Use: Emergency contraceptive.
Nexterone. (Prism Pharmaceuticals) Amiodarone hydrochloride. **Inj., Soln.: 50 mg/mL:** 3 mL, 10 mL, 30 mL single-dose vials; 3 mL prefilled syringe.
1.5 mg/mL and 1.8 mg/mL: Premixed in dextrose. Single-dose *Galaxy* containers. 100 mL, 200 mL. *Rx.*
Use: Cardiovascular agent, antiarrhythmic agent.
N.G.T. (Geneva) Triamcinolone acetonide 0.1%, nystatin 100,000 units/g. Cream. Tube 15 g. *Rx.*
Use: Antifungal; corticosteroid, topical.
NG-29.
Use: Diagnostic aid. [Orphan Drug]
Niacal. (Jones Pharma) Calcium lactate 324 mg, niacin 25 mg. Tab. Peppermint flavor. Bot. 100s, 1000s. *OTC.*
Use: Vasodilator; vitamin supplement.
•**niacin.** (NYE-uh-sin) *USP 34.*
Use: Antihyperlipidemic; vitamin, enzyme co-factor.
See: Niacal.
Niacin Flush-Free.
Niacin No Flush.
Niacor.
Niaspan.
Ni Cord XL.
Nicotinic Acid.
Slo-Niacin.
W/Combinations.
See: Lipo-Nicin.
Niacin Flush-Free. (Mason) Niacin 750 mg. Inositol 211.5 mg. Preservative free and sugar free. Cap. 50s. *OTC.*
Use: Water-soluble vitamin.
niacin/lovastatin.
Use: Antihyperlipidemic.
See: Advicor.
Niacin No Flush. (Windmill) Niacin 100 mg, 250 mg. Preservative free and sugar free. Tab. 60s. *OTC.*

Use: Water-soluble vitamin.
niacin/simvastatin.
Use: Antihyperlipidemic.
See: Simcor.
•**niacinamide.** (nye-ah-SIN-ah-mide) *USP 34.*
Use: Vitamin, enzyme co-factor.
niacinamide (nicotinamide). (Various Mfr.) Niacinamide (nicotinamide) 100 mg, 500 mg. Tab. Bot. 100s, 250s. *Rx-OTC.*
Use: Water-soluble vitamin.
Niacor. (Upsher-Smith) Niacin 500 mg. Lactose. Tab. Bot. 100s. *Rx.*
Use: Water-soluble vitamin.
Nialexo-C. (Roberts) Niacin 50 mg, vitamin C 30 mg. Tab. Bot. 100s. *OTC.*
Use: Vitamin supplement.
Niarb Super. (Miller Pharmacal Group) Magnesium 100 mg, vitamin C 200 mg, niacinamide 200 mg (as ascorbate). Tab. Bot. 100s. *OTC.*
Use: Mineral, vitamin supplement.
Niaspan. (Abbott) Niacin 500 mg, 750 mg, 1000 mg. ER Tab. Bot. 100s. *Rx.*
Use: Water-soluble vitamin.
Niazide. (Major) Trichlormethiazide 4 mg. Tab. Bot. 100s, 1000s. *Rx.*
Use: Diuretic.
niazo. Neotropin.
Use: Antiseptic, urinary.
•**nibroxane.** (nye-BROX-ane) USAN.
Use: Antimicrobial, topical.
nicamindon.
See: Nicotinamide.
•**nicardipine hydrochloride.** (NYE-CAR-dih-peen) USAN.
Tall Man: niCARdipine
Use: Calcium channel blocker.
See: Cardene IV.
Cardene SR.
nicardipine hydrochloride. (Teva) Nicardipine hydrochloride 2.5 mg/mL. Inj., Soln. Single-use vial. 10 mL. *Rx.*
Use: Cardiovascular agent, calcium channel blocking agent.
nicardipine hydrochloride. (Various Mfr.) Nicardipine hydrochloride 20 mg, 30 mg. Cap. Bot. 90s, 500s. *Rx.*
Use: Calcium channel blocker.
N'ICE. (Insight Pharmaceuticals) Menthol 5 mg. Sugar free. Assorted, cherry, menthol, orange, citrus, and honey lemon flavors. Loz. 24s. *OTC.*
Use: Anesthetic, local; cough suppressant.
N'ice 'n Clear. (GlaxoSmithKline) Menthol 5 mg, sorbitol. Loz. Pkg. 16s. *OTC.*
Use: Anesthetic, local.
•**nicergoline.** (nice-ERR-go-leen) USAN.
Use: Vasodilator.

Nichols Syphon Powder. (Last) Sodium bicarbonate, sodium Cl, sodium borate. Pouch 12.2 g (add to 32 oz. water to yield isotonic soln.).

•**niclosamide.** (nye-CLOSE-ah-mide) USAN.
Use: Anthelmintic.

nicobion.
See: Nicotinamide.

NicoDerm CQ. (GlaxoSmithKline Consumer) Nicotine 7 mg, 14 mg, 21 mg/day (dose absorbed in 24 hours). Transdermal system. Box 7s (21 mg only), 14s, original and clear patches. *OTC.*
Use: Smoking deterrent.

nicoduozide. A mixture of nicothazone and isoniazid.

•**nicorandil.** (NIH-CAR-an-dill) USAN.
Use: Coronary vasodilator.

Ni Cord XL Caps. (Scot-Tussin) Nicotinic acid 400 mg. Cap. Bot. 100s, 500s. *OTC.*
Use: Vitamin supplement.

Nicorette. (GlaxoSmithKline Consumer) Nicotine polacrilex. **Chewing gum:** 2 mg, 4 mg/square; orange, mint, and original flavors. Chewing gum. Box 48, 108, 168 pieces. **Lozenge:** 2 mg, 4 mg. Aspartame, mannitol, phenylalanine 3.4 mg. 72s. *OTC.*
Use: Smoking deterrent.

nicotamide.
See: Nicotinamide.

nicothazone. Nicotinal dehydethiose micarbazone.

nicotilamide.
See: Nicotinamide.

nicotinamide. Niacinamide, USP. Vitamin B_3, aminicotin, dipegyl, nicamindon, nicotamide, nicotilamide, nicotinic acid amide.

nicotinamide adenine dinucleotide.
Name used for Nadide.

nicotinamide with zinc-copper and folic acid. (Brookstone Pharmaceuticals) Nicotinamide 750 mg, zinc oxide 25 mg, cupric oxide 1.5 mg, folic acid 500 mcg. Tab. 60s. *Rx.*
Use: Multivitamin, mineral combination.

•**nicotine.** (NIK-oh-teen) USP 34.
Use: Smoking cessation adjunct.
See: Nicotine Inhalation System.
  Nicotine Nasal Spray.
  Nicotine Polacrilex.
  Nicotine Transdermal System.

nicotine gum. (Various Mfr.) Nicotine polacrilex 2 mg, 4 mg/square. Chewing gum. Box 48, 108 pieces. *OTC.*
Use: Smoking deterrent.

nicotine inhalation system.
Use: Smoking deterrent.
See: Nicotrol Inhaler.

nicotine nasal spray.
Use: Smoking deterrent.
See: Nicotrol NS.

•**nicotine polacrilex.** (NIK-oh-teen PAHL-ah-KRILL-ex) USP 34.
Use: Smoking cessation adjunct.
See: Commit.
  Nicorette.
  Nicotine Gum.
  Thrive.

nicotine polacrilex. (Perrigo) Nicotine (as polacrilex) 2 mg. Phenylalanine 3.4 mg, aspartame, mannitol. Mint flavor. Loz. 48s. *OTC.*
Use: Smoking deterrent.

nicotine resin complex.
See: Nicotine Polacrilex.

•**nicotine transdermal system.** (NIK-oh-teen) USP 34.
Use: Smoking cessation adjunct.

nicotine transdermal system.
Use: Smoking deterrent.
See: Habitrol.
  NicoDerm CQ.
  Nicotrol.
  Prostep.

nicotine transdermal system. (Various Mfr.) Nicotine 7 mg, 14 mg, 21 mg/day (dose absorbed in 24 hours). Transdermal system. Box 7s, 30s. *OTC.*
Use: Smoking deterrent.

nicotinic acid. Niacin, USP.

nicotinic acid. (Rugby) Nicotinic acid 1,000 mg. Gluten free, preservative free, sugar free. Tab., controlled release. 100s. *OTC.*
Use: Water-soluble vitamin.

nicotinic acid. (Various Mfr.) Nicotinic acid. **Tab.:** 50 mg, 100 mg, 250 mg, 500 mg. Bot. 100s, 250s (50 mg, 100 mg only), 1000s (500 mg only). **TR Tab.:** 250 mg, 500 mg. Bot. 100s, 250s (250 mg only), 1000s (500 mg only). **SR Tab.:** 500 mg. Bot. 100s. **ER Cap.:** 250 mg, 400 mg. Bot. 100s, 1000s (250 mg only). **SR Cap.:** 125 mg, 500 mg. Bot. 100s. **TR Cap.:** 250 mg, 500 mg. Bot. 100s, 1000s (500 mg only). *Rx-OTC.*
Use: Water-soluble vitamin.

nicotinic acid amide. Niacinamide, USP.
See: Niacinamide.

nicotinic acid with combinations.
See: Niacin w/Combinations.

•**nicotinyl alcohol.** (NIK-oh-TIN-ill AL-koe-hahl) USAN.
Use: Vasodilator, peripheral.

nicotinyl tartrate. 3-Pyridinemethanol tartrate.

Nicotrol. (Pharmacia) Nicotine 5 mg, 10 mg, 15 mg (released gradually over 16 hours). Trans. system. Box 7s, 14s. *OTC.*
Use: Smoking deterrent.

Nicotrol Inhaler. (Pharmacia) Nicotine 4 mg delivered (10 mg/cartridge). Inhaler Kit contains mouthpiece, storage trays each containing 6 cartridges, 1 plastic storage case, patient information leaflet. Box 42s, 168s. *Rx.*
Use: Smoking deterrent.

Nicotrol NS. (Pharmacia) Nicotine 0.5 mg per actuation (10 mg/mL). Parabens, EDTA. Spray pump. Bot. 10 mL. ($\approx$ 200 applications). Each unit has a glass container mounted with metered spray pump. *Rx.*
Use: Smoking deterrent.

nieraline.
See: Epinephrine.

Nifediac CC. (Teva) Nifedipine 30 mg, 60 mg, 90 mg. Lactose (except 30 mg). Film-coated. ER Tab. 100s, 300s (except 90 mg), 1000s (except 90 mg). *Rx.*
Use: Calcium channel blocker.

Nifedical XL. (Teva) Nifedipine 30 mg, 60 mg. Lactose. Film-coated. ER Tab. Bot. 100s, 300s. *Rx.*
Use: Calcium channel blocker.

•**nifedipine.** (nye-FED-ih-peen) *USP 34.*
Tall Man: NIFEdipine
Use: Calcium channel blocker; urinary tract agent. [Orphan Drug]
See: Adalat CC.
  Afeditab CR.
  Nifediac CC.
  Nifedical XL.
  Procardia.
  Procardia XL.

nifedipine. (Mylan) Nifedipine 30 mg, 60 mg, 90 mg. ER Tab. Bot. 100s, 300s (except 90 mg). *Rx.*
Use: Calcium channel blocker.

nifedipine. (Various Mfr.) Nifedipine 10 mg, 20 mg. May be liquid filled. Cap. 100s, 300s. *Rx.*
Use: Calcium channel blocker.

Niferex. (Schwarz Pharma) Polysaccharide iron complex. Iron 100 mg/5 mL, alcohol 10%, sorbitol. Dye free, sugar free. Elix. Bot. 237 mL. *OTC.*
Use: Mineral supplement.

Niferex. (Ther-Rx) Polysaccharide-iron complex. Iron 60 mg, lactose. Cap. UD 100s. *OTC.*
Use: Mineral supplement.

Niferex-150. (Ther-Rx) Elemental iron (from ferrous asparto glycinate and polysaccharide iron complex) 150 mg, vitamin C (calcium ascorbate and calcium threonate) 50 mg, succinic acid 50 mg. Cap. 90s. *OTC.*
Use: Mineral supplement.

Niferex-150 Forte. (Ther-Rx) Elemental iron (from ferrous asparto glycinate and polysaccharide-iron complex) 150 mg, vitamin C (as calcium ascorbate and calcium threonate) 60.8 mg, folic acid 1 mg, vitamin B_{12} 25 mcg. Cap. 90s. *Rx.*
Use: Mineral, vitamin supplement.

Niferex-PN. (Ther-Rx) Iron 60 mg, folic acid 1 mg, vitamins C 50 mg, B_{12} 3 mcg, A 4000 units, D 400 units, B_1 3 mg, B_2 3 mg, B_6 2 mg, B_3 10 mg, Zn 18 mg, Ca, sorbitol. Bot. 30s, 100s, 1000s. *Rx.*
Use: Mineral, vitamin supplement.

Niferex-PN Forte. (Ther-Rx) Calcium 250 mg, iron 60 mg, vitamins A 5000 units, D 400 units, E 30 mg, B_1 3 mg, B_2 3.4 mg, B_3 20 mg, B_6 4 mg, B_{12} 12 mcg, C 80 mg, folic acid 1 mg, Cu, I, Mg, Zn 25 mg. Bot. 100s. *Rx.*
Use: Mineral, vitamin supplement.

•**nifluridide.** (nye-FLURE-ih-DIDE) USAN.
Use: Ectoparasiticide.

•**nifungin.** (nih-FUN-jin) USAN. Substance derived from *Aspergillus giganteus.*

•**nifuradene.** (NYE-fyoor-ad-EEN) USAN.
Use: Anti-infective.

•**nifuraldezone.** (NYE-fer-AL-dee-zone) USAN. (Eaton Medical)
Use: Anti-infective.

•**nifuratel.** (NYE-fyoor-at-ell) USAN.
Use: Anti-infective; antifungal; antiprotozoal, trichomonas.

•**nifuratrone.** (nye-FYOOR-ah-trone) USAN.
Use: Anti-infective.

•**nifurdazil.** (NYE-fyoor-dazz-ill) USAN.
Use: Anti-infective.

nifurethazone.
Use: Anti-infective.

•**nifurimide.** (nye-FYOOR-ih-MIDE) USAN.
Use: Anti-infective.

•**nifurmerone.** (NYE-fyoor-MER-ohn) USAN.
Use: Antifungal.

nifuroxime.
Use: Antifungal; anti-infective, topical; antiprotozoal.
See: Micofur.

•**nifurpirinol.** (nye-fer-PIHR-ih-nole) USAN.
Use: Anti-infective.

• **nifurquinazol.** (NYE-fyoor-KWIN-azz-ole) USAN.
Use: Anti-infective.

• **nifurthiazole.** (NYE-fyoor-THIGH-ah-zole) USAN.
Use: Anti-infective.

nifurtimox.
Use: CDC anti-infective agent.
See: Lampit.

Nighttime Cold Softgels. (Goldline) Dextromethorphan HBr 10 mg, doxylamine succinate 6.25 mg, pseudoephedrine hydrochloride 30 mg, acetaminophen 250 mg. Alcohol free. Sorbitol. Softgels. 12s. *OTC.*
Use: Antitussive combination.

Nighttime Pamprin. (Chattem) Diphenhydramine hydrochloride 50 mg, acetaminophen 650 mg. Pow. Pkg. 4s. *OTC.*
Use: Sleep aid.

Nighttime Sleep Aid. (Rugby) Diphenhydramine hydrochloride 50 mg. Tab. Bot. 50s. *OTC.*
Use: Antihistamine, nonselective ethanolamine.

nigrin. Streptonigrin.
Use: Antineoplastic.

Niko-Mag. (Scruggs) Magnesium oxide 500 mg. Cap. Bot. 100s, 1000s. *OTC.*
Use: Antacid.

Nikotime TD Caps. (Major) Niacin 125 mg, 250 mg. TD Cap. Bot. 100s, 1000s. *OTC.*
Use: Vitamin supplement.

Nilandron. (Aventis) Nilutamide 50 mg, 150 mg, lactose. Tab. Bot. 90s (50 mg only), 30s (150 mg only). *Rx.*
Use: Antineoplastic; hormone, antiandrogen.

• **nilotinib.** (nye-LOE-ti-nib) USAN.
Use: Protein-tyrosine kinase inhibitor.
See: Tasigna.

Nilstat. (Lederle) Nystatin 100,000 units/mL. Cherry flavor. Susp. 60 mL, 473 mL. *Rx.*
Use: Antifungal.

Nilstat Powder. (Wyeth) Nystatin pow. 150 million, 1 billion, 2 billion units. Bot. *Rx.*
Use: Antifungal.

Nil Tuss. (Minnesota Pharm) Dextromethorphan HBr 10 mg, chlorpheniramine maleate 1.25 mg, phenylephrine hydrochloride 5 mg, ammonium Cl 83 mg/5 mL. Syr. Bot. Pt. *OTC.*
Use: Antihistamine; antitussive; decongestant; expectorant.

• **nilutamide.** (nye-LOO-tah-mide) USAN.
Use: Antineoplastic; hormone, antiandrogen.

See: Nilandron.

• **nilvadipine.** (NILL-vah-DIH-peen) USAN.
Use: Antagonist, calcium channel.

Nil Vaginal Cream. (Century) Sulfanilamide 15%, 9-aminoacridine hydrochloride 0.2%, allantoin 1.5%. Bot. 4 oz. w/applicator. *OTC.*
Use: Anti-infective, vaginal.

• **nimazone.** (nih-mah-ZONE) USAN.
Use: Anti-inflammatory.

Nimbex. (Abbott) Cisatracurium besylate 2 mg/mL, Vial 5 mL, 10 mL; 10 mg/mL, Vial 20 mL. Inj. *Rx.*
Use: Nondepolarizing neuromuscular blocker; muscle relaxant.

Nimbus. (Biomerica) Monoclonal antibody-based enzyme immunoassay. Screens for urinary chorionic gonadotropin. Pkg. 10s, 25s, 50s. *Rx.*
Use: Diagnostic aid.

• **nimodipine.** (NYE-MOE-dih-peen) *USP 34.*
Tall Man: niMODipine
Use: Vasodilator, calcium channel blocker

nimodipine. (Various Mfr.) Nimodipine 30 mg. Liquid filled. Cap. UD 30s, 100s. *Rx.*
Use: Calcium channel blocking agent.

Nion B Plus C. (Nion Corp.) Vitamins B_1 15 mg, B_2 10.2 mg, B_3 50 mg, B_5 10 mg, C 300 mg. Capl. Bot 100s. *OTC.*
Use: Vitamin supplement.

Niong. (US Ethicals) Nitroglycerin 2.6 mg, 6.5 mg. CR Tab. Bot. 100s. *Rx.*
Use: Antianginal.

Nipent. (Hospira) Pentostatin 10 mg/vial. Mannitol 50 mg/vial. Pow. for Inj. Vial. Single-dose. *Rx.*
Use: Antineoplastic.

Niratron. (Progress) Chlorpheniramine maleate 4 mg/5 mL. Bot. pt. *Rx.*
Use: Antihistamine.

Niravam. (Schwarz Pharma) Alprazolam 0.25 mg, 0.5 mg, 1 mg, 2 mg. Sucralose, sucrose. Orange flavor. Orally Disintegrating Tab. 100s. *Rx.*
Use: Antianxiety agent.

• **niridazole.** (nye-RIH-dah-ZOLE) USAN.
Use: Antischistosomal.

• **nisbuterol mesylate.** (NISS-BYOO-teh-role) USAN.
Use: Bronchodilator.

• **nisobamate.** (NYE-so-BAM-ate) USAN.
Use: Anxiolytic; hypnotic; sedative.

• **nisoldipine.** (nye-SOLE-dih-peen) USAN.
Use: Calcium channel blocker.
See: Sular.

nisoldipine. (Mylan) Nisoldipine 20 mg, 30 mg, 40 mg. Polydextrose. Film-coated ER Tab. 100s, 500s. *Rx.*
Use: Cardiovascular agent, calcium channel blocking agent.

•**nisoxetine.** (NISS-OX-eh-teen) USAN.
Use: Antidepressant.

•**nisterime acetate.** (nye-STEER-eem) USAN.
Use: Androgen.

•**nitarsone.** (NITE-AHR-sone) USAN.
Use: Antiprotozoal, histomonas.

•**nitazoxanide.** (nye-tah-ZOX-ah-nide)
Use: Antiprotozoals.
See: Alinia.

Nite Time Children's. (Topco) Pseudo-ephedrine hydrochloride 10 mg, chlor-pheniramine maleate 0.67 mg, dextro-methorphan HBr 5 mg per 5 mL. Su-crose, cherry flavor, alcohol free. Liq. Bot. 118 mL. *OTC.*
Use: Upper respiratory combination, de-congestant, antihistamine, antitus-sive.

Nite Time Cold Formula. (Alra) Pseudo-ephedrine hydrochloride 10 mg, doxyl-amine succinate 1.25 mg, dextrometh-orphan HBr 5 mg, acetaminophen 167 mg, alcohol 25%. Liq. Bot. 180 mL, 300 mL. *OTC.*
Use: Analgesic; antihistamine; antitus-sive; decongestant.

Nite Time Cold Formula for Adults. (Al-pharma) Dextromethorphan HBr 5 mg, doxylamine succinate 2.1 mg, pseudo-ephedrine hydrochloride 10 mg, aceta-minophen 167 mg per 5 mL. Alcohol 10%, saccharin, sucrose. Liq. Bot. 296 mL. *OTC.*
Use: Upper respiratory combination, an-titussive, antihistamine, deconges-tant, analgesic.

•**nitisinone.** (nit-IS-i-none) USAN.
Use: Tyrosinemia.
See: Orfadin.

•**nitralamine hydrochloride.** (nye-TRAL-ah-meen) USAN.
Use: Antifungal.

•**nitramisole hydrochloride.** (nye-TRAM-ih-sole) USAN.
Use: Anthelmintic.

nitrates.
Use: Vasodilator.
See: Amyl Nitrate.
Isosorbide Dinitrate.
Isosorbide Mononitrate.
Nitroglycerin.

•**nitrazepam.** (nye-TRAY-zeh-pam) USAN.
Use: Anticonvulsant; hypnotic; seda-tive.

Nitrek. (Bertek) Nitroglycerin 0.2 mg/h (22.4 mg), 0.4 mg/h (44.8 mg), 0.6 mg/h (67.2 mg). Transdermal Patch. Box 30s. *Rx.*
Use: Vasodilator.

•**nitrendipine.** (NIGH-TREN-dih-peen) USAN.
Use: Antihypertensive.

•**nitric acid.** (NYE-trick) *NF 29.*
Use: Pharmaceutic aid, acidifying agent.
See: Nitric Oxide.

nitric acid silver. Silver Nitrate.

nitric oxide.
Use: Respiratory inhalant; primary pul-monary hypertension agent. [Orphan Drug]
See: INOmax.

Nitro-Bid. (Savage) Nitroglycerin 2% in lanolin-white petrolatum base. Lactose. Oint. Tube 30 g, 60 g, UD 1 g. *Rx.*
Use: Vasodilator.

Nitrocap. (Freeport) Nitroglycerin 2.5 mg. TR Cap. Bot. 100s. *Rx.*
Use: Antianginal.

•**nitrocycline.** (NYE-troe-SIGH-kleen) USAN.
Use: Anti-infective.

•**nitrodan.** (NYE-troe-dan) USAN.
Use: Anthelmintic.

Nitrodisc. (Roberts) Nitroglycerin. Trans-dermal nitroglycerin discs releasing 16 mg, 24 mg, 32 mg. Patch. Ctn. 30s, 100s. *Rx.*
Use: Antianginal.

Nitro-Dur. (Key) Nitroglycerin 0.1 mg/h (20 mg), 0.2 mg/h (40 mg), 0.3 mg/h (60 mg), 0.4 mg/h (80 mg), 0.6 mg/h (120 mg), 0.8 mg/h (160 mg). Trans-dermal Patch. 30s, UD 30s. *Rx.*
Use: Vasodilator.

Nitrofan Caps. (Major) Nitrofurantoin 50 mg, 100 mg. Cap. Bot. 100s, 500s. *Rx.*
Use: Anti-infective, urinary.

nitrofurans.
See: Nitrofurantoin.

•**nitrofurantoin.** (nye-troe-FYOOR-an-toyn) *USP 34.*
Use: Anti-infective, urinary.
See: Furadantin.
Macrobid.
Macrodantin.

nitrofurantoin. (Various Mfr.) Nitrofuran-toin as macrocrystals 50 mg, 100 mg. Cap. Bot. 100s, 500s, 1000s. *Rx.*
Use: Anti-infective, urinary.

nitrofurantoin. (Various Mfr.) Nitrofuran-toin (as monohydrate/macrocrystals) 100 mg. Cap. 100s, 500s. *Rx.*
Use: Anti-infective, urinary.

•**nitrofurazone.** (nye-troe-FYOOR-a-zone) *USP 34.*
Use: Anti-infective, topical.
Nitrogard. (Forest) Transmucosal nitroglycerin 2 mg, 3 mg. Buccal CR Tab. Bot. 100s, UD 100s. *Rx.*
Use: Vasodilator.
•**nitrogen.** (NYE-troe-jen) *NF 29.*
Use: Pharmaceutic aid, air displacement.
nitrogen monoxide. Laughing Gas, Nitrous Oxide.
Use: Anesthetic, general; analgesic.
nitrogen mustard.
See: Mustargen.
nitrogen mustard derivatives.
See: Leukeran.
Mustargen.
Triethylenemelamine.
nitrogen mustards.
Use: Alkylating agents.
See: Chlorambucil.
Cyclophosphamide.
Ifosfamide.
Mechlorethamine Hydrochloride.
Melphalan.
•**nitroglycerin.** (nye-troe-GLH-suh-rin) *USP 34.*
Use: Vasodilator.
See: Minitran.
Niong.
Nitrek.
Nitro-Bid.
Nitrodisk.
Nitro-Dur.
Nitrogard.
Nitrolingual.
Nitro-Lyn.
NitroMist.
Nitrostat.
Nitro-Time.
Transderm-Nitro.
nitroglycerin. (Wilshire Pharmaceuticals) Nitroglycerin 0.4 mg per metered spray. Alcohol 20%, peppermint oil. Spray, lingual. 4.9 g and 12 g (60 and 200 metered doses). *Rx.*
Use: Vasodilator, nitrate.
nitroglycerin. (Various Mfr.) Nitroglycerin. **ER Cap.:** 2.5 mg, 6.5 mg, 9 mg. Bot. 30s (9 mg only), 60s, 100s, UD 60s (2.5 mg only), UD 100s. **Oint.:** 2%. Tube 30 g, 60 g. **Soln. for Inj.:** 5 mg/mL. Single-dose vials. 5 mL, 10 mL. **Sublingual Tab.:** 0.3 mg (¹⁄₂₀₀ gr), 0.4 mg (¹⁄₁₅₀ gr), 0.6 mg (¹⁄₁₀₀ gr). May contain lactose. 25s (0.4 mg only), 100s. *Rx.*
Use: Vasodilator.

•**nitroglycerin, diluted.** (nye-troe-GLIH-suh-rin) *USP 34. Formerly Glyceryl Trinitrate.*
Use: Vasodilator, coronary.
nitroglycerin in 5% dextrose. (Various Mfr.) Nitroglycerin 100 mcg/mL, 200 mcg/mL, 400 mcg/mL. Inj. Glass containers. 250 mL, 500 mL. *Rx.*
Use: Vasodilator.
nitroglycerin injection. (Abbott) Nitroglycerin 25 mg/mL. Vial 5 mL, 10 mL.
Use: Antianginal; vasodilator.
See: Tridil.
nitroglycerin, intravenous.
Use: Vasodilator.
nitroglycerin patch.
Use: Antianginal.
See: Nitrek.
nitroglycerin transdermal. (Mylan) Nitroglycerin 0.1 mg/h. Transdermal Patch. 30s. *Rx.*
Use: Vasodilator.
nitroglycerin transdermal. (Various Mfr.) Nitroglycerin 0.2 mg/h (16 mg to 62.5 mg), 0.4 mg/h (32 mg to 125 mg), or 0.6 mg/h (75 mg to 187.5 mg). Transdermal Patch. Box 30s. *Rx.*
Use: Vasodilator.
nitroglycerin transdermal system. (Hercon Laboratories, Inc.) Nitroglycerin 37.3 mg, 74.6 mg, 111.9 mg. Patch Pkg. 30s. *Rx.*
Use: Vasodilator.
nitroglycerol.
See: Nitroglycerin.
Nitrolan. (Elan) Protein 60 g, fat 40 g, carbohydrates 160 g, Na 690 mg, K 1.17 g/L, lactose free. With appropriate vitamins and minerals. Liq. In 237 mL *Tetra Pak* containers and 1000 mL *New Pak* closed systems with and without *Color Check. OTC.*
Use: Nutritional supplement.
Nitrolin. (Schein) Nitroglycerin 2.5 mg, 9 mg. SR Cap. **2.5 mg:** Bot. 100s. **9 mg:** Bot. 60s. *Rx.*
Use: Antianginal.
Nitrolingual. (Sciele Pharma) Nitroglycerin 0.4 mg/metered dose. Alcohol 20%, peppermint oil. Aerosol Spray, lingual. 4.9 g and 12 g (60 and 200 metered doses). *Rx.*
Use: Vasodilator.
Nitro-Lyn. (Lynwood) Nitroglycerin 2.5 mg. Cap. Bot. 100s. *Rx.*
Use: Antianginal.
nitromannite.
See: Mannitol Hexanitrate.
nitromannitol.
See: Mannitol Hexanitrate.

Nitromed. (US Ethicals) Nitroglycerin 2.6 mg, 6.5 mg. CR Tab. Bot. 100s. *Rx.*
Use: Antianginal.

• **nitromersol.** (nye-troe-MER-sole) *USP 34.*
Use: Anti-infective, topical.

• **nitromide.** (NYE-troe-mide) USAN.
Use: Anti-infective.

• **nitromifene citrate.** (nye-TROE-mih-feen) USAN.
Use: Antiestrogen.

NitroMist. (Akrimax Pharmaceuticals) Nitroglycerin 0.4 mg per spray. Aerosol spray, lingual. 8.5 g (230 metered doses). *Rx.*
Use: Vasodilator.

Nitronet. (US Ethicals) Nitroglycerin 2.6 mg, 6.5 mg. CR Tab. Bot. 100s. *Rx.*
Use: Antianginal.

Nitropress. (Hospira) Sodium nitroprusside 50 mg/2 mL. Vial. *Rx.*
Use: Antihypertensive.

nitroprusside sodium.
Use: Antihypertensive.
See: Nitropress (Abbott).
    Sodium Nitroprusside.

nitrosoureas.
Use: Alkylating agent; antineoplastic.
See: Carmustine.
    Lomustine.
    Streptozocin.

Nitrostat. (Parke-Davis) Nitroglycerin 0.3 mg (1/200 g), 0.4 mg (1/150 g), 0.6 mg (1/100 g). Lactose. Sublingual Tab. Bot. 25s (0.4 mg only), 100s. *Rx.*
Use: Vasodilator.

Nitrostat IV. (Parke-Davis) Nitroglycerin for infusion. **0.8 mg/mL:** Amp. 10 mL. **5 mg/mL:** Amp. 10 mL, Vial 10 mL. **10 mg/mL:** Vial 10 mL. *Rx.*
Use: Antianginal.

Nitro-Time. (Time-Cap Labs) Nitroglycerin 2.5 mg, 6.5 mg, 9 mg, lactose, sucrose. ER Cap. Bot. 60s, 90s, 100s. *Rx.*
Use: Vasodilator.

nitrous acid, sodium salt. Sodium Nitrite.

• **nitrous oxide.** (NYE-trus OX-ide) *USP 34.* Laughing Gas. Nitrogen Monoxide.
Use: Anesthesia, inhalation.

nitrous oxide. (Airgas) Nitrous oxide 100% (provided as a liquefied compressed gas). Gas, Inhal. Cylinder.
Use: General anesthetic, gas.

• **nivazol.** (NIH-vah-ZOLE) USAN.
Use: Corticosteroid, topical.

Nivea Moisturizing. (Beiersdorf) **Cream:** Mineral oil, petrolatum, lanolin alcohol, glycerin, microcrystalline wax, paraffin, magnesium sulfate, decyloleate, octyl dodecanol, aluminum stearate, citric acid, magnesium stearate. 120 g, 180 g, 300 g, 480 g. **Lot.:** Mineral oil, lanolin, isopropyl myristate, cetearyl alcohol, glyceryl stearate, acrylamide/sodium acrylate copolymer, simethicone, methychloroisothiazolinone, methylisothiazolinone. In 180 mL, 300 mL, 450 mL. *OTC.*
Use: Emollient.

Nivea Moisturizing Creme Soap. (Beiersdorf) Sodium tallowate, sodium cocoate, glycerin, petrolatum, titanium dioxide, NaCl, octyldodecanol, macadamia nut oil, aloe, sodium thiosulfate, lanolin alcohol, pentasodium pentetate, EDTA, BHT, beeswax. Bar 90 g, 150 g. *OTC.*
Use: Dermatologic, cleanser.

Nivea Oil. (Beiersdorf) Emulsion of neutral aliphatic hydrocarbons. **Liq.:** Bot. 2 oz, 4 fl oz, pt, qt. **Cream:** Tube 1 oz, 2⅓ oz, Jar 4 oz, 6 oz, 1 lb, 5 lb. tin. **Soap:** Bath or toilet size. *OTC.*
Use: Emollient.

Nivea Sun. (Beiersdorf) Octyl methoxycinnamate, octyl salicylate, benzophenone-3, 2-phenylbenzimidazole-5-sulfonic acid. Lot. Bot. 120 mL. *OTC.*
Use: Sunscreen.

• **nivimedone sodium.** (nih-VIH-meh-dohn) USAN.
Use: Antiallergic.

• **nivocasan.** (nye-VOE-ka-san) USAN.
Use: Apoptosis prevention during cell stress.

Nix Complete Lice Treatment System. (Insight) Permethrin 1%. Cetyl alcohol, isopropyl alcohol 20%, parabens. Liq., Top. 59 mL w/comb, gloves, cape, and drop cloth. *OTC.*
Use: Scabicide/pediculicide.

Nix Creme Rinse. (Insight) Permethrin 1%. Isopropyl alcohol 20%, cetyl alcohol, parabens. Liq. (cream rinse). 60 mL with comb. *OTC.*
Use: Pediculicide.

• **nizatidine.** (nye-ZAT-ih-deen) *USP 34.*
Use: Histamine H_2 antagonist.
See: Axid.
    Axid AR.
    Axid Pulvules.

nizatidine. (Various Mfr.) Nizatidine. **Cap.:** 150 mg, 300 mg. 30s (300 mg only), 60s (150 mg only), 100s, 500s, 1000s (150 mg only), UD 100s (150 mg only). **Soln.:** 15 mg/mL. Glycerin, parabens, saccharin, sucrose. Bubble gum flavor. 480 mL. *Rx.*
Use: Histamine H_2 antagonist.

Nizoral. (McNeil Consumer) Ketoconazole 2%. Shampoo. 120 mL. *Rx.*
Use: Antifungal agent; topical antiinfective.

Nizoral A-D. (McNeil Consumer) Ketoconazole 1%. Tetrasodium EDTA. Shampoo. Bot. 207 mL. *OTC.*
Use: Antifungal agent; topical antiinfective.

N-methyl-D-aspartate receptor antagonists.
Use: Treatment of Alzheimer dementia.
See: Memantine hydrochloride.

n-methylhydrazine.
Use: Antineoplastic.
See: Procarbazine Hydrochloride.

n-methylisatin beta-thiosemicarbazone. Under study.
Use: Smallpox protection.

n, n-diethylvanillamide.
See: Ethamivan.

No-Aspirin. (Walgreen) Acetaminophen 325 mg. Tab. Bot. 100s. *OTC.*
Use: Analgesic.

No-Aspirin Extra Strength. (Walgreen) Acetaminophen 500 mg. Tab. **Tab.:** Bot. 60s, 100s. **Cap.:** Bot. 50s, 100s. *OTC.*
Use: Analgesic.

•**noberastine.** (no-BER-ast-een) USAN.
Use: Antihistamine.

Noble Formula. (Ontos) Pyrithione zinc 0.25%. **Cream:** Alcohol, almond oil, rose hip oil, vitamin E. 120 mL. **Spray:** Alcohol. 120 mL. *OTC.*
Use: Dermatological agent.

•**nocodazole.** (no-KOE-DAH-zole) USAN.
Use: Antineoplastic.

Nodolor. (Macoven Pharmaceuticals) Acetaminophen 325 mg, dichloralphenazone 100 mg, isometheptene mucate 65 mg. Lactose. Cap. 100s. *c-IV.*
Use: Migraine combination.

No Drowsiness Allerest. (Novartis) Pseudoephedrine hydrochloride 30 mg, acetaminophen 500 mg. Tab. Bot. 20s. *OTC.*
Use: Analgesic; decongestant.

No Drowsiness Sinarest. (Medeva) Pseudoephedrine hydrochloride 30 mg, acetaminophen 500 mg. Tab. Bot. 24s. *OTC.*
Use: Analgesic; decongestant.

nofetumomab merpentan.
See: Verluma.

•**nogalamycin.** (no-GAL-ah-MY-sin) USAN.
Use: Antineoplastic.

NoHist. (Larken) Phenylephrine hydrochloride 20 mg, chlorpheniramine maleate 8 mg. ER Tab. 100s. *Rx.*
Use: Upper respiratory combination, decongestant and antihistamine.

NoHist-A. (Larken) Phenylephrine hydrochloride 5 mg, chlorpheniramine maleate 2.5 mg, phenyltoloxamine citrate 7.5 mg per 5 mL. Alcohol and sugar free. Saccharin, sorbitol. Cotton candy flavor. Liq. 473 mL. *Rx.*
Use: Upper respiratory combination, decongestant and antihistamine.

NoHist DMX. (Larken) Chlorpheniramine maleate 8 mg, dextromethorphan HBr 30 mg, phenylephrine hydrochloride 20 mg. ER Tab. 100s. *Rx.*
Use: Upper respiratory combination, antitussive combination.

NoHist EXT. (Larken) Chlorpheniramine maleate 8 mg, methscopolamine nitrate 2.5 mg. ER Tab. 100s. *Rx.*
Use: Upper respiratory combination, decongestant, antihistamine, and anticholinergic.

NoHist LQ. (Larken Labs) Chlorpheniramine maleate 4 mg, phenylephrine hydrochloride 10 mg. Edetate disodium, glycerin, parabens, propylene glycol, saccharin. Alcohol free and sugar free. Bubble gum flavor. Liq. 473 mL. *OTC.*
Use: Upper respiratory combination, decongestant and antihistamine.

NoHist-PDX. (Larken Labs) Chlorpheniramine maleate 0.75 mg, dextromethorphan hydrobromide 2.75 mg, phenylephrine hydrochloride 1.75 mg. Saccharin, sorbitol. Alcohol free. Cherry flavor. Drops. 30 mL w/dropper. *Rx.*
Use: Upper respiratory combination, antitussive combination.

NoHist-Plus. (Larken) Chlorpheniramine maleate 2 mg, methscopolamine nitrate 1.25 mg, phenylephrine hydrochloride 10 mg. Mannitol, saccharin, sugar. Chew. Tab. 100s. *Rx.*
Use: Upper respiratory combination, decongestant, antihistamine, anticholinergic combination.

Nokane. (Wren) Salicylamide 4 g, n-acetyl-p-aminophenol 4 g, caffeine 0.5 gr. Tab. Bot. 40s. *OTC.*
Use: Analgesic combination.

•**nolinium bromide.** (no-LIN-ee-uhm) USAN.
Use: Antisecretory; antiulcerative.

•**nomegestrol.** (NOE-me-JES-trol) USAN.
Use: Hormonal contraceptive.

•**nomegestrol acetate.** (NOE-me-JES-trol) USAN.
Use: Hormonal contraceptive.

Nometic. Diphenidol.
Use: Antiemetic.

•**nomifensine maleate.** (NO-mih-FEN-seen) USAN.
Use: Antidepressant.

Nomuc-PE. (Cypress) Pseudoephedrine hydrochloride 60 mg, guaifenesin 200 mg. Parabens. ER Cap. 100s. *Rx.*
Use: Upper respiratory combination, decongestant and expectorant combination.

Nonamin. (Western Research) Ca 100 mg, Cl 90 mg, Mg 50 mg, Zn 3.75 mg, Fe 4.5 mg, Cu 0.5 mg, I 37.5 mcg, K 49 mg, P 100 mg. Tab. Bot. 1000s. *OTC.*
Use: Mineral supplement.

Non-Aspirin Extra Strength. (Mason) Acetaminophen 500 mg. Tab. 100s. *OTC.*
Use: Analgesic.

nonbarbiturate sedative/hypnotic agents.
See: Sedative/Hypnotic Agents (Nonbarbiturate).

Non-Drowsy Allergy. (Major) Loratadine 10 mg. Lactose. Tab. 10s. *OTC.*
Use: Antihistamine, peripherally selective piperidine.

Non-Drowsy Allergy Relief. (Major) Loratadine 10 mg. Phenylalanine 0.9 mg, aspartame, lactose, mannitol. Cherry flavor. Orally Disintegrating Tab. 10s. *OTC.*
Use: Antihistamine, peripherally selective piperidine.

Non-Drowsy Allergy Relief for Kids. (Major) Loratadine 5 mg per 5 mL. Glycerin, sucrose. Fruit flavor. Syrup. 120 mL. *OTC.*
Use: Antihistamine, peripherally selective piperidine.

Non-Drowsy Contac Sinus. (Glaxo-SmithKline) Pseudoephedrine hydrochloride 30 mg, acetaminophen 500 mg. Cap. Bot. 24s. *OTC.*
Use: Analgesic; decongestant.

None. (Forest) Heparin sodium 1000 units/mL. No preservatives. Amps 5 mL. Box 25s. *Rx.*
Use: Anticoagulant.

Non-Habit Forming Stool Softener. (Rugby) Docusate sodium 100 mg, sorbitol, parabens. Cap. Bot. 100s, 1000s. *OTC.*
Use: Laxative.

nonnarcotic analgesic combinations.
See: Acetaminophen, Aspirin, Caffeine.
Acetaminophen, Butalbital.
Acetaminophen, Butalbital, and Caffeine.

Diclofenac Sodium/Misoprostol.
Naproxen/Lansoprazole.

nonnarcotic antitussives.
See: Benzonatate.
Carbetapentane Tannate.
Dextromethorphan Hydrobromide.
Dextromethorphan Hydrobromide/Benzocaine.
Diphenhydramine Hydrochloride.

non-nucleoside reverse transcriptase inhibitors. *Rx.*
Use: Antiretroviral.
See: Delavirdine Mesylate.
Efavirenz.
Efavirenz/Emtricitabine/Tenofovir Disoproxil Fumarate.
Etravirine.
Nevirapine.
Rescriptor.

nonoxynol. (Ortho-McNeil) *OTC.*
Use: Contraceptive, spermicide.

•**nonoxynol-15.** (NAHN-ox-sih-nahl) USAN.
Use: Pharmaceutic aid, surfactant.

•**nonoxynol-4.** (NAHN-ox-sih-nahl) USAN.
Use: Pharmaceutic aid, surfactant.

•**nonoxynol-9.** (NAHN-ox-sih-nahl) *USP 34.*
Use: Spermicide; pharmaceutic aid, wetting and solubilizing agent.
See: Conceptrol.
Delfen.
Encare.

•**nonoxynol-10.** (nahn-OCK-sih-nahl) *NF 29.*
Use: Pharmaceutic aid, surfactant.

•**nonoxynol-30.** (NAHN-ox-sih-nahl) USAN. Under study.
Use: Pharmaceutic aid, surfactant.

nonselective alkylamines.
Use: Antihistamine.
See: Alkylamines, nonselective.

nonselective ethanolamines.
Use: Antihistamine.
See: Ethanolamines, nonselective.

nonselective piperazines.
Use: Antihistamine.
See: Piperazines, nonselective.

nonselective piperidines.
Use: Antihistamine.
See: Piperidines, nonselective.

nonsteroidal anti-inflammatory agents.
See: Celecoxib.
Diclofenac Potassium.
Diclofenac Sodium.
Etodolac.
Fenoprofen Calcium.
Flurbiprofen.
Ibuprofen.

Indomethacin.
Ketoprofen.
Ketorolac Tromethamine.
Meclofenamate Sodium.
Mefenamic Acid.
Meloxicam.
Nabumetone.
Naproxen.
Oxaprozin.
Piroxicam.
Selective COX-2 Inhibitors.
Sulindac.
Tolmetin Sodium.

nonsteroidal anti-inflammatory agents, ophthalmic.
See: Bromfenac.
Diclofenac Sodium.
Flurbiprofen Sodium.
Ketorolac Tromethamine.
Nepafenac.
Suprofen.

nonsteroidal anti-inflammatory agents, topical.
See: Diclofenac.

nonylphenoxypolyethoxy ethanol.
Nonoxynol.
Use: Contraceptive, spermicide.
See: Delfen.

No Pain-HP. (Young Again Products) Capsaicin 0.075%. Roll-on. 60 mL. *OTC.*
Use: Analgesic, topical.

Nora-BE. (Watson) Norethindrone 0.35 mg. Lactose. Tab. 28s. *Rx.*
Use: Sex hormone, contraceptive hormone.

•**noracymethadol hydrochloride.** (nahr-ASS-ih-METH-ah-dole) USAN.
Use: Analgesic.

•**norbolethone.** (nahr-BOLE-eth-ohn) USAN.
Use: Anabolic.

Norcet Tablets. (Holloway) Hydrocodone bitartrate 5 mg, acetaminophen 500 mg. Tab. Bot. 100s. *c-III.*
Use: Analgesic combination; narcotic.

Norco. (Watson) Hydrocodone bitartrate 10 mg, acetaminophen 325 mg. Tab. Bot. 100s, 500s. *c-III.*
Use: Analgesic; narcotic.

Norco 5/325. (Watson) Hydrocodone bitartrate 5 mg, acetaminophen 325 mg, sucrose. Tab. Bot. 100s, 500s. *c-III.*
Use: Narcotic analgesic combination.

Norcuron. (Organon Teknika) Vecuronium bromide 10 mg/5 mL. **With diluent:** Vial 5 mL lyophilized powder and 5 mL Amp. of sterile water for injection. Box 10s. **Without diluent:** Vial 5 mL lyophilized powder. Box 10s. **Prefilled syringe:** Vial 10 mL lyophilized powder and 10 mL syringe w/bacteriostatic water for injection. Box 10s. *Rx.*
Use: Muscle relaxant.

norcycline.
Use: Anti-infective.

Nordette-28. (Barr/Duramed) Levonorgestrel 0.15 mg, ethinyl estradiol 30 mcg. Lactose. Tab. 28s with 7 inert tabs. *Rx.*
Use: Sex hormone, contraceptive hormone.

Norditropin. (Novo Nordisk) Somatropin. 5 mg/1.5 mL, 10 mg/1.5 mL, 15 mg/ 1.5 mL, 30 mg/3 mL. Histidine 1 mg (5 mg, 10 mg only), 1.7 mg (15 mg only), 3.3 mg (30 mg only); poloxamer 188; phenol 4.5 mg, 9 mg (30 mg only); mannitol 60 mg (5 mg, 10 mg only), 58 mg (15 mg only), 117 mg (30 mg only). Inj. *Nordiflex* prefilled pens and cartridges (5 mg, 15 mg only). *Rx.*
Use: Hormone, growth.

Norel EX. (US Pharm) Phenylephrine hydrochloride 40 mg (extended release), guaifenesin 800 mg (400 mg immediate release/400 mg extended release). Lactose. ER Tab. 100s. *Rx.*
Use: Upper respiratory combination, decongestant and expectorant.

norelgestromin/ethinyl estradiol.
Use: Sex hormone, contraceptive hormone.
See: Ortho Evra.

Norel LA. (US Pharm) Phenylephrine hydrochloride 40 mg, carbinoxamine maleate 8 mg. ER Tab. 100s. *Rx.*
Use: Decongestant and antihistamine.

Norel SR. (US Pharm) Phenylephrine hydrochloride 40 mg, chlorpheniramine maleate 8 mg, phenyltoloxamine citrate 50 mg, acetaminophen 325 mg. ER Tab. 100s. *Rx.*
Use: Upper respiratory combination, decongestant, antihistamine, and analgesic.

•**norepinephrine bitartrate.** (NOR-eh-pih-NEFF-reen bye-TAR-trate) *USP 34.*
Formerly levarterenol bitartrate.
Use: Adrenergic, vasoconstrictor, vasopressor.
See: Levophed.

norepinephrine bitartrate. (Abbott) Norepinephrine bitartrate (as base) 1 mg/ mL. Sodium metabisulfite 0.46 mg, sodium chloride 8.2 mg. Inj. Amps. 4 mL. *Rx.*
Use: Vasopressor.

•**norethindrone.** (nor-ETH-in-drone) *USP 34.*
Use: Progestin.

See: Jolivette.
  Micronor.
  Nor-Q.D.
  Ortho Micronor.
W/Ethinyl Estradiol.
  See: Aranelle.
  Balziva.
  Brevicon.
  Femcon Fe.
  GenCept.
  Heather.
  Jenest-28.
  Junel Fe 1/20.
  Junel Fe 1.5/30.
  Leena.
  Loestrin Fe 1/20.
  Loestrin Fe 1.5/30.
  Loestrin 21 1/20.
  Loestrin 21 1.5/30.
  Microgestin Fe 1/20.
  Microgestin Fe 1.5/30.
  Modicon.
  Norinyl 1 + 35.
  Nortrel 1/35.
  Nortrel 0.5/35.
  Ortho-Novum 1/35.
  Ortho-Novum 7/7/7.
  Ortho-Novum 10/11.
  Ovcon-50.
  Ovcon-35.
  Tri-Norinyl.
  Zenchent.
W/Mestranol.
  See: Necon 1/50.
  Norinyl.
  Norinyl 1 + 50.
  Ortho-Novum 1/50.
norethindrone. (Barr) Norethindrone
  acetate 5 mg. Tab. Bot. 50s. *Rx.*
  Use: Sex hormone, progestin.
norethindrone. (Glenmark Pharmaceuti-
  cals) Norethindrone 0.35 mg. Lactose.
  Tab. 28s. *Rx.*
  Use: Oral contraceptive, progestin-only
  product.
•**norethindrone acetate.** (nor-ETH-in-
  drone) *USP 34.*
  Use: Sex hormone, progestin.
  See: Aygestin.
W/Ethinyl Estradiol.
  See: Estrostep Fe.
  Femhrt.
  Jinteli.
  Junel 21 Day 1/20.
  Junel 21 Day 1.5/30.
  Loestrin 24 Fe.
  Tilia Fe.
  Tri-Legest.
W/Estradiol.
  See: Activella.

CombiPatch.
  Mimvey.
**norethindrone/ethinyl estradiol and
  ferrous fumarate.** (Watson) Ethinyl
  estradiol 0.025 mg, norethindrone
  0.8 mg. Lactose, mannitol, sucralose.
  Chew. Tab. 24s w/4 ferrous fumarate
  (75 mg) chewable tablets. *Rx.*
  Use: Oral monophasic contraceptive.
•**norethynodrel.** (nor-eh-THIGH-no-drell)
  USP 34.
  Use: Hormone, progestin.
  See: Enovid.
Norflex. (Graceway Pharmaceuticals)
  Orphenadrine citrate 30 mg/mL. So-
  dium bisulfite. Inj. Amp. 2 mL. *Rx.*
  Use: Muscle relaxant.
•**norfloxacin.** (nor-FLOX-uh-SIN) *USP 34.*
  Use: Anti-infective.
  See: Noroxin.
•**norflurane.** (nor-FLUR-ane) USAN. Un-
  der study.
  Use: Anesthetic, general.
•**norgestimate.** (nore-JEST-ih-mate)
  USAN. *Formerly Dexnorgestrel Ace-
  time.*
  Use: Hormone, progestin.
W/Estradiol.
  See: Prefest.
W/Ethinyl Estradiol.
  See: MonoNessa.
  Ortho-Cyclen.
  Ortho Tri-Cyclen.
  Previfem.
  Tri-Previfem.
•**norgestomet.** (nore-JESS-toe-met)
  USAN.
  Use: Hormone, progestin.
•**norgestrel.** (nor-JESS-trell) *USP 34.*
  Use: Contraceptive; hormone, progestin.
W/Ethinyl Estradiol.
  See: Lo/Ovral.
  Low-Ogestrel.
  Ogestrel.
  Ovral.
•**norgestrel and ethinyl estradiol tab-
  lets.** *USP 34.*
  Use: Contraceptive.
  See: Norinyl 1 + 35.
Norinyl. (Roche) Norethindrone 2 mg,
  mestranol 0.1 mg. Tab. *Memorette*
  Disp. of 20s. Refill folders of 20s. *Rx.*
  Use: Contraceptive.
Norinyl 1 + 50. (Watson) Norethindrone
  1 mg, mestranol 50 mcg. Lactose. Tab.
  Wallette 28s with 7 inert tabs. *Rx.*
  Use: Sex hormone, contraceptive hor-
  mone.
Norinyl 1 + 35. (Watson) Norethindrone
  1 mg, ethinyl estradiol 35 mcg. Lac-

tose. Tab. *Wallette* 28s with 7 inert tabs. *Rx.*
Use: Sex hormone, contraceptive hormone.

Norisodrine Aerosol. (Abbott) Norisodrine hydrochloride (isoproterenol hydrochloride) 0.25% (2.8 mg/mL) in inert chlorofluorohydrocarbon propellants, alcohol 33%, ascorbic acid 0.1% as preservative. Aerosol 15 mL. Box 12s. *Rx.*
Use: Bronchodilator.

Norisodrine/Calcium Iodide Syrup.
(Abbott) Isoproterenol sulfate 3 mg, calcium iodide, anhydrous 150 mg/5 mL, alcohol 6%. Bot. Pt. *Rx.*
Use: Bronchodilator.

Noritate. (Dermik Labs) Metronidazole 1%. Parabens, glycerin. Cream. Tubes. 30 g. *Rx.*
Use: Topical anti-infective; antibiotic.

Norlestrin Fe 1/50 Tablets. (Parke-Davis) Norethindrone acetate 1 mg, ethinyl estradiol 50 mcg. Compact 21 yellow Tab., 7 brown 75 mg ferrous fumarate Tab. Pkg. 5 compacts. Pkg. 5 refills; Ctn. 10 × 5 refills. *Rx.*
Use: Contraceptive.

Norlestrin Fe 2.5/50 Tablets. (Parke-Davis) Norethindrone acetate 2.5 mg, ethinyl estradiol 50 mcg. Compact 21 Tab., 7 brown 75 mg ferrous fumarate Tab. Pkg. 5 compacts. Pkg. 5 refills; Ctn. 10 × 5 refills. *Rx.*
Use: Contraceptive.

Norlestrin-28 1/50 Tablet. (Parke-Davis) Norethindrone acetate 1 mg, ethinyl estradiol 50 mcg. Compact 21 yellow, 7 white (inert) tablets. Pkg. 5 compacts. Pkg. 5 refills; Ctn. 10 × 5 refills. *Rx.*
Use: Contraceptive.

Norlestrin-21 1/50 Tablets. (Parke-Davis) Norethindrone acetate 1 mg, ethinyl estradiol 50 mcg. Compact 21s. Pkg. 5 compacts. Pkg. 5 refills; Ctn. 10 × 5 refills. *Rx.*
Use: Contraceptive.

Norlestrin-21 2.5/50 Tablets. (Parke-Davis) Norethindrone acetate 2.5 mg, ethinyl estradiol 50 mcg. Tab. Compact 21s. Pkg. 5 compacts. Pkg. 5 refills; Ctn. 10 × 5 refills. *Rx.*
Use: Contraceptive.

Normaderm Cream & Lotion. (Doak Dermatologics) Buffered lactic acid in vanishing bases. **Cream:** Jar 3 ¾ oz, 16 oz. **Lot.:** Bot. 4 oz, 16 oz, 128 oz. *OTC.*
Use: Dermatologic, emollient.

normal human serum albumin. Albumin Human.

normal human serum albumin. (Baxter Healthcare) Normal human serum albumin. **5% Inj.:** 50 mL, 250 mL, 500 mL **25% Inj.:** 20 mL, 50 mL, 100 mL. *Rx.*
Use: Blood volume supporter.

Normaline. (Apothecary Prods.) Sodium chloride 250 mg. Tab. Bot. 200s, 500s. *OTC.*
Use: Ophthalmic.

normal saline.
See: Sodium Chloride 0.9%.

Normol. (Alcon) Sterile, isotonic solution of thimerosal 0.004%, chlorhexidine gluconate 0.005%, edetate disodium 0.1%. Bot. 8 oz. *OTC.*
Use: Contact lens care.

Normosol-M. (Abbott) Na+ 40 mEq, K+ 13 mEq, Mg++ 3 mEq, Cl- 40 mEq, acetate 16 mEq, osmolarity 10% mOsm/L, pH ≈ 6. Soln. Single-dose container 1000 mL. *Rx.*
Use: Intravenous nutritional therapy, intravenous replenishment solution.

Normosol-M and 5% Dextrose.
(Hospira) Dextrose 50 g, calories 170, Na+ 40 mEq, K+ 13 mEq, Mg++ 3 mEq, Cl- 40 mEq, acetate 16 mEq, osmolarity 363 mOsm/L. Soln. Bot. 500 mL, 1000 mL. *Rx.*
Use: Intravenous nutritional therapy, intravenous replenishment solution.

Normosol-R. (Hospira) Na+ 140 mEq, K+ 5 mEq, Mg++ 3 mEq, Cl- 98 mEq, acetate 27 mEq, gluconate 23 mEq, osmolarity 294 mOsm/L, preservative free, ph ≈ 6. Soln. Single-dose container 500 mL, 1000 mL. *Rx.*
Use: Intravenous nutritional therapy, intravenous replenishment solution.

Normosol-R and 5% Dextrose. (Abbott) Dextrose 50 g, calories 185, Na+ 140 mEq, K+ 5 mEq, Mg++ 3 mEq, Cl- 98 mEq, acetate 27 mEq, gluconate 23 mEq, osmolarity 547 mOsm/L. Soln. Bot. 500 mL, 1000 mL. *Rx.*
Use: Intravenous nutritional therapy, intravenous replenishment solution.

Normosol-R pH 7.4. (Abbott) Na+ 140 mEq, K+ 5 mEq, Mg++ 3 mEq, Cl- 98 mEq, acetate 27 mEq, gluconate 23 mEq, osmolarity 295 mOsm/L, preservative free. Soln. Single-dose container 500 mL, 1000 mL. *Rx.*
Use: Intravenous nutritional therapy, intravenous replenishment solution.

Normotensin. (Marcen) Mucopolysaccharide 20 mg, sodium nucleate 25 mg, epinephrine-neutralizing factor 25 units, sodium citrate 10 mg, inositol 5 mg, phenol 0.5%/mL. IM Soln. for

Inj. Multi-dose vial 10 mL, 30 mL. *Rx.*
Use: Antihypertensive.

Norolon. (Sanofi-Synthelabo) Chloroquine phosphate. *Rx.*
Use: Antimalarial.

Noroxin. (Merck & Co.) Norfloxacin 400 mg. Tab. 100s, UD 20s. *Rx.*
Use: Urinary anti-infective, fluoroquinolone.

Norpace. (Pharmacia) Disopyramide phosphate 100 mg, 150 mg, lactose. Cap. Bot. 100s, 1000s. *Rx.*
Use: Antiarrhythmic.

Norpace CR. (Pharmacia) Disopyramide phosphate 100 mg, 150 mg, sucrose. ER Cap. Bot. 100s, 500s, UD 100s. *Rx.*
Use: Antiarrhythmic.

Norphyl. (Vita Elixir) Aminophylline 100 mg. Tab. *Rx.*
Use: Bronchodilator.

Norpramin. (Sanofi Aventis) Desipramine hydrochloride 10 mg, 25 mg, 50 mg, 75 mg, 100 mg, 150 mg. Mannitol, sucrose. Film-coated. Tab. 50s (150 mg only), 100s (except 150 mg). *Rx.*
Use: Antidepressant.

Nor-QD. (Watson) Norethindrone 0.35 mg. Lactose. Tab. 28s. *Rx.*
Use: Sex hormone, contraceptive hormone.

Nortemps Children's. (Ballay) Acetaminophen 160 mg/5 mL. Alcohol free. Butylparaben, corn syrup, sorbitol. Cotton candy flavor. Oral Susp. 118 mL. *OTC.*
Use: Analgesic.

Northyx. (Centrix) Methimazole 5 mg, 10 mg, 15 mg, 20 mg. Lactose. Tab. 100s. *Rx.*
Use: Thyroid drug, antithyroid agent.

Nortrel 1/35. (Barr) Ethinyl estradiol 35 mcg, norethindrone 1 mg. Lactose. Tab. Pkt. 21s, 28s (7 inert tabs.). *Rx.*
Use: Sex hormone, contraceptive hormone.

Nortrel 0.5/35. (Barr) Ethinyl estradiol 35 mcg, norethindrone 0.5 mg. Lactose. Tab. Pkt. 21s, 28s (7 inert tabs.). *Rx.*
Use: Sex hormone, contraceptive hormone.

nortriptyline. (Various Mfr.) Nortriptyline 10 mg, 25 mg, 50 mg, 75 mg. Cap. 100s, 500s. *Rx.*
Use: Antidepressant.

•**nortriptyline hydrochloride.** (nor-TRIP-tih-leen) *USP 34.*
Use: Antidepressant.
See: Aventyl Hydrochloride Pulvules. Pamelor.

nortriptyline hydrochloride. (Various Mfr.). **Soln.:** Nortriptyline base 10 mg/ 5 mL. Alcohol 4%, sorbitol. Bot. 480 mL. **Cap.:** Nortriptyline hydrochloride 10 mg, 25 mg, 50 mg, 75 mg. Bot. 100s, 500s, 1,000s; blister pack 25s (except 75 mg), 100s, 600s; UD 100s (except 75 mg). *Rx.*
Use: Antidepressant.

Norval. Docusate sodium.
Use: Laxative.

Norvasc. (Pfizer) Amlodipine. **2.5 mg:** Bot. 90s, 100s; **5 mg:** Bot. 90s, 100s, 300s, UD 100s; **10 mg:** Bot. 90s, 100s, UD 100s. *Rx.*
Use: Calcium channel blocker.

Norvir. (Abbott) Ritonavir. **Soft Gel Cap.:** 100 mg. Bot. 30s, 120s. **Oral Soln.:** 80 mg/mL. Saccharin, ethanol, peppermint and caramel flavors. Bot. 240 mL. **Tab.:** 100 mg. Film coated. Sorbitan. 30s. *Rx.*
Use: Antiretroviral, protease inhibitor.

Norwich Extra Strength. (Lee) Aspirin 500 mg. Tab. Bot. 150s. *OTC.*
Use: Analgesic.

Norwich Regular Strength. (Lee) Aspirin 325 mg. Coated. Tab. 100s. *OTC.*
Use: Analgesic.

Nosalt. (GlaxoSmithKline) Potassium Cl, potassium bitartrate, adipic acid, mineral oil, fumaric acid. Na < 10 mg/5 g (0.43 mEq/5 g), K 2502 mg/5 g (64 mEq/5 g). Pkg. 330 g. *OTC.*
Use: Salt substitute.

Nosalt Seasoned. (GlaxoSmithKline) Potassium Cl, dextrose, onion, and garlic, spices, lactose, cream of tartar, paprika, silica, disodium inosinate, disodium guanylate, turmeric. Na < 5 mg/ 5 g (0.2 mEq/5 g), K 1328 mg/5 g (34 mEq/5 g). Pkg. 240 g. *OTC.*
Use: Salt substitute.

•**noscapine.** (NAHS-kah-peen) *USP 34.*
Use: Antitussive.

noscapine hydrochloride. l-Narcotine-hydrochloride.
Use: Antitussive.
See: Noscaps.

Noscaps. (Table Rock) Noscapine 7.5 mg, chlorpheniramine maleate 1 mg, phenylephrine hydrochloride 5 mg, N-acetyl-p-aminophenol 150 mg, salicylamide 150 mg, vitamin C 20 mg. Cap. Bot. 100s, 500s. *OTC.*
Use: Analgesic; antihistamine; decongestant; vitamin C.

Nose Better. (Oakhurst) Allantoin 0.5%, camphor 0.75%, menthol 0.5%. Lanolin, methylparaben. Gel. Tube 12.9 g. *OTC.*
Use: Upper respiratory combination, topical.

Noskote. (Schering-Plough) Oxybenzone
3%, homosalate 8%. SPF 8. Cream
13.2 g, 30 g. *OTC.*
Use: Sunscreen.
Noskote Sunblock. (Schering-Plough)
Padimate O 8%, oxybenzone 3%, benzyl alcohol. SPF 15. Cream. Tube
30 g. *OTC.*
Use: Sunscreen.
Nostril. (Boehringer Ingelheim) Phenylephrine hydrochloride 0.25%, 0.5%,
benzalkonium Cl 0.004% in buffered
aqueous soln. Bot. 15 mL, pump spray.
OTC.
Use: Decongestant.
**Nöstrilla Complete Congestion Relief
12-Hour.** (Insight) Oxymetazoline
hydrochloride 0.05%. Benzalkonium
chloride, camphor, edetate disodium,
eucalyptol, menthol. Soln., Intranasal
Spray. 15 mL. *OTC.*
Use: Nasal decongestant, imidazoline.
**Nöstrilla Conditioning Double Mois-
ture.** (Insight) Oxymetazoline hydrochloride 0.05%. Benzalkonium chloride,
eucalyptol, sodium chloride, spearmint
oil, winter green oil. Soln., Intranasal
Spray. 15 mL. *OTC.*
Use: Nasal decongestant, imidazoline.
Nöstrilla 12-Hour. (Insight) Oxymetazoline hydrochloride 0.05%, benzalkonium chloride, glycine, sorbitol. Soln.
Spray bot. 15 mL. *OTC.*
Use: Nasal decongestant, imidazoline.
Notuss-AC. (SJ Pharmaceuticals) Chlorpheniramine maleate 2 mg, codeine
phosphate 10 mg per 5 mL. Saccharin,
sorbitol. Alcohol, dye, sugar, and gluten free. Cotton candy flavor. Liq.
473 mL. *c-v.*
Use: Upper respiratory combination, antitussive and antihistamine.
Notuss-DC. (SJ Pharmaceuticals) Codeine phosphate 10 mg, pseudoephedrine hydrochloride 30 mg per 5 mL. Alcohol, dye, sugar, and gluten free.
Saccharin, sorbitol. Bubble gum flavor.
Liq. 473 mL. *c-v.*
Use: Upper respiratory combination, antitussive and decongestant.
Notuss-Forte. (SJ Pharmaceutical)
Chlorpheniramine maleate 4 mg,
hydrocodone bitartrate 5 mg, pseudoephedrine hydrochloride 40 mg. Saccharin, sorbitol. Alcohol free, dye free,
gluten free, and sugar free. Vanilla flavor. Syr. 473 mL. *c-iii.*
Use: Upper respiratory combination, antitussive combination.
Notuss NX. (SJ Pharmaceuticals) Chlorcyclizine hydrochloride 9.375 mg, co-

deine phosphate 10 mg. Glycerin, propylene glycol, saccharin, sorbitol. Alcohol
free, dye free, gluten free, and sugar free.
Cherry flavor. Liq. 473 mL. *c-v.*
Use: Upper respiratory combination, antitussive combination.
Notuss NXD. (SJ Pharmaceuticals)
Chlorcyclizine hydrochloride 9.375 mg,
codeine phosphate 10 mg, pseudoephedrine hydrochloride 30 mg. Glycerin, propylene glycol, saccharin,
sorbitol. Alcohol free, dye free, gluten
free, and sugar free. Berry vanilla flavor.
Liq. 473 mL. *c-v.*
Use: Upper respiratory combination, antitussive combination.
Notuss-PE. (SJ Pharmaceuticals) Codeine phosphate 10 mg, phenylephrine
hydrochloride 10 mg per 5 mL. Saccharin, sorbitol. Alcohol free, dye free,
gluten free, and sugar free. Cotton
candy flavor. Liq. 473 mL. *c-v.*
Use: Upper respiratory combinations,
antitussive combination.
Nouriva Repair. (Ferndale) Petrolatum,
paraffin, mineral oil, sorbitan oleate,
carnauba wax, ceramide 3, cholesterol,
glycerin, oleic acid, palmitic acid, acry-
lates/C 10–30 albyl acrylate crosspolymer, tromethamine. Cream. 30 g. *OTC.*
Use: Emollient.
Novacort. (Primus) Hydrocortisone acetate 2%, pramoxine 1%. Alcohols, aloe,
glycerin. Gel. Tubes. 29 g. *Rx.*
Use: Anti-inflammatory agent.
Nova-Dec. (Rugby) Iron 18 mg, vitamins
A 5000 units, D 400 units, E 30 units,
B_1 1.7 mg, B_2 2 mg, B_3 20 mg, B_5
10 mg, B_6 3 mg, B_{12} 6 mcg, C 60 mg,
folic acid 0.4 mg, Ca, Cr, Cu, I, Mg, Mo,
Mn, P, Se, K, Zn 15 mg, vitamin K, Cl,
Ni, Sn, V, B, biotin 30 mcg. Tab. Bot.
130s. *OTC.*
Use: Mineral, vitamin supplement.
Novadyne Expectorant. (Various Mfr.)
Pseudoephedrine 30 mg, codeine
phosphate 10 mg, guaifenesin 100 mg/
5 mL, alcohol 7.5%. Bot. 120 mL, pt,
gal. *c-iii.*
Use: Antitussive; decongestant; expec-
torant.
Novagest Expectorant with Codeine.
(Major) Pseudoephedrine hydrochlo-
ride 30 mg, codeine phosphate 10 mg,
guaifenesin 100 mg per 5 mL. Alco-
hol 8.2%, sugar, menthol, parabens.
Liq. Bot. 118 mL, 473 mL. *c-v.*
Use: Upper respiratory combination, an-
titussive, decongestant, expectorant.
Novahistine DH. (Deston Therapeutics)
Dihydrocodeine bitartrate 7.25 mg,

chlorpheniramine maleate 2 mg, phenylephrine hydrochloride 5 mg per 5 mL. Alcohol and sugar free. EDTA, parabens, saccharin, sorbitol. Strawberry flavor. Liq. 473 mL. *c-iii*.
Use: Antitussive combination.

novamidon.
See: Aminopyrine.

Novamine. (Clintec Nutrition) Amino acid concentration 11.4%, for infusion. Nitrogen 1.8 g/100 mL. Essential amino acids (mg/100 mL): Isoleucine 570, leucine 790, lysine 900, methionine 570, phenylalanine 790, threonine 570, tryptophan 190, valine 730. Nonessential amino acids (mg/100 mL): Alanine 1650, arginine 1120, histidine 680, proline 680, serine 450, tyrosine 30, glycine 790, glutamic acid 570, aspartic acid 330, acetate 114 mEq/L, sodium metabisulfite 30 mg/100 mL. In 250 mL, 500 mL, 1 liter. *Rx.*
Use: Parenteral nutritional supplement.

Novamine Without Electrolytes.
(Clintec Nutrition) Amino acid concentration 8.5%, for infusion. Nitrogen 1.35 g/100 mL. Essential amino acids (mg/100 mL): Isoleucine 420, leucine 590, lysine 673, methionine 420, phenylalanine 590, threonine 420, tryptophan 140, valine 550. Nonessential amino acids (mg/100 mL): Alanine 1240, arginine 840, histidine 500, proline 500, serine 340, tyrosine 20, glycine 590, glutamic acid 420, aspartic acid 250, acetate 88 mEq/L, sodium bisulfite 30 mg/100 mL. In 500 mL, 1 liter. *Rx.*
Use: Nutritional supplement, parenteral.

Novantrone. (Serono) Mitoxantrone hydrochloride 2 mg free base/mL, sodium chloride 0.8%, sodium acetate 0.005%, acetic acid 0.046%, preservative free. Inj. Multi-dose Vial 10 mL. *Rx.*
Use: Antineoplastic; immunologic agent, immunomodulator; anthracenedione.

Novarel. (Ferring) Chorionic gonadotropin 10,000 units per vial with 10 mL diluent (1,000 units per mL), mannitol, benzyl alcohol 0.9%. Pow. for Inj. Vials. 10 mL. *Rx.*
Use: Ovulation stimulant.

NovaSource Renal. (Novartis Nutrition) Protein (sodium and calcium caseinates, arginine, taurine, carnitine) 74 g, carbohydrates (corn syrup, fructose, hydrolyzed corn starch) 200 g, fat (high oleic sunflower oil, corn oil, medium chain triglycerides, soy lecithin) 100 g/

L, vitamins A, B_1, B_2, B_3, B_5, B_6, B_{12}, C, D, E, K, folic acid, biotin, choline, Ca chloride, Cu, Fe, I, Mg, Mn, P, Se, Zn, Na 1000 mg (43.5 mEq)/L, Na 1600 mg/complete feeding *Brik* Paks) (70 mEq)/L (closed system), K 810 mg (20.8 mEq)/L, K 1100 mg/complete feeding *Brik* Paks (28.2 mEq)/L (closed system), H_2O 700 mOsm/kg (complete feeding *Brik* Paks), H_2O 960 mOsm/kg (closed system), 2 cal/mL, vanilla flavor. Liq. *Tetra Brik* Paks 237 mL (27s), closed system containers 1000 mL (6s). *OTC.*
Use: Enteral nutritional therapy.

novatropine.
See: Homatropine Methylbromide.

Novocain. (Abbott) Procaine hydrochloride 1%, 10%. Inj. *Uni-Amp* 2 mL. Single-dose amp. 6 mL w/acetone sodium bisulfite (1% only). Multidose vial 30 mL w/acetone sodium bisulfite, chlorobutanol (1% only). *Rx.*
Use: Anesthetic, local ester.

Novocain for Spinal Anesthesia. (Sanofi-Synthelabo) Procaine hydrochloride 10% soln. Amp. 2 mL. Box 25s. *Rx.*
Use: Anesthetic, spinal.

Novolin N. (Novo Nordisk) Human insulin (rDNA) 100 units/mL. Inj. Vials. 10 mL. *OTC.*
Tall Man: NovoLIN
Use: Antidiabetic, insulin.

Novolin N PenFill. (Novo Nordisk) Human insulin (rDNA) 100 units/mL. Cartridges. 5 × 1.5. Use with *NovoPen* and *Novolin Pen. OTC.*
Tall Man: NovoLIN
Use: Antidiabetic, insulin.

Novolin N Prefilled. (Novo Nordisk) Human insulin (rDNA) 100 units/mL. Inj. Prefilled syringes. 5 × 1.5 mL. *OTC.*
Tall Man: NovoLIN
Use: Antidiabetic, insulin.

Novolin R. (Novo Nordisk) Human insulin (rDNA) 100 units/mL. Inj. Vials. 10 mL. *OTC.*
Tall Man: NovoLIN
Use: Antidiabetic, insulin.

Novolin R PenFill. (Novo Nordisk) Human insulin (rDNA) 100 units/mL. Cartridges. 5 × 1.5. Use with *NovoPen* and *Novolin Pen. OTC.*
Tall Man: NovoLIN
Use: Antidiabetic, insulin.

Novolin R Prefilled. (Novo Nordisk) Human insulin (rDNA) 100 units/mL. Inj. Prefilled syringes. 5 × 1.5 mL. *OTC.*
Tall Man: NovoLIN
Use: Antidiabetic, insulin.

Novolin 70/30. (Novo Nordisk) Human insulin (rDNA) 100 units/mL. Inj. Vials. 10 mL. *OTC.*
Tall Man: NovoLIN
Use: Antidiabetic, insulin.
Novolin 70/30 PenFill. (Novo Nordisk) Human insulin (rDNA) 100 units/mL. Cartridges. 5 × 1.5 mL. Use with *Novo-Pen* and *Novolin Pen. OTC.*
Tall Man: NovoLIN
Use: Antidiabetic, insulin.
Novolin 70/30 Prefilled. (Novo Nordisk) Human insulin (rDNA) 100 units/mL. Inj. Prefilled syringes. 5 × 1.5 mL. *OTC.*
Tall Man: NovoLIN
Use: Antidiabetic, insulin.
NovoLog. (Novo Nordisk) Human insulin aspart 100 units/mL. Metacresol 1.72 mg/mL. Inj. *PenFill* cartridges. 3 mL. Vials. 10 mL. *FlexPen* prefilled syringes. 3 mL. *Rx.*
Tall Man: NovoLOG
Use: Antidiabetic, insulin.
NovoSeven RT. (Novo Nordisk) Coagulation factor VIIa, recombinant 1 mg, 2 mg, 5 mg, 8 mg. Preservative free. Inj., lyophilized Pow. for Soln. Single-use vial w/histidine diluent. *Rx.*
Use: Hematological agent, antihemophilic agent.
Noxafil. (Schering Corporation) Posaconazole 40 mg/mL. Polysorbate 80, simethicone, sodium benzoate, xanthan gum, glucose. Cherry flavored. Susp., Oral. 105 mL with calibrated dosing spoon. *Rx.*
Use: Antifungal agent, triazole antifungal.
Noxzema Antiseptic Cleanser Sensitive Skin Formula. (Noxell Corp.) Benzalkonium Cl 0.13%. Bot. 4 oz, 8 oz. *OTC.*
Use: Dermatologic, cleanser.
Noxzema Antiseptic Skin Cleanser. (Noxell Corp.) SD 40 alcohol 63%. Bot. 4 oz, 8 oz. *OTC.*
Use: Dermatologic, cleanser.
Noxzema Antiseptic Skin Cleanser Extra Strength Formula. (Noxell Corp.) SD 40 alcohol 36%, isopropyl alcohol 34%. Bot. 4 oz, 8 oz. *OTC.*
Use: Dermatologic, cleanser.
Noxzema Clear Ups. (Noxell Corp.) Salicylic acid 0.5% on pads. Jar 50s. *OTC.*
Use: Dermatologic, acne.
Noxzema Clear Ups Acne Medicine Maximum Strength Lotion. (Noxell Corp.) Benzoyl peroxide 10%. Bot. 1 oz. Vanishing formula. *OTC.*
Use: Dermatologic, acne.

Noxzema Clear Ups Maximum Strength. (Noxell Corp.) Salicylic acid 2% on pads. Jar. 50s. *OTC.*
Use: Dermatologic, acne.
Noxzema Medicated Skin Cream. (Noxell Corp.) Menthol, camphor, clove oil, eucalyptus oil, phenol. Jar 2.5 oz, 4 oz, 6 oz, 10 oz. Tube 4.5 oz. Bot. 6 oz., 14 oz. Pump Bottle 10.5 oz. *OTC.*
Use: Counterirritant.
Noxzema On-The-Spot. (Noxell Corp.) Benzoyl peroxide 10% in vanishing and tinted lotion. Bot. 0.25 oz. *OTC.*
Use: Dermatologic, acne.
Nplate. (Amgen) Romiplostim 250 mcg, 500 mcg. Mannitol, sucrose, L-histidine, polysorbate 20. Preservative free. Inj., lyophilized Pow. for Soln. Single-use vial. 250 mcg, 500 mcg. *Rx.*
Use: Hematopoietic agent, thrombopoietin mimetic agent.
NP Thyroid. (Acella Pharmaceuticals) Thyroid dessicated (porcine derived) 30 mg (½ gr), 60 mg (1 gr), 90 mg (1 ½ gr). Dextrose, maltodextrin, mineral oil. Tab. 100s. *Rx.*
Use: Thyroid hormone.
N-Trifluoroacetyladriamycin-14-valerate. (Anthra) *Rx.*
Use: Antineoplastic.
NTS Transdermal System. (Circa) Nitroglycerin transdermal system 5 mg/24 hours or 15 mg/24 hours. Box 30s. *Rx.*
Use: Antianginal.
NTZ Long-Acting. (Sanofi-Synthelabo) Oxymetazoline hydrochloride 0.05%, benzalkonium Cl, phenylmercuric acetate 0.002% as preservatives. Drops. Bot. 1 oz. Spray Bot. 1 oz. *OTC.*
Use: Decongestant.
Nubain. (Endo) Nalbuphine hydrochloride 10 mg/mL, 20 mg/mL. Parabens. Amp (available as sulfite/paraben free) 1 mL. Vial 10 mL. *Rx.*
Use: Narcotic agonist-antagonist analgesic.
Nu-Bolic. (Seatrace) Nandrolone phenpropionate 25 mg/mL. Vial 5 mL. *c-III.*
Use: Anabolic steroid.
nucite.
See: Inositol.
nucleoside analog reverse transcriptase inhibitor combinations.
Use: Antiretroviral.
See: Abacavir/Lamivudine.
Emtricitabine/Tenofovir/Disoproxil Fumarate.
Lamivudine And Zidovudine.

nucleoside reverse transcriptase inhibitors.
Use: Antiretroviral.
See: Abacavir Sulfate.
  Didanosine.
  Emtricitabine.
  Lamivudine.
  Stavudine.
  Telbivudine.
  Zalcitabine.
  Zidovudine.
nucleotide analog reverse transcriptase inhibitor.
Use: Antiretroviral.
See: Tenofovir Disoproxil Fumarate.
Nucofed. (Monarch) Codeine phosphate 20 mg, pseudoephedrine hydrochloride 60 mg. Lactose. Cap. Bot. 60s. *c-III.*
Use: Upper respiratory combination, antitussive combination.
NuCort. (WraSer) Hydrocortisone acetate 2%. Aloe, benzyl alcohol, camphor, cetyl alcohol, glycerin, glyceryl stearate, PEG-7. Lot. 60 mL. *Rx.*
Use: Anti-inflammatory agent; corticosteroid, topical.
Nucotuss Expectorant. (Alpharma) Pseudoephedrine hydrochloride 60 mg, codeine phosphate 20 mg, guaifenesin 200 mg per 5 mL. Alcohol 12.5%. Syrup. Bot. 473 mL. *c-III.*
Use: Upper respiratory combination, antitussive, decongestant, expectorant.
Nucotuss Pediatric Expectorant. (Alpharma) Pseudoephedrine hydrochloride 30 mg, codeine phosphate 10 mg, guaifenesin 100 mg per 5 mL. Alcohol 6%, strawberry flavor. Syrup. Bot. 473 mL. *c-v.*
Use: Upper respiratory combination, antitussive, decongestant, expectorant.
Nucynta. (PriCara) Tapentadol hydrochloride 50 mg, 75 mg, 100 mg. Film coated. Lactose. Tab. 100s, UD 10s. *Rx.*
Use: CNS agent, opioid analgesic.
Nuedexta. (Avanir) Dextromethorphan hydrobromide 20 mg/quinidine sulfate 10 mg. Lactose. Cap. 60s. *Rx.*
Use: Psychotherapeutic combination.
•**nufenoxole.** (NEW-fen-OX-ole) USAN.
Use: Antiperistaltic.
Nuhist. (Dayton) Phenylephrine tannate 5 mg, chlorpheniramine tannate 4.5 mg per 5 mL. Methylparaben, saccharin, sucrose. Susp. 473 mL. *Rx.*
Use: Decongestant and antihistamine.
Nu-Iron 150. (Merz) Polysaccharide-iron complex equivalent to 150 mg iron. Parabens, EDTA, castor oil, sucrose. Cap. Bot. 100s. *OTC.*
Use: Mineral supplement.

Nu-Iron Plus Elixir. (Merz) Polysaccharide iron complex 300 mg, folic acid 3 mg, vitamin B_{12} 75 mcg/15 mL. Bot. 237 mL. *Rx.*
Use: Mineral, vitamin supplement.
Nu-Iron-V. (Merz) Polysaccharide iron 60 mg, folic acid 1 mg, vitamins A 4000 units, C 50 mg, D 400 units, B_1 3 mg, B_2 3 mg, B_3 10 mg, B_6 2 mg, B_{12} 3 mcg, Ca. Tab. Bot. 100s. *Rx.*
Use: Mineral, vitamin supplement.
Nulecit. (Watson Labs) Elemental iron 12.5 mg/mL (as sodium ferric gluconate complex). Benzyl alcohol 9 mg/mL, sucrose 20%. Inj., Soln. Vial. 5 mL. *Rx.*
Use: Trace element.
NuLev. (Schwarz Pharma) L-hyoscyamine sulfate 0.125 mg, aspartame, mannitol, phenylalanine 1.7 mg, mint flavor. Orally disintegrating tab. Bot. 100s. *Rx.*
Use: Anticholinergic/antispasmodic.
Nul-Tach. (Davis & Sly) Potassium 16 mg, magnesium 13 mg, ascorbic acid 250 mg. Tab. Bot. 100s. *Rx.*
Use: Antiarrhythmic.
NuLYTELY. (Braintree) PEG 3350 420 g, sodium bicarbonate 5.72 g, sodium chloride 11.2 g, potassium chloride 1.48 g, cherry, lemon-lime, orange flavors. Pow. for Recon. Disp. Jugs 4 L. *Rx.*
Use: Laxative.
Numby Stuff. (Iomed) Lidocaine hydrochloride 2% for iontophoretic dermal delivery. Epinephrine 1:100,000 per 30 mL multiple-unit fliptop vial. *Rx.*
Use: Topical local anesthetic, amide local anesthetic.
Numoisyn. (Align) **Loz.:** Sorbitol 0.3 g, polyethylene glycol, malic acid, sodium citrate, calcium phosphate dibasic, hydrogenated cottonseed oil, citric acid, magnesium stearate, silicon dioxide. 100s. **Susp.:** Sorbitol, linseed (flaxseed) extract, *Chondrus crispus*, parabens, sodium benzoate, potassium sorbate, dipotassium phosphate. 30 mL, 300 mL. *Rx.*
Use: Saliva substitute.
Numotizine Cataplasm. (Hobart) Guaiacol 0.26 g, beechwood creosote 1.302 g, methyl salicylate 0.26 g/100 g. Jar 4 oz. *OTC.*
Use: Analgesic, topical.
Numotizine Cough Syrup. (Hobart) Guaifenesin 5 g, ammonium Cl 5 g, sodium citrate 20 g, menthol 0.04 g/fl oz. Bot. 3 oz, pt, gal. *OTC.*
Use: Expectorant.
Nu-Natal Advanced. (Rising) Ca 200 mg, Fe (as carbonyl iron) 90 mg,

vitamin D 400 units, E 30 units, B_1 3 mg, B_2 3.4 mg, B_3 20 mg, B_6 20 mg, B_{12} 12 mcg, C 120 mg, FA 1 mg, CU 2 mg, Mg, dioctyl sodium sulfosuccinate 50 mg, Zn 25 mg. Mineral oil. Film-coated. Tab. UD 90s. *Rx.*
Use: Multivitamin.

nunol.
See: Phenobarbital.

NuOx. (Gentex) Benzoyl peroxide 6%, sulfur 3%. Benzyl alcohol, disodium EDTA, glycerin. Gel. 43 g. *Rx.*
Use: Acne product combination.

Nupercainal. (Ciba Consumer) Dibucaine 1%. Acetone, sodium bisulfite, lanolin, mineral oil, white petrolatum. Oint. 30 g, 60 g. *OTC.*
Use: Topical local anesthetic.

Nuquin HP. (Stratus) **Cream:** 4% hydroquinone, octyl methoxycinnamate, glycerin, cetyl alcohol, cetostearyl alcohol, stearyl alcohol, sodium metabisulfite. Tube 14.2 g, 28.4 g, 56.7 g. **Gel:** 4% hydroquinone, 30 mg dioxybenzone per g. Alcohol, sodium metabisulfite, EDTA. Tube 14.2 g, 28.4 g. *Rx.*
Use: Dermatologic.

Nu-Salt. (Cumberland Packing Corp.) Potassium Cl, potassium bitartrate, calcium silicate, natural flavor derived from yeast. Sodium 0.85 mg/5 g (< 0.04 mEq/5 g), potassium 2640 mg/5 g (68 mEq/5 g). Pkg. 90 g. *OTC.*
Use: Salt substitute.

Nu-Tears. (Optopics) Polyvinyl alcohol 1.4%, EDTA, NaCl, benzalkonium chloride, potassium chloride. Soln. Bot. 15 mL. *OTC.*
Use: Artificial tears.

Nu-Tears II. (Optopics) Polyvinyl alcohol 1%, PEG-400 1%, EDTA, benzalkonium chloride. Soln. Bot. 15 mL. *OTC.*
Use: Artificial tears.

Nu-Thera. (Kirkman) Vitamins A 10,000 units, D 400 units, B_1 10 mg, B_2 5 mg, niacinamide 100 mg, B_6 1 mg, B_{12} 5 mcg, C 150 mg, Ca 103 mg, P 80 mg, Fe 10 mg, Mg 5.5 mg, Mn 1 mg, K 5 mg, Zn 1.4 mg. Cap. Bot. 100s. *OTC.*
Use: Mineral, vitamin supplement.

nutmeg oil.
Use: Pharmaceutic aid, flavor.

Nutracort. (Galderma) Hydrocortisone 1%. Cream Jar 4 oz. Tube 30 g, 60 g. *Rx.*
Use: Corticosteroid, topical.

Nutraderm. (Galderma) Oil-in-water emulsion. **Lot.:** Plastic bot. 8 oz, 16 oz. **Cream:** Tube 1.5 oz, 3 oz, Jar lb. *OTC.*
Use: Emollient.

Nutraderm Bath Oil. (Galderma) Mineral oil, PEG-4 dilaurate, lanolin oil, butylparaben, benzophenone-3, fragrance, D & C Green No. 6. Bot. 8 oz. *OTC.*
Use: Emollient.

Nutraloric. (Nutraloric) A chocolate, vanilla, or strawberry flavored liquid containing, when mixed with whole milk to make 1 L, 91.7 g protein, 175 g carbohydrates, 125 g fat, 875 mg Na, 3166.7 mg, K 2.2 calories/mL. Pow. Can 480 g. *OTC.*
Use: Nutritional supplement.

Nutrament Drink Box. (Drackett) Protein 10 g, fat 7 g, carbohydrate 35 g, vitamins, minerals/240 calories/8 oz. Liq. Drink Box. *OTC.*
Use: Nutritional supplement.

Nutrament Liquid. (Mead Johnson Nutritionals) Protein (calcium and sodium caseinates, skim milk, soy protein isolates [in all flavors except chocolate]) 44.5 g, carbohydrate (sugar, corn syrup) 144.6 g, fat (canola oil, high oleic sunflower oil, corn oil, soy lecithin) 27.8 g/L, vitamins A, B_1, B_2, B_3, B_5, B_6, B_{12}, C, D, E, K, biotin, folate, Ca, Cr, Cu, Fe, I, Mg, Mn, Mo, P, Se, Zn, Na 695 mg, K 1390 mg/L, 1 cal/mL, vanilla, strawberry, chocolate, banana, coconut, and eggnog flavors. Liq. Can. 12 oz. *OTC.*
Use: Nutritional supplement.

Nutramigen. (Bristol-Myers Squibb) Hypoallergenic formula that supplies 640 calories/qt. Protein 18 g, fat 25 g, carbohydrates 86 g, vitamins A 2000 units, D 400 units, E 20 units, C 52 mg, folic acid 100 mcg, B_1 0.5 mg, B_2 0.6 mg, niacin 8 mg, B_6 0.4 mg, B_{12} 2 mcg, biotin 50 mcg, pantothenic acid 3 mg, K-1 100 mcg, Cl 85 mg, inositol 30 mg, Ca 600 mg, P 400 mg, I 45 mcg, Fe 12 mg, Mg 70 mg, Cu 0.6 mg, Zn 5 mg, Mn 200 mcg, Cl 550 mg, K 700 mg, Na 300 mg/qt of formula (4.9 oz pow.). Liq. Can 16 oz, 390 mL concentrate, 1 qt ready-to-use. *OTC.*
Use: Nutritional supplement.

Nutramin. (Thurston) Vitamins A 666 units, D 66 units, B_1 666 mcg, B_2 333 mcg, niacinamide 2 mg, folic acid 0.0444 mcg, Ca 16.6 mg, P 8.33 mg, Fe 1.33 mg, I 0.15 mg. Tab. Bot. 200s, 500s, 1000s. *OTC.*
Use: Mineral, vitamin supplement.

Nutramin Granular. (Thurston) Vitamins A 333 units, D 333 units, B_1 3.3 mg, B_2 1.6 mg, niacinamide 10 mg, folic acid 0.133 mg, Ca 250 mg, P 115 mg, Fe

6.6 mg, I 0.15 mg/5 g. Bot. 10 oz, 32 oz. OTC.
Use: Mineral, vitamin supplement.

Nutraplus. (Valeant) Urea 10% in emollient cream base or lotion base with preservatives. **Cream:** Tube 3 oz, Jar lb. **Lot.:** Bot. 8 oz, 16 oz. OTC.
Use: Emollient.

Nutra-Soothe. (Pertussin) Colloidal oatmeal, light mineral oil. Emollient bath preparation. Pow. Pkts. 9s. OTC.
Use: Dermatologic.

Nutravance. (Breckenridge) Vitamins A 3,000 units, B_1 20 mg, B_2 5 mg, B_3 25 mg, B_5 15 mg, B_6 25 mg, B_{12} 50 mcg, C 300 mg, D_3 400 units, E 100 units, Cr, Cu, Mg, Mn, Se, Zn, alpha-lipoic acid 15 mg, biotin 100 mcg, lutein 5 mg. Film coated. PEG. Tab. 100s. *Rx.*
Use: Multivitamin with minerals (except iron).

Nutravims. (Health for Life Brands) Vitamins A 6000 units, D 1250 units, C 50 mg, E 5 units, B_{12} 5 mcg, B_1 3 mg, B_2 3 mg, B_6 0.5 mg, niacinamide 20 mg, calcium pantothenate 5 mg, Zn 1.5 mg, Mn 1 mg, I 0.15 mg, K 5 mg, Mg 4 mg, Fe 15 mg, Ca 59 mg, P 45 mg. Cap. Bot. 100s, 250s, 1000s. OTC.
Use: Mineral, vitamin supplement.

Nutren 1.5 Liquid. (Clintec Nutrition) Casein, maltodextrin, corn syrup, sucrose, MCT, corn oil, vitamins A, B_1, B_2, B_3, B_5, B_6, B_{12}, C, D, E, K, folic acid, biotin, choline, Ca, Cl, Cu, Fe, I, Mg, Mn, P, Zn. 250 mL. OTC.
Use: Nutritional supplement.

Nutren 1.0 Liquid. (Clintec Nutrition) Potassium and sodium caseinate, maltodextrin, sucrose, MCT, corn oil, lecithin, vitamins A, B_1, B_2, B_3, B_5, B_6, B_{12}, C, D, E, K, folic acid, biotin, choline, Ca, Cl, Cu, Fe, I, Mg, Mn, P, Zn. Can 250 mL. OTC.
Use: Nutritional supplement.

Nutren 2.0 Liquid. (Nestle Nutrition) Biotin 800 mcg, calcium 1,340 mg, calories 2,000 kcal/L, carbohydrate 196 g, chloride 1,876 mg, choline 900 mg, chromium 80 mcg, copper 2.8 mg, fat 104 g, golic acid 1,080 mcg, iodine 200 mcg, iron 24 mg, L-carnitine 160 mg, magnesium 536 mg, manganese 5.2 mg, molybdenum 240 mcg, pantothenic acid 28 mg, phosphorus 1,340, potassium 1,920 mg, protein 80 g/L, selenium 80 mcg, sodium 1,300 mg, taurine 160 mg, vitamin A 6,400 units, vitamin B_1 4 mg, vitamin B_2 4.8 mg, vitamin B_3 56 mg, vitamin B_6

8 mg, vitamin B_{12} 16 mcg, vitamin C 280 mg, vitamin D 532 units, vitamin E 56 units, vitamin K 100 mcg, zinc 28 mg per L. Gluten and lactose free. Corn syrup, maltodextrin, sucrose. Liq. 1,000 mL. OTC.
Use: Nutritional supplement.

Nutr-E-Sol. (Advanced Nutritional Therapy) Vitamin E 798 IU per 30 mL. Sugar and dye free. Liq. 473 mL. OTC.
Use: Vitamin supplement.

Nutrex. (Holloway) Ca 162 mg, Fe 27 mg, vitamins A 5000 units, D 400 units, E 30 mg, B_1 2.25 mg, B_2 2.6 mg, B_3 20 mg, B_5 10 mg, B_6 3 mg, B_{12} 9 mcg, C 90 mg, folic acid 0.4 mg, Cu, I, K, Mg, Mn, P, Zn 22.5 mg, biotin 45 mcg. Tab. Bot. 100s. OTC.
Use: Mineral, vitamin supplement.

Nutricon Tablets. (Taylor Pharmaceuticals) Ca 200 mg, Fe 20 mg, vitamins A 2500 units, D 200 units, E 15 mg, B_1 1.5 mg, B_2 1.5 mg, B_3 10 mg, B_5 5 mg, B_6 2 mg, B_{12} 5 mcg, C 50 mg, folic acid 0.4 mg, Cu, I, Mg, Zn 3.75 mg, biotin 150 mcg. Bot. 120s. OTC.
Use: Mineral, vitamin supplement.

NutriDox. (Advanced Vision Research) Doxycycline 75 mg. Cap. 30s, blister 1s, and convenience kits with *TheraTears Nutrition* softgels and *iHeat* portable warm compress system. *Rx.*
Use: Anti-infective agent, tetracycline.

Nutri-E. (Nutri Vention) Vitamin E.
Cream: 200 units/g. Jar 1 oz, 2 oz. **Oil:** 1 oz. **Oint.:** 200 units/g. Tube 1 oz, 1.5 oz. **Cap.:** 200 units. Bot. 80s; 400 units. Bot. 60s, 100s; 800 units. Bot. 55s. OTC.
Use: Vitamin supplement.

Nutrifac ZX. (Rising Pharmaceuticals) Vitamin A 5000 units, D_3 400 units, E (succinate) 50 units, B_1 20 mg, B_2 20 mg, B_3 100 mg, B_5 25 mg, B_6 25 mg, B_{12} 50 mcg, C 500 mg, folic acid 1 mg, Zn 20 mg, Ca, Cr, Cu, Mg, Mn, Se, biotin 200 mcg, tartrazine, mineral oil. Tab. 60s. *Rx.*
Use: Multivitamin.

NutriFocus. (Ross) Protein (Na caseinate, milk protein isolate, soy protein isolate, arginine) 61.7 g, carbohydrate (corn syrup, sugar, fructooligosaccharides) 212.3 g, fat (canola oil, high-oleic safflower oil, corn oil, lecithin) 48.8 g/L, vitamins A, B_1, B_2, B_3, B_5, B_6, B_{12}, C, D, E, K, folic acid 417 mcg/L, beta carotene, biotin, choline, Ca, chloride, Cr, Cu, Fe, I, Mg, Mn, Mo, P, Se, Zn, Na 917 mg, K 1668 mg/L, fiber 20.85 g/L, 1.5 cal/mL, lactose and gluten free,

chocolate and vanilla flavors. Liq. Can. 240 mL. *OTC.*
Use: Enteral nutritional therapy.

NutriHeal. (Nestle) Protein 62.4 g, carbohydrate 112.8 g, fat 33.2 g, Na 876 mg/L, K 1248 mg/L, cal 1/mL. Vitamins A, B_1, B_2, B_3, B_5, B_6, B_{12}, C, D, E, K, beta carotene, biotin, chloride, choline, folic acid, Ca, Cr, Cu, Fe, I, Mg, Mn, Mo, P, Se, Zn. Vanilla flavor. Liq. Can. 250 mL. *OTC.*
Use: Nutritional supplement.

Nutrilan. (Elan) A vanilla, chocolate, or strawberry flavored liquid containing 38 g protein, 37 g fat, 143 g carbohydrates, 632.5 mg Na, 1.073 g K/L. With appropriate vitamins and minerals. In 237 mL *Tetra Pak* containers. *OTC.*
Use: Nutritional supplement.

Nutrilipid. (McGaw) Soybean oil intravenous fat emulsion. **10%:** Calories 1.1/mL. Bot. 250 mL, 500 mL. **20%:** Calories 2/mL. Bot. 250 mL, 500 mL. *Rx.*
Use: Nutritional supplement, parenteral.

Nutrilyte. (American Regent) Na^+ 25 mEq, K^+ ≈ 40 mEq, Ca^{++} 5 mEq, Mg^{++} 8 mEq, Cl^- ≈ 33 mEq, acetate ≈ 41 mEq, gluconate 5 mEq/20 mL, osmolarity ≈ 7562 mOsm/L. Conc. Soln. Single-dose vial 20 mL, pharmacy bulk pkg. 100 mL. *Rx.*
Use: Intravenous nutritional therapy, intravenous replenishment solution.

Nutrilyte II. (American Regent) Na^+ 35 mEq, K^+ 20 mEq, Ca^{++} 4.5 mEq, Mg^{++} 5 mEq, Cl^- 35 mEq, acetate 29.5 mEq/20 mL, osmolarity ≈ 6212 mOsm/L. Conc. Soln. Single-dose vial 20 mL, pharmacy bulk pkg. Vial 100 mL. *Rx.*
Use: Intravenous nutritional therapy, intravenous replenishment solution.

Nutri-Plex Tablets. (Faraday) Vitamins B_1 5 mg, B_2 5 mg, B_6 5 mg, pantothenic acid 25 mg, B_{12} 12.5 mcg, niacinamide 50 mg, iron gluconate 30 mg, choline bitartrate 50 mg, inositol 50 mg, PABA 15 mg, C 150 mg/2 Tab. Bot. 100s, 250s. *OTC.*
Use: Mineral, vitamin supplement.

Nutrisource Modular System. (Novartis) Individual Nutrisource modules available: protein, amino acids, amino acids (high branched chain), carbohydrate, lipid (medium chain triglycerides), lipid (long branched chain triglycerides), vitamins, minerals. Cans of liquid. Packets of powder. *OTC.*
Use: Nutritional supplement.

Nutri-Val. (Marcen) Vitamins A 5000 units, D 500 units, B_1 10 mg, B_2

5 mg, B_{12} activity 5 mcg, B_6 5 mcg, C 50 mg, hesperidin 5 mg, niacinamide 15 mg, folic acid 0.2 mg, calcium pantothenate 50 mg, choline bitartrate 50 mg, betaine hydrochloride 25 mg, lipo-K 0.4 mg, duodenum substance 50 mg, pancreas substance 50 mg, inositol 25 mg, Cy-yeast hydrolysates 50 mg, rutin 5 mg, l-lysine hydrochloride 5 mg, E 5 units, Ossonate (glucuronic complex) 8 mg, glutamic acid 30 mg, lecithin 5 mg, Fe 20 mg, I 0.15 mg, Ca 50 mg, P 40 mg, B 0.1 mg, Cu 1 mg, Mn 1 mg, Mg 1 mg, K 5 mg, Zn 0.5 mg, biotin 0.02 mg. Cap. Bot. 100s, 500s, 1000s. *OTC.*
Use: Mineral, vitamin supplement.

Nutri-Vite Natural Multiple Vitamin and Minerals. (Faraday) Vitamins A 15,000 units, D 400 units, B_1 1.5 mg, B_2 3 mg, B_{12} 15 mcg, niacin 500 mcg, B_6 20 mcg, choline 1.75 mg, folic acid 13 mcg, pantothenic acid 50 mcg, p-aminobenzoic acid 12 mcg, inositol 1.72 mg, C 60 mg, citrus bioflavonoids 15 mg, E 50 units, iron gluconate 15 mg, Ca 192 mg, P 85 mg, I 0.15 mg, red bone marrow 30 mg/3 Tab. Protein-coated Tab. Bot. 100s, 250s. *OTC.*
Use: Mineral, vitamin supplement.

Nutrizyme. (Enzyme Process) Vitamins A 5000 units, D 400 units, C 60 mg, B_1 1.5 mg, B_2 1.7 mg, niacinamide 20 mg, B_6 2 mg, pantothenate 10 mg, B_{12} 6 mcg, E 30 units, Fe 10 mg, Cu 1 mg, Zn 1 mg, Folac in 0.025 mg. Tab. Bot. 90s, 250s. *OTC.*
Use: Mineral, vitamin supplement.

Nutropin. (Genentech) Somatropin 5 mg (≈ 15 units)/vial, 10 mg (≈ 30 units)/vial. Pow. for Inj. (lyophilized). **5 mg:** Mannitol 45 mg, glycine 1.7 mg. w/multiple-dose vial of diluent (Bacteriostatic water for injection w/benzyl alcohol 0.9%). **10 mg:** Mannitol 90 mg, glycine 3.4 mg. w/multiple-dose vials of diluent (Bacteriostatic water for injection w/benzyl alcohol 0.9%). *Rx.*
Use: Hormone, growth.

Nutropin AQ. (Genentech) Somatropin 10 mg (≈ 30 units)/vial 20 mg (≈ 60 units)/cartridge. Sodium chloride 17.4 mg, phenol 5 mg, polysorbate 20 4 mg, sodium citrate 10 mM. Inj. 2 mL vials and pen cartridges (10 mg). 2 mL pen cartridges (20 mg). *Rx.*
Use: Hormone, growth.

Nutropin AQ NuSpin 5. (Genetech) Somatropin 5 mg (≈ 15 units)/mL. Sodium chloride 17.4 mg, phenol 5 mg, polysorbate 20 (4 mg), sodium citrate

10 mM. Inj., Soln. Multidose, prefilled injection device. Rx.
Use: Growth hormone.

Nutropin AQ NuSpin 10. (Genetech) Somatropin 10 mg (≈ 30 units)/vial or cartridge. Sodium chloride 17.4 mg, phenol 5 mg, polysorbate 20 (4 mg), sodium citrate 10 mM. Inj., Soln. Multidose prefilled injection device. Rx.
Use: Growth hormone.

Nutropin AQ NuSpin 20. (Genetech) Somatropin 20 mg (≈ 60 units)/cartridge. Sodium chloride 17.4 mg, phenol 5 mg, polysorbate 20 (4 mg), sodium citrate 10 mM. Inj., Soln. Multidose, prefilled injection device. Rx.
Use: Growth hormone.

Nutrox Capsules. (Tyson) Vitamins A 10,000 units, E 150 units, B_1 25 mg, B_2 25 mg, B_3 50 mg, B_5 22 mg, C 80 mg, l-cysteine, taurine, glutathione, zinc oxide 15 mg, Se. Cap. Bot. 90s. OTC.
Use: Mineral, vitamin supplement.

NuvaRing. (Organon) Etonogestrel 0.12 mg, ethinyl estradiol 2.7 mg/sachet. Box 1s, 3s. Rx.
Use: Sex hormone, contraceptive hormone.

Nuvigil. (Cephalon) Armodafinil 50 mg, 150 mg, 250 mg. Lactose. Tab. 60s. c-iv.
Use: Central nervous system stimulant, analeptic.

Nuzine Ointment. (Hobart) Guaiacol 1.66 g, oxyquinoline sulfate 0.42 g, zinc oxide 2.5 g, glycerine 1.66 g, lanum (anhydrous) 43.76 g, petrolatum 50 g/100 g. Tube 1 oz. OTC.
Use: Anorectal preparation.

NXY-059.
Use: Investigational neuroprotectant.

Nycoff. (Dover Pharmaceuticals) Dextromethorphan HBr. Tab. UD Box 500s. Sugar, lactose, and salt free. OTC.
Use: Antitussive.

Nyco-White. (Whiteworth Towne) Nystatin, neomycin, gramicidin, triamcinolone. Cream. Tube 15 g, 30 g, 60 g. Rx.
Use: Anti-infective, topical.

Nyco-Worth. (Whiteworth Towne) Nystatin. Cream. Tube 15 g. Rx.
Use: Antifungal, topical.

Nydrazid. (Apothecon) Isoniazid 100 mg/mL, chlorobutanol 0.25%. Inj. Vial 10 mL. Rx.
Use: Antituberculosal.

• **nylestriol.** (NYE-less-TRY-ole) USAN.
Use: Estrogen.

NyQuil.
See: Vicks NyQuil.

Nyral. (Pal-Pak, Inc.) Cetylpyridinium Cl 0.5 mg, benzocaine 5 mg/Loz. w/parabens. Pkg. 100s, 1000s. OTC.
Use: Antiseptic.

• **nystatin.** (nye-STAT-in) USP 34.
Use: Antifungal.
See: Mycostatin.
Nilstat.
Nystop.
Pedi-Dri.
W/Diphenhydramine Hydrochloride, Hydrocortisone.
See: First Duke's Mouthwash.
W/Diphenhydramine Hydrochloride, Hydrocortisone, Tetracycline Hydrochloride.
See: First Mary's Mouthwash.

nystatin. (Paddock) Nystatin 50 million units, 150 million units, 500 million units, 1 billion units, 2 billion units, 5 billion units. Rx.
Use: Antifungal.

nystatin. (Various Mfr.) Nystatin. **Susp.:** 100,000 units/mL. 5 mL, 60 mL, 480 mL. **Tab.:** 500,000 units. Bot. 100s. **Vaginal Tab.:** 100,000 units. Pkg. 15s, 30s w/applicator(s). Rx.
Use: Antifungal.

nystatin and triamcinolone acetonide.
Use: Antifungal; anti-infective; corticosteroid, topical.
See: Mycolog.

nystatin and triamcinolone acetonide cream.
Use: Antifungal; corticosteroid, topical.

nystatin and triamcinolone acetonide ointment.
Use: Antifungal; corticosteroid, topical.

Nystop. (Paddock) Nystatin 100,000 units/g. Dispersed in talc. Pow. 15 g, 30 g. Rx.
Use: Antifungal.

Ny-Tannic. (Allegis Pharmaceuticals) Phenylephrine tannate 25 mg, chlorpheniramine tannate 9 mg. Tab. 100s. Rx.
Use: Upper respiratory combination, decongestant and antihistamine.

Nytcold Medicine. (Rugby) Pseudoephedrine hydrochloride 10 mg, doxylamine succinate 1.25 mg, dextromethorphan HBr 5 mg, acetaminophen 167 mg, alcohol 25%, glucose, saccharin, sucrose, cherry flavor. Liq. Bot. 177 mL. OTC.
Use: Analgesic; antihistamine; antitussive; decongestant.

Nytime Cold Medicine. (Rugby) Acetaminophen 1000 mg, doxylamine succinate 7.5 mg, pseudoephedrine hydrochloride 60 mg, dextromethorphan HBr

30 mg/30 mL, alcohol 25%. Bot. 6 oz,
10 oz. *OTC.*
Use: Analgesic; antihistamine; antitussive; decongestant.

Nytol. (Block Drug) Diphenhydramine hydrochloride 25 mg. Tab. Bot. 16s, 32s, 72s. *OTC.*
Use: Sleep aid.

Nytol Maximum Strength. (Block Drug) Diphenhydramine hydrochloride 50 mg, lactose. Tab. Bot. 8s. *OTC.*
Use: Sleep aid.

O

O.A.D. (Sween) Ostomy. Bot. 1.25 oz, 4 oz, 8 oz. *OTC.*
Use: Deodorant; ostomy.

Oasis. (Zitar) Artificial saliva. Bot. 6 oz. *OTC.*
Use: Antixerostomia agent.

•**oatmeal, colloidal.** *USP 34.*
Use: Antipruritic, topical.
See: Aveeno.

•**obatoclax mesylate.** (oh-BAT-oh-klax) USAN.
Use: Antineoplastic.

OB Complete. (Vertical) Vitamin A 2100 units, vitamin D_3 315 units, vitamin E 20 units, vitamin B_1 2 mg, vitamin B_2 3.4 mg, vitamin B_3 10 mg, vitamin B_6 10 mg, vitamin B_{12} 15 mcg, vitamin C 120 mg, folic acid 1.25 mg, zinc 10 mg, copper 1 mg, magnesium 15 mg, iron 50 mg. Sugar free. Tab. UD 100s. *Rx.*
Use: Multivitamin with minerals.

OB Complete with DHA. (Vertical) Vitamin D_3 400 units, vitamin E 30 units, vitamin B_1 2 mg, vitamin B_2 3.4 mg, vitamin B_6 10 mg, vitamin B_{12} 15 mcg, vitamin C 120 mg, folic acid 1.25 mg, DHA 200 mg, zinc 25 mg, copper 1 mg, iron 28 mg. Softgel Cap. 60s. *Rx.*
Use: Multivitamin with minerals.

Obepar. (Tyler) Vitamins A 3000 units, D 300 units, B_1 3 mg, B_2 2 mg, nicotinamide 10 mg, B_6 3 mg, calcium pantothenate 2 mg, B_{12} 3 mcg, C 37.5 mg, Ca 150 mg, Fe 5 mg, Mg 1 mg, Mn 0.1 mg, K 1 mg, Zn 0.15 mg. Cap. Bot. 100s. *OTC.*
Use: Mineral, vitamin supplement.

•**obeticholic acid.** (oh-BET-i-KOL-ik) USAN.
Use: Treatment of primary biliary cirrhosis.

Obe-Tite. (Scot-Tussin) Phendimetrazine tartrate 35 mg. Tab. Bot. 100s, 500s. *c-III.*
Use: Anorexiant.

Obezine. (Western Research) Phendimetrazine tartrate 35 mg. Tab. *Handi count* 28 (36 bags of 28s). *c-III.*
Use: Anorexiant.

•**obidoxime chloride.** (OH-bih-DOX-eem) USAN.
Use: Cholinesterase reactivator.

•**oblimersen sodium.** (ob-li-MER-sen) USAN.
Use: Anticancer therapy.

Obrical. (Canright) Calcium lactate 500 mg, vitamins D 400 units, ferrous sulfate exsiccated 35 mg, B_1 1 mg, B_2 1 mg, C 10 mg. Tab. Bot. 100s, 1000s. *OTC.*
Use: Mineral, vitamin supplement.

Obrical-F. (Canright) Ferrous sulfate 50 mg, calcium lactate 500 mg, vitamins D 400 units, B_1 1 mg, B_2 1 mg, C 10 mg, folic acid 0.67 mg. Tab. Bot. 100s, 1000s. *OTC.*
Use: Mineral, vitamin supplement.

Obrite. (Milton Roy) Contact lens and eye glass cleaner. Plastic spray Bot. 30 mL, 55 mL. *OTC.*
Use: Contact lens and eye glass care.

Obstetrix-100. (Seyer) Ca 250 mg, Fe 100 mg, vitamin A 2700 units, D_3 400 units, E (as dl-alpha tocopheryl) 30 units, B_1 3 mg, B_2 3.4 mg, B_3 20 mg, B_6 20 mg, B_{12} 12 mcg, C 250 mg, folic acid 1 mg, Zn 25 mg, sodium docusate 50 mg. Tab. UD 30s. *Rx.*
Use: Vitamin, mineral supplement.

OB-Tinic. (Roberts) Fe 65 mg, vitamins A 6000 units, D 400 units, E 30 units, B_1 1.1 mg, B_2 1.8 mg, B_3 15 mg, B_6 2.5 mg, B_{12} 5 mcg, C 60 mg, folic acid 1 mg, Ca Tab. Bot. 100s. *Rx.*
Use: Mineral, vitamin supplement.

Obtrex. (Pronova) Vitamin A 2700 units, E 18 mg, C 120 mg, selenium 65 mcg, D_3 400 units, folic acid 1 mg, zinc 25 mg, B_1 3 mg, B_2 3.4 mg, B_3 20 mg, B_6 40 mg, B_{12} 2 mcg, magnesium 30 mg, sodium docusate 50 mg. Tab. 60s. *Rx.*
Use: Vitamin, mineral supplement.

O-Cal f.a. (bPharmics) Tab.: Ca 200 mg, Fe 66 mg, vitamins A 5000 units, D 400 units, E 30 mg, B_1 3 mg, B_2 3 mg, B_3 20 mg, B_6 4 mg, B_{12} 12 mcg, C 90 mg, folic acid 1 mg, fluoride 1.1 mg, Mg, I, Cu, Zn 15 mg. Bot. 100s. *Rx.*
Use: Mineral, vitamin supplement.

O-Cal Prenatal. (Pharmics) Ca 200 mg, Fe 15 mg, vitamin A 2500 units, D 400 units, E 30 units, B_1 1.5 mg, B_2 1.6 mg, B_3 17 mg, B_6 12 mg, B_{12} 12 mcg, C 70 mg, folic acid 1 mg, Zn 15 mg, Cu, I, Mg. Tab. Bot. 100s. *Rx.*
Use: Multivitamin.

•**ocaperidone.** (oke-ah-PURR-ih-dohn) USAN.
Use: Antipsychotic.

Occlusal HP. (Medicis) Salicylic acid 17%. Soln. Bot. 10 mL. *OTC.*
Use: Keratolytic.

Occucoat. (Bausch & Lomb) Hydroxypropyl methylcellulose 2%. Soln. Syringe 1 mL with cannula. *Rx.*
Use: Ophthalmic.

Ocean. (Fleming & Co.) Sodium Cl

0.65%, benzalkonium chloride. Soln. Spray Bot. 45 mL, 473 mL. *OTC.*
Use: Nasal decongestant.

Ocean for Kids. (Fleming) Sodium chloride 0.65%. Alcohol free. Benzalkonium chloride, EDTA, glycerin. Nasal spray. 37.5 mL. *OTC.*
Use: Nasal decongestant.

Ocean Plus. (Fleming & Co.) Caffeine 2.5%, benzyl alcohol. Soln. Bot. 15 mL. *OTC.*
Use: Moisturizer, nasal.

Ocella. (Barr Laboratories) Drospirenone 3 mg, ethinyl estradiol 30 mcg. Lactose. Film coated. Tab. Blister packs 28s, w/7 inert tablets. *Rx.*
Use: Oral contraceptive, monophasic contraceptive.

• **ocfentanil hydrochloride.** (ock-FEN-tah-NILL) USAN.
Use: Analgesic, narcotic.

• **ocinaplon.** (oh-SIN-ah-plahn) USAN.
Use: Anxiolytic.

OCL. (Abbott Hospital Products) Sodium Cl 146 mg, sodium bicarbonate 168 mg, sodium sulfate decahydrate 1.29 g, potassium Cl 75 mg, PEG 3350 6 g, polysorbate 80 30 mg/100 mL. Oral Soln. Bot. 1500 mL (3 pack). *Rx.*
Use: Laxative.

• **ocrelizumab.** (oh-kre-LIZ-oo-mab) USAN.
Use: Rheumatoid arthritis.

• **ocriplasmin.** (OK-ri-PLAS-min) USAN.
Use: Cardiovascular agent.

• **ocrylate.** (AH-krih-late) USAN.
Use: Surgical aid, tissue adhesive.

• **octabenzone.** (OCK-tah-BEN-zone) USAN.
Use: Ultraviolet screen.

octadecanoic acid.
See: Stearic Acid.

octadecanoic acid, sodium salt.
See: Sodium Stearate.

octadecanoic acid, zinc salt.
See: Zinc Stearate.

octadecanol-l.
See: Stearyl Alcohol.

octafluoropropane.
Use: Radiopaque agent.
See: Definity.

• **octanoic acid.** (OCK-tah-NO-ik) USAN.
Use: Antifungal.

octapeptide sequence.
Use: Antiviral.
See: Flumadine.

Octarex. (Health for Life Brands) Vitamins A 5000 units, D 1000 units, B_1 1.5 mg, B_2 2 mg, B_6 0.1 mg, calcium pantothenate 1 mg, niacinamide 20 mg,

C 37.5 mg, E 1 unit, B_{12} 1 mcg. Cap. Bot. 100s, 1000s. *OTC.*
Use: Mineral, vitamin supplement.

Octavims. (Health for Life Brands) Vitamins A 6000 units, D 1250 units, C 50 mg, E 5 units, B_1 3 mg, B_2 3 mg, B_6 0.5 mg, niacinamide 20 mg, calcium pantothenate 5 mg, B_{12} 5 mcg, Ca 59 mg, P 45 mg. Cap. Bot. 100s, 250s, 1000s. *OTC.*
Use: Mineral, vitamin supplement.

• **octazamide.** (OCK-TAY-zah-mide) USAN.
Use: Analgesic.

• **octenidine hydrochloride.** (OCK-TEN-ih-deen) USAN.
Use: Anti-infective, topical.

• **octenidine saccharin.** (OCK-TEN-ih-deen SACK-ah-rin) USAN.
Use: Dental plaque inhibitor.

• **octicizer.** (OCK-tih-SIGH-zer) USAN. Santicizer 141.
Use: Pharmaceutic aid, plasticizer.

• **octinoxate.** (ok-TIN-ox-ate) *USP 34. Formerly octylmethoxycinnamate.*
Use: Sunscreen.
W/Combinations.
See: Keri Age Defy & Protect.
Lubriderm Daily Moisture with SPF 15.
TI-Screen Sports.

• **octisalate.** (ok-ti-SAL-ate) *USP 34. Formerly octyl salicylate.*
Use: Sunscreen.
W/Combinations.
See: Lubriderm Daily Moisture with SPF 15.
Scar Cream Maximum Strength.
TI-Screen Sports.
W/Avobenzone, Homosalate, Octocrylene, Oxybenzone.
See: Neutrogena Ultra Sheer Dry-Touch Sunblock.

Octocaine. (Septodont) Lidocaine hydrochloride 2%, epinephrine 1:100,000, sodium bisulfite. Inj. Cartridge 1.8 mL. *Rx.*
Use: Anesthetic, local.

• **octocrylene.** (OCK-toe-KRIH-leen) *USP 34.*
Use: Ultraviolet screen.
W/Avobenzone, Ecamsule.
See: Anthelios SX.
UV Protective.
W/Avobenzone, Ecamsule, Titanium Dioxide.
See: Capital Soleil 20.
W/Avobenzone, Homosalate, Oxybenzone, Octisalate.
See: Neutrogena Ultra Sheer Dry-Touch Sunblock.

●**octodrine.** (OCK-toe-DREEN) USAN.
Under study.
Use: Adrenergic, vasoconstrictor; anesthetic, local.

●**octoxynol 9.** (ock-TOXE-ih-nahl 9)
NF 29.
Use: Pharmaceutic aid, surfactant.

OctreoScan. (Mallinckrodt) Pentetreotide
10 mcg, indium In 111 chloride sterile
solution. Kit. Vials. 10 mL. *Rx.*
Use: Radiopaque agent.

●**octreotide.** (ock-TREE-oh-tide) USAN.
Use: Antisecretory, gastric.

●**octreotide acetate.** (ock-TREE-oh-tide)
USAN.
Use: Somatostatin analog.
See: Sandostatin.
Sandostatin LAR Depot.

octreotide acetate. (Various Mfr.) Octreotide acetate 0.05 mg/mL, 0.1 mg/
mL, 0.2 mg/mL, 0.5 mg/mL, 1 mg/mL.
Inj. Single-dose vials. 1 mL (except
0.2 mg/mL and 1 mg/mL). Multi-dose
vials. 5 mL (0.2 mg/mL and 1 mg/mL
only). *Rx.*
Use: Somatostatin analog.

●**octreotide pamoate.** (ock-TREE-oh-tide
PAM-oh-ate) USAN.
Use: Antineoplastic.

●**octriptyline phosphate.** (ock-TRIP-tih-leen) USAN.
Use: Antidepressant.

●**octrizole.** (OCK-TRY-zole) USAN.
Use: Ultraviolet screen.

●**octyldodecanol.** (OK-til-doe-DEK-a-nole) *NF 29.*
Use: Pharmaceutic aid, oleaginous vehicle.

octyl methoxycinnamate.
See: Octinoxate.

octylphenoxy polyethoxyethanol. (Antara) A mono-ether of a polyethylene
glycol. Igepal CA 630.

octyl salicylate.
See: Octisalate.

Ocufen. (Allergan) Flurbiprofen sodium
0.03%. Polyvinyl alcohol 1.4%, thimerosal 0.005%, EDTA. Ophth. Soln.
Bot. 2.5 mL w/dropper. *Rx.*
Use: NSAID, ophthalmic.

●**ocufilcon A.** (OCK-you-FILL-kahn A)
USAN.
Use: Contact lens material, hydrophilic.

●**ocufilcon B.** (OCK-you-FILL-kahn B)
USAN.
Use: Contact lens material, hydrophilic.

●**ocufilcon C.** (OCK-you-FILL-kahn C)
USAN.
Use: Contact lens material, hydrophilic.

●**ocufilcon D.** (OCK-you-FILL-kahn D)
USAN.
Use: Contact lens material, hydrophilic.

●**ocufilcon E.** (OCK-you-FILL-kahn E)
USAN.
Use: Contact lens material, hydrophilic.

●**ocufilcon F.** (OCK-you-FILL-kahn F)
USAN.
Use: contact lens material, hydrophilic.

Ocuflox. (Allergan) Ofloxacin 3 mg/mL,
benzalkonium chloride 0.005%. Soln.
Bot. 1 mL, 5 mL, 10 mL. *Rx.*
Use: Anti-infective, ophthalmic.

ocular lubricants.
Use: Ophthalmic.
See: Akwa Tears.
Artificial Tears.
Dry Eyes.
Duolube.
Duratears Naturale.
Hypotears.
Lacri-Lube NP.
Lacri-Lube S.O.P.
Lipo-Tears.
LubriTears.
OcuCoat PF.
Puralube.
Refresh PM.
Systane Nighttime.
Tears Renewed.
Vit-A-Drops.

Ocu-Lube. (Bausch & Lomb) Petrolatum
sterile, preservative and lanolin free.
Oint. Tube 3.5 g. *OTC.*
Use: Lubricant, ophthalmic.

Ocumeter.
See: Decadron Phosphate.

OCuSOFT. (OCuSOFT) PEG-80 sorbitan
laurate, sodium trideceth sulfate, PEG-
150 distearate, cocoamidopropyl hydroxy-sultaine, lauroamphocarboxyglycinate, sodium laureth-13 carboxylate, PEG-15 tallow polyamine, quaternium-15. Alcohol
and dye free. Soln. Pads UD 30s, Bot.
30 mL, 120 mL, 240 mL, Compliance kit
(120 mL and 100 pads). *OTC.*
Use: Cleanser, ophthalmic.

OCuSOFT VMS. (OCuSOFT) Vitamins A
5000 units, E 30 units, C 60 mg, Cu,
Se, Zn 40 mg. Tab. Bot. 60s. *OTC.*
Use: Mineral, vitamin supplement.

Ocutricin. (Bausch & Lomb) Polymyxin
B sulfate 10,000 units, bacitracin zinc
400 units, neomycin sulfate 3.5 mg.
Oint. Tube 3.5 g. *Rx.*
Use: Antibiotic, ophthalmic.

Ocuvite. (Bausch & Lomb) Vitamins A
5000 units, E 30 units, C 60 mg, Zn
40 mg, Cu, Se 40 mcg. Tab. Bot. 120s.
OTC.
Use: Mineral, vitamin supplement.

Ocuvite Extra. (Bausch & Lomb) Vitamin A 1000 units, C 300 mg, E 100 units, Zn 40 mg, B_3 40 mg, B_2 3 mg, Cu, Se, Mn, l-glutathione, lutein 2 mg. Tab. Bot. 50s. *OTC.*
Use: Vitamin supplement.

Ocuvite Lutein. (Bausch & Lomb) Vitamin E 30 units, C 60 mg, Zn 15 mg, Cu, lutein 6 mg. Lactose. Cap. 36s. *OTC.*
Use: Mineral, vitamin supplement.

Ocuvite PreserVision. (Bausch & Lomb) Vitamin A 7160 units, E 100 units, C 113 mg, Zn 17.4 mg, Cu. Lactose. Tab. 120s. *OTC.*
Use: Mineral, vitamin supplement.

oestergon.
See: Estradiol.

Oesto-Mins. (Tyson) Ascorbic acid 500 mg, Ca 250 mg, Mg 250 mg, K 45 mg, vitamin D 100 units/4.5 g. Pow. Bot. 200 g. *OTC.*
Use: Vitamin supplement.

oestradiol.
See: Estradiol.

oestrasid.
See: Dienestrol.

oestrin.
See: Estrone.

oestroform.
See: Estrone.

•**ofatumumab.** (OH-fa-TUE-mue-mab) USAN.
Use: Antineoplastic.

OFF-Ezy Corn & Callous Remover. (Del) Salicylic acid 17% in a collodion-like vehicle of 65% ether and 21% alcohol. Kit. 13.5 mL with callous smoother and 3 corn cushions. *OTC.*
Use: Keratolytic.

OFF-Ezy Corn Remover. (Del) Salicylic acid 13.57%, inflexible collodion base, ether 65%, alcohol 21%. Liq. Bot. 0.45 oz. *OTC.*
Use: Keratolytic.

OFF-Ezy Wart Remover. (Del) Salicylic acid 17% in flexible collodion base, ether 65%, alcohol 21%. Liq. Bot. 13.5 mL. *OTC.*
Use: Keratolytic.

Ofirmev. (Cadence Pharmaceuticals) Acetaminophen 10 mg/mL. Mannitol. Inj., Soln. Single-use vial. 100 mL. *Rx.*
Use: Analgesic.

•**ofloxacin.** (oh-FLOX-uh-SIN) *USP 34.*
Use: Anti-infective.
See: Floxin.
Ocuflox.

ofloxacin. (Pacific Pharma) Ofloxacin 0.3% (3 mg/mL). Benzalkonium chloride 0.005%. Ophth. Soln. 5 mL, 10 mL. *Rx.*
Use: Otic antibiotic.

ofloxacin. (Various Mfr.) Ofloxacin.
Soln.: 0.3% (3 mg/mL). Benzalkonium chloride 0.005%. Dropper bot. 5 mL, 10 mL. **Tab.:** 200 mg, 300 mg, 400 mg. 50s (except 400 mg), 100s. *Rx.*
Use: Otic preparation; anti-infective.

•**ofornine.** (ah-FAR-neen) USAN.
Use: Antihypertensive.

Oforta. (Sanofi-Aventis) Fludarabine phosphate 10 mg. Film coated. Lactose. Tab. UD 15s, UD 20s. *Rx.*
Use: Antimetabolite, purine analog and related agent.

Ogestrel 0.5/50. (Watson) Norgestrel 0.5 mg, ethinyl estradiol 50 mcg. Lactose. Tab. Pack 28s with 7 inert tabs. *Rx.*
Use: Sex hormone, contraceptive hormone.

•**oglufanide disodium.** (oh-GLOO-fa-nide) USAN. Previously Glufanide disodium.
Use: Immunomodulator; angiogenesis inhibitor (Kaposi sarcoma).

Oilatum Soap. (GlaxoSmithKline) Polyunsaturated vegetable oil 7.5%. Bar 120 g, 240 g. *OTC.*
Use: Dermatologic, cleanser.

oil of camphor with combinations.
See: Sloan's Liniment.

Oil of Olay Daily UV Protectant. (Procter & Gamble) SPF 15. **Cream:** Titanium dioxide, ethylhexyl p-methoxycinnamate, 2-phenylbenzimidazole-5-sulfonic acid, glycerin, triethanolamine, imidazolidinyl urea, parabens, carbomer, PEG-10, EDTA, castor oil, tartrazine. Scented and unscented. 51 g. **Lot.:** Ethylhexyl p-methoxycinnamate, 2-phenylbenzimidazole-5-sulfonic acid, titanium dioxide, cetyl alcohol, imidazolidinyl urea, parabens, EDTA, castor oil, tartrazine. Bot. 105 g, 157.7 g. *OTC.*
Use: Sunscreen.

Oil of Olay Foaming Face Wash. (Procter & Gamble) Potassium cocoyl hydrolyzed collagen, glycerin, EDTA. Liq. Bot. 90 mL, 210 mL. *OTC.*
Use: Dermatologic, acne.

oil of pine with combinations.
See: Sloan's Liniment.

ointment and lotion base.
See: Hydrocerin.

ointment base, washable.
See: Cetaphil.
Velvachol.

•**ointment, bland lubricating ophthalmic.** *USP 34.*
Use: Lubricant, ophthalmic.

- **ointment, hydrophilic.** *USP 34.*
  Use: Pharmaceutic aid, oil-in-water emulsion ointment base.
- **ointment, rose water.** *USP 34.*
  Use: Pharmaceutic aid, emollient, ointment base.
- **ointment, white.** *USP 34.*
  Use: Pharmaceutical aid, oleaginous ointment base.
- **ointment, yellow.** *USP 34.*
  Use: Pharmaceutic aid, ointment base.
- **olaflur.** (OH-lah-flure) USAN.
  Use: Dental caries agent.
  olamine.
  See: Ethanolamine.
- **olanexidine hydrochloride.** (OH-lan-EX-i-deen) USAN.
  Use: Antimicrobial.
- **olanzapine.** (oh-LAN-zah-PEEN) USAN.
  Tall Man: OLANZapine
  Use: Antipsychotic, dibenzapine derivative.
  See: Zyprexa.
    Zyprexa Relprevv.
    Zyprexa Zydis.
  W/Fluoxetine Hydrochloride.
  See: Symbyax.
- **olaratumab.** (oh-LAR-a-TUE-mab) USAN.
  Use: Antineoplastic.
- **olcorolimus.** (OL-kor-OH-li-mus) USAN.
  Use: Inhibition of smooth muscle cell proliferation.
  old tuberculin.
  See: Mono-Vacc Test O.T.
    Tuberculin, Old, Tine Test.
  oleandomycin phosphate. Phosphate of an antibacterial substance produced by *Streptomyces antibioticus.*
  Use: Anti-infective.
  oleandomycin, triacetyl. Troleandomycin, USP.
- **oleic acid.** (oh-LAY-ik) *NF 29.*
  Use: Pharmaceutic aid, emulsion adjunct.
- **oleic acid I 131.** (oh-LAY-ik) USAN.
  Use: Radiopharmaceutical.
- **oleic acid I 125.** (oh-LAY-ik) USAN.
  Use: Radiopharmaceutical.
  oleovitamin A.
  See: Vitamin A.
- **oleovitamin A and D.** (OH-lee-oh-VYE-ta-min) *USP 34.*
  Use: Vitamin supplement.
  See: Super D Perles.
  oleovitamin D, synthetic.
  Use: Vitamin supplement.
  Oleptro. (Labopharm) Trazodone hydrochloride 150 mg, 300 mg. Film coated.

PEG. ER Tab. 30s, 90s, 500s, UD 30s. *Rx.*
Use: Antidepressant.
- **oleyl alcohol.** (oh-LAY-il) *NF 29.*
  Use: Pharmaceutic aid, emulsifying agent, emollient.
  See: Pataday.
    Patanol.
- **olive oil.** *NF 29.*
  Use: Emollient, pharmaceutic aid, setting retardant for dental cements.
- **olmesartan.** (ole-mih-SAR-tan) USAN.
  Use: Antihypertensive.
- **olmesartan medoxomil.** (ole-mih-SAR-tan meh-DOX-oh-mill) USAN.
  Use: Antihypertensive.
  See: Benicar.
  W/Amlodipine Besylate.
  See: Azor.
  W/Hydrochlorothiazide.
  See: Benicar HCT.
- **olopatadine hydrochloride.** (oh-low-pat-AD-een) USAN.
  Use: Antiallergic, allergic rhinitis, urticaria, allergic conjunctivitis, asthma.
  See: Pataday.
    Patanase.
    Patanol.
  olopatadine hydrochloride. (Alcon) Olopatadine hydrochloride 0.2%. Benzalkonium chloride 0.01%, EDTA, povidone, dibasic sodium phosphate, sodium chloride, hydrochloric acid/sodium hydroxide. Soln., Ophth. 2.5 mL fill in 4 mL bottle. *Rx.*
  Use: Ophthalmic antihistamine.
- **olsalazine sodium.** (OLE-SAL-uh-zeen) USAN. *Formerly Sodium azodisalicylate, azodisal sodium.*
  Use: Maintenance of remission of ulcerative colitis in patients intolerant of sulfasalazine; anti-inflammatory, gastrointestinal.
  See: Dipentum.
  Olux. (GlaxoSmithKline) Clobetasol propionate 0.05%, ethanol 60%, cetyl alcohol, stearyl alcohol. Foam. Can. 50 g, 100 g. *Rx.*
  Use: Anti-inflammatory.
  Olux-E. (GlaxoSmithKline) Clobetasol propionate 0.5 mg. Cetyl alcohol, light mineral oil, white petrolatum. Foam. 100 g. *Rx.*
  Use: Anti-inflammatory.
- **olvanil.** (OLE-van-ill) USAN.
  Use: Analgesic.
  Omacor. (Ross) Eicosapentanaenoic acid (EPA) 465 mg, docosahexaenoic acid (DHA) 375 mg, α-tocopherol 4 mg.

Cap. 120s. *Rx.*
Use: Dietary supplement.
●**omadacycline.** (oh-MAD-a-SYE-kleen)
USAN.
Use: Antibiotic.
●**omadacycline tosylate.** (oh-MAD-a-
SYE-kleen) USAN.
Use: Antibiotic.
●**omalizumab.** (oh-mah-lie-ZOO-mab)
USAN.
Use: Monoclonal antibody.
See: Xolair.
omapatrilat.
Use: Vasopeptidase inhibitor.
●**omecamtiv mecarbil.** (OM-e-KAM-tiv
me-KAR-bil) USAN.
Use: Cardiovascular agent.
Omega Oil. (Block Drug) Methyl nicotin-
ate, methyl salicylate, capsicum oleo-
resin, histamine dihydrochloride, isopro-
pyl alcohol 44%. Bot. 2.5 oz, 4.85 oz.
OTC.
Use: Analgesic, topical.
●**omega-3-acid ethyl esters.** USAN.
Use: Hypolipidemic.
Omega 3 Complex. (ChronoHealth) DHA
192 mg, EPA 251 mg, vitamin E 11 units
(as mixed tocopherols) Cap., softgels.
Unit of use 1s. *OTC.*
Use: Fish oil.
**omega-3 (n-3) polyunsaturated fatty
acids.** From cold water fish oils.
Use: Dietary supplement to reduce risk
of coronary artery disease.
See: Animi-3.
Cardi-Omega 3.
Lovaza.
Max EPA.
Omacor.
Promega.
Sea-Omega 50.
SuperEPA.
●**omeprazole.** (oh-MEH-pray-ZAHL)
USP 34.
Use: Proton pump inhibitor.
See: Prilosec.
Prilosec OTC.
W/Sodium Bicarbonate.
See: Zegerid.
Zegerid OTC.
omeprazole. (Various Mfr.) Omeprazole
10 mg, 20 mg, 40 mg. May contain lac-
tose, sucrose (40 mg). Enteric-coated
granules. DR Cap. 30s (except 40 mg),
100s, 1,000s (40 mg), UD 30s (40 mg).
Rx.
Use: Proton pump inhibitor.
●**omeprazole sodium.** (oh-MEH-pray-
ZOLE) USAN.
Use: Antisecretory, gastric.

omeprazole/sodium bicarbonate.
(Various Mfr.) Omeprazole/sodium bi-
carbonate. **Cap.:** 20 mg/1,100 mg,
40 mg/1,100 mg. 30s, 500s. **Pow. for
Susp.:** 20 mg/1,680 mg, 40 mg/
1,680 mg. Sucrose, sucralose, xylitol.
UD 30s. *Rx.*
Use: Proton pump inhibitor combina-
tion.
OM 401.
Use: Sickle cell disease. [Orphan Drug]
●**omiganan pentahydrochloride.** (oh-me-
GAN-an PEN-ta-HYE-droe-KLOR-ide)
USAN.
Use: Antimicrobial.
Omnaris. (Nycomed) Ciclesonide
50 mcg/actuation. Edetate sodium.
Spray Susp. Intranasal. 125 g glass bot.
(120 actuations) with metered-dose
pump with oxygen absorber sachet. *Rx.*
Use: Respiratory inhalant, intranasal
steroid.
Omnicef. (Abbott) **Cap.:** Cefdinir 300 mg.
Bot. 60s. **Oral Susp.:** 125 mg/5 mL,
250 mg/5 mL. Sucrose, strawberry flavor. Bot. 60 mL, 100 mL. *Rx.*
Use: Anti-infective, cephalosporin.
Omnicol. (Delta Pharmaceutical Group)
Dextromethorphan HBr 15 mg, chlorpheniramine maleate 4 mg, phenyl-
ephrine hydrochloride 5 mg, pheninda-
mine tartrate 4 mg, salicylamide
227 mg, acetaminophen 100 mg, caf-
feine alkaloid 10 mg, ascorbic acid
25 mg. Tab. Bot. 100s. *OTC.*
Use: Antitussive, antihistamine, decon-
gestant, analgesic.
Omnihemin. (Delta Pharmaceutical
Group) Fe 110 mg, vitamins C 150 mg,
B_{12} 7.5 mcg, folic acid 1 mg, Zn 1 mg,
Cu 1 mg, Mn 1 mg, Mg 1 mg. Tab. or
Soln. 5 mL. **Tab.:** Bot. 100s. **Soln.:** Bot.
Pt. *Rx.*
Use: Mineral, vitamin supplement.
OmniHIB. (GlaxoSmithKline) Purified
Haemophilus influenzae type b capsu-
lar polysaccharide 10 mcg, tetanus tox-
oid 24 mcg/0.5 mL, sucrose 8.5%.
Pow. for Inj. (lyophilized). Vial w/0.6 mL
syringe of diluent. *Rx.*
Use: Immunization.
OMNIhist II L.A. (Dexo Pharma) Phenyl-
ephrine hydrochloride 25 mg, chlor-
pheniramine maleate 8 mg, meth-
scopolamine nitrate 2.5 mg. Dye free.
Tab. Bot. 100s. *Rx.*
Use: Upper respiratory combination, an-
ticholinergic, antihistamine, decon-
gestant combination.
Omninatal. (Delta Pharmaceutical
Group) Fe 60 mg, Cu 2 mg, Zn 15 mg,

vitamins A 8000 units, D 400 units, C 90 mg, Ca 200 mg, folic acid 1.5 mg, B_1 2.5 mg, B_2 3 mg, niacinamide 20 mg, pyridoxine hydrochloride 10 mg, pantothenic acid 15 mg, B_{12} 8 mcg. Tab. Bot. 100s. *Rx.*
Use: Mineral, vitamin supplement.

Omnipaque 140. (Nycomed) Iohexol 302 mg equivalent to iodine 140 mg/mL. EDTA. Inj. Vials. 50 mL, Bot. *Rx.*
Use: Radiopaque agent, parenteral.

Omnipaque 300. (Nycomed) Iohexol 647 mg equivalent to iodine 300 mg/mL. EDTA. Inj. Vials. 10 mL, 30 mL, 50 mL. Bot. 50 mL. Flex. Cont. 100 mL, 150 mL. Prefilled Syringes. 50 mL. 75 mL fill in 100 mL Bot. 100 mL fill in 100 mL Bot. 125 mL fill in 200 mL Bot. 150 mL fill in 200 mL Bot. 125 mL fill in 150 mL Flex. Cont. *Rx.*
Use: Radiopaque agent, parenteral.

Omnipaque 350. (Nycomed) Iohexol 755 mg equivalent to iodine 350 mg/mL. EDTA. Inj. Vials. 50 mL. Bot. 50 mL. Flex. Cont. 100 mL, 150 mL, 200 mL. Prefilled Syringes. 50 mL. 75 mL fill in 100 mL Bot., 100 mL fill in 100 mL Bot., 125 mL fill in 200 mL Bot., 150 mL fill in 200 mL Bot., 200 mL fill in 200 mL Bot., 250 mL fill in 300 mL Bot., 125 mL fill in 150 mL Flex. Cont. *Rx.*
Use: Radiopaque agent, parenteral.

Omnipaque 240. (Nycomed) Iohexol 518 mg equivalent to iodine 240 mg/mL. EDTA. Inj. Vials. 10 mL, 20 mL, 50 mL. Bot. 50 mL. Flex. Cont. 100 mL, 150 mL, 200 mL. Prefilled Syringes. 50 mL. 100 mL fill in 100 mL Bot. 150 mL fill in 200 mL Bot. 200 mL fill in 200 mL Bot. *Rx.*
Use: Radiopaque agent, parenteral.

Omnipen. (Wyeth) **Cap.:** Ampicillin anhydrous 250 mg, 500 mg. Bot. 100s, 500s. **Pow. for Oral Susp.:** Ampicillin trihydrate 125 mg, 250 mg/5 mL when reconstituted. Pow. for Oral Susp. Bot. 100 mL, 150 mL, 200 mL. *Rx.*
Use: Anti-infective, penicillin.

Omnipen-N. (Wyeth) Ampicillin sodium 125 mg, 250 mg, 500 mg, 1 g, 2 g, 10 g. Pow. for Inj. Vial, Piggyback and *ADD-Vantage* vials (only 500 mg, 1 g, 2 g). *Rx.*
Use: Anti-infective, penicillin.

Omnipred. (Alcon) Prednisolone 1% (as acetate). Susp., Ophth. Drop-Tainer (with benzalkonium chloride 0.01%, EDTA, polysorbate 80, glycerin, hydroxypropyl methylcellulose). 5 mL, 10 mL. *Rx.*
Use: Ophthalmic and otic agent, corticosteroid.

Omniscan. (GE Healthcare) Gadodiamide 287 mg/mL. Preservative free. Inj. Soln. Vials. 5 mL, 10 mL, 20 mL, 50 mL. Prefilled Syringes. 10 mL, 15 mL, 20 mL. *Rx.*
Use: Radiopaque agent, parenteral.

Omnitabs. (Halsey Drug) Vitamins A 5000 units, D 400 units, C 50 mg, B_1 3 mg, B_2 2.5 mg, niacin 20 mg, B_6 1 mg, B_{12} 1 mcg, pantothenic acid 0.9 mg Tab. Bot. 100s. *OTC.*
Use: Vitamin supplement.

Omnitabs with Iron. (Halsey Drug) Vitamins A 5000 units, D 400 units, B_1 3 mg, B_2 2.5 mg, B_6 1 mg, B_{12} 1 mcg, C 50 mg, niacinamide 20 mg, calcium pantothenate 1 mg, Fe 15 mg. Tab. Bot. 100s. *OTC.*
Use: Mineral, vitamin supplement.

Omnitrope. (Sandoz) Somatropin. **1.5 mg (≈ 4.5 units):** Glycine 27.6 mg. Vials with diluent (sterile water for injection). Pow. for Inj., lyophilized. **5.8 mg (≈ 17.4 units):** Glycine 27.6 mg. Vials with diluent (bacteriostatic water for injection containing benzyl alcohol 1.5% as a preservative). Pow. for Inj., lyophilized. **5 mg/ mL:** Poloxamer 188 3 mg, mannitol 52.5 mg, benzyl alcohol. Inj., Soln. Cartridges. *Rx.*
Use: Growth hormone.

•**omoconazole nitrate.** (oh-moe-KAHN-ah-zole) USAN.
Use: Antifungal.

•**omtriptolide sodium.** (ohm-TRIP-toe-lide) USAN.
Use: Antineoplastic.

•**onabotulinumtoxinA.** (ON-a-bot-u-lin-um-tox-in-a) USAN.
Use: Botulinum toxin.
See: Botox.
 Botox Cosmetic.

•**onamelatucel-L.** (ON-a-MEL-a-TOO-sel) USAN.
Use: Antineoplastic.

•**onartuzumab.** (ON-ar-TOOZ-oo-mab) USAN.
Use: Treatment of cancer.

Oncaspar. (Enzon) Pegaspargase 750 units/mL. Preservative free. Inj. Single-use vials. *Rx.*
Use: Antineoplastic agent.

Oncet. (Wakefield) Hydrocodone bitartrate 5 mg, acetaminophen 500 mg. Cap. Bot. 100s. *c-III.*
Use: Analgesic; antitussive.

OncoRad ov103.
Use: Antineoplastic. [Orphan Drug]

Oncovin. (Eli Lilly) Vincristine sulfate for inj. 1 mg/mL, 2 mg/2 mL, or 5 mg/5 mL.

Soln. Ctn. 10s. Hyporets 1 mg/Pkg 3s; 2 mg/Pkg 3s. *Rx.*
Use: Antineoplastic.

Oncovite. (Mission Pharmacal) Vitamin A 10,000 units, C 500 mg, D_3 400 units, E 200 units, B_1 0.37 mg, B_2 0.5 mg, B_6 25 mg, B_{12} 1.5 mcg, folate 0.4 mg, Zn 7.5 mg, sugar. Tab. Bot. 120s. *OTC.*
Use: Vitamin supplement.

• **ondansetron.** (ahn-DAN-SEH-trahn) *USP 34.*
Use: Antiemetic/antivertigo agent, 5-HT_3 receptor antagonist.
See: Zofran ODT.
Zuplenz.

ondansetron. (Sandoz) Ondansetron 4 mg, 8 mg. Aspartame, mannitol, parabens, phenylalanine < 0.3 mg. Strawberry flavor. Tab., orally disintegrating. UD 10s (8 mg), UD 30s. *Rx.*
Use: Antiemetic/antivertigo agent, 5-HT_3 receptor antagonist.

• **ondansetron hydrochloride.** (ahn-DAN-SEH-trahn) *USAN.*
Use: Anxiolytic; antiemetic; antischizophrenic.
See: Zofran.

ondansetron hydrochloride. (Sandoz) Ondansetron hydrochloride 4 mg, 8 mg. Phenylalanine < 0.3 mg, aspartame, mannitol, parabens. Strawberry flavor. Orally Disintegrating Tab. UD 10s (8 mg only), UD 30s. *Rx.*
Use: Antiemetic/antivertigo agent.

ondansetron hydrochloride. (Various Mfr.) Ondansetron hydrochloride. **Inj.:** 2 mg/mL. May contain parabens. Sodium chloride. Single-dose and multidose vials. 32 mg/50 mL. Preservative free. Citric acid 26 mg, dextrose 2,500 mg, sodium citrate 11.5 mg. Single-dose containers. 50 mL. **Soln.:** 4 mg/5 mL. May contain saccharin, sorbitol. Strawberry flavor. 50 mL. **Tab.:** 4 mg, 8 mg, 16 mg, 24 mg. Polydextrose (16 mg only), lactose. Filmcoated. 30s, 100s (8 mg, 16 mg only), 500s, UD 1s (24 mg only), UD 3s (except 16 mg, 24 mg), UD 100s (except 16 mg), blister card 1s (16 mg only). *Rx.*
Use: Antiemetic/antivertigo agent.

ondansetron hydrochloride and dextrose. (Hospira) Ondansetron hydrochloride (as hydrochloride dihydrate) 32 mg per 50 mL. Preservative free. Dextrose 2500 mg, citric acid 26 mg, sodium citrate 11.5 mg. Inj. Single-dose flexible plastic containers. *Rx.*
Use: Antiemetic/antivertigo agent.

Ondrox. (LSI) Ca 50 mg, vitamins A 6000 units, D 300 units, E 50 units, B_1 0.75 mg, B_2 0.75 mg, B_3 10 mg, B_5 5 mg, B_6 1 mg, B_{12} 3 mcg, C 125 mg, folic acid 200 mcg, biotin 15 mcg, I, Mg, Cu, P, vitamin K, Cr, Mn, Mo, Se, V, B, Si, Zn 7.5 mg, inositol, citrus bioflavonoids, N-acetylcysteine, l-methionine, l-glutamine, taurine. Tab. Bot. 60s, 180s. *OTC.*
Use: Mineral, vitamins supplements.

One-A-Day Essential. (Bayer Consumer Care) Vitamins A 5000 units, E 30 units, C 60 mg, folic acid 0.4 mg, B_1 1.5 mg, B_2 1.7 mg, B_3 20 mg, B_6 2 mg, B_{12} 6 mcg, B_5 10 mg, D 400 units. Tab. Sodium free. Bot. 75s, 130s. *OTC.*
Use: Vitamin supplement.

One-A-Day Extras Antioxidant. (Bayer Consumer Care) Vitamin E 200 units, C 250 mg, A 5000 units, Zn 7.5 mg, Cu, Se, Mn, tartrazine. Softgel Cap. Bot. 50s. *OTC.*
Use: Vitamin supplement.

One-A-Day Extras Vitamin E. (Bayer Consumer Care) Vitamin E 400 units. Softgel Cap. Bot. 60s. *OTC.*
Use: Vitamin supplement.

One-A-Day 55 Plus. (Bayer Consumer Care) Vitamin A 6000 units, C 120 mg, B_1 4.5 mg, B_2 3.4 mg, B_3 20 mg, D 400 units, E 60 units, B_6 6 mg, folic acid 0.4 mg, biotin 30 mcg, B_5 20 mg, K 25 mcg, Ca 220 mg, I, Mg, Cu, Zn 15 mg, Cr, Se, Mo, Mn, K, Cl. Tab. Bot. 50s, 80s. *OTC.*
Use: Mineral, vitamin supplement.

One-A-Day Kids. (Bayer Consumer Care) Vitamin A 5000 units, C 60 mg, D 400 units, E 30 units, B_1 1.5 mg, B_2 1.7 mg, B_3 20 mg, B_5 10 mg, B_6 2 mg, B_{12} 6 mcg, folic acid 400 mcg, biotin 40 mcg, calcium 100 mg, iron 18 mg, phosphorus 100 mg, iodine 150 mcg, magnesium 20 mg, zinc 15 mg, copper 2 mg, sorbitol, aspartame, phenylalanine. Chew. Tab. 50s. *OTC.*
Use: Vitamin, mineral supplement.

One-A-Day Kids Scooby-Doo! Fizzy Vites. (Bayer Consumer Care) Ca 50 mg, Fe (as ferrous fumarate) 9 mg, vitamin A 1500 units, D 200 units, E 15 units, B_1 0.75 mg, B_2 0.85 mg, B_3 7.5 mg, B_5 5 mg, B_6 1 mg, B_{12} 3 mcg, C 170 mg, FA 200 mcg, biotin 20 mcg, P, I, Mg, Zn, Cu, Na. Aspartame, phenylalanine, sucrose, vegetable oil. Chew. Tab. 60s. *OTC.*
Use: Multivitamin.

One-A-Day Maximum Formula. (Bayer Consumer Care) Fe 18 mg, vitamins A 5000 units, D 400 units, E 30 units,

B_1 1.5 mg, B_2 1.7 mg, B_3 20 mg, B_5 10 mg, B_6 2 mg, B_{12} 6 mcg, C 60 mg, folic acid 0.4 mg, Ca, Cl, Cr, Cu, I, K, Mg, Mn, Mo, P, Se, Zn 15 mg, biotin 30 mcg. Tab. Bot. 60s, 100s. *OTC.*
Use: Mineral, vitamin supplement.
One-A-Day Men's Vitamins. (Bayer Consumer Care) Vitamin A 5000 units, C 200 mg, B_1 2.25 mg, B_2 2.55 mg, B_3 20 mg, D 400 units, E 45 units, B_6 3 mg, folic acid 0.4 mg, B_{12} 9 mcg, B_5 10 mg. Tab. Bot. 60s, 100s. *OTC.*
Use: Mineral, vitamin supplement.
One-A-Day Weight Smart. (Bayer Consumer Care) Ca 300 mg, Fe (as ferrous fumarate) 18 mg, vitamin A 2500 units, D 400 units, B_1 1.9 mg, B_2 2.125 mg, B_3 25 mg, B_5 12.5 mg, B_6 2.5 mg, B_{12} 7.5 mcg, FA 400 mcg, vitamin K, Mg, Zn, Se, Cu, Mn, Cr, EGCG, dextrose, glucose. Tab. 50s, 100s. *OTC.*
Use: Multivitamin.
One-A-Day Women's Formula. (Bayer Consumer Care) Ca 450 mg, Fe 27 mg, vitamins A 5000 units, D 400 units, E 30 mg, B_1 1.5 mg, B_2 1.7 mg, B_3 20 mg, B_5 10 mg, B_6 2 mg, B_{12} 6 mcg, C 60 mg, folic acid 0.4 mg, Zn 15 mg, tartrazine. Tab. Bot. 60s, 100s. *Rx.*
Use: Mineral, vitamin supplement.
One-Daily. (Geri-Care) Fe 18 mg, vitamin A 5,000 units, D 400 units, B_1 2 mg, B_2 2.5 mg, B_3 20 mg, B_5 1 mg, B_6 1 mg, B_{12} 1 mcg, C 50 mg. PEG. Tab. 100s, 1,000s. *OTC.*
Use: Multivitamin with minerals.
One-Daily Multi-Vitamin with Minerals. (Geri-Care) Vitamins A 5,000 units, C 50 mg, D 400 units, B_1 2 mg, B_2 2.5 mg, B_3 20 mg, B_5 1 mg, B_6 1 mg, B_{12} 1 mcg, Ca 19 mg, Fe 4.5 mg, P, I, Zn, Cr, Mn, Mg, Se. Mineral oil, sucrose. Tab. 100s. *OTC.*
Use: Multivitamin.
1+1-F Creme. (Oxypure) Clioquinol 3%, hydrocortisone 1%, pramoxine hydrochloride 1%. Tube 30 g. *Rx.*
Use: Corticosteroid; anesthetic, local; antifungal, topical.
•**onercept.** (O-ner-sept) USAN.
Use: Anti-tumor-necrosis factor activity.
One-Tablet-Daily. (Various Mfr.) Vitamins A 5000 units, D 400 units, E 30 mg, B_1 1.5 mg, B_2 1.7 mg, B_3 20 mg, B_5 10 mg, B_6 2 mg, B_{12} 6 mcg, C 60 mg, folic acid 0.4 mg. Tab. Bot. 30s, 100s, 250s, 365s, 1000s. *OTC.*
Use: Vitamin supplement.

One-Tablet-Daily Plus Iron. (Various Mfr.) Iron 18 mg, vitamins A 5000 units, D 400 units, E 15 mg, B_1 1.5 mg, B_2 1.7 mg, B_3 20 mg, B_6 2 mg, B_{12} 6 mcg, C 60 mg, folic acid 0.4 mg. Tab. Bot. 100s, 250s, 365s. *OTC.*
Use: Mineral, vitamin supplement.
One-Tablet-Daily with Iron. (Ivax) Fe 18 mg, A 5000 units, D 400 units, E 30 mg, B_1 1.5 mg, B_2 1.7 mg, B_3 20 mg, B_5 10 mg, B_6 2 mg, B_{12} 6 mcg, C 60 mg, folic acid 0.4 mg. Tab. Bot. 100s. *OTC.*
Use: Mineral, vitamin supplement.
One-Tablet-Daily with Minerals. (Ivax) Fe 18 mg, vitamins A 5000 units, D 400 units, E 30 units, B_1 1.5 mg, B_2 1.7 mg, B_3 20 mg, B_5 10 mg, B_6 2 mg, B_{12} 6 mcg, C 60 mg, folic acid 0.4 mg, Ca, Cl, Cr, Cu, I, K, Mg, Mn, Mo, P, Se, Zn 15 mg, biotin 30 mcg. Tab. Bot. 100s, 1000s. *OTC.*
Use: Mineral, vitamin supplement.
1000-BC, IM, or IV. (Solvay) Vitamins B_1 25 mg, B_2 2.5 mg, B_6 5 mg, panthenol 5 mg, B_{12} 500 mcg, niacinamide 75 mg, C 100 mg/mL. Vial 10 mL. *Rx.*
Use: Vitamin supplement.
1-2-3 Ointment No. 20. (Durel) Burow's solution, lanolin, zinc oxide (Lassar's paste). Jar oz, 1 lb, 6 lb. *OTC.*
Use: Anti-inflammatory, topical.
1-2-3 Ointment No. 21. (Durel) Burow's solution 1 part, lanolin 2, zinc oxide (Lassar's paste) 1.5 oz, cold cream 1.5 oz. Jar oz, 1 lb, 6 lb. *OTC.*
Use: Anti-inflammatory, topical.
Onglyza. (Bristol-Myers Squibb) Saxagliptin 2.5 mg (equiv. to saxagliptin hydrochloride 2.79 mg), 5 mg (equiv. to saxagliptin hydrochloride 5.58 mg). Film coated. Lactose. Tab. 30s, 90s, 500s (5 mg only), UD 100s (5 mg only). *Rx.*
Use: Antidiabetic agent, dipeptidyl peptidase-4 inhibitor.
•**onobotulinumtoxinA.** USAN.
Use: Botulinum Toxin.
See: Botox.
Botox Cosmetic.
Onoton Tablets. (Sanofi-Synthelabo) Pancreatin, hemicellulose, ox bile extracts. *OTC.*
Use: Digestive aid.
Onset Forte Micro-Coated. (Medique) Phenylephrine hydrochloride 5 mg, chlorpheniramine maleate 2 mg, acetaminophen 162.5 mg. Tab. 100s, 500s. *OTC.*
Use: Upper respiratory combination, decongestant, antihistamine, and analgesic.

• **onsifocon A.** (on-si-FOE-kon A) USAN.
Use: Hydrophobic.

Onsolis. (Meda Pharmaceuticals) Fentanyl citrate 200 mcg, 400 mcg, 600 mcg, 800 mcg, 1,200 mcg per film. Saccharin, parabens, peppermint oil. Film, soluble; buccal. Foil package. 30s. *c-II.*
Use: CNS agent, opioid analgesic.

Ontak. (EISAI) Denileukin diftitox 150 mcg/mL. Soln. for Inj, frozen, EDTA. Single-use vial. *Rx.*
Use: Antineoplastic; biological resonse modifier.

• **ontazolast.** (ahn-TAH-zoe-last) USAN.
Use: Antiasthmatic, leukotriene antagonist.

Ontosein.
See: Orgotein.

Onxol. (Zenith-Goldline) Paclitaxel 6 mg/mL, polyoxyl 35 castor oil 527 mg/mL, dehydrated alcohol 49.7%. Inj. Multidose vial 5 mL, 25 mL, 50 mL. *Rx.*
Use: Antimitotic agent; taxoid.

Opana. (Endo Pharmaceuticals) Oxymorphone hydrochloride. **Inj., Soln.:** 1 mg/mL. Amps. 1 mL. **Tab.:** 5 mg, 10 mg. Lactose. Tab. 100s, UD 100s. *c-II.*
Use: Opioid analgesic.

Opana ER. (Endo Pharmaceuticals) Oxymorphone hydrochloride 5 mg, 10 mg, 20 mg, 30 mg, 40 mg. Lactose (40 mg only), methylparaben. Film-coated. ER Tab. 100s, UD 100s. *c-II.*
Use: Opioid analgesic.

Opcon. (Bausch & Lomb) Naphazoline hydrochloride 0.1%. Soln. Bot. 15 mL. *OTC.*
Use: Mydriatic; vasoconstrictor.

Opcon-A. (Bausch & Lomb) 0.027% nephazoline hydrochloride, 0.315% pheniramine maleate, 0.5% hydroxypropyl methylcellulose, 0.01% benzalkonium chloride, 0.1% EDTA, NaCl, boric acid, sodium buffers. Soln. Bot. 15 mL. *OTC.*
Use: Mydriatic; vasoconstrictor; antihistamine.

o,p'-DDD.
Use: Miscellaneous antineoplastic.
See: Lysodren

• **opebacan.** (oh-PE-bay-kan) USAN.
Use: Antimicrobial

Operand. (Aplicare) **Aerosol:** Iodine 0.5%. 90 mL. **Skin cleanser:** Iodine 1%. 90 mL. **Oint.:** Iodine 1%. 30 g, lb, packette 1.2 g, 2.7 g. **Perineal wash conc.:** Iodine 1%. 240 mL. **Prep soln.:** Iodine 1%. 60 mL, 120 mL, 240 mL, pt, qt. **Soln:** Prep pad 100s, swab stick 25s. **Surgical scrub:** Povidone-iodine 7.5%. 60 mL, 120 mL, 240 mL, pt, qt, gal, packette 22.5 mL. **Whirlpool conc.:** Iodine 1%. Gal. *OTC.*
Use: Antiseptic; antimicrobial.

Operand Douche. (Aplicare) Povidone-iodine. Soln. Bot. 60 mL, 240 mL, UD 15 mL. *OTC.*
Use: Vaginal agent.

o-phenylphenol.
W/Amyl complex, phenylmercuric nitrate.
See: Lubraseptic Jelly.

Ophthacet. (Vortech Pharmaceuticals) Sodium sulfacetamide 10%. Soln. 15 mL. *Rx.*
Use: Anti-infective, ophthalmic.

ophthalmic agents.
See: Alocril.
  Nedocromil Sodium.
  Pemirolast Potassium.

ophthalmic and otic agents.
See: Corticosteroids.
  Cycloplegic Mydriatics.
  Mast Cell Stabilizers.
  Nonsteroidal Anti-inflammatory Agents.
  Ophthalmic Antibiotics.
  Ophthalmic Antihistamines.
  Ophthalmic Antiviral Agents.
  Ophthalmic Decongestants.
  Ophthalmic Hyperosmolar Preparations.
  Ophthalmic Nonsurgical Adjuncts.
  Steroid Antibiotic Combinations.

ophthalmic antibiotics.
See: Erythromycin.
  Gatifloxacin.
  Levofloxacin.
  Moxifloxacin Hydrochloride.

ophthalmic antihistamines.
See: Alcaftadine.
  Azelastine.
  Emedastine Difumarate.
  Epinastine Hydrochloride.
  Ketotifen.
  Olopatadine Hydrochloride.

ophthalmic decongestant agents.
See: Naphazoline Hydrochloride.
  Oxymetazoline Hydrochloride.
  Phenylephrine Hydrochloride.
  Tetrahydrozoline Hydrochloride.

ophthalmic diagnostic products.
See: Fluorexon.
  Indocyanine Green.
  Lissamine Green.
  Rose Bengal.
  Tear Test Strips.

ophthalmic hyperosmolar preparations.
See: Sodium Chloride, Hypertonic.

ophthalmic nonsurgical adjuncts.
See: SteriLid.

ophthalmic phototherapy.
See: Verteporfin.
ophthalmic surgical adjuncts.
See: Botox.
Botulinum Toxin Type A.
Hydroxypropyl Methylcellulose.
Sodium Hyaluronate.
Trypan Blue.
Ophtha P/S. (Edwards) Prednisolone
acetate 0.5%, sodium sulfacetamide
10%, hydroxyethyl cellulose, EDTA,
polysorbate 80, sodium thiosulfate,
benzalkonium chloride 0.025%. Susp.
Bot. 5 mL. *Rx.*
Use: Corticosteroid; anti-infective, ophthalmic.
Ophtha P/S Ophthalmic Suspension.
(Edwards) Sodium sulfacetamide 10%,
prednisolone acetate 0.5%. Bot. 5 mL
w/dropper. *Rx.*
Use: Corticosteroid; anti-infective, oph-
thalmic.
Ophthetic. (Allergan) Proparacaine
hydrochloride 0.5%. Benzalkonium
chloride 0.01%, glycerin, sodium chloride, hydrochloride acid and/or sodium
hydroxide. Bot. 15 mL. *Rx.*
Use: Anesthetic, ophthalmic.
opioid agonists-antagonist analgesics.
See: Buprenorphine.
opioid analgesic combinations.
See: Acetaminophen, Caffeine,
Dihydrocodeine Bitartrate.
Acetaminophen, Oxycodone Hydro-
chloride.
Butalbital, Aspirin, Caffeine with Co-
deine Phosphate.
Hydrocodone Bitartrate, Ibuprofen.
Meperidine Hydrochloride, Prometha-
zine Hydrochloride.
opioid analgesics.
See: Alfentanil Hydrochloride.
Codeine.
Fentanyl Citrate.
Fentanyl Transdermal System.
Hydromorphone Hydrochloride.
Levomethadyl Acetate Hydrochloride.
Levorphanol Tartrate.
Meperidine Hydrochloride.
Methadone Hydrochloride.
Morphine Sulfate.
Opium.
Oxycodone Hydrochloride.
Oxymorphone Hydrochloride.
Propoxyphene Hydrochloride.
Propoxyphene Napsylate.
Remifentanil Hydrochloride.
Sufentanil Citrate.
Tapentadol Hydrochloride.
Tramadol Hydrochloride.

•**opipramol hydrochloride.** (oh-PIH-prah-
mole) USAN.
Use: Antipsychotic; antidepressant;
tranquilizer.
•**opium.** (OH-pee-uhm) *USP 34.*
Use: Opioid analgesic; pharmaceutic
necessity for powdered opium.
See: Opium Tincture, Deodorized.
Paregoric.
opium and belladonna. (Wyeth) Powdered opium 60 mg, extract of belladonna 15 mg. Supp. Box 20s. *c-II.*
Use: Analgesic, narcotic; anticholinergic; antispasmodic.
•**opium powdered.** (OH-pee-uhm)
USP 34.
Use: Pharmaceutical necessity for Paregoric.
opium tincture, camphorated.
Use: Antidiarrheal.
See: Paregoric
opium tincture, deodorized. (Ranbaxy)
Anhydrous morphine equivalent to
10 mg/mL. Alcohol 19%. Liq. Bot.
120 mL, 473 mL. *c-II.*
Use: Opioid analgesic.
•**oprelvekin.** (oh-PRELL-veh-kin) USAN.
Use: Hematopoietic, interleukin.
See: Neumega.
Optase. (Onset Therapeutics) Balsam
peru 87 mg, castor oil 788 mg, trypsin 0.12 mg. Oleth 10, safflower oil. Gel.
6 g, 95 g. *Rx.*
Use: Topical enzyme combination.
Opti-Bon Eye Drops. (Barrows) Phenylephrine hydrochloride, berberine sulfate, boric acid, sodium Cl, sodium bisulfite, glycerin, camphor, water, peppermint water, thimerosal 0.004%. Bot.
1 oz. *OTC.*
Use: Ophthalmic.
Opticaps. (Health for Life Brands) Vitamins A 32,500 units, D 3250 units, B_1
15 mg, B_2 5 mg, B_6 0.5 mg, C 150 mg,
E 5 units, calcium pantothenate 3 mg,
niacinamide 150 mg, B_{12} 20 mcg, Fe
11.26 mg, choline bitartrate 30 mg, inositol 30 mg, pepsin 32.5 mg, diastase
32.5 mg, Ca 30 mg, P 25 mg, Mg
0.7 mg, Fr. dicalcium phosphate
110 mg, Mn 1.3 mg, K 0.68 mg, Zn
0.45 mg, hesperidin compound 25 mg,
biotin 20 mcg, brewer's yeast 50 mg,
wheat germ oil 20 mg, hydrolyzed yeast
81.25 mg, protein digest 47.04 mg,
amino acids 34.21 mg. Cap. Bot. 30s,
60s, 90s, 1000s. *OTC.*
Use: Mineral, vitamin supplement.
Opticare PMS. (Standard Drug Co.)
Fe 2.5 mg, vitamins 2083 units, D

17 units, E 14 units, B_1 4.2 mg, B_2 4.2 mg, B_3 4.2 mg, B_5 4.2 mg, B_6 50 mg, B_{12} 10.4 mcg, C 250 mg, folic acid 0.03 mg, Cr, Cu, I, K, Mg, Mn, Se, Zn 4.2 mg, biotin 10.4 mcg, choline bitartrate, bioflavonoids, inositol, PABA, rutin, Ca, amylase activity, protease activity, lipase activity, betaine, tartrazine. Bot. 150s. *OTC.*
Use: Mineral, vitamin supplement.

Opti-Clean II Especially For Sensitive Eyes. (Alcon) EDTA 0.1%, polyquaternium 1 0.001%, polymeric cleaners, Tween 21. Thimerosal free. Bot. 12 mL, 20 mL. *OTC.*
Use: Contact lens care.

Opti-Clear. (Major) Tetrahydrozoline hydrochloride 0.05%. Benzalkonium chloride 0.01%, boric acid, EDTA, sodium borate, sodium chloride. Ophth. Soln. 15 mL. *OTC.*
Use: Ophthalmic decongestant.

Opti-Free. (Alcon) Citrate buffer, sodium chloride, EDTA 0.05%, polyquaternium 1 0.001%. Soln. Bot. 10 mL, 20 mL. *OTC.*
Use: Contact lens rewetting solution.

Opti-Free Express Multi-Purpose. (Alcon) Isotonic. Myristamidopropyl dimethylamine 0.0005%, polyquaternium-1 0.001%, citrate, sodium chloride, boric acid, sorbitol, EDTA. Soln. 118 mL. *OTC.*
Use: Soft contact lens disinfection system.

Opti-Free Non-Hydrogen Peroxide-Containing System. (Alcon) Isotonic. Citrate buffer, NaCl, EDTA 0.05%, polyquaternium-1 0.001%. Thimerosal free. Soln. 118 mL, 237 mL, 355 mL. *OTC.*
Use: Contact lens disinfection system.

Opti-Free Surfactant Cleaning Solution. (Alcon) EDTA 0.01%, polyquaternium 1 0.001%, microclens polymeric cleaners, Tween 21. Thimerosal free. Soln. Bot. 12 mL, 20 mL. *OTC.*
Use: Contact lens care.

Optigene. (Pfeiffer) Sodium chloride, mono- and dibasic sodium phosphate, benzalkonium chloride, EDTA. Soln. Bot. 118 mL. *OTC.*
Use: Irrigant, ophthalmic.

Optigene 3. (Pfeiffer) Tetrahydrozoline hydrochloride 0.05%. Benzalkonium chloride 0.01%, boric acid, EDTA 0.1%, sodium borate. Ophth. Soln. Bot. 15 mL. *OTC.*
Use: Mydriatic, vasoconstrictor; ophthalmic decongestant.

Optilets-500. (Abbott) Vitamins B_1

15 mg, B_2 10 mg, B_3 100 mg, B_5 20 mg, B_6 5 mg, C 500 mg, A 10,000 units, D 400 units, E 30 units, B_{12} 12 mcg. Filmtab. Bot. 120s. *OTC.*
Use: Mineral, vitamin supplement.

Optilets-M-500. (Abbott) Vitamins C 500 mg, B_3 100 mg, B_5 20 mg, B_1 15 mg, A 5000 units, B_2 10 mg, B_6 5 mg, D 400 units, B_{12} 12 mcg, E 30 units, Fe 20 mg, Mg, Zn 1.5 mg, Cu, Mn, I. Filmtab. Bot. 120s. *OTC.*
Use: Mineral, vitamin supplement.

OptiMARK. (Mallinckrodt) Gadoversetamide 330.9 mg/mL. Calcium versetamide sodium 28.4 mg, calcium chloride dihydrate 0.7 mg per mL. Preservative free. Inj., Soln. Vials. 5 mL, 10 mL, 15 mL, 20 mL. Syringes. 10 mL, 15 mL, 20 mL, 30 mL. *Rx.*
Use: Radiopaque agent, parenteral.

Optimental. (Ross) Protein 12.2 g, fat 6.7 g, carbohydrate 32.9 g, vitamin A 1950 units, D 67 units, E 50 units, K 20 mcg, C 50 mg, folic acid 135 mcg, B_1 0.5 mg, B_2 0.57 mg, B_6 0.67 mg, B_{12} 2 mcg, B_3 6.7 mg, choline 100 mg, biotin 100 mcg, B_5 3.4 mg, Na 250 mg, K 420 mg, chloride 320 mg, Ca 250 mg, P 250 mg, Mg 100 mg, I 38 mcg, Mn 0.84 mg, Cu 0.34 mg, Zn 3.8 mg, Fe 3 mg, Se 12 mcg, Cr 20 mcg, Mo 25 mcg, sucrose, canola oil, soy oil. Liq. Bot. 237 mL. *OTC.*
Use: Nutritional therapy, enteral.

Optimine. (Key) Azatadine maleate 1 mg, lactose. Tab. Bot. 100s. *Rx.*
Use: Antihistamine, nonselective piperidine.

Optimox Prenatal. (Optimox) Ca 100 mg, iron 5 mg, vitamins A 833 units, D 67 units, E 2 mg, B_1 0.5 mg, B_2 0.6 mg, B_3 6.7 mg, B_5 3.3 mg, B_6 0.73 mg, B_{12} 0.87 mcg, C 30 mg, folic acid 0.13 mg, Cr, Cu, I, K, Mg, Mn, Se, Zn 3.17 mg. Tab. Bot. 360s. *OTC.*
Use: Mineral, vitamin supplement.

Optimyd. (Schering-Plough) Prednisolone phosphate 0.5%, sodium sulfacetamide 10%, sodium thiosulfate. Sterile Soln. Drop Bot. 5 mL. *Rx.*
Use: Anti-infective; corticosteroid; ophthalmic.

Optinate Omega-3 L-Vcaps. (First Horizon) **Cap.:** Docosahexaenoic acid 250 mg. Blister packs of 5s. **Tab.:** Calcium 200 mg, iron 90 mg, vitamin D_3 400 units, E 10 units, B_1 3 mg, B_2 3.4 mg, niacinamide 20 mg, B_6 20 mg, B_{12} 12 mcg, C 120 mg, folate 1 mg, biotin 30 mcg, pantothenic acid 6 mg, copper 2 mg, zinc 15 mg, magnesium

30 mg, docusate sodium 50 mg. Lactose, sucrose. Film-coated. Blister packs of 5s. *Rx.*
Use: Multivitamin.

Opti-One. (Alcon) EDTA 0.05%, polyquaternium-1 0.001%, sodium chloride, citrate buffer. Soln. 10 mL. *OTC.*
Use: Contact lens rewetting solution.

Opti-One Multi-Purpose. (Alcon) EDTA 0.05%, polyquaternium-1 0.001%, sodium choride. Buffered, isotonic. Soln. Bot. 118 mL, 237 mL, 355 mL, 473 mL. *OTC.*
Use: Contact lens care.

Opti-One Rewetting. (Alcon) EDTA 0.05%, polyquaternium 1 0.001%, sodium chloride, citrate buffer, isotonic. Drops. Bot. 10 mL. *OTC.*
Use: Contact lens care.

OptiPranolol. (Bausch & Lomb) Metipranolol hydrochloride 0.3%, benzalkonium chloride 0.004%, glycerin, EDTA, povidone, hydrochloric acid, sodium chloride, sodium hydroxide and/or hydrochloric acid. Soln. Bot. 5 mL, 10 mL w/dropper. *Rx.*
Use: Antiglaucoma agent; beta-adrenergic blocker.

Optiray 160. (Mallinckrodt) Ioversol 339 mg, iodine 160 mg/mL. EDTA. Inj. Bot. 50 mL, 100 mL. *Rx.*
Use: Radiopaque agent, parenteral.

Optiray 300. (Mallinckrodt) Ioversol 636 mg, iodine 300 mg/mL. EDTA. Inj. Bot. 50 mL, 100 mL, 150 mL. 200 mL fill in 250 mL Bot. Hand-held syringe. 50 mL. Power injector syringe. 100 mL fill in 125 mL. *Rx.*
Use: Radiopaque agent, parenteral.

Optiray 350. (Mallinckrodt) Ioversol 741 mg, iodine 350 mg/mL. EDTA. Inj. Bot. 50 mL, 100 mL, 150 mL. 75 mL fill in 100 mL Bot., 200 mL fill in 250 mL Bot. Hand-held syringes. 30 mL, 50 mL. Power injector syringes. 50 mL fill in 125 mL, 75 mL fill in 125 mL, 100 mL fill in 125 mL. Power Injector Syringes. 125 mL. *Rx.*
Use: Radiopaque agent, parenteral.

Optiray 320. (Mallinckrodt) Ioversol 678 mg, iodine 320 mg/mL. EDTA. Inj. Vials. 20 mL, 30 mL. Bot. 50 mL, 100 mL, 150 mL. 75 mL fill in 150 mL Bot. 200 mL fill in 250 mL Bot. Hand-held syringes. 30 mL, 50 mL. Power injector syringes. 50 mL fill in 125 mL, 75 mL fill in 125 mL, 100 mL fill in 125 mL Power injector syringes. 125 mL. *Rx.*
Use: Radiopaque agent, parenteral.

Optiray 240. (Mallinckrodt) Ioversol 509 mg, iodine 240 mg/mL. EDTA. Inj. Bot. 50 mL, 100 mL, 150 mL, 200 mL fill in 250 mL Bot. Hand-held syringes. 50 mL. Power injector syringes. 125 mL. *Rx.*
Use: Radiopaque agent, parenteral.

Opti-Soft Especially for Sensitive Eyes. (Alcon) Buffered, isotonic. EDTA 0.1%, polyquaternium 1 0.001%, NaCl, borate buffer. For lenses w/≤ 45% water content. Soln. Bot. 118 mL, 237 mL, 355 mL. *OTC.*
Use: Contact lens care.

Optison. (GE Healthcare) Perflutren 0.22 ± 0.11 mg/mL. Protein type A microspheres 5 to 8×10^8, albumin human 10 mg, N-acetyltryptophan 0.2 mg, caprylic acid 0.12 mg. Preservative free. Inj., Susp. Single-use vials. 3 mL. *Rx.*
Use: Radiopaque agent, parenteral agent.

Optivar. (MedPointe Healthcare) Azelastine hydrochloride 0.05%. Benzalkonium chloride 0.125 mg, EDTA, dihydrate, hydroxypropylmethylcellulose, sodium hydroxide. Soln., Ophth. 6 mL w/dropper. *Rx.*
Use: Ophthalmic antihistamine.

Optive. (Allergan) Carboxymethylcellulose sodium 0.5%, glycerin 0.9%. Ophth. Soln. 15 mL. *OTC.*
Use: Artificial tear solution.

Optivite for Women. (Optimox) Vitamins A 2083 units, D 16.7 units, E 14 mg, B_1 4.2 mg, B_2 4.2 mg, B_3 4.2 mg, B_5 4.2 mg, B_6 50 mg, B_{12} 10.4 mcg, C 250 mg, Fe 2.5 mg, folic acid 0.03 mg, Zn 4.2 mg, choline 52 mg, inositol 10 mg, Cr, Cu, I, K, Mg, Mn, Se, citrus bioflavonoids, PABA, rutin, pancreatin, biotin. Tab. Bot. 180s. *OTC.*
Use: Mineral, vitamin supplement.

Optivite P.M.T. (Optimox) Vitamins A 2083 units, D, E 16.7 mg, B_1 4.2 mg, B_2 4.2 mg, B_3 4.2 mg, B_5 4.2 mg, B_6 50 mg, B_{12} 10.4 mcg, C 250 mg, Fe 2.5 mg, FA 0.03 mg, Zn 4.2 mg, choline, Ca, Cr, Cu, I, K, Mg, Mn, Se, bioflavonoids, betaine, PABA, rutin, pancreatin, biotin, inositol. Tab. Bot. 180s. *OTC.*
Use: Mineral, vitamin supplement.

OptiZen. (InnoZen) Polysorbate 80 0.5%. EDTA, NaCl, sodium phosphate, sorbic acid. Drops. 10 mL. *OTC.*
Use: Artificial tears.

Orabase. (Colgate) Benzocaine 20%. Paste, Dental. 5 g. *OTC.*
Use: Local anesthetic, topical; ester local anesthetic.

Orabase-B. (Colgate) Benzocaine 20%, mineral oil. Paste. 5 g, 15 g. *OTC.*
Use: Mouth and throat preparation.
Orabase Baby. (Colgate) Benzocaine 7.5%, alcohol free, fruit flavor. Gel. Tube 7.2 mL. *OTC.*
Use: Anesthetic, local.
Orabase HCA. (Colgate) Hydrocortisone acetate 0.5%, polyethylene 5%, mineral oil. Gel. Tube 5 mL. *Rx.*
Use: Corticosteroid, dental.
Orabase Lip. (Colgate) Benzocaine 5%, allantoin 1.5%, menthol 0.5%, petrolatum, lanolin, parabens, camphor, phenol/g. Cream. Tube 10 g. *OTC.*
Use: Anesthetic, local.
Orabase Plain. (Colgate) Gelatin, pectin & sodium carboxymethyl cellulose in polyethylene and mineral gel. Paste. Tube 5 g, 15 g. *OTC.*
Use: Mouth and throat preparation.
Oracea. (Galderma) Doxycycline 40 mg (30 mg immediate release and 10 mg delayed release). Sugar spheres. Cap. 30s. *Rx.*
Use: Tetracycline, anti-infective.
Oracit. (Carolina Medical Products) Sodium citrate 490 mg, citric acid 640 mg/ 5 mL, (sodium 1 mEq/mL equivalent to 1 mEq bicarbonate), alcohol 0.25%. Soln. Bot. Pt, UD 15 mL, 30 mL. *Rx.*
Use: Alkalinizer, systemic.
Oraderm Lip Balm. (Schattner) Sodium phenolate, sodium tetraborate, phenol, base containing an anionic emulsifier. ⅛ oz. *OTC.*
Use: Anesthetic; antiseptic, local.
ORA5. (McHenry Laboratories, Inc.) Copper sulfate, iodine, potassium iodide, alcohol 1.5%. Liq. Bot. 3.75 mL, 30 mL. *OTC.*
Use: Mouth preparation.
ORAfix Special. (Hogil) Tube 1.4 oz, 2.4 oz. *OTC.*
Use: Denture adhesive.
ORAfix Ultra. (Hogil) Tube 3.2 oz. *OTC.*
Use: Denture adhesive.
Oragrafin Calcium Granules. (Bristol-Myers Squibb) Ipodate calcium (61.7% iodine) 3 g/8 g Pkg. 25 × 1 dose pkg.
Use: Radiopaque agent.
Orahesive. (Colgate Oral) Gelatin, pectin, sodium carboxymethylcellulose. Pow. Bot. 25 g. *OTC.*
Use: Denture adhesive.
Orajel. (Del) Benzocaine 10% in a special base. Gel. Tube 0.2 oz, 0.5 oz. *OTC.*
Use: Anesthetic, local.
Orajel D. (Del) Benzocaine 10%, saccharin. Gel. Tube 9.45 mL. *OTC.*
Use: Anesthetic, local.

Orajel Mouth-Aid. (Del) Benzocaine 20%. **Liq.:** Cetylpyridinium chloride 0.1%, ethyl alcohol 70%, tartrazine, saccharin, 13.5 mL. **Gel:** Benzalkonium chloride 0.02%, zinc Cl 0.1%, EDTA, saccharin. 5.6 g, 10 g. *OTC.*
Use: Topical local anesthetic.
Orajel Perioseptic. (Del) Carbamide peroxide 15%, saccharin, methylparaben, EDTA, sorbitol, ethyl alcohol. Liq. Bot. 240 mL. *OTC.*
Use: Mouth and throat product.
Orajel P.M. Nighttime Formula Toothache Pain Relief. (Del) Benzocaine 20%, menthol, methyl salicylate, saccharin. Cream. 5.4 g. *OTC.*
Use: Mouth and throat product.
Orajel Regular Strength. (Church Dwight) Benzocaine 10%. PEG, saccharin. Gel. 5.1 g, 7.1 g, 9.4 g. *OTC.*
Use: Topical local anesthetic, ester local anesthetic.
Oral-B Muppets Fluoride Toothpaste. (Oral-B) Fluoride 0.22%. Pump 4.3 oz. *OTC.*
Use: Dental caries agent.
oral contraceptives.
See: Alesse.
Apri.
Aviane.
Beyaz.
Brevicon.
Caziant.
Desogen.
Enovid-E 21.
Estrostep Fe.
GenCept.
Gianvi.
Heather.
Jenest-28.
Levlen.
Levlite.
Levora.
Loestrin 21 1/20.
Loestrin 21 1.5/30.
Loestrin Fe 1/20.
Loestrin Fe 1.5/30.
Lo/Ovral.
Low-Ogestrel.
Microgestin Fe 1/20.
Microgestin Fe 1.5/30.
Micronor.
Mircette.
Modicon.
MonoNessa.
Necon 0.5/35.
Necon 1/35.
Necon 1/50.
Necon 10/11.
Nelulen.
Nordette.

Norinyl 1+35.
Norinyl 1+50.
Nor-QD.
Nortrel 0.5/35.
Nortrel 1/35.
Ocella.
Ogestrel 0.5/50.
Ortho Cept.
Ortho-Cyclen.
Ortho-Novum 1/35.
Ortho-Novum 1/50.
Ortho-Novum 7/7/7.
Ortho-Novum 10/11.
Ortho Tri-Cyclen.
Ovcon-35.
Ovcon-50.
Ovral.
Ovulen-21.
Ovulen-28.
Plan B.
Preven.
Seasonale.
Seasonique.
Tri-Levlen.
Tri-Norinyl.
Triphasil.
Trivora.
Yasmin.
Zovia 1/35E.
Zovia 1/50E.

Oral Drops/Canker Sore Relief. (Weeks & Leo) Carbamide peroxide 10% in anhydrous glycerin base. Bot. 30 mL. *OTC.*
Use: Mouth preparation.

oral rehydration salts.
Use: Electrolyte combination.

Oral Wound Rinse. (Carrington) Acemannan hydrogel. Fructose. Mouthwash. 7.4 g. *OTC.*
Use: Mouth and throat product.

OraMagic Plus. (MPM Medical) Benzocaine 10%. Maltodextrin, xylitol. Oral Rinse. 60 mL, 210 mL. *OTC.*
Use: Mouth and throat product.

OraMagicRx. (MPM Medical) *AloemannonPlus* (high molecular weight complex carbohydrates, mannons, and low molecular weight constituents extracted from aloe vera), citric acid, lemon/lime flavor, maltodextrin, potassium benzoate, potassium sorbate, xanthan, xylitol. Alcohol free. Pow. for Oral Rinse. 25 g, 37.5 g. *Rx.*
Use: Mouth and throat product.

Oramide. (Major) Tolbutamide 0.5 g. Tab. Bot. 100s, 1000s. *Rx.*
Use: Antidiabetic.

Oraminic II. (Vortech Pharmaceuticals) Brompheniramine maleate 10 mg/mL. Inj. Vial. 10 mL multidose. *Rx.*
Use: Antihistamine.

Oramorph SR. (AAIPharma) Morphine sulfate 15 mg, 30 mg, 60 mg, 100 mg (for use only in opioid-tolerant patients). Lactose. CR Tab. Bot. 50s (30 mg only), 100s, 250s (30 mg only), 500s (15 mg only), UD 25s (60 mg and 100 mg only), UD 100s (15 mg and 30 mg only). *c-II.*
Use: Opioid analgesic.

orange flower oil.
Use: Flavor; perfume; vehicle.

orange flower water.
Use: Flavor; perfume.

•**orange oil.** *NF 29.*
Use: Flavor.

•**orange peel tincture, sweet.** *NF 29.*
Use: Flavor.

•**orange spirit, compound.** *NF 29.*
Use: Flavor.

•**orange syrup.** *NF 29.*
Use: Flavored vehicle.

Orap. (Teva) Pimozide 1 mg, 2 mg, lactose. Tab. Bot. 100s. *Rx.*
Use: Antipsychotic.

Orapred. (Sciele) Prednisolone 15 mg (equiv. to prednisolone sodium phosphate 20.2 mg)/5 mL. Dye free, alcohol 2%, fructose, monammonium glycyrrhizinate, sorbitol, grape flavor. Oral Soln. Bot. 20 mL, 237 mL. *Rx.*
Use: Adrenocortical steroid, glucocorticoid.

Orapred ODT. (Sciele) Prednisolone 10 mg (equiv. to prednisolone sodium phosphate 13.4 mg), 15 mg (equiv. to prednisolone sodium phosphate 20.2 mg), 30 mg (equiv. to prednisolone sodium phosphate 40.3 mg). Mannitol, sucralose, sucrose. Grape flavor. Orally Disintegrating Tab. UD 48s. *Rx.*
Use: Andrenocortical steroid, glucocorticoid.

Oraqix. (Dentsply Pharmaceutical) Lidocaine 2.5%, prilocaine 2.5%. Gel. Single-use cartridge w/applicator 20s. 1.7 g. *Rx.*
Use: Topical local anesthetic combination.

OraQuick Advance Rapid HIV-1/2 Antibody Test. (OraSure Technologies) Collection kit: Test device, absorbent packet, developer solution vial, test stands, and specimen collection loops for 25 or 100 tests. Device for in vitro immunoassay. For professional use only.
Use: Diagnostic aid.

Orasept. (Pharmakon) Tannic acid 12.16%, methyl benzethonium hydrochloride 1.53%, ethyl alcohol 53.31%,

camphor, menthol, benzyl alcohol, spearmint oil, cassia oil. Liq. Bot. 15 mL. *OTC.*
Use: Mouth and throat preparation.

Orasept, Throat. (Pharmakon) Benzocaine 0.996%, methyl benzethonium Cl 1.037%, sorbitol 70%, menthol, peppermint, saccharin. Throat spray. 45 mL. *OTC.*
Use: Mouth and throat preparation.

Orasol. (Ivax) Benzocaine 6.3%, phenol 0.5%, alcohol 70%, povidone-iodine. Liq. Bot. 14.79 mL. *OTC.*
Use: Anesthetic, local.

OraSure HIV-1. (Epitope) Collection kit: Cotton fiber on a stick with collection vial. Device for oral specimen collection. For professional use only.
Use: Diagnostic aid.

OraVerse. (Novalar Pharmaceuticals) Phentolamine mesylate 0.4 mg per 1.7 mL. D-mannitol, edetate disodium. Preservative free. Inj., Soln. Dental cartridge. *Rx.*
Use: Agent for pheochromocytoma.

Oravig. (Par) Miconazole 50 mg. Lactose, milk protein concentrate. Tab., buccal. 14s. *Rx.*
Use: Antifungal agent, imidazole antifungal.

Oraxyl. (e5 Pharma) Doxycycline 20 mg (as hyclate). Cap. 100s. *Rx.*
Use: Tetracycline.

Orazinc. (Mericon Industries) Zinc sulfate 220 mg. Cap. Bot. 100s, 1000s. *OTC.*
Use: Mineral supplement.

orbenin. Sodium cloxacillin.
Use: Anti-infective.
See: Cloxapen.

Orbiferrous. (Orbit) Ferrous fumarate 300 mg, vitamins B$_{12}$ 12 mcg, C 50 mg, B$_1$ 3 mg, defatted desiccated liver 50 mg. Tab. Bot. 60s, 500s. *OTC.*
Use: Mineral, vitamin supplement.

Orbit. (Spanner) Vitamins A 6250 units, D 400 units, B$_1$ 3 mg, B$_2$ 3 mg, B$_6$ 2 mg, B$_{12}$ 5 mcg, C 75 mg, niacinamide 20 mg, calcium pantothenate 10 mg, E 15 units, biotin 15 mcg, Fe 20 mg. Tab. Bot. 100s. *OTC.*
Use: Mineral, vitamin supplement.

Orbivan. (Atley) Acetaminophen 300 mg, butalbital 50 mg, caffeine 40 mg. Cap. 100s. *Rx.*
Use: Nonnarcotic analgesic combination, nonnarcotic analgesic with barbiturates.

• **orbofiban acetate.** (ore-boe-FIE-ban) USAN.
Use: Fibrinogen receptor antagonist;

platelet aggregation inhibitor, antithrombotic.

• **orconazole nitrate.** (ahr-KOE-nah-zole) USAN.
Use: Antifungal.

• **oregovomab.** (oh-re-GOE-voe-mab) USAN.
Use: Monoclonal antibody (ovarian cancer).

Orencia. (Bristol-Myers Squibb) Abatacept 250 mg. Maltose 500 mg, monobasic sodium phosphate 17.2 mg, sodium chloride 14.6 mg. Pow. for Soln., Inj., lyophilized. Single-use vials with syringe. *Rx.*
Use: Immunomodulator, immunologic agent.

Orexin. (Roberts) Vitamins B$_1$ 8.1 mg, B$_6$ 4.1 mg, B$_{12}$ 25 mcg. Chew. Tab. Bot. 100s. *OTC.*
Use: Vitamin supplement.

Orfadin. (Rare Disease Therapeutics, Inc.) Nitisinone 2 mg, 5 mg, 10 mg. Cap. 60s. *Rx.*
Use: Tyrosinemia.

Organidin. (Wallace) **Tab.:** 30 mg. Bot. 100s. **Elix.:** 60 mg/5 mL. 21.75% alcohol, glucose, saccharin. Bot. Pt., gal. **Soln.:** 50 mg/mL. Bot. 30 mL w/dropper.
Use: Expectorant.

Organ-I NR. (Qualitest) Guaifenesin 200 mg. Maltodextrin. Tab. 100s. *OTC.*
Use: Expectorant.

Orglagen. (Ivax) Orphenadrine citrate 100 mg. Tab. Bot. 100s, 1000s. *Rx.*
Use: Muscle relaxant.

• **orgotein.** (OR-goe-teen) USAN. A group of soluble metalloproteins isolated from liver, red blood cells, and other mammalian tissues.
Use: Anti-inflammatory; antirheumatic.

orgotein. (Diagnostic Data) Pure watersoluble protein with a compact conformation maintained by 4 g atoms of chelated divalent metals, produced from bovine liver as a Cu-Zn mixed chelate having superoxide dismutase activity. Ontosein, Palosein.

oriental ginseng.
See: Ginseng, Asian.

Original Alka-Seltzer Effervescent. (Bayer Consumer Care) 1700 mg sodium bicarbonate, 325 mg aspirin, 1000 mg citric acid, 9 mg phenylalanine, 506 mg Na, aspartame. Tab. Pkg. 24s. *OTC.*
Use: Antacid.

Original Eclipse Sunscreen. (Tri Tec) Padimate O, glyceryl PABA, SPF 10.

Lot. Bot. 120 mL. *OTC.*
Use: Sunscreen.

Original Sensodyne. (Block Drug) Strontium chloride hexahydrate 10%, saccharin, sorbitol. Toothpaste. Tube 59.5 g. *OTC.*
Use: Mouth and throat preparation.

• **oritavancin diphosphate.** (or-IT-a-VAN-sin) USAN.
Use: Antibacterial.

• **orlistat.** (ORE-lih-stat) USAN.
Use: Inhibitor, pancreatic lipase.
See: Alli.
  Xenical.

• **ormaplatin.** (ORE-mah-PLAT-in) USAN.
Use: Antineoplastic.

• **ormetoprim.** (ore-MEH-toe-PRIM) USAN.
Use: Anti-infective.

Ornex No Drowsiness. (B.F. Ascher) Pseudoephedrine hydrochloride 30 mg, acetaminophen 325 mg. Lactose, PEG. Tab. Bot. 24s, 48s. *OTC.*
Use: Upper respiratory combination, analgesic, decongestant.

Ornex No Drowsiness Maximum Strength. (B.F. Ascher) Pseudoephedrine hydrochloride 30 mg, acetaminophen 500 mg. PEG. Tab. Bot. 24s. *OTC.*
Use: Upper respiratory combination, analgesic, decongestant.

• **ornidazole.** (ahr-NIH-DAH-zole) USAN.
Use: Anti-infective.

Ornidyl. (Hoechst) Eflornithine hydrochloride 200 mg/mL. Inj. Vial. 100 mL. *Rx.*
Use: Antiprotozoal.

• **ornithine phenylacetate.** (OR-ni-theen) USAN.
Use: Ammonia detoxifying agent.

• **orpanoxin.** (AHR-pan-OX-in) USAN.
Use: Anti-inflammatory.

Orpeneed VK. (Hanlon) Penicillin, buffered, 400,000 units. Tab. Bot. 100s. *Rx.*
Use: Anti-infective, penicillin.

• **orphenadrine citrate.** (ore-FEN-uh-dreen) *USP 34.*
Use: Antihistamine, muscle relaxant.
See: Banflex.
  Flexon.
  Myolin.
  Norflex.
W/Aspirin, Caffeine.
See: Orphenadrine Compound.
  Orphenadrine Compound-DS.

orphenadrine citrate. (Apothecon) Orphenadrine citrate 100 mg. Lactose. SR Tab. 100s, 500s. *Rx.*
Use: Muscle relaxant.

orphenadrine citrate. (Various Mfr.) Orphenadrine citrate. **Inj:** 30 mg/mL. Amps. 2 mL. Vials. 10 mL. **Tab.:** 100 mg. Bot. 30s, 100s, 500s, 1000s. *Rx.*
Use: Antihistamine; muscle relaxant.

Orphenadrine Compound. (Sandoz) Aspirin 385 mg, caffeine 30 mg, orphenadrine citrate 25 mg. Lactose. Tab. 100s. *Rx.*
Use: Skeletal muscle relaxant.

Orphenadrine Compound-DS. (Sandoz) Aspirin 770 mg, caffeine 60 mg, orphenadrine citrate 50 mg. Lactose. Tab. 100s. *Rx.*
Use: Skeletal muscle relaxant.

Orphengesic Forte. (Various Mfr.) Orphenadrine citrate 50 mg, aspirin 770 mg, caffeine 60 mg, lactose. Tab. Bot. 100s, 500s. *Rx.*
Use: Analgesic, muscle relaxant.

Ortac-DM. (ION Laboratories, Inc.) Dextromethorphan 10 mg, phenylephrine hydrochloride 5 mg, guaifenesin 100 mg/5 mL. Liq. Bot. 4 oz. *OTC.*
Use: Antitussive, decongestant, expectorant.

ortal sodium. Sodium 5-ethyl-5-hexylbarbiturate. Hexethal sodium.

ortedrine.
See: Amphetamines.

orthesin.
See: Benzocaine.

Ortho All-Flex Diaphragm. (Ortho-McNeil) Diaphragm kit (all flex arcing spring) in plastic compact, sizes 55, 60, 65, 70, 75, 80, 85, 90, 95 mm. *Rx.*
Use: Contraceptive.

orthocaine.
See: Orthoform.

Ortho-Cept. (Ortho-McNeil) Desogestrel 0.15 mg, ethinyl estradiol 30 mcg. Lactose. Tab. *Dialpak* and *Veridate* 28s with 7 inert tabs. *Rx.*
Use: Sex hormone, contraceptive hormone.

Orthoclone OKT3. (Ortho Biotech) Muromonab-CD3 5 mg/5 mL. Polysorbate 80 1 mg. Inj. Amps 5 mL. *Rx.*
Use: Immunosuppressant.

Ortho-Cyclen. (Ortho-McNeil) Norgestimate 0.25 mg, ethinyl estradiol 35 mcg. Lactose. Tab. *Dialpak* and *Veridate* 28s with 7 inert tabs. *Rx.*
Use: Sex hormone, contraceptive hormone.

Ortho Diaphragm. (Ortho-McNeil) Diaphragm kit, coil spring sizes 50, 55, 60, 65, 70, 75, 80, 85, 90, 95, 100, 105 mm. *Rx.*
Use: Contraceptive.

Ortho Diaphragm-White. (Ortho-McNeil) Diaphragm kit, flat spring sizes 55, 60, 65, 70, 75, 80, 85, 90, 95 mm. *Rx.*
Use: Contraceptive.

Ortho Dienestrol Vaginal Cream. (Ortho-McNeil) Dienestrol 0.01%. Cream. Tube 78 g with or without applicator. *Rx.*
Use: Estrogen.

Ortho Evra. (Ortho-McNeil) Norelgestromin 6 mg, ethinyl estradiol 0.75 mg/patch. Transdermal system. Box cycles (3 patches), single patches. *Rx.*
Use: Sex hormone, contraceptive hormone.

Orthoflavin. (Enzyme Process) Vitamins C 150 mg, E 25 mg. Tab. Bot. 100s, 250s. *OTC.*
Use: Vitamin supplement.

Orthoform. (Columbus) Tyrothricin 0.5 mg, tetracaine hydrochloride 0.5%, epinephrine 1/1000 Soln. 2%/g. Oint. Tube oz. *Rx.*
Use: Anti-infective, ophthalmic.

Ortho-Gynol Contraceptive. (Johnson & Johnson) Oxtoxynol 9. Gel. Tube. 75 g w/applicator and 75 g, 114 g refills. *OTC.*
Use: Contraceptive.

ortho-hydroxybenzoic acid. Salicylic Acid, USP.

orthohydroxyphenylmercuric chloride.
Use: Antiseptic.
W/Benzocaine, Parachlorometaxylenol, Benzalkonium Chloride, Phenol.
See: Unguentine.

Ortho Micronor. (Ortho-McNeil) Norethindrone 0.35 mg. Lactose. Tab. *Dialpak* 28s. *Rx.*
Use: Sex hormone, contraceptive hormone.

Ortho-Novum 1/50. (Ortho-McNeil) Norethindrone 1 mg, mestranol 50 mcg. Lactose. Tab. *Dialpak* 28s with 7 inert tabs. *Rx.*
Use: Sex hormone, contraceptive hormone.

Ortho-Novum 1/35. (Ortho-McNeil) Norethindrone 1 mg, ethinyl estradiol 35 mcg. Lactose. Tab. *Dialpak* and *Veridate* 28s with 7 inert tabs. *Rx.*
Use: Sex hormone, contraceptive hormone.

Ortho-Novum 7/7/7. (Ortho-McNeil) **Phase 1:** Norethindrone 0.5 mg, ethinyl estradiol 35 mcg. 7 tabs. **Phase 2:** Norethindrone 0.75 mg, ethinyl estradiol 35 mcg. 7 tabs. **Phase 3:** Norethindrone 1 mg, ethinyl estradiol 35 mcg. 7 tabs. Lactose. Tab. *Dialpak* and *Veridate* 28s with 7 inert tabs. *Rx.*

Use: Sex hormone, contraceptive hormone.

Ortho-Novum 10/11. (Ortho-McNeil) **Phase 1:** Norethindrone 0.5 mg, ethinyl estradiol 35 mcg. 10 tabs. **Phase 2:** Norethindrone 1 mg, ethinyl estradiol 35 mcg, 11 tabs. Lactose. Tab. *Dialpak* and *Veridate* 28s with 7 inert tabs. *Rx.*
Use: Sex hormone, contraceptive hormone.

Ortho Personal Lubricant. (Johnson & Johnson) Greaseless, water-soluble, and non-staining aqueous hydrocolloid gel. Acid buffered to vaginal pH. Tube 2 oz, 4 oz. *OTC.*
Use: Lubricant.

Ortho Tri-Cyclen. (Ortho-McNeil) **Phase 1:** Norgestimate 0.18 mg, ethinyl estradiol 35 mcg. 7 tabs. **Phase 2:** Norgestimate 0.215 mg, ethinyl estradiol 35 mcg. 7 tabs. **Phase 3:** Norgestimate 0.25 mg, ethinyl estradiol 35 mcg. 7 tabs. Lactose. Tab. *Dialpak* and *Veridate* 28s with 7 inert tabs. *Rx.*
Use: Sex hormone, contraceptive hormone.

Ortho Tri-Cyclen Lo. (Ortho-McNeil) **Phase 1:** Norgestimate 0.18 mg, ethinyl estradiol 25 mcg. 7 tabs. **Phase 2:** Norgestimate 0.215 mg, ethinyl estradiol 25 mcg. 7 tabs. **Phase 3:** Norgestimate 0.25 mg, ethinyl estradiol 25 mcg. 7 tabs. Talc, lactose. Tab. *Dialpak* and *Veridate* 28s with 7 inert tabs. *Rx.*
Use: Sex hormone, contraceptive hormone.

Orthovisc. (Anika) Hyaluronan 15 mg. Sodium chloride 9 mg/mL. Inj. Prefilled syringe. 2 mL. *Rx.*
Use: Physical adjunct.

OrthoWash. (Omnil Oral) Sodium fluoride (as acidulated phosphate solution) 0.044%. Grape flavor. Rinse. 480 mL. *Rx.*
Use: Prevention of dental caries.

orthoxine. Methoxyphenamine.

orticalm.
Use: Hypotensive; tranquilizer.

•**orvepitant.** (or-VEE-pi-tant) USAN.
Use: CNS agent.

•**orvepitant maleate.** (or-VEE-pi-tant) USAN.
Use: CNS agent.

orvus.
See: Gardinol Type Detergents.

Os-Cal Extra D. (GlaxoSmithKline) Vitamin D_3 500 units (as cholecalciferol), calcium 500 mg (as calcium carbonate). Alcohol, corn syrup, parabens, PEG,

sucrose. Gluten free. Tab. 60s, 120s. OTC.
Use: Nutritional combination product.

Os-Cal 500. (GlaxoSmithKline Consumer) Calcium carbonate 1250 mg (elemental calcium 500 mg). **Tab.:** Oyster shell powder, corn syrup, parabens. Bot. 75s. **Chew. Tab.:** Dextrose. Bot. 60s. OTC.
Use: Mineral supplement.

Os-Cal 500 + D. (GlaxoSmithKline Consumer) **Chew. Tab.:** Calcium 500 mg, vitamin D 400 units. Aspartame, phenylalanine, sorbitol, sucrose. Lemon chiffon flavor. 60s. **Tab.:** Calcium 500 mg, vitamin D 200 units, corn syrup, parabens, polydextrose. Bot. 75s, 160s. OTC.
Use: Mineral, vitamin supplement.

Os-Cal Fortified. (GlaxoSmithKline Consumer) Ca 250 mg, Fe (as ferrous fumarate) 5 mg, Mg, Mn, zinc 0.5 mg, D 125 units, B_1 1.7 mg, B_2 1.7 mg, B_3 15 mg, B_6 2 mg, C 50 mg, E 0.8 units, parabens, corn syrup solids, EDTA. Tab. Bot. 100s. OTC.
Use: Mineral, vitamin supplement.

Os-Cal Fortified Multivitamin & Minerals. (GlaxoSmithKline Consumer) Vitamins A 1668 units, D 125 units, E 0.8 units, B_1 1.7 mg, B_2 1.7 mg, B_3 15 mg, B_6 2 mg, C 50 mg, Fe 5 mg, Ca 250 mg, Zn 0.5 mg, Mn, Mg, EDTA, parabens. Tab. Bot. 100s. OTC.
Use: Mineral, vitamin supplement.

Os-Cal Plus. (GlaxoSmithKline Consumer) Ca 250 mg, vitamins D 125 units, A 1666 units, C 33 mg, B_2 0.66 mg, B_1 0.5 mg, B_6 0.5 mg, niacinamide 3.33 mg, Zn 0.75 mg, Mn 0.75 mg, Fe 16.6 mg. Tab. Bot. 100s. OTC.
Use: Mineral, vitamin supplement.

Os-Cal 250. (GlaxoSmithKline Consumer) Oyster shell powder as calcium 250 mg, vitamin D 125 units, and trace minerals (Cu, Fe, Mg, Mn, Zn, silica). Tab. Bot. 100s, 240s, 500s, 1000s. OTC.
Use: Mineral, vitamin supplement.

Os-Cal 250 + D. (GlaxoSmithKline Consumer) Calcium carbonate 625 mg, vitamin D 125 units. Tab. Bot. 100s. OTC.
Use: Mineral, vitamin supplement.

Os-Cal Ultra. (GlaxoSmithKline Consumer) Ca 600 mg, vitamin D 200 units, C 60 mg, E 15 units, Mg 20 mg, Zn 7.5 mg, Cu, Mn, boron 250 mcg. Lactose, sucrose. Tab. 120s. OTC.
Use: Nutritional supplement.

●**oseltamivir phosphate.** (oh-sel-TAM-i-vir) USAN.
Use: Antiviral.

See: Tamiflu.

Osmitrol. (Baxter PPI) Mannitol in water. **5%:** 1000 mL. **10%:** 500 mL, 1000 mL. **15%:** 150 mL, 500 mL. **20%:** 250 mL, 500 mL. Mannitol in 0.3% Na. **5%:** 1000 mL. Mannitol in 0.45% Na. **20%:** 500 mL. Rx.
Use: Diuretic.
See: Mannitol.

Osmolite. (Ross) Isotonic liquid food containing 1.06 calories/mL. Two quarts (2000 calories) provides 100% US RDA vitamins and minerals for adults and children. Osmolality: 300 mOsm/kg water. Ready-to-Use: Bot. Can 8 fl oz, 32 fl oz. OTC.
Use: Nutritional supplement.

Osmolite HN. (Ross) High nitrogen isotonic liquid food containing 1.06 calories/mL; 1400 calories provides 100% USRDA vitamins and minerals for adults and children. Osmolality: 300 mOsm/kg water. Ready-to-Use: Bot. 8 fl oz. Can 8 fl oz, 32 fl oz. OTC.
Use: Nutritional supplement.

OsmoPrep. (Salix Pharmaceuticals) Sodium phosphate 1.5 g (sodium phosphate monobasic monohydrate 1.102 g, sodium phosphate dibasic 0.398 g). Gluten free. 100s. Rx.
Use: Laxative.

osmotic diuretics.
See: Ismotic.
Mannitol.
Osmitrol.
Osmoglyn.
Ureaphil.

●**ospemifene.** (os-PEM-i-feen) USAN.
Use: Selective estrogen receptor modulator; post-menopausal vaginal atrophy.

ospolot.
Use: Anticonvulsant drug; pending release.

Ossonate. (Marcen) Cartilage mucopolysaccharide extract, chondroitin sulfate 50 mg. Cap. Bot. 100s, 500s, 1000s.

Ossonate-Plus. (Marcen) Ossonate mucopolysaccharide extract 50 mg, acetaminophen 300 mg, salicylamide 200 mg. Cap. Bot. 100s, 500s, 1000s. OTC.
Use: Antiarthritic.

Ossonate-Plus, Inj. (Marcen) Ossonate cartilage mucopolysaccharide extract 12.5 mg, case in hydrolysates 80 mg, sulfur 20 mg, sodium citrate 5 mg, benzyl alcohol 0.5%, phenol 0.5%/mL.

Multidose 10 mL vial. *Rx.*
Use: Muscle relaxant, pain reliever.

Ossonate-75. (Marcen) Chondroitin sulfate 37.5 mg, benzyl alcohol 0.5%, phenol 0.5%, sodium citrate 5 mg/mL. Vial 10 mL. *Rx.*
Use: Infantile and atopic eczemas; drug allergies; dermatoses associated with intestinal toxemias.

Osteo-D. (Teva)
See: Secalciferol.

Osteolate. (Fellows) Sodium thiosalicylate 50 mg, benzyl alcohol 2%/mL. Inj. Vial 30 mL. *Rx.*
Use: Analgesic.

Osteo-Mins. (Tyson) **Pow.:** Vitamin C 500 mg, Ca 250 mg, Mg 250 mg, K 45 mg, 100 units D/4.5 g, sugar free. 200 g. *OTC.*
Use: Vitamin supplement.

Osteon/D. (Taylor Pharmaceuticals) Ca 600 mg, P 400 mg, Mg 240 mg, vitamin D 400 units. Tab. Bot. 180s. *Rx.*
Use: Mineral, vitamin supplement.

Ostiderm Roll-On. (Pedinol Pharmacal) Aluminum chlorohydrate, camphor, alcohol, EDTA, diazolidinyl urea. Bot. 88.7 mL. *OTC.*
Use: Antipruritic; astringent, topical.

OstiGen Melts. (US Food & Pharmaceuticals) Vitamin D 150 units, Ca 350 mg, vitamin K, P, Mg, Cu, Na, K. Chocolate, chocolate mint, and caramel flavors. Sugar free. Orally Disintegrating Tab. 90s. *OTC.*
Use: Multivitamin.

Osto-K. (Parthenon) Potassium 1 mEq (39 mg from gluconate, Cl, and citrate), vitamin C 25 mg, sodium 0.52 mg. Tab. Bot. 60s. *OTC.*
Use: Mineral, vitamin supplement.

Otic Domeboro. (Bayer) Acetic acid 2%, aluminum acetate solution. Soln. 60 mL with dropper. *Rx.*
Use: Otic.

Otic Edge. (River's Edge) Antipyrine 5.4%, benzocaine 1.4%, policosanol 0.0097%. Acetic acid, glycerin. Soln., Otic. 14 mL w/dropper. *Rx.*
Use: Otic preparation.

Otic-HC. (Roberts) Chloroxylenol 1 mg, pramoxine hydrochloride 10 mg, hydrocortisone alcohol 10 mg, benzalkonium Cl 0.2 mg/mL. Bot. 12 mL. *Rx.*
Use: Otic.

Oticin. (Teral) Parachlorometaxylenol 0.01 g, proxazocain hydrochloride 0.1 g. Drops, otic. 10 mL w/dropper. *Rx.*
Use: Miscellaneous otic preparation.

Oticin HC. (Teral) Hydrocortisone 1 g, parachlormetaxylenol 0.01 g, proxazo-

caine hydrochloride 0.1 g. Edetate disodium. Drops, otic. 10 mL w/dropper. *Rx.*
Use: Miscellaneous otic preparation.

Otic-Neo-Cort Dome.
See: Neo-Cort Dome.

Otic-Plain. (Roberts) Chloroxylenol 1 mg, pramoxine hydrochloride 10 mg, benzalkonium Cl 0.2 mg/mL. Bot. 12 mL. *Rx.*
Use: Otic.

Otic Solution No. 1. (Foy Laboratories) Hydrocortisone alcohol 10 mg, pramoxine hydrochloride 10 mg, benzalkonium Cl 0.2 mg, acetic acid glacial 20 mg/mL w/propylene glycol q.s. Bot. *Rx.*
Use: Otic.

Otocain. (Abana) Benzocaine 20%, benzethonium chloride 0.1%, glycerin 1%, polyethylene glycol 300. Soln. Bot. 15 mL. *Rx.*
Use: Otic preparation.

Oto-End 10. (Larken Laboratories) Chloroxylenol 0.1%, hydrocortisone 1%, pramoxine hydrochloride 1%. Edetate disodium. Soln., Otic. 10 mL w/dropper. *Rx.*
Use: Ophthalmic and otic agent, otic preparation.

Otogesic HC Solution. (Lexis Laboratories) Polymyxin B sulfate 10,000 units, neomycin sulfate 3.5 mg, hydrocortisone 10 mg/mL, potassium metabisulfite 0.1%. Bot. 10 mL. *Rx.*
Use: Otic.

Otogesic HC Suspension. (Lexis Laboratories) Polymyxin B sulfate 10,000 units, neomycin sulfate 3.5 mg, hydrocortisone 10 mg/mL, benzalkonium Cl 0.01%. Bot. 10 mL. *Rx.*
Use: Otic.

Otomar-HC. (Marnel) Chloroxylenol 1 mg, hydrocortisone 10 mg, pramoxine hydrochloride 10 mg/mL. Otic Soln. Plastic dropper vials 10 mL. *Rx.*
Use: Otic preparation.

Otosporin. (Calmic) Hydrocortisone 1%, neomycin sulfate 5 mg, polymyxin B 10,000 units. Soln. 10 mL with dropper. *Rx.*
Use: Steroid and antibiotic combination.

Otrivin. (Novartis) Xylometazoline hydrochloride 0.1%, benzalkonium chloride, sodium chloride, EDTA. Soln. Dropper Bot. 25 mL. Spray Bot. 20 mL. *OTC.*
Use: Nasal decongestant, imidazoline.

Otrivin Pediatric Nasal. (Novartis) Xylometazoline hydrochloride 0.05%, benzalkonium chloride, EDTA. Soln. Drop-

per Bot. 25 mL. *OTC.*
Use: Nasal decongestant, imidazoline.

ouabain octahydrate. Ouabain, USP.

Ovace. (Tiber) Sodium sulfacetamide 10%. EDTA, lactic acid, methylparaben. Top. Foam. 50 g, 100 g. *Rx.*
Use: Topical anti-infective, antibiotic agent.

Ovace Plus. (Tiber) Sulfacetamide sodium 10%. **Cream:** Cetearyl alcohol, cetyl alcohol, disodium EDTA, glycerin, glyceryl monostearate, mineral oil, parabens, PEG-3, PEG-100. 45 g. **Wash, Soap:** Cetearyl alcohol, edetate disodium, glyceryl, methylparaben, PEG-3, PEG-6, PEG-150. 340 g. *Rx.*
Use: Anti-infective, topical; antibiotic agent.

Ovace Plus Shampoo. (Kylemore Pharmaceuticals) Sulfacetamide sodium 10%. PEG-150. Shampoo. 227 g. *Rx.*
Use: Topical anti-infective, antibiotic agent.

ovarian extract. Aqueous extract of whole ovaries of cattle.
Use: Estrogen.

ovarian substance. (Various Mfr.) Whole ovarian substance from cattle, sheep, or swine. *Rx.*
Use: Estrogen.

Ovastat. (Medac GmbH c/o Princeton Regulatory Assoc.)
See: Treosulfan.

Ovcon-50. (Warner Chilcott) Norethindrone 1 mg, ethinyl estradiol 50 mcg. Lactose. Tab. Pack 28s with 7 inert tabs. *Rx.*
Use: Sex hormone, contraceptive hormone.

Ovcon-35. (Warner Chilcott) Norethindrone 0.4 mg, ethinyl estradiol 35 mcg. Lactose. Tab. Pack 28s with 7 inert tabs. *Rx.*
Use: Sex hormone, contraceptive hormone.

•**ovemotide.** (oh-VEM-oh-tide) USAN.
Use: Melanoma peptide vaccine.

Overtime. (BDI) Caffeine 200 mg. Tab. Bot. 100s, 500s. *OTC.*
Use: CNS stimulant, analeptic.

Ovide. (Taro) Malathion 0.5%. In a vehicle of isopropyl alcohol 78%, terpineol, dipentene, and pine needle oil. Lot. Bot. 59 mL. *Rx.*
Use: Pediculicide, scabicide.

Ovidrel. (Serono) Choriogonadotropin alfa 250 mcg/0.5 mL, mannitol 28.1 mg, 85% O-phosphoric acid 505 mcg. Inj. Single-dose prefilled syringes. *Rx.*
Use: Sex hormone, ovulation stimulant.

ovifollin.
See: Estrone.

Ovlin. (Sigma-Tau) **Tab.:** Ethinyl estradiol 0.02 mg, conjugated estrogens 0.2 mg. Bot. 100s, 1000s. **Inj.:** Estrone 2 mg, ethinyl estradiol 0.05 mg, vitamin B_{12} 1000 mcg/mL. Vial 30 mL. *Rx.*
Use: Estrogen.

Ovocylin Dipropionate. (Novartis) Estradiol dipropionate. *Rx.*
Use: Estrogen.

Ovral. (Wyeth-Ayerst) Norgestrel 0.5 mg, ethinyl estradiol 50 mcg. Lactose. Tab. *Pilpak* 21s, 28s with 7 inert tabs. *Rx.*
Use: Sex hormone, contraceptive hormone.

ovulation stimulants.
See: Choriogonadotropin Alfa.
Chorionic Gonadotropin.
Clomiphene Citrate.
Gonadotropins.
Lutropin Alfa.
Menotropins.

ovulation tests.
See: Clearblue Easy Ovulation Test.
First Response Ovulation Predictor Test Kit.
Fortel Ovulation.

Ovulen-28. (Pharmacia) Ethynodiol diacetate 1 mg, mestranol 0.1 mg. Tab. w/7 inert Tab. *Compack* 28s: 21 active tab., 7 placebo tab. *Compack* dispenser 28s. Box 6 × 28. Refill 28s, Box 12 × 28. *Rx.*
Use: Contraceptive.

Ovulen-21. (Pharmacia) Ethynodiol diacetate 1 mg, mestranol 0.1 mg. Tab. *Compack* Disp. 21s, 6 × 21, 24 × 21. Refill 21s, 12 × 21. *Rx.*
Use: Contraceptive.

Ovustick Self-Test. (Monoclonal Antibodies) Home test for ovulation. Test kit 10s.
Use: Diagnostic aid.

Oxabid. (Jamieson-McKames) Magnesium oxide 140 mg or magnesium oxide heavy 400 mg. Cap. Bot. 100s. *OTC.*
Use: Antacid.

•**oxacillin sodium.** (ox-uh-SILL-in) USP 34.
Use: Anti-infective.

oxacillin sodium. (Various Mfr.) Oxacillin sodium 500 mg, 1 g, 2 g, 10 g. Pow. for Inj. Vial (except 10 g), piggyback vial (1 g, 2 g only), *ADD-Vantage* vials (1 g, 2 g only), Bulk Vial (10 g only). *Rx.*
Use: Anti-infective, penicillin.

oxadimedine hydrochloride.
Use: Antiarrhythmic.

oxafuradene. (OX-ah-FYOOR-ah-deen) Name used for Nifuradene.
Use: Platelet aggregation agent.

•**oxagrelate.** (OX-ah-greh-LATE) USAN.
Use: Platelet aggregation inhibitor.

oxaliplatin. (ocks-AL-ih-pla-tin)
Use: Antineoplastic. [Orphan Drug]
See: Eloxatin.

oxaliplatin. (Various Mfr.) Oxaliplatin. **Inj.; Soln, Conc.:** 5 mg/mL. Preservative free. Single-use vial. 10 mL, 20 mL. **Inj., lyophilized Pow. for Soln.:** 50 mg, 100 mg. May contain lactose. Preservative free. Single-use vial. *Rx.*
Use: Antineoplastic agent, platinum coordination complex.

oxalodinones.
Use: Anti-infective.
See: Linezolid.

•**oxamarin hydrochloride.** (OX-ah-mah-rin) USAN.
Use: Hemostatic.

•**oxamisole hydrochloride.** (ox-AM-ih-sole) USAN.
Use: Immunoregulator.

•**oxamniquine.** (ox-AM-nih-kwin) *USP 34.*
Use: Antischistosomal, treatment of schistosomiasis.

oxanamide.
Use: Anxiolytic.

Oxandrin. (Savient) Oxandrolone 2.5 mg, 10 mg, lactose. Tab. Bot. 100s (2.5 mg only), 60s (10 mg only). *c-III.*
Use: Anabolic steroid.

•**oxandrolone.** (ox-AN-droe-lone) *USP 34.*
Use: Anabolic steroid.
See: Oxandrin.

oxandrolone. (Sandoz) Oxandrolone 2.5 mg, 10 mg. Lactose. Tab. 100s, 1000s. *c-III.*
Use: Anabolic steroid.

•**oxantel pamoate.** (OX-an-tell PAM-oh-ate) USAN.
Use: Anthelmintic.

•**oxaprotiline hydrochloride.** (OX-ah-PRO-tih-leen) USAN.
Use: Antidepressant.

•**oxaprozin.** (OX-ah-pro-zin) *USP 34.*
Use: Nonsteroidal anti-inflammatory agent.
See: Daypro.
Daypro ALTA.

oxaprozin. (Eon Labs) Oxaprozin 600 mg. Film-coated. Tab. Bot. 100s, 500s, 1000s, blister 100s. *Rx.*
Use: Nonsteroidal anti-inflammatory agent.

•**oxarbazole.** (ox-AHR-bah-zole) USAN.
Use: Antiasthmatic.

•**oxatomide.** (ox-AT-ah-mid) USAN.
Use: Antiallergic, antiasthmatic.

•**oxazepam.** (ox-AZ-e-pam) *USP 34.*
Use: Anxiolytic, sedative.

oxazepam. (Various Mfr.) Oxazepam 10 mg, 15 mg, 30 mg. Cap. 100s, 500s, UD 100s. *c-IV.*
Use: Anxiolytic.

ox bile extract. Purified ox gall.
See: Bile Extract.

•**oxcarbazepine.** (OC-kar-BAZ-e-peen) USAN.
Tall Man: OXcarbazepine
Use: Anticonvulsant; antiepileptic.
See: Trileptal.

oxcarbazepine. (Sandoz) Oxcarbazepine 60 mg/mL. Ethanol, saccharin, sorbitol. Susp. 250 mL w/dosing syringe and adapter. *Rx.*
Use: Anticonvulsant.

oxcarbazepine. (Various Mfr.) Oxcarbazepine 150 mg, 300 mg, 600 mg. Tab. 30s, 100s, 500s, 1000s, UD 100s. *Rx.*
Use: Anticonvulsant.

•**oxelumab.** (ox-EL-ue-mab) USAN.
Use: Treatment of asthma.

•**oxendolone.** (ox-EN-doe-lone) USAN.
Use: Antiandrogen (benign prostatic hypertrophy).

•**oxethazaine.** (ox-ETH-a-zane) USAN.
Use: Anesthetic, local.

•**oxetorone fumarate.** (ox-EH-toe-rone) USAN.
Use: Antimigraine.

•**oxfendazole.** (ox-FEN-da-zole) USAN.
Use: Anthelmintic.

•**oxfenicine.** (ox-FEN-ih-seen) USAN.
Use: Vasodilator.

ox gall.
See: Ox Bile Extract.

•**oxibendazole.** (ox-ee-BEND-ah-zole) USAN.
Use: Anthelmintic.

•**oxiconazole nitrate.** (ox-ee-KAHN-ah-zole) USAN.
Use: Antifungal.
See: Oxistat.

oxidized bile acids.
See: Bile Acids, Oxidized.

oxidized cellulose. Absorbable cellulose. Cellulosic acid.
Use: Hemostatic.
See: Oxycel.
Surgicel.

•**oxidopamine.** (OX-ih-DOE-pah-meen) USAN.
Use: Adrenergic (ophthalmic).

•**oxidronic acid.** (OX-ih-DRAHN-ik)

USAN.
Use: Regulator (calcium).
Oxi-Freeda. (Freeda) Vitamin A 5000 units, E 150 mg, B_3 40 mg, C 100 mg, B_1 20 mg, B_2 20 mg, B_5 20 mg, B_6 20 mg, B_{12} 10 mcg, Zn 15 mg, Se, glutathione, L-cysteine. Tab. Bot. 100s, 250s. *OTC.*
Use: Mineral, vitamin supplement.
•**oxifungin hydrochloride.** (OX-ih-FUN-jin) USAN.
Use: Antifungal.
•**oxilorphan.** (ox-ih-LORE-fan) USAN.
Use: Narcotic antagonist.
•**oximonam.** (OX-ih-MOE-nam) USAN.
Use: Anti-infective.
•**oximonam sodium.** (OX-ih-MOE-nam) USAN.
Use: Anti-infective.
oxine.
See: Oxyquinoline Sulfate.
•**oxiperomide.** (ox-ih-PURR-oh-mide) USAN.
Use: Antipsychotic.
Oxipor VHC. (Medtech) Coal tar soln. 25% (equiv. to 5% coal tar), alcohol 79%. Lot. Bot. 56 mL. *OTC.*
Use: Antipsoriatic.
•**oxiramide.** (ox-EER-am-ide) USAN.
Use: Cardiovascular agent.
Oxistat. (Pharmaderm) Oxiconazole nitrate 1%. Cream. Tube 15 g, 30 g, 60 g; Lot. Bot. 30 mL. *Rx.*
Use: Antifungal, topical.
•**oxisuran.** (OX-ih-SUH-ran) USAN.
Use: Antineoplastic.
•**oxmetidine hydrochloride.** (ox-MEH-tih-DEEN) USAN.
Use: Antiulcerative.
•**oxmetidine mesylate.** (ox-MEH-tih-DEEN) USAN.
Use: Antiulcerative.
•**oxogestone phenpropionate.** (ox-oh-JESS-tone fen-PRO-pih-oh-nate) USAN.
Use: Hormone, progestin.
Oxolamine. (Arcum) Crystalline hydroxycobalamin 1000 mcg/mL. Vial 10 mL. *Rx.*
Use: Vitamin supplement.
•**oxolinic acid.** (ox-oh-LIH-nik acid) USAN.
Use: Anti-infective.
Oxothiazolidine Carboxylate. (Clintec Nutrition) Phase I restoration of glutathione depletion in HIV, ARC, AIDS; prevention of inflammation-induced HIV replication. *Rx.*
Use: Immunomodulator.

l-2-oxothiazolidine-4-carboxylic acid.
Use: Treatment of adult respiratory distress syndrome. [Orphan Drug]
See: Procysteine.
•**oxprenolol hydrochloride.** (ox-PREH-no-lole) *USP 34.* Under study.
Use: Beta-adrenergic receptor blocker, vasodilator (coronary).
Oxsoralen. (ICN Pharmaceuticals) Methoxsalen 1% (10 mg/mL), acetone, alcohol 71%. Lot. Bot. 30 mL. *Rx.*
Use: Dermatologic.
Oxsoralen-Ultra. (ICN Pharmaceuticals) Methoxsalen 10 mg. Soft Gelatin Cap. Bot. 50s. *Rx.*
Use: Dermatologic.
•**oxtriphylline.** (ox-TRY-fih-lin) *USP 34.*
Use: Bronchodilator.
W/Guaifenesin.
See: Brondecon.
•**oxybenzone.** (ox-ee-BEN-zone) *USP 34.*
Use: Ultraviolet screen.
W/Avobenzone, Homosalate, Octisalate, Octocrylene.
See: Neutrogena Ultra Sheer Dry-Touch Sunblock.
W/Dioxybenzone, Benzophenone.
See: Solbar.
W/Combinations.
See: Coppertone.
Keri Age Defy & Protect.
Lubriderm Daily Moisture with SPF 15.
Noskote.
Shade.
Super Shade.
TI-Screen Sports.
•**oxybutynin chloride.** (OX-ee-BYOO-tih-nin) *USP 34.*
Use: Anticholinergic.
See: Ditropan XL.
Gelnique.
Oxytrol.
oxybutynin chloride. (Various Mfr.) Oxybutynin chloride. **ER Tab.:** 5 mg, 10 mg, 15 mg. May contain lactose (15 mg). 100s, 500s (5 mg, 10 mg only). **Tab.:** 5 mg. Bot. 100s, 500s, 1000s, blister pack 25s, UD 100s. **Syr.:** 5 mg/5 mL. Bot. 473 mL. *Rx.*
Use: Antispasmodic; anticholinergic.
Oxycel. (Becton Dickinson & Co.) Cellulosic acid in absorbable hemostatic agent prepared from cellulose. Resembles ordinary surgical gauze or cotton. Pledget 2 × 1 × 1 inch. 10s. Pad 3 × 3 inch. 8 ply. 10s. Strip 5 × 0.5 inch. 4 ply. 18 × 2 inch. 4 ply. 10s. 36 × 0.5 inch. 4 ply. *Rx.*
Use: Hemostatic, topical.

Oxycet. (Halsey Drug) Oxycodone hydrochloride 5 mg, acetaminophen 325 mg. Tab. Bot. 100s, 500s, Hospital pack 250s. *c-II.*
Use: Narcotic analgesic combination.

Oxy-Chinol. (Ferndale) Potassium oxyquinoline sulfate 1 g. Tab. Bot. 100s, 1000s. *OTC.*
Use: Antimicrobial, deodorant.

•**oxychlorosene.** (OCK-sih-KLOR-ah-seen) USAN. Monoxychlorosene. Hydrocarbon derivative containing 14 carbons and hypochlorous acid. The hydrocarbon chain also has a phenyl substituent which in turn holds a sulfonic acid group.
Use: Anti-infective, topical.
See: Clorpactin WCS-90.

•**oxychlorosene sodium.** (OCK-sih-KLOR-ah-seen) USAN. Sodium salt of the complex derived from hypochlorous acid and tetradecylbenzene sulfonic acid. Action of active chlorine.
Use: Anti-infective, topical.

•**oxycodone.** (OX-ee-KOE-dohn) USAN.
Tall Man: oxyCODONE
Use: Analgesic, narcotic w/combinations.
See: Endocet.
W/Acetaminophen.
See: Primlev.

oxycodone and acetaminophen. (Mallinckrodt) Oxycodone hydrochloride/acetaminophen 7.5 mg/325 mg, 7.5 mg/500 mg, 10 mg/325 mg, 10 mg, 650 mg. Tab. 20s, 100s, 500s, 1,000s, UD 100s. *c-II.*
Use: Narcotic analgesic.

oxycodone and acetaminophen. (Various Mfr.) **Cap.:** Oxycodone hydrochloride 5 mg, acetaminophen 500 mg. Bot. 100s, 500s, 1000s, UD 25s. **Tab.:** Oxycodone hydrochloride 5 mg, acetaminophen 325 mg. Bot. 100s, 500s, 1000s, UD 25s. *c-II.*
Use: Analgesic combination, narcotic.

oxycodone and aspirin. (Various Mfr.) Oxycodone hydrochloride 4.5 mg, oxycodone terephthalate 0.38 mg, aspirin 325 mg. Tab. Bot. 100s, 500s, 1000s, UD 25s. *c-II.*
Use: Analgesic combination, narcotic.

•**oxycodone hydrochloride.** (OX-ee-KOE-dohn) *USP 34.*
Tall Man: oxyCODONE
Use: Opioid analgesic.
See: M-oxy.
OxyContin.
OxyFAST.
OxyIR.

Roxicodone.
Roxicodone Intensol.
W/Acetaminophen
See: Pimalev.
Xolox.
W/Combinations.
See: Endocet.
Magnacet.
Percocet.
Percodan.
Perloxx.
Tylox.

oxycodone hydrochloride. (Amide) Oxycodone hydrochloride 15 mg, 30 mg. Lactose. IR Tab. 100s, UD 100s. *c-II.*
Use: Opioid analgesic.

oxycodone hydrochloride. (Endo) Oxycodone hydrochloride 10 mg, 20 mg, 40 mg. CR Tab. 30s, 500s. *c-II.*
Use: Opioid analgesic.

oxycodone hydrochloride. (Ethex) Oxycodone hydrochloride. **Cap.:** 5 mg. Lactose. 100s, UD 100s. **Tab.:** 10 mg, 20 mg. 100s, UD 100s. *c-II.*
Use: Opioid analgesic.

oxycodone hydrochloride. (Teva) Oxycodone hydrochloride 80 mg. Lactose. Film-coated. ER Tab. 100s. *c-II.*
Use: Opioid analgesic.

oxycodone hydrochloride. (Various Mfr.) Oxycodone hydrochloride. **CR Tab.:** 80 mg. Lactose. 100s, 500s, 1,000s. **Oral Soln.:** 5 mg/5 mL. 500 mL. **Soln. Concentrate:** 20 mg/mL. 30 mL. **Tab.:** 5 mg, 15 mg, 30 mg. Bot. 100s, 500s (except 15 mg, 30 mg), UD 100s. *c-II.*
Use: Opioid analgesic, narcotic agonist.

oxycodone hydrochloride and ibuprofen. (Various Mfr.) Oxycodone hydrochloride 5 mg, ibuprofen 400 mg. May contain lactose, polydextrose. Film-coated. Tab. 30s, 100s, 500s. *c-II.*
Use: Narcotic analgesic.

•**oxycodone terephthalate.** (OX-ee-KOE-dohn teh-REFF-thah-late) *USP 34.*
Tall Man: oxyCODONE
Use: Analgesic, narcotic.

OxyContin. (Purdue) Oxycodone hydrochloride 10 mg, 15 mg, 20 mg, 30 mg, 40 mg, 60 mg, 80 mg. Lactose. CR Tab. Bot. 100s, UD 25s (except 15 mg, 30 mg, 60 mg). *c-II.*
Tall Man: OxyCONTIN
Use: Opioid analgesic.

Oxy Cover. (GlaxoSmithKline) Benzoyl peroxide 10%. Cream. 30 g. *OTC.*
Use: Dermatologic, acne.

oxyethylene oxypropylene polymer.
See: Poloxalkol.

W/Danthron, vitamin B₁, carboxymethyl cellulose.
See: Evactol.
OxyFAST. (Purdue Pharma LP) Oxycodone hydrochloride 20 mg/mL. Saccharin. Conc. Soln. Dropper Bot. 30 mL. *c-II.*
Use: Opioid analgesic.
•**oxyfilcon A.** (OX-ee-FILL-kahn A) USAN.
Use: Contact lens material (hydrophilic).
Oxy 5 Acne-Pimple Medication. (GlaxoSmithKline) Benzoyl peroxide 5% in lotion base. Lot. Bot. oz. *OTC.*
Use: Dermatologic, acne.
•**oxygen.** (OX-i-jen) *USP 34.*
Use: Gas, medicinal.
•**oxygen 93 percent.** (OX-i-jen) *USP 34.*
Use: Gas, medicinal.
OxyIR. (Purdue Pharma) Oxycodone hydrochloride 5 mg. Sucrose. Cap. Bot. 100s. *c-II.*
Use: Opioid analgesic.
OXY Medicated Cleanser and Maximum Strength Pads. (Mentholatum) Salicylic acid 2%, SD alcohol 44%, citric acid, menthol, propylene glycol. Cleanser. Bot. 120 mL. Pads 50s, 90s. *OTC.*
Use: Dermatologic, acne.
OXY Medicated Cleanser and Regular Strength Pads. (Mentholatum) Salicylic acid 0.5%, SD alcohol 28%, citric acid, menthol, propylene glycol. Cleanser. Bot. 120 mL. Pads 50s, 90s. *OTC.*
Use: Dermatologic, acne.
OXY Medicated Cleanser and Sensitive Skin Pads. (Mentholatum) Salicylic acid 0.5%, alcohol 22%, disodium lauryl sulfosuccinate, menthol, trisodium EDTA. Cleanser. Bot. 120 mL. Pads 50s, 90s. *OTC.*
Use: Dermatologic, acne.
OXY Medicated Soap. (Mentholatum) Triclosan 1%, bentonite, cocoamphodipropionate, iron oxides, glycerin, magnesium silicate, sodium borohydride, sodium cocoate, sodium tallowate, talc, EDTA, titanium dioxide. Bar. 97.5 g. *OTC.*
Use: Dermatologic, acne.
•**oxymetazoline hydrochloride.** (OX-ee-MET-azz-oh-leen) *USP 34.*
Use: Nasal decongestant, imidazoline; adrenergic (vasoconstrictor); mydriatic.
See: Afrin All Night No Drip.
Afrin Extra Moisturizing.
Afrin No-Drip 12-Hour.
Afrin No-Drip 12-Hour Extra Moisturizing.

Afrin Severe Congestion with Menthol.
Afrin Sinus 12 Hour Relief.
Afrin 12-Hour Original.
Dristan 12-Hr Nasal.
Duramist Plus 12-Hr Decongestant.
Duration.
Genasal.
Nasal Decongestant, Maximum Strength.
Nasal Relief.
Neo-Synephrine 12-Hour Extra Moisturizing.
Nōstrilla Complete Congestion Relief 12-Hour.
Nōstrilla Conditioning Double Moisture.
Nōstrilla 12-Hour.
12 Hour Nasal.
Twice-A-Day 12-Hour Nasal.
Vicks Sinex 12 Hour.
Vicks Sinex 12 Hour UltraFine Mist for Sinus Relief.
Visine LR.
oxymetazoline hydrochloride. (Various Mfr.) Oxymetazoline hydrochloride 0.05%. Soln. Spray Bot. 15 mL, 30 mL. *OTC.*
Use: Nasal decongestant, imidazoline.
•**oxymetholone.** (OCK-sih-METH-oh-lone) *USP 34.*
Use: Anabolic steroid.
See: Anadrol-50.
•**oxymorphone hydrochloride.** (ox-ee-MORE-fone) *USP 34.*
Use: Opioid analgesic.
See: Opana.
Opana ER.
oxymorphone hydrochloride. (Endo Pharmaceuticals) Oxymorphone hydrochloride 5 mg, 10 mg. Lactose. Tab. 100s, UD 100s. *c-II.*
Use: Opioid analgesic.
OXY Night Watch. (Mentholatum) Salicylic acid 1%, cetyl alcohol, silica, propylene glycol, stearyl alcohol, sodium laureth sulfate, parabens, EDTA. Lot. Bot. 60 mL. *OTC.*
Use: Dermatologic, acne.
OXY Night Watch Maximum Strength. (Mentholatum) Salicylic acid 2%, cetyl alcohol, EDTA, parabens, stearyl alcohol. Lot. Bot. 60 mL. *OTC.*
Use: Dermatologic, acne.
OXY Night Watch Sensitive Skin. (Mentholatum) Salicylic acid 1%, cetyl alcohol, EDTA, stearyl alcohol, parabens. Lot. Bot. 60 mL. *OTC.*
Use: Dermatologic, acne.
OXY Oil-Free Maximum Strength Acne Wash. (Mentholatum) Benzoyl peroxide

10%, parabens, diazolidinyl urea. Liq.
237 mL. *OTC.*
Use: Dermatologic, acne.
•**oxypertine.** (OX-ee-PURR-teen) USAN.
Integrin hydrochloride.
Use: Psychotherapeutic agent, antidepressant.
•**oxyphenbutazone.** (ox-ee-fen-BYOO-
tah-zone) *USP 34.*
Use: Analgesic, antiarthritic, anti-
inflammatory, antipyretic, antirheumatic.
•**oxyphenisatin acetate.** (OX-ee-fen-
EYE-sah-tin) USAN.
Use: Laxative.
See: Endophenolphthalein.
Isacen.
Prulet.
•**oxypurinol sodium.** (OX-ee-PYOO-ree-
nahl) USAN.
Use: Investigational xanthine oxidase
inhibitor.
•**oxyquinoline.** (OX-ih-KWIN-oh-lin)
USAN.
Use: Disinfectant.
oxyquinoline benzoate. (Merck & Co.)
Pkg. lb.
•**oxyquinoline sulfate.** (OX-ih-KWIN-oh-
lin) *NF 29.*
Use: Disinfectant, pharmaceutic aid
(complexing agent).
See: Chinositol.
W/Combinations.
See: Acid Jelly.
Fem ph.
Oxyzal Wet Dressing.
Rectal Medicone Unguent.
OXY-Scrub. (Mentholatum) Abradant
cleanser containing dissolving abradant
particles of sodium tetraborate deca-
hydrate. Tube 2.65 oz. *OTC.*
Use: Dermatologic, acne.
Oxysept 1. (Allergan) Microfiltered hydro-
gen peroxide 3% w/sodium tannate and
sodium nitrate, preservative free, buf-
fered. Soln. Bot. 355 mL. *OTC.*
Use: Contact lens care.
•**oxytetracycline.** (OX-i-TET-ra-SYE-
kleen) *USP 34.*
Use: Anti-infective.
See: Terramycin.
•**oxytetracycline and nystatin capsules.**
USP 34.
Use: Anti-infective, antifungal.
•**oxytetracycline and nystatin for oral
suspension.** *USP 34.*
Use: Anti-infective, antifungal.
•**oxytetracycline calcium.** (OX-i-TET-ra-
SYE-kleen) *USP 34.*
Use: Anti-infective.

•**oxytetracycline hydrochloride.** (OX-i-
TET-ra-SYE-kleen) *USP 34.* An antibiotic from *Streptomyces rimosus.*
Use: Anti-infective; antirickettsial.
•**oxytetracycline hydrochloride and
hydrocortisone acetate ophthalmic
suspension.** *USP 34.*
Use: Anti-infective, anti-inflammatory.
•**oxytetracycline hydrochloride and
hydrocortisone ointment.** *USP 34.*
Use: Anti-infective; anti-inflammatory.
•**oxytetracycline hydrochloride and
polymyxin B sulfate ointment.**
USP 34.
Use: Anti-infective.
•**oxytetracycline hydrochloride and
polymyxin B sulfate ophthalmic
ointment.** *USP 34.*
Use: Anti-infective.
•**oxytetracycline hydrochloride and
polymyxin B sulfate topical powder.**
USP 34.
Use: Anti-infective.
•**oxytetracycline hydrochloride and
polymyxin B sulfate vaginal inserts.**
USP 34.
Use: Anti-infective.
oxytetracycline-polymyxin B. Mix of
oxytetracycline hydrochloride and polymyxin B sulfate.
Use: Anti-infective.
•**oxytocin.** (ox-ih-TOE-sin) *USP 34.*
Use: Oxytocic.
See: Pitocin.
oxytocin. (Various Mfr.) Oxytocin
10 units/mL. Inj. Vials. 3 mL, 10 mL. *Rx.*
Use: Uterine active agent.
oxytocin nasal solution.
Use: Oxytocic.
oxytocin, synthetic.
See: Pitocin.
Oxytrol. (Watson) Oxybutynin 36 mg (de-
livers 3.9 mg/day over 3 to 4 days).
Transdermal Patch. 8s. *Rx.*
Use: Anticholinergic.
OXY Wash. (Mentholatum) Benzoyl per-
oxide 10%. Liq. Bot. 120 mL. *OTC.*
Use: Dermatologic, acne.
Oxyzal Wet Dressing. (Gordon Labora-
tories) Benzalkonium Cl 1:2000, oxy-
quinoline sulfate, distilled water. Drop-
per bot. 1 oz, 4 oz. *OTC.*
Use: Dermatologic, counterirritant.
Oysco D. (Rugby) Ca 250 mg, D
125 units. Tab. Bot. 100s, 250s, 1000s.
OTC.
Use: Mineral, vitamin supplement.
Oysco 500. (Rugby) Calcium carbonate
1250 mg (elemental calcium 500 mg),
as oyster shell calcium. Tab. Bot. 60s,

250s. *OTC.*
Use: Mineral supplement.
Oyst-Cal-D. (Ivax) Calcium 250 mg, vitamin D 125 units. Tab. Bot. 100s, 1000s. *OTC.*
Use: Mineral, vitamin supplement.
Oyst-Cal 500. (Goldline) Calcium carbonate 1250 mg (elemental calcium 500 mg), as oyster shell calcium. Preservative free. Tartrazine. Tab. Bot. 60s, 120s. *OTC.*
Use: Mineral supplement.
Oyster Calcium. (NBTY) Ca 275 mg, D 200 units, A 800 units. Tab. Bot. 100s. *OTC.*
Use: Mineral, vitamin supplement.
Oystercal-D. (NBTY) Calcium 250 mg, vitamin D 125 units. Tab. Bot. 100s, 250s. *OTC.*
Use: Mineral, vitamin supplement.

Oyster Shell Calcium. (Various Mfr.) Calcium carbonate 1250 mg (elemental calcium 500 mg). Tab. Bot. 60s, 150s, 300s, 1000s, UD 100s. *OTC.*
Use: Mineral supplement.
oyster shells.
See: Os-Cal.
Oysco 500.
Oyst-Cal 500.
•**ozolinone.** (oh-ZOE-lih-NOHN) USAN.
Use: Diuretic.
•**ozoralizumab.** (oh-ZOR-a-LIZ-oo-mab) USAN.
Use: Immunomodulator.
Ozurdex. (Allergan) Dexamethasone 0.7 mg. Implant, intravitreal. Pouch w/single-use applicator. *Rx.*
Use: Ophthalmic and otic agent, corticosteroid.

P

Pabalate-SF. (Wyeth) Potassium salicylate 300 mg, potassium aminobenzoate 300 mg. Tab. Bot. 100s, 500s. *OTC.*
Use: Antirheumatic.
PABA-Salicylate. (Various Mfr.) Sodium salicylate, p-aminobenzoate, vitamin C. Tab. Bot. 100s, 500s. *OTC.*
Use: Analgesic; vitamin combination.
PABA sodium. (Various Mfr.) Sodium p-aminobenzoate. *OTC.*
Use: Vitamin supplement.
Pabasone. (Pinex) Sodium salicylate 5 g, para-aminobenzoic acid 5 g, ascorbic acid 20 mg. Tab. Bot. 100s. *OTC.*
Use: Analgesic; vitamin supplement.
P-A-C. Preparations of phenacetin, aspirin, caffeine.
See: A.P.C. preparations.
  Empirin preparations.
P-A-C Analgesic. (Lee) Aspirin 400 mg, caffeine 32 mg. Tab. Bot. 100s, 1000s. *OTC.*
Use: Analgesic combination.
Pacemaker Prophylaxis Pastes with Fluoride. (Pacemaker) Silicone dioxide and diatomaceous earth, sodium fluoride 4.4%. Light abrasive, cinnamon/cherry. Medium abrasive, orange. Heavy abrasive, mint. Paste. Bot. 8 oz.
Use: Dental caries agent.
Pacerone. (Upsher Smith) Amiodarone hydrochloride 100 mg, 200 mg, 400 mg. Lactose. Tab. Bot. 30s (100 mg, 400 mg only), 60s (200 mg only), 90s (200 mg only), 100s (400 mg only), 500s (except 100 mg), UD 100s. *Rx.*
Use: Antiarrhythmic.
Paclin VK. (Armenpharm Ltd.) Penicillin phenoxymethyl 125 mg, 250 mg. Tab. Bot. 100s, 1000s. *Rx.*
Use: Anti-infective, penicillin.
•**paclitaxel.** (pak-lih-TAX-uhl) *USP 34.*
Tall Man: PACLitaxel
Use: Antineoplastic; antimitotic agent.
See: Abraxane.
  Onxol.
  Taxol.
paclitaxel. (SuperGen) Paclitaxel 6 mg/mL. Polyoxyethylated castor oil (*Cremophor EL*) 527 mg/mL, dehydrated alcohol 49.7%. Inj. Multidose vials. 5 mL, 16.7 mL. *Rx.*
Use: Antimitotic agent.
•**paclitaxel poliglumex.** (pak-lih-TAX-uhl pol-ee-GLOO-mex) USAN.
Tall Man: PACLitaxel
Use: Antineoplastic.
Pacnex HP. (Medimetriks Pharmaceuticals) Benzoyl peroxide 7%. Alcohol,

aloe, edetate disodium, glycerin, glyceryl, green tea, PEG, propylene glycol. Pad. UD 60s. *Rx.*
Use: Topical anti-infective, antibiotic.
Pacnex LP. (Medimetriks Pharmaceuticals) Benzoyl peroxide 4.25%. Alcohol, aloe, edetate disodium, glycerin, glyceryl, green tea, PEG, propylene glycol. Pad. UD 60s. *Rx.*
Use: Topical anti-infective, antibiotic.
P-A-C Revised Formula Analgesic. (Pharmacia) Aspirin 400 mg, caffeine 32 mg. Tab. Bot. 100s, 1000s. *OTC.*
Use: Analgesic.
•**padimate A.** (PAD-ih-mate A) USAN.
Use: Ultraviolet screen.
•**padimate O.** (PAD-ih-mate O) *USP 34.*
Use: Ultraviolet screen.
See: Coppertone.
  Eclipse.
  Shade.
  Super Shade.
  Tropical Blend.
W/Combinations.
See: Glyquin.
•**paflufocon A.** (PA-floo-FOE-kon A) USAN.
Use: Contact lens material, hydrophobic.
•**paflufocon B.** (PA-flo-FOE-kon B) USAN.
Use: Contact lens material, hydrophobic.
•**paflufocon C.** (PA-flo-FOE-kon C) USAN.
Use: Contact lens material, hydrophobic.
•**paflufocon D.** (PA-flo-FOE-kon D) USAN.
Use: Contact lens material, hydrophobic.
•**paflufocon D-hem-iberfilcon A.** (pafloo-FOE-kon eye-ber-FIL-kon A) USAN.
Use: Contact lens material, hybrid.
•**paflufocon E.** (PA-flo-FOE-kon E) USAN.
Use: Contact lens material, hydrophobic.
•**pafuramidine maleate.** (PA-fur-AM-i-deen) USAN.
Use: Anti-infective.
•**pagoclone.** (PAG-oh-klone) USAN.
Use: Anxiolytic.
PAH.
See: Sodium aminohippurate.
Painaid. (Zee Medical) Aspirin 162 mg, salicylamide 152 mg, acetaminophen 110 mg, caffeine 32.4 mg. Tab. 24s. *OTC.*
Use: Nonnarcotic analgesic.

Painaid BRF Back Relief Formula. (Zee Medical) Magnesium salicylate tetrahydrate 250 mg, acetaminophen 250 mg. Tab. 24s. *OTC.*
Use: Nonnarcotic analgesic.

Painaid ESF Extra-Strength Formula. (Zee Medical) Acetaminophen 250 mg, aspirin 250 mg, caffeine 65 mg. Tab. 24s. *OTC.*
Use: Nonnarcotic analgesic.

Painaid PMF Premenstrual Formula. (Zee Medical) Acetaminophen 500 mg, pamabrom 25 mg. Tab. 24s. *OTC.*
Use: Nonnarcotic analgesic.

Pain and Fever. (Rugby) Acetaminophen. **Tab.:** 325 mg. Bot. 100s. **Tab. and Capl.:** 500 mg. Bot. 100s, 1000s. *OTC.*
Use: Analgesic.

Pain and Fever Children's. (Rugby) Acetaminophen 80 mg. Aspartame, dextrose, phenylalanine, sugar. Fruit flavor. Chew. Tab. 30s *OTC.*
Use: Analgesic.

Pain and Fever Reliever Children's. (Rugby) Acetaminophen. **Soln., Conc., Oral:** 100 mg/mL. Alcohol free. Butylparaben, corn syr., sorbitol. Cherry flavor. 15 mL. **Soln., Oral:** 160 mg/5 mL. Sorbitol, sucrose. Cherry flavor. 118 mL. *OTC.*
Use: Analgesic.

Pain Bust-R II. (Continental Consumer Products) Methyl salicylate 17%, menthol 12%. Cream. Jar 90 g. *OTC.*
Use: Liniment.

Pain Doctor. (E. Fougera) Capsaicin 0.025%, methyl salicylate 25%, menthol 10%, parabens, propylene glycol. Cream. Tube 60 g. *OTC.*
Use: Anesthetic, local.

Pain Gel Plus. (Mentholatum Co.) Menthol 4%, aloe, vitamin E. Gel. Tube 57 g. *OTC.*
Use: Liniment.

Pain-gesic. (Mason Remedies) Phenyltoloxamine citrate 30 mg, acetaminophen 325 mg. Lactose. Tab. 100s. *OTC.*
Use: Upper respiratory combination, decongestant, antihistamine, and analgesic.

Pain Relief. (Walgreen) Methyl salicylate 15%, menthol 10%. Oint. Tube 1.5 oz, 3 oz. *OTC.*
Use: Analgesic, topical.

Pain Relief Extra Strength. (Basic) Acetaminophen 500 mg. Tab. Bot. 100s. *OTC.*
Use: Analgesic, local.

Pain Reliever. (Magno-Humphries) Acetaminophen 325 mg. Tab. 100s, 250s, 1000s. *OTC.*
Use: Analgesic.

Pain Reliever Extra Strength. (Magno-Humphries) Acetaminophen 500 mg. Tab. 100s, 250s, 1000. *OTC.*
Use: Analgesic.

Pain Relievers-Tension Headache Relievers. (Weeks & Leo) Acetaminophen 325 mg, phenyltoloxamine citrate 30 mg. Tab. Bot. 40s, 100s. *OTC.*
Use: Analgesic combination.

Pain Relieving Rub. (G & W Labs) Menthol 10%, methyl salicylate 15%. Cetyl alcohol, glycerin, glyceryl, triethanolamine. Cream. 114 g. *OTC.*
Use: Rub and liniment.

Paladin. (Pal Midwest Ltd.) Petrolatum, starch, lanolin, zinc oxide, mineral oil, boric acid, beeswax, vitamin A and D concentrate. Oint. 2 oz. *OTC.*
Use: Diaper rash products.

Palbar No. 2. (Roberts) Atropine sulfate 0.012 mg, scopolamine HBr 0.005 mg, hyoscyamine HBr 0.018 mg, phenobarbital 32.4 mg. Tab. Bot. 100s. *Rx.*
Use: Anticholinergic; antispasmodic; sedative; hypnotic.

Palcaps 10. (Breckenridge) Lipase 10,000 units, protease 37,500 units, amylase (porcine-derived enzymes) 33,200 units. Sucrose. Enteric-coated microspheres. DR Cap. 100s, 250s. *Rx.*
Use: Digestive enzyme.

•**paldimycin.** (pal-dih-MY-sin) USAN.
Use: Anti-infective.

palestrol.
See: Diethylstilbestrol.

Palgic. (Pamlab) Carbinoxamine maleate 4 mg/5 mL. Parabens. Sugar free. Bubble gum flavor. Liq. 118 mL, 473 mL. *Rx.*
Use: Antihistamine.

Palgic-D. (Pamlab) Pseudoephedrine hydrochloride 80 mg, carbinoxamine maleate 8 mg. Dye free. ER Tab. Bot. 100s. *Rx.*
Use: Upper respiratory combination, antihistamine, decongestant.

Palgic DS. (Pamlab) Carbinoxamine maleate 2 mg, pseudoephedrine hydrochloride 25 mg per 5 mL. Strawberry/pineapple flavor. Syr. Bot. 15 mL, 473 mL. *Rx.*
Use: Upper respiratory combination, antihistamine, decongestant.

•**palifermin.** (pal-ee-FER-min) USAN.
Use: Keratinocyte growth factor; mucositis.
See: Kepivance.

- **palifosfamide.** (pal-i-FOS-fa-mide) USAN.
  Use: Antineoplastic agent.
- **palinavir.** (pal-LIH-nah-veer) USAN.
  Use: Antiviral.
- **palinum.**
  Use: Hypnotic; sedative.
  See: Cyclobarbital calcium.
- **paliperidone.** (pal-ee-PER-i-done) USAN.
  Use: Antipsychotic, schizophrenia.
  See: Invega.
  Invega Sustenna.
- **paliperidone palmitate.** (pal-ee-PER-i-done PAL-mih-tate) USAN.
  Use: Antipsychotic, schizophrenia.
- **palivizumab.**
  Use: Antibody.
  See: Synagis.
- **palmoxirate sodium.** (pal-MOX-ihr-ate) USAN.
  Use: Antidiabetic.
- **Palomar "E".** (Pal Midwest) Vitamin E, boric acid, beeswax, lanolin, mineral oil, petroleum, starch, zinc oxide. Oint. 2 oz. *OTC.*
  Use: Emollient.
- **palonosetron hydrochloride.** (pal-oh-NO-seh-trahn) USAN.
  Use: 5-HT$_3$ receptor antagonist; anti-emetic/antivertigo agent.
  See: Aloxi.
- **palovarotene.** (PA-loe-VAR-oh-teen) USAN.
  Use: Treatment of emphysema.
- **PALS.** (Palisades Pharmaceuticals) Chlorophyllin copper complex 100 mg. Tab. Bot. 30s, 100s, 1000s, UD 30s. *OTC.*
  Use: Deodorant, systemic.
- **pamabrom.** (PAM-a-brom) USAN.
  See: Maximum Strength Aqua-Ban.
  W/Acetaminophen.
  See: Midol Teen Formula.
  Painaid PMF Premenstrual Formula.
  Women's Tylenol Multi-Symptom Menstrual Relief.
  W/Acetaminophen, Magnesium Salicylate.
  See: Pamprin Maximum Pain Relief.
  W/Acetaminophen, Pyrilamine Maleate.
  See: Midol Pre-Menstrual Syndrome.
  Pamprin Multi-Symptom Maximum Strength.
  Vitelle Lurline PMS.
- **pamapimod.** (pa-MAP-i-mod) USAN.
  Use: Treatment of rheumatoid arthritis.
- **pamaqueside.** (pam-ah-KWEH-side) USAN.
  Use: Antiatherosclerotic; hypocholesterolemic.

- **pamatolol sulfate.** (PAM-ah-TOE-lole) USAN.
  Use: Anti-adrenergic, β-receptor.
- **Pamelor.** (Mallinckrodt) Nortriptyline hydrochloride 10 mg, 25 mg, 50 mg, 75 mg. Benzyl alcohol, EDTA, parabens. Cap. 100s, 500s (25 mg only), UD 100s (except 75 mg). *Rx.*
  Use: Antidepressant.
- **pamidronate disodium.** (pam-IH-DROE-nate) USAN.
  Use: Bisphosphonate.
  See: Aredia.
- **pamidronate disodium.** (Faulding) Pamidronate disodium 6 mg/mL. Mannitol 400 mg. Inj. Vials. 10 mL. *Rx.*
  Use: Bisphosphonate.
- **pamidronate disodium.** (Sandoz) Pamidronate disodium 30 mg (mannitol 470 mg), 90 mg (mannitol 375 mg). Pow. for Inj., lyophilized. Vials. *Rx.*
  Use: Bisphosphonate.
- **pamidronate disodium.** (Various Mfr.) Pamidronate disodium 3 mg/mL, 9 mg/mL. May contain mannitol. Inj. Vials. 10 mL. *Rx.*
  Use: Bisphosphonate.
- **Pamine.** (Kenwood/Bradley) Methscopolamine bromide 2.5 mg. Tab. Bot. 100s, 500s. *Rx.*
  Use: Anticholinergic/antispasmodic.
- **Pamine Forte.** (Kenwood Therapeutics) Methscopolamine bromide 5 mg. Tab. 60s. *Rx.*
  Use: Anticholinergic/antispasmodic.
- **Pamine FQ Kit.** (Kenwood Therapeutics) Methscopolamine bromide 5 mg with *Flora-Q* capsules containing 8 million CFUs of *Lactobacillus acidophilus*, *L. paracasei, Bifidobacteriura*, and *Streptococcus thermophilus.* Gluten free. Tab. Packs of 60 methscopolamine bromide tablets and 30 *Flor-Q* capsules. *Rx.*
  Use: GI anticholinergic/antispasmodic, quaternary anticholinergic.
- **p-aminosalicylic acid salts.**
  See: Aminosalicylic acid salts.
- **Pamprin Extra Strength Multi-Symptom Relief Formula.** (Chattem) Acetaminophen 400 mg, pamabrom 25 mg, pyrilamine maleate 15 mg. Tab. Bot. 12s, 24s, 48s. *OTC.*
  Use: Analgesic combination.
- **Pamprin Maximum Cramp Relief Formula Caplets.** (Chattem) Acetaminophen 500 mg, pamabrom 25 mg, pyrilamine maleate 15 mg. Tab. Bot. 8s, 16s, 32s. *OTC.*
  Use: Analgesic combination.

Pamprin Maximum Pain Relief Caplets. (Chattem) Acetaminophen 250 mg, magnesium salicylate 250 mg, pamabrom 25 mg. Tab. Bot. 16s, 32s. *OTC.*
Use: Analgesic combination.

Pamprin Multi-Symptom Maximum Strength. (Chattem) Acetaminophen 500 mg, pamabrom 25 mg, pyrilamine maleate 15 mg. **Cap.:** Bot. 24s, 48s. **Tab.:** Bot. 12s, 24s, 48s. *OTC.*
Use: Analgesic combination.

•**panadiplon.** (pan-ad-IH-plone) USAN.
Use: Anxiolytic.

Panadol Extra Strength. (GlaxoSmith-Kline) Acetaminophen 500 mg. Tab. 30s, 60s. *OTC.*
Use: Analgesic.

Panadol, Infants'. (GlaxoSmithKline) Acetaminophen 100 mg/mL. Drops. Bot. 15 mL with 0.8 mL dropper. *OTC.*
Use: Analgesic.

Panadol, Jr. (GlaxoSmithKline) Acetaminophen 160 mg. Cap. Box. 30s. *OTC.*
Use: Analgesic.

Panafil White. (Rystan) Papain 10,000 units enzyme activity, hydrophilic base/g, urea 10%. Oint. Tube oz. *Rx.*
Use: Enzyme, topical.

Panalgesic. (ECR) Methyl salicylate 55.01%, menthol 1.25%, camphor 3.1%, in alcohol 22%, emollients, color. Liq. 4 oz, pt, 0.5 gal. *OTC.*
Use: Analgesic, topical.

Panasol. (Seatrace) Prednisone 5 mg. Tab. Bot. 100s. *Rx.*
Use: Corticosteroid.

Panatuss DXP. (Seyer) Dexbrompheniramine maleate 2 mg, dextromethorphan hydrobromide 20 mg, phenylephrine hydrochloride 10 mg. Aspartame, parabens, PEG, phenylalanine 15 mg per 5 mL, propylene glycol, sucrose. Alcohol free. Raspberry flavor. Syrup. 118 mL. *Rx.*
Use: Upper respiratory combination, antitussive combination.

Pan C-500. (Freeda) Hesperidin 100 mg, citrus bioflavonoids 100 mg, vitamin C 500 mg. Sodium and sugar free. Tab. Bot. 100s, 250s, 500s. *OTC.*
Use: Water-soluble vitamin.

Pancof. (Pan American) Dihydrocodeine bitartrate 7.5 mg, chlorpheniramine maleate 2 mg, pseudoephedrine hydrochloride 15 mg per 5 mL. Saccharin, sorbitol, alcohol free, dye free, sugar free. Syr. 473 mL. *c-III.*
Use: Antitussive combination.

Pancof-EXP. (Pan American) Dihydrocodeine bitartrate 7.5 mg, guaifenesin 100 mg, pseudoephedrine 15 mg per 5 mL. Saccharin, sorbitol, menthol. Alcohol and dye free. Syr. Bot. 25 mL, 473 mL. *Rx.*
Use: Upper respiratory combination, antitussive, expectorant, decongestant.

Pancof XP. (Pan American) Hydrocodone bitartrate 3 mg, guaifenesin 90 mg per 5 mL. Menthol, saccharin, sorbitol. Syr. 3700 mL. *c-III.*
Use: Antitussive with expectorant.

•**pancopride.** (PAN-koe-pride) USAN.
Use: Antiemetic, anxiolytic, peristaltic stimulant.

pancreatic enzyme.
See: Ox bile extract.
Pepsin.

pancreatic substance. Substance from fresh pancreas of hog or ox, containing the enzymes amylopsin, trypsin, steapsin.

•**pancreatin.** (PAN-kree-ah-tin) *USP 34.* Pancreatic enzymes obtained from hog or cattle pancreatic tissue.
Use: Enzyme (digestant adjunct).

•**pancrelipase.** (pan-KREE-lih-pace) *USP 34.* Preparation of hog pancreas with high content of steapsin and adequate amounts of pancreatic enzymes.
Use: Enzyme (digestant adjunct).
See: Ultrase.
Ultrase MT 18.
Ultrase MT 12.
Ultrase MT 20.
Viokase.

pancrelipase. (X-Gen Pharmaceuticals) Amylase 27,000 units, lipase 5000 units, protease 17,000 units. Enteric-coated beads. Cap., delayed release. 100s. *Rx.*
Use: Digestive enzyme.

pancrelipase. (Various Mfr.) Lipase 4,500 units, protease 25,000 units, amylase 20,000 units; lipase 16,000 units, protease 48,000 units, amylase 48,000 units. Cap. 100s, 250s. *Rx.*
Use: Digestive enzyme.

Pancretide. (Baxter PPI) Pancreatic polypeptide in normal saline.
Use: Fibrinolytic conditions.

pancuronium.
See: Pancuronium bromide.

•**pancuronium bromide.** (PAN-cue-ROW-nee-uhm) USAN.
Use: Neuromuscular blocker, muscle relaxant.

pancuronium bromide. (Various Mfr.) Pancuronium bromide. **1 mg/mL:** Vials 10 mL with benzyl alcohol. **2 mg/mL:** Benzyl alcohol. Vials 2 mL, 5 mL.

Amps with benzyl alcohol. *Rx.*
Use: Neuromuscular blocker, muscle relaxant.

Pandel. (Collagenex) Hydrocortisone probutate 0.1%, white petrolatum, light mineral oil, stearyl alcohol, parabens. Cream. Tube 15 g, 45 g, 80 g. *Rx.*
Use: Corticosteroid, topical.

P & S. (Ivax) Mineral oil, water, glycerin, fragrance, phenol, sodium chloride. Liq. 4 oz, 8 oz. *OTC.*
Use: Antiseborrheic.

P & S Shampoo. (Aero Pharmaceuticals) Salicylic acid 2%. Lactic acid, parabens, tetrasodium EDTA, triethanolamine, urea. Shampoo. 236 mL. *OTC.*
Use: Keratolytic agent.

Panfil G. (Pan American) **Cap.:** Dyphylline 200 mg, guaifenesin 100 mg, lactose. Bot. 100s. **Syr.:** Dyphylline 100 mg, guaifenesin 50 mg/5 mL, parabens, sorbitol, sucrose, vanilla flavor. Bot. 473 mL. *Rx.*
Use: Antiasthmatic; expectorant.

Panhematin. (Ovation) Hematin 301 mg/vial (equivalent to hematin 7 mg/mL) after reconstitution w/Sterile Water for Injection 43 mL, sorbitol 300 mg, preservative free. Pow. for Inj. Single-dose dispensing vial 100 mL. *Rx.*
Use: Hematinic.

Panitol. (Wesley) Allylisobutyl barbituric acid 15 mg, acetaminophen 300 mg. Tab. Bot. 100s, 1000s. *Rx.*
Use: Analgesic; hypnotic; sedative.

•**panitumumab.** (pan-i-TUE-moo-mab) USAN.
Use: Antineoplastic; monoclonal antibody.
See: Vectibix.

Panlor DC. (Pan American) Acetaminophen 356.4 mg, caffeine 30 mg, dihydrocodeine bitartrate 16 mg. Cap. Bot. 100s. *c-III.*
Use: Analgesic.

PanMist-DM. (Pan American) **Syr.:** Dextromethorphan HBr 15 mg, guaifenesin 100 mg, pseudoephedrine hydrochloride 40 mg per 5 mL. Strawberry flavor. Alcohol, sugar, and dye free. Bot. 15 mL, 473 mL. **ER Tab.:** Dextromethorphan HBr 32 mg, guaifenesin 595 mg, pseudoephedrine hydrochloride 48 mg. Bot. 100s. *Rx.*
Use: Upper respiratory combination, antitussive, expectorant, decongestant.

PanMist JR. (Pan American) Pseudoephedrine hydrochloride 48 mg, guaifenesin 595 mg, dye free. ER Tab. Bot. 100s. *Rx.*

Use: Upper respiratory combination, decongestant, expectorant.

PanMist LA. (Pan American) Pseudoephedrine hydrochloride 85 mg, guaifenesin 795 mg. ER Tab. Bot. 100s. *Rx.*
Use: Upper respiratory combination, decongestant, expectorant.

PanMist S. (Pan American) Pseudoephedrine hydrochloride 40 mg, guaifenesin 200 mg. Alcohol free, grape flavor. Syr. Bot. 15 mL, 473 mL. *Rx.*
Use: Upper respiratory combination, decongestant, expectorant.

Panmycin. (Pharmacia) Tetracycline hydrochloride 250 mg. Cap. Bot. 100s, 1000s. *Rx.*
Use: Anti-infective, tetracycline.

PanOxyl. (GlaxoSmithKline) Benzoyl peroxide. **Bar:** 10%. Cetostearyl alcohol, glycerin, castor oil, mineral oil in a rich lathering, mild surfactant cleansing base. Soap free. 113 g. **Liq.:** 2.5%. Cetearyl alcohol. Soap free. 156 g. **Wash:** 10%. Alcohol, methylparaben. 156 g. *OTC.*
Use: Dermatologic, acne.

PanOxyl AQ 2½, 5, 10. (GlaxoSmithKline) Benzoyl peroxide 2.5%, 5%, 10%, methylparaben, EDTA, glycerin. Gel. Tube 57 g, 113 g. *Rx.*
Use: Dermatologic, acne.

panparnit hydrochloride. Caramiphen hydrochloride.
Use: Antiparkinsonian.

Panretin. (Ligand) Alitretinoin 0.1%. Dehydrated alcohol. Gel. Tube 60 g. *Rx.*
Use: Second-generation retinoid.

Panscol. (Ivax) Salicylic acid 3%, lactic acid 2%, phenol (< 1%). **Oint.:** Jar 3 oz. **Lot.:** Bot. 4 oz. *OTC.*
Use: Emollient.

•**panthenol.** (PAN-theh-nahl) *USP 34.* Alcohol corresponding to pantothenic acid.
Use: Vitamin; emollient.
W/Combinations.
See: Lifer-B.

Panthoderm. (Aventis) Dexpanthenol 2% in water-miscible cream. Cream. Tube 1 oz. Jar 2 oz, lb. *OTC.*
Use: Emollient.

pantocaine.
See: Tetracaine hydrochloride.

Pantocrin-F. (Spanner) Plurigland, ovarian, anterior and posterior pituitary, adrenal, thyroid extracts. Vial 30 mL. *Rx.*
Use: Hormone.

•**pantoprazole.** (pan-TOE-pra-zole) USAN.
Use: Antiulcerative.

•**pantoprazole sodium.** (pahn-TOE-prazz-ole) USAN.
Use: Proton pump inhibitor.
See: Protonix.
    Protonix I.V.
pantoprazole sodium. (Teva) Pantoprazole 20 mg (as pantoprazole sodium 22.6 mg), 40 mg (as pantoprazole sodium 45.1 mg). May contain lactose. DR Tab. 90s. *Rx.*
Use: Proton pump inhibitor.
pantothenic acid.
Use: Vitamin B_5 supplement.
See: Calcium Pantothenate.
pantothenic acid salts.
See: Calcium pantothenate.
    Sodium pantothenate.
pantothenol.
See: Dexpanthenol.
pantothenyl alcohol.
See: Dexpanthenol.
pantothenylol.
See: Panthenol.
Panvitex Geriatric. (Forest) Safflower oil 340 mg, vitamins A 10,000 units, D 400 units, B_1 5 mg, B_6 1 mg, B_2 2.5 mg, B_{12} activity 2 mcg, C 75 mg, niacinamide 40 mg, calcium pantothenate 4 mg, E 2 units, inositol 15 mg, choline bitartrate 31.4 mg, Ca 75 mg, P 58 mg, Fe 30 mg, Mn 0.5 mg, K 2 mg, Zn 0.5 mg, Mg 3 mg. Cap. Bot. 100s, 1000s. *OTC.*
Use: Mineral, vitamin supplement.
Panvitex Plus Minerals. (Forest) Vitamins A 5000 units, D 400 units, B_1 3 mg, B_2 2.5 mg, niacinamide 20 mg, B_6 1.5 mg, calcium pantothenate 5 mg, B_{12} 2.5 mcg, C 50 mg, E 3 units, Ca 215 mg, P 166 mg, Fe 13.4 mg, Mg 7.5 mg, Mn 1.5 mg, K 5 mg, Zn 1.4 mg. Cap. Bot. 100s, 1000s. *OTC.*
Use: Mineral, vitamin supplement.
Panvitex Prenatal. (Forest) Ferrous fumarate 150 mg, cobalamin concentration 2 mcg, vitamins A 6000 units, D 400 units, B_1 1.5 mg, B_2 2.5 mg, niacinamide 15 mg, B_6 3 mg, C 100 mg, Ca 250 mg, calcium pantothenate 5 mg, folic acid 0.2 mg. Cap. Bot. 100s, 1000s. *OTC.*
Use: Mineral, vitamin supplement.
Panvitex T-M. (Forest) Vitamins A 10,000 units, D 400 units, B_1 10 mg, B_6 1 mg, B_2 5 mg, B_{12} 5 mcg, C 150 mg, niacinamide 100 mg, Ca 103 mg, P 80 mg, Fe 10 mg, Mn 1 mg, K 5 mg, Zn 1.4 mg, Mg 5.56 mg. Cap. Bot. 100s, 1000s. *OTC.*
Use: Mineral, vitamin supplement.
PAP. (Abbott Diagnostics) Enzyme immunoassay for measurement of prostatic acid phosphatase. Test kit 100s.
Use: Diagnostic aid.
Papadeine #3. (Vangard Labs, Inc.) Codeine phosphate 30 mg, acetaminophen 300 mg. Tab. Bot. 100s, 1000s. *c-III.*
Use: Analgesic combination; narcotic.
•**papain.** (pap-ANE) *USP 34.* A proteolytic substance derived from *Carica papaya.*
Use: Proteolytic enzyme.
W/Combinations.
See: Ziox 405.
Pap-a-Lix. (Freeport) n-acetyl-aminophenol 120 mg, alcohol 10%/ 5 mL. Bot. 4 oz, gal. *OTC.*
Use: Analgesic.
•**papaverine hydrochloride.** (pap-PAV-uhr-een) *USP 34.*
Use: Vasodilator.
See: Pavagen TD.
papaverine hydrochloride. (Various Mfr.) Papaverine hydrochloride. **Inj.:** 30 mg/mL. Vial 2 mL, multiple-dose vial 10 mL. **TR Cap.:** 150 mg. 100s, 1000s. *Rx.*
Use: Vasodilator.
papillomavirus vaccine, quadrivalent, human.
Use: Active immunization agent, viral vaccine.
See: Gardasil.
Paplex Ultra. (Medicis) Salicylic acid 26% in flexible collodion. Bot. 15 mL. *OTC.*
Use: Keratolytic.
para-aminobenzoic acid. (Various Mfr.) para-aminobenzoic acid. **Tab.:** 100 mg. Bot. 100s, 250s. **SR Tab.:** 100 mg. Bot. 100s. *OTC.*
Use: Sunscreen; agent for scleroderma.
para-aminobenzoic acid (PABA).
Use: Sunscreen; agent for scleroderma.
See: Potaba.
•**para-aminosalicylic acid.** *USP 34.* Aminosalicylic acid. *Rx.*
Use: Antituberculosis.
Parabaxin. (Parmed Pharmaceuticals, Inc.) Methocarbamol 500 mg, 750 mg. Tab. Bot. 100s. *Rx.*
Use: Muscle relaxant.
parabrom.
See: Pyrabrom.
parabromidylamine.
See: Brompheniramine.
    Dimetane Decongestant.
Paracaine. (Ocusoft) Proparacaine hydrochloride 0.5%. Soln. 15 mL. *Rx.*
Use: Ophthalmic local anesthetic.
paracarbinoxamine maleate. Carbinoxamine.

• **paracetaldehyde.** *USP 34.*
See: Parldehyde.

Paracet Forte. (Major) Chlorzoxazone, acetaminophen. Tab. Bot. 100s, 1000s. *Rx.*
Use: Muscle relaxant.

parachloramine hydrochloride. Meclizine hydrochloride.
See: Bonine.

parachlorometaxylenol.
Use: Phenolic antiseptic.
W/Pramoxine hydrochloride, hydrocortisone, benzalkonium Cl, acetic acid.
See: Rezamid.

• **parachlorophenol.** (PAR-a-KLOR-oh-FEE-nole) *USP 34.*
Use: Anti-infective, topical.

• **parachlorophenol, camphorated.** (PAR-a-KLOR-oh-FEE-nole) *USP 34.*
Use: Anti-infective, topical.

paracodin.
See: Dihydrocodeine.

Paraeusal Liquid. (Paraeusal) Liq. Bot. 2 oz, 6 oz, 12 oz.
Use: Minor skin irritations.

Paraeusal Solid. (Paraeusal) Oint. Jar 1 oz, 2 oz, 16 oz.
Use: Dermatologic, counterirritant.

• **paraffin.** (PAR-ah-fin) *NF 29.*
Use: Pharmaceutic aid (stiffening agent).

• **paraffin, synthetic.** (PAR-ah-fin) *NF 29.*
Use: Pharmaceutic aid (stiffening agent).

Paraflex. (McNeil Pharm.) Chlorzoxazone 250 mg. Tab. Bot. 100s. *Rx.*
Use: Muscle relaxant.

Parafon Forte DSC. (Janssen) Chlorzoxazone 500 mg. Cap. Bot. 100s, 500s, UD 100s. *Rx.*
Use: Muscle relaxant.

paraform. Paraformaldehyde (No Manufacturer Available).

paraformaldehyde.
Use: Essentially the same as formaldehyde.
See: Formaldehyde.
Trioxymethylene (an incorrect term for paraformaldehyde).

paraglycylarsanilic acid. N-carbamyl-methyl-p-aminobenzenearsonic acid, the free acid of tryparsamide.

Parahist HD. (Pharmics) Phenylephrine hydrochloride 5 mg, chlorpheniramine maleate 2 mg, hydrocodone bitartrate 1.67 mg, alcohol free. Liq. Bot. 473 mL. *c-III.*
Use: Antihistamine; antitussive; decongestant.

Para-Jel. (Health for Life Brands) Benzocaine 5%, cetyl dimethyl benzyl ammonium Cl. Tube 0.25 oz. *OTC.*
Use: Anesthetic, local.

• **paraldehyde.** (par-AL-deh-hide) *USP 34.*
Use: Hypnotic; sedative.

paramephrin.
See: Epinephrine.

• **paramethasone acetate.** (PAR-ah-meth-ah-zone) *USP 34.*
Use: Corticosteriod, topical.
See: Haldrone.

para-monochlorophenol.
See: Camphorated para-chlorophenol.

• **paranyline hydrochloride.** (PAR-ah-NYE-leen) USAN.
Use: Anti-inflammatory.

• **parapenzolate bromide.** (pa-rah-PEN-zoe-late) USAN.
Use: Anticholinergic.

Paraplatin. (Bristol-Myers Squibb) Carboplatin 50 mg, 150 mg, 450 mg. Mannitol. Inj., lyophilized Pow. for Soln. Single-use vial. *Rx.*
Use: Antineoplastic agent, platinum coordination complex.

pararosaniline embonate. Pararosaniline pamoate.

• **pararosaniline pamoate.** (par-ah-row-ZAN-ih-lin PAM-oh-ate) USAN.
Use: Antischistosomal.

parasympatholytic agents. Cholinergic blocking agents.
See: Anticholinergic agents.
Antispasmodics.
Mydriatics.
Parkinsonism agents.

parasympathomimetic agents.
See: Cholinergic agents.

• **parathyroid hormone.** (par-a-THYE-roid) USAN.
Use: Anti-osteoporotic.

Paratrol. (Walgreen) Pyrethrins 0.2%, piperonyl butoxide technical 2%, deodorized kerosene 0.8%. Liq. Bot. 2 oz. *OTC.*
Use: Pediculicide.

Parazone. (Henry Schein) Chlorzoxazone 250 mg, acetaminophen 300 mg. Tab. Bot. 100s, 1000s. *Rx.*
Use: Muscle relaxant; analgesic.

• **parbendazole.** (par-BEN-dah-ZOLE) USAN. Under study.
Use: Anthelmintic.

Parcillin. (Parmed Pharmaceuticals, Inc.) Crystalline potassium penicillin G 240 mg, 400,000 units. Tab. Bot. 100s, 1000s. Pow. for Syr. 400,000 units/5 mL. 80 mL. *Rx.*
Use: Anti-infective, penicillin.

• **parconazole hydrochloride.** (par-KOE-nah-zole) USAN.
Use: Antifungal.

Parcopa. (Azur Pharma) Carbidopa/levodopa 10 mg/100 mg (phenylalanine 3.4 mg), 25 mg/100 mg (phenylalanine 3.4 mg), 25 mg/250 mg (phenylalanine 8.4 mg). Aspartame, mannitol. Mint flavor. Orally Disintegrating Tab. 100s. *Rx.*
Use: Antiparkinson agent.

• **pardoprunox.** (par-doe-PRUE-nox) USAN.
Use: Parkinson disease; restless legs syndrome.

• **pardoprunox hydrochloride.** (par-doe-PRUE-nox) USAN.
Use: Parkinson disease; restless legs syndrome.

• **parecoxib.** (pa-re-KOX-ib) USAN.
Use: Anti-inflammatory; analgesic.

• **paregoric.** (par-eh-GORE-ik) *USP 34.*
Use: Antiperistaltic.

paregoric. (Various Mfr.) Morphine anhydrous equivalent 2 mg/5 mL. Alcohol 45%, may contain benzoic acid. Liq. Bot. 473 mL. *c-III.*
Use: Antiperistaltic; opioid analgesic.

Paremyd. (Akorn) Hydroxyamphetamine HBr 1%, tropicamide 0.25%. Soln. Bot. 5 mL, 15 mL. *Rx.*
Use: Cycloplegic, mydriatic.

parenabol. Boldenone undecylenate.

• **pareptide sulfate.** (PAR-epp-tide) USAN.
Use: Antiparkinsonian.

Par Estro. (Parmed Pharmaceuticals, Inc.) Conjugated estrogens 1.25 mg. Tab. Bot. 100s. *Rx.*
Use: Estrogen.

Par-F. (Pharmics) Fe 60 mg, Ca 250 mg, vitamins C 120 mg, A 5000 units, D 400 units, B_1 3 mg, B_2 3.4 mg, B_{12} 12 mcg, B_6 12 mg, B_3 20 mg, Cu, I, Mg, Zn 15 mg, E 30 units, folic acid 1 mg. Tab. Bot. 100s. *Rx.*
Use: Mineral, vitamin supplement.

Par Glycerol. (Par Pharmaceuticals) Iodinated glycerol 60 mg/5 mL. Alcohol 21.75%, peppermint oil, corn syr., saccharin. Caramel-mint flavor. Elix. Bot. Pt. *Rx.*
Use: Expectorant.

• **pargyline hydrochloride.** (PAR-jih-leen) *USP 34.*
Use: Antihypertensive.

• **paricalcitol.** (pah-ri-KAL-si-tole) *USP 34.*
Use: Hyperparathyroidism.
See: Zemplar.

Parkelp. (Phillip R. Park) Pacific sea kelp. **Tab.:** Bot. 100s, 200s, 500s, 800s.
Gran.: Bot. 2 oz, 7 oz, 1 lb, 3 lb. *OTC.*
Use: Nutritional supplement.

parkinsonism, agents for. Parasympatholytic agents.
See: Akineton.
Benztropine Mesylate.
Caramiphen Hydrochloride.
Cogentin.
Dopar.
Eldepryl.
Kemadrin.
Larodopa.
Lodosyn.
Parlodel.
Permax.
Sinemet.
Symmetrel.
Trihexyphenidyl Hydrochloride.
Trihexy-2.

Parlodel. (Novartis) Bromocriptine mesylate. Lactose. **Tab.:** 2.5 mg. Bot. 30s, 100s. **Cap.:** 5 mg. Bot. 30s, 100s. *Rx.*
Use: Antiparkinsonian.

Parmeth. (Parmed Pharmaceuticals, Inc.) Promethazine hydrochloride 50 mg. Cap. Bot. 100s, 1000s. *Rx.*
Use: Antiemetic; antihistamine; antivertigo.

parminyl. Salicylamide, phenacetin, caffeine, acetaminophen.

Par-Natal-FA. (Parmed Pharmaceuticals, Inc.) Vitamins A 4000 units, D 400 units, thiamine hydrochloride 2 mg, riboflavin 2 mg, pyridoxine hydrochloride 0.8 mg, ascorbic acid 50 mg, niacinamide 10 mg, I 0.15 mg, folic acid 0.1 mg, cobalamin concentrate 2 mcg, Fe 50 mg, Ca 240 mg. Cap. Bot. 100s, 1000s. *OTC.*
Use: Mineral, vitamin supplement.

Par-Natal Plus 1 Improved. (Parmed Pharmaceuticals, Inc.) Elemental calcium 200 mg, elemental iron 65 mg, vitamins A 4000 units, D 400 units, E 11 mg, B_1 1.5 mg, B_2 3 mg, B_3 20 mg, B_6 10 mg, B_{12} 12 mcg, C 120 mg, folic acid 1 mg, Zn 25 mg, Cu. Tab. Bot. 500s. *Rx.*
Use: Mineral, vitamin supplement.

Parnate. (GlaxoSmithKline) Tranylcypromine sulfate 10 mg. Lactose. Film-coated. Tab. Bot. 100s. *Rx.*
Use: Antidepressant, monoamine oxidase inhibitor.

parodyne.
See: Antipyrine.

paroleine.
See: Petrolatum Liquid.

• **paromomycin sulfate.** (par-oh-moe-MY-sin) *USP 34.* An antibiotic substance obtained from cultures of certain *Strep-*

tomyces species, one of which is *Streptomyces rimosus.*
Use: Antiamebic.
See: Humatin.

paromomycin sulfate. (Caraco Pharmaceutical Laboratories) Paromomycin 250 mg. Cap. 100s. *Rx.*
Use: Oral aminoglycoside.

parothyl. (Henry Schein) Meprobamate 400 mg, tridihexethyl Cl 25 mg. Tab. Bot. 100s. *c-iv.*
Use: Anticholinergic; anxiolytic; antispasmodic.

paroxetine. (Various Mfr.) Paroxetine hydrochloride 10 mg, 20 mg, 30 mg, 40 mg. Tab. 30s, 100s, 1000s, UD 100s. *Rx.*
Use: Antidepressant, selective serotonin reuptake inhibitor.

•**paroxetine hydrochloride.** (puh-ROX-eh-teen) *USP 34.*
Tall Man: PARoxetine
Use: Antidepressant, selective serotonin reuptake inhibitor.
See: Paxil.
  Paxil CR.

paroxetine hydrochloride. (Apotex USA) Paroxetine hydrochloride 10 mg/5 mL. Oral Susp. 250 mL. *Rx.*
Use: Antidepressant, selective serotonin reuptake inhibitor.

paroxetine hydrochloride. (Mylan) Paroxetine 12.5 mg, 25 mg, 37.5 mg. Lactose, PEG, polydextrose. Film-coated. CR Tab. 30s, 100s (12.5 and 25 mg only), 500s (12.5 and 25 mg only). *Rx.*
Use: Antidepressant, selective serotonin reuptake inhibitor.

•**paroxetine mesylate.** (puh-ROX-eh-teen) USAN.
Tall Man: PARoxetine
Use: Antidepressant, selective serotonin reuptake inhibitor.
See: Pexeva.

parpanit.
See: Caramiphen hydrochloride.

parsley concentrate. Garlic concentrate. *Rx.*

Par-Supp. (Parmed Pharmaceuticals, Inc.) Estrone 0.2 mg, lactose 50 mg. Vaginal Supp. Pkg. 12s.
Use: Estrogen.

•**partricin.** (PAR-trih-sin) USAN. Antibiotic produced by *Streptomyces aureofaciens.*
Use: Antifungal; antiprotozoal.

Partuss A.C. (Parmed Pharmaceuticals, Inc.) Guaifenesin 100 mg, pheniramine maleate 7.5 mg, codeine phosphate 10 mg, alcohol 3.5%/5 mL. Bot. 4 oz. *c-v.*

Use: Antihistamine; antitussive; expectorant.

Parvlex. (Freeda) Iron 100 mg, vitamins B_1 20 mg, B_2 20 mg, B_3 20 mg, B_5 1 mg, B_6 10 mg, B_{12} 50 mcg, C 50 mg, folic acid 0.1 mg, Cu, Mn. Tab. Bot. 100s, 250s. *OTC.*
Use: Mineral, vitamin supplement.

Pas-C. (Hellwig) Pascorbic. p-aminosalicylic acid 0.5 g with vitamin C. Tab. Bot. 1000s. *Rx.*
Use: Antituberculosal.

•**pascolizumab.** (pas-co-LIZ-oo-mab) USAN.
Use: Asthma.

Paser. (Jacobus Pharm) Aminosalicylic acid 4 g. Oral DR Gran. Pkt. *Rx.*
Use: Antituberculosis agent.

passiflora. Dried flowering and fruiting tops of *Passiflora incarnata.* Phenobarbital, valerian, hyoscyamus.

Pataday. (Alcon) Olopatadine hydrochloride 0.2%. Benzalkonium chloride. Ophth. Soln. 2.5 mL. *Rx.*
Use: Ophthalmic antihistamine.

Patanase. (Alcon Labs) Olopatadine 0.6% (equiv. to olopatadine hydrochloride 665 mcg). Benzalkonium chloride 0.01%, edetate disodium. Spray, Soln., Intranasal. Metered-dose manual spray pump and applicator. 30.5 g (240 actuations). *Rx.*
Use: Respiratory inhalant, intranasal antihistamine.

Patanol. (Alcon) Olopatadine hydrochloride 0.1%. Soln. *Drop-Tainer* 5 mL. *Rx.*
Use: Antihistamine, ophthalmic.

patent ductus arteriosus, agents for.
See: Alprostadil.
  Ibuprofen Lysine.
  Indomethacin Sodium.
  Indomethacin Sodium Trihydrate.

Path. (Parker) Buffered neutral formalin soln. 10%. Bot. 1 gal, 5 gal. Jar 4 oz.
Use: Tissue specimen fixative.

Pathocil. (Wyeth) Dicloxacillin sodium.
Cap.: 250 mg, 500 mg. Bot. 50s (500 mg only), 100s (250 mg only).
Pow. for Oral Susp.: 62.5 mg/5 mL. Bot. to make 100 mL. *Rx.*
Use: Anti-infective, penicillin.

•**paulomycin.** (PAW-low-MY-sin) USAN.
Use: Anti-infective.

Pavagen TD. (Rugby) Papaverine hydrochloride 150 mg. TR Cap. Bot. 100s, 500s, 1000s. *Rx.*
Use: Vasodilator.

Paxil. (Apotex) Paroxetine hydrochloride.
Tab.: 10 mg, 20 mg, 30 mg, 40 mg. Film-coated. Bot. 30s; 90s (20 mg only), SUP 100s (20 mg only). **Oral Susp.:**

10 mg/5 mL. Parabens, saccharin, sorbitol, orange flavor. Bot. 250 mL. *Rx.*
Use: Antidepressant, selective serotonin reuptake inhibitor.

Paxil CR. (Apotex) Paroxetine hydrochloride 12.5 mg, 25 mg, 37.5 mg. Lactose. Enteric-coated. CR Tab. Bot. 30s. *Rx.*
Use: Antidepressant, selective serotonin reuptake inhibitor.

•**pazinaclone.** (pah-ZIN-ah-klone) USAN.
Use: Anxiolytic.

Pazo Hemorrhoid. (Bristol-Myers Squibb) Zinc oxide 5%, ephedrine sulfate 0.2%, camphor 2% in lanolinpetrolatum base. Oint. Tube 28 g. *OTC.*
Use: Anorectal preparation.

•**pazopanib hydrochloride.** (paz-OH-panib) USAN.
Use: Antineoplastic.
See: Votrient.

•**pazoxide.** (pay-ZOX-ide) USAN.
Use: Antihypertensive.

PB-Hyos. (Kylemore) Atropine sulfate 0.0194 mg, hyoscyamine hydrobromide or sulfate 0.1037 mg, phenobarbital 16.2 mg, scopolamine hydrobromide 0.0065 mg. Alcohol 23%, glycerin, saccharin, sorbitol, sucrose. Grape flavor. Elix. 473 mL. *c-iv.*
Use: Gastrointestinal anticholinergic/antispasmodic, gastrointestinal anticholinergic combination.

PBM Allergy. (Boca Pharmacal) Brompheniramine maleate 3 mg, dextromethorphan HBr 15 mg, pseudoephedrine hydrochloride 30 mg per 5 mL. Alcohol and sugar free. Saccharin, sorbitol. Berry-vanilla flavor. Syr. 473 mL. *Rx.*
Use: Upper respiratory combination, antitussive combination.

PB 100. (Schlicksup) Phenobarbital 1.5 g. Tab. Bot. 1000s. *c-iv.*
Use: Hypnotic; sedative.

PBZ. (Novartis) Tripelennamine hydrochloride 25 mg, 50 mg. Tab. Bot. 100s. *Rx.*
Use: Antihistamine.

PBZ-SR. (Novartis) Tripelennamine hydrochloride 100 mg. SR Tab. Bot. 100s. *Rx.*
Use: Antihistamine.

PCE Dispertab. (Abbott) Erythromycin 333 mg (lactose), 500 mg. Polymer-coated particles. Tab. Bot. 60s (333 mg only), 100s (500 mg only). *Rx.*
Use: Anti-infective, erythromycin.

P Chlor DM. (SDA Labs) Chlorpheniramine maleate 1 mg, dextromethorphan hydrobromide 3 mg, phenylephrine hydrochloride 3.5 mg. Glycerin, sodium benzoate, sorbitol. Alcohol free and sugar free. Grape flavor. Drops. 30 mL. *Rx.*
Use: Upper respiratory combination, antitussive combination.

P Chlor GG. (Boca Pharmacal) Phenylephrine hydrochloride 2 mg, chlorpheniramine maleate 1 mg, guaifenesin 20 mg per 1 mL. Peach flavor. Drops. 30 mL with dropper. *Rx.*
Use: Upper respiratory combination, decongestant, antihistamine, and expectorant combination.

p-chlorometaxylenol. Benzocaine, benzyl alcohol, propylene glycol.
W/Hydrocortisone, pramoxine hydrochloride.
See: 20-Caine Burn Relief.

p-chlorophenol.
See: Parachlorophenol.

PCM. (Boca Pharmacal) Phenylephrine hydrochloride 10 mg, chlorpheniramine maleate 2 mg, methscopolamine nitrate 1.25 mg. Lactose, mannitol, sugar. Chew. Tab. 100s. *Rx.*
Use: Upper respiratory combination, decongestant, antihistamine, and anticholinergic.

PCMX.
See: Parachlorometaxylenol.

PC-Tar. (Geritrex) Coal tar 1%. EDTA. Shampoo. 180 mL. *OTC.*
Use: Photochemotherapy.

PDP Liquid Protein. (Wesley) Protein 15 g (from protein hydrolysates), cal 60/30 mL. Bot. Pt, qt, gal. *OTC.*
Use: Protein supplement.

Peacock's Bromides. (Natcon) **Liq.:** Potassium bromide 6 g, sodium bromide 6 g, ammonium bromide 3 g/5 mL. Bot. 8 oz. **Tab.:** Potassium bromide 3 g, sodium bromide 3 g, ammonium bromide 1.5 g. Bot. 100s. *Rx.*
Use: Hypnotic; sedative.

•**peanut oil.** (PEE-nut) *NF 29.*
Use: Pharmaceutic aid (solvent).

PE-CPM-MSN 8-2-0.75. (Kylemore) Chlorpheniramine maleate 2 mg, methscopolamine nitrate 0.75 mg, phenylephrine hydrochloride 8 mg. Glycerin, parabens, PEG, potassium, *Prosweet*, sorbate, sucrose, saccharin, sorbitol, sucralose. Grape flavor. Syrup. 473 mL. *Rx.*
Use: Upper respiratory combination; decongestant, antihistamine, and anticholinergic combination.

Pectamol. (British Drug House) Diethylaminoethoxyethyl-a,a-diethylphenylacetate citrate. Bot. 4 fl oz, 16 fl oz, 80 fl oz, 160 fl oz.
Use: Antitussive.

• **pectin.** (PECK-tin) *USP 34.*
Use: Protectant; pharmaceutic aid, suspending agent.
W/Benzocaine.
See: Cēpacol Sore Throat + Coating Relief Maximum Numbing.
W/Combinations.
See: Furoxone.
Kaopectate.

Pedenex. (Health for Life Brands) Caprylic acid, zinc undecylenate, sodium propionate. Tube 1.5 oz. Foot pow. spray 5 oz. *OTC.*
Use: Antifungal, topical.

PediaCare Children's Decongestant. (McNeil) Phenylephrine hydrochloride 2.5 mg/5 mL. EDTA, sorbitol, sucralose. Oral Soln. 118 mL. *OTC.*
Use: Nasal decongestant.

PediaCare Children's Long-Acting Cough. (McNeil) Dextromethorphan HBr 7.5 mg per 5 mL. Alcohol and sugar free. Saccharin, sorbitol. Grape flavor. Oral Soln. 120 mL. *OTC.*
Use: Nonnarcotic antitussive.

PediaCare Children's Multi-Symptom Cold. (McNeil) Phenylephrine hydrochloride 5 mg, dextromethorphan HBr 5 mg per 5 mL. Sorbitol, sodium 10 mg/5 mL. Grape flavor. Liq. Bot. 118 mL. *OTC.*
Use: Upper respiratory combination, decongestant, antihistamine, antitussive.

PediaCare Children's NightRest Multi-Symptom Cold. (McNeil) Phenylephrine hydrochloride 5 mg, diphenhydramine hydrochloride 12.5 per 5 mL. EDTA, sorbitol, sucralose. Grape flavor. Liq. 118 mL. *OTC.*
Use: Upper respiratory combination, decongestant and antihistamine.

PediaCare Children's NightTime Cough. (McNeil) Diphenhydramine 12.5 mg per 5 mL. Sucrose. Cherry flavor. Liq. Bot. 120 mL. *OTC.*
Use: Antitussive.

Pediacof. (Sanofi-Synthelabo) Codeine phosphate 5 mg, phenylephrine hydrochloride 2.5 mg, chlorpheniramine maleate 0.75 mg, potassium iodide 75 mg/5 mL, sodium benzoate 0.2%, alcohol 5%. Syr. Bot. 16 fl oz. *c-v.*
Use: Antihistamine; antitussive; decongestant; expectorant.

Pediaderm AF. (Arbor Pharmaceuticals) Nystatin 100,000 units/g. Aluminum hydroxide gel, medical antifoam AF emulsion, parabens, PEG 400, propylene glycol, titanium dioxide, white petrolatum. Cream. 30 g w/diaper defense cream (beeswax, light mineral oil, parabens, paraffin, PEG-30, vitamin E, white petrolatum, zinc oxide. *Rx.*
Use: Topical anti-infective, antifungal agent.

Pediaderm TA. (Arbor Pharmaceuticals) Triamcinolone acetonide 0.1%. Cetyl alcohol, glyceryl, cetyl esters wax, polysorbate 80, propylene glycol. Cream. 30 g w/protective emollient (petrolatum, glycerin, mineral oil, cetyl alcohol, parabens). *Rx.*
Use: Anti-inflammatory agent, topical corticosteroid.

Pediahist DM. (Boca Pharmacal) **Drops:** Pseudoephedrine hydrochloride 15 mg, brompheniramine maleate 1 mg, dextromethorphan hydrobromide 4 mg per 1 mL. Sorbitol. Grape flavor. 30 mL with dropper. **Syr.:** Pseudoephedrine hydrochloride 30 mg, brompheniramine maleate 2 mg, dextromethorphan hydrobromide 5 mg, guaifenesin 50 mg per 5 mL. Alcohol free. Corn syr. Grape flavor. 473 mL. *Rx.*
Use: Antitussive combination, antitussive and expectorant combination, upper respiratory combination.

Pedia-Lax. (Fleet) Magnesium hydroxide 400 mg. Watermelon flavor. Chew. Tab. 30s. *OTC.*
Use: Laxative.

Pedialyte. (Ross) Na 45 mEq, K 20 mEq, chloride 35 mEq, citrate 30 mEq, dextrose 25 g/L. 100 calories/L. **Plastic Bot.:** 8 fl oz. (unflavored), 32 fl oz. (unflavored, fruit). **Nursing Bot.:** Hospital use. Bot. 8 fl oz. *OTC.*
Use: Electrolytes, mineral supplement.

Pedialyte Electrolyte. (Ivax) Dextrose 25 g, K 20 mEq, Cl 35 mEq, Na 45 mEq, citrate 30 mEq, 100 cal/L. Oral Soln. Bot. 1 L. *OTC.*
Use: Electrolytes, mineral supplement.

Pedialyte Freezer Pops. (Ross) Na 45 mEq, K 20 mEq, Cl 35 mEq, citrate 30 mEq, dextrose 25 g/L, phenylalanine, aspartame. Liq. Ready-to-freeze pops. 2.1 fl oz. Box. 16s. *OTC.*
Use: Electrolytes, mineral supplement.

Pediamycin. (Ross) Erythromycin ethylsuccinate for oral suspension 100 mg/2.5 mL. Drops. Bot. 50 mL (Dropper enclosed). *Rx.*
Use: Anti-infective, erythromycin.

PediaPhyl D. (River's Edge) Phenylephrine tannate 10 mg, chlorpheniramine tannate 8 mg per 5 mL. Sugar free. Aspartame, methylparaben, phenylalanine, saccharin, sorbitol. Bubble gum flavor. Susp. 473 mL. *Rx.*

Use: Upper respiratory combination, decongestant and antihistamine.

Pediapred. (Celltech Pharmaceuticals) Prednisolone 5 mg/5 mL (equiv. to prednisolone sodium phosphate 6.7 mg/5 mL). Methylparaben, EDTA, sorbitol. Raspberry flavor. Oral Soln. Bot. 120 mL. *Rx.*
Use: Adrenocortical steroid, glucocorticoid.

Pedia Relief Cough-Cold. (Major) Chlorpheniramine maleate 1 mg, dextromethorphan hydrobromide 5 mg, pseudoephedrine hydrochloride 15 mg per 5 mL. Alcohol free. Cherry flavor. Liq. 118 mL. *OTC.*
Use: Upper respiratory combination, antitussive combination.

Pedia Relief Decongestant Plus Cough Infants'. (Major) Pseudoephedrine hydrochloride 9.375 mg, dextromethorphan HBr 3.125 mg per 1 mL. Sorbitol, cherry flavor, alcohol free. Drops. Bot. 15 mL w/dropper. *OTC.*
Use: Upper respiratory combination, decongestant, antitussive.

Pediarix. (GlaxoSmithKline) Diphtheria toxoid 25 Lf, tetanus toxoid 10 Lf, inactivated pertussis toxin 25 mcg, filamentous hemagglutinin 25 mcg, pertactin 8 mcg, hepatitis B surface antigen 10 mcg, D-antigen units type 1 poliovirus 40, DU type 2 poliovirus 8, DU type 3 poliovirus 32, sodium chloride 4.5 mg, aluminum adjuvant ($\leq$ 0.85 mg aluminum by assay). Preservative free. Vial. Single-dose, prefilled syringes. *Rx.*
Use: Vaccine.

PediaSure. (Abbott Nutrition) Protein 30 g (L-carnitine, milk protein concentrate, whey protein concentrate, taurine), carbohydrate 131 g (corn maltodextrin, sucrose), fat 38 g (high-oleic safflower oil, soy oil, medium chain triglycerides)/L. Na 380 mg/L, K 1310 mg/L, 480 (vanilla, strawberry, and banana cream), 540 (chocolate), 560 (orange cream) mOsm/kg H_2O, 1 cal/mL. Vitamins A, B_1, B_2, B_3, B_5, B_6, B_7, B_{12}, C, D, E, K, inositol, Cl$^-$, Cr, Ca, P, Mg, I, Mn, Cu, Se, Zn, Fe, folic acid. Gluten and lactose free. Vanilla, chocolate, strawberry, banana cream, orange cream flavors. Ready-to-use cans and bots. 240 mL. *OTC.*
Use: Infant food, enteral nutritional therapy.

PediaSure with Fiber. (Ross) Protein 30 g (sodium caseinate, low-lactose whey, carnitine, taurine), carbohydrate

113.5 g (maltodextrin, sucrose, soy fiber [total dietary fiber 5 g]), fat 49.7 g (high-oleic safflower oil, soy oil, medium chain triglyceride oil, lecithin)/L, vitamins A, B_1, B_2, B_3, B_6, B_{12}, C, D, E, K, folic acid, Ca, Fe, I, Mg, P, Se, Zn, Na 380 mg (16.5 mEq), K 1310 mg (33.5 mEq), cal 1/L, vanilla flavor, lactose and gluten free. Liq. Bot. 8 oz. *OTC.*
Use: Enteral nutritional therapy, defined formula diet.

PediaTan. (ProEthic) Chlorpheniramine (as tannate) 8 mg. Methylparaben, sodium saccharin, sorbitol. Sugar free. Bubble gum flavor. Oral Susp. 473 mL. *Rx.*
Use: Antihistamine.

Pediatex. (Zyber) Carbinoxamine maleate 1.67 mg/5 mL. Alcohol and dye free. Saccharin, sorbitol. Cotton candy flavor. Liq. 15 mL, 473 mL. *Rx.*
Use: Antihistamine, nonselective ethanolamine.

Pediatex-CT. (Zyber) Phenylephrine hydrochloride 5 mg, diphenhydramine hydrochloride 12.5 mg. Saccharin. Strawberry flavor. Chew. Tab. 100s. *Rx.*
Use: Upper respiratory combination, decongestant and antihistamine.

Pediatex-D. (Zyber) Pseudoephedrine hydrochloride 12.5 mg, carbinoxamine maleate 1.67 mg per 5 mL. Sugar, alcohol, and dye free. Cotton candy flavor. Liq. Bot. 20 mL, 473 mL. *Rx.*
Use: Upper respiratory combination, decongestant, antihistamine.

Pediatex-DM. (Zyber) Pseudoephedrine hydrochloride 15 mg, carbinoxamine maleate 2 mg, dextromethorphan HBr 15 mg per 1 mL. Saccharin, sorbitol, cotton candy flavor. Liq. Bot. 20 mL, 473 mL. *Rx.*
Use: Upper respiratory combination, decongestant, antihistamine, antitussive.

Pediatex HC. (Zyber) Pseudoephedrine hydrochloride 17.5 mg, chlorpheniramine maleate 2.5 mg, hydrocodone bitartrate 1.67 mg per 5 mL. Sugar free. Saccharin, sorbitol. Cotton candy flavor. Syr. 20 mL, 480 mL. *c-III.*
Use: Pediatric antitussive combination.

Pediatex 12. (Zyber) Carbinoxamine tannate 3.2 mg/5 mL. Methylparaben, saccharin, sucrose. Candy apple flavor. Oral Susp. 20 mL, 473 mL. *Rx.*
Use: Antihistamine.

Pediatex 12 D. (Zyber) Pseudoephedrine tannate 45.2 mg, carbinoxamine tannate 3.6 mg per 5 mL. Magnasweet,

methylparaben, saccharin, sucrose.
Candy apple flavor. Susp. Bot. 20 mL,
473 mL. *Rx.*
Use: Pediatric decongestant and antihistamine.
Pediatric Advil Drops. (Wyeth Consumer Healthcare) Ibuprofen 100 mg/
2.5 mL. EDTA, glycerin, sorbitol, su-
crose, grape flavor. Susp. Bot. 7.5 mL.
OTC.
Use: Anti-inflammatory.
Pediatric Cough. (Weeks & Leo)
Ammonium Cl 300 mg, sodium citrate
600 mg/oz. Syr. Bot. 4 oz. *OTC.*
Use: Expectorant.
Pediatric Cough & Cold. (Ivax) Dextromethorphan HBr 5 mg, chlorpheniramine maleate 1 mg, pseudoephedrine
hydrochloride 15 mg per 5 mL. Alcohol free. Liq. 120 mL. *OTC.*
Use: Upper respiratory combination, antitussive combination.
Pediatric Cough & Cold Medicine.
(Silarx) Dextromethorphan HBr 5 mg,
chlorpheniramine maleate 1 mg,
pseudoephedrine hydrochloride 15 mg
per 5 mL. Alcohol free. Sorbitol. Liq.
120 mL. *OTC.*
Use: Upper respiratory combination, antitussive combination.
Pediatric Electrolyte. (Ivax) Dextrose
25 g, K 20 mEq, Cl 35 mEq, Na
45 mEq, citrate 48 mEq, calories 100/
L. Soln. Bot. 1 L. *OTC.*
Use: Nutritional supplement, enteral.
Pediatric Maintenance Solution. (Abbott) IV solution w/dose calculated ac-
cording to age, weight, clinical condition. Bot. 250 mL. *Rx.*
Use: Electrolytes, nutrient replacement.
Pediatric Multiple Trace Element.
(American Regent) Zn (as sulfate)
0.5 mg, Cu (as sulfate) 0.1 mg, Mn (as
sulfate) 0.03 mg, Cr (as chloride)
1 mcg/mL. Soln. Vial 10 mL. *Rx.*
Use: Nutritional supplement, parenteral.
Pedi-Boot Mist Kit. (Pedinol Pharmacal)
Cetylpyridinium Cl, triacetin, chloroxyle-
nol. Bot. 2 oz. *OTC.*
Use: Antifungal; antiseptic; deodorant.
Pedicran with Iron. (Scherer) Vitamin
B$_{12}$ (crystallized) 25 mcg, ferric pyro-
phosphate, soluble (elemental iron
30 mg) 250 mg, thiamine mononitrate
10 mg, nicotinamide 10 mg, alcohol 1%/
5 mL. Bot. 4 oz, pt. *OTC.*
Use: Mineral, vitamin supplement.
pediculicides/scabicides.
See: Lindane.
Malathion.
Permethrin.

Pedi-Dri. (Pedinol Pharmacal) Nystatin
100,000 units/g, talc. Pow. Plastic Bot.
w/shaker cap. 56.7 g. *Rx.*
Use: Antifungal; antiperspirant; deodorant; foot powder.
Pediox. (Atley) Pseudoephedrine hydrochloride 15 mg, chlorpheniramine
maleate 2 mg. Aspartame, phenylalanine, mannitol, sorbitol, xylitol, grape
flavor. Chew. Tab. 100s. *Rx.*
Use: Decongestant and antihistamine.
Pediox-S. (Atley) Chlorpheniramine
maleate 4 mg/5 mL. Aspartame, methylparaben, phenylalanine 8.419 mg/
5 mL, sucralose. Cotton candy flavor.
Susp. 118 mL. *Rx.*
Use: Antihistamine, nonselective alkylamine.
Pedi-Pro. (Pedinol) Benzalkonium chloride, menthol. Pow. 56.7 g. *OTC.*
Use: Antifungal; antiperspirant;
deodorant.
Pedituss Cough. (Major) Phenylephrine
hydrochloride 2.5 mg, chlorpheniramine
maleate 0.75 mg, codeine phosphate
5 mg, potassium iodide 75 mg/5 mL, alcohol 5%, saccharin, sorbitol, sucrose.
Syr. Bot. Pt., gal. *c-v.*
Use: Antihistamine; antitussive; decongestant; expectorant.
Pedolatum. (King) Salicylic acid, sodium
salicylate. Oint. Pkg. 0.5 oz. *OTC.*
Use: Analgesic, topical.
Pedric Senior. (Pal-Pak, Inc.) Acetaminophen 320 mg. *OTC.*
Use: Analgesic.
PedvaxHIB. (Merck & Co.) Purified capsular polysaccharide of *Haemophilus
influenzae* type b, *Neisseria meningitidis* OMPC 250 mcg/dose when recon-
stituted, sodium chloride 0.9%, lactose
2 mg, thimerosal 1:20,000. Pow. for Inj.
or Soln. Single-dose vial with vial of
aluminum hydroxide diluent or single-
dose vial. *Rx.*
Use: Immunization.
•**pefloxacin.** (PEH-FLOX-ah-sin) USAN.
Use: Anti-infective.
•**pefloxacin mesylate.** (pe-FLOX-a-sin)
USAN.
Use: Anti-infective.
PEG. (Medco Lab) Polyethylene glycol.
Oint. Jar 16 oz. *OTC.*
Use: Pharmaceutical aid, ointment base.
•**pegademase bovine.** (peg-AD-ah-MASE
BOE-vine) USAN.
Use: Replacement therapy (adenosine
deaminase deficiency); modified en-
zyme for use in ADA deficiency.
[Orphan Drug]
See: Adagen.

- **pegadricase.** (peg-AD-ri-kase) USAN.
  Use: Treatment of hyperuricemia.
- **pegamotecan.** (peg-am-oh-TEE-kan) USAN.
  Use: Gastrointestinal.

Peganone. (Lundbeck) Ethotoin 250 mg.
Lactose. Tab. 100s. *Rx.*
Use: Anticonvulsant.

- **pegaptanib octasodium.** (pag-AP-ta-nib) USAN.
  Use: Age-related macular degeneration disease.
- **pegaptanib sodium.** (pag-AP-ta-nib) USAN.
  Use: Age-related macular degeneration disease.
  See: Macugen.
- **pegaspargase.** (peh-ASS-par-jase) USAN.
  Use: Antineoplastic.
  See: Oncaspar.

Pegasys. (Roche) Peginterferon alfa-2a 180 mcg. Inj. Single-use vials (sodium chloride 8 mg, polysorbate 80 0.05 mg, benzyl alcohol 10 mg) 1 mL; prefilled syringes (sodium chloride 4 mg, polysorbate 80 0.025 mg, benzyl alcohol 5 mg) 0.5 mL; available in vial (4 single-use vials, 4 1-mL syringes with needles, 8 alcohol swabs) and prefilled syringe (4 single-use prefilled syringes, 4 needles, and 4 alcohol swabs) monthly convenience packs. *Rx.*
Use: Immunologic agent, immunomodulator.

- **pegdinetanib.** (PEG-dye-NET-a-nib) USAN.
  Use: Antineoplastic.

pegfilgrastim.
Use: Hematopoietic, colony stimulating factor.
See: Neulasta.

PE/GG. (Kylemore) Guaifenesin 100 mg, phenylephrine hydrochloride 7.5 mg. Propylene glycol, propylparaben, saccharin, sodium benzoate, sorbitol. Orange flavor. Liq. 473 mL. *Rx.*
Use: Upper respiratory combination, decongestant and expectorant combination.

PEG-glucocerebrosidase. (Enzon)
Use: Treatment of Gaucher disease. [Orphan Drug]

- **peginesatide.** (PEG-in-ES-a-tide) USAN.
  Use: Treatment of anemia associated with chronic kidney disease.
- **peginesatide acetate.** (PEG-in-ES-a-tide) USAN.
  Use: Treatment of anemia associated with chronic kidney disease.

- **peginterferon alfa-2a.** (peg-IN-ter-FEER-ahn AL-fuh-2a) USAN.
  Use: Immunologic agent, immunomodulator.
  See: Pegasys.
- **peginterferon alfa-2b.** (peg-IN-ter-FEER-ahn AL-fuh-2b) USAN.
  Use: Immunologic agent, immunomodulator.
  See: PEG-Intron.
- **peginterferon lambda-1a.** (PEG-in-ter-FEER-on LAM-da) USAN.
  Use: Treatment of chronic hepatitis C infection.

PEG-interleukin-2. (Cetus)
Use: Immunomodulator. [Orphan Drug]

PEG-Intron. (Schering) Peginterferon alfa-2b 50 mcg/0.5 mL, 80 mcg/0.5 mL, 120 mcg/0.5 mL, 150 mcg/0.5 mL when reconstituted. Pow. for Inj., lyophilized. Vial 2 mL (contains dibasic and monobasic sodium phosphate 1.11 mg, polysorbate 80 0.074 mg, and sucrose 59.2 mg) with 1.25 mL diluent vial, 2 syringes, and 2 alcohol swabs and *Redipen* (contains dibasic and monobasic sodium phosphate 1.013 mg, polysorbate 80 0.0675 mg, and sucrose 54 mg) with 1 B-D needle and 2 alcohol swabs. *Rx.*
Use: Immunologic agent, immunomodulator.

PEG-L-asparaginase. (Enzon) *Rx.*
Use: Antineoplastic.

- **peglicol 5 oleate.** (PEG-lih-kahl 5 OH-lee-ate) USAN.
  Use: Pharmaceutic aid, emulsifying agent.
- **pegloticase.** (peg-LOE-ti-kase) USAN.
  Use: Gout.
  See: Krystexxa.
- **pegnivacogin.** (peg-NYE-va-KOG-in) USAN.
  Use: Anticoagulant.
- **pegorgotein.** (peg-AHR-gah-teen) USAN.
  Use: Free oxygen radical scavenger.
- **pegoterate.** (PEG-oh-TEER-ate) USAN.
  Use: Pharmaceutic aid, suspending agent.
- **pegoxol 7 stearate.** (peg-OX-ole 7 STEE-ah-rate) USAN.
  Use: Pharmaceutic aid, emulsifying agent.
- **pegsunercept.** (peg-SOO-ner-sept) USAN.
  Use: TNF-inhibitor; anti-inflammatory (Crohn disease, RA).

PEG 3350.
Use: Laxative.
See: Dulcolax Balance.
GlycoLax.
MoviPrep.
TriLyte.
W/Sodium Bicarbonate, Sodium Chloride, Potassium Chloride.
See: TriLyte.
W/Sodium Bicarbonate, Sodium Chloride, Sodium Sulfate, Potassium Chloride.
See: GaviLyte-C.
GaviLyte-G.

PEG-3350, sodium chloride, sodium bicarbonate, potassium chloride.
(Mylan) PEG 3350 420 g, sodium bicarbonate 5.72 g, sodium chloride 11.2 g, potassium chloride 1.48 g. Pow. for Soln. Disposable jug w/cherry, lemon lime, orange, and pineapple flavor packs. 4 L. *Rx.*
Use: Laxative, bowel evacuant.

•**pegvisomant.** (peg-VI-soe-mant) USAN.
Use: Acromegaly; proliferative diabetic retinopathy.

PE HCL-CPM-MSN 10-2-0.75. (Kylemore) Chlorpheniramine maleate 2 mg, methscopolamine nitrate 0.75 mg, phenylephrine hydrochloride 10 mg. Glycerin, parabens, propylene glycol, sodium benzoate, sucrose. Grape flavor. Syrup. 473 mL. *Rx.*
Use: Upper respiratory combination; decongestant, antihistamine, and anticholinergic combination.

PE-Hist DM. (Larkin) Chlorpheniramine maleate 2 mg, dextromethorphan hydrobromide 15 mg, phenylephrine hydrochloride 5 mg. Methylparaben, saccharin, sucrose. Alcohol free. Syrup. 473 mL. *Rx.*
Use: Upper respiratory combination, antitussive combination.

•**pelanserin hydrochloride.** (peh-LAN-ser-in) USAN.
Use: Antihypertensive; vasodilator (serotonin S_2 and α_1 adrenergic receptor blocker).

•**peldesine.** (PELL-deh-seen) USAN.
Use: Antineoplastic; antipsoriatic.

pelentan. Ethyl Biscoumacetate. (No Manufacturer Available).

PeleVerus Clear. (LTC Products) Zinc acetate 0.9%, beeswax, panthenol, petrolatum, vitamin E. Oint. 100 g. *OTC.*
Use: Miscellaneous skin protectant.

•**peliglitazar.** (pel-ee-GLI-ta-zar) USAN.
Use: Antidiabetic.

•**peliomycin.** (PEE-lee-oh-MY-sin) USAN.

An antibiotic derived from *Streptomycin luteogriseus.*
Use: Antineoplastic.

•**pelitinib.** (pel-i-TYE-nib) USAN.
Use: Antineoplastic.

•**pelitrexol.** (PEL-i-trex-ol) USAN.
Use: Antineoplastic.

•**pelretin.** (PELL-REH-tin) USAN.
Use: Antikeratinizer.

•**pelrinone hydrochloride.** (PELL-rih-nohn) USAN.
Use: Cardiovascular agent.

•**pemedolac.** (peh-MEH-doe-LACK) USAN.
Use: Analgesic.

•**pemerid nitrate.** (PEM-eh-rid) USAN.
Use: Antitussive.

pemetrexed. (pem-eh-TREX-ehd)
Use: Antimetabolite.
See: Alimta.

•**pemetrexed disodium.** (pem-eh-TREX-ehd) USAN.
Tall Man: PEMEtrexed
Use: Antineoplastic.

•**pemirolast potassium.** (peh-mihr-OH-last) USAN.
Use: Antiallergic; inhibitor (mediator release).
See: Alamast.

Penagen-VK. (Grafton) Penicillin V. **Tab.:** 250 mg. Bot. 100s. **Pow.:** 250 mg/100 mL. *Rx.*
Use: Anti-infective, penicillin.

•**penamecillin.** (PEN-ah-meh-SILL-in) USAN.
Use: Anti-infective.

•**penbutolol sulfate.** (pen-BYOO-toe-lole) USP 34.
Use: Antiadrenergic/sympatholytic, beta-adrenergic blocking agent.
See: Levatol.

•**penciclovir.** (pen-SIGH-kloe-VEER) USAN.
Use: Antiviral.
See: Denavir.

PENcream. (Humco) Caprylic/capric triglyceride, cetearyl alcohol, ceteareth 20, glyceryl stearate, isopropyl palmitate, PEG 100, propylene glycol, octyldodecanol, lecithin, ethylhextlglycerin, phenoxyethanol. Cream. 45 g. *OTC.*
Use: Ointment and lotion base.

Penecare. (Schwarz Pharma) **Cream:** Lactic acid, mineral oil, imidurea. Tube 120 g. **Lot.:** Lactic acid, imidurea. Bot. 240 mL. *OTC.*
Use: Emollient.

Penecort. (Allergan) Hydrocortisone 1%,

2.5%, benzyl alcohol, petrolatum, stearyl alcohol, propylene glycol, isopropyl myristate, polyoxyl 40 stearate, carbomer 934, sodium lauryl sulfate, edetate disodium w/sodium hydroxide to adjust pH, purified water. Cream. **1%:** Tube 30 g, 60 g. **2.5%:** Tube 30 g. *Rx.*
Use: Corticosteroid, topical.

•**penfluridol.** (pen-FLEW-rih-dahl) USAN.
Use: Antipsychotic.

•**penicillamine.** (PEN-ih-SILL-ah-meen) *USP 34.*
Use: Chelating agent; metal complexing agent, cystinuria, rheumatoid arthritis.
See: Cuprimine.
Depen.

penicillin. (pen-ih-SILL-in) Unless clarified, it means an antibiotic substance or substances produced by growth of the molds *Penicillium notatum* or *P. chrysogenum.*
Use: Anti-infective.

penicillin aluminum. *Rx.*
Use: Anti-infective, penicillin.

penicillinase-resistant penicillins.
Use: Anti-infective.
See: Dicloxacillin Sodium.
Nafcillin Sodium.
Oxacillin Sodium.

•**penicillin calcium.** (pen-ih-SILL-in) *USP 34. Rx.*
Use: Anti-infective, penicillin.

penicillin, dimethoxy-phenyl. Methicillin sodium.
Use: Anti-infective, penicillin.

penicillin G, aqueous.
Use: Anti-infective.
See: Penicillin G potassium.
Pfizerpen.

•**penicillin G benzathine.** (pen-ih-SILL-in G BENZ-ah-theen) *USP 34.*
Use: Anti-infective.
See: Bicillin L-A.
Permapen.

penicillin G benzathine/penicillin G procaine.
Use: Anti-infective.
See: Bicillin C-R.
Bicillin C-R 900/300.

•**penicillin G potassium.** (pen-ih-SILL-in) *USP 34.*
Use: Anti-infective.
See: Pfizerpen.

penicillin G potassium. (Baxter PPI) Penicillin G potassium 1,000,000 units, 2,000,000 units, 3,000,000 units. Premixed frozen Inj. Galaxy cont. 50 mL. *Rx.*
Use: Anti-infective, penicillin.

penicillin G potassium. (Marsam) Penicillin G potassium 1,000,000 units, 5,000,000 units, 10,000,000 units, 20,000,000 units/vial. Pow. for Inj. Vial. *Rx.*
Use: Anti-infective, penicillin.

•**penicillin G procaine.** (pen-ih-SILL-in G PRO-cane) *USP 34.*
Use: Anti-infective.

penicillin G procaine. (Monarch) Penicillin G procaine 600,000 units/vial. Inj. 1 mL *Tubex*; 1,200,000 units/vial. Inj. 2 mL *Tubex.* Parabens, povidone. *Rx.*
Use: Anti-infective, penicillin.

•**penicillin G procaine and dihydrostreptomycin sulfate intramammary infusion.** *USP 34.*
Use: Anti-infective.

•**penicillin G procaine and dihydrostreptomycin sulfate injectable suspension.** *USP 34.*
Use: Anti-infective.

•**penicillin G procaine and novobiocin sodium intramammary infusion.** *USP 34.*
Use: Anti-infective.

penicillin G procaine combinations.
See: Bicillin C-R.

•**penicillin G procaine, dihydrostreptomycin sulfate, and prednisolone injectable suspension.** *USP 34.*
Use: Anti-infective; anti-inflammatory.

•**penicillin G procaine, dihydrostreptomycin sulfate, chlorpheniramine maleate, and dexamethasone injectable suspension.** *USP 34.*
Use: Anti-infective; antihistamine; antiinflammatory.

•**penicillin G procaine, neomycin and polymyxin B sulfates, and hydrocortisone acetate topical suspension.** *USP 34.*
Use: Anti-infective; anti-inflammatory.

penicillin G procaine/penicillin G benzathine.
Use: Anti-infective.
See: Bicillin C-R.
Bicillin C-R 900/300.

penicillin G procaine, sterile. Sterile Susp., Intramammary infusion, Procaine Penicillin.
Use: Anti-infective.

penicillin G procaine w/aluminum stearate suspension, sterile.
Use: Anti-infective.

•**penicillin G sodium.** (PEN-ih-SILL-in G) *USP 34.*
Use: Anti-infective.

penicillin G sodium. (Marsam) Penicillin G sodium 5,000,000 units/Vial. Pow. for

Inj. Vial. *Rx.*
Use: Anti-infective, penicillin.
penicillin G sodium. (Sandoz) Penicillin G sodium 5,000,000 units. Sodium 1.68 mEq/million vials. Pow. for Inj. Vials. *Rx.*
Use: Anti-infective, penicillin.
•**penicillin G sodium for injection.** *USP 34.*
Use: Anti-infective.
penicillin hydrabamine phenoxymethyl.
Use: Anti-infective.
penicillin O chloroprocaine.
Use: Anti-infective, penicillin.
penicillin O, sodium. Allylmercaptomethyl penicillin.
Use: Anti-infective.
penicillin, phenoxyethyl.
Use: Anti-infective, penicillin.
penicillin phenoxymethyl benzathine.
Use: Anti-infective, penicillin.
See: Penicillin V benzathine.
penicillin phenoxymethyl hydrabamine.
Use: Anti-infective, penicillin.
See: Penicillin V hydrabamine.
penicillins.
Use: Anti-infective.
See: Aminopenicillins.
  Extended-Spectrum Penicillins.
  Natural Penicillins.
  Penicillinase-Resistant Penicillins.
penicillin S benzathine and penicillin G procaine suspension, sterile.
Use: Anti-infective.
penicillins, extended spectrum.
Use: Anti-infective.
See: Piperacillin Sodium.
  Piperacillin Sodium/Tazobactam Sodium.
  Ticarcillin/Clavulanate.
  Ticarcillin Disodium.
penicillins, natural.
Use: Anti-infective.
See: Penicillin G (Aqueous).
  Penicillin G Benzathine and Procaine Combined, Intramuscular.
  Penicillin G Benzathine, Intramuscular.
  Penicillin G Procaine, Injectable.
  Penicillin V (Phenoxymethyl Penicillin).
•**penicillin V.** (pen-ih-SILL-in V) *USP 34.* *Formerly Penicillin Phenoxymethyl.* A biosynthetic penicillin formed by fermentation, with suitable precursors of *Penicillin notatum.*
Use: Anti-infective.
See: Penicillin VK.
  Veetids.

•**penicillin V benzathine.** (pen-ih-SILL-in V BEN-zah-theen) *USP 34. Formerly Penicillin Benzathine Phenoxymethyl.*
Use: Anti-infective.
•**penicillin V hydrabamine.** (pen-ih-SILL-in V HIGH-drah-BAM-een) *USP 34. Formerly Penicillin Hydrabamine Phenoxymethyl.*
Use: Anti-infective.
Penicillin VK. (Various Mfr.) Penicillin v. **Tab.:** 250 mg, 500 mg. Bot. 100s, 500s (500 mg only), 1000s (250 mg only). **Pow. for Oral Soln.:** 125 mg/5 mL, 250 mg/5 mL when reconstituted. Bot. 100 mL, 200 mL. *Rx.*
Use: Anti-infective, penicillin.
•**penicillin V potassium.** (pen-ih-SILL-in) *USP 34. Formerly Penicillin Potassium Phenoxymethyl.*
Use: Anti-infective.
See: Beepen VK.
  Betapen VK.
  Bopen-VK.
  Pen-Vee K.
  Pfizerpen VK.
  Suspen.
  V-Cillin K.
penidural.
Use: Anti-infective.
Pen-Kera Creme with Keratin Binding Factor. (B.F. Ascher) Bot. 8 oz. *OTC.*
Use: Emollient.
Penlac Nail Lacquer. (Dermik Labs) Ciclopirox 8%. Isopropyl alcohol. Top. Soln. Bot. 3.3 mL, 6.6 mL w/brushes. *Rx.*
Use: Anti-infective, topical; antifungal.
Pennsaid. (Nuvo) Diclofenac 1.5% (1 mL contains diclofenac sodium 16.05 mg). Alcohol, glycerin. Soln. 15 mL, 150 mL. *Rx.*
Use: Anti-inflammatory agent; nonsteroidal anti-inflammatory drug, topical.
Penntuss. (Medeva) Codeine (as polistirex) 10 mg, chlorpheniramine maleate 4 mg/5 mL. Bot. Pt. *c-v.*
Use: Antitussive; antihistamine.
•**pentabamate.** (PEN-tah-BAM-ate) USAN.
Use: Anxiolytic.
Pentacarinat. (Aventis) Pentamidine isethionate 300 mg. Inj. Single-dose vial. *Rx.*
Use: Anti-infective.
Pentacel. (Sanofi Pasteur) Diphtheria toxoid 15 Lf, tetanus toxoid 5 Lf, pertussis toxin detoxified 20 mcg, filamentous hemagglutinin 20 mcg, pertactin 3 mcg, fimbriae types 2 and 3 five mcg, type 1 inactivated poliovirus (Mahoney)

40 D-antigen units, type 2 inactivated poliovirus (MEF-1) 8 D-antigen units, type 3 inactivated poliovirus (Saukett) 32 D-antigen units, lyophilized polyribosyl-ribilol-phosphate of *Haemophilus influenzae* type B 10 mcg bound to tetanus toxoid 24 mcg per 0.5 mL. Aluminum phosphate 1.5 mg (aluminum 0.33 mg), residual formaldehyde ≤ 5 mcg, residual glutaraldehyde < 50 ng, residual bovine serum albumin ≤ 50 ng, 2-phenoxyethanol 3.3 mg (0.6% v/v), neomycin < 4 pg, polymyxin B sulfate < 4 pg. Preservative free. Inj., Susp. Single-dose vial for reconstitution. *Rx.*
Use: Vaccine combination, diphtheria and tetanus toxoids and acellular pertussis adsorbed, inactivated poliovirus and *haemophilus influenzae* type B conjugate vaccine combined.

pentacosactride.
Use: Corticotrophic peptide.

● **pentaerythritol tetranitrate diluted.** (pen-tuh-eh-Rith-rih-tole teh-truh-NYE-trate) *USP 34.*
Use: Vasodilator.
See: Arcotrate No. 1.
Arcotrate No. 2.
Duotrate 45.
Pentetra Paracote.
Peritrate.
Petro-20 mg.
Tetratab.
Tetratab No. 1.
Vasolate.
Vasolate-80.
W/Combinations.
See: Arcotrate No. 3.
Bitrate.
Dimycor.

pentafluoropropane.
W/Tetraflluoroethane.
See: Gebauer's Spray and Stretch.

● **pentafilcon A.** (PEN-tah-FILL-kahn A) USAN.
Use: Contact lens material, hydrophilic.

● **pentalyte.** (PEN-tah-lite) USAN.
Use: Electrolyte combination.

● **pentamidine isethionate.** (pen-TAM-i-deen EYE-se-THYE-oh-nate) USAN.
Use: Anti-infective.
See: NebuPent.
Pentam 300.
Pentacarinat.

pentamidine isethionate. (Abbott) Pentamidine isethionate 300 mg. Pow. for Inj., lyophilized. Single-dose fliptop vials. *Rx.*
Use: Anti-infective.

● **pentamorphone.** (PEN-tah-MORE-fone)

USAN.
Use: Analgesic; narcotic.

pentamoxane hydrochloride.
Use: Anxiolytic.

Pentam 300. (American Pharmaceutical Partners) Pentamidine isethionate 300 mg. Single-dose vials. *Rx.*
Use: Anti-infective.

● **pentamustine.** (PEN-tah-MUSS-teen) USAN.
Use: Antineoplastic.

pentaphonate. Dodecyltriphenylphosphonium pentachlorophenolate.
Use: Anti-infective.

● **pentapiperium methylsulfate.** (PEN-tah-PIP-ehr-ee-uhm METH-ill-SULL-fate) USAN.
Use: Anticholinergic.

pentapyrrolidinium bitartrate.
See: Pentolinium tartrate.

Pentasa. (Shire US) Mesalamine 250 mg, 500 mg. Sugar. CR Cap. Bot. 120s (500 mg only), 240s (250 mg only), UD 80s. *Rx.*
Use: Anti-inflammatory.

pentasodium colistinmethanesulfonate. Sterile Colistimethate Sodium.

● **pentastarch.** (PEN-tah-starch) USAN.
Use: Leukopheresis adjunct, red cell sedimenting agent. [Orphan Drug]

Penta-Stress. (Penta) Vitamins A 10,000 units, D 500 units, B_1 10 mg, B_2 10 mg, B_6 1 mg, calcium pantothenate 5 mg, niacinamide 50 mg, C 100 mg, E 2 units, B_{12} 3.3 mcg. Cap. Bot. 90s, 1000s, Jar 250s. *OTC.*
Use: Mineral, vitamin supplement.

Penta-Viron. (Penta) Calcium carbonate 500 mg, ferrous fumarate 100 mg, vitamins C 50 mg, D 167 units, A 3.333 units, B_1 3.3 mg, B_2 3.3 mg, B_6 2 mg, calcium pantothenate 1.6 mg, niacinamide 16.7 mg, E 2 units. Cap. Bot. 100s, 1000s, Jar 250s. *OTC.*
Use: Mineral, vitamin supplement.

Pentazine. (Century) Promethazine 50 mg/mL. Inj. Vial 10 mL. *Rx.*
Use: Antihistamine.

Pentazine VC w/Codeine. (Century) Promethazine hydrochloride 6.25 mg, codeine phosphate 10 mg. Liq. Bot. 118 mL, pt, gal. *c-v.*
Use: Antihistamine; antitussive.

Pentazine w/Codeine. (Century) Promethazine expectorant. Bot. 4 oz, 16 oz, gal.
Use: Antihistamine.

● **pentazocine.** (pen-TAZ-oh-seen) *USP 34.*

Use: Narcotic agonist-antagonist analgesic.
See: Talwin.

• **pentazocine and aspirin.** (pen-TAZ-oh-seen and AS-pir-in) *USP 34. Formerly pentazocine hydrochloride and aspirin.*
Use: Analgesic.

• **pentazocine and naloxone.** (pen-TAZ-oh-seen and NAL-ox-one) *USP 34. Formerly pentazocine and naloxone hydrochloride.*
Use: Analgesic.

pentazocine and naloxone. (Royce) Pentazocine 50 mg, naloxone hydrochloride 0.5 mg. Tab. Box. 100s, 500s, 1000s. *Rx.*
Use: Analgesic.

• **pentazocine hydrochloride.** (pen-TAZ-oh-seen) *USP 34.*
Use: Analgesic.
W/Acetaminophen.
See: Talacen.

pentazocine hydrochloride and acetaminophen. (Watson) Pentazocine hydrochloride 25 mg, acetaminophen 650 mg. Tab. Bot. 100s, 500s, 1000s. *c-IV.*
Use: Analgesic combination.

• **pentazocine injection.** (pen-TAZ-oh-seen) *USP 34. Formerly pentazocine lactate injection.*
Use: Analgesic.
See: Talwin.

• **pentetate calcium trisodium.** (PEN-teh-tate KAL-see-uhm try-SO-dee-uhm) USAN.
Use: Chelating agent, plutonium.

pentetate calcium trisodium. (Akorn) Pentetate calcium trisodium 200 mg/mL. Inj. 5 mL single-use ampules. *Rx.*
Use: Chelating agent, plutonium, americium, or curium.

• **pentetate calcium trisodium Yb 169.** (PEN-teh-tate) USAN.
Use: Radiopharmaceutical.

• **pentetate indium disodium In 111.** (PEN-teh-tate IN-dee-uhm) USAN.
Use: In vivo diagnostic aid, radiopharmaceutical.
See: Indium DTPA In 111.

pentetate zinc trisodium.
Use: Detoxification agent, chelating agent.

pentetate zinc trisodium. (Akorn) Pentetate zinc trisodium 200 mg/mL. Inj. 5 mL single-use ampules. *Rx.*
Use: Detoxification agent, chelating agent.

• **pentetic acid.** (PEN-teh-tick) *USP 34.*
Use: Diagnostic aid.

Pentetra-Paracote. (Paddock) Pentaerythritol tetranitrate 30 mg, 80 mg. Cap. Bot. 100s, 500s, 1000s. *Rx.*
Use: Antianginal.

pentetreotide.
Use: Radiopaque agent, parenteral.
See: OctreoScan.

• **pentiapine maleate.** (pen-TIE-ah-PEEN) USAN.
Use: Antipsychotic.

• **pentigetide.** (pent-EYE-jeh-TIDE) USAN.
Use: Antiallergic.

Pentina. (Freeport) Rauwolfia serpentina, 100 mg. Tab. Bot. 1000s. *Rx.*
Use: Antihypertensive.

• **pentisomicin.** (pent-IH-so-MY-sin) USAN.
Use: Anti-infective.

• **pentizidone sodium.** (pen-TIH-ZIH-dohn) USAN.
Use: Anti-infective.

• **pentobarbital.** (pen-toe-BAR-bih-tahl) *USP 34.*
Tall Man: PENTobarbital
Use: Hypnotic; sedative.
See: Nembutal.
W/Combinations
See: Cafergot PB.

• **pentobarbital sodium.** (pen-toe-BAR-bih-tahl) *USP 34.*
Tall Man: PENTobarbital
Use: Hypnotic; sedative.
See: Nembutal Sodium.
W/Ergotamine tartrate, caffeine alkaloid, bellafoline.
See: Cafergot PB.

pentobarbital sodium. (Wyeth) Pentobarbital sodium 50 mg/mL. Inj. *Tubex* 2 mL. *c-II.*
Use: Hypnotic; sedative.

pentobarbital, soluble.
See: Pentobarbital Sodium.

pentolinium tartrate. Pentamethylene-1:5-bis (1'-methylpyrrolidinium bitartrate).
Use: Antihypertensive.

Pentol Tabs. (Major) Pentaerythritol tetranitrate. **Tab.: 10 mg:** Bot. 1000s. **20 mg:** Bot. 100s, 1000s. **SA Tab.: 80 mg:** Bot. 250s, 1000s. *Rx.*
Use: Antianginal.

• **pentomone.** (PEN-toe-MONE) USAN.
Use: Prostate growth inhibitor.

• **pentopril.** (PEN-toe-prill) USAN.
Use: Enzyme inhibitor, angiotensin-converting.

• **pentosan polysulfate sodium.** (PEN-toe-san PAHL-in-SULL-fate) USAN.
Use: Anti-inflammatory, interstitial cystitis.
See: Elmiron.

- **pentostatin.** (PEN-toe-STAT-in) USAN.
  Use: Potentiator; leukemia; antineoplastic. [Orphan Drug]
  See: Nipent.
pentostatin. (Bedford) Pentostatin 10 mg. Mannitol 50 mg. Inj., Lyophilized Pow. for Soln., Conc. Single-dose vials. *Rx.*
  Use: Antimetabolite, purine analogs and related agent.
Pentothal. (Abbott) Thiopental sodium 400 mg/g. Rectal Susp. 2 g syringe. *Rx.*
  Use: Anesthetic.
- **pentoxifylline.** (pen-TOX-IH-fill-in) *USP 34.*
  Use: Hemorrheologic agent.
  See: Trental.
pentoxifylline. (Copley) Pentoxifylline 400 mg. Film-coated. CR Tab. Bot. 100s, 500s, bulk pack 5000s. *Rx.*
  Use: Hemorrheologic agent.
pentoxifylline extended-release. (Purepac) Pentoxifylline 400 mg. ER Tab. Bot. 100s, 500s, 1000s. *Rx.*
  Use: Hemorrheologic agent.
Pentrax. (Medicis) Coal tar extract 5%. Shampoo. Bot. 236 mL. *OTC.*
  Use: Antiseborrheic.
- **pentrinitrol.** (pen-TRY-nye-TROLE) USAN.
  Use: Vasodilator, coronary.
Pent-T-80. (Mericon Industries) Pentaerythritol tetranitrate 80 mg. TD Cap. Bot. 100s, 1000s. *Rx.*
  Use: Antianginal.
Pen-V. (Ivax) Penicillin 250 mg, 500 mg. Tab. Bot. 100s, 1000s. *Rx.*
  Use: Anti-infective, penicillin.
Pen-Vee K. (Wyeth) Penicillin V 250 mg, 500 mg Tab. Bot. 100s, 500s, UD 100s. *Rx.*
  Use: Anti-infective, penicillin.
Pen-Vee K for Oral Solution. (Wyeth) Penicillin V 125 mg/5 mL, 250 mg/5 mL. Bot. 100 mL, 150 mL (250 mg/5 mL only), 200 mL. *Rx.*
  Use: Anti-infective, penicillin.
Pepcid. (Merck) Famotidine. **Tab.:** 20 mg, 40 mg. Film-coated. Bot. 1000s, 10,000. Unit-of-use 30s, 90s, 100s. UD 100s. *Uniblister* 31s. **Pow. for Oral Susp.:** 40 mg/5 mL when reconstituted. Parabens, sucrose. Cherry, banana, mint flavors. Bot. 400 mg. *Rx.*
  Use: Histamine H$_2$ antagonist.
Pepcid AC. (J & J Merck) Famotidine. **Chew. Tab.:** 10 mg. Phenylalanine 1.4 mg, lactose, aspartame, mannitol. Pkg. 6s, 18s, 30s, 50s, 60s, 68s. **Gelcap:** 10 mg. Bot. 30s, 50s, 60s, 90s.

Tab.: 10 mg. Pkg. 2s, 6s, 18s, 30s, 60s, 90s. *OTC.*
  Use: Histamine H$_2$ antagonist.
Pepcid AC Maximum Strength. (J & J Merck) Famotidine 20 mg. Tab. 25s. *OTC.*
  Use: Histamine H$_2$ antagonist.
Pepcid AC Maximum Strength EZ Chews. (J & J Merck) Famotidine 20 mg. Dextrose, lactose, sucralose. Cool mint, berry, and cream flavors. Tab. 25s, 50s. *OTC.*
  Use: Gastrointestinal agent, histamine H$_2$ antagonist.
Pepcid Complete. (J & J Merck) Famotidine 10 mg, calcium carbonate 800 mg, magnesium hydroxide 165 mg. Lactose, sugar. Mint flavor. Chew. Tab. Bot. 5s, 15s, 25s, 50s. *OTC.*
  Use: Histamine H$_2$ antagonist combination.
Pepcid RPD. (Merck) Famotidine 20 mg, 40 mg. Aspartame, mint flavor, mannitol, phenylalanine 1.05 mg (20 mg only), 2.1 mg (40 mg only). Orally disintegrating Tab. UD 30s, 100s. *Rx.*
  Use: Histamine H$_2$ antagonist.
- **peplomycin sulfate.** (PEP-low-MY-sin) USAN.
  Use: Antineoplastic.
- **peppermint.** *NF 29.*
  Use: Pharmaceutic aid, flavor, perfume; antitussive; expectorant; nasal decongestant.
- **peppermint oil.** *NF 29.*
  Use: Pharmaceutic aid, flavor.
- **peppermint spirit.** *USP 34.*
  Use: Pharmaceutic aid, flavor, perfume.
- **peppermint water.** *NF 29.*
  Use: Pharmaceutic aid, vehicle, flavored.
Pepsamar. (Sanofi-Synthelabo) **Liq.:** Aluminum hydroxide. **Susp.:** Aluminum hydroxide, magnesium hydroxide, sorbitol. **Tab.:** Aluminum hydroxide. *OTC.*
  Use: Antacid.
Pepsamar Comp. Tablets. (Sanofi-Synthelabo) Aluminum hydroxide, magnesium hydroxide. *OTC.*
  Use: Antacid.
Pepsamar Esp. (Sanofi-Synthelabo) **Liq.:** Aluminum hydroxide, glycerin. **Tab.:** Aluminum hydroxide, magnesium hydroxide, mannitol powder. *OTC.*
  Use: Antacid.
Pepsamar HM. (Sanofi-Synthelabo) Aluminum hydroxide, starch. Tab. *OTC.*
  Use: Antacid.
Pepsicone. (Sanofi-Synthelabo) **Gel:** Aluminum hydroxide, magnesium

hydroxide, simethicone. **Tab.:** Aluminum hydroxide, magnesium hydroxide, simethicone. *OTC.*
Use: Antacid; antiflatulent.

pepsin.
Use: Digestive aid.
W/Combinations
See: Biloric.

• **pepstatin.** (pep-STAT-in) USAN.
Use: Enzyme inhibitor, pepsin.

Peptamen. (Clintec Nutrition) Enzymatically hydrolyzed whey proteins, maltodextrin, starch, MCT, sunflower oil, lecithin, vitamins A, B_1, B_2, B_3, B_5, B_6, B_{12}, C, D, E, K, folic acid, biotin, choline, Ca, Cl, Cu, Fe, I, Mg, Mn, P, Zn. Liq. Can 500 mL. *OTC.*
Use: Nutritional supplement.

Peptenzyme. (Schwarz Pharma) Alcohol 16%. Pleasantly aromatic. Bot. Pt.
Use: Pharmaceutic aid.

Peptic Relief. (Rugby) Bismuth subsalicylate. **Chew. Tab.:** 262 mg, dextrose, sorbitol. Bot. 30s. **Liq.:** 87.3 mg/5 mL, saccharin, sorbitol. Bot. 237 mL. *OTC.*
Use: Antidiarrheal.

Peptinex. (Novartis Nutrition) Protein (whey protein hydrolysate, taurine, L-carnitine) 50 g, carbohydrate (hydrolyzed cornstarch) 160 g, fat (soybean oil, medium chain triglycerides, soy lecithin) 17 g/L, vitamins A, B_1, B_2, B_3, B_5, B_6, B_{12}, C, D, E, K, biotin, choline, folic acid, Ca, Cl, Cr, Cu, Fe, I, Mg, Mn, Mo, P, Se, Zn, Na 1010 mg (44 mEq), K 1490 mg (38 mEq)/L, H_2O 320 mOsm/kg, 1 cal/mL, vanilla flavor. Liq. *Tetra Brik* Paks 8 oz. *OTC.*
Use: Enteral nutritional therapy.

Peptinex DT. (Novartis Nutrition) Protein (casein hydrolysate, amino acids) 50 g, carbohydrate (maltodextrin, modified cornstarch) 164 g, fat (medium chain triglycerides, soybean oil) 17.4 g/L, vitamins A, B_1, B_2, B_3, B_5, B_6, B_{12}, C, D, E, K, biotin, choline, folic acid, Ca, Cl, Cr, Cu, Fe, I, Mg, Mn, Mo, P, Se, Zn, Na 1700 mg (74 mEq), K 800 mg (21 mEq)/L, H_2O 460 mOsm/kg, 1 cal/mL, lactose and gluten free. Liq. Can 250 mL; closed system containers 1 L, 1.5 L. *OTC.*
Use: Enteral nutritional therapy.

Pepto-Bismol. (Procter & Gamble) **Chew. Tab.:** Bismuth subsalicylate 262.5 mg. Pkg. 24s, 42s. **Liq.:** Bismuth subsalicylate 262 mg/15 mL. Bot. 4 oz, 8 oz, 12 oz, 16 oz. **Tab.:** Bismuth subsalicylate 262 mg, < 2 mg sodium. Capl. Sugar free. Bot. 24s, 40s. *OTC.*
Use: Antidiarrheal.

Pepto-Bismol Maximum Strength. (Procter & Gamble) 524 mg/15 mL. Liq. Bot. 120 mL, 240 mL, 360 mL. *OTC.*
Use: Antidiarrheal.

Pepto Children's. (Procter & Gamble) Calcium carbonate 400 mg (elemental calcium 160 mg). Mannitol, sorbitol, sugar. Sodium free. Bubble gum and watermelon flavors. Chew. Tab. 24s. *OTC.*
Use: Mineral.

• **peramivir.** (per-AM-i-vir) USAN.
Use: Neuromindase inhibitor.

Perandren Phenylacetate. (Novartis) Testosterone phenylacetate. *c-III.*
Use: Androgen.

percaine.
Use: Local anesthetic.
See: Dibucaine hydrochloride.

perchloroethylene.
See: Tetrachloroethylene.

Percocet. (Endo) Oxycodone hydrochloride/acetaminophen 2.5 mg/325 mg, 5 mg/325 mg, 7.5 mg/325 mg, 7.5 mg/500 mg, 10 mg/325 mg, 10 mg/650 mg. Tab. Bot. 100s, 500s (except 7.5 mg/325 mg), UD 100s (except 7.5 mg/325 mg). *c-II.*
Use: Analgesic combination; narcotic.

Percodan. (Endo Pharmaceuticals) Oxycodone hydrochloride 4.5 mg, oxycodone terephthalate 0.38 mg, aspirin 325 mg. Tab. Bot. 100s, 500s, 1000s, UD 250s. *c-II.*
Use: Analgesic combination; narcotic.

Percogesic. (Medtech) Acetaminophen 325 mg, diphenhydramine hydrochloride 12.5 mg. Mineral oil, PEG. Tab. 90s. *OTC.*
Use: Upper respiratory combination, analgesic, antihistamine.

Percogesic Extra Strength. (Medtech) Diphenhydramine hydrochloride 12.5 mg, acetaminophen 500 mg. Tab. Bot. 60s. *OTC.*
Use: Upper respiratory combination, antihistamine, analgesic.

Percomorph Liver Oil. May be blended with 50% other fish liver oils; each g contains vitamins A 60,000 units, D 8500 units.

Percy Medicine. (Merrick Medicine) Bismuth subnitrate 959 mg, calcium hydroxide 21.9 mg/10 mL, alcohol 5%. *OTC.*
Use: Antidiarrheal.

Perdiem. (Novartis) Blend of psyllium 82%, senna 18% as active ingredients in granular form. Sodium content (0.08 mEq) 1.8 mg/rounded tsp. (6 g). Can. 100 g, 250 g, UD 6 g. *OTC.*
Use: Laxative.

Perdiem Fiber Therapy. (Novartis) Psyllium 4.03 g, sodium 1.8 mg, potassium 36.1 mg, 4 cal/6 g, sucrose, dye free, mint flavor. Gran. Can. 100 g, 250 g. *OTC.*
Use: Laxative.

Pere-Diosate. (Towne) Docusate sodium 100 mg, casanthranol 30 mg. Cap. Bot. 100s. *OTC.*
Use: Laxative.

Perestan. (Henry Schein) Docusate sodium 100 mg, casanthranol 30 mg. Cap. Bot. 100s, 1000s. *OTC.*
Use: Laxative.

• **perfilcon A.** (per-FILL-kahn A) USAN.
Use: Contact lens material, hydrophilic.

• **perflenapent.** (per-FLEN-ah-pent) USAN.
Use: Diagnostic aid, ultrasound contrast agent.

• **perflexane.** (per-FLEKS-ane) USAN.
Use: Diagnostic aid, ultrasound contrast agent.

• **perflisopent.** (per-FLYE-soh-pent) USAN.
Use: Diagnostic aid, ultrasound contrast agent.

• **perflubrodec.** (per-FLOO-broe-deck) USAN.
Use: Anemia.

• **perflubron.** (per-FLEW-brahn) *USP 34.*
Use: Contrast agent; blood substitute.

• **perflubutane.** (per-FLOO-bue-tane) USAN.
Use: Ultrasound contrast agent.

• **perflutren.** (per-FLOO-tren) *USP 34.*
Use: Radiopaque agent, parenteral.
See: Definity.

• **perflutren protein-type A microspheres injectable suspension.** (per-FLOO-tren PROE-teen) *USP 34.* Formerly perflutren protein-type A microspheres for injection.
Use: Diagnostic aid.
See: Optison.

Perforomist. (Dey) Formoterol fumarate 20 mcg/2 mL. Inh. Soln. Unit-dose vials. Cartons of 60s. *Rx.*
Use: Bronchodilator.

• **perfosfamide.** (per-FOSS-fam-ide) USAN.
Use: Antineoplastic. [Orphan Drug]

• **pergolide mesylate.** (PURR-go-lide) *USP 34.*
Use: Antiparkinson agent.

Pergrava. (Arcum) Vitamins A 2000 units, D 300 units, B_1 2 mg, B_2 2 mg, nicotinamide 10 mg, B_6 2 mg, B_{12} 5 mcg, C 60 mg, Ca 40 mg. Cap. Bot. 100s, 1000s. *OTC.*
Use: Mineral, vitamin supplement.

Pergrava No. 2. (Arcum) Vitamins A 2000 units, D 300 units, B_1 2 mg, B_2 2 mg, nicotinamide 10 mg, B_6 2 mg, C 60 mg, calcium lactate monohydrate 200 mg, ferrous gluconate 31 mg, folic acid 0.1 mg. Cap. Bot. 100s, 1000s. *OTC.*
Use: Mineral, vitamin supplement.

perhexiline. (per-HEX-ih-leen)
Use: Antianginal.

• **perhexiline maleate.** (per-HEX-ih-leen) USAN.
Use: Vasodilator, coronary.

perhydrol.
See: Hydrogen Peroxide 30%.

Peri-Care. (Sween) Vitamins A and D in petroleum ointment base. Tube 0.5 oz, 1.75 oz. Jar 2 oz, 5 oz, 8 oz. *OTC.*
Use: Emollient.

Peri-Colace. (Purdue) Docusate sodium 50 mg, sennosides 8.6 mg. Tab. 10s, 30s, 60s. *OTC.*
Use: Laxative.

Peridex. (Procter & Gamble) Chlorhexidine gluconate 0.12%, alcohol 11.6%, glycerin, PEG-40 sorbitan diisostearate, flavor, sodium saccharin, FD&C blue No. 1, water. Bot. 480 mL. *Rx.*
Use: Mouth preparation.

Peridin-C. (Beutlich) Hesperidin methyl cholcone (bioflavonoids) 50 mg, hesperidin complex 150 mg, ascorbic acid 200 mg. Tab. Bot. 100s, 500s. *OTC.*
Use: Water-soluble vitamin.

Peries. (Xttrium) Medicated pads w/witch hazel, glycerin. Jar pad 40s. *OTC.*
Use: Hygienic wipe and local compress.

Periguard. (DermaRite) Aloe vera, lanolin, mineral oil, parabens, vitamin A, vitamin D, vitamin E. Oint. 100 g. *OTC.*
Use: Dermatological agent, protectant.

• **perindopril.** (per-IN-doe-prill) USAN.
Use: ACE inhibitor.

• **perindopril erbumine.** (per-IN-doe-prill ehr-BYOO-meen) USAN.
Use: Angiotensin-converting enzyme inhibitor.
See: Aceon.

perindopril erbumine. (Roxane) Perindopril erbumine 2 mg, 4 mg, 8 mg. May contain lactose. Tab. 30s, 100s, 500s (except 2 mg). *Rx.*
Use: Renin angiotensin antagonist, angiotensin-converting enzyme inhibitor.

PerioChip. (Adria) Chlorhexidine gluconate 2.5 mg. Chip Blister pack 10s. *Rx.*
Use: Anesthetic.

Perio-Eze 20. (Moyco Union Broach Division) Oral paste.
Use: Analgesic, topical.

PerioGard. (Colgate Oral) Chlorhexidine gluconate 0.12%, alcohol 11.6%, glycerin, PEG-40, sorbitol diisostearnate, saccharin. Rinse. Bot. 473 mL w/15 mL dose cup. *Rx.*
Use: Anesthetic.

PerioMed. (Omnii Oral) Stannous fluoride concentrate 0.64%. Alcohol-free. Tropical fruit, mint, and cinnamon flavor. Rinse. 283.5 g. *Rx.*
Use: Prevention of dental caries.

Periostat. (CollaGenex) Doxycycline hyclate 20 mg. Lactose. Tab. Bot. 60s, 100s, 1000s. *Rx.*
Use: Anti-infective; mouth and throat product.

Peri Sofcap. (Alton) Docusate sodium with peristim. Bot. 100s, 1000s. *OTC.*
Use: Laxative.

Peritrate. (Parke-Davis) Pentaerythritol tetranitrate. **Tab.: 10 mg:** Bot. 100s, 1000s. **20 mg:** Bot. 100s, 1000s, UD 100s. **40 mg:** Bot. 100s. *Rx.*
Use: Antianginal.

Peritrate S.A. (Parke-Davis) Pentaerythritol tetranitrate 80 mg (20 mg in immediate-release layer, 60 mg in sustained-release base). Tab. Bot. 100s, 1000s, UD 100s. *Rx.*
Use: Antianginal.

Peri-Wash. (Sween) Bot. 4 oz, 8 oz, 1 gal., 5 gal., 30 gal., 55 gal.
Use: Anorectal preparation.

Peri-Wash II. (Sween) Bot. 4 oz, 8 oz, 1 gal., 5 gal., 30 gal., 55 gal.
Use: Anorectal preparation.

Perlane. (Medicis) Hyaluronic acid 20 mg/mL. Inj., Gel. Single-use, prefilled syringes. *Rx.*
Use: Physical adjunct.

Perlane-L. (Medicis Aesthetics) Hyaluronic acid 20 mg/mL. Lidocaine 0.3%. Inj., gel. Single-use, prefilled syringe. *Rx.*
Use: Physical adjunct.

•**perlapine.** (PURR-lah-peen) USAN.
Use: Hypnotic; sedative.

Perlatan.
See: Estrone.

Perloxx. (Athlon Pharmaceuticals) Oxycodone hydrochloride/acetaminophen 2.5 mg/300 mg, 5 mg/300 mg, 7.5 mg/300 mg. Tab. 100s. *c-ii.*
Use: Narcotic analgesic.

•**permanganic acid, potassium salt.** USP 34. Potassium permanganate.

Permapen. (Roerig) Penicillin G benzathine 1,200,000 units/dose with polyvinylpyrrolidone, parabens. Inj. *Isoject* 2 mL. *Rx.*
Use: Anti-infective, penicillin.

•**permethrin.** (per-METH-rin) USAN. Synthetic pyrethrin.
Use: Pediculicide for treatment of head lice, ectoparasiticide.
See: Acticin.
Elimite.
Nix.
Nix Complete Lice Treatment System.

permethrin. (Various Mfr.) Permethrin. **Cream:** 5%. 60 g. **Lot.:** 1%. 60 mL with comb. *OTC.*
Use: Scabicide, pediculicide.

Permitil. (Schering) Fluphenazine hydrochloride. **Concentrate:** 5 mg/mL, alcohol 1%, parabens. Dropper Bot. 118 mL. **Tab.:** 2.5 mg, 5 mg, 10 mg, lactose. Bot. 100s (except 10 mg), 1000s (10 mg only). *Rx.*
Use: Antipsychotic.

Pernox. (Bristol-Myers Squibb) Microfine granules of polyethylene 20%, sulfur 2%, salicylic acid 2% in a combination of soapless cleansers and wetting agents. Lot. Bot. 6 oz. *OTC.*
Use: Dermatologic, acne.

Pernox Lathering Abradant Scrub. (Ranbaxy) Sulfur, salicylic acid. Lot. Bot. 141 g. *OTC.*
Use: Dermatologic, acne.

Pernox Medicated Lathering Scrub Cleanser. (Bristol-Myers Squibb) Polyethylene granules 26%, sulfur 2%, salicylic acid 1.5% w/soapless surface-active cleansers and wetting agents. Regular or lemon. Tube 2 oz, 4 oz. *OTC.*
Use: Dermatologic, acne.

Pernox Scrub for Oily Skin. (Ranbaxy) Sulfur, salicylic acid, EDTA. Cleanser. 56 g, 113 g. *OTC.*
Use: Dermatologic, acne.

Pernox Shampoo. (Bristol-Myers Squibb) Sodium laureth sulfate, water, lauramide DEA, quaternium 22, PEG-75 lanolin/hydrolyzed animal protein, fragrance, sodium Cl, lactic acid, sorbic acid, disodium EDTA, FD&C yellow No. 6 and blue No. 1. Bot. 8 oz. *OTC.*
Use: Cleanser; conditioner.

peroxidase.
W/Glucose oxidase, potassium, iodide.
See: Diastix Reagent Strips.

peroxide, dibenzoyl. Benzoyl Peroxide, Hydrous.

peroxides.
See: Carbamide Peroxide.
Hydrogen Peroxide.
Urea Peroxide.

Peroxyl. (Colgate Oral) Hydrogen peroxide 1.5% in a mint-flavored base. Gel. Tube 15 mL. *OTC.*
Use: Mouth preparation.

Peroxyl Dental Rinse. (Colgate Oral) Hydrogen peroxide 1.5% in mint-flavored base, alcohol 6%. Bot. 240 mL, pt. *OTC.*
Use: Mouth preparation.

• **perphenazine.** (per-FEN-uh-ZEEN) *USP 34.*
Use: Antiemetic; antipsychotic; anxiolytic.

perphenazine. (Various Mfr.) Perphenazine 2 mg, 4 mg, 8 mg, 16 mg. Tab. Bot. 100s, 500s (4 mg, 8 mg only), 1000s, UD 100s. *Rx.*
Use: Antipsychotic.

perphenazine/amitriptyline.
See: Etrafon-A.
Etrafon Forte.
Etrafon 2-25.

perphenazine/amitriptyline. (Various Mfr.) Perphenazine/amitriptyline 2 mg/ 10 mg, 2 mg/25 mg, 4 mg/10 mg, 4 mg/25 mg, 4 mg/50 mg. Tab. Bot. 21s (2 mg/10 mg only), 100s, 250s (4 mg/ 10 mg and 4 mg/50 mg only), 500s (except 4 mg/50 mg), 800s (4 mg/25 mg only), 1000s (except 4 mg/50 mg).
Use: Miscellaneous psychotherapeutic.

Persangue. (Arcum) Ferrous gluconate 192 mg, vitamins C 150 mg, B$_1$ 3 mg, B$_2$ 3 mg, B$_{12}$ 50 mcg. Cap. Bot. 100s, 500s. *OTC.*
Use: Mineral, vitamin supplement.

Persantine. (Boehringer Ingelheim) Dipyridamole 25 mg, 50 mg, 75 mg. Tab. **25 mg, 50 mg:** Bot. 100s, 1000s, UD 100s. **75 mg:** Bot. 100s, 500s, UD 100s. *Rx.*
Use: Antiplatelet.

• **persic oil.** (PER-sik) *NF 29.*
Use: Vehicle.

pertechnetic acid, sodium salt. Sodium Pertechnetate Tc-99m Solution.

Pertscan-99m. (Abbott Diagnostics) Radiodiagnostic. Inj. Tc-99m.
Use: Diagnostic aid.

Pertussin. (Pertussin) Dextromethorphan HBr 15 mg/5 mL, alcohol 9.5%. Syr. Bot. 3 oz, 6 oz. *OTC.*
Use: Antitussive.

Pertussin All-Night PM. (Pertussin) Acetaminophen 167 mg, doxylamine succinate 1.25 mg, pseudoephedrine hydrochloride 10 mg, dextromethorphan HBr 5 mg/5 mL, alcohol 25%. Liq. Bot. 240 mL. *OTC.*
Use: Analgesic; antihistamine; antitussive; decongestant.

Pertussin CS. (Pertussin) Dextromethorphan HBr 3.5 mg, guaifenesin 25 mg/ 5 mL, 8.5% alcohol. Bot. 90 mL. *OTC.*
Use: Antitussive; expectorant.

Pertussin ES. (Pertussin) Dextromethorphan HBr 15 mg/5 mL, alcohol 9.5%, sugar, sorbitol. Liq. Bot. 120 mL. *OTC.*
Use: Antitussive.

• **pertussis immune globulin.** (per-TUSS-iss) *USP 34.* Formerly Pertussis Immune Human Globulin.
Use: Immunization.

pertussis vaccine. (Michigan Department of Health) Vial 5 mL.
Use: Immunization.

• **pertussis vaccine acellular.** *USP 34.*
Use: Immunization.
W/Diphtheria and tetanus toxoids.
See: Adacel.
Boostrix.
Daptacel.
Infanrix.
Tripedia.

pertussis vaccine, acellular, and diphtheria and tetanus toxoids, adsorbed.
Use: Immunization.
See: Adacel.
Boostrix.
Daptacel.
Infanrix.
Tripedia.

• **pertussis vaccine adsorbed.** *USP 34.*
Use: Immunization.

• **pertuzumab.** (per-TUE-zue-mab) USAN.
Use: Antineoplastic.

Peruvian balsam.
Use: Local protectant, rubefacient.
W/Benzocaine, Zinc Oxide Bismuth Subgallate, Boric Acid.
See: Hemorrhoidal Ointment.
W/Lidocaine, Bismuth Subgallate, Zinc Oxide, Aluminum Subacetate.
See: Xylocaine.

• **perzinfotel.** (per-zin-FOE-tel) USAN.
Use: NMDA receptor antagonist.

peson. Sodium Lyapolate. Polyethylene sulfonate sodium.
Use: Anticoagulant.

PE Tann/CP Tann. (Brighton Pharmaceuticals) Phenylephrine tannate 20 mg, chlorpheniramine tannate 4 mg per 5 mL. Aspartame, methylparaben, phenylalanine 5 mg, saccharin, sorbitol. Alcohol free. Bubble gum flavor. Susp. 473 mL. *Rx.*
Use: Upper respiratory combination, decongestant and antihistamine.

Peterson's Ointment. (Peterson) Carbolic acid, camphor, tannic acid, zinc

oxide. Tube w/pipe 1 oz. Jar 16 oz. Can 1.4 oz, 3 oz. *OTC.*
Use: Anorectal preparation.
Pethadol. (Halsey Drug) Meperidine hydrochloride 50 mg, 100 mg. Tab. Bot. 100s, 1000s. *c-II.*
Use: Analgesic; narcotic.
pethidine hydrochloride.
See: Meperidine Hydrochloride.
PETN.
See: Pentaerythritol Tetranitrate.
petrichloral. Pentaerythritol chloral.
Use: Sedative.
•**petrolatum.** (pe-troe-LAY-tum) *USP 34.*
Use: Pharmaceutic aid (ointment base).
See: Aloe Vesta.
petrolatum gauze.
Use: Surgical aid.
•**petrolatum, hydrophilic.** (pe-troe-LAY-tum hye-droe-FIL-ik) *USP 34.*
Use: Pharmaceutic aid, absorbent, ointment base; topical protectant.
•**petrolatum, liquid.** (pe-troe-LAY-tum) *USP 34.* Mineral Oil, Light Mineral Oil, Adepsine Oil, Glymol, Liquid Paraffin, Parolein, White Mineral Oil, Heavy Liquid Petrolatum.
Use: Laxative.
See: Fleet Mineral Oil.
Mineral Oil.
Saxol.
petrolatum, liquid, emulsion.
Use: Lubricant, laxative.
W/Irish Moss, Casanthranol.
See: Haley's M. O.
petrolatum, red veterinarian. (AstraZeneca) Also known as RVP.
W/Zinc Oxide, 2-ethoxyethyl p-methoxycinnamate.
See: RVPaque.
•**petrolatum, white.** (pe-troe-LAY-tum) *USP 34.*
Use: Pharmaceutic aid, oleaginous ointment base; topical protectant.
See: Moroline.
Petro-Phylic Soap. (Doak Dermatologics) Hydrophilic Petrolatum. Cake 4 oz.
Use: Emollient; anti-infective, topical.
Petro-20. (Foy Laboratories) Pentaerythritol tetranitrate 20 mg. Tab. Bot. 100s, 1000s. *Rx.*
Use: Antianginal.
•**pexelizumab.** (peks-e-li-ZOO-mab) USAN.
Use: Monoclonal antibody.
Pexeva. (Synthon) Paroxetine mesylate 10 mg, 20 mg, 30 mg, 40 mg. Tab. 30s, 100s (20 mg only), 500s (20 mg only). *Rx.*

Use: Antidepressant, selective serotonin reuptake inhibitor.
Pfeiffer's Cold Sore. (Pfeiffer) Gum benzoin 7%, camphor, menthol, thymol, eucalyptol, alcohol 85%. Lot. Bot. 15 mL. *OTC.*
Use: Cold sores; fever blisters; moisturizer.
PF4RIA. (Abbott Diagnostics) Platelet factor 4 radioimmunoassay for the quantitative measurement of total PF4 levels in plasma.
Use: Diagnostic aid.
Pfizerpen. (Pfizer) Penicillin G potassium 5,000,000 units, 20,000,000 units/vial, sodium ≈ 6.8 mg (0.3 mEq), potassium 65.6 mg (1.68 mEq)/million units. Pow. for Inj. Vial. *Rx.*
Use: Anti-infective, penicillin.
Pfizerpen VK. (Pfizer) Penicillin V potassium. Tab. **250 mg:** Bot. 1000s.
500 mg: Bot. 100s. *Rx.*
Use: Anti-infective, penicillin.
PGA.
See: Folic Acid.
PGE.
Use: Prostaglandin.
See: Alprostadil.
pH acid. (Ivax) Bot. 8 oz.
Use: Dermatologic.
Phadiatop RIA Test. (Pharmacia) Determination of IgE antibodies specific to inhalant allergens in human serum. Kit 60s.
Use: Diagnostic aid.
Phanatuss Cough. (Pharmakon) Dextromethorphan HBr 10 mg, guaifenesin 85 mg, potassium citrate 75 mg, citric acid 35 mg/5 mL, sorbitol, menthol. Syr. Bot. 118 mL. *OTC.*
Use: Antitussive; expectorant.
Phanatuss DM. (Pharmakon) Dextromethorphan HBr 10 mg, guaifenesin 100 mg per 5 mL. Parabens, saccharin, menthol, alcohol free, sugar free. Syr. Bot. 118 mL. *OTC.*
Use: Upper respiratory combination, antitussive, expectorant.
pH Antiseptic Skin Cleanser. (Walgreen) Alcohol 63%. Bot. 16 oz. *OTC.*
Use: Astringent; cleanser.
Pharazine. (Halsey Drug) Bot. 4 oz, pt, gal.
Use: A series of cough and cold products.
Pharmadine. (Sherwood Davis & Geck) Povidone-iodine. **Oint.:** Pkt. 1 g, 1.5 g, 2 g, 30 g, 1 lb. **Perineal wash:** 240 mL. **Skin cleanser:** 240 mL. **Soln.:** 15 mL, 120 mL, 240 mL, pt, qt. **Soln., swabs:** 100s. **Soln., swabsticks:** 1 or

3/packet in 250s. **Spray:** 120 g. **Surgical scrub:** 30 mL, pt, qt, gal, foil-pack 15 mL. **Surgical scrub sponge/brush:** 25s. **Swabsticks, lemon glycerin:** 100s. **Whirlpool soln.:** Gal. *OTC.*
Use: Antiseptic.

Pharmaflur. (Pharmics) Sodium fluoride 2.21 mg. Tab. Bot. 1000s. *Rx.*
Use: Dental caries agent.

Pharmalgen Hymenoptera Venoms. (ALK) Freeze-dried venom or venom protein. Vials of 120 mcg, 1100 mcg for each of honey bee, white-faced hornet, yellow hornet, yellow jacket, or wasp. Vials of 360 mcg, 3300 mcg for mixed vespids (white-faced hornet, yellow hornet, yellow jacket). Diagnostic kit: 5 × 1 mL vial. Treatment kit: 6 × 1 mL vial or 1 × 1.1 mg multiple-dose vial. Starter Kit: 6 × 1 mL, prediluted 0.01 mcg to 100 mcg/mL.
Use: Antivenom.

Pharmalgen Standardized Allergenic Extracts. (ALK) 100,000 allergenic units. Vial. Box 5 × 1 mL.
Use: Diagnostic aid.

Phazyme. (GlaxoSmithKline) Simethicone. **Cap.:** 180 mg. 12s. **Drops:** 40 mg/0.6 mL, saccharin. Bot. 30 mL w/dropper. **Tab.:** 60 mg. Bot. 50s, 100s, 1000s. *OTC.*
Use: Antiflatulent.

Phazyme 95. (GlaxoSmithKline) Simethicone 95 mg. Tab. Bot. 100s. *OTC.*
Use: Antiflatulent.

Phazyme 125. (GlaxoSmithKline) Simethicone 125 mL. Cap. Bot. 50s. *OTC.*
Use: Antiflatulent.

Phazyme Quick Dissolve. (GlaxoSmithKline) Simethicone 125 mg. Phenylalanine 0.4 mg, aspartame, mannitol, sorbitol. Mint flavor. Chew. Tab. 18s, 48s. *OTC.*
Use: Antiflatulent.

•**phemfilcon A.** (FEM-fill-kahn A) USAN.
Use: Contact lens material, hydrophilic.

Phenabid. (GIL) Phenylephrine hydrochloride 20 mg, chlorpheniramine maleate 8 mg. Dye and sugar free. ER Tab. 100s. *Rx.*
Use: Upper respiratory combination, decongestant and antihistamine.

Phenabid DM. (GIL) Dextromethorphan HBr 30 mg, chlorpheniramine maleate 8 mg, phenylephrine hydrochloride 20 mg. Sugar, dye, and preservative free. ER Tab. 100s, 500s, 1000s. *Rx.*
Use: Upper respiratory combination, antitussive combination.

phenacaine hydrochloride.
Use: Anesthetic, local.

Phenacal. (NeuroGenesis/Matrix Tech.) D,l-phenylalanine 500 mg, l-glutamine 15 mg, l-tyrosine 25 mg, l-carnitine 10 mg, l-arginine pyroglutamate 10 mg, l-ornithine/l-aspartate 10 mg, Cr 0.033 mg, Se 0.012 mg, vitamin B_1 0.33 mg, B_2 5 mg, B_3 3.3 mg, B_5 0.33 mg, B_6 0.33 mg, B_{12} 1 mcg, E 5 units, biotin 0.05 mg, folic acid 0.066 mg, Fe 1 mg, Zn 2.5 mg, Ca 35 mg, I 0.25 mg, Cu 0.33 mg, Mg 25 mg. Cap. Bot. 42s, 180s. *OTC.*
Use: Nutritional supplement.

phenacetin. Acetophenetidin. Ethoxyacetanilide.
Note: This drug has been withdrawn from the market because of liver and kidney toxicity. This drug is no longer official in the USP.
Use: Antipyretic; analgesic.

Phenadex Senior. (Alra) Dextromethorphan HBr 10 mg, guaifenesin 200 mg/5 mL. Liq. Bot. 118 mL. *OTC.*
Use: Antitussive; expectorant.

Phenadoz. (Paddock) Promethazine hydrochloride 12.5 mg, 25 mg. Cocoa butter. Supp. 12s. *Rx.*
Use: Antihistamine, nonselective phenothiazine.

phenamazoline hydrochloride.
Use: Vasoconstrictor.

Phenameth. (Major) Promethazine 25 mg. Tab. Bot. 1000s. *Rx.*
Use: Antiemetic; antihistamine.

Phenameth DM. (Major) Promethazine hydrochloride 6.25 mg, dextromethorphan HBr 15 mg/5 mL, alcohol. Syr. Bot. 120 mL. *Rx.*
Use: Antihistamine; antitussive.

Phenameth VC w/Codeine. (Major) Phenylephrine hydrochloride 5 mg, promethazine hydrochloride 6.25 mg, codeine phosphate 10 mg/5 mL, alcohol 7%. Syr. Bot. Pt, gal. *c-v.*
Use: Antihistamine; antitussive; decongestant.

Phenameth w/Codeine. (Major) Promethazine hydrochloride 6.25 mg, codeine phosphate 10 mg/5 mL, alcohol 7%. Syr. Bot. 4 oz, pt, gal. *c-v.*
Use: Antihistamine; antitussive.

phenantoin. Mephenytoin.

Phenapap. (Rugby) Pseudoephedrine hydrochloride 30 mg, acetaminophen 325 mg. Tab. Bot. 100s. *OTC.*
Use: Upper respiratory combination, decongestant, analgesic.

Phenapap Sinus Headache & Congestion. (Rugby) Pseudoephedrine hydrochloride 30 mg, chlorpheniramine 2 mg, acetaminophen 325 mg. Tab. Bot.

30s, 100s, 1000s. *OTC.*
Use: Analgesic; antihistamine; decongestant.

phenaphthazine. Sodium dinitro phenylazonaphthol disulfonate.

phenarsone sulfoxylate. Methanesulfinic acid disodium salt.
Use: Antiamebic.

Phenaseptic. (Rugby) Phenol 1.4%, saccharin, cherry flavor. Throat spray. Bot. 177 mL. *OTC.*
Use: Mouth and throat product.

Phenaspirin Compound. (Davis & Sly) Phenobarbital 0.25 g, aspirin 3.5 g. Cap. Bot. 1000s. *Rx.*
Use: Analgesic; hypnotic; sedative.

PhenaVent D. (Ethex) Phenylephrine hydrochloride 40 mg, guaifenesin 1200 mg. Film-coated. ER Tab. 100s. *Rx.*
Use: Decongestant and expectorant combination, upper respiratory combination.

PhenaVent LA. (Ethex) Phenylephrine hydrochloride 30 mg, guaifenesin 600 mg. Film-coated. Tab. 100s. *Rx.*
Use: Decongestant, expectorant.

phenazocine hydrobromide.
Use: Analgesic.

PhenazoForte Plus. (Creekwood Pharmaceutical) Butalbital 15 mg, hyoscyamine hydrobromide 300 mcg, phenazopyridine hydrochloride 150 mg. Lactose, mineral oil, PEG. Tab. 30s. *Rx.*
Use: Renal and genitourinary agent, interstitial cystitis combination.

phenazone.
See: Antipyrine.

•**phenazopyridine hydrochloride.** (fen-AZZ-oh-PIH-rih-deen) *USP 34.*
Use: Analgesic, urinary.
See: AZO Standard.
   AZO Standard Maximum Strength.
   Baridium.
   Geridium.
   Prodium.
   Pyridium.
   Urogesic.
   UTI Relief.
W/Butalbital, Hyoscyamine Hydrobromide.
   See: PhenazoForte Plus.
W/Combinations.
   See: Phenazopyridine Plus.
   Pyridium Plus.
   Urisan-P.

phenazopyridine hydrochloride. (Various Mfr.) Phenazopyridine hydrochloride 100 mg, 200 mg. Tab. 100s, 1000s, UD 100s. *Rx.*
Use: Interstitial cystitis agent.

Phenazopyridine Plus. (Breckenridge) Phenazopyridine hydrochloride 150 mg, hyoscyamine hydrobromide 0.3 mg, butabarbital 15 mg. Tab. 30s. *Rx.*
Use: Interstitial cystitis agent.

•**phenbutazone sodium glycerate.** (fen-BYOO-tah-zone so-dee-uhm GLIH-seh-rate) *USAN.*
Use: Anti-inflammatory.

•**phencarbamide.** (FEN-car-BAM-id) *USAN.*
Use: Anticholinergic; spasmolytic.

Phencarb GG. (Boca Pharmacal) Carbetapentane citrate 20 mg, guaifenesin 100 mg, phenylephrine hydrochloride 10 mg per 5 mL. EDTA, sorbitol, sugar. Spearmint flavor. Syr. 473 mL. *Rx.*
Use: Antitussive and expectorant combination, upper respiratory combination.

Phenchlor-Eight. (Freeport) Chlorpheniramine maleate 8 mg. TR Cap. Bot. 1000s. *Rx.*
Use: Antihistamine.

Phenchlor-Twelve. (Freeport) Chlorpheniramine maleate 12 mg. TR Cap. Bot. 1000s. *Rx.*
Use: Antihistamine.

•**phencyclidine hydrochloride.** (fen-SIGH-klih-deen) *USAN.*
Use: Anesthetic.

phendimetrazine. (Various Mfr.) Phendimetrazine tartrate 35 mg. Tab. Bot. 100s, 1000s, 5000s. *c-III.*
Use: CNS stimulant, anorexiant.

•**phendimetrazine tartrate.** (fen-die-MEH-trah-zeen) *USP 34.*
Use: CNS stimulant, anorexiant.
See: Anorex.
   Bontril PDM.
   Bontril Slow Release.
   Delcozine.
   Di-Ap-Trol.
   Elphemet.
   Melfiat-105 Unicelles.
   Obe-Tite.
   Phendimetrazine.
   Phen-70.
   Prelu-2.
   Reducto, Improved.
   Rexigen Forte.
   Slim-Tabs.

phendimetrazine tartrate. (Sandoz) Phendimetrazine tartrate 105 mg. Sucrose. ER Cap. 100s, 1000s. *c-III.*
Use: Anorexiant.

Phendry. (LuChem Pharmaceuticals, Inc.) Diphenhydramine hydrochloride

12.5 mg/5 mL, alcohol 14%. Elix. Bot. Pt, gal. *OTC.*
Use: Antihistamine.

Phendry Children's Allergy Medicine. (LuChem Pharmaceuticals, Inc.) Diphenhydramine hydrochloride 12.5 mg/5 mL, alcohol 14%. Elix. Bot. 120 mL. *OTC.*
Use: Antihistamine.

phenelzine dihydrogen sulfate.
See: Nardil.

•**phenelzine sulfate.** (FEN-uhl-zeen) *USP 34.*
Use: Antidepressant.
See: Nardil.

phenelzine sulfate. (Gavis Pharmaceuticals) Phenelzine sulfate 15 mg. Film coated. Edetate disodium, mannitol, PEG. Tab. 60s. *Rx.*
Use: Antidepressant, monoamine oxidase inhibitor.

Phenergan. (Wyeth) Promethazine hydrochloride. **Inj.:** 25 mg/mL, 50 mg/mL. EDTA, sodium metabisulfite 0.25 mg/mL. Inj. Amp. 1 mL. **Supp.:** 12.5 mg, 25 mg. Cocoa butter. Box. 12s. **Tab.:** 12.5 mg, 25 mg, 50 mg. Saccharin (except 50 mg), lactose. Bot. 100s. 10 blister strips of 10 (25 mg only). *Rx.*
Use: Antihistamine, nonselective phenothiazine.

Phenergan with Codeine. (Wyeth) Promethazine hydrochloride 6.25 mg, codeine phosphate 10 mg/5 mL. Bot. 4 oz, 6 oz, 8 oz, pt, gal. *c-v.*
Use: Antihistamine; antitussive.

Phenergan with Dextromethorphan. (Wyeth) Promethazine hydrochloride 6.25 mg, dextromethorphan HBr 15 mg/5 mL, alcohol 7%. Bot. 4 oz, 6 oz, pt, gal. *Rx.*
Use: Antihistamine; antitussive.

pheneridine.
Use: Analgesic.

i-phenethylbiguanide monohydrochloride. Phenformin hydrochloride.

Phenex-1. (Ross) Protein 15 g, fat 23.9 g, carbohydrates 46.3 g, linoleic acid 1800 mg, Fe 9 mg, Na 190 mg, K 675 mg, Cal 480/100 g. With appropriate vitamins and minerals. Phenylalanine free. Pow. Can 350 g. *OTC.*
Use: Nutritional supplement.

Phenex-2. (Ross) Protein 30 g, fat 15.5 g, carbohydrates 30 g, Na 880 mg, K 1370 mg, Cal 410/mL. With appropriate vitamins and minerals. Phenylalanine free. Pow. Can 325 g. *OTC.*
Use: Nutritional supplement.

Phenflu G. (AMBI) Dextromethorphan

HBr 30 mg, guaifenesin 600 mg, phenylephrine hydrochloride 15 mg, acetaminophen 500 mg. Dye free. Tab. 100s. *Rx.*
Use: Upper respiratory combination, antitussive and expectorant combination.

phenformin hydrochloride. *Rx.*
Note: Withdrawn from market in 1977. Available under IND exemption.
Use: Hypoglycemic.

Phenhist DH w/Codeine. (Rugby) Pseudoephedrine hydrochloride 30 mg, chlorpheniramine maleate 2 mg, codeine phosphate 10 mg/5 mL, alcohol 5%. Liq. Bot. 120 mL, 480 mL. *c-v.*
Use: Antihistamine; antitussive; decongestant.

Phenhist Expectorant. (Rugby) Pseudoephedrine hydrochloride 30 mg, codeine phosphate 10 mg, guaifenesin 100 mg/5 mL, alcohol 7.5%. Liq. Bot. 118 mL, pt, gal. *c-v.*
Use: Antihistamine; antitussive; decongestant.

•**phenindamine tartrate.** (fen-IN-dah-meen) USAN.
Use: Antihistamine, nonselective piperidine.

W/Phenylephrine Hydrochloride, Aspirin, Caffeine, Aluminum Hydroxide, Magnesium Carbonate.
See: Dristan.

W/Phenylephrine Hydrochloride, Caramiphen Ethanedisulfonate.
See: Dondril.

W/Phenylephrine Hydrochloride, Chlorpheniramine Maleate, Belladonna Alkaloids.
See: Comhist LA.

W/Phenylephrine Hydrochloride, Chlorpheniramine Maleate, Drytane.
See: Comhist.

W/Phenylephrine Hydrochloride, Pyrilamine Maleate, Chlorpheniramine Maleate, Dextromethorphan HBr.
See: Histalet.

pheniodol.
See: Iodoalphionic acid.

pheniprazine hydrochloride.
Use: Antihypertensive.

•**pheniramine maleate.** (fen-IR-a-meen) *USP 34.*
Use: Antihistamine.
See: Citra Forte.
  Partuss AC.
  Tritussin.

W/Acetaminophen, Phenylephrine Hydrochloride.
See: Theraflu Cold & Sore Throat.
  Theraflu Flu & Sore Throat.
  Theraflu Nighttime Severe Cold.

W/Caffeine Citrate, Phenylephrine Hydrochloride, Sodium Salicylate.
See: Scot-Tussin Original Multi-Action Cold and Allergy.
W/Dextromethorphan Hydrobromide, Phenylephrine Hydrochloride.
See: Theraflu Cold & Cough.
W/Naphazoline Hydrochloride.
See: Naphcon-A.
Opcon-A.
Visine-A.
•**phenmetrazine hydrochloride.** (fen-MEH-trah-zeen) *USP 34.*
Use: Anorexic.
•**phenobarbital.** (fee-no-BAR-bih-tahl) *USP 34.*
Tall Man: PHENobarbital
Use: Anticonvulsant; hypnotic; sedative.
See: Luminal Sodium.
Solfoton.
W/Atropine Sulfate.
See: Antrocol.
W/Atropine Sulfate, Hyoscyamine Hydrobromide or Sulfate, Scopolamine Hydrobromide.
See: Antispasmodic.
Donnatal.
Donnatal Extentabs.
PB-Hyos.
Quadrapax.
phenobarbital. (Pharmaceutical Associates) Phenobarbital 15 mg/5 mL. Elix. Bot. Pt, UD 5 mL, 10 mL, 20 mL. *c-iv.*
Use: Anticonvulsant; hypnotic; sedative.
phenobarbital. (Various Mfr.) Phenobarbital. **Tab.: 15 mg, 30 mg:** Bot. 100s, 1000s, 5000s, UD 100s. **60 mg:** Bot. 100s, 1000s, UD 100s. **100 mg:** 100s, 1000s. **Elix.:** 20 mg/5 mL. Bot. Pt, gal, UD 5 mL, UD 7.5 mL.
Use: Anticonvulsant; hypnotic; sedative.
phenobarbital and theobromine combinations.
See: Theobromine w/phenobarbital combinations.
•**phenobarbital sodium.** (fee-no-BAR-bih-tahl) *USP 34.*
Tall Man: PHENobarbital
Use: Anticonvulsant; hypnotic; sedative.
See: Luminal Injection.
phenobarbital sodium. (Wyeth) Phenobarbital sodium Inj. **30 mg/mL, 60 mg/mL:** *Tubex* 1 mL. **65 mg/mL:** Vial 1 mL. *c-iv.*
Use: Anticonvulsant; hypnotic; sedative.
phenobarbital sodium in propylene glycol. (Vitarine) Amp. 0.13 g: 1 mL,

Box 25s, 100s. *c-iv.*
Use: Anticonvulsant; hypnotic; sedative.
phenobarbital with aminophylline.
See: Aminophylline.
phenobarbital with central nervous system stimulants.
See: Arcotrate No. 3.
Spabelin.
phenobarbital with homatropine methylbromide.
See: Homatropine methylbromide and phenobarbital combinations.
phenobarbital with hyoscyamus.
See: Hyoscyamus products and phenobarbital combinations.
phenobarbital with mannitol hexanitrate.
Use: Anticonvulsant; sedative; hypnotic.
See: Mannitol hexanitrate with phenobarbital combinations.
phenobarbital with theophylline.
See: Theophylline with phenobarbital combinations.
Pheno-Bella. (Ferndale) Belladonna extract 10.8 mg, phenobarbital 16.2 mg. Tab. Bot. 100s, 1000s. *Rx.*
Use: Anticholinergic; antispasmodic; hypnotic; sedative.
•**phenol.** (FEE-nole) *USP 34.*
Use: Pharmaceutical aid, preservative; topical antipruritic; mouth and throat product.
See: Chloraseptic Kids Sore Throat.
Chloraseptic Sore Throat.
Green Throat Spray.
Phenaseptic.
Red Throat Spray.
Triaminic Sore Throat Spray.
W/Benzocaine.
See: Anbesol.
W/Lidocaine.
See: Skeeter Stik.
W/Resorcinol, Boric Acid, Basic Fuchsin, Acetone.
See: Castellani's Paint.
•**phenolate sodium.** (FEEN-oh-late) USAN.
Use: Disinfectant.
Phenolax. (Pharmacia) Phenolphthalein 64.8 mg. Wafer. Bot. 100s. *OTC.*
Use: Laxative.
•**phenol, camphorated topical gel.** (FEE-nole) *USP 34.*
Use: Topical antipruritic.
•**phenol, liquefied.** (FEE-nole) *USP 34.*
Use: Topical antipruritic.
•**phenolphthalein.** (fee-nahl-THAY-leen) *USP 34.*
Use: Indicator.

phenolsulfonates.
See: Sulfocarbolates.
phenolsulfonic acid. Sulfocarbolic acid. Used in Sulphodine. (Strasenburgh).
phenoltetrabromophthalein. Disulfonate Disodium.
See: Sulfobromophthalein Sodium.
Pheno Nux. (Pal-Pak, Inc.) Phenobarbital 16.2 mg, nux vomica extract 8.1 mg, calcium carbonate 194.4 mg. Tab. Bot. 1000s. *c-iv.*
Use: Sedative; hypnotic; antacid.
phenothiazine. Thiodiphenylamine.
phenothiazine derivatives.
See: Chlorpromazine Hydrochloride.
　Fluphenazine.
　Mesoridazine.
　Perphenazine.
　Prochlorperazine.
　Thioridazine Hydrochloride.
　Trifluoperazine Hydrochloride.
phenothiazines, nonselective.
See: Promethazine Hydrochloride.
Phenoturic. (Truett) Phenobarbital 40 mg/5 mL. Elix. Bot. Pt, gal. *c-iv.*
Use: Hypnotic; sedative.
●**phenoxybenzamine hydrochloride.** (fen-ox-ee-BEN-zuh-meen) *USP 34.*
Use: Antihypertensive.
See: Dibenzyline.
phenoxymethyl penicillin.
See: Penicillin V.
phenoxymethyl penicillin potassium.
See: Penicillin V potassium.
phenoxynate. Mixture of phenylphenols 17% to 18%, octyl and related alkylphenols 2% to 3%.
●**phenprocoumon.** (fen-PRO-koo-mahn) USAN.
Use: Anticoagulant.
Phen-70. (Parmed Pharmaceuticals, Inc.) Phendimetrazine tartrate 70 mg. Tab. Bot. 100s, 1000s. *c-iii.*
Use: Anorexiant.
Phental. (Armenpharm Ltd.) Belladonna alkaloids, phenobarbital 0.25 g. Tab. Bot. 1000s. *c-iv.*
Use: Anticholinergic; antispasmodic; hypnotic; sedative.
Phentamine. (Major) Phentermine hydrochloride 30 mg. Cap. (equivalent to 24 mg base). Bot. 100s. *c-iv.*
Use: Anorexiant.
●**phentermine.** (FEN-ter-meen) USAN.
Use: Anorexic.
See: Adipex-P.
　Wilpowr.
phentermine as resin complex.
See: Ionamin.

●**phentermine hydrochloride.** (FEN-ter-meen) *USP 34.*
Use: CNS stimulant, anorexiant.
See: Adipex-P.
　Pro-Fast HS.
　Pro-Fast SR.
phentermine hydrochloride. (Various Mfr.) **Tab.:** Phentermine hydrochloride 8 mg, 37.5 mg (equivalent to 30 mg phentermine base). Bot. 100s (37.5 mg only), 1000s. **Cap.:** Phentermine resin 15 mg. Bot. 100s, 1000s. Phentermine hydrochloride 18.75 mg (equivalent to 15 mg phentermine base), 30 mg (equivalent to 24 mg phentermine base), 37.5 mg (equivalent to 30 mg phentermine base). Bot. 100s (except 18.75 mg), 1000s. *c-iv.*
Use: CNS stimulant, anorexiant.
phentetiothalein sodium. Iso-Iodeikon.
Use: Radiopaque agent.
phentolamine hydrochloride.
Use: Antihypertensive.
●**phentolamine mesylate.** (fen-TOLE-uh-meen) *USP 34.* Formerly Phentolamine Methanesulfonate.
Use: Agent for Pheochromocytoma.
See: OraVerse.
phentolamine mesylate for injection. (Bedford) Phentolamine mesylate 5 mg. Mannitol. Pow. for Inj. Vial 2 mL. *Rx.*
Use: Antiadrenergic.
phentolamine methanesulfonate. Phentolamine mesylate.
Phentolox w/APAP. (Global Source) Phenyltoloxamine citrate 30 mg, acetaminophen 325 mg. Tab. Bot. 1000s. *Rx.*
Use: Antihistamine; analgesic.
phentydrone.
Use: Systemic fungicide.
Phenydex. (Roxmar) Dextromethorphan HBr 20 mg, guaifenesin 200 mg, phenylephrine hydrochloride 10 mg, pyrilamine maleate 25 mg per 5 mL. Sugar, alcohol, and dye free. Phenylalanine. Cherry menthol flavor. Liq. 118 mL. *Rx.*
Use: Antitussive and expectorant.
Phenydex Pediatric. (Roxmar) Phenylephrine hydrochloride 2.5 mg, dextromethorphan HBr 5 mg, guaifenesin 50 mg per 5 mL. Phenylalanine, tutti frutti flavor. Liq. 118 mL. *Rx.*
Use: Pediatric antitussive and expectorant.
n-phenylacetamide.
See: Acetanilid.
●**phenylalanine.** (fen-ill-AL-ah-NEEN) *USP 34.*
Use: Amino acid.

W/Combinations.
See: Amoxicillin.
Amoxil.
Benadryl Children's Allergy Fastmelt.
Pepcid AC.
phenylalanine ammonia-lyase.
Use: Hyperphenylalaninemia. [Orphan Drug]
phenylalanine mustard.
See: Melphalan.
•**phenyl aminosalicylate.** (FEN-ill ah-MEE-no-sah-LIH-sih-late) USAN.
Use: Anti-infective.
phenylazo. (A.P.C.) Phenylazodiaminopyridine hydrochloride 1.5 g. Tab. Bot. 1000s. *Rx.*
Use: Analgesic, urinary.
phenylazodiaminopyridine.
See: Phenazopyridine.
phenylazodiaminopyridine hydrobromide.
See: Phenazopyridine Hydrobormide.
phenylazodiaminopyridine hydrochloride.
See: Phenazopyridine Hydrochloride.
phenylazo sulfisoxazole. (A.P.C.) Sulfisoxazole 0.5 g, phenylazopyridine 50 mg. Tab. Bot. 1000s. *Rx.*
Use: Anti-infective, sulfonamide.
phenylbenzimidazole sulfonic acid.
See: Ensulizole.
•**phenylbutazone.** (fen-ill-BYOO-tah-zone) *USP 34.*
Use: Antirheumatic.
phenylbutylpiperadine derivatives.
Use: Antipsychotic.
See: Haloperidol.
Pimozide.
phenylcarbinol.
See: Benzyl Alcohol, NF.
Phenyl Chlor-Tan Pediatric. (Hi-Tech) Phenylephrine tannate 5 mg, chlorpheniramine tannate 4.5 mg per 5 mL. Methylparaben, saccharin, sucrose. Susp. 473 mL. *Rx.*
Use: Decongestant and antihistamine, upper respiratory combination.
phenylcinchoninic acid. Name used for cinchophen.
•**phenylephrine bitartrate.** *USP 34.*
W/Aspirin, Chlorpheniramine Maleate.
See: Alka-Seltzer Plus Cold.
Alka-Seltzer Plus Sparkling Original Cold Formula.
W/Aspirin, Dextromethorphan Hydrobromide.
See: Alka-Seltzer Plus Day & Night Cold.
W/Aspirin, Dextromethorphan Hydrobromide, Doxylamine Succinate.
See: Alka-Seltzer Plus Day & Night Cold.

Alka-Seltzer Plus Night Cold.
phenylephrine CM. (Boca Pharmacal) Phenylephrine hydrochloride 40 mg, chlorpheniramine maleate 8 mg, methscopolamine nitrate 2.5 mg. ER Tab. 30s, 100s. *Rx.*
Use: Decongestant, antihistamine, and anticholinergic, upper respiratory combination.
Phenylephrine Complex. (Breckenridge) Brompheniramine maleate 4 mg, dextromethorphan hydrochloride 15 mg, phenylephrine hydrochloride 7.5 mg per 5 mL. Saccharin, sodium benzoate, sorbitol, glycerin. Alcohol free, dye free, sugar free. Strawberry flavor. Liq. 473 mL. *Rx.*
Use: Upper respiratory combination, antitussive combination.
•**phenylephrine hydrochloride.** (fen-ill-EFF-rin) *USP 34.*
Use: Adrenergic; mydriatic; sympathomimetic; vasoconstrictor; nasal decongestant, arylalkylamine.
See: AH-Chew.
AK-Dilate.
Alconefrin.
Altafrin.
Anu-Med.
Formulation R.
4-Way Fast Acting.
4-Way Menthol.
Isopto Frin.
Little Colds for Infants and Children.
Little Noses Gentle Formula, Infants & Children.
Lusonal.
Mydfrin 2.5%.
Neofrin.
Neo-Synephrine.
Neo-Synephrine Extra Strength.
Neo-Synephrine Mild Strength.
Neo-Synephrine Regular Strength.
PediaCare Children's Decongestant.
Refresh Redness Relief.
Relief.
Rhinall.
Sudafed PE.
Sudafed PE Maximum Strength Nasal Decongestant.
Super-Anahist Nasal Spray.
Triaminic Thin Strips Cold.
Vicks Sinex.
Vicks Sinex UltraFine Mist for Sinus Relief.
Zincfrin.
W/Acetaminophen.
See: Alka-Seltzer Plus Sinus.
Comtrex Maximum Strength Day & Night Flu Therapy.

Comtrex Maximum Strength Day &
Night Severe Cold & Sinus.
Contac Cold + Flu Day.
Dilotab II.
Excedrin Sinus Headache.
Mapap Sinus Congestion and Pain
Maximum Strength.
Sine-Off Non-Drowsy Maximum
Strength.
Sinutab Sinus.
Sudafed PE Sinus Headache.
Vicks DayQuil Sinex.
W/Acetaminophen, Chlorpheniramine
Maleate.
See: Alka-Seltzer Plus Fast Crystal
Packs.
Comtrex Maximum Strength Day &
Night Flu Therapy.
Comtrex Maximum Strength Day &
Night Severe Cold & Sinus.
Contac Cold + Flu.
Contac Cold + Flu Night.
Dristan Cold Multi-Symptom Formula.
Dryphen Multi-Symptom Formula.
Medicidin-D.
Onset Forte Micro-Coated.
Pyrroxate Extra Strength.
Sine Off Sinus/Cold.
Tylenol Allergy Multi-Symptom.
Tylenol Allergy Multi-Symptom Conve-
nience Pack.
Tylenol Plus Children's Cold.
Tylenol Sinus Congestion & Pain
Nighttime.
W/Acetaminophen, Chlorpheniramine
Maleate, Dextromethorphan Hydrobro-
mide.
See: Alka-Seltzer Plus Cold & Cough.
Comtrex Maximum Strength Day &
Night Cold & Cough.
Comtrex Maximum Strength Night-
time Cold & Cough.
Robitussin Cough, Cold & Flu Night-
time.
Theraflu Nighttime Severe Cold.
Tylenol Cold Head Congestion Night-
time.
Tylenol Cold Multi-Symptom Night-
time.
Tylenol Plus Children's Flu.
Tylenol Plus Children's Multi-
Symptom Cold.
W/Acetaminophen, Dexbromphenir-
amine.
See: Sinadrin PE.
W/Acetaminophen, Dextromethorphan
Hydrobromide.
See: Alka-Seltzer Plus Day & Night
Cold.
Alka-Seltzer Plus Day Cold.
Alka-Seltzer Plus Day Non-Drowsy
Cold.

Comtrex Maximum Strength Day &
Night Cold & Cough.
Mapap Cold Formula Multi-Symptom.
Theraflu Daytime Severe Cold &
Cough.
Theraflu Warming Relief Daytime
Multi-Symptom Cold.
Tylenol Cold Head Congestion Day-
time.
Tylenol Cold Multi-Symptom Daytime.
Vicks DayQuil Multi-Symptom Cold/
W/Acetaminophen, Dextromethorphan
Hydrobromide, Diphenhydramine
Hydrochloride.
See: Respa C & C.
W/Acetaminophen, Dextromethorphan
Hydrobromide, Doxylamine Succinate.
See: Alka-Seltzer Plus Day & Night
Cold.
Alka-Seltzer Plus Night Cold Formula.
Tylenol Cold Multi-Symptom Night-
time.
W/Acetaminophen, Dextromethorphan
Hydrobromide, Guaifenesin.
See: Phenflu G.
Sine-Off Cough/Cold.
Sudafed PE Multi-Symptom Cold and
Cough.
W/Acetaminophen, Diphenhydramine
Hydrochloride.
See: Benadryl Allergy & Cold.
Benadryl Allergy & Sinus Headache.
Benadryl Severe Allergy & Sinus
Headache Maximum Strength.
Sudafed PE Multi-Symptom Severe
Cold.
Sudafed PE Nighttime Cold Maxi-
mum Strength.
Theraflu Nighttime Severe Cough &
Cold.
Theraflu Sugar-Free Nighttime Se-
vere Cough & Cold.
Theraflu Warming Relief Flu & Sore
Throat.
Tylenol Allergy Multi-Symptom Conve-
nience Pack.
Tylenol Allergy Multi-Symptom Night-
time.
W/Acetaminophen, Doxylamine Succi-
nate.
See: Vicks NyQuil Sinex.
W/Acetaminophen, Guaifenesin.
See: Coldonyl.
Duratuss A.
Sine-Off Multi Symptom Relief.
Tylenol Sinus Congestion & Pain Se-
vere Daytime.
W/Acetaminophen, Pheniramine Maleate.
See: Theraflu Cold & Sore Throat.
Theraflu Flu & Sore Throat.

Theraflu Nighttime Severe Cold.
W/Antipyrine, Benzocaine.
See: Ear-Gesic.
W/Benzalkonium Chloride.
See: Mydfrin Ophthalmic.
Rhinall.
W/Brompheniramine Maleate.
See: Alacol.
Alenaze-D.
Alenaze-D NR.
BröveX PB.
Cenhist.
Dimetapp Children's Cold & Allergy.
LoHist PEB.
Respahist-II.
Seradex-LA.
Tanabid SR.
VaZol-D.
Vazotab.
Zotex-PE.
W/Brompheniramine Maleate, Carbeta-
pentane Citrate.
See: V-Cof.
W/Brompheniramine Maleate, Codeine
Phosphate.
See: BröveX PB C.
BröveX PB CX.
M-End PE.
Poly-Tussin AC.
W/Brompheniramine Maleate, Dextro-
methorphan Hydrobromide.
See: Alahist DM.
BröveX PB DM.
BröveX PEB DM.
Balacall DM.
BPM PE DM.
BROM/PE/DM.
Children's Dimaphen DM.
LoHist-DM.
Phenylephrine Complex.
TGQ 7.5PEH/4BRM/15DM.
TL-Hist DM.
Tusdec-DM.
W/Brompheniramine Maleate, Dextro-
methorphan Hydrobromide, Guai-
fenesin.
See: AccuHist PDX.
Bromhist-PDX.
W/Brompheniramine Maleate, Dihydroco-
deine Bitartrate.
See: Poly-Tussin DHC.
W/Caffeine Citrate, Pheniramine Maleate,
Sodium Salicylate.
See: Scot-Tussin Original Multi-Action
Cold and Allergy.
W/Carbetapentane Citrate, Dexchlor-
pheniramine Maleate.
See: Corzall-PE.
W/Carbetapentane Citrate, Diphenhydra-
mine Tannate.
See: D-Tann CD.

W/Carbetapentane Citrate, Guaifenesin.
See: Albatussin.
Carbatab-12.
Carbatuss.
Extendryl GCP.
Gentex 30.
Levall.
Phencarb GG.
Zinx GCP.
W/Carbinoxamine Maleate.
See: Histamax D.
XiraHist Pediatric.
W/Carbinoxamine Maleate, Dextrometh-
orphan Hydrobromide.
See: XiraHist DM Pediatric.
W/Chlorcyclizine Hydrochloride, Codeine
Phosphate.
See: Nasotuss.
W/Chlorpheniramine Maleate.
See: AMBI 10PEH/4CPM.
Actifed Cold & Allergy.
Allerest PE.
Ceron.
C-Phen.
Dallergy.
Dallergy-Jr.
Ed A-Hist.
Extendryl PEM.
Nasohist.
NoHist.
NoHist LQ.
Phenabid.
Rescon-Jr.
Sonahist.
W/Chlorpheniramine Maleate, Codeine
Phosphate.
See: Endal CD.
W/Chlorpheniramine Maleate, Dextro-
methorphan Hydrobromide.
See: AMBI 10PEH/4CPM/20DM.
Bronkids.
Centergy DM.
Ceron-DM.
Corfen-DM.
CP DEC-DM.
C-Phen DM.
DM/PE/CPM.
Donatussin DM.
Ed-A-Hist DM.
Father John's Medicine Plus.
Maxichlor PEH DM.
Nasohist DM.
Neo DM.
NoHist DMX.
NoHist-PDX.
P Chlor DM.
PE-Hist DM.
Phenabid DM.
Relahist-DM.
Rondec-DM.
Rondex-DM.

Sonahist DM.
TGQ 15DM/5PEH/2CPM.
Trigofen DM.
Trital DM.
Z-Dex 12D.
ZoDen DM.
W/Chlorpheniramine Maleate, Dextro-
methorphan Hydrobromide, Guai-
fenesin.
  See: Chlordex GP.
  DM/CPM/PE/GG.
  Donatussin.
W/Chlorpheniramine Maleate, Dihydroco-
deine Bitartrate.
  See: DiHydro-PE.
  Duohist DH.
W/Chlorpheniramine Maleate, Guai-
fenesin.
  See: P Chlor GG.
W/Chlorpheniramine Maleate, Hydro-
codone Bitartrate.
  See: Histinex HC.
  Neo HC.
  Notuss-Forte.
  Relacon-HC.
  Vanex-HD.
W/Chlorpheniramine Maleate, Meth-
scopolamine Nitrate.
  See: AeroHist Plus.
  AeroKid.
  Ah-Chew Ultra.
  CPM 8/PE 20/MSC 1.25.
  Dallergy.
  Dallergy PE.
  Dehistine.
  Denaze.
  DriHist SR.
  Drysec.
  Duradryl.
  Extendryl.
  NoHist-Plus.
  OMNIhist II LA.
  PCM.
  PE-CPM-MSN 8-2-0.75.
  PE HCL-CPM-MSN 10-2-0.75.
  Phenylephrine CM.
  QV Allergy.
  Ralix.
  Rescon.
  Rescon-MX.
  SymPak.
  SymPak PDX.
  Zinx PCM.
W/Chlorpheniramine Maleate, Phenyl-
toloxamine Citrate.
  See: Nalex-A.
  NoHist-A.
  Rhinacon A.
W/Chlorpheniramine Maleate, Pyrilamine
Maleate.
  See: MyHist-PD.

Polyhist PD.
Pyrichlor PE.
Triplex AD.
W/Codeine Phosphate.
  See: Alahist AC.
  Notuss-PE.
W/Codeine Phosphate, Dexchlorphenir-
amine Maleate.
  See: Dexphen W/C.
W/Codeine Phosphate, Diphenhydramine
Hydrochloride.
  See: Airacof.
W/Codeine Phosphate, Guaifenesin.
  See: Giltuss Ped-C.
W/Codeine Phosphate, Promethazine
Hydrochloride.
  See: Promethazine VC w/Codeine.
W/Codeine Phosphate, Pyrilamine
Maleate.
  See: Pro-Red AC.
  Zotex-C.
W/Dexbrompheniramine Maleate, Dextro-
methorphan Hydrobromide.
  See: Panatuss DXP.
W/Dexchlorpheniramine Maleate.
  See: NalDex.
W/Dexchlorpheniramine Maleate, Meth-
scopolamine Nitrate.
  See: Extendryl.
  Dexphen M.
W/Dextromethorphan Hydrobromide.
  See: Dimetapp Toddler's Decongestant
    Plus Cough.
  Little Colds Decongestant Plus
    Cough.
  PediaCare Children's Multi-Symptom
    Cold.
  Safetussin CD.
  Theraflu Thin Strips Daytime Cough
    & Cold.
  Triaminic Children's Thin Strips Day
    Time Cold & Cough.
  Triaminic Daytime Cold & Cough.
  Vicks Formula 44D Cough & Head
    Congestion Relief.
W/Dextromethorphan Hydrobromide,
Guaifenesin.
  See: AMBI 10PEH/400GFN/20DM.
  Biobron SF.
  Biogil.
  BioGtuss.
  Bio T Pres.
  Bio T Pres Pediatric.
  Biotuss.
  Bio-Tussi.
  Broncotron-D.
  Brontuss DX.
  Dacex PE.
  Deconex DM.
  Deconex DMX.
  Despec NR.

Dynatuss EX.
Endacon.
ExeCof.
ExeTuss-DM.
GFN 1200/DM 20/PE 40.
Giltuss.
Giltuss Pediatric.
Giltuss TR.
Guaifen.
Maxiphen DM.
NeoTuss-D.
Phlemex Forte.
Phlemex-PE.
Robitussin Children's Cough &
  Cold CF.
SINUtuss DM.
TriTuss.
TriTuss ER.
Tussi-Pres.
Tussi-Pres Pediatric.
Tusso DM.
Tusso DMR.
Tusso XR.
Z-Dex.
Z-Dex Pediatric.
Zotex.
Zotex-D.
Zotex Pediatric.
W/Dextromethorphan Hydrobromide,
  Pheniramine Maleate.
  See: Theraflu Cold & Cough.
W/Dextromethorphan Hydrobromide,
  Pyrilamine Maleate.
  See: Albutussin.
  Aldex DM Tannate.
  Codal-DM.
  Codimal DM.
  MyHist-DM.
  Poly Hist DM.
  Pyril DM.
  Reme Hist DM.
  Theraflu Cold & Cough.
  Triplex DM.
W/Dihydrocodeine Bitartrate.
  See: Alahist DHC.
W/Dihydrocodeine Bitartrate, Guai-
  fenesin.
  See: Donatuss DC.
  Poly-Tussin EX.
W/Dihydrocodeine Bitartrate, Pyrilamine
  Maleate.
  See: Poly Hist DHC.
W/Diphenhydramine Hydrochloride.
  See: Alahist LQ.
  Aldex-CT.
  Benadryl-D Allergy & Sinus.
  PediaCare Children's NightRest Multi-
    Symptom Cold.
  Pediatex-CT.
  Robitussin Pediatric Cough & Cold
    Nighttime.

Sudafed PE Nighttime Nasal Decon-
  gestant.
Theraflu Thin Strips Nighttime Cold &
  Cough.
Triaminic Children's Thin Strips Night
  Time Cold & Cough.
Triaminic Night Time Cold & Cough.
W/Diphenhydramine Hydrochloride.
  See: Sudafed PE Day & Night.
W/Guaifenesin.
  See: AMBI 10PEH/400GFN.
  Crantex.
  Deconex.
  Deconsal II.
  Despec.
  Donatussin.
  D-Phen 1000.
  D-Tab.
  Duratuss.
  Duratuss GP.
  Dynex LA.
  ED Bron GP.
  Entex LA.
  Entex LQ.
  ExeTuss.
  ExeTuss GP.
  Extendryl G.
  Gentex LA.
  GFN 600/Phenylephrine 20.
  Gilphex TR.
  Guaifed.
  Guaifed-PD.
  Guaifen PE.
  Guaphenyl LA.
  J-Max.
  Liquibid-D.
  Liquibid-PD.
  Liquibid PD-R.
  Medent-PE.
  Mucinex Cold for Kids.
  MucusRelief Sinus.
  MyDex.
  Nasex.
  Nasex-G.
  Nariz.
  Norel EX.
  PE/GG.
  PhenaVent D.
  PhenaVent LA.
  Reluri.
  Rescon 66.
  Robitussin PE Head and Chest Con-
    gestion.
  Sil-Tex.
  Simuc-GP.
  Sinutab Non-Drying.
  SINUtab PE.
  Sitrex.
  Sitrex PD.
  Sudafed PE Non-Drying Sinus.
  SymPak.

Triaminic Chest & Nasal Congestion.
Tussbid.
Tussbid PD.
Visonex.
Zinx GP.
Zotex GPX.
W/Hydrocodone Bitartrate, Pyrilamine
Maleate.
  See: Tussplex.
W/Methscopolamine Nitrate.
  See: Extendryl PEM.
W/Pyrilamine Maleate.
  See: Deconsal CT.
phenylephrine hydrochloride. (Various
Mfr.) Phenylephrine hydrochloride.
Ophth. Soln.: 2.5%, 10%. 2.5 mL, 5 mL
(10% only), 15 mL (2.5% only). **Soln.:**
1%. Bot. 480 mL. *Rx-OTC.*
  Use: Nasal decongestant, arylalkyl-
amine.
phenylephrine hydrochloride. (Various
Mfr.) Phenylephrine hydrochloride.
Ophth. Soln. 2.5%: Bot. 15 mL. **10%:**
Bot. 2 mL, 5 mL. **Inj.:** 1% (10 mg/mL).
Vials. 1 mL, 5 mL. *Rx.*
  Use: Adrenergic, mydriatic, sympathomimetic, vasoconstrictor.
**phenylephrine hydrochloride/brom-
pheniramine maleate.** (Brighton) ER
Cap. Phenylephrine hydrochloride/
brompheniramine maleate. **7.5 mg/
6 mg:** Parabens, sucrose. 100s.
15 mg/12 mg: Sugar. 100s. *Rx.*
  Use: Upper respiratory combination, decongestant and antihistamine.
**phenylephrine hydrochloride/guai-
fenesin.** (Brighton) Phenylephrine
hydrochloride/guaifenesin 15 mg/
600 mg, 25 mg/1200 mg. Dye free
(25 mg/1200 mg only). ER Tab. 100s.
Rx.
  Use: Decongestant and expectorant
combination, upper respiratory combination.
**phenylephrine hydrochloride/guai-
fenesin.** (Prasco) Phenylephrine
hydrochloride 30 mg, guaifenesin
1200 mg. Dye free. ER Tab. 100s. *Rx.*
  Use: Decongestant and expectorant
combination, upper respiratory combination.
**phenylephrine hydrochloride/guai-
fenesin.** (River's Edge) Phenylephrine
hydrochloride 40 mg, guaifenesin
600 mg. ER Tab. 100s. *Rx.*
  Use: Upper respiratory combination, decongestant and expectorant combination.
phenylephrine tannate.
W/Brompheniramine Tannate.
  See: BröveX ADT.

GTan Plus Oral Suspension.
J-Tan D.
Relhist.
W/Brompheniramine Tannate, Carbeta-
pentane Tannate.
  See: Vazotan Tannate.
W/Brompheniramine Tannate, Dextro-
methorphan Tannate.
  See: Dur-Tan DM.
  Neo DM.
W/Carbetapentane Tannate.
  See: Levall 12.
  Zinx D-Tuss.
W/Carbetapentane Tannate, Chlorphenir-
amine Tannate.
  See: D-Tann CT.
  Dytan CS.
  XiraTuss.
W/Carbetapentane Tannate, Chlorphenir-
amine Tannate, Ephedrine Tannate.
  See: Quad-Tuss Tannate Pediatric.
  Rynatuss.
  Rynatuss Pediatric.
W/Carbetapentane Tannate, Diphen-
hydramine Tannate.
  See: D-Tann CT.
  Dytan-CS.
W/Carbetapentane Tannate, Pyrilamine
Tannate.
  See: C-Tanna 12D.
  Tannate-12D S.
  Tannihist-12 D.
  Tussi-12D.
  Tussi-12D S.
W/Chlorpheniramine Tannate.
  See: AlleRx.
  BP Allergy Junior.
  Ed Chlor-Ped D.
  Ny-Tannic.
  PediaPhyl D.
  PE Tann/CP Tann.
  Phenyl Chlor-Tan Pediatric.
  R-Tanna.
  Rynatan.
  Rynatan Pediatric.
  Ry-Tann.
  TanalHist-D Pediatric.
  Tannate Pediatric.
W/Chlorpheniramine Tannate, Meth-
scopolamine Nitrate.
  See: AH-Chew.
  AH-Chew Ultra.
  Redur-PCM.
W/Chlorpheniramine Tannate, Pyrilamine
Tannate.
  See: Conal.
  Triotann Pediatric.
  Triple Tannate Pediatric.
W/Pyrilamine Tannate.
  See: Rynesa 12S.

phenylephrine tannate, chlorpheniramine tannate and pyrilamine tannate. (Ivax) Phenylephrine tannate 25 mg, chlorpheniramine tannate 8 mg, pyrilamine tannate 25 mg. Tab. Bot. 100s, 500s. Rx.
Use: Antihistamine; decongestant.

phenylephrine tannate/chlorpheniramine tannate/pyrilamine tannate pediatric. (Duramed) Phenylephrine tannate 5 mg, pyrilamine tannate 12.5 mg, chlorpheniramine tannate 2 mg/5 mL. Methylparaben, saccharin, sucrose, strawberry-blackberry-currant flavor. Susp. Unit of use 118 mL, Bot. 473 mL. Rx.
Use: Upper respiratory combination, decongestant, antihistamine.

•phenylethyl alcohol. (fen-ill-ETH-ill) USP 34.
Use: Pharmaceutic aid, antimicrobial.

phenyl-ethyl-hydrazine, beta. Phenelzine dihydrogen sulfate.
See: Nardil.

phenylethylmalonylurea.
See: Phenobarbital.

Phenyl-Free 1. (Mead Johnson Nutritionals) Corn syr. solids 49.2%, casein hydrolysate 18.7% (enzymic digest of casein containing amino acids and small peptides), corn oil 18%, modified tapioca starch 9.57%, protein equivalent 15%, fat 18%, carbohydrate 60%, minerals (ash) 3.6%, phenylalanine 75 mg/100 g pow., vitamins A 1600 units, D 400 units, E 10 units, C 52 mg, folic acid 100 mcg, B_1 0.5 mg, B_2 0.6 mg, niacin 8 mg, B_6 0.4 mg, B_{12} 2 mcg, biotin 0.05 mg, pantothenic acid 3 mg, vitamin K-1 100 mcg, choline 85 mg, inositol 30 mg, Ca 600 mg, P 450 mg, I 45 mcg, Fe 12 mg, Mg 70 mg, Cu 0.6 mg, Zn 4 mg, Mn 1 mg, C 450 mg, K 650 mg, Na 300 mg/qt. at normal dilution of 20 k cal/fl oz, Can 2 1/2 lb. OTC.
Use: Nutritional supplement.

Phenylgesic. (Ivax) Phenyltoloxamine citrate 30 mg, acetaminophen 325 mg. Tab. Bot. 100s, 1000s. OTC.
Use: Upper respiratory combination, analgesic, antihistamine.

Phenylhistine DH. (Qualitest) Chlorpheniramine maleate 2 mg, codeine phosphate 10 mg, pseudoephedrine hydrochloride 30 mg. Alcohol 5%, saccharin, sorbitol, sucrose. Liq. 118 mL, 473 mL. c-v.
Use: Upper respiratory combination, antitussive combination.

phenylic acid.
See: Phenol.

phenylketonuria agents.
See: Dihydrochloride.
Sapropterin.

•phenylmercuric acetate. (fen-ill-mer-CURE-ik ASS-eh-tate) NF 29.
Use: Pharmaceutic aid, antimicrobial; preservative, bacteriostatic.
W/Benzocaine, chlorothymol, resorcin.
See: Lanacane.

phenylmercuric acetate. (Various Mfr.) Phenylmercuric acetate. Bot. 1 lb, 5 lb, 10 lb.
Use: Pharmaceutic aid, antimicrobial; preservative, bacteriostatic.

phenylmercuric borate. (F. W. Berk) Pkg. Custom packed.
W/Benzyl alcohol, benzocaine, butyl p-aminobenzoate.
See: Dermathyn.

phenylmercuric chloride. Chlorophenylmercury.

•phenylmercuric nitrate. (fen-ill-mer-CURE-ik) NF 29.
Use: Pharmaceutic aid, antimicrobial; preservative, bacteriostatic.
W/Amyl, phenylphenol complex.
See: Lubraseptic Jelly.

phenylmercuric nitrate. (A.P.L.) Phenylmercuric nitrate. Oint. 1:1500: 1 oz, 4 oz, lb. (Chicago Pharm) Loz. w/benzocaine. Bot. 100s, 1000s. Ophth. Oint., 1:3000: Tube ⅛ oz. Soln. 1:20,000: Bot. pt, gal. Vaginal supp., 1:5000: Box 12s.
Use: Pharmaceutic aid, antimicrobial; preservative, bacteriostatic.

phenylmercuric picrate.
Use: Antimicrobial.

phenylphenol-o.
W/Amyl complex, phenylmercuric nitrate.
See: Lubraseptic.

phenylpropylmethylamine hydrochloride. Vonedrine hydrochloride.

phenyl salicylate.
See: Salol.
W/Atropine Sulfate, Benzoic Acid, Hyoscyamine Sulfate, Methenamine, Methylene Blue.
See: Uritact DS.
W/Hyoscyamine Sulfate, Methenamine, Methylene Blue, Sodium Biphosphate.
See: Urimax.
W/Hyoscyamine Sulfate, Methenamine, Methylene Blue, Sodium Phosphate Monobasic.
See: Uticap.
Utrona-C.

phenyl-tert-butylamine.
See: Phentermine.

phenylthilone.
Use: Anticonvulsant.

•**phenyltoloxamine citrate.** USP 34.
Use: Antihistamine.
W/Acetaminophen.
See: Aceta-Gesic.
BP Poly-650.
Flextra-DS.
Lagesic.
Pain-gesic.
Phenylgesic.
Relagesic.
Staflex.
Zflex.
W/Acetaminophen, Aspirin, Caffeine, Salicylamide.
See: Levacet.
W/Acetaminophen, Caffeine, Magnesium Salicylate.
See: Durabac Forte.
W/Acetaminophen, Caffeine, Salicylamide.
See: Durabac.
W/Acetaminophen, Salicylamide.
See: Duraxin.
Ed-Flex.
W/Amylase, Cellulase, Hyoscyamine Sulfate, Lipase, Protease.
See: Digex.
W/Chlorpheniramine Maleate, Phenylephrine Hydrochloride.
See: Nalex-A.
NoHist-A.
Rhinacon A.
W/Hyoscyamine Sulfate.
See: Digex NF.

phenyltoloxamine PE CPM. (Boca Pharmacal) Phenylephrine hydrochloride 5 mg, chlorpheniramine maleate 2.5 mg, phenyltoloxamine citrate 7.5 mg. Alcohol and sugar free. Cotton candy flavor. Liq. 473 mL. Rx.
Use: Upper respiratory combination, decongestant and antihistamine.

phenyltoloxamine resin w/combinations.
See: Tussionex.

Phenylzin. (Ciba Vision) Zinc sulfate 0.25%, phenylephrine hydrochloride 0.12%. Bot. 15 mL. Rx.
Use: Decongestant, ophthalmic.

•**phenyramidol hydrochloride.** (FEN-ih-RAM-ih-dole) USAN.
Use: Analgesic; muscle relaxant.

Phenytek. (Mylan) Phenytoin extended 200 mg, 300 mg. Cap. 30s, 100s. Rx.
Use: Anticonvulsant, hydantoin.

•**phenytoin.** (FEN-ih-toe-in) USP 34. Formerly Diphenylhydantoin.
Use: Anticonvulsant.
See: Dilantin.

Dilantin-125.
Phenytek.
phenytoin. (Various Mfr.) Phenytoin 125 mg per 5 mL. May contain alcohol, sucrose, sodium benzoate, glycerin. Susp. 240 mL. Rx.
Use: Anticonvulsant, hydantoin.

•**phenytoin sodium.** (FEN-ih-toe-in) USP 34. Formerly Diphenylhydantoin Sodium.
Use: Anticonvulsant; cardiac depressant, antiarrhythmic.
See: Dilantin.
W/Phenobarbital.
See: Dilantin with Phenobarbital Kapseals.

phenytoin sodium. (Caraco) Phenytoin sodium 200 mg, 300 mg. ER Cap. 30s, 100s, 500s. Rx.
Use: Anticonvulsant, hydantoin.

phenytoin sodium. (Wockhardt USA) Phenytoin sodium 30 mg. ER Cap. 100s, 1,000s. Rx.
Use: Anticonvulsant, hydantoin.

phenytoin sodium. (Various Mfr.) Phenytoin sodium. **ER Cap.:** 30 mg, 100 mg. May contain lactose, mannitol, sugar (100 mg). 100s, 1,000s (30 mg); 30s, 100s, 500s, 1,000s, UD 100s (100 mg). **Inj., Soln.:** 50 mg/mL. May contain alcohol, propylene glycol. 2 mL, 5 mL. Rx.
Use: Anticonvulsant, hydantoin.

pheochromocytoma, agents for.
See: Metyrosine.
Phenoxybenzamine Hydrochloride.
Phentolamine Mesylate.

Pherazine DM. (Halsey Drug) Promethazine 6.25 mg, dextromethorphan HBr 15 mg, alcohol 7%/5 mL. Bot. 4 oz, 6 oz, pt, gal. Rx.
Use: Antihistamine; antitussive.

Pherazine VC. (Halsey Drug) Phenylephrine hydrochloride 5 mg, promethazine hydrochloride 6.25 mg, alcohol 7%/5 mL. Syr. Bot. Pt, gal. Rx.
Use: Antihistamine; decongestant.

Pherazine VC with Codeine. (Halsey Drug) Phenylephrine hydrochloride 5 mg, promethazine hydrochloride 6.25 mg, codeine phosphate 10 mg, alcohol 7%/5 mL. Syr. Bot. Pt, gal. c-v.
Use: Antihistamine; antitussive; decongestant.

Pherazine w/Codeine. (Halsey Drug) Promethazine hydrochloride 6.25 mg, codeine phosphate 10 mg/5 mL, alcohol 7%, sorbitol, sucrose. Syr. Bot. 120 mL, pt, gal. c-v.
Use: Antihistamine; antitussive.

phethenylate. Also sodium salt.

Phicon. (T.E. Williams Pharmaceuticals) Pramoxine hydrochloride 0.5%, vitamin A 7500 units, E 2000 units/30 g. Cream. Tube 60 g. *OTC.*
Use: Emollient.

Phicon F. (T.E. Williams Pharmaceuticals) Undecylenic acid 8%, pramoxine hydrochloride 0.05%. Cream. 60 g. *OTC.*
Use: Anesthetic, local; antifungal.

Phillips'. (Bayer Consumer Care) Magnesium (as magnesium oxide) 500 mg. Polyvinyl alcohol. Tab. 24s. *OTC.*
Use: Laxative.

Phillips' Chewable. (Bayer Consumer Care) Magnesium hydroxide 311 mg. Tab. 100s, 200s.
Use: Laxative, antacid.

Phillips' LaxCaps. (Bayer Consumer Care) Docusate sodium 83 mg, phenolphthalein 90 mg. Cap. Bot. 8s, 24s, 48s. *OTC.*
Use: Laxative.

Phillips' Liqui-Gels. (Bayer Consumer Care) Docusate sodium 100 mg, parabens, sorbitol. Softgel Cap. Bot. 10s, 30s, 50s. *OTC.*
Use: Laxative.

Phillips' Milk of Magnesia. (Bayer Consumer Care) Magnesium hydroxide 400 mg/5 mL, saccharin (mint), sorbitol, sugar (cherry), mint, cherry, regular flavors. Susp. Bot. 120 mL, 360 mL, 780 mL. *OTC.*
Use: Laxative; antacid.

Phillips' Milk of Magnesia Concentrated. (Bayer Consumer Care) Magnesium hydroxide 800 mg/5 mL, sorbitol, sugar, strawberry creme flavor. Susp. Bot. 240 mL. *OTC.*
Use: Laxative; antacid.

Phish Omega. (Pharmics) Natural salmon oil concentrate containing EPA 120 mg, DHA 100 mg. Cap. Bot. 60s. *OTC.*
Use: Vitamin supplement.

Phish Omega Plus. (Pharmics) Natural fish oil concentrate containing EPA 300 mg, DHA 200 mg. Cap. Bot. 60s. *OTC.*
Use: Vitamin supplement.

pHisoDerm. (Chattem) Sodium octoxynol-2 ethane sulfonate, white petrolatum, water, mineral oil (with lanolin alcohol and oleyl alcohol), sodium benzoate, octoxynol-3, tetrasodium EDTA, methylcellulose, cocamide MEA, imidazolidinyl urea. **Regular:** 150 mL, 270 mL, 480 mL, gal. **Oily skin:** 150 mL, 480. *OTC.*
Use: Dermatologic, cleanser.

pHisoDerm for Baby. (Chattem) Sodium octoxynol-2 ethane sulfonate, petrolatum, octoxynol-3, mineral oil (with lanolin alcohol and oleyl alcohol), cocamide MEA, imidazolidinyl urea, sodium benzoate, tetrasodium EDTA, methylcellulose, hydrochloric acid. Liq. Bot. 150 mL, 270 mL. *OTC.*
Use: Dermatologic, cleanser.

pHisoHex. (Sanofi-Synthelabo) Entsufon sodium, hexachlorophene 3%, petrolatum, lanolin cholesterols, methylcellulose, polyethylene glycol, polyethylene glycol monostearate, lauryl myristyl diethanolamine, sodium benzoate, water, pH adjusted with hydrochloric acid. Emulsion, Bot. 5 oz, pt, gal. Wall dispensers pt. Unit packets 0.25 oz. Box 50s, Pedal operated dispenser 30 oz. *OTC.*
Use: Antimicrobial, antiseptic.

pHisoMed. (Sanofi-Synthelabo) Hexachlorophene. *OTC.*
Use: Antimicrobial; antiseptic.

pHisoPuff. (Sanofi-Synthelabo) Nonmedicated cleansing sponge. Box sponge 1s. *OTC.*
Use: Dermatologic, cleanser.

P-Hist. (Midlothian Laboratories) Dextromethorphan HBr 5 mg, pyrilamine maleate 5 mg, dexchlorpheniramine maleate 1.25 mg, phenylephrine hydrochloride 5 mg per 5 mL. Saccharin, sorbitol. Grape flavor. Syr. 473 mL. *Rx.*
Use: Antitussive combination, upper respiratory combination.

P-Hist DM. (Midlothian Laboratories) Dextromethorphan HBr 5 mg, brompheniramine maleate 1 mg, pseudoephedrine hydrochloride 12 mg per 1 mL. Alcohol and dye free. Magnasweet, menthol, sucrose. Grape flavor. Concentrate Soln. 30 mL with dropper. *Rx.*
Use: Pediatric antitussive combination.

Phlemex Forte. (Cypress) Dextromethorphan HBr 30 mg, guaifenesin 1200 mg, phenylephrine hydrochloride 30 mg. Dye free. ER Tab. 100s. *Rx.*
Use: Upper respiratory combination, antitussive and expectorant combination.

Phlemex-PE. (Cypress) Phenylephrine hydrochloride 20 mg, dextromethorphan HBr 20 mg, guaifenesin 800 mg. ER Tab. 100s. *Rx.*
Use: Antitussive and expectorant combination, upper respiratory combination.

PhosChol. (American Lecithin) Phosphatidylcholine (highly purified lecithin).

Softgel: 565 mg, 900 mg. Bot. 100s, 300s. **Liq. Conc.:** 3000 mg/5 mL. Bot. 240 mL, 480 mL. *OTC.*
Use: Nutritional supplement.
phoscolic acid.
Use: Adjuvant.
Phos-Flur Oral Rinse Supplement.
(Colgate Oral Pharmaceuticals) Acidulated phosphate sodium fluoride 0.05%, fluoride 1 mL/5 mL. Bot. 250 mL, 500 mL, gal. *Rx.*
Use: Dental caries preventative.
PhosLo. (Fresenius) Calcium acetate.
Cap.: 667 mg (elemental calcium 169 mg). Polyethylene glycol 8000. 200s. **Gelcap:** 667 mg (elemental calcium 169 mg). Polyethylene glycol 8000. 200s. *Rx.*
Use: Mineral supplement.
PHOS-NaK. (Cypress) Potassium 280 mg, phosphorus 250 mg, sodium 160 mg/packet, fruit flavor. Pow. Packets. 1.5 g (100s). *OTC.*
Use: Phosphorus replacement.
phosphate.
See: Potassium Phosphate.
Sodium Phosphate.
phosphate binders.
Use: Phosphate reduction.
See: Lanthanum Carbonate.
Sevelamer Carbonate.
Sevelamer Hydrochloride.
Phospha 250 Neutral. (Rising Pharmaceuticals) Dibasic sodium phosphate 852 mg, monobasic potassium phosphate 155 mg, monobasic sodium phosphate 130 mg (contains potassium 1.1 mEq, sodium 13 mEq). Filmcoated. Tab. 100s. *Rx.*
Use: Urinary acidifier, acid phosphate.
phosphentaside. Adenosine-5-monophosphate. Adenylic acid.
phosphocysteamine.
Use: Cystinosis. [Orphan Drug]
phosphodiesterase type 5 inhibitors.
Use: Impotence agents.
See: Sildenafil Citrate.
Tadalafil.
Vardenafil Hydrochloride.
phosphonoformic acid.
See: Foscarnet sodium.
phosphorated carbohydrate solution.
See: Emetrol.
Nausea Relief.
Nausatrol.
Nausetrol.
•**phosphoric acid.** (fos-FORE-ik) *NF 29.*
Use: Pharmaceutic aid, solvent.
W/Dextrose, Fructose.
See: Emetrol.
Nausatrol.

Nausea Relief.
Nausetrol.
phosphoric acid, diluted.
Use: Pharmaceutic aid, solvent.
phosphorus.
Use: Phosphorus replacement.
See: K-Phos Neutral.
PHOS-NaK.
Uro-KP-Neutral.
W/Calcium Glycerophosphate.
See: Prelief.
Phospho-Soda. (C.B. Fleet) Sodium biphosphate 48 g, sodium phosphate 18 g/100 mL. Bot. 1.5 oz, 3 oz, 8 oz. Flavored, unflavored. *OTC.*
Use: Laxative.
Phosphotec. (Bristol-Myers Squibb) Technetium Tc-99m pyrophosphate kit. 10 vials/kit.
Use: Radiodiagnostic.
photochemotherapy.
See: Aminolevulinic acid hydrochloride.
Methoxasalen.
Methyl Aminolevulinate.
Psoralens.
Tar-containing preparations.
photochemotherapy, ophthalmic.
See: Verteporfin.
Visudyne.
Photofrin. (Pinnacle Biologics) Porfimer sodium 75 mg. Preservative free. Freeze-dried cake or Pow. for Inj. Vial. *Rx.*
Use: Antineoplastic.
Photoplex Sunscreen. (Allergan) Butyl methoxydibenzoylmethane 3%, padimate O 7%. Lot. 120 mL. *OTC.*
Use: Sunscreen.
Phrenilin Forte. (Valeant) Acetaminophen 650 mg, butalbital 50 mg, benzyl alcohol, parabens, EDTA. Cap. Bot. 100s, 500s. *Rx.*
Use: Analgesic; hypnotic; sedative.
Phrenilin w/Caffeine and Codeine.
(Valeant) Codeine phosphate 30 mg, acetaminophen 325 mg, caffeine 40 mg, butalbital 50 mg. Cap. 100s. *c-III.*
Use: Narcotic analgesic.
Phresh 3.5 Finnish Cleansing Liquid.
(3M) Water, cocamidopropyl betaine, lactic acid, polyoxyethylene distearate, polyoxyethylene monostearate, hydroxyethyl cellulose, sodium phosphate, methylparaben. Bot. 6 oz. *OTC.*
Use: Soapless cleansing agent.
pH-Stabil. (Healthpoint Medical) Skin protection cream. Bot. 8 oz. Cream. Tube 2 oz. *OTC.*
Use: Dermatologic.
Phthalamaquin. (Penick) Quinetolate.
Use: Antiasthmatic.

phthalazine, i-hydrazino-, monohydro-chloride. Hydralazine hydrochloride.
phthalazinones, peripherally selective.
Use: Antihistamine.
See: Azelastine Hydrochloride.
phylcardin.
See: Aminophylline.
phyllindon.
See: Aminophylline.
Phylorinol. (Schaffer) Phenol 0.6%, boric acid, strong iodine solution, sorbitol 70% solution, sodium copper chlorophyll. Liq. Bot. 240 mL. *OTC.*
Use: Mouth and throat preparation.
Phylorinol Mouthwash. (Schaffer) Phenol 0.6%, methyl salicylate, sorbitol. Bot. 240 mL. *OTC.*
Use: Mouth and throat preparation.
physical adjuncts.
See: Calcium Hydroxylapatite.
Hyaluronic Acid Derivatives.
Hyaluronidase.
Poly-l-lactic Acid.
physiological irrigating solution.
See: Physiolyte.
Physiosol.
TIS-U-SOL.
Physiolyte. (McGaw) Sodium Cl 530 mg, sodium acetate 370 mg, sodium gluconate 500 mg, potassium Cl 37 mg, magnesium Cl 30 mg/100 mL. Soln. Bot. 500 mL, 2 L, 4 L. *Rx.*
Use: Irrigant, ophthalmic.
Physiosol Irrigation. (Hospira) Bot. 250 mL, 500 mL, 1000 mL glass or Aqualite (semirigid) containers. *Rx.*
Use: Irrigant, ophthalmic.
•**physostigmine salicylate.** (FYE-soe-STIG-meen) *USP 34.*
Use: Anticholinergic.
See: Antilirium.
physostigmine salicylate. (Akorn) Physostigmine salicylate 1 mg/mL. Benzyl alcohol 2%, sodium metabisulfite 0.1%. Inj. Amp. 2 mL. *Rx.*
Use: Cholinergic, antidote.
•**physostigmine sulfate.** (FYE-soe-STIG-meen) *USP 34.*
Use: Cholinergic, ophthalmic.
•**phytate persodium.** (FIE-tate per-SO-dee-uhm) USAN.
Use: Pharmaceutic aid.
•**phytate sodium.** (FYE-tate) USAN. Sodium salt of inositol hexaphosphoric acid.
Use: Chelating agent, calcium.
phytic acid. Inositol hexophosphoric acid.
•**phytonadione.** (fye-toe-nuh-DIE-ohn) *USP 34.*

Use: Fat-soluble vitamin.
See: Vitamin K.
phytonadione. (Hospira) Vitamin K 2 mg/mL, 10 mg/mL. Dextrose, benzyl alcohol 9 mg. Inj. Emulsion. Ampuls. 0.5 mL (2 mg/mL only), 1 mL (10 mg/mL only). *Rx.*
Use: Fat-soluble vitamin.
•**piboserod hydrochloride.** (pi-BOE-ser-od) USAN.
Use: Irritable bowel syndrome.
•**picenadol hydrochloride.** (pih-SEN-AID-ole) USAN.
Use: Analgesic.
•**piclamilast.** (pih-KLAM-ill-ast) USAN.
Use: Antiasthmatic, type IV phosphodiesterase inhibitor.
•**picoplatin.** (PI-koe-PLA-tin) USAN.
Use: Antineoplastic.
•**picotrin diolamine.** (PIH-koe-trin die-OH-lah-meen) USAN.
Use: Keratolytic.
picrotoxin. Cocculin.
Use: Respiratory.
•**picumeterol fumarate.** (PIKE-you-MEH-teh-role) USAN.
Use: Bronchodilator.
•**pifarnine.** (pih-FAR-neen) USAN.
Use: Antiulcerative, gastric.
pigment agent combinations.
See: Solage.
Tri-Luma.
pigment agents.
See: Dihydroxyacetone.
Hydroquinone.
Monobenzone.
•**pilocarpine.** (PYE-loe-KAR-peen) *USP 34.*
Use: Antiglaucoma; ophthalmic cholinergic; miotic.
•**pilocarpine hydrochloride.** (PYE-loe-KAR-peen) *USP 34.*
Use: Cholinergic, ophthalmic; topically as a miotic, xerostomia and keratoconjunctivitis sicca; mouth and throat product. [Orphan Drug]
See: Isopto Carpine.
Piloptic.
Salagen.
pilocarpine hydrochloride. (Actavis Elizabeth) Pilocarpine hydrochloride 5 mg, 7.5 mg. Film-coated. Tab. 100s. *Rx.*
Use: Mouth and throat products.
pilocarpine hydrochloride. (Sandoz) Pilocarpine hydrochloride 5 mg. Tab. 100s. *Rx.*
Use: Treatment of dry mouth.
pilocarpine hydrochloride. (Various Mfr.) Pilocarpine hydrochloride. **0.5%:**

15 mL, 30 mL. **1%:** 2 mL, 15 mL, 30 mL, UD 1 mL. **2%, 4%:** 2 mL, 15 mL, 30 mL. **6%:** 15 mL.
Use: Cholinergic, ophthalmic; topically as a miotic, xerostomia and keratoconjunctivitis sicca. [Orphan Drug]

• **pilocarpine nitrate.** (PYE-loe-KARpeen) *USP 34.*
Use: Cholinergic, ophthalmic.

Pilopine HS. (Alcon) Pilocarpine hydrochloride 4%. Gel. Tube 3.5 g. *Rx.*
Use: Antiglaucoma.

Piloptic. (Optopics) Pilocarpine hydrochloride 0.5%, 1%, 2%, 3%, 4%, 6%. Soln. Bot. 15 mL. *Rx.*
Use: Antiglaucoma.

Pilostat. (Bausch & Lomb) Pilocarpine hydrochloride 0.5%, 1%, 2%, 3%, 4%, 6%. Soln. Bot. 15 mL, twinpack 2 × 15 mL. *Rx.*
Use: Antiglaucoma.

Pima. (Fleming & Co.) Potassium iodide 325 mg/5 mL. Sugar. Black-raspberry flavor. Syrup. Pt., gal. *Rx.*
Use: Thyroid drug.

• **pimagedine hydrochloride.** (pih-MAHjeh-deen) USAN.
Use: Inhibitor (advanced glycosylation end-product formation inhibitors).

• **pimecrolimus.** (PIM-e-KROE-li-mus) USAN.
Use: Immunomodulator, topical.
See: Elidel.

• **pimetine hydrochloride.** (PIM-eh-teen) USAN.
Use: Antihyperlipoproteinemic.

piminodine esylate.
Use: Analgesic.

piminodine ethanesulfonate.
Use: Analgesic; narcotic.

• **pimobendan.** (pie-MOE-ben-dan) USAN.
Use: Cardiovascular agent.

• **pimozide.** (pih-moe-ZIDE) *USP 34.*
Use: Antipsychotic.
See: Orap.

• **pinacidil.** (pie-NASS-ih-DILL) USAN.
Use: Antihypertensive.

• **pinadoline.** (pih-nah-DOE-leen) USAN.
Use: Analgesic.

• **pindolol.** (PIN-doe-lahl) *USP 34.*
Use: Antiadrenergic/sympatholytic, beta-adrenergic blocking agent, vasodilator.
See: Visken.

pindolol. (Various Mfr.) Pindolol 5 mg, 10 mg. Tab. Bot. 100s, 500s, 1000s. *Rx.*
Use: Antiadrenergic/sympatholytic, beta-adrenergic blocker.

pine needle oil.
Use: Perfume; flavor.

pine tar.
Use: Local antieczematic; rubefacient.

pine tar oil.
See: Grandpa's Wonder Pine Tar Conditioner.

Pinex Concentrate Cough. (Last) Dextromethorphan HBr 7.5 mg/5 mL (after diluting 3 oz. concentrate to make 16 oz. solution). Syr. Bot. 3 oz. *OTC.*
Use: Antitussive.

Pinex Cough. (Last) Dextromethorphan HBr 7.5 mg/5 mL. Syr. Bot. 3 oz, 6 oz. *OTC.*
Use: Antitussive.

Pinex Regular. (Last) Potassium guaiacolsulfonate, oil of pine and eucalyptus, extract of grindelia, alcohol 3%/30 mL. Syr. Bot. 3 oz, 8 oz. Also cherry flavored 3 oz. Super and concentrated 3 oz. *OTC.*
Use: Expectorant.

Pink Bismuth. (Ivax) Pink bismuth 130 mg/15 mL. Liq. Bot. 240 mL. *OTC.*
Use: Antidiarrheal.

• **pinoxepin hydrochloride.** (pih-NOX-eh-PIN) USAN.
Use: Antipsychotic.

Pin-Rid. (Apothecary Prods.) Pyrantel pamoate 180 mg (equivalent to 62.5 mg pyrantel base). Cap., soft gel. 24s. *OTC.*
Use: Anthelmintic.

Pin-X. (Effcon) **Chew. Tab.:** Pyrantel pamoate 720.5 mg (equiv. to pyrantel base 250 mg). Dextrose, maltodextrin, sorbitol. Orange flavor. 12s. **Susp.:** Pyrantel pamoate 50 mg/mL. Parabens, sorbitol. Caramel flavor. 30 mL. *OTC.*
Use: Anthelmintic.

• **pioglitazone hydrochloride.** (PIE-oh-GLIH-tah-zone) USAN.
Use: Antidiabetic.
See: Actos.
W/Glimepiride.
See: Duetact.
W/Metformin Hydrochloride.
See: ActoPlus Met.
ActoPlus Met XR.

• **pipamperone.** (pih-PAM-peer-OHN) USAN. *Formerly Floropipamide.*
Use: Antipsychotic.

• **pipazethate.** (pip-AZZ-eh-thate) USAN.
Use: Cough suppressant; antitussive.

pipazethate hydrochloride.
Use: Antitussive.

• **piperacetazine.** (pih-PURR-ah-SET-ah-zeen) USAN.
Use: Antipsychotic.

•**piperacillin.** (PI-per-a-SIL-in) *USP 34.*
Use: Anti-infective.

•**piperacillin sodium.** (PI-per-a-SIL-in)
USP 34.
Use: Anti-infective.

piperacillin sodium. (American Pharmaceutical Partners) Piperacillin sodium (as base) 2 g, 3 g, 4 g, 40 g. Contains sodium 1.85 mEq (42.5 mg) per g. Pow. for Inj. Vials (except 40 g). Pharmacy bulk vials (40 g only). *Rx.*
Use: Extended-spectrum penicillin.

piperacillin sodium and tazobactam sodium.
Use: Anti-infective.
See: Zosyn.

piperacillin/tazobactam. (Various Mfr.)
Piperacillin/tazobactam (as piperacillin sodium/tazobactam sodium) 2 g/0.25 g, 3 g/0.375 g, 4 g/0.5 g. Sodium 108 mg (2 g/0.25 g), 162 mg (3 g/0.375 g), 216 mg (4 g/0.5 g). Preservative free. Inj., Pow. for Soln., concentrate. Single-dose vial. *Rx.*
Use: Penicillin, extended-spectrum penicillin.

•**piperamide maleate.** (PIH-per-ah-mid) USAN.
Use: Anthelmintic.

•**piperazine.** (pi-PER-a-zeen) *USP 34.*
Use: Anthelmintic.

•**piperazine citrate.** (pi-PER-a-zeen)
USP 34. Piperazine Citrate Telra Hydrous Tripiperazine Dicitrate.
Use: Anthelmintic.
See: Bryrel.
Ta-Verm.

•**piperazine edetate calcium.** (pi-PER-a-zeen) USAN.
Use: Anthelmintic.

piperazine estrone sulfate.
See: Estropipate.

piperazine hexahydrate. Tivazine.

piperazine phosphate.
Use: Anthelmintic.

piperazines, peripherally selective.
Use: Antihistamine.
See: Cetirizine Hydrochloride.
Dihydrochloride.
Levocetirizine Dihydrochloride.

piperazines, nonselective.
Use: Antihistamine.
See: Hydroxyzine.

piperidine phosphate.
Use: Psychiatric drug.

piperidines, nonselective.
Use: Antihistamine.
See: Cyproheptadine.
Phenindamine Tartrate.

piperidines, peripherally selective.
Use: Antihistamine.
See: Desloratidine.
Fexofenadine Hydrochloride.
Loratadine.

piperidolate hydrochloride.
Use: Anticholinergic.

piperoxan hydrochloride. Fourneau 933. Benzodioxane. Diagnosis of hypertension.
Use: Diagnostic aid.

pipethanate hydrochloride.
Use: Anxiolytic.

•**piposulfan.** (PIP-oh-SULL-fan) USAN.
Use: Antineoplastic.

•**pipotiazine palmitate.** (PIP-oh-TIE-ah-zeen PAL-mih-tate) USAN.
Use: Antipsychotic.

•**pipoxolan hydrochloride.** (pih-POX-oh-lan) USAN.
Use: Muscle relaxant.

•**piprozolin.** (PIP-row-ZOE-lin) USAN.
Use: Choleretic.

•**piquindone hydrochloride.** (PIH-kwin-dohn) USAN.
Use: Antipsychotic.

•**piquizil hydrochloride.** (PIH-kwih-zill) USAN.
Use: Bronchodilator.

•**piracetam.** (pir-A-se-tam) USAN.
Use: Cognition adjuvant; cerebral stimulant, myoclonus. [Orphan Drug]

•**pirandamine hydrochloride.** (pih-RAN-dah-meen) USAN.
Use: Antidepressant.

•**pirazmonam sodium.** (pihr-AZZ-moe-nam) USAN.
Use: Antimicrobial.

•**pirazolac.** (PIHR-AZE-oh-lack) USAN.
Use: Antirheumatic.

•**pirbenicillin sodium.** (pihr-ben-IH-SILL-in) USAN.
Use: Anti-infective.

•**pirbuterol acetate.** (pihr-BUE-ter-ol) USAN.
Use: Bronchodilator, sympathomimetic.
See: Maxair Autohaler.

•**pirbuterol hydrochloride.** (pihr-BUE-ter-ol) USAN.
Use: Bronchodilator.

•**pirenperone.** (PIHR-en-PURR-ohn) USAN.
Use: Anxiolytic.

•**pirenzepine hydrochloride.** (PIHR-en-zeh-PEEN) USAN.
Use: Antiulcerative.

•**piretanide.** (pihr-ETT-ah-nide) USAN.
Use: Diuretic.

•**pirfenidone.** (PEER-FEN-ih-dohn)
USAN.
Use: Analgesic; anti-inflammatory; antipyretic.
Piridazol.
See: Sulfapyridine.
•**piridicillin sodium.** (pihr-RIH-dih-SILL-
in) USAN.
Use: Anti-infective.
•**piridronate sodium.** (pihr-IH-DROE-
nate) USAN.
Use: Regulator, calcium.
•**piriprost.** (PIR-i-prost) USAN.
Use: Antiasthmatic.
•**piriprost potassium.** (PIR-i-prost)
USAN.
Use: Antiasthmatic.
piriton.
See: Chlorpheniramine.
•**piritrexim isethionate.** (pih-rih-TREX-im
eye-seh-THIGH-oh-nate) USAN.
Use: Antiproliferative. [Orphan Drug]
•**pirlimycin hydrochloride.** (PIHR-lih-MY-
sin) USAN.
Use: Anti-infective.
•**pirmagrel.** (PIHR-mah-GRELL) USAN.
Use: Inhibitor, thromboxane synthetase.
•**pirmenol hydrochloride.** (PIHR-MEH-
nahl) USAN.
Use: Cardiovascular agent, antiarrhythmic.
•**pirnabine.** (PIHR-NAH-bean) USAN.
Use: Antiglaucoma agent.
•**piroctone.** (pir-OK-tone) USAN.
Use: Antiseborrheic.
•**piroctone olamine.** (pir-OK-tone OLE-a-
meen) USAN.
Use: Antiseborrheic.
•**pirodavir.** (pih-ROW-dav-ihr) USAN.
Use: Antiviral.
•**pirogliride tartrate.** (PIHR-oh-GLIE-ride)
USAN.
Use: Antidiabetic.
•**pirolate.** (PIHR-oh-late) USAN.
Use: Antiasthmatic.
•**pirolazamide.** (PIHR-ole-aze-ah-mide)
USAN.
Use: Cardiovascular agent, antiarrhythmic.
•**piroxantrone hydrochloride.** (PIH-row-
ZAN-trone) USAN.
Use: Antineoplastic.
•**piroxicam.** (phr-OX-i-kam) *USP 34.*
Use: Anti-inflammatory.
See: Feldene.
piroxicam. (Various Mfr.) Piroxicam
10 mg, 20 mg. Cap. Bot. 100s; 500s,
1000s, UD 100s (10 mg only). *Rx.*

Use: Nonsteroidal anti-inflammatory
agent.
•**piroxicam betadex.** (phr-OX-i-kam BAY-
ta-dex) USAN.
Use: Analgesic; anti-inflammatory; antirheumatic.
•**piroxicam cinnamate.** (phr-OX-i-kam
SIN-a-mate) USAN.
Use: Anti-inflammatory.
•**piroxicam olamine.** (phr-OX-i-kam OLE-
a-meen) USAN.
Use: Anti-inflammatory; analgesic.
•**piroximone.** (PIHR-ox-ih-MONE) USAN.
Use: Cardiovascular agent.
•**pirprofen.** (pihr-PRO-fen) USAN.
Use: Anti-inflammatory.
•**pirquinozol.** (PIHR-KWIN-oh-zole)
USAN.
Use: Antiallergic.
•**pirsidomine.** (pihr-SIH-doe-meen)
USAN.
Use: Vasodilator.
pitavastatin.
Use: HMG-CoA Reductase Inhibitor.
See: Livalo.
Pitayine.
See: Quinidine.
Pitocin. (JHP Pharmaceuticals) Oxytocin.
Inj. 1 mL amps (chlorobutanol 0.5%),
1 mL *Steri-Dose* disposable syringes,
1 mL *Steri-Vials.* 10 units/mL. *Rx.*
Use: Oxytocic.
Pitressin Synthetic. (JHP Pharm) Vaso-
pressin 20 pressor units/mL. Chlorobu-
tanol 0.5%. Inj., Soln. 1 mL vial. *Rx.*
Use: Posterior pituitary hormone, vaso-
pressin.
Pitts Carminative. (Del) Bot. 2 oz.
Use: Antiflatulent.
pituitary, anterior. The anterior lobe of
the pituitary gland supplies protein hor-
mones classified under following head-
ings.
See: Corticotropin.
Gonadotropin.
Growth hormone.
Thyrotropic Principle.
Pituitary Function Test.
See: Metopirone.
pituitary, posterior, hormones.
See: Desmopressin Acetate.
Vasopressin.
Oxytocin.
Pitocin.
Pitressin.
•**pituitary, posterior, injection.** *USP 34.*
Use: Hormone, antidiuretic.
•**pivampicillin hydrochloride.** (piv-AM-pi-
SIL-in) USAN.
Use: Anti-infective.

- **pivampicillin pamoate.** (piv-AM-pi-SIL-in PAM-oh-ate) USAN.
  Use: Anti-infective.
- **pivampicillin probenate.** (piv-AM-pi-SIL-in PROE-be-nate) USAN.
  Use: Anti-infective.
- **pivopril.** (PIH-voe-PRILL) USAN.
  Use: Antihypertensive.
- **pixantrone.** (PIX-an-trone) USAN.
  Use: Antineoplastic.
- **pixantrone dimaleate.** (PIX-an-trone) USAN.
  Use: Treatment of non-Hodgkin lymphoma.

pix carbonis.
  See: Coal tar.

Pix Juniperi.
  Use: Sunscreen; moisturizer.
  See: Juniper tar.

- **pizotyline.** (pih-ZOE-tih-leen) USAN.
  Use: Anabolic; antidepressant; serotonin inhibitor, migraine.

placebo capsules. (Cowley) No. 3 orange red; No. 4 yellow. Bot. 1000s.
  Use: Placebo.

placebo tablets. (Cowley) 1 g white; 2 g white; 3 g white, red or yellow, pink, orange; 4 g white; 5 g white. Bot. 1000s.
  Use: Placebo.

Plan B. (Teva) Levonorgestrel 0.75 mg. Lactose. Tab. Blister pack 2s. *OTC.*
  Use: Sex hormone, contraceptive hormone.

Plan B One-Step. (Duramed) Levonorgestrel 1.5 mg. Lactose. Tab. 1s. *OTC.*
  Use: Emergency contraceptive.

Planocaine.
  See: Procaine hydrochloride.

planochrome.
  See: Merbromin.

plantago, ovata coating.
  See: Konsyl.
  Metamucil.

- **plantago seed.** (PLAN-tah-go seed) *USP 34.*
  Use: Laxative.

Plasbumin-5. (Talecris) Normal serum albumin (human) 5% USP fractionated from normal serum plasma, heat treated against hepatitis virus. Albumin 12.5 g/250 mL. Inj. Vial 50 mL. Bot. with IV set 250 mL, 500 mL. *Rx.*
  Use: Plasma protein fraction.

Plasbumin-25. (Talecris) Normal serum albumin (human) 25% USP fractionated from normal serum plasma, heat treated against hepatitis virus. Albumin 12.5 g/50 mL. Inj. Vial 20 mL. Bot. with IV set 50 mL, 100 mL. *Rx.*
  Use: Plasma protein fraction.

plasma expanders or substitutes.
  See: Dextran 6% and LMD 10%.
  Macrodex.

Plasma-Lyte A ph 7.4. (Baxter PPI) Na 140 mEq, K 5 mEq, Mg 3 mEq, Cl 98 mEq, acetate 27 mEq, gluconate 23 mEq, osmolarity 294 mOsm/L, pH 7.4. Soln. Plastic Bot. 500 mL, 1000 mL. *Rx.*
  Use: Intravenous nutritional therapy, intravenous replenishment solution.

Plasma-Lyte 56 and 5% Dextrose. (Baxter PPI) Na 40 mEq, K 13 mEq, Mg 3 mEq, Cl 40 mEq, acetate 16 mEq, dextrose 50 g, calories 170, osmolarity 363 mOsm/L. Soln. Plastic Bot. 500 mL, 1000 mL. *Rx.*
  Use: Intravenous nutritional therapy, intravenous replenishment solution.

Plasma-Lyte 56 in Water. (Baxter PPI) Na 40 mEq, K 13 mEq, Mg 3 mEq, Cl 40 mEq/L, acetate 16 mEq/L. Plastic Bot. 500 mL, 1000 mL. *Rx.*
  Use: Nutritional supplement, parenteral.

Plasma-Lyte M and 5% Dextrose. (Baxter PPI) Na 40 mEq, K 16 mEq, Ca 5 mEq, Mg 3 mEq, Cl 40 mEq, acetate 12 mEq, lactate 12 mEq, dextrose 50 g, calories 180, osmolarity 377 mOsm/L. Soln. Plastic Bot. 500 mL, 1000 mL. *Rx.*
  Use: Intravenous nutritional therapy, intravenous replenishment solution.

Plasma-Lyte 148. (Baxter PPI) Na 140 mEq, K 5 mEq, Mg 3 mEq, Cl 98 mEq, acetate 27 mEq, gluconate 23 mEq, osmolarity 294 mOsm/L, ph ≈ 5.5. Soln. Bot. 500 mL, 1000 mL. *Rx.*
  Use: Intravenous nutritional therapy, intravenous replenishment solution.

Plasma-Lyte 148 and 5% Dextrose. (Baxter PPI) Dextrose 50 g, calories 190, Na 140 mEq, K 5 mEq, Mg 3 mEq, Cl 98 mEq, acetate 27 mEq, osmolarity 547 mOsm, gluconate 23 mEq/L. Soln. Bot. 500 mL, 1000 mL. *Rx.*
  Use: Intravenous nutritional therapy, intravenous replenishment solution.

Plasma-Lyte R. (Baxter PPI) Na 140 mEq, K 10 mEq, Ca 5 mEq, Mg 3 mEq, Cl 103 mEq, acetate 47 mEq, lactate 8 mEq, osmolarity 312 mOsm/L, ph ≈ 5.5. Soln. Bot. 1000 mL. *Rx.*
  Use: Intravenous nutritional therapy, intravenous replenishment solution.

Plasma-Lyte R and 5% Dextrose. (Baxter PPI) Dextrose 50 g, calories 180, Na^+ 140 mEq, K^+ 10 mEq, Ca^{++} 5 mEq, Mg^{++} 3 mEq, Cl^- 103 mEq, lactate 8 mEq, acetate 47 mEq, osmolarity 564 mOsm/L, sodium bisulfite. Soln.

Bot. 1000 mL. *Rx.*
Use: Intravenous nutritional therapy, intravenous replenishment solution.

Plasma-Lyte R Injection. (Baxter PPI) Na 140 mEq, K 10 mEq, Ca 5 mEq, Mg 3 mEq, Cl 103 mEq, acetate 47 mEq, lactate 8 mEq/L. Bot. 1000 mL. *Rx.*
Use: Nutritional supplement, parenteral.

Plasmanate. (Talecris) Plasma protein fraction (human) 5%. USP Vial 50 mL. Bot. 250 mL, 500 mL with set. *Rx.*
Use: Plasma protein fraction.

Plasma-Plex. (Centeon) Plasma protein fraction 5%. Inj. Vial 250 mL, 500 mL. *Rx.*
Use: Plasma protein fraction.

•**plasma protein fraction.** *USP 34.* Formerly *Plasma Protein Fraction, Human.*
Use: Blood-volume supporter.
See: Plasmanate.
  Plasma-Plex.
  Plasmatein.
  Protenate.

plasma protein fraction. (Baxter PPI) For the plasma protein preparation obtained from human plasma using the Cohn fractionation technique. Bot. 250 mL.
Use: Blood volume supporter.

Plasmatein. (Alpha Therapeutic) Plasma protein fraction 5%. Inj. Vial w/injection set 250 mL, 500 mL. *Rx.*
Use: Plasma protein fraction.

plasmochin naphthoate. Pamaquine naphthoate.
Use: Antimalarial.

•**platelet concentrate.** *USP 34.*
Use: Platelet replenisher.

Platelet Factor 4. (Abbott Diagnostics) Radioimmunoassay for quantitative measurement of total PF4 levels in plasma. Test kit 100s.
Use: Diagnostic aid.

platinum coordination complex.
Use: Antineoplastic.
See: Carboplatin.
  Oxaliplatin.

Plavix. (Bristol-Myers Squibb) Clopidogrel 75 mg (equiv. to clopidogrel bisulfate 97.875 mg), 300 mg (equiv to clopidogrel bisulfate 391.5 mg). Castor oil, lactose, mannitol. Film-coated. Tab. Bot. 30s, 90s, 500s (75 mg only), UD 4s (300 mg only), UD 30s (300 mg only), UD 100s. *Rx.*
Use: Antiplatelet, aggregation inhibitor.

Plax. (McNeil-PPC) Sorbitol solution, alcohol 8.7%, tetrasodium pyrophosphate, benzoic acid, poloxamer 407, sodium benzoate, sodium lauryl sulfate,

sodium saccharin, xanthan gum. Original, mint, sensation, and softmint flavors. Mouthwash. 118 mL, 237 mL, 473 mL, 710 mL. *OTC.*
Use: Anti-infective.

•**plecanatide.** (ple-KAN-a-tide) USAN.
Use: Gastrointestinal agent.

•**pleconaril.** (pleh-KOE-nah-rill) USAN.
Use: Antiviral.

PledgaClin. (JSJ Pharmaceuticals) Clindamycin phosphate 1%. Isopropyl alcohol 50%, propylene glycol. Pledget. 69s. *Rx.*
Use: Topical anti-infective, antibiotic agent.

Plegisol. (Hospira) Calcium Cl dihydrate 17.6 mg, magnesium Cl hexahydrate 325.3 mg, potassium Cl 119.3 mg, sodium Cl 643 mg/100 mL. Approximately 260 mOsm/L. Single-dose container 1000 mL without sodium bicarbonate. *Rx.*
Use: Cardiovascular agent.

•**plerixafor.** (pler-IX-a-fore) USAN.
Use: Stem cell mobilizer.
See: Mozobil.

Pletal. (Otsuka America Pharmaceutical) Cilostazol 50 mg. Tab. Bot. 60s. *Rx.*
Use: Antiplatelet.

Plewin. (Sanofi-Synthelabo) Glycobiarsol, chloroquine phosphate. Tab. *Rx.*
Use: Amebicide.

Plexion. (Medicis) Sulfur 5%, sodium sulfacetamide 10%, cetyl alcohol, stearyl alcohol, EDTA, parabens. Cleanser. Bot. 170 g, 340 g. *Rx.*
Use: Keratolytic.

Plexion Cleansing Cloths. (Medicis) Sulfur 5%, sodium sulfacetamide 10%. Glycerine, glyceryl stearate, propylene glycol, propylene glycol oleate, alcohols, EDTA, parabens. Cloths. 30s. *Rx.*
Use: Keratolytic agent.

Plexion SCT. (Medicis) Sulfur 5%, sodium sulfacetamide 10%, witch hazel, benzyl alcohol. Cream. Tube 120 g. *Rx.*
Use: Keratolytic.

Plexion TS. (Medicis) Sulfur 5%, sodium sulfacetamide 10%. Mineral oil, glyceryl stearate, propylene glycol, propylene glycol oleate, alcohols, EDTA, sodium thiosulfate, coco-glycerides. Susp. Topical. 30 g. *Rx.*
Use: Keratolytic agent.

Plexolan. (Last) Zinc oxide, lanolin. Cream. Tube 1.25 oz, 3 oz. Jar 16 oz. *OTC.*
Use: Dermatologic.

Plexon. (Sigma-Tau) Testosterone 10 mg, estrone 1 mg, liver 2 mcg, pyri-

doxine hydrochloride 10 mg, panthenol 10 mg, inositol 20 mg, choline Cl 20 mg, vitamin B_2 2 mg, B_{12} 100 mcg, procaine hydrochloride 1%, niacinamide 100 mg/mL. Vial 10 mL.
Use: Hormone; mineral, vitamin supplement.

Pliagel. (Alcon) NaCl, KCl, poloxamer 407, sorbic acid 0.25%, EDTA 0.5%. Soln. Bot. 25 mL. *OTC.*
Use: Contact lens care.

Pliaglis. (ZARS) Lidocaine 7%, tetracaine 7%. Parabens, petrolatum, polyvinyl alcohol. Cream 30 g. *Rx.*
Use: Topical local anesthetic.

•**plinabulin.** (PLIN-a-BUE-lin) USAN.
Use: Antineoplastic.

•**plomestane.** (PLOE-mess-TANE) USAN.
Use: Antineoplastic, aromatase inhibitor.

Plova. (Washington Ethical) Psyllium mucilloid. Pow. (flavored) 12 oz., (plain) 10 0.5 oz. *OTC.*
Use: Laxative.

•**plovamer.** (PLOE-va-mer) USAN.
Use: Treatment of multiple sclerosis.

•**plovamer acetate.** (PLOE-va-mer) USAN.
Use: Treatment of multiple sclerosis.

Pluravit. (Sanofi-Synthelabo) Multivitamin. Drops.
Use: Vitamin supplement.

PMB 400. (Wyeth) Conjugated estrogens 0.45 mg, meprobamate 400 mg, lactose, sucrose. Tab. Bot. 100s. *Rx.*
Use: Anxiolytic, estrogen.

PMB 200. (Wyeth) Conjugated estrogens 0.45 mg, meprobamate 200 mg, lactose, sucrose. Tab. Bot. 60s. *Rx.*
Use: Anxiolytic, estrogen.

P.M.P. Compound. (Mericon Industries) Chlorpheniramine maleate 4 mg, phenylephrine hydrochloride 15 mg, salicylamide 300 mg, scopolamine methylnitrate 0.8 mg. Tab. Bot. 100s, 1000s. *Rx.*
Use: Analgesic; antihistamine; decongestant.

P.M.P. Expectorant. (Mericon Industries) Codeine phosphate 10 mg, phenylephrine hydrochloride 10 mg, guaifenesin 40 mg, chlorpheniramine maleate 2 mg/5 mL. Bot. Gal. *c-v.*
Use: Antihistamine; antitussive; decongestant; expectorant.

pneumococcal 7-valent conjugate vaccine.
Use: Immunization.
See: Prevnar.

pneumococcal vaccine, polyvalent.
Use: Agent for active immunization, bacterial vaccine.
See: Pneumovax 23.

Pneumomist. (ECR) Guaifenesin 600 mg. SR Tab. Bot. 100s. *Rx.*
Use: Expectorant.

Pneumotussin. (ECR) Hydrocodone bitartrate 2.5 mg, guaifenesin 300 mg. Dye free. Tab. Bot. 100s. *c-III.*
Use: Upper respiratory combination, antitussive, expectorant.

Pneumotussin HC. (ECR) Hydrocodone bitartrate 5 mg, guaifenesin 100 mg/ 5 mL. Syr. Bot. 120 mL, 480 mL. *c-III.*
Use: Antitussive; expectorant.

Pneumovax 23. (Merck) 23 polysaccharide isolates 25 mcg each/0.5 mL dose. Phenol 0.25%. Inj. Vials. 1-dose, 5-dose. *Rx.*
Use: Agent for active immunization, bacterial vaccine.

PNS Unna Boot. (Pedinol Pharmacal) Nonsterile gauze bandage 10 yds × 3". Box 12s.
Use: Ambulatory procedure in treatment of leg ulcers and varicosities.

PNV-DHA Plus. (Acella) Vitamins E 30 units, B_6 25 mg, B_{12} 1 mcg, C 40 mg, folate 1.4 mg, Ca 75 mg, Fe 27 mg, DHA 250 mg. Glycerin, lecithin oil, vegetable oil. Gluten free, lactose free, sugar free. Cap., softgel. 30s. *Rx.*
Use: Prenatal vitamin with minerals.

PNV-Iron. (Acella) Vitamins B_1 3 mg, B_2 3.4 mg, B_3 20 mg, B_5 7 mg, B_6 2.6 mg, B_{12} 500 mcg, C 80 mg, D_3 400 units, E 30 units (as dl-alpha-tocopheryl acetate), biotin 30 mcg, L-methylfolate Ca 1 mg, Ca 200 mg, Cu, Fe 29 mg, folic acid 0.4 mg, Mg, Zn. Gluten free and lactose free. Tab. 90s. *Rx.*
Use: Prenatal vitamin with minerals.

•**pobilukast edamine.** (poe-BIH-loo-kast EH-dah-meen) USAN.
Use: Antiasthmatic, leukotriene antagonist.

pochlorin. Prophyrinic and chlorophyllic compound.
Use: Antihypercholesterolemic agent.

Pod-Ben-25. (C & M Pharmacal) Podophyllin 25% in benzoin tincture. Bot. 1 oz. *Rx.*
Use: Keratolytic.

Podoben. (American Pharmaceutical) Podophyllum resin extract 25%. Bot. 5 mL. *Rx.*
Use: Keratolytic.

Podocon-25. (Paddock) Podophyllum resin 25% in benzoin tincture. Soln.

15 mL. *Rx.*
Use: Keratolytic.

•**podofilox.** (pah-dah-FILL-ox) USAN.
Use: Antimitotic.
See: Condylox.

podofilox. (Various Mfr.) Podofilox 0.5%. Alcohol 95%. Top. Soln. 3.5 mL. *Rx.*
Use: Antimitotic.

podophyllin.
See: Podophyllum resin.

•**podophyllum.** (pode-oh-FIL-um) *USP 34.*
Use: Pharmaceutic necessity.

•**podophyllum resin.** (pode-oh-FIL-um REZ-in) *USP 34.*
Use: Caustic.
See: Podoben.

podophyllum resin. (Various Mfr.) Podophyllin. Pkg. 1 oz, 0.25 lb, 1 lb.
Use: Caustic.

Point-Two Mouthrinse. (Colgate Oral Pharmaceuticals) Sodium fluoride 0.2% in a flavored neutral liquid. Bot. 120 mL. *Rx.*
Use: Dental caries agent.

•**poison ivy extract, alum precipitated.** (poy-zuhn EYE-vee EX-tract, AL-uhm pree-SIP-ih-tay-tehd) USAN.
Use: Ivy poisoning counteractant.

•**polacrilin.** (POL-a-KRILL-in) USAN. Methacrylic acid with divinylbenzene. A synthetic ion-exchange resin, supplied in the hydrogen or free acid form. Amberlite IRP-64.
Use: Pharmaceutic aid.

•**polacrilin potassium.** (POL-a-KRILL-in) *NF 29.* A synthetic ion-exchange resin, prepared through the polymerization of methacrylic acid and divinylbenzene, further neutralized with potassium hydroxide to form the potassium salt of methacrylic acid and divinylbenzene. Supplied as a pharmaceutical-grade ion-exchange resin in a particle size of 100- to 500-mesh.
Use: Pharmaceutic aid, tablet disintegrant.
See: Amberlite IRP-88.

Poladex Tabs. (Major) Dexchlorpheniramine maleate. Tab. **4 mg:** Bot. 100s, 250s, 1000s. **6 mg:** Bot. 100s, 1000s. *Rx.*
Use: Antihistamine.

polamethene resin caprylate. The physiochemical complex of the acid-binding ion exchange resin, polyamine-methylene resin and caprylic acid.

Polaramine. (Schering-Plough) Dexchlorpheniramine maleate, lactose. **Tab.:** 2 mg, lactose. Bot. 100s. **Syr.:**

2 mg/5 mL alcohol 6%, sorbitol, menthol, parabens, sugar, orange-like flavor. Bot. 473 mL. *Rx.*
Use: Antihistamine, nonselective alkylamine.

Polaramine Expectorant. (Schering-Plough) Dexchlorpheniramine maleate 2 mg, pseudoephedrine sulfate 20 mg, guaifenesin 100 mg/5 mL, alcohol 7.2%, menthol, sorbitol, sugar. Liq. Bot. 473 mL. *Rx.*
Use: Upper respiratory combination, antihistamine, decongestant, expectorant.

Polaramine Repetabs. (Schering-Plough) Dexchlorpheniramine maleate 4 mg, 6 mg, parabens, lactose, sugar. TR Tab. Bot. 100s. *Rx.*
Use: Antihistamine, nonselective alkylamine.

Poldeman. (Sanofi-Synthelabo) Kaolin. Susp. *OTC.*
Use: Antidiarrheal.

Poldeman AD. (Sanofi-Synthelabo) Kaolin. Susp. *OTC.*
Use: Antidiarrheal.

Poldemicina. (Sanofi-Synthelabo) Kaolin. Susp. *OTC.*
Use: Antidiarrheal.

•**poldine methylsulfate.** (POLE-deen METH-ill-SULL-fate) *USP 34.*
Use: Anticholinergic.

•**policapram.** (PAH-lee-CAP-ram) USAN.
Use: Pharmaceutic aid, tablet binder.

Polident Dentu-Grip. (Block Drug) Carboxymethylcellulose gum, ethylene oxide polymer. Pkg. 0.675 oz, 1.75 oz, 3.55 oz. *OTC.*
Use: Denture adhesive.

•**polifeprosan 20.** (pahl-ee-FEH-pro-SAHN 20) USAN.
Use: Pharmaceutic aid, biodegradable polymer for controlled drug delivery.

•**poligeenan.** (PAHL-ih-JEE-nan) USAN. Polysaccharide produced by extensive hydrolysis of carragheen from red algae.
Use: Pharmaceutic aid, dispersing agent.

•**poliglecaprone 90.** (POL-ee-GLEK-a-prone 90) USAN.
Use: Surgical aid, surgical suture coating (absorbable).

•**poliglecaprone 25.** (POL-ee-GLEK-a-prone 25) USAN.
Use: Surgical aid, surgical suture material (absorbable).

•**poliglusam.** (pahl-ee-GLUE-sam) USAN.
Use: Antihemorrhagic, hemostatic; dermatologic, wound therapy.

•**polignate sodium.** (poe-LIG-nate) USAN.
Use: Enzyme inhibitor, pepsin.

Poli-Grip. (Block Drug) Karaya gum, magnesium oxide in petrolatum mineral oil base, peppermint and spearmint flavor. Tube 0.75 oz, 1.5 oz, 2.5 oz. *OTC.*
Use: Denture adhesive.

poliomyelitis vaccine, inactivated. (Aventis Pasteur) (Purified, Salk Type IPV) Poliovirus vaccine, inactivated. Amp. 5 × 1 mL. Vial 10 dose. *Rx.*
Use: Immunization.
See: IPOL.
Poliovirus Vaccine, Inactivated

•**poliovirus vaccine, inactivated.** (POE-lee-oh-VYE-russ) *USP 34.* Formerly *Poliomyelitis Vaccine.*
Use: Immunization.
See: IPOL.

poliovirus vaccine, inactivated. (Aventis Pasteur) Amp. 1 mL. Box 5s. Vial 10 dose. Subcutaneous administration.
Use: Agent for immunization, active.

poliovirus vaccine, inactivated, diphtheria and tetanus toxoids and acellular pertussis adsorbed, hepatitis B (recombinant), combined.
Use: Active immunization, toxoid.
See: Diphtheria and Tetanus Toxoids and Acellular Pertussis Adsorbed, Hepatitis B (Recombinant), Inactivated Poliovirus Vaccine Combined.

•**polipropene 25.** (pahl-ee-PRO-peen 25) USAN.
Use: Pharmaceutic aid, tablet excipient.

•**polixetonium chloride.** (pahl-ix-eh-TOE-nee-uhm) USAN.
Use: Pharmaceutic aid, preservative.

Polocaine. (APP Pharmaceutical) Mepivacaine hydrochloride. **1%, 2%:** Mannitol. Inj. Multidose vial 50 mL. **3%:** Sodium bisulfite. Inj. Dental cartridge 1.8 mL. *Rx.*
Use: Anesthetic, local amide.

Polocaine MPF. (APP Pharmaceutical) Mepivacaine hydrochloride. **1%, 1.5%:** Inj. Methylparaben. Single-dose vial 30 mL. **2%:** Inj. Single-dose vial 20 mL. *Rx.*
Use: Anesthetic, local amide.

Poloris Poultices. (Block Drug) Benzocaine 7.5 mg, capsicum 4.6 mg in poultice base. Pkg. 5 unit, 12 unit. *Rx.*
Use: Anesthetic, local.

•**poloxalene.** (PAHL-OX-ah-leen) *USP 34.* Liquid nonionic surfactant polymer of polyoxypropylene polyoxyethylene type.
Use: Pharmaceutic aid, surfactant.

poloxalkol. Polyoxyethylene polyoxypropylene polymer.

•**poloxamer.** (pahl-OX-ah-mer) *NF 29.*
Use: Pharmaceutic aid (ointment and suppository base, surfactant, tablet binder and coating agent, emulsifying agent).

poloxamer-iodine.
See: Prepodyne.

poloxamer 188.
Use: Cathartic; sickle cell crisis; severe burns. [Orphan Drug]

poloxamer 188 lf.
Use: Pharmaceutic aid, surfactant.

poloxamer 182 d.
Use: Pharmaceutic aid, surfactant.

poloxamer 182 lf.
Use: Food additive; pharmaceutic aid.

poloxamer 331.
Use: Food additive, surfactant; AIDS-related toxoplasmosis. [Orphan Drug]

polyamine resin.
See: Polyamine-Methylene Resin.

polyanhydroglucose. Polyanhydroglucuronic acid.

Polybase. (Paddock) Preblended polyethylene glycol suppository base for incorporation of medications where a water-soluble base is indicated. Jar 1 lb, 5 lb.
Use: Pharmaceutical aid, suppository base.

polybenzarsol. Benzocal.

Poly-Bon Drops. (Barrows) Vitamins A 3000 units, D 400 units, C 60 mg, B_1 1 mg, B_2 1.2 mg, niacinamide 8 mg/0.6 mL. Bot. 50 mL. *OTC.*
Use: Vitamin supplement.

•**polybutester.** (PAHL-ee-byoot-ESS-ter) USAN.
Use: Surgical aid, surgical suture material.

•**polybutilate.** (PAHL-ee-BYOO-tih-late) USAN.
Use: Surgical aid, surgical suture coating.

•**polycarbophil.** (POL-ee-KAR-boe-fil) *USP 34.*
Use: Laxative.
See: Bulk Forming Fiber Laxative.
Equalactin.
FiberCon.
Fiber-Lax.
FiberNorm.
Konsyl Fiber.

Polycillin. (Bristol-Myers Squibb) Ampicillin trihydrate. **Cap.: 250 mg:** Bot. 100s, 500s, 1000s, UD 100s. **Cap.: 500 mg:** Bot. 100s, 500s, UD 100s. **Pediatric Drops:** 100 mg/mL. Dropper

bot. 20 mL. **Susp.: 125 mg/5 mL:** Bot.
80 mL, 100 mL, 150 mL, 200 mL,
UD 5 mL. **Susp.: 250 mg/5 mL:** Bot.
80 mL, 100 mL, 150 mL, 200 mL,
UD 5 mL. **Susp.: 500 mg/5 mL:** Bot.
100 mL, UD 5 mL. *Rx.*
Use: Anti-infective, penicillin.

Polycitra K Crystals. (McNeil) Potassium
citrate monohydrate 3300 mg, citric acid
1002 mg, potassium ion 30 mEq, equivalent to 30 mEq bicarbonate. UD pkg.
Sugar free. Box 100s. *Rx.*
Use: Alkalinizer, systemic.

polycosanol.
W/Acetic Acid, Antipyrine, Benzocaine.
See: AABP.
Auralgan.

Polycose. (Ross) Glucose polymers derived from controlled hydrolysis of corn
starch. Calories 380, carbohydrate
94 g, water 6 g, Na 110 mg, K 10 mg,
Cl 223 mg, Ca 30 mg, P 5 mg/100 g.
Pow. Can 12.3 oz. Case 6s. *OTC.*
Use: Nutritional supplement.

•**polydextrose.** (PAH-lee-DEX-trose)
USAN.
Use: Food additive.

polydimethylsiloxane (silicone oil).
Use: Ophthalmic.
See: AdatoSil 5000.

Polydine. (Century) Povidone-iodine in
ointment base. Oint. Jar 1 oz, 4 oz, lb.
OTC.
Use: Anti-infective, topical.

Polydine. (Century) Povidone-iodine solution. Soln. Bot. 1 oz, 4 oz, 8 oz, pt,
gal. *OTC.*
Use: Antiseptic.

Polydine Scrub. (Century) Povidone-
iodine in scrub solution. Bot. 1 oz, 4 oz,
8 oz, pt, gal. *OTC.*
Use: Antiseptic.

•**polydioxanone.** (PAHL-ee-die-OX-ah-
nohn) USAN.
Use: Surgical aid, surgical suture material (absorbable).

Poly ENA Test System for RNP and SM.
(Wampole) Qualitative identification of
auto antibodies to extractable nuclear
antigens in human serum by gel precipitation technique. Aid in the diagnosis
of SLE, MCTD, PSS, SS. Box test 48s.
Use: Diagnostic aid.

**Poly ENA Test System for RNP, SM,
SSA, and SSB.** (Wampole) Qualita-
tive identification of auto antibodies to
extractable nuclear antigens in human
serum by gel precipitation techniques.
Aid in the diagnosis of SLE, MCTD,
PSS, SS. Box test 96s.
Use: Diagnostic aid.

**Poly ENA Test System for SSA and
SSB.** (Wampole) Qualitative identification of auto antibodies to extractable
nuclear antigens in human serum by
gel precipitation techniques. Aid in the
diagnosis of SLE, MCTD, PSS, SS.
Box test 48s.
Use: Diagnostic aid.

polyene antifungals.
See: Amphotericin B Desoxycholate.
Amphotericin B, Lipid-Based.
Nystatin.

•**polyethadene.** (PAHL-ee-ETH-ah-
DEEN) USAN.
Use: Antacid.

•**polyethylene excipient.** (POL-ee-ETH-i-
leen) *NF 29.*
Use: Pharmaceutic aid, stiffening agent.

•**polyethylene glycol.** (POL-ee-ETH-i-
leen GLYE-kol) *NF 29.*
Use: Pharmaceutic aid (ointment and
suppository base, tablet excipient,
solvent, tablet and capsule lubricant).
See: Dulcolax Balance.
GaviLAX.
GlycoLax.
MiraLax.
Zanfel.

polyethylene glycol. (Braintree) PEG
3350 255 g, 527 g. Pow. for Oral Soln.
16 oz (255 g only), 32 oz (527 g only).
Rx.
Use: Laxative.

polyethylene glycol and electrolytes.
Use: Rehydration; bowel evacuant.
See: Colyte.
GoLYTELY.
NuLYTELY.
OCL.

•**polyethylene glycol monomethyl ether.**
(POL-ee-ETH-i-leen GLYE-kol) *NF 29.*
Use: Pharmaceutic aid, excipient.

**polyethylene glycol 3350 and electro-
lytes.** (Mylan) PEG 3350 236 g, sodium sulfate 22.74 g, sodium bicarbonate 6.74 g, NaCl 5.86 g, KCl 2.97 g.
Pow. for Soln. Disposable jug. *Rx.*
Use: Laxative, bowel evacuant.

•**polyethylene granules.** (POL-ee-ETH-i-
leen)
Use: Poison ivy treatment.
See: Zanfel.
Zanfel Wash.

•**polyethylene oxide.** (POL-ee-ETH-i-leen
OX-ide) *NF 29.*
Use: Pharmaceutic aid, suspending and
viscosity agent, tablet binder.

•**polyferose.** (PAHL-ee-feh-rohs) USAN.
An iron carbohydrate chelate containing approximately 45% of iron in which

the metallic (Fe) ion is sequestered within a polymerized carbohydrate derived from sucrose.
Use: Hematinic.

Poly-F Fluoride. (Major) Fluoride 0.5 mg, vitamins A 1500 units, D 400 units, E 5 mg, B_1 0.5 mg, B_2 0.6 mg, B_3 8 mg, B_6 0.4 mg, B_{12} 2 mcg, C 35 mg/mL. Drops. Bot. 50 mL. *Rx.*
Use: Mineral, vitamin supplement.

•**polyglactin 910.** (POL-ee-GLAK-tin 910) USAN.
Use: Surgical aid, surgical suture coating (absorbable).

•**polyglactin 370.** (POL-ee-GLAK-tin 370) USAN. Lactic acid polyester with glycolic acid.
Use: Surgical aid, surgical suture coating (absorbable).

•**polyglycolic acid.** (PAHL-ee-glie-KAHL-ik) USAN.
Use: Surgical aid, surgical suture material.

•**polyglyconate.** (PAHL-ee-GLIE-koe-nate) USAN.
Use: Surgical aid, surgical suture material (absorbable).

Poly Hist DHC. (Poly Pharmaceuticals) Dihydrocodeine bitartrate 7.5 mg, phenylephrine hydrochloride 5 mg, pyrilamine maleate 7.5 mg. Glycerin, propylene glycol, saccharin, sorbitol. Alcohol free, dye free, gluten free, and sugar free. Fruit gum flavor. Liq. 473 mL. *c-III.*
Use: Upper respiratory combination, antitussive combination.

Poly-Hist DM. (Poly Pharmaceuticals) Dextromethorphan HBr 15 mg, pyrilamine maleate 12.5 mg, phenylephrine hydrochloride 7.5 mg per 5 mL. Sugar, alcohol, and dye free. Saccharin, sorbitol. Grape flavor. Liq. 20 mL, 473 mL. *Rx.*
Use: Antitussive combination, upper respiratory combination.

Poly Hist NC. (Poly Pharmaceuticals) Codeine phosphate 10 mg, pseudoephedrine hydrochloride 15 mg, triprolidine hydrochloride 1.25 mg. Glycerin, propylene glycol, saccharin, sorbitol. Alcohol free, dye free, and sugar free. Cotton candy flavor. Liq. 473 mL. *c-v.*
Use: Upper respiratory combination, antitussive combination.

Poly-Hist PD. (Poly Pharmaceuticals) Phenylephrine hydrochloride 7.5 mg, chlorpheniramine maleate 2 mg, pyrilamine maleate 12.5 mg per 5 mL. Sugar, alcohol, and dye free. Saccharin, sorbitol. Bubble gum flavor. Susp. 473 mL. *Rx.*
Use: Decongestant and antihistamine, upper respiratory combination.

poly I; poly C12U.
Use: AIDS; antineoplastic. [Orphan Drug]

Poly-Iron 150. (Cypress) Polysaccharide iron complex 150 mg. PEG, tartrazine. Cap. 100s. *OTC.*
Use: Trace element.

poly-l-lactic acid.
Use: Restoration/correction of facial fat loss in individuals with HIV.
See: Sculptra.

•**polymacon.** (PAHL-ee-MAY-kahn) USAN.
Use: Contact lens material, hydrophilic.

polymeric oxygen.
Use: Sickle cell disease. [Orphan Drug]

polymeric phosphate binders.
Use: Treatment of hyperphosphatemia.
See: Sevelamer hydrochloride.

•**polymetaphosphate P 32.** (pahl-ee-met-ah-FOSS-fate) USAN.
Use: Radiopharmaceutical.

Polymox. (Bristol-Myers Squibb) Amoxicillin trihydrate. **Cap.:** 250 mg. Bot. 100s, 500s, UD 100s; 500 mg. Bot. 50s, 100s, 500s, UD 100s. **Oral Susp.:** 125 mg, 250 mg/5 mL. Bot. 80 mL, 100 mL, 150 mL. **Ped. Drops:** 50 mg/mL. Bot. 15 mL. *Rx.*
Use: Anti-infective, penicillin.

polymyxin B. (Various Mfr.) Antimicrobial substances produced by *Bacillus polymyxa.*

•**polymyxin B sulfate.** (POL-ee-MIX-in) USP 34.
Use: Anti-infective.
W/Bacitracin Zinc.
See: Double Antibiotic.
  Polysporin.
W/Combinations.
See: AK-Poly-Bac Oint.
  Cortisporin.
  Maxitrol.
  Mycitracin.
  Neomycin and Polymyxin B Sulfates and Bacitracin Zinc Ophthalmic Ointment.
  Neosporin G.U. Irrigant.
  Neosporin Maximum Strength.
  Neosporin Ophthalmic Ointment.
  Neosporin Ophthalmic Solution.
  Neotal.
  Neo-Thrycex.
  Ocutricin.
  Poly-Pred Liquifilm Ophthalmic Suspension.

Polytrim Ophthalmic Solution.
Pyocidin-Otic.
Terak.
Terramycin w/Polymyxin B Sulfate.
Tigo.
Trimethoprim Sulfate and Polymyxin B Sulfate Ophthalmic.
Trimixin.
Triple Antibiotic.
W/Neomycin, Bacitracin Zinc.
See: Neosporin Original Triple Antibiotic.
W/Neomycin, Bacitracin Zinc, Lidocaine.
See: Lanabiotic.
W/Neomycin, Bacitracin Zinc, Pramoxine Hydrochloride.
See: Neosporin Plus Pain Relief.
Tri-Biozene.
W/Neomycin, Pramoxine Hydrochloride.
See: Neosporin Plus Pain Relief.
polymyxin B sulfate and bacitracin zinc.
Use: Anti-infective, topical.
See: Betadine First Aid Antibiotics Plus Moisturizer.
Double Antibiotic.
Polysporin.
polymyxin B sulfate and hydrocortisone.
Use: Anti-infective; anti-inflammatory, otic.
•**polymyxin B sulfate and trimethoprim ophthalmic solution.** (POL-ee-MIX-in) USP 34.
Use: Anti-infective, ophthalmic.
polymyxin-neomycin-bacitracin. (Various Mfr.) Oint. OTC.
Use: Anti-infective, topical.
polynoxylin. Anaflex.
polyoxyethylene 8 stearate.
See: Polyoxyl 8 Stearate.
polyoxyethylene 50 stearate.
See: Polyoxyl 50 stearate.
polyoxyethylene 40 monostearate.
See: Polyoxyl 40 stearate.
Myrj 52 & M2S.
polyoxyethylene lauryl ether.
W/Benzoyl Peroxide, Ethyl Alcohol.
See: Benzagel.
Desquam-X.
polyoxyethylene nonyl phenol.
W/Sodium Edetate, Docusate Sodium, 9-Aminoacridine Hydrochloride.
See: Vagisec Plus.
polyoxyethylene sorbitan monolaurate. Polysorbate 20.
W/Ferrous Gluconate, Vitamins.
See: Simron Plus.
polyoxyethylene 20 sorbitan monoleate.
See: Polysorbate 80.

polyoxyethylene 20 sorbitan trioleate.
Tween 85. (Zeneca Pharmaceuticals), Polysorbate 85.
polyoxyethylene 20 sorbitan tristearate. Tween 65. (Zeneca Pharmaceuticals), Polysorbate 65.
•**polyoxyl 8 stearate.** (POL-ee-OX-il 8 STEER-ate) USAN.
Use: Pharmaceutic aid, surfactant.
See: Myrj 45.
polyoxyl 50 stearate. Formerly Polyoxyethylene 50 stearate.
Use: Pharmaceutic aid, surfactant, emulsifying agent.
•**polyoxyl 40 hydrogenated castor oil.** (POL-ee-OX-il 40 hye-DROJ-en-AYted KAS-tor) NF 29.
Use: Pharmaceutic aid, surfactant, emulsifying agent.
•**polyoxyl 40 stearate.** (POL-ee-OX-il 40 STEER-ate) NF 29. Macrogic Stearate 2000 (I.N.N.) Polyoxyethylene 40 monostearate.
Use: Pharmaceutic aid; hydrophilic oint., surfactant; surface-active agent.
See: Myrj 52 & M2S.
•**polyoxyl 10 oleyl ether.** (POL-ee-OX-il 10 oh-LAY-il EE-ther) NF 29.
Use: Pharmaceutic aid, surfactant.
•**polyoxyl 35 castor oil.** (POL-ee-OX-il 35 KAS-tor) NF 29.
Use: Pharmaceutic aid, surfactant, emulsifying agent.
•**polyoxyl 20 cetostearyl ether.** (POL-ee-OX-il 20 SEE-toe-STEER-il EE-ther) NF 29.
Use: Pharmaceutic aid, surfactant.
•**polyoxypropylene 15 stearyl ether.** (POL-ee-OX-ee-PROE-pi-leen 15 STEER-il EE-ther) USAN. Formerly PPG-15 Stearyl Ether.
Use: Pharmaceutic aid, solvent.
Poly-Pred Liquifilm. (Allergan) Prednisolone acetate 0.5%, neomycin sulfate equivalent to 0.35% neomycin base, polymyxin B sulfate 10,000 units/mL, polyvinyl alcohol 1.4%, thimerosal 0.001%, polysorbate 80, propylene glycol, sodium acetate. Ophth. Susp. Bot. 5 mL, 10 mL. Rx.
Use: Anti-infective; corticosteroid, ophthalmic.
polypropylene glycol. An addition polymer of propylene oxide and water.
Use: Pharmaceutic aid, suspending agent.
polysaccharide-iron complex.
Use: Mineral supplement.
See: EZFE 200.
Ferrex 150.

iFerex 150.
Myferon.
Niferex.
Nu-Iron 150.
Poly-Iron 150.
W/Ferrous Fumarate.
See: Tandem.
polysaccharide iron complex. (Various Mfr.) Iron (as polysaccharide iron complex) 150 mg. Cap. Bot. 100s. *OTC.*
Use: Mineral supplement.
polysonic lotion. (Parker) Multipurpose ultrasound lotion with high coupling efficiency. Bot. 8.5 oz, gal.
Use: Diagnostic aid, therapeutic aid.
•**polysorbate 80.** (POL-ee-SOR-bate 80) *NF 29.*
Use: Pharmaceutic aid, surfactant; artificial tears.
See: OptiZen.
W/Glycerin.
See: Refresh Dry Eye Therapy.
•**polysorbate 85.** (POL-ee-SOR-bate 85) USAN.
Use: Pharmaceutic aid, surfactant.
•**polysorbate 40.** (POL-ee-SOR-bate 40) *NF 29.*
Use: Pharmaceutic aid, surfactant.
•**polysorbate 60.** (POL-ee-SOR-bate 60) *NF 29.*
Use: Pharmaceutic aid, surfactant.
•**polysorbate 65.** (POL-ee-SOR-bate 65) USAN.
Use: Pharmaceutic aid, surfactant.
•**polysorbate 20.** (POL-ee-SOR-bate 20) *NF 29.*
Use: Pharmaceutic aid, surfactant.
Polysporin. (Pfizer) Polymyxin B sulfate 10,000 units, bacitracin zinc 500 units per g. White petrolatum base. Oint. Tubes. ≈ 15 g, ≈ 30 g. *OTC.*
Use: Anti-infective, antibiotic, topical.
polysulfides. Polythionate.
Polytabs-F Chewable Vitamin. (Major) Fluoride 1 mg, vitamins A 2500 units, D 400 units, E 15 mg, B_1 1.05 mg, B_2 1.2 mg, B_3 13.5 mg, B_6 1.05 mg, B_{12} 4.5 mcg, C 60 mg, folic acid 0.3 mg. Chew. Tab. Bot. 100s, 1000s. *Rx.*
Use: Mineral, vitamin supplement.
Poly Tan DM. (Poly) Dextromethorphan tannate 30 mg, dexbrompheniramine tannate 4 mg, pyrilamine maleate 3.5 mg, phenylephrine tannate 25 mg per 5 mL. Alcohol and sugar free. Aspartame, parabens, phenylalanine 7 mg per 5 mL. Candy apple flavor. Susp. 15 mL, 473 mL. *Rx.*
Use: Upper respiratory combination, antitussive combination.

Polytar Shampoo. (GlaxoSmithKline) Polytar 4.5% (coal tar soln., solubilized crude coal tar equiv. to 0.5% coal tar). Lanolin. 177 mL, 355 mL. *OTC.*
Use: Antiseborrheic.
Polytar Soap. (GlaxoSmithKline) Coal tar soln. 2.5% (equiv. to coal tar 0.5%). Glycerin, ethyl alcohol, peanut oil. 113 g. *OTC.*
Use: Dermatologic.
•**polytef.** (PAHL-ee-teff) USAN.
Use: Prosthetic aid.
Polytinic. (Pharmics) Elemental iron 100 mg, vitamin C 300 mg, folic acid 1 mg. tab. Bot. 100s. *Rx.*
Use: Mineral, vitamin supplement.
Polytrim. (Allergan) Polymyxin B sulfate 10,000 units, trimethoprim 1 mg/mL, benzalkonium chloride 0.04 mg/mL, sodium chloride, sodium hydroxide. Bot. 5 mL, 10 mL. *Rx.*
Use: Anti-infective, ophthalmic.
Polytuss-DM. (Rhode) Dextromethorphan HBr 15 mg, chlorpheniramine maleate 1 mg, guaifenesin 25 mg/5 mL. Bot. 4 oz, 8 oz. *OTC.*
Use: Antihistamine; antitussive; expectorant.
Poly-Tussin AC. (Poly Pharmaceuticals) Brompheniramine maleate 2 mg, codeine phosphate 10 mg, phenylephrine hydrochloride 7.5 mg per 5 mL. Saccharin, sorbitol. Alcohol free. Raspberry-bubblegum flavor. Liq. 473 mL. *c-v.*
Use: Upper respiratory combination, antitussive combination.
Poly-Tussin DHC. (PolyPharmaceuticals) Brompheniramine maleate 4 mg, dihydrocodeine bitartrate 3 mg, phenylephrine hydrochloride 7.5 mg per 5 mL. PEG, saccharin. Grape flavor. Liq. 473 mL. *c-v.*
Use: Upper respiratory combination, antitussive combination.
Poly-Tussin EX. (Poly Pharmaceuticals) Dihydrocodeine bitartrate 7.5 mg, guaifenesin 50 mg, phenylephrine hydrochloride 7.5 mg. Glycerin, propylene glycol, saccharin, sorbitol. Alcohol free, dye free, gluten free, and sugar free. Grape flavor. Liq. 473 mL. *c-III.*
Use: Upper respiratory combination, antitussive and expectorant combination.
•**polyurethane foam.** (PAHL-ih-you-ree-thane foam) USAN.
Use: Prosthetic aid, internal bone splint.
Poly-Vent DM. (Poly Pharmaceuticals) Dextromethorphan hydrobromide 15 mg, guaifenesin 400 mg, pseudoephedrine hydrochloride 45 mg. Tab.

60s. *OTC.*
Use: Upper respiratory combination, antitussive and expectorant combination.
Poly-Vent Plus. (Poly Pharmaceuticals) Acetaminophen 500 mg, guaifenesin 200 mg, pseudoephedrine hydrochloride 45 mg. Tab. 100s. *OTC.*
Use: Upper respiratory combination, decongestant and expectorant.
polyvidone. *Name previously used for Povidone.*
Poly-Vi-Flor 1 mg. (Bristol-Myers Squibb) Vitamins A 2500 units, D 400 units, E 15 units, C 60 mg, B_1 1.05 mg, B_2 1.2 mg, B_3 13.5 mg, B_6 1.05 mg, B_{12} 4.5 mcg, fluoride 1 mg, folic acid 0.3 mg, sucrose. Chew. Tab. Bot. 100s, 1000s. **With Iron:** Above formula plus Fe 12 mg, Cu 1 mg, Zn 10 mg. Tab. *Rx.*
Use: Mineral, vitamin supplement; dental caries agent.
Poly-Vi-Flor 0.5 mg. (Bristol-Myers Squibb) **Chew. Tab.:** Vitamins A 2500 units, D 400 units, E 15 units, C 60 mg, B_1 1.05 mg, B_2 1.2 mg, B_3 13.5 mg, B_6 1.05 mg, B_{12} 4.5 mcg, fluoride 0.5 mg, folic acid 0.3 mg. Bot. 100s. **Chew. Tab. With Iron:** Above formula plus Fe 12 mg, Cu, Zn 10 mg. Tab. Bot. 100s. **Drops:** Vitamins A 1500 units, D 400 units, E 5 units, C 35 mg, B_1 0.5 mg, B_2 0.6 mg, B_6 0.4 mg, niacin 8 mg, B_{12} 2 mcg, fluoride 0.5 mg/mL. Dropper Bot. 30 mL, 50 mL. **Tab.:** Fluoride 0.5 mg, vitamins A 2500 units, D 400 units, E 15 mg, $B_1$1.05 mg, B_2 1.2 mg, B_3 13.5 mg, B_6 1.05 mg, B_{12} 4.5 mcg, C 60 mg, folic acid 0.3 mg, Cu, Fe 12 mg, Zn 10 mg, sucrose. Bot. 100s. *Rx.*
Use: Mineral, vitamin supplement; dental caries agent.
Poly-Vi-Flor 0.5 mg w/Iron. (Bristol-Myers Squibb) **Drops:** Vitamins A 1500 units, D 400 units, E 5 units, C 35 mg, B_1 0.5 mg, B_2 0.6 mg, B_3 8 mg, B_6 0.4 mg, fluoride 0.5 mg, Fe 10 mg/mL. Dropper Bot. 50 mL. **Chew. Tab.:** Vitamins A 2500 units, D 400 units, E 15 units, B_1 1.05 mg, B_2 1.2 mg, B_3 13.5 mg, B_6 1.05 mg, B_{12} 4.5 mcg, C 60 mg, folic acid 0.3 mg, fluoride 0.5 mg, Fe 12 mg, Cu, Zn 10 mg, lactose, sucrose. Bot. 100s. *Rx.*
Use: Mineral, vitamin supplement; dental caries agent.
Poly-Vi-Flor 0.25 mg. (Bristol-Myers Squibb) **Drops:** Vitamins A 1500 units, D 400 units, E 5 units, C 35 mg, B_1

0.5 mg, B_2 0.6 mg, B_6 0.4 mg, B_3 8 mg, B_{12} 2 mcg, fluoride 0.25 mg/mL. Dropper Bot. 50 mL. **Chew. Tab.:** Vitamins A 2500 units, D 400 units, E 15 units, B_1 1.05 mg, B_2 1.2 mg, B_3 13.5 mg, B_6 1.05 mg, B_{12} 4.5 mcg, C 60 mg, folic acid, 0.3 mg, fluoride 0.25 mg, lactose, sucrose. Bot. 100s. *Rx.*
Use: Mineral, vitamin supplement; dental caries agent.
Poly-Vi-Flor 0.25 mg w/Iron. (Bristol-Myers Squibb) **Drops:** Vitamins A 1500 units, D 400 units, E 5 units, C 35 mg, B_1 0.5 mg, B_2 0.6 mg, B_6 0.4 mg, niacin 8 mg, fluoride 0.25 mg, Fe 10 mg/mL. Bot. 50 mL. **Chew. Tab.:** Vitamins A 2500 units, D 400 units, E 15 units, B_1 1.05 units, B_2 1.2 mg, B_3 13.5 mg, B_6 1.05 mg, B_{12} 4.5 mcg, C 60 mg, folic acid 0.3 mg, fluoride 0.25 mg, Cu, Fe 12 mg, Zn 10 mg, lactose, sucrose. Bot. 100s. *Rx.*
Use: Mineral, vitamin supplement; dental caries agent.
•**polyvinyl acetate phthalate.** (POL-ee-VYE-nil ASS-e-tate THAL-ate) *NF 29.*
Use: Pharmaceutic aid, coating agent.
•**polyvinyl alcohol.** (POL-ee-VYE-nil) *USP 34.* Ethanol, homopolymer.
Use: Pharmaceutic aid, viscosity-increasing agent.
See: Liquifilm Forte.
Puralube Tears.
W/Hydroxypropyl Methylcellulose.
See: Liquifilm Wetting.
polyvinylpyrrolidone. *Name previously used for Povidone.*
Poly-Vi-Sol. (Bristol-Myers Squibb) **Drops:** Vitamins A 1500 units, D 400 units, C 35 mg, B_1 0.5 mg, B_2 0.6 mg, E 5 units, B_6 0.4 mg, B_3 8 mg, B_{12} 2 mcg/mL. Bot. 50 mL. **Chew. Tab.:** Vitamins A 2500 units, E 15 units, D 400 units, C 60 mg, B_1 1.05 mg, B_2 1.2 mg, B_3 13.5 mg, B_6 1.05 mg, B_{12} 4.5 mcg, folic acid 0.3 mg. Bot. 100s. **Chew. Tab. With Iron:** Above formula plus Fe 12 mg, Zn 8 mg. Tab. Bot. 100s. Circus shape Tab. Bot. 100s. *OTC.*
Use: Vitamin supplement.
Poly-Vi-Sol w/Iron. (Bristol-Myers Squibb) **Chew. Tab.:** Fe 12 mg, vitamins A 2500 units, D 400 units, E 15 mg, B_1 1.05 mg, B_2 1.2 mg, B_3 13.5 mg, B_6 1.05 mg, B_{12} 4.5 mcg, C 60 mg, folic acid 0.3 mg, Cu, Zn 8 mg, sugar. Bot. 100s. **Drops:** Vitamins A 1500 units, D 400 units, E 5 units, C 35 mg, B_1 0.5 mg, B_2 0.6 mg, B_3 8 mg,

B_6 0.4 mg, Fe 10 mg/mL. Bot. 50 mL. *OTC.*
Use: Mineral, vitamin supplement.
Poly-Vi-Sol w/Minerals. (Bristol-Myers Squibb) Fe 12 mg, vitamins A 2500 units, D 400 units, E 15 mg, B_1 1.05 mg, B_2 1.2 mg, B_3 13.5 mg, B_6 1.06 mg, B_{12} 4.5 mcg, C 60 mg, folic acid 0.3 mg, Cu, Zn 8 mg. Chew. Tab. Bot. 60s, 100s. *OTC.*
Use: Mineral, vitamin supplement.
Poly-Vitamin Drops. (Schein) Vitamins A 1500 units, D 400 units, E 5 units, B_1 0.5 mg, B_2 0.6 mg, B_3 8 mg, B_6 0.4 mg, B_{12} 1.5 mcg, C 35 mg/mL. Dropper. Bot. 50 mL. *OTC.*
Use: Vitamin supplement.
Polyvitamin Drops with Iron. (Various Mfr.) Fe 10 mg, vitamins A 1500 units, D 400 units, E 5 mg, B_1 0.5 mg, B_2 0.6 mg, B_3 8 mg, B_6 0.4 mg, C 35 mg/mL. Bot. 50 mL. *OTC.*
Use: Mineral, vitamin supplement.
Polyvitamin Drops w/Iron and Fluoride. (Various Mfr.) Fluoride 0.25 mg, Vitamins A 1500 units, D 400 units, E 5 units, B_1 0.5 mg, B_2 0.6 mg, B_3 8 mg, B_6 0.4 mg, C 35 mg, Fe 10 mg. Bot. 50 mL. *Rx.*
Use: Mineral, vitamin supplement; dental caries agent.
Polyvitamin Fluoride. (Various Mfr.) Fluoride 0.25 mg, vitamins A 1500 units, D 400 units, E 5 units, B_1 0.5 mg, B_2 0.6 mg, B_3 8 mg, B_6 0.4 mg, B_{12} 2 mcg, C 35 mg/mL. Dropper. Bot. 50 mL. *Rx.*
Use: Mineral, vitamin supplement; dental caries agent.
Polyvitamin Fluoride w/Iron. (Various Mfr.) Fluoride 1 mg, vitamins A 2500 units, D 400 units, E 15 mg, B_1 1.05 mg, B_2 1.2 mg, B_3 13.5 mg, B_6 1.05 mg, B_{12} 4.5 mcg, C 60 mg, folic acid 0.3 mg, Fe 12 mg, Cu, Zn 10 mg. Tab. Bot. 100s, 1000s. *Rx.*
Use: Mineral, vitamin supplement; dental caries agent.
Poly-Vitamins w/Fluoride. (Various Mfr.) Fluoride 1 mg, vitamins A 2500 units, D 400 units, E 15 mg, B_1 1.05 mg, B_2 1.2 mg, B_3 13.5 mg, B_6 1.05 mg, B_{12} 4.5 mcg, C 60 mg, folic acid 0.3 mg. Chew. Tab. Bot. 100s, 1000s. *Rx.*
Use: Mineral, vitamin supplement; dental caries agent.
Poly-Vitamins w/Fluoride 0.5 mg. (Various Mfr.) **Drops:** Fluoride 0.5 mg, vitamins A 1500 units, D 400 units, E 5 units, B_1 0.5 mg, B_2 0.6 mg, B_3 8 mg, B_6 0.4 mg, B_{12} 2 mcg, C 35 mg/mL. Bot. 50 mL. **Tab.:** Fluoride 0.5 mg, vita-

mins A 2500 units, D 400 units, E 15 mg, B_1 1 mg, B_2 1.2 mg, B_3 13.5 mg, B_6 1 mg, B_{12} 4.5 mcg, C 60 mg, folic acid 0.3 mg. Bot. 100s, 1000s. *Rx.*
Use: Mineral, vitamin supplement; dental caries agent.
Polyvitamin w/Fluoride. (Rugby) Fluoride 0.5 mg, vitamins A 1500 units, D 400 units, E 5 mg, B_1 0.5 mg, B_2 0.6 mg, B_3 8 mg, B_6 0.4 mg, B_{12} 2 mcg, C 35 mg/mL. Dropper Bot. 50 mL. *Rx.*
Use: Mineral, vitamin supplement; dental caries agent.
Polyvite with Fluoride. (Geneva) Fluoride 0.25 mg, vitamins A 1500 units, D 400 units, E 5 mg, B_1 0.5 mg, B_2 0.6 mg, B_3 8 mg, B_6 0.4 mg, B_{12} 2 mcg, C 35 mg/mL. Dropper Bot. 50 mL. *Rx.*
Use: Mineral, vitamin supplement; dental caries agent.
•**pomaglumetad methionil.** (POE-ma-GLOO-me-tad) USAN.
Use: CNS agent.
•**ponalrestat.** (poe-NAHL-ress-TAT) USAN.
Use: Antidiabetic.
Ponaris. (Jamol Lab Inc.) Nasal emollient of mucosal lubricating and moisturizing botanical oils. Cajeput, eucalyptus, peppermint in iodized cottonseed oil. Bot. 1 oz w/dropper. *OTC.*
Use: Moisturizer, nasal.
•**ponatinib.** (poe-NA-ti-nib) USAN.
Use: Antineoplastic.
•**ponatinib hydrochloride.** (poe-NA-ti-nib) USAN.
Use: Antineoplastic.
•**ponezumab.** (poe-NEZ-oo-mab) USAN.
Use: CNS agent.
Ponstel. (Sciele Pharma) Mefenamic acid 250 mg. Lactose. Cap. Bot. 100s. *Rx.*
Use: Nonsteroidal anti-inflammatory agent.
Pontocaine. (Sanofi-Synthelabo) **Cream:** Tetracaine hydrochloride 1%, glycerin, light mineral oil, methylparaben, sodium metabisulfite. Tube 28.35 g. **Oint.:** Tetracaine 0.5%, menthol, white petrolatum. Tube 28.35 g. *OTC.*
Use: Anesthetic, topical.
Pontocaine Hydrochloride. (Hospira) Tetracaine hydrochloride. **Inj. 0.2%:** Dextrose 6%. Amp 2 mL. **0.3%:** Dextrose 6%. Amp 5 mL. **1%:** Acetone sodium bisulfite. Amp 2 mL. **Pow. for reconstitution:** *Niphanoid* (instantly soluble). Amp. *Rx.*
Use: Anesthetic, injectable local.

Pontocaine 2% Aqueous Solution.
(Sanofi-Synthelabo) Tetracaine hydrochloride 20 mg, chlorobutanol 4 mg/mL
of 2% soln. Bot. 30 mL, Box 12s. Bot.
118 mL, Box 6s. *Rx.*
Use: Anesthetic, local.

Po-Pon-S. (Shire US) Vitamins A
2000 units, D 100 units, E 5 mg,
B_1 5 mg, B_2 3 mg, B_3 35 mg, B_5 15 mg,
B_6 4 mg, B_{12} 6 mcg, C 100 mg, Ca, P.
Tab. Bot. 60s, 240s. *OTC.*
Use: Vitamin, mineral supplement.

poppy-seed oil. The ethyl ester of the
fatty acids of the poppy w/iodine.

poractant alfa.
Use: Lung surfactant.
See: Curosurf.

**porcine islet preparation, encapsu-
lated.**
Use: For type I diabetes patients already on immunosuppression.
[Orphan Drug]

•**porfimer sodium.** (PORE-fih-muhr)
USAN.
Use: Antineoplastic.
See: Photofrin.

•**porfiromycin.** (par-FIH-row-MY-sin)
USAN.
Use: Anti-infective; antineoplastic.

Pork NPH Iletin II. (Eli Lilly) Purified pork
insulin 100 units/mL in isophane insulin
suspension (insulin w/protamine and
zinc). Inj. Bot. 10 mL.
Use: Antidiabetic.

Pork Regular Iletin II. (Eli Lilly) Insulin
100 units/mL. Purified pork. Inj. Vial
10 mL.
Use: Antidiabetic.

•**porofocon A.** (POR-oh-FOE-kon A)
USAN.
Use: Contact lens material, hydro-
phobic.

•**porofocon B.** (POR-oh-FOE-kon B)
USAN.
Use: Contact lens material, hydro-
phobic.

Portabiday. (Washington Ethical) Concentrated soln. of alkylamine lauryl sulfate, a mild detergent with pH approx.
6 for use with *Portabiday* Vaginal
Cleansing Kit. Bot. 3 oz. *OTC.*
Use: Vaginal agent.

Portagen. (Bristol-Myers Squibb) A nutritionally complete dietary powder containing as a % of the calories protein
14% as caseinate, fat 41% (medium
chain triglycerides 86%, corn oil 14%),
carbohydrate 45% as corn syr. solids
and sucrose, vitamins A 5000 units, D
500 units, E 20 units, C 52 mg, B_1

1 mg, B_2 1.2 mg, B_6 1.4 mg, B_{12} 4 mcg,
niacin 13 mg, folic acid 0.1 mg, choline 83 mg, biotin 0.05 mg, Ca 600 mg,
P 450 mg, Mg 133 mg, Fe 12 mg, I
47 mcg, Cu 1 mg, Zn 6 mg, Mn 0.8 mg,
Cl 550 mg, Na 300 mg, K 800 mg,
pantothenic acid 6.7 mg, K-1 0.1 mg/
qt. 20 Kcal/fl oz. Can 1 lb. *OTC.*
Use: Nutritional supplement, enteral.

Portia. (Barr) Levonorgestrel 0.15 mg,
ethinyl estradiol 30 mcg. Lactose. Film-
coated. Tab. Packs. 21s, 28s (with 7 inert
tabs. [lactose]. *Rx.*
Use: Sex hormone, contraceptive hormone.

porton asparaginase.
See: Erwinia L-asparaginase.

•**posaconazole.** (poe-sa-KONE-a-zole)
USAN.
Use: Antifungal.
See: Noxafil.

**positive and negative hCG urine con-
trols.** (Wampole) Positive and negative human urine controls for urine pregnancy tests. 1 set, 1 vial each.
Use: Diagnostic aid.

Poslam Psoriasis Ointment. (Last) Sulfur 5%, salicylic acid 2%. Jar 1 oz.
Use: Antipsoriatic.

posterior pituitary hormones.
See: Concentraid.
DDAVP.
Desmopressin Acetate.
Stimate.
Vasopressin.

posterior pituitary injection.
Use: Hormone, antidiuretic.

postlobin-o.
See: Pituitary, Posterior, Hormones.

postlobin-v.
See: Pituitary, Posterior, Hormones.

Posture. (Iverness Medical) Elemental
calcium 600 mg. Preservative free.
Tab. Bot. 90s. *OTC.*
Use: Mineral supplement, calcium.

Posture D 600. (Wyeth) Calcium phos-
phate 600 mg, vitamin D 125 units.
Tab. Bot. 60s. *OTC.*
Use: Mineral supplement.

Potaba. (Glenwood) Aminobenzoate potassium. **Cap.:** 500 mg. Bot. 250s,
1000s. **Tab.:** 500 mg. Bot. 100s, 1000s.
Envule (Pow.): 2 g. Box 50s. *Rx.*
Use: Water-soluble vitamin.

Potachlor 10%. (Rosemont) Potassium
and chloride 20 mEq/15 mL. Alcohol
5%. Bot. Pt, gal. Alcohol 3.8%. Bot. Pt,
gal, UD 15 mL, 30 mL. *Rx.*
Use: Electrolyte supplement.

Potachlor 20%. (Rosemont) Potassium
and chloride 40 mEq/15 mL. Alcohol

free. Liq. Bot. pt, gal. *Rx.*
Use: Electrolyte supplement.

•**potash, sulfurated.** (PTO-ash SUL-fur-AY-ted) *USP 34.*
Use: Source of sulfide.

potassic saline lactated injection.
Use: Electrolyte replacement.

•**potassium acetate.** (poe-TASS-ee-um) *USP 34.* Acetic acid, potassium salt.
Use: Electrolyte replacement; to avoid Cl when high concentration of potassium is needed.

potassium acetate. (Various Mfr.) Potassium acetate 40 mEq. Inj. 20 mL in 50 mL Vial.
Use: Electrolyte replacement; to avoid Cl when high concentration of potassium is needed.

potassium acid phosphate.
See: K-Phos.

potassium acid phosphate/sodium acid phosphate.
Use: Genitourinary.
See: K-Phos M.F.
K-Phos No. 2.

•**potassium aspartate and magnesium aspartate.** (poe-TASS-ee-um a-SPAR-tate and mag-NEE-zee-um a-SPAR-tate) USAN.
Use: Nutrient.

•**potassium benzoate.** (poe-TASS-ee-um BEN-zoe-ate) *NF 29.*
Use: Pharmaceutic aid, preservative.

•**potassium bicarbonate.** (poe-TASS-ee-um bye-KAR-bo-nate) *USP 34.*
Use: Pharmaceutic necessity; electrolyte replacement.
W/Citric Acid, Sodium Bicarbonate.
See: Alka-Seltzer Gold.

•**potassium bicarbonate and potassium chloride effervescent tablets for oral solution.** *USP 34.*
Use: Electrolyte supplement.

•**potassium bicarbonate and potassium chloride for effervescent oral solution.** *USP 34.*
Use: Electrolyte supplement.

•**potassium bicarbonate and sodium bicarbonates and citric acid effervescent tablets for oral solution.** *USP 34.*
Use: Electrolyte supplement.

•**potassium bicarbonate effervescent tablets for oral solution.** *USP 34.*
Use: Electrolyte supplement.

•**potassium bitartrate.** *USP 34.*
Use: Cathartic.

•**potassium carbonate.** *USP 34.*
Use: Potassium therapy; pharmaceutic aid, alkalizing agent.

potassium channel blockers.
See: Dalfampridine.

potassium citrate.
Use: Urinary alkalinizer.
See: Urocit-K.

potassium citrate. (Rising Pharmaceuticals) Potassium citrate 5 mEq, 10 mEq. ER Tab. 100s. *Rx.*
Use: Urinary alkalinizer.

•**potassium chloride.** *USP 34.*
Use: Electrolyte replacement; potassium deficiency, hypopotassemia.
See: Cena-K.
Choice 10.
Choice 20.
Kaochlor.
Kaochlor-Eff.
Kaon Cl.
Kaon Cl-10.
Kaon Cl 20%.
K-Lor.
Klor-Con.
Klorvess.
Klotrix.
K-Lyte/Cl.
K-Lyte/Cl 50.
K-Tab.
Micro-K Extencaps.
Ten-K.
W/PEG 3350, Sodium Bicarbonate, Sodium Chloride.
See: TriLyte.
W/PEG 3350, Sodium Bicarbonate, Sodium Chloride, Sodium Sulfate.
See: GaviLyte-C.
GaviLyte-G.

potassium chloride. (Abbott) Potassium chloride. **Ampules:** 20 mEq, 10 mL; 40 mEq, 20 mL. **Pintop Vials:** 10 mEq, 5 mL in 10 mL; 20 mEq, 10 mL in 20 mL; 30 mEq, 12.5 mL in 30 mL; 40 mEq, 12.5 mL in 30 mL. **Fliptop Vials:** 20 mEq, 10 mL in 20 mL; 40 mEq, 20 mL in 50 mL. **Univ. Add. Syr.:** 5 mEq/5 mL, 20 mEq/10 mL, 30 mEq/20 mL, 40 mEq/20 mL (Eli Lilly and Co.) Amp. (40 mEq) 20 mL, 6s, 25s. *Rx.*
Use: Nutritional therapy.

potassium chloride. (KV Pharmaceutical Co.) Microencapsulated potassium chloride 600 mg equivalent to 8 mEq. ER Cap. 100s, 500s. *Rx.*
Use: Electrolyte.

potassium chloride. (Major) Potassium 20 mEq/15 mL. Glycerin, saccharin, sodium benzoate, sorbitol. Sugar free. Cherry flavor. Soln. 473 mL. *Rx.*
Use: Electrolyte.

potassium chloride. (Roxane) Potassium chloride. **Oral soln.:** Sugar free. 40 mEq/30 mL. Bot. 6 oz, 500 mL, 1 L,

5 L 20%. 80 mEq/30 mL. Bot. 500 mL, 1 L, 5 L. **Pow.:** 20 mEq/4 g. Pkt. 30s, 100s. *Rx.*
Use: Electrolyte supplement.

potassium chloride. (Various Mfr.) Microencapsulated potassium chloride 1500 mg equivalent to potassium 20 mEq. ER Tab. 100s, 500s, 1000s, UD 100s. *Rx.*
Use: Electrolyte.

potassium chloride. (Wyeth) Potassium Cl 10%, 20%. Sugar free. Soln. Bot. 16 oz, gal. *Rx.*
Use: Electrolyte supplement.

•**potassium chloride in dextrose and sodium chloride injection.** *USP 34.*
Use: Electrolyte supplement.

potassium chloride in 5% dextrose. (Various Mfr.) Dextrose 50 g; calories 170; K⁺ 10, 20, 30, or 40 mEq; Cl⁻ 10, 20, 30, or 40 mEq, osmolarity ≈ 272, 292 to 295, 310 to 312, or 330 to 333 mOsm/L. Soln. Bot. 500 mL (330 to 333 mOsm only), 1000 mL. *Rx.*
Use: Intravenous nutritional therapy, intravenous replenishment solution.

potassium chloride in 5% dextrose and lactated Ringer's. (Baxter Healthcare) Dextrose 50 g, calories 170, Na⁺ 130 mEq, K⁺ 24 or 44 mEq, Ca⁺⁺ 3 mEq, Cl⁻ 129 or 149 mEq, lactate 28 mEq, osmolarity 565 or 605 mOsm/L. Soln. Bot. 1000 mL. *Rx.*
Use: Intravenous nutritional therapy, intravenous replenishment solution.

potassium chloride in 5% dextrose and lactated Ringer's. (Hospira) Dextrose 50 g, kcal 179, Na+ 130 mEq, K+ 24 mEq, Ca++ 2.7 mEq, Cl− 129 mEq, lactate 28 mEq, 563 mOsm per liter. Inj. 1000 mL. *Rx.*
Use: Intravenous nutritional therapy.

potassium chloride in 5% dextrose and 0.45% sodium chloride. (Various Mfr) Dextrose 50 g; calories 170; Na⁺ 77 mEq, K⁺ 10, 20, 30, or 40 mEq, Cl⁻ 87, 97, 107, or 117 mEq; osmolarity ≈ 425, 445 to 447, ≈ 465, or 487 to 490 mOsm/L. Soln. Bot. 500 mL (445 to 447 mOsm only); 1000 mL. *Rx.*
Use: Intravenous nutritional therapy, intravenous replenishment solution.

potassium chloride in 5% dextrose and 0.9% sodium chloride. (Various Mfr) Dextrose 50 g; calories 170; Na⁺ 154 mEq; K⁺ 20 or 40 mEq, Cl⁻ 174 or 194 mEq; osmolarity ≈ 600 or 640 mOsm/L. Soln. Bot. 1000 mL. *Rx.*
Use: Intravenous nutritional therapy, intravenous replenishment solution.

potassium chloride in 5% dextrose and 0.33% sodium chloride. (Various Mfr) Dextrose 50 g; calories 170; Na⁺ 56 mEq; K⁺ 20, 30, or 40 mEq, Cl⁻ 76, 86, or 96 mEq; osmolarity 405, 425, or 446 mOsm/L. Soln. Bot. 500 mL (405 mOsm only); 1000 mL. *Rx.*
Use: Intravenous nutritional therapy, intravenous replenishment solution.

potassium chloride in 5% dextrose and 0.2% sodium chloride. (Various Mfr) Dextrose 50 g; calories 170; Na⁺ 34 mEq; K⁺ 10, 20, 30, or 40 mEq, Cl⁻ 44, 54, 64, or 74 mEq; osmolarity ≈ 340, 360, 380, or 400 mOsm/L. Soln. Bot. 250 mL, 500 mL (≈ 360 mOsm only); 1000 mL. *Rx.*
Use: Intravenous nutritional therapy, intravenous replenishment solution.

•**potassium chloride in lactated Ringer's and dextrose injection.** *USP 34.*
Use: Electrolyte supplement.

•**potassium chloride in sodium chloride injection.** *USP 34.*
Use: Electrolyte supplement.

potassium chloride in 10% dextrose and 0.2% sodium chloride. (B. Braun) Dextrose 100 g, calories 340, Na⁺ 34 mEq; K⁺ 20 mEq, Cl⁻ 54 mEq; osmolarity 615 mOsm/L. Soln. Bot. 250 mL. *Rx.*
Use: Intravenous nutritional therapy, intravenous replenishment solution.

potassium chloride in 3.3% dextrose and 0.3% sodium chloride. (B. Braun) Dextrose 33 g, calories 110, Na⁺ 51 mEq, K⁺ 20 mEq, Cl⁻ 71 mEq, osmolarity 310 mOsm/L. Soln. Bot. 1000 mL. *Rx.*
Use: Intravenous nutritional therapy, intravenous replenishment solution.

potassium chloride in 0.9% sodium chloride. (Various Mfr.) Na⁺ 154 mEq, K⁺ 20 or 40 mEq, Cl⁻ 174 or 194 mEq, osmolarity ≈ 350 or 390 mOsm/L. Soln. Bot. 1000 mL. *Rx.*
Use: Intravenous nutritional therapy, intravenous replenishment solution.

•**potassium chloride K 42.** (poe-TASS-ee-um K 42) USAN.
Use: Radiopharmaceutical.

potassium chloride, sodium chloride, and calcium carbonate.
Use: Salt replacement.
See: Sustain.

potassium chloride with potassium gluconate.
Use: Electrolyte supplement.

•**potassium citrate.** (poe-TASS-ee-um SIT-rate) *USP 34.* Tripotassium citrate.

Use: Alkalizer. [Orphan Drug]
See: Urocit-K.
W/Citric Acid, Sodium Citrate.
See: Cytra.
Polycitra K Crystals.
W/Dextromethorphan Hydrobromide,
Guaifenesin.
See: Sorbutuss NR.
W/Sodium citrate.
See: Bicitra.
potassium citrate monohydrate.
W/Citric Acid Monohydrate.
See: Taron-Crystals.
potassium clavulanate/amoxicillin.
Use: Anti-infective, penicillin.
See: Amoclan.
Amoxicillin and potassium clavula-
nate.
Augmentin.
potassium clavulanate/ticarcillin.
Use: Anti-infective, penicillin.
See: Ticarcillin and clavulanate potas-
sium.
• **potassium glucaldrate.** (poe-TASS-ee-
um gloo-KAL-drate) USAN.
Use: Antacid.
• **potassium gluconate.** (poe-TASS-ee-
um GLOO-koe-nate) USP 34.
Use: Electrolyte replacement.
See: Kaon.
potassium gluconate. (Various Mfr.) Potassium 40 mEq provided by potassium
gluconate 9.36 g/30 mL, alcohol 5%.
Elix. Bot. Pt, Patient-Cup 15 mL. *Rx.*
Use: Electrolyte supplement.
• **potassium gluconate and potassium
chloride for oral solution.** USP 34.
Use: Replacement therapy.
• **potassium gluconate and potassium
chloride solution.** USP 34.
Use: Replacement therapy.
• **potassium gluconate and potassium
citrate oral solution.** USP 34.
Use: Electrolyte supplement.
• **potassium gluconate, potassium citrate, and ammonium chloride oral
solution.** USP 34.
Use: Electrolyte supplement.
potassium glutamate. The monopotassium salt of l-glutamic acid.
potassium G penicillin.
See: Penicillin G potassium.
• **potassium guaiacolsulfonate.** (poe-
TASS-ee-um GWYE-a-kol-SUL-foe-
nate) USP 34. Sulfoguaiacol. Potassium
Hydroxymethoxybenzene sulfonate.
Used in many cough preps.
Use: Expectorant.
See: Pinex Regular.

W/Dextromethorphan Hydrobromide.
See: Prolex DM.
Prolex DMX.
• **potassium hydroxide.** (poe-TASS-ee-
um hye-DROX-ide) NF 29.
Use: Pharmaceutic aid, alkalinizing
agent.
potassium in sodium chloride. (Various
Mfr.) Potassium Cl 0.15%, 0.22%, 0.3%
in sodium Cl 0.9%. Soln. for Inj.
1000 mL. *Rx.*
Use: Intravenous replenishment solu-
tion, nutritional supplement.
• **potassium iodide.** (poe-TASS-ee-um
EYE-oh-dide) USP 34.
Use: Expectorant; antifungal; supple-
ment, iodine; thyroid drug.
See: Iosat.
Pima.
ThyroSafe.
ThyroShield.
W/Combinations.
See: Diastix Reagent Strips.
Elixophyllin-KI.
KIE.
Mudrane.
Mudrane-2.
W/Iodine.
See: Strong Iodine Solution (Lugol's So-
lution).
potassium iodide. (Roxane) Potassium
iodide 1 g/mL. Soln. 30 mL, 240 mL.
Rx.
Use: Thyroid drug.
potassium iodide. (Various Mfr.) Potas-
sium iodide 1 g/mL. Soln. 30 mL,
240 mL, pt. *Rx.*
Use: Thyroid drug.
• **potassium metabisulfite.** (poe-TASS-
ee-um MET-a-bye-SUL-fite) NF 29.
Use: Pharmaceutic aid, antioxidant.
• **potassium metaphosphate.** (poe-TASS-
ee-um MET-a-FOS-fate) NF 29.
Use: Pharmaceutic aid, buffering agent.
• **potassium nitrate.** (poe-TASS-ee-um
NYE-trate) USP 34.
W/Silver Nitrate.
See: Grafco.
potassium p-aminobenzoate.
See: Potaba.
W/Potassium salicylate.
See: Pabalate-SF.
potassium penicillin G.
Use: Anti-infective, penicillin.
See: Penicillin G, Potassium.
potassium penicillin V.
Use: Anti-infective, penicillin.
See: Phenoxymethyl penicillin potas-
sium.

•**potassium permanganate.** (poe-TASS-ee-um per-MAN-ga-nate) *USP 34.* Permanganic acid, potassium salt.
Use: Anti-infective, topical.

potassium phenethicillin. Phenethicillin potassium.
Use: Anti-infective.

potassium phenoxymethyl penicillin.
Use: Anti-infective.
See: Penicillin V potassium.

potassium phosphate. (Various Mfr.) Phosphate 3 mM, potassium 4.4 mEq per mL. Inj. Vials. 5 mL, 10 mL, 15 mL, 30 mL, 50 mL. *Rx.*
Use: Intravenous nutritional therapy, mineral.

•**potassium phosphate, dibasic.** (poe-TASS-ee-um FOS-fate) *USP 34.*
Use: Calcium regulator.

•**potassium phosphate, monobasic.** (poe-TASS-ee-um FOS-fate) *NF 29.* Dipotassium hydrogen phosphate.
Use: Pharmaceutic aid, buffering agent; source of potassium.
W/Dibasic Sodium Phosphate, Monobasic Sodium Phosphate.
See: Phospha 250 Neutral.

potassium phosphate, monobasic. (Abbott) Potassium phosphate monobasic 15 mM, 5 mL in 10 mL vial; 45 mM, 15 mL in 20 mL/Inj. vial.
Use: Pharmaceutic aid, buffering agent; source of potassium.

potassium reagent strips. (Bayer Consumer Care) Quantitative dry reagent strip test for potassium in serum or plasma. Bot. 50s.
Use: Diagnostic aid.

potassium-removing resins.
See: Sodium Polystyrene Sulfonate.

potassium rhodanate.
See: Potassium Thiocyanate.

potassium salicylate.
See: Neocylate.
W/Potassium P-Aminobenzoate.
See: Pabalate-SF.

potassium salt.
See: Potassium sorbate.

•**potassium sodium tartrate.** (poe-TASS-ee-um SOE-dee-um TAR-trate) *USP 34.*
Use: Laxative.

•**potassium sorbate.** (poe-TASS-ee-um SOR-bate) *NF 29.*
Use: Pharmaceutic aid, antimicrobial.

•**potassium sulfate.** (poe-TAS-ee-um) USAN.
Use: Bowel evacuant.
W/Magnesium Sulfate, Sodium Sulfate.
See: Suprep Bowel Prep.

potassium sulfocyanate. Potassium Rhodanate.
See: Potassium thiocyanate.

potassium thiocyanate. Potassium sulfocyanate, potassium rhodanate.

potassium thiphencillin.
Use: Anti-infective.

potassium troclosene. (Monsanto) Potassium dichloroisocyanurate.
Use: Anti-infective.

•**povidone.** (POE-vi-done) *USP 34.* Formerly Polyvidone, Polyvinylpyrrolidone.
Use: Pharmaceutic aid, dispersing and suspending agent.

•**povidone-iodine.** *USP 34.*
Use: Anti-infective, topical.
See: Betadine.
 Betadine PrepStick.
 Betadine PrepStick Plus.
 Massengill Medicated.
W/Lidocaine Hydrochloride.
See: ProTech First-Aid Stik.

povidone-iodine complex.
See: Betadine.

•**povidone I 131.** (POE-vi-done) USAN.
Use: Radiopharmaceutical.

•**povidone I 125.** (POE-vi-done) USAN.
Use: Radiopharmaceutical.

PowerMate. (Green Turtle Bay Vitamin Co.) Vitamins A 5000 units, E 100 units, B_3 12.5 mg, C 250 mg, Zn 2.5 mg, Se 7.5 mcg, n-acetyl-L-cysteine 25 mg, glutathione 5 mg, gingko biloba 5 mg, green tea extract 100 mg, pine bark extract 5 mg, echinacea 50 mg, golden seal root 20 mg, coenzyme Q10 2 mg, yeast free. Tab. Bot. 50s. *OTC.*
Use: Amino acid

PowerSleep. (Green Turtle Bay Vitamin Co.) L-glutamine 250 mg, 5-HTP 25 mg, melatonin 0.25 mg, vitamin B_3 25 mg, B_6 5 mg, inositol 100 mg, Ca 25 mg, passion flower extract 100 mg, valerian powder 75 mg. Tab. Bot. 60s. *OTC.*
Use: Amino acid.

PowerVites. (Green Turtle Bay Vitamin Co.) Vitamin A 2500 units, D 150 units, E 12.5 units, C 125 mg, B_1 6.3 mg, B_2 6.3 mg, B_3 25 mg, B_5 25 mg, B_6 12.5 mg, B_{12} 6.3 mcg, biotin, folic acid 0.15 mg, B, Ca, Mg, Cu, Zn 2.5 mg, Cr, Mn, K, Se, betaine, hesperidin. Tab. Bot. 40s, 100s, 200s. *OTC.*
Use: Mineral, vitamin supplement.

Poyaliver Stronger. (Forest) Liver inj. (equivalent to 10 mcg B_{12}), vitamin B_{12} 100 mcg, folic acid 10 mcg, niacinamide 1%/mL. Vial 10 mL. *Rx.*
Use: Nutritional supplement, parenteral.

Poyamin Jel Injection. (Forest) Cyanocobalamin 1000 mcg/mL. Vial 10 mL.
Use: Nutritional supplement, parenteral.
Poyaplex. (Forest) Vitamins B₁ 100 mg, niacinamide 100 mg, B₆ 10 mg, B₂ 1 mg, panthenol 10 mg, B₁₂ 5 mcg/mL. Vial 10 mL, 30 mL. *Rx.*
Use: Nutritional supplement, parenteral.
•**pozanicline.** (poe-ZAN-i-kleen) USAN.
Use: CNS agent.
•**pozanicline tartrate.** (poe-ZAN-i-kleen) USAN.
Use: CNS agent.
P.P.D. tuberculin.
See: Tuberculin Purified Protein Derivative.
P.P. factor. Pellagra preventive factor.
See: Nicotinic Acid.
ppg-15 stearyl ether.
Use: Pharmaceutic aid, surfactant.
PR. (PruGen) Cyclomethicone, dimethicone, hexyl laurate, polyglyceryl-4-isostearate, propylparaben. Dye free. Cream. 56.7 g kit w/*PruDrate* moisturizing cream. *Rx.*
Use: Emollient.
•**practolol.** (PRAK-toe-lole) USAN.
Use: Antiadrenergic, β-receptor.
Pradaxa. (Boehringer Ingelheim Pharmaceuticals) Dabigatran etexilate 75 mg (equiv. to dabigatran etexilate mesylate 86.48 mg), 150 mg (equiv. to dabigatran etexilate mesylate 172.95 mg). Cap. 60s, UD 60s. *Rx.*
Use: Anticoagulant, thrombin inhibitor.
•**pradefovir mesylate.** (prad-e-FOE-veer) USAN.
Use: Antiviral.
•**pralatrexate.** (PRAL-a-TREX-ate) USAN.
Tall Man: PRALAtrexate
Use: Folic acid antagonist.
See: Folotyn.
•**pralidoxime chloride.** (PRAL-i-DOX-eem) *USP 34.*
Use: Cholinesterase reactivator; antidote.
See: Protopam Chloride.
pralidoxime chloride. (Survival Technical) Pralidoxime chloride 600 mg, benzyl alcohol, aminocaproic acid. Inj. Vial 2 mL. *Rx.*
Use: Antidote.
pralidoxime chloride/atropine.
Use: Detoxification agent, antidote.
See: DuoDote.
•**pralidoxime iodide.** (PRAL-i-DOX-eem EYE-oh-dide) USAN.
Use: Cholinesterase reactivator.
•**pralidoxime mesylate.** (PRAL-i-DOX-eem) USAN.
Use: Cholinesterase reactivator.

pralidoxime methiodide.
See: Pralidoxime Iodide.
•**pralmorelin dihydrochloride.** (pral-more-ELL-in die-HIGH-droe-KLOR-ide) USAN.
Use: Growth hormone-releasing factor.
•**pralnacasan.** (PRAL-na-ka-san) USAN.
Use: Rheumatoid arthritis.
PrameGel. (Bioglan) Pramoxine hydrochloride 1%. Emollient base with menthol 0.5%, benzyl alcohol, SD alcohol 40. Gel. Bot. 118 mL. *OTC.*
Use: Topical local anesthetic.
•**pramiconazole.** (PRAM-i-KON-a-zole) USAN.
Use: Antifungal.
Pramilet FA. (Ross) Vitamins A 4000 units, B₁ 3 mg, B₂ 2 mg, B₆ 3 mg, B₁₂ 3 mcg, C 60 mg, D 400 units, B₅ 1 mg, B₃ 10 mg, Ca 250 mg, Cu, I, Fe 40 mg, Mg, Zn, folic acid 1 mg. Filmtab. Bot. 100s. *Rx.*
Use: Mineral, vitamin supplement.
•**pramipexole dihydrochloride.** (pram-ih-PEX-ole) USAN.
Use: Antiparkisonian; antischizophrenic; antidepressant.
See: Mirapex.
Mirapex XR.
pramipexole dihydrochloride. (Various Mfr.) Pramipexole dihydrochloride 0.125 mg, 0.25 mg, 0.5 mg, 0.75 mg, 1 mg, 1.5 mg. May contain mannitol. Tab. 30s, 63s, 90s, 500s, 5,000s, 6,000s, UD 100s (0.125 mg); 30s, 90s, 500s, 5,500s, UD 100s (0.25 mg); 30s, 90s, 500s, 4,000s, UD 100s (0.5 mg); 30s, 90s, 500s, 2,500s, UD 100s (0.75 mg); 30s, 90s, 500s, 2,500s, UD 100s (1 mg); 30s, 90s, 500s, 1,500s, UD 100s (1.5 mg). *Rx.*
Use: Dopaminergic, nonergot dopamine receptor agonist.
•**pramiracetam hydrochloride.** (PRAM-i-RA-se-tam) USAN. *Formerly Amacetam Hydrochloride.*
Use: Cognition adjuvant.
•**pramiracetam sulfate.** (PRAM-i-RA-se-tam) USAN. *Formerly Amacetam Sulfate.*
Use: Cognition adjuvant.
•**pramlintide acetate.** (PRAM-lin-tide) USAN.
Use: Antidiabetic agent, amylin analog.
See: Symlin.
Pramosone Cream 1%. (Ferndale) Hydrocortisone acetate 1%, pramoxine hydrochloride 1% in cream base. Tube 1 oz, 4 oz. Jar 4 oz, lb. *Rx.*
Use: Corticosteroid; anesthetic, local.

Pramosone Cream 2.5%. (Ferndale) Hydrocortisone acetate 2.5%, pramoxine hydrochloride 1% in cream base. Tube 1 oz, 4 oz. Jar lb. *Rx.*
Use: Corticosteroid; anesthetic, local.

Pramosone Cream 0.5%. (Ferndale) Hydrocortisone acetate 0.5%, pramoxine hydrochloride 1% in cream base. Tube 1 oz, 4 oz. Jar 4 oz, lb.
Use: Corticosteroid; anesthetic, local.

Pramosone E. (Ferndale) Hydrocortisone acetate 2.5%, pramoxine 1%. *Hydrolipid* base. Cetostearyl alcohol, mineral oil, propylparaben, triethanolamine, white petrolatum. Cream. 28.4 g, 57 g. *Rx.*
Use: Topical corticosteroid combination.

Pramosone Lotion 1%. (Ferndale) Hydrocortisone acetate 1%, pramoxine hydrochloride 1% in lotion base. Bot. 2 oz, 4 oz, 8 oz. *Rx.*
Use: Corticosteroid; anesthetic, local.

Pramosone Lotion 2.5%. (Ferndale) Hydrocortisone acetate 2.5%, pramoxine hydrochloride 1% in lotion base. Bot 2 oz, gal. *Rx.*
Use: Corticosteroid; anesthetic, local.

Pramosone Lotion 0.5%. (Ferndale) Hydrocortisone acetate 0.5%, pramoxine hydrochloride 1% in lotion base. Bot. 1 oz, 4 oz, 8 oz. *Rx.*
Use: Corticosteroid; anesthetic, local.

Pramosone Ointment 1%. (Ferndale) Hydrocortisone acetate 1%, pramoxine hydrochloride 1% in ointment base. Tube 1 oz, 4 oz. Jar 4 oz, lb. *Rx.*
Use: Corticosteroid; anesthetic, local.

•**pramoxine hydrochloride.** (pram-OX-een) *USP 34.*
Use: Anesthetic, topical.
See: Campho-Phenique Cold Sore Treatment and Scab Relief.
Itch-X.
PrameGel.
Prax.
ProctoFoam NS.
Sarna Sensitive Anti-Itch.
Sarna Ultra.
Tronothane Hydrochloride.
Tucks.
W/Bacitracin Zinc, Neomycin, Polymyxin B Sulfate.
See: Neosporin Plus Pain Relief.
Tri-Biozene.
W/Benzalkonium Chloride.
See: Bactine Pain Relieving Cleansers.
W/Benzalkonium Chloride, Chloroxylenol, Hydrocortisone.
See: Cortic-ND.
Mediotic-HC.

W/Calamine.
See: Aveeno Anti-Itch.
Caladryl.
W/Chloroxylenol, Glycerin, Zinc Acetate Dihydrate.
See: Zinotic.
Zinotic ES.
W/Chloroxylenol, Hydrocortisone.
See: Oto-End 10.
Zoto-HC.
W/Chloroxylenol, Zinc Acetate Dihydrate.
See: ZinOtic ES.
W/Clioquinol, Hydrocortisone.
See: 1 + 1-F Creme.
W/Dimethicone.
See: Gold Bond Intensive Healing.
W/Hydrocortisone Acetate.
See: Analpram-E.
EndaRoid.
HC Pram 1%.
HC Pramoxine.
HC Pram 2.5%.
Pramosone E.
Proctofoam-HC.
ZyPram.
W/Neomycin, Polymyxin B Sulfate.
See: Neosporin Plus Pain Relief.

PrandiMet. (Novo Nordisk) Repaglinide 1 mg/metformin hydrochloride 500 mg, repaglinide 2 mg/metformin hydrochloride 500 mg. PEG, sorbitol. Tab. 20s, 100s. *Rx.*
Use: Antidiabetic agent, antidiabetic combination product.

Prandin. (Novo Nordisk) Repaglinide 0.5 mg, 1 mg, 2 mg. Tab. Bot. 100s, 500s, 1000s. *Rx.*
Use: Antidiabetic, meglitinide.

•**pranolium chloride.** (pray-NO-lee-uhm) USAN.
Use: Cardiovascular agent, antiarrhythmic.

•**prasugrel hydrochloride.** (pra-SOO-grel) USAN.
Use: Platelet antagonist.
See: Effient.

Pravachol. (Bristol-Myers Squibb) Pravastatin sodium 10 mg, 20 mg, 40 mg, 80 mg. Lactose. Tab. Bot. 90s, 500s (80 mg only), 1000s (20 mg only), UD 100s (except 10 mg). *Rx.*
Use: Antihyperlipidemic, HMG-CoA reductase inhibitor.

•**pravadoline maleate.** (pray-AH-doe-leen) USAN.
Use: Analgesic.

•**pravastatin sodium.** (PRUH-vuh-stuh-tin) USAN.

Use: Antihyperlipidemic, HMG-CoA reductase inhibitor.
See: Pravachol.

pravastatin sodium. (Various Mfr.) Pravastatin sodium 10 mg, 20 mg, 40 mg, 80 mg. May contain lactose. Tab. 30s (except 80 mg), 90s, 100s, 500s, 1000s. *Rx.*
Use: Antihyperlipidemic agent, HMG-CoA reductase inhibitor.

Prax. (Ferndale) Pramoxine hydrochloride 1%. **Cream:** Hydrophilic base with glycerin, cetyl alcohol, white petrolatum. 30 g, 113.4 g, 1 lb. **Lot.:** Hydrophilic base with potassium sorbate 0.1%, sorbic acid 0.1%, mineral oil, cetyl alcohol, glycerin, lanolin. Bot. 15 mL, 120 mL, 240 mL. *OTC.*
Use: Topical local anesthetic.

praziquantel.
Use: Anthelmintic.
See: Biltricide.

•**prazosin hydrochloride.** (PRAY-zoe-sin) *USP 34.*
Use: Antihypertensive, antiadrenergic.
See: Minipress.

prazosin hydrochloride. (Various Mfr.) Prazosin hydrochloride 1 mg, 2 mg, 5 mg. Cap. Bot. 100s, 250s, 500s, 1000s (except 5 mg).
Use: Antihypertensive, antiadrenergic.

Pre-Attain. (Sherwood Davis & Geck) Sodium caseinate, maltodextrin, corn oil, soy lecithin, vitamins A, B_1, B_2, B_3, B_5, B_6, B_{12}, C, D, E, K, folic acid, Ca, Cl, Cu, Fe, I, Mg, Mn, P, Zn. Liq. Can 250 mL, closed system 1000 mL. *OTC.*
Use: Nutritional supplement.

PreCare. (Ther-Rx) Vitamin C 50 mg, Ca 250 mg, Fe 40 mg, D_3 6 mcg, E 3.5 mg, B_6 2 mg, folic acid 1 mg, Mg, Zn 15 mg, Cu, mannitol, sucrose, vanilla flavor. Chew. Tab. UD 100s. *Rx.*
Use: Vitamin, mineral supplement.

PreCare Conceive. (Ther-Rx) Vitamin C 60 mg, Ca 200 mg, Fe 30 mg, E 30 units, thiamin 3 mg, riboflavin 3.4 mg, niacin 20 mg, pyridoxine 50 mg, folic acid 1 mg, Mg, cyanocobalamin 12 mcg, Zn 15 mg, Cu, lactose. Tab. UD 100s. *Rx.*
Use: Vitamin, mineral supplement.

PreCare Premier. (Thera-Rx) Vitamin C 50 mg, D_3 240 units, E 3.5 units, B_1 3 mg, B_2 3.4 mg, B_3 20 mg, B_6 50 mg, folic acid 1 mg, B_{12} 12 mcg, calcium 250 mg, sumalate iron 30 mg, magnesium 25 mg, zinc 15 mg, copper 2 mg, docusate sodium 50 mg, succinic acid 35 mg. Lactose, PEG, poly-

dextrose, sucrose, vegetable oil. Tab. 30s. *Rx.*
Use: Nutritional supplement.

PreCare Prenatal. (Ther-Rx) Ca 250 mg, Fe (as ferrous fumarate) 40 mg, E (dl-alpha tocopheryl acetate) 3.5 mg, D_3 6 mcg, B_1 3 mg, B_2 3.4 mg, B_3 20 mg, B_6 12 mcg, C 50 mg, folic acid 1 mg, Mg, Zn 15 mg, Cu. Dye free. Tab. UD 100s. *Rx.*
Use: Vitamin, mineral supplement.

Precedex. (Abbott) Dexmedetomidine hydrochloride 100 mcg/mL, sodium chloride 9 mg, preservative free. Inj. Vial 2 mL. *Rx.*
Use: Sedative; hypnotic (nonbarbiturate).

Precef for Injection. (Bristol-Myers Squibb) Ceforanide 500 mg, 1 g/Vial or piggyback. *Rx.*
Use: Anti-infective, cephalosporin.

Precision High Nitrogen Diet. (Novartis) Vanilla flavor: Maltodextrin, pasteurized egg white solids, sucrose, natural and artificial flavors, medium chain triglycerides, partially hydrogenated soybean oil, polysorbate 80, mono- and diglycerides, vitamins, minerals. Pow. Packet 2.93 oz. *OTC.*
Use: Nutritional supplement.

Precision LR Diet. (Novartis) Orange flavor: Maltodextrin, pasteurized egg white solids, sucrose, medium chain triglycerides, partially hydrogenated soybean oil with BHA, citric acid, natural and artificial flavors, mono- and diglycerides, polysorbate 80, FD&C Yellow No. 5 and No. 6, vitamins, minerals. Pow. Packet 3 oz. *OTC.*
Use: Nutritional supplement.

Precose. (Bayer) Acarbose 25 mg, 50 mg, 100 mg. Tab. Bot. 100s, UD 100s (except 25 mg). *Rx.*
Use: Antidiabetic.

Predamide Ophthalmic. (Maurry) Sodium sulfacetamide 10%, prednisolone acetate 0.5%, hydroxyethyl cellulose, polysorbate 80, sodium thiosulfate, benzalkonium Cl 0.025%. Bot. 5 mL, 15 mL. *Rx.*
Use: Anti-infective; corticosteroid, ophthalmic.

Pred Forte. (Allergan) Prednisolone acetate 1%. Benzalkonium chloride, EDTA, polysorbate 80, hydroxypropyl methylcellulose, sodium bisulfite, boric acid, sodium chloride, sodium citrate. Ophth. Susp. Bot. 1 mL, 5 mL, 10 mL, 15 mL. *Rx.*
Use: Corticosteroid, ophthalmic.

Pred-G. (Allergan) **Oint.:** Prednisolone

acetate 0.6%, gentamicin sulfate 0.3%, chlorobutanol 0.5%. Oint. Tube 3.5 g.
Ophth. Susp.: Prednisolone acetate 1%, gentamicin sulfate 0.3%, benzalkonium chloride 0.005%, polyvinyl alcohol 1.4%, EDTA, hydrochloric acid, hydroxypropyl methylcellulose, sodium chloride, polysorbate 80, sodium citrate dihydrate, sodium hydroxide. Bot. 2 mL, 5 mL, 10 mL. *Rx.*
Use: Corticosteroid; anti-infective, ophthalmic.
Predicort-AP. (Oxypure) Prednisolone sodium phosphate 20 mg, prednisolone acetate 80 mg/mL. Vial 10 mL. *Rx.*
Use: Corticosteroid.
Predicort-RP. (Oxypure) Prednisolone sodium phosphate equivalent to prednisolone phosphate 20 mg, niacinamide 25 mg/mL. Vial 10 mL. *Rx.*
Use: Corticosteroid.
Pred Mild. (Allergan) Prednisolone acetate 0.12%. Benzalkonium chloride, EDTA, polysorbate 80, hydroxypropyl methylcellulose, sodium bisulfite, boric acid, sodium chloride, sodium citrate. Ophth. Susp. Bot. 5 mL, 10 mL. *Rx.*
Use: Corticosteroid, ophthalmic.
•**prednazate.** (PRED-nah-zate) USAN.
Use: Anti-inflammatory.
•**prednicarbate.** (PRED-nih-CAR-bate) USAN.
Use: Corticosteroid, topical.
See: Dermatop.
prednicarbate. (Fougera) Prednicarbate 0.1%. Cetostearyl alcohol, EDTA, lanolin alcohols, mineral oil, white petrolatum. Cream. 15 g, 60 g. *Rx.*
Use: Anti-inflammatory agent, topical corticosteroid.
prednicarbate. (Fougera) Prednicarbate 0.1%. Glyceryl, white petrolatum. Oint. 15 g, 60 g. *Rx.*
Use: Anti-inflammatory agent; corticosteroid, topical.
•**prednimustine.** (PRED-nih-MUSS-teen) USAN.
Use: Antineoplastic. [Orphan Drug]
•**prednisolone.** (pred-NIS-oh-lone) *USP 34.* Metacortandralone.
Tall Man: prednisoLONE
Use: Corticosteroid; adrenocortical steroid, glucocorticoid.
See: AsmalPred Plus.
  Cordrol.
  Millipred.
  Orapred.
  Orapred ODT.
  Prelone.
  Veripred 20.

prednisolone. (Halsey Drug) Prednisolone 15 mg/5 mL, alcohol 5%. Syr. Bot. 236 mL, 473 mL. *Rx.*
Use: Corticosteroid.
prednisolone. (Various Mfr.) Prednisolone. **Syr.:** 15 mg/mL. Sucrose. 240 mL, 480 mL. **Tab.:** 5 mg. 100s, 1000s, 5000s. *Rx.*
Use: Adrenocortical steroid, glucocorticoid.
•**prednisolone acetate.** (pred-NIS-oh-lone) *USP 34.*
Tall Man: prednisoLONE
Use: Corticosteroid, topical; adrenocortical steroid, glucocorticoid.
See: Flo-Pred.
  Omnipred.
  Pred.
  Pred Forte.
  Pred Mild.
  Predicort-AP.
  Sigpred.
  Steraject.
W/Combinations.
See: Blephamide.
  Blephamide Ophthalmic Ointment.
  Metimyd.
  Poly-Pred Liquifilm.
  Pred-G.
  Pred-G S.O.P.
prednisolone acetate. (Various Mfr.) Prednisolone acetate 1%. Benzalkonium chloride 0.01%, EDTA, polysorbate 80, glycerin, hypromellose, dibasic sodium phosphate. Ophth. Susp. Bot. 5 mL, 10 mL, 15 mL. *Rx.*
Use: Corticosteroid, ophthalmic.
prednisolone acetate and prednisolone sodium phosphate. (Various Mfr.) Prednisolone acetate 80 mg, prednisolone sodium phosphate 20 mg/mL. Inj. Vial 10 mL. *Rx.*
Use: Corticosteroid.
prednisolone butylacetate.
Use: Corticosteroid.
prednisolone cyclopentylpropionate.
Use: Corticosteroid.
•**prednisolone hemisuccinate.** (pred-NIS-oh-lone HEM-ee-SUX-i-nate) *USP 34.*
Tall Man: prednisoLONE
Use: Corticosteroid, topical.
•**prednisolone sodium metazoate.** (pred-NIS-oh-lone) USAN.
Use: Gastrointestinal agent.
•**prednisolone sodium phosphate.** (pred-NIS-oh-lone) *USP 34.*
Tall Man: prednisoLONE
Use: Corticosteroid, topical; adrenocortical steroid, glucocorticoid.

See: AsmalPred Plus.
Orapred.
Orapred ODT.
Pediapred.
Prednisol.
W/Prednisolone acetate.
See: Optimyd.
Vasocidin Ophthalmic Solution.
prednisolone sodium phosphate.
(Bausch & Lomb) Prednisolone sodium
phosphate 1%. Hypromellose, monobasic and dibasic sodium phosphate,
sodium chloride, EDTA, benzalkonium
chloride 0.01%. Ophth. Soln. 5 mL,
10 mL, 15 mL. *Rx.*
Use: Ophthalmic corticosteroid.
prednisolone sodium phosphate. (Upstate Pharma) Prednisolone sodium
phosphate 6.75 mg (prednisolone 5 mg)
per 5 mL. Oral Soln. 120 mL. *Rx.*
Use: Adrenocortical steroid, glucocorticoid.
prednisolone sodium phosphate.
(Various Mfr.) Prednisolone sodium
phosphate 0.125%, 1%. Soln. Bot.
5 mL, 10 mL, 15 mL. *Rx.*
Use: Corticosteroid, topical.
prednisolone sodium phosphate.
(Various Mfr.) Prednisolone sodium
phosphate 20.2 mg (prednisolone
15 mg) per 5 mL. Oral Soln. 237 mL.
Rx.
Use: Adrenocortical steroid, glucocorticoid.
•**prednisolone sodium succinate for
injection.** *USP 34.*
Tall Man: prednisoLONE
Use: Corticosteroid, topical.
•**prednisolone tebutate.** (pred-NIS-oh-
lone TEB-ue-tate) *USP 34.*
Tall Man: prednisoLONE
Use: Corticosteroid, topical.
See: Metalone.
prednisolone tertiary-butylacetate.
See: Prednisolone Tebutate.
•**prednisone.** (PRED-nih-sone) *USP 34.*
Tall Man: predniSONE
Use: Corticosteroid; adrenocortical steroid, glucocorticoid.
prednisone. (Roxane) Prednisone. **Oral
Soln.:** 5 mg/5 mL. Alcohol 5%, EDTA,
fructose, saccharin. 120 mL, 500 mL,
UD 5 mL. **Tab.:** 1 mg, 2.5 mg. Lactose.
100s, 1000s (1 mg only), UD 100s. *Rx.*
Use: Glucocorticoid, adrenocortical steroid.
prednisone. (Various Mfr.) Prednisone
5 mg, 10 mg, 20 mg, 50 mg. Tab. Bot.
100s, 500s (except 50 mg), 1000s,
5000s (5 mg only), UD 100s. *Rx.*

Use: Adrenocortical steroid, glucocorticoid.
Prednisone Intensol. (Roxane) Prednisone 5 mg/mL. Alcohol 30%. Oral Soln.
Bot. 30 mL w/calibrated dropper. *Rx.*
Use: Adrenocortical steroid, glucocorticoid.
•**prednival.** (PRED-nih-val) USAN.
Use: Corticosteroid.
Predsulfair. (Bausch & Lomb) **Drops:**
Prednisolone acetate 0.5%, sodium
sulfacetamide 10%, hydroxypropyl
methylcellulose, polysorbate 80 0.5%,
sodium thiosulfate, benzalkonium Cl
0.01%. Bot. 5 mL, 15 mL. **Oint.:** Prednisolone acetate 0.5%, sodium sulfacetamide 10%, mineral oil, white petrolatum, lanolin, parabens. 3.5 g. *Rx.*
Use: Anti-infective; corticosteroid, ophthalmic.
Prefest. (Barr/Duramed) Estradiol 1 mg;
estradiol 1 mg/norgestimate 0.09 mg.
Lactose. Tab. Blister card 30s (15 each
tablet). *Rx.*
Use: Sex hormone, estrogen and progestin combination.
**Preflex Daily Cleaning Especially for
Sensitive Eyes.** (Alcon) Isotonic,
aqueous solution of sorbic acid, sodium
phosphates, sodium Cl, tyloxapol,
hydroxyethyl cellulose, polyvinyl alcohol, EDTA. Bot. 30 mL. *OTC.*
Use: Contact lens care.
•**pregabalin.** (preh-GAB-ah-lin) USAN.
Use: Anticonvulsant.
See: Lyrica.
Pregestimil. (Bristol-Myers Squibb) Protein hydrolysate formula supplies
640 calories/qt. protein 18 g, fat 26 g,
carbohydrate 86 g, vitamins A 2000 units,
D 400 units, E 15 units, C 52 mg, folic acid 100 mcg, thiamine hydrochloride
0.5 mg, riboflavin 0.6 mg, niacin 8 mg,
B_6 0.4 mg, B_{12} 2 mcg, biotin 0.05 mg,
pantothenic acid 3 mg, K-1 100 mcg,
choline 85 mg, inositol 30 mg, Ca
600 mg, P 400 mg, I 45 mcg, Fe 12 mg,
Mg 70 mg, Cu 0.6 mg, Zn 4 mg, Mn
0.2 mg, Cl 550 mg, K 700 mg, Na
300 mg/qt. (20 Kcal/fl oz.). Pow. Can
lb. *OTC.*
Use: Nutritional supplement, enteral.
**Pregnaslide Latex hCG Test with Fast
Trak Slides.** (Wampole) Latex agglutination slide test for the qualitative detection of hCG in urine. Test 24s. Test kit
96s.
Use: Diagnostic aid.
pregneninolone.
See: Ethisterone.

pregnenolone.
Use: Treatment of rheumatoid arthritis.
•**pregnenolone succinate.** (preg-NEN-oh-lone) USAN.
Use: Nonhormonal sterol derivative.
Pregnosis Slide Test. (Roche) Latex agglutination inhibition slide test. 50s, 200s.
Use: Diagnostic aid.
Pregnyl. (Organon) Chorionic gonadotropin 10,000 units/vial with diluent 10 mL (1000 units per mL), benzyl alcohol 0.9%. Vial 10 mL. *Rx.*
Use: Ovulation stimulant.
Preject Preinjection Topical Anesthetic. (Colgate Oral) Benzocaine 20% in polyethylene glycol base. Jar 2 oz. *OTC.*
Use: Anesthetic, local.
Prelestrin. (Taylor Pharmaceuticals) Conjugated estrogens 0.625 mg, 1.25 mg. Tab. Bot. 100s, 1000s. *Rx.*
Use: Estrogen.
Prelief. (AKPharma) Calcium glycerophosphate 65 mg, phosphorus 50 mg. Tab. 120s. *OTC.*
Use: Antacid.
Prelone. (Aero) Prednisolone 15 mg/5 mL. Alcohol 5%, saccharin, sucrose. Cherry flavor. Syr. 240 mL. *Rx.*
Use: Adrenocortical steroid, glucocorticoid.
Prelu-2. (Roxane) Phendimetrazine tartrate 105 mg, sucrose. Cap. Bot. 100s. *c-III.*
Use: CNS stimulant, anorexiant.
Premarin. (Wyeth-Ayerst) Conjugated estrogens. 0.3 mg, 0.45 mg, 0.625 mg, 0.9 mg, 1.25 mg. Lactose, sucrose. Tab. Bot. 100s (except 0.625 mg), 1000s (except 0.45 mg, 0.9 mg), UD 100s (0.45 mg, 0.625 mg only). *Rx.*
Use: Estrogen, sex hormone.
Premarin Intravenous. (Wyeth-Ayerst) Conjugated estrogens 25 mg. Inj. *Secules* each with 5 mL sterile diluent. Lactose 200 mg, simethicone 0.2 mg, sodium citrate 12.2 mg, benzyl alcohol 2%. *Rx.*
Use: Estrogen.
Premarin Vaginal. (Wyeth-Ayerst) Conjugated estrogens 0.625 mg/g in a nonliquefying base. Benzyl alcohol, cetyl alcohol, mineral oil. Cream. Tube with or without calibrated applicator 42.5 g. *Rx.*
Use: Estrogen, sex hormone.
Premarin w/Meprobamate.
See: PMB 400.
PMB 200.
Premphase. (Wyeth-Ayerst) Conjugated estrogens 0.625 mg. Medroxyprogesterone acetate 5 mg/conjugated estrogens 0.625 mg. Lactose, sucrose. Tab. Dial pack 28s (14 of each tablet). *Rx.*
Use: Sex hormone, estrogen, progestin combination.
Prempro. (Wyeth-Ayerst) Conjugated estrogen 0.3 mg/medroxyprogesterone acetate 1.5 mg, conjugated estrogen 0.45 mg/medroxyprogesterone acetate 1.5 mg, conjugated estrogen 0.625 mg/medroxyprogesterone acetate 2.5 mg (lactose, sucrose), conjugated estrogen 0.625 mg/medroxyprogesterone acetate 5 mg (lactose, sucrose). Tab. Dial pack 28s (except 0.45 mg/1.5 mg), *EZ Dial* 28s (0.45 mg/1.5 mg only). *Rx.*
Use: Sex hormone, estrogen, progestin combination.
Prēmsyn PMS. (Chattem) Acetaminophen 500 mg, pamabrom 25 mg, pyrilamine maleate 15 mg. Cap. Bot. 20s, 40s. *OTC.*
Use: Analgesic; antihistamine; diuretic.
•**prenalterol hydrochloride.** (PREE-NAL-teh-role) USAN.
Use: Adrenergic.
Prenatabs RX. (Cypress) Ca 200 mg, Fe (as carbonyl iron) 29 mg, vitamin A 4000 units, D 400 units, E (dl-alpha tocopheryl acetate) 30 units, B_1 3 mg, B_2 3 mg, B_3 20 mg, B_5 7 mg, B_6 3 mg, B_{12} 8 mcg, C 120 mg, folic acid 1 mg, biotin 30 mcg, Zn 15 mg, Cu, I, Mg. Tab. Bot. 90s. *Rx.*
Use: Mineral, vitamin supplement.
Prenatal AD. (Cypress) Ca 200 mg, Fe (carbonyl iron) 90 mg, vitamin A 2700 units, D_3 400 units, E (dl-alpha tocopheryl acetate) 30 units, B_1 3 mg, B_2 3.4 mg, B_3 20 mg, B_6 20 mg, B_{12} 12 mcg, C 120 mg, folic acid 1 mg, Zn 25 mg, Cu, Mg, docusate sodium 50 mg. Tab. Bot. 90s. *Rx.*
Use: Mineral, vitamin supplement.
Prenatal Folic Acid + Iron. (Everett) Vitamins, minerals, folic acid 1 mg. Tab. Bot. 100s. *Rx.*
Use: Mineral, vitamin supplement.
Prenatal H.P. (Mission Pharmacal) Vitamins A 4000 units, C 100 mg, D_3 400 units, B_1 4 mg, B_2 2 mg, B_3 10 mg, B_5 1 mg, B_6 20 mg, B_{12} 2 mcg, folate 0.8 mg, Ca 50 mg, Fe 30 mg, sugar. Tab. Bot. 100s. *OTC.*
Use: Mineral, vitamin supplement.
Prenatal Maternal. (Ethex) Ca 250 mg, Fe 4 mg, B_2 60 mg, vitamins A 5000 units, D 400 units, E 30 mg, B_1 2.9 mg, B_2 3.4 mg, B_3 20 mg, B_5 10 mg, B_6 12.2 mg, B_{12} 12 mcg, C 100 mg, fo-

lic acid 1 mg, Cr, Cu, I, Mg, Mn, Mo, Zn 25 mg, biotin 30 mcg. Tab. Bot. 100s. *Rx.*
Use: Mineral, vitamin supplement.

Prenatal 19. (Cypress) Ca 200 mg, Fe 29 mg, vitamin A 1000 units, D 400 units, E (dl-alpha tocopheryl acetate) 30 units, B_1 3 mg, B_2 3 mg, B_3 15 mg, B_5 7 mg, B_6 20 mg, B_{12} 12 mcg, C 100 mg, folic acid 1 mg, Zn 20 mg, docusate sodium 25 mg. Tab. Bot. 100s. *Rx.*
Use: Mineral, vitamin supplement.

Prenatal 19 Chewable. (Cypress) Ca 200 mg, Fe 29 mg, vitamin A 1000 units, D 400 units, E (dl-alpha tocopheryl acetate) 30 units, B_1 3 mg, B_2 3 mg, B_3 15 mg, B_5 7 mg, B_6 20 mg, B_{12} 12 mcg, C 100 mg, folic acid 1 mg, Zn 20 mg, docusate sodium 25 mg, orange flavor. Tab. Bot. 100s. *Rx.*
Use: Mineral, vitamin supplement.

Prenatal PC 40. (Integrity) Ca 250 mg, Fe (as ferrous fumarate and carbonyl iron) 40 mg, vitamin D_3 6 mcg, E (dl-alpha tocopheryl acetate) 3.5 mg, B_1 3 mg, B_2 3.4 mg, B_3 20 mg, B_6 20 mg, B_{12} 12 mcg, C 50 mg, folic acid 1 mg, Zn 15 mc, CU, Mg, polydextrose. Tab. UD 100s. *Rx.*
Use: Multivitamin.

Prenatal Plus. (Ivax) Vitamins A (as acetate and carotene) 4000 units, D 400 units, E 22 mg, C 120 mg, folic acid 1 mg, B_1 1.84 mg, B_2 3 mg, B_3 20 mg, B_6 10 mg, B_{12} 12 mcg, Ca 200 mg, Fe 65 mg, Cu 2 mg, Zn 25 mg. Tab. Bot. 100s. *Rx.*
Use: Mineral, vitamin supplement.

Prenatal Plus Iron. (Major) Vitamins A 4000 units, D 400 units, E 22 mg, C 120 mg, folic acid 1 mg, B_1 1.84 mg, B_2 3 mg, niacinamide 20 mg, B_6 10 mg, B_{12} 12 mcg, Ca 200 mg, Cu 2 mg, Fe 27 mg, Zn 25 mg. Tab. Bot. 100s. *Rx.*
Use: Vitamin, mineral supplement.

Prenatal Rx with Beta Carotene. (Various Mfr.) Ca 200 mg, Fe 60 mg, vitamins A 4000 units, D 400 units, E 15 mg, B_1 1.5 mg, B_2 1.6 mg, B_3 17 mg, B_5 7 mg, B_6 4 mg, B_{12} 2.5 mcg, C 80 mg, folic acid 1 mg, biotin 30 mcg, Cu, Mg, Zn 25 mg. Tab. Bot. 100s, 500s. *Rx.*
Use: Mineral, vitamin supplement.

Prenatal-S. (Goldline) Ca 200 mg, iron 27 mg, vitamins A 4000 units, D 400 units, E 11 units, B_1 1.84 mg, B_2 1.7 mg, B_6 2.6 mg, B_{12} 4 mcg, C 100 mg, niacin 18 mg, folate 800 mcg, Zn 25 mg. Tab. Bot. 100s. *OTC.*
Use: Mineral, vitamin supplement.

Prenatal with Folic Acid. (Geneva) Ca 200 mg, Fe 60 mg, vitamins A 4000 units, D 400 units, E 11 mg, B_1 1.5 mg, B_2 1.7 mg, B_3 18 mg, B_6 2.6 mg, B_{12} 4 mcg, C 100 mg, folic acid 0.8 mg, Zn 25 mg. Tab. Bot. 100s. *OTC.*
Use: Mineral, vitamin supplement.

Prenatal with Folic Acid. (Eon Labs) Vitamins A 6000 units, D 400 units, E 30 units, folic acid 1 mg, C 60 mg, B_1 1.1 mg, B_2 1.8 mg, B_6 2.5 mg, B_{12} 5 mcg, niacin 15 mg, Ca 125 mg, Fe 65 mg. Tab. Bot. 100s, 1000s. *Rx.*
Use: Mineral, vitamin supplement.

Prenatal Z. (Ethex) Ca 300 mg, Fe 65 mg, vitamins A 5000 units, D 400 units, E 30 mg, B_1 3 mg, B_2 3 mg, B_3 20 mg, B_6 12.2 mg, B_{12} 12 mcg, C 80 mg, folic acid 1 mg, Zn 20 mg, I, Mg. Tab. Bot. 100s. *Rx.*
Use: Mineral, vitamin supplement.

Prenate Elite. (Sciele) Vitamins A 2500 units, C 80 mg, D_3 400 units, E 10 units, B_1 3 mg, B_2 3.4 mg, B_5 6 mg, B_6 20 mg, B_{12} 12 mcg, folate 1 mg, biotin 300 mcg, Ca 120 mg, Fe 27 mg, I, Cu, Mg, Zn. Hydrogenated soybean oil, hydrogenated vegetable oil, polyvinyl alcohol, povidone, sucrose. Tab. 90s. *Rx.*
Use: Nutritional combination product, prenatal vitamin with minerals.

Prenate 90. (Sanofi-Synthelabo) Vitamins A 4000 units, D 400 units, E 30 mg, C 120 mg, folic acid 1 mg, B_1 3 mg, B_2 3.4 mg, B_6 20 mg, B_{12} 12 mcg, B_3 20 mg, DSS, Ca 250 mg, I, Fe 90 mg, Cu, Zn 20 mg. FC Tab. Bot. 100s, 1000s. *Rx.*
Use: Mineral, vitamin supplement.

PreNate Plus. (Boca) Vitamins A 4,000 units, D 400 units, E 22 units, B_1 1.84 mg, B_2 3 mg, B_3 20 mg, B_6 10 mg, B_{12} 12 mcg, C 120 mg, Cu, Zn, folate 1 mg, Ca 200 mg, Fe 27 mg. Maltodextrin, mineral oil, sucrose. Tab. 100s. *Rx.*
Use: Prenatal vitamin with minerals.

Prenavite. (Rugby) Ca 200 mg, Fe 60 mg, vitamins A 4000 units, D 400 units, E 11 mg, B_1 1.5 mg, B_2 1.7 mg, B_3 18 mg, B_6 2.6 mg, B_{12} 4 mcg, C 100 mg, folic acid 0.8 mg, Zn 25 mg. Tab. Bot. 100s, 500s. *OTC.*
Use: Mineral, vitamin supplement.

PreNexa. (Upsher-Smith) Vitamins B_6 25 mg, C 28 mg, D_3 400 units, E (as d-alpha tocopherol acetate) 30 units, folic acid 1.25 mg, Ca 160 mg, Fe 27 mg,

DHA 300 mg, docusate sodium 55 mg. Glycerin, palm kernel oil, sodium benzoate, soybean oil, sunflower oil. Cap. 30s. *Rx.*
Use: Prenatal vitamin with minerals.

• **prenylamine.** (PREH-nill-ah-meen) USAN. Segontin; synadrin lactate.
Use: Coronary vasodilator.

Preparation H. (Wyeth Consumer Health) **Cream:** Glycerin 14.4%, phenylephrine hydrochloride 0.25%, pramoxine hydrochloride 1%, white petrolatum 15%. Aloe, cetyl alcohol, EDTA, mineral oil, parabens, stearyl alcohol. 15 g, 26 g. **Oint.:** Petrolatum 71.9%, mineral oil 14%, shark liver oil 3%, phenylephrine hydrochloride 0.25%, corn oil, glycerin, lanolin, lanolin alcohol, parabens, tocopherol. 30 g, 60 g. **Supp.:** Shark liver oil 3%, cocoa butter 79%, corn oil, EDTA, parabens, tocopherol. 12s, 24s, 36s, 48s. *OTC.*
Use: Anorectal preparation.

Preparation H Cooling. (Wyeth Consumer Health) Witch hazel 50%, phenylephrine hydrochloride 0.25%, alcohol 7.5%, EDTA, parabens. Gel. Tube 51 g. *OTC.*
Use: Anorectal preparation.

Prepcat. (Mallinckrodt) Barium sulfate 1.5%. Simethicone, sorbitol, strawberry flavor. Susp. Bot. 450 mL. *Rx.*
Use: Radiopaque agent, GI contrast agent.

Prepcat 2000. (Lafayette) Barium sulfate 1.2% w/w suspension. Bot. 2000 mL, Case Bot. 4s.
Use: Radiopaque agent.

Prepcort. (Whitehall-Robins) Hydrocortisone 0.5%. Cream. Tube 0.5 oz, 1 oz.
Use: Corticosteroid.

Pre-Pen. (ALK-Abelló) Benzylpenicilloyl polylysine 6 × 10^{-5} per 25 mL. Inj., Soln. Single-dose amp. *Rx.*
Use: In vivo diagnostic aid.

Prepidil. (Pharmacia) Dinoprostone 0.5 mg. Gel. Syringes (with 2 shielded catheters 10 and 20 mm tip) 3 g. *Rx.*
Use: Cervical ripening.

Prepodyne. (West) Titratable iodine.
Soln.: 1%. Bot. Pt, gal. **Scrub:** 0.75%. Bot. 6 oz, gal. **Swabs:** Saturated with soln. Pkt. 1s, Box 100s. **Swabsticks:** Saturated with soln. Pkt. 1s, Box 50s. Pkt. 3s, Box 75s.
Use: Antiseptic, topical.

Presalin. (Roberts) Aspirin 260 mg, salicylamide 120 mg, acetaminophen 120 mg, aluminum hydroxide 100 mg. Tab. Bot. 50s. *OTC.*
Use: Analgesic combination; antacid.

Prescription Strength Desenex. (Novartis Consumer Health) **Spray Liq.:** Miconazole nitrate 2%. SD alcohol 40-B 15%. 105 mL. **Spray Pow.:** Miconazole nitrate 2%. SD alcohol 40-B 10%, aloe vera gel. 90 mL. *OTC.*
Use: Antifungal, topical.

Preservative Free Moisture Eyes. (Bausch & Lomb) Propylene glycol 0.95%, boric acid, NaCl, KCl, sodium borate, EDTA. Soln. UD 32s. *OTC.*
Use: Artificial tear solution.

PreserVision Lutein. (Bausch & Lomb) Vitamin C 226 mg, E 200 units, Cu 0.8 mg, lutein 5 mg, Zn 34.75 mg. Softgel Cap. 50s. *OTC.*
Use: Nutritional combination product, multivitamin with minerals.

pressor agents.
See: Sympathomimetic agents.

Pressorol. (Baxter PPI) Metaraminol bitartrate 10 mg/mL. Inj. Vial 10 mL. *Rx.*
Use: Vasoconstrictor.

PreSun Active. (Bristol-Myers Squibb) Octyl methoxycinnamate, oxybenzone, octyl salicylate, 69% SD alcohol 40. PABA free. Waterproof. SPF 15, 30. Gel. 120 g. *OTC.*
Use: Sunscreen.

PreSun 8 Creamy. (Bristol-Myers Squibb) Padimate O 5%, oxybenzone 2%. Waterproof. SPF 8. Bot. 4 oz. *OTC.*
Use: Sunscreen.

PreSun 8 Lotion. (Bristol-Myers Squibb) Padimate O 7.3%, oxybenzone 2.3%, SD alcohol 40 60%. SPF 8. Bot. 4 oz. *OTC.*
Use: Sunscreen.

PreSun 15 Creamy. (Bristol-Myers Squibb) Padimate O 8%, oxybenzone 3%, benzyl alcohol. Waterproof. SPF 15. Bot. 4 oz. *OTC.*
Use: Sunscreen.

PreSun 15 Facial Sunscreen. (Bristol-Myers Squibb) Padimate O (octyl dimethyl PABA) 8%, oxybenzone 3%. SPF 15. Bot. 2 oz. *OTC.*
Use: Sunscreen.

PreSun 15 Facial Sunscreen Stick. (Bristol-Myers Squibb) Octyl dimethyl PABA 8%, oxybenzone 3%. SPF 15. Stick 0.42 oz. *OTC.*
Use: Sunscreen.

PreSun 15 Lip Protector. (Bristol-Myers Squibb) Padimate O 8%, oxybenzone 3%. SPF 15. Stick 4.5 g. *OTC.*
Use: Sunscreen.

PreSun 15 Lotion. (Bristol-Myers Squibb) Padimate O 5%, PABA 5%, oxybenzone 3%, SD alcohol 40 58%.

SPF 15. Bot. 4 oz. *OTC.*
Use: Sunscreen.

PreSun 15 Sensitive Skin Sunscreen. (Bristol-Myers Squibb) Octyl methoxycinnamate, oxybenzone, octyl salicylate, cetyl alcohol, PABA free, waterproof, SPF 15. Cream. Bot. 120 mL. *OTC.*
Use: Sunscreen.

PreSun for Kids. (Bristol-Myers Squibb) **Cream:** Octyl methoxycinnamate, oxybenzone, octyl salicylate, cetyl alcohol, PABA free. Waterproof. SPF 29. Bot. 120 mL. **Liq.:** Padimate O, octyl methoxycinnamate, oxybenzone, octyl salicylate, SD alcohol 40 19%. Waterproof. SPF 23. Spray Bot. 105 mL. *OTC.*
Use: Sunscreen.

PreSun 4 Creamy. (Bristol-Myers Squibb) Padimate O 1.4%, alcohol, titanium dioxide. Waterproof. Lot. SPF 4. Bot. 4 oz. *OTC.*
Use: Sunscreen.

PreSun Moisturizing. (Bristol-Myers Squibb) Octyl dimethyl PABA, oxybenzone, cetyl alcohol, diazolidinyl urea. SPF 46. Lot. Bot. 120 mL. *OTC.*
Use: Sunscreen.

PreSun Moisturizing Sunscreen with Keri, SPF 15. (Bristol-Myers Squibb) Octyl dimethyl PABA, oxybenzone, cetyl alcohol, diazolidinyl urea. Waterproof. Lot. Bot. 120 mL. *OTC.*
Use: Sunscreen.

PreSun Moisturizing Sunscreen with Keri, SPF 25. (Bristol-Myers Squibb) Octyl methoxycinnamate, oxybenzone, octyl salicylate, petrolatum, cetyl alcohol, diazolidinyl urea. Waterproof. Lot. Bot. 120 mL. *OTC.*
Use: Sunscreen.

PreSun Spray Mist. (Bristol-Myers Squibb) Octyl dimethyl PABA, octyl methoxycinnamate, oxybenzone, octyl salicylate, 19% SD alcohol 40, C12-15 alcohols benzoate. Waterproof. SPF 23. Liq. Bot. 120 mL. *OTC.*
Use: Sunscreen.

PreSun 39 Creamy Sunscreen. (Bristol-Myers Squibb) Padimate O, oxybenzone, cetyl alcohol. Waterproof. SPF 39. Cream Bot. 120 mL. *OTC.*
Use: Sunscreen.

PreSun 29 Sensitive Skin Sunscreen. (Bristol-Myers Squibb) Octyl methoxycinnamate, oxybenzone, octyl salicylate. Waterproof. SPF 29. Bot. 4 oz. *OTC.*
Use: Sunscreen.

PreSun 23. (Bristol-Myers Squibb) Padimate O, octyl methoxycinnamate, oxybenzone, octyl salicylate, SD alcohol 40 19%. Waterproof. SPF 23. Spray mist. Bot. 105 mL. *OTC.*
Use: Sunscreen.

PreSun Ultra. (Bristol-Myers Squibb) Avobenzone 3%, octyl methoxycinnamate 7.5%, octyl salicylate 5%, oxybenzone 6%. SPF 30. SD alcohol 65.5%. Gel. 120 mL. *OTC.*
Use: Sunscreen.

Pretend-U-Ate. (Vitalax) Enriched candy-appetite pacifier. Pkg. 20s. *OTC.*
Use: Dietary aid.

prethcamide. Mixture of crotethamide and cropropamide.
See: Micoren.

Pretts Diet Aid. (Milance Laboratories, Inc.) Alginic acid 200 mg, sodium carboxymethylcellulose 100 mg, sodium bicarbonate 70 mg. Chew. Tab. Bot. 60s. *OTC.*
Use: Dietary aid.

Pretty Feet & Hands. (B.F. Ascher) Paraffin, triethanolamine, parabens. Cream 90 g. *OTC.*
Use: Emollient.

Pretz Irrigation. (Parnell) Sodium chloride, yerba santa. Soln. Spray bot. 273 mL. *OTC.*
Use: Nasal decongestant.

Pretz Moisturizing. (Parnell) Sodium chloride, glycerin, yerba santa. Soln. Spray bot. 50 mL. *OTC.*
Use: Nasal decongestant.

Prevacid. (Takeda Pharmaceuticals) Lansoprazole. **DR Cap.:** 15 mg, 30 mg. Enteric-coated granules, sugar spheres, sucrose. Bot. 100s (30 mg only), 1000s, unit-of-use 30s, (15 mg only) UD 100s. **Gran. for DR Oral Susp.:** 15 mg, 30 mg. Enteric-coated granules, sugar, mannitol, docusate sodium, strawberry flavor. UD 30s. **Orally Disintegrating DR Tab.:** 15 mg (phenylalanine 2.5 mg), 30 mg (phenylalanine 5.1 mg). Mannitol, lactose, aspartame, strawberry flavor. Enteric-coated granules. UD 30s. *Rx.*
Use: Proton pump inhibitor.

Prevacid SoluTab. (TAP) Lansoprazole 15 mg (phenylalanine 2.5 mg), 30 mg (phenylalanine 5.1 mg). Mannitol, lactose, aspartame, strawberry flavor. DR Orally Disintegrating Tab. UD 30s. *Rx.*
Use: Proton pump inhibitor.

Prevacid 24 Hour. (Novartis) Lansoprazole 15 mg (contains enteric-coated granules). PEG, sugar spheres, sucrose. Cap., delayed release. 14s, 28s,

42s. *OTC.*
Use: Proton pump inhibitor.

Prevalite. (Upsher Smith) Cholestyramine 4 g (as anhydrous cholestyramine resin)/5.5 g powder. Aspartame, phenylalanine 14.1 mg/5.5 g, orange flavor. Pow. for Oral Susp. 5.5 g packets. 42s, 60s. Cans. 231 g (42 doses). *Rx.*
Use: Antihyperlipidemic; bile acid sequestrant.

PreviDent 5000 Plus. (Colgate Oral) Sodium fluoride 1.1%, sorbitol, saccharin, spearmint and fruit flavors. Dental Cream. Tube 51 g (1s, 2s). *Rx.*
Use: Caries prevention.

PreviDent Rinse. (Colgate Oral) Neutral sodium fluoride 0.2%, alcohol 6%, mint flavor. Sol. Bot. 250 mL, gal (w/pump dispenser). *Rx.*
Use: Dental caries agent.

Preview. (Lafayette) Barium sulfate 60% w/v suspension. Bot. 355 mL, Case 24 bot.
Use: Radiopaque agent.

Preview 2000. Barium sulfate 60% w/v suspension. Bot. 2000 mL, Case 4 Bot.
Use: Radiopaque agent.

Previfem. (Qualitest) Ethinyl estradiol 35 mcg, norgestimate 0.25 mg. Lactose. Tab. 28s w/7 white inert tablets. *Rx.*
Use: Oral contraceptive, monophasic contraceptive.

Prevision. Mestranol, USP.

Prevnar. (Wyeth Lederle Vaccines) 6 polysaccharide isolates 2 mcg each, 1 polysaccharide isolate 4 mcg per 0.5 mL, aluminum 0.125 mg/dose. Inj. Prefilled syringe. 0.5 mL. *Rx.*
Use: Immunization.

Prevnar 13. (Wyeth) Total saccharides 30.8 mcg (each 0.5 mL dose contains ≈ 2.2 mcg of each of *Streptococcus pneumonia* serotypes 1, 3, 4, 5, 6A, 7F, 9V, 14, 18C, 19A, 19F, and 23F saccharides; and 4.4 mcg of serotype 6B saccharides) per 0.5 mL dose. Inj., Susp. Single-dose, prefilled syringe (also contains CRM_{197} carrier protein 34 mcg, 100 mcg of polysorbate 80, succinate buffer 295 mcg, aluminum 125 mcg as aluminum phosphate adjuvant per dose). 0.5 mL. *Rx.*
Use: Agent for active immunization, bacterial vaccine.

Prevpac. (Takeda Pharmaceuticals) Two *Prevacid* (lansoprazole) 30 mg Cap. Four *Trimox* (amoxicillin) 500 mg Cap. Two *Biaxin* (clarithromycin) 500 mg. Tab. Daily administration pack.
Use: H. pylori eradication.

Prexonate. (Tennessee Pharmaceutic) Vitamins A acetate 5000 units, D 500 units, B_6 2 mg, B_1 5 mg, B_2 2 mg, C 100 mg, B_{12} 2.5 mcg, calcium pantothenate 1 mg, niacinamide 15 mg, folic acid 1 mg, Fe 45 mg, Ca 500 mg, intrinsic factor 3 mg. Tab. Bot. 100s, 1000s. *Rx.*
Use: Mineral, vitamin supplement.

•**prezatide copper acetate.** (PREH-zat-IDE KAH-per) USAN.
Use: Immunomodulator.

Prezista. (Tibotec Therapeutics) Darunavir ethanolate 75 mg, 150 mg, 400 mg, 600 mg. Film-coated. Tab. 60s (400 mg and 600 mg), 240s (150 mg), 480s (75 mg). *Rx.*
Use: Antiretroviral, protease inhibitor.

Prialt. (Azur Pharma) Ziconotide 25 mcg/mL (used only for ziconotide-naive pump priming), 100 mcg/mL. Preservative free. L-methionine. Inj. Single-use vials. 1 mL, 2 mL, 5 mL (100 mcg/mL only); 20 mL (25 mcg/mL only). *Rx.*
Use: Management of severe chronic pain.

•**pridefine hydrochloride.** (PRIH-deh-FEEN) USAN.
Use: Antidepressant.

•**pridopidine.** (pri-DOE-pi-deen) USAN.
Use: CNS agent.

•**pridopidine hydrochloride.** (pri-DOE-pi-deen) USAN.
Use: CNS agent.

Prid Salve. (Walker) Ichthammol, Phenol, Lead Oleate, Rosin, Beeswax, Lard. Tin 20 g. *OTC.*
Use: Drawing salve.

•**prifelone.** (PRIH-feh-LONE) USAN.
Use: Anti-inflammatory, dermatologic.

Priftin. (Aventis) Rifapentine 150 mg. EDTA, polyethylene glycol. Tab. Bot. 32s. *Rx.*
Use: Antituberculosal.

•**priliximab.** (prih-LICK-sih-mab) USAN.
Use: Monoclonal antibody (autoimmune lymphoproliferative diseases, organ transplantation).

•**prilocaine.** (PRIL-oh-kane) USAN.
Use: Anesthetic, local.
W/Lidocaine.
See: EMLA.
EMLA Anesthetic.
Oraqix.

•**prilocaine and epinephrine injection.** USP 34.
Use: Anesthetic, local.

•**prilocaine hydrochloride.** (PRIL-oh-kane) USP 34.
Use: Anesthetic, local amide.

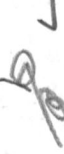

See: Citanest Forte.
  Citanest Plain.
Prilosec. (AstraZeneca) Omeprazole. **DR
  Cap.:** 10 mg, 20 mg, 40 mg. Lactose,
  mannitol. Enteric-coated granules. 100s
  (40 mg only), 1000s, unit-of-use 30s.
  DR Susp.: 2.5 mg, 10 mg. Dextrose,
  sugar spheres. UD 30s. *Rx.*
  Tall Man: PriLOSEC
  Use: Proton pump inhibitor.
Prilosec OTC. (Proctor and Gamble)
  Omeprazole magnesium 20 mg. Su-
  crose, talc. DR Tab. 14s, 28s, 42s.
  OTC.
  Tall Man: PriLOSEC
  Use: Proton pump inhibitor.
primacaine.
  Use: Anesthetic, local.
•**primaquine phosphate.** (PRIM-uh-
  kween) *USP 34.*
  Use: Antimalarial.
primaquine phosphate. (Sanofi-
  Synthelabo) Primaquine phosphate
  26.3 mg. Tab. Bot. 100s.
  Use: Antimalarial.
primaquine phosphate. (Sanofi-
  Synthelabo)
  Use: Treatment of AIDS-associated
  PCP. [Orphan Drug]
Primatene. (Wyeth Consumer Health-
  care) Ephedrine hydrochloride
  12.5 mg, guaifenesin 200 mg. Tab. 24s,
  60s. *OTC.*
  Use: Upper respiratory combination, de-
  congestant and expectorant combina-
  tion.
Primatene M. (Wyeth Consumer Health-
  care) Theophylline 118 mg, ephedrine
  hydrochloride 24 mg, pyrilamine
  maleate 16.6 mg. Tab. Bot. 24s, 60s.
  OTC.
  Use: Antihistamine, bronchodilator.
Primatene Mist. (Wyeth Consumer
  Healthcare) Epinephrine 0.22 mg/spray.
  Alcohol 34%, chlorofluorocarbon. Aer.
  Bot. 15 mL w/mouthpiece or 15 mL refills. *OTC.*
  Use: Bronchodilator, sympathomimetic;
  vasopressor.
Primatene Mist Suspension. (Wyeth
  Consumer Healthcare) Epinephrine bi-
  tartrate 0.3 mg. Bot. 10 mL w/mouth-
  piece. Spray. *OTC.*
  Use: Bronchodilator.
Primatene P. (Wyeth Consumer Health-
  care) Theophylline 118 mg, ephedrine
  hydrochloride 24 mg, phenobarbital
  8 mg. Tab. Bot. 24s, 60s. *OTC.*
  Use: Bronchodilator; hypnotic; sedative.

Primatuss Cough Mixture 4. (Rugby)
  Doxylamine succinate 3.75 mg, dex-
  tromethorphan HBr 7.5 mg/5 mL, alco-
  hol 10%. Liq. Bot. 180 mL. *OTC.*
  Use: Antihistamine; antitussive.
Primatuss Cough Mixture 4D. (Rugby)
  Pseudoephedrine hydrochloride 20 mg,
  dextromethorphan HBr 10 mg, guaifenesin 67 mg/5 mL, alcohol 10%. Liq.
  Bot. 120 mL. *OTC.*
  Use: Antitussive; decongestant; expectorant.
Primaxin I.M. (Merck) Imipenem 500 mg,
  cilastatin 500 mg. Sodium 1.4 mEq.
  Pow. for Inj. Vials. *Rx.*
  Use: Anti-infective.
Primaxin I.V. (Merck) Imipenem 250 mg,
  cilastatin 250 mg, sodium 0.8 mEq. Imi-
  penem 500 mg, cilastatin 500 mg, so-
  dium 1.6 mEq. Pow. for Inj. Vials, infu-
  sion bottles, *ADD-Vantage* vials. *Rx.*
  Use: Anti-infective.
•**primidolol.** (prih-MID-oh-lahl) USAN.
  Use: Antianginal; antihypertensive; cardiovascular agent, antiarrhythmic.
•**primidone.** (PRIM-ih-dohn) *USP 34.*
  Use: Anticonvulsant.
  See: Mysoline.
primidone. (Lannett) Primidone 50 mg.
  Tab. 100s, 500s, 1000s. *Rx.*
  Use: Anticonvulsant.
primidone. (Various Mfr.) Primidone
  250 mg. Tab. Bot. 100s, 500s, 1000s.
  Rx.
  Use: Anticonvulsant.
Primlev. (Atley) Acetaminophen/oxy-
  codone hydrochloride 300 mg/5 mg,
  300 mg/7.5 mg, 300 mg/10 mg. Tab.
  100s. *c-ii.*
  Use: Opioid analgesic combination.
primostrum. A prep. of primiparous co-
  lostrum.
Primsol. (Ascent Pediatrics) Trimetho-
  prim 50 mg/5 mL, parabens, sorbitol,
  alcohol free, bubble gum flavor. Oral
  Soln. Bot. 473 mL. *Rx.*
  Use: Anti-infective.
•**prinaberel.** (prin-a BER-el) USAN.
  Use: Anti-inflammatory.
Principen. (Geneva) Ampicillin trihydrate.
  Cap.: 250 mg, 500 mg, lactose. Bot.
  100s, 500s, UD 100s. **Pow. for Oral
  Susp.:** 125 mg/5 mL, 250 mg/5 mL, su-
  crose, fruit flavor. Bot. 100 mL, 150 mL
  (125 mg/5 mL only), 200 mL. *Rx.*
  Use: Anti-infective, penicillin.
Principen with Probenecid. (Bristol-
  Myers Squibb) Ampicillin (as trihydrate)
  3.5 g, probenecid 1 g/regimen. Single-
  dose Bot. 9s. *Rx.*
  Use: Anti-infective, penicillin.

Prinivil. (Merck) Lisinopril 10 mg, 20 mg. Mannitol. Tab. Bot. Unit-of-use 90s. *Rx.*
Use: Renin angiotensin antagonist, angiotensin-converting enzyme inhibitor.

•**prinomastat.** (pri-NOE-ma-stat) USAN.
Use: Antineoplastic; antiangiogenic; retinal and subfoveal choroidal neovascularization.

•**prinomide tromethamine.** (PRIH-no-MIDE troe-METH-ah-meen) USAN.
Use: Antirheumatic.

•**prinoxodan.** (prin-OX-oh-dan) USAN.
Use: Cardiovascular agent.

Prinzide. (Merck) Lisinopril/hydrochlorothiazide 10 mg/12.5 mg, 20 mg/12.5 mg, 20 mg/25 mg. Tab. Unit-of-use 30s (20 mg/25 mg only), unit-of-use 100s. *Rx.*
Use: Antihypertensive.

Pristiq. (Wyeth) Desvenlafaxine 50 mg (equiv. to desvenlafaxine succinate 76 mg), 100 mg (equiv. to desvenlafaxine succinate 152 mg). Dextrose. ER Tab. 14s, 30s, 90s, 10 blisters of 10s. *Rx.*
Use: Antidepressant, serotonin and norepinephrine reuptake inhibitor.

Privigen. (CSL Behring) Immune globulin (human) 10% (100 mg/mL). Preservative free. Inj., Soln. Single-use vials. 5 g, 10 g, 20 g. *Rx.*
Use: Immune globulin.

Privine. (Insight) Naphazoline hydrochloride, benzalkonium chloride, EDTA. Soln. Dropper bot. 25 mL. Spray bot. 20 mL. *OTC.*
Use: Nasal decongestant, imidazoline.

•**prizidilol hydrochloride.** (PRIH-zie-DILL-ole) USAN.
Use: Antihypertensive.

Pro-Acet Douche Concentrate. (Pro-Acet) Lactic, citric, and acetic acids, sodium lauryl sulfate, lactose, dextrose, sodium acetate. Pkg. polyethylene envelope 10 mL. Contents of 1 envelope to be diluted with 2 quarts of water. Douche 6 oz, 12 oz. Travel Packet 10 mL. *OTC.*
Use: Vaginal agent.

•**proadifen hydrochloride.** (pro-AD-ih-fen) USAN.
Use: Synergist, nonspecific.

ProAir HFA. (Ivax) Albuterol (as sulfate) 90 mcg/actuation. Contains no chlorofluorocarbons. Aerosol. 8.5 g (200 inhalations). *Rx.*
Use: Bronchodilator; sympathomimetics.

ProAmatine. (Shire) Midodrine hydrochloride 2.5 mg, 5 mg, 10 mg. Tab.

Bot. 100s. *Rx.*
Use: Orthostatic hypotension; vasopressor.

Probarbital Sodium. 5-Ethyl-5-isopropyl-barbiturate sodium.

Probax. (Fischer) Propolis 2%, petrolatum, mineral oil, lanolin. Gel. Tube 3.5 g. *OTC.*
Use: Mouth and throat preparation.

Probec-T. (Roberts) Vitamins B_1 12.2 mg, B_2 10 mg, B_3 100 mg, B_5 18.4, B_6 4.1 mg, B_{12} 5 mcg, C 600 mg. Tab. Bot. 60s. *OTC.*
Use: Mineral, vitamin supplement.

Proben-C. (Rugby) Probenecid 500 mg, colchicine 0.5 mg. Tab. Bot. 100s, 1000s. *Rx.*
Use: Antigout agent.

•**probenecid.** (pro-BEN-uh-sid) *USP 34.*
Use: Uricosuric.
W/Ampicillin.
See: Principen w/Probenecid.

probenecid and colchicine.
Use: Agent for gout.

probenecid and colchicine. (Various Mfr.) Probenecid 500 mg, colchicine 0.5 mg. Tab. Bot. 100s, 1000s. *Rx.*
Use: Agent for gout.

•**probicromil calcium.** (pro-BYE-KROE-mill) USAN.
Use: Antiallergic, prophylactic.

Pro-Bionate. (NaTREN) *Lactobacillus acidophilus* strain NAS 2 billion units/g. **Pow.:** 52.5 g, 90 g. **Cap.:** Bot. 30s, 60s. *OTC.*
Use: Antidiarrheal; nutritional supplement.

Probiotic Formula. (Rugby) *Lactobacillus acidophilus* 2 billion CFU, *L. salivarius* 2 billion CFU, *L. plantarum* 2 billion CFU, *L. casei* 2 billion CFU, *Bifidobacterium lactis* 2 billion CFU. Cap. 30s. *OTC.*
Use: Nutritional supplement, probiotic.

•**probucol.** (PRO-byoo-kahl) *USP 34.*
Use: Antihyperlipidemic.
See: Lorelco.

•**probutate.** (pro-BYOO-tate) USAN. Formerly buteprate.
Use: Radical.

•**procainamide hydrochloride.** (pro-CANE-uh-mide) *USP 34.*
Use: Cardiovascular agent, antiarrhythmic.

procainamide hydrochloride. (Hospira) Procainamide hydrochloride 100 mg/mL. Methylparaben. Inj. Soln. Vials. 10 mL. *Rx.*
Use: Antiarrhythmic agent.

procainamide hydrochloride. (Various Mfr.) Procainamide hydrochloride 500 mg/mL. Inj. Vial. 2 mL. *Rx.*
Use: Antiarrhythmic.

•**procaine and tetracaine hydrochlorides and levonordefrin injection.** *USP 34.*
Use: Anesthetic, local.

procaine base.
Use: Anesthetic, local.
See: Anucaine.

•**procaine hydrochloride.** (pro-CANE) *USP 34.* Bernocaine, Chlorocaine, Ethocaine, Irocaine, Kerocaine, Syncaine.
Use: Anesthetic, injectable local.
See: Novocain.

procaine hydrochloride. (Various Mfr.) Procaine hydrochloride 1%, 2%, may contain sodium metabisulfite. Inj. Multiple-dose vials. 30 mL.
Use: Anesthetic, injectable local.

•**procaine hydrochloride and epinephrine injection.** *USP 34.*
Use: Anesthetic, local.

procaine hydrochloride and levonordefrin injection.
Use: Anesthetic, local.

procaine, penicillin G suspension, sterile.
Use: Anti-infective, penicillin.
See: Penicillin G Procaine.
Pfizerpen.

procaine, penicillin G w/aluminum stearate suspension, sterile.
Use: Anti-infective, penicillin.
See: Penicillin G Procaine with Aluminum Stearate Suspension, Sterile.

procaine, tetracaine and nordefrin hydrochlorides injection.
Use: Anesthetic, local.

procaine, tetracaine and phenylephrine hydrochlorides injection.
Use: Anesthetic.

Pro-Cal. (Pro-Biotiks) Ca 750 mg, Mg 160 mg, P 580 mg, vitamin D 400 units, C 30 mg. Levulose. Tab. 120s, 240s. *OTC.*
Use: Nutritional supplement, vitamin.

ProcalAmine Injection. (McGaw) Injection of amino acid 3%, glycerin 3%, electrolytes. Bot. 1000 mL. *Rx.*
Use: Nutritional supplement, parenteral.

•**procarbazine hydrochloride.** (pro-CAR-buh-ZEEN) *USP 34.* (Roche) Natulan.
Use: Cytostatic; antineoplastic.
See: Matulane.

Procardia. (Pfizer) Nifedipine 10 mg, 20 mg. Saccharin (10 mg only). Liquid filled. Cap. Bot. 100s, 300s (10 mg only). *Rx.*
Use: Calcium channel blocker.

Procardia XL. (Pfizer) Nifedipine. Film-coated. ER Tab. **30 mg, 60 mg:** Bot. 100s, 300s, 5000s, UD 100s. **90 mg:** Bot 100s, UD 100s. *Rx.*
Use: Calcium channel blocker.

•**procaterol hydrochloride.** (PRO-CAT-ehr-ole) USAN.
Use: Bronchodilator.

ProCentra. (FSC Laboratories) Dextroamphetamine sulfate 5 mg per 5 mL. Saccharin, sorbitol. Bubble gum flavor. Soln. 473 mL. *c-ii.*
Use: Amphetamine.

Proception Sperm Nutrient Douche. (Milex) Ringer type glucose douche. Bot. sufficient for 10 douches. *OTC.*
Use: Vaginal agent.

•**prochlorperazine.** (PROE-klor-PER-a-zeen) *USP 34.*
Use: Antiemetic, antipsychotic.
See: Compro.

prochlorperazine. (Various Mfr.) Prochlorperazine. **Inj.:** 5 mg/mL. Vials. 10 mL. **Supp.:** 2.5 mg, 5 mg, 25 mg. 12s. *Rx.*
Use: Antiemetic, antipsychotic.

prochlorperazine. (Various Mfr.) Prochlorperazine maleate 5 mg, 10 mg, 25 mg. Tab. 12s (5 mg only), 30s (except 25 mg), 100s, 1000s, UD 32s (10 mg only), UD 100s. *Rx.*
Use: Antiemetic.

prochlorperazine. (Wyeth-Ayerst) Prochlorperazine edisylate 5 mg/mL. Inj. Amps. 2 mL. Vials. 2 mL, 10 mL. *Rx.*
Use: Antiemetic.

•**prochlorperazine edisylate.** (PROE-klor-PER-a-zeen e-DIS-i-late) *USP 34.*
Use: Antipsychotic; antiemetic.
See: Compazine.

prochlorperazine edisylate. (Various Mfr.) Prochlorperazine edisylate 5 mg/mL. Inj. 2 mL vials. *Rx.*
Use: Antipsychotic.

prochlorperazine ethanedisulfonate. Prochlorperazine Edisylate, USP.
Use: Anxiolytic.

prochlorperazine/isopropamide. (Various Mfr.) Isopropamide iodide 5 mg, prochlorperazine maleate 10 mg. Cap. Bot. 100s, 500s, 1000s, UD 100s. *Rx.*
Use: Anticholinergic; antispasmodic; antiemetic; antivertigo.

•**prochlorperazine maleate.** (PROE-klor-PER-a-zeen) *USP 34.*
Use: Antiemetic; antipsychotic.
See: Compazine.

prochlorperazine maleate. (Various Mfr.) Prochlorperazine maleate 5 mg, 10 mg. Tab. Bot. 100s, 500s, 1000s, UD 100s. Blister packs. 25s. *Rx.*
Use: Antipsychotic.

•**procinonide.** (pro-SIN-oh-nide) USAN.
Use: Adrenocortical steroid.

Pro-Clear. (ProPharma) Codeine phosphate 9 mg, guaifenesin 200 mg. Maltodextrin, tartrazine. Cap. 100s. *c-v.*
Use: Upper respiratory combination, antitussive with expectorant.

•**proclonol.** (PRO-klah-nole) USAN. Under study.
Use: Anthelmintic; antifungal.

Pro Comfort Athlete's Foot Spray. (Scholl) Tolnaftate 1%. Aer. Can 4 oz. *OTC.*
Use: Antifungal, topical.

Pro Comfort Jock Itch Spray Powder. (Scholl) Tolnaftate 1%. Aer. Can 3.5 oz. *OTC.*
Use: Antifungal, topical.

ProCoMycin. (Physicians Science and Nature) Polymyxin B sulfate 10,000 units/g, neomycin 3.5 mg/g, bacitracin zinc 500 units/g, lidocaine 40 mg. Aloe, avocado oil, cetearyl alcohol, parabens. Oint. 15 g. *OTC.*
Use: Topical anti-infective, antibiotic combination.

Procort. (Roberts) Hydrocortisone 1%. **Cream:** Tube 30 g. **Spray:** Can. 45 mL. *OTC.*
Use: Corticosteroid, topical.

Procrit. (Ortho Biotech) Epoetin alfa, recombinant 2000 units/mL, 3000 units/mL, 4000 units/mL, 10,000 units/mL, 20,000 units/mL, 40,000 units/mL. Inj. Soln. Single-dose vials. 1 mL, preservative free with albumin (human) 2.5 mg/mL (except 20,000 units/mL). Multidose vials. 1 mL (20,000 units/mL only) and 2 mL (10,000 units only), preserved with benzyl alcohol 1% and with albumin (human) 2.5 mg/mL. *Rx.*
Use: Hematopoietic.

Proctocort. (Salix) Hydrocortisone. Cream 30 g w/rectal applicator. Hydrocortisone acetate 30 mg. Supp. Box. 12s. *Rx.*
Use: Corticosteroid.

ProctoCream-HC 2.5%. (Schwarz Pharma) Hydrocortisone 2.5%, glyceryl monostearate, glycerin, stearyl alcohol, benzyl alcohol. Cream. Tube 30 g. *Rx.*
Use: Corticosteroid.

ProctoFoam. (Alaven Pharmaceutical) Pramoxine hydrochloride 1%. Aer. Foam. Bot. 15 g w/applicator. *OTC.*
Use: Topical local anesthetic.

ProctoFoam-HC. (Alaven) Hydrocortisone acetate 1%, pramoxine hydrochloride 1% in hydrophilic foam base. Bot. aerosol container, Aerosol foam 10 g w/applicator. *Rx.*
Use: Corticosteroid; anesthetic, local.

Pro-Cute. (Ferndale) Silicone, hexachlorophene, lanolin. Cream. 2 oz, lb. *OTC.*
Use: Emollient.

ProCycle Gold. (Cyclin) Vitamins A 833.3 units, D 66.7 units, E 66.7 units, C 30 mg, B_1 1.7 mg, B_2 1.7 mg, B_3 3.3 mg, B_5 1.7 mg, B_6 3.3 mg, B_{12} 21 mcg, folic acid 66.7 mg, Ca 166.7 mg, Fe 3 mg, Zn 2.5 mg, B, Cu, Cr, I, Mg, Mn, Se, PABA, inositol, rutin, biotin, hesperidin, pancreatin, betaine. Tab. Sugar free. Bot. 100s. *OTC.*
Use: Mineral, vitamin supplement.

•**procyclidine hydrochloride.** (pro-SIklih-deen) *USP 34.*
Use: Muscle relaxant; antiparkinsonian.

Procysteine. (Free Radical Sciences)
See: L_2-Oxothiazolidine$_4$-carboxylic acid.

Proderm Topical Dressing. (Dow Hickam) Castor oil 650 mg, Peruvian balsam 72.5 mg/0.82 mL. Aer. 4 oz. *OTC.*
Use: Dermatologic, wound therapy.

•**prodilidine hydrochloride.** (pro-DIH-lih-deen) USAN.
Use: Analgesic.

Prodium. (Breckenridge) Phenazopyramide hydrochloride 95 mg. Tab. 12s, 30s. *OTC.*
Use: Analgesic.

•**prodolic acid.** (PRO-dole-ik acid) USAN.
Use: Anti-inflammatory.

Prodrin. (Gentex Pharma) Acetaminophen 500 mg, caffeine 20 mg, isometheptene mucate 130 mg. Tab. 50s. *Rx.*
Use: Agent for migraine, migraine combination.

Pro-Est. (Burgin-Arden) Progesterone 25 mg, estrogenic substance 25,000 units, sodium carboxymethylcellulose 1 mg, sodium Cl 0.9%, benzalkonium Cl 1:10,000, sodium phosphate dibasic 0.1% in water. *Rx.*
Use: Estrogen, progestin combination.

•**profadol hydrochloride.** (PRO-fah-dahl) USAN.
Use: Analgesic.

Profamina.
See: Amphetamine.

Pro-Fast HS. (American Pharmaceutical) Phentermine hydrochloride 18.75 mg (equivalent to 15 mg phentermine base), EDTA, benzyl alcohol, parabens. Cap. Bot. 100s. *c-iv.*
Use: CNS stimulant, anorexiant.

Pro-Fast SR. (American Pharmaceutical) Phentermine hydrochloride 37.5 mg (equivalent to 30 mg phentermine base), sugar, tartrazine, EDTA, benzyl alcohol, parabens. Cap. Bot. 100s. *c-iv.*
Use: CNS stimulant, anorexiant.

Profen Forte. (Ivax) Pseudoephedrine hydrochloride 90 mg, guaifenesin 800 mg. ER Tab. Bot. 100s *Rx.*
Use: Upper respiratory combination; decongestant, expectorant.

Profen Forte DM. (Ivax) Pseudoephedrine hydrochloride 90 mg, dextromethorphan HBr 60 mg, guaifenesin 800 mg. SR Tab. Bot. 100s. *Rx.*
Use: Upper respiratory combination, antitussive, decongestant, expectorant.

Profen II. (Ivax) Pseudoephedrine hydrochloride 45 mg, guaifenesin 800 mg. ER Tab. Bot. 100s. *Rx.*
Use: Upper respiratory combination, decongestant, expectorant.

Profen II DM. (Ivax) Pseudoephedrine hydrochloride 45 mg, guaifenesin 800 mg, dextromethorphan HBr 30 mg. ER Tab. Bot. 100s. *Rx.*
Use: Upper respiratory combination, antitussive, decongestant, expectorant.

Professional Care Lotion, Extra Strength. (Walgreen) Zinc oxide 0.25% in a lotion base. Lot. Bot. 16 oz. *OTC.*
Use: Astringent; antiseptic, dermatologic.

Profiber. (Sherwood Davis & Geck) Sodium caseinate, dietary fiber from soy, calcium caseinate, hydrolyzed cornstarch, corn oil, soy lecithin, vitamins A, B_1, B_2, B_3, B_5, B_6, B_{12}, C, D, E, K, folic acid, biotin, choline, Ca, Cl, Cr, Cu, Fe, I, Mg, Mn, Mo, P, Se, Zn. Liq. Can 250 mL, closed system 1000 mL. *OTC.*
Use: Nutritional supplement.

Profilnine SD. (Grifols) Factor IX, II, X, and low amounts of VII (human). Preservative free. Solvent/detergent treated. Inj., lyophilized Pow. for Soln. Inj. Kit w/single-dose vials and sterile water for injection. *Rx.*
Use: Antihemophilic agent.

proflavine dihydrochloride. 3,6-Diaminoacridine dihydrochloride.

proflavine sulfate. 3,6-Diaminoacridine sulfate.

• **progabide.** (pro-GAB-ide) USAN.
Use: Anticonvulsant, muscle relaxant.

Progens. (Major) Conjugated estrogens. Tab. **0.625 mg:** Bot. 100s, 1000s. **1.25 mg:** Bot. 1000s. **2.5 mg:** Bot. 100s, 1000s. *Rx.*
Use: Estrogen.

Pro-Gesic. (Nastech) Trolamine salicylate 10%, propylene glycol, methylparahydroxybenzoic acid, propyl parahydroxybenzoic acid, EDTA. Liq. Bot. 75 mL. *OTC.*
Use: Liniment.

• **progesterone.** (pro-JESS-ter-ohn) *USP 34.* Flavolutan, Luteogan, Luteosan, Lutren.
Use: Hormone, progestin.
W/Oil.
See: Crinone.
Endometrin.
Prochieve.
Prometrium.

progesterone. (Various Mfr.) Progesterone Pow. 1 g, 10 g, 25 g, 100 g, 1000 g.
Use: Hormone, progestin.

progesterone in oil. (Various Mfr.) Progesterone 50 mg/mL. May contain sesame oil, benzyl alcohol. Inj. Multidose vials. 10 mL. *Rx.*
Use: Sex hormone, progestin.

progestins. Progesterone.
Use: Sex hormone.
See: Estrogens and Progestins Combined.
Hydroxyprogesterone Caproate.
Medroxyprogesterone Acetate.
Megestrol Acetate.
Micronor.
Norethindrone.
Norethindrone Acetate.
Nor-QD.
Progesterone.

• **proglumide.** (pro-GLUE-mid) USAN. (Wallace)
Use: Anticholinergic.

Proglycem. (Baker Norton) **Cap.:** Diazoxide 50 mg. Bot. 100s. **Oral Susp.:** Diazoxide 50 mg/mL. Alcohol 7.25%, parabens, sorbitol. Chocolate-mint flavor. 30 mL w/calibrated dropper. *Rx.*
Use: Hyperglycemic.

Prograf. (Astellas) Tacrolimus. **Cap.:** 0.5 mg, 1 mg, 5 mg. Lactose. 100s, blister cards of 10s. **Inj.:** 5 mg/mL. Polyoxyl 60 hydrogenated castor oil (HCO-60) 200 mg/mL, dehydrated alcohol 80%. Amp. 1 mL. *Rx.*
Use: Immunosuppressant.

proguanil hydrochloride.
See: Chloroguanide hydrochloride.

W/Atovaquone.
See: Malarone.
Malarone Pediatric.

ProHance. (Bracco Diagnostics) Gadoteridol 279.3 mg/mL. Preservative free. Inj. Soln. Single-dose vials. 5 mL fill in 15 mL; 10 mL, 15 mL, 20 mL fill in 30 mL. Prefilled syringes. 10 mL and 17 ml fill in 20 mL. *Rx.*
Use: Radiopaque agent, parenteral.

ProHIBiT. (Aventis Pasteur) Purified capsular polysaccharide of *Haemophilus influenzae* type b 25 mcg, conjugated diphtheria toxoid protein 18 mcg/0.5 mL dose. Also called PRP-D. Inj. Vial 0.5 mL, 2.5 mL, 5 mL. Syr. 0.5 mL. *Rx.*
Use: Immunization.

Prohist CF. (Poly Pharmaceuticals) Chlophedianol hydrochloride 25 mg, triprolidine hydrochloride 2.5 mg. Glycerin, propylene glycol, saccharin, sorbitol. Grape flavor. Liq. 473 mL. *Rx.*
Use: Upper respiratory combination, antitussive combination.

Prohist DM. (ProEthic) Dextromethorphan HBr 5 mg, brompheniramine maleate 1 mg, pseudoephedrine hydrochloride 12 mg per 1 mL. Alcohol and dye free. Magnasweet, menthol, saccharin, sucrose. Grape flavor. Drops. 30 mL with dropper. *Rx.*
Use: Upper respiratory combination, antitussive combination.

• **proinsulin human.** (PRO-in-suh-LIN HYOO-muhn) USAN.
Use: Antidiabetic.

Prolactin RIA. (Abbott Diagnostics) Quantitative measurement of total circulating human prolactin. Test unit 50s, 100s.
Use: Diagnostic aid.

Prolactin RIAbead. (Abbott Diagnostics) Radioimmunoassay for the quantitative measurement of prolactin in human serum and plasma.
Use: Diagnostic aid.

proladyl. Pyrrobutamine.
Use: Antihistamine.

prolase. Proteolytic enzyme from *Carica papaya.*
See: Papain.

Prolastin. (Bayer) Alpha$_1$-proteinase inhibitor 500 mg, 1000 mg ($\geq$ 20 mg alpha$_1$-PI/mL when reconstituted). Preservative free w/polyethylene glycol, sucrose and small amounts of other plasma proteins. Pow. for Inj., lyophilized. Single-dose vial w/20 mL diluent (500 mg only), w/40 mL diluent (1000 mg only). *Rx.*
Use: Alpha$_1$-proteinase inhibitor.

Proleukin. (Prometheus) Aldesleukin (interleukin-2) 22 $\times$ 10^6 IU/vial (18 million IU [1.1 mg] per mL when reconstituted). Mannitol 50 mg, sodium dodecyl sulfate 0.18 mg, monobasic 0.17 mg and dibasic 0.89 mg sodium phosphate. Preservative free. Pow. for Inj., lyophilized. Single-use vials. *Rx.*
Use: Biological response modifiers.

Prolex DM. (Blansett) Dextromethorphan hydrobromide 15 mg, potassium guaiacolsulfonate 300 mg per 5 mL. Alcohol free and sugar free. Pineappleorange flavor. Liq. 473 mL. *Rx.*
Use: Upper respiratory combination, antitussive with expectorant.

Prolex DMX. (Blansett Pharmacal) Dextromethorphan hydrobromide 15 mg, potassium guaiacolsulfonate 100 mg per 5 mL. Benzoic acid, menthol, propylene glycol, saccharin, sorbitol. Alcohol free and sugar free. Pineappleorange flavor. Liq. 473 mL. *Rx.*
Use: Upper respiratory combination, antitussive with expectorant.

Prolia. (Amgen) Denosumab 60 mg/mL. Sorbitol 4.7%. Preservative free. Inj., Soln. Single-use, prefilled syringe and vial. *Rx.*
Use: Monoclonal antibody.

• **proline.** (PRO-leen) *USP 34.*
Use: Amino acid.

• **prolintane hydrochloride.** (pro-LIN-tane) USAN.
Use: Antidepressant.

Proloprim. (GlaxoSmithKline) Trimethoprim 100 mg. Tab. Bot. 100s, UD 100s (in sesame oil with benzyl alcohol). *Rx.*
Use: Anti-infective, urinary.

Promacet. (MCR American) Acetaminophen 650 mg, butalbital 50 mg. Tab. 100s. *Rx.*
Use: Nonnarcotic analgesic.

Promachlor. (Geneva) Chlorpromazine hydrochloride 10 mg, 25 mg, 50 mg, 100 mg, 200 mg. Tab. Bot. 100s, 1000s. *Rx.*
Use: Antiemetic; antivertigo; antipsychotic.

Promacta. (GlaxoSmithKline) Eltrombopag 25 mg, 50 mg. Mannitol. Filmcoated. Tab. 30s. *Rx.*
Use: Hematopoietic agent, thrombopoietin receptor agonist.

Promega. (Parke-Davis) Omega-3 (N-3) polyunsaturated fatty acids 1000 mg, containing EPA 350 mg, DHA 150 mg, vitamins E (3% RDA), A, B$_1$, B$_2$, B$_3$, Ca, Fe (< 2% RDA). Cap., cholesterol and sodium free. Bot. 30s. *OTC.*
Use: Mineral, vitamin supplement.

Promega Pearls. (Parke-Davis) EPA 168 mg, DHA 72 mg, cholesterol < 2 mg, E 1 units, < 2% RDA of A, B_1, B_2, B_3, Fe, Ca. Cap. Bot. 60s, 90s. *OTC.*
Use: Vitamin supplement.

Prometa. (Muro) Metaproterenol sulfate 10 mg/5 mL, with saccharin and sorbitol, strawberry flavor. Syr. Bot. 480 mL. *Rx.*
Use: Bronchodilator.

promethazine. (Alpharma) Promethazine 25 mg, hard fat. Supp. 12s. *Rx.*
Use: Antihistamine, nonselective phenothiazine.

• **promethazine hydrochloride.** (pro-METH-uh-zeen) *USP 34.*
Use: Antiemetic; antihistamine, nonselective phenothiazine.
See: Pentazine.
Phenadoz.
Phenergan.
Promethegan.
Sigazine.
W/Codeine Phosphate, Phenylephrine Hydrochloride.
See: Promethazine VC w/Codeine.
W/Dextromethorphan Hydrobromide.
See: Promethazine w/Dextromethorphan Cough.
W/Meperidine Hydrochloride.
See: Meprozine.
W/Phenylephrine Hydrochloride.
See: Promethazine VC.
Prometh VC Plain.

promethazine hydrochloride. (Able Labs) Promethazine hydrochloride 12.5 mg. May contain lactose. Tab. 30s, 100s, 500s, 1000s. *Rx.*
Use: Antihistamine.

promethazine hydrochloride. (Ivax) Promethazine hydrochloride 12.5 mg. May contain hard fat. Supp. 12s. *Rx.*
Use: Antihistamine.

promethazine hydrochloride. (Various Mfr.) Promethazine hydrochloride. **Tab.:** 25 mg, 50 mg. May contain lactose. Bot. 30s, 100s, 500s, 1000s. **Syr.:** 6.25 mg/5 mL. Alcohol. Bot. 473 mL. **Supp.:** 25 mg, 50 mg. May contain hard fat (25 mg only). Pkg. 12s. **Inj.:** 25 mg/mL, 50 mg/mL. May contain EDTA. Amp. 1 mL. *Rx.*
Use: Antiemetic; antihistamine, nonselective phenothiazine; sedative.

promethazine hydrochloride and phenylephrine hydrochloride. (Various Mfr.) Phenylephrine hydrochloride 5 mg, promethazine hydrochloride 6.25 mg/5 mL. Alcohol 7%, may contain sorbitol, sugar, parabens.

Syr. Bot. 118 mL, 473 mL, 3.8 L. *Rx.*
Use: Upper respiratory combination, decongestant, antihistamine.

promethazine hydrochloride, phenylephrine hydrochloride, and codeine phosphate. (Alpharma) Codeine phosphate 10 mg, promethazine hydrochloride 6.25 mg, phenylephrine hydrochloride 5 mg per 5 mL. Alcohol 7%, parabens, sucrose, saccharin, sugar. Strawberry flavor. Syr. 118 mL, 237 mL, 473 mL. *c-v.*
Use: Antitussive combination, upper respiratory combination.

promethazine hydrochloride w/codeine. (Various Mfr.) Codeine phosphate 10 mg, promethazine hydrochloride 6.25 mg per 5 mL. May contain corn syr., parabens, saccharin. Syr. Bot. 118 mL, 473 mL. *c-v.*
Use: Upper respiratory combination, antitussive combination.

Promethazine VC. (Various Mfr.) Phenylephrine hydrochloride 5 mg, promethazine hydrochloride 6.25 mg per 5 mL. May contain alcohol 7%, menthol, parabens, saccharin sucrose. Syr. Bot. 118 mL, 237 mL, 473 mL. *Rx.*
Use: Antihistamine and decongestant, upper respiratory combination.

Promethazine VC w/Codeine. (Qualitest) Promethazine hydrochloride 6.25 mg, phenylephrine hydrochloride 5 mg, codeine phosphate 10 mg per 5 mL. Alcohol 7%, menthol, parabens, saccharin, sucrose. Strawberry flavor. Syr. Bot. 118 mL. *c-v.*
Use: Upper respiratory combination, antitussive combination.

promethazine w/dextromethorphan cough. (Morton Grove) Dextromethorphan HBr 15 mg, promethazine hydrochloride 6.25 mg per 5 mL. Alcohol 7.1%, EDTA, methylparaben, sugar. Syr. Bot. 118 mL, 473 mL. *Rx.*
Use: Upper respiratory combination, antitussive combination.

Promethegan. (G & W) Promethazine hydrochloride 12.5 mg, 25 mg, 50 mg. Supp., Rectal. 12s, 1000s. *Rx.*
Use: Antihistamine, nonselective phenothiazine.

promethestrol dipropionate.
Use: Estrogen.

Prometh VC Plain. (Alpharma) Phenylephrine hydrochloride 5 mg, promethazine hydrochloride 6.25 mg/5 mL. Alcohol 7%. Syr. Bot. 3.8 L. *Rx.*
Use: Upper respiratory combination, antihistamine, decongestant.

Prometh VC w/Codeine Cough. (Alpharma) Codeine phosphate 10 mg, promethazine hydrochloride 6.25 mg, phenylephrine hydrochloride 5 mg per 5 mL. Alcohol 7%, parabens, sugar, saccharin. Syr. Bot. 118 mL, 237 mL, 473 mL, 3.8 L. *c-v.*
Use: Upper respiratory combination, antitussive, antihistamine, decongestant.

Prometh w/Codeine Cough. (Alpharma) Codeine phosphate 10 mg, promethazine hydrochloride 6.25 mg per 5 mL. Alcohol 7%, corn syr., parabens, saccharin. Syr. Bot. 118 mL. *c-v.*
Use: Upper respiratory combination, antitussive, antihistamine.

Prometh w/Dextromethorphan. (Alpharma) Dextromethorphan HBr 15 mg, promethazine hydrochloride 6.25 mg per 5 mL. Alcohol 7%, parabens, saccharin, lemon/mint flavor. Syr. Bot. 118 mL, 237 mL, 473 mL, 3.8 L. *Rx.*
Use: Upper respiratory combination, antitussive, antihistamine.

Prometol. (Viobin) Concentrated wheat germ oil. **3 min/Cap.:** Bot. 100s, 250s. **10 min/Cap.:** Bot. 100s. *OTC.*
Use: Supplement.

Prometrium. (Solvay) Progesterone 100 mg, 200 mg. Peanut oil. Cap. Micronized Soft Gel. Bot. 100s. *Rx.*
Use: Progestin, sex hormone.

prominal.
See: Mephobarbital.

Promine. (Major) Procainamide 250 mg, 375 mg, 500 mg. Cap. Bot. 100s, 250s, 1000s, UD 100s (375 mg/Cap. w/500s instead of 250s). *Rx.*
Use: Antiarrhythmic.

Promine S.R. (Major) Procainamide. **SR Tab.:** 250 mg. Bot. 100s, 250s; 500 mg. Bot. 100s, 250s, 1000s; 750 mg. **SR Cap.:** 250 mg, 375 mg, 500 mg. Bot. 100s, 250s. *Rx.*
Use: Antiarrhythmic.

Promiseb. (Promius Pharma) Castor oil, disodium EDTA, PEG-30. Cream. 30 g. *Rx.*
Use: Emollient.

Promist HD. (UCB) Hydrocodone bitartrate 2.5 mg, pseudoephedrine hydrochloride 30 mg, chlorpheniramine maleate 2 mg/5 mL, alcohol 5%, menthol, saccharin, sorbitol. Bot. Pt. *c-iii.*
Use: Antihistamine; antitussive; decongestant.

Promist LA. (UCB) Pseudoephedrine hydrochloride 120 mg, guaifenesin 500 mg. Tab. Bot. 100s. *Rx.*
Use: Decongestant; expectorant.

Pro-Mix R.D.P. (Navaco) Protein 15 g (from whey protein), fat 0.8 g, carbohydrate 1 g, Na 46 mg, K 165 mg, Cl 46 mg, Ca 73.6 mg, P 64.4 mg, Fe 0.3 mg, Cr, Cu, Mg, Mn, Mo, Se, Zn, 72 Cal./5 Tbsp. (20 g). Pow. Packet 20 g, can 300 g. *OTC.*
Use: Nutritional supplement.

Promylin Enteric Coated Microzymes. (Shear/Kershman) Enteric-coated pancrelipase. Lipase 4000 units, amylase 20,000 units, protease 25,000 units. *Rx.*
Use: Digestive enzymes.

Pro-Nasyl. (Progonasyl) o-Iodobenzoic acid 0.5%, triethanolamine 5.5% in a special neutral hydrophilic base compounded from oleic acid, mineral oil, vegetable oil. Bot. 15 mL, 60 mL.
Use: Treatment of sinusitis.

Pronemia Hematinic. (Wyeth) Iron 115 mg, B$_{12}$ 15 mcg, IFC 75 mg, C 150 mg, folic acid 1 mcg. Cap. Bot. 30s. *Rx.*
Use: Iron w/B$_{12}$ and intrinsic factor.

Pronto. (Del) Pyrethrins 0.33%, piperonyl butoxide 4%, benzyl alcohol, decyl alcohol, isopropyl alcohol. Shampoo. 60 mL, 120 mL with comb. *OTC.*
Use: Pediculicide.

Propac. (Biosearch Medical Products) Protein 3 g (from whey protein), carbohydrate 0.2 g, fat 0.3 g, Cl 3 mg, K 20 mg, Na 9 mg, Ca 24 mg, P 12 mg, 16 Cal/Tbsp. (4 g). Pow. Packet 19.5 g, Can 350 g. *OTC.*
Use: Nutritional supplement.

Propacet 100. (Teva) Propoxyphene napsylate 100 mg, acetaminophen 650 mg. Tab. Bot. 100s, 500s. *c-iv.*
Use: Analgesic combination; narcotic.

propaesin. (Various Mfr.) Propyl p-Aminobenzoate.

•**propafenone hydrochloride.** (pro-pah-FEN-ohn) *USP 34.*
Use: Antiarrhythmic agent.
See: Rythmol.
    Rythmol SR.

propafenone hydrochloride. (Par Pharmaceuticals) Propafenone hydrochloride 225 mg, 325 mg, 425 mg. Lactose. ER Cap. 60s, 90s, 100s, 500s, 1,000s. *Rx.*
Use: Antiarrhythmic agent.

propafenone hydrochloride. (Various Mfr.) Propafenone 150 mg, 225 mg, 300 mg. Tab. Bot. 100s, 500s (except 300 mg). *Rx.*
Use: Antiarrhythmic agent.

Propagon-S. (Spanner) Estrone 2 mg, 5 mg/mL. Vial 10 mL. *Rx.*
Use: Estrogen.

Propain HC. (Springbok) Acetaminophen 500 mg, hydrocodone bitartrate 5 mg. Cap. Bot. 100s, 500s. *c-III.*
Use: Analgesic combination; narcotic.

•**propane.** (PROE-pane) *NF 29.*
Use: Aerosol propellant.

propanediol diacetate, 1,2.
See: VoSoL.

1,2,3-propanetriol, trinitrate. Nitroglycerin Tab., USP.

•**propanidid.** (pro-PAN-ih-did) USAN.
Use: Anesthetic, intravenous.

propanolol. Propranolol.

•**propantheline bromide.** (pro-PAN-thuh-leen) *USP 34.*
Use: Anticholinergic.

propantheline bromide. (Various Mfr.) Propantheline bromide 15 mg. Tab. 100s, 500s, 1000, UD 100s. *Rx.*
Use: Anticholinergic.

PROPApH Astringent Cleanser Maximum Strength. (Del) Salicylic acid 2%, aloe vera gel, SD alcohol 40-2 55.1%. Liq. Bot. 355 mL. *OTC.*
Use: Dermatologic, acne.

PROPApH Cleansing for Oily Skin. (Del) Salicylic acid 0.6%, SD alcohol 40, EDTA, menthol. Lot. Bot. 180 mL. *OTC.*
Use: Dermatologic, acne.

PROPApH Cleansing for Sensitive Skin. (Del) Salicylic acid 0.5%, SD alcohol 40, aloe vera gel, EDTA, menthol. Pads. In 45s. *OTC.*
Use: Dermatologic, acne.

PROPApH Cleansing Lotion for Normal/Combination Skin. (Del) Salicylic acid 0.5%, SD alcohol 40, EDTA. Lot. Bot. 180 mL. Pads. 45s. *OTC.*
Use: Antiacne.

PROPApH Cleansing Maximum Strength. (Del) Salicylic acid 2%, SD alcohol 40, aloe vera gel, EDTA, propylene glycol, menthol. Pads. In 45s. *OTC.*
Use: Dermatologic, acne.

PROPApH Cleansing Pads. (Del) Salicylic acid 0.5%, SD alcohol 40, EDTA, menthol. Pads. 45s. *OTC.*
Use: Dermatologic, acne.

PROPApH Foaming Face Wash. (Del) Salicylic acid 2%, aloe vera gel, EDTA, menthol. Alcohol, oil and soap free. Liq. Bot. 180 mL. *OTC.*
Use: Dermatologic, acne.

PROPApH Maximum Strength Acne Cream. (Del) Salicylic acid 2%, acetylated lanolin alcohol, cetearyl alcohol, stearyl alcohol, EDTA, menthol. Tube 19.5 g. *OTC.*
Use: Dermatologic, acne.

PROPApH Medicated Acne Cream with Aloe. (Del) Salicylic acid 2%. Tube 1 oz. *OTC.*
Use: Dermatologic, acne.

PROPApH Medicated Acne Stick with Aloe. (Del) Salicylic acid 2%. Stick 0.05 oz. *OTC.*
Use: Dermatologic, acne.

PROPApH Medicated Cleansing Pads with Aloe. (Del) Salicylic acid 0.5%, SD alcohol 40 25%, aloe. Jar containing 45 pads. *OTC.*
Use: Dermatologic, acne.

PROPApH Peel-Off Acne Mask. (Del) Salicylic acid 2%, tartrazine, parabens, polyvinyl alcohol, vitamin E acetate, SD alcohol 40. Mask. 60 mL. *OTC.*
Use: Dermatologic, acne.

PROPApH Skin Cleanser with Aloe. (Del) Salicylic acid USP 0.5%, SD alcohol 40 25%. Liq. Bot. 6 oz, 10 oz. *OTC.*
Use: Dermatologic, acne.

•**proparacaine hydrochloride.** (pro-PAR-ah-cane) *USP 34.*
Use: Anesthetic local, ophthalmic.
See: Alcaine.
Ophthetic.
Paracaine.
W/Fluorescein Sodium.
See: Flucaine.
Fluoracaine.

proparacaine hydrochloride. (Various Mfr.) Proparacaine hydrochloride 0.5%. Soln. 15 mL. *Rx.*
Use: Anesthetic local, ophthalmic.

proparacaine hydrochloride and fluorescein sodium. (Various Mfr.) Proparacaine hydrochloride 0.5%, fluorescein sodium 0.25%. Povidone, glycerin, EDTA, thimerosal 0.01%. Soln. Bot. 5 mL with dropper. *Rx.*
Use: Anesthetic local, ophthalmic.

proparacaine hydrochloride/procaine hydrochloride.
Use: Anesthetic.

•**propatyl nitrate.** (PRO-pah-till) USAN. Investigational drug in US but available in England.
Use: Coronary vasodilator.

Propecia. (Merck) Finasteride 1 mg, lactose. Film-coated. Tab. Unit-of-use 30s, *ProPak* carton of 3 unit-of-use bottles of 30. *Rx.*
Use: Androgen hormone inhibitor; hair growth.

•**propenzolate hydrochloride.** (pro-PEN-zoe-late) USAN.
Use: Anticholinergic.

propesin. Name used for *Risocaine.*

Prophene 65. (Halsey Drug) Propoxyphene hydrochloride 65 mg. Cap. Bot. 100s, 500s, 1000s. *c-IV.*
Use: Analgesic; narcotic.

prophenpyridamine maleate.
See: Pheniramine maleate.
W/Combinations
See: Trimahist.
Vasotus.

Pro-Phree. (Ross) Fat 31 g, carbohydrate 60 g, linoleic acid 2250 mg, Fe 11.9 mg, Na 250 mg, K 875 mg, with appropriate vitamins and minerals, 520 Cal/100 g. Protein free. Pow. Can 350 g. *OTC.*
Use: Nutritional supplement.

Prophyllin. (Rystan) Sodium propionate 5%, chlorophyll derivatives 0.0125%. Tube 1 oz. *Rx.*
Use: Anti-infective, topical.

•**propikacin.** (PRO-pih-KAY-sin) USAN.
Use: Anti-infective.

Propimex-1. (Ross) Protein 15 g, fat 23.9 g, carbohydrate 46.3 g, linoleic acid 1800 mg, Fe 9 mg, Na 190 mg, K 675 mg, with appropriate vitamins and minerals, 480 Cal/100 g. Methionine and valine free. Pow. Can 350 g. *OTC.*
Use: Nutritional supplement.

Propimex-2. (Ross) Protein 30 g, fat 15.5 g, carbohydrate 30 g, Na 880 mg, K 1370 mg, with appropriate vitamins and minerals, 410 Cal/mL. Methionine and valine free. Pow. Can 325 g. *OTC.*
Use: Nutritional supplement for propionic or methylmalonic acidemia.

•**propiolactone.** (PRO-pee-oh-LACK-tone) USAN.
Use: Disinfectant, sterilizing agent of vaccines and tissue grafts.

•**propionic acid.** (pro-pee-AHN-ik) *NF 29.*
Use: Antimicrobial; pharmaceutic aid, acidifying agent.

propionyl erythromycin lauryl sulfate.
See: Erythromycin Propionate Lauryl Sulfate.

•**propiram fumarate.** (PRO-pih-ram) USAN.
Use: Analgesic.

Propisamine.
See: Amphetamine.

propitocaine. Prilocaine.

Proplex. (Baxter PPI) Plasma derived concentrate of clotting Factors II, VII, IX, X. Actual number of units shown on each bottle. Heat treated. Heparin. Pow. for Inj. Vial 30 mL w/diluent, needles. *Rx.*
Use: Antihemophilic.

•**propofol.** (PRO-puh-FOLE) *USP 34.*
Use: Anesthetic, intravenous.
See: Diprivan.
Fresenius Propoven.

propofol. (Baxter Healthcare) Propofol 10 mg/mL, soybean oil 100 mg/mL, glycerol 22.5 mg/mL, egg yolk phospholipid 12 mg/mL, sodium metabisulfite 0.25 mg/mL, ph = 4.5 to 6.4. Inj. Emulsion. Single-use vial 20 mL; Single-use infusion vial 50 mL, 100 mL. *Rx.*
Use: Anesthetic.

Propoquin. Amopyroquin hydrochloride.
Use: Antimalarial.

•**propoxycaine and procaine hydrochlorides and levonordefrin injection.** *USP 34.*
Use: Anesthetic, local.

•**propoxycaine and procaine hydrochlorides and norepinephrine bitartrate injection.** *USP 34.*
Use: Anesthetic, local.

•**propoxycaine hydrochloride.** (pro-POX-ih-cane) *USP 34.*
Use: Anesthetic, local.

propoxychlorinol. Toloxychlorinol.

•**propoxyphene hydrochloride.** (proe-POX-i-feen) *USP 34.*
Use: Analgesic.
See: Darvon Pulvules.
Dolene Plain.
Pro-Gesic.
W/Combinations.
See: Darvon Compound-65 Pulvules.
Darvon Compound-32 Pulvules.
Dolene, AP-65.
Dolene Compound-65.

propoxyphene hydrochloride. (Various Mfr.) Propoxyphene hydrochloride 65 mg. Cap. Bot. 100s. *c-IV.*
Use: Opioid analgesic.

propoxyphene hydrochloride and acetaminophen tablets. (Various Mfr.) Propoxyphene hydrochloride 65 mg, acetaminophen 650 mg. Tab. Bot. 500s. *c-IV.*
Use: Analgesic.

•**propoxyphene hydrochloride, aspirin, and caffeine capsules.** *USP 34.*
Use: Analgesic.

•**propoxyphene napsylate.** (proe-POX-i-feen NAP-si-late) *USP 34.*
Use: Analgesic.
W/Acetaminophen.
See: Trycet.

propoxyphene napsylate and acetaminophen. (Pliva) Propoxyphene napsylate 100 mg, acetaminophen 500 mg. Lactose. Tab. 100s. *c-IV.*
Use: Narcotic analgesic.

propoxyphene napsylate and acetaminophen. (Various Mfr.) Propoxyphene napsylate 50 mg, acetamino-

phen 325 mg. Tab. Bot. 100s, 500s, 550s, 1000s, UD 100s. Propoxyphene napsylate 100 mg, acetaminophen 650 mg. Tab. Bot. 30s, 50s, 100s, 500s, 1000s, UD 100s. *c-IV.*
Use: Analgesic.

•**propoxyphene napsylate and aspirin tablets.** *USP 34.*
Use: Analgesic.

•**propranolol hydrochloride.** (pro-PRAN-oh-lahl) *USP 34.*
Use: Antiadrenergic/sympatholytic, beta-adrenergic blocker.
See: Inderal LA.
InnoPran XL.
Propranolol Intensol.

propranolol hydrochloride. (Various Mfr.) Propranolol hydrochloride. **Tab.:** 10 mg, 20 mg, 40 mg, 60 mg, 80 mg. May contain lactose. 30s, 100s, 1000s. **ER Cap.:** 60 mg, 80 mg, 120 mg, 160 mg. 100s, 500s, 1000s. **Inj.:** 1 mg/mL. Vial 1 mL. *Rx.*
Use: Antiadrenergic/sympatholytic, beta-adrenergic blocker.

propranolol hydrochloride solution. (Roxane) Propranolol hydrochloride 4 mg/mL, 8 mg/mL, parabens, saccharin, sorbitol, dye free, strawberry-mint flavor. Oral Soln. 500 mL. *Rx.*
Use: Antiadrenergic/sympatholytic, beta-adrenergic blocker.

propranolol/hydrochlorothiazide. (Various Mfr.) Propranolol hydrochloride/hydrochlorothiazide 40 mg/25 mg, 80 mg/25 mg. Bot. 100s, 1000s (80 mg/25 mg only). *Rx.*
Use: Antihypertensive.

propranolol intensol. (Roxane) Propranolol hydrochloride 80 mg/mL, alcohol and dye free. Concentrated Oral Soln. Bot. 30 mL with dropper. *Rx.*
Use: Antiadrenergic/sympatholytic, beta-adrenergic blocker.

•**propylene carbonate.** (PRO-pi-leen CAR-boe-nate) *NF 29.*
Use: Pharmaceutic aid, gelling agent.

•**propylene glycol.** (PRO-pi-leen GLYE-kol) *USP 34.*
Use: Pharmaceutic aid, humectant, solvent, suspending agent.

•**propylene glycol alginate.** (PRO-pi-leen GLYE-kol AL-ji-nate) *NF 29.*
Use: Pharmaceutic aid, suspending, viscosity-increasing agent.

propylene glycol diacetate.
Use: Pharmaceutic aid, solvent.

•**propylene glycol monostearate.** (PRO-pi-leen GLYE-kol mon-oh-STEER-ate) *NF 29.*

Use: Pharmaceutic aid, emulsifying agent.

•**propyl gallate.** (PRO-pill GAL-ate) *NF 29.*
Use: Pharmaceutic aid; antioxidant.

•**propylhexedrine.** (pro-pill-HEX-ih-dreen) *USP 34.*
Use: Adrenergic, vasoconstrictor; appetite suppressant; antihistamine.

•**propyliodone.** (pro-pill-EYE-oh-dohn) *USP 34.*
Use: Diagnostic aid, radiopaque medium.
See: Dionosil Oily.

propylnoradrenaline-iso.
See: Isoproterenol.

propyl p-aminobenzoate. (Various Mfr.) Propaesin.
Use: Anesthetic, local.

•**propylparaben.** (PROE-pil-PAR-a-ben) *NF 29.* Propyl Chemosept (Chemo Puro).
Use: Pharmaceutic aid, antifungal agent.

•**propylparaben sodium.** (PROE-pil-PAR-a-ben) *NF 29.*
Use: Pharmaceutic aid, antimicrobial preservative.

•**propylthiouracil.** (pro-puhl-thigh-oh-YOU-rah-sill) *USP 34.*
Use: Antithyroid agent.

propylthiouracil. (Various Mfr.) Propylthiouracil 50 mg. Tab. Bot. 100s, 1000s. *Rx.*
Use: Antithyroid agent.

Pro-Q. (CollaGenex) Dimethicone, glycerin, parabens. Foam. 76 mL, 161 mL. *OTC.*
Use: Protectant.

ProQuad. (Merck & Co.) Mixture of 4 viruses: $\geq 3.00 \log_{10}$ $TCID_{50}$ (50% tissue culture infectious dose) of measles virus; $4.3 \log_{10}$ $TCID_{50}$ of mumps virus; $3.00 \log_{10}$ $TCID_{50}$ of rubella virus; and $\geq 3.99 \log_{10}$ plaque-forming units of varicella virus per 0.5 mL. Also contains sucrose, hydrolyzed gelatin, sodium chloride, sorbitol, monosodium L-glutamate, sodium phosphate dibasic, human albumin, sodium bicarbonate, potassium phosphate monobasic, potassium chloride, potassium phosphate dibasic, residual components of MRC-5 cells including DNA and protein, neomycin, bovine calf serum. Preservative free. Pow. for Inj., lyophilized. Single-dose vials. 1s with diluent. *Rx.*
Use: Agent for immunization.

•**proquazone.** (PRO-kwah-zone) USAN.
Use: Anti-inflammatory.

Proquin XR. (Esprit) Ciprofloxacin (as ciprofloxacin hydrochloride) 500 mg. ER Tab. Film-coated. 30s, 50s, UD 3s. *Rx.*
Use: Fluoroquinolones.

Pro-Red AC. (Pro-Pharma) Codeine phosphate 9 mg, pyrilamine maleate 8.33 mg, phenylephrine hydrochloride 5 mg. Alcohol free and sugar free. Glycerin, saccharin, sorbitol. Cotton candy flavor. Syr. 473 mL. *c-v.*
Use: Upper respiratory combination, antitussive combination.

•**prorenoate potassium.** (pro-REN-oh-ate) USAN.
Use: Aldosterone antagonist.

Prorone. (Sigma-Tau) Progesterone 25 mg/mL. Aqueous or oil susp. Vial 10 mL. *Rx.*
Use: Hormone, progestin.

•**proroxan hydrochloride.** (pro-ROCK-san) USAN. *Formerly Pyrroxane, Pirrousan.*
Use: Antiadrenergic, α-receptor.

Proscar. (Merck) Finasteride 5 mg, lactose. Tab. 1000s, Unit-of-use 30s, 100s, UD 100s. *Rx.*
Use: Androgen hormone inhibitor.

•**proscillaridin.** (pro-sih-LARE-ih-din) USAN. Talusin, Tradenal.
Use: Cardiovascular agent.

Prosed/DS. (Ferring) Methenamine 81.6 mg, phenyl salicylate 36.2 mg, methylene blue 10.8 mg, benzoic acid 9 mg, hyoscyamine sulfate 0.12 mg. Sugar. Sugar coated. Tab. 100s. *Rx.*
Use: Anti-infective, urinary.

ProSight Lutein. (Major) Ca 22 mg, vitamin E 30 units, C 60 mg, Zn 15 mg, Cu 2 mg. Cap. Bot. 36s. *OTC.*
Use: Nutritional combination product.

Pro Skin. (Marlyn Nutraceuticals) Vitamins A 6250 units, E 100 units, C 100 mg, B_5 10 mg, Zn 10 mg, Se. Cap., Bot. 60s. *OTC.*
Use: Mineral, vitamin supplement.

ProSobee. (Bristol-Myers Squibb) Milk free formula supplies 640 cal/qt, protein 19.2 g, fat 34 g, carbohydrate 64 g, vitamins A 2000 units, D 400 units, E 20 units, C 52 mg, folic acid 100 mcg, B_1 0.5 mg, B_2 0.6 mg, niacin 8 mg, B_6 0.4 mg, B_{12} 2 mcg, biotin 50 mg, pantothenic acid 3 mg, K-1 100 mcg, choline 50 mg, inositol 30 mg, Ca 600 mg, P 475 mg, I 65 mcg, Fe 12 mg, Mg 70 mg, Cu 0.6 mg, Zn 5 mg, Mn 1.6 mg, Cl 530 mg, K 780 mg, Na 230 mg/Qt. (20 Kcal/fl oz). Concentrated liq. can 13 fl oz; Ready-to-Use Liq. Can 8 fl oz,

32 fl oz. Pow., Can 14 oz. *OTC.*
Use: Nutritional supplement.

ProSobee Concentrate. (Bristol-Myers Squibb) P-soy protein isolate, l-methionine. CHO. Corn syr. solids, soy and coconut oil, lecithin, mono- and diglycerides. Protein 20.3 g, CHO 65.4 g, fat 33.6 g, Fe 12 mg, 640 cal/serving. Concentrate 390 mL. *OTC.*
Use: Nutritional supplement.

Pro-Sof w/Casanthranol SG. (Vangard Labs, Inc.) Casanthranol 30 mg, docusate sodium 100 mg. Cap. Bot. 100s, 1000s.
Use: Laxative.

prostacyclin analog.
Use: Vasodilator.
See: Iloprost.

prostaglandin agonist.
Use: Antiglaucoma agent.
See: Bimatoprost.
　　Latanoprost.
　　Lumigan.
　　Travatan.
　　Travoprost.

prostaglandin E_2.
See: Dinoprostone.

prostaglandins.
Use: Abortifacient; agent for impotence; agent for cervical ripening; patent ductus arteriosus; antiulcerative.
See: Carboprost Tromethamine.
　　Dinoprostone.
　　Misoprostol.

•**prostalene.** (PRAHST-ah-leen) USAN.
Use: Prostaglandin.

ProstaScint. (Cytogen) Each kit contains capromab pendetide 0.5 mg/mL of sodium phosphate buffered saline and 1 vial of sodium acetate 82 mg in 2 mL sterile water for inj. Preservative free. Includes 1 sterile 0.22 mcm *Millex GV filter,* prescribing information, and 2 identification labels. *Rx.*
Use: In vivo diagnostic aid.

Pro-Stat 101. (Medical Nutrition) Protein 15 g/30 mL (collagen hydrolysate, amino acids [including histidine, isoleucine, leucine, lysine, methionine, phenylalanine, threonine, tryptophan, valine, alanine, arginine, aspartic acid, cystine, glutamic acid, glycine, proline, serine, tyrosine, hydroxylysine, hydroxyproline]). Fructose, potassium sorbate, sodium 14.5 mg/30 mL, sucralose, xylitol. Gluten free and lactose free. Natural, butter pecan, and wild cherry flavors. Liq. 887 mL. *OTC.*
Use: Nutritional supplement.

Pro-Stat 64. (Medical Nutrition) Protein 15 g/30 mL (collagen hydrolysate,

amino acids [including histidine, isoleucine, leucine, lysine, methionine, phenylalanine, threonine, tryptophan, valine, alanine, arginine, aspartic acid, cystine, glutamic acid, glycine, proline, serine, tyrosine, hydroxylysine, hydroxyproline]). Acesulfame-K, glycerin, potassium sorbate, sodium 14.5 mg/ 30 mL, sucralose, xylitol. Gluten free, lactose free, and sugar free. Natural, grape, and wild cherry punch flavors. Liq. 887 mL. *OTC.*
Use: Nutritional supplement.

Prosteon. (Theralogix) Vitamin D$_3$ 500 units, K 25 mcg, B, Ca, Mg, Sr. Tab. 240s. *OTC.*
Use: Multivitamin with minerals.

ProStep. (Wyeth) Transdermal nicotine 11 mg, 22 mg/day. Patch 7s. *Rx.*
Use: Smoking deterrent.

Prostigmin. (Valeant) Neostigmine methylsulfate 1:4000 (0.25 mg/mL), 1:2000 (0.5 mg/mL), 1:1000 (1 mg/mL). Inj. Amps. 1 mL with 0.2% methyl- and propylparabens (except 1:1000). Multidose vials. 10 mL with phenol 0.45%, sodium acetate 0.2 mg (except 1:4000). *Rx.*
Use: Muscle stimulant; urinary cholinergic.

Prostigmin Bromide. (AstraZeneca) Neostigmine bromide 15 mg. Tab. Bot. 100s, 1000s. *Rx.*
Use: Muscle stimulant.

Prostin E2. (Pfizer) Dinoprost 20 mg. Supp. Containers of 1 each. *Rx.*
Use: Abortifacient.

Prostin VR Pediatric. (Pfizer) Alprostadil 500 mcg/mL. Amp. 1 mL. *Rx.*
Use: Arterial patency agent.

Prostonic. (Seatrace) Thiamine hydrochloride 10 mg, alanine 130 mg, glutamic acid 130 mg, amino-acetic acid 130 mg. Cap. Bot. 100s. *Rx.*
Use: Palliative relief of benign prostatic hypertrophy.

Protabolin. (Taylor Pharmaceuticals) Methandriol dipropionate 50 mg/mL. Vial 10 mL. *Rx.*
Use: Hormone.

•**protamine sulfate.** (PRO-tuh-meen) *USP 34.*
Use: Coagulant, heparin antagonist.
W/Insulin Lispro.
See: Humalog Mix 50/50.
  Humalog Mix 75/25.

protamine sulfate. (Various Mfr.) Protamine sulfate 10 mg/mL. Preservative free. Inj. Vials 5 mL, 25 mL.
Use: Coagulant, heparin antagonist.

protargin mild.
See: Silver Protein, Mild.

Protargol. (Sterwin) Strong silver protein. Pow. Bot. 25 g. *Rx.*
Use: Antiseptic.

protease.
W/Amylase, Cellulase, Hyoscyamine Sulfate, Lipase, Phenyltoloxamine Citrate.
See: Digex.
W/Amylase, Lipase.
See: Creon.
  Palcaps 10.
  Pancrelipase.
  Tri-Pase 8.
  Tri-Pase 16.
  Zenpep.

protease inhibitors.
Use: Antiretroviral.
See: Atazanavir Sulfate.
  Darunavir Ethanolate.
  Fosamprenavir Calcium.
  Indinavir Sulfate.
  Lopinavir/Ritonavir.
  Nelfinavir Mesylate.
  Ritonavir.
  Saquinavir Mesylate.
  Tipranavir.

proteasome inhibitors.
See: Bortezomib.

ProTech First-Aid Stik. (Triton) Lidocaine hydrochloride 2.5%, povidone iodine 10%. Liq. 14 mL dab-on applicator. *OTC.*
Use: Topical local anesthetic combination.

Protectol Medicated Powder. (Jones Pharma) Calcium undecylenate 15%. Bot. 2 oz. *OTC.*
Use: Diaper rash preparation.

Protegra Softgels. (Wyeth) Vitamins E 200 units, C 250 mg, beta-carotene 3 mg, Zn 7.5 mg, Cu, Se, Mn. Cap. Bot. 50s. *OTC.*
Use: Vitamin supplement.

proteinase inhibitor, alpha 1.
See: Prolastin.

protein C concentrate (human).
Use: Thrombolytic agent, human protein C.
See: Ceprotin.

protein C1 inhibitors.
See: C1 Inhibitor (Human).

•**protein hydrolysate injection.** (PROEteen hye-DROL-i-sate) *USP 34.*
Use: Fluid, nutrient replacement.
See: Amigen.
  Aminogen.
  Lacotein.

protein hydrolysates oral.
Use: Enteral nutritional supplement.
See: Nutramigen.

Pregestimil.

W/Vitamin B₁₂.
See: Stuart Amino Acids and B₁₂.

protein-tyrosine kinase inhibitor.
See: Dasatinib.
Imatinib.
mTOR Inhibitor.
Nilotinib.
Sunitinib Malate.

Protenate. (Baxter PPI) Plasma protein fraction (Human) 5%. Inj. Vial 250 mL, 500 mL w/administration set. Rx.
Use: Plasma protein fraction.

Prothers. (ICN) Soap free. White petrolatum, disodium cocamido MIPA-sulfosuccinate, pentane, ammonium laureth sulfate, PEG-150 distearate, hydroxypropyl methylcellulose, imidazolidinyl urea, parabens, propylene glycol stearate, hydrogenated soy glyceride, sodium stearyl lactylate. Liq. Bot. 180 mL. OTC.
Use: Dermatologic, cleanser.

prothipendyl hydrochloride.
Use: Sedative.

Proticuleen. (Spanner) Vitamin B₁₂ activity 10 mcg, folic acid 10 mg, B₁₂ crystalline 50 mcg, niacinamide 75 mg/mL. Multiple-dose vial 10 mL. IM Inj. Rx.
Use: Nutritional supplement, parenteral.

Protonix. (Wyeth-Ayerst) Pantoprazole sodium. **DR Susp.:** 40 mg (as pantoprazole sodium sesquihydrate 45.1 mg). Enteric-coated gran. UD 30s. **DR Tab.:** 20 mg (as pantoprazole sodium sesquihydrate 22.6 mg), 40 mg (as pantoprazole sodium sesquihydrate 45.1 mg). Mannitol. Tab. Bot. 90s, UD 100s (40 mg only). Rx.
Use: Proton pump inhibitor.

Protonix I.V. (Wyeth-Ayerst) Pantoprazole sodium 40 mg. EDTA. Inj., freeze-dried, Pow. for Soln. Vials. Rx.
Use: Proton pump inhibitor.

proton pump inhibitors.
See: Esomeprazole Magnesium.
Lansoprazole.
Omeprazole.
Omeprazole/Sodium Bicarbonate.
Pantoprazole Sodium.
Rabeprazole Sodium.

Protopam Chloride. (Wyeth-Ayerst) Pralidoxime chloride 1 g. Pow. for Inj. Single-use vial. 20 mL. Rx.
Use: Antidote.

Protopic. (Astellas Pharma) Tacrolimus 0.03%, 0.1%. Mineral oil, white petrolatum. Oint. Tube 30 g, 60 g, 100 g. Rx.
Use: Immunomodulator, topical.

Protosan. (Recsei) Protein 87.5%, lactose 0.5%, fat 1.3%, ash 3.5%, Na 0.02%. Jar 1 lb, 5 lb. OTC.
Use: Nutritional supplement.

Prot-O-Sea. (Barth's) Protein 90%, containing amino acids and minerals. Bot. 100s, 500s. OTC.
Use: Nutritional supplement.

Protostat. (Ortho-McNeil) Metronidazole. Tab. **250 mg:** Bot. 100s. **500 mg:** Bot. 50s. Rx.
Use: Anti-infective.

Protran Plus. (Vangard Labs, Inc.) Meprobamate 150 mg, ethoheptazine citrate 75 mg, aspirin 250 mg. Tab. Bot. 100s. 500s. Rx.
Use: Analgesic, anxiolytic combination.

•**protriptyline hydrochloride.** (pro-TRIP-tih-leen) USP 34.
Use: Antidepressant.
See: Vivactil.

protriptyline hydrochloride. (Various Mfr.) Protriptyline hydrochloride 5 mg, 10 mg. Tab. Bot. 100s, 1000s. Rx.
Use: Antidepressant.

Provenge. (Dendreon Corporation) Sipuleucel-T 50 million autologous CD54⁺ cells (activated with prostatic acid phosphatase linked to granulocyte-macrophage colony-stimulating factor). Inj., Susp. Patient-specific infusion bags. 250 mL. Rx.
Use: Miscellaneous antineoplastic.

Proventil HFA. (Key) Albuterol sulfate 90 mcg/actuation. Aer. Can. 6.7 g/ (200 inhalations). Contains no chlorofluorocarbons (CFCs). Rx.
Use: Bronchodilator, sympathomimetic.

Provera. (Pharmacia & Upjohn) Medroxyprogesterone acetate 2.5 mg, 5 mg, 10 mg. Lactose, sucrose. Tab. Bot. 30s, 100s; 500s, UD 10s (10 mg only). Rx.
Use: Sex hormone, progestin.

Provigil. (Cephalon) Modafinil 100 mg, 200 mg, lactose, talc. Tab. Bot. 100s. c-IV.
Use: CNS stimulant, analeptic.

ProVisc. (Alcon) Sodium hyaluronate 10 mg/mL. Sodium chloride 8.4 mg/mL. Inj. Disposable syringe. 0.4 mL, 0.55 mL, 0.85 mL. Rx.
Use: Ophthalmic surgical adjunct.

Provocholine. (Methapharm) Methacholine Cl 100 mg/5 mL. Soln. for Inhalation. Vial 5 mL. Rx.
Use: Diagnostic aid.

Prox/APAP. (Forest) Propoxyphene hydrochloride 65 mg, acetaminophen 650 mg. Tab. Bot. 100s, 500s. c-IV.
Use: Analgesic combination; narcotic.

•**proxazole.** (PROX-a-zole) USAN.
Use: Analgesic; anti-inflammatory; muscle relaxant.

•**proxazole citrate.** (PROX-a-zole) USAN.
  Use: Relaxant, smooth muscle; analgesic; anti-inflammatory.
•**proxicromil.** (prox-ih-KROE-mill) USAN.
  Use: Antiallergic.
Proxigel. (Schwarz Pharma) Carbamide peroxide 10% in a water-free gel base. Tube 34 g w/applicator. *OTC.*
  Use: Antiseptic, cleanser.
•**proxorphan tartrate.** (PROX-ahr-fan TAR-trate) USAN.
  Use: Analgesic; antitussive.
Proxy 65. (Parmed Pharmaceuticals, Inc.) Propoxyphene hydrochloride 65 mg, acetaminophen 650 mg. Tab. Bot. 100s, 500s. *c-iv.*
  Use: Analgesic combination; narcotic.
Prozac. (Eli Lilly/Dista) Fluoxetine hydrochloride. **Pulvules:** 10 mg, 20 mg, 40 mg. Bot. 30s (except 10 mg); 100s (except 40 mg); 2000s, blister card 31s (20 mg only). **Oral Soln.:** 20 mg/5 mL. Alcohol 0.23%, sucrose, mint flavor. Bot. 120 mL. *Rx.*
  Tall Man: PROzac
  Use: Antidepressant, selective serotonin reuptake inhibitor.
Prozac Weekly. (Eli Lilly/Dista) Fluoxetine hydrochloride 90 mg. Sucrose, sugar spheres. Enteric-coated pellets. DR Cap. Blister 4s. *Rx.*
  Tall Man: PROzac
  Use: Antidepressant, selective serotonin reuptake inhibitor.
prucalopride hydrochloride.
  Use: Constipation.
prucalopride succinate.
  Use: Constipation.
PruClair. (PruGen) *Butyrospermum parkii,* glyceryl stearate, glycyrrhetinic acid, PEG-100 stearate, alcohols, allantoin, DMDM hydantoin, disodium EDTA, ethylhexylglycerin, sodium hyaluronate, tocopheryl acetate. Cream. 100 g. *Rx.*
  Use: Miscellaneous topical combination.
Prudents. (Bariatric) Acetylphenylisatin 5 mg. Chewable protein and amino acid. Tab. Bot. 30s, 100s. *OTC.*
  Use: Laxative.
Prudoxin. (Healthpoint Medical) Doxepin hydrochloride 5%. Cream, Top. 45 g. *Rx.*
  Use: Topical antihistamine preparation.
Prulet. (Mission Pharmacal) White phenolphthalein 60 mg. Tab. Strips 12s, 40s. *OTC.*
  Use: Laxative.
PruMyx. (PruGen) Olive oil, glycerin, palm glycerides, vegetable oil, lecithin,

squalane, betaine, palmitamide MEA, sarcosine, acetamide MEA, hydroxyethyl cellulose, sodium carbomer, carbomer, xanthan gum. Preservative free and fragrance free. Cream. 140 g. *Rx.*
  Use: Miscellaneous topical combination.
prune powder concentrated dehydrated.
  See: Diacetyl-dihydroxyphenylisatin.
Prurilo. (Whorton Pharmaceuticals, Inc.) Menthol 0.25%, phenol 0.25%, calamine lotion in special lubricating base. Bot. 4 oz, 8 oz. *OTC.*
  Use: Dermatologic, counterirritant.
•**prussian blue insoluble.** (PRUSH-un) USAN.
  Use: Antidote.
prussian blue oral.
  Use: Chelating agents; detoxification agent.
  See: Radiogardase.
•**pruveranserin.** (prue-VAN-ser-in) USAN.
  Use: 5-HT$_2$ receptor antagonist; insomnia.
•**pruvanserin hydrochloride.** (prue-VAN-ser-in) USAN.
  Use: 5-HT$_2$ receptor antagonist; insomnia.
PSE BPM. (Boca Pharmacal) Pseudoephedrine hydrochloride 60 mg, brompheniramine maleate 4 mg. Alcohol, sugar, and dye free. Cherry flavor. Liq. 473 mL. *Rx.*
  Use: Decongestant and antihistamine, upper respiratory combination.
PSE Brom DM. (Boca Pharmacal) Dextromethorphan HBr 30 mg, brompheniramine maleate 4 mg, pseudoephedrine hydrochloride 60 mg per 5 mL. Alcohol and sugar free. Sorbitol. Syr. 473 mL. *Rx.*
  Use: Upper respiratory combination, antitussive combination.
PSE CPM. (Boca Pharmacal) Pseudoephedrine hydrochloride 15 mg, chlorpheniramine maleate 2 mg. Aspartame, sugar, mannitol, phenylalanine. Grape flavor. Chew. Tab. 100s. *Rx.*
  Use: Decongestant and antihistamine, upper respiratory combination.
PSE 15/CPM 2. (Cypress) Pseudoephedrine hydrochloride 15 mg, chlorpheniramine maleate 2 mg. Aspartame, phenylalanine 1.7 mg. Chew. Tab. 100s. *Rx.*
  Use: Upper respiratory combination, decongestant and antihistamine.
PSE 120/MSC 2.5. (Cypress) Pseudoephedrine hydrochloride 120 mg, meth-

scopolamine nitrate 2.5 mg. Dye free. ER Tab. Bot. 60s. *Rx.*
Use: Upper respiratory combination, decongestant, antihistamine, and anticholinergic.

Pseudo Carb DM Pediatric. (Boca Pharmacal) Dextromethorphan HBr 15 mg, carbinoxamine maleate 3 mg, pseudoephedrine hydrochloride 12.5 mg per 5 mL. Alcohol, sugar, and dye free. Liq. 118 mL, 473 mL. *Rx.*
Use: Upper respiratory combination, antitussive combination.

Pseudo Carb Pediatric. (Boca Pharmacal) Pseudoephedrine hydrochloride 12.5 mg, carbinoxamine maleate 2 mg. Alcohol, sugar, and dye free. Liq. 118 mL, 473 mL. *Rx.*
Use: Upper respiratory combination, decongestant and antihistamine.

Pseudo-Car DM. (Geneva) Pseudoephedrine hydrochloride 60 mg, carbinoxamine maleate 4 mg, dextromethorphan HBr 15 mg/5 mL, alcohol < 0.6%. Bot. Pt, gal. *Rx.*
Use: Antihistamine; antitussive; decongestant.

Pseudo-Chlor. (Various Mfr.) Pseudoephedrine hydrochloride 120 mg, chlorpheniramine maleate 8 mg. Cap. Bot. 100s, 250s. *Rx.*
Use: Antihistamine; decongestant.

Pseudo Cough. (Boca Pharmacal) Dextromethorphan HBr 15 mg, guaifenesin 175 mg, pseudoephedrine hydrochloride 32 mg per 5 mL. Alcohol free. Acesulfame K, saccharin, sorbitol. Grape flavor. Liq. 118 mL, 473 mL. *Rx.*
Use: Upper respiratory combination, antitussive and expectorant combination.

• **pseudoephedrine hydrochloride.** (SOO-doe-e-FED-rin) *USP 34.*
Use: Adrenergic, vasoconstrictor.
See: Congestaid.
   Dimetapp, Maximum Strength 12-Hour Non-Drowsy.
   ElixSure Children's Congestion.
   Genaphed.
   Kid Kare.
   Nasal Decongestant, Children's Non-Drowsy.
   Nasal Decongestant Oral.
   Simply Stuffy.
   Sinustop.
   Sudafed.
   Sudafed Children's Non-Drowsy.
   Sudafed Non-Drowsy, Maximum Strength.
   Sudafed Non-Drowsy 12 Hour Long-Acting.

   Sudafed Non-Drowsy 24 Hour Long-Acting.
   SudoGest Non-Drowsy.
   Triaminic AM Decongestant Formula.
   Unifed.
W/Acetaminophen.
See: Dilotab II.
   Mapap Sinus Maximum Strength.
   Ornex No Drowsiness.
   Ornex No Drowsiness Maximum Strength.
W/Acetaminophen, Chlorpheniramine Maleate.
See: Advil Allergy Sinus.
   BC Allergy, Sinus, Headache.
W/Acetaminophen, Dextromethorphan Hydrobromide, Guaifenesin.
See: Duraflu.
   Flutabs.
   Maxiflu DM.
   Maxiflu G.
   Tylenol Cold Severe Congestion.
W/Acetaminophen, Guaifenesin.
See: Poly-Vent Plus.
   Tylenol Sinus Severe Congestion.
W/Belladonna Alkaloids, Chlorpheniramine Maleate.
See: Respa A.R.
W/Brompheniramine Maleate.
See: Bidhist-D.
   BPM Pseudo 6/45 mg.
   Bromaline.
   Bromhist-NR.
   Bromhist Pediatric.
   Brotapp.
   BröveX PSB.
   BröveX SR.
   Histex SR.
   J-Tan D PD.
   Lodrane.
   Lodrane LD.
   Lodrane 12 D.
   Lodrane 24 D.
   LoHist-LQ.
   LoHist PSB.
   LoHist 12D.
   PSE-BPM.
   Q-Tapp.
   Respahist.
   Sildec.
   Sinuhist.
   SymPak II.
   Touro Allergy.
   ULTRAbrom.
   ULTRAbrom PD.
W/Brompheniramine Maleate, Chlophedianol Hydrochloride.
See: Dicel CD.
W/Brompheniramine Maleate, Codeine Phosphate.
See: CPB WC.

Mar-Cof BP.
M-End WC.
Mesehist WC.
W/Brompheniramine Maleate, Dextro-
methorphan Hydrobromide.
See: AccuHist DM Pediatric.
Anaplex-DM Cough.
Bromaline DM.
Bromdex D.
Brometane-DX Cough.
Bromfed DM.
Bromhist-DM.
Bromhist PDX.
Bromphenex DM.
Brotapp DM.
BröveX PSB DM.
Dallergy DM.
Dimaphen DM Cough, Cold & Allergy.
Dimetane DX.
DM/PSE/BPM.
Myphetane DX Cough.
Neo DM.
PBM Allergy.
Pediahist DM.
Prohist DM.
PSE Brom DM.
Q-Tapp DM Cold and Cough.
Rondec DM.
Sildec-DM.
TGQ 50PSE/3BRM/30DM.
TGQ 40PSE/4BRM/20DM.
TGQ 30PSE/3BRM/15DM.
W/Brompheniramine Maleate, Dextro-
methorphan Hydrobromide, Guai-
fenesin.
See: Bromhist DM Pediatric.
Histacol DM Pediatric.
Pediahist DM.
W/Brompheniramine Maleate, Dihydroco-
deine Bitartrate.
See: J-COF DHC.
W/Carbetapentane Citrate.
See: Corzall.
W/Carbetapentane Citrate, Guaifenesin.
See: Exall-D.
W/Carbetapentane Citrate, Pyrilamine
Maleate.
See: Corzall Plus.
W/Carbinoxamine Maleate.
See: Cordron-D.
Cordron-D NR.
Palgic-DS.
Pseudo Carb Pediatric.
Rondec TR.
Sildec.
W/Cetirizine Hydrochloride.
See: All Day Allergy-D.
W/Chlophedianol Hydrochloride.
See: Clofera.

W/Chlophedianol Hydrochloride, Guai-
fenesin.
See: Vanacof Dx.
W/Chlorcyclizine Hydrochloride, Codeine
Phosphate.
See: Notuss NXD.
W/Chlorpheniramine Maleate.
See: AccuHist.
Allerest Maximum Strength.
AMBI 60PSE/4CPM.
CPM PSE.
Colfed-A.
Deconamine.
Deconomed SR.
Duratuss DA.
Genaphed Plus.
Histex.
LoHist-D.
Neutrahist.
PSE CPM.
PSE 15/CPM 2.
RE2+30.
Sudafed Sinus & Allergy.
SudaHist.
Sudal-12 Tannate.
SudoGest Sinus & Allergy Maximum
Strength.
Zinx Chlor-D.
W/Chlorpheniramine Maleate, Codeine
Phosphate.
See: Phenylhistine DH.
Zodry DAC 80.
Zodry DAC 50.
Zodry DAC 40.
Zodry DAC 60.
Zodry DAC 30.
Zodry DAC 35.
Zodry DAC 25.
W/Chlorpheniramine Maleate, Dextro-
methorphan Hydrobromide.
See: AccuHist PDX.
Allres DS.
AMBI 60PSE/4CPM/20DM.
CPM/PSE DM.
Dicel DM.
Esocor P.
KidKare Children's Cough/Cold.
Mesehist DM.
Neutrahist PDX.
Pedia Relief Cough-Cold.
Pediatric Cough & Cold.
Pediatric Cough & Cold Medicine.
Rescon DM.
Triaminic-D Children's.
W/Chlorpheniramine Maleate, Dihydroco-
deine Bitartrate.
See: DiHydro-CP.
Pancof.
Tricof.

W/Chlorpheniramine Maleate, Guaifene-
sin, Hydrocodone Bitartrate.
See: ZTuss Expectorant.
W/Chlorpheniramine Maleate, Hydro-
codone Bitartrate.
See: Notuss-Forte.
  Pediatex HC.
  Tussend.
W/Chlorpheniramine Maleate, Meth-
scopolamine Nitrate.
See: CPM 8/PSE 90/MSC 2.5.
  DryMax.
  Relcof PSE.
  Time-Hist QD.
W/Codeine Phosphate.
See: EndaCof-DC.
  Notuss-DC.
  Nucofed.
W/Codeine Phosphate, Guaifenesin.
See: Cheratussin DAC.
  Guiatuss DAC.
  Lortuss EX.
  Mytussin DAC.
  Tusnel C.
  Zodryl DEC 80.
  Zodryl DEC 50.
  Zodryl DEC 40.
  Zodryl DEC 60.
  Zodryl DEC 30.
  Zodryl DEC 35.
  Zodryl DEC 25.
W/Codeine Phosphate, Triprolidine
Hydrochloride.
See: Poly Hist NC.
W/Dexchlorpheniramine Maleate.
See: HexaFed.
W/Dexchlorpheniramine Maleate, Dextro-
methorphan Hydrobromide.
See: TanaCof-DM.
  Tanafed DMX.
  Tannate DMP-DEX.
W/Dexchlorpheniramine Maleate, Meth-
scopolamine Nitrate.
See: D-Hist D.
  Histatab D.
W/Dextromethorphan Hydrobromide.
See: Robitussin Pediatric Cough & Cold
  Formula.
W/Dextromethorphan Hydrobromide,
Acetaminophen.
See: 666 Cold Preparation Maximum
  Strength.
W/Dextromethorphan Hydrobromide,
Doxylamine Succinate.
See: Lortuss DM.
W/Dextromethorphan Hydrobromide,
Guaifenesin.
See: Aldex GS DM.
  Ambifed-G DM.
  AMBI 60/580/30.
  AMBI 60PSE/400GFN/20DM.

  AMBI 40PSE/400GFN/20DM.
  Bionel.
  Bionel Pediatric.
  Capmist DM.
  Despec.
  Donatussin DM.
  ExeFen DMX.
  GFN 600/PSE 60/DM 30.
  Liquicough DM.
  Maxifed DM.
  Maxifed DMX.
  Medent DMI.
  PanMist-DM.
  Poly-Vent DM.
  Pseudo Cough.
  Q-Tussin CF.
  Relacon DM NR.
  Relasin DM.
  Robaben CF.
  Robitussin Cough & Cold D.
  Sudafed Multi-Symptom Cold &
  Cough.
  TGQ 30PSE/150GFN/15DM.
  Tidafen DM.
  TL-DEX DM.
  Touro CC-LD.
  Tusnel.
  Tusnel-DM Pediatric.
  Tusnel Pediatric.
  Z-Cof DMX.
  Z-Cof 8DM.
  Z-Cof I.
W/Dextromethorphan Hydrobromide,
Pyrilamine Maleate.
See: Viravan-PDM.
W/Dihydrocodeine, Guaifenesin.
See: Despec-EXP.
  Pancof-EXP.
W/Diphenhydramine Hydrochloride.
See: Respa-SA.
  Tekral.
W/Doxylamine Succinate.
See: Lortuss LQ.
W/Guaifenesin.
See: Altarussin-PE.
  Ambifed.
  Ambifed-G.
  AMBI 40PSE/400GFN.
  AMBI 60/580.
  AMBI 60PSE/400GFN.
  Coldmist JR.
  Coldmist LA.
  Congestac.
  Dynex.
  Entex PSE.
  GFN-PSE.
  Guaifenex GP.
  Guaifenex PSE.
  Guaifenex PSE 85.
  Guaifenex PSE 60.
  GuaiMAX-D.

Iosal II.
LEV/PSE/GG.
Maxifed.
Maxifed-G.
Mucinex D.
Mucinex D Maximum Strength.
Nasatab LA.
Nomuc-PE.
Respa-1st.
Respaire-120 SR.
Respaire-60 SR.
Severe Congestion Tussin.
Stamoist E.
Sudafed Maximum Strength Non-
Drowsy Non-Drying Sinus.
SudaTex G.
Tenar PSE.
Touro LA.
Triacting.
W/Ibuprofen.
See: Advil Cold & Sinus.
Children's Motrin Cold.
W/Methscopolamine Nitrate.
See: AllePak Dose Pack.
Allergy DN.
AlleRx-D.
AlleRx Dose Pack.
Amdry-D.
PSE 120/MSC 2.5.
W/Naproxen Sodium.
See: Aleve-D Sinus & Cold.
W/Pyrilamine Maleate.
See: Viravan-P.
W/Triprolidine Hydrochloride.
See: Allerfrim.
Altafed.
Aprodine.
Genac.
Silafed.
Tripohist D.
pseudoephedrine hydrochloride.
(Ohm) Pseudoephedrine hydrochloride
120 mg. Castor oil. ER Tab. 10s. *OTC.*
Use: Nasal decongestant, arylalkyl-
amine.
pseudoephedrine hydrochloride.
(Various Mfr.) Pseudoephedrine hydro-
chloride. **Tab.:** 30 mg, 60 mg. Bot. 24s
(30 mg only), 100s, 1000s, blister pack
100s. **Liq.:** 30 mg/5 mL. Bot. 120 mL,
473 mL. *OTC.*
Use: Nasal decongestant, arylalyl-
amine.
**pseudoephedrine hydrochloride and
triprolidine hydrochloride.** (Various
Mfr.) Pseudoephedrine hydrochloride
60 mg, triprolidine hydrochloride
2.5 mg. Tab. Bot. 100s, 1000s, UD
100s. *Rx.*
Use: Antihistamine; decongestant.

• **pseudoephedrine hydrochloride, carbinoxamine maleate, and dextromethorphan hydrobromide oral solution.** *USP 34.*
Use: Decongestant, antihistamine, antitussive.
**pseudoephedrine hydrochloride/chlor-
pheniramine maleate.** (Brighton)
Pseudoephedrine hydrochloride
100 mg, chlorpheniramine maleate
12 mg. Sugar. ER Cap. 100s. *Rx.*
Use: Upper respiratory combination, decongestant and antihistamine.
**pseudoephedrine hydrochloride/guai-
fenesin.** (River's Edge) Pseudoephedrine hydrochloride/guaifenesin 45 mg/
800 mg, 50 mg/1200 mg, 60 mg/
500 mg, 90 mg/800 mg. ER Tab. 30s
(50 mg/1200 mg only), 100s. *Rx.*
Use: Upper respiratory combination, decongestant and expectorant combination.
**pseudoephedrine hydrochloride/guai-
fenesin.** (Various Mfr.) Pseudoephedrine hydrochloride 45 mg, guaifenesin
800 mg. Tab. 100s. *Rx.*
Use: Upper respiratory combination, decongestant and expectorant combination.
**pseudoephedrine hydrochloride/guai-
fenesin LA.** (URL) Pseudoephedrine
hydrochloride 85 mg, guaifenesin
795 mg. ER Tab. 100s. *Rx.*
Use: Decongestant and expectorant
combination, upper respiratory combination.
**pseudoephedrine hydrochloride/guai-
fenesin SR.** (URL) Pseudoephedrine
hydrochloride 48 mg, guaifenesin
595 mg. ER Tab. 100s. *Rx.*
Use: Decongestant and expectorant
combination, upper respiratory combination.
• **pseudoephedrine polistirex.** (SOO-
doe-e-FED-rin POL-ee-SYE-rex)
USAN.
Use: Decongestant, nasal.
W/Combinations.
See: Atuss-12 DM.
• **pseudoephedrine sulfate.** (SOO-doe-e-
FED-rin) *USP 34.*
Use: Bronchodilator.
See: Afrinol Repetabs.
W/Desloratadine.
See: Clarinex-D 24 Hour.
W/Dexbrompheniramine Maleate.
See: Drixoral Cold & Allergy.
W/Loratadine.
See: Alavert Allergy & Sinus D-12 Hour.
Allergy Relief & Nasal Decongestant.
Claritin-D 12 Hour.

Claritin-D 24 Hour.
Clear-Atadine D.
Loratadine D.
pseudoephedrine tannate.
W/Brompheniramine Tannate.
See: Brovex PD.
B-Vex PD.
Lodrane D.
W/Carbetapentane Tannate.
See: Carb Pseudo-Tan.
Respi-Tann.
Respi-Tann Pd.
W/Carbinoxamine Tannate, Dextromethorphan Tannate.
See: Carb PSE 12 DM.
W/Chlorpheniramine Tannate, Dextromethorphan Tannate.
See: Atuss DS Tannate.
W/Dexchlorpheniramine Tannate, Dextromethorphan Tannate.
See: Indamix DM.
W/Dexchlorpheniramine Tannate, Pyrilamine Tannate.
See: Nalfrx.
Pseudo-Gest. (Major) Pseudoephedrine hydrochloride 30 mg, 60 mg. Tab. Bot. 24s, 100s. *OTC.*
Use: Decongestant.
Pseudo-Gest Plus. (Major) Pseudoephedrine hydrochloride 60 mg, chlorpheniramine maleate 4 mg. Tab. Bot. 24s, 100s, 200s. *OTC.*
Use: Antihistamine; decongestant.
Pseudo-Hist. (Holloway) Pseudoephedrine hydrochloride 30 mg, chlorpheniramine maleate 10 mg. Cap. Bot. 100s. *OTC.*
Use: Antihistamine; decongestant.
Pseudo-Hist Expectorant. (Holloway) Pseudoephedrine 15 mg, hydrocodone bitartrate 2.5 mg, guaifenesin 100 mg, alcohol 5%. Bot. 480 mL. *c-III.*
Use: Antitussive; decongestant; expectorant.
pseudomonas test.
Use: Urine test.
pseudomonic acid A.
Use: Anti-infective, topical.
See: Bactroban.
Pseudo Plus. (Weeks & Leo) Pseudoephedrine hydrochloride 60 mg, chlorpheniramine maleate 4 mg. Tab. Bot. 40s. *OTC.*
Use: Antihistamine; decongestant.
Pseudo Syrup. (Major) Pseudoephedrine 30 mg/5 mL. Liq. Bot. 120 mL, pt, gal. *OTC.*
Use: Decongestant.
psoralens.
See: Methoxsalen.
Psor-a-set. (Hogil) Salicylic acid 2%.

Soap. Bar 97.5 g. *OTC.*
Use: Keratolytic.
Psorcon E. (Dermik) Diflorasone diacetate 0.05%. **Oint.:** Emollient, occlusive base, lanolin alcohol, white petrolatum. Tube 15 g, 30 g, 60 g. **Cream:** Hydrophilic base, stearyl alcohol, cetyl alcohol, mineral oil. Tube 15 g, 30 g, 60 g. *Rx.*
Use: Corticosteroid, topical.
Psorent. (NeoStrata) Coal tar solution 15% (equiv. to coal tar 2.3%). Soln. 100 mL. *OTC.*
Use: Miscellaneous tar-containing product.
Psorinail. (Summers) Coal tar solution w/ isopropyl alcohol 2.5%, 3-butylene glycol I, acetyl mandelic acid. Liq. Bot. 30 mL. *OTC.*
Use: Antipsoriatic, topical.
Psorion. (ICN) Betamethasone dipropionate 0.05%, mineral oil, white petrolatum, propylene glycol. Cream. Tube 15 g, 45 g. *Rx.*
Use: Corticosteroid, topical.
psychotherapeutic agents.
See: Atomoxetine Hydrochloride.
Fluoxetine Hydrochloride.
Olanzapine.
Sodium Oxybate.
Tranquilizers.
psychotherapeutic combinations.
See: Dextromethorphan Hydrobromide/
Quinidine Sulfate.
Olanzapine/Fluoxetine Hydrochloride.
psyllium.
Use: Laxative.
See: Fiberall Natural Flavor
Fiberall Orange Flavor.
Fiberall Tropical Fruit Flavor.
Genfiber.
Genfiber, Orange Flavor.
Geri-Mucil.
Hydrocil Instant.
Konsyl.
Konsyl-D.
Konsyl Easy Mix Formula.
Konsyl-Orange.
Konsyl Orange Sugar Free.
Metamucil.
Metamucil Orange Flavor, Original Texture.
Metamucil Orange Flavor, Smooth Texture.
Metamucil Original Texture.
Metamucil, Sugar Free, Orange Flavor, Smooth Texture.
Metamucil, Sugar Free, Smooth Texture.
Natural Fiber Laxative.
Natural Psyllium Fiber.

Perdiem Fiber Therapy.
Reguloid.
Reguloid, Orange.
Reguloid, Sugar Free Orange.
Reguloid, Sugar Free Regular.
Serutan.
Syllact.
W/Sennosides.
See: Senna Prompt.

•**psyllium hemicellulose.** (SIL-ee-um
HEM-ee-SEL-ue-lose) *USP 34.*
Use: Laxative.

•**psyllium husk.** (SIL-ee-um) *USP 34.*
Use: Laxative, cathartic.

psyllium hydrocolloid.
Use: Laxative.

psyllium seed gel.
Use: Laxative.

pteroic acid. The compound formed by
the linkage of carbon 6 of 2-amine-4-
hydroxypteridine by means of a methylene group with the nitrogen of p-
aminobenzoic acid.

pteroylglutamic acid.
See: Folic acid.

pteroylmonoglutamic acid. Pteroylglutamic acid.
See: Folic acid.

P-Tex. (Poly Pharmaceuticals) Brompheniramine tannate 10 mg/5 mL. Alcohol and sugar free. Peach flavor. Oral
Susp. 480 mL. *Rx.*
Use: Antihistamine.

PTFE. (Ethicon) Polytef.

PTU.
See: Propylthiouracil.

Pulexn DM. (Ballay Pharmaceuticals)
Dextromethorphan HBr 10 mg, guaifenesin 100 mg per 5 mL. Saccharin,
sorbitol. Syr. 473 mL. *Rx.*
Use: Antitussive with expectorant.

Pulmicort Flexhaler. (AstraZeneca)
Budesonide 90 mcg (each actuation
delivers ≈ 80 mcg/metered dose),
180 mcg (each actuation delivers
≈ 160 mcg/metered dose). Lactose.
Inh. Pow. 60 dose *Flexhaler* (90 mcg
only), 120 dose *Flexhaler* (180 mcg
only). *Rx.*
Use: Corticosteroid.

Pulmicort Respules. (AstraZeneca)
Budesonide 0.25 mg/2 mL, 0.5 mg/
2 mL, 1 mg/2 mL. EDTA. Inh. Susp.
Single-dose envelopes. 30s. *Rx.*
Use: Respiratory inhalant, corticoste-
roid.

Pulmocare. (Abbott Nutrition) Protein
62.6 g (L-carnitine, taurine), carbohydrate 105.7 g (corn maltodextrin, sucrose), fat 93.3 g (canola oil, corn oil,
high oleic safflower oil, medium chain

triglycerides, soy lecithin)/L. Sodium
1310 mg/L, potassium 1960 mg/L,
475 mOsm/kg H_2O, 1.5 cal/mL. Vita-
mins A, B_1, B_2, B_3, B_5, B_6, B_7, B_{12}, C, D,
E, K, Ca, choline, Cl^-, Cr, Cu, Fe, fo-
lic acid, I, Mg, Mn, Mo, P, Se, Zn. Gluten and lactose free. Vanilla and strawberry flavors and unflavored. Liq.
240 mL, 1 L. *OTC.*
Use: Enteral nutritional therapy, defined
formula diet.

pulmonary surfactant replacement.
(Scios Nova)
Use: Diagnostic aid, thyroid. [Orphan
Drug]

**pulmonary surfactant replacement,
porcine.**
Use: Diagnostic aid, thyroid. [Orphan
Drug]
See: Curosurf.

Pulmosin. (Spanner) Guaiacol 0.1 g, eucalyptol 0.08 g, camphor 0.05 g, iodoform 0.02 g/2 mL. Multiple-dose vial
30 mL. IM. Inj. *Rx.*

Pulmozyme. (Genentech) Dornase alfa
1 mg, calcium chloride dihydrate
0.15 mg, NaCl 8.77 mg/mL. Soln. for
Inh. Amps. Single-use 2.5 mL. *Rx.*
Use: Anti-infective.

•**pumice.** (PUM-iss) *USP 34.*
Use: Abrasive, dental.

punctum plug. (Eagle Vision) Silicone
plug. 0.5 mm, 0.6 mm, 0.7 mm,
0.8 mm. Pkg. 2 plugs, 1 inserter tool.
Rx.
Use: Punctal plug.

Puralube. (Fera Pharmaceuticals) White
petrolatum 85%, mineral oil 15%. Oint.,
Ophth. 3.5 g, UD 1 g (20s). *OTC.*
Use: Ocular lubricant.

Puralube Tears. (E. Fougera) Polyvinyl
alcohol 1%, polyethylene glycol 400
1%, EDTA, benzalkonium Cl. Soln. Bot.
15 mL. *OTC.*
Use: Lubricant, ophthalmic.

Puresept Murine Saline. (Ross) **Disinfecting soln.:** Sterile hydrogen peroxide solution 3%, sodium stannate, sodium nitrate, phosphate buffers, thimerosal free. 237 mL. **Murine Saline
Soln.:** Buffered isotonic solution w/bo-
rate buffers, NaCl, sorbic acid 0.1%,
EDTA 0.1%. 60, 237, 355 mL. Includes
cups and lens holder. *OTC.*
Use: Contact lens care.

Puri-Clens. (Sween) UD 2 oz. Bot. 8 oz.
Use: Dermatologic, wound therapy.

purified oxgall.
See: Bile Extract, Ox.

purified protein derivative of tuber-culin.
Use: Mantoux TB test.
See: Aplisol.
Aplitest.
Tubersol.

purified type II collagen.
Use: Juvenile rheumatoid arthritis.
[Orphan Drug]

purine analogs and related agents.
Use: Antimetabolite.
See: Allopurinol.
Cladribine.
Clofarabine.
Fludarabine Phosphate.
Mercaptopurine.
Pentostatin.
Rasburicase.
Thioguanine.

Purinethol. (Gate Pharmaceuticals) Mercaptopurine 50 mg. Tab. Bot. 25s, 250s. *Rx.*
Use: Antineoplastic.

•**puromycin.** (PURE-oh-MY-sin) USAN.
Use: Antineoplastic; antiprotozoal, try-panosoma.

•**puromycin hydrochloride.** USAN.
Use: Antineoplastic; antiprotozoal, try-panosoma.

purple foxglove.
See: Digitalis.

Purpose Shampoo. (Johnson & Johnson) Water, amphoteric-19, PEG-44 sorbitan laurate, PEG-150 distea-rate, sorbitan laurate, boric acid, fra-grance, benzyl alcohol. Bot. 8 oz. *OTC.*
Use: Dermatologic.

Purpose Soap. (Johnson & Johnson) Sodium tallowate, sodium cocoate, gly-cerin, NaCl, BHT, EDTA. Bar 108 g, 180 g. *OTC.*
Use: Dermatologic, cleanser.

Pursettes Premenstrual. (DEP Corp.) Acetaminophen 500 mg, pamabrom 25 mg, pyrilamine maleate 15 mg. Tab. Bot. 24s. *OTC.*
Use: Analgesic; antihistamine; diuretic.

PVP-I. (Day-Baldwin) Povidone-iodine. Oint. Tube 1 oz, Jar lb, Foilpac 1.5 g. *OTC.*
Use: Antiseborrheic; antiseptic.

Py-Co-Pay Tooth Powder. (Block Drug) Sodium Cl, sodium bicarbonate, cal-cium carbonate, magnesium carbonate, tricalcium phosphate, eugenol, methyl salicylate. Can 7 oz. *OTC.*
Use: Dentifrice.

Pylera. (Axcan) Bismuth subcitrate po-tassium 140 mg/metronidazole 125 mg/ tetracycline hydrochloride 125 mg.

Cap. 120s. *Rx.*
Use: Helicobacter pylori agent.

Pyocidin-Otic. (Forest) Hydrocortisone 5 mg, polymyxin B sulfate 10,000 USP units/mL in a vehicle containing water and propylene glycol. Otic Soln. Bot. 10 mL w/sterile dropper. *Rx.*
Use: Anti-infective; corticosteroid; otic.

•**pyrabrom.** (PEER-ah-brahm) USAN.
Use: Antihistamine.

Pyracol. (Davis & Sly) Pyrathyn hydro-chloride 0.08 g, ammonium Cl 0.778 g, citric acid 0.52 g, menthol 0.006 g/fl oz. Bot. pt.

pyraminyl.
See: Pyrilamine maleate.

pyranilamine maleate.
See: Pyrilamine maleate.

pyranisamine bromotheophyllinate.
See: Pyrabrom.

pyranisamine maleate.
See: Pyrilamine maleate.

•**pyrantel pamoate.** (pi-RAN-tel PAM-oh-ate) *USP 34.*
Use: Anthelmintic.
See: Pin-Rid.
Pin-X.

•**pyrantel tartrate.** (pi-RAN-tel) USAN.
Use: Anthelmintic.

•**pyrazinamide.** (peer-uh-ZIN-uh-mide) *USP 34.* Aldinamide, Zinamide.
Use: Antituberculosis agent.

pyrazinamide. (Various Mfr.) Pyrazin-amide 500 mg. Tab. 60s, 90s, 100s, 500s, UD 100s.
Use: Anti-tuberculosis agent.

pyrazinecarboxamide.
See: Pyrazinamide.

•**pyrazofurin.** (pihr-AZZ-oh-FYOO-rin) USAN.
Use: Antineoplastic.

pyrazoline.
See: Antipyrine.

pyrbenzindole.
See: Benzindopyrine Hydrochloride.

•**pyrethrum extract.** (pye-REE-thrum) *USP 34.*
Use: Pediculicide.

Pyribenzamine.
See: PBZ.

Pyrichlor PE. (Breckenridge) Chlor-pheniramine maleate 2 mg, phenyl-ephrine hydrochloride 10 mg, pyril-amine maleate 10 mg per 5 mL. Gly-cerin, saccharin, sodium benzoate, sorbitol. Alcohol free and sugar free. Grape flavor. Liq. 473 mL. *Rx.*
Use: Upper respiratory combination, de-congestant and antihistamine.

Pyridamole. (Major) Dipyridamole. Tab.
25 mg: Bot. 1000s, 2500s. **50 mg,**
75 mg: 100s, 1000s. *Rx.*
Use: Antianginal; antiplatelet.
Pyridene. (Health for Life Brands)
Phenylazo Diamino Pyridine hydrochloride 100 mg. Tab. Bot. 24s, 100s,
1000s. *Rx.*
Use: Analgesic, urinary.
Pyridium. (Warner Chilcott) Phenazo-
pyridine hydrochloride 100 mg, 200 mg.
Sucrose, lactose. Tab. Bot. 100s,
1000s, UD 100s. *Rx.*
Use: Interstitial cystitis agent.
Pyridium Plus. (Warner Chilcott) Phenazopyridine hydrochloride 150 mg, hyo-
scyamine HBr 0.3 mg, butabarbital
15 mg, lactose. Tab. Bot. 30s, 100s. *Rx.*
Use: Interstitial cystitis agent.
•**pyridostigmine bromide.** (pihr-id-oh-
STIG-meen) *USP 34.*
Use: Cholinergic.
See: Mestinon.
pyridostigmine bromide. (Various Mfr.)
Pyridostigmine bromide 60 mg. Tab.
100s, 500s. *Rx.*
Use: Cholinergic.
Pyridox. (Oxford Pharmaceutical Ser-
vices) **No. 1:** Pyridoxine hydrochloride
100 mg. Tab. **No. 2:** Pyridoxine hydro-
chloride 200 mg. Tab. Bot. 100s. *OTC.*
Use: Vitamin supplement.
pyridoxal. Vitamin B$_6$. *OTC.*
Use: Vitamin supplement.
pyridoxamine. Vitamin B$_6$. *OTC.*
Use: Vitamin supplement.
See: Pyridoxine Hydrochloride.
•**pyridoxine hydrochloride.** (peer-ih-
DOX-een) *USP 34.*
Use: Enzyme co-factor vitamin, water-
soluble vitamin.
See: Aminoxin.
Vitamin B$_6$.
W/Combinations.
See: Vitelle Lurline PMS.
pyridoxine hydrochloride. (Various Mfr.)
Pyridoxine hydrochloride 100 mg/mL.
Chorobutanol anhydrous 5 mg. Inj. Vi-
als. 1 mL. *Rx.*
Use: Enzyme co-factor vitamin, water-
soluble vitamin.
pyridoxol.
See: Pyridoxine Hydrochloride.
Vitamin B$_6$.
pyrilamine bromotheophyllinate.
See: Bromaleate.
Pyrabrom.
•**pyrilamine maleate.** (peer-IL-a-meen)
USP 34.
Use: Antihistamine.

W/Acetaminophen, Caffeine.
See: Midol Menstrual Complete.
W/Acetaminophen, Pamabrom.
See: Pamprin Multi-Symptom Maximum
Strength.
W/Carbetapentane Citrate, Pseudo-
ephedrine Hydrochloride.
See: Corzall Plus.
W/Chlorpheniramine Maleate, Phenyl-
ephrine Hydrochloride.
See: MyHist-PD.
Polyhist PD.
Pyrichlor PE.
W/Codeine Phosphate, Phenylephrine
Hydrochloride.
See: Pro-Red AC.
Zotex-C.
W/Dextromethorphan Hydrobromide,
Phenylephrine Hydrochloride.
See: Albutussin.
Aldex DM Tannate.
Codal-DH.
Codimal DM.
MyHist-DM.
Poly Hist DM.
Pyril DM.
Reme Hist DM.
Triplex DM.
W/Dextromethorphan Hydrobromide,
Pseudoephedrine Hydrochloride.
See: Viravan-PDM.
W/Dihydrocodeine Bitartrate, Phenyl-
ephrine Hydrochloride.
See: Poly Hist DHC.
W/Hydrocodone Bitartrate, Phenylephrine
Hydrochloride.
See: Tussplex.
W/Phenylephrine Hydrochloride.
See: Deconsal CT.
W/Zinc Oxide.
See: Z-Xtra.
pyrilamine tannate.
Use: Antihistamine.
W/Carbetapentane Tannate, Phenyl-
ephrine Tannate.
See: C-Tanna 12D.
Tannate-12D S.
Tannihist-12 D.
Tussi-12D.
Tussi-12D S.
W/Chlorpheniramine Tannate, Phenyl-
ephrine Tannate.
See: Conal.
Triotann Pediatric.
Triple Tannate Pediatric.
W/Dexchlorpheniramine Tannate,
Pseudoephedrine Tannate.
See: Nalfrx.
W/Dextromethorphan Hydrobromide,
Pseudoephedrine Hydrochloride.
See: Viravan-T.

W/Phenylephrine Tannate.
See: AllanVan-S B.I.D.
R-Tanna 12.
Ryna-12.
Rynesa 12S.
RY-T-12.
W/Pseudoephedrine Hydrochloride.
See: Viravan-P.
Pyril DM. (Macoven) Dextromethorphan hydrobromide 15 mg, phenylephrine hydrochloride 5 mg, pyrilamine maleate 16 mg. Glycerin, methylparaben, sucrose, sucralose. Grape flavor. Susp. 473 mL. Rx.
Use: Upper respiratory combination, antitussive combination.
•**pyrimethamine.** (pihr-ih-METH-ah-meen) USP 34.
Use: Antimalarial.
See: Daraprim.
pyrimidine analogs.
Use: Antimetabolite.
See: Capecitabine.
Cytarabine.
Floxuridine.
Fluorouracil.
Gemcitabine Hydrochloride.
pyrimidine antagonist, topical.
Use: Dermatologic agent.
See: Fluorouracil.
•**pyrinoline.** (PIHR-ih-NO-leen) USAN.
Use: Cardiovascular agent, antiarrhythmic.
Pyrinyl Plus. (Rugby) Pyrethrins 0.33%, piperonyl butoxide 4%, benzyl alcohol. Shampoo. 59 mL. OTC.
Use: Pediculicide.
pyrithen.
See: Chlorothen Citrate.
•**pyrithione sodium.** (PEER-ih-THIGH-ohn) USAN.
Use: Antimicrobial, topical.
•**pyrithione zinc.** (PEER-ih-THIGH-ohn zingk) USAN. Zinc Omadine.
Use: Antifungal; anti-infective; antiseborrheic.
See: Denorex Everyday Dandruff.
Dermazine.
DHS Zinc.
Head & Shoulders.
Noble Formula.
Zincon.
ZNP Bar.

W/Ketoconazole.
See: Xolegel Duo Convenience Pack.
Pyrogallic Acid. (Gordon Laboratories) Pyrogallic acid 25%, chlorobutanol. Oint. Jar 1 oz, 1 lb.
Use: Dermatologic, wart therapy.
pyrogallol. Pyrogallic acid.
Pyrohep. (Major) Cyproheptadine hydrochloride 4 mg. Tab. Bot. 250s, 500s. Rx.
Use: Antihistamine.
•**pyrovalerone hydrochloride.** (PIE-row-val-EH-rone) USAN.
Use: Central stimulant.
•**pyroxamine maleate.** (pihr-OX-ah-meen) USAN.
Use: Antihistamine.
•**pyroxylin.** (pihr-OX-ih-lin) USP 34.
Soluble gun cotton. Cellulose nitrate.
Use: Pharmaceutic necessity for collodion.
pyrrobutamine phosphate.
Use: Antihistamine.
•**pyrrocaine.** (PIHR-oh-cane) USAN.
Use: Anesthetic, local.
pyrrocaine hydrochloride.
Use: Anesthetic, local.
pyrrocaine hydrochloride and epinephrine injection.
Use: Anesthetic, local.
•**pyrroliphene hydrochloride.** (pihr-OLE-ih-feen) USAN.
Use: Analgesic.
•**pyrrolnitrin.** (pihr-OLE-nye-trin) USAN. Under study.
Use: Antifungal.
Pyrroxate Extra-Strength. (Lee) Phenylephrine hydrochloride 10 mg, chlorpheniramine maleate 4 mg, acetaminophen 650 mg. PEG. Tab. 24s. OTC.
Use: Decongestant, antihistamine, and analgesic, upper respiratory combination.
•**pyrvinium pamoate.** (pihr-VIN-ee-uhm PAM-oh-ate) USP 34.
Use: Anthelmintic.
PYtest. (Tri-Med) 1 mCi^{14}-C-urea. Cap. UD 1s, 10s, 100s. Rx.
Use: Diagnostic aid.
PYtest Kit. (Tri-Med) Breath test for detecting H. pylori. Kit. 1 PYtest Cap. and breath collection equipment. Rx.
Use: Diagnostic aid.

Q

QB. (Major) Theophylline 150 mg, guaifenesin 90 mg. Liq. Bot. Pt, gal. *Rx.*
Use: Bronchodilator, expectorant.

QDALL. (Atley) Pseudoephedrine hydrochloride 100 mg, chlorpheniramine maleate 12 mg. Sucrose. Cap. 100s. *Rx.*
Use: Decongestant and antihistamine.

QDALL AR. (Atley) Chlorpheniramine (as maleate) 12 mg. Sucrose. ER Cap. 100s. *Rx.*
Use: Antihistamine.

Q-dryl. (Qualitest Pharmaceuticals) Diphenhydramine hydrochloride 12.5 mg per 5 mL. Glycerin, saccharin, sodium 5 mg, sucrose. Alcohol free. Cherry flavor. Liq. 237 mL. *OTC.*
Use: Antihistamine, nonselective ethanolamine.

Q-Pap. (Qualitest) Acetaminophen 325 mg. Tab. 100s. *OTC.*
Use: Analgesic.

Q-Pap Children's. (Qualitest) Acetaminophen. **Elix.:** 160 mg/5 mL. Alcohol free. Sorbitol, sucrose. Grape flavor. 118 mL, 3785 mL. **Liq.:** 160 mg/5 mL. Alcohol free. Sorbitol, sucrose. Cherry and grape flavors. 118 mL, 473 mL, 3785 mL. **Oral Susp.:** 160 mg/5 mL. Alcohol free. Butylparaben, corn syrup, sorbitol. Grape and bubble gum flavors. 118 mL. *Rx.*
Use: Analgesic.

Q-Pap Extra Strength. (Qualitest) Acetaminophen 500 mg. Tab. 100s. *OTC.*
Use: Analgesic.

Q-Pap Infants. (Qualitest) Acetaminophen 100 mg/mL. Alcohol free. Butylparaben, saccharin. Fruit flavor. Soln., Conc., Oral. 15 mL. *OTC.*
Use: Analgesic.

Q-Tapp. (Qualitest) Pseudoephedrine hydrochloride 15 mg, brompheniramine maleate 1 mg per 5 mL. Alcohol free. Corn syrup, saccharin, sorbitol. Grape flavor. Elix. 237 mL. *OTC.*
Use: Upper respiratory combination, decongestant and antihistamine.

Q-Tapp DM Cold & Cough. (Qualitest) Dextromethorphan HBr 5 mg, brompheniramine maleate 1 mg, pseudoephedrine hydrochloride 15 mg per 5 mL. Alcohol free. Corn syrup, saccharin, sorbitol. Grape flavor. Elixir. 118 mL. *OTC.*
Use: Upper respiratory combination, antitussive combination.

Q.T. Quick Tanning Suntan by Coppertone. (Schering-Plough) Ethylhexyl p-methoxycinnamate, dihydroxyacetone. SPF 2. Lot. Bot. 120 mL. *OTC.*
Use: Sunscreen.

Qua-Bid. (Quaker City Pharmacal) Papaverine hydrochloride 150 mg. TR Cap. Bot. 100s, 1000s. *OTC.*
Use: Vasodilator.

•**quadazocine mesylate.** (kwad-AZE-oh-SEEN) USAN.
Use: Opioid antagonist.

Quadramet. (DuPont) Samarium SM 153 lexidronam 1850 MBq/mL (50 mCi/mL) at calibration. Inj. Frozen, single-dose vial. 10 mL. In 2 mL fill (3700 MBq), 3 mL fill (5550 MBq). *Rx.*
Use: Treatment for bone lesions.

Quadrapax. (Acella Pharmaceuticals) Atropine sulfate 0.0194 mg, scopolamine hydrobromide 0.0065 mg, hyoscyamine hydrobromide or sulfate 0.1037 mg. Alcohol 23%, glycerin, saccharin, sorbitol, sucrose. Grape flavor. Elix. 473 mL. *c-IV.*
Use: Gastrointestinal anticholinergic combination.

quadruple sulfonamides.
See: Sulfonamides.

Quad-Tuss Tannate Pediatric. (Hi-Tech) Carbetapentane tannate 30 mg, chlorpheniramine tannate 4 mg, phenylephrine tannate 5 mg, ephedrine tannate 5 mg per 5 mL. Methylparaben, saccharin, sucrose. Susp. 473 mL. *Rx.*
Use: Upper respiratory combination, antitussive combination.

Qualaquin. (AR Scientific) Quinine sulfate 324 mg. Cap. 30s, 100s, 500s, 1,000s. *Rx.*
Use: Antimalarial.

Qual-Tussin. (Pharmaceutical Associates) Dextromethorphan HBr 7.5 mg, guaifenesin 100 mg, phenylephrine hydrochloride 10 mg, chlorpheniramine maleate 2 mg per 5 mL. Parabens, saccharin, sucrose. Fruit flavor. Syrup. 473 mL. *Rx.*
Use: Antitussive and expectorant.

Quasense. (Watson Pharma) Ethinyl estradiol 30 mcg, levonorgestrel 0.15 mg. Lactose. Tab. 91s with 7 inert tablets (lactose). *Rx.*
Use: Contraceptive hormone, sex hormone.

quaternary anticholinergics.
See: Glycopyrrolate.

•**quazepam.** (KWAZ-e-pam) *USP 34.*
Use: Sedative/hypnotic, nonbarbiturate.
See: Doral.

•**quazinone.** (KWAZ-i-none) USAN.
Use: Cardiovascular agent.

•**quazodine.** (KWAZ-oh-deen) USAN.
Use: Cardiovascular agent.

•**quazolast.** (KWAZ-oh-last) USAN.
Use: Antiasthmatic mediator release inhibitor.

Quelicin. (Hospira) Succinylcholine Cl. **Inj. 20 mg/mL:** Fliptop vial 10 mL, *Abboject* Syringe 5 mL. **100 mg/mL:** Amp. 10 mL. **Quelicin-500:** 5 mL in Pintop vial 10 mL. **Quelicin-1000:** 100 mg/mL. Parabens. Preservative free, single-use vial. 5 mL, 10 mL. Multidose vial. 20 mL. *Rx.*
Use: Muscle relaxant.

Quelidrine Cough. (Abbott) Dextromethorphan HBr 10 mg, chlorpheniramine maleate 2 mg, ephedrine hydrochloride 5 mg, phenylephrine hydrochloride 5 mg, ammonium Cl 40 mg, ipecac fluid extract 0.005 mL, ethyl alcohol 2%/ 5 mL. Syrup. Bot. 4 oz. *Rx.*
Use: Antihistamine; antitussive; bronchodilator; decongestant; expectorant.

Quercetin. (Freeda) Quercetin (from eucalyptus) 50 mg, 250 mg. Sugar and sodium free. Tab. Bot. 100s, 250s. *OTC.*
Use: Water-soluble vitamin.

Quertine.
Use: Bioflavonoid supplement.

Questran. (Par) Anhydrous cholestyramine resin 4 g per 9 g powder. Sucrose. Pow. for Oral Susp. Packets. 9 g (60s). Cans. 378 g. *Rx.*
Use: Antihyperlipidemic; bile acid sequestrant.

Questran Light. (Par) Anhydrous cholestyramine resin 4 g per 6.4 g powder. Maltodextrin, aspartame, phenylalanine 28.1 mg per 6.4 g, orange vanilla flavor. Pow. for Oral Susp. Packets. 6.4 g (60s). Cans. 268 g. *Rx.*
Use: Antihyperlipidemic; bile acid sequestrant.

•**quetiapine fumarate.** (cue-TIE-ah-peen) USAN.
Tall Man: QUEtiapine
Use: Antipsychotic, dibenzapine derivative.
See: Seroquel.
Seroquel XR.

Quiagel. (Rugby) Kaolin 6 g, pectin 142.8 mg, hyoscyamine sulfate 0.1037 mg, atropine sulfate 0.0194 mg, scopolamine HBr 0.0065 mg/30 mL. Susp. Bot. Pt, gal. *Rx.*
Use: Antidiarrheal.

Quibron Plus. (Bristol-Myers Squibb) Ephedrine hydrochloride 25 mg, theophylline (anhydrous) 150 mg, buta-barbital 20 mg, guaifenesin 100 mg. Cap. Bot. 100s. *Rx.*
Use: Antiasthmatic combination.

Quibron Plus Elixir. (Bristol-Myers Squibb) Theophylline 150 mg, ephedrine hydrochloride 25 mg, guaifenesin 100 mg, butabarbital 20 mg, alcohol 15%. Elix. Bot. Pt. *Rx.*
Use: Antiasthmatic combination.

Quick-K. (Western Research) Potassium bicarbonate 650 mg (potassium 6.5 mEq). Tab. Bot. 30s, 100s. *Rx.*
Use: Electrolyte supplement.

Quick Melts Children's Non-Aspirin. (Marlex) Acetaminophen 80 mg. Bubble gum flavor (gluten free, mannitol, sorbitol, sucralose, sugar), grape flavor (gluten and sugar free, corn syrup, mannitol, sorbitol, sucralose), watermelon flavor (gluten and sugar free, mannitol, sorbitol, sucralose). Tab., disintegrating. 30s. *OTC.*
Use: Analgesic.

Quick Melts Jr. Strength Non-Aspirin. (Marlex) Acetaminophen 160 mg. Bubble gum flavor (gluten free, mannitol, sorbitol, sucralose, sugar), grape flavor (gluten and sugar free, corn syrup, mannitol, sorbitol, sucralose). Tab., disintegrating. 30s. *OTC.*
Use: Analgesic.

Quiebar. (Nevin) Butabarbital sodium. **Spantab.** 1.5 gr. TR Spantab. Bot. 50s, 500s. **Elix.:** 30 mg/5 mL. Bot. Pt, gal. **Tab.:** 15 mg. Bot. 100s, 1000s; 30 mg. Bot. 1000s. **A.C. Cap.:** Bot. 100s, 500s. *c-III.*
Use: Hypnotic; sedative.

Quiebel. (Nevin) Butabarbital sodium 15 mg, belladonna extract 15 mg. Cap. Bot. 100s, 1000s. Elix. Pt, gal. *c-III.*
Use: Anticholinergic; antispasmodic; hypnotic; sedative.

Quiecof. (Nevin) Dextromethorphan HBr 7.5 mg, chlorpheniramine maleate 0.75 mg, guaiacol glyceryl ether 25 mg/ 5 mL. Bot. 4 oz, pt, gal. *OTC.*
Use: Antitussive; antihistamine; expectorant.

Quiet Night. (Rosemont) Pseudoephedrine hydrochloride 10 mg, doxylamine succinate 1.25 mg, dextromethorphan HBr 5 mg, acetaminophen 167 mg/ 5 mL. Liq. Bot. 180 mL, 300 mL. *OTC.*
Use: Analgesic; antihistamine; antitussive; decongestant.

Quiet Time. (Whiteworth Towne) Acetaminophen 600 mg, ephedrine sulfate 8 mg, dextromethorphan HBr 15 mg, doxylamine succinate 7.5 mg, alcohol 25 mg/30 mL. Bot. 180 mL. *OTC.*

Use: Analgesic; antihistamine; antitussive; decongestant.

●**quiflapon sodium.** (KWIH-flap-ahn) USAN.
Use: Antiasthmatic; inflammatory bowel disease suppressant.

Quik-Cept. (Laboratory Diagnostics) Slide test for pregnancy, rapid latex inhibition test. Kit 25s, 50s, 100s.
Use: Diagnostic aid.

Quik-Cult. (Laboratory Diagnostics) Slide test for fecal occult blood. Kit 150s, 200s, 300s, and tape test.
Use: Diagnostic aid.

●**quilostigmine.** (Kwill-oh-STIG-meen) USAN.
Use: Cholinergic, cholinesterase inhibitor; treatment of Alzheimer disease.

Quinaglute Dura-Tabs. (Berlex) Quinidine gluconate 324 mg. Tab. Bot. 100s, 250s, 500s, UD 100s. Unit-of-use 90s, 120s. *Rx.*
Use: Antiarrhythmic.

●**quinaldine blue.** (kwin-AL-deen) USAN.
Use: Diagnostic agent, obstetrics.

●**quinaprilat.** (KWIN-ah-PRILL-at) *USP 34.*
Use: Antihypertensive; enzyme inhibitor, angiotensin-converting.

●**quinapril hydrochloride.** (KWIN-uh-PRILL) USAN.
Use: Antihypertensive; enzyme inhibitor, angiotensin-converting.
See: Accupril.
W/Hydrochlorothiazide.
See: Accuretic.
Quinaretic.

quinapril hydrochloride. (Various Mfr.) Quinapril hydrochloride 5 mg, 10 mg, 20 mg, 40 mg. May contain lactose. Tab. 90s, 500s. *Rx.*
Use: Angiotensin-converting enzyme inhibitor.

quinapril hydrochloride/hydrochlorothiazide. (Greenstone) Hydrochlorothiazide/quinapril hydrochloride 12.5 mg/10 mg, 12.5 mg/20 mg, 25 mg/20 mg. Lactose. Film-coated. Tab. 90s. *Rx.*
Use: Antihypertensive combination.

Quinaretic. (Amide) Hydrochlorothiazide/quinapril hydrochloride 12.5 mg/20 mg, 25 mg/20 mg. Film-coated. Tab. 30s, 100s, 500s. *Rx.*
Use: Antihypertensive combination.

●**quinazosin hydrochloride.** (kwin-AZZ-oh-sin) USAN.
Use: Antihypertensive.

●**quinbolone.** (KWIN-bole-ohn) USAN.
Use: Anabolic.

●**quindecamine acetate.** (kwin-DECK-ah-meen) USAN.
Use: Anti-infective.

●**quindonium bromide.** (kwin-DOE-nee-um) USAN.
Use: Cardiovascular agent, antiarrhythmic.

●**quinelorane hydrochloride.** (kwih-NELL-oh-RANE) USAN.
Use: Antihypertensive; antiparkinsonian.

●**quinetolate.** (Kwin-EH-toe-late) USAN.
Use: Muscle relaxant.

●**quinfamide.** (KWIN-fah-mide) USAN.
Use: Antiamebic.

●**quingestanol acetate.** (kwin-JESS-tan-ahl) USAN.
Use: Hormone, progestin.

●**quingestrone.** (kwin-JESS-trone) USAN.
Use: Hormone, progestin.

quinidine.
Tall Man: quiNIDine
Use: Antiarrhythmic.
See: Quinidine Gluconate.
Quinidine Sulfate.

●**quinidine gluconate.** (KWIN-ih-deen) *USP 34.*
Tall Man: quiNIDine
Use: Cardiovascular agent, antiarrhythmic.

quinidine gluconate. (Lilly) Quinidine gluconate 80 mg/mL (50 mg/mL quinidine), EDTA 0.005%, phenol 25%. Inj. Vials. 10 mL multidose. *Rx.*
Use: Antiarrhythmic.

quinidine gluconate. (Various Mfr.) Quinidine gluconate 324 mg. SR Tab. Bot. 100s, 250s, 500s. *Rx.*
Use: Antiarrhythmic.

●**quinidine sulfate.** (KWIN-ih-deen) *USP 34.*
Tall Man: quiNIDine
Use: Cardiovascular agent, antiarrhythmic.

quinidine sulfate. (Mutual) Quinidine sulfate 100 mg (equiv. to 83 mg base). Tab. 50s, 100s, 250s, 500s, 1000s. *Rx.*
Use: Antiarrhythmic agent, quinidine.

quinidine sulfate. (Various Mfr.) Quinidine sulfate. **Tab.:** 200 mg, 300 mg. Bot. 100s, 1000s. **SR Tab.:** 300 mg. 100s, 250s. *Rx.*
Use: Cardiovascular agent, antiarrhythmic.

quinine and urea hydrochloride.
Use: Sclerosing agent.

●**quinine ascorbate.** (KWIE-nine ass-CORE-bate) USAN. *Formerly quinine biascorbate.*

Tall Man: quiNINE
Use: Smoking deterrent.
quinine bisulfate.
Use: Analgesic; antimalarial; antipyretic.
quinine dihydrochloride.
Use: Antimalarial.
quinine ethylcarbonate.
See: Euquinine.
quinine glycerophosphate. Quinine
compound with glycerol phosphate.
•**quinine sulfate.** (KWIE-nine) *USP 34.*
Tall Man: quiNINE
Use: Antimalarial.
W/Dextromethorphan Hydrobromide.
See: Nuedexta.
quinisocaine.
See: Dimethisoquin Hydrochloride.
quinolinone derivatives.
Use: Antipsychotic.
See: Aripiprazole.
quinophan.
See: Cinchophen.
Quinora. (Key) Quinidine sulfate 300 mg.
Tab. Bot. 100s, 1000s, UD 100s. *Rx.*
Use: Antiarrhythmic.
quinoxyl.
See: Chiniofon.
•**quinpirole hydrochloride.** (KWIN-pihr-
ole) USAN.
Use: Antihypertensive.
quinprenaline. Quinterenol sulfate.
Quin-Release. (Major) Quinidine gluco-
nate 324 mg. SR Tab. Bot. 100s, 250s,
500s, UD 100s. *Rx.*
Use: Antiarrhythmic.
Quinsana Plus. (Stephan) Tolnafate 1%,
cornstarch, talc. Pow. In 90 g. *OTC.*
Use: Antifungal, topical.
Quintabs. (Freeda) Vitamins A
10,000 units, D 400 units, E 29 mg,
B_1 25 mg, B_2 25 mg, B_3 100 mg,
B_5 25 mg, B_6 25 mg, B_{12} 25 mcg,
C 300 mg, folic acid 0.1 mg, inositol,
PABA. Tab. Bot. 100s, 250s. *OTC.*
Use: Vitamin supplement.
Quintabs-M. (Freeda) Iron 15 mg, Vitamins A 10,000 units, D 400 units, E
50 mg, B_1 30 mg, B_2 30 mg, B_3 150 mg,
B_5 30 mg, B_6 30 mg, B_{12} 30 mcg, C
300 mg, folic acid 0.4 mg, Ca, Cu, K,

Mg, Mn, Se, Zn 30 mg, PABA. Tab. Bot.
100s, 250s, 500s. *OTC.*
Use: Mineral, vitamin supplement.
•**quinterenol sulfate.** (kwin-TER-en-ahl)
USAN.
Use: Bronchodilator.
•**quinuclium bromide.** (kwih-NEW-klee-
uhm) USAN.
Use: Antihypertensive.
•**quinupristin.** (kwih-NEW-priss-tin)
USAN.
Use: Anti-infective.
W/Dalfopristin
See: Synercid.
•**quipazine maleate.** (KWIP-ah-zeen)
USAN.
Use: Antidepressant; oxytocic.
quipenyl naphthoate.
See: Plasmochin Naphthoate.
Quixin. (Santen) Levofloxacin 0.5%
(5 mg/mL), benzalkonium chloride
0.005%. Soln. Bot. 2.5 mL, 5 mL. *Rx.*
Use: Antibiotic.
•**quizartinib.** (kwiz-AR-ti-nib) USAN.
Use: Antineoplastic.
•**quizartinib dihydrochloride.** (kwiz-AR-
ti-nib) USAN.
Use: Antineoplastic.
Qutenza. (NeurogesX) Capsaicin 8%.
Patch. Single-use patch w/cleansing
gel. *Rx.*
Use: Dermatological agent, counterirritant.
QV-Allergy. (Pharmaceutical Associates)
Phenylephrine hydrochloride 10 mg,
chlorpheniramine maleate 2 mg, methscopolamine nitrate 0.625 mg per
5 mL. Sucrose. Grape flavor. Syrup.
473 mL. *Rx.*
Use: Upper respiratory combination, decongestant, antihistamine, and anticholinergic combination.
QVAR. (Ivax) Beclomethasone dipropionate 40 mcg, 80 mcg per actuation.
Aer. Can. 7.3 g (100 actuations w/ac-
tuator). *Rx.*
Use: Respiratory inhalant, corticosteroid.

R

RabAvert. (Chiron) Rabies antigen ≥ 2.5 IU/mL. Freeze-dried, fixed virus strain Flury LEP grown in cultures of chicken fibroblasts. With human albumin < 0.3 mg, processed bovine gelatin < 12 mg, potassium glutamate 1 mg, sodium EDTA 0.3 mg, neomycin < 1 mcg, chlortetracycline < 20 ng, amphotericin B < 2 ng, ovalbumin < 3 ng per dose. Inj., Lyophilized Pow. for Reconstitution. Single-dose vial with 1 vial diluent, 1 disposable syringe, 1 longer needle for reconstitution, and 1 smaller needle for injection. *Rx.*
Use: Active immunization, viral vaccine.

•**rabeprazole sodium.** (rab-EH-pray-zahl) USAN.
Tall Man: RABEprazole
Use: Proton pump inhibitor.
See: AcipHex.

rabies antigen.
Use: Immunization.

•**rabies immune globulin.** (RAY-beez ih-MYOON GLAB-byoo-lin) *USP 34.*
Use: Immunization.
See: HyperRab S/D.
Imogam Rabies-HT.

rabies immune globulin (RIG), human.
See: Rabies immune globulin.

•**rabies vaccine.** (RAY-beez vaccine) *USP 34.*
Use: Active immunization agent, viral vaccine.
See: Imovax Rabies.
RabAvert.

•**racemethionine.** (RAY-see-meh-THIGH-oh-neen) *USP 34. Formerly Methionine.*
Use: Acidifier, urinary.

racemic calcium pantothenate.
See: Calcium Pantothenate, Racemic.

racemic desoxynorephedrine. Amphetamine.

racemic ephedrine hydrochloride. Racephedrine hydrochloride.

racemic pantothenic acid.
See: Calcium Pantothenate.

•**racephedrine hydrochloride.** (RAYSE-e-FED-rin) USAN.
Use: Vasoconstrictor; decongestant, nasal.

racephedrine hydrochloride. (Pharmacia) Racephedrine hydrochloride **Cap.:** ⅜ gr. Bot. 40s, 250s, 1000s. **Soln.:** 1%. Bot. 1 fl oz, pt, gal.
Use: Vasoconstrictor; decongestant, nasal.

•**racephenicol.** (race-FEN-ih-KAHL) *USP 34.*
Use: Anti-infective.

•**racepinephrine hydrochloride.** (race-epp-ih-NEFF-rin) *USP 34.*
Use: Bronchodilator; vasopressor.
See: MicroNefrin.
Nephron.
S2.

•**raclopride C11.** (RACK-low-pride) *USP 34.*
Use: Radiopharmaceutical.

•**radafaxine hydrochloride.** (rad-a-FAX-een) USAN.
Use: Antidepressant, antianxiety.

•**radezolid.** (ra-DEZ-oh-lid) USAN.
Use: Antibacterial agent.

•**radezolid hydrochloride.** (ra-DEZ-oh-lid) USAN.
Use: Antibacterial agent.

RadiaPlexRx. (MPM Medical) Aloe vera, diazolidinyl urea and iodopropynyl butylcarbamate, EDTA, glycerin, glyceryl stearate, isopropyl palmitate, lipowax, mineral oil, myritol, phenoxyethanol, polydimethylsiloxane fluid, sodium hyaluronate, triethanolamine. Top. Gel. 170 g. *Rx.*
Use: Flexible hydroactive dressing.

Radiesse. (Bioform Medical) Calcium hydroxylapatite (particle size range is 25 to 45 microns). Implant, Subcutaneous. Single-use prefilled syringes. 0.3 mL, 1.3 mL. *Rx.*
Use: Physical adjunct.

radioactive isotopes.
See: Albumin, Aggregated Iodinated.
Chlormerodrin Hg 197.
Chlormerodrin Hg 203.
Cyanocobalamin Co 57.
Cyanocobalamin Co 60.
Radio-Iodinated Serum Albumin.
Selenomethionine Se 75.
Sodium Chromate Cr 51.
Sodium Iodide I 131.
Sodium Iodide I 125.
Sodium Phosphate P 32.
Sodium Radio Chromate.
Sodium Radio Iodide.
Sodium Radio Phosphate.
Strontium Nitrate Sr 85.
Technetium Tc 99m.
Triolein I 131.
Xenon Xe 133.

Radiogardase. (HEYL Chemisch-pharmazeutische Fabrik GmbH & Co.) Prussian blue oral 0.5 g (blue powder in gelatin capsules). Cap. 30s. *Rx.*
Use: Chelating agent; detoxification agent.

radiogold (^{198}Au) solution. Gold Au-198 injection.
Use: Irradiation therapy.
radio-iodide (^{131}I), sodium.
Use: Radiopharmaceutical.
See: Iodotope.
radio-iodinated (^{131}I) serum albumin. (Human) Iodinated I-131 albumin.
radio-iodinated (^{125}I) serum albumin.
See: (Human) Iodinated I-125 albumin.
radiopaque agents.
See: Gastrointestinal Contrast Agents (Iodinated).
Gastrointestinal Contrast Agents (Miscellaneous).
Radiopaque Agents, Miscellaneous.
radiopaque agents, miscellaneous.
See: Diatrizoate Meglumine.
Diatrizoate Meglumine 52% and Diatrizoate Sodium 8%.
Diatrizoate Meglumine 52.7% and Iodipamide Meglumine 26.8%.
Diatrizoate Meglumine 66% and Diatrizoate Sodium 10%.
Ethiodized Oil.
Ferumoxides.
Gadobenate Dimeglumine.
Gadodiamide.
Gadopentetate Dimeglumine.
Gadoteridol.
Gadoversetamide.
Iodipamide Meglumine 52%.
Iodixanal.
Iohexol.
Iopamidol.
Iopromide.
Iosulfan Blue.
Iothalamate Meglumine.
Ioversol.
Ioxaglate Meglumine 39.3% and Ioxaglate Sodium 19.6%.
Mangafodipir Trisodium.
Pentetreotide.
Perflutren.
Perflutren, Protein Based.
Technetium Tc-99m Mebrofenin.
radiopaque polyvinyl chloride.
Use: Radiopaque agent, GI contrast agent.
See: Sitzmarks.
radio-phosphate (^{32}P), sodium.
Use: Radiopharmaceutical.
radioselenomethionine 75 Se. Selenomethionine Se 75.
radiotolpovidone I-131. Tolpovidone I-131.
●**rafoxanide.** (ray-FOX-ah-nide) USAN.
Use: Anthelmintic.
Ragus. (Miller Pharmacal Group) Mg 27 mg, vitamins C 100 mg, Ca 580 mg, P 450 mg, l-lysine 25 mg, dl-methionine

50 mg, A 5000 units, D 400 units, E 10 mg, B$_1$ 20 mg, B$_2$ 3 mg, B$_6$ 5 mg, B$_{12}$ 9 mcg, niacinamide 80 mg, pantothenic acid 5 mg, Fe 20 mg, Cu 1 mg, Mn 2 mg, K 10 mg, Zn 2 mg, I 0.1 mg/3 Tab. Bot. 100s. *OTC.*
Use: Mineral, vitamin supplement.
●**ralitoline.** (rah-LIT-oh-leen) USAN.
Use: Anticonvulsant.
Ralix. (Cypress) Phenylephrine hydrochloride 40 mg, chlorpheniramine maleate 8 mg, methscopolamine nitrate 2.5 mg. ER Tab. 100s. *Rx.*
Use: Decongestant, antihistamine, and anticholinergic, upper respiratory combination.
R A Lotion. (Medco Lab) Resorcinol 3%, alcohol 43%. Lot. Plastic Bot. 120 mL, 240 mL, 480 mL. *OTC.*
Use: Dermatologic, acne.
●**raloxifene hydrochloride.** (ral-OX-ih-FEEN) USAN. *Formerly Keoxifene Hydrochloride.*
Use: Antiestrogen.
See: Evista.
●**raltegravir.** (ral-TEG-ra-vir) USAN.
Use: Antiretroviral agent, integrase inhibitor.
See: Isentress.
●**raltegravir potassium.** (ral-TEG-ra-vir) USAN.
Use: Antiviral.
●**raltitrexed.** (ral-tih-TREX-ehd) USAN.
Use: Advanced colorectal cancer treatment (thymidylate synthase inhibitor), antineoplastic.
●**raluridine.** (ral-YOUR-ih-deen) USAN.
Use: Antiviral.
●**ramelteon.** (ram-EL-tee-on) USAN.
Use: Sleep disorders.
See: Rozerem.
●**ramipril.** (ruh-MIH-prill) USAN.
Use: Antihypertensive, enzyme inhibitor (angiotensin-converting), congestive heart failure.
See: Altace.
ramipril. (Actavis) Ramipril 1.25 mg, 2.5 mg, 5 mg, 10 mg. Tab. 100s, 500s, 1,000s (except 1.25 mg). *Rx.*
Use: Renin angiotensin system antagonists, angiotensin-converting enzyme inhibitor.
ramipril. (Cobalt) Ramipril 1.25 mg, 2.5 mg, 5 mg, 10 mg. Cap. 30s (1.25 mg only), 100s, 500s (except 1.25 mg), 1000s (10 mg only). *Rx.*
Use: Renin angiotensin system antagonist, angiotensin-converting enzyme inhibitor.

- **ramoplanin.** (ram-oh-PLAN-in) USAN.
  Use: Investigational anti-infective.
- **ramucirumab.** (RA-mue-SIR-ue-mab) USAN.
  Use: Antineoplastic.
  ranestol. Triclofenol piperazine.
  Use: Anthelmintic.
  Ranexa. (Gilead Sciences) Ranolazine 500 mg, 1,000 mg. Lactose (1,000 mg only), PEG (500 mg only). Film-coated. ER Tab. 60s, 500s. *Rx.*
  Use: Miscellaneous antianginal agent.
- **ranibizumab.** (ra-NIB-i-ZUE-mab) USAN.
  Use: Age-related macular degeneration.
  See: Lucentis.
  Raniclor. (Ranbaxy) Cefaclor 125 mg (phenylalanine 2.8 mg), 187 mg (phenylalanine 4.2 mg), 250 mg (phenylalanine 5.6 mg), 375 mg (phenylalanine 8.4 mg). Aspartame, mannitol, tartrazine. Fruity flavor. Chew. Tab. 20s, 30s (125 mg and 250 mg only), 250s, UD 100s. *Rx.*
  Use: Antibiotic.
- **ranimycin.** (ran-ih-MY-sin) USAN.
  Use: Anti-infective.
- **ranitidine.** (ra-NI-ti-deen) USAN.
  Use: Histamine H$_2$ antagonist.
  See: Zantac.
  Zantac Efferdose.
  Zantac 150 Maximum Strength.
  Zantac 75.
  ranitidine. (Various Mfr.) Ranitidine (as base). **Cap.:** 150 mg, 300 mg. 30s (300 mg only), 60s (150 mg only), 100s (300 mg only), 500s (150 mg only). **Inj.:** 25 mg/mL. Single-dose vials. 2 mL. Multidose vials. 6 mL with phenol 5 mg/mL. **Tab.:** 75 mg, 150 mg, 300 mg. Bot. 10s (75 mg only); 20s (75 mg only); 30s (except 150 mg); 60s (except 300 mg); 100s (except 75 mg); 250s (300 mg only); 500s (150 mg only); 1000s, 5000s, UD 100s (150 mg only). *Rx-OTC.*
  Use: Histamine H$_2$ antagonist.
- **ranitidine hydrochloride.** (ra-NI-ti-deen) USP 34.
  Use: Histamine H$_2$ antagonist.
  ranitidine hydrochloride. (Various Mfr.) Ranitidine 15 mg/mL. May contain alcohol, parabens, saccharin, sorbitol. Peppermint flavor. Soln. 473 mL. *Rx.*
  Use: Histamine H$_2$ antagonist.
- **ranolazine.** (RAY-no-lah-ZEEN) USAN.
  Use: Antianginal agent, miscellaneous.
  See: Ranexa.
  Rapaflo. (Watson Pharma) Silodosin 4 mg, 8 mg. Cap. 30s, 100s (4 mg);

30s, 90s, 1,000s (8 mg). *Rx.*
  Use: Antiadrenergic agent—peripherally acting, alpha-1-adrenergic blocker.
  Rapamune. (Wyeth Laboratories) Sirolimus. **Oral Soln.:** 1 mg/mL. Ethanol. 60 mL glass bot. with oral syringe adaptor. **Tab.:** 0.5 mg, 1 mg, 2 mg. Lactose, PEG, sucrose. 100s, *Redipak* UD 100s. *Rx.*
  Use: Immunologic, immunosuppressive.
  Rapid B-12 Energy. (Mason) Cyanocobalamin 200 mcg per spray. Glycerin, potassium sorbate. Peppermint flavor. Spray, Soln.; sublingual. 30 mL. *OTC.*
  Use: Water-soluble vitamin.
  Rapid Test Strep. (SmithKline Diagnostics) Latex slide agglutination test for identification of group A streptococci. Box. 25s, 100s.
  Use: Diagnostic aid.
  rasagiline.
  Use: Antiparkinson agent.
  See: Azilect.
- **rasagiline mesylate.** (rass-AH-jih-leen) USAN.
  Use: Antiparkinson agent.
- **rasburicase.** (raz-BYORR-ih-kays) USAN.
  Use: Antimetabolite.
  See: Elitek.
  rastinon. Tolbutamide.
  Use: Antidiabetic.
  rattlesnake bite therapy.
  See: Antivenin (Crotalidae).
  Rauneed. (Hanlon) Rauwolfia 50 mg, 100 mg. Tab. Bot. 100s. *Rx.*
  Use: Antihypertensive.
  Raunescine. (Penick) An alkaloid of rauwolfia serpentina. Under study.
  Use: Antihypertensive.
  Raunormine. (Penick) 11-Desmethoxy reserpine. *Rx.*
  Use: Antihypertensive.
  Raurine. (Westerfield) Reserpine. **Tab.:** 0.1 mg. Bot. 100s. **Delayed-Action Cap.:** 0.5 mg. Bot. 100s. *Rx.*
  Use: Antihypertensive.
  Rauserfia. (New Eng. Phr. Co.) Rauwolfia serpentina 50 mg, 100 mg. Tab. Bot. 100s. *Rx.*
  Use: Antihypertensive.
  Rautina. (Fellows) Rauwolfia serpentina whole root 50 mg, 100 mg. Tab. Bot. 1000s. *Rx.*
  Use: Antihypertensive.
  Rauval. (Pal-Pak, Inc.) Rauwolfia whole root 50 mg, 100 mg. Tab. Bot. 100s, 500s, 1000s. *Rx.*
  Use: Antihypertensive.

rauwolfia/bendroflumethiazide.
(Various Mfr.) Bendroflumethiazide
4 mg, powdered rauwolfia serpentina
50 mg. Tab. Bot. 100s. *Rx.*
Use: Antihypertensive.
•**rauwolfia serpentina.** (rah-WOOL-fee-ah ser-pen-TEE-nah) *USP 34.*
Use: Antihypertensive.
See: Rauneed.
Rauval.
Rawfola.
T-Rau.
**rauwolfia serpentina active principles
(alkaloids).** Deserpidine, rescinnamone.
See: Reserpine.
rauwolscine. An alkaloid of Rauwolfia
canescens. Under study.
Use: Antihypertensive.
Ravocaine. (Cook-Waite Laboratories,
Inc.) Propoxycaine hydrochloride 4 mg,
procaine 20 mg, norepinephrine bitartrate equivalent to 0.033 mg levophed
base, sodium Cl 3 mg, acetone sodium
bisulfite not more than 2 mg. Cartridge
1.8 mL. *Rx.*
Use: Anesthetic, local.
ravuconazole.
Use: Antifungal.
Rawfola. (Foy Laboratories) Rauwolfia
serpentina 50 mg. Tab. Bot. 1000s. *Rx.*
Use: Antihypertensive.
Rawl Vite. (Rawl) Vitamins A
10,000 units, D 500 units, B$_1$ 10 mg, B$_2$
5 mg, B$_6$ 1 mg, calcium pantothenate
5 mg, nicotinamide 50 mg, C 125 mg, E
2.5 units. Tab. Bot. 100s. *OTC.*
Use: Mineral, vitamin supplement.
Rawl Whole Liver Vitamin B Complex.
(Rawl) Whole liver 500 mg, amino acids found in the whole liver, vitamins B$_1$
1 mg, B$_2$ 2 mg, niacinamide 5 mg, choline Cl 12 mg, B$_6$ 0.2 mg, calcium
pantothenate 0.2 mg, inositol 5 mg,
biotin 0.6 mcg, B$_{12}$ 0.3 mcg. Cap. Bot.
100s, 500s. *OTC.*
Use: Mineral, vitamin supplement.
•**raxibacumab.** (RAX-ee-BAK-ue-mab)
USAN.
Use: Anthrax infection.
Ray Block. (Del-Ray) Octyl dimethyl
PABA 5%, benzophenone-3 3%, SD alcohol. Lot. Bot. 118.3 mL. *OTC.*
Use: Sunscreen.
Ray-D. (Nion Corp.) Vitamin D 400 units,
thiamine mononitrate 1 mg, riboflavin
2 mg, niacin 10 mg, I 0.1 mg, Ca
375 mg, P 300 mg/6 Tab. In base of
brewer's yeast. Bot. 100s, 500s. *OTC.*
Use: Mineral, vitamin supplement.

•**rayon, purified.** (RAY-ahn) *USP 34.*
Use: Surgical aid.
raythesin. (Raymer)
See: Propyl p-Aminobenzoate.
Razadyne. (Janssen) Galantamine hydrobromide. **Tab.:** 4 mg, 8 mg, 12 mg.
Lactose. Film-coated. Bot. 60s. **Oral
Soln.:** 4 mg/mL. Saccharin. Bot.
100 mL with calibrated pipette. *Rx.*
Use: Cholinesterase inhibitor.
Razadyne ER. (Janssen) Galantamine
hydrobromide (as base) 8 mg, 16 mg,
24 mg. Sucrose. ER Cap. 30s. *Rx.*
Use: Cholinesterase inhibitor.
•**razaxaban hydrochloride.** (ra-ZAX-a-ban) USAN.
Use: Anticoagulant.
Razepam. (Major) Temazepam 15 mg,
30 mg. Cap. Bot. 100s. *c-iv.*
Use: Hypnotic; sedative.
•**razupenem.** (RAZ-u-PEN-em) USAN.
Use: Antibiotic.
RCF. (Ross) Carbohydrate free low iron
soy protein formula base. Carbohydrate and water must be added. For infants unable to tolerate the amount or
type of carbohydrate in conventional
formulas. Can 14 fl oz. (Concentrated
liq.). *OTC.*
Use: Nutritional supplement.
Reabilan. (Elan) Protein 31.5 g, fat 39 g,
carbohydrates 131.5 g, Na 702 mg, K
1.252 g/L, lactose free. With appropriate
vitamins and minerals. Liq. Bot.
375 mL. *OTC.*
Use: Nutritional supplement.
Reabilan HN. (Elan) Protein 58.2 g, fat
52 g, carbohydrates 158 g, Na
1000 mg, K 1661 mg/L, lactose free.
With appropriate vitamins and minerals.
Liq. Bot. 375 mL. *OTC.*
Use: Nutritional supplement.
Readi-Cat. (EZ EM) Barium sulfate 1.3%,
2.1%. Saccharin, sorbitol. Orange flavor and vanilla flavor. Susp. 450 mL,
900 mL, 1,900 mL. *Rx.*
Use: Radiopaque agent, miscellaneous
gastrointestinal contrast agent.
Readi-Cat 2. (EZ EM) Barium sulfate 2%.
Saccharin, sorbitol. Apple flavor, banana flavor, berry flavor, vanilla flavor.
Susp. 250 mL, 450 mL, 900 mL,
1,900 mL. *Rx.*
Use: Radiopaque agent, miscellaneous
gastrointestinal contrast agent.
Rea-Lo. (Whorton Pharmaceuticals, Inc.)
Urea in water-soluble moisturizing oil
base. **Lot.:** 15%. Bot. 4 oz, pt. **Cream:**
30%. Jar 2 oz, 16 oz. *OTC.*
Use: Emollient.

RE Benzoyl Peroxide. (River's Edge) Benzoyl peroxide 3.5%, 5.5%, 8.5%. Cetearyl alcohol, cetyl alcohol, glycerin, glyceryl, parabens, PEG-3, stearyl alcohol. Cream. In 45 g. *Rx.*
Use: Anti-infective, antibiotic.

Rebetol. (Schering) Ribavirin. **Cap.:** 200 mg. Lactose. Bot 42s, 56s, 70s, 84s. **Oral Soln.:** 40 mg/mL. Glycerin, propylene glycol, sodium benzoate, sorbitol, sucrose. Bubble gum flavor. 100 mL. *Rx.*
Use: Antiviral.

Rebif. (Serono) Interferon beta-1a 8.8 mcg/0.2 mL (2.4 million units) (human albumin 0.8 mg, mannitol 10.9 mg, sodium acetate 0.16 mg in water for injection), 22 mcg/0.5 mL (6 million units) (human albumin 2 mg, mannitol 27.3 mg, sodium acetate 0.4 mg), 44 mcg/0.5 mL (12 million units) (human albumin 4 mg, mannitol 27.3 mg, sodium acetate 0.4 mg). Preservative free. Inj. Prefilled single-use syringes. Box. 1s, 12s (except 8.8 mcg). *Titration Packs* 6s (8.8 mcg only). *Rx.*
Use: Immunologic, immunomodulator.

•**rebimastat.** (re-BIM-a-stat) USAN.
Use: Antineoplastic.

reboxetine mesylate.
Use: Antidepressant.

•**recainam hydrochloride.** (reh-CANE-am) USAN.
Use: Cardiovascular agent, antiarrhythmic.

•**recainam tosylate.** (reh-CANE-am TAH-sill-ate) USAN.
Use: Cardiovascular agent, antiarrhythmic.

Recal D. (River's Edge) Vitamin B 250 mcg, Ca citrate 1,342 mg, folic acid 1 mcg, Mg 50 mg, B_6 10 mg, B_{12} 125 mcg, D_3 300 units. Maltodextrin, sugar. Chocolate flavor. Wafer, Chew. 60s. *Rx.*
Use: Multivitamin.

RE Chlordiazepoxide/Clidinium. (River's Edge) Chlordiazepoxide hydrochloride 5 mg, clidinium bromide 2.5 mg. Lactose. Cap. 100s. *Rx.*
Use: GI anticholinergic combination.

Reclast. (Novartis) Zoledronic acid 5 mg/100 mL (as zoledronic acid monohydrate 5.33 mg). Mannitol 4,950 mg. Inj., Soln. 100 mL. *Rx.*
Use: Bisphosphonate.

•**reclazepam.** (reh-CLAY-zeh-pam) USAN.
Use: Hypnotic; sedative.

Reclipsen. (Watson) Ethinyl estradiol 30 mcg, desogestrel 0.15 mg. Lactose.

Tab. 28s with 7 inert tablets. *Rx.*
Use: Contraceptive hormone, sex hormone.

Reclomide. (Major) Metoclopramide hydrochloride 10 mg. Tab. Bot. 100s, 500s, 1000s, UD 100s. *Rx.*
Use: Antiemetic, gastrointestinal stimulant.

recombinant human activated protein C.
Use: Thrombolytic agent.
See: Drotrecogin Alfa (Activated). Protein C Concentrate (Human).

recombinant human erythropoietin.
Use: Hemotopoietic.
See: Darbepoetin Alfa. Epoetin Alfa, Recombinant.

recombinant human insulin-like growth factor I.
Use: Antibody-mediated growth hormone resistance. [Orphan Drug]

recombinant soluble human CD4. rCD4.
Use: Antiviral, HIV. [Orphan Drug]

recombinant tissue plasminogen activator. *Rx.*
See: Activase.

Recombinate. (Baxter) Recombinant antihemophilic factor 250 units, 500 units, 1,000 units. Albumin (human) ≤ 12.5 mg/mL, histidine, PEG 3350, sodium, von Willebrand Factor ≤ 2 mg per AHF unit. Preservative free. Monoclonal antibody purified. Inj., lyophilized Pow. for Soln. Single-dose Bot. and diluent (sterile water for injection 10 mL). *Rx.*
Use: Antihemophilic agent.

Recombivax HB. (Merck) Hepatitis B vaccine recombinant. Hepatitis B surface antigen. **Pediatric/Adolescent:** 5 mcg/0.5 mL, preservative free. Inj. Single-dose vial 0.5 mL. **Adult:** 10 mcg/mL, thimerosal 50 mcg/mL. Inj. Single-dose vial 1 mL, multi-dose vial 3 mL, prefilled, single-dose syringe 1 mL. **Dialysis:** 40 mcg/mL, thimerosal 50 mcg/mL. Inj. Single-dose vial 1 mL. *Rx.*
Use: Immunization, viral vaccine.

Recortex 10X in Oil. (Forest) 1000 mcg/mL. Vial 10 mL. *Rx.*

Recothrom. (Zymo Genetics) Thrombin (recombinant) 1,000 units/mL. PEG. Preservative free. Pow. for Soln., lyophilized, Top. 5,000 and 20,000 unit single-use vials; 20,000 unit spray applicator kit. *Rx.*
Use: Hemostatic.

Recover. (Dermik) Bot. 2.25 oz. *OTC.*
Use: Dermatologic.

Rectagene. (Pfeiffer) Live yeast cell derivative supplying 2000 units Skin Respiratory Factor/oz, shark liver oil in a cocoa butter base. Supp. 12s. *OTC.*
Use: Anorectal preparation.

Rectagene Medicated Rectal Balm. (Pfeiffer) Live yeast cell derivative that supplies 2000 units Skin Respiratory Factor/30 g, refined shark liver oil 3%, white petrolatum, lanolin, thyme oil, 1:10,000 phenylmercuric nitrate. Oint. Tube. 56.7 g. *OTC.*
Use: Anorectal preparation.

Rectal Medicone. (Medicore) Benzocaine 2 g, balsam peru 1 g, hydroxyquinoline sulfate 0.25 g, menthol ⅓ g, zinc oxide 3 g. Supp. Box 12s, 24s. *OTC.*
Use: Anesthetic; antiseptic, topical.

Rectal Medicone Unguent. (Medicore) Benzocaine 20 mg, oxyquinoline sulfate 5 mg, menthol 4 mg, zinc oxide 100 mg, balsam peru 12.5 mg, petrolatum 625 mg, lanolin 210 mg/g. Tube 1.5 oz. *OTC.*
Use: Anorectal preparation.

red blood cells. Human red blood cells given by IV infusion.
Use: Blood replenisher.

red cell tagging solution.
See: A-C-D.

Red Cross Toothache Kit. (Mentholatum Co.) Eugenol 85%, sesame oil. Drops. Bot. 3.7 mL w/cotton pellets and tweezers. *OTC.*
Use: Anesthetic, local.

red ferric oxide.
Use: Pharmaceutic aid (color).

Reditemp-C. (Wyeth) Ammonium nitrate, water, and special additives. Pkg. Large and small sizes. 4 × 10s. *OTC.*
Use: Cold compress.

Red Throat Spray. (Clay-Park Labs) Phenol 1.4%. Glycerin, saccharin. Alcohol free. Throat spray. 177 mL. *OTC.*
Use: Mouth and throat product.

Reducto, Improved. (Arcum) Phendimetrazine bitartrate 35 mg. Tab. Bot. 100s, 1000s. *c-III.*
Use: Anorexiant.

Reese's Pinworm. (Reese) Pyrantel pamoate. **Cap., soft gel:** 180 mg (equiv. to pyrantel base 62.5 mg). 24s. **Oral Susp.: 50 mg/mL:** 30 mL. **144 mg/mL:** Equiv. to 50 mg/mL of pyrantel base. Glycerin, saccharin, sodium 4 mg per 5 mL, sorbitol. Banana flavor. 30 mL w/measuring cup. **Tab.:** 180 mg (equiv. to pyrantel base 62.5 mg). 24s. *OTC.*
Use: Anthelmintic.

ReFacto. (Wyeth) Recombinant antihemophilic factor 250 units, 500 units, 1,000 units, 2,000 units. L-histidine, sodium, sucrose. Preservative free and albumin free. Inj., lyophilized Pow. for Soln. Single-use vials and diluent (sodium chloride 0.9% 4 mL). *Rx.*
Use: Antihemophilic agent.

Refenesen Plus Severe Strength Cough & Cold Medicine. (Reese) Pseudoephedrine hydrochloride 60 mg, guaifenesin 400 mg. Tab. Pkg. 16s. *OTC.*
Use: Upper respiratory combination, decongestant, expectorant.

Refludan. (Hoechst-Marion Roussel) Lepirudin 50 mg, mannitol. Pow. for Inj. Boxes of 10s. *Rx.*
Use: Thrombin inhibitor.

Refresh Classic. (Allergan) Polyvinyl alcohol 1.4%, povidone 0.6%, sodium Cl. UD 30s, 50s (0.3 mL single-dose container). *OTC.*
Use: Artificial tears.

Refresh Dry Eye Therapy. (Allergan) Glycerin 1%, polysorbate 80 1%. Preservative free. Castor oil. Ophth. Drops. Single-use containers. 0.4 mL. *OTC.*
Use: Artificial tear solution.

Refresh Lacri-Lube. (Allergen Optical) White petrolatum 56.8%, mineral oil 42.5%, chlorobutanol, lanolin alcohols. Oint.; Ophth. 3.5 g, 7 g. *OTC.*
Use: Ocular lubricant.

Refresh Liquigel. (Allergan) Carboxymethylcellulose sodium 1%, boric acid, calcium chloride, magnesium chloride, potassium chloride, sodium borate, sodium chloride. Soln.; Ophth. 15 mL, 30 mL. *OTC.*
Use: Ophthalmic agent, artificial tear solution.

Refresh Plus. (Allergan) Carboxymethylcellulose sodium 0.5%, sodium chloride. Preservative free. Soln. 0.3 mL/single-use container 4s, 30s. *OTC.*
Use: Artificial tears.

Refresh PM. (Allergan) White petrolatum 56.8%, mineral oil 41.5%, lanolin alcohol, sodium Cl. Tube 3.5 g. *OTC.*
Use: Lubricant, ophthalmic.

Refresh Redness Relief. (Allergan) Phenylephrine hydrochloride 0.12%. Benzalkonium chloride, edetate disodium, polyvinyl alcohol 1.4%. Soln., Ophth. 15 mL. *OTC.*
Use: Ophthalmic decongestant.

Refresh Tears. (Allergan) Carboxymethylcellulose 0.5%. Drops. Bot. 15 mL w/dropper. *OTC.*
Use: Artificial tears.

• **regadenoson.** (re-ga-DEN-oh-son)
USAN.
Use: In vivo diagnostic aid.
See: Lexiscan.

Regain. (NCI Medical Foods) Protein
15 g, carbohydrates 52 g, fat 7 g,
Na 45 mg, K 75 mg, Ca 200 mg, P
100 mg, Ca, Fe, vitamin B$_{12}$, Mg, folic
acid, fructose. With dietary fiber. 300
calories. Lactose free. Vanilla, strawberry, and malt flavors. Bar 85 g. *OTC.*
Use: Nutritional supplement.

Regenecare HA. (MPM Medical) Lidocaine hydrochloride 2%. Aloe vera gel,
glycerin, parabens. Gel. 85 g. *OTC.*
Use: Topical local anesthetic, amide
local anesthetic.

Regenecare Wound. (MPM Medical)
Lidocaine hydrochloride 2%. Aloe,
collagen. Gel. 14 g. *Rx.*
Use: Local anesthetic, topical; amide
local anesthetic.

Reglan. (Schwarz Pharma) Metoclopramide (as monohydrochloride monohydrate) 5 mg, 10 mg. Lactose (5 mg
only). Tab. Bot. 100s, 500s, (10 mg
only), *Dis-Co* UD 100s. *Rx.*
Use: Antiemetic, gastrointestinal stimulant.

Reglan. (Wyeth-Ayerst) Metoclopramide
(as monohydrochloride monohydrate)
5 mg/mL. Preservative free. Inj. Amps.
2 mL, 10 mL. Vials. 2 mL, 10 mL,
30 mL. *Rx.*
Use: Antiemetic, gastrointestinal stimulant.

• **regramostim.** (reh-GRAH-moe-STIM)
USAN.
Use: Biological response modifier; antineoplastic adjunct; antineutropenic;
hematopoietic stimulant.

Regranex. (Johnson & Johnson Wound
Management) Becaplermin 0.01%.
Parabens. Gel. Tube. 2 g, 15 g. *Rx.*
Use: Diabetic neuropathic ulcers.

**Regular Strength Bayer Enteric Coated
Caplets.** (Bayer Consumer Care) Aspi-
rin 325 mg. Bot. 50s, 100s. EC Tab.
OTC.
Use: Analgesic.

Reguloid. (Rugby) Psyllium husk fiber
95% pure 3.4 g/5 mL, dextrose, 14 cal/
tsp. Pow. Can. 369 g, 540 g. *OTC.*
Use: Laxative.

Reguloid, Orange. (Rugby) Psyllium mucilloid 3.4 g, sucrose, orange flavor/
tbsp. Pow. Can. 369 g, 540 g. *OTC.*
Use: Laxative.

Reguloid, Sugar Free Orange. (Rugby)
Psyllium hydrophilic mucilloid 3.4 g, aspartame, phenylalanine 30 mg/rounded

tsp. Pow. Can. 284 g, 426 g. *OTC.*
Use: Laxative.

Reguloid, Sugar Free Regular. (Rugby)
Psyllium hydrophilic mucilloid 3.4 g,
aspartame, phenylalanine 6 mg/dose.
Pow. Can. 284 g, 426 g. *OTC.*
Use: Laxative.

Rehydralyte. (Ross) Sodium 75 mEq,
potassium 20 mEq, chloride 65 mEq,
citrate 30 mEq, dextrose 25 g/L, 100
calories/L. Ready-to-use Bot. 8 oz. *Rx.*
Use: Fluid, electrolyte replacement.

• **relacatib.** (REL-a-ka-tib) USAN.
Use: Osteoporosis.

Relacon-DM NR. (Cypress) Dextromethorphan HBr 15 mg, guaifenesin 200 mg,
pseudoephedrine hydrochloride 32 mg
per 5 mL. Alcohol free. Saccharin,
sorbitol. Grape flavor. Liq. 473 mL. *Rx.*
Use: Upper respiratory combination,
antitussive and expectorant combination.

Relacon-HC. (Cypress) Hydrocodone bitartrate 3.5 mg, chlorpheniramine
maleate 2.5 mg, phenylephrine hydrochloride 10 mg per 5 mL. Alcohol,
sugar, and dye free. Raspberry flavor.
Liq. 473 mL. *c-III.*
Use: Upper respiratory combination, antitussive combination.

Relagesic. (International Ethical) Phenyltoloxamine citrate 50 mg, acetaminophen 650 mg. Tab. 100s. *Rx.*
Use: Antihistamine and analgesic.

Relagesic Liquid. (International Ethical)
Acetaminophen 160 mg, phenyltoloxamine citrate 5 mg per 5 mL. Parabens,
sucralose. Alcohol free, dye free, and
sugar free. Grape flavor. Liq. 118 mL.
Rx.
Use: Nonnarcotic analgesic combination.

Relahist-DM. (Cypress) Chlorpheniramine maleate 1 mg, dextromethorphan
HBr 3 mg, phenylephrine hydrochloride 2 mg per 1 mL. Saccharin, sorbitol. Orange vanilla flavor. Conc. Soln.
30 mL. *Rx.*
Use: Upper respiratory combination; antitussive, decongestant, antihistamine.

Relasin DM. (Cypress) Dextromethorphan HBr 15 mg, guaifenesin 175 mg,
pseudoephedrine hydrochloride 32 mg
per 5 mL. Alcohol free. Menthol, saccharin, sorbitol. Grape flavor. Liq.
473 mL. *Rx.*
Use: Upper respiratory combination, antitussive and expectorant combination.

relaxin. A purified ovarian hormone of
pregnancy (obtained from sows) re-

sponsible for pubic relaxation or separation of the symphysis pubis in mammals.

RelCof CPM. (Burel) Chlorpheniramine maleate 8 mg, methscopolamine nitrate 2.5 mg. ER Tab. 100s. *Rx.*
Use: Upper respiratory combination; decongestant, antihistamine, and anticholinergic combination.

RelCof DN PE. (Burel) *RelCof PE:* Chlorpheniramine maleate 8 mg, methscopolamine nitrate 2.5 mg, phenylephrine hydrochloride 20 mg. CR Tab. 10s. *RelCof CPM:* Chlorpheniramine maleate 8 mg, methscopolamine nitrate 2.5 mg. CR Tab. 10s. *Rx.*
Use: Upper respiratory combination; decongestant, antihistamine, and anticholinergic combination.

RelCof DN PSE. (Burel) *RelCof PSE:* Chlorpheniramine maleate 8 mg, methscopolamine nitrate 2.5 mg, pseudoephedrine hydrochloride 120 mg. Lactose. CR Tab. 10s. *RelCof CPM:* Chlorpheniramine maleate 8 mg, methscopolamine nitrate 2.5 mg. CR Tab. 10s. *Rx.*
Use: Upper respiratory combination; decongestant, antihistamine, and anticholinergic combination.

RelCof PSE. (Burel) Pseudoephedrine hydrochloride 120 mg, chlorpheniramine maleate 8 mg, methscopolamine nitrate 2.5 mg. lactose. ER Tab. 100s. *Rx.*
Use: Upper respiratory combination, decongestant, antihistamine, and anticholinergic combination.

Relenza. (GlaxoSmithKline) Zanamivir 5 mg. Lactose 20 mg. Pow. for Inh. Blister. Box 4 blisters w/ 5 *Rotadisks* and 1 *Disk-haler. Rx.*
Use: Antiviral.

Relhist. (Burel Pharmaceuticals) Brompheniramine tannate 6 mg/phenylephrine tannate 15 mg. Orange flavor. Chew. Tab. 60s. *Rx.*
Use: Upper respiratory combination, decongestant and antihistamine.

Reliable Gentle Laxative. (Goldline Consumer) Bisacodyl. 5 mg, lactose, sugar. EC, DR Tab. Bot. 100s, 1000s. 10 mg. Supp. Bot. 100s, 1000s. *OTC.*
Use: Laxative.

Relief Solution. (Allergan) Phenylephrine hydrochloride 0.12%, antipyrine 0.1%. Soln. Bot. 20 mL. *OTC.*
Use: Decongestant combination, ophthalmic.

Reli on Ketone Test Strips. (Bayer) Reagent strips for urine tests. 50s. *OTC.*

Use: Diagnostic aid.

Relistor. (Wyeth) Methylnaltrexone bromide 12 mg per 0.6 mL. Edetate calcium disodium 0.24 mg, sodium chloride 3.9 mg. Inj., Soln. Single-use vials. *Rx.*
Use: Detoxification agent, antidote.

• **relomycin.** (REE-low-MY-sin) USAN. A macrolide antibiotic produced by a variant strain of *Streptomyces hygroscopicus.*
Use: Anti-infective.

Relpax. (Pfizer) Eletriptan HBr 24.2 mg, 48.5 mg, lactose. Tab. Blistercard. 12s. *Rx.*
Use: Antimigraine agent, serotonin 5-HT$_1$ receptor agonist.

Reluri. (Cypress) Phenylephrine hydrochloride 30 mg, guaifenesin 1200 mg. Dye free. ER Tab. 100s. *Rx.*
Use: Upper respiratory combination, decongestant and expectorant combination.

• **remacemide hydrochloride.** (rem-ASS-eh-MIDE) USAN.
Use: Anticonvulsant (neuroprotective).

Rem Cough Medicine. (Last) Dextromethorphan HBr 5 mg/5 mL. Bot. 3 oz, 6 oz. *OTC.*
Use: Antitussive.

Remedy. (Medline) Benzalkonium chloride 0.12%. Aloe barbadensis, citrus oils, glycerin, parabens, tetrasodium EDTA, urea. Cleanser. 236 mL. *OTC.*
Use: Anti-infective, topical; antiseptic and germicide.

Remedy Calazime. (Medlline) Menthol 0.2%, zinc oxide 20%. Beeswax, carthamus tinctorious seed oil, citrus oils, glycerin, glycine, methylparaben, olea europaea fruit oil, PEG-8, white petrolatum, zea mays oil. Oint. 113 g. *OTC.*
Use: Miscellaneous protectant.

Remegel Soft Chewable Antacid. (Warner Lambert) Aluminum hydroxide-magnesium carbonate 476.4 mg. Chew. Tab. Pkg. 8s, 24s. *OTC.*
Use: Antacid.

Reme Hist DM. (River's Edge) Dextromethorphan HBr 15 mg, pyrilamine maleate 12.5 mg, phenylephrine hydrochloride 7.5 mg per 5 mL. Sugar, alcohol, and dye free. Saccharin, sorbitol. Grape flavor. Liq. 473 mL. *Rx.*
Use: Upper respiratory combination, antitussive combination.

Remeron. (Organon) Mirtazapine 15 mg, 30 mg, 45 mg. Lactose. Film coated. Tab. 30s. *Rx.*
Use: Antidepressant, tetracyclic compound.

Remeron SolTab. (Organon) Mirtazapine 15 mg, 30 mg, 45 mg. Aspartame, mannitol, sucrose, phenylalanine 2.6 mg (15 mg), 5.2 mg (30 mg), and 7.8 mg (45 mg). Orange flavor. Orally Disintegrating Tab. UD 30s. *Rx.*
Use: Antidepressant, tetracyclic compound.

•**remestemcel-L.** (REM-e-STEM-sel-l) USAN.
Use: Immunomodulator.

Remicade. (Centocor) Infliximab 100 mg. Sucrose 500 mg. Preservative free. Inj., lyophilized, Pow. for Soln. Single-use vials. 20 mL. *Rx.*
Use: Immunologic agent; immunomodulator.

•**remifentanil hydrochloride.** (reh-mih-FEN-tah-nill) USAN.
Use: Opioid analgesic.
See: Ultiva.

•**remiprostol.** (reh-mih-PROSTE-ole) USAN.
Use: Antiulcerative.

Remivox. (Janssen) Lorcainide hydrochloride. *Rx.*
Use: Antiarrhythmic.

Remodulin. (United Therapeutics) Treprostinil sodium 1 mg/mL, 2.5 mg/mL, 5 mg/mL (sodium chloride 5.3 mg), 10 mg/mL (sodium chloride 4 mg). Inj. Multi-use vials. 20 mL. *Rx.*
Use: Vasodilator.

•**remogliflozin etabonate.** (re-MOE-gli-FLOE-zin) USAN.
Use: Antidiabetic agent.

•**remoxipride.** (reh-MOX-ih-PRIDE) USAN.
Use: Antipsychotic.

•**remoxipride hydrochloride.** (reh-MOX-ih-PRIDE) USAN.
Use: Antipsychotic.

Remular-S. (Inter. Ethical) Chlorzoxazone 250 mg. Tab. Bot. 100s. *Rx.*
Use: Muscle relaxant.

RE MultiVit with Fluoride. (River's Edge) **1 mg:** Fluoride 1 mg, folate 0.3 mg (as folic acid), vitamins A 2,500 units, B_1 1.05 mg, B_2 1.2 mg, B_3 13.5 mg, B_6 1.05 mg, B_{12} 4.5 mcg, C 60 mg, D 400 units, E 15 units. **0.5 mg:** Fluoride 0.5 mg, folate 0.3 mg, vitamins A 2,500 units, B_1 1.05 mg, B_2 1.2 mg, B_3 13.5 mg, B_6 1.05 mg, B_{12} 4.5 mcg, C 60 mg, D 400 units, E 15 units. **0.25 mg:** Fluoride 0.25 mg, folate 0.3 mg, vitamins A 2,500 units, $B_1$1.05 mg, $B_2$1.2 mg, $B_3$13.5 mg, $B_6$1.05 mg, B_{12}4.5 mcg, C 60 mg, D 400 units, E 15 units. PEG, sugar (0.25 mg only).Chew. Tab. 100s.
Use: Nutritional supplement, multivitamin with fluoride.

ReNaf. (River's Edge) Fluoride 0.25 mg, 0.5 mg, 1 mg. Sugar free. Vanilla, grape, and cherry flavors. Chew. Tab. 120s, 1,000s. *Rx.*
Use: Trace element.

Renagel. (Genzyme) Sevelamer hydrochloride 400 mg, 800 mg. Film-coated. Tab. Bot. 180s (800 mg only), 360s (400 mg only). *Rx.*
Use: Phosphate binder.

renanolone. *Rx.*
Use: Steroid anesthetic.

Renax. (Everett) Vitamin E (as d-alpha tocopheryl succinate) 35 units, B_1 3 mg, B_2 2 mg, B_3 20 mg, B_5 10 mg, B_6 15 mg, B_{12} 12 mg, C 50 mg, folic acid 2.5 mg, Zn 20 mg, biotin 300 mcg, Cr, Se. Capl. Bot. 90s. *Rx.*
Use: Vitamin, mineral supplement.

Renbu. (Wren) Butabarbital sodium 32.4 mg. Tab. Bot. 100s, 1000s. *c-III.*
Use: Hypnotic; sedative.

renin angiotensin system antagonists.
See: Angiotensin-Converting Enzyme Inhibitors.
Angiotensin II Receptor Antagonists.
Direct Renin Inhibitors.
Selective Aldosterone Receptor Antagonists.

renin inhibitors, direct.
See: Aliskirin.

RenoCal-76. (Bracco Diagnostics) Diatrizoate meglumine 660 mg, diatrizoate sodium 100 mg, iodine 370 mg/mL. EDTA. Inj. Vials. 50 mL. Bot. 100 mL, 150 mL, 200 mL. *Rx.*
Use: Radiopaque agent.

renoform.
See: Epinephrine.

Renografin-60. (Bracco Diagnostics) Diatrizoate meglumine 520 mg, diatrizoate sodium 80 mg, iodine 292.5 mg/mL. EDTA. Inj. Vials. 10 mL, 50 mL. Bot. 100 mL. *Rx.*
Use: Radiopaque agent.

Reno-M Dip. (Bracco Diagnostics) Diatrizoate meglumine 300 mg, iodine 141 mg/mL. Inj. Bot. 300 mL. *Formerly Renografin-Dip. Rx.*
Use: Radiopaque agent.

Renormax. (Novartis) Spirapril 3 mg, 6 mg, 12 mg, 24 mg. Tab. *Rx.*
Use: ACE inhibitor.

Reno-Sed. (Vita Elixir) Methenamine 2 g, salol 0.5 g, methylene blue 1/10 g, benzoic acid 1/8 g, atropine sulfate 1/1000 g, hyoscyamine sulfate 1/2000 g. Tab. *Rx.*
Use: Anti-infective, urinary.

Renova. (Ortho Dermatological) Tretinoin 0.02%, 0.05%, stearyl alcohol, EDTA; parabens, benzyl alcohol, cetyl alcohol (0.02% only); methylparabens (0.05% only). Cream. Tube. 20 g (0.05% only), 40 g, 60 g (0.05% only). *Rx.*
Use: Retinoid.

Renovist. (Bracco Diagnostics) Diatrizoate methylglucamine 34.3%, diatrizoate sodium 35%, iodine 37%. Inj. Vial 50 mL, Box 25s.
Use: Radiopaque agent.

Renovist II. (Bracco Diagnostics) Diatrizoate sodium 29.1%, meglumine diatrizoate 28.5%, iodine 31%. Inj. Vial 30 mL, 60 mL, Box 25s.
Use: Radiopaque agent.

Renovue-Dip. (Bracco Diagnostics) Iodamide meglumide 24%, iodine 11.1%. Infusion Bot. 300 mL.
Use: Radiopaque agent.

Renovue-65. (Bracco Diagnostics) Iodamide meglumide 65%, organically bound iodine 30%, edetate disodium. Vial 50 mL.
Use: Radiopaque agent.

Rentamine Pediatric. (Major) Phenylephrine tannate 5 mg, chlorpheniramine tannate 4 mg, carbetapentane tannate/5 mL, saccharin, sucrose. Syr. Bot. Pt. *Rx.*
Use: Antihistamine, antitussive, decongestant.

ReNu Multi-Purpose. (Bausch & Lomb) Isotonic. Sodium chloride, sodium borate, boric acid, poloxamine, polyaminopropyl biguanide 0.00005%, EDTA 0.01%. Soln. Bot. 118 mL, 237 mL, 355 mL. *OTC.*
Use: Contact lens disinfection system.

ReNu Saline. (Bausch & Lomb) Isotonic buffered soln. of sodium Cl, boric acid, polyaminopropyl biguanide 0.00003%, EDTA. Soln. Bot. 355 mL. *OTC.*
Use: Contact lens care.

Renvela. (Genzyme) Sevelamer (as sevelamer carbonate). **Tab.:** 800 mg. Film-coated. 30s, 270s. **Pow. for Susp.:** 0.8 g, 2.4 g per packet. Sucralose. Citrus cream flavor. 90s. *Rx.*
Use: Phosphate binder.

ReoPro. (Lilly) Abciximab 2 mg/mL in buffered solution of sodium phosphate 0.01 M, sodium chloride 0.15 M. Preservative free. Inj. Single-use vials. 5 mL. *Rx.*
Use: Antiplatelet, glycoprotein IIb/IIIa inhibitor.

•**repaglinide.** (re-PAG-li-nide) *USP 34.*
Use: Antidiabetic, meglitinide.
See: Prandin.

Repan. (Everett) Butalbital 50 mg, caffeine 40 mg, acetaminophen 325 mg. Tab. Bot. 100s. *Rx.*
Use: Analgesic; hypnotic; sedative.

Repan CF. (Everett) Acetaminophen 650 mg, butalbital 50 mg. Tab. Bot. 100s. *Rx.*
Use: Analgesic combination.

•**reparixin.** (RE-pa-RIX-in) USAN.
Use: Immunosuppressive.

•**repifermin.** (re-pi-FER-min) USAN.
Use: Mucositis; wound healing.

•**repirinast.** (reh-PIRE-ih-nast) USAN.
Use: Antiallergic; antiasthmatic.

Replete. (Clintec Nutrition) K caseinate, Ca caseinate, maltodextrin, sucrose, corn oil, lecithin, vitamins A, B_1, B_2, B_3, B_5, B_6, B_{12}, C, D, E, K, folic acid, biotin, choline, Ca, Cl, Cu, Fe, I, Mg, Mn, P, Zn. Liq. Bot. 250 mL. *OTC.*
Use: Nutritional supplement.

Reprexain. (Hawthorn) Hydrocodone bitartrate/ibuprofen 2.5 mg/200 mg, 5 mg/200 mg, 10 mg/200 mg. PEG, polydextrose (2.5 mg/200 mg only). Film coated. Tab. 60s (5 mg/200 mg), 100s (2.5 mg/200 mg and 10 mg/ 200 mg). *c-III.*
Use: Opioid analgesic combination.

Reprieve. (Mayer Lab) Caffeine 32 mg, salicylamide 225 mg, vitamin B_1 50 mg, homatropine methylbromide 0.5 mg. Tab. Bot. 8s, 16s. *Rx.*
Use: Analgesic combination.

•**repromicin.** (rep-ROW-MY-sin) USAN.
Use: Anti-infective.

Repronex. (Ferring) Follicle-stimulating hormone and luteinzing hormone 75 units or 150 units. Pow. or pellet for inj., lyophilized. Vial with diluent. *Rx.*
Use: Sex hormone, ovulation stimulant.

•**reproterol hydrochloride.** (re-PROE-ter-ol) USAN.
Use: Bronchodilator.

Reptilase-R. (Abbott Diagnostics) Diagnostic for the investigation of fibrin formation and disturbances in fibrin formation due to causes other than thrombin inhibition.
Use: Diagnostic aid.

Requa's Charcoal. (Requa, Inc.) Wood charcoal 10 g. Tab. Pkg. 50s. Can 125s. *OTC.*
Use: Antiflatulent.

Requip. (GlaxoSmithKline) Ropinirole hydrochloride 0.25 mg, 0.5 mg, 1 mg, 2 mg, 3 mg, 4 mg, 5 mg. Lactose, PEG. Film-coated. Tab. Bot. 100s. *Rx.*
Use: Antiparkinson agent.

Requip XL. (GlaxoSmithKline) Ropinirole 2 mg, 4 mg, 6 mg, 8 mg, 12 mg. Lactose, maltodextrin, mannitol, PEG. Film coated. ER Tab. 30s, 90s (except 12 mg). *Rx.*
Use: Antiparkinson agent.

Resa. (Vita Elixir) Reserpine 0.25 mg. Tab. Bot. *Rx.*
Use: Antihypertensive.

Resaid. (Geneva) Phenylpropanolamine hydrochloride 75 mg, chlorpheniramine maleate 12 mg. Cap. Bot. 100s, 1000s. *Rx.*
Use: Antihistamine, decongestant.

Resaid S.R. (Geneva) Phenylpropanolamine hydrochloride 75 mg, chlorpheniramine maleate 12 mg. SR Cap. Bot. 100s, 1000s. *Rx.*
Use: Antihistamine, decongestant.

Rescaps-D S.R. (Geneva) Phenylpropanolamine hydrochloride 75 mg, caramiphen edisylate 40 mg. Cap. Bot. 100s. *Rx.*
Use: Antitussive, decongestant.

Rescon. (Capellon) Chlorpheniramine maleate 12 mg, methscopolamine nitrate 1.25 mg, phenylephrine hydrochloride 40 mg. Lactose. SR Tab. 90s. *Rx.*
Use: Upper respiratory combination; decongestant, antihistamine, and anticholinergic combination.

Rescon-DM. (Capellon) Dextromethorphan HBr 10 mg, pseudoephedrine hydrochloride 30 mg, chlorpheniramine maleate 2 mg per 5 mL. Alcohol, sugar, and dye free. Parabens, saccharin, sorbitol, fruit punch flavor. Liq. Bot. 118 mL, 473 mL. *OTC.*
Use: Upper respiratory combination, antitussive combination.

Rescon-GG. (Capellon) Phenylephrine hydrochloride 5 mg, guaifenesin 100 mg/5 mL. Alcohol and dye free. Parabens, sorbitol, sugar. Cherry flavor. Liq. Bot 118 mL, 473 mL. *OTC.*
Use: Upper respiratory combination, decongestant, expectorant.

Rescon-JR. (Capellon) Dexchlorpheniramine maleate 3 mg, phenylephrine hydrochloride 20 mg. ER Tab. 90s. *Rx.*
Use: Upper respiratory combination, decongestant and antihistamine.

Rescon-MX. (Capellon) Dexchlorpheniramine maleate 6 mg, phenylephrine hydrochloride 40 mg. Tab. 90s. *Rx.*
Use: Upper respiratory combination; decongestant, antihistamine, anticholinergic.

Rescriptor. (Agouron) Delavirdine mesylate 100 mg, 200 mg, lactose. Tab. Bot. 180s (200 mg only), 360s (100 mg only). *Rx.*
Use: Antiretroviral, non-nucleoside reverse transcriptase inhibitor.

Reserpaneed. (Hanlon) Reserpine 0.25 mg. Tab. Bot. 100s, 1000s. *Rx.*
Use: Antihypertensive.

• **reserpine.** (reh-SER-peen) *USP 34.*
Use: Antihypertensive.
See: Broserpine.
De Serpa.
Elserpine.
Raurine.
Reserpaneed.
Sertabs.
Zepine.

• **reserpine, hydralazine hydrochloride, and hydrochlorothiazide tablets.** *USP 34.*
Use: Antihypertensive.

resiquimod.
Use: Antiviral; antitumor.

• **reslizumab.** (res-li-ZOO-mab) USAN.
Use: Bronchial asthma.

• **resocortol butyrate.** (reh-so-CORE-tole BYOO-tih-rate) USAN.
Use: Corticosteroid; anti-inflammatory, topical.

Resol. (Wyeth) Na 50 mEq, K 20 mEq, Cl 50 mEq, citrate 34 mEq, Ca 4 mEq, Mg 4 mEq, phosphate 5 mEq, glucose 20 g/L. Contains 80 calories/L. Ctn. 32 fl oz. *Rx.*
Use: Fluid, electrolyte replacement.

Resolve/GP Daily Cleaner. (Allergan) Buffered solution with cocoamphocarboxyglycinate, sodium lauryl sulfate, hexylene glycol, alkyl ether sulfate, fatty acid amide surfactant cleaning agents, preservative free. Soln. Bot. 30 mL. *OTC.*
Use: Contact lens care.

Resonium-A. (Sanofi-Synthelabo) Sodium polystyrene sulfonate. *Rx.*
Use: Potassium removing resin.

resorcin.
See: Resorcinol.
W/Benzocaine.
See: Vagisil.

• **resorcinol.** (reh-SORE-sih-nole) *USP 34.*
Use: Keratolytic.
W/Benzocaine.
See: Unguentine Maximum Strength.
Vagisil.
Vagisil Maximum Strength.
W/Combinations.
See: Adult Acnomel.
Bicozene.
Black and White.

Clearasil Adult Care.
Rezamid.

•**resorcinol and sulfur lotion.** (reh-SORE-sih-nole) *USP 34.*
Use: Antifungal; parasiticide; scabicide.

•**resorcinol and sulfur topical suspension.** (reh-SORE-sih-nole) *USP 34.*
Use: Antifungal; parasiticide; scabicide.

•**resorcinol monoacetate.** (re-SORE-sih-nole) *USP 34.*
Use: Antiseborrheic; keratolytic.

resorcinolphthalein sodium.
Use: Antiseborrheic, topical.
See: Fluorescein Sodium.

Resource. (Novartis Nutrition) Ca and Na caseinates, soy protein isolate 37 g, sugar, hydrolyzed cornstarch 140 g, corn oil, soy lecithin 37 g, Na 890 mg, K 1600 mg, A, B_1, B_2, B_3, B_5, B_6, B_{12}, C, D, E, K, Ca, P, I, Fe, Mg, Cu, Zn, Mn, Cl, gluten free, vanilla, chocolate, strawberry flavor. Liq. Bot. 237 mL. *OTC.*
Use: Nutritional supplement.

Resource Diabetic. (Novartis Nutrition) Protein (sodium and calcium caseinates, soy protein isolates, carnitine, taurine) 63 g, carbohydrate (hydrolyzed cornstarch, fructose) 99 g, fat (high oleic sunflower oil, soybean oil) 47 g/L, vitamins A, B_1, B_2, B_3, B_5, B_6, B_{12}, C, D, E, K, biotin, choline, folic acid, m-inositol, Ca, chloride, Cr, Cu, Fe, I, Mg, Mn, Mo, P, Se, Zn, Na 970 mg (42 mEq), K 1100 mg (29 mEq), H_2O 450 mOsm/Kg, 1.06 cal/mL, fiber 13 g/L, lactose free, french vanilla, chocolate, strawberry, flavors. Liq. *Tetra Brik* Paks 237 mL (27s), closed system containers 1000 mL, 1500 mL (6s). *OTC.*
Use: Enteral nutritional therapy.

Resource Fruit Beverage. (Novartis Nutrition) Protein (whey protein concentrates) 38 g, carbohydrates (sugar, hydrolyzed cornstarch) 150 g/L, vitamins A, B_1, B_2, B_3, B_5, B_6, B_{12}, C, D, E, K, biotin, choline, folic acid, Ca, chloride, Cu, Fe, I, Mg, Mn, P, Zn, Na < 295 mg (< 13 mEq), K < 93 mg (< 2.4 mEq), H_2O 700 mOsm/Kg, 0.76 cal/mL, lactose free, orange, peach and wild berry flavors. Liq. *Tetra Brik* Paks 237 mL (27s). *OTC.*
Use: Enteral nutritional therapy.

Resource Instant Crystals. (Novartis Nutrition) Maltodextrin, sucrose, hydrogenated soy oil, sodium caseinate, calcium caseinate, soy protein isolate, potassium citrate, polyglycerol estersof fatty acids, vanilla and artificial flavors, vitamins and minerals. Instant Crystals. Pkt. 1.5 oz., 2 oz. *OTC.*
Use: Nutritional supplement.

Resource Just for Kids. (Novartis Nutrition) Protein (sodium and calcium caseinates, whey protein concentrate, carnitine, taurine) 30 g, carbohydrate (hydrolyzed cornstarch, sucrose) 110 g, fat (high oleic sunflower oil, soybean oil, medium chain triglycerides oil) 50 g, vitamins A, B_1, B_2, B_3, B_5, B_6, B_{12}, C, D, E, K, biotin, choline, folic acid, m-inositol, Ca, chloride, Cr, Cu, Fe, I, Mg, Mn, Mo, P, Se, Zn, Na 380 mg (17 mEq)/L, K 1300 mg (33 mEq)/L, H_2O 390 mOsm/Kg, 1 cal/mL, lactose free, french vanilla, chocolate, strawberry flavors. Liq. *Tetra Brik Paks* 237 mL (27s). *OTC.*
Use: Enteral nutritional therapy.

Resource Plus. (Novartis Nutrition) Ca and Na caseinates, soy protein isolate 54.9 g, maltodextrin, sucrose 200 g, corn oil, lecithin 53.3 g, Na 899 mg, K 1740 mg, A, B_1, B_2, B_3, B_5, B_6, B_{12}, C, D, E, K, biotin, choline, Ca, P, I, Fe, Mg, Cu, Zn, Cl, Mn, gluten free, vanilla, chocolate, strawberry flavors. Liq. Bot. 8 oz. *OTC.*
Use: Nutritional supplement.

Respa A.R. (Respa) Pseudoephedrine hydrochloride 90 mg, chlorpheniramine maleate 8 mg, belladonna alkaloids (atropine, hyoscyamine, scopolamine) 0.24 mg. Dye and sugar free. ER Tab. 100s. *Rx.*
Use: Upper respiratory combination, decongestant, antihistamine, and anticholinergic.

Respa C & C. (Respa) Acetaminophen 575 mg, dextromethorphan hydrobromide 30 mg, diphenhydramine hydrochloride 37.5 mg, phenylephrine hydrochloride 18 mg. Tab. 100s. *Rx.*
Use: Upper respiratory combination, antitussive combination.

Respa-DM. (Respa) Dextromethorphan HBr 28 mg, guaifenesin 600 mg. Dye free. ER Tab. 100s. *Rx.*
Use: Upper respiratory combination, antitussive with expectorant.

Respa-1st. (Respa) Pseudoephedrine hydrochloride 58 mg, guaifenesin 600 mg. ER Tab. 100s. *Rx.*
Use: Upper respiratory combination, decongestant and expectorant combination.

Respahist. (Respa) Pseudoephedrine hydrochloride 60 mg, brompheniramine maleate 6 mg. Sucrose. ER Cap. 100s.

Rx.
Use: Upper respiratory combination, decongestant and antihistamine.

Respahist-II. (Respa) Brompheniramine maleate 6 mg, phenylephrine hydrochloride 19 mg. ER Tab. 100s. *Rx.*
Use: Upper respiratory combination, decongestant and antihistamine.

Respaire-120 SR. (Laser) Pseudoephedrine hydrochloride 120 mg (extended release), guaifenesin 250 mg (immediate release). Corn starch, sugar. ER Cap. Bot. 100s. *Rx.*
Use: Upper respiratory combination, decongestant, expectorant.

Respaire-60 SR. (Laser) Pseudoephedrine hydrochloride 60 mg, guaifenesin 200 mg. Corn starch, sugar. ER Cap. Bot. 100s. *Rx.*
Use: Upper respiratory combination, decongestant and expectorant combination.

Respalor. (Bristol-Myers Squibb) Protein 75 g, carbohydrate 146 g, fat 70 g, Na 1248 mg, K 1456 mg, Fe 12.5 mg, cal/L 1498. Lactose free. Vanilla flavor. With appropriate vitamins and minerals. Liq. Bot. 237 mL. *OTC.*
Use: Nutritional supplement.

Respa-SA. (Respa Pharmaceuticals) Diphenhydramine hydrochloride 37.5 mg, pseudoephedrine hydrochloride 58 mg. Tab. 100s. *Rx.*
Use: Upper respiratory combination, decongestant and antihistamine.

Resperal. (Cypress) Dextromethorphan HBr 5 mg, pyrilamine maleate 5 mg, dexchlorpheniramine maleate 1.25 mg, phenylephrine hydrochloride 5 mg per 5 mL. Alcohol, sugar, dye, and gluten free. Saccharin, sorbitol. Grape flavor. Syrup. 473 mL. *Rx.*
Use: Upper respiratory combination, antitussive combination.

Respihaler Decadron Phosphate. (Merck & Co.)
See: Decadron Phosphate.

Respiracult. (Orion) Culture test for group A beta-hemolytic streptococci. In 10s.
Use: Diagnostic aid.

Respiralex. (Orion) Latex agglutination test to detect group A streptococci in throat and nasopharynx. Kit 1s.
Use: Diagnostic aid.

respiratory enzymes.
See: Alpha$_1$-Proteinase Inhibitor.

respiratory gases.
See: Nitric Oxide.

respiratory inhalant combinations.
See: Budesonide/Formoterol.

Fluticasone Propionate/Salmeterol.

respiratory inhalants.
See: Corticosteroids.
Intranasal Antihistamines.
Intranasal Steroids.
Mast Cell Stabilizers.
Mucolytics.
Respiratory Gases.

respiratory syncytial virus immune globulin (human) (RSV-IG).
Use: Prophylaxis against respiratory tract infection.

Respi-Tann. (Teamm) Carbetapentane citrate 20 mg (as carbetapentane tannate 25 mg), pseudoephedrine hydrochloride 30 mg (as pseudoephedrine tannate 75 mg). Dye free. Saccharin, sugar. Cherry flavor. Chew. Tab. 1s, 100s. *Rx.*
Use: Upper respiratory combination, antitussive combination.

Respi-Tann Pd. (Teamm) Carbetapentane citrate 7.5 mg (as carbetapentane tannate 15 mg), pseudoephedrine hydrochloride 30 mg (as pseudoephedrine tannate 60 mg) per 5 mL. Magnasweet, methylparaben. Grape bubble gum flavor. Susp. 15 mL, 473 mL. *Rx.*
Use: Upper respiratory combination, antitussive combination.

Restasis. (Allergan) Cyclosporine emulsion 0.05%, glycerin, castor oil, polysorbate 80, preservative free. Single-use vials. 0.4 mL. *Rx.*
Use: Immunologic agent.

Rest Easy. (Walgreen) Acetaminophen 1000 mg, pseudoephedrine hydrochloride 60 mg, dextromethorphan HBr 30 mg, doxylamine succinate 7.5 mg/30 mL. Bot. 6 oz, 16 oz. *OTC.*
Use: Analgesic; antihistamine; antitussive; decongestant.

Restoril. (Mallinckrodt) Temazepam 7.5 mg, 15 mg, 22.5 mg, 30 mg. Lactose. Cap. Bot. 30s (7.5 mg and 22.5 mg only), 100s, 500s (15 mg and 30 mg only). *c-IV.*
Use: Sedative/hypnotic, nonbarbiturate.

Restylane. (Medicis Aesthetics) Hyaluronic acid 20 mg/mL. Gel for Inj. Single-use prefilled syringes. *Rx.*
Use: Physical adjunct.

Restylane-L. (Medicis Aesthetics) Hyaluronic acid 20 mg/mL. Lidocaine 0.3%. Inj., gel. Single-use, prefilled syringe. *Rx.*
Use: Physical adjunct.

Re-Tann. (Midlothian Labs) Carbetapentane tannate 25 mg, pseudoephedrine tannate 75 mg per 5 mL.

Aspartame, parabens, phenylalanine. Cherry flavor. Susp. 473 mL. *Rx.*
Use: Antitussive combination.

• **retapamulin.** (re-TAP-a-MUE-lin) USAN.
Use: Antibiotic.
See: Altabax.

• **retaspimycin.** (RET-asp-i-MY-sin) USAN.
Use: Antineoplastic agent.

• **retaspimycin hydrochloride.** (RET-asp-i-MY-sin) USAN.
Use: Antineoplastic agent.

Retavase. (Centocor) Reteplase 10.4 units (18.1 mg). Pow. for Inj., lyophilized. Preservative-free. Kits with package insert, 2 single-use reteplase vials of 10.4 U (18.1 mg), 2 single-use diluent vials for reconstitution (10 mL sterile water for injection), 2 sterile 10 mL syringes, 2 sterile dispensing pins, 4 sterile needles, and 2 alcohol swabs. Half kits with package insert, 1 single-use reteplase vial 10.4 U (18.1 mg), 1 single-use diluent vial for reconstitution (10 mL sterile water for injection), and a sterile dispensing pin. *Rx.*
Use: Management of acute myocardial infarction.

• **reteplase, recombinant.** (RE-te-plase) USAN.
Use: Management of acute myocardial infarction; plasminogen activator.
See: Retavase.

• **retigabine.** (re-TIG-a-been) USAN.
Use: Antiepileptic.

Retin-A. (Ortho) **Cream:** Tretinoin 0.1%, 0.05%, 0.025%, stearyl alcohol (0.1% only). Cream. Tube 20 g, 45 g. **Gel:** Tretinoin 0.01%, 0.025%, alcohol 90%. Gel. Tube 15 g, 45 g. *Rx.*
Use: Dermatologic, acne; retinoid.

Retin-A Micro. (Ortho) Tretinoin 0.04%, 0.1%, glycerin, propylene glycol, benzyl alcohol, EDTA. Gel. Tube 20 g, 45 g. *Rx.*
Use: Dermatologic, acne; retinoid.

retinoic acid. Tretinoin.
Use: Keratolytic.
See: Retin A.

9-cis-retinoic acid.
Use: Acute promyelocytic leukemia. [Orphan Drug]

retinoids.
See: Adapalene.
Retinoids, First Generation.
Retinoids, Second Generation.
Tazarotene.

retinoids, first generation.
See: Isotretinoin.

Tretinoin.

retinoids, second generation.
See: Acitretin.
Alitretinoin.

Retinol. (NBTY) Vitamin A 100,000 units, glycol stearate, mineral oil, propylene glycol, lanolin oil, propylene glycol stearate SE, lanolin alcohol, retinol, parabens, EDTA. Cream. Tube 60 g. *OTC.*
Use: Emollient.

Retinol-A. (Young Again Products) Vitamin A palmitate 300,000 units/30 g. Cream. Tube 60 g. *OTC.*
Use: Emollient.

Retisert. (Bausch & Lomb) Fluocinolone acetonide 0.59 mg. Ophth. Implant. Individual cartons. *Rx.*
Use: Corticosteroid, ophthalmic.

Retrovir. (GlaxoSmithKline) Zidovudine. **Tab.:** 300 mg. Bot. 60s. **Cap:** 100 mg. Bot. 100s. UD 100s. **Syrup:** 50 mg/5 mL, sodium benzoate 0.2%, sucrose, strawberry flavor. Bot. 240 mL. **Inj:** 10 mg/mL. Single-use Vial 20 mL. *Rx.*
Use: Antiretroviral, nucleoside reverse transcriptase inhibitor.

RE2+30. (River's Edge) Pseudoephedrine hydrochloride 30 mg, chlorpheniramine maleate 2 mg per 5 mL. Saccharin, sorbitol. Grape flavor. Syrup. 118 mL. *Rx.*
Use: Upper respiratory combination, decongestant and antihistamine.

RE-U40. (River's Edge) Urea (carbamide) 40%. Colloidal oatmeal, glycerin, parabens. Aer. Foam. Aerosolized canister. 70 g. *Rx.*
Use: Emollient.

RE Urea 50. (River's Edge) Urea 50%. Cetyl alcohol, disodium EDTA, glycerin, lactic acid, mineral oil PEG-6, titanium dioxide. Soln., Top. Prefilled applicator. 4 mL.
Use: Emollient.

• **revaprazan hydrochloride.** (re-VA-prazan) USAN.
Use: Agent for GERD.

Revatio. (Pfizer) Sildenafil citrate. **Tab.:** 20 mg. Lactose. Film-coated. 90s. **Inj., Soln.:** 10 mg per 12.5 mL. Dextrose 50.5 mg/mL. Single-use vial. 12.5 mL. *Rx.*
Use: Treatment of pulmonary arterial hypertension to improve exercise ability.

Reversol. (Organon Teknika) Edrophonium chloride 10 mg/mL. Inj. Vial. 10 mL. *Rx.*
Use: Muscle stimulant.

ReVia. (Duramed) Naltrexone hydrochloride 50 mg. Film-coated. Tab. Bot. 30s,

100s. *Rx.*
Use: Antidote.
Revlimid. (Celgene) Lenalidomide 5 mg, 10 mg, 15 mg, 25 mg. Lactose. Cap. 28s (except 15 mg, 25 mg), 21s (15 mg, 25 mg only), 25s (25 mg only), 100s. *Rx.*
Use: Immunomodulator.
Revonto. (US Worldmeds) Dantrolene sodium 20 mg/vial. Mannitol 3 g/vial. Inj., lyophilized Pow. for Soln. Vial. 65 mL. *Rx.*
Use: Skeletal muscle relaxants, direct acting.
Revs Caffeine T.D. (Eon Labs) Caffeine 250 mg. Cap. Bot. 100s, 1000s. *OTC.*
Use: CNS stimulant.
Rexahistine. (Econo Med Pharmaceuticals) Phenylephrine hydrochloride 5 mg, chlorpheniramine maleate 1 mg, menthol 1 mg, sodium bisulfite 0.1%, alcohol 5%/5 mL. Bot. Gal. *OTC.*
Use: Antihistamine, decongestant.
Rexahistine DH. (Econo-Rx) Codeine phosphate 10 mg, phenylephrine hydrochloride 10 mg, chlorpheniramine maleate 2 mg, menthol 1 mg, alcohol 5%/5 mL. Bot. Gal. *c-v.*
Use: Antihistamine, antitussive, decongestant.
Rexahistine Expectorant. (Econo-Rx) Codeine phosphate 10 mg, phenylephrine hydrochloride 10 mg, chlorpheniramine maleate 2 mg, guaifenesin 100 mg, menthol 1 mg, alcohol 5%/5 mL. Bot. Gal. *c-v.*
Use: Antihistamine, antitussive, decongestant, expectorant.
Rexigen Forte. (ION Laboratories, Inc.) Phendimetrazine tartrate 105 mg. SR Cap. Bot. 100s. *c-III.*
Use: Anorexiant.
rexinoids.
See: Bexarotene.
Reyataz. (Bristol-Myers Squibb) Atazanavir sulfate (as base) 100 mg, 150 mg, 200 mg, 300 mg. Lactose, alcohols, simethicone. Cap. 30s (300 mg only), 60s (except 300 mg). *Rx.*
Use: Antiretroviral, protease inhibitor.
Rezamid. (Summers) Sulfur 5%, resorcinol 2%, SD alcohol 40 28%. Lot. Bot. 56.7 mL. *OTC.*
Use: Dermatologic; acne.
•**rezatomidine.** (RE-za-TOE-mi-deen) USAN.
Use: Treatment of chronic pain.
Rezine. (Marnel) Hydroxyzine hydrochloride 10 mg, 25 mg. Tab. Bot. 100s. *Rx.*
Use: Anxiolytic.

ReZyst IM. (Zyber) *Lactobacillus* and *Bifidobacterium* 150 mg. Sorbitol, sucralose, xylitol. Berry flavor. Chew. Tab. 60s. *OTC.*
Use: Oral nutritional supplement, probiotic.
RF Latex Test. (Laboratory Diagnostics) Rapid latex agglutination test for the qualitative screening and semi-quantitative determination of rheumatoid factor. Kit 100s.
Use: Diagnostic aid.
R-Frone. (Serono)
See: Interferon Beta.
R-Gen. (Ivax) Iodinated glycerol 60 mg/5 mL, alcohol 21.75%. Elix. Bot. Pt. *Rx.*
Use: Expectorant.
R-Gene 10. (Pharmacia & Upjohn) Arginine hydrochloride 1 g per 10 mL. Chloride ion 47.5 mEq per 100 mL. Preservative free. Inj., Soln. 300 mL. *Rx.*
Use: In vivo diagnostic aid.
R-HCTZ-H. (Wyeth) Reserpine 0.1 mg, hydrochlorothiazide 15 mg, hydralazine hydrochloride 25 mg. Tab. Bot. 100s, 500s. *Rx.*
Use: Antihypertensive.
Rheomacrodex. (Medisan) Dextran 40 10% in sodium Cl 0.9% or in dextrose 5%. Soln. Bot. 500 mL. *Rx.*
Use: Plasma expander.
Rheumatex. (Wampole) Latex agglutination test for the qualitative detection and quantitative determination of rheumatoid factor in serum. Kit 100s.
Use: Diagnostic aid.
Rheumaton. (Wampole) Two-minute hemagglutination slide test for the qualitative and quantitative determination of rheumatoid factor in serum or synovial fluid. Test kit 20s, 50s, 150s.
Use: Diagnostic aid.
Rheumatrex Dose Pack. (STADA Pharm) Methotrexate 2.5 mg. Tab. Pkg. 5 mg, 7.5 mg, 10 mg, 12.5 mg, 15 mg/week dose packs. *Rx.*
Use: Antipsoriatic; antirheumatic; antimetabolite.
Rhinabid. (Breckenridge) Phenylephrine hydrochloride 15 mg, brompheniramine maleate 12 mg. Sugar. ER Cap. 100s. *Rx.*
Use: Decongestant and antihistamine.
Rhinabid PD. (Breckenridge) Phenylephrine hydrochloride 7.5 mg, brompheniramine maleate 6 mg. Sugar. ER Cap. 100s. *Rx.*
Use: Pediatric decongestant and antihistamine.

Rhinacon A. (Breckenridge) Phenylephrine hydrochloride 20 mg, chlorpheniramine maleate 4 mg, phenyltoloxamine citrate 40 mg. ER Tab. 100s. *Rx.*
Use: Upper respiratory combination, decongestant and antihistamine.

Rhinall. (Scherer) Phenylephrine hydrochloride 0.25%, sodium bisulfite, chlorobutanol, benzalkonium chloride. Soln. Spray Bot. 40 mL. Dropper Bot. 30 mL. *OTC.*
Use: Nasal decongestant, arylalkylamine.

Rhinall 10. (Scherer) Phenylephrine hydrochloride 0.2%. Drop. Bot. oz. *OTC.*
Use: Decongestant.

Rhinaris. (PharmaScience) Sodium chloride. **Gel, intranasal:** 0.2%. Benzalkonium chloride, PEG, propylene glycol. 28.4 g. **Soln., intranasal:** 0.2%. Benzalkonium chloride, PEG, propylene glycol. Spray. 30 mL. *OTC.*
Use: Nasal decongestant.

Rhinaris Lubricating Mist. (Pharmascience) Polyethylene glycol 15%, propylene glycol 5% (spray only) 20% (gel only), benzalkonium chloride, sodium chloride. Soln. Spray Bot. 30 mL. Gel Tube. 28.35 g. *OTC.*
Use: Nasal decongestant.

Rhinatate. (Major) Phenylephrine tannate 25 mg, chlorpheniramine tannate 8 mg, pyrilamine tannate 25 mg. Tab. Bot. 100s, 250s. *Rx.*
Use: Antihistamine, decongestant.

Rhinatate-NF Pediatric. (Major) Phenylephrine tannate 5 mg, chlorpheniramine tannate 4.5 mg per 5 mL. Methylparaben, saccharin, sucrose. Susp. Bot. 473 mL. *Rx.*
Use: Upper respiratory combination, decongestant, antihistamine.

Rhinatate Pediatric. (Major) Phenylephrine tannate 5 mg, chlorpheniramine tannate 2 mg, pyrilamine tannate 12.5 mg/5 mL, methylparaben, saccharin, sucrose, strawberry-blackberry-currant flavor. Susp. Bot. 473 mL *Rx.*
Use: Upper respiratory combination, decongestant, antihistamine.

Rhinocort Aqua. (AstraZeneca) Budesonide 32 mcg/actuation. Dextrose, polysorbate 80, EDTA. Spray, Intranasal. Bot. 8.6 g (120 metered sprays) with metered-dose pump. *Rx.*
Use: Respiratory inhalant, intranasal steroid.

Rhinolar-EX. (McGregor Pharmaceuticals, Inc.) Phenylpropanolamine hydrochloride 75 mg, chlorpheniramine maleate 8 mg. SR Cap. Dye free. Bot. 60s. *Rx.*
Use: Antihistamine, decongestant.

Rhinolar-EX 12. (McGregor Pharmaceuticals, Inc.) Phenylpropanolamine hydrochloride 75 mg, chlorpheniramine maleate 12 mg. SR Cap. Dye free. Bot. 60s. *Rx.*
Use: Antihistamine, decongestant.

Rhinosyn. (Great Southern) Pseudoephedrine hydrochloride 60 mg, chlorpheniramine maleate 4 mg/5 mL, alcohol 0.45%, sucrose. Liq. Bot. 120 mL, 473 mL. *OTC.*
Use: Antihistamine, decongestant.

Rhinosyn DM. (Great Southern) Pseudoephedrine hydrochloride 30 mg, chlorpheniramine maleate 2 mg, dextromethorphan HBr 15 mg/5 mL, alcohol 1.4%, sucrose. Liq. Bot. 120 mL. *OTC.*
Use: Antihistamine, antitussive, decongestant.

Rhinosyn DMX. (Great Southern) Dextromethorphan HBr 15 mg, guaifenesin 100 mg/5 mL, alcohol 1.4%. Syr. Bot. 120 mL. *OTC.*
Use: Antitussive, expectorant.

Rhinosyn-PD. (Great Southern) Pseudoephedrine hydrochloride 30 mg, chlorpheniramine maleate 2 mg/5 mL. Liq. Bot. 120 mL. *OTC.*
Use: Antihistamine, decongestant.

Rhinosyn-X. (Great Southern) Pseudoephedrine hydrochloride 30 mg, dextromethorphan HBr 10 mg, guaifenesin 100 mg/5 mL, alcohol 7.5%. Liq. Bot. 120 mL. *OTC.*
Use: Antitussive, decongestant, expectorant.

rhodanate.
See: Potassium Thiocyanate.

rhodanide. More commonly Rhodanate, same as thiocyanate.
See: Potassium Thiocyanate.

•**RH$_o$(D) immune globulin.** (RH$_o$D ih-MYOON GLAB-byoo-lin) *USP 34.*
Use: Immunization.
See: BayRho-D Full Dose.
　Gamulin Rh.
　MICRh$_o$GAM.
　HyperRHO S/D Mini-Dose.
　RhoGAM.
　Rhophylac.
　WinRho SD.
　WinRho SDF.

RH$_o$(D) immune globulin intravenous (human). (RH$_o$D ih-MYOON GLAB-byoo-lin) *Formerly RH$_o$ Immune Human Globulin.*

Use: Immune thrombocytopenic purpura, immunizing agent (passive). [Orphan Drug]
See: WinRho SDF.

RhoGAM. (Ortho-Clinical Diagnostics) $Rh_o(D)$ immune globulin 5% ± 1% gamma globulin. Sodium chloride 2.9 mg, polysorbate 80 0.01%, glycine 15 mg/mL. Preservative free. Filtrated. Soln. for Inj. Pkg. Prefilled single-dose syringe, package insert, control form, patient ID card. 5s, 25s, 100s. *Rx.*
Use: Immunization.

RhoGAM Ultra Filtered Plus. (Ortho-Clinical Diagnostics) $Rh_o(D)$ immune globulin 300 mcg (1,500 units). Glycine 15 mg/mL, polysorbate 80 0.01%, sodium chloride 2.9 mg/mL. Preservative free. Inj., Soln. Package w/single-dose syringe, control form, and patient ID card. 1s, 5s, 25s. *Rx.*
Use: Biologic and immunological agent, immune globulin.

Rhophylac. (CSL Behring) $Rh_o(D)$ immune globulin IV (human) 1,500 units (300 mcg). Glycine, sodium chloride. Preservative free. Inj. Soln. Prefilled syringes. 2 mL. *Rx.*
Use: Immunization.

Rhythmin. (Sidmak) Procainamide 250 mg, 500 mg. SR Tab. Bot. 100s, 500s, 1000s. *Rx.*
Use: Antiarrhythmic.

RiaSTAP. (CSL Behring) Fibrinogen concentrate (human) ≈ 1 g (900 to 1,300 mg). Albumin 400 to 700 mg. Preservative free. Inj., Lyophilized Pow. for Soln. Single-use vial. *Rx.*
Use: Hemostatic, systemic.

• **ribaminol.** (rye-BAM-ih-nahl) USAN.
Use: Memory adjuvant.

RibaPak. (Par) Ribavirin 400 mg, 600 mg. Lactose, PEG 3350. Film-coated. Tab. UD 14s. Also available in a 400 mg and 600 mg combination package (1000 mg/day). *Rx.*
Use: Antiviral agent.

Ribasphere. (Three Rivers) Ribavirin. **Cap.:** 200 mg. Lactose. Pellet filled. 42s, 56s, 70s, 84s, 140s, 168s, 180s. **Tab.:** 200 mg, 400 mg, 600 mg. Lactose, PEG 3350. Film-coated. 56s (except 200 mg), 168s (200 mg only), 250s (600 mg only), 500s (except 600 mg); *RibaPak* 800 and 1,000 dose packs (400 mg only), *RibaPak* 1,000 and 1,200 dose packs (600 mg only) (Each *RibaPak* 800 dose pack contains 14 ribavirin 400 mg tablets. Each *RibaPak* 1,000 dose pack contains 7 ribavirin 400 mg tablets and 7 ribavirin

600 mg tablets. Each *RibaPak* 1,200 dose pack contains 14 ribavirin 600 mg tablets.). *Rx.*
Use: Antiviral agents.

Ribatab. (PRX Pharmaceuticals) Ribavirin 400 mg, 600 mg. Lactose, PEG 3350. Film-coated. Tab. UD 14s. Also available in a 400 mg and 600 mg combination package (1000 mg/day). *Rx.*
Use: Antiviral agent.

• **ribavirin.** (rye-buh-VIE-rin) USP 34.
Use: Antiviral.
See: Copegus.
   Rebetol.
   Ribasphere.
   RibPak.
   Ribatab.
   Virazole.

ribavirin. (Various Mfr.) Ribavirin. **Cap.:** 200 mg. 42s, 56s, 70s, 84s, 140s, 168s, 180s, 1,000s, UD 100s. **Tab.:** 200 mg. 168s 180s, 1,000s, UD 100s. *Rx.*
Use: Antiviral agent.

ribavirin. (Zydus) Ribavirin 400 mg, 500 mg. PEG. Film-coated. Tab. 28s, 56s, 60s. *Rx.*
Use: Antiviral agent.

ribavirin and interferon alfa-2b, recombinant.
Use: Antineoplastic.

• **riboflavin.** (RYE-boh-FLAY-vin) USP 34.
Use: Vitamin (enzyme co-factor), water-soluble vitamin.
See: B_2-400.
   Cyto B2.
   Vitamin B_2.

riboflavin. (Various Mfr.) Riboflavin 50 mg, 100 mg. Tab. Bot. 100s, 250s. *OTC.*
Use: Water-soluble vitamin.

• **riboflavin 5'-phosphate sodium.** (RYE-boh-FLAY-vin) USP 34.
Use: Vitamin.

• **riboprine.** (RYE-boe-PREEN) USAN.
Use: Antineoplastic.

Ribozyme. (Fellows) Riboflavin-5-phosphate sodium 50 mg/mL Inj. Vial 10 mL. *Rx.*

ricin (blocked) conjugated murine mca. (ImmunoGen)
Use: Antineoplastic. [Orphan Drug]

Ricolon Solution. (Sanofi-Synthelabo) Ricolon concentrate. Soln. *Rx.*
Use: Leucocytotic preparation.

RID. (Bayer) Pyrethrins 0.33%, piperonyl butoxide 4%. SD alcohol. Shampoo. 60 mL, 120 mL, 240 mL, and 120 mL kits containing gel, comb, and lice control spray. *OTC.*
Use: Pediculicide.

•**ridaforolimus.** (rid-a-for-OH-li-mus)
USAN.
Use: Antineoplastic.
Rid•a•Pain•HP. (Pfeiffer) Capsaicin
0.075%, alcohols, parabens. Cream.
Tube. 45 g. *OTC.*
Use: Analgesic.
Ridaura. (GlaxoSmithKline) Auranofin
3 mg. Cap. Bot. 60s. *Rx.*
Use: Antirheumatic.
Rid Lice Control Spray. (Pfizer) Syn-
thetic pyrethroids 0.5%, related com-
pounds 0.065%, aromatic petroleum hy-
drocarbons 0.664%. Spray. Can 5 oz.
OTC.
Use: Pediculicide.
Rid Lice Elimination System. (Pfizer)
Rid lice killing shampoo, nit removal
comb, Rid lice control spray and instruc-
tion booklet/unit. *OTC.*
Use: Pediculicide.
•**ridogrel.** (RYE-doe-grell) USAN.
Use: Thromboxane synthetase
inhibitor.
•**rifabutin.** (RIFF-uh-BYOO-tin) *USP 34.*
Use: Anti-infective (antimycobacterial),
MAC disease; antituberculosal.
See: Mycobutin.
Rifadin. (Aventis) Rifampin. **150 mg/**
Cap.: Bot. 30s. **300 mg/Cap.:** Bot. 30s,
60s, 100s. **Pow. for Inj.:** 600 mg. Vi-
als. *Rx.*
Use: Antituberculous.
•**rifalazil.** (RIFF-ah-lah-zill) USAN.
Use: Antibacterial.
Rifamate. (Aventis) Rifampin 300 mg,
isoniazid 150 mg. Cap. Bot. 60s. *Rx.*
Use: Antituberculosal.
•**rifametane.** (RIFF-ah-met-ane) USAN.
Use: Anti-infective.
•**rifamexil.** (riff-ah-MEX-ill) USAN.
Use: Anti-infective.
•**rifamide.** (RIFF-am-ide) USAN.
Use: Anti-infective.
•**rifampin.** (RIFF-am-pin) *USP 34.* Rifampin, isoniazid, and pyrazinamide. Tablets.
Use: Anti-infective, antituberculostatic.
See: Rifadin.
Rifater.
Rimactane.
rifampin. (Akorn-Strides) Rifampin
600 mg. Lyophilized Pow. for Inj. Vial.
Rx.
Use: Anti-infective agent, antituberculosis agent.
rifampin. (Various Mfr.) Rifampin 150 mg,
300 mg. Cap. Bot. 30s, 60s (300 mg
only), 100s, 500s (300 mg only). *Rx.*
Use: Antituberculosal.

•**rifampin and isoniazid.** *USP 34.*
Use: Anti-infective (tuberculostatic).
See: IsonaRif.
Rifamate.
•**rifampin, isoniazid, and pyrazinamide.**
USP 34.
Use: Anti-infective (tuberculostatic).
See: Rifater.
•**rifampin, isoniazid, pyrazinamide, and**
ethambutol hydrochloride. *USP 34.*
Use: Anti-infective (tuberculostatic).
•**rifamycin.** (RIF-a-MYE-sin) USAN.
Use: Treatment of traveler's diarrhea.
•**rifamycin sodium.** (RIF-a-MYE-sin)
USAN.
Use: Treatment of traveler's diarrhea.
•**rifapentine.** (RIFF-ah-pen-teen) USAN.
Use: Anti-infective, antituberculosal.
See: Priftin.
rifapentine.
Use: Pulmonary tuberculosis; *mycobac-*
terium avium complex in AIDS pa-
tients. [Orphan Drug]
Rifater. (Aventis) Rifampin 120 mg, iso-
niazid 50 mg, pyrazinamide 300 mg.
Tab. Bot. 60s. *Rx.*
Use: Antituberculosal.
•**rifaximin.** (riff-AX-ih-min) USAN.
Use: Anti-infective.
See: Xifaxan.
r-IFN-beta. Recombinant interferon beta.
RIG. Rabies immune globulin.
Use: Immunization, rabies.
See: Imogam.
•**rilapladib.** (ri-LAP-la-dib) USAN.
Use: Atherosclerosis.
•**rilonacept.** (ri-LON-a-sept) USAN.
Use: Immunomodulator.
See: Arcalyst.
•**rilotumumab.** (ril-oh-TOOM-ue-mab)
USAN.
Use: Antineoplastic.
•**rilpivirine.** (RIL-pi-VIR-een) USAN.
Use: Treatment of HIV infection.
•**rilpivirine hydrochloride.** (RIL-pi-VIR-
een) USAN.
Use: Treatment of HIV infection.
Rilutek. (Aventis) Riluzole 50 mg. Tab.
Rx.
Use: Amyotrophic lateral sclerosis
agent.
•**riluzole.** (RILL-you-zole) USAN.
Use: Amyotrophic lateral sclerosis
agent. [Orphan Drug]
See: Rilutek.
•**rimabotulinumtoxinB.** (RIM-a-BOT-ue-
LYE-num-TOX-in-BEE) USAN.
Use: Botulinum toxin.

Rimactane. (Novartis) Rifampin 300 mg. Cap. Bot. 30s, 60s, 100s. *Rx.*
Use: Antituberculous.

Rimadyl. (Roche) *Rx.*
Use: Analgesic, NSAID.
See: Carprofen.

•**rimantadine hydrochloride.** (rih-MAN-tuh-deen) *USP 34.*
Use: Antiviral.
See: Flumadine.

rimantadine hydrochloride. (Various Mfr.) Rimantadine hydrochloride 100 mg. Tab. 100s, 1,000s. *Rx.*
Use: Antiviral agent.

•**rimcazole hydrochloride.** (RIM-kazz-OLE) *USAN.*
Use: Antipsychotic.

•**rimexolone.** (rih-MEX-oh-lone) *USAN.*
Use: Ophthalmic corticosteroid.
See: Vexol.

•**rimiterol hydrobromide.** (RIH-mih-TER-ole) *USAN.*
Use: Bronchodilator.

•**rimonabant.** (RIM-oh-nab-ant) *USAN.*
Use: Investigational selective cannabinoid type 1 receptor blocker; weight loss.

Rimso-50. (Research Industries) Dimethyl sulfoxide in a 50% aqueous soln. Bot. 50 mL. *Rx.*
Use: Interstitial cystitis agent.

Rinade. (Econo Med Pharmaceuticals) Chlorpheniramine maleate 8 mg, phenylephrine hydrochloride 20 mg, methscopolamine nitrate 2.5 mg. Cap. Bot. 120s. *Rx.*
Use: Anticholinergic; antihistamine, decongestant.

•**rindopepimut.** (RIN-doe-PEP-i-mut) *USAN.*
Use: Immunotherapeutic agent.

Ringer's in 5% dextrose. (Various Mfr.) Dextrose 50 g, calories 170, Na$^+$ $\approx$ 147 mEq, K$^+$ 4 mEq, Ca^{++} $\approx$ 4.5 mEq, Ca$^-$ $\approx$ 4.5 mEq, Cl$^-$ $\approx$ 156 mEq, osmolarity $\approx$ 560 mOsm/L. Soln. Bot. 500 mL. 1000 mL. *Rx.*
Use: Intravenous nutritional therapy, intravenous replenishment solution.

•**Ringer's injection.** *USP 34.*
Use: Fluid, electrolyte replacement; irrigant, ophthalmic.

Ringer's injection. (Various Mfr.) Na$^+$ $\approx$ 147 mEq, K$^+$ 4 mEq, Ca^{++} $\approx$ 4 mEq, Cl$^-$ $\approx$ 156 mEq, osmolarity $\approx$ 310 mOsm/L. Soln. Bot. 500 mL. 1000 mL. *Rx.*
Use: Intravenous nutritional therapy, intravenous replenishment solution.

Ringer's injection, lactated. *USP 34.*
Use: Fluid, electrolyte replacement.

Ringer's irrigation. (Various Mfr.) Sodium chloride 0.86 g, potassium chloride 0.03 g, calcium chloride 0.033 g/ 100 mL. Bot. 1 liter. *Rx.*
Use: Irrigant, ophthalmic.

Rinnovi Nail System. (Quinnova) Urea 50%. EDTA. Stick. In 6s with nail and cuticle cleanser and protectant sprays. *Rx.*
Use: Emollient.

•**rintatolimod.** (RIN-ta-TOL-i-mod) *USAN.*
Use: Antiviral.

Riomet. (Ranbaxy) Metformin hydrochloride 500 mg/5 mL. Saccharin, cherry flavor. Oral Soln. Bot. 120 mL, 480 mL. *Rx.*
Use: Antidiabetic agent, biguanide.

Riopan Plus Double Strength Suspension. (Wyeth) Magaldrate 1080 mg, simethicone 40 mg/5 mL. Bot. 360 mL. *OTC.*
Use: Antacid; antiflatulent.

Riopan Plus Double Strength Tablets. (Wyeth) Magaldrate 1080 mg, simethicone 20 mg. Chew. Tab. Bot. 60s. *OTC.*
Use: Antacid; antiflatulent.

Riopan Plus Tablets. (Wyeth) Magaldrate 480 mg, simethicone 20 mg. Chew. Tab. Bot. 50s, 100s. *OTC.*
Use: Antacid; antiflatulent.

•**rioprostil.** (RYE-oh-PRAHS-till) *USAN.*
Use: Gastric antisecretory.

•**ripazepam.** (rip-AZE-eh-pam) *USAN.*
Use: Anxiolytic.

•**risedronate sodium.** (riss-ED-row-nate) *USAN.*
Use: Bisphosphonate.
See: Actonel.
Atelvia.
W/Calcium Carbonate.
See: Actonel with Calcium.

•**rismorelin porcine.** (riss-more-ELL-in PORE-sine) *USAN.*
Use: Hormone, growth hormone-releasing.

•**risocaine.** (RIZZ-oh-cane) *USAN.*
Use: Anesthetic, local.

•**risotilide hydrochloride.** (rih-SO-tih-LIDE) *USAN.*
Use: Cardiovascular agent (antiarrhythmic).

Risperdal. (Janssen) Risperidone. **Tab.:** 0.25 mg, 0.5 mg, 1 mg, 2 mg, 3 mg, 4 mg. Lactose. Bot. 60s, 500s (except 4 mg), UD 100s. **Oral Soln.:** 1 mg/mL. Bot. 30 mL w/calibrated pipette. *Rx.*
Tall Man: RisperDAL
Use: Antipsychotic, benzisoxazole derivative.

Risperdal Consta. (Janssen) Risperidone 12.5 mg, 25 mg, 37.5 mg, 50 mg. Inj., Pow. for Soln., ER. Vials/Kits. Dose pack contains prefilled syringe and 2 mL of diluent. *Rx.*
Tall Man: RisperDAL
Use: Antipsychotic, benzisoxazole derivatives.

Risperdal M-Tab. (Janssen) Risperidone 0.5 mg (phenylalanine 0.14 mg), 1 mg (phenylalanine 0.28 mg), 2 mg (phenylalanine 0.42 mg), 3 mg (phenylalaine 0.63 mg), 4 mg (phenylalanine 0.84 mg). Aspartame, mannitol, peppermint oil. Orally disintegrating tab. UD 28s, UD 30s (0.5 mg, 1 mg only). *Rx.*
Tall Man: RisperDAL
Use: Antispychotic, benzisoxazole derivative.

• **risperidone.** (RISS-PURR-ih-dohn) USAN.
Tall Man: risperiDONE
Use: Antipsychotic, neuroleptic, benzisoxazole deriative.
See: Risperdal.
Risperdal Consta.
Risperdal M-Tab.

risperidone. (Dr. Reddy's Laboratories) Risperidone 0.5 mg, 1 mg, 2 mg, 3 mg, 4 mg. Aspartame, mannitol, phenylalanine 2.1 mg (0.5 mg), 4.21 mg (1 mg), 8.4 mg (2, 3, and 4 mg). Orally disintegrating Tab. UD 30s and 100s. *Rx.*
Use: Antipsychotic agent, benzisoxazole derivative.

risperidone. (Teva) Risperidone. **Tab.:** 0.25 mg, 0.5 mg, 1 mg, 2 mg, 3 mg, 4 mg. Lactose, PEG. Film coated. 60s, 500s (except 4 mg). **Soln.:** 1 mg/mL. Sorbitol. 30 mL w/calibrate pipette. *Rx.*
Use: Antipsychotic agent, benzisoxazole derivative.

risperidone. (Various Mfr.) Risperidone 1 mg/mL. Soln. Bot. w/calibrated pipette. 30 mL. *Rx.*
Use: Antipsychotic agent, benzisoxazole derivative.

• **ristianol phosphate.** (riss-TIE-ah-NOLE) USAN.
Use: Immunoregulator.

Ritalin. (Novartis) Methylphenidate hydrochloride 5 mg, 10 mg, 20 mg. Lactose (except 20 mg), sucrose (20 mg only), talc (20 mg only). Tab. Bot. 100s. *c-II.*
Use: Central nervous system stimulant.

Ritalin LA. (Novartis) Methylphenidate hydrochloride 10 mg, 20 mg, 30 mg, 40 mg. Sugar spheres, talc. ER Cap. Bot. 100s. *c-II.*
Use: Central nervous system stimulant.

Ritalin-SR. (Novartis) Methylphenidate hydrochloride 20 mg, lactose, cetostearyl alcohol, mineral oil, color-additive free. SR Tab. Bot. 100s. *c-II.*
Use: Central nervous system stimulant.

• **ritanserin.** (rih-TAN-ser-in) USAN.
Use: Serotonin antagonist.

• **ritodrine.** (RIH-toe-DREEN) USAN.
Use: Muscle relaxant.

• **ritolukast.** (rih-tah-LOO-kast) USAN.
Use: Antiasthmatic (leukotriene antagonist).

• **ritonavir.** (rih-TON-a-veer) USAN.
Use: Antiretroviral, protease inhibitor.
See: Norvir.

ritonavir/lopinavir.
Use: Antiretroviral, protease inhibitor.
See: Kaletra.

Rituxan. (Biogen Idec/Genentech) Rituximab 10 mg/mL. Polysorbate 80 0.7 mg/mL. Preservative free. Inj. Single-use vial. 10 mL, 50 mL. *Rx.*
Use: Antineoplastic; monoclonal antibody.

• **rituximab.** (rih-TUCK-sih-mab) USAN.
Tall Man: riTUXimab
Use: Antineoplastic (microtubule inhibitor); monoclonal antibody.
See: Rituxan.

• **rivanicline galactarate.** (rye-VAN-i-kleen gal-AK-tar-ate) USAN.
Use: Ulcerative colitis; nicotinic receptor agonist.

rivastigmine tartrate.
Use: Cholinesterase inhibitor.
See: Exelon.

rivastigmine tartrate. (Dr. Reddy's Laboratories) Rivastigmine 1.5 mg, 3 mg, 4.5 mg, 6 mg. Cap. 30s, 60s, 100s, 500s. *Rx.*
Use: Cholinesterase inhibitor.

• **rizatriptan benzoate.** (rye-zah-TRIP-tan BENZ-oh-ate) USAN.
Use: Antimigraine, serotonin 5-HT$_1$ receptor agonist.
See: Maxalt.
Maxalt-MLT.

• **rizatriptan sulfate.** (rye-zah-TRIP-tan) USAN.
Use: Antimigraine.

RMS. (Upsher-Smith) Morphine sulfate 5 mg, 10 mg, 20 mg, 30 mg. Rectal. Supp. Box 12s. *c-II.*
Use: Opioid analgesic.

Robafen. (Major) Guaifenesin 100 mg/5 mL, alcohol 3.5%. Syr. Bot. 118 mL, 240 mL, pt, gal. *OTC.*
Use: Expectorant.

Robafen AC Cough. (Major) Guaifenesin 100 mg, codeine phosphate 10 mg/

5 mL, alcohol 3.5%, parabens. Syrup. Bot. 473 mL. *c-v.*
Use: Antitussive; expectorant, narcotic.

Robafen CF. (Major) Psuedoephedrine hydrochloride 30 mg, dextromethorphan HBr 10 mg, guaifenesin 100 mg per 5 mL. Saccharin, sorbitol, alcohol free. Liq. Bot. 237 mL. *OTC.*
Use: Upper respiratory combination, antitussive and expectorant combination.

Robafen DAC. (Major) Pseudoephedrine 30 mg, codeine phosphate 10 mg, guaifenesin 100 mg/5 mL, alcohol 1.4%. Liq. Bot. Pt. *c-v.*
Use: Antitussive, decongestant, expectorant.

Robafen DM. (Major) Dextromethorphan HBr 10 mg, guaifenesin 100 mg/5 mL, alcohol 1.4%. Syrup. Bot. 473 mL. *OTC.*
Use: Antitussive; expectorant.

Robafen DM Max. (Major) Dextromethorphan hydrobromide 10 mg, guaifenesin 200 mg. Glycerin, menthol, PEG, propylene glycol, saccharin, sorbitol. Alcohol free and sugar free. Liq. 118 mL. *OTC.*
Use: Upper respiratory combination, antitussive with expectorant.

Robafen PE. (Major) Pseudoephedrine hydrochloride 30 mg, guaifenesin 100 mg/5 mL, glucose, corn syrup, saccharin, alcohol free. Liq. Bot. 118 mL. *OTC.*
Use: Upper respiratory combination, decongestant, expectorant.

robanul.
See: Robinul.

RoBathol Bath Oil. (Pharmaceutical Specialties) Cottonseed oil, alkyl aryl polyether alcohol. Lanolin free. Oil. Bot. 240 mL, 480 mL, gal. *OTC.*
Use: Dermatologic.

•**robatumumab.** (ROE-ba-TOOM-ue-mab) USAN.
Use: Antineoplastic.

Robaxin. (Schwarz Pharma) Methocarbamol 500 mg. Saccharin. Tab. Bot. 100s, 500s, *Disco-Pak* 100s. *Rx.*
Use: Muscle relaxant.

Robaxin. (Wyeth-Ayerst) Methocarbamol 100 mg/mL in a soln. of polyethylene glycol 300. Inj. Vial 10 mL. *Rx.*
Use: Muscle relaxant.

Robaxin-750. (Schwarz Pharma) Methocarbamol 750 mg. Saccharin. Tab. Bot. 100s, 500s, *Disco-Pak* 100s. *Rx.*
Use: Muscle relaxant.

Robimycin. (Wyeth) Erythromycin 250 mg. Tab. Bot. 100s, 500s. *Rx.*
Use: Anti-infective, erythromycin.

Robinul. (Sciele) Glycopyrrolate 1 mg, lactose. Tab. Bot. 100s. *Rx.*
Use: Anticholinergic.

Robinul Forte. (Sciele) Glycopyrrolate 2 mg, lactose. Tab. Bot. 100s. *Rx.*
Use: Anticholinergic.

Robinul Injectable. (Baxter) Glycopyrrolate 0.2 mg/mL, benzyl alcohol 0.9%. Vial 1 mL, 2 mL, 5 mL, 20 mL. *Rx.*
Use: Anticholinergic.

Robitussin Children's Cough & Cold CF. (Pfizer Consumer Healthcare) Dextromethorphan hydrobromide 5 mg, guaifenesin 50 mg, phenylephrine hydrochloride 2.5 mg. Glycerin, propylene glycol, sodium 3 mg, sodium benzoate, sorbitol, sucralose. Liq. 118 mL. *Rx.*
Use: Upper respiratory combination, antitussive and expectorant combination.

Robitussin Cough & Cold D. (Wyeth Consumer Healthcare) Dextromethorphan hydrobromide 15 mg, guaifenesin 200 mg, pseudoephedrine hydrochloride 30 mg per 5 mL. Menthol, PEG, sodium 4 mg, sorbitol, sucralose. Liq. 118 mL. *OTC.*
Use: Upper respiratory combination, antitussive and expectorant combination.

Robitussin Cough & Congestion. (Wyeth Consumer) Dextromethorphan 10 mg, guaifenesin 200 mg per 5 mL. Alcohol free. Corn syrup, menthol, PEG, saccharin, sorbitol. Liq. 118 mL. *OTC.*
Use: Upper respiratory combination, antitussive with expectorant.

Robitussin Cough, Cold & Flu Nighttime. (Wyeth Consumer) Dextromethorphan HBr 5 mg, chlorpheniramine maleate 1 mg, phenylephrine hydrochloride 2.5 mg, acetaminophen 160 mg per 5 mL. Alcohol free. Menthol, sodium 2 mg/5 mL, sorbitol, sucralose. Syrup. 118 mL. *OTC.*
Use: Upper respiratory combination, antitussive combination.

Robitussin Cough DM. (Wyeth Consumer) Dextromethorphan HBr 10 mg, guaifenesin 100 mg per 5 mL. Alcohol free. Glycerin, corn syrup, menthol, saccharin sodium. Liq. 118 mL. *OTC.*
Use: Upper respiratory combination, antitussive with expectorant.

Robitussin Cough Drops. (Wyeth Consumer) Menthol 7.4 mg, 10 mg, eucalyptus oil, sucrose, corn syrup. Loz. Pkg. 9s, 25s, menthol 10 mg, eucalyptus oil, sucrose, corn syrup, honey-lemon flavor. Loz. Pkg. 9s, 25s. *OTC.*
Use: Antitussive.

Robitussin CoughGels. (Wyeth Consumer) Dextromethorphan HBr 15 mg. Sorbitol. Liquid-filled. Cap. 20s. *OTC.*
Use: Nonnarcotic antitussive.

Robitussin Cough Long-Acting. (Wyeth Consumer) Dextromethorphan HBr 15 mg/5 mL. Alcohol, glucose, corn syrup, saccharin, cherry flavor. Liq. Bot. 118 mL, 237 mL. *OTC.*
Use: Nonnarcotic antitussive.

Robitussin Cough Sugar-Free DM. (Wyeth Consumer) Dextromethorphan HBr 10 mg, guaifenesin 100 mg per 5 mL. Sugar and alcohol free. Acesulfame K, methylparaben, PEG, saccharin. Liq. Bot. 118 mL. *OTC.*
Use: Upper respiratory combination, antitussive with expectorant.

Robitussin Night Time Pediatric Cough & Cold. (Wyeth Consumer) Diphenhydramine hydrochloride 6.25 mg, phenylephrine hydrochloride 2.5 mg per 5 mL. Alcohol free. Sodium 3 mg/5 mL, sorbitol, sucralose. Liq. Bot. 118 mL. *OTC.*
Use: Upper respiratory combination, antitussive combination.

Robitussin Pediatric Cough. (Wyeth Consumer) Dextromethorphan HBr 7.5 mg/5 mL. Alcohol and sugar free. Saccharin, sorbitol, cherry flavor. Syrup. Bot. 118 mL. *OTC.*
Use: Nonnarcotic antitussive.

Robitussin Pediatric Cough & Cold CF. (Wyeth Consumer) Dextromethorphan HBr 2 mg, guaifenesin 40 mg, phenylephrine hydrochloride 1 mg per 1 mL. Alcohol free. PEG, sorbitol, sucralose. Drops. 30 mL with oral dosing device. *OTC.*
Use: Upper respiratory combination, antitussive and expectorant combination.

Robitussin Pediatric Cough & Cold Long-Acting. (Wyeth Consumer) Dextromethorphan HBr 7.5 mg, chlorpheniramine maleate 1 mg per 5 mL. Sodium 3 mg/5 mL, sorbitol, sucralose. Liq. 118 mL. *OTC.*
Use: Upper respiratory combination, antitussive combination.

Robitussin PE Head and Chest Congestion. (Wyeth Consumer) Phenylephrine hydrochloride 5 mg, guaifenesin 100 mg per 5 mL. Menthol, sorbitol, sucralose. Liq. 118 mL. *OTC.*
Use: Upper respiratory combination, decongestant and expectorant combination.

Robomol/ASA. (Major) Methocarbamol w/ASA. Tab. Bot. 100s, 500s. *Rx.*
Use: Muscle relaxant; analgesic.

Rocaltrol. (Validus) Calcitriol. **Cap.:** 0.25 mcg, 0.5 mcg, sorbitol, parabens. Bot. 30s (0.25 mcg only), 100s. **Oral Soln.:** 1 mcg/mL. Bot. with dispensers. 15 mL. *Rx.*
Use: Antihypocalcemic; vitamin.

•**rocastine hydrochloride.** (row-KASS-teen) USAN.
Use: Antihistamine.

Rocephin. (Genentech) Ceftriaxone sodium (as base). **Pow. for Inj.:** 500 mg, 1 g, 2 g. **500 mg:** Vials. **1 g, 2 g:** Vials, piggyback vials, ADD-Vantage vials. **Inj.:** 1 g, 2 g. Dextrose. Frozen Premixed. 50 mL plastic containers. *Rx.*
Use: Anti-infective; cephalosporin.

•**rocuronium bromide.** (row-kuhr-OH-nee-uhm) USAN.
Use: Neuromuscular blocker, muscle relaxant.
See: Zemuron.

rocuronium bromide. (Various Mfr.) Rocuronium bromide 10 mg/mL. Inj., Soln. Multidose vial 5 mL, 10 mL. *Rx.*
Use: Muscle relaxant—adjunct to anesthesia, nondepolarizing neuromuscular blocker.

•**rodocaine.** (ROW-doe-cane) USAN.
Use: Anesthetic, local.

roentgenography.
See: Iodine Products, Diagnostic.

•**roflumilast.** (roe-FLUE-mi-last) USAN.
Use: Bronchial asthma; chronic obstructive pulmonary disease.
See: Daliresp.

•**roflurane.** (row-FLEW-rane) USAN.
Use: Anesthetic, general.

Rogaine. (Pfizer Consumer Health) Minoxidil 2%. Topical Soln. Bot. 60 mL w/ multiple applicators. *OTC.*
Use: Antialopecia agent.

Rogaine Extra Strength for Men. (Pfizer Consumer Health) Minoxidil 5%. Alcohol. Soln. Bot. 60 mL w/dropper and sprayer applicators. 2s. *OTC.*
Use: Antialopecia agent.

Rogaine Men's Extra Strength. (Pfizer Consumer Health) Minoxidil 5%. Cetyl alcohol, SD alcohol, stearyl alcohol. Aer. Foam, Top. 60 g. *OTC.*
Use: Antialopecia agent.

•**rogletimide.** (row-GLETT-ih-MIDE) USAN.
Use: Antineoplastic (aromatase inhibitor).

Rolaids. (Pfizer Consumer Healthcare) Magnesium hydroxide 110 mg, calcium carbonate 550 mg. Dextrose, sucrose. Peppermint, spearmint, and cherry fla-

vors. Chew. Tab. 12s, 36s, 150s, 250s, 300s. *OTC.*
Use: Antacid.

Rolaids Calcium Rich. (Pfizer Consumer Healthcare) Calcium carbonate 412 mg, magnesium hydroxide 80 mg. Chew. Tab. Bot. 12s, 36s, 75s, 150s. *OTC.*
Use: Antacid.

Rolaids Extra Strength. (Pfizer Consumer Healthcare) Magnesium hydroxide 135 mg, calcium carbonate 675 mg. Dextrose, sucrose. Cool strawberry, freshmint, fruit, tropical punch flavors. Chew. Tab. 10s, 30s, 100s. *OTC.*
Use: Antacid.

Rolaids Extra Strength Plus Gas Relief. (Pfizer Consumer Healthcare) Calcium carbonate 1177 mg, simethicone 80 mg. Corn syrup, maltodextrin, sodium 2 mg, sorbitol, sucrose. Chew. Tab. 6s, 12s, 36s. *OTC.*
Use: Antacid.

Rolaids Extra Strength Softchews. (Pfizer Consumer Healthcare) Calcium carbonate 1,177 mg (elemental calcium 470.8 mg). Corn syrup, corn syrup solids, nonfat dry milk, sucrose. Vanilla creme and wild cherry flavors. Chew. Tab. 18s. *OTC.*
Use: Mineral supplement; antacid.

Rolaids Multi-Symptom. (Pfizer Consumer Healthcare) Magnesium hydroxide 135 mg, calcium carbonate 675 mg, simethicone 60 mg, dextrose, sucrose. Cool mint and berry flavors. Chew. Tab. 10s, 30s, 100s. *OTC.*
Use: Antacid.

Rolatuss Expectorant. (Huckaby Pharmacal) Phenylephrine hydrochloride 5 mg, chlorpheniramine maleate 2 mg, codeine phosphate 9.85 mg, ammonium Cl 33.3 mg/5 mL, alcohol 5%. Bot. 480 mL. *c-v.*
Use: Antihistamine, antitussive, decongestant, expectorant.

Rolatuss Plain. (Major) Phenylephrine hydrochloride 5 mg, chlorpheniramine maleate 2 mg/5 mL. Liq. Bot. 473 mL. *OTC.*
Use: Antihistamine, decongestant.

Rolatuss w/Hydrocodone. (Major) Phenylpropanolamine hydrochloride 3.3 mg, phenylephrine hydrochloride 5 mg, pyrilamine maleate 3.3 mg, pheniramine maleate 3.3 mg, hydrocodone bitartrate 1.67 mg/5 mL. Liq. Bot. 480 mL. *c-III.*
Use: Antihistamine, antitussive, decongestant.

●**roletamide.** (row-LET-am-ide) USAN.
Use: Hypnotic; sedative.

●**rolgamidine.** (role-GAM-ih-deen) USAN.
Use: Antidiarrheal.

Rolicap. (Arcum) Vitamins A acetate 5000 units, D_2 400 units, B_1 3 mg, B_2 2.5 mg, B_6 10 mg, C 50 mg, niacinamide 20 mg, B_{12} 1 mcg. Chew. Tab. Bot. 100s, 1000s. *OTC.*
Use: Vitamin supplement.

●**rolicyprine.** (ROW-lih-SIGH-preen) USAN.
Use: Antidepressant.

●**rolipram.** (ROLE-ih-pram) USAN.
Use: Anxiolytic.

●**rolitetracycline.** (ROW-li-tet-rah-SIGH-kleen) USAN.
Use: Anti-infective.

●**rolitetracycline nitrate.** (ROW-li-tet-rah-SIGH-kleen) USAN. Tetrim.
Use: Anti-infective.

●**rolodine.** (ROW-low-deen) USAN.
Use: Muscle relaxant.

Romach Antacid. (Last) Magnesium carbonate 400 mg, sodium bicarbonate 250 mg. Tab. Strip pack 60s, 500s. *OTC.*
Use: Antacid.

●**romazarit.** (row-MAZZ-ah-rit) USAN.
Use: Anti-inflammatory; antirheumatic.

Romazicon. (Hoffman-La Roche) Flumazenil 0.1 mg/mL, parabens, EDTA. Inj. Vials 5 mL, 10 mL. *Rx.*
Use: Antidote.

Romex. (A.P.C.) **Troche:** Polymyxin B sulfate 1000 units, benzocaine 5 mg, cetalkonium Cl 2.5 mg, gramicidin 100 mcg, chlorpheniramine maleate 0.5 mg, tyrothricin 2 mg. Pkg. 10s.
Liq.: Guaifenesin 200 mg, dextromethorphan HBr 60 mg, chlorpheniramine maleate 12 mg, phenylephrine hydrochloride 30 mg/fl oz. Bot. 4 oz. *Rx.*
Use: Antihistamine, antitussive, decongestant, expectorant; anti-infective.

Romex Cough & Cold Capsules. (A.P.C.) Guaifenesin 65 mg, dextromethorphan HBr 10 mg, chlorpheniramine maleate 1.5 mg, pyrilamine maleate 12.5 mg, phenylephrine hydrochloride 5 mg, acetaminophen 160 mg. Cap. Bot. 21s. *OTC.*
Use: Antihistamine, antitussive, decongestant, expectorant.

Romex Cough & Cold Tablets. (A.P.C.) Dextromethorphan HBr 7.5 mg, phenylephrine hydrochloride 2.5 mg, ascorbic acid 30 mg. Tab. Box 15s. *OTC.*
Use: Antitussive, decongestant.

•**romidepsin.** (ROE-mi-DEP-sin) USAN.
Tall Man: romiDEPsin
Use: Cutaneous T-cell lymphoma.
See: Istodax.

Romilar AC. (Scot-Tussin) Codeine phosphate 10 mg, guaifenesin 100 mg per 5 mL. Menthol, aspartame, parabens, phenylalanine. Sugar, dye, and alcohol free. Liq. Bot. 473 mL. *c-v.*
Use: Upper respiratory combination, antitussive, expectorant.

•**romiplostim.** (roe-MIP-loe-stim) USAN.
Tall Man: romiPLOStim
Use: Hematopoietic agent, thrombopoietin mimetic agent.
See: Nplate.

•**ronacaleret hydrochloride.** (ROE-na-KAL-er-et) USAN.
Use: Antiviral.

Rondamine-DM. (Major) **Drops:** Pseudoephedrine 25 mg, carbinoxamine maleate 2 mg, dextromethorphan HBr 4 mg/mL. Bot. 30 mL. **Syrup:** Dextromethorphan HBr 15 mg, brompheniramine maleate 4 mg, pseudoephedrine hydrochloride 60 mg per 5 mL. Alcohol < 0.2%, grape flavor. Bot. 120 mL. 473 mL, 3.8 L. *Rx.*
Use: Upper respiratory combination, antihistamine, antitussive, decongestant.

Rondec-DM. (Alliant) Dextromethorphan HBr 15 mg, chlorpheniramine maleate 4 mg, phenylephrine hydrochloride 12.5 mg per 5 mL. Alcohol and sugar free. Saccharin, sorbitol. Grape flavor. Syr. Bot. 20 mL, 118 mL, 473 mL. *Rx.*
Use: Upper respiratory combination; antitussive combination.

Rondex DM. (Pack) Dextromethorphan HBr 3 mg, chlorpheniramine maleate 1 mg, phenylephrine hydrochloride 3.5 mg per 1 mL. Alcohol and sugar free. Saccharin, sorbitol. Grape flavor. Oral Drops. 30 mL with dropper. *Rx.*
Use: Upper respiratory combination, antitussive combination.

•**ronidazole.** (row-NYE-dazz-OLE) USAN.
Use: Antiprotozoal.

•**ronnel.** (RAHN-ell) USAN. Fenchlorphos.
Use: Insecticide (systemic).

•**rontalizumab.** (RON-ta-LIZ-ue-mab) USAN.
Use: Treatment of systemic lupus erythematosus.

•**ropidoxuridine.** (roe-PYE-dox-URE-i-deen) USAN.
Use: Treatment of cancer.

ropinirole. (Various Mfr.) Ropinirole hydrochloride 0.25 mg, 0.5 mg, 1 mg, 2 mg, 3 mg, 4 mg, 5 mg. May contain lactose, PEG. Tab. 100s, 1,000s. *Rx.*
Use: Antiparkinson agent, dopaminergic.

•**ropinirole hydrochloride.** (row-PIN-ih-role) USAN.
Tall Man: rOPINIRole
Use: Antiparkinsonian (D_2 receptor agonist).
See: Requip.
Requip XL.

•**ropitoin hydrochloride.** (ROW-pih-toe-in) USAN.
Use: Cardiovascular agent (antiarrhythmic).

ropivacaine hydrochloride.
Use: Anesthetic, local injectable.
See: Naropin.

•**ropizine.** (row-PIH-zeen) USAN.
Use: Anticonvulsant.

•**roquinimex.** (row-KWIH-nih-mex) USAN.
Use: Biological response modifier; immunomodulator; antineoplastic.

•**rosabulin.** (ROE-za-BUE-lin) USAN.
Use: Antineoplastic.

Rosaderm Kit. (River's Edge) Sodium sulfacetamide 10%, sulfur 5%. Disodium EDTA, mineral oil, parabens. Soap. 170 g, 340 g, kits w/*RE Cleansing Lotion.* *Rx.*
Use: Acne product, combination.

Rosanil. (Galderma) Sulfur 5%, sodium sulfacetamide 10%, EDTA, light mineral oil, parabens. Cleanser. 170 g. *Rx.*
Use: Keratolytic agent.

rosaniline dyes.
See: Fuchsin, Basic.
Methylrosaniline Cl.

•**rosaramicin.** (row-ZAR-ah-MY-sin) USAN. *Formerly Rosamicin.*
Use: Anti-infective.

•**rosaramicin butyrate.** (row-ZAR-ah-MY-sin BYOO-tih-rate) USAN. *Formerly Rosamicin Butyrate.*
Use: Anti-infective.

•**rosaramicin propionate.** (row-ZAR-ah-MY-sin PRO-pee-oh-nate) USAN. *Formerly Rosamicin Propionate.*
Use: Anti-infective.

•**rosaramicin sodium phosphate.** (row-ZAR-ah-MY-sin) USAN. *Formerly Rosamicin Sodium Phosphate.*
Use: Anti-infective.

•**rosaramicin stearate.** (row-ZAR-ah-MY-sin STEE-ah-rate) USAN. *Formerly Rosamicin Stearate.*
Use: Anti-infective.

rose bengal.
Use: Ophthalmic diagnostic product.

rose bengal. (Akorn) Rose bengal 1%. Bot. 5 mL.
Use: Diagnostic, tissue staining.

rose bengal. (Barnes-Hind) Rose bengal 1.3 mg. Strip. Box 100s. *OTC.*
Use: Diagnostic aid.

•**rose bengal sodium I 131 injection.** (rose BEN-gal) *USP 34.*
Use: Diagnostic aid (hepatic function), radiopharmaceutical.

•**rose bengal sodium I 125.** (rose BEN-gal) USAN.
Use: Radiopharmaceutical.

Rose-C. (Barth's) Vitamin C 300 mg, rose hip extract/5 mL. Liq. Dropper Bot. 2 oz, 8 oz. *OTC.*
Use: Vitamin supplement.

rose hips. (Burgin-Arden) Vitamin C 300 mg, in base of sorbitol. Bot. 4 oz, 8 oz. *OTC.*
Use: Vitamin supplement.

rose hips vitamin C. (Kirkman) Vitamin C 100 mg, 250 mg, 500 mg. Tab. Bot. 100s, 250s, 500s (except 100 mg). *OTC.*
Use: Vitamin supplement.

•**rose oil.** (rose) *NF 29.*
Use: Pharmaceutic aid; perfume.

rose water ointment.
Use: Emollient, ointment base.

•**rose water, stronger.** (rose) *NF 29.*
Use: Pharmaceutic aid; perfume.

•**rosiglitazone maleate.** (roe-sih-GLIH-tah-sone) USAN.
Use: Antidiabetic, thiazolidinedione.
See: Avandia.
W/Glimepiride.
See: Avandaryl.
W/Metformin.
See: Avandamet.

•**rosin.** (ROZZ-in) *USP 34.*
Use: Stiffening agent, pharmaceutical necessity.

•**rosoxacin.** (row-SOX-ah-sin) USAN.
Use: Anti-infective.

Ross SLD. (Ross) Low-residue nutritional supplement for patients restricted to a clear liquid feeding or with fat malabsorption disorders. Packet 1.35 oz. Ctn. 6s. Case 4 ctn. Can 13.5 oz. Case 6s. *OTC.*
Use: Nutritional supplement.

•**rostaporfin.** (roe-sta-POR-fin) USAN.
Use: Cutaneous carcinomas; Kaposi sarcomas; choroidal neovascularization.

Rosula. (Pharmaderm) **Gel:** Sodium sulfacetamide 10%, sulfur 5% in a 10% urea vehicle. Benzyl alcohol, cetyl alcohol, EDTA, mineral oil, PEG 100, stea-

rate. Tube. 45 mL. **Foam:** Sodium sulfacetamide 10%, sulfur 4%. Cetyl alcohol, lactic acid, parabens, propylene glycol, stearyl alcohol. 100 g. *Rx.*
Use: Acne product combination.

Rosula Clarifying Wash. (Pharmaderm) Sodium sulfacetamide 10%, sulfur 4%. EDTA, parabens, PEG 100, stearyl alcohol, urea 10%. Top. Liq. 473 mL. *Rx.*
Use: Keratolytic agent, acne product combination.

Rosula NS. (Pharmaderm) Sodium sulfacetamide 10% urea vehicle. EDTA, sodium thiosulfate. Pads. 30s. *Rx.*
Use: Keratolytic agent.

•**rosuvastatin calcium.** (roe-SOO-va-statin) USAN.
Use: Antihyperlipidemic agent, HMG-CoA reductase inhibitor.
See: Crestor.

Rotalex Test. (Orion) Latex slide agglutination test for detection of rotavirus in feces. Kit 1s.
Use: Diagnostic aid.

Rotarix. (GlaxoSmithKline) Rotavirus human 89–12 strain (G1P[8] type); at least 10^6 cell culture infective dose per 1 mL (after reconstitution). Preservative free. Dextran, glucose, sorbitol, sucrose. Pow. for Susp., Lyophilized, Oral. Vials with 1 mL prefilled liquid diluent and transfer adapter for reconstitution. *Rx.*
Use: Agent for active immunization.

RotaTeq. (Merck) Rotavirus outer capsid protein (2.2 × 10^6 infectious units of G1, 2.8 × 10^6 infectious units of G2, 2.2 × 10^6 infectious units of G3, 2 × 10^6 infectious units of G4, 2.3 × 10^6 infectious units of rotavirus attachment protein P1A[8]) per 2 mL. Preservative free. Sucrose. Oral Susp. Single-dose tubes. 2 mL (10s). *Rx.*
Use: Immunization.

rotavirus vaccine live.
Use: Immunization.
See: Rotarix.
RotaTeq.

Rotazyme II. (Abbott Diagnostics) Enzyme immunoassay for detection of rotavirus antigen in feces. Test kit 50s.
Use: Diagnostic aid.

•**rotigaptide.** (roe-ti-GAP-tide) USAN.
Use: Antiarrhythmic agent.

•**rotigotine.** (ROE-ti-goe-tine) USAN.
Use: Antiparkinson agent, dopaminergic.

•**rotoxamine.** (row-TOX-ah-meen) USAN.
Use: Antihistamine.

•**rovelizumab.** (roe-ve-LYE-zue-mab) USAN.
Use: Immunomodulator.

Rowasa. (Alaven) Mesalamine 4 g/
60 mL. EDTA, potassium metabisulfite,
white petrolatum. Enema. 7s and 28s
with lubricated applicator tip in disposable bots. *Rx.*
Use: Anti-inflammatory.

•**roxadimate.** (rox-AD-ih-mate) USAN.
Use: Sunscreen.

Roxanol. (aaiPharma) Morphine sulfate
20 mg/mL. Oral Soln., concentrate.
Bot. 30 mL, 120 mL w/calibrated dropper. *c-ii.*
Use: Opioid analgesic.

Roxanol 100. (aaiPharma) Morphine sulfate 100 mg/5 mL. Oral Soln., concentrate. Bot. 240 mL with calibrated
spoon. *c-ii.*
Use: Opioid analgesic.

Roxanol T. (aaiPharma) Morphine sulfate 20 mg/mL. Flavored. Oral Soln.,
concentrate. Bot. 30 mL, 120 mL with
calibrated dropper. *c-ii.*
Use: Opioid analgesic.

•**roxarsone.** (ROX-AHR-sone) USAN.
Use: Anti-infective.

•**roxatidine acetate.** (ROX-ah-tih-DEEN)
USAN.
Use: Antiulcer.

Roxicet. (Roxane) **Oral Soln.:** Oxycodone hydrochloride 5 mg, acetaminophen 325 mg/5 mL. Bot. UD 5 mL,
500 mL. **Tab.:** Oxycodone hydrochloride 5 mg, acetaminophen 325 mg,
0.4% alcohol. Bot. 100s, 500s, UD
100s. *c-ii.*
Use: Analgesic combination, narcotic.

Roxicet 5/500. (Roxane) Oxycodone
hydrochloride 5 mg, acetaminophen
500 mg. Cap. Bot. 100s, UD 100s. *c-ii.*
Use: Analgesic combination, narcotic.

Roxicodone. (aaiPharma) **Oral Soln.:**
Oxycodone hydrochloride 5 mg/5 mL.
Sorbitol. Bot. 500 mL, UD 5 mL. **Tab.:**
Oxycodone hydrochloride 5 mg, 15 mg,
30 mg. Lactose (15 mg, 30 mg only).
Bot. 100s, UD 100s. *c-ii.*
Use: Opioid analgesic.

Roxicodone Intensol. (aaiPharma) Oxycodone hydrochloride 20 mg/mL. Conc.
Soln. Bot. 30 mL with calibrated dropper. *c-ii.*
Use: Opioid analgesic.

•**roxifiban acetate.** (rox-ih-FIE-ban)
USAN.
Use: Antithrombotic, fibrinogen recep-
tor antagonist.

Roxilox. (Roxane) Oxycodone hydro-
chloride 5 mg, acetaminophen 500 mg.
Cap. Bot. 100s. *c-ii.*
Use: Narcotic analgesic combination.

Roxiprin. (Roxane) Oxycodone hydrochloride 4.5 mg, oxycodone terephthalate 0.38 mg, aspirin 325 mg. Tab. Bot.
100s, 1000s, UD 100s. *c-ii.*
Use: Analgesic combination, narcotic.

•**roxithromycin.** (ROX-ith-row-MY-sin)
USAN.
Use: Anti-infective.

Rozerem. (Takeda Pharmaceutical) Ramelteon 8 mg. Lactose. Tab. Bot. 30s,
100s, 500s. *Rx.*
Use: Insomnia.

Rozex. (Galderma) Metronidazole 0.75%.
Top. Emulsion. Tube. 60 g. *Rx.*
Use: Anti-inflammatory, dermatologic.

•**rozrolimupab.** (ROZ-roe-LIM-ue-pab)
USAN.
Use: Recombinant polyclonal antibody.

R/S. (Summers) Sulfur 5%, resorcinol
2%, alcohol 28%. Lot. Bot. 56.7 mL.
OTC.
Use: Dermatologic; acne.

R-Tanna. (Prasco) Phenylephrine tannate 25 mg, chlorpheniramine tannate
9 mg. Tab. 100s. *Rx.*
Use: Upper respiratory combination, decongestant and antihistamine.

R-Tannamine. (Qualitest) Phenylephrine
tannate 25 mg, chlorpheniramine tannate 8 mg, pyrilamine tannate 25 mg.
Tab. Bot. 100s. *Rx.*
Use: Antihistamine; decongestant.

R-Tannamine Pediatric. (Qualitest)
Phenylephrine tannate 5 mg, chlorpheniramine tannate 2 mg, pyrilamine
tannate 12.5 mg/5 mL, 120 mL,
473 mL. *Rx.*
Use: Antihistamine; decongestant.

R-Tanna S Pediatric. (Prasco) Phenylephrine tannate 5 mg, chlorpheniramine tannate 4.5 mg per 5 mL. Methylparaben, saccharin, sucrose, grape
flavor. Susp. 118 mL. *Rx.*
Use: Decongestant and antihistamine.

R-Tannate. (Various Mfr.) Phenylephrine
tannate 25 mg, chlorpheniramine tannate 8 mg, pyrilamine tannate 25 mg.
Tab. Bot. 100s. *Rx.*
Use: Antihistamine; decongestant.

R-Tannate Pediatric. (Various Mfr.)
Phenylephrine tannate 5 mg, chlor-
pheniramine tannate 2 mg, pyrilamine
tannate 12.5 mg/5 mL, saccharin. Susp.
Bot. 473 mL. *Rx.*
Use: Antihistamine; decongestant.

R-Tanna 12. (Duramed) Phenylephrine
tannate 5 mg, pyrilamine tannate
30 mg/5 mL. Saccharin, sucrose, methylparaben, strawberry-currant flavor.
Susp. Unit of use 118 mL with oral syringe. *Rx.*

Use: Upper respiratory combination, decongestant, antihistamine.

R-3 Screen Test. (Wampole) A three-minute latex-eosin slide test for the qualitative detection of rheumatoid factor activity in serum. Kit 100s.
Use: Diagnostic aid.

rt-PA.
Use: Tissue plasminogen.
See: Activase.

RII retinamide.
Use: Myelodysplastic syndromes.
[Orphan Drug]

Rubacell. (Abbott Diagnostics) Passive hemagglutination (PHA) test for the detection of antibody to rubella virus in serum or recalcified plasma.
Use: Diagnostic aid.

Rubacell II. (Abbott Diagnostics) Passive hemagglutination (PHA) test to detect antibody to rubella in serum or recalcified plasma. In 100s, 1000s.
Use: Diagnostic aid.

Rubaquick Diagnostic Kit. (Abbott Diagnostics) Rapid passive hemagglutination (PHA) for the detection of antibodies to rubella virus in serum specimens.
Use: Diagnostic aid.

Ruba-Tect. (Abbott Diagnostics) Hemagglutination inhibition test for the detection and quantitation of rubella antibody in serum. In 100s.
Use: Diagnostic aid.

Rubatrope-57. (Bristol-Myers Squibb) Cyanocobalamin Co 57 Capsules; Soln U.S.P. 24. *OTC.*
Use: Vitamin supplement.

Rubazyme. (Abbott Diagnostics) Enzyme immunoassay for 1 gG antibody to rubella virus. Test kit 100s, 1000s.
Use: Diagnostic aid.

Rubazyme-M. (Abbott Diagnostics) Enzyme immunoassay for IgM antibody to rubella virus in serum. Test kit 50s.
Use: Diagnostic aid.

•**rubella virus vaccine, live.** (roo-BELL-ah) *USP 34.*
Use: Immunization.

Rubex. (Bristol-Myers Squibb Oncology/Virology) Doxorubicin hydrochloride 100 mg, lactose 500 mg, preservative free. Pow. for Inj. lyophilized. Vial. *Rx.*
Use: Antibiotic.

•**rubidium chloride Rb 86.** (roo-BIH-dee-uhm) USAN.
Use: Radiopharmaceutical.

•**rubidium chloride Rb 82 injection.** (roo-BIH-dee-uhm) *USP 34.*
Use: Diagnostic aid (radioactive, cardiac disease), radiopharmaceutical.

•**rubitecan.** USAN.
Use: Antineoplastic.

ruboxistaurin.
Use: Investigational protein kinase C beta inhibitor.

•**rucaparib.** (roo-KAP-a-rib) USAN.
Use: Antineoplastic.

•**rufinamide.** (roo-FIN-a-mide) USAN.
Use: Antiepileptic.
See: Banzel.

RU 486.
Use: Antiprogesterone.

Ru-lets M 500. (Rugby) Vitamin C 500 mg, B_3 100 mg, B_5 20 mg, B_1 15 mg, B_2 10 mg, B_6 5 mg, A 10,000 units, B_{12} 12 mcg, D 400 units, E 30 mg, Mg, Fe 20 mg, Cu, Zn 1.5 mg, Mn, I. Tab. Bot. 100s. *OTC.*
Use: Mineral, vitamin supplement.

RuLox Plus. (Rugby) **Susp.:** Aluminum hydroxide 500 mg, magnesium hydroxide 450 mg, simethicone 40 mg/5 mL. Bot. 355 mL. **Tab.:** Aluminum hydroxide 200 mg, magnesium hydroxide 200 mg, simethicone 25 mg. Chew. Bot. 50s. *OTC.*
Use: Antacid; antiflatulent.

RuLox Suspension. (Rugby) Aluminum hydroxide 225 mg, magnesium hydroxide 200 mg/5 mL. Parabens, saccharin, sorbitol. Susp. 360 mL, 769 mL, gal. *OTC.*
Use: Antacid.

•**rupintrivir.** (roo-PIN-tri-veer) USAN.
Use: Antiviral.

•**ruplizumab.** (rue-PLYE-zue-mab) USAN.
Use: Immune thrombocytopenic purpura; systemic lupus erythematosus.

•**rusalatide acetate.** (roo-SAL-a-tide) USAN.
Use: Tissue and bone repair.

rust inhibitor.
See: Sodium Nitrite.

•**rutamycin.** (ROO-tah-MY-sin) USAN. From strain of *Streptomyces rutgersensis.* Under study.
Use: Antifungal.

rutgers 612.
See: Ethohexadiol.

rutin. (Various Mfr.) 3-Rhamnoglucoside of 5,7,3',4-tetrahydroxyflavonol. Eldrin, globulariacitrin, myrticalorin, oxyritin, phytomelin, rutoside, sophorin. Tab. 20 mg, 50 mg, 60 mg, 100 mg. *Rx.*
Use: Vascular disorders.

rutoside.
See: Rutin.

Ru-Tuss II. (Knoll) Phenylpropanolamine hydrochloride 75 mg, chlorpheniramine maleate 12 mg. Cap. Bot. 100s. *Rx.*
Use: Antihistamine, decongestant.

• **ruxolitinib.** (RUX-oh-LI-ti-nib) USAN.
Use: Antineoplastic.

• **ruxolitinib phosphate.** (RUX-oh-LI-ti-nib) USAN.
Use: Antineoplastic.

RVPaque. (ICN) Red petrolatum, zinc oxide, cinoxate, in water-resistant base. Tube 15 g, 37.5 g. *OTC.*
Use: Sunscreen.

Rx Support Heartburn & Acid Reflux. (Mason Vitamins) Ca, folic acid 400 mcg, vitamins B_6 10 mg, B_{12} 200 mcg, D 1,000 units (as cholecalciferol). PEG. Tab. 60s. *OTC.*
Use: Multivitamin with minerals (except iron).

Rx Support Heartburn & Acid Reflux Plus Aloe. (Mason Vitamins) Aloe vera powder 100 mg, Ca, folic acid 400 mcg, vitamins D 1,000 units (as cholecalciferol), B_6 10 mg, B_{12} 200 mcg. PEG. Tab. 60s. *OTC.*
Use: Multivitamin with minerals (except iron).

Rybix ODT. (Victory Pharma) Tramadol hydrochloride 50 mg. Aspartame, mannitol. Mint flavor. Tab., orally disintegrating. UD 30s. *Rx.*
Use: Opioid analgesic.

Rymed. (Edwards) **Cap.:** Pseudoephedrine hydrochloride 30 mg, guaifenesin 250 mg. Cap. Bot. 100s. **Liq.:** Pseudoephedrine hydrochloride 30 mg, guaifenesin 100 mg/5 mL, alcohol 1.4%. Bot. Pt. *OTC.*
Use: Decongestant, expectorant.

Rymed-TR. (Edwards) Phenylpropanolamine hydrochloride 75 mg, guaifenesin 400 mg. Tab. Bot. 100s. *OTC.*
Use: Decongestant, expectorant.

Ryna-CX. (Wallace) Guaifenesin 100 mg, pseudoephedrine hydrochloride 30 mg, codeine phosphate 10 mg, alcohol 7.5%, saccharin, sorbitol/5 mL. Bot. 4 oz, pt. *c-v.*
Use: Antitussive, decongestant, expectorant.

Rynatan. (Medpointe) Phenylephrine tannate 25 mg, chlorpheniramine tannate 9 mg. Tab. 100s. *Rx.*
Use: Decongestant and antihistamine, upper respiratory combination.

Rynatan Pediatric. (Medpointe) **Chew. Tab.:** Phenylephrine tannate 5 mg, chlorpheniramine tannate 4.5 mg. Maltodextrin, saccharin, sucrose. Grape flavor. 30s. **Susp.:** Phenylephrine tannate 5 mg, chlorpheniramine tannate 4.5 mg per 5 mL. Tartrazine, methylparaben, saccharin, sucrose, strawberry-currant flavor. Bot. 473 mL. *Rx.*

Use: Upper respiratory combination, decongestant and antihistamine.

Rynatan-S Pediatric. (Wallace) Phenylephrine tannate 5 mg, chlorpheniramine tannate 2 mg, pyrilamine tannate 12.5 mg/5 mL. Susp. Bot. 120 mL w/ syringe. *Rx.*
Use: Antihistamine, decongestant.

Rynatuss. (Medpointe) Carbetapentane tannate 60 mg, chlorpheniramine tannate 5 mg, ephedrine tannate 10 mg, phenylephrine tannate 10 mg. Tab. Bot. 100s. *Rx.*
Use: Upper respiratory combination, antitussive combination.

Rynatuss Pediatric. (Medpointe) Carbetapentane tannate 30 mg, chlorpheniramine tannate 4 mg, ephedrine tannate 5 mg, phenylephrine tannate 5 mg per 5 mL. Saccharin, tartrazine, methylparaben, sucrose. Strawberry-currant flavor. Susp. Bot. 237 mL, 473 mL. *Rx.*
Use: Upper respiratory combination, antitussive combination.

Ryna-12. (Mena Pharmaceuticals) Phenylephrine tannate 25 mg, pyrilamine tannate 60 mg. Tab. 100s. *Rx.*
Use: Upper respiratory combination, decongestant and antihistamine.

Ryna-12X. (Medpointe) **Susp.:** Phenylephrine tannate 5 mg, pyrilamine tannate 30 mg, guaifenesin 100 mg per 5 mL. Methylparaben, saccharin, sucrose. Grape flavor. 120 mL. **Tab.:** Phenylephrine tannate 25 mg, pyrilamine tannate 60 mg, guaifenesin 200 mg. 30s. *Rx.*
Use: Upper respiratory combination, decongestant, antihistamine, and expectorant.

Rynesa 12S. (Amneal Pharmaceuticals) Pyrilamine tannate 30 mg, phenylephrine tannate 5 mg per 5 mL. Methylparaben, saccharin, sucrose. Cherry berry flavor. Susp. 118 mL, 473 mL. *Rx.*
Use: Upper respiratory combination, decongestant and antihistamine.

Ryneze. (SJ Pharmaceuticals) Chlorpheniramine maleate 4 mg, scopolamine 1.25 mg per 5 mL. Saccharin, sorbitol. Alcohol free, dye free, gluten free, and sugar free. Grape flavor. Liq. 473 mL. *Rx.*
Use: Upper respiratory combination; decongestant, antihistamine, and anticholinergic combination.

Ry-Tann. (Midlothian) Chlorpheniramine tannate 9 mg, phenylephrine tannate 25 mg. Lactose. Tab. 100s. *Rx.*

Use: Upper respiratory combination, decongestant and antihistamine.

Rythmol. (GlaxoSmithKline) Propafenone hydrochloride 150 mg, 225 mg. Film-coated. Tab. 100s, UD 100s. *Rx.*
Use: Antiarrhythmic agent.

Rythmol SR. (GlaxoSmithKline) Propafenone hydrochloride 225 mg, 325 mg, 425 mg. ER Cap. 100s. *Rx.*
Use: Antiarrhythmic agent.

RY-T-12. (Hi-Tech) Phenylephrine tannate 5 mg, pyrilamine tannate 30 mg per 5 mL. Methylparaben, saccharin, sucrose. Strawberry-currant flavor. Susp. 118 mL, 473 mL. *Rx.*
Use: Upper respiratory combination, decongestant and antihistamine.

Ryzolt. (Purdue) Tramadol hydrochloride 100 mg, 200 mg, 300 mg. ER Tab. 30s, 90s. *Rx.*
Use: Opioid analgesic.

S

Saave+. (NeuroGenesis/Matrix Tech.)
Vitamin D 40 mg, L-phenylalanine,
L-glutamine 25 mg, vitamins A
333.3 units, B_1 2.417 mg, B_2 0.85 mg,
B_3 33 mg, B_5 15 mg, B_6 3 mg, B_{12}
5 mcg, folic acid 0.067 mg, C 100 mg,
E 5 units, biotin 0.05 mg, Ca 25 mg,
Cr 0.01 mg, Fe 1.5 mg, Mg 25 mg,
Zn 2.5 mg. Cap. Yeast and preserva-
tive free. Bot. 42s, 180s. *OTC.*
Use: Mineral, vitamin supplement.

•**sabcomeline hydrochloride.** (sab-KOE-
meh-leen) USAN.
Use: Treatment of Alzheimer disease.

•**sabeluzole.** (sah-BELL-you-zole) USAN.
Use: Anticonvulsant; antihypoxic.

Sabril. (Lundbeck) Vigabatrin. **Pow. for
Soln.:** 500 mg. 500 mg packets. 50s.
Tab.: 500 mg. Film-coated. 100s. *Rx.*
Use: Anticonvulsant.

•**saccharin.** (SACK-ah-rin) *NF 29.*
Use: Pharmaceutic aid (flavor).

saccharin. (Merck & Co.) Saccharin.
Pow. Pkg. 1 oz, 0.25 lb, 1 lb. (Bristol-
Myers Squibb) Tab. 0.25 g, 0.5 g. Bot.
500s, 1000s; 1 g. Bot. 1000s.
Use: Pharmaceutic aid (flavor).

•**saccharin calcium.** (SACK-ah-rin)
USP 34.
Use: Non-nutritive sweetener.

•**saccharin sodium.** (SACK-ah-rin)
USP 34.
Use: Sweetener (non-nutritive).
See: Sweeta.

saccharin sodium. (Various Mfr.) Saccharin sodium. Pow., Bot. 1 oz, 0.25 lb,
1 lb. Tab.
Use: Sweetener (non-nutritive).

saccharin soluble.
See: Saccharin Sodium.

Sac-500. (Western Research) Vitamin C
500 mg. TR Cap. Bot. 1000s. *OTC.*
Use: Vitamin supplement.

sacrosidase.
Use: Nutritional therapy.
See: Sucraid.

Saf-Clens. (Calgon Vestal Laboratories)
Meroxapol 105, NaCl, potassium sorbate NF, DMDM hydantoin. Spray. Bot.
177 mL. *OTC.*
Use: Dermatologic, wound therapy.

Safeskin. (C & M Pharmacal) A dermato-
logically acceptable detergent for patients who are sensitive to ordinary detergents. No whiteners, brighteners,
or other irritants. Bot. qt.
Use: Laundry detergent for sensitive
skin.

Safe Suds. (Ar-Ex) Hypoallergenic, all-
purpose detergent for patients whose
hands or respiratory membranes are ir-
ritated by soaps or detergents. pH 6.8.
No enzymes, phosphates, lanolin, fill-
ers, bleaches. Bot. 22 oz.
Use: Detergent.

Safetussin CD. (Kramer) Dextromethorphan HBr 15 mg, phenylephrine hydrochloride 2.5 mg per 5 mL. Menthol,
parabens. Liq. 120 mL. *OTC.*
Use: Upper respiratory combination, antitussive combination.

Safetussin DM. (Kramer) Guaifenesin
100 mg, dextromethorphan HBr 15 mg
per 5 mL. Aspartame, menthol, parabens, phenylalanine 4.2 mg/5 mL. Mint
flavor. Liq. Bot. 120 mL. *OTC.*
Use: Upper respiratory combination, antitussive, expectorant.

Safety-Coated Arthritis Pain Formula.
(Whitehall-Robins) Enteric coated aspi-
rin 500 mg. Tab. Bot. 24s, 60s. *OTC.*
Use: Analgesic.

•**safflower oil.** (SAF-low-er) *USP 34.*
Use: Pharmaceutic aid (vehicle, oleaginous).

safflower oil.
Use: Nutritional supplement.
See: Microlipid.

•**safingol.** (saff-IN-gole) USAN.
Use: Antineoplastic (adjunct); antipsoriatic.

•**safingol hydrochloride.** (saff-IN-gole)
USAN.
Use: Antineoplastic (adjunct); antipsori-
atic.

Safyral. (Bayer) Drospirenone 3 mg, ethinyl estradiol (as betadex clathrate)
30 mcg. Film coated. Lactose, levomefolate calcium 0.451 mg, PEG. Tab.
21s w/7 tablets (levomefolate calcium
0.451 mg). *Rx.*
Use: Oral monophasic contraceptive.

•**sagopilone.** (sa-GOP-i-lone) USAN.
Use: Antineoplastic.

Saizen. (Serono) Somatropin 5 mg
($\approx$ 15 units)/vial, 8.8 mg ($\approx$ 26.4 units)/
vial. Sucrose. Pow. for Inj., lyophilized.
Vial w/diluent (bacteriostatic water for
injection w/benzyl alcohol 0.9%). *Click-
easy* cartridge w/diluent (bacteriostatic
water for injection and metacresol
0.3%) (8.8 mg only). *Rx.*
Use: Hormone, growth.

SalAc Cleanser. (Medicis) Salicylic acid
2%, benzyl alcohol, glyceryl cocoate.
Liq. Bot. 177 mL. *OTC.*
Use: Dermatologic, acne.

salacetin.
See: Acetylsalicylic Acid.
Salacid 60%. (Gordon Laboratories) Salicylic acid 60% in ointment base. Jar 2 oz. *OTC.*
Use: Keratolytic.
Salacid 25%. (Gordon Laboratories) Salicylic acid 25% in ointment base. Jar 2 oz, lb. *OTC.*
Use: Keratolytic.
Salactic Film. (Pedinol Pharmacal) Salicylic acid 16.7% in flexible collodion w/ color. Liq. Applicator Bot. 15 mL. *OTC.*
Use: Keratolytic.
Salacyn. (Stratus) Salicylic acid 6%. Cetearyl alcohol, cetyl alcohol, disodium EDTA, glycerin, mineral oil, parabens, PEG-3, PEG-100. **Cream:** 400 g. **Lot.:** 414 mL. *Rx.*
Use: Keratolytic agent.
Salagen. (Eisai) Pilocarpine hydrochloride 5 mg, 7.5 mg. Tab. Bot. 100s. *Rx.*
Use: Mouth and throat product.
Salazide. (Major) Hydroflumethiazide 50 mg, reserpine 0.125 mg. Tab. Bot. 100s, 500s, 1000s. *Rx.*
Use: Antihypertensive combination.
Salazide-Demi. (Major) Hydroflumethiazide 25 mg, reserpine 0.125 mg. Tab. Bot. 100s. *Rx.*
Use: Antihypertensive combination.
salbutamol.
See: Albuterol.
• **salcaprozate sodium.** (sal-KAP-roe-zate) USAN.
Use: Oral absorption promoter.
Salcegel. (Apco) Sodium salicylate 5 g, calcium ascorbate 25 mg, calcium carbonate 1 g, dried aluminum hydroxide gel 2 g. Tab. Bot. 100s. *OTC.*
Use: Analgesic.
Sal-Clens Acne Cleanser. (C & M Pharmacal) Salicylic acid 2%. Gel. Tube 240 g. *OTC.*
Use: Dermatologic, acne.
• **salcolex.** (SAL-koe-lex) USAN.
Use: Analgesic; anti-inflammatory; antipyretic.
Salese With Xylitol. (Nuvora) Eucalyptus oil, glyceryl, sucralose, lemon oil, peppermint oil, wintergreen oil, xylitol, zinc. Alcohol free and sugar free. Peppermint, wintergreen, and mild lemon flavors. Loz. 12s. *OTC.*
Use: Mouth and throat product.
• **salethamide maleate.** (sal-ETH-ah-MIDE) USAN. Under study.
Use: Analgesic.
saletin.
See: Acetylsalicylic Acid.

Saleto. (Mallard) Aspirin 210 mg, acetaminophen 115 mg, salicylamide 65 mg, caffeine 16 mg. Tab. Bot. 100s, 1000s, *Sani-Pak* 1000s. *OTC.*
Use: Analgesic.
Saleto-200. (Roberts) Ibuprofen 200 mg. Tab. Bot. 1000s, UD 50s. *OTC.*
Use: Analgesic; NSAID.
Salex. (Coria) Salicylic acid. **Cream.:** 6%. Alcohols, glycerin, parabens. Bot. 400 g. **Lot.:** 6%. Alcohols, EDTA, glycerin, mineral oil, parabens, PEG 100. 414 mL. **Shampoo:** 6%. Cetearyl alcohol, EDTA, glycerin, parabens. 177 mL. *Rx.*
Use: Keratolytic agent.
Salflex. (Carnrick) Salsalate 500 mg, 750 mg. Tab. Bot. 100s. *Rx.*
Use: Analgesic.
• **salicyl alcohol.** (SAL-ih-sill AL-koe-hahl) USAN. Formerly Saligenin, Saligenol, Salicain.
Use: Anesthetic, local.
• **salicylamide.** (SAL-i-SIL-a-mide) *USP 34.*
Use: Analgesic.
W/Acetaminophen, Aspirin, Caffeine.
See: Medi-First Extra Strength Pain Relief.
W/Acetaminophen, Caffeine, Phenyltoloxamine Citrate.
See: Durabac.
W/Aspirin, Caffeine.
See: BC Powder Arthritis Strength.
Stanback Headache Powders.
W/Combinations.
See: Anodynos.
Dapco.
Duraxin.
Ed-Flex.
Levacet.
Nokane.
Painaid.
P.M.P. Compound.
Presalin.
Saleto.
Salipap.
Salocol.
Sinulin.
Sleep Tablets.
salicylanilide.
Use: Antifungal.
salicylated bile extract. Chologestin.
• **salicylate meglumine.** (suh-LIH-sih-late) USAN.
Use: Antirheumatic; analgesic.
salicylates.
See: Aspirin
Aspirin, Buffered.
Diflunisal.

Magnesium Salicylate.
Salsalate.
Sodium Thiosalicylate
salicylazosulfapyridine.
See: Sulfasalazine.
•**salicylic acid.** (sal-ih-SILL-ik) *USP 34.*
Use: Keratolytic.
See: Calicylic.
Compound W for Kids.
Compound W One Step Wart Remover for Kids.
Hydrisalic.
Keralyt.
Maximum Strength Wart Remover.
MG217 Sal-Acid.
OFF-Ezy Corn & Callous Remover.
P & S.
PROPApH Astringent Cleanser Maximum Strength.
Psor-a-set.
Salactic Film.
Salacyn.
Salex.
Sal-Plant.
Salvax.
SA 6%.
Scalpicin.
Sebulex with Conditioners.
Virasal.
Wart-Off.
W/Benzoyl Peroxide/Tocopherol.
See: Inova 8/2 Acne Control Therapy.
Inova 4/1 Acne Control Therapy.
W/Combinations.
See: Aveenobar Medicated.
Akne Drying Lotion.
Bensal HP.
Clearasil Clearstick for Sensitive Skin, Maximum Strength.
Clearasil Clearstick, Maximum Strength.
Clearasil Clearstick, Regular Strength.
Clearasil Double Clear.
Clearasil Double Textured Pads.
Clearasil Medicated Deep Cleanser.
Duofilm.
Duo-WR.
Ionax Astringent Cleanser.
Ionil.
Ionil T.
MG217 Medicated Tar Free.
MG217 Sal-Acid.
Neutrogena T/Sal.
Occlusal HP.
Oxy Clean Medicated Pads for Sensitive Skin.
Oxy Night Watch.
Pernox.
PROPApH.
Salicylic Acid Cleansing Bar.
Salicylic Acid & Sulfur Soap.

Sebulex with Conditioners.
W/Sulfur.
See: Exoderm.
salicylic acid. (Brookstone) Salicylic acid 6%. Glycerin, parabens, polysorbate 20, polysorbate 80, propylene glycol, tolamine. Aer., Foam. 70 g. *Rx.*
Use: Keratolytic agent.
salicylic acid. (Kylemore Pharmaceuticals) Salicylic acid 6%. EDTA, SD alcohol. Gel. 40 g. *Rx.*
Use: Keratolytic agent.
salicylic acid. (River's Edge) Salicylic acid 6%. EDTA, SD alcohol 40–2. Gel. 40 g. *Rx.*
Use: Keratolytic agent.
salicylic acid & sulfur soap. (GlaxoSmithKline) Salicylic acid 3%, sulfur 10%, EDTA. Cake 116 g. *OTC.*
Use: Antiseborrheic; keratolytic.
salicylic acid cleansing bar. (GlaxoSmithKline) Salicylic acid 2%, EDTA. Cake 113 g. *OTC.*
Use: Antiseborrheic; keratolytic.
salicylic acid shampoo. (Hi Tech Pharmacal) Salicylic acid 6%. Edetate disodium, glycerin, parabens. Shampoo. 177 mL. *Rx.*
Use: Keratolytic agent.
salicylic acid topical foam.
Use: Keratolytic.
salicylsalicylic acid. Salsalate.
Use: Analgesic.
See: Disalcid.
salicylsulphonic acid. Sulfosalicylic acid.
Saligenin. (City Chemical Corp.) Salicyl alcohol. Bot. 25 g, 100 g. *OTC.*
Saline. (Bausch & Lomb) Buffered isotonic. Thimerosal 0.001%, boric acid, NaCl, EDTA. Soln. Bot. 355 mL. *OTC.*
Use: Contact lens care.
saline laxatives.
See: Epsom Salt.
Fleet Phospho-soda.
Magnesium Citrate.
Milk of Magnesia.
Milk of Magnesia-Concentrated.
Phillips' Milk of Magnesia.
Phillips' Milk of Magnesia, Concentrated.
Saline Solution. (Akorn) Saline solution, isotonic, preserved. Bot. 12 oz. *OTC.*
Use: Contact lens care, soaking.
Saline Spray. (Akorn) Isotonic nonpreserved saline aerosol soln. Bot. 2 oz, 8 oz, 12 oz. *OTC.*
Use: Contact lens care.
SalineX. (Muro) Sodium chloride 0.4%, benzalkonium chloride, propylene glycol, polyethylene glycol, EDTA. Soln.

Dropper bot. 15 mL. Mist bot. 50 mL.
OTC.
Use: Nasal decongestant.

Salipap. (Freeport) Salicylamide 5 g, acetaminophen 5 g. Tab. Bot. 1000s. *OTC.*
Use: Analgesic.

Salithol. (Madland) Balm of methyl salicylate, menthol, camphor. Liq. Bot. pt, gal. Oint. Jar 1 lb, 5 lb. *OTC.*
Use: Analgesic, topical.

Salivart. (Gebauer) Sodium carboxymethylcellulose, sorbitol, sodium chloride, potassium chloride, calcium chloride, magnesium chloride, dibasic potassium phosphate, and nitrogen (as propellant). Preservative free. Soln. Aerosol spray can 75 mL. *OTC.*
Use: Saliva substitute.

Saliva Substitute. (Roxane) Sorbitol, sodium carboxymethylcellulose, methylparaben. Soln. Bot. 120 mL. *OTC.*
Use: Saliva substitute.

saliva substitutes.
Use: Mouth and throat product.
See: Entertainer's Secret.
　Moi-Stir.
　Moi-Stir Swabsticks.
　MouthKote.
　Numoisyn.
　Salivart.
　Saliva Substitute.

SalivaSure. (Scandinavian Formulas) Apple acid, citric acid, dibasic calcium phosphate, xylitol. Citrus flavor. Loz. 90s. *OTC.*
Use: Mouth and throat product.

Salkera. (Onset Therapeutics) Salicylic acid 6%. Aloe, cetostearyl alcohol, edetate disodium, parabens, white petrolatum. Top. Foam. 60 g. *Rx.*
Use: Keratolytic agent.

Salk vaccine.
See: IPOL.
　Poliovirus Vaccine, Inactivated.

•**salmeterol xinafoate.** (sal-MEH-teh-role zin-AF-oh-ate) USAN.
Use: Bronchodilator, sympathomimetic.
See: Serevent Diskus.

salmeterol xinafoate/fluticasone propionate.
Use: Bronchodilator, sympathomimetic.
See: Advair Diskus.
　Advair HFA.

•**salnacedin.** (sal-NAH-seh-din) USAN.
Use: Anti-inflammatory, topical.

Salocol. (Roberts) Acetaminophen 115 mg, aspirin 210 mg, salicylamide 65 mg, caffeine 16 mg. Tab. Bot. 1000s. *Rx.*
Use: Analgesic combination.

Salpaba w/Colchicine. (Madland) Sodium salicylate 0.25 g, para-aminobenzoic acid 0.25 g, vitamin C 20 mg, colchicine 0.25 mg. Tab. Bot. 100s, 1000s. *Rx.*
Use: Antigout.

Sal-Plant. (Pedinol Pharmacal) Salicylic acid 17% in flexible collodion vehicle. Gel. Tube 14 g. *OTC.*
Use: Keratolytic.

•**salsalate.** (SAL-sah-late) *USP 34.*
Use: Analgesic; anti-inflammatory.
See: Marthritic.

Salsitab. (Upsher-Smith) Salsalate 500 mg, 750 mg. Tab. Bot. 100s, 500s, UD 100s. *Rx.*
Use: Analgesic.

Salten. (Wren) Salicylamide 10 g. Tab. Bot. 100s, 1000s. *OTC.*
Use: Analgesic.

salt replacement products.
See: Slo-Salt-K.
　Sodium Chloride.

salts, rehydration, oral.
Use: Electrolyte combination.

salt substitutes.
Use: Sodium-free seasoning agent.
See: Adolph's Salt Substitute.
　Adolph's Seasoned Salt Substitute.
　Morton Salt Substitute.
　Morton Seasoned Salt Substitute.
　NoSalt.
　Nu-Salt.

salt tablets. (Cross) Sodium Cl 650 mg. Tab. Dispenser 500s. *OTC.*
Use: Salt replenisher.

Sal-Tropine. (Hope) Atropine sulfate 0.4 mg. Tab. Bot. 100s. *Rx.*
Use: Anticholinergic/antispasmodic.

Salvarsan.
Use: Antisyphilitic.

Salvax. (Quinnova) Salicylic acid 6%. Dimethicone, glycerin, parabens, polysorbate 80, povidone, propylene glycol, trolamine. Aer. Foam. Kit w/150 g *Hydro 35* foam. 70 g, 200 g. *Rx.*
Use: Keratolytic agent.

Salvax Duo. (Quinnova) Salicylic acid 6%, urea 40%, glycerin, parabens. Foam. 70 g. *Rx.*
Use: Miscellaneous topical combination.

Salvite-B. (Faraday) Sodium chloride 7 g, dextrose 3 g, vitamin B$_1$ 1 mg. Tab. Bot. 100s, 1000s. *OTC.*

•**samalizumab.** (SA-ma-LIZ-oo-mab) USAN.
Use: Antineoplastic.

•**samarium Sm 153 lexidronam injection.** (sah-MARE-ee-uhm Sm 153 lex-

lH-drah-nam) *USP 34.*
Use: Antineoplastic; radiopharmaceutical.
• **samarium Sm 153 lexidronam pentasodium.** (sah-MARE-ee-uhm Sm 153 lex-lH-drah-nam) USAN.
Use: Antineoplastic; radiopharmaceutical.
See: Quadramet.
Samsca. (Otsuka America) Tolvaptan 15 mg, 30 mg. Lactose. Tab. UD 10s. *Rx.*
Use: Vasopressin receptor antagonist.
Sanctura. (Various Mfr.) Trospium chloride 20 mg. Lactose, sucrose. Tab. 60s, 500s. Blister 14s. *Rx.*
Use: Anticholinergic.
Sanctura XR. (Allergan) Trospium chloride 60 mg. Sugar spheres. ER Cap. 30s. *Rx.*
Use: Anticholinergic.
Sancura. (Thompson Medical) Benzocaine, chlorobutanol, chlorothymol, benzoic acid, salicylic acid, benzyl alcohol, cod liver oil, lanolin in a washable petrolatum base. Oint. 30 g, 90 g.
Use: Anesthetic, local.
Sancuso. (ProStrakan) Granisetron 3.1 mg per 24 hours (34.3 mg per 52 cm^2). Patch, Transdermal. 1s. *Rx.*
Use: Antiemetic/antivertigo agent, 5-HT$_3$ receptor antagonist.
• **sancycline.** (SAN-SIGH-kleen) USAN.
Use: Anti-infective.
Sandimmune. (Novartis) Cyclosporine. **Oral soln.:** 100 mg/mL. Alcohol 12.5%. Bot. 50 mL with syringe. **Inj.:** 50 mg/mL. Polyoxyethylated castor oil 650 mg/mL, alcohol 32.9%. Amp. 5 mL. **Soft Gelatin Cap.:** 25 mg, 100 mg. Sorbitol, dehydrated alcohol ≤ 12.7%. UD 30s. *Rx.*
Tall Man: SandIMMUNE
Use: Immunosuppressant.
sandoptal. Isobutyl allylbarbituric acid.
See: Butalbital.
W/Caffeine, Aspirin, Phenacetin.
See: Fiorinal.
W/Caffeine, Aspirin, Phenacetin, Codeine Phosphate.
See: Fiorinal w/Codeine.
Sandostatin. (Novartis) Octreotide acetate. **0.05 mg/mL, 0.1 mg/mL, 0.5 mg/mL:** Inj. Amp 1 mL. **0.2 mg/mL, 1 mg/mL:** Inj. 5 mL multidose vials. *Rx.*
Tall Man: SandoSTATIN
Use: Somatostatin analog.
Sandostatin LAR Depot. (Novartis) Octreotide acetate 10 mg per 5 mL, 20 mg per 5 mL, 30 mg per 5 mL. Pow. for Inj. Susp. Kits with 2 mL diluent,

1½" 20-gauge needles and instruction booklet. *Rx.*
Tall Man: SandoSTATIN
Use: Somatostatin analog.
Sanestro. (Sandia) Estrone 0.7 mg, estradiol 0.35 mg, estriol 0.14 mg. Tab. Bot. 100s, 1000s. *Rx.*
Use: Estrogen.
• **sanfetrinem cilexetil.** (san-FEH-trih-nem sigh-LEX-eh-till) USAN.
Use: Anti-infective.
• **sanfetrinem sodium.** (san-FEH-trih-nem) USAN.
Use: Anti-infective.
SangCya. (SangStat) Cyclosporine 100 mg/mL, alcohol 10.5%. Oral Soln. Bot. 50 mL. *Rx.*
Use: Immunosuppressive.
• **sanguinarium chloride.** (san-gwih-NARE-ee-uhm) USAN. *Formerly Sanguinarine Chloride.*
Use: Antimicrobial; anti-inflammatory; antifungal.
Sanguis. (Sigma-Tau) Liver 10 mcg, vitamin B$_{12}$ 100 mcg, folic acid 1 mcg/mL. Vial 10 mL. *Rx.*
Use: Nutritional supplement.
Sani-Supp. (G & W) Glycerin. Supp. **Adults:** Box 10s, 25s, 50s. **Pediatric:** Box 10s, 25s. *OTC.*
Use: Laxative.
sanluol.
See: Arsphenamine.
Sanstress. (Sandia) Vitamins A 25,000 units, D 400 units, B$_1$ 10 mg, B$_2$ 5 mg, niacinamide 100 mg, B$_6$ 1 mg, B$_{12}$ 5 mcg, C 150 mg, Ca 103 mg, P 80 mg, Fe 10 mg, Cu 1 mg, I 0.1 mg, Mg 5.5 mg, Mn 1 mg, K 5 mg, Zn 1.4 mg. Cap. Bot. 100s, 1000s. *OTC.*
Use: Mineral, vitamin supplement.
Santiseptic. (Santiseptic) Menthol, phenol, benzocaine, zinc oxide, calamine. Lot. Bot. 4 oz. *OTC.*
Use: Dermatologic, counterirritant.
Santyl. (Knoll) Proteolytic enzyme derived from *Clostridium histolyticum* 250 units/g. Oint. Tube. 15 g, 30 g. *Rx.*
Use: Enzyme, topical.
• **sapacitabine.** (SAP-a-SYE-ta-been) USAN.
Use: Antineoplastic.
• **saperconazole.** (SAP-ehr-KOE-nah-zole) USAN.
Use: Antifungal.
Saphris. (Schering-Plough) Asenapine 5 mg, 10 mg. Mannitol, sucralose (black cherry flavor only). Unflavored or black cherry flavor. Tab., sublingual. 60s, UD 100s. *Rx.*

Use: Antipsychotic agent, dibenzapine derivative.

saponated cresol solution.
See: Cresol.

• **saprisartan potassium.** (sap-rih-SAHR-tan) USAN.
Use: Antihypertensive.

• **sapropterin dihydrochloride.** (SAP-roe-TER-in) USAN.
Use: Phenylketonuria (PKU).
See: Kuvan.

• **saquinavir mesylate.** (sack-KWIN-uh-vihr) *USP 34.*
Use: Antiviral.
See: Invirase.

• **saracatinib.** (SAR-a-KA-ti-nib) USAN.
Use: Antineoplastic.

• **saracatinib difumarate.** (SAR-a-KA-ti-nib) USAN.
Use: Antineoplastic.

Sarafem. (Warner Chilcott) Fluoxetine hydrochloride. **Pulvule:** 10 mg, 20 mg. Blister 28s. **Tab.:** 10 mg, 15 mg, 20 mg. 4 blister cards of 7 tablets. *Rx.*
Use: Antidepressant, selective serotonin reuptake inhibitor.

• **sarafloxacin hydrochloride.** (sa-rah-FLOX-ah-SIN) USAN.
Use: Anti-infective (DNA gyrase inhibitor).

• **saralasin acetate.** (sare-AL-ah-sin) USAN.
Use: Antihypertensive.

Saratoga. (Blair) Boric acid, zinc oxide, eucalyptol, white petrolatum. Oint. Tube 1 oz, 2 oz. *OTC.*
Use: Dermatologic, counterirritant.

l-sarcolysin. Melphalan.
Use: Antineoplastic.

Sardo Bath & Shower. (Schering-Plough) Mineral oil, tocopherol. Oil. Bot. 112.5 mL. *OTC.*
Use: Emollient.

Sardo Bath Oil Concentrate. (Schering-Plough) Mineral oil, isopropyl palmitate. Bot. 3.75 oz, 7.75 oz. *OTC.*
Use: Emollient.

Sardoettes. (Schering-Plough) Mineral oil, tocopherol, beta-carotene. Towelettes. Box 25s. *OTC.*
Use: Emollient.

Sardoettes Moisturizing Towelettes. (Schering-Plough) Mineral oil, isopropyl palmitate, impregnated towelling material. Individual packets. Box 25s. *OTC.*
Use: Emollient.

• **sargramostim.** (sar-GRUH-moe-STIM) USAN.
Use: Antineutropenic; hematopoietic stimulant; leukopoietic (granulocyte macrophage colony-stimulating factor).
See: Leukine.

Sarisol No. 2. (Halsey Drug) Butabarbital sodium 30 mg. Tab. Bot. 100s, 1000s. *c-III.*
Use: Hypnotic; sedative.

• **sarizotan hydrochloride.** (sar-i-ZOE-tan) USAN.
Use: Antiparkinson agent.

• **sarmoxicillin.** (sar-MOX-ih-SILL-in) USAN.
Use: Anti-infective.

Sarna. (GlaxoSmithKline) Triclosan 0.2%. Benzyl alcohol, parabens, PEG-75, stearyl alcohol. Fragrance free. Wash. 237 mL. *OTC.*
Use: Anti-infective, topical; antiseptic and germicide.

Sarna Anti-Itch. (GlaxoSmithKline) Camphor 5%, menthol 5%, carbomer 940, cetyl alcohol, DMDM hydantoin. Foam. Bot. 105 mL. *OTC.*
Use: Emollient.

Sarna Sensitive Anti-Itch. (GlaxoSmithKline) Pramoxine hydrochloride 1%. Benzyl alcohol, cetyl alcohol, petrolatum. Fragrance free. Lot. 222 mL. *OTC.*
Use: Topical local anesthetic.

Sarna Ultra. (GlaxoSmithKline) Pramoxine hydrochloride 1%, menthol 0.5%, petrolatum 30%, benzyl alcohol. Cream. 56.6 g. *OTC.*
Use: Topical local anesthetic.

• **sarpicillin.** (sahr-PIH-SILL-in) USAN.
Use: Anti-infective.

SA 6%. (River's Edge) Salicylic acid 6%. **Cream:** Alcohol, ammonium lactate, cetyl alcohol, dimethicone, disodium EDTA, glycerin, glyceryl, mineral oil, parabens, PEG-3, PEG-100, trolamine. 454 g in kit w/cleanser. **Lotion:** Alcohol, disodium EDTA, glycerin, glyceryl, mineral oil, parabens, PEG-100, trolamine. 237 mL in kit w/cleanser. *Rx.*
Use: Keratolytic agent.

SAStid soap. (GlaxoSmithKline) Salicylic acid 3%, sulfur 5%. EDTA, HEDTA. Soap. 100 g. *OTC.*
Use: Dermatologic, acne.

Savella. (Forest) Milnacipran hydrochloride 12.5 mg, 25 mg, 50 mg, 100 mg. PEG. Tab. Film-coated. 60s, 180s (except 12.5 mg), UD 5s (12.5 mg), UD 8s (25 mg), UD 42s (50 mg), UD 100s. *Rx.*
Use: Antidepressant, serotonin and norepinephrine reuptake inhibitor.

• **saxagliptin.** (SAX-a-GLIP-tin) USAN.
Use: Antidiabetic.

See: Onglyza.
W/Metformin Hydrochloride.
   See: Kombiglyze XR.
saxol.
   See: Petrolatum.
saw palmetto.
   Use: Dietary supplement.
scabicides/pediculicides.
   See: Crotamiton.
   Lindane.
   Malathion.
   Permethrin.
   Spinosad.
Scalacort DK. (Avidas Pharmaceuticals)
   Hydrocortisone 2%. Benzalkonium
   chloride, isopropyl alcohol. Lot. 29.6 mL
   and shampoo. Rx.
   Use: Anti-inflammatory agent, topical
   corticosteroid.
Scalpicin. (Combe) Salicylic acid 3%,
   menthol, SD alcohol 40. Shampoo. Bot.
   45 mL, 75 mL, 120 mL. OTC.
   Use: Corticosteroid, topical.
Scan. (Parker) Water-soluble gel. Bot.
   8 oz, gal.
   Use: Ultrasound aid.
Scandonest. (Septodont) Mepivacaine
   hydrochloride 3%. Sodium chloride
   6 mg. Inj., Soln. Dental cartridge.
   1.7 mL. Rx.
   Use: Injectable local anesthetic, amide
   local anesthetic.
Scandonest L. (Septodont) Mepivacaine
   hydrochloride 2% w/levonordefrin
   1:20,000. Edetate disodium, sodium
   chloride 4 mg. Inj., Soln. Dental cartridge. 1.7 mL. Rx.
   Use: Injectable local anesthetic, amide
   local anesthetic.
Scar Cream Maximum Strength. (Clay-
   Park Labs) Octyl methoxycinnamate
   7.5%, octyl salicylate 5%. Alcohols, mineral oil, parabens, urea. Cream. 28 g.
   OTC.
   Use: Sunscreen.
Scarlet Red Ointment Dressings. (Sherwood Davis & Geck) 5% scarlet red,
   lanolin, olive oil, petrolatum. Gauze.
   5" × 9" strips. Rx.
   Use: Dermatologic, wound therapy.
Schamberg's. (C & M Pharmacal) Men-
   thol 0.15%, phenol 1%, zinc oxide, pea-
   nut oil, lime water. Bot. Pt, gal. OTC.
   Use: Antipruritic; counterirritant.
•Schick test control. USP 34. Formerly
   Diphtheria Toxin, Inactivated Diagnostic.
   Use: Diagnostic aid (dermal reactivity
   indicator).
Schirmer Tear Test. (Various Mfr.) Ster-
   ile tear flow test strips. 250s. Rx.
   Use: Diagnostic aid, ophthalmic.

Schlesinger's Solution.
   See: Morphine Hydrochloride.
Sclerex. (Miller Pharmacal Group) Inositol 2 g, magnesium complex 34 mg,
   vitamins C 100 mg, calcium succinate
   25 mg, A 2500 units, D 200 units, E
   100 units, B₁ 5 mg, B₂ 5 mg, B₆ 5 mg,
   B₁₂ 5 mcg, niacin 10 mg, niacinamide
   30 mg, pantothenic acid 7.5 mg, folic
   acid 0.1 mg, Fe 10 mg, Cu 1 mg, Mn
   2 mg, Zn 9 mg, I 0.10 mg/3 Tab. Bot.
   60s. OTC.
   Use: Mineral, vitamin supplement.
Scleromate. (Glenwood) Morrhuate so-
   dium 50 mg/mL. Inj. Multiple-use vial.
   30 mL. Rx.
   Use: Sclerosing agent.
sclerosing agents.
   Use: Treatment of varicose veins.
   See: Ethanolamine Oleate.
   Morrhuate Sodium.
   Sodium Tetradecyl Sulfate.
Sclerosol. (Bryan) Talc 4 g. Aerosol.
   Single-use aluminum canister with
   2 delivery tubes of 15 cm and 25 cm.
   Rx.
   Use: Antineoplastic.
Scopace. (Hope Pharm) Scopolamine
   0.4 mg. Tab. Bot. 100s. Rx.
   Use: Antiparkinson; antiemetic/antiver-
   tigo agent; GI anticholinergic/anti-
   spasmodic.
•scopafungin. (SKOE-pah-FUN-jin)
   USAN.
   Use: Antifungal; anti-infective.
Scope. (Procter & Gamble) Cetylpyri-
   dinium Cl, tartrazine, saccharin, SD al-
   cohol 38F 67.9%. Liq. Bot. 90 mL,
   180 mL, 360 mL, 720 mL, 1080 mL,
   1440 mL. OTC.
   Use: Mouthwash.
•scopolamine hydrobromide. (skoe-
   PAHL-uh-meen) USP 34. Formerly
   Hyoscine Hydrobromide. Hyoscine, l-
   Scopolamine, Epoxytropine tropate.
   Use: Anticholinergic (ophthalmic); cy-
   cloplegic; hypnotic; mydriatic; seda-
   tive; GI anticholinergic/antispasmodic.
   See: Scopace.
   Transderm-Scōp.
W/Atropine Sulfate, Hyoscyamine Hydro-
   bromide or Sulfate, Phenobarbital.
   See: Antispasmodic.
   Donnatal.
   Donnatal Extentabs.
   PB-Hyos.
   Quadrapax.
W/Combinations.
   See: Belladonna.
   Belladonna Alkaloids.

Respa A.R.
Stahist.

scopolamine hydrobromide. (Glaxo-SmithKline) Scopolamine HBr 0.86 mg/mL. Inj. Vials. 1 mL. *Rx.*
Use: Amnestic; anxiolytic; sedative; GI anticholinergic/antispasmodic.

scopolamine hydrobromide. (Invenex) Scopolamine HBr 0.3 mg/mL. Inj. Vial 1 mL. *Rx.*
Use: Amnestic; anxiolytic; sedative.

scopolamine hydrobromide. (Various Mfr.) Scopolamine HBr 0.3 mg/mL, 0.4 mg/mL, 1 mg/mL. Inj. Amps. 0.5 mL (0.4 mg/mL only). Vials. 1 mL. *Rx.*
Use: GI anticholinergic/antispasmodic.

scopolamine methobromide.
See: Methscopolamine Bromide.

scopolamine methyl nitrate.
See: Methscopolamine Nitrate.

scopolamine salts.
See: Belladonna.

Scotavite. (Scot-Tussin) Vitamins A 25,000 units, D 400 units, B_1 10 mg, B_2 10 mg, B_6 5 mg, B_{12} 5 mcg, niacinamide 100 mg, calcium pantothenate 20 mg, C 200 mg, d-alpha tocopheryl 15 units, acid succinate iodine 0.15 mg. Tab. Bot. 100s, 500s. *OTC.*
Use: Mineral, vitamin supplement.

Scotcil. (Scot-Tussin) **Tab.:** Potassium penicillin 400,000 units w/calcium carbonate. Bot. 100s, 500s. **Pow.:** 80 mL, 150 mL. *Rx.*
Use: Anti-infective, penicillin.

Scotonic. (Scot-Tussin) Vitamins B_1 10 mg, B_2 5 mg, B_6 1 mg, niacinamide 50 mg, choline Cl 100 mg, inositol 100 mg, B_{12} 25 mcg, Ca 19 mg, Fe 50 mg, folic acid 0.15 mg, alcohol 15%, sodium benzoate 0.1%/45 mL. Bot. Pt, gal. *OTC.*
Use: Mineral, vitamin supplement.

Scott's Emulsion. (GlaxoSmithKline) Vitamins A 1,250 units, D 1,400 units/4 tsp. Bot. 6.25 oz, 12.5 oz. *OTC.*
Use: Vitamin supplement.

Scot-Tussin Allergy Relief Formula Clear. (Scot-Tussin) Diphenhydramine hydrochloride 12.5 mg/5 mL. Alcohol and dye free. Parabens, menthol. Cherry-strawberry flavor. Liq. Bot. 118 mL. *OTC.*
Use: Antihistamine, nonselective ethanolamine.

Scot-Tussin DM. (Scot-Tussin) Dextromethorphan HBr 15 mg, chlorpheniramine maleate 2 mg per 5 mL. Sugar and alcohol free. Magnasweet, menthol, parabens. Liq. Bot. 118 mL. *OTC.*

Use: Upper respiratory combination, antitussive combination.

Scot-Tussin DM Cough Chasers. (Scot-Tussin) Dextromethorphan HBr 5 mg. Peppermint oil, sorbitol. Sugar and dye free. Loz. Box 20s. *OTC.*
Use: Nonnarcotic antitussive.

Scot-Tussin Expectorant. (Scot-Tussin) Guaifenesin 100 mg/5 mL. Parabens, phenylalanine, menthol, aspartame. Alcohol and dye free. Grape flavor. Liq. Bot. 118 mL. *OTC.*
Use: Expectorant.

Scot-Tussin Hayfebrol. (Scot-Tussin) Pseudoephedrine hydrochloride 30 mg, chlorpheniramine maleate 2 mg/5 mL. Parabens, menthol, alcohol and dye free. Liq. Bot. 120 mL. *OTC.*
Use: Upper respiratory combination, decongestant, antihistamine.

Scot-Tussin Original Multi-Action Cold and Allergy. (Scot-Tussin) Phenylephrine hydrochloride 4 mg, pheniramine maleate 13 mg, sodium salicylate 83 mg, caffeine citrate 25 mg/5 mL. Saccharin, parabens, cherry-strawberry flavor. Sugar, alcohol, and dye free. Syrup. Liq. Bot. 118 mL, 473 mL, 3.8 L. *OTC.*
Use: Upper respiratory combination, decongestant, antihistamine, analgesic.

Scot-Tussin Pharmacal Allergy. (Scot-Tussin) Diphenhydramine hydrochloride 12.5 mg/5 mL, parabens, menthol. Liq. Dye free, sugar free. Bot. 120 mL. *OTC.*
Use: Antihistamine.

Scot-Tussin Pharmacal DM. (Scot-Tussin) Dextromethorphan HBr 15 mg, chlorpheniramine maleate 2 mg/5 mL, alcohol 10%, sugar free. Liq. Bot. 4 oz, 8 oz. *OTC.*
Use: Antihistamine.

Scot-Tussin Pharmacal DM Cough Chasers. (Scot-Tussin) Dextromethorphan HBr 2.5 mg, dye free, sorbitol. Loz. Pkg. 20s. *OTC.*
Use: Antitussive.

Scot-Tussin Pharmacal DM2. (Scot-Tussin) Dextromethorphan HBr 15 mg, guaifenesin 100 mg, alcohol 1.4%/5 mL. Syrup. Bot. 120 mL, 240 mL. *OTC.*
Use: Antitussive; expectorant.

Scot-Tussin Pharmacal Expectorant. (Scot-Tussin) Guaifenesin 100 mg/5 mL, menthol, aspartame, phenylalanine, parabens, alcohol and dye free. Liq. Bot. 30 mL, 118.3 mL, 240 mL. *OTC.*
Use: Expectorant.

Scot-Tussin Pharmacal Sugar-Free.
(Scot-Tussin) Dextromethorphan HBr
15 mg, chlorpheniramine maleate
2 mg/5 mL. Bot. 4 oz, 8 oz, 16 oz, gal.
OTC.
Use: Antitussive; antihistamine.
**Scot-Tussin Pharmacal Sugar-Free
Expectorant.** (Scot-Tussin) Guaifene-
sin 100 mg/5 mL w/alcohol 3.5%. Dye,
sodium free, and sugar free. *OTC.*
Use: Expectorant.
Scot-Tussin Pharmacal with Sugar.
(Scot-Tussin) Phenylephrine hydrochlo-
ride 4.17 mg, pheniramine maleate
13.3 mg, sodium citrate 83.33 mg, sodium salicylate 83.33 mg, caffeine cit-
rate 25 mg/5 mL. Bot. 4 oz, 8 oz, 16 oz,
gal. *OTC.*
Use: Analgesic combination; antihista-
mine; decongestant.
Scot-Tussin Senior Clear. (Scot-Tussin)
Guaifenesin 200 mg, dextromethorphan
HBr 15 mg per 5 mL. Parabens, phenylalanine, aspartame, menthol, alcohol
free, sugar free. Liq. Bot. 118 mL. *OTC.*
Use: Upper respiratory combination,
antitussive, expectorant.
Sculptra. (Dermik Laboratories) Poly-l-
lactic acid (freeze dried). Pow. for Inj.
Single-use vials. *Rx.*
Use: Restoration/correction of facial fat
loss in individuals with HIV.
scurenaline.
See: Epinephrine.
scuroforme.
See: Butyl Aminobenzoate.
S.D.M. #50. (AstraZeneca) Isosorbide
dinitrate 50% in lactose. *Rx.*
Use: Vasodilator.
S.D.M. #5. (AstraZeneca) Mannitol hexa-
nitrate 7% in lactose. *Rx.*
Use: Vasodilator.
S.D.M. #40. (AstraZeneca) Isosorbide
dinitrate 25% in lactose. *Rx.*
Use: Vasodilator.
S.D.M. #17. (AstraZeneca) Nitroglycerin
10% in lactose. *Rx.*
Use: Vasodilator.
S.D.M. #35. (AstraZeneca) Pentaerythri-
tol tetranitrate 35% in mannitol. *Rx.*
Use: Vasodilator.
S.D.M. #37. (AstraZeneca) Nitroglycerin
10% in ethanol. *Rx.*
Use: Vasodilator.
S.D.M. #27. (AstraZeneca) Nitroglycerin
10% in propylene glycol. *Rx.*
Use: Vasodilator.
S.D.M. #23. (AstraZeneca) Pentaerythri-
tol tetranitrate 20% in lactose. *Rx.*
Use: Vasodilator.

Sea & Ski Baby Lotion Formula.
(Carter-Wallace) Octyl-dimethyl PABA.
SPF 2. Lot. Bot. 120 mL. *OTC.*
Use: Sunscreen.
Sea & Ski Golden Tan. (Carter-Wallace)
Padimate O. SPF 4. Lot. Bot. 120 mL.
OTC.
Use: Sunscreen.
Sea Greens. (Modern Aids Inc.) Iodine
0.25 mg. Tab. Bot. 220s, 460s. *OTC.*
Sea Master. (Barth's) Vitamins A
10,000 units, D 400 units. Cap. Bot.
100s, 500s. *OTC.*
Use: Vitamin supplement.
Sea-Omega 50. (Rugby) Omega-3 poly-
unsaturated fatty acid 1000 mg. Cap.
containing EPA 300 mg, DHA 200 mg,
vitamin E 1 unit. Bot. 30s, 50s. *OTC.*
Use: Nutritional supplement.
Sea-Omega 30. (Rugby) N-3 fat content
(mg) EPA 180, DHA 140. 100s. *OTC.*
Use: Nutritional supplement.
Seasonale. (Duramed) Levonorgestrel
0.15 mg, ethinyl estradiol 30 mcg. Lac-
tose. Film-coated. Tab. 91s w/7 white
inert tabs. *Rx.*
Use: Contraceptive hormone, sex hor-
mone.
Seasonique. (Duramed) **Phase 1:** Levonorgestrel 0.15 mg, ethinyl estradiol
10 mcg. Lactose. Film-coated. Tab. 84s.
Phase 2: Ethinyl estradiol 10 mcg.
Lactose. Film-coated. Tab. 7s. *Rx.*
Use: Contraceptive hormone, sex hor-
mone.
Seba-Lo. (Whorton Pharmaceuticals,
Inc.) Acetone-alcohol cleanser. Bot.
4 oz. *OTC.*
Use: Skin cleanser.
Sebana. (Bristol-Myers Squibb) Salicylic
acid 2%. Shampoo. Bot. 4 oz, 8 oz, pt,
qt, 0.5 gal. *OTC.*
Use: Antiseborrheic.
Sebanatar. (Bristol-Myers Squibb) Sali-
cylic acid 2%, liquor carbonis deter-
gens 3%. Shampoo. Bot. 4 oz, 8 oz, pt,
qt, 0.5 gal, gal. *OTC.*
Use: Antiseborrheic.
Seba-Nil Cleansing Mask. (Galderma)
Astringent face mask containing SD
alcohol 40, sulfated castor oil, methyl-
paraben. Tube 105 g. *OTC.*
Use: Dermatologic, acne.
Seba-Nil Liquid. (Galderma) Alcohol
49.7%, acetone, polysorbate 20. Liq.
Bot. 240 mL, pt. *OTC.*
Use: Dermatologic, acne.
Seba-Nil Oily Skin Cleanser. (Gal-
derma) SD alcohol, acetone. Liq. Bot.
240 mL, 473 mL. *OTC.*
Use: Dermatologic, acne.

Sebasorb. (Summers) Activated attapulgite 10%, salicylic acid 2%. Lot. Bot. 45 mL. *OTC.*
Use: Dermatologic, acne.

SE BPO. (Seton Pharmaceuticals) Benzoyl peroxide 3%, 6%, 9%. Cetyl alcohol, glycerin, sodium hyaluronate, zinc. Cloths, topical. UD 60s. *Rx.*
Use: Topical anti-infective, antibiotic agent.

SE BPO 7%. (Seton Pharmaceuticals) Benzoyl peroxide 7%. Castor oil, dimethicone, edetate disodium, glycerin, methylparaben, PEG-15, PEG-40. Soap. 180 g. *Rx.*
Use: Topical anti-infective, antibiotic agent.

Seb-Prev. (Perrigo) Sulfacetamide sodium 10%. EDTA, methylparaben. Gel. 30 g, 60 g. *Rx.*
Use: Topical anti-infective.

Seb-Prev. (Glades) Sodium sulfacetamide 10%. Propylene glycol, EDTA, methylparaben. Lot. 118 mL. *Rx.*
Use: Dermatologic agent, acne product.

Seb-Prev Wash. (Perrigo) Sulfacetamide sodium 10%. Edetate disodium, PEG-6, PEG-60, PEG-150, methylparaben. Soap. 170 mL, 340 mL. *Rx.*
Use: Topical anti-infective.

Sebulex with Conditioners. (Bristol-Myers Squibb) Sulfur 2%, salicylic acid 2%. Bot. 4 oz, 8 oz. *OTC.*
Use: Antiseborrheic.

• **secalciferol.** (seh-kal-SIFF-eh-ROLE) USAN.
Use: Regulator (calcium); treatment of familial hypophosphatemic rickets. [Orphan Drug]
See: Osteo-D.

• **seclazone.** (SEK-lah-zone) USAN.
Use: Anti-inflammatory; uricosuric.

• **secobarbital.** (see-koe-BAR-bih-tahl) *USP 34.*
Use: Hypnotic; sedative.
W/Combinations.
See: Monosyl.

secobarbital elixir.
See: Seconal.

• **secobarbital sodium.** (see-koe-BAR-bih-tahl) *USP 34.*
Use: Hypnotic; sedative.

secobarbital sodium. (Wyeth) Secobarbital sodium 50 mg/mL. Inj. *Tubex* 2 mL. *c-II.*
Use: Hypnotic; sedative.

secobarbital sodium and amobarbital sodium capsules.
Use: Hypnotic; sedative.

See: Tuinal.

Seconal Sodium Pulvules. (Marathon) Secobarbital sodium 100 mg. Cap. Bot. 100s, UD 100s. *c-II.*
Use: Hypnotic; sedative.

Secran. (Scherer) Vitamins B_1 10 mg, B_3 10 mg, B_{12} 25 mcg, alcohol 17%. Liq. Bot. 480 mL. *OTC.*
Use: Vitamin supplement.

secretin.
Use: Diagnostic aid, gastrointestinal function test.
See: ChiRhoStim.

Sectral. (Reddy Pharmaceuticals) Acebutolol hydrochloride 200 mg, 400 mg. Cap. Bot. 100s, *Redipak* 100s (200 mg only). *Rx.*
Use: Antiadrenergic/sympatholytic, beta-adrenergic blocker.

• **secukinumab.** (SEK-ue-KIN-ue-mab) USAN.
Use: Uveitis, rheumatoid arthritis, psoriasis.

sedaform.
See: Chlorobutanol.

Sedamine. (Health for Life Brands) Phosphorated carbohydrate soln. Bot. 4 oz. *OTC.*
Use: Antinauseant.

Sedamine. (Oxypure) Hyoscyamine sulfate 0.1037 mg, atropine sulfate 0.0194 mg, hyoscine HBr 0.0065 mg, phenobarbital 16.2 mg. Tab. Bot. 100s, 1000s. *Rx.*
Use: Antispasmodic; sedative.

Sedapap. (Merz) Acetaminophen 650 mg, butalbital 50 mg. Tab. Bot. 100s. *Rx.*
Use: Analgesic.

Sedapar. (Parmed Pharmaceuticals, Inc.) Atropine sulfate 0.0195 mg, hyoscine HBr 0.0065 mg, hyoscyamine sulfate 0.104 mg, phenobarbital 0.25 g. Tab. Bot. 1000s. *Rx.*
Use: Antispasmodic; sedative.

sedative/hypnotic agents.
See: Barbiturates.
Bromides.
Butisol Sodium.
Carbamide Compounds.
Chloral Hydrate.
Chlorobutanol.
Paraldehyde.
Phenergan.
Triazolam.

sedative/hypnotic agents, nonbarbiturate.
See: Benzodiazepines.
Chloral Hydrate.
Dexmedetomidine Hydrochloride.
Eszopiclone.

Imidazopyridines.
Melatonin Receptor Agonists.
Paraldehyde.
Propiomazine Hydrochloride.
Pyrazolopyrimidine.
sedeval.
See: Barbital.
•**sedoxantrone trihydrochloride.** (sed-OX-an-trone try-HIGH-droe-KLOR-ide) USAN.
Use: Antineoplastic (DNA topoisomerase II inhibitor).
Sedral. (Vita Elixir) Phenobarbital ⅛ g, theophylline 2 g, ephedrine g. Tab. *Rx.*
Use: Bronchodilator; sedative.
•**seglitide acetate.** (SEH-glih-TIDE) USAN.
Use: Antidiabetic.
selective aldosterone receptor antagonists.
See: Eplerenone.
selective COX-2 inhibitors.
Use: Anti-inflammatory; nonsteroidal anti-inflammatory agent.
See: Celecoxib.
selective estrogen receptor modulator.
Use: Sex hormone.
See: Raloxifene Hydrochloride.
selective factor Xa inhibitor.
Use: Anticoagulant.
See: Fondaparinux Sodium.
selective phosphodiesterase 4 inhibitors.
See: Roflumilast.
selective serotonin reuptake inhibitors.
Use: Antidepressant.
See: Citalopram Hydrobromide.
Escitalopram Oxalate.
5-HT$_{1A}$ Receptor Agonists.
Fluoxetine Hydrochloride.
Fluvoxamine Maleate.
Paroxetine Hydrochloride.
Sertraline Hydrochloride.
selective vascular endothelial growth factor antagonist.
See: Pegaptanib Sodium.
Ranibizumab.
•**selegiline hydrochloride.** (se-LE-ji-leen) USAN.
Use: Antiparkinson agent.
See: Carbex.
Eldepryl.
Emsam.
Zelapar.
selegiline hydrochloride. (Various Mfr.) Selegiline 5 mg. May contain lactose. **Cap.:** 60s, 500s, 1,000s. **Tab.:** 60s, 500s. *Rx.*
Use: Antiparkinson agent.

Selenicel. (Taylor Pharmaceuticals) Selenium yeast complex 200 mcg, vitamins C 100 mg, E 100 mg. Cap. Bot. 90s. *OTC.*
Use: Vitamin supplement.
•**selenious acid.** (seh-LEE-nee-us) *USP 34.*
Use: Supplement (trace mineral).
selenium. (Nion Corp.) Selenium 50 mcg. Tab. Bot. 100s. *Rx.*
Use: Nutritional supplement, parenteral.
selenium disulfide.
See: Selenium Sulfide.
•**selenium sulfide.** (seh-LEE-nee-uhm SULL-fide) *USP 34.*
Use: Antidandruff; antifungal; antiseborrheic.
See: Head & Shoulders Intensive Treatment.
Selenos.
Selsun.
selenium sulfide. (Kylemore) Selenium sulfide 2.25%. Caprylic/capric triglyceride, edetate disodium, parabens, propylene glycol, urea, zinc. Shampoo, Susp. 180 mL. *Rx.*
Use: Antipsoriatic agent.
selenium sulfide. (Various Mfr.) Selenium sulfide. **Lot./Shampoo:** 1%. 210 mL. **Lot.:** 2.5%. 120 mL. *Rx-OTC.*
Use: Antidandruff; antiseborrheic.
•**selenomethionine Se 75.** (seh-LEE-no-meh-THIGH-oh-neen Se 75) USAN.
Use: Diagnostic aid (pancreas function determination), radiopharmaceutical.
See: Sethotope.
Selenos. (Breckenridge Pharmaceutical) Selenium sulfide 2.25%. Caprylic/capric triglyceride, edetate disodium, parabens, propylene glycol, urea, zinc. Shampoo, Susp. 180 mL. *Rx.*
Use: Anti-psoriatic agent.
•**seletracetam.** (SEL-e-TRA-se-tam) USAN.
Use: Antieplectic.
Selfemra. (Teva) Fluoxetine hydrochloride 10 mg, 20 mg. Cap. 28s. *Rx.*
Use: Antidepressant, selective serotonin reuptake inhibitor.
•**selfotel.** (SELL-fah-tell) USAN.
Use: NMDA antagonist.
•**selodenoson.** (sel-oh-DEN-oh-son) USAN.
Use: Cardiovascular agent.
Selora. (Sanofi-Synthelabo) Potassium Cl. Pow. *OTC.*
Use: Salt substitute.
Selsun. (Abbott) Selenium sulfide 2.5%. Lot. 120 mL. *Rx.*
Use: Antiseborrheic.

Selsun Blue Medicated Treatment.
(Chattem) Selenium sulfide 1%. Menthol. Lot./Shampoo. 325 mL. *OTC.*
Use: Antiseborrheic.

•**selumetinib.** (SEL-ue-ME-ti-nib) USAN.
Use: Antineoplastic.

•**selumetinib sulfate.** (SEL-ue-ME-ti-nib) USAN.
Use: Antineoplastic.

Selzentry. (ViiV Healthcare) Maraviroc 150 mg, 300 mg. Film-coated. Tab. Bot. 60s. *Rx.*
Use: Antiretroviral, cellular chemokine receptor antagonist.

•**semaglutide.** (SEM-a-GLOO-tide) USAN.
Use: Treatment of type 2 diabetes.

•**sematilide hydrochloride.** (SEH-may-tih-LIDE) USAN.
Use: Cardiovascular agent (antiarrhythmic).

•**semaxanib.** (sem-AX-an-ib) USAN.
Use: Antineoplastic.

•**semduramicin.** (sem-DER-ah-MY-sin) USAN.
Use: Coccidiostat.

•**semduramicin sodium.** (sem-DER-ah-MY-sin) USAN.
Use: Coccidiostat.

Semicid. (Whitehall-Robins) Nonoxynol-9 100 mg. Vag. Supp. Box 9s, 18s. *OTC.*
Use: Contraceptive.

Semprex-D. (Celltech) Acrivastine 8 mg, pseudoephedrine hydrochloride 60 mg. Lactose. Cap. Bot. 100s. *Rx.*
Use: Upper respiratory combination, decongestant, antihistamine.

•**semuloparin.** (SEM-ue-loe-PAR-in) USAN.
Use: Antithrombotic.

•**semuloparin sodium.** (SEM-ue-loe-PAR-in) USAN.
Use: Antithrombotic.

•**semustine.** (SEH-muss-teen) USAN.
Use: Antineoplastic.

Senexon. (Rugby) Sennosides. **Liq.:** 8.8 mg/mL. Parabens, sucrose. 237 mL. **Tab.:** 8.6 mg. Lactose. Bot. 100s, 1000s. *OTC.*
Use: Laxative.

•**senicapoc.** (SEN-i-KAY-pok) USAN.
Use: Sickle cell disease.

Senilavite. (Defco) Vitamins A 5,000 units, C 100 mg, B_1 2.5 mg, B_2 2 mg, nicotinamide 10 mg, B_6 1 mg, calcium pantothenate 5 mg, B_{12} w/intrinsic factor concentrate 0.133 units, ferrous fumarate 150 mg, glutamic acid

hydrochloride 150 mg, docusate sodium 50 mg. Cap. Bot. 100s. *OTC.*
Use: Nutritional supplement.

Senilezol. (Edwards) Vitamins B_1 0.42 mg, B_2 0.42 mg, $B_3$1.67 mg, B_5 0.83 mg, B_6 0.17 mg, B_{12} 0.83 mcg, ferric pyrophosphate 3.3 mg/15 mL, alcohol 15%. Liq. Bot. 473 mL. *OTC.*
Use: Mineral, vitamin supplement.

•**senna.** (SEN-ah) *USP 34.*
Use: Laxative.
W/Docusate Sodium.
See: Dok Plus.
Senna Plus.
Senna-S.

senna. (Pharmaceutical Associates) Senna leaf extract 176 mg per 5 mL. Glycerin, parabens, sucrose. Syrup. 237 mL. *OTC.*
Use: Laxative.

senna. (SDA Labs) Sennosides 8.8 mg/5 mL. Parabens, sucrose. Syrup. 236 mL. *OTC.*
Use: Laxative, irritant or stimulant laxative.

senna concentrate, standardized.
Use: Cathartic.
See: Senexon.
Senokot.
W/Docusate Sodium.
See: Senokot-S.
W/Psyllium.
See: Perdiem.

senna fruit extract, standardized.
Use: Cathartic.
See: Dosaflex.
Senokot.

Senna-Gen. (Ivax) Sennosides 8.6 mg, lactose. Tab. Bot. 100s, 1000s. *OTC.*
Use: Laxative.

Senna Plus. (Contract Pharmacal) Docusate sodium 50 mg, senna concentrate (as sennosides) 8.6 mg. Tartrazine. Tab. 100s. *OTC.*
Use: Laxative.

Senna Prompt. (Konsyl) Sennosides 9 mg, psyllium 500 mg. Cap. 90s. *OTC.*
Use: Laxative.

Senna-S. (Akyma) Docusate sodium 50 mg, sennosides 8.6 mg. Tab. 1000s. *OTC.*
Use: Laxative.

Senna Smooth. (Novartis Consumer Health) Sennosides 15 mg. Sucrose. Tab. 24s. *OTC.*
Use: Laxative.

•**sennosides.** (SEN-oh-sides) *USP 34.*
Use: Laxative.
See: Agoral.
Black Draught.
Dr. Edwards' Olive.

Evac-U-Gen.
ex-lax.
ex-lax chocolated.
Fletcher's Castoria.
Gentle Nature Natural Vegetable Laxative.
Lax-Pills.
Little Tummys Laxative.
Maximum Relief ex-lax.
Senexon.
Senna.
Senna-Gen.
Senna Smooth.
Senokot.
SenokotXTRA.
W/Docusate Sodium.
See: Dok Plus.
   ex-lax Gentle Strength.
   PeriColace.
   Senna Plus.
   Senna-S.
W/Psyllium.
See: Senna Prompt.

Senokot. (Purdue) **Gran.:** Sennosides 15 mg/5 mL, sucrose. Can. 56 g, 170 g, 340 g. **Tab.:** Sennosides 8.6 mg, lactose. Bot. 10s, 20s, 50s, 100s, 1000s. UD 100s. **Syr.:** Sennosides 8.8 mg/5 mL, alcohol free, parabens, sucrose. Bot. 59 mL, 237 mL. *OTC.*
Use: Laxative.

Senokot-S. (Purdue) Docusate sodium 50 mg, senna concentrate 8.6 mg, lactose. Tab. Bot. 10s, 30s, 60s, 1000s, UD 100s. *OTC.*
Use: Laxative.

Senokot Suppositories. (Purdue) Standardized senna concentrate. Supp. Pkg. 6s. *OTC.*
Use: Laxative.

SenokotXTRA. (Purdue) Sennosides 17 mg, lactose. Tab. Bot. 12s, 36s. *OTC.*
Use: Laxative.

Sensi-Care Moisturizing Body. (ConvaTec) Dimethicone 1%, petrolatum 30%, cetyl alcohol, glycerin, urea. Cream. 85 g. *OTC.*
Use: Emollient.

Sensipar. (Amgen) Cinacalcet hydrochloride (as base) 30 mg, 60 mg, 90 mg. Film-coated. Tab. 30s. *Rx.*
Use: Calcium receptor agonist.

Sensitive Eyes. (Bausch & Lomb) Sorbic acid 0.1%, EDTA 0.025%, NaCl, boric acid, sodium borate. Soln. Bot. 118 mL, 237 mL, 355 mL. *OTC.*
Use: Contact lens care.

Sensitive Eyes Daily Cleaner. (Bausch & Lomb) Sorbic acid 0.25%, EDTA 0.5%, NaCl, hydroxypropyl methylcellulose, poloxamine, sodium borate. Soln. Bot. 20 mL. *OTC.*
Use: Contact lens care.

Sensitive Eyes Drops. (Bausch & Lomb) Buffered. Sorbic acid 0.1%, EDTA 0.025%, sodium chloride, boric acid, sodium borate. Soln. Bot. 30 mL. *OTC.*
Use: Contact lens rewetting solution.

Sensitive Eyes Plus. (Bausch & Lomb) Boric acid, sodium borate, KCl, NaCl, polyaminopropyl biguanide 0.00003%, EDTA 0.025%. Soln. Bot. 118 mL, 355 mL. *OTC.*
Use: Contact lens care.

Sensitive Eyes Saline. (Bausch & Lomb) NaCl, borate buffer, sorbic acid 0.1%, EDTA. Soln. Bot. 118 mL, 237 mL, 355 mL. *OTC.*
Use: Contact lens care.

Sensitive Eyes Saline/Cleaning Solution. (Bausch & Lomb) Isotonic solution w/borate buffer, NaCl, poloxamine, sorbic acid 0.15%, sodium borate, boric acid, EDTA 0.1%. Soln. Bot. 237 mL. *OTC.*
Use: Contact lens care.

Sensodyne Fresh Mint Toothpaste. (Block Drug) Potassium nitrate 5%, sodium monofluorophosphate 0.76%, saccharin, sorbitol. Mint flavor. Tube 2.4 oz, 4.6 oz. *OTC.*
Use: Dentifrice.

Sensodyne-SC Toothpaste. (Block Drug) Glycerin, sorbitol, sodium methylcocoyl taurate, PEG-40 stearate, strontium Cl hexahydrate 10%, methyl- and propylparabens. Tinted. Tube 2.1 oz, 4 oz. *OTC.*
Use: Dentifrice.

SensoGARD. (Block Drug) Benzocaine 20%, parabens. Gel. Tube 9.4 g. *OTC.*
Use: Anesthetic, local.

Sensorcaine. (APP Pharmaceuticals) Bupivacaine hydrochloride 0.25% or 0.5%. Bupivacaine hydrochloride 0.25% or 0.5%, epinephrine 1:200,000, methylparaben 1 mg/mL. Inj. Multidose vial 50 mL. *Rx.*
Use: Anesthetic, local amide.

Sensorcaine MPF. (APP Pharmaceuticals) Bupivacaine hydrochloride 0.25%, 0.5%, 0.75%. Inj. Single-dose amp. 30 mL (except 0.5%). Single-dose vials 10 mL, 30 mL. Bupivacaine hydrochloride 0.25%, 0.5%, or 0.75% with epinephrine 1:200,000. Inj. Single-dose amp. 5 mL (0.5% only), 30 mL (except 0.5%). Single-dose vials 10 mL, 30 mL. *Rx.*
Use: Anesthetic, local amide.

Sensorcaine-MPF Spinal. (APP Pharmaceuticals) Bupivacaine hydrochloride 0.75%, dextrose 8.25%. Inj. Amp. 2 mL. *Rx.*
Use: Anesthetic, local amide.

•**sepazonium chloride.** (SEP-ah-ZOE-nee-uhm) USAN.
Use: Anti-infective, topical.

•**seperidol hydrochloride.** (seh-PURR-ih-dahl) USAN.
Use: Neuroleptic; antipsychotic.

•**seprilose.** (SEH-prih-LOHS) USAN.
Use: Antirheumatic.

•**seproxetine hydrochloride.** (sep-ROX-eh-teen) USAN.
Use: Antidepressant.

Septi-Chek. (Roche) Blood culture and simultaneous sub-culture system with three media to support clinically significant pathogens. Quick and easy assembly forms a closed system to protect sub-cultures from contamination.
Use: Diagnostic aid.

Septiphene. (SEP-tih-feen) (Monsanto)
Use: Disinfectant.

Septo. (Vita Elixir) Methylbenzethonium Cl, ethanol 2%, menthol. *OTC.*
Use: Antimicrobial; antiseptic.

Septra DS. (Monarch) Trimethoprim 160 mg, sulfamethoxazole 800 mg. Tab. 20s, 100s, 500s. *Rx.*
Use: Anti-infective.

•**seractide acetate.** (seer-ACK-tide) USAN.
Use: Corticotrophic peptide, hormone (adrenocorticotrophic).

Seradex-LA. (Allegis Pharmaceuticals) Brompheniramine maleate 6 mg, phenylephrine hydrochloride 19 mg. ER Tab. 100s. *Rx.*
Use: Upper respiratory combination, decongestant and antihistamine.

Ser-A-Gen. (Ivax) Hydrochlorothiazide 15 mg, reserpine 0.1 mg, hydralazine hydrochloride 25 mg. Tab. Bot. 100s, 1000s. *Rx.*
Use: Antihypertensive combination.

Seralyzer. (Bayer Consumer Care) A system for the measurement of enzymes, potassium levels, blood chemistries, and therapeutic drug assays consisting of a reflectance photometer and a series of solid-phase reagent strips.
Use: Diagnostic aid.

•**seratrodast.** (seh-RAH-troe-dast) USAN.
Use: Anti-inflammatory (non-antihistaminic); antiasthmatic (thromboxane receptor antagonist).

•**serazapine hydrochloride.** (ser-AZE-ah-PEEN) USAN.
Use: Anxiolytic.

Sereen. (Foy Laboratories) Chlordiazepoxide hydrochloride 10 mg. Cap. Bot. 500s, 1000s. *c-IV.*
Use: Anxiolytic.

Sereine Cleaning Solution. (Optikem) Cocoamphodiacetate and glycols, EDTA 0.1%, benzalkonium Cl 0.01%. Soln. Bot. 60 mL. *OTC.*
Use: Contact lens care.

Sereine Wetting/Soaking Solution. (Optikem) EDTA 0.1%, benzalkonium Cl 0.01%. Soln. Bot. 120 mL. *OTC.*
Use: Contact lens care, soaking, wetting.

Sereine Wetting Solution. (Optikem) EDTA 0.1%, benzalkonium chloride 0.01%. Soln. Bot. 60 mL, 120 mL. *OTC.*
Use: Contact lens care.

Serene. (Health for Life Brands) Salicylamide 2 g, scopolamine aminoxide HBr 0.2 mg. Cap. Bot. 24s, 60s. *Rx.*
Use: Analgesic; sedative.

Serevent Diskus. (GlaxoSmithKline) Salmeterol xinafoate 50 mcg, lactose. Pow. for Inh. Blisters 28s, 60s. *Rx.*
Use: Bronchodilator, sympathomimetic.

•**sergliflozin.** (SER-gli-FLOE-zin) USAN.
Use: Antidiabetic.

•**sergolexole maleate.** (SER-go-LEX-ole) USAN.
Use: Antimigraine.

sericinase. A proteolytic enzyme.

•**serine.** (SER-een) *USP 34.*
Use: Amino acid.

•**serlopitant.** (ser-LOE-pi-tant) USAN.
Use: Genitourinary agent.

•**sermetacin.** (ser-MET-ah-sin) USAN.
Use: Anti-inflammatory.

•**sermorelin acetate.** (SER-moe-REH-lin) USAN.
Use: Growth hormone-releasing factor, diagnostic aid. [Orphan Drug]

Seromycin Pulvules. (Dura) Cycloserine 250 mg. Cap. Bot. 40s. *Rx.*
Use: Antituberculosis agent.

Serophene. (Serono) Clomiphene citrate 50 mg. Tab. Bot. 10s, 30s. *Rx.*
Use: Ovulation inducer; sex hormone.

Seroquel. (AstraZeneca) Quetiapine (as quetiapine fumarate) 25 mg, 50 mg, 100 mg, 200 mg, 300 mg, 400 mg. Lactose. Film-coated. Tab. Bot. 60s (300 mg only), 100s (except 300 mg), 1000s (25 mg and 50 mg only), UD 100s. *Rx.*
Tall Man: SEROquel
Use: Antipsychotic, dibenzapine derivative.

Seroquel XR. (AstraZeneca) Quetiapine 50 mg (equiv. to quetiapine fumarate 58 mg), 150 mg (equiv. to quetiapine fumarate 173 mg), 200 mg (equiv. to quetiapine fumarate 230 mg), 300 mg (equiv. to quetiapine fumarate 345 mg), 400 mg (equiv. to quetiapine fumarate 461 mg). Lactose. Film-coated. 60s, 500s (50 mg and 150 mg only), UD 100s. *Rx.*
Tall Man: SEROquel
Use: Antipsychotic, dibenzapine derivative.

Serostim. (Serono) Somatropin 4 mg/vial ($\approx$ 12 units), 5 mg/vial ($\approx$ 15 units), 6 mg/vial ($\approx$ 18 units), 8.8 mg/vial ($\approx$26.4 units). Sucrose. Inj. lyophilized Pow. for Soln. Single-use vial w/diluent (except 8.8 mg/vial). Multidose vial w/diluent (8.8 mg/vial only). *Rx.*
Use: Hormone, growth.

serotonin and norepinephrine reuptake inhibitors.
Use: Antidepressant.
See: Desvenlafaxine Succinate.
Duloxetine Hydrochloride.
Venlafaxine Hydrochloride.

serotonin 5-HT$_1$ receptor agonists.
Use: Antimigraine agents.
See: Almotriptan Malate.
Eletriptan Hydrobromide.
Frovatriptan Succinate.
Naratriptan Hydrochloride.
Rizatriptan Benzoate.
Sumatriptan Succinate.
Zolmitriptan.

serotonin reuptake inhibitors, selective.
Use: Antidepressant.
See: Citalopram Hydrochloride.
Escitalopram.
Fluoxetine Hydrochloride.
Fluvoxamine Maleate.
Paroxetine.
Sertraline Hydrochloride.

Serpasil-Apresoline. (Novartis)
#1: Reserpine 0.1 mg, hydralazine hydrochloride 25 mg. Tab. Bot. 100s.
#2: Reserpine 0.2 mg, hydralazine hydrochloride 50 mg. Tab. Bot. 100s. *Rx.*
Use: Antihypertensive combination.

Serpasil-Esidrix. (Novartis) **#1:** Reserpine 0.1 mg, hydrochlorothiazide 25 mg. Tab. **#2:** Reserpine 0.1 mg, hydrochlorothiazide 50 mg. Tab. Bot. 100s, 1000s. *Rx.*
Use: Antihypertensive combination.

Serpazide. (Major) Reserpine 0.1 mg, hydralazine hydrochloride 25 mg, hydrochlorothiazide 15 mg. Tab. Bot.

100s, 1000s. *Rx.*
Use: Antihypertensive combination.

Serratia marcescens extract (polyribosomes).
Use: Primary brain malignancies. [Orphan Drug]

Sertabs. (Table Rock) Reserpine 0.25 mg, 0.5 mg. Tab. Bot. 100s, 500s. *Rx.*
Use: Antihypertensive.

sertaconazole nitrate. (SIR-tah-KAHN-uh-zole)
Use: Antifungal agent, topical anti-infective.
See: Ertaczo.

Sertina. (Fellows) Reserpine 0.25 mg. Tab. Bot. 1000s, 5000s. *Rx.*
Use: Antihypertensive.

• **sertindole.** (ser-TIN-dole) USAN.
Use: Antipsychotic.

• **sertraline hydrochloride.** (SIR-truh-leen) USAN.
Use: Antidepressant, selective serotonin reuptake inhibitor.
See: Zoloft.

sertraline hydrochloride. (Ranbaxy Pharmaceuticals) Sertraline 20 mg/mL (as base). Alcohol 15.8%, menthol. Mint flavor. Oral Concentrate. Soln. Bot. 60 mL with calibrated droppers. *Rx.*
Use: Antidepressant, selective serotonin reuptake inhibitor.

sertraline hydrochloride. (Various Mfr.) Sertraline hydrochloride (as base) 25 mg, 50 mg, 100 mg. May contain lactose, polydextrose. Tab. 30s, 50s, 60s, 90s, 100s, 180s, 480s (except 25 mg), 500s, 1000s, 3000s (50 mg only), 5000s, UD 100s (except 25 mg). *Rx.*
Use: Antidepressant, selective serotonin reuptake inhibitor.

serum, albumin, human, radioiodinated.
See: Albumin Injection.

serum, albumin, normal human.
See: Albumin Human.

serum, globulin (human), immune.
Use: Immunization.

Serutan. (GlaxoSmithKline) Psyllium 2.5 g, sodium < 0.03 g/heaping tsp, saccharin, sugar. Gran. Can. 170 g, 540 g. *OTC.*
Use: Laxative.

• **sesame oil.** (SES-a-me) *NF 29.*
Use: Pharmaceutic aid (solvent; vehicle, oleaginous).

Sesame Street Complete. (McNeil Consumer) Ca 80 mg, Fe 10 mg, vitamins A 2750 units, D 200 units, E 10 mg, B$_1$

0.75 mg, B_2 0.85 mg, B_3 10 mg, B_5 5 mg, B_6 0.7 mg, B_{12} 3 mcg, C 40 mg, folic acid 0.2 mg, biotin 15 mg, Cu, I, Mg, Zn 8 mg. Lactose. Tab. Bot. 50s. *OTC.*
Use: Mineral, vitamin supplement.

Sesame Street Plus Iron. (McNeil Consumer) Fe 10 mg, vitamins A 2750 units, D 200 units, E 10 units, B_1 0.75 mg, B_2 0.85 mg, B_3 10 mg, B_5 5 mg, B_6 0.7 mg, B_{12} 3 mcg, C 40 mg, folic acid 0.2 mg. Chew. Tab. Bot. 50s. *OTC.*
Use: Mineral, vitamin supplement.

Sesame Street Vitamins. (McNeil Consumer) **For ages 4 and older:** Vitamins A 5,000 units, B_1 1.5 mg, B_{12} 6 mcg, C 60 mg, D 400 units, E 30 units, folic acid 400 mcg, biotin 300 mcg. Chew. Tab. Bot. 60s. **For ages 2 to 3:** Vitamins A 2,500 units, B_1 0.7 mg, B_2 0.8 mg, B_3 9 mg, B_5 5 mg, B_6 0.7 mg, B_{12} 3 mcg, C 40 mg, D 400 units, E 10 units, folic acid 200 mcg, biotin 150 mcg. Chew. Tab. Bot. 60s. *OTC.*
Use: Vitamin supplement.

Sesame Street Vitamins and Minerals. (McNeil Consumer) **For ages 4 and older:** Vitamins A 5,000 units, B_1 1.5 mg, B_2 1.7 mg, B_3 20 mg, B_5 10 mg, B_6 2 mg, B_{12} 6 mcg, C 60 mg, D 400 units, E 30 units, folic acid 400 mcg, biotin 300 mcg, Ca 100 mg, Fe 18 mg, I 150 mcg, Zn 15 mg, Cu 2 mg. Chew. Tab. Bot. 60s. **For ages 2 to 3:** Vitamins A 2,500 units, B_1 0.7 mg, B_{12} 3 mcg, C 40 mg, D 400 units, E 10 units, folic acid 200 mcg, biotin 150 mcg, Ca 80 mg, Fe 10 mg, I 70 mcg, Zn 8 mg, Cu 1 mg. Chew. Tab. Bot. 60s. *OTC.*
Use: Mineral, vitamin supplement.

Sethotope. (Bristol-Myers Squibb) Selenomethionine selenium 75; available as 0.25, 1 mCi.
Use: Diagnostic imaging.

• **setileuton.** (set-i-LOO-ton) USAN.
Use: Treatment of asthma.

• **setoperone.** (SEE-toe-per-OHN) USAN.
Use: Antipsychotic.

• **sevelamer carbonate.** (se-VEL-a-mer) USAN.
Use: Phosphate binder.
See: Renvela.

• **sevelamer hydrochloride.** (se-VEL-a-mer) USAN.
Use: Phosphate binder.
See: Renagel.

Severe Congestion Tussin. (AmerisourceBergen) Pseudoephedrine hydrochloride 30 mg, guaifenesin 200 mg. Sorbitol. Softgel. Pkg. 12s. *OTC.*
Use: Upper respiratory combination, decongestant, expectorant.

• **sevirumab.** (seh-VIE-roo-mab) USAN.
Use: Monoclonal antibody (antiviral).

• **sevoflurane.** (SEE-voe-FLEW-rane) USAN.
Use: Anesthetic, general, volatile liquid.
See: Sojourn.
Ultane.

sex hormones.
See: Anabolic Steroids.
Androgen Hormone Inhibitor.
Androgens.
Contraceptive Hormones.
Danazol.
Esterified Estrogens.
Estradiol.
Estradiol Cypionate.
Estradiol Topical Emulsion.
Estradiol Transdermal System.
Estradiol Valerate.
Estrogen and Androgen Combinations.
Estrogens.
Estrogens and Progestins Combined.
Estrogens, Conjugated.
Estrogens, Miscellaneous Topical.
Estrogens, Miscellaneous Vaginal.
Estrogens, Synthetic.
Estropipate.
Gonadotropin-Releasing Hormone Antagonists.
Gonadotropin-Releasing Hormones.
Ovulation Stimulants.
Progestins.
Raloxifene Hydrochloride.
Selective Estrogen Receptor Modulator.

• **sezolamide hydrochloride.** (seh-ZOLE-ah-MIDE) USAN.
Use: Carbonic anhydrase inhibitor.

SF 5000 Plus. (Cypress Pharmaceutical) Fluoride 1.1%. Glycerin, saccharin, sorbitol. Cream, dental. 51 g. *Rx.*
Use: Trace element.

SF 1.1%. (Cypress) Fluoride 0.5% Parabens, saccharin, sorbitol. Mint flavor. Gel, dental. 56 g. *Rx.*
Use: Trace element.

sfRowasa. (Alaven) Mesalamine 4 g per 60 mL. Edetate disodium. Sulfite free. Susp. 7s, 14s, 28s. *Rx.*
Use: Gastrointestinal agent.

Shade. (Schering-Plough) SPF 15. Contains one or more of the following ingredients: Padimate O, oxybenzone, ethylhexyl-p-methoxycinnamate. Bot.

118 mL, 120 mL, 240 mL. *OTC.*
Use: Sunscreen.
Shade Cream. (O'Leary) Jar 0.25 oz.
OTC.
Use: Contouring cream.
Shade Sunblock Gel, 15 SPF. (Schering-Plough) Ethylhexyl p-methoxycinnamate, octyl salicylate, oxybenzone, SD alcohol 40. PABA free. SPF 15. Waterproof. Gel. Bot. 120 mL. *OTC.*
Use: Sunscreen.
Shade Sunblock Gel, 30 SPF. (Schering-Plough) Ethylhexyl p-methoxycinnamate, homosalate, oxybenzone, 73% SD alcohol 40. Bot. 120 mL. *OTC.*
Use: Sunscreen.
Shade Sunblock Gel, 25 SPF. (Schering-Plough) Ethylhexyl p-methoxycinnamate, octyl salicylate, homosalate, oxybenzone, SD alcohol 40. PABA free. Gel. Bot. 120 mL. *OTC.*
Use: Sunscreen.
Shade Sunblock Lotion, 15 SPF.
(Schering-Plough) Ethylhexyl p-methoxycinnamate, oxybenzone, benzyl alcohol, phenethyl alcohol. PABA free. Waterproof. Lot. Bot. 120 mL. *OTC.*
Use: Sunscreen.
Shade Sunblock Lotion, 45 SPF.
(Schering-Plough) Ethylhexyl p-methoxycinnamate, oxybenzone, 2-ethylhexyl salicylate, benzyl alcohol, phenethyl alcohol. PABA free. Waterproof. Lot. Bot. 120 mL. *OTC.*
Use: Sunscreen.
Shade Sunblock Lotion, 30 SPF.
(Schering-Plough) Ethylhexyl p-methoxycinnamate, 2-ethylhexyl salicylate, homosalate, oxybenzone, benzyl alcohol, phenethyl alcohol. PABA free. Waterproof. Lot. Bot. 120 mL. *OTC.*
Use: Sunscreen.
Shade Sunblock Stick, 30 SPF.
(Schering-Plough) Ethylhexyl p-methoxycinnamate, oxybenzone, 2-ethylhexyl salicylate, homosalate. PABA free. Waterproof. Stick. 18 g. *OTC.*
Use: Sunscreen.
Shade UVA Guard. (Schering-Plough) Octyl methoxycinnamate 7.5%, avobenzone 3%, oxybenzone 3%. Waterproof. SPF 15. Lot. 120 mL. *OTC.*
Use: Sunscreen.
Sheik Elite. (Durex) Condom with nonoxynol-9 15%. 3s, 12s, 24s, 36s. *OTC.*
Use: Contraceptive.
•**shellac.** (she-LAK) *NF 29.*
Use: Pharmaceutic aid (tablet coating agent).

Shellgel. (Cytosol Ophthalmics) Sodium hyaluronate 12 mg/mL, sodium chloride 9 mg/mL. Inj. Disposable syringes. 0.8 mL. *Rx.*
Use: Ophthalmic surgical adjunct.
Shepard's Cream Lotion. (Dermik) Creamy lotion with no lanolin or mineral oil, for entire body. Scented or unscented. Bot. 8 oz, 16 oz. *OTC.*
Use: Emollient.
Sherhist. (Sheryl) Phenylephrine hydrochloride, pyrilamine maleate. Tab. Bot. 100s. Liq. Bot. Pt.
Use: Decongestant; antihistamine.
Shernatal. (Sheryl) Phosphorus free calcium, non-irritating iron, trace minerals and essential vitamins. Tab. Bot. 100s. *OTC.*
Use: Mineral, vitamin supplement.
Shohl's solution. Sodium Citrate and Citric Acid. Oral Soln.
Use: Alkalizer, systemic.
short chain fatty acid solution.
Use: Ulcerative colitis. [Orphan Drug]
Shur-Clens. (GlaxoSmithKline) Poloxamer 188 20%. Soln. Bot. UD 100 mL, 200 mL. *OTC.*
Use: Dermatologic.
Shur Seal Gel. (Milex) Nonoxynol-9 2. 24 UD gel paks. *OTC.*
Use: Contraceptive, spermicide.
Sibelium. (Janssen) Flunarizine hydrochloride. *Rx.*
Use: Vasodilator.
•**sibenadet hydrochloride.** (si-BEN-a-det) USAN.
Use: Chronic obstructive pulmonary disease.
•**sibopirdine.** (sih-BOE-pihr-deen) USAN.
Use: Nootropic; cognition enhancer (Alzheimer disease).
•**sibrafran.** (sib-rah-FIE-ban) USAN.
Use: Antithrombotic; fibrinogen receptor antagonist; platelet aggregation inhibitor.
•**sibutramine hydrochloride.** (sih-BYOO-trah-meen) USAN.
Use: Antidepressant, CNS stimulant, anorexic.
See: Meridia.
sickle cell test.
Use: Diagnostic aid.
See: Sickledex.
Sickledex. (Ortho-Clinical Diagnostics) Test kit 12s, 100s.
Use: Diagnostic aid to detect hemoglobin S.
•**sifalimumab.** (SYE-fa-LIM-ue-mab) USAN.
Use: Monoclonal antibody.

Sigamine. (Sigma-Tau) Cyanocobalamin injection 1000 mcg/mL. Vial 10 mL, 30 mL. Also Sigamine L.A. Vial 10 mL. *Rx.*
Use: Vitamin supplement.

Sigazine. (Sigma-Tau) Promethazine hydrochloride 50 mg/mL. Vial 10 mL. *Rx.*
Use: Antihistamine.

Signa Creme. (Parker) Conductive cosmetic quality electrolyte cream. Bot. 5 oz, 2 L, 4 L. *OTC.*
Use: Diagnostic aid.

Signa Gel. (Parker) Conductive saline electrode gel. Tube 250 g.
Use: Diagnostic aid, gel.

Signa Pad. (Parker) Premoistened electrode pads.
Use: Diagnostic aid, pad.

Signatal C. (Sigma-Tau) Ca 230 mg, Fe 49.3 mg, vitamins A 4,000 units, D 400 units, B_1 2 mg, B_2 2 mg, B_6 1 mg, B_{12} 2 mcg, folic acid 0.1 mg, niacinamide 10 mg, C 50 mg, I 0.15 mg. SC Tab. Bot. 100s, 1000s. *OTC.*
Use: Mineral, vitamin supplement.

Signate. (Sigma-Tau) Dimenhydrinate 50 mg, propylene glycol 50%, benzyl alcohol 5%/mL. Vial 10 mL. *Rx.*
Use: Antiemetic; antivertigo.

Signef "Supps". (Fellows) Hydrocortisone 15 mg. Supp. 12s. w/ or w/o applicator. *Rx.*
Use: Corticosteroid, vaginal.

Sigpred. (Sigma-Tau) Prednisolone acetate. Vial 10 mL. *Rx.*
Use: Corticosteroid.

Sigtab. (Roberts) Vitamins A 5,000 units, D 400 units, B_1 10.3 mg, B_2 10 mg, C 333 mg, B_3 100 mg, B_6 6 mg, B_5 20 mg, folic acid 0.4 mg, B_{12} 18 mcg, E 15 mg. Tab. Bot. 90s, 500s. *OTC.*
Use: Vitamin supplement.

Sigtab-M. (Roberts) Vitamins A 6000 units, D_3 400 units, E 45 mg, C 100 mg, B_3 25 mg, B_1 5 mg, B_2 5 mg, B_6 3 mg, folic acid 400 mcg, B_5 0.015 mg, biotin 45 mcg, Ca 200 mg, P, Fe 18 mg, Mg, Cu, Zn 15 mg, Mn, K, Cl, Mo, Se, Cr, Ni, Sn, V, Si, B, vitamin K, I. Tab. Bot. 100s. *OTC.*
Use: Mineral, vitamin supplement.

Silace. (Silarx) Docusate sodium. **Liq.:** 10 mg/mL. Parabens. 473 mL. **Syrup:** 60 mg/15 mL. Alcohol ≤ 1%. Bot. 473 mL. *OTC.*
Use: Laxative.

Siladryl. (Silarx) Diphenhydramine hydrochloride 12.5 mg/5 mL. Black cherry flavoring, parabens, propylene glycol, saccharin, sorbitol. Alcohol free

and sugar free. Liq. 118 mL, 237 mL. *OTC.*
Use: Antihistamine, nonselective ethanolamine.

Silafed. (Silarx) Pseudoephedrine hydrochloride 30 mg, triprolidine hydrochloride 1.25 mg/5 mL. Methylparaben, sucrose, saccharin. Syrup. Bot. 118 mL. *OTC.*
Use: Upper respiratory combination, antihistamine and decongestant combination.

•**silafilcon A.** (SIH-lah-FILL-kahn A) USAN.
Use: Contact lens material (hydrophilic).

•**silafocon A.** (SIH-lah-FOH-kahn A) USAN.
Use: Contact lens material (hydrophobic).

•**silandrone.** (sil-AN-drone) USAN.
Use: Androgen.

Silapap Children's. (Silarx) Acetaminophen. **Elix.:** 160 mg/5 mL. Alcohol free. Bot. 237 mL. **Liq.:** 160 mg/5 mL. Alcohol and sugar free. Methylparaben, saccharin. 118 mL, 237 mL, 473 mL. *OTC.*
Use: Analgesic.

Silapap Infant's. (Silarx) Acetaminophen 100 mg/mL. Alcohol free. Soln., Conc., Oral. 15 mL, 30 mL. *OTC.*
Use: Analgesic.

Sildec. (Silarx) **Drops:** Pseudoephedrine hydrochloride 15 mg, carbinoxamine maleate 1 mg per 1 mL. Saccharin, sorbitol. 30 mL with dropper. **Syrup:** Pseudoephedrine hydrochloride 15 mg, brompheniramine maleate 4 mg. Saccharin, sorbitol. Raspberry flavor. 120 mL, 480 mL. *Rx.*
Use: Upper respiratory combination, decongestant and antihistamine.

Sildec-DM. (Silarx) Pseudoephedrine hydrochloride 45 mg, dextromethorphan HBr 15 mg, brompheniramine maleate 4 mg per 5 mL. Saccharin, sorbitol, grape flavor. Syrup. Bot. 118 mL, 473 mL. *Rx.*
Use: Upper respiratory combination, antihistamine, antitussive, decongestant.

•**sildenafil citrate.** (sill-DEN-ah-fil SIH-trate) USAN.
Use: Anti-impotence agent.
See: Revatio.
   Viagra.

Silenor. (Somaxon Pharmaceuticals) Doxepin 3 mg (equiv. to doxepin hydrochloride 3.39 mg), 6 mg (equiv. to doxepin hydrochloride 6.78 mg). Tab.

30s, 100s, 500s, UD 30s. *Rx.*
Use: Antidepressant, tricyclic compound.

• **silica, dental-type.** (SILL-ih-kah) *NF 29.*
Use: Pharmaceutic aid.

• **siliceous earth, purified.** (sih-LIH-shus) *NF 29.*
Use: Pharmaceutic aid (filtering medium).

• **silicon dioxide.** (SILL-ih-kahn die-OX-ide) *NF 29. Formerly Silica Gel.*
Use: Pharmaceutic aid (dispersing and suspending agent).
W/Calcium Chloride, Dibasic Sodium Phosphate, Monobasic Sodium Phosphate, Sodium Chloride, Sodium Bicarbonate.
See: NeutraSal.

• **silicon dioxide, colloidal.** (SILL-ih-kahn die-OX-ide) *NF 29.*
Use: Pharmaceutic aid (tablet/capsule diluent, suspending and thickening agent).

Silicone. (Dow Hickam) Dimethicone. Liq., Bot. oz. Bulk Pkg. Oint.

silicone oil.
See: Polydimethylsiloxane (Silicone Oil).

silicone ointment. Dimethicone Dimethyl Polysiloxane.

silicone powder. (Gordon Laboratories) Talc with silicone. Pkg. 4 oz, 1 lb, 5 lb. *OTC.*
Use: Dusting powder.

silodosin. (sil-OH-doe-sin)
Use: Antiadrenergic agent, peripherally acting; alpha-1–adrenergic blocker.
See: Rapaflo.

• **silodrate.** (SILL-oh-drate) *USAN.*
Use: Antacid.

Silphen Cough. (Silarx) Diphenhydramine hydrochloride 12.5 mg/5 mL, alcohol 5%, menthol, sucrose, parabens, strawberry flavor. Syr. Bot. 118 mL. *OTC.*
Use: Antihistamine.

Silphen DM. (Silarx) Dextromethorphan HBr 10 mg/5 mL. Alcohol 5%, menthol, methylparaben, sucrose. Syrup. Bot. 118 mL. *OTC.*
Use: Nonnarcotic antitussive.

Sil-Tex. (Silarx) Phenylephrine hydrochloride 7.5 mg, guaifenesin 100 mg per 5 mL. Alcohol, sugar, and dye free. Saccharin, sorbitol. Punch flavor. Liq. 473 mL. *Rx.*
Use: Upper respiratory combination, decongestant and expectorant combination.

Siltussin DAS. (Silarx) Guaifenesin 100 mg/5 mL. Strawberry flavor. Liq. 118 mL. *OTC.*
Use: Expectorant.

Siltussin DM. (Silarx) Dextromethorphan HBr 10 mg, guaifenesin 100 mg/5 mL. Saccharin, sucrose, methylparaben, menthol. Alcohol free. Liq. Bot. 118 mL, 237 mL, 473 mL. *OTC.*
Use: Upper respiratory combination, antitussive, expectorant.

Siltussin DM Cough. (Silarx) Dextromethorphan HBr 10 mg, guaifenesin 100 mg per 5 mL. Alcohol free. Sucrose, saccharin, methylparaben. Syrup. 118 mL. *OTC.*
Use: Antitussive with expectorant.

Siltussin SA. (Silarx) Guaifenesin 100 mg/5 mL, strawberry flavor. Liq. 118 mL, 237 mL, 473 mL. *OTC.*
Use: Expectorant.

• **siltuximab.** (sil-TUX-i-mab) *USAN.*
Use: Antineoplastic.

Silvadene. (Hoechst Marion Roussel) Silver sulfadiazine 10 mg/g in a water–miscible base. Contains white petrolatum, stearyl alcohol, methylparaben 0.3%. Cream. 20 g, 50 g, 85 g, 400 g, 1000 g. *Rx.*
Use: Anti-infective, topical.

silver.
See: Elta SilverGel.

silver compounds.
See: Silver Nitrate.
Silver Protein, Mild.
Silver Protein, Strong.

• **silver nitrate.** (SILL-ver NYE-trate) *USP 34.*
Use: Anti-infective, topical.
W/Potassium Nitrate.
See: Grafco.

• **silver nitrate, toughened.** (SILL-ver NYE-trate) *USP 34.*
Use: Caustic.

silver protein, mild. Argentum Vitellinum, Cargentos, Mucleinate Mild, Protargin Mild.

silver protein, strong.
See: Protargol.

silver sulfadiazine. (SILL-ver SULL-fah-DIE-ah-zeen)
Use: Anti-infective, topical.
See: Silvadene.
SSD.
SSD AF.
Thermazene.

Simcor. (Abbott) Niacin (extended release)/simvastatin 500 mg/20 mg, 500 mg/40 mg, 750 mg/20 mg, 1,000 mg/40 mg. Lactose, PEG.

ER Tab. 90s. *Rx.*
Use: Antihyperlipidemic.

•**simenepag.** (sye-MEN-e-pag) USAN.
Use: Ophthalmic agent.

•**simenepag isopropyl.** (sye-MEN-e-pag) USAN.
Use: Ophthalmic agent.

•**simeprevir.** (sim-E-pre-vir) USAN.
Use: Treatment of hepatitis C.

•**simethicone.** (sih-METH-ih-cone)
USP 34. Mixture of liquid dimethyl polysiloxanes with silica aerogel.
Use: Antiflatulent.
See: Baby Gas-X Infant.
   Bicarsim.
   Bicarsim Forte.
   Gas Relief.
   Gas-X Extra Strength.
   Gas-X Thin Strips.
   Mylanta Gas.
   Mylanta Gas, Maximum Strength.
   Mylicon.
   Mylicon-80.
   Phazyme.
   Phazyme Quick Dissolve.
W/Aluminum Hydroxide, Magnesium Hydroxide.
See: Maalox Advanced Maximum Strength.
   Maalox Advanced Regular Strength.
   Mi-Acid Maximum Strength.
W/Calcium Carbonate.
See: Maalox Junior.
   Rolaids Extra Strength Plus Gas Relief.
W/Citric Acid, Sodium Bicarbonate.
See: E-Z Gas II.
W/Combinations.
See: Di-Gel.
   Gas-Ban.
   Gas-X with Maalox Extra Strength.
   Mintox.
   Mylanta Maximum Strength.
   Mylanta Regular Strength.
   Rolaids Multi-Symptom.
   Trial AG.
W/Loperadmide Hydrochloride.
See: Imodium Multi-Symptom Relief.

Similac Human Milk Fortifier. (Ross) Protein (nonfat milk, whey protein concentrate) 1 g, carbohydrate (corn syrup solids) 1.8 g, fat (fractionated coconut oil [medium chain triglycerides], soy lecithin) 0.36 g per 4 packets (3.6 g), with vitamins A, B_1, B_2, B_3, B_5, B_6, B_{12}, C, D, E, K, folic acid (folacin), biotin, Ca, chloride, Cu, Fe, Mg, Mn, P, Zn, Na 15 mg, K 63 mg, 14 cal/3.6 g. Add to breast milk. Pow. Pkt. 0.9 g (50s). *OTC.*
Use: Enteral nutritional therapy.

Similac Low-Iron Liquid & Powder. (Ross) Protein 14.3 g, carbohydrates 72 g, fat 36 g, Fe 1.5 mg, with appropriate vitamins and minerals. **Liq.:** 390 mL concentrate, 240 mL and 1 qt. ready-to-use, 120 mL and 240 mL nursettes. **Pow.:** 1 lb. *OTC.*
Use: Nutritional supplement.

Similac Natural Care Human Milk Fortifier. (Ross) Liquid fortifier designed to be mixed with human milk or fed alternately with human milk to low-birth-weight infants. Supplied as 24 Cal/fl oz. Bot. 4 fl oz. *OTC.*
Use: Nutritional supplement.

Similac PM 60/40. (Ross) Milk-based formula ready-to-feed or powder with 60:40 whey to casein ratio (20 Cal/fl oz). **Bot.:** Hospital use 4 fl oz. ready-to-feed. **Pow.:** Can lb. *OTC.*
Use: Nutritional supplement.

Similac Special Care 20. (Ross) Infant formula ready-to-feed (20 Cal/fl oz). Bot. 4 fl oz. *OTC.*
Use: Nutritional supplement.

Similac Special Care 24. (Ross) Infant formula ready-to-feed (24 Cal/fl oz). Bot. 4 fl oz. *OTC.*
Use: Nutritional supplement.

Similac 13/Similac 13 with Iron. (Ross) Milk-based infant formula ready-to-feed containing 13 calories/fl oz, 1.8 mg Fe/100 calories. Bot. 4 fl. oz. *OTC.*
Use: Nutritional supplement.

Similac 24 LBW. (Ross) Low-iron infant formula, ready-to-feed, 24 calories/fl oz. Bot. 4 fl oz. *OTC.*
Use: Nutritional supplement.

Similac 24/Similac 24 with Iron. (Ross) Milk-based infant formula ready-to-feed (24 cal/fl oz), Fe 1.8 mg/100 calories. Bot. 4 fl oz. *OTC.*
Use: Nutritional supplement.

Similac 27. (Ross) Milk-based ready-to-feed infant formula (27 cal/fl oz). Bot. 4 fl oz. *OTC.*
Use: Nutritional supplement.

Similac 20/Similac with Iron 20. (Ross) Milk-based infant formula. Standard dilution (20 cal/fl oz). Similac with iron: Fe 1.8 mg/100 cal. **Pow.:** Can lb. **Concentrated Liq.:** Can 13 fl oz. **Ready-to-feed:** Can 8 fl oz, 32 fl oz. Bot. 4 fl oz, 8 fl oz. *OTC.*
Use: Nutritional supplement.

•**simotaxel.** (sim-oh-TAX-el) USAN.
Use: Antineoplastic.

Simplet. (Major) Pseudoephedrine hydrochloride 60 mg, chlorpheniramine maleate 4 mg, acetaminophen 650 mg. Tab. Bot. 100s. *OTC.*

Use: Upper respiratory combination, analgesic, antihistamine, decongestant.

Simply Cough. (McNeil) Dextromethorphan HBr 5 mg/5 mL. Corn syrup, sucralose, alcohol free, cherry berry flavor. Liq. 120 mL. *OTC.*
Use: Nonnarcotic antitussive.

Simply Saline. (Blairex) Sodium chloride. Soln. Spray bot. 44 mL. *OTC.*
Use: Nasal decongestant.

Simply Sleep. (McNeil) Diphenhydramine hydrochloride 25 mg. Tab. 24s, 48s. *OTC.*
Use: Nonprescription sleep aid.

Simply Stuffy. (McNeil) Pseudoephedrine hydrochloride 30 mg. Lactose. Tab. Pkg. 24s. *OTC.*
Use: Nasal decongestant, arylalkylamine.

Simponi. (Centocor Ortho Biotech) Golimumab 50 mg per 0.5 mL. Preservative free. Inj., Soln. Single-dose prefilled syringe, prefilled *SmartJect* autoinjector (needle cover on the prefilled syringe and on the prefilled syringe in the autoinjector contains dry natural rubber, a derivative of latex). *Rx.*
Use: Immunologic agent, immunomodulator.

Simron Plus. (GlaxoSmithKline) Fe 10 mg, vitamins B_{12} 3.33 mcg, C 50 mg, B_6 1 mg, folic acid 0.1 mg. Cap. Parabens. Bot. 100s. *OTC.*
Use: Mineral supplement.

• **simtrazene.** (SIM-trah-seen) USAN.
Use: Antineoplastic.

Simuc-GP. (Cypress) Phenylephrine hydrochloride 25 mg, guaifenesin 1200 mg. ER Tab. 100s. *Rx.*
Use: Upper respiratory combination, decongestant and expectorant combination.

Simulect. (Novartis) Basiliximab 200 mg, sucrose, mannitol, potassium phosphate, sodium chloride, preservative free. Pow. for Inj., lyophilized. Single-use vial. *Rx.*
Use: Immunologic, immunosuppressive.

• **simvastatin.** (SIM-vuh-STAT-in) *USP 34.*
Formerly Synvinolin.
Use: Antihyperlipidemic, HMG-CoA reductase inhibitor.
See: Zocor.

simvastatin. (Synthon Pharmaceuticals) Simvastatin 10 mg, 20 mg, 40 mg, 80 mg. Sucralose. Tab., Disintegrating. 30s, 90s. *Rx.*
Use: Antihyperlipidemic agent, HMG-CoA reductase inhibitors.

simvastatin. (Various Mfr.) Simvastatin 5 mg (film-coated), 10 mg, 20 mg, 40 mg, 80 mg. May contain lactose. Tab. 30s, 60s (5 mg only); 90s (5 mg, 80 mg only); 500s (5 mg only); 1000s (5 mg, 80 mg only); unit-of-use 30s (80 mg only); UD 100s (except 5 mg, 80 mg). *Rx.*
Use: Antihyperlipidemic, HMG-CoA reductase inhibitor.

simvastatin/ezetimibe.
Use: Antihyperlipidemic.
See: Vytorin.

simvastatin/niacin.
Use: Antihyperlipidemic.
See: Simcor.

Sinadrin PE. (Reese) Acetaminophen 650 mg, dexbrompheniramine 2 mg, phenylephrine hydrochloride 10 mg. Dye free. Tab. 30s. *OTC.*
Use: Upper respiratory combination; decongestant, antihistamine, and analgesic combination.

• **sinapultide.** (si-na-PUL-tide) USAN.
Use: Treatment of respiratory distress syndrome (pulmonary surfactant).

Sinarest Decongestant. (Novartis) Oxymetazoline hydrochloride 0.05%. Spray. Bot. 0.5 oz. *OTC.*
Use: Decongestant.

Sinarest Extra-Strength. (Novartis) Acetaminophen 500 mg, chlorpheniramine maleate 2 mg, pseudoephedrine hydrochloride 30 mg. Tab. 24s. *OTC.*
Use: Analgesic; antihistamine; decongestant.

Sinarest No Drowsiness. (Novartis) Pseudoephedrine hydrochloride 30 mg, acetaminophen 500 mg. Tab. Pkg. 20s. *OTC.*
Use: Analgesic; decongestant.

Sinarest Sinus. (Novartis) Acetaminophen 325 mg, chlorpheniramine maleate 2 mg, pseudoephedrine hydrochloride 30 mg. Tab. Pkg. 20s, 40s, 80s. *OTC.*
Use: Analgesic; antihistamine; decongestant.

Sinarest 12 Hour. (Novartis) Oxymetazoline hydrochloride 0.05%. Nasal Spray Bot. 15 mL. *OTC.*
Use: Decongestant.

Sina-12X. (MedPointe) **Oral Susp.:** Phenylephrine tannate 5 mg, guaifenesin 100 mg per 5 mL. Methylparaben, saccharin, sucrose. Grape flavor. 118 mL. **Tab.:** Phenylephrine tannate 25 mg, guaifenesin 200 mg. 30s. *Rx.*
Use: Upper respiratory combination, decongestant and expectorant combination.

• **sincalide.** (SIN-kah-lide) USAN.
Use: Choleretic, diagnostic aid, gastro-intestinal function test.
See: Kinevac.

Sine-Aid IB. (McNeil Consumer) Pseudo-ephedrine 30 mg, ibuprofen 200 mg. Capl. Pkg. 20s. *OTC.*
Use: Analgesic; decongestant.

Sine-Aid Sinus Headache. (McNeil Consumer) Acetaminophen 325 mg, pseudoephedrine hydrochloride 30 mg. Tab. Bot. 24s, 50s, 100s. *OTC.*
Use: Analgesic; decongestant.

Sine-Aid Sinus Headache, Extra Strength. (McNeil Consumer) Aceta-minophen 500 mg, pseudoephedrine hydrochloride 30 mg. Capl. Bot. 24s, 50s. *OTC.*
Use: Analgesic; decongestant.

• **sinefungin.** (sih-neh-FUN-jin) USAN.
Use: Antifungal.

Sinemet CR. (Merck Sharp & Dohme) Carbidopa 25 mg, 50 mg, levodopa 100 mg, 200 mg. ER Tab. Bot. 100s, 500s, UD 100s. *Rx.*
Use: Antiparkinson agent.

Sinemet 10/100. (Merck Sharp & Dohme) Carbidopa 10 mg, levodopa 100 mg. Tab. Bot. 100s, UD 100s. *Rx.*
Use: Antiparkinson agent.

Sinemet 25/100. (Merck Sharp & Dohme) Carbidopa 25 mg, levodopa 100 mg. Tab. Bot. 100s, UD 100s. *Rx.*
Use: Antiparkinson agent.

Sinemet 25/250. (Merck Sharp & Dohme) Carbidopa 25 mg, levodopa 250 mg. Tab. Bot. 100s, UD 100s. *Rx.*
Use: Antiparkinson agent.

Sine-Off Cough/Cold. (Hogil) Phenyl-ephrine hydrochloride 5 mg, dextro-methorphan HBr 15 mg, guaifenesin 200 mg, acetaminophen 325 mg. Tab. 24s. *OTC.*
Use: Upper respiratory combination, de-congestant, antihistamine, and expec-torant combination.

Sine-Off Multi Symptom Relief Severe Cold. (Hogil) Acetaminophen 325 mg, guaifenesin 200 mg, phenylephrine hydrochloride 5 mg. Tab. 24s. *OTC.*
Use: Upper respiratory combination, an-titussive and expectorant combina-tion.

Sine-Off Non-Drowsy Maximum Strength. (Hogil) Phenylephrine hydro-chloride 5 mg, acetaminophen 325 mg. Tab. Pkg. 12s. *OTC.*
Use: Upper respiratory combination, de-congestant, analgesic.

Sine-Off Sinus/Cold. (Hogil) Phenyl-ephrine hydrochloride 5 mg, chlor-pheniramine maleate 2 mg, acetamino-phen 500 mg. Tab. 24s. *OTC.*
Use: Upper respiratory combination, de-congestant, antihistamine, and anal-gesic combination.

Sinequan. (Roerig) Doxepin hydrochlo-ride. **Cap.:** 10 mg, 25 mg, 50 mg, 75 mg, 100 mg, 150 mg. 50s (150 mg only), 100s (except 150 mg), 500s (150 mg only), 1000s (except 150 mg), 5000s (25 mg, 50 mg only). **Oral Conc.:** 10 mg/mL. Parabens, pepper-mint oil, sorbitol. 118 mL w/calibrated dropper. *Rx.*
Tall Man: SINEquan
Use: Antidepressant.

Singlet for Adults. (GlaxoSmithKline) Pseudoephedrine hydrochloride 60 mg, chlorpheniramine maleate 4 mg, aceta-minophen 650 mg, sucrose. Tab. Bot. 100s. *OTC.*
Use: Upper respiratory combination, an-algesic, antihistamine, decongestant.

Singulair. (Merck) Montelukast. **Chew. Tab.:** 4 mg (equiv. to montelukast so-dium 4.2 mg), 5 mg (equiv. to mon-telukast sodium 5.2 mg). Aspartame, mannitol, phenylalanine 0.674 mg (4 mg only), 0.842 mg (5 mg only), cherry flavor. Unit-of-use 30s, 90s, UD 100s. **Gran.:** 4 mg/packet (equiv. to montelukast sodium 4.2 mg). Mannitol. 30 packets. **Tab.:** 10 mg (equiv. to montelukast sodium 10.4 mg). Lactose. Film-coated. Unit-of-use 30s, 90s, UD 100s, 8000s. *Rx.*
Use: Leukotriene receptor antagonist.

Sino-Eze MLT. (Global Source) Salicyl-amide 3.5 g, acetaminophen 100 mg, phenylephrine hydrochloride 5 mg, chlorpheniramine maleate 2 mg. Tab. Bot. 1000s. *Rx.*
Use: Upper respiratory combination, an-algesic, antihistamine, decongestant.

Sinografin. (Bracco Diagnostics) Dia-trizoate meglumine 527 mg, iodipamide meglumine 268 mg, iodine 380 mg/mL. EDTA. Inj. Vials. 10 mL. *Rx.*
Use: Radiopaque agent.

Sinufed Timecelle. (Roberts) Pseudo-ephedrine hydrochloride 60 mg, guai-fenesin 300 mg. Cap. Bot. 100s. *Rx.*
Use: Upper respiratory combination, de-congestant, expectorant.

Sinuhist. (Dexo) Brompheniramine maleate 6 mg, pseudoephedrine hydro-chloride 45 mg. Dye free. Tab. 100s. *Rx.*
Use: Upper respiratory combination, de-congestant and antihistamine.

Sinumist-SR. (Roberts) Guaifenesin 600 mg. Tab. Bot. 100s. *Rx.*
Use: Upper respiratory combination, expectorant.

Sinupan. (ION Laboratories, Inc.) Phenylephrine hydrochloride 40 mg, guaifenesin 200 mg. SR Cap. Bot. 100s. *Rx.*
Use: Upper respiratory combination, decongestant, expectorant.

Sinus Excedrin Extra Strength. (Bristol-Myers Squibb) Pseudoephedrine hydrochloride 30 mg, acetaminophen 500 mg. Tab or Cap. Bot. 50s. *OTC.*
Use: Upper respiratory combination, decongestant, analgesic.

Sinus Headache & Congestion. (Rugby) Pseudoephedrine hydrochloride 30 mg, chlorpheniramine maleate 2 mg, acetaminophen 500 mg. Tab. Bot. 100s, 1000s. *OTC.*
Use: Upper respiratory combination, decongestant, antihistamine, analgesic.

Sinus Pain Formula Allerest. (Medeva) Pseudoephedrine hydrochloride 30 mg, chlorpheniramine maleate 2 mg, acetaminophen 500 mg. **Cap.:** Bot. 24s, 50s. **Gelcap:** Bot. 20s, 40s. *OTC.*
Use: Upper respiratory combination, analgesic, antihistamine, decongestant.

Sinus Relief. (Major) Pseudoephedrine hydrochloride 30 mg, acetaminophen 325 mg. Tab. Bot. 24s, 100s, 1000s. *OTC.*
Use: Upper respiratory combination, decongestant, analgesic.

Sinus-Relief Maximum Strength. (Major) Pseudoephedrine hydrochloride 30 mg, acetaminophen 500 mg, dextrose. Tab. Pkg. 24s. *OTC.*
Use: Upper respiratory combination, decongestant, analgesic.

Sinus Tablets. (Walgreen) Acetaminophen 325 mg, chlorpheniramine maleate 2 mg, pseudoephedrine hydrochloride mg. Tab. Bot. 30s. *OTC.*
Use: Upper respiratory combination, analgesic, antihistamine, decongestant.

Sinustop. (Nature's Way) Pseudoephedrine hydrochloride 60 mg, echinacea purpura, ginger, goldenseal root. Cap. Pkg. 20s. *OTC.*
Use: Nasal decongestant, arylakylamine.

Sinutab Maximum Strength Sinus Allergy. (J&J Consumer) Acetaminophen 500 mg, pseudoephedrine hydrochloride 30 mg, chlorpheniramine maleate 2 mg. Tab. or Capl. 24s. *OTC.*
Use: Upper respiratory combination, analgesic, antihistamine, decongestant.

Sinutab Non-Drying. (McNeil) Phenylephrine hydrochloride 5 mg, guaifenesin 200 mg. Cap. 24s. *OTC.*
Use: Upper respiratory combination, decongestant and expectorant combination.

Sinutab Sinus. (Pfizer) Phenylephrine hydrochloride 5 mg, acetaminophen 325 mg. PEG. Tab. Pkg. 24s. *OTC.*
Use: Upper respiratory combination, decongestant, analgesic.

Sinutab Sinus Maximum Strength Without Drowsiness Formula. (Pfizer) Acetaminophen 500 mg, pseudoephedrine hydrochloride 30 mg. Tab or Cap. Pack 24s. *OTC.*
Use: Upper respiratory combination, analgesic, decongestant.

Sinutab Sinus Regular Strength Without Drowsiness. (Pfizer) Pseudoephedrine hydrochloride 30 mg, acetaminophen 325 mg. Tab. Bot. 24s. *OTC.*
Use: Upper respiratory combination, analgesic, decongestant.

Sinutab Sinus Without Drowsiness Regular Strength. (Pfizer) Pseudoephedrine hydrochloride 30 mg, acetaminophen 325 mg. Tab. Pkg. 24s. *OTC.*
Use: Upper respiratory combination, decongestant, analgesic.

SINUtuss DM. (Dexo Pharma) Dextromethorphan HBr 30 mg, guaifenesin 600 mg, phenylephrine hydrochloride 15 mg. Tab. 100s. *Rx.*
Use: Upper respiratory combination, antitussive and expectorant combination.

SINUvent PE. (WE Pharm) Phenylephrine hydrochloride 15 mg, guaifenesin 600 mg. ER Tab. 100s. *Rx.*
Use: Upper respiratory combination, decongestant and expectorant combination.

•**siplizumab.** (sip-LIZ-oo-mab) USAN.
Use: Monoclonal antibody.

•**sipuleucel-T.** (SYE-pul-oo-sel) USAN.
Use: Investigational antineoplastic.

Siroil. (Siroil) Mercuric oleate, cresol, vegetable and mineral oil. Emulsion Bot. 8 oz. *OTC.*
Use: Antiseptic.

sir-o-lene.
Use: Emollient.

•**sirolimus.** (SER-oh-lih-muss) USAN. *Formerly Rapamycin.*
Use: Immunologic, immunosuppressive.
See: Rapamune.

•**sirukumab.** (si-RUK-ue-mab) USAN.
Use: Antirheumatic agent.

•**sisomicin.** (SIS-oh-MY-sin) USAN.
Use: Anti-infective.
•**sisomicin sulfate.** (SIS-oh-MY-sin)
USP 34.
Use: Anti-infective.
Sitabs. (Canright) Lobeline sulfate
1.5 mg, benzocaine 2 mg, aluminum
hydroxide-magnesium carbonate co-
dried gel 150 mg. Loz. Bot. 100s. *OTC.*
Use: Smoking deterrent.
•**sitafloxacin.** (si-ta-FLOKS-a-sin) USAN.
Use: Antibacterial.
•**sitagliptin phosphate.** (sit-a-GLIP-tin)
USAN.
Tall Man: sitaGLIPtin
Use: Antidiabetic.
See: Januvia.
W/Metformin Hydrochloride.
See: Janumet.
•**sitaxsentan sodium.** (SYE-tax-EN-tan)
USAN.
Use: Congestive heart failure; ischemic
deficits; hypertension; prostate can-
cer; investigational endothelin recep-
tor antagonist.
•**sitogluside.** (SIGH-toe-GLUE-side)
USAN.
Use: Antiprostatic hypertrophy.
Sitrex. (Vindex) Phenylephrine hydro-
chloride 20 mg, guaifenesin 1200 mg.
Dye free. ER Tab. 100s. *Rx.*
Use: Upper respiratory combination, de-
congestant and expectorant combination.
Sitrex PD. (Vindex) Phenylephrine hydrochloride 7.5 mg, guaifenesin 75 mg per
5 mL. Alcohol, sugar, and dye free.
Punch flavor. Liq. 473 mL. *Rx.*
Use: Upper respiratory combination, de-
congestant and expectorant combina-
tion.
Sitzmarks. (Konsyl) Radiopaque polyvinyl chloride radiopaque rings 24 (1 mm
× 4.5 mm). Cap. Box. 10s. *Rx.*
Use: Radiopaque agent, miscellaneous
GI contrast agent.
•**sivelestat.** (si-VEL-es-tat) USAN.
Use: Acute respiratory distress syndrome.
•**sivelestat sodium.** (si-VEL-es-tat)
USAN.
Use: Acute respiratory distress syndrome.
Sixameen. (Spanner) Vitamins B,
100 mg, B$_6$ 100 mg/mL. Vial 10 mL.
OTC.
Use: Vitamin supplement.
**666 Cold Preparation, Maximum
Strength.** (Monticello) Dextromethorphan HBr 3.3 mg, pseudoephedrine

hydrochloride 10 mg, acetaminophen
108.3 mg per 5 mL. Saccharin, sucrose,
sodium 23.5 mg/5 mL. Liq. Bot.
118 mL, 177 mL. *OTC.*
Use: Upper respiratory combination, an-
titussive combination.
Skeeter Stik. (Triton) Lidocaine 4%, phe-
nol 2%, isopropyl alcohol base. Liq.
14 mL. *OTC.*
Use: Topical local anesthetic.
Skelaxin. (King) Metaxalone 800 mg.
Tab. Bot. 100s, 500s. *Rx.*
Use: Muscle relaxant.
skeletal muscle relaxants.
See: Baclofen.
Carisoprodol.
Chlorphenesin Carbamate.
Chlorzoxazone.
Cyclobenzaprine Hydrochloride.
Dantrolene Sodium.
Diazepam.
Metaxalone.
Methocarbamol.
Orphenadrine Citrate.
Tizanidine Hydrochloride.
Skelid. (Sanofi-Aventis) Tiludronate
200 mg (equiv. to tiludronate disodium
240 mg). Lactose. Tab. 56s. *Rx.*
Use: Bisphosphonates.
Skin Degreaser. (Health & Medical Tech-
niques) Freon 100%. Bot. 2 oz, 4 oz.
OTC.
Use: Dermatologic, degreaser.
skin protectants.
See: Zinc Oxide.
Skin Shield. (Del) Dyclonine hydrochlo-
ride 0.75%, benzethonium Cl 0.2%, ac-
etone, amyl acetate, castor oil, SD al-
cohol 40 10%. Waterproof. Liq. Bot.
13.3 mL. *OTC.*
Use: Dermatologic, protectant.
skin test antigen, multiple.
See: T.R.U.E. Test.
SK 110679. (GlaxoSmithKline)
Use: Hormone, growth. [Orphan Drug]
Sleep Cap. (Weeks & Leo) Diphenhydra-
mine hydrochloride 50 mg. Cap. Bot.
25s, 50s. *OTC.*
Use: Sleep aid.
Sleep-Eze. (Whitehall-Robins) Diphen-
hydramine hydrochloride 25 mg. Tab.
Pkg. 12s, 26s, 52s. *OTC.*
Use: Sleep aid.
Sleep Tablets. (Towne) Scopolamine
aminoxide HBr 0.2 mg, salicylamide
250 mg. Tab. Bot. 36s, 90s. *Rx.*
Use: Sleep aid.
Sleep II. (Walgreen) Diphenhydramine
hydrochloride 25 mg. Tab. Bot. 16s,
32s, 72s. *OTC.*
Use: Sleep aid.

Sleepwell 2-Nite. (Rugby) Diphenhydramine hydrochloride 25 mg. Tab. Bot. 72s. *OTC.*
Use: Sleep aid.

Slender. (Carnation) Skim milk, vegetable oils, caseinates, vitamins, minerals. **Liq.:** 220 Cal/10 oz. Can. **Pow.:** 173 or 200 Cal mixed w/6 oz skim or low fat milk. Pkg 1 oz. *OTC.*
Use: Dietary aid.

Slim-Fast. (Thompson Medical) Meal replacement powder mixed with milk to replace 1, 2 or 3 meals a day. *OTC.*
Use: Dietary aid.

Slim-Line. (Thompson Medical) Benzocaine, dextrose. Chewing gum. Box 24s. *OTC.*
Use: Dietary aid.

Slim-Tabs. (Wesley) Phendimetrazine tartrate 35 mg. Tab. Bot. 1000s. *c-III.*
Use: Anorexiant.

Sloan's Liniment. (Warner Lambert) Capsicum oleoresin 0.62%, methyl salicylate 2.66%, oil of camphor 3.35%, turpentine oil 46.76%, oil of pine 6.74%. Bot. 2 oz, 7 oz. *OTC.*
Use: Analgesic, topical.

Slo-Niacin. (Upsher-Smith) Niacin. 250 mg, 500 mg, 750 mg. Sugar free. CR Tab. Bot. 100s. *OTC.*
Use: Water-soluble vitamin.

Slo-Salt-K. (Mission Pharmacal) KCl 150 mg, NaCl 410 mg. Tab. Bot. 1000s. Strip 100s. *OTC.*
Use: Salt substitute.

Slow FE. (Ciba) Ferrous sulfate 142 mg (iron 45 mg). Ascorbic acid, PEG. ER Tab. 30s, 60s, 90s. *OTC.*
Use: Mineral supplement.

Slow Fe Slow Release Iron With Folic Acid. (Novartis) Fe 50 mg, folic acid 0.4 mg. SR Tab. Bot. 20s. *OTC.*
Use: Mineral, vitamin supplement.

Slow-Mag. (Purdue) Magnesium 143 mg, calcium 238 mg, chloride 405 mg, sodium 5 mg. Maltodextrin, mineral oil. Tab. 60s. *OTC.*
Use: Mineral.

Slow Release Iron. (Cardinal Health) Ferrous sulfate exsiccated (dried) 160 mg (iron 50 mg). Maltodextrin, mineral oil. SR Tab. 30s. *OTC.*
Use: Mineral supplement.

SLT Tablets. (Western Research) Sodium levothyroxine 0.1 mg, 0.2 mg, 0.3 mg. Bot. 1000s.
Use: Hormone, thyroid.

Small Fry Chewable Tabs. (Health for Life Brands) Vitamins A 5000 units, D 1000 units, B$_{12}$ 5 mcg, B$_1$ 3 mg, B$_2$ 2.5 mg, B$_6$ 1 mg, C 50 mg, niacinamide 20 mg, calcium pantothenate 1 mg, E 1 unit, l-lysine 15 mg, biotin 10 mg. Chew. Tab. Bot. 100s, 250s, 365s. *OTC.*
Use: Mineral, vitamin supplement.

•**smallpox vaccine.** (SMAWL-pox-VAXeen) *USP 34.*
Use: Immunization.

smoking deterrents.
See: Bupropion hydrochloride.
Nicotine.
Nicotine Gum.
Nicotine Inhalation System.
Nicotine Nasal Spray.
Nicotine Polacrilex.
Nicotine Transdermal System.
Varenicline Tartrate.

snakebite antivenins.
See: Antivenin (Crotalidae) Polyvalent.
Antivenin (Micurus fulvius).

snake venom.
Use: Trypanosomiasis.

Snaplets-D. (Baker Norton) Pseudoephedrine hydrochloride 6.25 mg, chlorpheniramine maleate 1 mg. Pkt., taste free. Granules 30s. *OTC.*
Use: Antihistamine; decongestant.

Snaplets-FR. (Baker Norton) Acetaminophen 80 mg. Pkt. Granules. 32s packets. *OTC.*
Use: Analgesic.

Snootie by Sea & Ski. (Carter-Wallace) Padimate O. SPF 10. Lot. Bot. 30 mL. *OTC.*
Use: Sunscreen.

Snooze Fast. (BDI) Diphenhydramine hydrochloride 50 mg. Tab. Bot. 36s. *OTC.*
Use: Sleep aid.

SN-13, 272.
See: Primaquine Phosphate.

Soakare. (Allergan) Benzalkonium Cl 0.01%, edetate disodium, NaOH to adjust pH, purified water. Bot. 4 fl oz. *OTC.*
Use: Contact lens care.

•**soap, green.** *USP 34.*
Use: Detergent.

soaps, germicidal.
See: Fostex.
pHisoHex.
Thylox.

soap substitutes.
See: Lowila Cake.
pHisoDerm.

•**sobetirome.** (SOE-be-TYE-rome) USAN.
Use: Dyslipidemia.

Sochlor. (OcuSoft) Sodium chloride, hypertonic. **Soln.:** 5%. Hydroxypropyl methylcellulose 2906, propylene glycol, methylparaben 0.023%, propylparaben 0.01%, boric acid. 15 mL. **Oint.:** 5%.

Mineral oil, white petrolatum, lanolin oil. 3.5 g. *OTC.*
Use: Ophthalmic agent, ophthalmic hyperosmolar preparation.

•**soda lime.** (SOE-da-lyme) *NF 29.*
Use: Carbon dioxide absorbent.

Soda Mint. (Eli Lilly) Sodium bicarbonate 5 g, peppermint oil q.s. Tab. Bot. 100s. *OTC.*
Use: Antacid.

Sodasone. (Fellows) Prednisolone sodium phosphate 20 mg, niacinamide 25 mg/mL. Vial 10 mL. *Rx.*
Use: Corticosteroid.

SodiPhluor. (Kylemore) Fluoride 0.5 mg per mL (from 1.1 mg of sodium fluoride). Methylparaben, sucralose. Sugar free. Peach flavor. Drops. 50 mL. *Rx.*
Use: Trace element.

•**sodium acetate.** (SOE-dee-um ASS-eh-tate) *USP 34.*
Use: Pharmaceutic aid (in dialysis solutions).

•**sodium acetate C 11 injection.** (SOE-dee-um ASS-eh-tate) *USP 34.*
Use: Radiopharmaceutical.

sodium acetosulfone. (SOE-dee-um ah-SEE-toe-sull-FONE)
Use: Leprostatic agent.

sodium acid phosphate.
See: Sodium Biphosphate.

sodium actinoquinol. (SOE-dee-um ack-TIH-no-kwin-OLE)
Use: Treatment of flash burns (ophthalmic).

•**sodium alginate.** (SOE-dee-um AL-jih-nate) *NF 29.*
Use: Pharmaceutic aid (suspending agent).

sodium aminobenzoate.
Use: Dermatomyositis and scleroderma.

sodium aminopterin. Aminopterin sodium.

sodium aminosalicylate.
See: Aminosalicylate Sodium.

sodium amobarbital. Amobarbital Sodium, USP.

•**sodium amylosulfate.** (SOE-dee-um AM-ill-oh-sull-fate) USAN.
Use: Enzyme inhibitor.

sodium anazolene. (SOE-dee-um an-AZE-oh-leen)
Use: Diagnostic aid.

sodium antimony gluconate. (Pentostam)
Use: Anti-infective.

•**sodium arsenate As 74.** (SOE-dee-um AHR-seh-nate) USAN.
Use: Radiopharmaceutical.

•**sodium ascorbate.** (SOE-dee-um ass-CORE-bate) *USP 34.*
Use: Water-soluble vitamin.
W/Ascorbic Acid.
See: Chewable Vitamin C.
Chew-C.
Fruit C 500.
Fruit C 100.
Fruit C 200.
Sunkist Vitamin C.
Vicks Vitamin C Drops.

sodium aurothiomalate.
See: Gold Sodium Thiosulfate.

•**sodium benzoate.** (SOE-dee-um BEN-zoe-ate) *NF 29.*
Use: Pharmaceutic aid (antifungal, preservative); antihyperammonemic.

sodium benzylpenicillin. Penicillin G Sodium, USP. Sodium Penicillin G. *Rx.*
Use: Anti-infective; penicillin.

•**sodium bicarbonate.** (SOE-dee-um by-CAR-boe-nate) *USP 34.*
Use: Alkalizer, systemic; antacid; electrolyte replacement.
W/Aspirin, Citric Acid.
See: Alka-Seltzer Extra Strength with Aspirin.
Alka-Seltzer Lemon Lime.
Alka-Seltzer Original.
Zee-Seltzer.
W/Calcium Chloride, Dibasic Sodium Phosphate, Monobasic Sodium Phosphate, Silicon Dioxide, Sodium Chloride.
See: NeutraSal.
W/Citric Acid.
See: Alka-Seltzer Heartburn Relief.
W/Citric Acid, Potassium Bicarbonate.
See: Alka-Seltzer Gold.
W/Citric Acid, Simethicone.
See: E-Z Gas II.
W/Omeprazole.
See: Zegerid.
Zegerid OTC.
W/PEG 3350, Sodium Chloride, Potassium Chloride.
See: Trilyte.
W/PEG 3350, Sodium Chloride, Sodium Sulfate, Potassium Chloride.
See: GaviLyte-C.
GaviLyte-G.
W/Potassium Bitartrate.
See: Ceo-Two.
W/Sodium Carboxymethylcellulose, Alginic Acid.
See: Pretts Diet Aid.

sodium bicarbonate. (Hospira) Sodium bicarbonate. Inj. 4.2% (5 mEq). Infant 10 mL Syringe. 7.5% (44.6 mEq). 50 mL Syringe or 50 mL Amp. 8.4% (10 mEq). Pediatric 10 mL Syringe or (50 mEq). 50 mL Syringe or 50 mL Vial.

Use: Alkalizer, systemic; antacid; electrolyte replacement.
sodium biphosphate.
Use: Cathartic.
See: Sodium Phosphate Monobasic.
W/Ammonium Biphosphate, Sodium Acid Pyrophosphate.
See: Ammonium Biphosphate, Sodium Biphosphate and Sodium Acid Pyrophosphate.
W/Hyoscyamine Sulfate, Methylene Blue, Methenamine, Phenyl Salicylate.
See: Urimax.
sodium bismuth tartrate.
See: Bismuth Sodium Tartrate.
sodium bisulfite. Sulfurous acid, monosodium salt. Monosodium sulfite.
Use: Antioxidant.
•**sodium borate.** (SO-dee-um) NF 29.
Use: Pharmaceutic aid (alkalizing agent).
sodium butabarbital.
See: Butabarbital Sodium.
Sodium Butyrate.
•**sodium butyrate.** (SO-dee-um) USP 34.
sodium calcium edetate.
See: Calcium Disodium Versenate.
•**sodium carbonate.** (SO-dee-um) NF 29.
Use: Pharmaceutic aid (alkalizing agent).
sodium carboxymethylcellulose.
Carboxymethylcellulose Sodium, USP. CMC. Cellulose Gum.
sodium cellulose glycolate.
See: Carboxymethylcellulose Sodium.
sodium cephalothin. (SO-dee-um SEFF-ah-low-thin) Cephalothin Sodium, USP.
Use: Anti-infective.
•**sodium chloride.** (SO-dee-um KLOR-ide) USP 34.
Use: Pharmaceutic aid (tonicity agent); bronchodilator, diluent; nasal decongestant.
See: Afrin Moisturizing Saline Mist.
Ayr Saline.
Breathe Free.
Entsol.
HuMist.
Mycinaire Saline Mist.
NaSal.
Nasal Moist.
Nasal Spray.
Normaline.
Ocean.
Ocean for Kids.
Pretz Irrigation.
Pretz Moisturizing.
Rhinaris.
Simply Saline.

W/Calcium Chloride, Dibasic Sodium Phosphate, Monobasic Sodium Phosphate, Silicon Dioxide, Sodium Bicarbonate.
See: NeutraSal.
W/Dextrose.
See: Dextrose 5% with 0.45% Sodium Chloride.
Dextrose 5% with 0.9% Sodium Chloride.
Dextrose 5% with 0.3% Sodium Chloride.
Dextrose 5% with 0.33% Sodium Chloride.
Dextrose 5% with 0.2% Sodium Chloride.
Dextrose 5% and 0.225% Sodium Chloride.
Dextrose 10% with 0.45% Sodium Chloride.
Dextrose 10% and 0.9% Sodium Chloride.
Dextrose 10% with 0.2% Sodium Chloride.
Dextrose 10% with 0.225% Sodium Chloride.
Dextrose 3.3% and 0.3% Sodium Chloride.
Dextrose 2.5% with 0.45% Sodium Chloride.
W/Dextrose, Potassium Chloride.
See: Potassium Chloride in 5% Dextrose and 0.45% Sodium Chloride.
Potassium Chloride in 5% Dextrose and 0.9% Sodium Chloride.
Potassium Chloride in 5% Dextrose and 0.33% Sodium Chloride.
Potassium Chloride in 5% Dextrose and 0.2% Sodium Chloride.
Potassium Chloride in 10% Dextrose and 0.2% Sodium Chloride.
Potassium Chloride in 3.3% Dextrose and 0.3% Sodium Chloride.
W/Dibasic Sodium Phosphate, Monobasic Sodium Phosphate, Calcium Chloride.
See: Cephosol.
W/PEG 3350, Sodium Bicarbonate, Potassium Chloride.
See: TriLyte.
W/PEG 3350, Sodium Bicarbonate, Sodium Sulfate, Potassium Chloride.
See: GaviLyte-C.
GaviLyte-G.

sodium chloride. (Various Mfr.) Sodium chloride 0.9%. May contain benzyl alcohol 9 mg. Inj. Vial 1 mL, 2 mL, 2.5 mL, 5 mL, 10 mL, 30 mL. Rx.
Use: Bronchodilator, diluent; intravenous nutritional therapy, electrolyte.

sodium chloride, calcium carbonate, and potassium chloride.
Use: Salt replacement.
See: Sustain.
sodium chloride diluents.
Use: Intravenous nutritional therapy, electrolyte.
See: Sodium Chloride 0.45%.
Sodium Chloride 0.9%.
sodium chloride, 5%. (Various Mfr.) Sodium 855 mEq/L, chloride 855 mEq/L, osmolarity 1710 mOsm/L. 500 mL. *Rx.*
Use: Intravenous nutritional therapy, electrolyte.
sodium chloride, hypertonic.
See: Sochlor.
•**sodium chloride injection.** (SOE-dee-um KLOR-ide) *USP 34.*
Use: Fluid and irrigation; electrolyte replacement; isotonic vehicle.
sodium chloride injection. (Abbott) Normal saline 0.9% in 150 mL, 250 mL, 500 mL, 1000 mL cont. **Partial-fill:** 50 mL in 200 mL, 50 mL in 300 mL, 100 mL in 300 mL. **Fliptop vial:** 10 mL, 20 mL, 50 mL, 100 mL. **Bacteriostatic vial:** 10 mL, 20 mL, 30 mL; 50 mEq, 20 mL in 50 mL fliptop or pintop vial; 100 mEq, 40 mL in 50 mL fliptop vial; sodium Cl 0.45%, 500 mL, 1000 mL; sodium Cl 5%, 500 mL; sodium Cl irrigating solution, 250 mL, 500 mL, 1000 mL, 3000 mL; (Pharmacia & Upjohn) sodium Cl 9 mg/mL w/benzyl alcohol 9.45 mg. Vial 20 mL (Sanofi Winthrop Pharmaceuticals). **Carpuject:** 2 mL fill cartridge, 22-gauge, 1¼-inch needle or 25-gauge, ⅝-inch needle. *Rx.*
Use: Fluid and irrigation; electrolyte replacement; isotonic vehicle.
sodium chloride injection. (Various Mfr.) Sodium chloride 14.6%, 23.4%. Inj. 20 mL (14.6% only), 30 mL (23.4% only), 40 mL (14.6% only), 100 mL (23.4% only), 200 mL. *Rx.*
Use: Intravenous nutritional therapy, electrolyte.
sodium chloride intravenous infusions for admixtures.
Use: Intravenous nutritional therapy, electrolyte.
See: Sodium Chloride, 5%.
Sodium Chloride, 3%.
Sodium Chloride, 0.45% (Half Normal Saline).
Sodium Chloride, 0.9% (Normal Saline).
•**sodium chloride Na 22.** (So-dee-um KLOR-ide) USAN.
Use: Radioactive agent.

sodium chloride substitutes.
See: Salt Substitutes.
sodium chloride tablets. (Parke-Davis) Sodium Cl 15 ½ g. Tab. Bot. 1000s. *OTC.*
Use: Normal saline.
sodium chloride, 3%. (Various Mfr.) Sodium 513 mEq/L, chloride 513 mEq/L. Osmolarity 1030 mOsm/L. 500 mL. *Rx.*
Use: Intravenous nutritional therapy, electrolyte.
sodium chloride 0.45%. (Dey) Sodium chloride 0.45%. Preservative free. Soln. Single-use vial 3 mL, 5 mL. *OTC.*
Use: Bronchodilator, diluent; intravenous nutritional therapy, electrolyte.
sodium chloride, 0.45% (half normal saline). (Various Mfr.) Sodium 77 mEq/L, chloride 77 mEq/L. Osmolarity ≈ 155 mOsm/L. 25 mL, 50 mL, 150 mL, 250 mL, 500 mL, 1000 mL. *Rx.*
Use: Intravenous nutritional therapy, electrolyte.
sodium chloride 0.9%. (Dey) Sodium chloride 0.9%. Preservative free. Soln. Vial 3 mL, 5 mL, 15 mL. *OTC.*
Use: Bronchodilator, diluent; intravenous nutritional therapy, electrolyte.
sodium chloride, 0.9% (normal saline). (Various Mfr.) Sodium 154 mEq/L, chloride 154 mEq/L. Osmolarity ≈ 310 mOsm/L. 2 mL, 3 mL, 5 mL, 10 mL, 20 mL, 25 mL, 30 mL, 50 mL, 100 mL, 150 mL, 250 mL, 500 mL, 1000 mL, 2 mL fill in 3 mL. *Rx.*
Use: Intravenous nutritional therapy, electrolyte.
sodium chlorothiazide for injection. (SOE-dee-um KLOR-oh-thigh-AZZ-ide) Chlorothiazide Sodium for Injection, USP.
Use: Diuretic.
•**sodium chromate Cr 51 injection.** (SOE-dee-um KROE-mate) *USP 34.*
Use: Diagnostic aid (blood volume determination); radiopharmaceutical.
•**sodium citrate.** (SOE-dee-um SIH-trate) *USP 34.*
Use: Alkalizer, systemic.
See: Anticoagulant Citrate Dextrose Solution.
Anticoagulant Citrate Phosphate Dextrose Solution.
sodium citrate and citric acid. Shohl's Solution.
Use: Alkalinizer, systemic.
sodium citrate/citric acid. (Pharmaceutical Associates) Sodium citrate 500 mg/citric acid 334 mg per 5 mL (sodium 1 mEq equiv. to bicarbonate 1 mEq/mL). Sugar free. Soln. 473 mL.

Rx.
Use: Systemic alkalinizer; urinary alkalinizer.

sodium cloxacillin. (SOE-dee-um CLOX-ah-SILL-in)
See: Cloxacillin Sodium.

sodium colistimethate. Colistimethate Sodium, Sterile. Antibiotic produced by *Aerobacillus colistinus.*

sodium colistin methanesulfonate. Colistimethane Sodium, USP. The sodium methanesulfonate salt of an antibiotic substance elaborated by *Aerobacillus colistinus.*
Use: Anti-infective.

•**sodium dehydroacetate.** (SO-dee-um) *NF 29.*
Use: Pharmaceutic aid (antimicrobial preservative).

sodium dextrothyroxine. (SOE-dee-um DEX-troe-thigh-ROCK-seen)
Use: Anticholesteremic.

sodium diatrizoate. Diatrizoate Sodium, USP.
Use: Radiopaque medium.

sodium dichloroacetate.
Use: Treatment of lactic acidosis and familial hypercholesterolemia. [Orphan Drug]

sodium dicloxacillin. (SOE-dee-um DIE-klox-uh-SILL-in) Dicloxacillin Sodium, USP.
Use: Anti-infective.

sodium dicloxacillin monohydrate.
Use: Anti-infective.
See: Pathocil.

sodium dihydrogen phosphate.
See: Sodium Biphosphate.

sodium dimethoxyphenyl penicillin.
See: Methicillin Sodium.

sodium dioctyl sulfosuccinate.
See: Docusate Sodium.

sodium diphenylhydantoin. Phenytoin Sodium, USP. Diphenylhydantoin Sodium.
Use: Anticonvulsant.

sodium edetate. (SOE-dee-um eh-deh-TATE) Edetate Disodium, USP. Tetrasodium ethylenediaminetetraacetate.
Use: Chelating agent.
See: Vagisec Plus.

sodium ethacrynate. Ethacrynate Sodium for Injection, USP.
Use: Diuretic.

•**sodium ethasulfate.** (SOE-dee-um ETH-ah-SULL-fate) USAN.
Use: Detergent.

sodium ethyl-mercuri-thio-salicylate.
See: Merthiolate.
Thimerosal.

•**sodium ferric gluconate complex.** (FER-ik GLOO-koe-nate) USAN.
Use: Iron product.
See: Ferrlecit.
Nulecit.

•**sodium fluorescein.** (SO-dee-um) *USP 34.* Fluorescein Sodium, USP; Resorcinolphthalein sodium.
Use: Diagnostic aid (corneal trauma indicator).

•**sodium fluoride.** (SOE-dee-um) *USP 34.*
Use: Dental caries agent.
See: ControlRx.
DentaGel.
EtheDent.
Fluor-A-Day.
Fluoride.
Flura-Drops.
Flura-Loz.
Karidium.
Karigel.
Listerine Tooth Defense.
Luride.
NaFeen.
OrthoWash.
PreviDent 5000 Plus.
T-Fluoride.
W/Vitamins.
See: Mulvidren-F.
W/Vitamins A, D, C.
See: Tri-Vi-Flor.

sodium fluoride. (Breckenridge) Fluoride 0.25 mg (from 0.55 mg of sodium fluoride) Sucralose, xylitol. Orange flavor. Chew. Tab. 120s. *Rx.*
Use: Trace element.

sodium fluoride. (Hi-Tech) Fluoride 0.5 mg per mL (from sodium fluoride 1.1 mg). Peach flavor. Drops. 50 mL. *Rx.*
Use: Prevention of dental caries.

•**sodium fluoride and phosphoric acid gel.** *USP 34.*
Use: Dental caries agent.

•**sodium fluoride F 18.** (SOE-dee-um) *USP 34.*
Use: Radiopharmaceutical.

sodium folate. Monosodium folate.
Use: Water-soluble, hematopoietic vitamin.

•**sodium formaldehyde sulfoxylate.** (SOE-dee-um) *NF 29.*
Use: Pharmaceutic aid (preservative).

•**sodium gluconate.** (SOE-dee-um) *USP 34.*
Use: Electrolyte, replacement.

sodium glucosulfone injection.
Use: Leprostatic.

sodium glycerophosphate. Glycerol phosphate sodium salt.
Use: Pharmaceutic necessity.

sodium glycocholate.
See: Bile Salts.

•**sodium heparin.** (SO-dee-um) *USP 34.* Heparin Sodium.
Use: Anticoagulant.

sodium hexobarbital.
Use: Intravenous general anesthetic.

sodium hyaluronate.
Use: Ophthalmic.
See: Amvisc.
Amvisc Plus.
Euflexxa.
Healon.
Healon5.
Hyalgan.
HyGel.
Hylira.
ProVisc.
Shellgel.
Supartz.
W/Chondroitin Sulfate.
See: DisCoVisc.
Viscoat.

sodium hyaluronate. (River's Edge) Sodium hyaluronate. **Lot.:** 0.1%. Parabens. 340 g, 1,000 g. **Gel:** 0.2%. Parabens. 30 g. *Rx.*
Use: Physical adjunct.

•**sodium hydroxide.** (SOE-dee-um) *NF 29.*
Use: Pharmaceutic aid (alkalizing agent).

•**sodium hypochlorite solution.** (SOE-dee-um high-poe-KLOR-ite) *USP 34.*
Use: Anti-infective, local; disinfectant.
See: Antiformin.
Dakin's Solution.
Hyclorite.

sodium hypophosphite. Sodium phosphinate.
Use: Pharmaceutic necessity.

sodium hyposulfite.
See: Sodium Thiosulfate.

•**sodium iodide.** (SOE-dee-um) *USP 34.*
Use: Nutritional supplement.

•**sodium iodide I 131.** (SOE-dee-um) *USP 34.*
Use: Antineoplastic; diagnostic aid (thyroid function determination); radiopharmaceutical; antithyroid agent.
See: Hicon.

sodium iodide I 131 therapeutic. (Mallinckrodt) **Cap.:** 0.75 to 100 mCi per capsule. **Oral Soln.:** 3.5 to 150 mCi per vial. *Rx.*
Use: Antithyroid agent.

•**sodium iodide I 125.** (SOE-dee-um) USAN.
Use: Diagnostic aid (thyroid function determination); radiopharmaceutical.

•**sodium iodide I 123.** (SOE-dee-um) *USP 34.*
Use: In vivo diagnostic aid, thyroid function test.

sodium iodide I-123. (Mallinckrodt Medical) Sodium iodide I^{123} 3.7 MBq, 7.4 MBq. Sucrose. Cap. Pkg. 1s, 3s, 5s. *Rx.*
Use: In vivo diagnostic aid, thyroid function test.

sodium iodipamide.
Use: Radiopaque medium.

•**sodium iodomethane sulfonate.** (SO-dee-um) *USP 34.* Methiodal Sodium.

•**sodium iothalamate.** (SOE-dee-um) *USP 34.* Iothalmate Sodium Inj.
Use: Radiopaque medium.

•**sodium ipodate.** (SOE-dee-um EYE-poe-date) *USP 34.* Ipodate Sodium.
Use: Radiopaque.

sodium isoamylethylbarbiturate.
See: Amytal Sodium.

•**sodium lactate injection.** (SOE-dee-um LACK-tate) *USP 34.*
Use: Fluid and electrolyte replacement.

sodium lactate injection. (Abbott) Sodium lactate 1/6 Molar, 250 mL, 500 mL, 1,000 mL; 50 mEq, 10 mL in 20 mL fliptop vial. *Rx.*
Use: Electrolyte replacement.

sodium lactate solution.
Use: Electrolyte replacement.

•**sodium lauryl sulfate.** (SOE-dee-um LAH-rill SULL-fate) *NF 29.* Sulfuric acid monododecyl ester sodium salt. Sodium monododecyl sulfate.
Use: Pharmaceutic aid (surfactant).
See: Duponol.
W/Hydrocortisone.
See: Nutracort.

sodium levothyroxine. Levothyroxine Sodium.
Use: Hormone, thyroid.
See: Synthroid.

sodium liothyronine. Liothyronine Sodium, USP.
Use: Hormone, thyroid.

sodium l-thyroxine.
See: Synthroid.

sodium lyapolate. (SOE-dee-um LIE-app-OLE-ate) Polyethylene sulfonate sodium. Peson (Hoechst Marion Roussel.)
Use: Anticoagulant.

sodium malonylurea.
See: Barbital Sodium.

sodium mercaptomerin. Mercaptomerin
Sodium, USP.
Use: Diuretic.
•**sodium metabisulfite.** (SOE-dee-um)
NF 29.
Use: Pharmaceutic aid (antioxidant).
sodium methiodal. Methiodal Sodium,
USP. Sodium monoiodomethanesulfo-
nate. Sodium Iodomethanesulfonate,
Inj.
Use: Radiopaque medium.
sodium methohexital for injection.
Methohexital Sodium for Injection, USP.
Use: Anesthetic, general.
See: Brevital Sodium.
sodium methoxycellulose. Mixture of
methylcellulose and sodium.
•**sodium monofluorophosphate.** (SOE-
dee-um mahn-oh-flure-oh-FOSS-fate)
USP 34.
Use: Dental caries agent.
See: Biotene Dry Mouth.
**sodium monomercaptoundecahydro-
closo-dodecaborate.**
Use: Treatment of glioblastoma multiforme. [Orphan Drug]
sodium morrhuate, injection. Morrhuate Sodium Inj., USP.
Use: Sclerosing agent.
sodium nafcillin. (SOE-dee-um naff-
SILL-in) Nafcillin Sodium, USP.
Use: Anti-infective.
sodium nicotinate. (Various Mfr.)
Use: IV nicotinic acid therapy.
•**sodium nitrite.** (SOE-dee-um NYE-trite)
USP 34.
Use: Antidote to cyanide poisoning, antioxidant. Vasodilator and antidote-
cyanide.
See: Cyanide Antidote Pkg.
sodium nitrite. (Hope) Sodium nitrite
30 mg/mL. Inj. Vials. 10 mL. *Rx.*
Use: Antidote, cyanide.
•**sodium nitroprusside.** (SOE-dee-um
NYE-troe-PRUSS-ide) *USP 34.*
Use: Antihypertensive.
See: Nitropress.
sodium nitroprusside. (Wyeth) Sodium
nitroprusside. 50 mg. Pow. for Inj.
5 mL. *Rx.*
Use: Antihypertensive.
sodium novobiocin. Sodium salt of antibacterial substance produced by *Streptomyces niveus.* Novobiocin monosodium salt.
Use: Anti-infective.
sodium ortho-iodohippurate. Iodohippurate Sodium, I 131 Injection, USP.
See: Hipputope.

•**sodium oxybate.** (SOE-dee-um OX-ee-
bate) USAN.
Use: Psychotherapeutic agent, miscellaneous.
See: Xyrem.
sodium pantothenate.
Use: Orally, dietary supplement.
sodium para-aminohippurate injection.
Use: IV, to determine kidney tubular excretion function.
sodium penicillin G. Penicillin G Sodium, Sterile, USP. Sodium benzylpenicillin.
sodium pentobarbital. Pentobarbital Sodium, USP.
Use: Hypnotic.
•**sodium perborate monohydrate.** (SOE-
dee-um) USAN.
sodium peroxyborate.
See: Sodium Perborate Monohydrate.
sodium peroxyhydrate.
See: Sodium Perborate Monohydrate.
•**sodium pertechnetate Tc 99m injection.** (SOE-dee-um per-TEK-neh-tate)
USP 34. Pertechnetic acid, sodium salt.
Use: Radiopharmaceutical.
See: Minitec.
sodium phenobarbital. Phenobarbital
Sodium, USP.
Use: Anticonvulsant; hypnotic.
•**sodium phenylacetate.** (SOE-dee-um
FEN-ill-ASS-eh-tate) USAN.
Use: Antihyperammonemic.
W/Sodium Benzoate.
See: Ammonul.
Ucephan.
**sodium phenylacetate and sodium
benzoate.**
Use: Antihyperammonemic. [Orphan
Drug]
•**sodium phenylbutyrate.** (SOE-dee-um
fen-ill-BYOOT-ih-rate) USAN.
Use: Antihyperammonemic. Treatment
of blood disorders. [Orphan Drug]
See: Buphenyl.
sodium phenylethylbarbiturate. Pheno-
barbital Sodium, USP.
sodium phosphate.
Use: Buffering agent; source of phos-
phate; laxative.
See: OsmoPrep
W/Gentamicin Sulfate, Monosodium
Phosphate, Sodium Chloride, Benzal-
konium Chloride.
See: Garamycin Ophthalmic.
W/Sodium Biphosphate.
See: Fleet Enema.
Phospho-Soda.
sodium phosphate. (Abbott) Disodium
hydrogen phosphate. 3 mM P and

4 mEq sodium. 15 mL in 30 mL fliptop vial. *Rx.*
Use: Intravenous nutritional therapy, mineral.

sodium phosphate. (Various Mfr.) Phosphate 3 mM, sodium 4 mEq per mL. Inj. Vials. 5 mL, 15 mL, 50 mL. *Rx.*
Use: Intravenous nutritional therapy, mineral.

•**sodium phosphate, dibasic.** (SOE-dee-um FOSS-fate) *USP 34.*
Use: Laxative.
See: Visicol.
W/Calcium Chloride, Monobasic Sodium Phosphate, Silicon Dioxide, Sodium Chloride, Sodium Bicarbonate.
See: NeutraSal.
W/Calcium Chloride, Monobasic Sodium Phosphate, Sodium Chloride.
See: Caphosol.
W/Monobasic Potassium Phosphate, Monobasic Sodium Phosphate Monohydrate, Phosphorus.
See: Phospha 250 Neutral.

•**sodium phosphate, dried.** (SO-dee-um) *USP 34.*
Use: Cathartic.

•**sodium phosphate, monobasic.** (SOE-dee-um FOSS-fate) *USP 34.*
Use: Cathartic.
See: Visicol.
W/Calcium Chloride, Dibasic Sodium Phosphate, Silicon Dioxide, Sodium Chloride, Sodium Bicarbonate.
See: NeutraSal.
W/Calcium Chloride, Dibasic Sodium Phosphate, Sodium Chloride.
See: Cephosol.
W/Dibasic Sodium Phosphate, Monobasic Potassium Phosphate, Phosphorus.
See: Phospha 250 Neutral.
W/Gentamicin Sulfate, Disodium Phosphate, Sodium Cl, Benzalkonium Cl.
See: Garamycin.
W/Hyoscyamine Sulfate, Methenamine, Methylene Blue, Phenyl Salicylate.
See: UtiCap.
Utrona-C.
W/Methenamine.
See: Uro-Phosphate.
Utac.
W/Methenamine, Phenyl Salicylate, Methylene Blue, Hyoscyamine, Alkaloid.
See: Fleet Enema.
Phospho-Soda.

•**sodium phosphate P 32 solution.** (SOE-dee-um FOSS-fate) *USP 34.*
Use: Antineoplastic; antipolycythemic; diagnostic aid (neoplasm); radiopharmaceutical.

•**sodium phosphates rectal solution.** (SO-dee-um) *USP 34.*

sodium phytate. (SOE-dee-um FYE-tate) Nonasodium phytate: Sodium cyclohexanehexyl (hexaphosphate).
Use: Chelating agent.

•**sodium polyphosphate.** (SOE-dee-um pahl-ee-FOSS-fate) USAN.
Use: Pharmaceutic aid.

•**sodium polystyrene sulfonate.** (SOE-dee-um pah-lee-STYE-reen SULL-fuh-nate) *USP 34.*
Use: Ion exchange resin (potassium).
See: Kayexalate.
Kionex.
SPS.

sodium polystyrene sulfonate. (Crookes-Barnes) Sodium polystyrene sulfonate 5% Soln. Eye drops. *Lacrivial* 15 mL. *Rx.*
Use: Ion exchange resin (potassium).

sodium polystyrene sulfonate. (Various Mfr.) Sodium polystyrene sulfonate (finely ground) Pow. for Susp. (oral or rectal). 454 g. *Rx.*
Use: Potassium-removing resin.

•**sodium propionate.** (SOE-dee-um PRO-pee-oh-nate) *NF 29.*
Use: Pharmaceutic aid (preservative).
W/Chlorophyll "A".
See: Prophyllin.

sodium psylliate.
Use: Sclerosing agent.

•**sodium pyrophosphate.** (SOE-dee-um pie-row-FOSS-fate) USAN.
Use: Pharmaceutic aid.

sodium radio chromate injection. Sodium Chromate Cr 51 Inj., USP.

sodium radio iodide solution. Sodium Iodide I-131 Solution, USP.
Use: Thyroid tumors; hyperthyroidism; cardiac dysfunction.

sodium radio-phosphate, P-32. Radio-Phosphate P 32 Solution. Sodium phosphate P-32 Solution, USP.

sodium rhodanate.
See: Sodium Thiocyanate.

sodium rhodanide.
See: Sodium Thiocyanate.

sodium saccharin. Saccharin Sodium, USP.
Use: Noncaloric sweetener.

•**sodium salicylate.** (SOE-dee-um) *USP 34.*
Use: Analgesic; IV, gout.
W/Combinations.
See: Apcogesic.
Bisalate.
Bufosal.

W/Phenylephrine Hydrochloride, Pheniramine Maleate, Caffeine Citrate.
See: Scot-Tussin Original Multi-Action Cold and Allergy.
sodium salicylate, natural.
Use: Analgesic.
sodium secobarbital. Secobarbital Sodium, USP.
Use: Hypnotic.
sodium secobarbital and sodium amobarbital.
Use: Sedative.
See: Tuinal.
•**sodium starch glycolate.** (SOE-deeum) *NF 29.*
Use: Pharmaceutic aid (tablet excipient).
•**sodium stearate.** (SOE-dee-um) *NF 29.*
Use: Pharmaceutic aid (emulsifying and stiffening agent).
•**sodium stearyl fumarate.** (SO-dee-um) *NF 29.*
Use: Pharmaceutic aid (tablet/capsule lubricant).
sodium stibogluconate.
Use: CDC anti-infective agent.
sodium succinate.
Use: Alkalinize urine & awaken patients following barbiturate anesthesia.
sodium sulamyd.
Use: Sulfonamide, ophthalmic.
See: Sodium Sulamyd Ophthalmic.
Sodium Sulamyd Ophthalmic Oint. 10% Sterile. (Schering-Plough) Sulfacetamide sodium 10%. Ophth. Oint. Tube 3.5 g. *Rx.*
Use: Anti-infective, ophthalmic.
Sodium Sulamyd Ophthalmic Soln. 10% Sterile. (Schering-Plough) Sulfacetamide sodium 10%. Ophth. Soln. Bot. 5 mL, 15 mL. *Rx.*
Use: Anti-infective, ophthalmic.
Sodium Sulamyd Ophthalmic Soln. 30% Sterile. (Schering-Plough) Sulfacetamide sodium 30%. Ophth. Soln. Bot. 15 mL. Box 1s. *Rx.*
Use: Anti-infective, ophthalmic.
sodium sulfabromomethazine.
Use: Anti-infective.
sodium sulfacetamide.
See: Ovace.
 Rosula NS.
 Seb-Prev.
 Sulfacetamide Sodium.
W/Sulfur.
See: Avar-e Emollient.
 Avar-e Green.
 Avar-e LS.
 Avar-e LS cleanser.
 BP Cleansing Wash.
 Cerisa.
 Clarifoam EF.
 Claris.
 Clenia.
 Plexion Cleansing Cloths.
 Plexion TS.
 Rosaderm Kit.
 Rosula Clarifying Wash.
 SulfaCleanse 8/4.
 Sumaxin.
 Sumaxin TS.
 Sumaxin Wash.
 Zencia.
sodium sulfacetamide. (Acella Pharmaceuticals) Sodium sulfacetamide 10%. Disodium EDTA, methylparaben, PEG. Soap. 473 mL. *Rx.*
Use: Topical anti-infective, antibiotic.
sodium sulfacetamide/sulfur. (Acella Pharmaceuticals) Sodium sulfacetamide/sulfur. **Soap:** 8%/4%. Alcohols, aloe, butylated hydroxytoluene, disodium EDTA, glycerol, green tea, parabens, PEG, white petrolatum. 473 mL. **Wash:** 9%/4%. Aloe, cetyl alcohol, disodium EDTA, glycerol, parabens, PEG-100, stearyl alcohol, white petrolatum. 473 mL. *Rx.*
Use: Acne product combination.
sodium sulfacetamide/sulfur. (Brookstone Pharmaceuticals) Sodium sulfacetamide 10%, sulfur 4%. Aloe, cetyl alcohol, disodium EDTA, glycerin, green tea, parabens, PEG-100, sodium metabisulfate, sodium thiosulfate, stearyl alcohol. Pad. 60s. *Rx.*
Use: Acne product combination.
sodium sulfacetamide/sulfur. (Fougera) Sodium sulfacetamide 10%/sulfur 4%. Alcohol, butylated hydroxytoluene, disodium EDTA, glyceryl, parabens, PEG. Soap. 473 mL. *Rx.*
Use: Acne product combination.
sodium sulfacetamide/sulfur. (Kylemore) Sodium sulfacetamide/sulfur. **Aer. Foam:** 10%/5%. Cetearyl alcohol, glycerin. 60 g. **Soap:** 10%/4%. Alcohols, BHT, disodium EDTA, parabens, PEG, urea 10%. 473 mL. *Rx.*
Use: Acne product combination.
sodium sulfacetamide/sulfur. (River's Edge) Sodium sulfacetamide/sulfur 10%/5%. **Gel:** Benzyl alcohol, cetyl alcohol, dimethicone, disodium EDTA, glyceryl, methylparaben, mineral oil, PEG-100, propylene glycol, stearyl alcohol, urea 10%. 45 mL. **Wash:** Cetyl alcohol, disodium EDTA, glyceryl, parabens, PEG-100, stearyl alcohol, urea 10%. 355 mL. *Rx.*
Use: Acne product combination.

sodium sulfacetamide 10%.
(A. Aarons.) Sodium sulfacetamide
10%, urea 10%. EDTA. Top. Pads. 30s.
Rx.
Use: Keratolytic agent, acne product.
sodium sulfadiazine.
See: Sulfadiazine Sodium.
sodium sulfamerazine.
See: Sulfamerazine Sodium.
•**sodium sulfate.** (SOE-dee-um SULL-
fate) *USP 34.*
Use: Calcium regulator.
W/Magnesium Sulfate, Potassium Sul-
fate.
See: Suprep Bowel Prep.
W/PEG 3350, Sodium Bicarbonate, So-
dium Chloride, Potassium Chloride.
See: GaviLyte-C.
GaviLyte-G.
•**sodium sulfate S 35.** (SOE-dee-um
SULL-fate) USAN.
Use: Radiopharmaceutical.
•**sodium sulfide.** (SO-dee-um) *USP 34.*
•**sodium sulfide gel.** (SO-dee-um)
USP 34.
sodium sulfobromophthalein. Sulfobromophthalein Sodium, USP.
Use: Diagnostic aid (hepatic function
determination).
sodium sulfocyanate.
See: Sodium Thiocyanate.
sodium sulfoxone. Sulfoxone Sodium,
USP. Disodium sulfonyl-bis (p-
phenyleneimino) dimethanesulfonate.
sodium suramin.
See: Suramin Hexasodium.
sodium taurocholate.
See: Bile Salts.
sodium tetradecyl sulfate.
Use: Sclerosing agent.
See: Sotradecol.
sodium tetraiodophenolphthalein.
See: Iodophthalein Sodium.
sodium thiamylal for injection. Thiamylal Sodium for Injection, USP.
Use: Anesthetic, general.
sodium thiocyanate. Sodium Sulfocyanate. Sodium Rhodanide.
sodium thiopental.
See: Thiopental Sodium.
•**sodium thiosulfate.** (SOE-dee-um thigh-
oh-SULL-fate) *USP 34.*
Use: For argyria, cyanide, and iodine
poisoning, arsphenamine reactions;
prevention of spread of ringworm of
feet; antidote to cyanide poisoning.
W/Salicylic Acid, Alcohol.
See: Versiclear.
W/Sodium Nitrite, Amyl Nitrite.
See: Cyanide Antidote Pkg.

sodium tolbutamide. Tolbutamide Sodium, USP.
Use: Diagnostic aid (diabetes).
sodium triclofos. (SOE-dee-um TRY-
kloe-foss) Sodium trichloroethylphos-
phate.
Use: Sedative; hypnotic.
•**sodium trimetaphosphate.** (SOE-dee-
um try-met-AH-FOSS-fate) USAN.
Use: Pharmaceutic aid.
sodium valproate.
See: Valproate Sodium.
sodium vinbarbital injection.
Use: Sedative.
sodium warfarin. Warfarin Sodium, USP.
Use: Anticoagulant.
Sod-Late 10. (Schlicksup) Sodium salicylate 10 g. Tab. Bot. 1000s. *OTC.*
Use: Analgesic.
Sodol Compound. (Major) Carisoprodol
200 mg, aspirin 325 mg. Tab. Bot.
100s, 500s. *Rx.*
Use: Muscle relaxant.
Sofcaps. (Alton) Docusate sodium
100 mg, 250 mg. Cap. Bot. 100s,
1000s. *OTC.*
Use: Laxative.
•**sofinicline.** (soe-FIN-i-kleen) USAN.
Use: CNS agent.
•**sofinicline benzenesulfonate.** (soe-FIN-
i-kleen) USAN.
Use: CNS agent.
Sof-Lax. (Fleet) Docusate sodium
100 mg. Softgel Cap. 60s. *OTC.*
Use: Laxative.
Sof/Pro-Clean. (Sherman Pharmaceuticals, Inc.) Buffered, hypertonic solution with thimerosal 0.004%, EDTA
0.1%, ethylene and propylene oxide,
octylphenoxypolyethoxyethanol, lauryl
sulfate salt of imidazoline. Soln. Bot.
30 mL. *OTC.*
Use: Contact lens care.
Sof/Pro Clean SA. (Sherman Pharmaceuticals, Inc.) Hypertonic solution: salt
buffers, copolymers of ethylene and
propylene oxide, octylphenoxypolyethoxyethanol, lauryl sulfate salt of imidazoline, sodium bisulfite 0.1%, sorbic acid 0.1%, trisodium EDTA 0.25%,
thimerosal free. Bot. 30 mL. *OTC.*
Use: Contact lens care.
Soft'n Soothe. (B.F. Ascher) Benzocaine, menthol, moisturizers. Tube 50 g.
OTC.
Use: Anesthetic, local.
Soft Sense. (Bausch & Lomb) **Hand
Lot.:** Petrolatum, vitamin E, aloe, parabens. Non-greasy. Bot. 444 mL. **Body
Lot.:** Petrolatum, vitamin E, parabens.

Non-greasy. Bot. 444 mL. *OTC.*
Use: Emollient.
SoftWear. (Ciba Vision) Isotonic, sodium Cl, boric acid, sodium borate, sodium perborate (generating up to 0.006% hydrogen peroxide stabilized with phosphoric acid). Soln. Bot. 120 mL, 240 mL, 360 mL. *OTC.*
Use: Contact lens care.
Sojourn. (Meridian) Sevoflurane. Liq. Inh. 250 mL. *Rx.*
Use: General anesthetic, volatile liquid.
•**solabegron hydrochloride.** (soe-la-BEG-ron) USAN.
Use: Antidiabetic.
Solaneed. (Hanlon) Vitamin A 25,000 units. Cap. Bot. 100s. *Rx.*
Use: Vitamin supplement.
•**solanezumab.** (SOE-la-NEZ-ue-mab) USAN.
Use: Alzheimer disease.
Solaquin. (ICN) Hydroquinone 2% with sunscreens. Tube. 28.4 g. *OTC.*
Use: Dermatologic.
Solaquin Forte. (ICN) Hydroquinone 4%, dioxybenzone, padimate O, oxybenzone, EDTA, sodium metabisulfite, cetearyl alcohol, stearyl alcohol, lactic acid. **Cream:** Vanishing cream base. Tube. 28.4 g. **Gel:** Padimate O, dioxybenzone, EDTA, alcohol, sodium metbisulfite. Tube. 28.4 g. *Rx.*
Use: Dermatologic.
Solar. (Doak Dermatologics) PABA, titanium dioxide, magnesium stearate in a flesh-colored, water-repellent base. Cream. Tube oz. *OTC.*
Use: Sunscreen.
Solaraze. (Pharmaderm) Diclofenac 3% (diclofenac sodium 30 mg/g). Benzyl alcohol. Gel. Tubes. 25 g, 50 g. *Rx.*
Use: Nonsteroidal anti-inflammatory drug, topical.
Solarcaine. (Schering-Plough) **Lot.:** Benzocaine, triclosan, mineral oil, alcohol, aloe extract, tocopheryl acetate, menthol, camphor, parabens, EDTA. 120 mL. **Aerosol:** Benzocaine 20% with triclosan 0.13%, SD alcohol 40 35%, tocopheryl acetate. 90 mL, 120 mL. *OTC.*
Use: Topical local anesthetic, ester local anesthetic.
Solarcaine Aloe Extra Burn Relief. (Schering-Plough) **Cream:** Lidocaine 0.5%. Aloe, EDTA, lanolin oil, lanolin, camphor, propylparaben, eucalyptus oil, menthol, tartrazine. 120 g. **Gel:** Lidocaine 0.5%. Aloe vera gel, glycerin, EDTA, isopropyl alcohol, menthol, diazolidinyl urea, tartrazine. 120 g, 240 g.

Spray: Lidocaine 0.5%. Aloe vera gel, glycerin, EDTA, diazolidinyl urea, vitamin E, parabens. 135 mg. *OTC.*
Use: Topical local anesthetic, amide local anesthetic.
Solarcaine Medicated First-Aid. (Schering-Plough) Benzocaine 20%. Triclosan 0.13%, alcohol. Spray. 90 mL. *OTC.*
Use: Topical local anesthetic, ester local anesthetic.
solargentum.
See: Silver Protein, Mild.
Solar Shield 15 SPF. (Akorn) Ethylhexyl p-methoxy-cinnamate 7.5%, oxybenzone in a moisturizing base 5%. PABA free. Waterproof. Lot. Bot. 120 mL. *OTC.*
Use: Sunscreen.
Solar Shield 30 SPF. (Akorn) Ethylhexyl p-methoxycinnamate 7.5%, oxybenzone 6%, 2-ethylhexyl salicylate 5%, 3-diphenylacrylate 7.5%, 2-ethylhexyl-2-cyano-3 in a moisturizing base, PABA free. Waterproof. Lot. Bot. 120 mL. *OTC.*
Use: Sunscreen.
SolBar PF 15. (Person and Covey) Octyl methoxycinnamate 7.5%, oxybenzone 5%. SPF 15. Cream. Bot. 1 oz, 4 oz. *OTC.*
Use: Sunscreen.
SolBar PF 50. (Person and Covey) Oxybenzone, octyl methoxycinnamate, octocrylene, PABA free. Waterproof. SPF 50. Cream. Tube 120 g. *OTC.*
Use: Sunscreen.
SolBar PF Liquid. (Person and Covey) Octyl methoxycinnamate 7.5%, oxybenzone 6%, SD alcohol 40 76%, PABA free. SPF 30. Liq. Bot. 120 mL. *OTC.*
Use: Sunscreen.
SolBar PF Paba Free 15. (Person and Covey) Oxybenzone 5%, octyl methoxycinnamate 7.5%. SPF 15. Cream. Tube 2.5 oz. *OTC.*
Use: Sunscreen.
SolBar Plus 15. (Person and Covey) Padimate 6%, oxybenzone 4%, dioxybenzone 2%. SPF 15. Cream. Tube 1 oz, 4 oz. *OTC.*
Use: Sunscreen.
Solfoton. (ECR) Phenobarbital 16 mg. Tab. or Cap. Bot. 100s, 500s. *c-IV.*
Use: Hypnotic; sedative.
Solfoton S/C. (ECR) Phenobarbital 16 mg. SC Tab. Bot. 100s. *c-IV.*
Use: Hypnotic; sedative.
Solia. (Prasco) Ethinyl estradiol 30 mcg, desogestrel 0.15 mg. Lactose. Tab. Blister cards. 28s with 7 inert tabs. *Rx.*
Use: Contraceptive hormone, sex hormone.

•**solifenacin succinate.** (sol-i-FEN-a-cin)
USAN.
Use: Anticholinergic.
See: VESIcare.

Soliris. (Alexion) Eculizumab 10 mg/mL.
Preservative free. Inj. Soln., Concentrate. Single-use vials. 30 mL. *Rx.*
Use: Monoclonal antibody.

•**solithromycin.** (soe-LITH-roe-MYE-sin)
USAN.
Use: Antibiotic.

Soliwax. Docusate Sodium, USP. Docusate Sodium, Solasulfone (I.N.N.).

Solodyn. (Medicis) Minocycline hydrochloride (as base) 45 mg, 65 mg,
90 mg, 115 mg, 135 mg. Lactose. Film-coated. ER Tab. 30s, 100s (except
65 mg and 115 mg). *Rx.*
Use: Tetracycline.

Sŏltice Quick-Rub. (Oakhurst) Menthol
5.1%, camphor 5.1%, eucalyptus oil,
glycerin, methyl salicylate. Oint. 37 g,
85 g. *OTC.*
Use: Rub and liniment.

Solu-Barb 0.25. (Forest) Phenobarbital
0.25 g. Tab. Bot. 24s. *c-IV.*
Use: Hypnotic; sedative.

**soluble complement receptor
(recombinant human) type 1.**
Use: Prevention or reduction of adult
respiratory distress syndrome.
[Orphan Drug]

Soluclenz Rx. (Obagi Medical Products)
Benzoyl peroxide 5%. Benzyl benzoate. Gel. 27 mL. *Rx.*
Use: Topical anti-infective, antibiotic
agent.

Solu-Cortef. (Pfizer) Hydrocortisone sodium succinate. Preservative free. Inj.,
Pow. for Soln. **100 mg:** Single-dose
Act-O-Vial. 2 mL. **250 mg:** Single-dose
Act-O-Vial. 2 mL. **500 mg:** Single-dose
Act-O-Vial. 4 mL. **1,000 mg:** Single-
dose *Act-O-Vial.* 8 mL. *Rx.*
Tall Man: Solu-CORTEF
Use: Corticosteroid.

Solu-Eze. (Forest) Hydroxyquinoline
0.12%, carbitol acetate 12.10%. Liq.
Bot. 3 oz. *Rx.*
Use: Dermatologic.

Solu-Medrol. (Pfizer) **40 mg/vial:**
Methylprednisolone sodium succinate.
Sodium phosphate anhydrous (monobasic 1.6 mg, dibasic 17.5 mg), lactose,
benzyl alcohol 9 mg. *Act-O-Vials.* 1 mL.
125 mg/vial: Methylprednisolone sodium succinate. Sodium phosphate anhydrous (monobasic 1.6 mg, dibasic
17.4 mg), benzyl alcohol ≈ 18 mg.
Act-O-Vials. 2 mL. **500 mg/vial:** Methylprednisolone sodium succinate.

Sodium phosphate anhydrous (monobasic 6.4 mg, dibasic 69.6 mg). May
contain benzyl alcohol 36 mg to
70.2 mg. Vials. 8 mL. Vials w/diluent.
8 mL. **1 g/vial:** Methylprednisolone sodium succinate. Sodium phosphate anhydrous (monobasic 12.8 mg, dibasic
139.2 mg). May contain benzyl alcohol
66.8 mg to 141 mg. Vials. 1 g. Vials
with diluent. 1 g. *Act-O-Vials.* 8 mL. **2 g/
vial:** Methylprednisolone sodium succinate. Vials with diluent. 2 g. Inj., Pow.
for Soln. *Rx.*
Tall Man: Solu-MEDROL
Use: Adrenocortical steroid, glucocorticoid.

Solumol. (C & M Pharmacal) Petrolatum, mineral oil, cetylstearyl alcohol, sodium lauryl sulfate, glycerin, propylene glycol, sorbic acid, purified water.
Jar lb. *OTC.*
Use: Pharmaceutical aid, ointment
base.

Soluvite C.T. (Pharmics) Vitamins A
2500 units, D 400 units, B_1 1.05 mg,
B_2 1.2 mg, B_6 1.05 mg, B_{12} 4.5 mcg,
C 60 mg, B_3 13.5 mg, E 15 units, fluoride 1 mg, folic acid 0.3 mg. Tab. Bot.
100s, 1000s. *Rx.*
Use: Mineral, vitamin supplement.

Solvisyn-A. (Towne) Water-soluble vitamin A 10,000 units, 25,000 units,
50,000 units. Cap. Bot. 100s, 1000s.
Rx-OTC.
Use: Vitamin supplement.

•**solypertine tartrate.** (SAHL-ee-PURR-
teen) USAN.
Use: Antiadrenergic.

Soma. (Wallace) Carisoprodol 350 mg.
Tab. Bot. 100s, 500s, UD 500s. *Rx.*
Use: Muscle relaxant.

Somagard. (Roberts)
See: Deslorelin.

•**somantadine hydrochloride.** (sah-
MAN-tah-deen) USAN.
Use: Antiviral.

somatostatin.
Use: Digestive aid. [Orphan Drug]

somatostatin analogs.
See: Lanreotide.
Octreotide Acetate.

•**somatropin.** (SO-muh-TROE-pin)
USAN. Growth hormone derived from
the anterior pituitary gland.
Use: Hormone, growth.
See: Accretropin.
Genotropin.
Genotropin MiniQuick.
Humatrope.
HumatroPen.
Norditropin.

Nutropin.
Nutropin AQ.
Nutropin AQ NuSpin 5.
Nutropin AQ NuSpin 10.
Nutropin AQ NuSpin 20.
Omnitrope.
Saizen.
Serostim.
Tev-Tropin.
Somatuline Depot. (Tercica) Lanreotide 60 mg (equiv. to lanreotide acetate 79.8 mg), 90 mg (equiv. to lanreotide acetate 116.4 mg), 120 mg (equiv. to lanreotide acetate 155.5 mg). Inj. Soln., ER. Single-use prefilled syringes. *Rx.*
Use: Somatostatin analog.
Somavert. (Pfizer) Pegvisomant 10 mg, 15 mg, 20 mg, mannitol 36 mg. Pow. for Inj., lyophilized. Vials. Single-dose. *Rx.*
Use: Acromegaly.
Sominex. (GlaxoSmithKline) Diphenhydramine hydrochloride. **Tab.:** 25 mg. Blister pack 16s, 32s, 72s. **Capl.:** 50 mg. Blister pack 8s, 16s, 32s. *OTC.*
Use: Sleep aid.
Sominex Pain Relief Formula. (GlaxoSmithKline) Diphenhydramine hydrochloride 25 mg, acetaminophen 500 mg. Tab. Blister pack 16s. Bot. 32s. *OTC.*
Use: Sleep aid; analgesic.
Somnote. (Breckenridge) Chloral hydrate 500 mg. Cap. 50s, UD 50s. *c-iv.*
Use: Sedative and hypnotic, nonbarbiturate.
Sonacide. (Wyeth) Potentiated acid glutaraldehyde. Bot. 1 gal, 5 gal. *OTC.*
Use: Disinfectant; sterilizing agent.
Sonahist. (River's Edge) Chlorpheniramine maleate 1 mg, phenylephrine hydrochloride 2 mg/mL. Parabens, saccharin, sorbitol. Orange-vanilla flavor. Drops. 30 mL. *Rx.*
Use: Upper respiratory combination, decongestant and antihistamine.
Sonahist DM. (Kylemore Pharmaceuticals) Chlorpheniramine maleate 1 mg, dextromethorphan hydrobromide 3 mg, phenylephrine hydrochloride 2 mg per mL. Glycerin, parabens, saccharin, sorbitol. Sweet orange vanilla flavor. Drops. 30 mL. *Rx.*
Use: Upper respiratory combination, antitussive combination.
Sonata. (King) Zaleplon 5 mg, 10 mg, lactose, tartrazine. Cap. Bot. 100s. *c-iv.*
Use: Sedative; hypnotic.
Sonekap. (Eastwood) Cap. Bot. 100s.
soneryl.
See: Butethal.

Soothaderm. (Pharmakon) Pyrilamine maleate 2.07 mg, benzocaine 2.08 mg, zinc oxide 41.35 mg/mL, camphor, menthol. Lot. Bot. 118 mL. *OTC.*
Use: Antihistamine; anesthetic, local.
Soothe. (Walgreen) Bismuth subsalicylate 100 mg. Tsp. Bot. 9 oz. *OTC.*
Use: Antidiarrheal.
Soothe & Cool. (Medline) Dimethicone 5%, zinc oxide 5%, lanolin, cetyl alcohol, vitamins A, D, and E. Cream. 118 mL. *OTC.*
Use: Diaper rash product.
Soothe XP. (Bausch & Lomb) Mineral oil 4.5%, light mineral oil 1%. EDTA, polysorbate 80, sodium chloride, sodium hydroxide and/or hydrochloride acid, sodium phosphate dibasic, sodium phosphate monobasic, octoxynol-40. Ophth. Soln. 15 mL. *OTC.*
Use: Artificial tears.
Soquette. (PBH Wesley Jessen) Polyvinyl alcohol w/benzalkonium Cl 0.01%, EDTA 0.2%. Bot. 4 fl oz. *OTC.*
Use: Contact lens care.
• **sorafenib.** (soe-RAF-e-nib) USAN.
Tall Man: SORAfenib
Use: Multikinase inhibitor.
See: Nexavar.
• **sorafenib tosylate.** (soe-RAF-e-nib) USAN.
Tall Man: SORAfenib
Use: Antineoplastic.
• **sorbic acid.** (SORE-bik) *NF 29.*
Use: Pharmaceutic aid (antimicrobial).
See: Clear Eyes Contact Lens Relief.
Sorbide T.D. (Merz) Isosorbide dinitrate 40 mg. TR Cap. Bot. 100s. *Rx.*
Use: Antianginal.
Sorbidon Hydrate. (Gordon Laboratories) Water-in-oil ointment. Jar 2 oz, 0.5 oz, 1 lb, 5 lb. *OTC.*
Use: Emollient.
sorbimacrogol oleate 300.
See: Polysorbate 80.
• **sorbinil.** (SORE-bih-nill) USAN.
Use: Enzyme inhibitor (aldose reductase).
• **sorbitan monolaurate.** (SORE-bih-tan MAHN-oh-LORE-ate) *NF 29.*
Use: Pharmaceutic aid (surfactant).
See: Span 20.
• **sorbitan monooleate.** (SORE-bih-tan MAHN-oh-OH-lee-ate) *NF 29.*
Use: Pharmaceutic aid (surfactant).
See: Span 80.
sorbitan monooleate polyoxyethylene derivatives.
See: Polysorbate 80.

• **sorbitan monopalmitate.** (SORE-bih-tan MAHN-oh-PAL-mih-tate) *NF 29.*
Use: Pharmaceutic aid (surfactant).
See: Span 40.

• **sorbitan monostearate.** (SORE-bih-tan MAHN-oh-STEE-ah-rate) *NF 29.*
Use: Pharmaceutic aid (surfactant).
See: Span 60.

sorbitans.
See: Polysorbate 80.

• **sorbitan sesquioleate.** (SORE-bih-tan SESS-kwih-OH-lee-ate) *NF 29.*
Use: Pharmaceutic aid (surfactant).
See: Arlacel C.

• **sorbitan trioleate.** (SORE-bih-tan TRY-OH-lee-ate) *NF 29.*
Use: Pharmaceutic aid, surfactant.
See: Span 85.

• **sorbitan tristearate.** (SORE-bih-tan TRY-STEE-ah-rate) USAN.
Use: Pharmaceutic aid; surfactant.
See: Span 65.

• **sorbitol.** (SOR-bi-tol) *NF 29.*
Use: Diuretic; dehydrating agent; humectant; pharmaceutic aid (sweetening agent, tablet excipient, flavor).
See: Numoisyn.
Sorbo.
W/Mannitol.
See: Sorbitol-Mannitol.

sorbitol. (B. Braun Medical) Sorbitol 3.3% (183 mOsm/L). Soln. 2,000 mL. *Rx.*
Use: Genitourinary irrigant, hexitol irrigant.

sorbitol. (Travenol) Sorbitol 3% (165 mOsm/L). Soln. 1,500 mL, 3,000 mL. *Rx.*
Use: Genitourinary irrigant, hexitol irrigant.

Sorbitol-Mannitol. (Hospira) Mannitol 0.54 g, sorbitol 2.7 g. Liq. Bot. 100 mL, 1500 mL, 3000 mL. *Rx.*
Use: Irrigant, genitourinary.

• **sorbitol solution.** (SOR-bi-tol) *USP 34.*
Use: Pharmaceutic aid (flavor, tablet excipient).

sorbitol solution. (Various Mfr.) 70% w/D-sorbitol. Soln. 454 mL. *OTC.*
Use: Laxative.

Sorbo. (AstraZeneca) Sorbitol Solution, USP.

Sorbsan. (Dow Hickam) Calcium alginate fiber 2 × 2, 3 × 3, 4 × 4, 4 × 8 inch. Box 1s. Wound packing fibers-calcium alginate fiber ¼ × 12 inch. Box 1s. *Rx.*
Use: Dermatologic, wound therapy.

Sorbutuss NR. (Teral) Dextromethorphan hydrobromide 15 mg, guaifenesin 150 mg, potassium citrate 127.5 mg per 7.5 mL. Parabens, sorbitol, sucralose. Alcohol free, dye free, and sugar free. Grape flavor. Liq. 474 mL. *OTC.*
Use: Upper respiratory combination, antitussive with expectorant.

sorethytan (20) monooleate.
See: Polysorbate 80.

Soriatane. (GlaxoSmithKline) Acitretin 10 mg, 17.5 mg, 22.5 mg, 25 mg. Capsule shells contain gelatin, iron oxide, titanium dioxide, may also contain benzyl alcohol. Cap. 30s. *Rx.*
Use: Retinoid, second generation.

Soriatane CK. (Stiefel) **Cap.:** Acitretin 10 mg. Maltodextrin, gelatin, iron oxide, titanium dioxide. May contain benzyl alcohol. 30s. **Foam:** Cetyl alcohol, mineral oil, petrolatum. 94 g. *Rx.*
Use: Retinoid (dermatologic), second-generation retinoid.

Sorilux. (Stiefel) Calcipotriene 0.005%. Alcohol, edetate disodium, light mineral oil, propylene glycol, white petrolatum. Topical Foam. 60 g, 120 g. *Rx.*
Use: Antipsoriatic agent.

Sosegon. (Sanofi-Synthelabo) Pentazocine. Soln., Susp., Tab. *c-IV.*
Use: Analgesic.

Soss-10. (Roberts) Sodium sulfacetamide 10%. Soln. Bot. 15 mL. *Rx.*
Use: Anti-infective, ophthalmic.

• **sotalol hydrochloride.** (SOTT-uh-lahl) *USP 34.*
Use: Antiadrenergic/sympatholytic, beta-adrenergic blocker.
See: Betapace.
Betapace AF.

sotalol hydrochloride. (Academic Pharmaceutical) Sotalol hydrochloride 15 mg/mL. Inj., Soln., Conc. Vial. 10 mL.
Use: Antiadrenergic/sympatholytic, beta-adrenergic blocking agent.

sotalol hydrochloride. (Various Mfr.) Sotalol hydrochloride 80 mg, 120 mg, 160 mg, 240 mg, lactose. Tab. Bot. 100s, 500s, 1000s. *Rx.*
Use: Antiadrenergic/sympatholytic; beta-adrenergic blocker.

sotalol hydrochloride AF. (Apotex) Sotalol hydrochloride 80 mg, 120 mg, 160 mg. Tab. 100s. *Rx.*
Use: Beta-adrenergic blocking agent.

• **sotatercept.** (soe-TAT-er-sept) USAN.
Use: Chemotherapy-induced anemia.

• **soterenol hydrochloride.** (so-TER-en-ole) USAN.
Use: Bronchodilator.

• **sotirimod.** (soe-TIR-i-mod) USAN.
Use: Dermatalogic agent.

Sotradecol. (AngioDynamics) Sodium tetradecyl sulfate 10 mg/mL, 30 mg/mL. Benzyl alcohol 0.02 mL. Inj. Vials. 2 mL. *Rx.*
Use: Sclerosing agent.

• **sotrastaurin.** (so-tra-STAW-rin) USAN.
Use: Immunomodulator.

• **sotrastaurin acetate.** (so-tra-STAW-rin) USAN.
Use: Immunomodulator.

Sotret. (Ranbaxy) Isotretinoin 10 mg, 20 mg, 30 mg, 40 mg. Parabens, EDTA. Softgel Cap. 30s, 100s. *Rx.*
Use: Retinoid, first generation.

Soxa-Forte. (Vita Elixir) Sulfisoxazole 0.5 g, phenazopyridine 50 mg. Tab. *Rx.*
Use: Anti-infective.

Soyalac. (Mt. Vernon Foods, Inc.) Infant formula based on an extract from whole soybeans containing all-essential nutrients. **Ready to Serve Liq.:** Can 32 fl oz. **Double Strength Conc.:** Can 13 fl oz. **Pow.:** Can 14 oz. *OTC.*
Use: Nutritional supplement.

Soyalac-I. (Mt. Vernon Foods, Inc.) Soy protein isolate infant formula containing no corn derivatives and a negligible amount of soy carbohydrates. Contains all essential nutrients in various forms. **Ready to Serve Liq.:** Can 32 fl oz. **Double Strength Conc.:** Can 13 fl oz. *OTC.*
Use: Nutritional supplement.

soya lecithin. Soybean extract. 100s.
Use: Phosphorus therapy.

• **soybean oil.** (SOI-been) *USP 34.*
Use: Pharmaceutic aid.
See: Intralipid 30%.
Intralipid 20%.
Liposyn III.

Spabelin. (Arcum) Hyoscyamine sulfate 81 mcg, atropine sulfate 15 mcg, scopolamine HBr 5 mcg, phenobarbital 16.2 mg/5 mL. Elix. Bot. 16 oz, gal. *Rx.*
Use: Anticholinergic; antispasmodic; hypnotic; sedative.

Spabelin No. 1. (Arcum) Phenobarbital 15 mg, belladonna powdered extract ⅛ g. Tab. Bot. 100s, 1000s. *Rx.*
Use: Hypnotic; sedative.

Spabelin No. 2. (Arcum) Phenobarbital 30 mg, belladonna powdered extract ⅛ g. Tab. Bot. 100s, 1000s. *Rx.*
Use: Hypnotic; sedative.

Span C. (Freeda) Citrus bioflavonoids 300 mg, vitamin C (ascorbic acid and rose hips) 200 mg. Sugar free. Calcium carbonate, calcium stearate. Tab. Bot.
100s, 250s, 500s. *OTC.*
Use: Water-soluble vitamin.

Span 80. (AstraZeneca) Sorbitan monooleate, *NF 20.*

Span 85. (AstraZeneca) Sorbitan trioleate. Mixture of oleate esters of sorbitol and its anhydrides.
Use: Surface active agent.

Span 40. (AstraZeneca) Sorbitan Monopalmitate, *NF 20.*

Span-PD. (Lexis Laboratories) Phentermine hydrochloride 37.5 mg. Cap. Bot. 100s. *c-IV.*
Use: Anorexiant.

Span-RD. (Lexis Laboratories) d-methamphetamine hydrochloride 12 mg, dl-methamphetamine hydrochloride 6 mg, butabarbital 30 mg. Tab. Bot. 100s, 1000s. *c-III.*
Use: Amphetamine; hypnotic; sedative.

Span 60. (AstraZeneca) Sorbitan Monostearate.

Span 65. (AstraZeneca) Sorbitan tristearate. Mixture of stearate esters of sorbitol and its anhydrides.
Use: Surface active agent.

Span 20. (AstraZeneca) Sorbitan Monolaurate.

• **sparfosate sodium.** (spar-FOSS-ate) USAN.
Use: Antineoplastic.

Sparkles Effervescent Granules. (Lafayette) Sodium bicarbonate 2000 mg, citric acid 1500 mg, simethicone. Pkt. Bot. UD 50s. *OTC.*
Use: Antacid.

Sparkles Granules. (Lafayette) Effervescent granules 4 g/Packet or 6 g/Packet. Each 6 g produces 500 mL of carbon dioxide gas. Ctn. 25 packets. Pkg. 2.
Use: Diagnostic aid.

Sparkles Tablets. (Lafayette) Effervescent tablets. Each 4.3 g of tablets produces 250 mL of carbon dioxide gas. Bot. 43 g (10 doses).
Use: Diagnostic aid.

• **sparsomycin.** (SPAR-so-MY-sin) USAN.
Use: Antineoplastic.

• **sparteine sulfate.** (SPAR-teh-een SULL-fate) USAN.
Use: Oxytocic.
W/Sodium Cl.
See: Tocosamine.

Spasmatol. (Pharmed) Homatropine MBr 3 mg, pentobarbital 12 mg, mephobarbital 8 mg. Tab. Bot. 100s, 1000s. *Rx.*
Use: Anticholinergic; antispasmodic; hypnotic; sedative.

Spasmolin. (Various Mfr.) Phenobarbital 16.2 mg, hyoscyamine HBr sulfate

0.1037 mg, atropine sulfate 0.0194 mg, scopolamine HBr 0.0065 mg. Tab. Bot. 100s, 1000s. *Rx.*
Use: Gastrointestinal anticholinergic combination.

spasmolytic agents.
See: Antispasmodics.

Spasno-Lix. (Freeport) Phenobarbital 16.2 mg, hyoscyamine sulfate 0.1037 mg, atropine sulfate 0.0194 mg, hyoscine HBr 0.0065 mg, alcohol 21% to 23%/5 mL. Bot. 4 oz. *Rx.*
Use: Anticholinergic; antispasmodic; hypnotic; sedative.

S.P.B. (Sheryl) Therapeutic B complex formula with ascorbic acid 300 mg. Tab. Bot. 100s. *OTC.*
Use: Vitamin supplement.

SPD. (A.P.C.) Methyl salicylate, methyl nicotinate, dipropylene glycol salicylate, oleoresin capsicum, camphor, menthol. Cream. Bot. 4 oz, Tube 1.5 oz. *OTC.*
Use: Analgesic, topical.

spearmint.
Use: Flavor.

spearmint oil.
Use: Flavor.

Special Shampoo. (Del-Ray) Non-medicated shampoo. *OTC.*
Use: Cleanser.

Spectazole. (Ortho Pharm Corp.) Econazole nitrate 1%. Water-miscible base, mineral oil. Cream. Tube 15 g, 30 g, 85 g. *Rx.*
Use: Antifungal, topical anti-infective.

spectinomycin. (speck-TIN-oh-MY-sin) *Formerly Actinospectocin.* An antibiotic isolated from broth cultures of *Streptomyces spectabilis. Rx.*
Use: Anti-infective.

•**spectinomycin hydrochloride, sterile.** (speck-TIN-oh-MY-sin) *USP 34.*
Use: Anti-infective.

Spectracef. (Cornerstone) Cefditoren pivoxil 200 mg, 400 mg. Mannitol. Film-coated. Tab. Bot. 20s, 28s (400 mg only), 60s (200 mg only). *Rx.*
Use: Antibiotic, cephalosporin.

Spectra 360. (Parker) Salt-free electrode gel. Tube 8 oz.
Use: T.E.N.S. application, ECG pediatric, and long-term procedures.

Spectrobid. (Roerig) Bacampicill hydrochloride 400 mg (equiv. to 280 mg ampicillin), lactose. Tab. 100s. *Rx.*
Use: Anti-infective, penicillin.

Spectro-Biotic. (A.P.C.) Bacitracin 400 units, neomycin sulfate 5 mg, polymyxin B sulfate 5000 units/g Oint. Tube 0.5 oz, 1 oz. *OTC.*
Use: Anti-infective, topical.

Spectro-Jel. (Recsei) Soap free. Iodomethylcellulose, carboxypolymethylene, cetyl alcohol, sorbitan monooleate, fumed silica, triethanolamine stearate, glycol polysiloxane, propylene glycol, glycerin, isopropyl alcohol 5%. Gel. Bot. 127.5 mL, pt, gal. *OTC.*
Use: Dermatologic, cleanser.

Spec-T Sore Throat Anesthetic. (Apothecon) Benzocaine 10 mg. Loz. Box 10s. *OTC.*
Use: Anesthetic, local.

spermaceti.
Use: Stiffening agent; pharmaceutic necessity for cold cream.

spermine. Diaminopropyltetramethylene.

Sperti. (Whitehall-Robins) Live yeast cell derivative supplying 2000 units skin respiratory factor/g w/shark liver oil 3%, phenylmercuric nitrate 1:10,000. Oint. Tube oz. *OTC.*
Use: Dermatologic, wound therapy.

spider-bite antivenin.
See: Antivenin (Latrodectus Mactans).

Spider-Man Children's Chewable Vitamin. (NBTY) Vitamins A 2500 units, D 400 units, E 15 mg, B_1 1.05 mg, B_2 1.2 mg, B_3 13.5 mg, B_6 1.05 mg, B_{12} 4.5 mcg, C 60 mg, folic acid 0.3 mg, xylitol, sorbitol. Chew. Tab. Bot. 75s, 130s. *OTC.*
Use: Vitamin supplement.

•**spinosad.** (SPIN-oh-sad) USAN.
Use: Scabicide/Pediculicide.
See: Natroba.

•**spiperone.** (spih-per-OHN) USAN.
Use: Antipsychotic.

•**spiradoline mesylate.** (spy-RAH-doe-leen) USAN.
Use: Analgesic.

•**spiramycin.** (SPIH-rah-MY-sin) USAN. Antibiotic substance from cultures of *Streptomyces ambofaciens.*
Use: Anti-infective.

•**spiraprilat.** (SPY-rah-PRILL-at) USAN.
Use: ACE inhibitor.

•**spirapril hydrochloride.** (SPY-rah-prill) USAN.
Use: ACE inhibitor.
See: Renormax.

Spiriva. (Boehringer Ingelheim) Tiotropium bromide 18 mcg (equiv. to tiotropium bromide 22.5 mcg). Lactose. Pow. for Inh. UD 5s, 30s, 90s, w/*HandiHaler* device. *Rx.*
Use: Bronchodilator, anticholinergic.

- **spirogermanium hydrochloride.** (SPY-row-JER-MAY-nee-uhm) USAN.
  Use: Antineoplastic.
- **spiromustine.** (SPY-row-MUSS-teen) USAN. *Formerly Spirohydantoin Mustard.*
  Use: Antineoplastic.

spironazide. (Schein) Spironolactone 25 mg, hydrochlorothiazide 25 mg. Tab. 100s, 1,000s, UD 100s. *Rx.*
  Use: Diuretic combination.
- **spironolactone.** (SPEER-oh-no-LAK-tone) *USP 34.*
  Use: Diuretic, aldosterone antagonist.
  See: Aldactone.
  W/Hydrochlorothiazide.
  See: Aldactazide.

spironolactone. (Various Mfr.) Spironolactone. Tab. **25 mg:** 60s, 100s, 500s, 1,000s. **50 mg:** 30s, 60s, 100s, 500s, 1,000s. **100 mg:** 100s, 500s. *Rx.*
  Use: Diuretic.

spironolactone w/hydrochlorothiazide. (Various Mfr.) Spironolactone 25 mg, hydrochlorothiazide 25 mg. Tab. Bot. 30s, 60s, 100s, 250s, 500s, 1000s, UD 32s, 100s. *Rx.*
  Use: Diuretic combination.
- **spiroplatin.** (SPY-row-PLAT-in) USAN.
  Use: Antineoplastic.

spirotriazine hydrochloride.
  Use: Anthelmintic.
- **spiroxasone.** (spy-ROX-ah-sone) USAN.
  Use: Diuretic.

Spirozide. (Rugby) Spironolactone 25 mg, hydrochlorothiazide 25 mg. Tab. Bot. 100s, 500s, 1000s. *Rx.*
  Use: Diuretic combination.

SPL-Serologic Types I and III. (Delmont) *Staphylococcus aureus* 120 to 180 million units, *Staphylococcus bacteriophage* plaque-forming 100 to 1000 million units/mL. Soln. Amp. 1 mL, Vial 10 mL. *Rx.*
  Use: Anti-infective.

Sporanox. (Janssen) Itraconazole 100 mg, sucrose, sugar. Bot. 30s, UD 30s, *PulsePak* 28s. *Rx.*
  Use: Antifungal, triazole.

Sporanox. (Ortho Biotech) Itraconazole 10 mg/mL. Saccharin, sorbitol. Cherry/caramel flavor. Oral Soln. Bot. 150 mL. *Rx.*
  Use: Antifungal, triazole.

Sportscreme. (Thompson Medical) Triethanolamine salicylate 10% in a nongreasy base. Cream. 37.5 g, 90 g. *OTC.*
  Use: Analgesic, topical.

Sports Spray Extra Strength. (Mentholatum Co.) Methyl salicylate 35%, menthol 10%, camphor 5%, alcohol 58%, isobutane. Spray. 90 mL. *OTC.*
  Use: Analgesic, topical.

Spray Skin Protectant. (Morton International) Isopropyl alcohol, polyvinylpyrrolidone, vinyl alcohol, plasticizer & propellant. Aer. Can 6 oz. *OTC.*
  Use: Dermatologic, protectant.

Sprayzoin. (Geritrex) Benzoin compound, ethyl alcohol. Spray. 118 mL. *OTC.*
  Use: Protectant.

spreading factor.
  See: Hyaluronidase.

Sprintec. (Barr) Norgestimate 0.25 mg, ethinyl estradiol 35 mcg. Lactose. Tab. 28s with 7 inert tabs. *Rx.*
  Use: Sex hormone, contraceptive hormone.

Sprix. (Roxro) Ketorolac tromethamine 15.75 mg/spray. Edetate disodium. Preservative free. Spray, Soln.; Intranasal. 1 single-day or 5 single-day 1.7 g bottles (delivers 8 sprays for a total of 126 mg of ketorolac). *Rx.*
  Use: Nonsteroidal anti-inflammatory agent.
- **sprodiamide.** (sprah-DIE-ah-mide) USAN.
  Use: Diagnostic aid (paramagnetic).

SPRX-105. (Reid-Provident) Phendimetrazine tartrate 105 mg. SR Cap. Bot. 28s, 500s. *c-III.*
  Use: Anorexiant.

Sprycel. (Bristol-Myers Squibb) Dasatinib 20 mg, 50 mg, 70 mg, 80 mg, 100 mg, 140 mg. Film-coated. Lactose. Tab. 30s (80 mg, 100 mg, 140 mg), 60s (20 mg, 50 mg, 70 mg). *Rx.*
  Use: Protein-tyrosine kinase inhibitor; treatment of leukemia.

SPS. (Carolina Medical Products) Sodium polystyrene sulfonate 15 g, sorbitol solution 21.5 mL, alcohol 0.3%/60 mL, propylene glycol, sodium saccharin, methylparaben, propylparaben. Cherry flavor. Susp. Bot. 120 mL, 473 mL, UD 60 mL. *Rx.*
  Use: Potassium-removing resin.
- **squalamine lactate.** (SKWAH-la-meen) USAN.
  Use: Antineoplastic.
- **squalane.** (SKWAH-lane) *NF 29.*
  Use: Pharmaceutic aid (vehicle, oleaginous).

SRC Expectorant. (Edwards) Hydrocodone bitartrate 5 mg, pseudoephedrine hydrochloride 60 mg, guaifenesin 200 mg w/alcohol 12.5%. Bot. Pt. *c-III.*
  Use: Antitussive; decongestant; expectorant.

Sronyx. (Watson Pharma) Ethinyl estradiol 20 mcg, levonorgestrel 0.1 mg. Lactose. Tab. 28s with 7 inert tablets (lactose). *Rx.*
Use: Contraceptive hormone, sex hormone.

SSD. (Dr. Reddy's Labs) Silver sulfadiazine 10 mg/g in a water-miscible base. Cetyl alcohol, white petrolatum, stearyl alcohol, methylparaben 0.3%. Cream. 25 g, 50 g, 85 g, 400 g, 1000 g. *Rx.*
Use: Topical anti-infective.

SSD AF. (Dr. Reddy's Labs) Silver sulfadiazine 10 mg/g in a water-miscible base. White petrolatum, stearyl alcohol, methylparaben 0.3%. Cream. Tube 50 g, 400 g, 1000 g. *Rx.*
Use: Topical anti-infective.

SSKI. (Upsher-Smith) Potassium iodide 1 g/mL. Soln. 30 mL, 240 mL. *Rx.*
Use: Thyroid drug.

S-Spas. (Southern States) Pentobarbital 16.2 mg, atropine sulfate 0.0194 mg, hyoscyamine sulfate 0.1037 mg, hyoscine HBr 0.0065 mg. **Liq.:** 5 mL. Bot. Pt. **Tab.:** Bot. 100s, 1000s. *Rx.*
Use: Anticholinergic; antispasmodic; hypnotic; sedative.

S.S.S. High Potency Vitamin. (S.S.S. Company) Vitamins C 300 mg, B_1 7.5 mg, B_2 7.5 mg, B_3 50 mg, Ca 100 mg, Fe 27 mg, E 50 units, B_6 2.5 mg, folic acid 200 mcg, B_{12} 12.5 mg, Mg 50 mg, Zn 12 mg, Cu 1.5 mg, biotin 22.5 mcg, pantothenic acid 10 mg. Tab. Bot. 20s, 40s, 80s. *OTC.*
Use: Vitamin, mineral supplement.

S.S.S. Vitamin and Mineral Supplement. (S.S.S. Company) Vitamins A 833 units, C 20 mg, E 10 units, B_1 1.7 mg, B_2 0.57 mg, niacinamide 6.7 mg, B_6 0.67 mg, B_{12} 2 mcg, D_3 133 units, biotin 100 mcg, pantothenic acid 3 mg, I 50 mcg, Fe 3 mg, Zn 1 mg, Ma 0.8 mg, Cr 8 mcg, Mo 8 mcg/5 mL, alcohol 6.6%, sugar. Liq. Bot. 236 mL. *OTC.*
Use: Vitamin, mineral supplement.

Stadol. (Bristol-Myers Squibb) Butorphanol tartrate 1 mg/mL; Vial 1 mL. 2 mg/mL; Vial 1 mL, 2 mL, 10 mL (with benzethonium chloride 0.1 mg/mL). *c-IV.*
Use: Analgesic.

Staflex. (Magna) Phenyltoloxamine citrate 55 mg, acetaminophen 500 mg. Tab. 100s. *Rx.*
Use: Nonnarcotic analgesic combination.

Staftabs. (Modern Aids Inc.) Fine bone flour containing calcium, phosphorus, iron, iodine, vitamin D, magnesium. Tab. Bot. 85s, 160s. *OTC.*
Use: Mineral, vitamin supplement.

Stagesic. (Magna) Hydrocodone bitartrate 5 mg, acetaminophen 500 mg. Cap. Bot. 100s. *c-III.*
Use: Analgesic combination, narcotic.

Stahist. (Magna) Chlorpheniramine maleate 8 mg, hyoscyamine sulfate 0.19 mg, atropine sulfate 0.04 mg, scopolamine HBr 0.01 mg, pseudoephedrine hydrochloride 90 mg. Dye free. ER Tab. Bot. 100s. *Rx.*
Use: Upper respiratory combination, antihistamine, anticholinergic, decongestant.

stainless iodized ointment. (Day-Baldwin) Jar lb.

stainless iodized ointment with methyl salicylate 5%. (Day-Baldwin) Jar lb.

Stalevo 50. (Novartis) Carbidopa 12.5 mg, levodopa 50 mg, entacapone 200 mg, mannitol, sucrose. Tab. 100s, 250s. *Rx.*
Use: Antiparkinson agent.

Stalevo 100. (Novartis) Carbidopa 25 mg, levodopa 100 mg, entacapone 200 mg, mannitol, sucrose. Tab. 100s, 250s. *Rx.*
Use: Antiparkinson agent.

Stalevo 150. (Novartis) Carbidopa 37.5 mg, levodopa 150 mg, entacapone 200 mg, mannitol, sucrose. Tab. 100s, 250s. *Rx.*
Use: Antiparkinson agents.

Stalevo 125. (Novartis) Carbidopa 31.25 mg, entacapone 200 mg, levodopa 125 mg. Mannitol, sucrose. Film-coated. Tab. 100s. *Rx.*
Use: Antiparkinson agent.

Stalevo 75. (Novartis) Carbidopa 18.75 mg, entacapone 200 mg, levodopa 75 mg. Mannitol, sucrose. Film-coated. Tab. 100s. *Rx.*
Use: Antiparkinson agent.

Stalevo 200. (Novartis) Carbidopa 50 mg, levodopa 200 mg, entacapone 200 mg. Mannitol, sucrose. Film-coated. Tab. 100s. *Rx.*
Use: Antiparkinson agent.

•**stallimycin hydrochloride.** (stal-IH-MY-sin) USAN.
Use: Anti-infective.

Stamoist E. (Magna) Pseudoephedrine hydrochloride 45 mg, guaifenesin 600 mg. ER Tab. Bot. 100s. *Rx.*
Use: Upper respiratory combination, decongestant and expectorant.

•**stamulumab.** (sta-MUL-ue-mab) USAN.
Use: Muscular dystrophy.

Stamyl. (Sanofi-Synthelabo) Pancreatin. Tab.
Use: Digestive aid.

Stanback Headache. (Glaxo-SmithKline Consumer Healthcare) Aspirin 845 mg, caffeine 65 mg. Lactose, potassium 55 mg per packet. Pow. 2s, 6s, 50s. *OTC.*
Use: Nonnarcotic analgesic combination.

•**stannous chloride.** (STAN-uhs KLOR-ide) USAN.
Use: Pharmaceutic aid.

•**stannous fluoride.** (STAN-uhs FLOR-ide) *USP 34.*
Use: Dental caries agent.
See: Just For Kids.
     PerioMed.

stannous fluoride. (Cypress) **Gel:** Stannous fluoride 0.4%, parabens, mint flavor. Tube 122 g. **Conc. Oral Rinse:** Stannous fluoride 0.63%, mint flavor. Bot. 283 g. *Rx-OTC.*
Use: Trace element.

•**stannous pyrophosphate.** (STAN-uhs PIE-row-FOSS-fate) USAN.
Use: Diagnostic aid (skeletal imaging).

•**stannous sulfur colloid.** (STAN-uhs SULL-fer KAHL-oyd) USAN.
Use: Diagnostic aid (bone, liver, and spleen imaging).

•**stanozolol.** (stan-OH-zoe-lole) *USP 34.*
Use: Anabolic steroid.

staphage lysate (SPL).
Use: Anti-infective.
See: SPL-Serologic Types I and III.

StaphAseptic. (Tec Labs) Benzethonium chloride 0.2%, lidocaine hydrochloride 2.5%. Disodium EDTA, glycerin, polyoxyl 35 castor oil, tea tree oil, white thyme oil. Gel. 56.7 g. *OTC.*
Use: Local anesthetic, topical; local anesthetic, topical combination.

staphylococcus bacteriophage lysate.
See: Staphage Lysate.

•**starch.** (stahrch) *NF 29.*
Use: Dusting powder; pharmaceutic aid.

starch glycerite.
Use: Emollient.

•**starch, pregelatinized.** (stahrch pree-jel-AT-inized) *NF 29.*
Use: Pharmaceutic aid (tablet excipient).

•**starch, topical.** (stahrch) *USP 34.*
Use: Dusting powder.

Starlix. (Novartis) Nateglinide 60 mg, 120 mg. Lactose. Tab. Bot. 100s, 500s. *Rx.*
Use: Antidiabetic, meglitinide.

Star-Otic. (Stellar) Burrows soln. nonaqueous, acetic acid, boric acid, propylene glycol. Drop Bot. 15 mL. *OTC.*
Use: Otic preparation.

•**statolon.** (STAY-toe-lone) USAN. Antiviral agent derived from *Penicillium stoloniferum.*
Use: Antiviral.

Statomin Maleate II. (Jones Pharma) Chlorpheniramine maleate 2 mg, acetaminophen 324 mg, caffeine 32 mg. Tab. Bot. 1000s. *Rx.*
Use: Antihistamine; analgesic.

•**stavudine.** (STAHV-you-deen) USAN.
Use: Antiretroviral.
See: Zerit.

stavudine. (Mylan) Stavudine 15 mg, 20 mg, 30 mg, 40 mg. Lactose. Cap. 60s, 100s, 500s. *Rx.*
Use: Antiretroviral agent, nucleoside reverse transcriptase inhibitor.

Stavzor. (Noven Therapeutics) Valproic acid 125 mg, 250 mg, 500 mg. Delayed release Cap. 100s. *Rx.*
Use: Anticonvulsant.

Sta-Wake Dextabs. (Health for Life Brands) Caffeine 1.5 g, dextrose 3 g. Tab. Bot. 36s, 1000s. *OTC.*
Use: CNS stimulant.

Staxyn. (Schering-Plough) Vardenafil 10 mg (equiv. to vardenafil hydrochloride 11.85 mg). Aspartame, mannitol, phenylalanine 1.01 mg, sorbitol. Tab., orally disintegrating. UD 4s, 40s. *Rx.*
Use: Impotence agent, phosphodiesterase type 5 inhibitor.

Stay Alert. (Apothecary Prods.) Caffeine 200 mg. Tab. Bot. 24s, 48s. *OTC.*
Use: CNS stimulant

Stay Awake. (Major) Caffeine 200 mg, dextrose. Tab. Bot. 16s. *OTC.*
Use: CNS stimulant, analeptic.

Stay-Brite. (Sherman Pharmaceuticals, Inc.) EDTA 0.25%, benzalkonium Cl 0.01%. Spray. Bot. 30 mL. *OTC.*
Use: Contact lens care.

Stay Moist Lip Conditioner. Padimate O, oxybenzone, aloe vera, vitamin E, tropical fruit flavor. SPF 15. Lip Balm 48 g. *OTC.*
Use: Emollient.

Stay-Wet. (Sherman Pharmaceuticals, Inc.) Polyvinyl alcohol, hydroxyethylcellulose, povidone, sodium Cl, potassium Cl, sodium carbonate, benzalkonium Cl 0.01%, EDTA 0.025%. Soln. Bot. 30 mL. *OTC.*
Use: Contact lens care.

Stay-Wet Rewetting. (Sherman Pharmaceuticals, Inc.) Polyvinyl alcohol, hydroxyethycellulose, povidone, NaCl,

KCl, sodium carbonate, benzalkonium Cl 0.01%, EDTA 0.025%. Soln. Bot. *OTC.*
Use: Lubricant-ophthalmic.

Stay-Wet 3 Wetting. (Sherman Pharmaceuticals, Inc.) Polyvinyl alcohol, hydroxyethycellulose, povidone, sodium Cl, potassium Cl, sodium carbonate, benzalkonium Cl 0.01%, EDTA 0.025%. Soln. 30 mL. *OTC.*
Use: Lubricant, ophthalmic.

Staze. (Del) Karaya gum. Tube 1.75 oz, 3.5 oz. *OTC.*
Use: Denture adhesive.

S-T Cort Cream. (Scot-Tussin) Hydrocortisone 0.5%, water-washable base, parabens. 120 g. *Rx.*
Use: Corticosteroid, topical.

S-T Cort Lotion. (Scot-Tussin) Hydrocortisone 0.5%, water-washable, lanolin alcohol, mineral oil base. 60 mL, 120 mL. *Rx.*
Use: Corticosteroid, topical.

• **stearic acid.** (STEER-ik) *NF 29.* Octadecanoic acid.
Use: Pharmaceutic aid (emulsion adjunct, tablet/capsule lubricant).

• **stearyl alcohol.** (STEE-rill AL-koe-hahl) *NF 29.*
Use: Pharmaceutic aid (emulsion adjunct).

• **steffimycin.** (steh-fih-MY-sin) USAN.
Use: Anti-infective; antiviral.

Stelara. (Centocor Ortho Biotech) Ustekinumab 90 mg per 1 mL. Sucrose 76 mg, L-histidine 1 mg, 0.04 mg of polysorbate 80. Preservative free. Inj., Soln. Single-use vial. *Rx.*
Use: Immunologic agent, immunomodulator.

stem cell mobilizers.
See: Plerixafor.

• **stenbolone acetate.** (STEEN-bow-lone) USAN.
Use: Anabolic.

Steraject. (Merz) Prednisolone acetate 25 mg, 50 mg/mL. Inj. Vial 10 mL. *Rx.*
Use: Corticosteroid.

sterculia gum.
See: Karaya Gum.

Stericol. (Alton) Isopropyl alcohol 91%. Soln. Bot. 16 oz, 32 oz, gal. *OTC.*
Use: Anti-infective, topical.

sterile erythromycin gluceptate.
Erythromycin monoglucoheptonate (salt). Erythromycin glucoheptonate (1:1) (salt).
Use: Anti-infective.

Sterile Lens Lubricant. (Blairex) Isotonic w/borate buffer system, sodium Cl,

hydroxypropyl methylcellulose, glycerin, sorbic acid 0.25%, EDTA 0.1%, thimerosal free. Soln. Bot. 15 mL. *OTC.*
Use: Lubricant, ophthalmic.

Sterile Saline. (Bausch & Lomb) Sodium Cl, borate buffer, EDTA, thimerosal free. Soln. Bot. 60 mL. *OTC.*
Use: Lubricant, ophthalmic.

Sterile Talc Powder. (Bryan) Talc 5 g. Pow. Glass Bot. 100 mL. *Rx.*
Use: Antineoplastic.

sterile thiopental sodium. Thiopental sodium, USP.
See: Pentothal.

sterile water for irrigation. (Various Mfr.) Sterile water for irrigation 0.45%, 0.9%. Soln. Bot. 150 mL, 250 mL, 500 mL, 1000 mL, 1500 mL, 2000 mL, 4000 mL. *Rx.*
Use: Irrigant, genitourinary.

SteriLid. (Advanced) Allantoin, boric acid, cocamidopropyl betadine, etidronic acid, hepes acetate, linalool oil, panthenol, PEG-80, PEG-150, sodium laureth-13 carboxylate, sodium lauroampho acetate, sodium perborate monohydrate, sodium trideceth sulfate, sorbitan laurate, tea tree oil, tris-EDTA. Soap, foam; Ophth. 48 mL. *Rx.*
Use: Ophthalmic agent, ophthalmic nonsurgical adjunct.

Steri-Unna Boot. (Pedinol Pharmacal) Glycerin, gum acacia, zinc oxide, white petrolatum, amylum in an oil base. 10 yds. × 3.5 in. sterilized bandage.
Use: Treatment of leg ulcers, varicosities, sprains, strains & to reduce swelling after surgery.

steroid antibiotic combinations.
Use: Anti-inflammatory; otic preparations.
See: AntibiOtic.
  Antibiotic Ear Solution.
  Ciprodex.
  Cipro HC Otic.
  Coly-Mycin S Otic.
  Cortisporin.
  Cortisporin Otic.
  Cortisporin-TC Otic.
  Ear-Eze.
  LazerSporin-C.
  Maxitrol.
  Octicair.
  Otosporin.
  Neomycin and Polymyxin B Sulfates and Dexamethasone.
  Neomycin/Polymyxin B Sulfates, Hydrocortisone Otic.
  Pediotic.
  Poly-Pred Liquifilm.
  Pred-G.

TobraDex.
Tobramycin and Dexamethasone.
steroids, intranasal.
See: Beclomethasone Dipropionate.
Budesonide.
Ciclesonide.
Flunisolide.
Fluticasone.
Mometasone Furoate Monohydrate.
Triamcinolone Acetonide.
S-T Forte 2. (Scot-Tussin) Hydrocodone bitartrate 2.5 mg, chlorpheniramine maleate 2 mg per 5 mL. Menthol, parabens. Sugar, alcohol, and dye free. Liq. Bot. 473 mL, 3.8 L. *c-III.*
Use: Upper respiratory combination, antitussive, antihistamine.
stilbamidine isethionate.
Use: Antiprotozoal.
•**stilbazium iodide.** (still-BAY-zee-uhm EYE-oh-dide) USAN.
Use: Anthelmintic.
stilbestrol.
See: Diethylstilbestrol Dipropionate.
stilbestronate.
See: Diethylstilbestrol Dipropionate.
stilboestrol.
See: Diethylstilbestrol Dipropionate.
Stilboestrol DP.
See: Diethylstilbestrol Dipropionate.
•**stilonium iodide.** (STILL-oh-nee-uhm EYE-oh-dide) USAN.
Use: Antispasmodic.
Stilronate.
See: Diethylstilbestrol Dipropionate.
Stimate. (CSL Behring) Desmopressin acetate 1.5 mg/mL. Spray, Soln., intranasal. 2.5 mL (25 sprays of 150 mcg each). *Rx.*
Use: Hormone.
stimulant laxatives.
See: Agoral.
Aromatic Cascara Fluidextract.
Bisac-Evac.
Bisacodyl.
Bisacodyl Uniserts.
Black Draught.
Cascara Aromatic.
Cascara Sagrada.
Correctol.
Dulcolax.
ex•lax.
ex•lax Chocolated.
Feen-a-mint.
Fleet Laxative.
Fletcher's Castoria.
Maximum Relief ex•lax.
Modane.
Reliable Gentle Laxative.
Senexon.
Senna-Gen.

Sennosides.
Senokot.
SenokotXTRA.
Women's Gentle Laxative.
Sting-Eze. (Wisconsin Pharmacal Co.) Diphenhydramine hydrochloride, camphor, phenol, benzocaine, eucalyptol. Liq. Bot. 15 mL. *OTC.*
Use: Antihistamine, topical.
•**stinging nettle.** *USP 34.*
Use: Dietary supplement.
Sting-Kill. (Randob Labs) **Swab:** Benzocaine 20%, menthol 1%. Isopropyl alcohol 15%. 0.5 mL. **Wipes:** Benzocaine 20%, menthol 1%. Isopropyl alcohol 15%. 8s. *OTC.*
Use: Topical local anesthetic.
•**stiripentol.** (STY-rih-PEN-tole) USAN.
Use: Anticonvulsant.
•**St. John's wort, powdered extract.** *USP 34.*
Use: Dietary supplement.
St. Joseph Adult Chewable Aspirin. (Schering-Plough) Aspirin 81 mg, saccharin. Chew. Tab. Bot. 36s. *OTC.*
Use: Analgesic.
St. Joseph Aspirin for Adults. (Schering-Plough) Aspirin 5 g. Tab. Bot. 36s, 100s, 200s. *OTC.*
Use: Analgesic.
St. Joseph Aspirin-Free Elixir for Children. (Schering-Plough) Acetaminophen 160 mg/5 mL. Alcohol free. Elix. Bot. 2 oz, 4 oz. *OTC.*
Use: Analgesic.
St. Joseph Aspirin-Free for Children Chewable. (Schering-Plough) Acetaminophen 80 mg, fruit flavor. Chew. Tab. Bot. 30s. *OTC.*
Use: Analgesic.
St. Joseph Aspirin-Free Infant. (Schering-Plough) Acetaminophen 100 mg/mL. Aspirin and sugar free. Drops. Bot. w/dropper. 0.5 oz. *OTC.*
Use: Analgesic.
St. Joseph Aspirin-Free Tablets for Children. (Schering-Plough) Acetaminophen 80 mg. Tab. Bot. 30s. *OTC.*
Use: Analgesic.
St. Joseph Cough Suppressant. (Schering-Plough) Dextromethorphan HBr 7.5 mg/5 mL, alcohol free, sucrose, cherry flavor. Liq. Bot. 60 mL, 120 mL. *OTC.*
Use: Antitussive.
St. Joseph Cough Syrup for Children. (Schering-Plough) Dextromethorphan HBr 7.5 mg/5 mL. Syr. Bot. 2 oz, 4 oz. *OTC.*
Use: Antitussive.

Stomal. (Foy Laboratories) Phenobarbital 16.2 mg, hyoscyamine sulfate 0.1037 mg, atropine sulfate 0.0194 mg, scopolamine HBr 0.0065 mg. Tab. Bot. 1000s. *Rx.*
Use: Anticholinergic; antispasmodic; hypnotic; sedative.

Stool Softener. (Apothecary Prods.) Docusate calcium 240 mg. Cap. Bot. 50s. *OTC.*
Use: Laxative.

Stool Softener. (Rugby) Docusate sodium. **Cap.:** 100 mg, 250 mg lactose, tartrazine. Bot. 1000s. **Soft gel Cap.:** 250 mg, sorbitol, parabens. Bot. 100s, 1000s. *OTC.*
Use: Laxative.

Stool Softener DC. (Rugby) Docusate calcium 240 mg, sorbitol, parabens. Cap. Bot. 100s, 500s, 1000s. *OTC.*
Use: Laxative.

Stop. (Oral-B) Stannous fluoride 0.4%. Tube 2 oz. *Rx.*
Use: Dental caries agent.

Stopayne Capsules. (Springbok) Codeine phosphate 30 mg, acetaminophen 357 mg. Cap. Bot. 100s, 500s, UD 100s. *c-III.*
Use: Analgesic; antitussive.

Stopayne Syrup. (Springbok) Acetaminophen 120 mg, codeine phosphate 12 mg/5 mL. Syr. Bot. 4 oz, 16 oz. *c-v.*
Use: Analgesic; antitussive.

Stop-Zit. (Purepac) Denatonium benzoate in a clear nail polish base. Bot. 0.75 oz. *OTC.*
Use: Nail-biting deterrent.

•**storax.** (STORE-ax) *USP 34.*
Use: Pharmaceutic necessity for benzoin tincture compound.

Stovarsol.
Use: Trichomonas vaginalis vaginitis; amebiasis; Vincent's angina.

Strattera. (Eli Lilly) Atomoxetine hydrochloride (as base) 10 mg, 18 mg, 25 mg, 40 mg, 60 mg, 80 mg, 100 mg. Cap. 30s. *Rx.*
Use: Psychotherapeutic agent.

Stren-Tab. (Barth's) Vitamins C 300 mg, B_1 10 mg, B_2 10 mg, niacin 33 mg, B_6 2 mg, pantothenic acid 20 mg, B_{12} 4 mcg. Tab. Bot. 100s, 300s, 500s. *OTC.*
Use: Vitamin supplement.

streptococcus immune globulin, group B.
Use: Immunization. [Orphan Drug]

streptokinase.
Use: Thrombolytic.

Streptolysin O Test. (Laboratory Diagnostics) Reagent 6 x 10 mL, buffer

6 × 40 mL, Control Serum, 6 × 10 mL, or Kit.
Use: Diagnosis of "group A" streptococcal infections.

streptomycin calcium chloride. Streptomycin Calcium Chloride Complex.

streptomycin sulfate.
Use: Antituberculosis agent.

streptomycin sulfate. (Pharma-Tek) Streptomycin sulfate 1 g. Cake, lyophilized. Vial. *Rx.*
Use: Antituberculosis agent.

Streptonase B. (Wampole) Tube test for determination of streptococcal infection by serum DNase-B antibodies. Kit 1.
Use: Diagnostic aid.

•**streptonicozid.** (STREP-toe-nih-KOE-zid) USAN.
Use: Anti-infective.

•**streptonigrin.** (strep-toe-NYE-grin) USAN. Antibiotic isolated from both filtrates of *Streptomyces flocculus.*
Use: Antineoplastic.
See: Nigrin.

streptovaricin. An antibiotic composed of several related components derived from cultures of *Streptomyces variabilis.*

•**streptozocin.** (STREP-toe-ZOE-sin) USAN.
Use: Antineoplastic.
See: Zanosar.

Streptozyme. (Wampole) Rapid hemagglutination slide test for the qualitative detection and quantitative determination of streptococcal extracellular antigens in serum, plasma, and peripheral blood. Kit 15s, 50s, 150s.
Use: Diagnostic aid, streptococcus.

Stress B-Complex. (H.L. Moore Drug Exchange) Vitamins E 30 units, B_1 15 mg, B_2 15 mg, B_3 100 mg, B_5 20 mg, B_6 20 mg, B_{12} 12 mcg, C 500 mg, folic acid 0.4 mg, Zn 23.9 mg, Cu, biotin 45 mcg. Tab. Bot. 60s. *OTC.*
Use: Mineral, vitamin supplement.

Stress B Complex with Vitamin C. (Mission Pharmacal) Vitamins B_1 13.8 mg, B_2 10 mg, B_3 50 mg, B_6 4.1 mg, C 300 mg, Zn 15 mg. Tab. Bot. 60s. *OTC.*
Use: Mineral, vitamin supplement.

Stress-Bee. (Rugby) Vitamins B_1 10 mg, B_2 10 mg, B_3 100 mg, B_5 20 mg, B_6 2 mg, B_{12} 6 mcg, C 300 mg. Cap. Bot. 100s. *OTC.*
Use: Vitamin supplement.

Stress Formula. (Various Mfr.) Vitamins E 30 mg, B_1 15 mg, B_2 15 mg, B_3 100 mg, B_5 20 mg, B_6 5 mg, B_{12} 12 mcg, C 600 mg, folic acid 0.4 mg, biotin 45 mcg. Cap., Tab. **Cap.:** Bot.

60s, 100s, 1000s. **Tab.**: Bot. 30s, 60s, 100s, 250s, 300s, 400s, 1000s, UD 100s. *OTC.*
Use: Vitamin supplement.

Stress Formula 600. (Vangard Labs, Inc.) Vitamins E 30 units, B_1 15 mg, B_2 10 mg, B_3 100 mg, B_5 20 mg, B_6 5 mg, B_{12} 12 mcg, C 500 mg, folic acid 0.4 mg, biotin 45 mcg. Tab. Bot. UD 100s. *OTC.*
Use: Vitamin supplement.

Stress Formula "605". (NBTY) Vitamins E 30 mg, B_1 15 mg, B_2 15 mg, B_3 100 mg, B_5 20 mg, B_6 5 mg, B_{12} 12 mcg, C 605 mg, folic acid 0.4 mg, biotin 45 mg. Tab. Bot. 60s. *OTC.*
Use: Vitamin supplement.

Stress Formula "605" with Zinc. (NBTY) Vitamins E 30 mg, B_1 20 mg, B_2 10 mg, B_3 100 mg, B_5 25 mg, B_6 5 mg, B_{12} 12 mcg, C 605 mg, folic acid 0.4 mg, Zn 23.9 mg, Cu, biotin 45 mcg. Tab. Bot. 60s. *OTC.*
Use: Mineral, vitamin supplement.

Stress Formula 600 Plus Iron. (Schein) Iron 27 mg, vitamins E 30 units, B_1 15 mg, B_2 15 mg, B_3 100 mg, B_5 20 mg, B_6 5 mg, B_{12} 12 mcg, C 600 mg, folic acid 0.4 mg, biotin 45 mcg. Tab. Bot. 60s, 250s. *OTC.*
Use: Mineral, vitamin supplement.

Stress Formula 600 Plus Zinc. (Schein) Vitamins E 30 mg, B_1 20 mg, B_2 10 mg, B_3 100 mg, B_5 25 mg, B_6 5 mg, B_{12} 12 mcg, C 600 mg, folic acid 0.4 mg, zinc 23.9 mg, Cu, Mg, biotin 45 mcg. Tab. Bot. 60s, 250s. *OTC.*
Use: Mineral, vitamin supplement.

Stress Formula Vitamins. (Various Mfr.) Vitamins E 30 mg, B_1 10 mg, B_2 10 mg, B_3 100 mg, B_5 20 mg, B_6 5 mg, B_{12} 12 mcg, C 500 mg, folic acid 0.4 mg, biotin 45 mcg. Cap. Bot. 100s. Tab. Bot. 60s. *OTC.*
Use: Vitamin supplement.

Stress Formula with Iron. (NBTY) Vitamins C 500 mg, B_1 10 mg, B_2 10 mg, B_3 100 mg, B_5 20 mg, B_6 5 mg, B_{12} 12 mcg, E 30 units, Fe 27 mg, folic acid 0.4 mg, biotin 45 mcg. Tab. Bot. 60s. *OTC.*
Use: Mineral, vitamin supplement.

Stress Formula with Zinc. (Towne) Vitamins E 45 units, C 600 mg, folic acid 400 mcg, B_1 20 mg, B_2 10 mg, niacinamide 100 mg, B_6 10 mg, B_{12} 25 mcg, biotin 40 mcg, pantothenic acid 25 mg, Cu 3 mg, Zn 23.9 mg. Tab. Bot. 60s. *OTC.*
Use: Mineral, vitamin supplement.

Stress Formula w/Zinc. (Various Mfr.) Vitamins E 30 units, B_1 10 mg, B_2 10 mg, B_3 100 mg, B_5 20 mg, B_6 5 mg, B_{12} 12 mcg, C 500 mg, folic acid 0.4 mg, biotin 45 mcg, Zn 23.9 mg, Cu. Tab. Bot. 60s. *OTC.*
Use: Mineral, vitamin supplement.

Stress "1000". (NBTY) Vitamins E 22 mg, B_1 15 mg, B_2 15 mg, B_3 100 mg, B_5 20 mg, B_6 5 mg, B_{12} 12 mcg, C 1000 mg. Tab. Bot. 60s. *OTC.*
Use: Vitamin supplement.

Stress 600 w/Zinc. (Nion Corp.) Vitamins E 45 units, B_1 20 mg, B_2 10 mg, B_3 100 mg, B_5 25 mg, B_6 10 mg, B_{12} 25 mcg, C 600 mg, folic acid 0.4 mg, Zn 5.5 mg, Cu, biotin 45 mcg. Tab. Bot. 60s. *OTC.*
Use: Mineral, vitamin supplement.

Stresstabs. (Wyeth) Vitamins E 30 mg, B_1 10 mg, B_2 10 mg, B_3 100 mg, B_5 20 mg, B_6 5 mg, B_{12} 12 mcg, C 500 mg, folic acid 0.4 mg, biotin 45 mcg. Tab. Bot. 60s. *OTC.*
Use: Vitamin supplement.

Stresstabs + Iron. (Wyeth) Fe 18 mg, E 30 units, B_1 10 mg, B_2 10 mg, B_3 100 mg, B_5 20 mg, B_6 5 mg, B_{12} 12 mcg, C 500 mg, folic acid 0.4 mg, biotin 45 mcg. Tab. Bot. 60s. *OTC.*
Use: Mineral, vitamin supplement.

Stresstabs + Zinc. (Wyeth) Vitamins E 30 mg, B_1 10 mg, B_2 10 mg, B_3 100 mg, B_5 20 mg, B_6 5 mg, B_{12} 12 mcg, C 500 mg, folic acid 0.4 mg, Zn 23.9 mg, Cu, biotin 45 mcg. Tab. Bot. 60s. *OTC.*
Use: Mineral, vitamin supplement.

Stresstabs 600. (Wyeth) Vitamins B_1 15 mg, B_2 10 mg, B_6 5 mg, B_{12} 12 mcg, C 600 mg, niacinamide 100 mg, vitamin E 30 units, biotin 45 mcg, folic acid 400 mcg, calcium pantothenate 20 mg. Tab. Bot. 30s, 60s, UD 10 x 10s. *OTC.*
Use: Vitamin supplement.

Stresstabs 600 with Iron. (Wyeth) Ferrous fumarate 27 mg, vitamins E 30 units, B_1 15 mg, B_2 15 mg, B_3 100 mg, B_5 20 mg, B_6 5 mg, B_{12} 12 mcg, C 600 mg, folic acid 0.4 mg, biotin 45 mcg. Tab. Bot. 30s, 60s. *OTC.*
Use: Mineral, vitamin supplement.

Stresstabs 600 with Zinc. (Wyeth) Vitamins B_1 15 mg, B_2 10 mg, B_3 100 mg, B_5 20 mg, B_6 5 mg, B_{12} 12 mcg, C 600 mg, E 30 units, folic acid 0.4 mg, biotin 45 mcg, Cu, Zn 23.9 mg. Tab. Bot. 30s, 60s. *OTC.*
Use: Mineral, vitamin supplement.

Stresstein. (Novartis) Maltodextrin, medium chain triglycerides, l-leucine, soy-

bean oil, l-isoleucine, l-valine, l-glutamic acid, l-arginine, l-lysine acetate, l-alanine, l-threonine, l-phenylalanine, l-aspartic acid, l-histidine, l-methionine, glycine, polyglycerol esters of fatty acids, l-serine, l-proline, sodium Cl, l-tryptophan, l-cysteine, sodium citrate, vitamins and minerals. Powder 3.4 oz. packets. *OTC.*
Use: High-protein, branched chain enriched tube feeding.

Striant. (Columbia) Testosterone 30 mg. Lactose. Buccal system. Blister packs of 10 systems. *Rx.*
Use: Androgen, sex hormone.

Stri-dex Antibacterial Cleansing. (Bayer Consumer Care) Triclosan 1%, acetylated lanolin alcohol, EDTA. Bar. 105 g. *OTC.*
Use: Dermatologic, acne.

Stri-dex B.P. (Bayer Consumer Care) Benzoyl peroxide 10%. in greaseless, vanishing cream base. *OTC.*
Use: Dermatologic, acne.

Stri-dex Clear. (Bayer Consumer Care) Salicylic acid 2%, SD alcohol 9.3%, EDTA. Gel. Tube. 30 g. *OTC.*
Use: Dermatologic, acne.

Stri-dex Face Wash. (Bayer Consumer Care) Triclosan 1%, glycerin, EDTA, alcohol free. Soln. Bot. 237 mL. *OTC.*
Use: Dermatologic, acne.

Stri-dex Lotion. (Bayer Consumer Care) Salicylic acid 0.5%, alcohol 28%, sulfonated alkyl benzenes, citric acid, sodium carbonate, simethicone, water. Bot. 4 oz. *OTC.*
Use: Dermatologic, acne.

Stri-dex Maximum Strength. (Bayer Consumer Care) Salicylic acid 2%, SD alcohol 44%, citric acid, menthol. Pad. Box 55s, 90s, dual-textured 32s. *OTC.*
Use: Antiacne.

Stri-dex Oil Fighting Formula. (Bayer Consumer Care) Salicylic acid 2%, citric acid, menthol, SD alcohol 54%. Super Scrub Pads. Box 55s. *OTC.*
Use: Dermatologic, acne.

Stri-dex Regular Strength. (Bayer Consumer Care) Salicylic acid 0.5%, SD alcohol 28%, citric acid, menthol. Pad. Box 55s. *OTC.*
Use: Dermatologic, acne.

Stri-dex Sensitive Skin. (Bayer Consumer Care) Salicylic acid 0.5%, citric acid, aloe vera gel, menthol, SD alcohol 28%. Pad. Box 50s, 90s. *OTC.*
Use: Dermatologic, acne.

Stromectol. (Merck & Co.) Ivermectin 3 mg. Tab. UD 20s. *Rx.*
Use: Anthelmintic.

strong iodine solution (Lugol's Solution). (Various Mfr.) Iodine 5% (50 mg/mL)/potassium iodide 10% (100 mg/mL). Soln. 120 mL, 437 mL, gal. *Rx.*
Use: Thyroid drug.

strong iodine tincture. (Various Mfr.) Iodine 7%, potassium iodide 5%, alcohol 83%. Soln. Bot. 500 mL, 4000 mL. *OTC.*
Use: Antimicrobial; antiseptic.

StrongStart. (Savage) Ca 200 mg, Fe 29 mg, vitamin A 1000 units, D 400 units, E 30 units, B_1 3 mg, B_2 3 mg, B_3 15 mg, B_5 7 mg, B_6 20 mg, B_{12} 12 mcg, C 100 mg, folic acid 1 mg, Zn 20 mg; docusate sodium 25 mg (Tab only). Tab., Chew. Tab. Bot. 30s, 100s. *Rx.*
Use: Vitamin, mineral supplement

strontium bromide. (Various Mfr.) Strontium bromide Cryst. or Granule, Bot. 0.25 lb, 1 lb. Amp. 1 g/10 mL. *Rx.*
Use: Antiepileptic; sedative.

•**strontium chloride Sr 85.** (STRAHN-shee-uhm) USAN.
Use: Radiopharmaceutical.

•**strontium chloride Sr 89 injection.** (STRAHN-shee-uhm) *USP 34.*
Use: Antineoplastic; radiopharmaceutical.
See: Metastron.

•**strontium nitrate Sr 85.** (STRAHN-shee-uhm) USAN.
Use: Radiopharmaceutical.

strontium Sr 85 injection.
Use: Diagnostic aid (bone scanning).

Strovite. (Everett) Vitamins B_1 15 mg, B_2 15 mg, B_3 100 mg, B_5 18 mg, B_6 4 mg, B_{12} 5 mcg, C 500 mg, folic acid 0.5 mg. Tab. Bot. 100s. *OTC.*
Use: Mineral, vitamin supplement.

Strovite Advance. (Everett) Vitamin D_3 400 units, E 100 units, B_1 20 mg, B_2 5 mg, B_3 25 mg, B_5 15 mg, B_6 25 mg, B_{12} 50 mcg, C 300 mg, folic acid 1 mg, Zn 25 mg, carotenoids 3000 units, biotin 100 mcg, alpha lipoic acid 15 mg, lutein 1 mg, Cr, Cu, Mg, Mn, Se, mineral oil. Tab. Bot. 100s. *Rx.*
Use: Vitamin, mineral supplement.

Strovite Forte. (Everett) Fe 10 mg, vitamins A 3000 units, A 1000 units (beta-carotene), E 60 units, D_3 400 units, folic acid 1 mg, C 500 mg, B_1 20 mg, B_2 20 mg, B_6 25 mg, B_{12} 50 mcg, B_3 100 mg, biotin 0.15 mg, B_5 25 mg, Se 50 mcg, Mg 50 mg, Zn 15 mg, Mo 20 mcg, Cu 3 mg, Cr 0.05 mg. Tab. Bot. 100s. *Rx.*
Use: Vitamin, mineral supplement.

Strovite One. (Everett Labs) Vitamin A (as carotenoids) 3,000 units, E 100 units, D₃ 1,000 units, C 300 mg, B₁ 20 mg, B₂ 5 mg, B₃ 25 mg, B₆ 25 mg, B₁₂ 50 mcg, biotin 100 mcg, folic acid 1 mcg, alpha-lipoic acid 15 mg, lutein 5 mg, pantothenic acid 15 mg, Cr, Cu, Mg, Mn, Se, Zn. Maltodextrin, soybean oil, sucrose. Tab. 90s. *Rx.*
Use: Multivitamin with minerals.

Strovite Plus. (Everett) Vitamins A 5000 units, E 30 mg, B₁ 20 mg, B₂ 20 mg, B₃ 100 mg, B₅ 25 mg, B₆ 25 mg, B₁₂ 50 mcg, C 500 mg, Fe 9 mg, folic acid 0.8 mg, Zn 22.5 mg, biotin 150 mcg, Cr, Cu, Mg, Mn. Bot. 100s. *OTC.*
Use: Mineral, vitamin supplement.

S.T. 37. (Numark Labs) Hexylresorcinol 0.1% in glycerin aqueous soln. Bot. 5.5 oz, 12 oz. *OTC.*
Use: Antiseptic, topical.

Stuart Formula. (J & J Merck Consumer Pharm.) Vitamins A 5000 units, B₁ 1.5 mg, B₂ 1.7 mg, B₃ 20 mg, B₆ 1 mg, B₁₂ 3 mcg, C 50 mg, D 400 units, E 10 units, Fe 5 mg, Cu, folic acid 0.4 mg, Ca, I, Tab. Bot. 100s. *OTC.*
Use: Mineral, vitamin supplement.

StuartNatal Plus 3. (Integrity) Ca 200 mg, Fe (as ferrous fumarate) 28 mg, vitamin A 3000 units, D 400 units, E (as dl-alpha tocopheryl acetate) 22 mg, B₁ 1.8 mg, B₂ 4 mg, B₃ 20 mg, B₆ 25 mg, B₁₂ 12 mcg, C 120 mg, folic acid 1 mg, Cu, Mg, Zn 25 mg. Tab. Bot. 100s. *Rx.*
Use: Vitamin, mineral supplement.

Stuart Prenatal. (Integrity) Vitamins A (100% as beta carotene) 4000 units, B₁ 1.8 mg, B₂ 1.7 mg, B₃ 20 mg, B₆ 2.6 mg, B₁₂ 8 mcg, C 120 mg, D 400 units, E (dl-alpha tocopheryl acetate) 30 units, Fe (as ferrous fumarate) 28 mg, Ca 200 mg, Zn 25 mg, folic acid 800 mcg. Tab. Bot. 100s. *OTC.*
Use: Mineral, vitamin supplement.

Stulex. (Jones Pharma) Docusate sodium 250 mg. Tab. Bot. 100s, 1000s. *OTC.*
Use: Fecal softener.

S2. (Nephron) Racepinephrine hydrochloride 2.25% (epinephrine base 1.125%). Edetate disodium. Soln. for Inh. Single-use vial. 0.5 mL. *OTC.*
Use: Bronchodilator, sympathomimetic; vasopressor.

Stye. (Del) White petrolatum 57.7%, mineral oil 31.9%. Wheat germ oil. Ophth. Oint. Bot. 3.5 g. *OTC.*
Use: Lubricant, ophthalmic.

Stypt-Aid. (Pharmakon) Benzocaine 28.71 mg, methylbenzethonium hydrochloride 9.95 mg, aluminum Cl hexahydrate 55.43 mg, ethyl alcohol 70.97%/mL in a glycerin, menthol base. Spray. 60 mL. *OTC.*
Use: Anesthetic, local.

styptirenal.
See: Epinephrine.

Stypto-Caine. (Pedinol Pharmacal) Hydroxyquinoline sulfate, tetracaine hydrochloride, aluminum Cl, aqueous glycol base. Soln. Bot. 2 oz. *Rx.*
Use: Hemostatic solution.

styrene polymer, sulfonated, sodium salt. Sodium Polystyrene Sulfonate, USP.

styronate resins. Ammonium and potassium salts of sulfonated styrene polymers.
Use: Conditions requiring sodium restriction.

Sublingual B Total. (Pharmaceutical Labs) Vitamins B₂ 1.7 mg, B₃ 20 mg, B₅ 30 mg, B₆ 2 mg, B₁₂ 1000 mcg, C 60 mg. Liq. Bot. 30 mL. *OTC.*
Use: Vitamin supplement.

Suboxone. (Reckitt Benckiser) Buprenorphine base 2 mg/naloxone 0.5 mg, buprenorphine base 8 mg/naloxone 2 mg, lactose, acesulfame K, lemon/lime flavor. Tab, Sublingual. Bot. 30s. *c-III.*
Use: Analgesic.

substituted ureas.
Use: Antisickling agent.
See: Hydrea.
Hydroxyurea.

Subutex. (Reckitt Benckiser) Buprenorphine hydrochloride 2 mg, 8 mg, lactose. Tab, Sublingual. Bot. 30s. *c-III.*
Use: Analgesic.

•**succimer.** (SUX-ih-mer) USAN.
Use: Diagnostic aid; cystine kidney stones, mercury and lead poisoning. [Orphan Drug]
See: Chemet.

succinimides.
Use: Anticonvulsant
See: Methsuximide.

•**succinobucol.** (sux-in-oh-BUE-kol) USAN.
Use: Cardiovascular agent.

•**succinylcholine chloride.** (suck-sin-ill-KOE-leen KLOR-ide) *USP 34.*
Use: Neuromuscular blocker.
See: Anectine.
Quelicin.
Sucostrin.

succinylsulfathiazole.
Use: Anti-infective, intestinal.

Sucostrin. (Apothecon) Succinylcholine Cl 20 mg/mL Inj. Vial 10 mL. *Rx.*
Use: Neuromuscular blocker.

Sucostrin Chloride. (Marsam) Succinylcholine Cl 20 mg/mL w/methylparaben 0.1%, propylparaben 0.01%. Vial 10 mL; High potency 100 mg/mL. Vial 10 mL. *Rx.*
Use: Muscle relaxant.

Sucraid. (Orphan Medical) Sacrosidase 8500 units/mL. Soln. Bot. 118 mL. *Rx.*
Use: Nutritional therapy.

• **sucralfate.** (sue-KRAL-fate) *USP 34.*
Use: Antiulcerative; oral complications of chemotherapy. [Orphan Drug]
See: Carafate.

sucralfate. (Precision Dose) Sucralfate 1 g/10 mL. Methylparaben, sorbitol. Susp. Unit dose cups. 10 mL. *Rx.*
Use: Antiulcerative.

sucralfate. (Various Mfr.) Sucralfate 1 g. Tab. Bot. 100s, 500s. *Rx.*
Use: Antiulcerative.

Sucrets Children's Formula. (Insight) Dyclonine hydrochloride 1.2 mg. Corn syrup, sucrose, cherry flavor. Loz. Tin 24s. *OTC.*
Use: Sore throat treatment for children 3 years and older.

Sucrets Complete. (Insight) Dyclonine hydrochloride 3 mg, menthol 6 mg. Acesulfame K, corn syrup, sucrose. Cherry and cool citrus flavors. Loz. 18s. *OTC.*
Use: Mouth and throat product.

Sucrets DM Cough Formula. (Insight) Dextromethorphan HBr 10 mg. Corn syrup, hydrogenated palm oil, sugar (honey lemon flavor only); menthol, sucrose (cherry flavor only). Honey lemon and cherry flavors. Loz. 18s. *OTC.*
Use: Nonnarcotic antitussive.

Sucrets DM Cough Suppressant. (Insight) Dextromethorphan HBr 10 mg. Corn syrup, menthol, sucrose. Cherry flavor. Loz. 6s. *OTC.*
Use: Nonnarcotic antitussive.

Sucrets Maximum Strength Sore Throat. (Insight) Dyclonine hydrochloride 3 mg. Loz. Corn syrup, menthol, sucrose. Loz. Tin 24s, 48s, 55s. *OTC.*
Use: Mouth and throat preparation.

Sucrets Original Formula Sore Throat. (Insight) Hexylresorcinol 2.4 mg. Corn syrup, menthol, sucrose. Mint flavor. Loz. 18s. *OTC.*
Use: Mouth and throat preparation.

Sucrets Original Formula Sore Throat Wild Cherry. (Insight) Dyclonine hydrochloride 2 mg. Corn syrup, menthol, sucrose. Cherry flavor. Loz. 24s. *OTC.*
Use: Mouth and throat product.

Sucrets Throat Spray. (Insight) Dyclonine hydrochloride 0.1%, alcohol 10%, sorbitol. Spray. Bot. 90 mL, 120 mL. *OTC.*
Use: Mouth and throat preparation.

• **sucrose.** (SUE-krose) *NF 29.*
Use: IV; diuretic & dehydrating agent; pharmaceutic aid (flavor, tablet excipient).

• **sucrose octaacetate.** (SUE-krose) *NF 29.*
Use: Pharmaceutic aid (alcohol denaturant).

• **sucrosofate potassium.** (sue-KROE-so-FATE) *USAN.*
Use: Antiulcerative.

Sudafed. (McNeil) Pseudoephedrine hydrochloride. 30 mg, 60 mg. **30 mg:** Box 24s, 48s. Bot. 100s, 1000s. **60 mg:** Bot. 100s, 1000s. *OTC.*
Use: Decongestant.

Sudafed Children's Non-Drowsy. (McNeil) Pseudoephedrine hydrochloride 15 mg/5 mL, EDTA, saccharin, sorbitol, grape flavor, alcohol free. Liq. 118 mL. *OTC.*
Use: Nasal decongestant, arylalkylamine.

Sudafed Cold & Sinus Non-Drowsy. (McNeil) Pseudoephedrine hydrochloride 30 mg, acetaminophen 325 mg, sorbitol. Liqui-Caps. Pkg. 10s, 20s. *OTC.*
Use: Upper respiratory combination, decongestant, analgesic.

Sudafed Maximum Strength Non-Drowsy Non-Drying Sinus. (McNeil) Pseudoephedrine hydrochloride 30 mg, guaifenesin 200 mg. Glycerin, PEG, sorbitol. Cap. 24s. *OTC.*
Use: Upper respiratory combination, decongestant and expectorant combination.

Sudafed Multi-Symptom Cold & Cough. (McNeil) Dextromethorphan HBr 10 mg, guaifenesin 100 mg, pseudoephedrine hydrochloride 30 mg, acetaminophen 250 mg, sorbitol. Liquicaps. Pkg. 20s. *OTC.*
Use: Upper respiratory combination, antitussive, expectorant, decongestant, analgesic.

Sudafed Non-Drowsy Maximum Strength. (McNeil) Pseudoephedrine hydrochloride 30 mg, lactose, sucrose. Tab. Bot. 24s, 96s. *OTC.*
Use: Nasal decongestant, arylalkylamine.

Sudafed Non-Drowsy 12 Hour Long-Acting. (McNeil) Pseudoephedrine hydrochloride 120 mg. ER Tab. Pkg. 10s. *OTC.*
Use: Nasal decongestant, arylalkylamine.

Sudafed Non-Drowsy 24 Hour Long-Acting. (McNeil) Pseudoephedrine hydrochloride 240 mg (immediate-release 60 mg, controlled-release 180 mg). CR Tab. Pkg. 10s. *OTC.*
Use: Nasal decongestant, arylalkylamine.

Sudafed PE. (McNeil) Phenylephrine hydrochloride 10 mg. Acesulfame K. Tab. 18s. *OTC.*
Use: Nasal decongestant.

Sudafed PE Day & Night. (McNeil Consumer) Tab. **Day:** Phenylephrine hydrochloride 10 mg. PEG. 18s. **Night:** Diphenhydramine hydrochloride 25 mg, phenylephrine hydrochloride 10 mg. PEG. 12s. *OTC.*
Use: Upper respiratory combination, decongestant and antihistamine.

Sudafed PE Maximum Strength Nasal Decongestant. (McNeil) Phenylephrine hydrochloride 10 mg. Acesulfame K, PEG. Tab. 18s, 36s, 72s. *OTC.*
Use: Nasal decongestant.

Sudafed PE Multi-Symptom Cold and Cough. (McNeil) Dextromethorphan HBr 10 mg, guaifenesin 100 mg, phenylephrine hydrochloride 5 mg, acetaminophen 325 mg. PEG. Tab. 20s. *OTC.*
Use: Antitussive and expectorant combination, upper respiratory combination.

Sudafed PE Multi-Symptom Severe Cold. (McNeil) Phenylephrine hydrochloride 5 mg, diphenhydramine hydrochloride 12.5 mg, acetaminophen 325 mg. PEG. Tab. 12s, 24s. *OTC.*
Use: Decongestant, antihistamine, and analgesic, upper respiratory combination.

Sudafed PE Nighttime Cold Maximum Strength. (McNeil) Phenylephrine hydrochloride 5 mg, diphenhydramine hydrochloride 25 mg, acetaminophen 325 mg. Tab. 20s. *OTC.*
Use: Decongestant, antihistamine, and analgesic combination, upper respiratory combination.

Sudafed PE Nighttime Nasal Decongestant. (McNeil) Phenylephrine hydrochloride 10 mg, diphenhydramine hydrochloride 25 mg. PEG. Tab. 12s. *OTC.*
Use: Upper respiratory combination, decongestant and antihistamine.

Sudafed PE Non-Drying Sinus. (McNeil) Phenylephrine hydrochloride 5 mg, guaifenesin 200 mg. PEG. Caps. Pkg. 24s. *OTC.*
Use: Upper respiratory combination, decongestant, expectorant.

Sudafed PE Sinus Headache Maximum Strength. (McNeil) Phenylephrine hydrochloride 5 mg, acetaminophen 325 mg. PEG. Tab. 24s, 48s, 72s. *OTC.*
Use: Decongestant and analgesic combination.

Sudafed Sinus & Allergy. (McNeil) Pseudoephedrine hydrochloride 60 mg, chlorpheniramine maleate 4 mg. Lactose. Pkg. 24s. *OTC.*
Use: Upper respiratory combination, decongestant, antihistamine.

Sudafed 12 Hour. (McNeil) Pseudoephedrine hydrochloride 120 mg. SA Cap. Box 10s, 20s, 40s. *OTC.*
Use: Decongestant.

SudaHist. (Larken Laboratories) Chlorpheniramine maleate 12 mg, pseudoephedrine hydrochloride 120 mg. Lactose. ER Tab. 100s. *Rx.*
Use: Upper respiratory combination, decongestant and antihistamine.

Sudal-DM. (Atley) Dextromethorphan HBr 30 mg, guaifenesin 500 mg, dye free. SR Tab. Bot. 100s. *Rx.*
Use: Upper respiratory combination, antitussive, expectorant.

Sudal 120/600. (Atley) Pseudoephedrine hydrochloride 120 mg, guaifenesin 600 mg. SR Tab. Bot. 100s. *Rx.*
Use: Upper respiratory combination, decongestant, expectorant.

Sudal-12 Tannate. (Atley) **Chew. Tab.:** Pseudoephedrine hydrochloride 60 mg, chlorpheniramine maleate 4 mg. Acesulfame K, magnasweet, mannitol, sucralose, aspartame, phenylalanine 25 mg. Grape flavor. 100s. **ER Susp.:** Pseudoephedrine polistirex (equiv. to pseudoephedrine hydrochloride 30 mg), chlorpheniramine polistirex (equiv. to chlorpheniramine maleate 6 mg) per 5 mL. Corn syrup, parabens. Strawberry flavor. 473 mL. *Rx.*
Use: Decongestant and antihistamine.

Sudanyl. (Dover Pharmaceuticals) Pseudoephedrine hydrochloride. Tab. Sugar, lactose, and salt free. UD Box 500s.
Use: Decongestant.

SudaTex G. (Larken) Guaifenesin 400 mg, pseudoephedrine hydrochloride 40 mg. Maltodextrin. Tab. 100s. *OTC.*

Use: Upper respiratory combination, decongestant and expectorant combination.

Sudatuss-2 DF. (PGD) Codeine phosphate 10 mg, guaifenesin 100 mg, pseudoephedrine hydrochloride 30 mg per 5 mL. Alcohol free. Parabens, aspartame, phenylalanine. Cherry flavor. Liq. 473 mL. *c-v.*
Use: Antitussive and expectorant.

Sudden Tan Lotion. (Schering-Plough) Padimate O, dihydroxyacetone, Bot. 4 oz. *OTC.*
Use: Artificial tanning; moisturizer; sunscreen.

SudoGest Non-Drowsy. (Major) Pseudoephedrine hydrochloride 30 mg. PEG, sugar. Tab. 100s. *Rx.*
Use: Nasal decongestant, arylalkylamine.

SudoGest Sinus & Allergy Maximum Strength. (Major Pharmaceuticals) Chlorpheniramine maleate 4 mg, pseudoephedrine hydrochloride 60 mg. Lactose. Tab. 48s. *OTC.*
Use: Upper respiratory combination, decongestant and antihistamine.

SudoGest Sinus Maximum Strength. (Major) Pseudoephedrine hydrochloride 30 mg, acetaminophen 500 mg, dextrose. Tab. Pkg. 24s. *OTC.*
Use: Upper respiratory combination, decongestant, analgesic.

•**sudoxicam.** (sue-DOX-ih-kam) USAN.
Use: Anti-inflammatory.

Sudrin. (Jones Pharma) Pseudoephedrine hydrochloride 30 mg. Tab. Bot. 100s, 1000s. *OTC.*
Use: Decongestant.

Sufenta. (Akorn) Sufentanil citrate (as base) 50 mcg/mL. Preservative free. Inj. Amp. 1 mL, 2 mL, 5 mL. *c-ii.*
Use: Opioid analgesic.

•**sufentanil.** (sue-FEN-tuh-nill) USAN.
Tall Man: SUFentanil
Use: Analgesic.

•**sufentanil citrate.** (sue-FEN-tuh-nill SIH-trate) *USP 34.*
Tall Man: SUFentanil
Use: Opioid analgesic.
See: Sufenta.

•**sufentanil citrate injection.** (sue-FEN-tuh-nill SIH-trate) *USP 34.*
Tall Man: SUFentanil
Use: Analgesic; narcotic.

•**sufotidine.** (sue-FOE-tih-DEEN) USAN.
Use: Antiulcerative.

Sufrex. (Janssen) Ketanserin tartrate. *Rx.*
Use: Serotonin antagonist.

•**sugammadex sodium.** (soo-GAM-ma-dex) USAN.
Use: CNS agent.

•**sugar, compressible.** (SHUG-er) *NF 29.*
Use: Pharmaceutic aid (flavor; tablet excipient).

•**sugar, confectioner's.** (SHUG-er) *NF 29.*
Use: Pharmaceutic aid (flavor; tablet excipient).

•**sugar, invert, injection.** (SHUG-er) *USP 34.*
Use: Replenisher (fluid and nutrient).

•**sugar spheres.** (SHUG-er) *NF 29.*
Use: Pharmaceutic aid (vehicle, solid carrier).

•**sulamserod hydrochloride.** (sul-AM-se-rod) USAN.
Use: Urge incontinence; atrial fibrillations.

Sular. (Sciele Pharma) Nisoldipine 8.5 mg, 17 mg, 25.5 mg, 34 mg. Tartrazine (17 mg only), lactose. Film-coated. ER Tab. 100s. *Rx.*
Use: Calcium channel blocker.

•**sulazepam.** (sull-AZE-eh-pam) USAN.
Use: Anxiolytic.

Sulazo. (Freeport) Sulfisoxazole 500 mg, phenylazodiaminopyridine hydrochloride 50 mg. Tab. Bot. 1000s. *Rx.*
Use: Analgesic; anti-infective.

•**sulbactam benzathine.** (sull-BACK-tam BENZ-ah-theen) USAN.
Use: Synergistic (penicillin/cephalosporin); inhibitor (β-lactamase).

•**sulbactam pivoxil.** (sull-BACK-tam pihv-OX-ill) USAN.
Use: Inhibitor (β-lactamase); synergist (penicillin/cephalosporin).

sulbactam sodium/ampicillin sodium.
Use: Anti-infective; penicillin.
See: Unasyn.

•**sulbactam sodium sterile.** (sull-BACK-tam) *USP 34.*
Use: Inhibitor (β-lactamase); synergist (penicillin/cephalosporin).

•**sulconazole nitrate.** (SULL-CONE-ah-zole) *USP 34.*
Use: Antifungal.
See: Exelderm.

•**sulesomab.** (sue-LEH-so-mab) USAN.
Use: Monoclonal antibody (diagnostic aid for detection of infectious lesions).

•**sulfabenz.** (SULL-fah-benz) USAN.
Use: Anti-infective.

•**sulfabenzamide.** (SULL-fah-BENZ-ah-mid) *USP 34.*
Use: Anti-infective.

sulfabromethazine sodium.
Use: Anti-infective.
Sulfacet. (Dermik)
See: Sulfacetamide.
• **sulfacetamide.** (sull-fah-SEE-tah-mide)
USP 34.
Use: Anti-infective.
W/Combinations.
See: Acet-Dia-Mer Sulfonamides.
Chero-Trisulfa-V.
Sulfa-10 Ophthalmic.
• **sulfacetamide sodium.** (sull-fah-SEE-tah-mide) *USP 34.*
Use: Anti-infective.
See: AK-Sulf.
Bleph 10.
Carmol Scalp Treatment.
Isopto Cetamide.
Klaron.
Klaron 10%.
Ovace Plus.
Ovace Plus Wash.
Seb-Prev.
Seb-Prev Wash.
Sodium Sulamyd Ophthalmic.
Sulf-15.
Sulf-10.
W/Prednisolone Acetate.
See: Blephamide S.O.P.
Metimyd.
W/Sulfur.
See: Novacet.
Plexion.
Plexion SCT.
Rosanil.
Rosula.
Sulfacet-R.
Vanocin.
Zetacet.
sulfacetamide sodium. (Various Mfr.)
Sulfacetamide sodium. **Lot.:** 10%. May
contain disodium EDTA, PEG 400,
methylparaben, urea. 89g, 118 mL.
Soln.: 10%. Bot. 15 mL. **Oint.:** 10%.
Tube 3.5 g.
Use: Anti-infective.
sulfacetamide sodium and prednisolone acetate.
Use: Anti-infective; anti-inflammatory,
ophthalmic.
See: Blephamide.
Metimyd.
Predsulfair.
Vasocidin.
sulfacetamide sodium and prednisolone sodium phosphate. (Schein)
Sulfacetamide sodium 10%, prednisolone sodium phosphate 0.25%. Soln.
5 mL, 10 mL. *Rx.*
Use: Anti-infective, ophthalmic.

sulfacetamide sodium 10%. (Fougera)
Sulfacetamide sodium 100 mg per mL.
Methylparaben, EDTA. Top. Susp.
118 mL. *Rx.*
Use: Acne product.
**sulfacetamide sodium 10% and sulfur
5%.** (Glades) Sulfur 5%, sodium sulfacetamide 10%, cetyl alcohol, benzyl alcohol, EDTA. Bot. 25 mL. Tube 30 mL.
Rx.
Use: Dermatologic, acne.
sulfacetamide, sulfadiazine, and sulfamerazine.
See: Acet-Dia-Mer-Sulfonamide.
Sulfacet-R. (Dermik) Sulfur 5%, sulfacetamide sodium 10%, parabens. Lot. Bot.
25 mL. *Rx.*
Use: Dermatologic, acne.
SulfaCleanse 8/4. (PruGen) Sodium sulfacetamide 8%, sulfur 4%. Alcohols,
aloe, butylated hydroxytoluene, edetate
disodium, glyceryl, green tea, parabens, PEG. Soap. 473 mL. *Rx.*
Use: Acne product combination.
• **sulfacytine.** (SULL-fah-SIGH-teen)
USAN.
Use: Anti-infective.
sulfadiasulfone sodium. Acetosulfone
sodium.
• **sulfadiazine.** (SULL-fah-DIE-ah-zeen)
USP 34.
Tall Man: sulfADIAZINE
Use: Anti-infective. [Orphan Drug]
W/Combinations.
See: Acet-dia-mer-sulfonamide.
Chemozine.
Chero-Trisulfa-V.
Meth-Dia-Mer Sulfonamides.
Silvadene.
Triple Sulfa.
sulfadiazine. (Sandoz) Sulfadiazine
500 mg. Tab. 100s, 1000s. *Rx.*
Use: Anti-infective.
sulfadiazine and sulfamerazine. Citrasulfas.
• **sulfadiazine, silver.** (sull-fah-DIE-ah-zeen) *USP 34.*
Tall Man: sulfADIAZINE
Use: Anti-infective, topical.
• **sulfadiazine sodium.** (SULL-fah-DIE-ah-zeen) *USP 34.*
Tall Man: sulfADIAZINE
Use: Anti-infective.
sulfadiazine, sulfamerazine, and sulfacetamide.
See: Acet-Dia-Mer-sulfonamide.
Coco Diazine.
• **sulfadimethoxine.** (SUL-fa-DYE-meth-OX-een) *USP 34.*

●**sulfadimethoxine sodium.** (SUL-fa-DYE-meth-OX-een) *USP 34.*

sulfadimidine.
See: Sulfamethazine.

sulfadine.
See: Sulfadimidine.
Sulfamethazine.
Sulfapyridine.

●**sulfadoxine.** (SULL-fah-DOX-een) *USP 34.*
Use: Anti-infective.

sulfaguanidine.
Use: GI tract infections.

Sulfair 15. (Bausch & Lomb) Sodium sulfacetamide 15%. Soln. Bot. 15 mL. *Rx.*
Use: Anti-infective, ophthalmic.

●**sulfalene.** (SULL-fah-leen) USAN.
Use: Anti-infective.

●**sulfamerazine.** (sull-fah-MER-ah-zeen)
Use: Anti-infective.
W/Combinations
See: Chemozine.
Chero-Trisulfa-V.

sulfamerazine sodium.
Use: Anti-infective.

sulfamerazine, sulfadiazine, and sulfamethazine.
Use: Anti-infective.
See: Meth-Dia-Mer Sulfonamides.

sulfamerazine, sulfadiazine, and sulfathiazole.
Use: Anti-infective.

●**sulfameter.** (SULL-fam-EE-ter) USAN.
Use: Anti-infective.

●**sulfamethazine.** (sull fa-METH-ah-zeen) *USP 34.*
Use: Anti-infective.
W/Sulfadiazine, Sulfamerazine.
See: Triple Sulfa.

●**sulfamethizole.** (sul-fa-METH-i-zole) USAN.
Use: Anti-infective.

sulfamethoprim. (Par Pharmaceuticals) Sulfamethoxazole 400 mg, trimethoprim 80 mg. Tab. Bot. 100s, 500s. *Rx.*
Use: Anti-infective.

●**sulfamethoxazole.** (sull-fah-meth-OX-ah-zole) *USP 34.*
Use: Anti-infective.
W/Trimethoprim.
See: Bactrim.
Septra DS.

sulfamethoxazole and phenazopyridine hydrochloride.
Use: Anti-infective, urinary.

●**sulfamethoxazole and trimethoprim injection.** (SULL-fah-meth-OX-ah-zole and try-METH-oh-prim) *USP 34.*
Use: Anti-infective, urinary.

sulfamethoxazole and trimethoprim oral suspension. (Various Mfr.) Trimethoprim 40 mg, sulfamethoxazole 200 mg/5 mL. Bot. 150 mL, 200 mL, 480 mL. *Rx.*
Use: Anti-infective, urinary.

sulfamethoxazole and trimethoprim tablets. (Various Mfr.) Trimethoprim 80 mg, sulfamethoxazole 400 mg. Tab. Bot. 100s, 500s. *Rx.*
Use: Anti-infective, urinary.

sulfamethoxazole/trimethoprim DS. (Various Mfr.) Trimethoprim 160 mg, sulfamethoxazole 800 mg. Tab, double-strength. Bot. 100s, 500s. *Rx.*
Use: Anti-infective.

sulfamethoxydiazine. Sulfameter.
Use: Anti-infective.

sulfamethoxypyridazine acetyl.
Use: Anti-infective.

sulfamethylthiadiazole.
Use: Anti-infective.

sulfametin. *Formerly Sulfamethoxydiazine.*
Use: Anti-infective.

sulfamezanthene.
Use: Anti-infective.
See: Sulfamethazine.

Sulfamide. (Rugby) Prednisolone acetate 0.5%, sodium sulfacetamide, hydroxypropyl methylcellulose, polysorbate 80, sodium thiosulfate, benzalkonium Cl 0.01%. Susp. Bot. 5 and 15 mL. *Rx.*
Use: Anti-infective, ophthalmic.

●**sulfamonomethoxine.** (SULL-fah-mahn-oh-meh-THOCK-seen) USAN.
Use: Anti-infective.

●**sulfamoxole.** (sull-fah-MOX-ole) USAN.
Use: Anti-infective.

p-sulfamoylbenzylamine hydrochloride. Sulfbenzamide.

Sulfamylon. (UDL) **Cream:** Mafenide 85 mg/g (as acetate). EDTA, cetyl alcohol, stearyl alcohol, parabens, sodium metabisulfite. 56.7 g, 113.4 g, 453.6 g. **Top. Soln.:** Mafenide acetate 5%. Packets. 50 g for reconstitution. *Rx.*
Use: Topical anti-infective.

2-sulfanilamidopyridine. Sulfadiazine, USP.
Use: Anti-infective.

●**sulfanilate zinc.** (sull-FAN-ih-late) USAN.
Use: Anti-infective.

n-sulfanilylacetamide.
Use: Anti-infective.
See: Sulfacetamide.

sulfanilylbenzamide.
Use: Anti-infective.
See: Sulfabenzamide.

- **sulfanitran.** (SULL-fah-NYE-tran) USAN.
  Use: Anti-infective.
- **sulfapyridine.** (sull-fah-PEER-ih-deen) *USP 34.*
  Use: Dermatitic herpetiformis suppressant. [Orphan Drug]
- **sulfasalazine.** (SULL-fuh-SAL-uh-zeen) *USP 34.* Formerly *Salicylazosulfapyridine.*
  Tall Man: sulfaSALAzine
  Use: Anti-infective; antirheumatic.
  See: Azulfidine.
     Azulfidine EN-tabs.
  sulfasalazine. (Greenstone) Sulfasalazine 500 mg. Enteric coated. DR Tab. 100s, 300s. *Rx.*
  Use: Anti-infective; antirheumatic.
  sulfasalazine. (Various Mfr.) Sulfasalazine 500 mg. Tab. Bot. 50s, 100s, 500s, 1000s. *Rx.*
  Use: Anti-infective; antirheumatic.
- **sulfasomizole.** (SULL-fah-SAHM-ih-zole) USAN.
  Use: Antibacterial; anti-infective; sulfonamide.
  sulfasymasine.
  Use: Anti-infective sulfonamide.
  Sulfa-10 Ophthalmic. (Maurry) Sodium sulfacetamide 10%, hydroxyethylcellulose, sodium borate, boric acid, disodium edetate, sodium metabisulfite, sodium thiosulfate 0.2%, chlorobutanol 0.2%, methylparaben 0.015%. Bot. 15 mL. *Rx.*
  Use: Anti-infective, ophthalmic.
  Sulfa-Ter-Tablets. (A.P.C.) Trisulfapyrimidines. Tab. Bot. 1000s.
- **sulfathiazole.** (sull-fah-THIGH-ah-zole) *USP 34.*
  Use: Anti-infective.
  Sulfatrim. (Activis MidAtlantic) Trimethoprim 40 mg, sulfamethoxazole 200 mg/5 mL. Alcohol < 0.5%, parabens, saccharin, sucrose. Fruit licorice and cherry flavors. Susp. 473 mL. *Rx.*
  Use: Anti-infective.
  Sulfatrim DS. (Ivax) Trimethoprim 800 mg, sulfamethoxazole 160 mg. Tab. Bot. 100s, 500s. *Rx.*
  Use: Anti-infective.
  Sulfatrim SS. (Ivax) Trimethoprim 400 mg, sulfamethoxazole 80 mg. Tab. Bot. 100s. *Rx.*
  Use: Anti-infective.
  Sulfa-Trip. (Major) Sulfathiazole 3.42%, sulfacetamide 2.86%, sulfabenzamide 3.7%, urea 0.64%. Cream. Tube 82.5 g. *Rx.*
  Use: Anti-infective, vaginal.

Sulfa Triple No. 2. (Global Source) Sulfadiazine 162 mg, sulfamerazine 162 mg, sulfamethazine 162 mg. Tab. Bot. 1000s. *Rx.*
Use: Anti-infective.
- **sulfazamet.** (sull-FAZE-ah-MET) USAN.
  Use: Anti-infective.
  Sulf-15. (Ciba Vision) Sodium sulfacetamide 15%. Soln. Bot. 5 mL, 15 mL. *Rx.*
  Use: Anti-infective, ophthalmic.
- **sulfinalol hydrochloride.** (SULL-FIN-ah-lahl) USAN.
  Use: Antihypertensive.
- **sulfinpyrazone.** (sull-fin-PEER-uh-zone) *USP 34.*
  Use: Uricosuric.
- **sulfisoxazole.** (sull-fih-SOX-uh-zole) *USP 34.*
  Tall Man: sulfiSOXAZOLE
  Use: Anti-infective.
  See: Gantrisin Pediatric.
     Soxa.
     Sulfisoxazole.
- **sulfisoxazole, acetyl.** (sull-fih-SOX-uh-zole, ASS-eh-till) *USP 34.*
  Tall Man: sulfiSOXAZOLE
  Use: Anti-infective.
  sulfisoxazole diethanolamine. Sulfisoxazole Diolamine.
- **sulfisoxazole diolamine.** (sull-fih-SOX-uh-zole die-OLE-ah-meen) *USP 34.*
  Tall Man: sulfiSOXAZOLE
  Use: Anti-infective.
  Sulfoam. (Doak) Sulfur 2%, parabens. Shampoo. Bot. 237 mL. *OTC.*
  Use: Control dandruff.
  sulfobromophthalein sodium. *USP 34.*
  Use: Liver function test.
  sulfocarbolates. Salts of Phenolsulfonic Acid, Usually Ca, Na, K, Cu, Zn.
- **sulfocon B.** (sul-FOE-kon) USAN.
  Use: Hydrophobic.
  sulfocyanate.
  See: Potassium Thiocyanate.
  Sulfo-Ganic. (Marcen) Thioglycerol 20 mg, sodium citrate 5 mg, phenol 0.5%, benzyl alcohol 0.5%/mL. Inj. Vial 10 mL, 30 mL.
  Use: Antiarthritic.
  Sulfolax. (Major) Docusate calcium 240 mg. Parabens, sorbitol. Soft Gel Cap. Bot. 100s. *OTC.*
  Use: Laxative.
  Sulfo-Lo. (Whorton Pharmaceuticals, Inc.) Sublimed sulfur, freshly precipitated polysulfides of zinc, potassium, sulfate, and calamine in aqueous-alcoholic suspension. **Lotion:** Bot. 4 oz,

8 oz. **Soap:** 3 oz. *OTC.*
Use: Dermatologic, acne.
•**sulfomyxin.** (SULL-foe-MIX-in) USAN.
Use: Anti-infective.
sulfonamides.
Use: Anticonvulsants.
See: Sulfacetamide Sodium.
Sulfadiazine.
Sulfamethoxazole.
Sulfisoxazole.
Sulfisoxazole Diolamine.
Zonisamide.
sulfonamides, triple.
See: Acet-Dia-Mer Sulfonamide.
Meth-Dia-Mer Sulfonamides.
sulfones.
See: Dapsone.
Glucosulfone Sodium.
•**sulfonterol hydrochloride.** (sull-FAHN-teer-ole) USAN.
Use: Bronchodilator.
sulfonylureas.
See: Chlorpropamide.
Glimepiride.
Glipizide.
Glyburide.
Tolazamide.
Tolbutamide.
Sulforcin. (Galderma) Sulfur 5%, resorcinol 2%, SD alcohol 40 11.65%, methylparaben. Lot. Bot. 120 mL. *OTC.*
Use: Dermatologic.
sulformethoxine. *Name used for Sulfadoxine.*
sulforthomidine. *Name used for Sulfadoxine.*
sulfosalicylate with methenamine.
See: Hexalen.
sulfosalicylic acid. Salicylsulphonic acid.
Sulfoxyl Regular. (Stiefel) Benzoyl peroxide 5%, sulfur 2%, stearic acid, zinc laurate. Lot. Bot. 59 mL. *Rx.*
Use: Dermatologic, acne.
Sulf-10. (Novartis Ophthalmic) Sodium sulfacetamide 10%. Bot. 15 mL; *Dropperette* 1 mL. *Rx.*
Use: Anti-infective, ophthalmic.
sulfur.
Use: Antiseborrheic.
See: Sulfoam.
W/Benzocaine.
See: Chigg Away.
W/Benzoyl Peroxide.
See: NuOx.
W/Salicylic Acid.
See: Exoderm.
W/Sodium Sulfacetamide.
See: Avar-e Emollient.
Avar-e Green.
Avar-e LS.

Avar LS Cleanser.
BP Cleansing Wash.
Cerisa.
Clarifoam EF.
Claris.
Rosaderm Kit.
Rosula Clarifying Wash.
SulfoCleanse 8/4.
Sumaxin.
Sumaxin TS.
Sumaxin Wash.
Zencia.
sulfurated lime topical solution. Vleminckx Lotion.
Use: Scabicide; parasiticide.
sulfur combinations.
See: Aveenobar Medicated.
Acnomel.
Acnotex.
Adult Acnomel.
Akne.
Avar.
Avar-e Emollient.
Avar-e Green.
Clearasil Adult Care.
Clenia.
Liquimat.
Pernox.
Plexion.
Plexion Cleansing Cloths.
Plexion SCT.
Plexion TS.
Rezamid.
SAStid Soap.
Sebulex with Conditioners.
Sulfacet-R.
Sulfo-lo.
Sulforcin.
Sulfur-8.
Sulpho-Lac.
Vanocin.
•**sulfur dioxide.** (SULL-fer die-OX-ide) *NF 29.*
Use: Pharmaceutic aid (antioxidant).
Sulfur-8 Hair & Scalp Conditioner.
(Schering-Plough) Sulfur 2%, menthol 1%, triclosan 0.1%. Cream. Jar 2 oz, 4 oz, 8 oz. *OTC.*
Use: Antiseborrheic.
Sulfur-8 Light Formula Hair & Scalp Conditioner. (Schering-Plough) Sulfur, triclosan, menthol. Cream. Jar 2 oz, 4 oz. *OTC.*
Use: Antiseborrheic.
Sulfur-8 Shampoo. (Schering-Plough) Triclosan 0.2%. Bot. 6.85 oz, 10.85 oz. *OTC.*
Use: Antiseborrheic.
•**sulfur hexafluoride.** (SUL-fur) USAN.
Use: Diagnostic aid (ultrasound).

•**sulfuric acid.** *NF 29.*
Use: Pharmaceutic aid (acidifying agent).

sulfuric acid/sulfonated phenolics.
Use: Mouth and throat product.
See: Debacterol.

sulfur ointment.
Use: Scabicide; parasiticide.

•**sulfur, precipitated.** (SUL-fur pree-SIP-a-TAY-ted) *USP 34.*
Use: Scabicide; parasiticide.
See: SAStid Soap.
  Sulfur Soap.

sulfur, salicyl diasporal. (Doak Dermatologics)
See: Diasporal.

sulfur soap. (GlaxoSmithKline) Precipitated sulfur 10%, EDTA. Cake 116 g. *OTC.*
Use: Dermatologic, acne.

•**sulfur, sublimed.** (SUL-fur) *USP 34.*
Flowers of Sulfur.
Use: Parasiticide; scabicide.

sulfur, topical.
See: Thylox.

•**sulindac.** (sull-IN-dak) *USP 34.*
Use: Nonsteroidal anti-inflammatory agent.
See: Clinoril.

sulindac. (Various Mfr.) Sulindac 150 mg, 200 mg. Tab. Bot. 100s, 500s, 1000s, UD 100s. *Rx.*
Use: Anti-inflammatory; NSAID.

•**sulisobenzone.** (sul-EYE-so-BEN-zone) USAN.
Use: Ultraviolet screen.
See: Uvinul MS-40.

•**sulmarin.** (SULL-mah-rin) USAN.
Use: Hemostatic.

Sulmasque. (C & M Pharmacal) Sulfur 6.4%, isopropyl alcohol 15%, methylparaben. Mask 150 g. *OTC.*
Use: Dermatologic, acne.

Sulnac. (Alra) Sulfathiazole 3.42%, sulfacetamide 2.86%, sulfabenzamide 3.7%, urea 0.64% in cream base. Tube 2.75 oz. *Rx.*
Use: Anti-infective.

•**sulnidazole.** (sull-NIH-dah-zole) USAN.
Use: Antiprotozoal (trichomonas).

•**suloctidil.** (sull-OCK-tih-dill) USAN.
Use: Vasodilator (peripheral).

•**sulofenur.** (SUE-low-FEN-ehr) USAN.
Use: Antineoplastic.

•**sulopenem.** (soo-loe-PEN-em) USAN.
Use: Anti-infective.

•**sulopenem etzadroxil.** (soo-loe-PEN-em et-za-DROX-il) USAN.
Use: Antibiotic.

•**sulotroban.** (suh-LOW-troe-ban) USAN.
Use: Treatment of glomerulonephritis.

•**suloxifen oxalate.** (sull-OX-ih-fen OX-ah-late) USAN.
Use: Bronchodilator.

suloxybenzone. (Wyeth)

sulphabenzide.
See: Sulfabenzamide.

Sulpho-Lac Acne Medication. (Doak Dermatologics) Sulfur 5%, zinc sulfate 27%, Vleminckx's Soln. 53%. Cream. Tube 28.35 g, 50 g. *OTC.*
Use: Dermatologic, acne.

Sulpho-Lac Soap. (Doak Dermatologics) Sulfur 5%, a coconut and tallow oil soap base. Bar 85 g. *OTC.*
Use: Dermatologic, acne.

•**sulpiride.** (SULL-pih-ride) USAN.
Use: Antidepressant.

•**sulprostone.** (sull-PRAHST-ohn) USAN.
Use: Prostaglandin.

Sul-Ray Acne. (Last) Sulfur 2% in cream base. Cream. Jar 1.75 oz, 6.75 oz, 20 oz. *OTC.*
Use: Dermatologic, acne.

Sul-Ray Aloe Vera Analgesic Rub. (Last) Camphor 3.1%, menthol 1.25%. Bot. 4 oz, 8 oz. *OTC.*
Use: Analgesic, topical.

Sul-Ray Aloe Vera Skin Protectant. (Last) Zinc oxide 1%, allantoin 0.5%. Cream. Jar 1 oz. *OTC.*
Use: Dermatologic, protectant.

Sul-Ray Shampoo. (Last) Sulfur shampoo 2%. Bot. 8 oz. *OTC.*
Use: Antidandruff.

Sul-Ray Soap. (Last) Sulfur soap. Bar 3 oz. *OTC.*
Use: Dermatologic, acne.

•**sultamicillin.** (SULL-TAM-ih-sill-in) USAN.
Use: Anti-infective.

•**sulthiame.** (sull-THIGH-aim) USAN.
Use: Anticonvulsant.

•**sulukast.** (suh-LOO-kast) USAN.
Use: Antiasthmatic (leukotriene antagonist).

Sumacal. (Biosearch Medical Products) CHO 95 g, 380 Cal., Na 100 mg, chloride 210 mg, K < 39 mg, Ca 20 mg/100 g. Pow. Bot. 400 g. *OTC.*
Use: Glucose polymer.

•**sumarotene.** (sue-MAHR-oh-teen) USAN.
Use: Keratolytic.

•**sumatriptan.** (SUE-muh-TRIP-tan) *USP 34.*
Tall Man: SUMAtriptan
Use: Agent for migraine, serotonin

5-HT$_1$ receptor agonist.
See: Imitrex.

sumatriptan. (Sandoz) Sumatriptan 5 mg, 20 mg. Soln., intranasal. 100 mcL unit-dose spray device. 6s. *Rx.*
Use: Agent for migraine, serotonin 5-HT$_1$ receptor agonist.

sumatriptan. (Teva) Sumatriptan 25 mg, 50 mg, 100 mg. Lactose, PEG. Film-coated. Tab. 9s. *Rx.*
Use: Agent for migraine, serotonin 5-HT$_1$ receptor agonist.

• **sumatriptan succinate.** (SUE-muh-TRIP-tan SOOS-in-ate) USAN.
Tall Man: SUMAtriptan
Use: Antimigraine agent, serotonin 5-HT$_1$ receptor agonist.
See: Imitrex.
  Sumavel DosePro.

sumatriptan succinate. (Sandoz) Sumatriptan. Inj., Soln. **6 mg per 0.5 mL:** Sodium chloride 3.5 mg. Single-dose pre-filled syringe cartridge. 6 mg. **4 mg per 0.5 mL:** Sodium chloride 3.8 mg. Single-dose vial. 4 mg. *Rx.*
Use: Agent for migraine, serotonin 5-HT$_1$ receptor agonist.

Sumavel DosePro. (Zogenix) Sumatriptan succinate 6 mg per 0.5 mL. Sodium chloride 3.5 mg. Inj., Soln. 6 mg single-dose vials in a prefilled, disposable, needle-free subcutaneous delivery system. *Rx.*
Use: Agent for migraine, serotonin 5-HT$_1$ receptor agonist.

Sumaxin. (Medimetriks) Sodium sulfacetamide 10%, sulfur 4%. Aloe, cetyl alcohol, edetate disodium, glycerin, glyceryl stearate, green tea, parabens, PEG-100, stearyl alcohol. Pad. 60s. *Rx.*
Use: Acne product combination.

Sumaxin TS. (Medimetriks) Sodium sulfacetamide 8%, sulfur 4%. Aloe, cetyl alcohol, edetate disodium, glyceryl, green tea, parabens, PEG-100, stearyl alcohol. Susp., topical. 473 mL. *Rx.*
Use: Acne product combination.

Sumaxin Wash. (Medimetriks) Sodium sulfacetamide 9%, sulfur 4%. Aloe, cetyl alcohol, edetate disodium, glyceryl, green tea, parabens, PEG-100, stearyl alcohol. Liq. 473 mL. *Rx.*
Use: Acne product combination.

Summer's Eve Disposable Douche. (C.B. Fleet) **Soln.:** Vinegar. 135 mL (1s, 2s). **Soln. Reg.:** Citric acid, sodium benzoate. **Soln. Scented:** Citric acid, sodium benzoate, octoxynol-9, EDTA. 135 mL (1s, 2s, 4s). *OTC.*
Use: Douche.

Summer's Eve Disposable Douche Extra Cleansing. (C.B. Fleet) Vinegar, sodium Cl, benzoic acid. Soln. 135 mL (1s, 2s, 4s). *OTC.*
Use: Douche.

Summer's Eve Feminine Bath. (C.B. Fleet) Ammonium laureth sulfate, EDTA. Liq. Bot. 45 mL, 345 mL. *OTC.*
Use: Vaginal preparation.

Summer's Eve Feminine Powder. (C.B. Fleet) Cornstarch, octoxynol-9, benzethonium chloride. Pow. Bot. 30 g, 210 g. *OTC.*
Use: Vaginal preparation.

Summer's Eve Feminine Wash. (C.B. Fleet) **Wipes:** Octoxynol-9, EDTA. Box 16s. **Liq.:** Ammonium laureth sulfate, PEG-75, lanolin, EDTA. Bot. 60 mL, 240 mL, 450 mL. *Rx.*
Use: Vaginal preparation.

Summer's Eve Medicated Disposable Douche. (C.B. Fleet) Contains povidone-iodide 0.3%. Single or twin 135 mL disposable units. *OTC.*
Use: Temporary relief of minor vaginal irritation and itching.

Summer's Eve Post Menstrual Disposable Douche. (C.B. Fleet) Sodium lauryl sulfate, parabens, monosodium and disodium phosphates, EDTA. Soln. 135 mL (2s). *OTC.*
Use: Douche.

Summit Extra Strength. (Pfeiffer) Acetaminophen 250 mg, aspirin 250 mg, caffeine 65 mg. Capl. Bot. 50s. *OTC.*
Use: Analgesic combination.

Sumycin '500'. (Par) Tetracycline hydrochloride 500 mg, mineral oil, lactose. Cap. Bot. 100s, 500s. *Rx.*
Use: Anti-infective; tetracycline.

Sumycin Syrup. (Par) Tetracycline hydrochloride 125 mg/5 mL, saccharin, sodium metabisulfite, sorbitol, sucrose, fruit flavor. Oral Susp. Bot. 473 mL. *Rx.*
Use: Anti-infective; tetracycline.

Sumycin '250'. (Par) Tetracycline hydrochloride 250 mg, mineral oil, lactose. Bot. 100s, 1000s. *Rx.*
Use: Anti-infective; tetracycline.

• **suncillin sodium.** (SUN-SILL-in SOE-dee-um) USAN.
Use: Anti-infective.

Sundown. (Johnson & Johnson) A series of products marketed under the Sundown name including: **Moderate:** (SPF 4) Padimate O, oxybenzone. **Extra:** (SPF 6) Oxybenzone, padimate O. **Maximal:** (SPF 8) Oxybenzone, padimate O. **Ultra:** (SPF 15, 30) oxybenzone, padimate O, octyl methoxy-

cinnamate. *OTC.*
Use: Sunscreen.

Sundown Sport Sunblock. (Johnson & Johnson) Titanium dioxide, zinc oxide. PABA free. Waterproof. SPF 15. Lot. 90 mL. *OTC.*
Use: Sunscreen.

Sundown Sunblock Cream Ultra SPF 24. (Johnson & Johnson) Padimate O, oxybenzone. *OTC.*
Use: Sunscreen.

Sundown Sunblock Stick SPF 15. (Johnson & Johnson) Octyl dimethyl PABA, oxybenzone. Stick 0.35 oz. *OTC.*
Use: Sunscreen.

Sundown Sunblock Stick SPF 20. (Johnson & Johnson) Octyl dimethyl PABA, octyl methoxycinnamate, oxybenzone, titanium dioxide. *OTC.*
Use: Sunscreen.

Sundown Sunblock Ultra Lotion 30 SPF. (Johnson & Johnson) Octyl methoxycinnamate, octyl salicylate, oxybenzone, titanium dioxide, cetyl alcohol, PABA free. Waterproof. Lot. Bot. 120 mL. *OTC.*
Use: Sunscreen.

Sundown Sunblock Ultra SPF 20. (Johnson & Johnson) Octyl dimethyl PABA, octyl methoxycinnamate, oxybenzone, titanium dioxide. *OTC.*
Use: Sunscreen.

Sundown Sunscreen Stick SPF 8. (Johnson & Johnson) Octyl dimethyl PABA, oxybenzone. Stick 0.35 oz. *OTC.*
Use: Sunscreen.

Sundown Sunscreen Ultra. (Johnson & Johnson) Octyl methoxycinnamate, octyl salicylate, oxybenzone, titanium dioxide, stearyl alcohol, cetyl alcohol, PABA free. Waterproof. SPF 15. Cream. Tube 60 g. *OTC.*
Use: Sunscreen.

•**sunepitron hydrochloride.** (soo-NE-pi-tron) USAN.
Use: Anxiolytic; antidepressant.

Sunice. (Citroleum) Allantoin 0.25%, menthol 0.25%, methyl salicylate 10%. Cream. Jar 3 oz. *OTC.*
Use: Burn therapy.

•**sunitinib malate.** (sue-NIH-tih-nib) USAN.
Tall Man: SUNItinib
Use: Protein-tyrosine kinase inhibitor.
See: Sutent.

Sunkist Multivitamins Complete, Children's. (Novartis) Fe 18 mg, vitamin A 5000 units, D_3 400 units, E 30 units, B_1 1.5 mg, B_2 1.7 mg, B_3 20 mg, B_5 10 mg, B_6 2 mg, B_{12} 6 mcg, C 60 mg, folic acid 400 mcg, Ca 100 mg, Cu, I, K,

Mg, Mn, P, Zn 10 mg, biotin 40 mcg, K_1 10 mcg. Sorbitol, aspartame, phenylalanine, tartrazine. Chew. Tab. Bot. 60s. *OTC.*
Use: Mineral, vitamin supplement.

Sunkist Multivitamins + Extra C, Children's. (Novartis) Vitamin A 2500 units, E 15 units, D_3 400 units, B_1 1.05 mg, B_2 1.2 mg, B_3 13.5 mg, B_6 1.05 mg, B_{12} 4.5 mcg, C 250 mg, folic acid 0.3 mg, vitamin K 5 mcg, sorbitol, aspartame, phenylalanine. Chew. Tab. Bot. 60s. *OTC.*
Use: Vitamin supplement.

Sunkist Vitamin C. (Novartis) Vitamin C (as ascorbic acid and sodium ascorbate) 60 mg, 250 mg, 500 mg. Fructose (except 60 mg), sorbitol, sucrose, lactose, orange flavor. Chew. Tab. Bot. 11s (60 mg only), 60s (250 mg only), 75s (500 mg only). *OTC.*
Use: Water-soluble vitamin.

SUNPRuF 15. (C & M Pharmacal) Octyl methoxycinnamate 7.5%, benzopherone-3 5%. PABA free. Waterproof. SPF 15. Lot. Bot. 240 mL. *OTC.*
Use: Sunscreen.

SUNPRuF 17. (C & M Pharmacal) Octyl methoxycinnamate 7.8%, octyl salicylate 5.2%, oil-free, water-resistant. SPF 17. Lot. Bot. 120 g. *OTC.*
Use: Sunscreen.

Sunshine Chewable Tablets. (Fibertone) Fe 5 mg, vitamins A 5000 units, D 400 units, E 67 mg, B_1 15 mg, B_2 15 mg, B_3 25 mg, B_5 20 mg, B_6 15 mg, B_{12} 15 mcg, C 150 mg, folic acid 0.1 mg, Ca, Cu, Mn, Zn, K, iodide, biotin, betaine, PABA, choline bitartrate, inositol, lecithin, hesperidin, rutin, bioflavonoids. Sorbitol, aspartame. Citrus flavor. Bot. 60s. *OTC.*
Use: Mineral, vitamin supplement.

Sunstick. (Rydelle) Lip and face protectant containing digalloyl trioleate 2.5% in emollient base. Stick Plas. swivel container 0.14 oz. *OTC.*
Use: Lip protectant.

SU-101.
Use: Malignant glioma. [Orphan Drug]

Supartz. (Smith & Nephew) Sodium hyaluronate 10 mg/mL. Inj. Prefilled syringes. 2.5 mL. *Rx.*
Use: Physical adjunct.

Super Aytinal. (Walgreen) Vitamins A 7000 units, B_1 5 mg, B_2 5 mg, B_5 10 mg, B_6 3 mg, B_{12} 9 mcg, C 90 mg, pantothenic acid 10 mg, D 400 units, E 30 units, niacin 30 mg, biotin 55 mcg, folic acid 0.4 mg, Fe 30 mg, Ca 162 mg, P 125 mg, I 150 mcg, Cu 3 mg, Mn

7.5 mg, Mg 100 mg, K 7.7 mg, Zn 24 mg, Cl 7 mg, Cr 15 mcg, Se 15 mcg, choline bitartrate 1000 mcg, inositol 1000 mcg, PABA 1000 mcg, rutin 1000 mcg, yeast 12 mg. Bot. 50s, 100s, 365s. *OTC.*
Use: Mineral, vitamin supplement.

Super-B. (Towne) Vitamins B₁ 50 mg, B₂ 20 mg, B₆ 5 mg, B₁₂ 15 mcg, C 300 mg, liver desiccated 100 mg, dried yeast 100 mg, niacinamide 25 mg, Ca pantothenate 5 mg, Fe 10 mg. Captab. Bot. 50s, 100s, 150s, 250s. *OTC.*
Use: Mineral, vitamin supplement.

Super Calicaps M-Z. (Nion Corp.) Ca 1200 mg, Mg 400 mg, Zn 15 mg, vitamins A 5000 units, D 400 units, Se 15 mcg. 3 Tabs. Bot. 90s. *OTC.*
Use: Mineral, vitamin supplement.

Super Calcium 1200. (Schiff Products/Weider Nutrition Intl.) Calcium carbonate 1512 mg (600 mg calcium). Cap. Bot. 60s, 120s. *OTC.*
Use: Mineral supplement.

Superdophilus. (NaTREN) *Lactobacillus acidophilus* strain DDS 1.2 billion/g Pow. 37.5 g, 75 g, 135 g. *OTC.*
Use: Antidiarrheal; nutritional supplement.

Super D Perles. (Pharmacia) Vitamins A 10,000 units, D 400 units. Cap. Bot. 100s. *OTC.*
Use: Vitamin supplement.

SuperEPA. (Advanced Nutritional Technology) Omega-3 polyunsaturated fatty acids 1200 mg. Cap. containing EPA 360 mg, DHA 240 mg. Bot. 60s, 90s. *OTC.*
Use: Nutritional supplement.

SuperEPA 2000. (Advanced Nutritional Technology) EPA 563 mg, DHA 312 mg, vitamin E 20 units. Cap. Bot. 30s, 60s, 90s. *OTC.*
Use: Nutritional supplement.

Supere-Pect. (Barth's) Alpha tocopherol 400 units, apple pectin 100 mg. Cap. Bot. 50s, 100s, 250s. *OTC.*
Use: Nutritional supplement.

Super Hi Potency. (Nion Corp.) Vitamins A 10,000 units, D 400 units, E 150 units, B₁ 75 mg, B₂ 75 mg, B₃ 75 mg, B₅ 75 mg, B₆ 75 mg, B₁₂ 75 mcg, C 250 mg, folic acid 0.4 mg, Zn 15 mg, betaine, biotin 75 mcg, Ca, Fe, hesperidin, I, K, Mg, Mn, Se. Tab. Bot. 100s. *OTC.*
Use: Mineral, vitamin supplement.

Super Hydramin Protein Powder. (Nion Corp.) Protein 41%, carbohydrate 21.8%, fat 1% in powder form. Can 1 lb. *OTC.*
Use: Nutritional supplement.

superinone. Tyloxapol.
Super Nutri-Vites. (Faraday) Vitamins A 36,000 units, D 400 units, B₁ 25 mg, B₂ 25 mg, B₆ 50 mg, B₁₂ 50 mcg, niacinamide 50 mg, Ca pantothenate 12.5 mg, choline bitartrate 150 mg, inositol 150 mg, betaine hydrochloride 25 mg, PABA 15 mg, glutamic acid 25 mg, desiccated liver 50 mg, C 150 mg, E 12.5 units, Mn gluconate 6.15 mg, bone meal 162 mg, Fe gluconate 50 mg, Cu gluconate 0.25 mg, Zn gluconate 2.2 mg, K iodide 0.1 mg, Ca 53.3 mg, P 24.3 mg, Mg gluconate 7.2 mg. Protein-coated Tab. Bot. 60s, 100s. *OTC.*
Use: Mineral, vitamin supplement.

superoxide dismutase (recombinant human).
Use: Protection of donor organ tissue. [Orphan Drug]

Super Plenamins Multiple Vitamins and Minerals. (Rexall Group) Vitamins A 8000 units, D₂ 400 units, vitamins B₁ 2.5 mg, B₂ 2.5 mg, C 75 mg, niacinamide 20 mg, B₆ 1 mg, B₁₂ 3 mcg, biotin 20 mcg, E 10 units, pantothenic acid 3 mg, liver conc. 100 mg, Fe 30 mg, Ca 75 mg, P 58 mg, I 0.15 mg, Cu 0.75 mg, Mn 1.25 mg, Mg 10 mg, Zn 1 mg. Tab. Bot. 36s, 72s, 144s, 288s, 365s. *OTC.*
Use: Mineral, vitamin supplement.

Superplex T. (Major) Vitamins B₁ 15 mg, B₂ 10 mg, B₃ 100 mg, B₅ 20 mg, B₆ 5 mg, B₁₂ 10 mcg, C 500 mg. Tab. Bot. 100s. *OTC.*
Use: Vitamin supplement.

Super Poli-Grip/Wernet's Cream. (Block Drug) Carboxymethylcellulose gum, ethylene oxide polymer, petrolatum-mineral oil base. Tube 0.7 oz, 1.4 oz, 2.4 oz. *OTC.*
Use: Denture adhesive.

Super Quints-50. (Freeda) Vitamins B₁ 50 mg, B₂ 50 mg, B₃ 50 mg, B₅ 50 mg, B₆ 50 mg, B₁₂ 50 mcg, folic acid 0.4 mg, PABA 30 mg, d-biotin 50 mcg, inositol 50 mg. Tab. Bot. 100s, 250s, 500s. *OTC.*
Use: Vitamin supplement.

Super Shade SPF-25. (Schering-Plough) Ethylhexyl p-methoxycinnamate, padimate O oxybenzone. SPF 25. Lot. Bot. 4 fl. oz. *OTC.*
Use: Sunscreen.

Super Shade Sunblock Stick SPF-25. (Schering-Plough) Ethylhexyl p-methoxycinnamate, oxybenzone, padimate O in stick. SPF 25. Tube 0.43 oz. *OTC.*
Use: Sunscreen.

Super Strength D-2000 IU. (Nature's Bounty) Vitamin D_3 (cholecalciferol) 2,000 units. Calcium 142 mg. Gluten free, preservative free, and sugar free. Tab. 100s. *OTC.*
Use: Fat-soluble vitamin.

Super Stress. (Towne) Vitamins C 600 mg, E 30 units B_1 15 mg, B_2 15 mg, niacin 100 mg, B_6 5 mg, B_{12} 12 mcg, pantothenic acid 20 mg. Tab. Bot. 60s. *OTC.*
Use: Vitamin supplement.

Super Troche. (Weeks & Leo) Benzocaine 5 mg, cetalkonium Cl 1 mg. Loz. Bot. 15s, 30s. *OTC.*
Use: Mouth and throat preparation.

Super Troche Plus. (Weeks & Leo) Benzocaine 10 mg, cetalkonium Cl 2 mg. Loz. Bot. 12s. *OTC.*
Use: Mouth and throat preparation.

Super-T with Zinc. (Towne) Vitamins A 10,000 units, D 400 units, E 15 units, C 200 mg, B_1 10 mg, B_2 10 mg, B_6 5 mg, B_{12} 6 mcg, niacinamide 50 mg, Fe 18 mg, I 0.1 mg, Cu 2 mg, Mn 1 mg, Zn 15 mg. Cap. Bot. 130s. *OTC.*
Use: Mineral, vitamin supplement.

Supervim. (US Ethicals) Vitamins and minerals. Tab. Bot. 100s.
Use: Mineral, vitamin supplement.

Super Wernet's Powder. (Block Drug) Carboxymethylcellulose gum, ethylene oxide polymer. Bot. 0.63 oz, 1.75 oz, 3.55 oz. *OTC.*
Use: Denture adhesive.

Suplena. (Abbot Nutrition) Protein (L-carnitine, milk protein, taurine) 45 g, carbohydrates (corn maltodextrin, maltitol syrup, sucrose) 205 g, fat (fructooligosaccharides, high oleic safflower oil, canola oil, soy lecithin) 96/L. Sodium 785 mg/L, potassium 1120 mg/L, 600 mOsm/kg H_2O, 1.8 cal/mL. Vitamins A, B_1, B_2, B_3, B_5, B_6, B_7, B_{12}, C, D, E, K, Ca, choline, Cl^-, Cr, Cu, Fe, folic acid, I, Mg, Mn, Mo, P, Se, Zn. Gluten and lactose free. Vanilla flavor. Liq. 240 mL. *OTC.*
Use: Enteral nutritional therapy, defined formula diets.

Suplical. (Parke-Davis) Calcium 600 mg/Square. Bot. 30s, 60s. *OTC.*
Use: Mineral supplement.

Supprelin LA. (Indevus) Histrelin acetate 50 mg. Implant, Subcutaneous. In carton with implantation kit. *Rx.*
Use: Hormone, gonadotropin-releasing hormone analog.

Suppress. (Ferndale) Dextromethorphan HBr 7.5 mg. Loz. 1000s. *OTC.*
Use: Antitussive.

Supra Min. (Towne) Vitamins A 10,000 units, D 400 units, E 30 units, C 250 mg, folic acid 0.4 mg, B_1 10 mg, B_2 10 mg, niacin 100 mg, B_6 5 mg, B_{12} 6 mcg, pantothenic acid 20 mg, I 150 mcg, Fe 100 mg, Mg 2 mg, Cu 20 mg, Mn 1.25 mg. Tab. Bot. 130s. *OTC.*
Use: Mineral, vitamin supplement.

Suprane. (Baxter) Desflurane. 240 mL. Volatile Liq. Bot. *Rx.*
Use: Anesthetic, general.

Suprarenal. Dried, partially defatted and powdered adrenal gland of cattle, sheep, or swine.

Suprax. (Lupin Pharma) Cefixime 100 mg/5 mL, 200 mg/5 mL. Sucrose. Strawberry flavored. Pow. for Oral Susp. 25 mL (200 mg/5 mL only), 37.5 mL (200 mg/5 mL), 50 mL, 75 mL, 100 mL. *Rx.*
Use: Anti-infective, cephalosporin.

Suprazine. (Major) Trifluoperazine 1 mg, 2 mg, 5 mg, 10 mg. Tab. Bot. 100s, 250s, 1000s, UD 100s (2 mg only). *Rx.*
Use: Anxiolytic.

Suprep Bowel Prep. (Braintree Labs) Sodium sulfate 17.5 g, potassium sulfate 3.13 g, magnesium sulfate 1.6 g per 180 mL. Sodium benzoate, sucralose. Soln. Kit w/2s and mixing container. *Rx.*
Use: Laxative, miscellaneous bowel evacuant.

Suprins. (Towne) Vitamins A palmitate 10,000 units, D 400 units, B_1 10 mg, B_2 10 mg, B_6 5 mg, B_{12} 6 mcg, C 250 mg, calcium pantothenate 20 mg, niacinamide 100 mg, biotin 25 mcg, E 15 units, Ca 103 mg, P 80 mg, Fe 10 mg, I 0.1 mg, Cu 1.0 mg, Zn 20 mg, Mn 1.25 mg. Captab. Bot. 100s. *OTC.*
Use: Mineral, vitamin supplement.

•**suproclone.** (SUH-pro-klone) USAN.
Use: Sedative; hypnotic.

•**suprofen.** (sue-PRO-fen) *USP 34.*
Use: Anti-inflammatory.

•**suramin hexasodium.** (SOOR-ah-min hex-ah-SOE-dee-um) USAN.
Use: Antineoplastic.

Surbex Filmtab. (Abbott) Vitamins B_1 6 mg, B_2 6 mg, B_3 30 mg, B_6 2.5 mg, B_5 10 mg, B_{12} 5 mcg. Filmtab. Bot. 100s. *OTC.*
Use: Mineral, vitamin supplement.

Surbex 750 with Iron. (Abbott) Vitamins B_1 15 mg, B_2 15 mg, B_6 25 mg, B_{12} 12 mcg, C 750 mg, B_5 20 mg, E 30 units, B_3 100 mg, Fe 27 mg, folic acid 0.4 mg. Tab. Bot. 50s. *OTC.*
Use: Mineral, vitamin supplement.

Surbex 750 with Zinc. (Abbott) B_1 15 mg, B_2 15 mg, B_6 20 mg, B_{12} 12 mcg, C 750 mg, E 30 units, B_5 20 mg, niacin 100 mg, folic acid 0.4 mg, Zn 22.5 mg. Tab. Bot. 50s. *OTC*.
Use: Mineral, vitamin supplement.

Surbex-T Filmtab. (Abbott) Vitamins B_1 15 mg, B_2 10 mg, B_3 100 mg, B_6 5 mg, B_{12} 10 mcg, B_5 20 mg, C 500 mg. Filmtab. Bot. 100s. *OTC*.
Use: Mineral, vitamin supplement.

Surbex with C Filmtabs. (Abbott) Vitamins B_1 6 mg, B_2 6 mg, B_3 30 mg, B_5 10 mg, B_6 2.5 mg, B_{12} 5 mg, C 500 mg. Film-coated. Tab. Bot. 100s. *OTC*.
Use: Vitamin supplement.

Surbu-Gen-T. (Ivax) Vitamins B_1 15 mg, B_2 10 mg, B_3 100 mg, B_5 20 mg, B_6 5 mg, B_{12} 10 mcg, C 500 mg. Tab. Bot. 100s. *OTC*.
Use: Vitamin supplement.

SureCell HCG-Urine Test. (Kodak Dental) Polyclonal/monoclonal antibody sandwich-based ELISA to detect human chorionic gonadotropin in urine. Kit 10s, 25s, 100s.
Use: Diagnostic aid.

SureCell Herpes (HSV) Test. (Kodak Dental) Monoclonal antibody-based ELISA to detect HSV 1 & 2 antigens from lesions. Kit 10s, 25s.
Use: Diagnostic aid.

SureCell Strep A Test. (Kodak Dental) ELISA to detect group A streptococci. Kit 10s, 25s, 100s.
Use: Diagnostic aid.

SureLac. (Caraco) 3000 FCC lactase units, sorbitol, mannitol. Chew. Tab. Bot. 60s. *OTC*.
Use: Nutritional supplement.

surface active extract of saline lavage of bovine lungs.
Use: Respiratory failure in preterm infants. [Orphan Drug]

surfactant, natural lung.
Use: Surfactant replacement therapy in neonatal respiratory distress syndrome. *See:* Survanta.

surfactant, synthetic lung.
Use: Surfactant replacement therapy in neonatal respiratory distress syndrome.

Surfak. (Pharmacia) Docusate calcium. 240 mg, sorbitol, parabens. Soft Gel Cap. Bot. 10s, 30s, 100s, 500s, UD 100s. *OTC*.
Use: Laxative.

Surfak Stool Softener. (Chattem) Docusate calcium 240 mg. Corn oil, glycerin, propylene glycol, sorbitol. Cap., soft gel. 10s. *OTC*.

Use: Laxative, fecal softener/surfactant.

•**surfilcon A.** (SER-FILL-kahn A) USAN.
Use: Hydrophilic contact lens material.

Surfol Post-Immersion Bath Oil. (Stiefel) Mineral oil, isopropyl myristate, isostearic acid, PEG-40, sorbitan peroleate. Bot. 8 oz. *OTC*.
Use: Dermatologic.

•**surfomer.** (SER-foe-mer) USAN.
Use: Hypolipidemic.

Surgasoap. (Wade) Castile vegetable oils. Bot. Qt., gal. *OTC*.
Use: Dermatologic, cleanser.

Surgel. (Ulmer Pharmacal) Propylene glycol, glycerin. Gel. Bot. 120 mL, 240 mL, gal. *OTC*.
Use: Lubricant.

Surgel Liquid. (Ulmer Pharmacal) Patient lubricant fluid. Bot. 4 oz, 8 oz, gal.
Use: Lubricant.

•**surgibone.** (SER-jih-bone) USAN. Bone and cartilage obtained from bovine embryos and young calves.
Use: Prosthetic aid (internal bone splint).

Surgical Simplex P. (Howmedica) Methyl methacrylate 20 mL poly 6.7 g, methyl methacrylate-styrene copolymer 33.3 g. **Pow.:** 40 g. **Liq.:** 20 mL. Bot.
Use: Bone cement.

Surgical Simplex P Radiopaque. (Howmedica) Methyl methacrylate 20 mL, poly 6 g, methyl methacrylate-styrene copolymer 30 g. **Pow.:** 40 g. **Liq.:** 20 mL. Bot.
Use: Bone cement.

Surgicel. (Johnson & Johnson) Sterile absorbable knitted fabric prepared by controlled oxidation of regenerated cellulose. Sterile strips 2×14, 4×8, 2×3, 0.5×2 inches. Surgical Nu-knit: 1×1, 3×4, 6×9 inches. Box 1s. *Rx*.
Use: Hemostatic.

Surgidine. (Continental Consumer Products) Iodine 0.8% in iodine complex. Germicide. Bot. 8 oz, gal. Foot operated dispenser 8 oz, gal. *OTC*.
Use: Antiseptic.

Surgi-Kleen. (Sween) Bot. 2 oz, 8 oz, 16 oz, 21 oz, gal, 5 gal, 30 gal, 55 gal.
Use: Dermatologic, cleanser.

Surgilube. (E. Fougera) Sterile surgical lubricant. Foilpac 3 g, 5 g. Tube 5 g, 2 oz, 4.25 oz.
Use: Lubricant.

Surgilube. (Savage) Chlorhexidine gluconate. Jelly; vaginal. 5 g, 120.49 g. *OTC*.

Use: Miscellaneous vaginal preparation.

•**suricainide maleate.** (ser-ih-CANE-ide) USAN.
Use: Cardiovascular agent (antiarrhythmic).

•**suritozole.** (suh-RIH-tah-ZOLE) USAN.
Use: Antidepressant.

Surmontil. (Barr/Duramed) Trimipramine maleate 25 mg, 50 mg, 100 mg. Lactose. Cap. Bot. 100s, UD 100s (50 mg only). *Rx.*
Use: Antidepressant.

surofene. Hexachlorophene.

•**suronacrine maleate.** (SUE-row-NAH-kreen) USAN.
Use: Cholinergic; cholinesterase inhibitor.

Surpass. (Wrigley) Calcium carbonate 300 mg (elemental calcium 120 mg). Aspartame, sorbitol, phenylalanine 3.9 mg. Wintergreen flavor. Gum. Box. 10s. *OTC.*
Use: Mineral supplement; antacid.

Surpass Extra Strength. (Wrigley) Calcium carbonate 450 mg (elemental calcium 180 mg). Aspartame, sorbitol, phenylalanine 3.9 mg. Fruit flavor. Gum. Box. 10s. *OTC.*
Use: Mineral supplement; antacid.

Survanta. (Ross Labs) Beractant 25 mg/mL, sodium chloride solution 0.9%, triglycerides 0.5 to 1.75 mg, free fatty acids 1.4 to 3.5 mg, protein < 1 mg/mL. Susp. Single-use vial containing 8 mL suspension. *Rx.*
Use: Lung surfactant.

Suspen. (Circle) Penicillin V potassium 250 mg/5 mL. Bot. 100 mL. *Rx.*
Use: Anti-infective, penicillin.

•**suspension structured vehicle.** *NF 29.*
Use: Pharmaceutical vehicle.

Sustacal Basic. (Bristol-Myers Squibb) A vanilla, strawberry, or chocolate flavored liquid containing 36.6 g protein, 34.6 g fat, 145.8 g carbohydrate, 833 mg Na, 1583 mg K/L. 1.04 Cal/mL, with appropriate vitamin and mineral levels to meet 100% of the US RDAs. Liq. Can 240 mL. *OTC.*
Use: Nutritional supplement.

Sustacal HC. (Bristol-Myers Squibb) High calorie nutritionally complete food. Protein 16%, fat 34%, carbohydrate 50%. Can 8 oz. Vanilla, chocolate, or eggnog. *OTC.*
Use: Nutritional supplement.

Sustacal Plus. (Bristol-Myers Squibb) A vanilla, eggnog, or chocolate flavored liquid containing 61 g protein, 58 g fat,

190 g carbohydrate, 15.2 mg Fe, 850 mg Na, 1480 mg K, 1520 cal/L, with appropriate vitamin and mineral levels to meet 100% of the US RDAs. Liq. Bot. 237 mL, 960 mL. *OTC.*
Use: Nutritional supplement.

Sustacal Powder. (Bristol-Myers Squibb) Caloric distribution and nutritional value when added to milk are similar to that of Sustacal liquid except lactose. Contains vanilla: Pow. 1.9 oz. packets 4s, 1 lb. can; Chocolate 1.9 oz. packets 4s. *OTC.*
Use: Nutritional supplement.

Sustacal Pudding. (Bristol-Myers Squibb) Ready-to-eat fortified pudding containing at least 15% of the US RDAs for protein, vitamins and minerals, in a 240 calorie serving. As a % of the calories, protein 11%, fat 36%, carbohydrate 53%. Flavors: Chocolate, vanilla, and butterscotch. Tins, 5 oz, 110 oz. *OTC.*
Use: Nutritional supplement.

Sustagen. (Bristol-Myers Squibb) High-calorie, high-protein supplement containing as a % of the calories, 24% protein, 8% fat, 68% carbohydrate. Contains all known essential vitamins and minerals. Prepared from nonfat milk, corn syrup solids, powdered whole milk, calcium caseinate, and dextrose. Vanilla: Can 1 lb, 5 lb. Chocolate: Can 1 lb. *OTC.*
Use: Nutritional supplement.

Sustain. (Zee Medical) Sodium chloride 220 mg, calcium carbonate 18 mg, potassium chloride 15 mg. Tab. 24s. *Rx.*
Use: Salt replacement.

Sustiva. (Bristol-Myers Squibb) Efavirenz. **Cap:** 50 mg, 200 mg. Lactose. Bot. 30s (50 mg), 90s (200 mg). **Tab:** 600 mg. Lactose. Bot. 30s. *Rx.*
Use: Antiretroviral, non-nucleoside reverse transcriptase inhibitor.

Sutent. (Pfizer) Sunitinib malate (as base) 12.5 mg, 25 mg, 50 mg. Cap. 30s. *Rx.*
Use: Protein-tyrosine kinase inhibitor.

•**suture, absorbable surgical.** (SOO-chur) *USP 34.*
Use: Surgical aid.

•**suture, nonabsorbable surgical.** (SOO-chur) *USP 34.*
Use: Surgical aid.

Suvaplex. (Tennessee Pharmaceutic) Vitamins A 5000 units, D 500 units, B_1 2.5 mg, B_2 2.5 mg, B_6 0.5 mg, B_{12} 1 mcg, C 37.5 mg, Ca pantothenate 5 mg, niacinamide 20 mg, folic acid

0.1 mg. Tab. Bot. 100s. *OTC.*
Use: Mineral, vitamin supplement.

•**suvorexant.** (SOO-voe-REX-ant) USAN.
Use: CNS agent.

•**suxemerid sulfate.** (sux-EM-er-rid)
USAN.
Use: Antitussive.

swamp root. Compound of various organic roots in an alcohol base.
Use: Diuretic to the kidney.

Sween-A-Peel. (Sween) Wafer 4 × 4.
Box 5s, 20s; Sheets 1212. Box 2s,
12s. *OTC.*
Use: Dermatologic, protectant.

Sween Cream. (Coloplast) Beeswax, cetyl alcohol, cod liver oil (vitamins A and D), lanolin oil, stearyl alcohol. Cream.
340 g. *OTC.*
Use: Emollient.

Sween Kind Lotion. (Sween) Bot. 21 oz,
gal. *OTC.*
Use: Dermatologic, cleanser.

Sween Prep. (Sween) Box wipes 54s.
Dab-o-matic 2 oz. Spray Top 4 oz. *OTC.*
Use: Dermatologic, protectant, medicated.

Sween Soft Touch. (Sween) Bot. 2 oz,
16 oz, 21 oz, 32 oz, 1 gal., 5 gal. *OTC.*
Use: Dermatologic, protectant, medicated.

Sweeta. (Bristol-Myers Squibb) Saccharin sodium, sorbitol. Bot. 24 mL, 2 oz,
4 oz. *OTC.*
Use: Sweetening agent.

Sweetaste. (Purepac) Saccharin 0.25 g,
0.5 g, 1 g. Tab. w/Sodium bicarbonate.
Bot. 1000s. *OTC.*
Use: Sugar substitute.

sweetening agents.
See: Saccharin.
Sweetaste.

Swiss Kriss. (Modern Aids Inc.) Senna leaves, herbs. Coarse cut mixture. Can
1.5 oz, 3.25 oz, Tab. 24s, 120s, 250s.
OTC.
Use: Laxative.

Syllact. (Wallace) Psyllium seed husks
3.3 g, 14 cal/rounded tsp, dextrose,
parabens, fruit flavor, saccharin. Pow.
Bot. 284 g. *OTC.*
Use: Laxative.

Symax Duotab. (Capellon) L-hyoscyamine sulfate 0.375 mg (0.125 mg immediate release, 0.25 mg extended release). ER Tab. 90s. *Rx.*
Use: Gastrointestinal anticholinergic/
antispasmodic.

Symax FasTab. (Capellon) Hyoscyamine sulfate 0.125 mg. Lactose, mannitol.
Peppermint flavor. Orally Disintegrating
Tab. 100s. *Rx.*

Use: Gastrointestinal anticholinergic/
antispasmodic.

Symax-SL. (Capellon) L-hyoscyamine
sulfate 0.125 mg. Sublingual Tab. Bot.
100s. *Rx.*
Use: Anticholinergic, antispasmodic,
belladonna alkaloid.

Symax-SR. (Capellon) L-hyoscyamine
sulfate 0.375 mg. SR Tab. Bot. 100s.
Rx.
Use: Anticholinergic, antispasmodic,
belladonna alkaloid.

Symbicort. (AstraZeneca) Budesonide/
formoterol 80 mcg/4.5 mcg, 160 mcg/
4.5 mcg per actuation. Formoterol
3.7 mcg as the free base, equiv. to formoterol fumarate dihydrate 4.5 mcg.
Inh. Aerosol. Canisters 6 g (60 actuations) (160 mcg/4.5 mcg) 6.9 g (60 actuations) (80 mcg/4.5 mcg), 10.2 g
(120 actuations) with actuator. *Rx.*
Use: Respiratory agent.

Symbyax. (Eli Lilly) Olanzapine/fluoxetine hydrochloride 3 mg/25 mg, 6 mg/
25 mg, 6 mg/50 mg, 12 mg/25 mg,
12 mg/50 mg. Cap. 30s; 100s, 1000s,
blister UD 100s (except 3 mg/25 mg).
Rx.
Use: Psychotherapeutic agent.

•**symclosene.** (SIM-kloe-seen) USAN.
Use: Anti-infective, topical.

•**symetine hydrochloride.** (SIM-eh-teen)
USAN.
Use: Antiamebic.

Symlin. (Amylin Pharmaceuticals, Inc.)
Pramlintide acetate 0.6 mg/mL, 1 mg/
mL. Soln. for Inj. Vials. 5 mL (0.6 mg/mL
only). Multidose pen injectors (1 mg/
mL only). 1.5 mL, 2.7 mL. *Rx.*
Use: Antidiabetic agent, amylin analog.

Symmetrel. (Endo) Amantadine hydrochloride. **Tab:** 100 mg. Bot. 100s,
500s. **Syrup:** 50 mg/5 mL. Sorbitol,
parabens. Bot. 480 mL. *Rx.*
Use: Antiviral; antiparkinsonian; treatment of drug-induced extrapyramidal symptoms.

SymPak. (Dexo) Tab. **Day (Sinuvent
PE):** Guaifenesin 600 mg, phenylephrine hydrochloride 15 mg. Carton
w/blister card of 14-day dosing regimen.
Night (Omnihist II LA): Chlorpheniramine maleate 8 mg, methscopolamine
nitrate 2.5 mg, phenylephrine hydrochloride 25 mg. Carton w/blister card of
14-day dosing regimen. *Rx.*
Use: Upper respiratory combination; decongestant, antihistamine, and expectorant combination.

SymPak PDX. (Dexo) Tab. **Day (Ah-
Chew Ultra):** Chlorpheniramine

maleate 2 mg (as chlorpheniramine tannate), methscopolamine nitrate 1.5 mg, phenylephrine hydrochloride 10 mg (as phenylephrine tannate). Saccharin, sugar. Blister card for 14-day dosing regimen. 2s. **Night (Dexodryl):** Chlorpheniramine maleate 2 mg (as chlorpheniramine tannate), methscopolamine nitrate 1.5 mg. Saccharin, sugar. Blister card for 14-day dosing regimen. 2s. *Rx.*
Use: Upper respiratory combination; decongestant, antihistamine, and anticholinergic combination.

SymPak II. (Dexo) Tab. **Day (Sinuhist):** Brompheniramine maleate 6 mg, pseudoephedrine hydrochloride 45 mg. Blister card for 14-day dosing regimen. 2s. **Night (Omnihist II LA):** Chlorpheniramine maleate 8 mg, methscopolamine nitrate 2.5 mg, phenylephrine hydrochloride 25 mg. Blister card for 14-day dosing regimen. 2s. *Rx.*
Use: Upper respiratory combination; decongestant, antihistamine, and anticholinergic combination.

sympatholytic agents.
See: Antiadrenergics/sympatholytics.

sympathomimetic agents.
See: Albuterol.
Arfomoterol Tartrate.
Bitolterol Mesylate.
Ephedrine Sulfate.
Epinephrine.
Formoterol Fumarate.
Isoetharine Hydrochloride.
Isoproterenol Hydrochloride.
Levalbuterol Hydrochloride.
Metaproterenol Sulfate.
Pirbuterol Acetate.
Salmeterol Xinafoate.
Terbutaline Sulfate.

Syna-Clear. (Pruvo) Decongestant plus Vitamin C. 25 mg. Tab. Bot. 12s, 30s.
Use: Decongestant.

Synacort. (Roche) Hydrocortisone cream. **1%:** Tube 15 g, 30 g, 60 g. **2.5%:** Tube 30 g. *Rx.*
Use: Corticosteroid, topical.

Synagis. (MedImmune) Palivizumab 100 mg/mL. Preservative free. Inj., Soln. Single-dose vial. 0.5 mL (w/histidine 1.9 mg, glycine 0.06 mg/mL), 1 mL (histidine 3.9 mg, glycine 0.1mg/mL). *Rx.*
Use: Monoclonal antibody.

Synalgos-DC. (Leitner) Dihydrocodeine bitartrate 16 mg, aspirin 356.4 mg, caffeine 30 mg. Cap. Bot. 100s, 500s. *c-III.*
Use: Analgesic combination; narcotic.

Synarel. (Pfizer) Nafarelin acetate 2 mg/mL (as nafarelin base). Nasal solution. Bot. 10 mL with metered pump spray. *Rx.*
Use: Endometriosis.

SynBiotics-3. (NutraCea) *Bifidobacterium longum* 4.5 billion CFU, *Lactobacillus rhamnosus* A, *L. plantarum, Saccharomyces boulardii.* Maltodextrin. Cap. 60s, UD 200s. *OTC.*
Use: Nutritional supplement.

Syncaine.
See: Procaine Hydrochloride.

Syncort.
See: Desoxycorticosterone Acetate.

Syncortyl.
See: Desoxycorticosterone Acetate.

Synemol. (Roche) Fluocinolone acetonide 0.025% in water-washable aqueous emollient base. Tube 15 g, 30 g, 60 g, 120 g. *Rx.*
Use: Corticosteroid, topical.

Synera. (Ferndale Labs) Lidocaine 70 mg, tetracaine 70 mg. Polyvinyl alcohol, parabens, sorbitan monopalmitate. Patch. 2s, 10s. *Rx.*
Use: Topical local anesthetic.

Synercid. (Monarch) Quinupristin 150 mg, dalfopristin 350 mg/10 mL. Inj. lyophilized. Vial 10 mL. *Rx.*
Use: Streptogramin.

Synophylate. (Schwarz Pharma) Theophylline sodium glycinate. **Elix.:** Theophylline 165 mg/15 mL w/alcohol 20%. Bot. Pt, gal. **Tab.:** Theophylline 165 mg. Tab. Bot. 100s, 1000s. *Rx.*
Use: Bronchodilator.

Syn-Rx. (Medeva) **AM:** Pseudoephedrine hydrochloride 60 mg, guaifenesin 600 mg. CR Tab. Bot. 28s. **PM:** Guaifenesin 600 mg. CR Tab. Bot. 28s. In 14-day treatment regimen of 56 tablets. *Rx.*
Use: Upper respiratory combination, decongestant, expectorant.

Synsorb Pk.
Use: Verocytotoxogenic *E. coli* infections. [Orphan Drug]

Synthaloids. (Buffington) Benzocaine, calcium-iodine complex. Loz. Salt free. Bot. 100s, 1000s. Unit boxes 8s, 16s. Box 24s. *Dispens-a-Kit* 500s. *Aidpaks* 100s. *Medipaks* 200s. *OTC.*
Use: Sore throat relief.

synthetic conjugated estrogens, A.
Use: Estrogen.
See: Cenestin.

•**synthetic conjugated estrogens, B.** (ES-troe-jens) USAN.
Use: Hormone replacement therapy, estrogen therapy.

synthetic lung surfactant.
See: Exosurf Neonatal.
synthoestrin.
See: Diethylstilbestrol Dipropionate.
Synthroid. (Abbott) Sodium levothyrox-ine 0.025 mg, 0.05 mg, 0.075 mg, 0.088 mg, 0.1 mg, 0.112 mg, 0.125 mg, 0.137 mg, 0.15 mg, 0.175 mg, 0.2 mg, 0.3 mg. Lactose, sugar. Tab. Bot. 100s, 1000s, UD 100s (0.05 mg, 0.075 mg, 0.1 mg, 0.125 mg, 0.15 mg, 0.2 mg). *Rx.*
Use: Hormone, thyroid.
Synthroid Injection. (Abbott) Lyophilized sodium levothyroxine 200 mcg, 500 mcg. Vial. 10 mL (100 mcg/mL when reconstituted.) *Rx.*
Use: Hormone, thyroid.
Synvisc. (Genzyme) Hylan polymers 8 mg/mL. Inj. Prefilled syringe. 2 mL. *Rx.*
Use: Physical adjunct.
Synvisc-One. (Genzyme) Hylan poly-mers 8 mg/mL. Sodium chloride 8.5 mg/ mL. Inj. Prefilled syringe. 6 mL. *Rx.*
Use: Physical adjunct.
Syphilis (FTA-ABS) Fluoro Kit. (Clinical Sciences)
Use: Test for syphilis.
Syprine. (Aton Pharma) Trientine hydro-chloride 250 mg. Cap. Bot. 100s. *Rx.*
Use: Chelating agent.
Syracol CF. (Roberts) Dextromethorphan HBr 15 mg, guaifenesin 200 mg. Tab.

Bot. 500s. *OTC.*
Use: Antitussive; expectorant.
Syroxine. (Major) Sodium levothyroxine 0.1 mg, 0.2 mg, 0.3 mg. Tab. Bot. 100s, 250s, 1000s, UD 100s. (3 mg 1000s). *Rx.*
Use: Hormone, thyroid.
Syrpalta. (Emerson) Syr. containing comb. of fruit flavors. Bot. Pt, gal. *OTC.*
Use: Pharmaceutical aid.
•**syrup.** (SIR-up) *NF 29.*
Use: Pharmaceutic aid (flavor).
Syrvite. (Various Mfr.) Vitamins A 2500 units, D 400 units, E 15 mg, B_1 1.05 mg, B_2 1.2 mg, B_3 13.5 mg, B_6 1.05 mg, B_{12} 4.5 mcg, C 60 mg/5 mL Liq. Bot. 480 mL. *OTC.*
Use: Vitamin supplement.
Systane. (Alcon) PEG-400 0.4%, propyl-ene glycol 0.3%. Soln., Ophth. 20 mL. *OTC.*
Use: Artificial tear solution.
Systane Balance. (J & J Healthcare) Propylene glycol 0.6%, boric acid, edetate disodium, mineral oil, polyquaternium-1 0.001%. Soln., Ophth. 10 mL. *OTC.*
Use: Artificial tears.
Systane Nighttime. (Alcon) Mineral oil 3%, white petrolatum 94%. Lanolin. Preservative free. Oint., Ophth. 3.5 g. *OTC.*
Use: Ocular lubricant.

T

TA. (C & M Pharmacal) Triamcinolone acetonide 0.025%, 0.05%. Cream. Jar 2 oz, 8 oz, 1 lb. *Rx.*
Use: Corticosteroid, topical.

TA. (Wampole) Antithyroid antibodies by IFA. Test 48s.
Use: Diagnostic aid, thyroid.

•**tabalumab.** (ta-BAL-ue-mab) USAN.
Use: Autoimmune diseases and B cell malignancies.

Tabasyn. (Freeport) Chlorpheniramine maleate 2 mg, phenylephrine hydrochloride 10 mg, acetaminophen 5 g, salicylamide 5 g. Tab. Bot. 1000s. *Rx.*
Use: Analgesic, antihistamine, decongestant.

Tab-A-Vite. (Major) Vitamins A 5000 units, D 400 units, E 30 units, B_1 1.5 mg, B_2 1.7 mg, B_3 20 mg, B_5 10 mg, B_6 2 mg, B_{12} 6 mcg, C 60 mg, FA 0.4 mg. Tab. Bot. 30s, 100s, 250s, 1000s, UD 100s. *OTC.*
Use: Mineral, vitamin supplement.

Tab-A-Vite Maximum. (Major) Vitamins A 2,500 units, D 400 units, E 30 units, B_1 1.5 mg, B_2 1.7 mg, B_3 20 mg, B_5 10 mg, B_6 2 mg, B_{12} 6 mcg, C 60 mg, K, Fe 18 mg, Ca 162 mg, folate 0.4 mg, B, Cl, Cr, Cu, I, K, Mg, Mn, Mo, Ni, P, Se, Si, Sn, V, Zn, biotin. Lactose free and sugar free. Tab. 60s. *OTC.*
Use: Multivitamin.

Tab-A-Vite + Iron. (Major) Fe 18 mg, vitamins A 5000 units, D 400 units, E 30 units, B_1 1.5 mg, B_2 1.7 mg, B_3 20 mg, B_5 10 mg, B_6 2 mg, B_{12} 6 mcg, C 60 mg, FA 0.4 mg, tartrazine. Tab. Bot. 100s. *OTC.*
Use: Mineral, vitamin supplement.

Tab-A-Vite Women's. (Major) Vitamins A 2,500 units, D 400 units, E 30 units, B_1 15 mg, B_2 1.7 mg, B_3 10 mg, B_5 5 mg, B_6 2 mg, B_{12} 6 mcg, C 60 mg, Fe 18 mg, Ca 450 mg, folate 0.4 mg, Mg, Zn. Mannitol. Lactose free, preservative free, and sugar free. Tab. 60s. *OTC.*
Use: Multivitamin.

Tabloid. (GlaxoSmithKline) Thioguanine 40 mg. Lactose. Tab. 25s. *Rx.*
Use: Antineoplastic.

Tacaryl. (Bristol-Myers Squibb) Methdilazine 3.6 mg. Chew. Tab. Bot. 100s. *Rx.*
Use: Antipruritic.

•**tacedinaline.** (ta-see-DYE-na-leen) USAN.
Use: Cancer agent.

TachoSil. (Baxter) Fibrinogen/thrombin (fibrinogen sealant, human) 337.4 mg/

123.1 units (9.5 cm × 4.8 cm), 170.5 mg/62.2 units (4.8 cm × 4.8 cm), 55.5 mg/20.3 units (3 cm × 2.5 cm). Patch (each fibrin sealant patch contains per cm^2: human fibrinogen range, 3.6 to 7.4 mg (5.5 mg); human thrombin range, 1.3 to 2.7 units (2 units); equine collagen and human albumin. 1s (except 170.5 mg/62.2 units), 2s (170.5 mg/62.2 units only), 5s (55.5 mg/20.3 units only). *Rx.*
Use: Topical hemostatic.

tachysterol.
See: Dihydrotachysterol.

Tacitin. (Novartis) Under study. Benzoctamine, B.A.N.

•**taclamine hydrochloride.** (TACK-lahmeen) USAN.
Use: Anxiolytic.

Taclonex. (Leo Pharma) Calcipotriene 0.005%, betamethasone dipropionate 0.064%. Mineral oil, white petrolatum. Oint. 60 g, 100 g. *Rx.*
Use: Antipsoriatic agent.

Taclonex Scalp. (Leo Pharma) Calcipotriene hydrate 0.005%, betamethasone dipropionate 0.064%. Castor oil, mineral oil. Susp. 15 g, 30 g, 60 g. *Rx.*
Use: Antipsoriatic agent.

•**tacrine hydrochloride.** (TACK-reen) USAN.
Use: Cognition adjuvant.
See: Cognex.

•**tacrolimus.** (tak-ROE-li-mus) USAN.
Use: Immunomodulator, topical; immunologic agent; immunosuppressive.
See: Prograf.
Protopic.

tacrolimus. (Sandoz) Tacrolimus 0.5 mg, 1 mg, 5 mg. Lactose. Cap. 100s. *Rx.*
Use: Immunologic agent, immunosuppressive.

Tac-3. (Allergan) Triamcinolone acetonide 3 mg/mL. Susp. Vial 5 mL. *Rx.*
Use: Corticosteroid.

•**tadalafil.** (tah-DA-la-fil) USAN.
Use: Erectile dysfunction.
See: AdCirca.
Cialis.

•**tafamidis.** (TA-fam-id-is) USAN.
Use: Transthyretin-associated amyloidosis.

•**tafamidis meglumine.** (TA-fam-id-is) USAN.
Use: Transthyretin-associated amyloidosis.

•**tafluprost.** (TA-floo-prost) USAN.
Use: Ophthalmic agent.

Tagamet. (GlaxoSmithKline) Cimetidine. Tab. **400 mg:** Bot. 60s. **800 mg:** Bot.

30s. *Rx.*
Use: Histamine H$_2$ antagonist.
Tagamet HB 200. (GlaxoSmithKline Consumer) Cimetidine 200 mg. Tab. Bot. 6s, 30s, 50s. *OTC.*
Use: Histamine H$_2$ antagonist.
•**talabostat.** (tal-AB-oh-stat) USAN.
Use: Antineoplastic.
•**talabostat mesylate.** (tal-AB-oh-stat) USAN.
Use: Antineoplastic.
Talacen Caplets. (Sanofi-Synthelabo) Pentazocine hydrochloride 25 mg, acetaminophen 650 mg. Tab. Bot. 100s. UD 250s. (10 × 25s). *c-iv.*
Use: Analgesic combination, narcotic.
•**talactoferrin alfa.** (ta-LAK-toe-FER-in) USAN.
Use: Anti-infective.
•**talampicillin hydrochloride.** (TAL-AM-pih-sill-in) USAN.
Use: Anti-infective.
•**talaporfin sodium.** (tal-a-PORE-fin) USAN.
Use: Photosensitizer.
•**talc.** (talk) *USP 34.* A native hydrous magnesium silicate.
Use: Dusting powder, pharmaceutic aid (tablet/capsule lubricant).
W/Zinc Oxide.
See: Caldesene.
talc powder, sterile.
Use: Antineoplastic.
See: Sclerosol.
•**taleranol.** (TAL-ehr-ah-nole) USAN.
Use: Enzyme inhibitor (gonadotropin).
•**taliglucerase alfa.** (TAL-i-GLOO-ser-ase AL-fa) USAN.
Use: Gaucher disease.
•**talimogene laherparepvec.** (tal-IM-oh-jeen la-HER-pa-REP-vek) USAN.
Use: Antineoplastic.
•**talisomycin.** (TAL-i-soe-MYE-sin) USAN.
Formerly Tallysomycin A.
Use: Antineoplastic.
•**talizumab.** (tal-IZ-ue-mab) USAN.
Use: Anaphylaxis.
•**talmetacin.** (TAL-MET-ah-sin) USAN.
Use: Analgesic, antipyretic, anti-inflammatory.
•**talniflumate.** (tal-NYE-FLEW-mate) USAN.
Use: Anti-inflammatory, analgesic.
•**talopram hydrochloride.** (TAY-low-pram) USAN.
Use: Potentiator (catecholamine).
•**talosalate.** (TAL-oh-SAL-ate) USAN.
Use: Analgesic, anti-inflammatory.

•**talotrexin ammonium.** (tal-oh-TREX-in) USAN.
Use: Antineoplastic.
•**talsaclidine fumarate.** (tale-SACK-lih-deen) USAN.
Use: Alzheimer disease treatment (muscarinic M$_1$-agonist).
•**taltobulin.** (tal-toe-BUE-lin) USAN.
Use: Antineoplastic.
Talwin. (Abbott Hospital Products) Pentazocine lactate 30 mg/mL. Inj. **Vials:** With acetone sodium bisulfite 2 mg and methylparaben 1 mg/mL. 10 mL. **Uni-Amps:** 1 mL. **Uni-Nest amps:** 1 mL. **Carpujects:** With acetone sodium bisulfite 1 mg. 1 mL, 2 mL. *c-iv.*
Use: Narcotic agonist-antagonist analgesic.
Tambocor. (Graceway Pharmaceuticals) Flecainide acetate 50 mg, 100 mg, 150 mg. Tab. Bot. 100s, UD 100s (except 150 mg). *Rx.*
Use: Antiarrhythmic agent.
•**tametraline hydrochloride.** (tah-MET-rah-leen) USAN.
Use: Antidepressant.
Tamiflu. (Genentech) Oseltamivir phosphate. **Cap.:** 30 mg, 45 mg, 75 mg. UD 10s. **Pow. for Oral Susp.:** 12 mg/mL after reconstitution. Sorbitol, saccharin, tutti-frutti flavor. Bot. 25 mL w/bottle adapter and oral dispenser. *Rx.*
Use: Antiviral.
•**tamoxifen citrate.** (ta-MOX-ih-fen) *USP 34.*
Use: Treatment of mammary carcinoma, antiestrogen.
tamoxifen citrate. (Various Mfr.) Tamoxifen citrate (as base) 10 mg, 20 mg. Tab. Bot. 60s, 180s, 500s, 1000s, UD 100s (10 mg only); 30s, 90s, 100s, 500s, 1000s, UD 100s (20 mg only). *Rx.*
Use: Antineoplastic, antiestrogen.
•**tampramine fumarate.** (TAM-prah-MEEN) USAN.
Use: Antidepressant.
Tamp-R-Tel. (Wyeth) A tamper-resistant package for narcotic drugs which includes the following: **Codeine phosphate:** 30 mg, 60 mg/mL. **Hydromorphone hydrochloride:** 1 mg, 2 mg, 3 mg, 4 mg/*Tubex.* **Meperidine hydrochloride:** 25 mg/mL. **Promethazine hydrochloride:** 25 mg/mL, 2 mL. **Meperidine hydrochloride:** 25 mg/mL, 50 mg/mL, 75 mg/mL, 100 mg/mL. **Morphine Sulfate:** 2 mg, 4 mg, 8 mg, 10 mg, 15 mg/mL. **Pentobarbital, Sodium:** 100 mg/2 mL. **Phenobarbital, Sodium:** 30 mg, 60 mg, 130 mg/mL.

Secobarbital, Sodium: 100 mg/2 mL.
•**tamsulosin hydrochloride.** (tam-SOO-loe-sin) USAN.
Use: Benign prostatic hyperplasia therapy; antiadrenergic.
See: Flomax.
W/Dutasteride.
See: Jalyn.
tamsulosin hydrochloride. (Various Mfr.) Tamsulosin hydrochloride 0.4 mg. May contain sugar spheres. Cap. 30s, 100s, 500s, 1,000s, UD 16s, UD 30s. *Rx.*
Use: Antiadrenergic agent, peripherally acting; alpha-1 adrenergic blocker.
Tanabid SR. (Portal Pharmaceutical) Brompheniramine maleate 6 mg, phenylephrine hydrochloride 30 mg. Tab. 100s. *Rx.*
Use: Upper respiratory combination, decongestant and antihistamine.
Tanac Gel. (Del) Dyclonine hydrochloride 1%, allantoin 0.5%, petrolatum, lanolin. Tube 9.45 mL. *OTC.*
Use: Cold sores, fever blisters, moisturizer.
Tanac Liquid. (Del) Benzalkonium chloride 0.12%, benzocaine 10%, tannic acid 6%. Saccharin. Bot. 13 mL. *OTC.*
Use: Mouth and throat preparation.
TanaCof-DM. (Larken) Dextromethorphan tannate 25 mg, dexchlorpheniramine tannate 2.5 mg, pseudoephedrine tannate 75 mg per 5 mL. Parabens, aspartame, phenylalanine. Cotton candy flavor. Susp. 118 mL, 473 mL. *Rx.*
Use: Antitussive combination.
Tanac Stick. (Del) Benzocaine 7.5%, tannic acid 6%, octyl dimethyl PABA 0.75%, allantoin 0.2%, benzalkonium chloride. 7.5%. Saccharin. Stick 0.1 oz. *OTC.*
Use: Cold sores, fever blisters, moisturizer.
Tanadex. (Del) Tannic acid 2.86%, phenol 1.05%, benzocaine 0.47%. Liq. Bot. 3 oz. *OTC.*
Use: Throat preparation.
Tan-a-Dyne. (Archer-Taylor) Tannic acid compound w/iodine. Liq. Bot. 4 oz., pt., gal. *OTC.*
Use: Gargle.
Tanafed DMX. (First Horizon) Dextromethorphan tannate 25 mg, dexchlorpheniramine tannate 2.5 mg, pseudoephedrine tannate 75 mg per 5 mL. Methylparaben, saccharin, sucrose, cotton candy flavor. Susp. 20 mL, 118 mL, 473 mL. *Rx.*
Use: Antitussive combination.

Tanafed DP. (First Horizon) Pseudoephedrine tannate 75 mg, dexchlorpheniramine tannate 2.5 mg/5 mL, methylparaben, saccharin, sucrose, strawberry-banana flavor. Susp. 20 mL, 118 mL, 473 mL. *Rx.*
Use: Decongestant and antihistamine.
TanaHist-D Pediatric. (Larken Laboratories) Chlorpheniramine tannate 2 mg, phenylephrine tannate 6 mg per mL. Methylparaben, saccharin, sorbitol. Cotton candy flavor. Soln., Conc. 60 mL w/dropper. *Rx.*
Use: Upper respiratory combination, decongestant and antihistamine.
TanaHist PD. (Larken Laboratories) Chlorpheniramine tannate 2 mg/mL.
Susp.: Methylparaben, saccharin, sorbitol. Cotton candy flavor. 60 mL.
Drops: Glycerin, methylparaben, saccharin, sodium benzoate, sorbitol. Cotton Candy flavor. 59 mL w/dropper. *Rx.*
Use: Antihistamine, nonselective alkylamine.
•**tanaproget.** (tan-a-PRO-jet) USAN.
Use: Contraceptive.
Tanavan. (Scientific Laboratories) Phenylephrine tannate 12.5 mg, pyrilamine tannate 30 mg per 5 mL. Grape flavor. Susp. 118 mL, 473 mL. *Rx.*
Use: Decongestant and antihistamine.
tanbismuth.
See: Bismuth Tannate.
•**tandamine hydrochloride.** (TAN-dah-meen) USAN.
Use: Antidepressant.
Tandem. (US Pharmaceutical) Elemental Fe 106 mg (ferrous fumarate 162 mg, polysaccharide iron complex 115.2 mg). Cap. Blister pack 90s. *Rx.*
Use: Dietary supplement.
Tandem DHA. (US Pharmaceutical) Vitamin B_6 25 mg, C 20 mg, folic acid 1 mg, Fe 30 mg, DHA 215.2 mg, EPA 53.46 mg. Cap. 90s. *Rx.*
Use: Multivitamin with iron.
Tandem F. (US Pharmaceutical) Fe 106 mg, folic acid 1 mg. Cap. 90s. *Rx.*
Use: Iron with vitamins.
Tandem OB. (US Pharmaceutical) Vitamin B_1 10 mg, B_2 6 mg, B_3 30 mg, B_5 10 mg, B_6 5 mg, B_{12} 15 mcg, C 200 mg, folic acid 1 mg, Cu 0.8 mg, Fe 106 mg, Mg 6.9 mg, Mn 1.3 mg, Zn 18.2 mg. Cap. 90s. *Rx.*
Use: Multivitamin with iron and other mineral.
Tandem Plus. (US Pharmaceutical) Vitamin B_1 10 mg, B_2 6 mg, B_3 30 mg, B_5 10 mg, B_6 5 mg, B_{12} 15 mcg, C 200 mg, folic acid 1 mg, Cu 0.8 mg, Fe 106 mg,

Mn 1.3 mg, Zn 18.2 mg. Cap. 90s. *Rx.*
Use: Multivitamin with iron and other minerals.

•**tandospirone citrate.** (TAN-doe-SPYE-rone) USAN.
Use: Anxiolytic.

•**tandutinib.** (tan-DOO-ti-nib) USAN.
Use: Cardiovascular agent.

Tannate Pediatric. (Amneal Pharmaceuticals) Chlorpheniramine tannate 4.5 mg, phenylephrine tannate 5 mg per 5 mL. Methylparaben, saccharin, sucrose. Susp. 118 mL, 473 mL. *Rx.*
Use: Upper respiratory combination, antihistamine and decongestant.

Tannate-12D S. (Hi-Tech) Carbetapentane tannate 30 mg, pyrilamine tannate 30 mg, phenylephrine tannate 5 mg per 5 mL. Methylparaben, saccharin, sucrose. Susp. 118 mL. *Rx.*
Use: Upper respiratory combination, antitussive combination.

•**tannic acid.** (TAN-ik) *USP 34.* Gallotannic acid. Glycerite. Tannin.
Use: Astringent.
See: Zilactin Medicated.

Tannic Spray. (Gebauer) Tannic acid 4.5%, chlorobutanol 1.3%, menthol < 1%, benzocaine < 1%, propylene glycol 33%, ethanol 60%. Liq. Bot. 2 oz. 4 oz. *OTC.*
Use: Relief of sunburn and other minor burns.

Tannic-12. (Cypress) Carbetapentane tannate 60 mg, chlorpheniramine tannate 5 mg. Tab. 100s. *Rx.*
Use: Upper respiratory combination, antitussive combination.

Tannic-12 S. (Cypress) Carbetapentane tannate 30 mg, chlorpheniramine tannate 4 mg per 5 mL. Methylparaben, saccharin, sucrose. Strawberry flavor. Susp. 118 mL. *Rx.*
Use: Upper respiratory combination, antitussive combination.

Tannihist-12 D. (Morton Grove) Carbetapentane tannate 30 mg, pyrilamine tannate 30 mg, phenylephrine tannate 5 mg per 5 mL. Methylparaben, saccharin, tartrazine. Strawberry-black current flavor. Susp. 118 mL, 473 mL. *Rx.*
Use: Upper respiratory combination, antitussive combination.

•**tanomastat.** (ta-NOE-ma-stat) USAN.
Use: Osteoarthritis; oncology.

Tanoral. (Pharmed) Phenylephrine tannate 25 mg, chlorpheniramine tannate 8 mg, pyrilamine tannate 25 mg. Tab. Bot. 100s. *Rx.*
Use: Antihistamine, decongestant.

Tapar. (Warner Chilcott) Acetaminophen 325 mg. Tab. Bot. 100s. *OTC.*
Use: Analgesic.

Tapazole. (Monarch) Methimazole 5 mg, 10 mg. Tab. Bot. 100s. *Rx.*
Use: Hyperthyroidism.

•**tape, adhesive.** (tape) *USP 34.*
Use: Surgical aid.

•**tapentadol.** (ta-PEN-ta-dol) USAN.
Use: Analgesic.
See: Nucynta.

Ta-Poff. (Ulmer Pharmacal) Adhesive tape remover. Liq. Bot. 1 pt. Aerosol. Can 6 oz. *OTC.*

•**taprenepag.** (ta-PREN-e-pag) USAN.
Use: Ophthalmic agent.

•**taprenepag isopropyl.** (ta-PREN-e-pag) USAN.
Use: Ophthalmic agent.

Tapuline. (Wesley) Activated attapulgite 600 mg, pectin 60 mg, homatropine methylbromide 0.5 mg. Chew. Tab. Bot. 100s, 1000s. *OTC.*
Use: Antidiarrheal.

tar.
See: Coal Tar.

Tarabine PFS. (Adria) Cytarabine 20 mg/mL, preservative free. Inj. Single vial 5 mL, bulk package vial 50 mL. *Rx.*
Use: Antimetabolite.

Taraphilic. (Medco) Coal tar distillate 1%, stearyl alcohol, petrolatum, parabens. Oint. 454 g. *OTC.*
Use: Dermatologic.

Tarceva. (Genentech Inc.) Erlotinib 25 mg, 100 mg, 150 mg. Lactose. Film-coated. Tab. 30s. *Rx.*
Use: Epidermal growth factor receptor inhibitor.

tar-containing products.
Use: Dermatologic.
See: Balnetar.
　Coal Tar.
　Cutar Emulsion.
　Doak Tar.
　Fototar.
　Medotar.
　MG 217 Medicated Tar.
　Oxipor VHC.
　Packer's Pine Tar.
　Pine Tar Oils.
　Polytar.
　PsoriGel.
　Taraphilic.

tar derivatives, shampoo.
Use: Dermatologic.
See: Creamy Tar.
　DHS Tar.
　Doak Tar.
　Ionil T Plus.

MG 217 Medicated Tar.
Neutrogena T/Gel Original.
Polytar.
Zetar.
Targretin. (Eisai) Bexarotene. **Soft Gelatin Cap.:** 75 mg. Bot. 100s. **Gel:** 1%, dehydrated alcohol. Tube 60 g. *Rx.*
Use: Rexinoid.
•**tariquidar.** (tar-I-kwi-dar) USAN.
Use: Chemotherapeutic aid.
Tarka. (Abbott) Trandolapril maleate/verapamil hydrochloride 1 mg/240 mg, 2 mg/180 mg, 2 mg/240 mg, 4 mg/240 mg. Lactose. Film-coated. Tab. Bot. 100s. *Rx.*
Use: Antihypertensive.
Tarnphilic. (Medco Lab) Coal tar 1%, polysorbate 0.5% in aquaphilic base. Jar 16 oz. *OTC.*
Use: Dermatologic.
Taron-Crystals. (Trigen) Potassium citrate monohydrate 3,300 mg, citric acid monohydrate 1,002 mg per packet (potassium 30 mEq and bicarbonate 30 mEq per reconstituted packet). Sucralose. Blueberry flavor. Pow. for Soln., oral. UD 4.32 g packet. *Rx.*
Use: Systemic alkalinizer.
Tarpaste. (Doak Dermatologics) Coal tar distilled 5% in zinc paste. Tube 1 oz, Jar 4 oz, w/Hydrocortisone 0.5%. Tube 1 oz. *OTC.*
Use: Dermatitis.
Tarsum Shampoo/Gel. (Summers) Coal tar 10%, salicylic acid 5% in shampoo base. Bot. 4 oz. *OTC.*
Use: Antiseborrheic, dermatologic, hair, and scalp.
tartar emetic.
See: Antimony Potassium Tartrate.
•**tartaric acid.** (tar-TAR-ik-AS-id) *NF 29.*
Use: Pharmaceutic aid (buffering agent).
Tashan. (Block Drug) Skin Cream. Vitamins A palmitate, D_2, D-panthenol, E. Tube 1 oz. *OTC.*
Use: Emollient.
•**tasidotin hydrochloride.** (TA-si-DOE-tin) USAN.
Use: Antineoplastic.
Tasigna. (Novartis) Nilotinib 150 mg, 200 mg (as nilotinib hydrochloride). Lactose. Cap. UD 28s. *Rx.*
Use: Protein-tyrosine kinase inhibitor.
Tasmar. (Roche) Tolcapone 100 mg, 200 mg, lactose. Tab. Bot. 90s. *Rx.*
Use: Antiparkinson agent.
•**tasosartan.** (tass-OH-sahr-tan) USAN.
Use: Antihypertensive.

•**taspoglutide.** (tas-poe-GLUE-tide) USAN.
Use: Antidiabetic.
Taste Function Test, Accusens T. (Westport Pharmaceuticals, Inc.) Tastant 60 mL. Kit. 15 Bot.
Use: Diagnostic aid.
Ta-Verm. (Table Rock) Piperazine citrate 100 mg/mL Syr. Bot. 1 pt, 1 gal. 500 mg Tab. Bot. 100s, 500s. *Rx.*
Use: Anthelmintic.
Tavilen Plus. (Table Rock) Liver solution 1 g, ferric pyrophosphate soluble 500 mg, vitamins B_1 6 mg, B_2 7.2 mg, B_6 3 mg, B_{12} 24 mcg, panthenol 3 mg, niacinamide 60 mg, l-lysine hydrochloride 300 mg, 5% alcohol/mL. Bot. 16 oz., 1 gal. *OTC.*
Use: Hematinic.
Tavist. (Novartis) Clemastine fumarate. **Tab.:** 2.68 mg. Bot. 100s. **Syrup:** 0.67 mg/5 mL. Bot. 118 mL. *Rx.*
Use: Antihistamine.
Tavist Allergy. (Novartis Consumer Health) Clemastine fumarate 1.34 mg, lactose.Tab. Pkg. 8s. *OTC.*
Use: Antihistamine, nonselective ethanolamine.
Tavist Allergy/Sinus/Headache. (Novartis) Pseudoephedrine hydrochloride 30 mg, clemastine fumarate 0.335 mg, acetaminophen 500 mg, methylparaben. Tab. Bot. 24s, 48s. *OTC.*
Use: Upper respiratory combination, decongestant, antihistamine, analgesic.
Tavist Sinus Maximum Strength. (Novartis) Pseudoephedrine hydrochloride 30 mg, acetaminophen 500 mg, lactose, dextrose, methylparaben. Tab. Pkg. 24s. *OTC.*
Use: Upper respiratory combination, decongestant, analgesic.
taxoids.
Use: Antimitotic.
See: Cabazitaxel.
Docetaxel.
Paclitaxel.
Taxol. (Bristol-Myers Squibb) Paclitaxel 6 mg/mL, polyoxyethylated castor oil (Cremophor EL) 527 mg/mL, dehydrated alcohol 49.7%. Inj. Multiple-dose Vial 5 mL, 16.7 mL, 50 mL. *Rx.*
Use: Antineoplastic; antimitotic, taxoid.
Taxotere. (Aventis) Docetaxel 20 mg/0.5 mL, 80 mg/2 mL. Polysorbate 80 1040 mg/mL, ethanol 13% in water for injection. Inj. Single-dose vial with 1.5 mL diluent (20 mg only) and 6 mL diluent (80 mg only). *Rx.*
Use: Antimitotic, taxoid.

•**tazadolene succinate.** (TAZZ-ah-DOE-leen) USAN.
Use: Analgesic.

•**tazarotene.** (tazz-AHR-oh-teen) USAN.
Use: Antiacne, antipsoriatic, retinoid.
See: Tazorac.

Tazicef. (Hospira) Ceftazidime. **Inj.:** 1 g, 2 g. *Galaxy* containers. **Pow. for Inj.:** 1 g, 2 g, 6 g. Sodium 2.3 mEq/g. Vials. *ADD-Vantage* vials. Piggyback vials (1 g, 2 g only). Bulk package (6 g only). *Rx.*
Use: Anti-infective, cephalosporin.

Tazidime. (Eli Lilly) Ceftazidime (as pentahydrate with L-arginine) 1 g, 2 g, 6 g. Pow. for Inj. *ADD-Vantage* vials (1 g, 2 g only). Vials. 20 mL (1 g only), 50 mL (2 g only), 100 mL. *Rx.*
Use: Anti-infective, cephalosporin.

•**tazifylline hydrochloride.** (TAY-zih-FIH-lin) USAN.
Use: Antihistamine.

•**tazobactam.** (TAZZ-oh-BACK-tam) USAN.
Use: Inhibitor (beta-lactamase).

•**tazobactam sodium.** (TAZZ-oh-BACK-tam) USAN.
Use: Inhibitor (beta-lactamase).

tazobactam sodium/piperacillin.
Use: Extended-spectrum penicillin.
See: Zosyn.

•**tazofelone.** (TAY-zah-feh-lone) USAN.
Use: Suppressant (inflammatory bowel disease).

•**tazolol hydrochloride.** (TAY-zoe-lole) USAN.
Use: Cardiotonic.

•**tazomeline citrate.** (tazz-OH-meh-leen) USAN.
Use: Alzheimer disease treatment (cholinergic agonist).

Tazorac. (Allergan) Tazarotene. **Cream:** 0.05%, 0.1%, benzyl alcohol 1%, EDTA, medium chain triglycerides, mineral oil. Cream. Tube 15 g, 30 g, 60 g. **Gel:** 0.05%, 0.1%, benzyl alcohol 1%, EDTA. Tube. 30 g, 100 g. *Rx.*
Use: Antiacne, antipsoriatic, retinoid.

Taztia XT. (Andrx Pharmaceuticals) Diltiazem hydrochloride 120 mg, 180 mg, 240 mg, 300 mg, 360 mg. ER Cap. 30s, 90s. *Rx.*
Use: Calcium channel blocker.

TBA-Pred. (Keene Pharmaceuticals) Prednisolone tebutate 10 mg/mL Susp. Vial 10 mL. *Rx.*
Use: Corticosteroid.

TC Suspension. (Aventis) Aluminum hydroxide 600 mg, magnesium hydroxide 300 mg/5 mL, sorbitol, sodium

0.8 mg/5 mL. Liq. In UD 15 mL, 30 mL (100s). *OTC.*
Use: Antacid.

T/Derm Tar Emollient. (Neutrogena) Neutar solubilized coal tar extract 5% in oil base. Bot. 4 oz. *OTC.*
Use: Antipsoriatic, antipruritic.

T-Dry. (Jones Pharma) Pseudoephedrine hydrochloride 120 mg, chlorpheniramine maleate 12 mg. SR Cap. Bot. 100s. *Rx.*
Use: Antihistamine, decongestant.

T-Dry Jr. (Jones Pharma) Pseudoephedrine hydrochloride 60 mg, chlorpheniramine maleate 4 mg. SR Cap. Bot. 100s. *OTC.*
Use: Antihistamine, decongestant.

TDX Cortisol. (Abbott Diagnostics) Fluorescence polarization immunoassay for the quantitative determination of cortisol in serum, plasma, or urine.
Use: Diagnostic aid.

TDX Thyroxine. (Abbott Diagnostics) Automated assay for quantitation of unsaturated thyroxine-binding sites in serum or plasma.
Use: Diagnostic aid.

TDX Total Estriol. (Abbott Diagnostics) Fluorescence polarization immunoassay for the quantitative determination of total estriol in serum, plasma, or urine.
Use: Diagnostic aid.

TDX Total T3. (Abbott Diagnostics) Automated assay for quantitation of total circulating triiodothyronine (T3) in serum or plasma.
Use: Diagnostic aid.

TDX T-Uptake. (Abbott Diagnostics) Automated assay for the determination of thyroxine-binding capacity in serum or plasma.
Use: Diagnostic aid.

Te Anatoxal Berna. (Berna) Tetanus toxoid adsorbed, 10 Lf units/0.5 mL. Vial 5 mL, Syringe. 0.5 mL. *Rx.*
Use: Immunization.

Tear Drop. (Parmed Pharmaceuticals, Inc.) Benzalkonium chloride 0.01%, polyvinyl alcohol, NaCl, EDTA. Soln. Drops. Bot. 15 mL. *OTC.*
Use: Artificial tears.

Tearisol. (Novartis Ophthalmic) Hydroxypropyl methylcellulose 0.5%, edetate disodium, benzalkonium chloride 0.01%, boric acid, potassium chloride. Bot. 15 mL. *OTC.*
Use: Artificial tears.

Tears Again. (OcuSOFT) Hydroxypropyl methylcellulose 0.3%, boric acid, phosphoric acid, potassium chloride, sodium chloride *Dissipate* as a preserva-

tive. Soln., Ophth. 15 mL. *OTC.*
Use: Artificial tears.

Tears Again MC. (OcuSOFT) Hydroxypropyl methylcellulose 0.3%, boric
acid, phosphoric acid, potassium chloride, sodium chloride *Dissipate* as a
preservative. Drops. 15 mL. *OTC.*
Use: Artificial tears.

Tears Naturale. (Alcon) Dextran 70
0.1%, benzalkonium chloride 0.01%,
hydroxypropyl methylcellulose 0.3%,
sodium chloride, EDTA, hydrochloric
acid, sodium hydrochloride, potassium
chloride. Soln. Bot. 15 mL, 30 mL. *OTC.*
Use: Artificial tears.

Tears Naturale Forte. (Alcon) Dextran
70 1%, hydroxypropyl methylcellulose
0.3%, glycerin 0.2%, polyquaternium-1
0.001%, NaCl, KCl, sodium borate.
Soln. 15 mL, 30 mL. *OTC.*
Use: Artificial tears.

Tears Naturale Free. (Alcon) Hydroxypropyl methylcellulose 2910 0.3%, dextran 70 0.1%, NaCl, KCl, sodium borate. Soln. Single-use containers
0.6 mL. *OTC.*
Use: Artificial tears.

Tears Naturale II. (Alcon) Dextran 70
0.1%, hydroxypropyl methylcellulose
2910 0.3%, polyquaternium-1 0.001%,
sodium chloride, potassium chloride,
sodium borate. Soln. *Drop-tainer* 15 mL,
30 mL. *OTC.*
Use: Artificial tears.

Tears Plus. (Allergan) Polyvinyl alcohol
1.4%, NaCl, povidone 0.6%, chlorobutanol 0.5%. *OTC.*
Use: Artificial tears.

tear test strips.
Use: Ophthalmic diagnostic product.
See: Schirmer Tear Test.

tea tree oil. (Metabolic Prod.) Australian
oil of Melaleuca alternifolia 100% pure.
Bot. 1 oz, 4 oz, 8 oz, 16 oz. **Cream:**
Bot. 8 oz. **Oint.:** Tube 1 oz, 3 oz. *OTC.*
Use: Antiseptic, antifungal, topical.

•**tebanicline tosylate.** (te-BAN-i-kleen)
USAN.
Use: Analgesic.

•**tebufelone.** (teh-BYOO-feh-LONE)
USAN.
Use: Analgesic, anti-inflammatory.

•**tebuquine.** (TEH-buh-KWIN) USAN.
Use: Antimalarial.

T.E.C. (Invenex) Zn 1 mg, Cu 0.4 mg, Cr
4 mcg, Mn 0.1 mg. Vial 10 mL. *Rx.*
Use: Trace element supplement.

•**tecadenoson.** (tek-a-DEN-o-son) USAN.
Use: Cardiovascular agent.

•**tecalcet hydrochloride.** (TE-kal-set)
USAN.
Use: Hyperparathyroidism.

•**tecarfarin.** (TEK-ar far-in) USAN.
Use: Anticoagulant.

•**tecarfarin sodium.** (TEK-ar far-in)
USAN.
Use: Anticoagulant.

•**tecastemizole.** (tek-a-STEM-mi-zole)
USAN.
Use: Antihistamine.

•**teceleukin.** (teh-see-LOO-kin) USAN.
Use: Immunostimulant.

Techneplex. (Bristol-Myers Squibb)
Technetium Tc 99m pentetate kit. 10 vi-
als/kit.
Use: Radiopaque agent.

TechneScan MAA. (Mallinckrodt) Aggre-
gated albumin (human).
Use: Preparation of Tc 99m Aggregated
Albumin (Human).

•**technetium Tc 99m albumin aggregated injection.** (tek-NEE-shee-uhm Tc
99m al-BYOO-min AGG-reh-GAY-tuhd)
USP 34.
Use: Diagnostic aid (lung imaging), radioactive agent.

•**technetium Tc 99m albumin colloid in-
jection.** (tek-NEE-shee-uhm Tc 99m al-
BYOO-min) *USP 34.*
Use: Radiopharmaceutical.

•**technetium Tc 99m albumin injection.**
(tek-NEE-shee-uhm Tc 99m al-BYOO-
min) *USP 34.*
Use: Radiopharmaceutical.

•**technetium Tc 99m albumin microaggregated.** (tek-NEE-shee-uhm Tc 99m
al-BYOO-min) USAN.
Use: Radiopharmaceutical.

**technetium Tc 99m antimelanoma mu-
rine monoclonal antibody.**
Use: Diagnostic aid. [Orphan Drug]

•**technetium Tc 99m antimony trisulfide
colloid.** (tek-NEE-shee-uhm) USAN.
Use: Radiopharmaceutical.

•**technetium Tc 99m apcitide.** (tek-NEE-
shee-uhm APP-sih-tide) *USP 34.*
Use: Radiopharmaceutical.

•**technetium Tc 99m arcitumomab injection.** (tek-NEE-shee-uhm AR-si-TOOM-
oh-mab) USAN.
Use: Radiopharmaceutical.

•**technetium Tc 99m bicisate.** (tek-NEE-
shee-uhm Tc 99m bye-SIS-ate) USAN.
Use: Diagnostic aid (brain imaging),
radiopharmaceutical.

•**technetium Tc 99m depreotide injection.** (tek-NEE-shee-uhm) *USP 34.*
Use: Radiopharmaceutical.

• **technetium Tc 99m disofenin injection.** (tek-NEE-shee-uhm) *USP 34.*
Use: Radiopharmaceutical; diagnostic aid (hepatobiliary function determination).

• **technetium Tc 99m etidronate injection.** (tek-NEE-shee-uhm) *USP 34.*
Use: Radiopharmaceutical.

• **technetium Tc 99m exametazime injection.** (tek-NEE-shee-uhm Tc 99m ex-ah-MET-ah-zeem) *USP 34.*
Use: Radiopharmaceutical.

• **technetium Tc 99m fanolesomab.** (tek-NEE-shee-uhm fa-noe-LES-oh-mab) USAN.
Use: Diagnostic aid (polymorphonuclear neutrophil accumulation); radiopharmaceutical.

technetium Tc 99m ferpentetate injection.
Use: Radiopharmaceutical.

• **technetium Tc 99m furifosmin.** (tek-NEE-shee-uhm Tc 99m fyoor-ih-FOSS-min) USAN.
Use: Diagnostic aid (radioactive, cardiac disease), radiopharmaceutical.

technetium Tc 99m generator solution. (New England Nuclear) Pertechnetate sodium Tc 99m.
Use: Radiopharmaceutical, radiopaque agent.

• **technetium Tc 99m glucepate injection.** (tek-NEE-shee-uhm) *USP 34.*
Formerly Technetium Tc 99m Sodium Gluceptate.
Use: Radiopharmaceutical.

• **technetium Tc 99m lidofenin injection.** (tek-NEE-shee-uhm) *USP 34.*
Use: Radiopharmaceutical.

• **technetium Tc 99m mebrofenin injection.** (tek-NEE-shee-uhm) *USP 34.*
Use: Radiopharmaceutical.
See: Choletec.

technetium Tc-99m mebrofenin. (CIS-US) Mebrofenin 45 mg. When sodium pertechnetate Tc-99m injection is added to the vial, the diagnostic agent technetium Tc-99m mebrofenin is formed containing up to 3,700 MBq (100 millicuries) of Tc-99m. Also contains stannous fluoride dihydrate (minimum) and total tin 1.03 mg maximum (as stannous fluoride dihydrate). May contain parabens. Inj., Lyophilized Pow. for Soln. Kits of 5 and 30 multidose vials. *Rx.*
Use: Radiopaque agent.

• **technetium Tc 99m medronate disodium.** (tek-NEE-shee-uhm) USAN.
Use: Radiopharmaceutical.

• **technetium Tc 99m medronate injection.** (tek-NEE-shee-uhm) *USP 34.*
Use: Diagnostic aid (skeletal imaging), radiopharmaceutical.
See: Macrotec.

• **technetium Tc 99m mertiatide injection.** (tek-NEE-shee-uhm Tc 99m MEER-TIE-ah-tide) *USP 34.*
Use: Diagnostic aid (renal function); radiopharmaceutical.

technetium Tc 99m murine monoclonal antibody (IgG2a) to B cell.
Use: Diagnostic aid. [Orphan Drug]

technetium Tc 99m murine monoclonal antibody to hCG.
Use: Diagnostic aid. [Orphan Drug]

technetium Tc 99m murine monoclonal antibody to human alpha-fotoprotein.
Use: Diagnostic aid. [Orphan Drug]

• **technetium Tc 99m nitridocade.** (tek-NEE-shee-uhm Tc 99m nye-TRID-oh-kade) USAN.
Use: Diagnostic aid (coronary artery disease); radiopharmaceutical.

• **technetium Tc 99m nofetumomab merpentan injection.** (tek-NEE-shee-uhm Tc 99m no-fe-TUE-mo-mab) *USP 34.*
Use: Radiopharmaceutical.

• **technetium Tc 99m oxidronate injection.** (tek-NEE-shee-uhm) *USP 34.*
Use: Diagnostic aid (skeletal imaging), radiopharmaceutical.

• **technetium Tc 99m pentetate calcium trisodium.** (tek-NEE-shee-uhm KAL-see-uhm try-so-dee-uhm) USAN.
Use: Radiopharmaceutical.

• **technetium Tc 99m pentetate injection.** (tek-NEE-shee-uhm) *USP 34. Formerly Technetium Tc 99m Pentetate Sodium.*
Use: Radiopharmaceutical.

• **technetium Tc 99m (pyro- and trimeta-) phosphates injection.** (tek-NEE-shee-uhm) *USP 34.*
Use: Radiopharmaceutical.

• **technetium Tc 99m pyrophosphate injection.** (tek-NEE-shee-uhm) *USP 34.*
Use: Radiopharmaceutical.

• **technetium Tc 99m red blood cells injection.** (tek-NEE-shee-uhm) *USP 34.*
Use: Radiopharmaceutical.

• **technetium Tc 99m sestamibi.** (tek-NEE-shee-uhm SES-ta-MIB-ee) *USP 34.*
Use: Diagnostic aid (radiopaque medium, cardiac perfusion); radiopharmaceutical.

• **technetium Tc 99m siboroxime.** (tek-NEE-shee-uhm Tc 99m sih-boe-ROX-

eem) USAN.
Use: Diagnostic aid (brain imaging), radiopharmaceutical.

•**technetium Tc 99m succimer injection.** (tek-NEE-shee-uhm) *USP 34.*
Use: Radiopharmaceutical, diagnostic aid (renal function determination).

•**technetium Tc 99m sulfur colloid injection.** (tek-NEE-shee-uhm) *USP 34.*
Use: Radiopharmaceutical.

technetium Tc 99m sulfur colloid kit.
Use: Radiopharmaceutical.
See: Tesuloid.

•**technetium Tc 99m teboroxime.** (tek-NEE-shee-uhm Tc 99m teh-boe-ROX-eem) USAN.
Use: Diagnostic aid (radiopaque medium, cardiac perfusion), radiopharmaceutical.

•**technetium Tc 99m tilmanocept.** (tek-NEE-shee-um til-MAN-oh-sept) USAN.
Use: Radiopharmaceutical.

teclosine. Under study.
Use: Amebicide.

•**teclozan.** (TEH-kloe-zan) USAN.
Use: Antiamebic.
See: Falmonox.

Tecnu Outdoor Skin Cleanser. (Tec Labs) Deodorized mineral spirits, propylene glycol, octylphenoxypolyethoxy-ethanol, mixed fatty acid soap. Lot. 118 mL, 355 mL. *OTC.*
Use: Poison ivy prevention.

•**tecogalan sodium.** (TEE-koe-gay-lan) USAN.
Use: Antineoplastic adjunct.

•**tecovirimat.** (tek-oh-VIR-i-mat) USAN.
Use: Treatment of smallpox.

•**tedisamil.** (te-DIS-a-mil) USAN.
Use: Investigational antiarrhythmic agent.

•**tedisamil sesquifumarate.** (te-DIS-a-mil SES-kwi-FUE-ma-rate) USAN.
Use: Antiarrhythmic agent.

•**tedizolid.** (TED-eye-ZOE-lid) USAN.
Use: Antibiotic.

•**tedizolid phosphate.** (TED-eye-ZOE-lid) USAN.
Use: Treatment of complicated skin and skin structure infections.

Tedral. (Parke-Davis) **Elix.:** Theophylline 32.5 mg, ephedrine hydrochloride 6 mg, phenobarbital 2 mg/5 mL. Alcohol 15%. Pediatric. Bot. Pt. **Tab.:** Theophylline 118 mg, ephedrine hydrochloride 24 mg, phenobarbital 8 mg. Tab. Bot. 24s, 100s, 1000s. UD 100s. **Susp. (Pediatric Pharmaceuticals):** Theophylline 65 mg, ephedrine hydrochloride

12 mg, phenobarbital 4 mg/5 mL. Bot. 8 oz. *Rx.*
Use: Antiasthmatic.

Tedral-SA. (Parke-Davis) Theophylline 180 mg, ephedrine hydrochloride 48 mg, phenobarbital 25 mg. SA Tab. Bot. 100s, 1000s. *Rx.*
Use: Antiasthmatic.

•**teduglutide.** (te-DUE-gloo-tide) USAN.
Use: Gastrointestinal disease.

Teebacin. (CMC) Sod. p-aminosalicylate. **Tab.:** 0.5 g Bot. 1000s. **Pow.:** Bot. lb. *Rx.*
Use: Antituberculosal.

Teebaconin. (CMC) Isoniazid 50 mg, 100 mg, 300 mg. Tab. Bot. 100s, 1000s. *Rx.*
Use: Antituberculosal.

Teebaconin w/Vitamin B₆. (CMC) Isoniazid 100 mg, 10 mg pyridoxine hydrochloride. Tab. Bot. 100s, 500s, 1000s. Isoniazid 300 mg, 30 mg pyridoxine hydrochloride. Tab. Bot. 100s, 1000s. *Rx.*
Use: Antituberculosal.

Teev. (Keene Pharmaceuticals) Estradiol valerate 4 mg, testosterone enanthate 90 mg/mL. Inj. Vial 10 mL. *Rx.*
Use: Androgen, estrogen combination.

•**tefibazumab.** (tef-ee-BA-zoo-mab) USAN.
Use: Anti-infective.

Teflaro. (Forest Pharmaceuticals) Ceftaroline fosamil (as ceftaroline fosamil monoacetate) 400 mg, 600 mg. Inj., Pow. for Soln. Single-use vial. *Rx.*
Use: Anti-infective, cephalosporin and related antibiotic.

•**teflurane.** (TEH-flew-rane) USAN.
Use: Anesthetic, general.

tegacid.
See: Glyceryl Monostearate.

•**tegafur.** (TEH-gah-fer) USAN.
Use: Antineoplastic.

Tegamide. (G & W) Trimethobenzamide hydrochloride 100 mg, 200 mg. Supp. Box. 10s, 50s. *Rx.*
Use: Antiemetic.

•**tegaserod maleate.** (teg-a-SER-od) USAN.
Note: Available through investigational limited access program.
Use: Gastrointestinal motility disorders.

•**teglarinad chloride.** (teg-LAR-i-nad kloride) USAN.
Use: Antineoplastic.

•**tegobuvir.** (TEG-oh-BUE-vir) USAN.
Use: Hepatitis C.

Tegretol. (Novartis) Carbamazepine. **Tab.:** 200 mg. Bot. 100s. **Chew. Tab.:**

100 mg. Sucrose. Bot. 100s. UD 100s.
Susp.: 100 mg/5 mL. Sorbitol, sucrose. Citrus/vanilla flavor. Bot. 450 mL. *Rx.*
Tall Man: TEGretol
Use: Anticonvulsant.

Tegretol-XR. (Novartis) Carbamazepine 100 mg, 200 mg, 400 mg. Mannitol. Film-coated. ER Tab. Bot. 100s. *Rx.*
Tall Man: TEGretol
Use: Anticonvulsant.

Tegrin. (Block Drug) Allantoin 2%, coal tar extract 5% in cream base. Cream. Tube 2 oz, 4.4 oz. *OTC.*
Use: Antipsoriatic.

T.E.H. Compound. (Various Mfr.) Theophylline 130 mg, ephedrine sulfate 25 mg, hydroxyzine hydrochloride 10 mg. Tab. Bot. 100s, 500s. *Rx.*
Use: Antiasthmatic.

•**teicoplanin.** (teh-kah-PLAN-in) USAN.
Use: Anti-infective.

Tekamlo. (Novartis) Amlodipine besylate/aliskiren (as aliskiren hemifumarate) 5 mg/150 mg, 10 mg/150 mg, 5 mg/300 mg, 10 mg/300 mg. Film coated. PEG. Tab. 30s, 90s, UD 100s. *Rx.*
Use: Antihypertensive combination.

Tekral. (Capellon Pharmaceutical) Diphenhydramine hydrochloride 100 mg, pseudoephedrine hydrochloride 120 mg. Lactose. Tab. 90s. *Rx.*
Use: Upper respiratory combination, decongestant, antihistamine.

Tekturna. (Novartis) Aliskiren 150 mg, 300 mg. Film-coated. Tab. 30s, 90s, UD 100s. *Rx.*
Use: Renin angiotensin system antagonist, direct renin inhibitor.

Tekturna HCT. (Novartis) Aliskirin/hydrochlorothiazide 150 mg/12.5 mg, 150 mg/25 mg, 300 mg/12.5 mg, 300 mg/25 mg. Lactose. Film-coated. Tab. 30s, 90s, blister pack 100s. *Rx.*
Use: Antihypertensive combination.

Telachlor TD Caps. (Major) Chlorpheniramine maleate 8 mg, 12 mg. TD Tab. Bot. 1000s. *Rx.*
Use: Antihistamine.

•**telapristone acetate.** (TEL-a-PRIS-tone) USAN.
Use: Female reproductive disorders.

•**telavancin hydrochloride.** (tel-a-VAN-sin) USAN.
Use: Antibacterial agent.
See: Vibativ.

•**telbivudine.** (tel-BI-vyoo-deen) USAN.
Use: Antiretroviral, nucleoside reverse transcriptase inhibitor.
See: Tyzeka.

•**telcagepant.** (tel-KA-je-pant) USAN.
Use: Treatment of migraine.

•**telcagepant potassium.** (tel-KA-je-pant) USAN.
Use: Treatment of migraine.

•**telinavir.** (teh-LIN-ah-veer) USAN.
Use: Antiviral.

•**telithromycin.** (tel-ITH-roe-MYE-sin) USAN.
Use: Anti-infective.
See: Ketek.

•**telmisartan.** (tell-mih-SAHR-tan) USAN.
Use: Angiotensin II receptor antagonist; antihypertensive.
See: Micardis.
W/Hydrochlorothiazide.
See: Micardis HCT.

•**telotristat.** (tel-OH-tri-stat) USAN.
Use: Carcinoid syndrome.

•**telotristat ethyl.** (tel-OH-tri-stat) USAN.
Use: Carcinoid syndrome.

•**telotristat etiprate.** (tel-OH-tri-stat) USAN.
Use: Carcinoid syndrome.

•**teloxantrone hydrochloride.** (teh-LOX-an-trone) USAN.
Use: Antineoplastic.

•**teludipine hydrochloride.** (teh-LOO-dih-peen) USAN.
Use: Antihypertensive, calcium channel antagonist.

•**temafloxacin hydrochloride.** (teh-mah-FLOX-ah-SIN) USAN.
Use: Anti-infective (microbial DNA topoisomerase inhibitor).

•**temanogrel.** (tem-AN-oh-grel) USAN.
Use: Anti-platelet agent.

•**temanogrel hydrochloride.** (tem-AN-oh-grel) USAN.
Use: Anti-platelet agent.

•**tematropium methylsulfate.** (teh-mah-TROE-pee-UHM METH-ill-SULL-fate) USAN.
Use: Anticholinergic.

•**temazepam.** (tem-AZE-uh-pam) *USP 34.*
Use: Sedative/hypnotic, nonbarbiturate.
See: Restoril.

temazepam. (Various Mfr.) Temazepam 7.5 mg, 15 mg, 22.5 mg, 30 mg. Lactose. Cap. 30s (22.5 mg only); 100s (except 22.5 mg only); 500s (15 mg and 30 mg only). *c-iv.*
Use: Sedative/hypnotic, nonbarbiturate.

•**temelastine.** (teh-mell-ASS-teen) USAN.
Use: Antihistamine.

•**temocapril hydrochloride.** (teh-MOE-cap-RILL) USAN.
Use: Antihypertensive.

•**temocillin.** (TEE-moe-SIH-lin) USAN.
Use: Anti-infective.

Temodar. (Schering) Temozolomide.
Cap.: 5 mg, 20 mg, 100 mg, 140 mg,
180 mg, 250 mg. Lactose. 5s, 14s (except 250 mg). **Inj., lyophilized Pow.
for Soln.:** 100 mg. Single-use vial. *Rx.*
Use: Antineoplastic.

•**temoporfin.** (teh-moe-PORE-fin) USAN.
Use: Antineoplastic.

Temovate. (Pharmaderm) **Cream:** Clobetasol propionate 0.05%. Tube 15 g,
30 g, 45 g. **Emollient:** Clobetasol propionate 0.05%. Tube 15 g, 30 g, 60 g.
Gel: Clobetasol propionate 0.05%.
Tube 15 g, 30 g, 60 g. **Oint.:** Clobetasol propionate 0.05%. Tube 15 g, 30 g,
45 g. *Rx.*
Use: Corticosteroid, topical.

•**temozolomide.** (TEM-oh-ZOE-loe-mide)
USAN.
Use: Antineoplastic.
See: Temodar.

Tempo. (Thompson Medical) Calcium
carbonate 414 mg, aluminum hydroxide
133 mg, magnesium hydroxide 81 mg,
simethicone 20 mg. Chew. Tab. Bot.
10s, 30s, 60s. *OTC.*
Use: Antacid, antiflatulent.

Temporary Punctal/Canalicular Collagen Implant. (Eagle Vision) 0.2 mm,
• 0.3 mm, 0.4 mm, 0.5 mm, 0.6 mm. Box
72s. *Rx.*
Use: Collagen implant, ophthalmic.

Temp Tab. (National Vitamin) Chloride
(as sodium and potassium chloride)
287 mg, sodium (as chloride) 180 mg,
potassium (as chloride) 15 mg. Tab.
Preservative-free. 100s. *OTC.*
Use: Electrolyte.

•**temsirolimus.** (TEM-sir-OH-li-mus)
USAN.
Use: Antineoplastic, protein-tyrosine kinase inhibitor, mTor inhibitor.
See: Torisel.

•**temurtide.** (teh-MER-TIDE) USAN.
Use: Vaccine adjuvant.

Tenar PSE. (Centrix) Guaifenesin
200 mg, pseudoephedrine hydrochloride 40 mg. Sorbitol, sucralose. Grape
flavor. Liq. 473 mL. *Rx.*
Use: Upper respiratory combination, decongestant and expectorant combination.

Tencet. (Roberts) Acetaminophen
500 mg, butalbital 50 mg, caffeine
40 mg. Cap. Bot. 100s, UD 1000s. *Rx.*
Use: Analgesic, hypnotic, sedative.

Tencon. (International Ethical Labs)
Acetaminophen 650 mg, butalbital

50 mg. Tab. Bot. 100s. *Rx.*
Use: Analgesic, hypnotic, sedative.

•**tenecteplase.** (teh-NECK-teh-place)
USAN.
Use: Thrombolytic agent, tissue plasminogen activator.
See: TNKase.

•**teneliximab.** (ten-el-IKS-i-mab) USAN.
Use: Monoclonal antibody.

Tenex. (Promius Pharma) Guanfacine
hydrochloride 1 mg, 2 mg. Lactose. Tab.
100s, 500s (1 mg only). *Rx.*
Use: Antihypertensive.

•**tenifatecan.** (TEN-i-fa-TEK-an) USAN.
Use: Antineoplastic.

•**teniposide.** (TEN-ih-POE-side) USAN.
Use: Antineoplastic. [Orphan Drug]
See: Vumon.

•**tenivastatin calcium.** (te-NI-va-sta-tin)
USAN.
Use: Antihyperlipidemic; HMG-CoA reductase inhibitor.

Ten-K. (Novartis) Potassium chloride
750 mg (10 mEq). CR Cap. Bot. 100s,
500s. UD, blister pak 100s. *Rx.*
Use: Electrolyte supplement.

•**tenofovir.** (te-NOE-fo-veer) USAN.
Use: Antiviral.

•**tenofovir disoproxil fumarate.** (te-NOE-fo-veer dye-soe-PROX-il) USAN.
Use: Antiretroviral, nucleotide analog
reverse transcriptase inhibitor.
See: Viread.
W/Emtricitabine.
See: Truvada.
W/Emtricitabine, Efavirenz.
See: Atripla.

Tenol. (Vortech Pharmaceuticals) **Liq.:**
Acetaminophen 120 mg, NAPA alcohol 7%/5 mL. Bot. 3 oz, 4 oz, gal. **Tab.:**
Acetaminophen 325 mg. Bot. 1000s.
OTC.
Use: Analgesic.

Tenol-Plus. (Vortech Pharmaceuticals)
Acetaminophen 250 mg, aspirin
250 mg, caffeine 65 mg. Tab. Bot.
1000s. *OTC.*
Use: Analgesic.

Tenoretic. (AstraZeneca) Atenolol/chlorthalidone 50 mg/25 mg, 100 mg/25 mg.
Tab. Bot. 100s. *Rx.*
Use: Antihypertensive, diuretic.

Tenormin. (AstraZeneca) Atenolol
25 mg, 50 mg, 100 mg. Tab. 100s. *Rx.*
Use: Antiadrenergic/sympatholytic,
beta-adrenergic blocker.

•**tenoxicam.** (ten-OX-ih-kam) USAN.
Use: Anti-inflammatory.

Tensive Conductive Adhesive Gel.
(Parker) Nonflammable conductive ad-

hesive electrode gel, eliminates tape and tape irritation. Tube 60 g.
Use: Therapeutic aid.

Tensocaine. (Sanofi-Synthelabo) Acetaminophen. Tab. *OTC.*
Use: Analgesic.

Tensolate. (Apco) Phenobarbital 0.25 g, hyoscyamine sulfate 0.1037 mg, atropine sulfate 0.0194 mg, hyoscine HBr 0.0065 mg. Tab. Bot. 100s. *Rx.*
Use: Antispasmodic.

Tensolax. (Sanofi-Synthelabo) Chlormezanone. Tab. *Rx.*
Use: Muscle relaxant.

Tensopin. (Apco) Phenobarbital 0.25 g, homatropine methylbromide 2.5 mg. Tab. Bot. 100s. *Rx.*
Use: Antispasmodic.

T.E.P. (Geneva) Phenobarbital 8 mg, theophylline 130 mg, ephedrine hydrochloride 24 mg. Tab. Bot. 100s. *Rx.*
Use: Antiasthmatic combination.

Tepanil. (3M) Diethylpropion hydrochloride 25 mg. Tab. Bot. 100s. *c-iv.*
Use: Anorexiant.

Tepanil Ten-Tab. (3M) Diethylpropion 75 mg. Tab. Bot. 30s, 100s, 250s. *c-iv.*
Use: Anorexiant.

•**tepoxalin.** (teh-POX-ah-lin) USAN.
Use: Antipsoriatic.

•**teprotide.** (TEH-pro-tide) USAN.
Use: Angiotensin-converting enzyme inhibitor.

•**teprotumumab.** (TEP-roe-TOOM-oo-mab) USAN.
Use: Antineoplastic.

tequinol sodium. *Name used for Actinoquinol Sodium.*

Tera-Gel. (Geritrex) Coal tar 0.5%. EDTA, parabens. Shampoo. 114 mL. *OTC.*
Use: Photochemotherapy.

Terak. (Akorn) Polymyxin B sulfate 10,000 units/g, oxytetracycline hydrochloride 5 mg/g, white and liquid petrolatum. Ophth. Oint. Tube 3.5 g. *Rx.*
Use: Anti-infective, ophthalmic.

Terazol 7. (Ortho-McNeil) Terconazole 0.4%, cetyl alcohol, stearyl alcohol. Vag. Cream. Tube 45 g w/1 measured-dose applicator. *Rx.*
Use: Antifungal, vaginal.

Terazol 3. (Ortho-McNeil) **Cream, vaginal:** Terconazole 0.8%. Tube 20 g with 1 measured-dose applicator. **Supp., vaginal:** Terconazole 80 mg, coconut oil/palm kernel oil. 2.5 g. 3s. *Rx.*
Use: Antifungal, vaginal.

•**terazosin hydrochloride.** (ter-AZ-oh-sin) USP 34.

Use: Antihypertensive, antiadrenergic.
See: Hytrin.

terazosin hydrochloride. (Geneva) Terazosin 1 mg, 2 mg, 5 mg, 10 mg (as base). Tab. Bot. 100s, 1000s. *Rx.*
Use: Antiadrenergic.

terazosin hydrochloride. (Various Mfr.) Terazosin hydrochloride 1 mg, 2 mg, 5 mg, 10 mg (as base), may contain lactose. Cap. Bot. 100s, 500s. *Rx.*
Use: Antiadrenergic.

•**terbinafine.** (TER-bin-ah-feen) USAN.
Use: Antifungal.
See: Terbinex.

terbinafine hydrochloride.
Use: Antifungal, allylamine.
See: Lamisil.
Lamisil AT.

terbinafine hydrochloride. (Taro) Terbinafine hydrochloride 1%. Benzyl alcohol, cetyl alcohol, stearyl alcohol. Cream. 24 g. *OTC.*
Use: Topical anti-infective, antifungal agent.

terbinafine hydrochloride. (Various Mfr.) Terbinafine hydrochloride 250 mg. May contain lactose. Tab. 30s, 90s, 100s, 500s. *Rx.*
Use: Antifungal agent, allylamine antifungal.

Terbinex. (JSJ Pharmaceuticals) Terbinafine 250 mg. Tab. Kit w/ 42 tablets and 12 mL topical Eco Formula.
Use: Antifungal agent, allylamine antifungal.

•**terbutaline sulfate.** (ter-BYOO-tuh-leen) USP 34.
Use: Bronchodilator, sympathomimetic.

terbutaline sulfate. (Various Mfr.) Terbutaline sulfate 1 mg/mL. Inj. Vials. 1 mL single-use. *Rx.*
Use: Bronchodilator, sympathomimetic.

terbutaline sulfate. (Global) Terbutaline sulfate 2.5 mg, 5 mg. Tab. Bot. 100s. *Rx.*
Use: Bronchodilator, sympathomimetic.

Tercodryl. (Health for Life Brands) Codeine phos. 0.75 g, pyrilamine maleate 25 mg/fl. oz. Bot. 4 oz. *c-v.*
Use: Antihistamine, antitussive.

•**terconazole.** (ter-CONE-uh-zole) USAN.
Formerly triaconazole.
Use: Antifungal.
See: Terazol 7.
Terazol 3.

terconazole. (Perrigo) Terconazole 80 mg. Vag. Supp. 3s with applicator. *Rx.*
Use: Vaginal antifungal agent.

terconazole. (Various Mfr.) Terconazole 0.4%, 0.8%. Alcohols. Vaginal cream.

Tube. 20 g (0.8 % only), 45 g (0.4% only). *Rx.*
Use: Vaginal antifungal agent.

Terg-A-Zyme. (Alconox) Detergent with enzyme action. Box 4 lb Ctn. 9 × 4 lb, 25 lb, 50 lb, 100 lb, 300 lb. *OTC.*
Use: Biodegradable detergent and wetting agent.

Teridol Jr. (Health for Life Brands) Terpin hydrate, cocillana, potassium guaiacol sulfonate, ammonium chloride. Bot. 3 oz. *OTC.*
Use: Expectorant.

•**teriparatide.** (ter-i-PAR-a-tide) USAN.
Use: Parathyroid hormone.
See: Forteo.

•**terlakiren.** (ter-lah-KIE-ren) USAN.
Use: Antihypertensive.

•**terlipressin.** (TER-li-PRES-in) USAN.
Use: Investigational posterior pituitary hormone; treatment of bleeding esophageal varices; vasoconstrictor. [Orphan Drug]
See: Glypressin.

Terocin. (Alexso) Capsaicin 0.025%, lidocaine 2.5%, menthol 10%, methyl salicylate 25%. Aloe, borago seed oil, cetyl alcohol, parabens, PEG, propylene glycol, triethanolamine. Lot. 120 mL. *OTC.*
Use: Topical local anesthetic combination.

•**terodiline hydrochloride.** (TEH-row-DIE-leen) USAN.
Use: Vasodilator, coronary.

•**teroxalene hydrochloride.** (ter-OX-ah-leen) USAN.
Use: Antischistosomal.

•**teroxirone.** (TER-OX-ih-rone) USAN.
Use: Antineoplastic.

Terpex Jr. (Health for Life Brands) d-Methorphan 25 mg, terpin hydrate, potassium guaiacol sulfonate, cocillana, ammonium chloride. Bot. 4 oz. *OTC.*
Use: Expectorant.

Terphan. (Pal-Pak, Inc.) Terpin hydrate 85 mg, dextromethorphan hydrobromide 10 mg/5 mL w/alcohol 40% Elix. Bot. Gal. *OTC.*
Use: Antitussive, expectorant.

•**terpin hydrate and codeine oral solution.** (TER-pin) *USP 34.*
Use: Expectorant, antitussive.

•**terpin hydrate oral solution.** (TER-pin) *USP 34.*
Use: Expectorant.

Terra-Cortril. (Pfizer) Hydrocortisone 1.5%, oxytetracycline hydrochloride 0.5%. Ophth. Susp. Bot. 5 mL. *Rx.*
Use: Anti-infective, corticosteroid, ophthalmic.

Terramycin w/Polymyxin B Sulfate. (Pfizer) Polymyxin B sulfate 10,000 units/g, oxytetracycline hydrochloride 5 mg/g, white and liquid petrolatum. Ophth. Oint. Tube 3.5 g. *Rx.*
Use: Anti-infective.

Terrell. (Minrad) Isoflurane. Liq. for Inh. 100 mL, 250 mL. *Rx.*
Use: General anesthetic.

Tersaseptic. (Doak Dermatologics) DEA-lauryl sulfate, lauramide DEA, propylene glycol, ethoxydiglycol, PEG-12 distearate, EDTA, triclosan, citric acid/ Shampoo/cleanser. Soapless. 473 mL. *OTC.*
Use: Dermatologic, acne.

tersavid.
Use: Monoamine oxidase inhibitor.

tertiary amyl alcohol.
See: Amylene Hydrate.

•**tesamorelin.** (TES-ah-moe-REL-in) USAN.
Use: Growth hormone–releasing factor.
See: Egrifta.

•**tesicam.** (TESS-ih-kam) USAN.
Use: Anti-inflammatory.

•**tesimide.** (TESS-ih-mide) USAN.
Use: Anti-inflammatory.

Tesogen. (Sigma-Tau) Testosterone 25 mg, estrone 2 mg/mL. Vial 10 mL. *c-III.*
Use: Androgen.

Tesogen L.A. (Sigma-Tau) Testosterone enanthate 180 mg, 90 mg, 50 mg, estradiol valerate 8 mg, 4 mg, 2 mg, respectively/mL. Vial 10 mL. *Rx.*
Use: Androgen, estrogen combination.

tespa.
Use: Antineoplastic.
See: Thiotepa.

Tessalon. (Pfizer) Benzonatate 200 mg. Parabens. Cap. Bot. 100s, 500s. *Rx.*
Use: Nonnarcotic antitussive.

Tessalon Perles. (Pfizer) Benzonatate 100 mg. Parabens. Cap. Bot. 100s, 500s. *Rx.*
Use: Nonnarcotic antitussive.

Testamone. (Oxypure) Testosterone 100 mg/mL. Inj. Vial 10 mL. *c-III.*
Use: Androgen.

Testex. (Taylor Pharmaceuticals) Testosterone propionate 50 mg, 100 mg/mL in sesame oil. Vial 10 mL. *c-III.*
Use: Androgen.

Testim. (Auxilium Pharm) Testosterone 1%. Ethanol 74%, glycerin. Gel. 5 g. *c-III.*
Use: Sex hormone, androgen.

Testoject-50. (Merz) Testosterone 50 mg/mL. Vial 10 mL. *c-III.*
Use: Androgen.

Testoject-LA. (Merz) Testosterone cypionate 200 mg/mL in oil. Vial 10 mL. *c-III.*
Use: Androgen.

•**testolactone.** (TESS-toe-LAK-tone) *USP 34.*
Use: Antineoplastic; sex hormone, androgen.

Testolin. (Taylor Pharmaceuticals) Testosterone suspension 25 mg, 50 mg, 100 mg/mL. Vial 10 mL 25 mg/mL. Vial 30 mL. *c-III.*
Use: Androgen.

Testopel. (Slate Pharmaceuticals) Testosterone 75 mg for subcutaneous administration. Pellets. 1 Pellet/Vial. Box 3s, 10s, 100s. *c-III.*
Use: Sex hormone, androgen.

•**testosterone.** (tess-TAHS-ter-ohn) *USP 34.*
Use: Androgen, sex hormone.
See: Androderm.
  AndroGel 1%.
  Andronaq-50.
  Fortesta.
  Homogene-S.
  Malotrone.
  Striant.
  Testim.
  Testolin.
  Testopel.
W/Combinations.
See: Andesterone.
  Angen.
  Tesogen.

testosterone. 2%. Oint.
Use: Vulvar dystrophies. [Orphan Drug]

testosterone, buccal.
Use: Androgen, sex hormone.
See: Striant.

testosterone cyclopentane propionate.
Testosterone Cypionate.

•**testosterone cypionate.** (tess-TAHS-ter-ohn) *USP 34.*
Use: Androgen, sex hormone.
See: Depo-Testosterone.
W/Combinations.
See: Depo-Testadiol.
  Menoject L.A.

testosterone cypionate. (Sandoz) Testosterone cypionate 100 mg/mL. Benzyl alcohol 9.45 mg, benzyl benzoate 0.1 mL, cottonseed oil 736 mg. Inj. Vials. 10 mL. *c-III.*
Use: Sex hormone, androgen.

testosterone cypionate. (Various Mfr.) Testosterone cypionate 200 mg/mL. Benzyl alcohol, cottonseed oil. Inj. Vials. 1 mL, 10 mL. *c-III.*
Use: Sex hormone, androgen.

•**testosterone enanthate.** (tess-TAHS-ter-ohn) *USP 34.*
Use: Sex hormone, androgen.
See: Delatestryl.
W/Estradiol Valerate.
See: Valertest.

testosterone enanthate. (Paddock) Testosterone enanthate 200 mg/mL. Sesame oil. Inj. Multiple-dose vials. 5 mL. *c-III.*
Use: Androgen, sex hormone.

testosterone heptanoate.
Use: Androgen.
See: Testosterone Enanthate.

•**testosterone ketolaurate.** (tess-TAHS-ter-ohn KEY-toe-LORE-ate) USAN.
Use: Androgen.

•**testosterone phenylacetate.** (tess-TAHS-ter-ohn fen-ill-ASS-ah-tate) USAN. Perandren phenylacetate.
Use: Androgen.

•**testosterone propionate.** (tess-TAHS-ter-ohn) *USP 34.*
Use: Androgen.

testosterone, transdermal.
Use: Sex hormone, androgen.
See: Androderm.

•**testosterone undecanoate.** (tess-TAHS-ter-ohn un-DEK-a-NOE-ate) USAN.
Use: Androgen.

Testred. (Valeant) Methyltestosterone 10 mg. Cap. Bot. 100s. *c-III.*
Use: Sex hormone, androgen.

Testuria. (Wyeth) Combination kit containing 5 × 20 sterile dip strips and 5 × 20 culture trays of trypticase soy agar.
Use: Diagnostic aid.

Tesuloid. (Bristol-Myers Squibb) Technetium Tc 99m sulfur colloid. 5 Vials. Kit.
Use: Radiopaque agent.

•**tetanus and diphtheria toxoids adsorbed for adult use.** (TET-ah-nus and diff-THEER-ee-uh TOX-oyds) *USP 34.*
Use: Immunization.
See: Decavac.

tetanus and diphtheria toxoids adsorbed purogenated. (Wyeth) Tetanus and diphtheria toxoids adsorbed purogenated. Adult *Lederject* disposable syringe 10 × 0.5 mL. Vial 5 mL, new package. *Rx.*
Use: Immunization.

tetanus and diphtheria toxoids and acellular pertussis vaccine, adsorbed.
Use: Immunization.
See: Adacel.
  Boostrix.
  Daptacel.

Infanrix.
TriHIBit.
Tripedia.

tetanus, diphtheria, acellular pertussis, Haemophilus influenzae type B conjugate vaccine.
Use: Immunization.
See: TriHIBit.

tetanus, diphtheria toxoids, and aluminum phosphate adsorbed. (Wyeth) Tetanus, diphtheria toxoids, and aluminum phosphate adsorbed. Inj. Vial 5 mL, *Tubex* 0.5 mL. *Rx.*
Use: Immunization.

•**tetanus immune globulin.** (TET-ah-nus ih-MYOON GLAH-byoo-lin) *USP 34. Formerly Tetanus Immune Human Globulin.* Gamma globulin fraction of the plasma of persons who have been hyperimmunized with tetanus toxoid, 16.5%. Vial 250 units.
Use: Prophylaxis of injured, against tetanus (passive immunizing agent).

•**tetanus toxoid.** (TET-n-us TOX-oyd) *USP 34.*
Use: Immunization.

•**tetanus toxoid, adsorbed.** (TET-n-us TOX-oyd) *USP 34.*
Use: Immunization.

tetanus toxoid, aluminum phosphate adsorbed. *Rx.*
Use: Immunization.

Tetcaine. (Ocusoft) Tetracaine hydrochloride 0.5%. Chlorobutanol 0.4%, sodium chloride 0.75%. Soln. 15 mL. *Rx.*
Use: Ophthalmic local anesthetic.

tetiothalein sodium.
See: Iodophthalein Sodium.

Tetrabead. (Abbott Diagnostics) Solid phase radioimmunoassay for the quantitative measurement of total circulating serum thyroxine.
Use: Diagnostic aid.

Tetrabead-125. (Abbott Diagnostics) T-3 uptake radioassay for the measurement of thyroid function by indirectly determining the degree of saturation of serum thyroxine binding globulin (TBG).
Use: Diagnostic aid.

tetrabenazine.
See: Xenazine.

•**tetracaine.** (TEH-trah-cane) *USP 34.*
Use: Anesthetic (topical).
W/Lidocaine.
See: Pliaglis.
Synera.

tetracaine. (Akorn) Tetracaine hydrochloride 1%. Sodium chloride 7.5 mg. Preservative free. Inj., Soln. Amp. 2 mL. *Rx.*

Use: Injectable local anesthetic, ester local anesthetic.

tetracaine and menthol ointment.
Use: Anesthetic, local.

•**tetracaine hydrochloride.** (TEH-trahcane) *USP 34.*
Use: Anesthetic, injectable local ester; ophthalmic local anesthetic.
See: Altacaine.
Pontocaine.
Pontocaine Hydrochloride.
W/Benzocaine, Butamben, Benzalkonium Chloride.
See: Cetacaine.

tetracaine hydrochloride. (Various Mfr.) Tetracaine hydrochloride 0.5%. Soln. 1 mL, 2 mL, 15 mL. *Rx.*
Use: Anesthetic; ophthalmic.

Tetracap. (Circle) Tetracycline hydrochloride 250 mg. Cap. Bot. 100s. *Rx.*
Use: Anti-infective, tetracycline.

tetrachlorethylene. Perchlorethylene, tetrachlorethylene.
Use: Anthelmintic (hookworms and some trematodes).

Tetracon. (Professional Pharmacal) Tetrahydrozoline hydrochloride 0.5 mg, disodium edetate 1 mg, boric acid 12 mg, benzalkonium chloride 0.1 mg, sodium chloride 2.2 mg, sodium borate 0.5 mg/mL w/water. Liq. Bot. 15 mL. *OTC.*
Use: Anti-irritant; ophthalmic.

tetracyclic compounds.
Use: Antidepressant.
See: Maprotiline Hydrochloride.
Mirtazapine.

•**tetracycline and amphotericin B.** (tehtrah-SIGH-kleen) *USP 34.*

•**tetracycline hydrochloride.** (teh-trahSIGH-kleen) *USP 34.*
Use: Anti-infective; antiamebic; antirickettsial.
See: Bicycline.
Cyclopar.
Panmycin.
Sumycin.
Tetracap.
Tetracyn.
W/Bismuth Subcitrate Potassium, Metronidazole.
See: Pylera.
W/Diphenhydramine Hydrochloride, Hydrocortisone, Nystatin.
See: First Mary's Mouthwash.

tetracycline hydrochloride. (Various Mfr.) Tetracycline hydrochloride 250 mg. 500 mg. Cap. Bot. 100s, 1000s, UD 100s. *Rx.*
Use: Anti-infective, antiamebic, antirickettsial.

•**tetracycline oral suspension.** (teh-trah-SIGH-kleen) *USP 34.*
Use: Anti-infective, tetracycline.

•**tetracycline phosphate complex.** (teh-trah-SIGH-kleen) *USP 34.*
Use: Anti-infective.

tetracyclines.
See: Demeclocycline Hydrochloride.
Doxycycline.
Minocycline Hydrochloride.
Oxytetracycline.
Tetracycline Hydrochloride.

tetracycline with n-acetyl-para-amino-phenol, phenyltoloxamine citrate.
(Roberts) Paltet, Cap.
Use: Anti-infective, tetracycline.

Tetracyn. (Pfizer) Tetracycline hydrochloride. Cap. **250 mg:** Bot. 1000s. **500 mg:** Bot. 100s. *Rx.*
Use: Anti-infective, tetracycline.

tetradecyl sulfate, sodium.
Use: Sclerosing agent.
See: Sotradecol.

tetraethyl ammonium bromide (TEAB).
Use: Diagnostic & therapeutic agent in peripheral vascular disorders. Diagnostic in hypertension.

tetraethylammonium chloride.
Use: Ganglionic blocking.

tetraethylthiuram disulfide.
See: Disulfiram.

•**tetrafilcon A.** (teh-trah-FILL-kahn) USAN.
Use: Contact lens material (hydrophilic).

tetrafluoroethane.
W/Pentafluoropropane.
See: Gebauer's Spray and Stretch.

Tetra-Formula. (Reese Pharm) Dextromethorphan HBr 10 mg, benzocaine 15 mg. Sucrose, glucose, dextrose. Loz. Pkg. 10s. *OTC.*
Use: Nonnarcotic antitussive.

tetrahydroaminoacridine.
Use: Cholinergic agent for Alzheimer disease.
See: Cognex.

tetrahydrophenobarbital calcium.
See: Cyclobarbital Calcium.

tetrahydroxyquinone. *Name used for tetroquinone.*

•**tetrahydrozoline hydrochloride.** (teh-trah-high-DRAHZ-ah-leen) *USP 34.*
Use: Adrenergic (vasoconstrictor); nasal decongestant, imidazoline; ophthalmic decongestant.
See: Altazine.
Murine Plus.
Opti-Clear.
Optigene 3.
Tyzine.
Tyzine Pediatric.
Visine.
Visine Advanced Relief.
Visine Allergy Relief.
Visine Maximum Redness Relief.

tetrahydrozoline hydrochloride.
(Various Mfr.) Tetrahydrozoline hydrochloride 0.05%. Ophth. Soln. 15 mL. *OTC.*
Use: Ophthalmic decongestant.

tetraiodophenolphthalein sodium.
See: Iodophthalein Sodium.

tetraiodophthalein sodium.
See: Iodophthalein Sodium.

tetramethylene dimethanesulfonate.
Busulfan.

tetramethylthiuram disulfide. Thiram.
Use: Anti-infective; antifungal.

•**tetramisole hydrochloride.** (teh-TRAM-ih-sole) USAN.
Use: Anthelmintic.

Tetraneed. (Hanlon) Pentaerythritol tetranitrate 80 mg. Time Cap. Bot. 100s. *Rx.*
Use: Antianginal.

tetrantoin.
Use: Anticonvulsant.

Tetratab. (Freeport) Pentaerythritol tetranitrate 10 mg. Tab. Bot. 1000s. *Rx.*
Use: Antianginal.

Tetratab No. 1. (Freeport) Pentaerythritol tetranitrate 20 mg. Tab. Bot. 1000s. *Rx.*
Use: Antianginal.

•**tetraxetan.** (te-TRAX-e-tan) USAN.
Use: Chelating agent.

•**tetrazolast meglumine.** (teh-TRAZZ-oh-last meh-GLUE-meen) USAN.
Use: Antiallergic; antiasthmatic.

Tetrazyme. (Abbott Diagnostics) Test kit 100s, 500s.
Use: Enzyme immunoassay for quantitative measurement of total circulating serum thyroxine (free and protein bound).

Tetrix. (Coria) Aluminum magnesium hydroxide stearate, cetyl dimethicone copolyol, cyclomethicone, dimethicone, hexyl laurate, polyglyceryl-4 isostearate, sodium chloride. Propylparabens. Cream. Kit w/two 56.7 g tubes and two 56.7 g tubes of *CaraVe* moisturizing cream. *Rx.*
Use: Miscellaneous topical combination.

•**tetrofosmin.** (teh-troe-FOSS-min) USAN.
Use: Diagnostic aid.

•**tetroquinone.** (TEH-troe-kwih-NOHN) USAN.
Use: Treat keloids, keratolytic (systemic).

•**tetroxoprim.** (tet-ROX-oh-prim) USAN.
Use: Anti-infective.

•**tetrydamine.** (teh-TRID-ah-meen) USAN.
Use: Analgesic; anti-inflammatory.

Tetterine. (S.S.S. Company) Miconazole nitrate 2%. Petrolatum. Oint. 28.4 g. *OTC.*
Use: Topical anti-infective, antifungal agent.

Teveten. (Abbott) Eprosartan mesylate 400 mg, 600 mg. Lactose, PEG. Film-coated. Tab. 100s. *Rx.*
Use: Antihypertensive.

Teveten HCT. (Abbott Laboratories) Eprosartan/hydrochlorothiazide 600 mg/12.5 mg. Lactose. Film-coated. Tab. 100s. *Rx.*
Use: Antihypertensive.

Tev-Tropin. (Gate) Somatropin 5 mg (≈ 15 units)/vial. Mannitol 30 mg. Pow. for Inj., lyophilized. Vials w/5 mL diluent (bacteriostatic sodium chloride 0.9% for injection w/benzyl alcohol 0.9%). *Rx.*
Use: Growth hormone.

Texacort. (Tiber Labs) Hydrocortisone 2.5%. Alcohol. Lipid free. Soln. 30 mL. *Rx.*
Use: Corticosteroid.

tezacitabine.
Use: Antineoplastic.

•**tezampanel.** (tez-AM-pan-el) USAN.
Use: Treatment of migraines.

tezosentan.
Use: Dual endothelin receptor antagonist.

T-Fluoride. (Tennessee Pharmaceutic) Sodium fluoride 2.21 mg. Tab. Bot. 100s, 1000s. *Rx.*
Use: Dental caries preventative.

T4. Levothyroxine Sodium.

T4 endonuclease V, liposome encapsulated.
Use: Xeroderma pigmentosum. [Orphan Drug]

T-4 RIA (PEG). (Abbott Diagnostics) Diagnostic kit 50s, 100s, 500s. *Rx.*
Use: For quantitative measurement of total circulating serum thyroxine.

T4, soluble, human recombinant. (Biogen) Phase I/II HIV.
Use: Antiviral.

TG.
Use: Antineoplastic.
See: Thioguanine.

T/Gel Scalp. (Neutrogena) Neutar coal tar extract 2%, salicylic acid 2%. Soln. Bot. 2 oz. *OTC.*
Use: Antipsoriatic; antiseborrheic.

T/Gel Therapeutic Conditioner. (Neutrogena) Neutar coal tar extract 1.5% in oil free conditioner base. Liq. Bot. 1.4 oz. *OTC.*
Use: Antipsoriatic; antiseborrheic.

T/Gel Therapeutic Shampoo. (Neutrogena) Neutar coal tar extract 2% in mild shampoo base. Bot. 4.4 oz., 8.5 oz. *OTC.*
Use: Antipsoriatic; antiseborrheic.

T-Gesic. (T.E. Williams Pharmaceuticals) Hydrocodone bitartrate 5 mg, acetaminophen 500 mg. Cap. Bot. 100s. *c-III.*
Use: Analgesic combination; narcotic; hypnotic; sedative.

TGQ 15DM/5PEH/2CPM. (TG United Pharmaceuticals) Chlorpheniramine maleate 2 mg, dextromethorphan hydrobromide 15 mg, phenylephrine hydrochloride 5 mg. Parabens, potassium citrate, potassium sorbate, propylene glycol, sorbitol, sucralose. Strawberry flavor. Liq. 473 mL. *Rx.*
Use: Upper respiratory combination, antitussive combination.

TGQ 50PSE/3BRM/30DM. (TG United Pharmaceuticals) Brompheniramine maleate 3 mg, dextromethorphan hydrobromide 30 mg, pseudoephedrine hydrochloride 50 mg per 5 mL. Parabens, potassium sorbate, propylene glycol, sorbitol, sucralose. Berry-vanilla flavor. Syrup. 473 mL. *Rx.*
Use: Upper respiratory combination, antitussive combination.

TGQ 40PSE/4BRM/20DM. (TG United Pharmaceuticals) Brompheniramine maleate 4 mg, dextromethorphan hydrobromide 20 mg, pseudoephedrine hydrochloride 40 mg. Tab. 100s. *Rx.*
Use: Upper respiratory combination, antitussive combination.

TGQ 7.5PEH/4BRM/15DM. (TG United Pharmaceuticals) Brompheniramine maleate 4 mg, dextromethorphan hydrobromide 15 mg, phenylephrine hydrochloride 7.5 mg per 5 mL. Parabens, potassium sorbate, propylene glycol, sorbitol, sucralose. Strawberry flavor. Liq. 473 mL. *Rx.*
Use: Upper respiratory combination, antitussive combination.

TGQ 30PSE/150GFN/15DM. (TG United Pharmaceuticals) Dextromethorphan hydrobromide 15 mg, guaifenesin 150 mg, pseudoephedrine hydrochloride 30 mg. Saccharin, sorbitol. Alcohol free. Mint flavor. Liq. 30 mL, 473 mL. *Rx.*
Use: Upper respiratory combination, antitussive and expectorant combination.

TGQ 30PSE/3BRM/15DM. (TG United Pharmaceuticals) Brompheniramine

maleate 3 mg, dextromethorphan hydrobromide 15 mg, pseudoephedrine hydrochloride 30 mg per 5 mL. Parabens, potassium sorbate, propylene glycol, sorbitol, sucralose. Berry-vanilla flavor. Liq. 473 mL. *Rx.*
Use: Upper respiratory combination, antitussive combination.

•**thalidomide.** (the-LID-oh-mide) USAN.
Use: Anti-infective; hypnotic; sedative; immunomodulator.
See: Thalomid.

Thalitone. (Monarch) Chlorthalidone 15 mg. Lactose. Tab. Bot. 100s. *Rx.*
Use: Diuretic.

•**thallous chloride Tl 201 injection.** (THAL-uhs) *USP 34.*
Use: Diagnostic aid (radiopaque medium); radioactive agent.

Thalomid. (Celgene) Thalidomide 50 mg, 100 mg, 200 mg. Cap. Blister packs. 28s, 84s (200 mg only), 140s (100 mg only), 280s (50 mg only). *Rx.*
Note: Available only to be prescribed and dispensed under the terms of the System for Thalidomide Education and Prescribing Safety (S.T.E.P.S.) restricted distribution program.
Use: Immunomodulator.

Tham. (Abbott) Tromethamine 18 g, acetic acid 2.5 g single-dose container. Soln. *Rx.*
Use: Nutritional supplement.

Tham-E. (Abbott) Tromethamine 36 g, NaCl 30 mEq/L, KCl 5 mEq/L, Cl 35 mEq/L. Total osmolarity 367 mOsm/L. Single-dose container 150 mL. *Rx.*
Use: Nutritional supplement.

theamin. Monoethanolamine salt of theophylline.

thenalidine tartrate.
Use: Antihistamine; antipruritic.

thenyldiamine hydrochloride.
Use: Antihistamine.

theobroma oil. Cocoa Butter.
Use: Pharmaceutical aid; suppository base.

theobromine sodium acetate. Theobromine calcium salt mixture with calcium salicylate.
Use: Diuretic; muscle relaxant.

Theochron. (Forest) Theophylline 100 mg, 200 mg, 300 mg, 450 mg. ER Tab. 100s. 500s (200 mg, 300 mg, 450 mg), 1,000s. *Rx.*
Use: Bronchodilator.

•**theofibrate.** (thee-oh-FYE-brate) USAN.
Use: Antihyperlipoproteinemic.

Theogen. (Sigma-Tau) Conjugated estrogens 2 mg/mL. Vial 10 mL, 30 mL. *Rx.*
Use: Estrogen.

Theogen I.P. (Sigma-Tau) Estrone 2 mg, potassium estrone sulfate 1 mg/mL. Inj. Vial 10 mL. *Rx.*
Use: Estrogen.

Theophenyllin. (H.L. Moore Drug Exchange) Theophylline 130 mg, ephedrine hydrochloride 24 mg, phenobarbital 8 mg. Tab. Bot. 1000s. *Rx.*
Use: Antiasthmatic.

•**theophylline.** (thee-AHF-ih-lin) *USP 34.*
Use: Bronchodilator; coronary vasodilator, diuretic; pharmaceutic necessity for Aminophylline Injection.
See: Elixophyllin.
    Theo-24.
    Theochron.
    Uniphyl.
W/Combinations.
See: Ceepa.
    Co-Xan.
    Neoasma.
    Quibron Plus.
    Tedral SA.
W/Guaifenesin.
See: Ed-Bron G.

theophylline. (Inwood) Theophylline 125 mg, 200 mg. ER Cap. 100s. *Rx.*
Use: Bronchodilator.

theophylline. (Various Mfr.) Theophylline 100 mg, 200 mg, 300 mg, 450 mg. ER Tab. 100s, 500s (200 mg, 300 mg), 1,000s (200 mg, 450 mg). *Rx.*
Use: Bronchodilator.

theophylline aminoisobutanol. Theophylline w/2-amino-2-methyl-1-propanol.
See: Butaphyllamine.

theophylline, 8-chloro, diphenhydramine. Dimenhydrinate.
See: Dramamine.

theophylline ethylenediamine.
See: Aminophylline.

theophylline in dextrose 5%. (Various Mfr.) Theophylline 0.8 mg/mL, 1.6 mg/mL, 2 mg/mL, 3.2 mg/mL, 4 mg/mL. Inj., Soln. 50 mL (4 mg/mL), 100 mL (2 mg/mL, 4 mg/mL), 250 mL (1.6 mg/mL, 3.2 mg/mL), 500 mL (0.8 mg/mL, 1.6 mg/mL), 1,000 mL (0.8 mg/mL). *Rx.*
Use: Bronchodilator.

theophylline olamine. Theophylline compound with 2-amino-ethanol (1:1).
Use: Bronchodilator.

theophylline reagent strips. (Bayer Consumer Care) Seralyzer reagent strip. Bot. 25s.
Use: Diagnostic aid; theophylline.

•**theophylline sodium glycinate.** (thee-AHF-ih-lin) *USP 34.*

Use: Bronchodilator.
See: Synophylate.

Theo-24. (UCB Pharma) Theophylline 100 mg, 200 mg, 300 mg, 400 mg. Sucrose. ER Cap. Bot. 100s, 500s (200 mg and 300 mg only). *Rx.*
Use: Antiasthmatic; bronchodilator.

Thera Bath. (Walgreen) Mineral oil 90%. Bot. 16 oz. *OTC.*
Use: Emollient.

Thera Bath with Vitamin E. (Walgreen) Mineral oil 91%, Vit. E 2000 units/ 16 oz. *OTC.*
Use: Emollient.

Therabid. (Mission Pharmacal) Vitamins C 500 mg, B_1 15 mg, B_2 10 mg, B_3 100 mg, B_5 20 mg, B_6 10 mg, B_{12} 5 mcg, A 5000 units, D 200 units, E 30 mg. Tab. Bot. 60s. *OTC.*
Use: Mineral, vitamin supplement.

Therabrand. (Health for Life Brands) Vitamins A 25,000 units, D 1000 units, B_1 10 mg, B_2 10 mg, niacinamide 100 mg, C 200 mg, B_6 5 mg, calcium pantothenate 20 mg, B_{12} 5 mcg. Cap. Bot. 100s, 1000s. *OTC.*
Use: Mineral, vitamin supplement.

Therabrand-M. (Health for Life Brands) Vitamins A 25,000 units, D 1000 units, C 200 mg, B_1 10 mg, B_2 10 mg, B_6 5 mg, niacinamide 100 mg, calcium pantothenate 20 mg, E 5 units, B_{12} 5 mcg, I 0.15 mg, Fe 15 mg, Cu 1 mg, Ca 125 mg, Mn 1 mg, Mg 6 mg, Zn 1.5 mg. Cap. Bot. 100s, 1000s. *OTC.*
Use: Mineral, vitamin supplement.

Theracap. (Arcum) Vitamins A 10,000 units, D 400 units, B_1 10 mg, B_2 5 mg, niacinamide 150 mg, C 150 mg. Cap. Bot. 100s, 1000s. *OTC.*
Use: Vitamin supplement.

Thera-Combex H-P. (Parke-Davis) Vitamins C 500 mg, B_1 25 mg, B_2 15 mg, B_{12} 5 mcg, niacinamide 100 mg, panthenol 20 mg. Cap. Bot. 100s. *OTC.*
Use: Vitamin supplement.

TheraCys. (Sanofi Pasteur) BCG live (for intravesical administration) 10.5 ± 8.7 × 10^8 CFU (equivalent to ≈ 81 mg dry weight). Monosodium glutamate. Preservative free. Inj., Lyophilized, Pow. for Susp. Vials. 81 mg w/3 mL diluent vial. *Rx.*
Use: Biological response modifier.

Theraflu Cold & Cough. (Novartis Consumer) Dextromethorphan HBr 20 mg, pheniramine maleate 20 mg, phenylephrine hydrochloride 10 mg. Acesulfame K, maltodextrin, sodium 43 mg. Pow. Pkt. 6s. *Rx.*

Use: Upper respiratory combination, antitussive combination.

Theraflu Cold & Sore Throat. (Novartis) Phenylephrine hydrochloride 10 mg, pheniramine maleate 20 mg, acetaminophen 325 mg. Acesulfame K, sucrose, sodium 44 mg. Lemon flavor. Pow. 6s. *OTC.*
Use: Upper respiratory combination, decongestant, antihistamine, and analgesic.

Theraflu Daytime Severe Cold & Cough. (Novartis) **Cap.:** Acetaminophen 325 mg, dextromethorphan HBr 10 mg, phenylephrine hydrochloride 5 mg. PEG. 24s. **Pow.:** Acetaminophen 650 mg, dextromethorphan hydrobromide 20 mg, phenylephrine hydrochloride 10 mg. Acesulfame K, aspartame, maltodextrin, phenylalanine 14 mg, sucrose. Berry infused with menthol and green tea flavor. 6s. *OTC.*
Use: Upper respiratory combination, analgesic, antitussive, decongestant combination.

Theraflu Flu & Chest Congestion. (Novartis) Guaifenesin 400 mg, acetaminophen 1,000 mg. Acesulfame K, aspartame, maltodextrin, phenylalanine 24 mg/packet, sodium 15 mg/packet, sucrose. Citrus flavor. Pow. 6s. *OTC.*
Use: Upper respiratory combination, expectorant with analgesic combination.

Theraflu Flu & Sore Throat. (Novartis) Phenylephrine hydrochloride 10 mg, pheniramine maleate 20 mg, acetaminophen 650 mg. Acesulfame K, sucrose, sodium 51 mg. Apple cinnamon flavor. Pow. 6s. *OTC.*
Use: Upper respiratory combination, decongestant, antihistamine, and analgesic.

Theraflu Nighttime Severe Cold. (Novartis) Acetaminophen 325 mg, chlorpheniramine maleate 2 mg, dextromethorphan HBr 10 mg, phenylephrine hydrochloride 5 mg. Acesulfame potassium, PEG. Tab. 24s. *OTC.*
Use: Upper respiratory combination, decongestant, analgesic, antihistamine, antitussive combination.

Theraflu Nighttime Severe Cough & Cold. (Novartis) Acetaminophen 650 mg, diphenhydramine hydrochloride 25 mg, phenylephrine hydrochloride 10 mg. Acesulfame K, aspartame, maltodextrin, phenylalanine 13 mg, sucrose. Honey lemon flavor infused with chamomile and white tea. Pow. 6s. *OTC.*

Use: Upper respiratory combination; decongestant, antihistamine, and analgesic combination.

Thera-Flur. (Colgate Oral Pharmaceuticals) Fluoride 0.5% (from sod. fluoride 1.1%). pH 4.5. Gel-Drops. Bot. 24 mL, 60 mL. *Rx.*
Use: Dental caries agent.

Thera-Flur-N. (Colgate Oral Pharmaceuticals) Neutral sodium fluoride 1.1%. Liq. Bot. 24 mL, 60 mL. *Rx.*
Use: Dental caries agent.

Theraflu Sugar-Free Nighttime Severe Cough & Cold. (Novartis) Acetaminophen 650 mg, diphenhydramine hydrochloride 25 mg, phenylephrine hydrochloride 10 mg. Acesulfame K, aspartame, maltodextrin, phenylalanine 13 mg. Sugar free. Honey lemon flavor. Pow. 6s. *OTC.*
Use: Upper respiratory combination; decongestant, antihistamine, and analgesic combination.

Theraflu Thin Strips Daytime Cough & Cold. (Novartis) Dextromethorphan HBr 20 mg, phenylephrine hydrochloride 10 mg. Alcohol < 5%, mannitol, sucralose. Cherry menthol flavor. Oral Strips. 12s. *OTC.*
Use: Upper respiratory combination, antitussive combination.

Theraflu Thin Strips Multi Symptom. (Novartis) Diphenhydramine hydrochloride 25 mg. Alcohol (less than 5%), sorbitol, sucralose. Cherry flavor. Orally Disintegrating Strips. 12s. *OTC.*
Use: Nonnarcotic antitussive.

Theraflu Thin Strips Nighttime Cold & Cough. (Novartis) Diphenhydramine hydrochloride 25 mg, phenylephrine hydrochloride 10 mg. Alcohol (less than 5%), mannitol, PEG, sucralose. Peppermint flavor. Orally Disintegrating Strips. 12s. *OTC.*
Use: Upper respiratory combination, decongestant and antihistamine.

Theraflu Warming Relief Daytime Multi-Symptom Cold. (Novartis) Acetaminophen 325 mg, dextromethorphan hydrobromide 10 mg, phenylephrine hydrochloride 5 mg. Benzoic acid, menthol, PEG, sucralose. Tab. 24s. *OTC.*
Use: Upper respiratory combination, antitussive combination.

Theraflu Warming Relief Flu & Sore Throat. (Novartis) Acetaminophen 108.3 mg, diphenhydramine hydrochloride 4.16 mg, phenylephrine hydrochloride 1.67 mg. Acesulfame K, alcohol 10%, edetate disodium, glycerin, malti-

tol, propylene glycol, sodium 2.3 mg, sodium benzoate. Cherry flavor. Liq. 245.5 mL. *OTC.*
Use: Upper respiratory combination; decongestant, antihistamine, and analgesic combination.

Therafortis. (General Vitamin) Vitamins A 12,500 units, D 1000 units, B_1 5 mg, B_2 5 mg, B_6 1 mg, B_{12} 3 mcg, niacinamide 50 mg, pantothenic acid salt 10 mg, C 150 mg, folic acid 0.5 mg. Cap. Bot. 100s, 1000s. *OTC.*
Use: Vitamin supplement.

Theragenerix. (Ivax) Vitamins A 5500 units, D 400 units, E 30 mg, B_1 3 mg, B_2 3.4 mg, B_3 30 mg, B_5 10 mg, B_6 3 mg, B_{12} 9 mcg, C 120 mg, folic acid 0.4 mg, biotin 15 mcg, beta-carotene 2500 units. Tab. Bot. 130s, 1000s. *OTC.*
Use: Vitamin supplement.

Theragenerix-H. (Ivax) Fe 66.7 mg, vitamins A 8333 units, D 133 units, E 5 units, B_1 3.3 mg, B_2 3.3 mg, B_3 33.3 mg, B_5 11.7 mg, B_6 3.3 mg, B_{12} 50 mcg, C 100 mg, folic acid 0.33 mg, Cu, Mg. Tab. Bot. 100s, 1000s. *OTC.*
Use: Mineral, vitamin supplement.

Theragenerix-M. (Ivax) Fe 27 mg, vitamins A 5000 units, D 400 units, E 30 mg, B_1 3 mg, B_2 3.4 mg, B_3 30 mg, B_5 10 mg, B_6 3 mg, B_{12} 9 mcg, C 120 mg, folic acid 0.4 mg, Ca, Cl, Cr, Cu, I, K, biotin 15 mcg, Mg, Mn, Mo, P, Se, Zn 15 mg, beta-carotene 2500 units. Tab. Bot. 130s, 1000s. *OTC.*
Use: Mineral, vitamin supplement.

Thera-Gesic. (Mission Pharmacal) Methyl salicylate, menthol. Balm. Tube 90 g, 150 g. *OTC.*
Use: Analgesic, topical.

Theragran. (Bristol-Myers Squibb) **Capl.:** Vitamins A 5000 units, D 400 units, E 30 units, B_1 3 mg, B_2 3.4 mg, B_3 20 mg, B_5 10 mg, B_6 3 mg, B_{12} 9 mcg, C 90 mg, folic acid 0.4 mg, biotin 30 mcg. Bot. 100s. **Liq.:** Vitamins A 5000 units, D 400 units, B_1 10 mg, B_2 10 mg, B_3 100 mg, B_5 21.4 mg, B_6 4.1 mg, B_{12} 5 mcg, C 200 mg/5 mL. Liq. Bot. 120 mL. *OTC.*
Use: Vitamin supplement.

Theragran AntiOxidant. (Bristol-Myers Squibb) Vitamins A 5000 units, C 250 mg, E 200 units, Mn, Cu, Zn, Se. Softgel Cap. Bot. 50s. *OTC.*
Use: Mineral, vitamin supplement.

Theragran Jr. with Iron. (Bristol-Myers Squibb) Fe 18 mg, vitamins A 5000 units, D 400 units, E 30 mg, B_1 1.5 mg, B_2 1.7 mg, B_3 20 mg, B_6 2 mg, B_{12} 6 mcg, C 60 mg, folic acid 0.4 mg

w/tartrazine. Tab. Bot. 75s. *OTC.*
Use: Mineral, vitamin supplement.

Theragran Stress Formula. (Bristol-Myers Squibb) Fe 27 mg, vitamins E 30 units, B_1 15 mg, B_2 15 mg, B_3 100 mg, B_5 20 mg, B_6 25 mg, B_{12} 12 mcg, C 600 mg, folic acid 0.4 mg, biotin 45 mcg. Tab. Bot. 75s. *OTC.*
Use: Mineral, vitamin supplement.

Thera Hematinic. (Major) Fe 66.7 mg, A 8333 units, D 133 units, E 5 units, B_1 3.3 mg, B_2 3.3 mg, B_3 33.3 mg, B_5 11.7 mg, B_6 3.3 mg, B_{12} 50 mcg, C 100 mg, folic acid 0.33 mg, Cu, Mg. Tab. Bot. 250s, 1000s. *OTC.*
Use: Mineral, vitamin supplements.

Thera-Hist Cold & Allergy. (Major) Pseudoephedrine hydrochloride 15 mg, chlorpheniramine maleate 1 mg/5 mL, sorbitol, sucrose. Syr. Bot. 118 mL. *OTC.*
Use: Upper respiratory combination, decongestant, antihistamine.

Thera-Hist Cold & Cough. (Major) Pseudoephedrine hydrochloride 15 mg, chlorpheniramine maleate 1 mg, dextromethorphan HBr 5 mg per 5 mL. Sorbitol, sucrose, cherry flavor. Syr. Bot. 118 mL. *OTC.*
Use: Upper respiratory combination, decongestant, antihistamine, antitussive.

Thera-M. (Various Mfr.) Vitamins A 5000 units, B_1 3 mg, B_2 3.4 mg, B_3 20 mg, B_5 10 mg, B_6 3 mg, B_{12} 9 mcg, C 90 mg, D 400 units, E 30 units, Fe 27 mg, folic acid 0.4 mg, biotin 30 mcg, P, Ca, Cu, Cr, Se, Mo, K, Cl, I, Mg, Mn, Zn 15 mg. Tab. Bot. 130s, 1000s. *OTC.*
Use: Mineral, vitamin supplement.

Thera Multi-Vitamin. (Major) Vitamins A 10,000 units, D 400 units, B_1 10 mg, B_2 10 mg, B_3 100 mg, B_5 21.4 mg, B_6 4.1 mg, B_{12} 5 mcg, C 200 mg/5 mL. Liq. Bot. 118 mL. *OTC.*
Use: Vitamin supplement.

Theraneed. (Hanlon) Vitamins A 16,000 units, B_1 10 mg, B_2 10 mg, B_6 2 mg, C 300 mg, calcium pantothenate 10 mg, niacinamide 10 mg, B_{12} 10 mcg. Cap. Bot. 100s. *OTC.*
Use: Mineral, vitamin supplement.

Therapals. (Faraday) Vitamins A 25,000 units, D 400 units, B_1 10 mg, B_2 5 mg, niacinamide 150 mg, B_6 0.5 mg, E 5 units, C 150 mg, B_{12} 10 mcg, Ca 103 mg, cobalt 0.1 mg, Cu 1 mg, K 0.15 mg, Mg 6 mg, Mn 1 mg, Mo 0.2 mg, P 80 mg, K 5 mg, Zn 1.2 mg. Tab. Bot. 100s, 250s, 1000s. *OTC.*
Use: Mineral, vitamin supplement.

TheraPatch Cold Sore. (LecTec) Lidocaine hydrochloride 4%, camphor 0.5%, aloe vera, eucalyptus oil, glycerin. Patch. Box 21s. *OTC.*
Use: Anesthetic, local.

TheraPatch Vapor Patch for Kids Cough Suppressant. (LecTec Corp.) Camphor 4.7%, menthol 2.6%. Glycerin, cherry scent. Patch. Box. 7s. *OTC.*
Use: Upper respiratory combination, topical.

Therapeutic. (Ivax) Vitamins A 5000 units, D 400 units, E 30 units, B_1 3 mg, B_2 3.4 mg, B_3 20 mg, B_5 10 mg, B_6 3 mg, B_{12} 9 mcg, C 90 mg, folic acid 0.4 mg, d-biotin 30 mcg. Tab. Bot. 100s, 130s. *OTC.*
Use: Vitamin supplement.

Therapeutic-H. (Ivax) Fe 66.7 mg, A 8333 units, D 133 units, E 5 units, B_1 3.3 mg, B_2 3.3 mg, B_3 33.3 mg, B_5 11.7 mg, B_6 3.3 mg, B_{12} 50 mcg, C 100 mg, folic acid 0.33 mg, Cu, Mg. Tab. Bot. 100s. *OTC.*
Use: Mineral, vitamin supplement.

Therapeutic-M. (Ivax) Fe 27 mg, vitamins A 5000 units, D 400 units, E 30 units, B_1 3 mg, B_2 3.4 mg, B_3 20 mg, B_5 10 mg, B_6 3 mg, B_{12} 9 mcg, C 90 mg, folic acid 0.4 mg, Ca, Cl, Cr, Cu, I, K, Mg, Mn, Mo, P, Se, Zn 15 mg, biotin 30 mcg. Tab. Bot. 1000s. *OTC.*
Use: Mineral, vitamin supplement.

Therapeutic Mineral Ice. (Novartis Consumer Health) Menthol 2%, ammonium hydroxide, carbomer 934, cupric sulfate, isopropyl alcohol, magnesium sulfate, thymol. Gel. Tube 105 mL, 240 mL, 480 mL. *OTC.*
Use: Liniment.

Therapeutic V & M. (Whiteworth Towne) Vitamins A 10,000 units, D 400 units, B_1 10 mg, B_2 10 mg, B_6 5 mg, B_{12} 5 mcg, niacinamide 100 mg, calcium pantothenate 20 mg, C 200 mg, E 15 units, I 0.15 mg, Fe 12 mg, Cu 2 mg, Mn 1 mg, Mg 60 mg, Zn 1.5 mg. Tab. *OTC.*
Use: Mineral, vitamin supplement.

Theraphon. (Health for Life Brands) Vitamins A 25,000 units, D 1000 units, B_1 10 mg, B_2 5 mg, C 150 mg, niacinamide 150 mg. Cap. Bot. 100s, 1000s. *OTC.*
Use: Vitamin supplement.

Thera-Plus. (Hi-Tech) Vitamins A 5,000 units, D 400 units, B_1 10 mg, B_2 10 mg, B_3 100 mg, B_5 21.4 mg, B_{12} 5 mcg, C 200 mg per 5 mL. Cherry flavoring, glycerin, methylparaben,

sodium benzoate, sugar. Liq. 118 mL. *OTC.*
Use: Nutritional supplement, vitamin.

Therapy Ice. (Major) Menthol 2%. Isopropyl alcohol. Gel. 226.8 g. *OTC.*
Use: Emollient.

TheraTears. (Advanced Vision Research) Carboxymethylcellulose sodium 1%, KCl, sodium bicarbonate, NaCl, sodium phosphate. Gel. UD 28s. *OTC.*
Use: Artificial tears.

Theravee Hematinic Vitamin. (Vangard Labs, Inc.) Fe 66.7 mg, A 8333 units, D 133 units, E 5 units, B_1 3.3 mg, B_2 3.3 mg, B_3 33.3 mg, B_5 11.7 mg, B_6 3.3 mg, B_{12} 50 mcg, C 100 mg, folic acid 0.33 mg, Cu, Mg. Tab. Bot. UD 100s. *OTC.*
Use: Mineral, vitamin supplement.

Theravee-M. (Vangard Labs, Inc.) Fe 27 mg, vitamins A 5000 units, D 400 units, E 30 units, B_1 3 mg, B_2 3.4 mg, B_3 30 mg, B_5 10 mg, B_6 3 mg, B_{12} 9 mcg, C 120 mg, folic acid 0.4 mg, Ca, Cl, Cr, Cu, K, I, Mg, Mn, Mo, Se, Zn 15 mcg, biotin 15 mcg, beta-carotene 2500 units. Tab. Bot. 100s, 1000s, UD 100s. *OTC.*
Use: Mineral, vitamin supplement.

Theravee Vitamin. (Vangard Labs, Inc.) Vitamins A 5500 units, D 400 units, E 30 units, B_1 3 mg, B_2 3.4 mg, B_3 30 mg, B_5 10 mg, B_6 3 mg, B_{12} 9 mcg, C 120 mg, folic acid 0.4 mg, biotin 15 mcg. Tab. Bot. 100s. UD 100s. *OTC.*
Use: Vitamin supplement.

Theravim. (NBTY) Vitamins A 5000 units, D 400 units, E 30 units, B_1 3 mg, B_2 3.4 mg, B_3 30 mg, B_5 10 mg, B_6 3 mg, B_{12} 9 mcg, C 90 mg, folic acid 0.4 mg, beta-carotene 1250 units, biotin 35 mcg. Tab. Bot. 130s. *OTC.*
Use: Vitamin supplement.

Theravim-M. (NBTY) Fe 27 mg, vitamins A 5000 units, D 400 units, E 30 mg, B_1 3 mg, B_2 3.4 mg, B_3 20 mg, B_5 10 mg, B_6 3 mg, B_{12} 9 mcg, C 90 mg, folic acid 0.4 mg, Ca, Cl, Cr, Cu, I, K, Mg, Mn, Mo, P, Se, Zn 15 mg, biotin 30 mcg. Tab. Bot. 130s. *OTC.*
Use: Mineral, vitamin supplement.

Theravite. (Alra) Vitamins A 10,000 units, D 400 units, B_1 10 mg, B_2 10 mg, B_3 100 mg, B_5 21.4 mg, B_6 4.1 mg, B_{12} 5 mcg, C 200 mg/5 mL. Liq. Bot. 118 mL. *OTC.*
Use: Vitamin supplement.

Therems. (Rugby) Vitamins A 5000 units, D 400 units, E 30 mg, B_1 3 mg, B_2 3.4 mg, B_3 30 mg, B_5 10 mg, B_6 3 mg, B_{12} 9 mcg, C 120 mg, folic acid 0.4 mg, beta-carotene 1250 units, biotin 15 mcg. Tab. Bot. 130s, 1000s. *OTC.*
Use: Vitamin supplement.

Therems-H. (Rugby) Vitamins A 1,400 units, C 100 mg, D 140 units, E 5 units, B_1 3.3 mg, B_2 3.3 mg, B_3 33.3 mg, B_5 11.7 mg, B_6 3.3 mg, B_{12} 50 mcg, folic acid 330 mcg, sodium 12 mg, Ca 130 mg, Fe, Mg, Cu. Film coated. PEG, mineral oil. Tab. 90s. *OTC.*
Use: Multivitamin.

Therems-M. (Rugby) Vitamins A 5,000 units, C 90 mg, D 400 units, E 60 units, K 28 mcg, B_1 3 mg, B_2 3.4 mg, B_3 20 mg, B_5 10 mg, B_6 6 mg, B_{12} 12 mcg, biotin 30 mcg, folic acid 400 mcg, Ca 40 mg, Fe, P, I, Mg, Zn, Se, Cu, Mn, Cr, Mo, Cl, K, B, Ni, Sn, V, Tn. Mannitol, sucrose, soy. Tab. 130s, 1,000s. *OTC.*
Use: Multivitamin.

Therevac. (Jones Pharma) Docusate potassium 283 mg, benzocaine 20 mg w/ soft soap in PEG 400 and glycerin base. Unit 4 mL, Cap. Pkgs. 4s, 12s, 50s. *OTC.*
Use: Bowel evacuant.

Therevac Plus. (Jones Pharma) Docusate sodium 283 mg, benzocaine 20 mg, glycerin 275 mg in a base of soft soap, polyethylene glycol, per 4 mL ampule. Disposable enema. Box 50s, UD 30s. *OTC.*
Use: Laxative.

Therevac-SB. (Jones Pharma) Docusate sodium 283 mg in a base of soft soap, polyethylene glycol, glycerin 275 mg per 4 mL ampule. Disposable enema. UD 30s. *OTC.*
Use: Laxative.

Therex-M. (Halsey Drug) Vitamins A 10,000 units, D 400 units, E 15 units, C 200 mg, B_1 10 mg, B_2 10 mg, niacinamide 100 mg, B_6 5 mg, B_{12} 5 mcg, calcium pantothenate 20 mg, I 150 mcg, Fe 12 mg, Mg 65 mg, Cu 2 mg, Zn 1.5 mg, Mn 1 mg. Tab. Bot. 100s. *OTC.*
Use: Mineral, vitamin supplement.

Therex No. 1. (Halsey Drug) Vitamins A 10,000 units, D 400 units, E 15 units, C 200 mg, B_1 10 mg, B_2 10 mg, niacinamide 100 mg, B_6 5 mg, B_{12} 5 mcg, calcium pantothenate 20 mg. Tab. Bot. 100s. *OTC.*
Use: Vitamin, mineral supplement.

Therex-Z. (Halsey Drug) Vitamins A 10,000 units, D 400 units, E 15 units, C 200 mg, B_1 10 mg, B_2 10 mg, niacinamide 100 mg, B_{12} 5 mcg, B_6 5 mg,

Ca pantothenate 20 mg, I 150 mcg, Cu 2 mg, Fe 12 mg, Zn 22.5 mg. Tab. Bot. 100s. *OTC.*
Use: Mineral, vitamin supplement.

Therma-Kool. (Nortech Laboratories) Compresses in following sizes: 3" × 5", 4" × 9", 8.5" × 10.5".
Use: Cold, hot compress.

Thermazene. (Ascend Labs) Silver sulfadiazine 10 mg/g in a water-miscible base. White petrolatum, stearyl alcohol, methylparaben 0.3%. Cream. Tube 50 g, 400 g, 1000 g. *Rx.*
Use: Topical anti-infective.

Thermodent. (Mentholatum Co.) Strontium chloride 10%. Tube. *OTC.*
Use: Dentrifice.

Theroal. (Vangard Labs, Inc.) Theophylline 24 mg, ephedrine hydrochloride 24 mg, phenobarbital 8 mg. Tab. Bot. 100s, 1000s. *Rx.*
Use: Antiasthmatic combination.

Theroxide Wash. (Medicis) Benzoyl peroxide 10%. Liq. Bot. 120 mL. *Rx.*
Use: Dermatologic, acid.

ThexForte. (KM Lee) Vitamins B$_1$ 25 mg, B$_2$ 15 mg, B$_3$ 100 mg, B$_5$ 10 mg, B$_6$ 5 mg, C 500 mg. Cap. Bot. 75s. *OTC.*
Use: Vitamin supplement.

Thia. (Sigma-Tau) Thiamine hydrochloride 100 mg/mL. Inj. Vial 30 mL. *Rx.*
Use: Vitamin supplement.

•**thiabendazole.** (THIGH-uh-BEND-uh-zole) *USP 34.*
Use: Anthelmintic.

thiacetarsamide sodium. Sodium mercaptoacetate S, S-diester with p-carbamoyl dithiobenzene arsonous acid.
Use: Antitrichomonal.

Thia-Dia-Mer-Sulfonamides. Sulfadiazine w/sulfamerazine & sulfathiazole.

Thiamilate. (Tyson) Thiamin (B$_1$) 20 mg. Enteric-coated Tab. Bot. 100s. *OTC.*
Use: Water-soluble vitamin.

thiamin (B$_1$).
Use: Water-soluble vitamin.
See: Thiamilate.
Thiamine Hydrochloride.

•**thiamine hydrochloride.** (THIGH-uh-min) *USP 34.*
Use: Enzyme co-factor vitamin.
See: Betalin S.
Thia.

thiamine hydrochloride. (Various Mfr.) Thiamin (B$_1$). **Tab.:** 50 mg, 100 mg, 250 mg. Bot. 100s, 250s; 1000s, UD 100s (100 mg only). **Inj.:** 100 mg/mL. Benzyl alcohol ≤ 9 mg. *Tubex* 1 mL in 2 mL. Multiple-dose vials. 2 mL. *Rx-OTC.*
Use: Water-soluble vitamin.

•**thiamine mononitrate.** (THIGH-uh-min) *USP 34.*
Use: Enzyme cofactor vitamin.

•**thiamiprine.** (thigh-AM-ih-preen) USAN.
Use: Antineoplastic.

•**thiamphenicol.** (THIGH-am-FEN-ih-kahl) USAN.
Use: Anti-infective.

•**thiamylal.** (thigh-AM-ih-lahl) *USP 34.*
Use: Anesthetic (intravenous).

•**thiamylal sodium for injection.** (thigh-AM-ih-lahl) *USP 34.*
Use: Anesthetic (intravenous).

thiazesim.
Use: Antidepressant.

•**thiazesim hydrochloride.** (thye-AZ-e-sim) USAN.
Use: Antidepressant.

•**thiazinamium chloride.** (THIGH-ah-ZIN-am-ee-uhm) USAN.
Use: Antiallergic.

thiazolidinediones.
Use: Antidiabetic.
See: Pioglitazone Hydrochloride.
Rosiglitazone Maleate.

thiethylene thiophosphoramide.
See: Thiotepa.

•**thiethylperazine.** (THIGH-eth-ill-PURR-ah-zeem) USAN.
Use: CNS depressant; antiemetic.

•**thiethylperazine maleate.** (THIGH-eth-ill-PURR-ah-zeen) *USP 34.*
Use: Antiemetic.

thihexinol methylbromide.
Use: Anticholinergic.

•**thimerfonate sodium.** (thigh-MER-foe-nate) USAN.
Use: Anti-infective, topical.

•**thimerosal.** (thigh-MER-oh-sal) *USP 34.*
Use: Anti-infective, topical; pharmaceutic aid (preservative).
W/Trifluridine.
See: Viroptic.

thiocarbanidin. Under study.
Use: Tuberculosis.

thiocyanate sodium. Sodium thiocyanate.
Use: Antihypertensive.

thiodinone. Name used for Nifuratel.

thiodiphenylamine.
See: Phenothiazine.

thioglycerol.
W/Sodium Citrate, Phenol, Benzyl Alcohol.
See: Sulfo-ganic.

•**thioguanine.** (THIGH-oh-GWAHN-een) *USP 34.*
Use: Antineoplastic.
See: Tabloid.

thiohexamide.
Use: Blood sugar-lowering compound.
thioisonicotinamide. Under study.
Use: Antituberculosal.
Thiola. (Mission Pharmacal) Tiopronin
100 mg. Tab. Bot. 100s. *Rx.*
Use: Anticholelithiasis.
•**thiopental sodium.** (thigh-oh-PEN-tahl)
USP 34.
Use: Anesthetic (intravenous); anticon-
vulsant.
See: Pentothal.
thiopental sodium. (I.M.S., Ltd.) Thio-
pental sodium. Pow. for Inj. **20 mg/mL:**
400 mg *Min-I-Mix* vial w/injector.
25 mg/mL: 250 mg, 500 mg *Min-I-Mix*
vials w/injector; 500 mg, 1 g, 2.5 g, 5 g,
10 g kits. *Rx.*
Use: Anesthetic, general.
thiophosphoramide.
See: Thiotepa.
Thioplex. (Amgen) Thiotepa 15 mg.
Powd. for Inj. Vials. *Rx.*
Use: Antineoplastic.
thiopropazate hydrochloride.
Use: Anxiolytic.
thioproperazine mesylate.
Use: CNS depressant; antiemetic.
•**thioridazine.** (THIGH-oh-RID-uh-zeen)
USP 34.
Use: Antipsychotic; hypnotic; sedative.
•**thioridazine hydrochloride.** (THIGH-oh-
RID-ah-zeen) *USP 34.*
Use: Antipsychotic; hypnotic; sedative.
**thioridazine hydrochloride concen-
trate.** (Various Mfr.) Thioridazine
hydrochloride. **30 mg/mL:** Bot. 120 mL.
100 mg/mL: Bot. 120 mL, 3.4 mL (UD
100s). *Rx.*
Use: Antipsychotic.
thioridazine hydrochloride tablets.
(Various Mfr.) Thioridazine hydrochloride 10 mg, 15 mg, 25 mg, 50 mg,
100 mg, 150 mg, 200 mg. Bot. 60s (except 15 mg, 150 mg, 200 mg), 100s,
1000s, UD 100s (except 150 mg,
200 mg). *Rx.*
Use: Antipsychotic.
•**thiosalan.** (THIGH-oh-sal-AN) USAN.
Use: Disinfectant.
•**thiotepa.** (thigh-oh-TEP-uh) *USP 34.*
Use: Antineoplastic.
See: Thioplex.
thiotepa. (Bedford) Thiotepa 15 mg. Pow.
for Inj, lyophilized. Single-dose vial. *Rx.*
Use: Antineoplastic.
thiotepa. (Sicor) Thiotepa 30 mg. Pow.
for Inj., lyophilized. Single-dose vials.
Rx.
Use: Antineoplastic.

thiotepa. (Wyeth) Thiotepa powder
15 mg, sodium chloride 80 mg, sodium
bicarbonate 50 mg. Vial. Pow. for Recon. Vial 15 mg. *Rx.*
Use: Antineoplastic.
•**thiothixene.** (THIGH-oh-THIX-een)
USP 34.
Use: Antipsychotic.
See: Navane.
thiothixene. (Various Mfr.) Thiothixene
1 mg, 2 mg, 5 mg, 10 mg. May contain lactose. Cap. 100s, 1000s, UD
100s (2 mg, 5 mg only). *Rx.*
Use: Antipsychotic.
•**thiothixene hydrochloride.** (THIGH-oh-
THIX-een) *USP 34.*
Use: Antipsychotic.
thiouracil. 2-Thiouracil.
Use: Treatment of hyperthyroidism, antianginal, congestive heart failure.
thioxanthene derivatives.
See: Thiothixene.
•**thiphenamil hydrochloride.** (thigh-FEN-
ah-mill) USAN.
Use: Muscle relaxant.
•**thiphencillin potassium.** (thigh-fen-
SILL-in) USAN.
Use: Anti-infective.
•**thiram.** (THIGH-ram) USAN.
Use: Antifungal.
Thixo-Flur. (Colgate Oral) Acidulated
phosphate sodium fluoride in gel base
1.2%. Gel. Bot. 4 oz, 8 oz., 32 oz.
Use: Dental caries agent.
•**thonzonium bromide.** (thahn-ZOE-nee-
uhm) *USP 34.*
Use: Detergent.
W/Colistin Base, Neomycin Base, Hydrocortisone Acetate, Polysorbate 80, Acetic Acid, Sodium Acetate.
See: Coly-Mycin-S.
Cortisporin-TC.
•**thonzylamine hydrochloride.** (thon-ZIL-
a-meen) USAN.
Use: Antihistamine.
Thorets. (Buffington) Benzocaine lozenge. *Dispens-A-Kits* 500s. Sugar, lactose, and salt free. *OTC.*
Use: Sore throat relief.
Thor-Prom. (Major) Chlorpromazine
10 mg, 25 mg, 50 mg, 100 mg, 200 mg.
Tab. Bot. 100s, 1000s (except
200 mg). Tab. Bot. 250s, 1000s
(200 mg only). *Rx.*
Use: Antiemetic; antipsychotic.
•**thozalinone.** (thoe-ZAL-ah-nohn) USAN.
Use: Antidepressant.
357 HR Magnum. (BDI) Caffeine 200 mg.
Tab. Bot. 36s, 100s, 500s. *OTC.*
Use: CNS stimulant, analeptic.

•**threonine.** (THREE-oh-neen) *USP 34.*
Use: Amino acid.
See: Threostat.
l-threonine.
Use: Antispasmodic. [Orphan Drug]
threonine. (Various Mfr.) Threonine
500 mg. Tab. 100s, 250s. *OTC.*
Use: Nutritional supplement.
Threostat. (Tyson) *Rx.*
Use: Antispasmodic.
See: Threonine.
Thrive. (Novartis) Nicotine polacrilex
2 mg, 4 mg. Acesulfame K, glycerin,
maltitol, saccharin, sodium 11 mg,
sorbitol. Mint flavor. Gum. 110s. *OTC.*
Use: Smoking deterrent, nicotine.
Throat Discs. (GlaxoSmithKline) Capsi-
cum, peppermint, mineral oil, sucrose.
Box 60s. *OTC.*
Use: Throat preparation.
Throat-Eze. (Faraday) Cetylpyridinium
chloride 1:3000, cetyl dimethylbenzyl
ammonium chloride 1:3000, benzocaine
10 mg. Wafer. Loz., foil wrapped. Vial
15. *OTC.*
Use: Anesthetic, local.
Thrombate III. (Talecris) Antithrombin III
(human) 500 units, 1000 units. Pow. for
Inj., lyophilized. Single-use vial w/
10 mL (500 mL units only), 20 mL
(1000 units only). Sterile water for in-
jection. *Rx.*
Use: Antithrombin.
Thrombi-Gel 40. (King Pharmaceuticals)
Thrombin (bovine origin) 1,000 units.
Residual formaldehyde ≤ 0.2 mg. Pre-
servative free. Pad, lyophilized; top.
Single-use 5s. *Rx.*
Use: Topical hemostatic.
Thrombi-Gel 100. (King Pharmaceuti-
cals) Thrombin (bovine origin)
20,000 units. Residual formaldehyde
≤ 0.2 mg. Preservative free. Pad, ly-
ophilized; top. Single-use 5s. *Rx.*
Use: Topical hemostatic.
Thrombi-Gel 10. (King Pharmaceuticals)
Thrombin (bovine origin) 1,000 units.
Residual formaldehyde ≤ 0.2 mg. Pre-
servative free. Pad, lyophilized; top.
Single-use 10s. *Rx.*
Use: Topical hemostatic.
•**thrombin.** (THROM-bin) *USP 34.* Throm-
bin, topical, mammalian origin.
Use: Hemostatic.
See: Evithrom.
Recothrom.
Thrombi-Gel 40.
Thrombi-Gel 100.
Thrombi-Gel 10.
Thrombin-JMI.
Thrombi-Pad 3 × 3.

•**thrombin alfa.** (THROM-bin AL-fa)
USAN.
Use: Hemostatic.
thrombin inhibitors.
Use: Anticoagulant.
See: Argatroban.
Bivalirudin.
Dabigatrin Etexilate.
Desirudin.
Lepirudin.
Thrombin-JMI. (King Pharmaceuticals)
Thrombin 1,000 units/mL. Preserva-
tive free. Pow. for Soln., lyophilized; top.
5,000 unit vials and Epistaxis Kit w/
diluent; 20,000 unit vials, Pump Spray
Kit, and Syringe Spray Kit w/diluent.
Rx.
Use: Topical hemostatic.
Thrombi-Pad 3 × 3. (King Pharmaceuti-
cals) Thrombin (bovine origin)
200 units. Preservative free. Pad, ly-
ophilized; top. Single-use 1s. *Rx.*
Use: Topical hemostatic.
thrombolytic agents.
See: Human Protein C.
Tissue Plasminogen Activators.
Thrombolytic Enzymes.
thrombolytic enzymes.
See: Streptokinase.
Urokinase.
thromboplastin.
Use: Diagnostic aid (prothrombin esti-
mation).
thrombopoietin receptor agonists.
See: Eltrombopag.
Thylox. (C.S. Dent & Co.) Medicated bar
soap w/absorbable sulfur. Bar 3.4 oz.
OTC.
Use: Cleanser.
•**thymalfasin.** (thigh-MAL-fah-sin) USAN.
Formerly Thymosin.
Use: Antineoplastic; vaccine enhance-
ment; hepatitis, infectious disease
treatment.
Thymoglobulin. (SangStat) Antithymocyte globulin (rabbit) 25 mg. Glycine
50 mg, mannitol 50 mg, sodium chloride 10 mg. Pow. for Inj., lyophilized. Vial
7 mL w/diluent vial 5 mL. *Rx.*
Use: Immune globulin.
•**thymol.** (THIGH-mole) *NF 29.*
Use: Antifungal; anti-infective; anesthetic, local; antitussive; decongestant; pharmaceutic aid (stabilizer).
W/Combinations.
See: Listerine Antiseptic.
Listerine, Natural Citrus.
Listerine, Tartar Control.
thymol. (Various Mfr.) Thymol 0.25 lb,
1 lb.

Use: Antifungal; anti-infective; anesthetic, local; antitussive; decongestant; pharmaceutic aid (stabilizer).

thymol iodide.
Use: Antifungal; anti-infective.

•**thymopentin.** (THIGH-moe-PEN-tin) USAN. *Formerly Thymopoietin 32-36.*
Use: Immunoregulator.

thyodatil. *Name used for nifuratel.*

Thyrogen. (Genzyme) Thyrotropin alfa 1.1 mg (4 to 12 units/mg). Mannitol 36 mg, sodium phosphate 5.1 mg, sodium chloride 2.4 mg. Inj., Lyophilized, Pow. for Soln. Kits. 2 vials (2 vials of thyrotropin alfa 1.1 mg), 4 vials (2 vials of thyrotropin alfa 1.1 mg and two 10 mL vials of sterile water for injection). *Rx.*
Use: In vivo diagnostic aid, thyroid function test.

•**thyroid.** (THIGH-royd) *USP 34.*
Use: Hormone, thyroid.
See: Arco Thyroid.

thyroid combinations.
See: Henydin.

thyroid desiccated.
Use: Hormone, thyroid.
See: Armour Thyroid.
 Bio-Throid.
 Nature Throid.
 Thyroid USP.
 Westhroid.

thyroid drugs.
See: Antithyroid agents.
 Methimazole.
 Potassium Iodide.
 Propylthiouracil.
 Sodium Iodide I 131.

thyroid function tests.
Use: In vivo diagnostic aid.
See: Sodium Iodide I 123.
 Sodium Iodide I 125.
 Sodium Iodide I 131.
 Thyrogen.
 Thyrotropin Alfa.
 Thytropar.

thyroid hormones.
See: Levothyroxine Sodium.
 Liothyronine Sodium.
 Liotrix.
 Thyroid Desiccated.

Thyroid USP. (Various Mfr.) Thyroid desiccated 32.5 mg (½ gr), 65 mg (1 gr), 130 mg (2 gr), 195 mg (3 gr). Tab. Bot. 100s, 1000s. *Rx.*
Use: Hormone, thyroid.

Thyrolar. (Forest) Liotrix 0.25 gr, 0.5 gr, 1 gr, 2 gr, 3 gr, lactose. Tab. Bot. 100s. *Rx.*
Use: Hormone, thyroid.

•**thyromedan hydrochloride.** (thigh-ROW-meh-dan) USAN.
Use: Thyromimetic.

thyropropic acid. (Warner Chilcott) Triopron.
Use: Anticholesteremic.

ThyroSafe. (Recip) Potassium iodide 65 mg. Lactose. Tab. 10s, 20s. *OTC.*
Use: Thyroid drug.

ThyroShield. (Fleming) Potassium iodide 65 mg/mL. Parabens, saccharin, sucrose. Black-raspberry flavor. Soln. 30 mL. *OTC.*
Use: Thyroid drug.

Thyro-Tabs. (Lloyd) Levothyroxine sodium 0.025 mg, 0.05 mg, 0.075 mg, 0.088 mg, 0.1 mg, 0.112 mg, 0.125 mg, 0.15 mg, 0.175 mg, 0.2 mg, 0.3 mg. Tab. Bot. 100s, 1000s. *Rx.*
Use: Hormone, thyroid.

thyrotropic hormone.
Use: In vivo diagnostic aid.
See: Thytropar.

thyrotropic principle of bovine anterior pituitary glands.
See: Thytropar.

thyrotropin.
Use: Diagnostic aid.
See: Thytropar.

•**thyrotropin alfa.** (thye-roh-TROH-pin) USAN.
Use: In vivo diagnostic aid, thyroid function test.
See: Thyrogen.

thyrotropin-releasing hormone.
Use: Diagnostic aid.

•**thyroxine I 131.** (thigh-ROX-een) USAN.
Use: Radiopharmaceutical.

•**thyroxine I 125.** (thigh-ROX-een) USAN.
Use: Radiopharmaceutical.

thyrozyme-II A. (Abbott Diagnostics) T-4 diagnostic kit. 100, 500 test units.
Use: Diagnostic aid, thyroid.

Thytropar. (Centeon) Thyrotropin from bovine anterior pituitary glands. Thyrotropin. Vial 10 units.
Use: Thyroid agent.

•**tiacrilast.** (TIE-ah-KRILL-ast) USAN.
Use: Antiallergic.

•**tiacrilast sodium.** (TIE-ah-KRILL-ast) USAN.
Use: Antiallergic.

•**tiagabine hydrochloride.** (tye-AG-a-been) USAN.
Tall Man: tiaGABine
Use: Anticonvulsant.
See: Gabitril.

•**tiamenidine.** (TIE-ah-MEN-ih-DEEN) USAN.
Use: Antihypertensive.

• **tiamenidine hydrochloride.** (TIE-ah-MEN-ih-DEEN) USAN.
Use: Antihypertensive.

• **tiapamil hydrochloride.** (tie-APP-ah-mill) USAN.
Use: Calcium antagonist.

• **tiaramide hydrochloride.** (TIE-ar-ah-MIDE) USAN.
Use: Antiasthmatic.

Tiazac. (Forest) Diltiazem hydrochloride 120 mg, 180 mg, 240 mg, 300 mg, 360 mg, 420 mg. Sucrose. ER Cap. Bot. 7s, 30s, 90s, 1000s. *Rx.*
Use: Calcium channel blocker.

• **tiazofurin.** (tye-AZ-oh-FURE-in) USAN.
Use: Antineoplastic.

TI-Baby Natural. (Fischer) Titanium dioxide 5%. SPF 16. Lot. Bot. 120 mL. *OTC.*
Use: Sunscreen.

• **tibenelast sodium.** (TIE-ben-ell-ast) USAN.
Use: Antiasthmatic; bronchodilator.

• **tibolone.** (TIH-bole-ohn) USAN.
Use: Menopausal symptoms suppressant.

• **tibric acid.** (TIE-brick) USAN.
Use: Antihyperlipoproteinemic.

• **tibrofan.** (TIE-broe-fan) USAN.
Use: Disinfectant.

• **ticabesone propionate.** (tie-CAB-eh-sone) USAN.
Use: Corticosteroid, topical.

• **ticarbodine.** (tie-CAR-boe-deen) USAN.
Use: Anthelmintic.

ticarcillin/clavulanate.
Use: Extended-spectrum penicillin.
See: Timentin.

• **ticarcillin cresyl sodium.** (tie-CAR-SIH-lin KREH-sill) USAN.
Use: Anti-infective.

• **ticarcillin disodium.** (tie-CAR-SIH-lin) *USP 34.*
Use: Extended-spectrum penicillin.

ticarcillin disodium and clavulanate potassium, sterile.
Use: Anti-infective; inhibitor (β-lactamase).
See: Timentin.

• **ticarcillin monosodium.** (tie-CAR-SIH-lin) *USP 34.*
Use: Anti-infective.

Tice BCG. (Organon) BCG live for intravesical administration. 1 to 8 × 10⁸ CFU (equivalent to ≈ 50 mg wet weight). Preservative free. Inj. Lyophilized. Pow. for Susp. Vials. ≈ 50 mg. *Rx.*
Use: Biological response modifier.

• **ticilimumab.** (tis-i-LIM-ue-mab) USAN.
Use: Antineoplastic.

• **ticlatone.** (TIE-klah-tone) USAN.
Use: Anti-infective; antifungal.

Ticlid. (Roche) Ticlopidine hydrochloride 250 mg. Tab. Bot. 30s, 60s, 500s. *Rx.*
Use: Antiplatelet.

• **ticlopidine hydrochloride.** (tie-KLOE-pih-DEEN) USAN.
Use: Platelet inhibitor.
See: Ticlid.

ticlopidine hydrochloride. (Various Mfr.) Ticlopidine hydrochloride 250 mg. Tab. Bot. 30s, 60s, 100s, 500s, 1000s. *Rx.*
Use: Platelet inhibitor.

• **ticolubant.** (tih-kahl-YOU-bant) USAN.
Use: Antipsoriatic.

Ticon. (Hauck) Trimethobenzamide hydrochloride 100 mg/mL, phenol. Inj. Vial 20 mL. *Rx.*
Use: Antiemetic; antivertigo.

• **ticrynafen.** (TIE-krin-ah-fen) USAN.
Use: Diuretic; uricosuric; antihypertensive.

Tidafen DM. (Tiber) Dextromethorphan HBr 60 mg, guaifenesin 800 mg, pseudoephedrine hydrochloride 90 mg. ER Tab. 100s. *Rx.*
Use: Upper respiratory combination, antitussive and expectorant combination.

tidembersat.
Use: Antimigraine.

Tidex. (Allison) Dextroamphetamine sulfate 5 mg. Tab. Bot. 100s, 1000s. *c-II.*
Use: Antiobesity agent.

Tidexsol. (Sanofi-Synthelabo) Acetaminophen. Tab. *OTC.*
Use: Analgesic.

• **tifurac sodium.** (TIE-fyoor-ak) USAN.
Use: Analgesic.

Tigan. (Monarch) Trimethobenzamide hydrochloride 300 mg. Cap. 100s. *Rx.*
Use: Antiemetic.

Tigan. (JHP Pharm) Trimethobenzamide hydrochloride 100 mg/mL. Amps (with methyl- and propylparabens). Inj. 2 mL. Vials (with phenol). 20 mL. Syringe (with phenol and EDTA). 2 mL. *Rx.*
Use: Antiemetic.

• **tigapotide triflutate.** (TYE-gah-POE-tide) USAN.
Use: Antineoplastic.

• **tigecycline.** (tye-ge-SYE-kleen) USAN.
Use: Anti-infective, glycylcycline.
See: Tygacil.

• **tigemonam dicholine.** (TIE-jem-OH-nam die-KOE-leen) USAN.
Use: Antimicrobial.

Tiger Balm. (Prince of Peace) Menthol 8%, camphor 11%. Cajuput oil, clove oil, mint oil, petrolatum. Oint. 18 g. *OTC.*
Use: Rub and liniment.

•**tigestol.** (tie-JESS-tole) USAN.
Use: Hormone, progestin.

Tigo. (Burlington) Polymyxin B sulfate 5000 units, zinc bacitracin 400 units, neomycin sulfate 5 mg/g Oint. Tube 0.5 oz. *OTC.*
Use: Anti-infective, topical.

Tihist-DP. (Vita Elixir) Dextromethorphan HBr 10 mg, pyrilamine maleate 16 mg, sodium citrate 3.3 g/5 mL. *OTC.*
Use: Antitussive; antihistamine.

Tihist Nasal Drops. (Vita Elixir) Pyrilamine maleate 0.1%, phenylephrine hydrochloride 0.25%, sodium bisulfite 0.2%, methylparaben 0.02%, propylparaben 0.01%/30 mL. Bot. *OTC.*
Use: Antihistamine; decongestant.

Tija. (Vita Elixir) Oxytetracycline hydrochloride. **Syrup:** 125 mg/5 mL. **Tab.:** 250 mg. *Rx.*
Use: Anti-infective, tetracycline.

Tikosyn. (Pfizer) Dofetilide 125 mcg, 250 mcg, 500 mcg. Cap. Bot. 14s, 60s, UD 40s. *Rx.*
Use: Antiarrhythmic.

•**tiletamine hydrochloride.** (tie-LET-ah-meen) *USP 34.*
Use: Anesthetic; anticonvulsant.

Tilia Fe. (Watson) **Phase 1:** Norethindrone acetate 1 mg, ethinyl estradiol 20 mcg (5 tabs.). **Phase 2:** Norethindrone acetate 1 mg, ethinyl estradiol 30 mcg (7 tabs.). **Phase 3:** Norethindrone acetate 1 mg, ethinyl estradiol 35 mcg (9 tabs.). Ferrous fumarate 75 mg (7 tabs.). Lactose. Tab. 28s. *Rx.*
Use: Sex hormone, contraceptive hormone.

•**tilidine hydrochloride.** (TIH-lih-DEEN) USAN.
Use: Analgesic.

TI-lite. (Fischer) Ethylhexyl p-methoxycinnamate 7.5%, titanium dioxide 2%, cetyl alcohol, phenethyl alcohol, parabens, EDTA. Cream 60 g. *OTC.*
Use: Sunscreen.

•**tilmacoxib.** (til-ma-KOX-ib) USAN.
Use: Cox-2 inhibitor.

•**tilomisole.** (TILL-oh-mih-sahl) USAN.
Use: Immunoregulator.

•**tilorone hydrochloride.** (TIE-lore-ohn) USAN.
Use: Antiviral.

•**tiludronate disodium.** (tie-LOO-droe-nate) USAN.
Use: Bisphosphonate.
See: Skelid.

•**timefurone.** (tie-MEH-fyoor-OHN) USAN.
Use: Antiatherosclerotic.

Time-Hist QD. (AMBI) Pseudoephedrine hydrochloride 120 mg, chlorpheniramine maleate 6 mg. PEG. ER Tab. Bot. 100s. *Rx.*
Use: Upper respiratory combination, decongestant, antihistamine, anticholinergic.

Timentin. (GlaxoSmithKline) **Inj., Pow. for Reconstitution:** Ticarcillin 3 g, clavulanic acid 0.1 g. Sodium 4.51 mEq, potassium 0.15 mEq/g. Vials. 3.1 g. *ADD-Vantage* vials. Pharmacy bulk pkg. (ticarcillin disodium 30 g, clavulanic acid 1 g). **Inj. Soln.:** Ticarcillin 3 g, clavulanic acid 0.1 g per 100 mL. Sodium 18.7 mEq, potassium 0.5 mEq/100 mL. Premixed, frozen *Galaxy* plastic cont. 100 mL. *Rx.*
Use: Extended-spectrum penicillin.

•**timobesone acetate.** (tie-MOE-beh-sone) USAN.
Use: Adrenocortical steroid, topical.

•**timolol.** (TI-moe-lahl) USAN.
Use: Antiadrenergic (β-receptor).

timolol/brimonidine tartrate.
Use: Agent for glaucoma.
See: Combigen.

•**timolol maleate.** (TI-moe-lahl) *USP 34.*
Use: Agent for glaucoma; antiadrenergic/sympatholytic, beta-adrenergic blocker.
See: Blocadren.
Betimol.
Istalol.
Timoptic.
Timoptic-XE.

timolol maleate. (Falcon Ophthalmics) Timolol maleate 0.25%, 0.5%. Gelforming Soln. Bot. 2.5 mL, 5 mL. *Rx.*
Use: Agent for glaucoma; betaadrenergic blocker.

timolol maleate. (Various Mfr.) Timolol maleate **Ophth. Soln.:** 0.25%, 0.5%. Bot. 2.5 mL, 5 mL, 10 mL, 15 mL. **Tab.:** 5 mg, 10 mg, 20 mg. Bot. 100s. *Rx.*
Use: Agent for glaucoma; antiadrenergic/sympatholytic; beta-adrenergic blocker.

timolol maleate/dorzolamide hydrochloride.
Use: Agent for glaucoma.
See: Cosopt.

timolol maleate ophthalmic. (Various Mfr.) Timolol maleate 3.4 mg/0.25 mL and 6.8 mg/0.5 mL. Soln. Bot. 2.5 mL, 5 mL, 10 mL, 15 mL. *Rx.*
Use: Antiglaucoma agent.

Timoptic. (Aton Pharma) Timolol maleate 0.25%, 0.5%. Ophth. Soln. *Ocumeter* 2.5 mL, 5 mL, 10 mL, 15 mL; *Ocudose*

UD 60s. *Rx.*
Use: Antiglaucoma agent; beta-adrenergic blocker.

Timoptic-XE. (Aton Pharma) Timolol maleate 0.25%, 0.5%. Gel-forming Soln. *Ocumeter* 2.5 mL, 5 mL. *Rx.*
Use: Antiglaucoma agent; beta-adrenergic blocker.

•**tinabinol.** (tie-NAB-ih-NOLE) USAN.
Use: Antihypertensive.

Tinactin. (Schering-Plough) **Soln. 1%:** Tolnaftate (10 mg/mL) w/butylated hydroxytoluene, in nonaqueous homogeneous PEG 400. Plastic squeeze bot. 10 mL. **Cream 1%:** Tolnaftate (10 mg/g) in homogeneous, nonaqueous vehicle of PEG-400, propylene glycol, carboxypolymethylene, monoamylamine, titanium dioxide, butylated hydroxytoluene. Tube 15 g, 30 g, UD 0.7 g. **Pow. 1%:** Tolnaftate w/corn starch, talc. Plastic container 45 g, 90 g. **Aerosol Pow. 1%:** Tolnaftate w/butylated hydroxytoluene, talc, polyethylene-polypropylene glycol monobutyl ether, denatured alcohol and inert propellant of isobutane. Spray Can 100 g. **Aerosol Liq. 1%:** Tolnaftate w/butylated hydroxytoluene, polyethylene-polyproplyene glycol monobutyl ether, 36% alcohol, and inert propellant of isobutane. Spray Can 120 mL. *OTC.*
Use: Antifungal.

Tinastat. (Vita Elixir) Sodium hyposulfite, benzethonium chloride/2 oz. *OTC.*
Use: Keratolytic.

Tinaval. (Pal-Pak, Inc.) Tolnaftate 1%. Pow. Bot. 45 g. *OTC.*
Use: Antifungal for jock itch, athlete's foot.

Tindamax. (Mission Pharmacal) Tinidazole 250 mg, 500 mg. Tab. 20s (500 mg only), 40s (250 mg only), 60s (500 mg only). *Rx.*
Use: Antiprotozoal.

tine test, old tuberculin. (Wyeth) Box of 25, 100, 250 test applicators.
See: Tuberculin Tine Test.

tine test, purified protein derivative. (Wyeth) Box of 25 or 100 test applicators.
See: Tuberculin Tine Test.

•**tin fluoride.** *USP 34.* Stannous Fluoride.

Ting. (Insight) Miconazole nitrate 2%. SD alcohol 40 10%, aloe vera gel. Spray Pow. Bot. 85 g. *OTC.*
Use: Anti-infective, antifungal, topical.

Ting. (Insight) Tolnaftate 1%. PEG-400, SD alcohol 40-B 41%. Spray, Liq., Top. 128 g. *OTC.*
Use: Anti-infective, topical; antifungal agent.

•**tinidazole.** (tie-NIH-dah-zole) USAN.
Use: Antiprotozoal.
See: Tindamax.

tinidazole. (BioComp Pharma) Tinidazole 250 mg, 500 mg. PEG, polydextrose. Tab. 20s (500 mg), 40s (250 mg), 60s (500 mg). *Rx.*
Use: Anti-infective agent, antiprotozoal.

Tinset. (Janssen) Oxatomide.
Use: Antiallergic; antiasthmatic.

•**tinzaparin sodium.** (tin-ZAP-ah-rin) USAN.
Use: Anticoagulant; low molecular weight heparin.
See: Innohep.

•**tioconazole.** (TIE-oh-KOE-nah-zole) *USP 34.*
Use: Antifungal.
See: Monistat 1.
Vagistat-1.

•**tiodazosin.** (TIE-oh-DAY-zoe-sin) USAN.
Use: Antihypertensive.

•**tiodonium chloride.** (TIE-oh-doe-nee-uhm) USAN.
Use: Anti-infective.

•**tiomolibdate diammonium.** (TYE-oh-moe-LIB-date) USAN.
Use: Alzheimer disease.

•**tioperidone hydrochloride.** (tie-oh-PURR-ih-dohn) USAN.
Use: Antipsychotic.

•**tiopinac.** (tie-OH-pin-ACK) USAN.
Use: Anti-inflammatory; analgesic, antipyretic.

tiopronin.
Use: Homozygous cystinuria. [Orphan Drug]
See: Thiola.

•**tiospirone hydrochloride.** (tie-OH-spih-rone) USAN.
Use: Antipsychotic.

•**tiotidine.** (TIE-OH-tih-deen) USAN.
Use: Antiulcerative.

tiotropium bromide.
Use: Bronchodilator, anticholinergic.
See: Spiriva.

•**tioxidazole.** (tie-OX-ih-DAH-zole) USAN.
Use: Anthelmintic.

•**tipapkinogene sovacivec.** (TIP-a-KIN-oh-jeen soe-VAS-i-vek) USAN.
Use: Antineoplastic.

•**tipelukast.** (TYE-pe-LOO-kast) USAN.
Use: Respiratory agent.

•**tipentosin hydrochloride.** (TIE-pin-toe-SIN) USAN.
Use: Antihypertensive.

•**tipifarnib.** (tip-ee-FAR-nib) USAN.
Use: Cancer.

•**tiplasinin.** (ti-PLAS-in-in) USAN.
Use: Hematologic.

Tipramine Tabs. (Major) Imipramine.
Tab. **10 mg:** Bot. 250s. **25 mg, 50 mg:**
Bot. 250s, 1000s. *Rx.*
Use: Antidepressant.

•**tipranavir.** (tip-RA-na-veer) USAN.
Use: Antiretroviral, protease inhibitor.
See: Aptivus.

•**tipredane.** (tie-PRED-ANE) USAN.
Use: Adrenocortical steroid, topical.

•**tiprenolol hydrochloride.** (tie-PREH-no-
lole) USAN.
Use: Antiadrenergic (β-receptor).

•**tiprinast meglumine.** (TIE-prih-nast
meh-GLUE-meen) USAN. Under study.
Use: Antiallergic.

•**tipropidil hydrochloride.** (TIE-PRO-pih-
dill) USAN.
Use: Vasodilator.

•**tiqueside.** (TIE-kweh-side) USAN.
Use: Antihyperlipidemic.

•**tiquinamide hydrochloride.** (tie-KWIN-
ah-mide) USAN.
Use: Anticholinergic (gastric).

•**tirapazamine.** (tie-rah-PAZZ-ah-meen)
USAN.
Use: Antineoplastic.

tiratricol.
Use: Antineoplastic. [Orphan Drug]

•**tirilazad mesylate.** (tie-RIH-lah-zad)
USAN.
Use: Antioxidant.
See: Freedox.

•**tirofiban hydrochloride.** (tie-rah-FIE-
ban) USAN.
Use: Antiplatelet, glycoprotein IIb/IIIa inhibitor.
See: Aggrastat.

Tl-Screen. (Pedinol Pharmacal) **Gel:**
SPF 20+, ethylhexyl p-methoxycinnamate
7.5%, oxybenzone 5%, 2-ethylhexyl salicylate 5%, SD alcohol 40 71%. 120 g.
Lip Balm: SPF 8+, ethylhexyl p-
methoxycinnamate 7.5%, oxybenzone
5%, petrolatum. 4.5 g. **Lot.:** SPF 8, ethylhexyl p-methoxycinnamate 6%, oxybenzone 2%. Bot. 120 mL. *OTC.*
Use: Sunscreen.

Tl-Screen Natural. (Pedinol Pharmacal)
Titanium dioxide 5%. Lot. Bot. 120 mL.
OTC.
Use: Sunscreen.

Tl-Screen Sports. (Pedinol) Octinoxate
7.5%, oxybenzone 6%, octisalate 5%,
avobenzone 2%. Alcohol 70%. Gel.
120 mL. *OTC.*
Use: Sunscreen.

Tl-Screen Sunless. (Pedinol Pharmacal)
Octyl methoxycinnamate 7.5%,

benzophene-3 3%, mineral oil, alcohols, PEG-100, parabens. SPF 17 or
23. Cream. Tube 118 mL. *OTC.*
Use: Sunscreen.

•**tisilfocon A.** (tih-sill-FOE-kahn) USAN.
Use: Contact lens material (hydrophobic).

Tisit. (Pfeiffer) **Gel:** Pyrethrins 0.3%, piperonyl butoxide 3%. 30 mL. **Lot.:**
Pyrethrins 0.3%, piperonyl butoxide 2%
(petroleum distillate and piperonyl
butoxide equiv. to 1.6% ether). 59 mL,
118 mL. **Shampoo:** Pyrethrins 0.33%,
piperonyl butoxide 4%. Bot. 59 mL,
118 mL. With comb. *OTC.*
Use: Pediculicide.

•**tisocalcitate.** (ti-soe-KAL-si-tate) USAN.
Use: Psoriasis.

TiSol. (Parnell) Benzyl alcohol 1%, menthol 0.04%, isotonic sodium chloride
0.9%, sorbitol, EDTA. Soln. Bot.
237 mL. *OTC.*
Use: Throat preparation.

tissue fixative and wash solution.
(Wampole) A modified Michel's tissue
fixative and buffered wash solution.
Use: Tissue specimen fixative.

tissue plasminogen activators.
See: Alteplase, Recombinant.
Reteplase, Recombinant.
Tenecteplase.

tissue respiratory factor (TRF). (International Hormone) RSF, SRF, LYCD,
PCO, Procytoxid marketed as
2000 units. Supplied as bulk liquid concentrate. *Rx.*
Use: Promotion of cellular oxidation.

Tis-U-Sol. (Baxter PPI) Pentalyte irrigation containing NaCl 800 mg, KCl
40 mg, magnesium sulfate 20 mg, sodium phosphate 8.75 mg, 6.25 mg
monobasic potassium phosphate/
100 mL. Bot. 250 mL, 1000 mL. *Rx.*
Use: Irrigant.

•**titanium dioxide.** (tie-TANE-ee-uhm die-
OX-ide) *USP 34.*
Use: Solar ray protectant, topical.
W/Avobenzone, Ecamsule, Octocrylene.
See: Capital Soleil 20.

Titralac. (3M) Calcium carbonate
420 mg, saccharin, Na 0.3 mg. Chew.
Tab. Bot. 40s, 100s, 1000s. *OTC.*
Use: Antacid.

Titralac Plus. (3M) **Chew. Tab.:** Calcium
carbonate 420 mg, simethicone 21 mg,
saccharin, sodium 1.1 mg. Bot. 100s.
Liq.: Calcium carbonate 500 mg, simethicone 20 mg, saccharin, sorbitol,
sodium 0.15 mg. Bot. 360 mL. *OTC.*
Use: Antacid.

●**tivozanib.** (ti-VOE-za-nib) USAN.
Use: Antineoplastic.

●**tixanox.** (TIX-ah-nox) USAN.
Use: Antiallergic.

●**tixocortol pivalate.** (tix-OH-kahr-tole PIH-vah-late) USAN.
Use: Anti-inflammatory, topical.

●**tizanidine hydrochloride.** (tie-ZAN-ih-deen) USAN.
Tall Man: tiZANidine
Use: Antispasmodic.
See: Zanaflex.

tizanidine hydrochloride. (Various Mfr.) Tizanidine 2 mg (equivalent to tizanidine hydrochloride 2.29 mg), 4 mg (equivalent to tizanidine hydrochloride 4.58 mg). Tab. 150s, 500s, 1,000s. *Rx.*
Use: Antispasmodic.

TL-DEX DM. (Trigen Labs) Dextromethorphan hydrobromide 15 mg, guaifenesin 200 mg, pseudoephedrine hydrochloride 32 mg per 5 mL. Potassium sorbate, parabens, propylene glycol, sorbitol, sucralose. Grape flavor. Liq. 473 mL. *Rx.*
Use: Upper respiratory combination, antitussive and expectorant combination.

TL 45%. (Trigen Labs) Urea 45%. Camphor, disodium EDTA, ethyl alcohol, eucalyptus oil, menthol. Lot. 473 g. *Rx.*
Use: Emollient.

TL-Hist CM. (Trigen Labs) Chlorpheniramine maleate 2 mg, codeine phosphate 10 mg per 5 mL. Sorbitol, sucralose, parabens, potassium citrate, potassium sorbate. Cotton candy flavor. Liq. 473 mL. *c-v.*
Use: Upper respiratory combination, antitussive combination.

TL-Hist DM. (Trigen Labs) Brompheniramine maleate 4 mg, dextromethorphan hydrobromide 15 mg, phenylephrine hydrochloride 7.5 mg per 5 mL. Parabens, potassium sorbate, propylene glycol, sorbitol, sucralose. Strawberry flavor. Liq. 473 mL. *Rx.*
Use: Upper respiratory combination, antitussive combination.

TL Icon. (Trigen Laboratories) Fe 110 mg, folic acid 0.5 mg, intrinsic factor 240 mg, vitamin B_{12} 15 mcg, vitamin C 75 mg. Cap. 60s. *Rx.*
Use: Trace element.

TMP-SMZ. Trimethoprim-Sulfamethoxazole. *Rx.*
Use: Anti-infective.
See: Bactrim.
  Bethaprim.
  Cotrim.
  Septra.
  Sulfatrim.

TNKase. (Genentech) Tenecteplase 50 mg. L-arginine 0.55 g, phosphoric acid 0.17 g, polysorbate 20 4.3 mg. Inj., Lyophilized, Pow. for Soln. Vial w/one 10-mL vial of Sterile Water for Injection and syringe. *Rx.*
Use: Thrombolytic agent; tissue plasminogen activator.

TOBI. (Novartis) Tobramycin 300 mg, NaCl 11.25 g/5 mL. Soln. for Inhalation. Single-use Amp. *Rx.*
Use: Cystic fibrosis.

●**toborinone.** (toe-BORE-ih-nohn) USAN.
Use: Cardiotonic.

Tobrades. (Alcon) Dexamethasone 0.1%, tobramycin 0.3%, thimerosal 0.001%, alcohol 0.5%, propylene glycol, polyoxyethylene, polyoxypropylene. Susp. 2.5 mL, 5 mL. *Rx.*
Use: Anti-infective; corticosteroid.

TobraDex. (Alcon) **Ophth. Oint.:** Dexamethasone 0.1%, tobramycin 0.3%, chlorobutanol 0.5%, mineral oil, white petrolatum. 3.5 g. **Ophth. Susp.:** Tobramycin 0.3%, dexamethasone 0.1%, benzalkonium chloride 0.01%, EDTA, hydroxyethyl cellulose, sodium chloride, sodium hydroxide tyloxapol. Drop-Tainers 2.5 mL, 5 mL, 10 mL. *Rx.*
Use: Anti-infective; corticosteroid; ophthalmic.

●**tobramycin.** (TOE-bruh-MY-sin) *USP 34.* An antibiotic obtained from cultures of *Streptomyces tenebrarius.*
Use: Anti-infective, ophthalmic.
See: AkTob.
  TOBI.
  Tobrex.

tobramycin. (Various Mfr.) Tobramycin 0.3%. Benzalkonium chloride 0.01%, boric acid. Soln. Bot. 5 mL. *Rx.*
Use: Anti-infective, ophthalmic.

tobramycin and dexamethasone. (Falcon) Dexamethasone 0.1%, tobramycin 0.3%. Benzalkonium chloride 0.01%, edetate disodium. Susp., Ophth. Drop-tainers. 2.5 mL, 5 mL, 10 mL. *Rx.*
Use: Ophthalmic and otic agent, steroid antibiotic combination.

●**tobramycin and dexamethasone ophthalmic ointment.** (TOE-bruh-MY-sin) *USP 34.*
Use: Anti-infective, ophthalmic.

tobramycin in 0.9% sodium chloride. (Hospira) Tobramycin (as sulfate) 0.8 mg/mL, 1.2 mg/mL. Inj. Single-dose flexible containers. 50 mL (1.2 mg/mL only), 100 mL (0.8 mg/mL only). *Rx.*
Use: Aminoglycoside.

•**tobramycin sulfate.** (TOE-bruh-MY-sin) *USP 34.*
Use: Anti-infective; aminoglycoside.

tobramycin sulfate. (American Pharmaceutical Partners) Tobramycin sulfate 1.2 g (40 mg/mL after reconstitution). Preservative free. Pow. for Inj. Pharmacy bulk package vial. 50 mL. *Rx.*
Use: Parenteral aminoglycoside.

tobramycin sulfate. (Various Mfr.) Tobramycin sulfate 40 mg/mL. Inj. Syringes: 1.5 mL, 2 mL. Vial 2 mL. Pediatric Inj. 10 mg/mL. Vial 2 mL. *Rx.*
Use: Aminoglycoside; anti-infective.

Tobrex. (Alcon) Tobramycin. Oint.: 3 mg/g. White petrolatum, mineral oil, chlorobutanol 0.05%. 3.5 g. Soln.: 0.3%. Benzalkonium chloride 0.01%, tyloxapol, boric acid. Bot. 5 mL *Drop-Tainer. Rx.*
Use: Anti-infective, ophthalmic.

•**tocamphyl.** (toe-KAM-fill) USAN.
Use: Choleretic.

•**tocilizumab.** (toe-si-LIZ-oo-mab) USAN.
Use: Immune globulin.
See: Actemra.

•**tocladesine.** (toe-CLA-de-seen) USAN.
Use: Antineoplastic; immunomodulator.

•**tocopherols excipient.** (toe-KAHF-ehr-ols) *NF 29.*
Use: Pharmaceutic aid (antioxidant).

•**tocophersolan.** (toe-KAHF-ehr-SO-lan) USAN.
Use: Vitamin supplement.

dl-alpha tocopheryl. Vitamin E.

dl-alpha tocopheryl acetate. Vitamin E.

Tocosamine. (Trent) Sparteine sulfate 150 mg, sodium chloride 4.5 mg/mL. Amps. 1 mL. Box 12s, 100s. *Rx.*
Use: Oxytocic.

•**tofacitinib.** (TOE-fa-SYE-ti-nib) USAN.
Use: Immunological disorders.

•**tofenacin hydrochloride.** (tah-FEN-ah-sin) USAN.
Use: Anticholinergic.

•**tofimilast.** (toe-FIM-i-last) USAN.
Use: Chronic obstructive disease; asthma.

•**tofogliflozin.** (TOE-foe-gli-FLOE-zin) USAN.
Use: Treatment of diabetes mellitus.

tofranazine. (Novartis) Combination of imipramine and promazine. Pending release.

Tofranil. (Novartis) Imipramine hydrochloride 10 mg, 25 mg, 50 mg. Tab. Bot. 100s. *Rx.*
Use: Antidepressant; antienuretic.

Tofranil-PM. (Novartis) Imipramine pamoate 75 mg, 100 mg, 125 mg, 150 mg, parabens. Cap. Bot. 30s, 100s. *Rx.*
Use: Antidepressant.

•**tolamolol.** (tahl-AIM-oh-lahl) USAN.
Use: Beta-adrenergic receptor blocker; coronary vasodilator; cardiovascular agent (antiarrhythmic).

•**tolazamide.** (tole-AZE-uh-mid) *USP 34.*
Tall Man: TOLAZamide
Use: Hypoglycemic; antidiabetic.

tolazamide. (Various Mfr.) Tolazamide 100 mg, 250 mg, 500 mg. Tab. 100s, 200s (250 mg only), 250s (except 250 mg), 500s (except 100 mg), 1000s (250 mg only). *Rx.*
Use: Antidiabetic.

•**tolbutamide.** (tole-BYOO-tuh-mide) *USP 34.*
Tall Man: TOLBUTamide
Use: Hypoglycemic; antidiabetic.

tolbutamide. (Various Mfr.) Tolbutamide 500 mg. Tab. 100s, 500s. *Rx.*
Use: Antidiabetic.

•**tolbutamide sodium.** (tole-BYOO-tuh-mide) *USP 34.*
Tall Man: TOLBUTamide
Use: In vivo diagnostic aid.

•**tolcapone.** (TOLE-kah-pone) USAN.
Use: Antiparkinsonian.
See: Tasmar.

•**tolciclate.** (tole-SIGH-klate) USAN.
Use: Antifungal.

Tolerex. (Procter & Gamble) Protein 20.6 g, carbohydrate 226.3 g, fat 1.45 g, Na 468 mg, K 1172 mg, mOsm/Kg H_2O 550, cal/mL 1, vitamins A, B_1, B_2, B_3, B_5, B_6, B_{12}, C, D, E, K, folic acid, biotin, choline, Ca, P, I, Fe, Mg, Cu, Zn, Mn, Se, Mo, Cr. Assorted flavors Pow. Pkts. 80 g. *OTC.*
Use: Mineral, vitamin supplement.

•**tolevamer potassium sodium.** (toe-LEV-a-mer) USAN.
Use: Antidiarrheal.

•**tolevamer sodium.** (toe-LEV-a-mer) USAN.
Use: Antidiarrheal.

•**tolfamide.** (TAHL-fah-MIDE) USAN.
Use: Enzyme inhibitor (urease).

Tolfrinic. (B.F. Ascher) Ferrous fumarate 200 mg, vitamins B_{12} 25 mcg, C 100 mg. Tab. Bot. 100s. *OTC.*
Use: Mineral, vitamin supplement.

•**tolgabide.** (TOLE-gah-bide) USAN.
Use: Antiepileptic (control of abnormal movements).

•**tolimidone.** (TAHL-IH-mih-dohn) USAN.
Use: Antiulcerative.

•**tolindate.** (TOLE-in-DATE) USAN.
Use: Antifungal.
•**tolmetin.** (TOLE-meh-tin) USAN.
Use: Anti-inflammatory.
•**tolmetin sodium.** (TOLE-meh-tin)
USP 34.
Use: Anti-inflammatory.
tolmetin sodium. (Various Mfr.) Tolmetin
sodium. **Tab.:** 200 mg, 600 mg. Bot.
100s, 500s (600 mg only), UD 100s
(600 mg only). **Cap.:** 400 mg. Bot.
100s, 500s, 1000s, UD 100s. *Rx.*
Use: Anti-inflammatory.
•**tolnaftate.** (tahl-NAFF-tate) *USP 34.*
Use: Antifungal.
See: Blis-To-Sol.
Breezee Mist Antifungal.
Lamisil AF Defense.
Dr. Scholl's.
Tinactin.
Ting.
•**tolofocon A.** (TOE-low-FOE-kahn A)
USAN.
Use: Contact lens material (hydro-
phobic).
toloxychlorinal.
Use: Sedative.
•**tolpovidone I 131.** (tahl-POE-vih-dohnl
131) USAN.
Use: Diagnostic aid (hypoalbuminemia);
radiopharmaceutical.
•**tolpyrramide.** (tole-PIR-a-mide) USAN.
Use: Oral hypoglycemic; antidiabetic.
•**tolterodine.** (tole-TEH-roe-deen) USAN.
Use: Treatment of urinary incontinence.
tolterodine tartrate.
Use: Anticholinergic.
See: Detrol.
Detrol LA.
•**tolu balsam.** (toe-LOO BALL-sam)
USP 34.
Use: Pharmaceutic necessity for Compound Benzoin Tincture; expectorant.
tolu balsam. (Eli Lilly) Syr. Bot. 16 fl. oz.
Use: Vehicle.
•**tolu balsam tincture.** (toe-LOO BALL-
sam) *NF 29.*
Use: Flavor.
toluidine blue o. Tolonium chloride.
Tolu-Sed. (Scherer) Codeine phosphate
10 mg, guaifenesin 100 mg/5 mL w/al-
cohol 10%. Sugar free. Bot. 4 oz., pt.
c-v.
Use: Antitussive; expectorant.
Tolu-Sed DM. (Scherer) Dextromethorphan HBr 10 mg, guaifenesin 100 mg
per 5 mL. Alcohol 10%. Sugar free. Liq.
Bot. 118 mL *OTC.*
Use: Upper respiratory combination, antitussive, expectorant.

•**tolvaptan.** (TOLE-vap-tan) USAN.
Use: Congestive heart failure; hyponatremia.
See: Samsca.
•**tomelukast.** (tah-MELL-you-KAST)
USAN.
Use: Antiasthmatic (leukotriene antagonist).
Tomocat. (Mallinckrodt) Barium sulfate
5%. Simethicone, sorbitol, strawberry
flavor. Conc. Susp. Bot. 145 mL
(480 mL for dilution), 225 mL (1000 mL
for dilution); enema kit in 110 mL with
480 mL bot. for dilution with flexible tubing, clamp, and enema tip. *Rx.*
Use: Radiopaque agent, miscellaneous
gastrointestinal contrast agent.
Tomocat 1000. (Lafayette) Barium sul-
fate suspension concentrate 5% w/v.
Bot. for dilution to 1.5% w/v at time of
use. Bot. 225 mL w/1000 mL dilution
Bot. Case 24 Bot. and 2 Dilution Bot.
Use: Radiopaque medium used to mark
the GI tract during CT scans.
•**tomopenem.** (TOE-moe-PEN-em)
USAN.
Use: Antibiotic.
tomoxetine hydrochloride. (TOE-MOX-
eh-teen)
See: Atomoxetine Hydrochloride.
**Tom's of Maine Natural Cough & Cold
Rub Cough Suppressant.** (Tom's of
Maine) Camphor 4.8%, menthol 2.6%.
Rub. Tube 92.4 g. *OTC.*
Use: Upper respiratory combination,
topical.
•**tonapofylline.** (TOE-na-POF-i-lin)
USAN.
Use: Heart failure.
Tonavite-M. (Ivax) Elix. Bot. 12 oz, pt.,
gal.
Use: Dietary supplement.
•**tonazocine mesylate.** (toe-NAZ-oh-
seen) USAN.
Use: Analgesic.
Tono-B Pediatric. (Pal-Pak, Inc.) Fe
5 mg, thiamine hydrochloride 0.167 mg,
riboflavin 0.133 mg. Tab. Bot. 1000s.
OTC.
Use: Mineral, vitamin supplement.
Tonopaque. (Mallinckrodt) Barium sul-
fate 95%. Simethicone. Pow. for Susp.
Kits. 340 g, 454 g. *Rx.*
Use: Radiopaque agent, GI contrast
agent.
Tonsiline. (Oakhurst) Alcohol 4%, glycerin, sucrose, iron chloride, magnesium carbonate, tolu balsam, sodium
saccharin. Mouthwash. 118 mL. *OTC.*
Use: Mouth and throat product.

Toothache Relief-3 in 1. (C.S. Dent & Co.) Toothache gum, toothache drops, benzocaine. Lot. *OTC.*
Use: Analgesic, topical.

Topamax. (Janssen) Topiramate **Tab.:** 25 mg, 50 mg, 100 mg. Lactose. Bot. 60s. **Sprinkle Cap.:** 15 mg, 25 mg. Sucrose. Bot. 60s. *Rx.*
Use: Anticonvulsant.

Top Brass ZP-11. (Revlon) Zinc pyrithione 0.5% in cream base. *OTC.*
Use: Antidandruff.

Top-Form. (Colgate Oral) Topical form-fitting gel applicators. Disposable trays for topical fluoride office treatments, plus permanent trays for topical fluoride home self-treatments. Box 100s. *Rx.*
Use: Topical fluoride applications in home or office.

Topic. (Roche) 5% benzyl alcohol in greaseless gel base containing camphor, menthol, w/30% isopropyl alcohol. Tube 2 oz. *OTC.*
Use: Antipruritic.

Topicaine. (ESBA Labs) Lidocaine hydrochloride 4%. Aloe vera oil, benzyl alcohol, EDTA, ethanol 35%, glycerin, glyceryl, jojoba oil. Gel. 10 g, 30 g, 113 g. *OTC.*
Use: Topical local anesthetic, amide local anesthetic.

Topicaine 5. (ESBA Labs) Lidocaine hydrochloride 5%. Aloe vera oil, benzyl alcohol, EDTA, ethanol, glycerin, glyceryl, jojoba oil, shea butter. Gel. 10 g, 30 g, 113 g. *OTC.*
Use: Topical local anesthetic, amide local anesthetic.

topical anesthetics, miscellaneous.
See: Ethyl Chloride.
   Fluro-Ethyl.

Topical Fluoride. (Pacemaker) Acidulated phosphate fluoride. Flavors: Orange, bubble gum, lime, raspberry, grape, cinnamon. Liq. Bot. 4 oz, pt. *Rx.*
Use: Corticosteroid, topical.

Topicort. (Taro) **Cream:** Desoximetasone 0.25% emollient cream consisting of isopropyl myristate, cetyl stearyl alcohol, white petrolatum, mineral oil, lanolin alcohol, purified water. Tube 15 g, 60 g, 120 g. **Gel:** Desoximetasone 0.05% in gel base. 20% alcohol. Tube 15 g, 60 g. **Oint.:** Desoximetasone 0.25% in ointment base. Tube 15 g, 60 g. *Rx.*
Use: Corticosteroid, topical.

Topicort LP. (Taro) Desoximetasone 0.05%. Cream. Tube 15 g, 60 g. *Rx.*
Use: Corticosteroid, topical.

Topiragen. (Upsher-Smith) Topiramate 25 mg, 50 mg, 100 mg, 200 mg. Lactose, PEG. Tab. 60s, 100s, 500s, 1,000s, UD 100s. *Rx.*
Use: Anticonvulsant.

•**topiramate.** (toe-PIRE-ah-MATE) USAN.
Use: Anticonvulsant.
See: Topamax.
   Topiragen.

topiramate. (Teva) Topiramate 15 mg, 25 mg. PEG, sugar. Cap. Sprinkle. 60s. *Rx.*
Use: Anticonvulsant.

topiramate. (Various Mfr.) Topiramate 25 mg, 50 mg, 100 mg, 200 mg. May contain lactose and PEG. Film-coated. Tab. 30s, 60s, 90s, 100s, 500s, 1,000s, UD 100s. *Rx.*
Use: Anticonvulsant.

•**topixantrone.** (toe-PIX-an-trone) USAN.
Use: Antineoplastic.

Toposar. (Gensia Sicor) Etoposide 20 mg, benzyl alcohol 30 mg, alcohol 30.5%/mL. Inj. Multiple–dose vial. 5 mL, 25 mL, 50 mL. *Rx.*
Use: Antineoplastic.

•**topotecan hydrochloride.** (toe-poe-TEE-kan) USAN.
Use: DNA topoisomerase inhibitor.
See: Hycamtin.

topotecan hydrochloride. (Various Mfr.) Topotecan hydrochloride 4 mg. May contain mannitol. Preservative free. Inj., lyophilized Pow. for Soln. Single-dose vial. *Rx.*
Use: Antineoplastic, DNA topoisomerase inhibitor.

Toprol XL. (AstraZeneca) Metoprolol succinate 23.75 mg (equivalent to metoprolol tartrate 25 mg), 47.5 mg (equivalent to metoprolol tartrate 50 mg), 95 mg (equivalent to metoprolol tartrate 100 mg), 190 mg (equivalent to metoprolol tartrate 200 mg). ER Tab. Bot. 100s. *Rx.*
Use: Antihypertensive; antiadrenergic/ sympatholytic, beta-adrenergic blocker.

•**topterone.** (TOP-ter-ohn) USAN.
Use: Antiandrogen.

•**toquizine.** (TOE-kwih-zeen) USAN.
Use: Anticholinergic.

•**toralizumab.** (toe-ra-LYE-zyoo-mab) USAN.
Use: Monoclonal antibody.

•**torapsel.** (tore-AP-sel) USAN.
Use: Hematologic agent.

•**torcetrapib.** (tore-SET-ra-pib) USAN.
Use: Cardiovascular agent.

●**torcitabine.** (tore-SITE-a-been) USAN.
Use: Polymerase inhibitor (hepatitis B).

●**toremifene citrate.** (TORE-EM-ih-feen)
USAN.
Use: Antiestrogen; antineoplastic.
See: Fareston.

●**torezolid.** (toe-REZ-oh-lid) USAN.
Use: Antibiotic.

●**torezolid phosphate.** (tore-EZ-oh-lid)
USAN.
Use: Antibiotic.

Torisel. (Wyeth) Temsirolimus 25 mg/mL.
Alcohol, polysorbate 80. Concentrated
Soln. for Inj. 2-vial kits. *Rx.*
Use: Antineoplastic, protein-tyrosine ki-
nase inhibitor, mTOR inhibitor.

●**torsemide.** (TORE-suh-MIDE) *USP 34.*
Use: Diuretic.
See: Demadex.

torsemide. (Teva) Torsemide 5 mg,
10 mg, 20 mg, 100 mg, lactose. Tab.
100s. *Rx.*
Use: Diuretic.

torula yeast, dried. Obtained by grow-
ing *Candida (torulopsis) utilis* yeast on
wood pulp wastes (Nutritional Labs)
Conc. 100 lb drums.
Use: Natural source of protein and Vitamin B-complex vitamins.

●**tosagestin.** (TOE-sa-jes-tin) USAN.
Use: Hormone replacement therapy.

●**tosedostat.** (toe-SED-oh-stat) USAN.
Use: Antineoplastic.

●**tosifen.** (TOE-sih-fen) USAN.
Use: Antianginal.

**tositumomab and iodine I 131 tositu-
momab.**
Use: Antineoplastic.
See: Bexxar.

●**tosufloxacin.** (toe-SUE-FLOX-ah-sin)
USAN.
Use: Anti-infective.

Totacillin. (GlaxoSmithKline) Ampicillin
trihydrate equivalent to: **Cap.:** 250 mg,
500 mg. Bot. 500s. **Pow. for Oral
Susp.:** 125 mg/5 mL, 250 mg/5 mL.
Bot. 100 mL, 200 mL. *Rx.*
Use: Anti-infective, penicillin.

Total. (Allergan) Polyvinyl alcohol, edetate disodium, benzalkonium chloride
in a sterile, buffered, isotonic solution.
Soln. Bot. 60 mL, 120 mL. *OTC.*
Use: Contact lens care.

TotalDay. (Nature's Blend) Vitamins A
25,000 units, D 1,000 units, E 100 units,
B_1 100 mg, B_2 100 mg, B_3 100 mg, B_5
100 mg, B_6 100 mg, B_{12} 100 mcg, C
500 mg, folate 1 mg, Fe 18 mg, Ca
250 mg, Cl, Cr, Cu, I, K, Mg, Mn, Mo,
P, Se, Zn, biotin, choline, citrus bioflavonoids complex, inositol, PABA, rutin.
Maltodextrin, polydextrose. Tab., timed
release. 120s. *OTC.*
Use: Multivitamin with minerals.

Total Eclipse Cooling Alcohol. (Novartis) Padimate O, oxybenzone, glyceryl
PABA, alcohol 77%. SPF 15. Lot. Bot.
120 mL. *OTC.*
Use: Sunscreen.

Total Eclipse Moisturizing. (Novartis)
Padimate O, oxybenzone, octyl salicy-
late. Moisturizing base. SPF 15. Lot.
Bot. 120 mL. *OTC.*
Use: Sunscreen.

**Total Eclipse Oil & Acne Prone Skin
Sunscreen.** (Novartis) Padimate O,
oxybenzone, glyceryl PABA, alcohol
77%. SPF 15. Lot. Bot. 120 mL. *OTC.*
Use: Sunscreen.

Total Formula. (Vitaline) Fe 20 mg, vitamins A 10,000 units, D 400 units, E
30 units, B_1 15 mg, B_2 15 mg, B_3
25 mg, B_5 25 mg, B_6 25 mg, B_{12}
25 mcg, C 100 mg, folic acid 0.4 mg,
Ca, Cr, Cu, I, K, Mg, Mn, Mo, P, Se, Si,
V, vitamin K, biotin 300 mcg, Zn
30 mg, choline, bioflavonoids, hesperidin, inositol, PABA, rutin. Tab. Bot. 90s,
100s. *OTC.*
Use: Mineral, vitamin supplement.

Total Formula-2. (Vitaline) Fe 20 mg, vitamins A 10,000 units, D 400 units, E
30 units, B_1 15 mg, B_2 15 mg, B_3
25 mg, B_5 25 mg, B_6 25 mg, B_{12}
25 mcg, C 100 mg, folic acid 0.4 mg,
Ca, Cr, Cu, I, K, Mg, Mn, Mo, P, Se, Si,
V, vitamin K, biotin 300 mcg, Zn
30 mg, choline, bioflavonoids, hesperidin, inositol, PABA, rutin. Tab. with boron. Bot. 60s. *OTC.*
Use: Mineral, vitamin supplement.

totaquine. Alkaloids from *Cinchona* bark,
7% to 12% quinine anhydrous, 70% to
80% total alkaloids (cinchonidine, cinchonine, quinidine & quinine).

Totect. (TopoTarget) Dexrazoxane
500 mg (equiv. to dexrazoxane hydrochloride 589 mg). Preservative free. Inj.
Lyophilized Pow. for Soln. Single-use
vials with 50 mL sodium lactate injection. *Rx.*
Use: Cytoprotective agent.

totomycin hydrochloride. Tetracycline.

Touro A & D. (Dartmouth) Chlorpheniramine maleate 4 mg, phenyltoloxamine
citrate 50 mg, phenylephrine hydrochloride 20 mg. SR Cap. Bot. 100s. *Rx.*
Use: Antihistamine; decongestant.

Touro Allergy. (Dartmouth) Pseudoephedrine hydrochloride 60 mg, brompheniramine maleate 5.75 mg. Su-

crose. ER Cap.100s. *Rx.*
Use: Upper respiratory combination, decongestant and antihistamine combination.
Touro CC. (Dartmouth) Guaifenesin
575 mg, pseudoephedrine hydrochloride 60 mg, dextromethorphan HBr
30 mg. Dye free. ER Tab. Bot. 100s.
Rx.
Use: Upper respiratory combination, antitussive and expectorant combination.
Touro CC-LD. (Dartmouth) Dextromethorphan HBr 30 mg, guaifenesin
575 mg, pseudoephedrine 25 mg. Dye
free. SR Tab. 100s. *Rx.*
Use: Antitussive and expectorant.
Touro DM. (Dartmouth) Dextromethorphan HBr 30 mg, guaifenesin 575 mg.
ER Tab. Bot. 100s. *Rx.*
Use: Upper respiratory combination, antitussive, expectorant.
Touro HC. (Dartmouth) Hydrocodone bitartrate 5 mg, guaifenesin 575 mg. Dye
free. ER Tab. 100s. *c-III.*
Use: Antitussive with expectorant.
Touro LA. (Dartmouth) Pseudoephedrine hydrochloride 120 mg, guaifenesin 525 mg. ER Tab. Bot. 100s. *Rx.*
Use: Upper respiratory combination, decongestant, expectorant.
Tovalt ODT. (Biovail) Zolpidem tartrate
5 mg, 10 mg. Acesulfame K, mannitol. Tab., Orally Disintegrating. UD 28s.
c-IV.
Use: Sedative/hypnotic, nonbarbiturate,
imidazopyridine.
Toviaz. (Pfizer) Fesoterodine fumarate
4 mg, 8 mg. Lactose, PEG, polyvinyl
alcohol. Film-coated. ER Tab. 30s, 90s,
UD 100s. *Rx.*
Use: Renal and genitourinary agent, an-
ticholinergic.
Toxo. (Wampole) *Toxoplasma* antibody
test system. Tests 120s.
Use: An IFA test system for the detec-
tion of antibodies to *Toxoplasma
gondii.*
toxoid, diphtheria.
Use: Immunization.
See: Diphtheria and Tetanus Toxoids,
Acellular Pertussis and Haemophi-
lus Influenzae Type B Conjugate
Vaccine.
Diphtheria and Tetanus Toxoids, Adult.
Diphtheria and Tetanus Toxoids, and
Acellular Pertussis Adsorbed,
Hepatitis B (Recombinant) and
Inactivated Poliovirus Vaccine Com-
bined.
Diphtheria and Tetanus Toxoids and

Acellular Pertussis Vaccine, Ad-
sorbed.
Diphtheria and Tetanus Toxoids, Pedi-
atric.
Tetanus and Diphtheria Toxoids Ad-
sorbed for Adult Use.
toxoid, tetanus. *Rx.*
Use: Immunization.
See: Diphtheria and Tetanus Toxoids,
Acellular Pertussis and Haemophi-
lus Influenzae Type B Conjugate
Vaccine.
Diphtheria and Tetanus Toxoids, Adult.
Diphtheria and Tetanus Toxoids and
Acellular Pertussis Adsorbed,
Hepatitis B (Recombinant) and
Inactivated Poliovirus Vaccine Com-
bined.
Diphtheria and Tetanus Toxoids and
Acellular Pertussis Vaccine, Ad-
sorbed.
Diphtheria and Tetanus Toxoids, Pedi-
atric.
Tetanus and Diphtheria Toxoids Ad-
sorbed for Adult Use.
Tetanus Toxoid.
Tetanus Toxoid, Adsorbed.
Tetanus Toxoid, Adsorbed, Puroge-
nated.
toxoplasmosis test.
Use: Diagnostic aid.
See: TPM Test.
•**tozasertib.** (TOE-za-SER-tib) USAN.
Use: Antineoplastic agent.
•**tozasertib lactate.** (TOE-za-SER-tib)
USAN.
Use: Antineoplastic agent.
t-PA.
Use: Tissue plasminogen activator.
See: Activase.
TPM-Test. (Wampole) Indirect hemagglu-
tination test for the qualitative and quan-
titative determination of antibodies to
Toxoplasma gondii in serum. Kit 120s.
Use: Diagnostic aid, toxoplasmosis.
TPN Electrolytes. (Hospira) Na⁺
35 mEq, K⁺ 20 mEq, Ca⁺⁺ 4.5 mEq,
Mg⁺⁺ 5 mEq, Cl⁻ 35 mEq, acetate
29.5 mEq/20 mL, osmolarity 6220
mOsm/L. Soln. Pharmacy bulk packaging vial 100 mL. *Rx.*
Use: Intravenous nutritional therapy,
intravenous replenishment solution.
TPN Electrolytes III. (Hospira) Na 25 Eq,
K 40.6 mEq, Ca 5 mEq, Mg 8 mEq, Cl
33.5 mEq, acetate 40.6 mEq, gluconate 5 mEq/20 mL, osmolarity 7520
mOsm/L. Soln. Pharmacy bulk pkg. Vial
100 mL. *Rx.*
Use: Intravenous nutritional therapy,
intravenous replenishment solution.

TPN Electrolytes II. (Hospira) Na 18 mEq, K 18 mEq, Ca 4.5 mEq, Mg 5 mEq, Cl 35 mEq, acetate 10.5 mEq/ 20 mL, osmolarity 4320 mOsm/L. Soln. Single-dose and additive syr. 20 mL *Rx.*
Use: Intravenous nutritional therapy, intravenous replenishment solution.

• **tracazolate.** (trak-AZ-oh-late) USAN.
Use: Sedative; hypnotic.

• **trabectedin.** (tra-BEK-te-din) USAN.
Use: Antineoplastic.

Trace. (Young Dental) Erythrosine conc. soln. Squeeze Bot. 30 mL, 60 mL. Dispenser Packets 200s. *OTC.*
Use: Diagnostic aid, disclose dental plaque.

trace elements.
Use: Mineral supplement.
See: Carbonyl Iron.
Complex Zinc Carbonates.
Ferrous Fumarate.
Ferrous Gluconate.
Ferrous Sulfate.
Ferrous Sulfate Exsiccated (Dried).
Fluoride.
Iron.
Iron Dextran.
Iron/Liver Combination.
Iron Sucrose.
Iron with Vitamin B_{12} and IFC.
Iron with Vitamin C.
Iron with Vitamins.
Manganese.
Polysaccharide-Iron Complex.
Sodium Ferric Gluconate Complex.
Zinc Acetate.
Zinc Gluconate.
Zinc Sulfate.

Trace Elements 4 Pediatric. (American Regent) Chromium (as chloride) 1 mcg, copper (as sulfate) 0.1 mg, manganese (as sulfate) 0.03 mg, zinc (as sulfate) 0.5 mg. Benzyl alcohol 0.9%. Inj. Multidose vial. 10 mL. *Rx.*
Use: Trace metal combination.

trace metals.
See: Chromic Chloride.
Zinc Sulfate.

Traceplex. (Enzyme Process) Fe 30 mg, I 0.1 mg, Cu 0.5 mg, Mg 40 mg, Zn 10 mg, B_{12} 5 mcg/4 Tabs. Bot. 100s, 250s. *OTC.*
Use: Mineral supplement.

Tracer bG. (Boehringer Mannheim) Reagent strips. Kit. 25s, 50s.
Use: Diagnostic aid.

Trace 28. (Young Dental) **Liq.:** FD&C Red No. 28 in aqueous soln. Bot. 30 mL, 60 mL. **Tab.:** FD&C Red No. 28. Box 30s, 180s, 700s. *OTC.*

Use: Diagnostic aid, disclose dental plaque.

Tracleer. (Actelion Pharm) Bosentan 62.5 mg, 125 mg. Tab. Bot. 60s. *Rx.*
Use: Vasodilator, endothelin receptor antagonist.

Tracrium Injection. (GlaxoSmithKline) Atracurium besylate 10 mg/mL Amp. 5 mL. Box 10s; 10 mL MDV. Box 10s. *Rx.*
Use: Muscle relaxant.

Tradjenta. (Boehringer Ingelheim) Linagliptin 5 mg. Film coated. Mannitol. Tab. 30s, 90s, 1,000s, UD 100s. *Rx.*
Use: Antidiabetic agent, dipeptidyl peptidase-4 inhibitor.

• **trafermin.** (trah-FUR-min) USAN.
Use: Treatment of stroke and coronary artery disease.

• **tragacanth.** (TRAG-ah-kanth) *NF 29.*
Use: Pharmaceutic aid (suspending agent).

• **tralokinumab.** (TRAL-oh-KIN-ue-mab) USAN.
Use: Respiratory agent.

• **tralonide.** (TRAL-oh-nide) USAN.
Use: Corticosteroid, topical.

tramadol. (Various Mfr.) Tramadol hydrochloride 50 mg. Tab. 100s, 500s, 1,000s. *Rx.*
Use: Opioid analgesic.

tramadol and acetaminophen. (Par) Tramadol hydrochloride 37.5 mg, acetaminophen 325 mg. Tab. 20s, 100s, 500s. *Rx.*
Use: Narcotic analgesic combination.

• **tramadol hydrochloride.** (TRAM-uh-dole) USAN.
Tall Man: traMADol
Use: Opioid analgesic.
See: Rybix ODT.
Ryzolt.
Ultram.
Ultram ER.
W/Acetaminophen.
See: Ultracet.

tramadol hydrochloride. (Various Mfr.) Tramadol hydrochloride 100 mg, 200 mg, 300 mg. ER Tab. 30s, 90s, 500s (except 300 mg). *Rx.*
Use: Opioid analgesic.

• **tramazoline hydrochloride.** (tram-AZ-oh-leen) USAN.
Use: Adrenergic.

• **tramiprosate.** (tram-IP-roe-sate) USAN.
Use: Alzheimer disease.

Trandate. (Faro Pharmaceuticals) Labetalol hydrochloride 100 mg, 200 mg, 300 mg. Tab. 100s, 500s, UD 100s. *Rx.*

Use: Antiadrenergic/sympatholytic, alpha/beta-adrenergic blocker.

trandolapril.
Use: Antihypertensive.
See: Mavik.
W/Verapamil Hydrochloride.
See: Tarka.

trandolapril. (Teva) Trandolapril 1 mg, 2 mg, 4 mg. Lactose. Tab. 100s. *Rx.*
Use: Antihypertensive.

trandolapril/verapamil hydrochloride. (Glenmark Pharmaceuticals) Trandolapril/verapamil hydrochloride 1 mg/240 mg, 2 mg/180 mg, 2 mg/240 mg, 4 mg/240 mg. Film coated. Lactose. ER Tab. 100s. *Rx.*
Use: Antihypertensive combination.

•**tranexamic acid.** (tran-ex-AM-ik) USAN.
Use: Hemostatic. [Orphan Drug]
See: Cyklokapron.
Lysteda.

•**tranilast.** (TRAN-ill-ast) USAN.
Use: Antiasthmatic.

tranquilizers.
See: Compazine.
Fenarol.
Librium.
Loxitane.
Meprobamate.
Miltown.
Permitil.
Prolixin.
Tranxene.
Trilafon.
Valium.
Vistaril.

Tranquils. (Halsey Drug) **Cap.:** Pyrilamine maleate 25 mg. Bot. 30s. **Tab.:** Acetaminophen 300 mg, pyrilamine maleate 25 mg. Bot. 30s. *OTC.*
Use: Sleep aid.

•**transcainide.** (trans-CANE-ide) USAN.
Use: Antiarrhythmic, cardiovascular agent.

Transderm-Nitro. (Summit) Nitroglycerin 12.5 mg, 25 mg, 50 mg, 75 mg, 100 mg. Patch. Box 30s, UD 30s (except 75 mg), 100s (except 75 mg, 100 mg). *Rx.*
Use: Antianginal.

Transderm-Scōp. (Baxter) Scopolamine 1.5 mg (delivers scopolamine ≈ 1 mg over 3 days). Transdermal Patch. 10s, 24s. *Rx.*
Use: Antiemetic/antivertigo agent.

transforming growth factor-beta 2. (Celtrix)
Use: Immunomodulator. [Orphan Drug]

Transthyretin EIA. (Abbott Diagnostics) Test kits 100s.
Use: Diagnostic aid.

Trans-Ver-Sal AdultPatch. (Doak Dermatologics) Salicylic acid 15%. Transdermal patch. 6 mm, 12 mm. 40s. Securing tape and cleaning file. *OTC.*
Use: Keratolytic.

Trans-Ver-Sal PediaPatch. (Doak Dermatologics) Salicylic acid 15%. Transdermal patch. 6 mm. 20s. Securing tape and cleaning file. *OTC.*
Use: Keratolytic.

Trans-Ver-Sal PlantarPatch. (Doak Dermatologics) Salicylic acid 15%. Transdermal patch. 20 mm patches, 25s. Securing tapes, cleaning file. *OTC.*
Use: Dermatologic, wart therapy.

Tranxene T-tab. (Ovation) Clorazepate dipotassium 3.75 mg, 7.5 mg, 15 mg. Tab. 100s, 500s, UD 100s. *c-iv.*
Use: Anxiolytic.

tranylcypromine. (Par) Tranylcypromine sulfate 10 mg. Film-coated. Tab. 100s. *Rx.*
Use: Antidepressant, monoamine oxidase inhibitor.

•**tranylcypromine sulfate.** (tran-ill-SIP-row-meen) *USP 34.*
Use: Antidepressant, monoamine oxidase inhibitor.
See: Parnate.

•**trastuzumab.** (tras-TOOZ-oo-mab) USAN.
Use: Monoclonal antibody.
See: Herceptin.

•**trastuzumab emtansine.** (tras-TOOZ-oo-mab em-TAN-seen) USAN.
Use: Antineoplastic.

Trasylol. (Bayer Consumer Care) Aprotinin 1.4 mg/mL. Inj. Vial 100 mL, 200 mL. *Rx.*
Use: Antihemophilic.

T-Rau. (Tennessee Pharmaceutic) Rauwolfia serpentina 50 mg or 100 mg. Tab. Bot. 100s, 1000s. *Rx.*
Use: Hypotensive.

Travamulsion 10% Intravenous Fat Emulsion. (Baxter PPI) 1.1 kcal/mL 270 mOsm/L. Bot. 500 mL. *Rx.*
Use: Nutritional supplement, parenteral.

Travamulsion 20% Intravenous Fat Emulsion. (Baxter PPI) 2 kcal/mL 300 mOsm/L. Bot. 500 mL. *Rx.*
Use: Nutritional supplement, parenteral.

Travasol. (Baxter Medication Delivery) Crystalline L-amino acids 8.5%. Inj. 500 mL, 1,000 mL, 2,000 mL. *Rx.*
Use: Nutritional supplement, parenteral.

Travasol 10%. (Baxter Medication Delivery) Crystalline L-amino acids 10%. Inj. Bot. 200 mL, 500 mL, 1000 mL, 2000 mL. *Rx.*
Use: Nutritional supplement, parenteral.

Travasol 3.5% M Injection with Electrolyte #45. (Baxter Medication Delivery) Crystalline L-amino acids 3.5%. Soln. Bot. IV 500 mL, 1000 mL. *Rx.*
Use: Nutritional supplement, parenteral.

Travasorb HN Peptide Diet. (Baxter PPI) High-nitrogen defined peptide 333 kcal. Pkt. 6 pkt. Carton. *OTC.*
Use: Nutritional supplement.

Travasorb MCT Liquid Diet. (Baxter PPI) Digestible protein medium-chain triglyceride diet. 89 g packets. *OTC.*
Use: Nutritional supplement.

Travasorb MCT Powder Diet. (Baxter PPI) Digestible protein medium-chain triglyceride diet 400 kcal. Pkt. 6 pkt. Carton. *OTC.*
Use: Nutritional supplement.

Travasorb Renal Diet. (Baxter PPI) 467 kcal. Pkt. 6 pkt. Carton. 112 g packets. *OTC.*
Use: Nutritional supplement.

Travasorb Standard Diet. (Baxter PPI) Defined peptide diet, 333 kcal. pkt. 6 packets. Ctn. *OTC.*
Use: Nutritional supplement.

Travasorb STD. (Clintec Nutrition) Enzymatically hydrolyzed lactalbumin 10 g, glucose oligosaccharides 63.3 g, MCT (fractioned coconut oil) 4.5 g, sunflower oil 4.5 g, Na 307 mg, K 390 mg, mOsm/560 Kg, H_2O, cal 333.3/mL, vitamins A, B_1, B_2, B_3, B_5, B_6, B_{12}, C, D, E, K, Ca, Cl, Cu, Fe, I, Mg, Mn, P, Zn. Gluten free. Pow. Pkts. 83.3 g. *OTC.*
Use: Nutritional supplement.

Travasorb Whole Protein Liquid Diet. (Baxter PPI) Lactose free complete nutrition 250 kcal. Can. 8 oz. *OTC.*
Use: Nutritional supplement.

Travatan Z. (Alcon) Travoprost 0.004%. Polyoxyl 40 hydrogenated castor oil, *sofZia* as a preservative. Ophth. Soln. *Drop-Tainers.* 2.5 mL, 5 mL. *Rx.*
Use: Agent for glaucoma; prostaglandin agonist.

Travel Aids. (Faraday) Dimenhydrinate 50 mg. Tab. Bot. 30s. *OTC.*
Use: Antiemetic; antivertigo.

Travel-Eze. (Health for Life Brands) Pyrilamine maleate 25 mg, hyoscine hydrobromide 0.325 mg. Tab. Pkg. 20s. *OTC.*
Use: Antiemetic; antivertigo.

Travel Sickness. (Walgreen) Dimenhydrinate 50 mg. Tab. Bot. 24s. *OTC.*
Use: Antiemetic; antivertigo.

Traveltabs. (Armenpharm Ltd.) Dimenhydrinate 50 mg. Tab. Bot. 100s. *OTC.*
Use: Antiemetic; antivertigo.

Travert. (Baxter PPI) Invert sugar injection 10% in water or saline. Plastic Bot.

500 mL, 1000 mL, electrolyte No. 2 Bot. 500 mL, 1000 mL, electrolyte No. 4 Bot. 250 mL, 500 mL Soln. (10%). *Rx.*
Use: Fluid, electrolyte replacement.

5% Travert and Electrolyte No. 2. (Baxter PPI) Invert sugar 50 g/L, calories 196 Cal/L, Na 56 mEq/L, K 25 mEq/L, Mg 6 mEq/L, Cl 56 mEq/L, phosphate 12.5 mEq/L, lactate 25 mEq/L, osmolarity 449 mOsm/L. 1000 mL. *Rx.*
Use: Nutritional supplement, parenteral.

10% Travert and Electrolyte No. 2. (Baxter PPI) Invert sugar 100 g/L, calories 384 Cal/L, Na 56 mEq/L, K 25 mEq/L, Mg 6 mEq/L, Cl 56 mEq/L, phosphate 12.5 mEq/L, lactate 25 mEq/L, osmolarity 726 mOsm/L. 1000 mL. *Rx.*
Use: Nutritional supplement, parenteral.

•**travoprost.** (TRA-voe-prost) USAN.
Use: Antiglaucoma; prostaglandin agonist.
See: Travatan Z.

•**trazodone hydrochloride.** (TRAY-zoe-dohn) *USP 34.*
Tall Man: traZODone
Use: Antidepressant.
See: Oleptro.

trazodone hydrochloride. (Barr) Trazodone hydrochloride 300 mg. Tab. Bot. 100s, 500s. *Rx.*
Use: Antidepressant.

trazodone hydrochloride. (Various Mfr.). Trazodone hydrochloride 50 mg, 100 mg, 150 mg. Tab. 100s, 500s, 1000s. UD 100s (except 150 mg). *Rx.*
Use: Antidepressant.

Treagan. (Trigen Labs) Antipyrine 5.4%, benzocaine 1.4%, u-polycosanol 410 0.0097%, acetic acid, glycerin. Soln., otic. 15 mL w/dropper. *Rx.*
Use: Miscellaneous otic preparation.

Treanda. (Cephalon) Bendamustine hydrochloride 25 mg, 100 mg. Preservative free. Mannitol 170 mg (100 mg), 42.5 mg (25 mg). Inj., Lyophilized, Pow. for Soln. Single-use vials. 20 mL (100 mg), 8mL (25 mg). *Rx.*
Use: Mechlorethamine derivative, ethylenimine/methylmelamine, alkylating agent.

•**trebenzomine hydrochloride.** (TRAY-BEN-zoe-meen) USAN.
Use: Antidepressant.

Trecator. (Wyeth) Ethionamide 250 mg. Film-coated. Tab. Bot. 100s. *Rx.*
Use: Antituberculosis agent.

•**trecovirsen sodium.** (treh-koe-VEER-sin) USAN.
Use: Antiviral.

•**trefentanil hydrochloride.** (treh-FEN-tah-nill) USAN.
Use: Analgesic.

•**treloxinate.** (trell-OX-ih-nate) USAN.
Use: Antihyperlipoproteinemic.

Trelstar. (Watson) Triptorelin pamoate 3.75 mg, 11.25 mg, 22.5 mg. Mannitol, polysorbate 80. Inj., lyophilized microgranules for Susp. Single-dose vial and in *Mixject* delivery system w/ 2 mL of diluent.

Trelstar Depot. (Watson) Triptorelin pamoate equivalent to 3.75 mg triptorelin peptide base, mannitol. Microgranules for Inj., lyophilized. Single-dose vial. *Rx.*
Use: Hormone; gonadotropin-releasing hormone analog.

Trelstar LA. (Watson) Triptorelin pamoate equivalent to 11.25 mg triptorelin peptide base, mannitol. Microgranules for Inj., lyophilized. Single-dose vial. *Rx.*
Use: Hormone; gonadotropin-releasing hormone analog.

Trental. (Hoechst Marion Roussel) Pentoxifylline 400 mg. Film-coated. CR Tab. Bot. 100s. Bulk pack. 5000s. *Rx.*
Tall Man: TRENtal
Use: Hemorrheologic agent.

Treo. (Biopharmaceutics) **SPF 8:** Octocrylene, octyl methoxycinnamate, benzophenone-3, octyl salicylate, isostearyl alcohol, diazolidinyl urea, propylparabens, citronella oil 0.05% (as insect repellant). Lot. Bot. 118 mL. **SPF 15:** Octocrylene, octyl methoxycinnamate, benzophenone-3, octyl salicylate, isostearyl alcohol, diazolidinyl urea, propylparaben, citronella oil 0.05% (as insect repellant). Lot. Bot. 118 mL. **SPF 30:** Octocrylene, octyl methoxycinnamate, benzophenone-3, octyl salicylate, isostearyl alcohol, diazolidinyl urea, propylparaben, citronella oil 0.05% (as insect repellant). Lot. Bot. 118 mL. *OTC.*
Use: Sunscreen.

treosulfan.
Use: Antineoplastic. [Orphan Drug]
See: Ovastat.

•**trepipam maleate.** (TREH-pih-pam MAL-ee-ate) USAN. *Formerly Trimopam Maleate.*
Use: Sedative; hypnotic.

•**treprostinil sodium.** (treh-PRAHST-in-ill SO-dee-uhm) USAN.
Use: Vasodilator.
See: Remodulin.
 Tyvaso.

•**trestolone acetate.** (TRESS-toe-lone) USAN.
Use: Antineoplastic; androgen.

trethocanoic acid.
Use: Anticholesteremic.

•**tretinoin.** (TREH-tih-NO-in) *USP 34.*
Use: Retinoid.
See: Atradin.
 Avita.
 Renova.
 Retin-A.
 Tretin-X.
W/Combinations.
See: Tri-Luma.
 Ziana.

tretinoin. (Alpharma, Spear Dermatology) Tretinoin 0.025%, may contain stearyl alcohol. Cream. Tube. 20 g, 45 g. *Rx.*
Use: Retinoid.

tretinoin. (Barr) Tretinoin 10 mg. Cap. 100s. *Rx.*
Use: Retinoid.

tretinoin. (Spear Dermatology.) Tretinoin. **Cream:** 0.05%, 0.1%, stearyl alcohol. Tube. 20 g, 45 g. **Gel:** 0.01%, 0.025%, alcohol. Tube. 15 g, 45 g. *Rx.*
Use: Retinoid.

Tretin-X. (Triax) Tretinoin. **Cream:** 0.025%, 0.05%, 0.1%. Hydrophilic vehicle. 35 g. **Gel:** 0.01%, 0.025%. Alcohol 90%. 35 g. *Rx.*
Use: Retinoid.

Trexall. (Barr) Methotrexate 5 mg, 7.5 mg, 10 mg, 15 mg, lactose. Film-coated. Tab. Bot. 30s, 60s, 100s. *Rx.*
Use: Antipsoriatic; antirheumatic; antimetabolite.

Trexan. (DuPont) Naltrexone hydrochloride 50 mg. Tab. Bot. 50s. *Rx.*
Use: Opioid antagonist.

Treximet. (GlaxoSmithKline) Naproxen sodium 500 mg, sumatriptan 85 mg. Dextrose, sodium 61.2 mg. Film-coated. Tab. 9s. *Rx.*
Use: Agent for migraine, migraine combination.

Trezix. (Wraser Pharmaceuticals) Acetaminophen 356.4 mg, caffeine 30 mg, dihydrocodeine bitartrate 16 mg. Cap. 100s. *c-III.*
Use: Opioid analgesic combination.

Triac. (Eon Labs) Triprolidine hydrochloride 2.5 mg, pseudoephedrine hydrochloride 60 mg. Tab. Bot. 100s, 1000s. *Rx.*
Use: Antihistamine; decongestant.

Triacet. (Teva) Triamcinolone acetonide 0.1%. Cream. Tube 15 g, 80 g. *Rx.*
Use: Corticosteroid, topical.

•**triacetin.** (try-ah-SEE-tin) *USP 34.* Formerly *glyceryl triacetate.*
Use: Antifungal, topical.
See: Fungacetin.

Triacin-C Cough. (Alpharma) Pseudoephedrine hydrochloride 30 mg, triprolidine hydrochloride 1.25 mg, codeine phosphate 10 mg per 5 mL. Alcohol 4.3%, methylparaben, caramel flavor. Syrup. Bot. 118 mL, 473 mL, 3.8 L. *c-v.*
Use: Upper respiratory combination, antihistamine, antitussive, decongestant.

Triact. (Sanofi-Synthelabo) Aluminum, magnesium hydroxide, simethicone. Liq., Tab. *OTC.*
Use: Antacid; antiflatulent.

Triacting. (Various Mfr.) Pseudoephedrine hydrochloride 15 mg, guaifenesin 50 mg/5 mL. May contain EDTA, sorbitol, sucrose. Liq. Bot. 118 mL. *OTC.*
Use: Upper respiratory combination, decongestant, expectorant.

Triacting Cold & Allergy. (Amerisource-Bergen) Pseudoephedrine hydrochloride 15 mg, chlorpheniramine maleate 1 mg/5 mL, sorbitol, sucrose, orange flavor, alcohol free. Liq. Bot. 118 mL. *OTC.*
Use: Upper respiratory combination, decongestant, antihistamine.

Tri-Acting Cold & Allergy. (Topco) Pseudoephedrine hydrochloride 15 mg, chlorpheniramine maleate 1 mg/5 mL, sorbitol, sucrose, orange flavor, alcohol free. Syr. Bot. 118 mL. *OTC.*
Use: Upper respiratory combination, decongestant, antihistamine.

Tri-Acting Cold & Cough. (Topco) Pseudoephedrine hydrochloride 15 mg, chlorpheniramine maleate 1 mg, dextromethorphan HBr 5 mg per 5 mL. Sorbitol, sucrose, cherry flavor, alcohol free. Syr. Bot. 118 mL. *OTC.*
Use: Upper respiratory combination, decongestant, antihistamine, antitussive.

Triad. (Forest) Butalbital 50 mg, acetaminophen 325 mg, caffeine 40 mg. Cap. Bot. 100s. *Rx.*
Use: Analgesic; hypnotic; sedative.

•**triafungin.** (TRY-ah-FUN-jin) USAN.
Use: Antifungal.

Trial AG. (Zee Medical) Aluminum hydroxide 200 mg, magnesium hydroxide 200 mg, simethicone 25 mg. Sucrose, mannitol. Lemon flavor. Tab. 20s. *OTC.*
Use: Antacid.

Trial Antacid. (Zee Medical) Calcium carbonate 420 mg (elemental calcium 168 mg). Sorbitol. Spearmint flavor. Chew. Tab. 24s. *OTC.*
Use: Mineral supplement; antacid.

•**triamcinolone.** (TRY-am-SIN-oh-lone) *USP 34.*
Use: Corticosteroid, topical.

•**triamcinolone acetonide.** (TRY-am-SIN-oh-lone ah-SEE-toe-nide) *USP 34.*
Use: Corticosteroid, topical; anti-inflammatory, topical; respiratory inhalant, corticosteroid; adrenocortical steroid, glucocorticoid; ophthalmic corticosteroid.
See: Azmacort.
Kenalog.
Nasacort AQ.
Triacet.
Triderm.
Triesence.
Tri-Nasal.
Trivaris.
W/Nystatin.
See: Mycolog-II.

triamcinolone acetonide. (Barr Labs) Triamcinolone acetonide 55 mcg/actuation. Benzalkonium chloride, dextrose, edetate disodium. Spray; Susp.; intranasal. Bot. w/ metered-dose pump unit and nasal adapter. 16.5 g (providing 120 actuations). *Rx.*
Use: Respiratory inhalant product, intranasal steroid.

triamcinolone acetonide. (Sandoz) Triamcinolone acetonide 10 mg/mL. Benzyl alcohol 0.9%. Inj., Susp. Multidose vial. 5 mL. *Rx.*
Use: Adrenocortical steroid, glucocorticoid.

triamcinolone acetonide. (Various Mfr.) Triamcinolone acetonide. **Cream: 0.025%, 0.1%:** Tube 15 g, 80 g, 454 g. **0.5%:** 15 g. **Lot.:** 0.025%, 0.1%. Bot. 60 mL. **Oint.: 0.025%, 0.1%:** Tube 15 g, 80 g, 454 g. **0.5%:** Tube 15 g. **Paste:** 0.1%.
Use: Corticosteroid, topical; anti-inflammatory, topical.

•**triamcinolone acetonide sodium phosphate.** (TRY-am-SIN-oh-lone ah-SEE-toe-nide) USAN.
Use: Corticosteroid, topical.

•**triamcinolone hexacetonide.** (TRY-am-SIN-ole-ohn HEX-ah-SEE-tone-ide) *USP 34.*
Use: Adrenocortical steroid, glucocorticoid.
See: Aristospan.

triamcinolone-16,17-acetonide.
See: Triamcinolone acetonide.

Triaminic AllerChews. (Novartis) Loratadine 10 mg. Mannitol. Orally Disintegrating Tab. 8s. *OTC.*
Use: Antihistamine, peripherally selective piperidine.

Triaminic AM Cough and Decongestant Formula. (Novartis) Pseudoephedrine hydrochloride 15 mg, dextromethorphan HBr 7.5 mg/5 mL, sorbitol, sucrose, orange flavor. Alcohol and dye free. Liq. Bot. 118 mL, 237 mL. *OTC.*
Use: Antitussive; decongestant.

Triaminic AM Decongestant Formula. (Novartis) Pseudoephedrine hydrochloride 15 mg/5 mL, sorbitol, sucrose, orange flavor, alcohol and dye free. Syr. Bot. 118 mL, 237 mL. *OTC.*
Use: Decongestant.

Triaminic AM Non-Drowsy Cough & Decongestant. (Novartis) Pseudoephedrine hydrochloride 15 mg, dextromethorphan HBr 7.5 mg per 5 mL. EDTA, sorbitol, sucrose, orange/strawberry flavor. Liq. Bot. 118 mL. *OTC.*
Use: Upper respiratory combination, decongestant, antitussive.

Triaminic Chest & Nasal Congestion. (Novartis Consumer Health) Phenylephrine hydrochloride 2.5 mg, guaifenesin 50 mg per 5 mL. Acesulfame K, sodium 3 mg. Tropical flavor. Liq. Bot. 118 mL. *OTC.*
Use: Upper respiratory combination, decongestant, expectorant.

Triaminic Children's Allergy. (Novartis Consumer Health) Diphenhydramine hydrochloride 12.5 mg. Alcohol < 5%, maltodextrin, PEG, propylene glycol, sorbitol, sucralose. Grape flavor. Strips, orally disintegrating. 14s. *OTC.*
Use: Antihistamine, nonselective ethanolamine.

Triaminic Children's Thin Strips Day Time Cold & Cough. (Novartis Consumer Health) Dextromethorphan HBr 5 mg, phenylephrine hydrochloride 2.5 mg. Alcohol < 0.5%. PEG, sucralose. Wild berry flavor. Oral Strips. 14s. *OTC.*
Use: Upper respiratory combination, antitussive combination.

Triaminic Children's Thin Strips Night Time Cold & Cough. (Novartis Consumer Health) Diphenhydramine hydrochloride 12.5 mg, phenylephrine hydrochloride 5 mg. Maltodextrin, mannitol, PEG, sucralose. Grape flavor. Oral Strips. 14s. *OTC.*
Use: Upper respiratory combination, decongestant and antihistamine.

Triaminic Cough & Runny Nose. (Novartis Consumer Health) **Orally Disintegrating Strips:** Diphenhydramine hydrochloride 12.5 mg. Alcohol less than 5%, sorbitol, sucralose. Grape flavor. 6s. **Soft-chews:** Chlorpheniramine maleate 1 mg, dextromethorphan hydrobromide 5 mg. Aspartame, maltodextrin, mannitol, phenylalanine 17.6 mg, sodium 5 mg, sorbitol, sucrose. Cherry flavor Tab., soft chews. 18s. *OTC.*
Use: Antihistamine, upper respiratory combination, antitussive combination.

Triaminic Cough & Sore Throat. (Novartis Consumer Health) **Liq.:** Dextromethorphan HBr 5 mg, acetaminophen 160 mg per 5 mL. EDTA, sucrose, sorbitol, sodium 5 mg/5 mL, grape flavor, alcohol free. Bot. 118 mL. **Soft-chews:** Dextromethorphan HBr 5 mg, acetaminophen 160 mg. Aspartame, mannitol, phenylalanine 28.1 mg, sodium 8 mg/5 mL, sorbitol, sucrose. Grape flavor. 18s. *OTC.*
Use: Upper respiratory combination, antitussive combination.

Triaminic Daytime Cold & Cough. (Novartis Consumer Health) Phenylephrine hydrochloride 2.5 mg, dextromethorphan HBr 5 mg per 5 mL. Sorbitol, sucrose, cherry flavor, alcohol free. Liq. Bot. 118 mL. *OTC.*
Use: Upper respiratory combination, antitussive combination.

Triaminic-D Children's. (Novartis Consumer Health) Chlorpheniramine maleate 1 mg, dextromethorphan hydrobromide 7.5 mg, pseudoephedrine hydrochloride 15 mg per 5 mL. Disodium edetate, propylene glycol, sodium 6 mg, sorbitol, sucrose. Alcohol free. Grape flavor. Syrup. 118 mL. *OTC.*
Use: Upper respiratory combination, antitussive combination.

Triaminic Flu, Cough & Fever. (Novartis Consumer Health) Chlorpheniramine maleate 1 mg, dextromethorphan HBr 7.5 mg, acetaminophen 160 mg per 5 mL. EDTA, sorbitol, sucrose, sodium 6 mg/5 mL. Bubble gum flavor. Liq. Bot. 118 mL. *OTC.*
Use: Upper respiratory combination, antitussive combination.

Triaminic Infants' Fever Reducer/Pain Reliever. (Novartis Consumer Health) Acetaminophen 100 mg/mL. Butylparaben, corn syrup, glycerin, propylene glycol, sodium benzoate, sorbitol. Alcohol free. Cherry and grape flavor. Soln., concentrate. 15 mL w/dropper.

OTC.
Use: CNS agent.
Triaminic Long Acting Cough. (Novartis Consumer Health) Dextromethorphan HBr 7.5 mg per 5 mL. Dye free. EDTA, sorbitol, sucrose. Berry punch flavor. Liq. 118 mL. *OTC.*
Use: Nonnarcotic antitussive.
Triaminic Night Time Cold & Cough. (Novartis Consumer Health) Diphenhydramine hydrochloride 6.25 mg, phenylephrine hydrochloride 2.5 mg per 5 mL. Alcohol free. Acesulfame K, EDTA, mannitol. Grape flavor. Liq. 118 mL with dosage cup. *OTC.*
Use: Upper respiratory combination, decongestant and antihistamine combination.
Triaminic Thin Strips Cold with Stuffy Nose. (Novartis Consumer Health) Phenylephrine hydrochloride 2.5 mg. Maltodextrin, sucralose. Raspberry flavor. Orally Disintegrating Strips. 16s. *OTC.*
Use: Nasal decongestant, arylalkylamine.
Triaminic Thin Strips Cough & Runny Nose. (Novartis Consumer Health) Diphenhydramine hydrochloride 12.5 mg. Alcohol (less than 5%), sorbitol, sucralose. Grape flavor. Orally Disintegrating Strips. 16s. *OTC.*
Use: Nonnarcotic antitussive.
Triaminic Thin Strips Long Acting Cough. (Novartis Consumer Health) Dextromethorphan hydrobromide 7.5 mg. Alcohol (less than 5%), sorbitol, sucralose. Cherry flavor. Orally Disintegrating Strips. 16s. *OTC.*
Use: Nonnarcotic antitussive.
Triamolone 40. (Forest) Triamcinolone diacetate 40 mg/mL. Vial 5 mL. *Rx.*
Use: Corticosteroid.
•**triampyzine sulfate.** (TRY-AM-pih-zeen) USAN.
Use: Anticholinergic.
•**triamterene.** (try-AM-tur-een) *USP 34.*
Use: Diuretic.
See: Dyrenium.
W/Hydrochlorothiazide
See: Dyazide.
triamterene/hydrochlorothiazide. (Various Mfr.) **Cap.:** Triamterene 37.5 mg, 50 mg, hydrochlorothiazide 25 mg, may contain lactose. Bot. 100s, 1000s. **Tab.:** Triamterene 37.5 mg, hydrochlorothiazide 25 mg. Bot. 100s, 500s, 1000s; triamterene 75 mg, hydrochlorothiazide 50 mg. Bot. 100s, 250s, 500s, 1000s. *Rx.*
Use: Diuretic combination.

Trianide. (Seatrace) Triamcinolone acetonide 40 mg/mL. Vial 5 mL. *Rx.*
Use: Corticosteroid.
Tri-A-Vite F. (Major) F_1 0.5 mg, vitamins A 1500 units, D 400 units, C 35 mg/mL Drops. Bot. 50 mL. *Rx.*
Use: Vitamin supplement.
Triaz. (Medicis) Benzoyl peroxide.
Cloths: 3%, 6%, 9%. Cetyl alcohol, glycerine, glycolic acid, zinc. 60s. **Gel:** 3%, 6%, 9%. Glycerin (except 9%), zinc lactase, EDTA, cetyl stearyl alcohol (except 3%), glycolic acid (9% only). Tube 42.5 g. **Lot.:** 3%, 6%, 10%. Glycerin, glycolic acid, petrolatum, menthol, zinc lactate. 85.1 g (10% only), 170.3 g, 340.2 g (except 10%). *Rx.*
Use: Antiacne.
triazenes.
Use: Alkylating agents.
See: Dacarbazine.
•**triazolam.** (trye-AZ-oh-lam) *USP 34.*
Use: Sedative/hypnotic, nonbarbiturate.
See: Halcion.
triazolam. (Various Mfr.) Triazolam 0.125 mg, 0.25 mg. Tab. Bot. 10s, 100s, 500s, UD 100s. *c-iv.*
Use: Sedative/hypnotic, nonbarbiturate.
triazole antifungals.
Use: Antifungal agents.
See: Fluconazole.
Itraconazole.
Posaconazole.
Voriconazole.
•**tribenoside.** (try-BEN-oh-SIDE) USAN. Not available in US.
Use: Sclerosing agent.
Tri-Biozene. (Reese) Polymyxin B sulfate 10,000 units, neomycin 3.5 mg, bacitracin zinc 500 units, pramoxine hydrochloride 10 mg per g. White petrolatum. Oint. Tubes. 15 g. *OTC.*
Use: Anti-infective, antibiotic, topical.
tribromoethanol.
Use: Anesthetic (inhalation).
tribromomethane. Bromoform.
•**tribromsalan.** (trye-BROM-sa-lan) USAN.
Use: Disinfectant.
tricalcium phosphate.
Use: Mineral supplement.
See: Calcium Phosphate, Tribasic.
•**tricetamide.** (trye-SET-a-mide) USAN.
Use: Hypnotic; sedative.
Tri-Chlor. (Gordon Laboratories) Trichloroacetic acid 80%. Bot. 15 mL. *Rx.*
Use: Cauterizing agent.
trichlorfon.
See: Metrifonate.

trichloroacetic acid. Acetic acid, trichloro.
Use: Topical, as a caustic.

trichlorobutyl alcohol.
See: Chlorobutanol.

• **trichloromonofluoromethane.** (try-klor-oh-mahn-oh-flure-oh-METH-ane) *NF 29.*
Use: Pharmaceutic aid (aerosol propellant).
W/Dichlorodifluoromethane.
See: Aerofreeze.

Trichotine. (Schwarz Pharma) **Pow.:** Sodium lauryl sulf., sod. perborate, monohydrate silica. Pkg. 150 g, 360 g. **Liq.:** Sodium lauryl sulfate, sodium borate, SD alcohol 40 8%, SD alcohol 23-A, EDTA. Bot. 120 mL, 240 mL. *OTC.*
Use: Feminine hygiene.

• **triciribine phosphate.** (TRY-SIH-bean) USAN. *Formerly Phosphate Salt of Tricyclic Nucleoside.*
Use: Antineoplastic.

• **tricitrates oral solution.** (TRY-SIH-trates) *USP 34.*
Use: Alkalizer (systemic, urinary); antiurolithic (cystine calculi, uric acid calculi); buffer (neutralizing).

triclobisonium. (Roche) Triburon, Oint.

triclobisonium chloride.
Use: Anti-infective, topical.

• **triclocarban.** (TRY-kloe-CAR-ban) USAN.
Use: Disinfectant.
See: Artra Beauty Bar.

• **triclofenol piperazine.** (TRY-kloe-FEE-nole pih-PURR-ah-zeen) USAN.
Use: Anthelmintic.

• **triclofos sodium.** (TRY-kloe-foss) USAN.
Use: Hypnotic; sedative.

• **triclonide.** (TRY-kloe-nide) USAN.
Use: Anti-inflammatory.

• **triclosan.** (TRY-kloe-san) *USP 34.*
Use: Anti-infective; disinfectant.
See: ASC Lotionized.
　Ca-Rezz.
　Clean and Clear Foaming Facial Cleanser.
　Clearasil Daily Face Wash.
　Sarna.
　Stridex Face Wash.

Tricodene Sugar Free Cough & Cold. (Pfeiffer) Chlorpheniramine maleate 2 mg, dextromethorphan HBr 10 mg per 5 mL. Alcohol and sugar free. Menthol, saccharin, sodium 12 mg/5 mL, sorbitol, mannitol. Liq. Bot. 120 mL. *OTC.*

Use: Upper respiratory combination, antitussive combination.

Tricodene Sugar Free. (Pfeiffer) Chlorpheniramine maleate 2 mg, dextromethorphan HBr 10 mg per 5 mL. Menthol, saccharin, sorbitol, mannitol, alcohol free, sugar free. Liq. Bot. 120 mL. *OTC.*
Use: Upper respiratory combination, antihistamine, antitussive.

Tricodene Syrup. (Pfeiffer) Pyrilamine maleate 4.17 mg, codeine phosphate 8.1 mg, terpin hydrate, menthol/5 mL. Syr. Bot. 120 mL. *c-v.*
Use: Antihistamine; antitussive.

Tricof. (Scientific Laboratories) Dihydrocodeine bitartrate 7.5 mg, chlorpheniramine maleate 2 mg, pseudoephedrine hydrochloride 15 mg per 5 mL. Sugar, alcohol, and dye free. Grape flavor. Syrup. 473 mL. *c-III.*
Use: Antitussive combination.

Tricof EXP. (Scientific Laboratories) Dihydrocodeine bitartrate 7.5 mg, guaifenesin 100 mg, pseudoephedrine hydrochloride 15 mg per 5 mL. Sugar and alcohol free. Vanilla-fruit flavor. Syrup. 473 mL. *c-III.*
Use: Antitussive and expectorant combination.

Tricof PD. (Scientific Laboratories) Dihydrocodeine bitartrate 3 mg, chlorpheniramine maleate 2 mg, phenylephrine hydrochloride 7.5 mg per 5 mL. Grape flavor. Syrup. 473 mL. *c-v.*
Use: Antitussive combination.

TriCor. (Abbott) Fenofibrate 48 mg, 145 mg. Lactose, sucrose. Tab. Bot. 90s. *Rx.*
Use: Antihyperlipidemic; fibric acid derivatives.

Tricosal. (Invamed) Choline magnesium trisalicylate 500 mg, 750 mg, 1000 mg. Tab. Bot. 100s, 500s. *Rx.*
Use: Salicylate.

tricyclic compounds.
Use: Antidepressant.
See: Amitriptyline Hydrochloride.
　Amoxapine.
　Clomipramine Hydrochloride.
　Desipramine Hydrochloride.
　Doxepin Hydrochloride.
　Imipramine Hydrochloride.
　Imipramine Pamoate.
　Nortriptyline Hydrochloride.
　Protriptyline Hydrochloride.
　Trimipramine Maleate.

Tridal. (Scientific Laboratories) Codeine phosphate 12.5 mg, guaifenesin 125 mg, phenylephrine hydrochloride 4 mg per 5 mL. Sugar, alcohol, and dye

free. Syrup. 473 mL. *c-v.*
Use: Antitussive and expectorant combination.

Tridal HD. (Scientific Laboratories) Hydrocodone bitartrate 2 mg, chlorpheniramine maleate 2 mg, phenylephrine hydrochloride 5 mg per 5 mL. Sugar and alcohol free. Cherry flavor. Susp. 473 mL. *c-III.*
Use: Antitussive combination.

Tridal HD Plus. (Scientific Laboratories) Hydrocodone bitartrate 3.5 mg, chlorpheniramine maleate 2 mg, phenylephrine hydrochloride 7.5 mg per 5 mL. Sugar free. Black raspberry flavor. Syrup. 473 mL. *c-III.*
Use: Antitussive combination.

Triderm. (Del-Ray) Triamcinolone acetonide 0.1%. Cream. Tube 30 g, 90 g. *Rx.*
Use: Corticosteroid.

Tridesilon Otic. (Bayer Consumer Care) Desonide 0.05%, acetic acid 2% in vehicle. Bot. 10 mL. *Rx.*
Use: Otic.

Tridrate Bowel Cleansing System. (Lafayette) Magnesium citrate 19 g. Bisacodyl tablets 5 mg each (3s). Bisacodyl suppository 10 mg (1s). Kit. *OTC.*
Use: Laxative.

• **trientine hydrochloride.** (TRY-en-TEEN) *USP 34.*
Use: Chelating agent; Wilson disease therapy adjunct.
See: Cuprid.
Syprine.

Triesence. (Alcon Laboratories) Triamcinolone acetonide 40 mg/mL. Sodium chloride, carboxymethylcellulose sodium 0.5%, polysorbate 80 0.015%, potassium chloride, sodium acetate, sodium citrate. Inj., Susp., Intravitreol. Single-use vials. 1 mL. *Rx.*
Use: Corticosteroid.

triethanolamine.
See: Trolamine.

triethanolamine salicylate.
See: Aspercreme.
Myoflex.

triethanolamine trinitrate biphosphate.
Trolnitrate Phosphate.

• **triethyl citrate.** (trye-ETH-il) *NF 29.*
Use: Pharmaceutic aid (plasticizer).

triethylenemelamine. Tretamine TEM.
Use: Antineoplastic.

triethylenethiophosphoramide.
See: Thiotepa.

Trifed-C. (Geneva) Pseudoephedrine hydrochloride 30 mg, triprolidine hydrochloride 1.25 mg, codeine phosphate 10 mg/5 mL, alcohol 4.3%. Syrup. Bot. Pt., gal. *c-v.*

Use: Antihistamine; antitussive; decongestant.

• **trifenagrel.** (try-FEN-ah-GRELL) USAN.
Use: Antithrombotic.

• **triflocin.** (try-FLOW-sin) USAN.
Use: Diuretic.

Tri-Flor-Vite with Fluoride. (Everett) Fluoride 0.25 mg, vitamins A 1500 units, D 400 units, C 35 mg/mL. Drops. 50 mL. *Rx.*
Use: Fluoride, vitamin supplement.

• **triflubazam.** (try-FLEW-bah-zam) USAN.
Use: Anxiolytic.

• **triflumidate.** (try-FLEW-mih-DATE) USAN.
Use: Anti-inflammatory.

• **trifluoperazine hydrochloride.** (try-flew-oh-PURR-uh-zeen) *USP 34.*
Use: Antipsychotic; anxiolytic; hypnotic; sedative.

trifluoperazine hydrochloride. (Various Mfr.) Trifluoperazine hydrochloride 1 mg, 2 mg, 5 mg, 10 mg. Tab. Bot. 100s, 500s, 1000s, UD 100s. *Rx.*
Use: Antipsychotic.

trifluorothymidine. *Rx.*
Use: Ophthalmic.
See: Viroptic.

• **trifluperidol.** (TRY-flew-PURR-ih-dahl) USAN.
Use: Antipsychotic.

• **trifluridine.** (try-FLEW-RIH-deen) *USP 34.*
Use: Antiviral used to treat herpes simplex eye infections.
See: Viroptic.

trifluridine. (Falcon Ophthalmics) Trifluridine 1%, in aqueous solution with NaCl, thimerosal 0.001%. Ophth. Soln. Bot. 7.5 mL. *Rx.*
Use: Antiviral.

Triglide. (Sciele Pharma) Fenofibrate 50 mg, 160 mg. Lactose. Tab. 90s. *Rx.*
Use: Antihyperlipidemic agent, fibric acid derivative.

triglyceride reagent strip. (Bayer Consumer Care) *Seralyzer* reagent strip. Bot. 25s.
Use: Diagnostic aid, triglycerides.

triglycerides, medium chain.
Use: Nutritional supplement.
See: MCT Oil.

Trigofen DM. (Trigen Laboratories) Chlorpheniramine maleate 1 mg, dextromethorphan hydrobromide 3 mg, phenylephrine hydrochloride 2 mg. Parabens, potassium citrate, potassium sorbate, propylene glycol, sorbitol, sucralose. Alcohol free, dye free, and sugar free. Orange-vanilla flavor. Liq.

30 mL w/dropper. *Rx.*
Use: Upper respiratory combination, antitussive combination.
Trihexane. (Rugby) Trihexyphenidyl
2 mg. Tab. Bot. 100s, 1000s. *Rx.*
Use: Anticholinergic; antiparkinsonian.
Trihexidyl. (Schein) Trihexyphenidyl
2 mg. Tab. Bot. 100s, 1000s. *Rx.*
Use: Anticholinergic; antiparkinsonian.
Trihexy-5. (Geneva) Trihexyphenidyl
5 mg. Tab. Bot. 100s, 1000s. *Rx.*
Use: Anticholinergic; antiparkinsonian.
•**trihexyphenidyl hydrochloride.** (try-hex-ee-FEN-in-dill) *USP 34.*
Use: Anticholinergic; antiparkinsonian.
trihexyphenidyl hydrochloride. (VersaPharm) Trihexyphenidyl hydrochloride 2 mg per 5 mL. Alcohol 5%, parabens, sorbitol. Lime-peppermint flavor. Elix. 473 mL. *Rx.*
Use: Antiparkinson agent.
Trihexy-2. (Geneva) Trihexyphenidyl
2 mg. Tab. Bot. 100s, 1000s. *Rx.*
Use: Anticholinergic; antiparkinsonian.
Tri-Histin. (Recsei) **Cap.:** Bot. 100s, 500s, 1000s. **Liq.:** Pyrilamine maleate 5 mg, chlorpheniramine maleate 0.5 mg/5 mL. Bot. Pt., gal. **SA Cap.: 100 mg:** Pyrilamine maleate 40 mg, pheniramine maleate 25 mg. **Tab.: 25 mg:** Pyrilamine maleate 10 mg, chlorpheniramine maleate 1 mg. Bot. 100s, 500s, 1000s. **50 mg:** Pyrilamine maleate 20 mg, methapyrilene hydrochloride 15 mg, chlorpheniramine maleate 2 mg. Bot. 1000s. *Rx-OTC.*
Use: Antihistamine combination.
Trihydroxyethylamine. Triethanolamine.
l-triiodothyronine sodium.
Use: Hormone, thyroid.
See: Cytomel.
  Liothyronine sodium.
Tri-K. (Century) Potassium acetate 0.5 g, potassium bicarbonate 0.5 g, potassium citrate 0.5 g/fl. oz. Saccharin. Bot. Pt., gal. *Rx.*
Use: Electrolyte supplement.
•**trikates oral solution.** (TRY-kates) *USP 34.*
Use: Replenisher (electrolyte).
Tri-Legest. (Barr) **Phase 1:** Norethindrone acetate 1 mg, ethinyl estradiol 20 mcg (5 tabs.). **Phase 2:** Norethindrone acetate 1 mg, ethinyl estradiol 30 mcg (7 tabs.). **Phase 3:** Norethindrone acetate 1 mg, ethinyl estradiol 35 mcg (9 tabs.). Ferrous fumarate 75 mg (7 tabs.). Lactose. Tab. 21s, 28s (with 7 inert tabs.). *Rx.*
Use: Sex hormone, contraceptive hormone.

Trileptal. (Novartis) Oxcarbazepine.
Tab.: 150 mg, 300 mg, 600 mg. Bot. 100s, UD 100s. **Susp.:** 60 mg/mL. Saccharin, sorbitol, ethanol. Bot. 250 mL with dosing syr. and adapter. *Rx.*
Use: Anticonvulsant.
Trilipix. (Abbott Laboratories) Fenofibrate 45 mg, 135 mg (as fenofibric acid). Cap., Delayed release. 90s. *Rx.*
Use: Antihyperlipidemic agent, fibric acid derivative.
•**trilostane.** (TRY-low-stane) USAN.
Use: Adrenocortical suppressant.
Tri-Luma. (Galderma) Fluocinolone acetonide 0.01%, hydroquinone 4%, tretinoin 0.05%, cetyl alcohol, glycerin, parabens, sodium metabisulfite, stearyl alcohol. Cream. Tube 30 g. *Rx.*
Use: Treatment of melasma.
TriLyte. (Alaven Pharmaceuticals) PEG 3350 420 g, sodium bicarbonate 5.72 g, sodium chloride 11.2 g, potassium chloride 1.48 g. Pow. for Soln. 4 L bot. with flavor packs. *Rx.*
Use: Laxative, bowel evacuant.
Trimagen. (Trigen Laboratories) Fe 70 mg, succinic acid 75 mg, vitamin C 152 mg (as calcium ascorbate and calcium threonate), vitamin B_{12} 10 mcg, desiccated stomach substance 50 mg. Film coated. Tab. 90s. *Rx.*
Use: Nutritional supplement.
Trimahist. (Tennessee Pharmaceutic) Phenylephrine hydrochloride 5 mg, prophenpyridamine maleate 12.5 mg, l-menthol 1 mg, alcohol 5%/5 mL. Elix. Bot. Pt., gal. *Rx.*
Use: Antihistamine; decongestant.
Trimax. (Sanofi-Synthelabo) Aluminum, magnesium hydroxide, simethicone. Gel. Tab. *OTC.*
Use: Antacid; antiflatulent.
trimazinol.
Use: Anti-inflammatory.
•**trimazosin hydrochloride.** (try-MAY-zoe-sin) USAN.
Use: Antihypertensive.
•**trimegestone.** (try-meh-JESS-tone) USAN.
Use: Hormone, progestin.
•**trimeprazine tartrate.** (trye-MEP-ra-zeen) USAN.
Use: Antipruritic.
trimetamide. Trimethamide.
trimethamide.
Use: Antihypertensive.
trimethobenzamide. (Various Mfr.) Trimethobenzamide hydrochloride 300 mg. Cap. Bot. 100s, 250s, 500s,

1,000s, UD 30s, UD 60s. *Rx.*
Use: Antiemetic/antivertigo agent.
•**trimethobenzamide hydrochloride.** (try-meth-oh-BEN-zuh-mide) *USP 34.*
Use: Antiemetic.
See: Tigan.
trimethobenzamide hydrochloride.
(Various Mfr.) Trimethobenzamide hydrochloride 100 mg/mL. Amp. 2 mL. Vials. 20 mL. *Rx.*
Use: Antiemetic/antivertigo agent.
•**trimethoprim.** (try-METH-oh-prim)
USP 34.
Use: Anti-infective.
See: Proloprim.
Trimpex.
W/Polymyxin B Sulfate.
See: Polytrim.
W/Sulfamethoxazole.
See: Bactrim.
Septra DS.
trimethoprim and sulfamethoxazole.
(Various Mfr.) **Tab.:** Trimethoprim 80 mg, sulfamethoxazole 400 mg. Bot. 100s, 500s. **Susp.:** Trimethoprim 40 mg, sulfamethoxazole 200 mg/5 mL. Alcohol 0.26%, methylparaben, saccharin, sorbitol. Grape and cherry flavors. 473 mL. **Inj.:** Sulfamethoxazole 80 mg/mL, trimethoprim 16 mg/mL. May contain alcohol, benzyl alcohol, metabisulfite. Single-use vial. 5 mL. Multiple-use vial. 10 mL, 30 mL. *Rx.*
Use: Anti-infective combination.
trimethoprim and sulfamethoxazole DS.
(Various Mfr.) Trimethoprim 160 mg, sulfamethoxazole 800 mg. Tab. Bot. 100s, 500s. *Rx.*
Use: Anti-infective combination.
trimethoprim hydrochloride.
Use: Anti-infective.
See: Primsol.
•**trimethoprim sulfate.** (try-METH-oh-prim) USAN.
Use: Anti-infective.
trimethoprim sulfate and polymyxin b sulfate ophthalmic. (Various Mfr.) Trimethoprim 1 mg, polymyxin B sulfate 10,000 units/mL. Soln. Bot. 10 mL. *Rx.*
Use: Anti-infective, ophthalmic.
trimethylene. Cyclopropane.
•**trimetozine.** (try-MET-oh-zeen) USAN.
Use: Hypnotic; sedative.
•**trimetrexate.** (TRY-meh-TREK-sate) USAN.
Use: Antineoplastic.
•**trimetrexate glucuronate.** (TRY-meh-TREK-sate glue-CURE-uh-nate) USAN.
Use: Antineoplastic.

•**trimipramine.** (TRY-MIH-prah-meen) USAN.
Use: Antidepressant.
•**trimipramine maleate.** (TRY-MIH-prah-meen) USAN.
Use: Antidepressant.
See: Surmontil.
Trimixin. (Hance) Bacitracin 200 units, polymyxin B sulfate 4000 units, neomycin sulfate 3 mg/g Oint. Tube 0.5 oz. *OTC.*
Use: Anti-infective, topical.
•**trimoprostil.** (TRY-moe-PRAHS-till) USAN.
Use: Gastric antisecretory.
Trimo-San. (Cooper Surgical) Oxyquinoline sulfate 0.025%, boric acid 1%, sodium borate 0.7%, sodium lauryl sulfate 0.1%, glycerin, methylparaben. Jelly. 120 g w/applicator, 120 g refill. *OTC.*
Use: Vaginal agent.
Trimox. (Sandoz) Amoxicillin 125 mg/5 mL when reconstituted. Sucrose. Raspberry-strawberry flavor. Pow. for Oral Susp. Bot. 80 mL, 100 mL, 150 mL. *Rx.*
Use: Penicillin, aminopenicillin.
•**trimoxamine hydrochloride.** (TRY-MOX-am-een) USAN.
Use: Antihypertensive.
Trimox Pediatric Drops. (Apothecon) Amoxicillin trihydrate 50 mg/mL when reconstituted, sucrose. Pow. for Oral Susp. Bot. 15 mL. *Rx.*
Use: Anti-infective, penicillin.
Trimpex. (Roche) *Tel-E-Dose* 100s. *Rx.*
Use: Anti-infective, urinary.
Trim-Qwik. (Columbia) Powder-based meal food supplement. Can 10 oz. *OTC.*
Use: Nutritional supplement.
Trimstat. (Laser) Phendimetrazine tartrate 35 mg. Tab. Bot. 100s, 1000s. *c-III.*
Use: Anorexiant.
Trim-Sulfa. *Rx.*
Use: Anti-infective.
See: Proloprim.
Trimethoprim.
Trimpex.
Trim Sulf D/S. (Lexis Laboratories) Sulfamethoxazole 800 mg, trimethoprim 160 mg. Tab. Bot. 100s, 500s. *Rx.*
Use: Anti-infective.
Trim Sulf S/S. (Lexis Laboratories) Sulfamethoxazole 400 mg, trimethoprim 80 mg. Tab. Bot. 100s, 500s. *Rx.*
Use: Anti-infective.

Tri-Nasal. (Muro) Triamcinolone acetonide 50 mcg/spray, EDTA, benzalkonium chloride 0.01%. Spray. Bot. 15 mL with triamcinolone acetonide 7.5 mg/bot. (120 metered sprays) with nasal applicator. *Rx.*
Use: Respiratory inhalant, intranasal steroid.

Trinate. (Cypress) Ca 200 mg, Fe 28 mg, vitamin A 3000 units, D 400 units, E (dl-alpha tocopheryl acetate) 22 mg, B$_1$ 1.8 mg, B$_2$ 4 mg, B$_3$ 20 mg, B$_6$ 25 mg, B$_{12}$ 12 mcg, C 120 mg, folic acid 1 mg, Zn 25 mg, Cu, Mg. Tab. Bot. 100s. *Rx.*
Use: Mineral, vitamin, supplement.

• **trinecol.** (TRI-ne-kol) USAN. (Pullus)
Use: Oral tolerance therapy.

TriNessa. (Watson) **Phase 1:** Norgestimate 0.18 mg, ethinyl estradiol 35 mcg. 7 tabs. **Phase 2:** Norgestimate 0.215 mg, ethinyl estradiol 35 mcg. 7 tabs.
Phase 3: Norgestimate 0.25 mg, ethinyl estradiol 35 mcg. 7 tabs. Tab. 28s with 7 inert tabs. *Rx.*
Use: Contraceptive hormone, sex hormone.

trinitrin tablets.
See: Nitroglycerin.

Tri-Norinyl. (Watson) **Phase 1:** Norethindrone 0.5 mg, ethinyl estradiol 35 mcg (7 tabs.). **Phase 2:** Norethindrone 1 mg, ethinyl estradiol 35 mcg (9 tabs.).
Phase 3: Norethindrone 0.5 mg, ethinyl estradiol 35 mcg (5 tabs.). Lactose. *Wallette* 28s with 7 inert tabs. *Rx.*
Use: Sex hormone, contraceptive hormone.

Trinotic. (Forest) Secobarbital 65 mg, amobarbital 40 mg, phenobarbital 25 mg. Tab. Bot. 1000s. *c-II.*
Use: Hypnotic.

Triofed. (Alra) Pseudoephedrine hydrochloride 30 mg, triprolidine hydrochloride 1.25 mg/5 mL. Syr. Bot. 118 mL, 473 mL. *OTC.*
Use: Antihistamine, decongestant.

• **triolein I 131.** (TRY-oh-leen) USAN.
Use: Radiopharmaceutical.

• **triolein I 125.** (TRY-oh-leen) USAN.
Use: Radiopharmaceutical.

Trionate. (Breckenridge) Carbetapentane tannate 60 mg, chlorpheniramine tannate 5 mg. Tab. Bot. 100s. *Rx.*
Use: Upper respiratory combination, antitussive combination.

Triostat. (JHP Pharmaceuticals) Liothyronine sodium 10 mcg/mL, w/ammonia 2.19 mg/mL, alcohol 6.8%. Inj. Vial 1 mL. *Rx.*
Use: Hormone, thyroid.

Triotann. (Various Mfr.) Phenylephrine tannate 25 mg, chlorpheniramine tannate 8 mg, pyrilamine tannate 25 mg. Tab. Bot. 100s, 500s. *Rx.*
Use: Antihistamine; decongestant.

Triotann Pediatric. (Prasco Laboratories) Phenylephrine tannate 5 mg, chlorpheniramine tannate 2 mg, pyrilamine tannate 12.5 mg/5 mL. Saccharin, sucrose, methylparaben, strawberry-blackberry-currant flavor. Susp. Bot. 473 mL. *Rx.*
Use: Upper respiratory combination, antihistamine, decongestant.

Triotann-S Pediatric. (Duramed) Phenylephrine tannate 5 mg, chlorpheniramine tannate 2 mg, pyrilamine tannate 12.5 mg/5 mL, methylparaben, saccharin, sucrose, strawberry-blackberry-currant flavor. Susp. Unit of use 118 mL. *Rx.*
Use: Upper respiratory combination, decongestant, antihistamine.

trioxane.
See: Trioxymethylene.

• **trioxifene mesylate.** (TRY-OX-ih-feen) USAN.
Use: Antiestrogen.

TriOxin. (Vertical Pharmaceuticals) Benzocaine 15 mg, chloroxylenol 1 mg, hydrocortisone acetate 10 mg per mL. Isopropyl alcohol, PEG-12, PEG-40. Susp., Otic. 15 mL. *Rx.*
Use: Ophthalmic and otic agent, miscellaneous otic preparation.

trioxymethylene. Name is incorrectly used to denote paraformaldehyde in some pharmaceuticals.
See: Paraformaldehyde.

Tri-Pain. (Ferndale) Acetaminophen 162 mg, aspirin 162 mg, salicylamide 162 mg, caffeine 16.2 mg. Tab. Bot. 100s. *OTC.*
Use: Analgesic combination.

• **tripamide.** (TRIP-ah-mide) USAN.
Use: Antihypertensive; diuretic.

Tri-Pase 8. (Acella) Lipase 8,000 units, protease 30,000 units, amylase 30,000 units. Lactose. Tab. 100s. *Rx.*
Use: Digestive enzyme.

Tri-Pase 16. (Acella) Lipase 16,000 units, protease 60,000 units, amylase 60,000 units. Lactose. Tab. 100s. *Rx.*
Use: Digestive enzyme.

Tripedia. (Aventis Pasteur) Diphtheria 6.7 Lf units, tetanus toxoid 5 Lf units, pertussis antigens 46.8 mcg/0.5 mL (pertussis toxin and hemagglutinin ≈ 23.4 mcg each). Formaldehyde, phenoxyethanol. Inj. Preservative-free single-dose vial with thimerosal (not

more than 0.3 mcg mercury/dose). *Rx.*
Use: Immunization.

• **tripelennamine citrate.** (trih-pell-EN-au-meen SIH-trate) *USP 34.*
Use: Antihistamine.

• **tripelennamine hydrochloride.** (trih-pell-EN-au-meen) *USP 34.*
Use: Antihistamine.
See: PBZ.
Pyribenzamine.

triphasic oral contraceptives.
See: Caziant.
Estrostep Fe.
Ortho-Novum 7/7/7.
Ortho Tri-Cyclen.
Tri-Levlen.
TriNessa.
Tri-Norinyl.
Triphasil.
Tri-Sprintec.
Trivora.

Triphasil. (Wyeth Labs) **Phase 1:** Levonorgestrel 0.05 mg, ethinyl estradiol 30 mcg (6 tablets). **Phase 2:** Levonorgestrel 0.075 mg, ethinyl estradiol 40 mcg (5 tablets). **Phase 3:** Levonorgestrel 0.125 mg, ethinyl estradiol 30 mcg (10 tablets). Lactose. Tab. 21s, 28s (with 7 inert tablets). *Rx.*
Use: Sex hormone, contraceptive hormone.

triphenylmethane dyes.
See: Fuchsin, Basic.
Methylrosaniline Chloride.

triphenyltetrazolium chloride. TTC.

tripiperazine dicitrate, hydrous.
See: Piperazine Citrate.

triple antibiotic. (Various Mfr.) Polymyxin B sulfate 5000 units, neomycin 3.5 mg, bacitracin zinc 400 units per g. Oint. Tubes. 15 g, 30 g, 454 g. *OTC.*
Use: Anti-infective, antibiotic, topical.

triple antibiotic ophthalmics. (Various Mfr.) Polymyxin B sulfate 10,000 units/g, neomycin sulfate 3.5 mg/g, bacitracin 400 units. Oint. 3.5 g. *Rx.*
Use: Anti-infective; ophthalmic.

triple barbiturate elixir. (CMC) Phenobarbital 0.25 g, butabarbital 0.125 g, pentobarbital g/5 mL. Bot. Pt., gal. *c-II.*
Use: Sedative.

Triple Cream. (Summers Labs) Avena sativa, beeswax, benzyl alcohol, white petrolatum. Cream. 114 g. OTC. Miscellaneous emollient.

Triple Dye. (Kerr Drug) Gentian violet, proflavine, hemisulfate, brilliant green in water. Dispensing Bot. 15 mL. Single-Use *Dispos-A-Swab* 0.65 mL. Box 10s. Case 10 × 50 Box.
Use: Antiseptic.

Triple Dye. (Xttrium) Brilliant green 2.29 mg, proflavine hemisulfate 1.14 mg, gentian violet 2.29 mg/mL. Bot. 30 mL.
Use: Disinfectant.

Triple-Gen. (Ivax) Hydrocortisone 1%, neomycin sulfate 0.35%, polymyxin B sulfate 10,000 units/mL, benzalkonium chloride, cetyl alcohol, glyceryl monostearate, polyoxyl 40 stearate, propylene glycol, mineral oil. Susp. Bot. 7.5 mL. *Rx.*
Use: Anti-infective; corticosteroid; ophthalmic.

Triplen. (Henry Schein) Tripelennamine hydrochloride 50 mg. Tab. Bot. 100s, 1000s. *Rx.*
Use: Antihistamine.

Triple Paste AF. (Summers) Miconazole nitrate 2%. Beeswax, lanolin, stearyl alcohol, white petrolatum, zinc oxide. Oint. 56.7 g. *OTC.*
Use: Topical antifungal agent.

• **triple sulfa.** (TRIP-el-SUL-fa) *USP 34.* Sulfathiazole, sulfacetamide, and sulfabenzamide.
Use: Anti-infective.

Triple Sulfoid. (Pal-Pak, Inc.) Sulfadiazine 167 mg, sulfamerazine 167 mg, sulfamethazine 167 mg/5 mL. Liq.: Bot. Pt., 2 oz. 12s. Tab.: Bot. 100s, 1000s. *Rx.*
Use: Anti-infective, sulfonamide.

triple sulfonamide. Dia-Mer-Thia Sulfonamides. Meth-Dia-Mer Sulfonamides.
Use: Anti-infective, sulfonamide.

Triple Tannate Pediatric. (Hi-Tech) Phenylephrine tannate 5 mg, chlorpheniramine tannate 2 mg, pyrilamine tannate 12.5 mg per 5 mL. Methylparaben, saccharin, sucrose. Susp. 473 mL. *Rx.*
Use: Upper respiratory combination, decongestant and antihistamine.

Triple Vita. (Rosemont) Vitamins A 1500 units, D 400 units, C 35 mg/mL, alcohol free. Drops. Bot. 50 mL. *OTC.*
Use: Vitamin supplement.

Triple Vita-Flor. (Rosemont) Fluoride 0.5 mg, vitamins A 1500 units, D 400 units, C 35 mg/mL, alcohol free. Drops. Bot. 50 mL. *Rx.*
Use: Dental caries agent; vitamin supplement.

Triple Vitamin ADC w/Fluoride. (Nilor Pharm) Fluoride 0.5 mg, vitamins A 1500 units, D 400 units, C 35 mg/mL. Drops. Bot. 50 mL. *Rx.*
Use: Mineral, vitamin supplement; dental caries agent.

Triple Vitamins w/Fluoride. (Major) Vitamin A 2500 units, D 400 units, C 60 mg, fluoride 1 mg, dextrose, sucrose. Chew. Tab. Bot. 100s. *Rx.*
Use: Vitamin supplement; dental caries agent.

Triplevite w/Fluoride. (Geneva) Fluoride. **0.25 mg/mL:** Vitamins A 1500 units, D 400 units, C 35 mg, alcohol free. Drops. Bot. 50 mL. **0.5 mg/mL:** Vitamins A 1500 units, D 400 units, C 35 mg/mL, alcohol free, cherry flavor. Drops. Bot. 50 mL. *Rx.*
Use: Dental caries agent; vitamin supplement.

Triplex DM. (Breckenridge) Dextromethorphan HBr 15 mg, pyrilamine maleate 12.5 mg, phenylephrine hydrochloride 7.5 mg per 5 mL. Alcohol, sugar, and dye free. Saccharin, sorbitol. Grape flavor. Liq. 473 mL. *Rx.*
Use: Upper respiratory combination, antitussive combination.

Tripodrine. (Schein) Pseudoephedrine hydrochloride 60 mg, triprolidine hydrochloride 2.5 mg. Tab. Bot. 100s, UD 100s. *Rx.*
Use: Antihistamine; decongestant.

Tripohist D. (Breckenridge) Pseudoephedrine hydrochloride 45 mg, triprolidine hydrochloride 1.25 mg per 5 mL. Alcohol and sugar free. Saccharin, sorbitol. Blueberry flavor. Liq. 473 mL. *Rx.*
Use: Upper respiratory combination, decongestant and antihistamine.

Triposed Syrup. (Halsey Drug) **Syr.:** Triprolidine hydrochloride 1.25 mg, pseudoephedrine hydrochloride 30 mg/5 mL. Bot. 120 mL, 240 mL, 473 mL, gal. **Tab.:** Triprolidine hydrochloride 2.5 mg, pseudoephedrine hydrochloride 60 mg. Bot. 100s, 1000s. *OTC.*
Use: Antihistamine; decongestant.

tripotassium citrate.
See: Potassium Citrate.

Tri-Previfem. (Qualitest) **Phase 1:** Norgestimate 0.18 mg, ethinyl estradiol 35 mcg. 7 tabs. **Phase 2:** Norgestimate 0.215 mg, ethinyl estradiol 35 mcg. 7 tabs. **Phase 3:** Norgestimate 0.25 mg, ethinyl estradiol 35 mcg. 7 tabs. Lactose. Tab. 28s with 7 inert tabs. *Rx.*
Use: Sex hormone, contraceptive hormone.

•**triprolidine hydrochloride.** (try-PRO-lih-deen) *USP 34.*
Use: Antihistamine, nonselective alkylamine.
See: Zymine.

W/Chlophedianol Hydrochloride.
See: ProHist CF.
W/Codeine Phosphate, Pseudoephedrine Hydrochloride.
See: Poly Hist NC.
W/Pseudoephedrine Hydrochloride.
See: Allerfrim.
Altafed.
Aprodine.
Genac.
Silafed.
Tripohist D.

triprolidine hydrochloride. (Centurion) Triprolidine 1.25 mg/5 mL. Alcohol and sugar free. Apple flavor. Liq. 473 mL. *Rx.*
Use: Antihistamine, nonselective alkylamine.

triprolidine hydrochloride and pseudoephedrine hydrochloride. (Various Mfr.) Triprolidine hydrochloride 1.25 mg, pseudoephedrine hydrochloride 30 mg/5 mL. Syr. Bot. 118 mL. *OTC.*
Use: Upper respiratory combination, antihistamine, decongestant.

triprolidine tannate.
Use: Antihistamine, nonselective alkylamine.
See: Zymine XR.
W/Pseudoephedrine Tannate.
See: Zyme DXR.

Triptifed. (Weeks & Leo) Triprolidine hydrochloride 2.5 mg, pseudoephedrine hydrochloride 60 mg. Tab. Bot. 36s, 100s. *Rx.*
Use: Antihistamine; decongestant.

Triptone. (Del Pharmaceuticals) Dimenhydrinate 50 mg. Tab. Bot. 12s. *OTC.*
Use: Antiemetic; antivertigo.

•**triptorelin.** (TRIP-toe-RELL-in) USAN.
Use: Antineoplastic.

•**triptorelin pamoate.** (TRIP-toe-RELL-in) USAN.
Use: Antineoplastic; hormone, gonadotropin-releasing hormone analog.
See: Trelstar.
Trelstar Depot.
Trelstar LA.

trisaccharides A and B.
Use: Hemolytic disease of the newborn. [Orphan Drug]

Trisenox. (Cephalon) Arsenic trioxide 1 mg/mL, preservative free. Inj. Box 10s. *Rx.*
Use: Antineoplastic.

trisodium citrate concentration.
Use: Leukapheresis procedures. [Orphan Drug]

Trisol. (Buffington) Borax, sodium chloride, boric acid. Irrig. Bot. oz, 4 oz. *OTC.*
Use: Artificial tears.

Trispec PSE. (Deliz) Dextromethorphan HBr 15 mg, guaifenesin 25 mg, pseudoephedrine hydrochloride 30 mg per 5 mL. Sugar, alcohol, and dye free. Saccharin, sorbitol. Grape flavor. Liq. 120 mL. *Rx.*
Use: Antitussive and expectorant combination.

Tri-Sprintec. (Barr) **Phase 1:** Norgestimate 0.18 mg, ethinyl estradiol 35 mcg. 7 tabs. **Phase 2:** Norgestimate 0.215 mg, ethinyl estradiol 35 mcg. 7 tabs. **Phase 3:** Norgestimate 0.25 mg, ethinyl estradiol 35 mcg. 7 tabs. Lactose. Tab. 28s. 7 inert tablets. *Rx.*
Use: Contraceptive hormone, sex hormone.

Tri-Statin. (Rugby) Triamcinolone acetonide 0.1%, neomycin sulfate 0.25%, gramicidin 0.25 mg, nystatin 100,000 units/g Cream. Tube 15 g, 30 g, 60 g, 120 g, 480 g. *Rx.*
Use: Anti-infective; corticosteroid, topical.

Tri-Statin II. (Rugby) Triamcinolone acetonide 0.1%, 100,000 units nystatin per g, white petrolatum, parabens. Cream. Tube 15 g, 30 g, 60 g, 120 g, 480 g. *Rx.*
Use: Antifungal; corticosteroid, topical.

trisulfapyridmines.
Use: Anti-infective, sulfonamide.
See: Triple Sulfa.

•**trisulfapyrimidines oral suspension.** (try-SOLL-fah-peer-IH-mih-deenz) *USP 34.*
Use: Anti-infective.
See: Meth-Dia-Mer Sulfonamides.

Tri-Super Flavons 1000. (Freeda) Bioflavonoids 1000 mg. Tab. Bot. 100s, 250s, 500s. *OTC.*
Use: Water-soluble vitamin.

Trital DM. (Breckenridge Pharmaceutical) Chlorpheniramine maleate 4 mg, dextromethorphan hydrobromide 15 mg, phenylephrine hydrochloride 10 mg. Sorbitol. Alcohol free, dye free, and sugar free. Grape flavor. Liq. 473 mL. *Rx.*
Use: Upper respiratory combination, antitussive combination.

Tritan. (Eon Labs) Phenylephrine tannate 25 mg, chlorpheniramine tannate 8 mg, pyrilamine tannate 25 mg. Tab. Bot. 100s, 250s, 1000s. *Rx.*
Use: Antihistamine; decongestant.

Tri-Tannate. (Rugby) Phenylephrine tannate 25 mg, chlorpheniramine tannate 8 mg, pyrilamine tannate 25 mg. Tab. Bot. 100s, 250s. *Rx.*
Use: Antihistamine; decongestant.

Tri-Tannate Pediatric. (Rugby) Phenylephrine tannate 5 mg, chlorpheniramine tannate 2 mg, pyrilamine tannate 12.5 mg. Susp. Bot. 473 mL. *Rx.*
Use: Antihistamine; decongestant.

Tri-Tannate Plus Pediatric Suspension. (Rugby) Phenylephrine tannate 5 mg, ephedrine tannate 5 mg, chlorpheniramine tannate 4 mg, carbetapentane tannate 30 mg/5 mL. Bot. 480 mL. *Rx.*
Use: Antihistamine; antitussive; decongestant.

•**tritiated water.** (TRIT-ee-ay-ted WA-ter) USAN.
Use: Radiopharmaceutical.

Tri-Tinic. (Vortech Pharmaceuticals) Liver desiccated 75 mg, stomach 75 mg, Vitamins B_{12} 15 mcg, Fe 110 mg, folic acid 1 mg, ascorbic acid 75 mg. Cap. Bot. 100s. *Rx.*
Use: Mineral, vitamin supplement.

TriTuss. (Everett) Dextromethorphan HBr 25 mg, guaifenesin 175 mg, phenylephrine hydrochloride 12.5 mg per 5 mL. Sugar and alcohol free. Saccharin, sorbitol. Strawberry flavor. Syrup. 473 mL. *Rx.*
Use: Upper respiratory combination, antitussive and expectorant combination.

TriTuss-A. (Everett) Phenylephrine hydrochloride 2 mg, carbinoxamine maleate 1 mg, dextromethorphan HBr 2 mg per 1 mL. Sugar free. Parabens, saccharin, sorbitol. Cherry flavor. Oral Drops. Bot. 30 mL with calibrated dropper. *Rx.*
Use: Pediatric antitussive combination.

TriTuss-ER. (Everett) Dextromethorphan HBr 30 mg, guaifenesin 600 mg, phenylephrine hydrochloride 10 mg. ER Tab. 100s. *Rx.*
Use: Upper respiratory combination, antitussive and expectorant combination.

Tritussin. (Scientific Laboratories) Hydrocodone bitartrate 5 mg, chlorpheniramine maleate 2 mg, phenylephrine hydrochloride 5 mg per 5 mL. Sugar and alcohol free. Candy apple flavor. Syrup. 473 mL. *c-III.*
Use: Antitussive combination.

Tritussin Cough. (Towne) Pyrilamine maleate 40 mg, pheniramine maleate 20 mg, citric acid 100 mg, codeine phosphate 58 mg/fl. oz. w/menthol and glycerin in flavored base. Syr. Bot. 4 oz. *c-v.*
Use: Antihistamine; antitussive; expectorant.

Trivaris. (Allergan) Triamcinolone acetonide 80 mg/mL. Sodium hyaluronate
2.3%. Preservative free. Inj., Gel Susp.
Single-use glass syringe. *Rx.*
Use: Adrenocortical steroid, glucocorticoid.

Tri-Vert. (T.E. Williams Pharmaceuticals)
Dimenhydrinate 25 mg, niacin 50 mg,
pentylenetetrazol 25 mg. Cap. Bot.
100s. *OTC.*
Use: Motion sickness.

Tri-Vi-Flor 1.0 mg. (Bristol-Myers
Squibb) Fluoride 1 mg, vitamins A
2500 units, D 400 units, C 60 mg, sucrose. Tab. Bot. 100s, 1000s. *Rx.*
Use: Dental caries agent; nutritional
supplement.

Tri-Vi-Flor 0.5 mg. (Bristol-Myers
Squibb) Fluoride 0.5 mg, vitamins A
1500 units, D 400 units, C 35 mg/mL.
Drops. Bot. 50 mL. *Rx.*
Use: Dental caries agent; nutritional
supplement.

Tri-Vi-Flor 0.25 mg. (Bristol-Myers
Squibb) Fluoride 0.25 mg, vitamins A
1500 units, D 400 units, C 35 mg/1 mL.
Drops. Bot. 50 mL. *Rx.*
Use: Dental caries agent; nutritional
supplement.

Tri-Vi-Flor 0.25 mg with Iron. (Bristol-
Myers Squibb) Fluoride 0.25 mg, vitamins A 1500 units, D 400 units, C
35 mg, Fe 10 mg/1 mL. Drops. Bot.
50 mL. *Rx.*
Use: Dental caries agent; nutritional
supplement.

Tri-Vi-Sol. (Bristol-Myers Squibb) Vitamin A 1500 units, D 400 units, C
35 mg/1 mL. Drops. Bot. 50 mL with
calibrated safety-dropper. *OTC.*
Use: Vitamin supplement.

Tri-Vi-Sol with Iron. (Bristol-Myers
Squibb) Vitamins A 1500 units, C
35 mg, D 400 units, Fe 10 mg/mL.
Drops. Bot. 50 mL. *OTC.*
Use: Mineral, vitamin supplement.

Trivitamin Fluoride. (Schein) **Drops:**
Fluoride 0.25 mg or 0.5 mg, vitamins A
1500 units, D 400 units, C 35 mg/mL.
Bot. 50 mL. **Chew. Tab.:** Fluoride
0.5 mg, vitamins A 2500 units, D
400 units, C 60 mg, sucrose. Bot. 100s.
Rx.
Use: Fluoride, vitamin supplement; dental caries agent.

Tri-Vitamin with Fluoride. (Rugby) Fluoride 0.5 mg, Vitamins A 1500 units, D
400 units, C 35 mg/mL Drops. Bot.
50 mL. *Rx.*
Use: Mineral, vitamin supplement.

Tri-Vite. (Foy Laboratories) Thiamine
hydrochloride 100 mg, pyridoxine
hydrochloride 100 mg, cyanocobalamin
1000 mcg/mL. Vial 10 mL. *Rx.*
Use: Vitamin supplement.

Trivora. (Watson) **Phase 1:** Levonorgestrel
0.05 mg, ethinyl estradiol 30 mcg (6 tablets). **Phase 2:** Levonorgestrel 0.075 mg,
ethinyl estradiol 40 mcg (5 tablets).
Phase 3: Levonorgestrel 0.125 mg, ethinyl estradiol 30 mcg (10 tablets). Lactose. Pack. 28s with 7 inert tablets. *Rx.*
Use: Sex hormone, contraceptive hormone.

Trizivir. (ViiV Healthcare) Abacavir sulfate 300 mg, lamivudine 150 mg, zidovudine 300 mg. Film-coated. Tab. Bot.
60s. *Rx.*
Use: Antiretroviral, nucleoside analog
reverse transcriptase inhibitor combination.

Trocaine. (Roberts) Benzocaine 10 mg.
Loz. UD 4s, 500s. *OTC.*
Use: Dietary aid.

Trocal. (Textilease) Dextromethorphan
HBr 7.5 mg. Cherry flavor. Loz. 10s,
50s, 500s. *OTC.*
Use: Nonnarcotic antitussive.

•**troclosene potassium.** (TROE-kloe-
seen) USAN.
Use: Anti-infective, topical.

•**trodusquemine.** (troe-DOO-skwe-meen)
USAN.
Use: Obesity.

•**troglitazone.** (TROE-glih-tazz-ohn)
USAN.
Use: Antidiabetic.

•**trolamine.** (TROLE-ah-meen) *NF 29.*
Formerly Triethanolamine.
Use: Pharmaceutic aid (alkalizing
agent), analgesic.

trolamine salicylate.
Use: Rub and liniment.
See: Analgesic Creme Rub.
Aspercreme with Aloe.
Flex-Power Performance Sports.

tromal.
Use: Analgesic; antidepressant agent.

•**tromethamine.** (TROE-meth-ah-meen)
USP 34.
Use: Alkalizer.

Tronolane. (Monticello) **Cream:** Pramoxine hydrochloride 1%, zinc oxide 5%,
cetyl alcohol, parabens. Tube 30 g,
60 g. **Supp.:** Hard fat 88.7%, phenylephrine hydrochloride 0.25%. Parabens. 12s. *OTC.*
Use: Anorectal preparation.

Tropamine+. (NeuroGenesis/Matrix Tech.)
Vitamins D 250 mg, l-phenylalanine,

l-tyrosine 150 mg, l-glutamine 50 mg, B_1 1.67 mg, B_2 2.5 mg, B_3 16.7 mg, B_5 15 mg, B_6 3.3 mg, B_{12} 5 mcg, folic acid 0.067 mg, C 100 mg, Ca 25 mg, Cr 0.01 mg, Fe 1.5 mg, Mg 25 mg, Zn 5 mg, yeast and preservative free. Cap. Bot. 42s, 180s. *OTC.*
Use: Nutritional supplement.

•**tropanserin hydrochloride.** (troe-PAN-ser-in) USAN.
Use: Serotonin receptor antagonist (specific in migraine).

TrophAmine Injection. (McGaw) Nitrogen 4.65 g, amino acids 30 g, protein 29 g/500 mL. Bot. 500 mL IV infusion. *OTC.*
Use: Nutritional supplement.

Troph-Iron. (GlaxoSmithKline Consumer) Vitamins B_{12} 25 mcg, B_1 10 mg, Fe 20 mg/5 mL. Saccharin. Bot. 4 fl. oz. *OTC.*
Use: Mineral, vitamin supplement.

Trophite (Iron). (Menley & James Labs, Inc.) Fe 60 mg, B_1 30 mg, B_{12} 75 mcg. Liq. Bot. 120 mL. *OTC.*
Use: Mineral, vitamin supplement.

Tropicacyl. (Akorn) Tropicamide solution 0.5%. 15 mL. 1% tropicamide. 2 mL, 15 mL. *Rx.*
Use: Cycloplegic; mydriatic.

Tropical Blend. (Schering-Plough) A series of products is marketed under the *Tropical Blend* name including: *Hawaii Blend Oil* SPF 2 (Bot. 8 oz.); *Hawaii Blend Lotion* SPF 2 (Bot. 8 oz.); *Rio Blend Oil* SPF 2 (Bot. 8 oz.); *Rio Blend Lotion* SPF 2 (Bot. 8 oz.); *Jamaica Blend Oil* SPF 2 (Bot. 8 oz.); *Jamaica Blend Lotion* SPF 2 (Bot. 8 oz.). All contain homosalate in various oil and lotion bases. *OTC.*
Use: Sunscreen.

Tropical Blend Dark Tanning. (Schering-Plough) **SPF 2:** Homosalate. **Oil:** Padimate O, oxybenzone. Bot. 180 mL, 240 mL. **Lot.:** Bot. 240 mL. **SPF 4:** Ethylhexyl p-methoxycinnamate, oxybenzone. Bot. 240 mL. *OTC.*
Use: Sunscreen.

Tropical Blend Dry Oil. (Schering-Plough) Homosalate, oxybenzone. Oil. Bot. 180 mL. *OTC.*
Use: Sunscreen.

Tropical Blend Tan Magnifier. (Schering-Plough) Triethanolamine salicylate. Oil. Bot. 240 mL. *OTC.*
Use: Sunscreen.

Tropical Gold Dark Tanning Lotion. (Ivax) SPF 4. Ethylhexyl p-methoxycinnamate, oxybenzone, benzyl alcohol, parabens, aloe extract, jojoba oil, vitamin E, EDTA. PABA free. Waterproof. Lot. Bot. 240 mL. *OTC.*
Use: Sunscreen.

Tropical Gold Dark Tanning Oil. (Ivax) SPF 2. Ethylhexyl p-methoxycinnamate, octyldimethyl PABA, mineral oil, coconut oil, cocoa butter, aloe, lanolin, eucalyptus oil, oils of plumeria, manako (mango), kuawa (guava), mikara (papaya), liliko (passion fruit), taro, kukui. Oil. Bot. 240 mL. *OTC.*
Use: Sunscreen.

Tropical Gold Sport Sunblock. (Ivax) SPF 15. Ethylhexyl p-methoxycinnamate, oxybenzone, diazolidinyl urea, parabens, aloe extract, jojoba oil, vitamin E, EDTA. PABA free. Perspiration-proof. Lot. Bot. 180 mL. *OTC.*
Use: Sunblock.

Tropical Gold Sunblock. (Ivax) **Lot: SPF 15:** Ethylhexyl p-methoxycinnamate, oxybenzone, vegetable oil, benzyl alcohol, parabens, imidazolidinyl urea, vitamin E, aloe extract, jojoba oil, EDTA. PABA free. Waterproof. Bot. 118 mL. **SPF 17:** Ethylhexyl p-methoxycinnamate, 2-ethylhexyl salicylate, homosalate, oxybenzone, aloe extract, vitamin E, vegetable and jojoba oils, benzyl alcohol, imidazolidinyl urea, parabens, EDTA. PABA free. Waterproof. Bot. 118 mL. **SPF 30:** Ethylhexyl p-methoxycinnamate, 2-ethylhexyl salicylate, homosalate, oxybenzone, aloe extract, vitamin E, vegetable and jojoba oils, benzyl alcohol, imidizolinyl urea, parabens, EDTA. PABA free. Waterproof. 118 mL. *OTC.*
Use: Sunblock.

Tropical Gold Sunscreen. (Ivax) SPF 8. Ethylhexyl p-methoxycinnamate, oxybenzone, benzyl alcohol, parabens, aloe extract, jojoba oil, vitamin E, EDTA. PABA free. Waterproof. Lot. Bot. 118 mL. *OTC.*
Use: Sunscreen.

•**tropicamide.** (troe-PIK-a-mide) *USP 34.*
Use: Anticholinergic (ophthalmic).
See: Mydral.
Mydriacyl.
Tropicacyl.

tropicamide. (Various Mfr.) Tropicamide 0.5%, 1%. Soln. Bot. 2 mL (0.5%), 15 mL.
Use: Anticholinergic (ophthalmic).

tropine benzhydryl ester methanesulfonate. Also named benztropine methane-sulfonate.

•**trospectomycin.** (TROE-speck-toe-MY-sin) USAN.
Use: Anti-infective.

•**trospium chloride.** (TROSE-pee-um) USAN.
Use: Anticholinergic.
See: Sanctura.
  Sanctura XR.

Trovit. (Sigma-Tau) Vitamins B$_2$ 0.3 mg, B$_6$ 1 mg, choline chloride 25 mg, panthenol 2 mg, dl-methionine 10 mg, inositol 20 mg, niacinamide 50 mg, vitamins B$_{12}$ 10 mcg/mL. Vial 30 mL. *Rx.*
Use: Vitamin B supplement.

T.R.U.E. Test. (GlaxoSmithKline) Allergen-containing patches. Test in multipak cartons (5s). *Rx.*
Use: Diagnostic aid, allergic.

Trusopt. (Merck) Dorzolamide (as base) 2%. Benzalkonium chloride 0.0075%, hydroxyethylcellulose, sodium hydroxide, mannitol. Soln. *Ocumeters.* 5 mL, 10 mL. *Rx.*
Use: Antiglaucoma.

Truvada. (Gilead) Emtricitabine 200 mg/ tenofovir disoproxil fumarate 300 mg (equiv. to tenofovir disoproxil 245 mg). Lactose. Film-coated. Tab. 30s. *Rx.*
Use: Antiretroviral.

Trycet. (Auriga) Propoxyphene napsylate 100 mg, acetaminophen 325 mg. Lactose. Film-coated. Tab. 100s. *c-IV.*
Use: Narcotic analgesic.

trypan blue.
Use: Ophthalmic surgery aid.
See: MembraneBlue.
  VisionBlue.

•**trypsin, crystallized.** (TRIP-sin) *USP 34.*
Use: Proteolytic enzyme.
W/Castor Oil.
See: Granulex.
W/Combinations.
See: Xenaderm.

tryptizol hydrochloride. Amitriptyline hydrochloride.

•**tryptophan.** (TRIP-toe-FAN) *USP 34.*
Use: Amino acid.

T/Scalp. (Neutrogena) Hydrocortisone 1%. Liq. Greaseless. Bot. 60 mL, 105 mL. *OTC.*
Use: Antipruritic; corticosteroid, topical.

TSPA.
Use: Antineoplastic.
See: Thiotepa.

TTC. Triphenyltetrazolium Chloride.

T-3 RIAbead. (Abbott Diagnostics) Test kit 50s, 100s.
Use: Diagnostic aid, thyroid.

tuaminoheptane sulfate.
Use: Adrenergic.

•**tuberculin.** (too-BURR-kyoo-lin) *USP 34.*
Use: Diagnostic aid (dermal reactivity indicator).

See: Aplisol.
  Aplitest.
  Tubersol.

Tuberculin, Mono-Vacc Test. (Lincoln Diagnostics) Mono-Vacc test is a sterile, disposable multiple puncture scarifier with liquid Old Tuberculin on the points. Box 25 tests. *Rx.*
Use: Diagnostic aid.

Tuberculin, Old Monovacc Test. (Wyeth) 5 TU activity test. Soln. of Old Tuberculin containing acacia 7%, lactose 8.5%. Test. Kits 25s, 100s, 250s. *Rx.*
Use: Diagnostic aid.

Tuberculin, Old, Tine Test. (Wyeth) 5 TY activity per test. Soln. of Old Tuberculin, containing acacia 7%, lactose 8.5%. Test. Kits 25s, 100s, 250s.
Use: Diagnostic aid.

tuberculin purified protein derivative.
Use: Diagnostic aid.
See: Aplisol.
  Tubersol.

tuberculin tests.
Use: Diagnostic aid.
See: Aplisol.
  Aplitest.
  Tine Test PPD.
  Tuberculin, Old MonoVacc Test.
  Tuberculin, Old, Tine Test.
  Tubersol.

tuberculin tine test. (Wyeth) **Old Tuberculin (OT):** Each disposable test unit consists of a stainless steel disc, with 4 tines (or prongs) 2 mm long, attached to a plastic handle. The tines have been dip-dried with antigenic material. The entire unit is sterilized by ethylene oxide gas. The test has been standardized by comparative studies, utilizing 0.05 mg US Standard Old Tuberculin 5 units or 0.0001 mg US Standard 5 units by the Mantoux technique. Reliability appears to be comparable to the standard Mantoux. Tests in a jar 25s. Package 100s. Bin Package 250s. **Purified Protein Derivative (PPD):** Equivalent to or more potent than 5 TU PPD Mantoux test. Tests in a jar 25s. Package 100s.
Use: Diagnostic aid.

tuberculosis vaccine.
Use: Immunization.
See: Tice BCG.

Tubersol. (Aventis Pasteur) Tuberculin purified protein derivative (Mantoux) 5 TU/0.1 mL, potassium and sodium phosphates, phenol 0.35%, polysorbate 80. Vial 1 mL (10 tests), 5 mL (50 tests). *Rx.*
Use: Diagnostic aid, tuberculosis.

•**tubocurarine chloride.** (too-boe-cure-AHR-een) *USP 34.*
Use: Neuromuscular blocker.

tubocurarine chloride, dimethyl. Dimethylether of d-tubocurarine chloride.

tubocurarine chloride hydrochloride pentahydrate. Tubocurarine Chloride.

tubocurarine iodide, dimethyl. Dimethyl ether of d-tubocurarine iodide.
Use: Muscle relaxant.

•**tubulozole hydrochloride.** (too-BYOO-lah-ZAHL) USAN.
Use: Antineoplastic (microtubule inhibitor).

Tucks. (Pfizer Consumer Health) Pramoxine hydrochloride 1%. Zinc oxide 12.5%, mineral oil 46.6%, cocoa butter. Oint. 30 g with applicator. *OTC.*
Use: Anorectal preparation.

Tucks Ointment. (Pfizer Consumer Health) Hydrocortisone 1%, diazolidinyl urea, parabens, mineral oil, sorbitan sesquioleate, white petrolatum. Oint. Tube 21 g. *OTC.*
Use: Corticosteroid, topical.

Tucks Suppositories. (Pfizer Consumer Health) Topical starch 51%, benzyl alcohol, soybean oil, tocopheryl acetate. Supp. Pkg. 12s. *OTC.*
Use: Anorectal preparation.

Tucks Take-Alongs. (Parke-Davis) Nonwoven wipes saturated with solution of witch hazel 50%, glycerine 10%, benzalkonium chloride 0.003%. Box 12s. *OTC.*
Use: Anorectal preparation.

•**tucotuzumab celmoleukin.** (TOO-koe-TOOZ-oo-mab SEL-moe-LOO-kin) USAN.
Use: Immune globulin.

Tuinal. (Eli Lilly) Equal parts Seconal Sod. & Amytal Sod. Pulvule. 100 mg, 200 mg. Bot. 100s. *c-II.*
Use: Hypnotic; sedative.

tumor necrosis factor-binding protein I. Serono *Rx.*
Use: Treatment of AIDS. [Orphan Drug]

tumor necrosis factor-binding protein II. Serono *Rx.*
Use: Treatment of AIDS. [Orphan Drug]

Tums Calcium for Life Bone Health. (GlaxoSmithKline Consumer) Calcium carbonate 1250 mg (elemental calcium 500 mg). Chew. Tab. Bot. 90s. *OTC.*
Use: Mineral supplement; antacid.

Tums Calcium for Life PMS. (GlaxoSmithKline Consumer) Calcium carbonate 750 mg (elemental calcium 300 mg). Sucrose. Strawberry flavor. Chew. Tab. Bot. 120s. *OTC.*
Use: Mineral supplement; antacid.

Tums Dual Action. (GlaxoSmithKline) Famotidine 10 mg, calcium carbonate 800 mg, magnesium hydroxide 165 mg. Aspartame, glyceryl, lactose, phenylalanine 2.2 mg, polysorbate 80. Berry flavor. Chew. Tab. 25s. *OTC.*
Use: Histamine H_2 antagonist combination.

Tums E-X. (GlaxoSmithKline Consumer) Calcium carbonate 750 mg (elemental calcium 300 mg). Sucrose, talc. Mixed berry, assorted fruit and sugar free orange (aspartame, phenylalanine < 1 mg, sorbitol) flavors. Chew. Tab. Bot. 96s. *OTC.*
Use: Mineral supplement; antacid.

Tums Kids. (GlaxoSmithKline Consumer) Calcium carbonate 750 mg (elemental calcium 300 mg). Dextrose, gluten, maltodextrin, sorbitol, sucrose. Cherry flavor. Chew. Tab. 36s. *OTC.*
Use: Mineral supplement; antacid.

Tums Plus. (GlaxoSmithKline) Calcium carbonate 500 mg, (elemental calcium 200 mg), simethicone 20 mg. Sucrose, sodium. Assorted fruit and mint flavors. Chew. Tab. Bot. 48s. *OTC.*
Use: Mineral supplement; antacid.

Tums Quik Pak. (GlaxoSmithKline Consumer) Calcium carbonate 1,000 mg. Dextrose, maltodextrin, sorbitol, sucrose. Berry flavor. Pow. 24s. *OTC.*
Use: Mineral supplement; antacid.

Tums Smooth Dissolve. (GlaxoSmithKline) Calcium carbonate 750 mg (elemental calcium 300 mg). Sorbitol, dextrose, sucrose (2 g sugar). Peppermint and assorted fruit flavors. Chew. Tab. 45s. *OTC.*
Use: Mineral supplement; antacid.

Tums Ultra. (GlaxoSmithKline Consumer) Calcium carbonate 1000 mg (elemental calcium 400 mg). Sucrose, talc. Mint flavor. Chew. Tab. Bot. 86s. *OTC.*
Use: Mineral supplement; antacid.

Tur-Bi-Kal Nasal Drops. (Emerson) Phenylephrine hydrochloride in a saline solution. Drops. Bot. oz., 12s. *OTC.*
Use: Decongestant.

Turbinaire.
See: Decadron Phosphate.

Turbinaire Decadron Phosphate. (Merck & Co.) Each metered spray delivers dexamethasone sodium phosphate equivalent to dexamethasone ≈ 84 mcg (170 sprays per cartridge), alcohol 2%. Aerosol. 12.6 g w/adapter or 12.6 g refill. *Rx.*
Use: Corticosteroid, topical.

•**turofexorate isopropyl.** (TUR-oh-FEX-
or-ate) USAN.
Use: Treatment of lipid disorders.
turpentine oil.
W/Combinations.
See: Sloan's Liniment.
Tusdec-DM. (Cypress) Dextromethorphan HBr 15 mg, brompheniramine
maleate 2 mg, phenylephrine hydrochloride 7.5 mg per 5 mL. Alcohol,
sugar, and dye free. Saccharin, sorbitol. Strawberry flavor. Liq. 473 mL. *Rx.*
Use: Upper respiratory combination,
antitussive combination.
Tusibron. (Kenwood) Guaifenesin
100 mg/5 mL, alcohol 3.5%. Liq. Bot.
118 mL. *OTC.*
Use: Expectorant.
Tusnel. (Llorens) Dextromethorphan HBr
15 mg, guaifenesin 200 mg, pseudoephedrine hydrochloride 30 mg per
5 mL. Alcohol, sugar, and dye free. Aspartame, parabens, phenylalanine
16.9 mg/5 mL. Liq. 178 mL. *Rx.*
Use: Upper respiratory combination, antitussive and expectorant combination.
Tusnel C. (Llorens) Codeine phosphate
10 mg, guaifenesin 100 mg, pseudoephedrine hydrochloride 30 mg per
5 mL. Alcohol 1.9%. Sugar free. Menthol, saccharin, sorbitol. Syrup. 473 mL.
c-v.
Use: Upper respiratory combination, antitussive and expectorant combination.
Tusnel-DM Pediatric. (Llorens) Dextromethorphan hydrobromide 2.5 mg,
guaifenesin 25 mg, pseudoephedrine
hydrochloride 7.5 mg. Glycerin, propylene glycol, saccharin, sodium benzoate. Drops. 60 mL. *OTC.*
Use: Upper respiratory combination, antitussive and expectorant combination.
Tusnel Pediatric. (Llorens) Dextromethorphan HBr 5 mg, guaifenesin 50 mg,
pseudoephedrine hydrochloride 15 mg
per 5 mL. Alcohol free. Aspartame,
corn syrup, parabens, phenylalanine.
Liq. 118 mL, 3780 mL. *Rx.*
Use: Upper respiratory combination, antitussive and expectorant combination.
Tussabar. (Tennessee Pharmaceutic)
Acetaminophen 400 mg, salicylamide
500 mg, potassium guaiacolsulfonate
120 mg, pyrilamine maleate 30 mg,
ammonium chloride 500 mg, sodium
citrate 500 mg, phenylephrine hydrochloride 30 mg/oz. Bot. Pt., gal. *Rx.*

Use: Analgesic; antihistamine; decongestant; expectorant.
Tussabid. (ION Laboratories, Inc.) Guaifenesin 200 mg, dextromethorphan HBr
30 mg. Cap. Bot. 24s, 100s. *OTC.*
Use: Antihistamine; expectorant.
Tussafed. (Everett) **Drops:** Carbinoxamine maleate 2 mg, pseudoephedrine
hydrochloride 25 mg, dextromethorphan HBr 4 mg/mL. Bot. 30 mL with
calibrated dropper. **Syrup:** Dextromethorphan HBr 15 mg, pseudoephedrine
hydrochloride 60 mg, carbinoxamine
maleate 4 mg per 5 mL. Menthol, grape
flavor, alcohol free, sugar free. Bot.
120 mL, 480 mL. *Rx.*
Use: Upper respiratory combination, antihistamine, antitussive, decongestant.
Tussafed EX. (Everett Laboratories) Dextromethorphan HBr 30 mg, guaifenesin
200 mg, phenylephrine hydrochloride
10 mg per 5 mL. EDTA, saccharin,
sorbitol, cherry-vanilla flavor, alcohol
free. Syr. Bot. 473 mL. *Rx.*
Use: Upper respiratory combination, antitussive, expectorant, decongestant.
Tussafin Expectorant. (Rugby) Pseudoephedrine hydrochloride 60 mg, hydrocodone bitartrate 5 mg, guaifenesin
200 mg/5 mL, alcohol 2.5%. Liq. Bot.
480 mL. *c-III.*
Use: Antitussive; decongestant; expectorant.
Tussall. (Everett) Dextromethorphan HBr
20 mg, dexbrompheniramine maleate
2 mg, phenylephrine hydrochloride
10 mg per 5 mL. EDTA, saccharin,
sorbitol. Strawberry flavor. Syrup.
473 mL. *Rx.*
Use: Upper respiratory combination, antitussive combination.
Tussall-ER. (Everett) Dextromethorphan
HBr 30 mg, dexbrompheniramine
maleate 6 mg, phenylephrine hydrochloride 20 mg. ER Tab. 100s. *Rx.*
Use: Upper respiratory combination, antitussive combination.
Tussanil DH. (Edwards) Phenylephrine
hydrochloride 10 mg, chlorpheniramine
maleate 4 mg, hydrocodone bitartrate
2.5 mg/5 mL w/alcohol 5%. Syrup. Bot.
Pt. *c-III.*
Use: Antihistamine; antitussive; decongestant.
Tussanil Expectorant. (Edwards) Hydrocodone bitartrate 2.5 mg, phenylephrine
hydrochloride 10 mg, guaifenesin
100 mg/5 mL w/alcohol 5%. Syrup. Bot.
Pt. *c-III.*
Use: Antitussive; decongestant; expectorant.

Tussanol. (Tyler) Pyrilamine maleate ¾ g, codeine phosphate 1 g, ammonium chloride 7.5 g, sodium citrate 5 g, menthol g/fl. oz. Bot. 4 fl. oz, pt, gal. *c-v.*
Use: Antihistamine; antitussive; expectorant.

Tussanol with Ephedrine. (Tyler) Ephedrine sulfate 2 g, pyrilamine maleate 0.75 g, codeine phosphate 1 g, ammonium chloride 7.5 g, sodium citrate 5 g, menthol g/30 mL. Bot. 16 fl. oz. *c-v.*
Use: Bronchodilator; antihistamine; antitussive; expectorant.

Tussar DM. (Aventis) Dextromethorphan HBr 15 mg, chlorpheniramine maleate 2 mg, phenylephrine hydrochloride 5 mg/5 mL w/methylparaben 0.1% Bot. 4 oz., pt. *Rx.*
Use: Antihistamine; antitussive; expectorant.

Tussar SF. (Aventis) Codeine phosphate 10 mg, guaifenesin 100 mg, pseudoephedrine hydrochloride 30 mg/5 mL, alcohol 2.5%. Bot. 120 mL, 473 mL. *c-v.*
Use: Antitussive; decongestant; expectorant.

Tussar-2. (Aventis) Codeine phosphate 10 mg, guaifenesin 100 mg, pseudoephedrine hydrochloride 30 mg/5 mL, alcohol 2.5%. Syrup. Bot. 473 mL. *c-v.*
Use: Antitussive; expectorant; decongestant.

Tussbid. (Breckenridge) Phenylephrine hydrochloride 15 mg, guaifenesin 400 mg. Sugar. ER Cap. 100s. *Rx.*
Use: Upper respiratory combination, decongestant and expectorant combination.

Tussbid PD. (Breckenridge) Phenylephrine hydrochloride 7.5 mg, guaifenesin 200 mg. ER Cap. 100s. *Rx.*
Use: Upper respiratory combination, decongestant and expectorant combination.

Tussend. (Monarch) **Syr.:** Hydrocodone bitartrate 2.5 mg, pseudoephedrine hydrochloride 30 mg, chlorpheniramine maleate 2 mg per 5 mL. Alcohol 5%, corn syrup, parabens, saccharin, sucrose, banana flavor. Bot. 473 mL. **Tab.:** Hydrocodone bitartrate 5 mg, chlorpheniramine maleate 4 mg, pseudoephedrine hydrochloride 60 mg. Lactose. Bot. 100s. *c-III.*
Use: Upper respiratory combination, antitussive, antihistamine, decongestant.

Tussgen. (Ivax) Pseudoephedrine hydrochloride 60 mg, hydrocodone bitartrate 5 mg/5 mL. Liq. Bot. 100s, 1000s. *c-III.*
Use: Antitussive; decongestant.

TUSSI-bid. (Capellon) Dextromethorphan HBr 60 mg, guaifenesin 1200 mg. ER Tab. Bot. 100s. *Rx.*
Use: Upper respiratory combination, antitussive, expectorant.

TussiCaps Full Strength. (Mallinckrodt) Chlorpheniramine maleate 8 mg (as chlorpheniramine polistirex), hydrocodone bitartrate 10 mg (as hydrocodone polistirex). Butyl alcohol, dehydrated alcohol, isopropyl alcohol, SDA3A alcohol, SD-45 alcohol. ER Cap. 20s, 100s. *c-III.*
Use: Upper respiratory combination, antitussive combination.

TussiCaps Half Strength. (Mallinckrodt) Chlorpheniramine maleate 4 mg (as chlorpheniramine polistirex), hydrocodone bitartrate 5 mg (as hydrocodone polistirex). Butyl alcohol, dehydrated alcohol, isopropyl alcohol, SDA3A alcohol, SD-45 alcohol. ER Cap. 20s, 100s. *c-III.*
Use: Upper respiratory combination, antitussive combination.

Tussigon. (Monarch) Hydrocodone bitartrate 5 mg, homatropine methylbromide 1.5 mg. Tab. Bot. 100s, 500s. *c-III.*
Use: Upper respiratory combination, antitussive combination.

TussiNATE. (Pediamed) Hydrocodone bitartrate 3.5 mg, diphenhydramine hydrochloride 12.5 mg, phenylephrine hydrochloride 5 mg per 5 mL. Alcohol free. Saccharin, sucrose. Black raspberry flavor. Syrup. 473 mL. *c-III.*
Use: Antitussive combination.

Tussionex Pennkinetic. (CellTech) Hydrocodone polistirex 10 mg, chlorpheniramine polistirex 8 mg per 5 mL. Parabens, sucrose, corn syrup, PEG. ER Susp. Bot. 473 mL. *c-III.*
Use: Upper respiratory combination, antitussive combination.

Tussi-Organidin DM-S NR. (Victory Pharma) Dextromethorphan HBr 10 mg, guaifenesin 300 mg per 5 mL. Alcohol and sugar free. Magnasweet, PEG, saccharin, sorbitol. Grape flavor. Liq. 118 mL with dosing syringe. *Rx.*
Use: Upper respiratory combination, antitussive with expectorant.

Tussi-Organidin NR. (Victory Pharma) Codeine phosphate 10 mg, guaifenesin 300 mg per 5 mL. Alcohol free. Saccharin, sorbitol, PEG. Liq. Bot. 473 mL. *c-v.*
Use: Upper respiratory combination, antitussive and expectorant combination.

Tussi-Organidin-S NR. (Victory Pharma) Codeine phosphate 10 mg, guaifenesin

300 mg per 5 mL. Alcohol and sugar free. PEG, saccharin, sorbitol. Liq. 118 mL with dosing syringe. *c-v.*
Use: Upper respiratory combination, antitussive with expectorant.

Tussi-Pres. (Kramer-Novis) Dextromethorphan hydrobromide 15 mg, guaifenesin 200 mg, phenylephrine hydrochloride 5 mg per 5 mL. Alcohol and sugar free. Phenylalanine 15 mg/5 mL, aspartame, parabens. Cherry flavor. Liq. 474 mL. *Rx.*
Use: Upper respiratory combination, antitussive and expectorant combination.

Tussi-Pres Pediatric. (Kramer-Novis) Phenylephrine hydrochloride 2.5 mg, dextromethorphan HBr 5 mg, guaifenesin 75 mg per 5 mL. Sugar, alcohol, and dye free. Parabens, aspartame, phenylalanine 14 mg per 5 mL. Orange flavor. Liq. 473 mL. *Rx.*
Use: Upper respiratory combination, antitussive and expectorant combination.

Tussi-12. (Meda Pharmaceuticals) **Susp.:** Carbetapentane tannate 30 mg, chlorpheniramine tannate 4 mg, phenylephrine tannate 5 mg/mL, glycerin, methylparaben, saccharin, sucrose. Bot. Pt. **Tab.:** Carbetapentane tannate 60 mg, chlorpheniramine tannate 5 mg. Bot. 100s. *Rx.*
Use: Upper respiratory combination, antihistamine, antitussive, decongestant.

Tussi-12 D. (Meda Pharmaceuticals) Carbetapentane tannate 60 mg, pyrilamine tannate 40 mg, phenylephrine tannate 10 mg. Tab. 100s. *Rx.*
Use: Antitussive combination.

Tussi-12D S. (Meda Pharmaceuticals) **Susp.:** Carbetapentane tannate 30 mg, pyrilamine tannate 30 mg, phenylephrine tannate 5 mg per 5 mL. Tartrazine, methylparaben, saccharin, sucrose, strawberry-currant flavor. 118 mL w/oral syringe. **Tab.:** Carbetapentane tannate 60 mg, pyrilamine tannate 40 mg, phenylephrine tannate 10 mg. 100s. *Rx.*
Use: Upper respiratory combination, antitussive combination.

Tussi-12 S. (Meda Pharmaceuticals) Chlorpheniramine tannate 4 mg, carbetapentane tannate 30 mg per 5 mL. Methylparaben, saccharin, sucrose, tartrazine, strawberry-currant flavor. Susp. Bot. 118 mL with syringe. *Rx.*
Use: Upper respiratory combination, antitussive combination.

Tussizone-12 RF. (Mallinckrodt) **Susp.:** Carbetapentane tannate 30 mg, chlorpheniramine tannate 4 mg per 5 mL. Tartrazine, methylparaben, saccharin, sucrose, strawberry currant flavor. 118 mL with oral syringe. *Rx.*
Use: Upper respiratory combination, antitussive combination.

Tuss-LA. (Hyrex) Pseudoephedrine hydrochloride 120 mg, guaifenesin 500 mg. LA Tab. Bot. 100s. *Rx.*
Use: Decongestant; expectorant.

Tusso-C. (Everett) Codeine phosphate 10 mg, guaifenesin 200 mg per 5 mL. Acesulfame K, aspartame, menthol, phenylalanine 0.03 mcg. Cherry vanilla flavor. Syr. 473 mL. *c-v.*
Use: Upper respiratory combination, antitussive with expectorant.

Tusso-DM. (Everett) Dextromethorphan HBr 23 mg (8 mg immediate release/ 15 mg extended release), guaifenesin 600 mg (200 mg immediate release/ 400 mg extended release), phenylephrine hydrochloride 9 mg (extended release). Lactose. ER Tab. 100s. *Rx.*
Use: Upper respiratory combination, antitussive with expectorant.

Tusso DMR. (Everett Labs) Dextromethorphan hydrobromide 14 mg, guaifenesin 288 mg, phenylephrine hydrochloride 7 mg. Maltodextrin. Cap. 100s. *Rx.*
Use: Upper respiratory combination, antitussive and expectorant combination.

Tusso XR. (Everett) Dextromethorphan HBr 20 mg, guaifenesin 100 mg, phenylephrine hydrochloride 10 mg per 5 mL. Acesulfame K, aspartame, methylparaben, phenylalanine 25.26 mg/ 5 mL. Grape flavor. Susp. 473 mL. *Rx.*
Use: Upper respiratory combination, antitussive and expectorant combination.

Tusso-ZMR. (Everett) Carbetapentane citrate 8 mg, guaifenesin 200 mg. Maltodextrin, tartrazine. Cap. 100s. *Rx.*
Use: Upper respiratory combination, antitussive with expectorant.

Tusso-ZR. (Everett) Carbetapentane citrate 7.5 mg, guaifenesin 150 mg per 5 mL. Saccharin, sorbitol, sucralose. Grape flavor. Syrup. 473 mL. *Rx.*
Use: Upper respiratory combination, antitussive with expectorant.

Tussplex. (Breckenridge) Hydrocodone bitartrate 6 mg, pyrilamine maleate 12 mg, phenylephrine hydrochloride 5 mg per 5 mL. Alcohol and sugar free. Saccharin, sorbitol. Black cherry flavor. Syrup. 473 mL. *c-III.*

Use: Upper respiratory combination, antitussive combination.

Tusstat. (Century) Diphenhydramine hydrochloride 12.5 mg/5 mL, alcohol 5%. Syrup. Bot. 30 mL, 118 mL, 473 mL, 3.8 L. *Rx.*
Use: Antihistamine, nonselective ethanolamine; antitussive.

Tusstat Expectorant. (Century) Diphenhydramine hydrochloride 80 mg, ammonium chloride 12 g, sodium citrate 5 g, menthol 0.13 g, alcohol 5%/oz. Bot. 4 fl. oz, pt, gal. *Rx.*
Use: Antihistamine; expectorant.

Tustan 12S. (Amneal Pharmaceuticals) Carbetapentane tannate 30 mg, chlorpheniramine tannate 4 mg per 5 mL. Methylparaben, saccharin, sucrose. Grape flavor. Susp. 118 mL, 473 mL. *Rx.*
Use: Upper respiratory combination, antitussive combination.

•**tuvirumab.** (tuh-VIE-roo-mab) USAN.
Use: Monoclonal antibody (antiviral).

T-Vites. (Freeda) Vitamins B_1 25 mg, B_2 25 mg, B_3 150 mg, B_5 25 mg, B_6 25 mg, C 100 mg, biotin 30 mcg, PABA, K, Mg, Mn carbonate 2 mg, Zn gluconate 20 mg. Tab. Bot. 100s. *OTC.*
Use: Mineral, vitamin supplement.

tween 20, 40, 60, 80. *NF 29.* (AstraZeneca) Polysorbates.
Use: Surface active agents.

12-Hour Antihistamine Nasal Decongestant. (United Research Laboratories) Pseudoephedrine sulfate 120 mg, dexbrompheniramine maleate 6 mg, sugar, sucrose. SR Tab. Bot. 10s. *OTC.*
Use: Decongestant.

12-Hour Cold. (Ivax) Dexbrompheniramine maleate 6 mg, pseudoephedrine sulfate 120 mg. SR Tab. Pkg. 10s, 20s. *OTC.*
Use: Antihistamine; decongestant.

12-Hour Nasal. (Various Mfr.) Oxymetazoline hydrochloride 0.05%. Soln. Spray Bot. 15 mL. *OTC.*
Use: Nasal decongestant, imidazoline.

Twelve Resin-K. (Key Company) Vitamin B_{12} 1,000 mcg on resin. Tab. 60s, 250s, 1000s. *OTC.*
Use: Water-soluble vitamin.

20% ProSol. (Baxter Healthcare) Amino acids 20 g, total nitrogen 3.21 g/ 100 mL, lysine acetate, glacial acetic acid. Sulfite free. Inj. *Vialflex* Cont. 500 mL, 1000 mL, 2000 mL. *Rx.*
Use: Nutritional therapy, intravenous.

20-20. (BDI) Caffeine 200 mg. Tab. Bot. 100s, 500s. *OTC.*
Use: CNS stimulant, analeptic.

20/20 Eye Drops. (S.S.S. Company) Naphazoline hydrochloride 0.012%. Benzalkonium chloride, EDTA, glycerin 0.2%. Ophth. Drops. 15 mL. *OTC.*
Use: Ophthalmic decongestant.

Twice-a-Day 12-Hour Nasal. (Major) Oxymetazoline 0.05%, EDTA, benzalkonium chloride, benzyl alcohol. Soln. Spray bot. 15 mL, 30 mL. *OTC.*
Use: Nasal decongestant, imidazoline.

Twilite. (Pfeiffer) Diphenhydramine hydrochloride 50 mg. Tab. 20s. *OTC.*
Use: Sleep aid.

Twinject. (Sciele) Epinephrine 1:1,000 (0.15 mg per 0.15 mL), 1:1,000 (0.3 mg per 0.3 mL). Chlorobutanol, sodium bisulfite. Latex free. Dual-dose autoinjector (contains a total of epinephrine 2 mL). *Rx.*
Use: Vasopressor used in shock.

Twinrix. (GlaxoSmithKline) Inactivated hepatitis A 720 ELU (ELISA [enzyme-linked immunosorbent assay] units), recombinant HBsAg (hepatitis B surface antigen) protein 20 mcg/mL. Preservative free. Inj. Single-dose vials. Single-dose prefilled, disposable *TIP-LOK* syringes. *Rx.*
Use: Active immunization, viral vaccine.

TwoCal HN High Nitrogen Liquid Nutrition. (Ross) High-nitrogen liquid nutrition (2 calories/mL). 1900 calories (1 quart), provides 100% US RDA for vitamins and minerals for adults and children over 4 yrs. Can 8 fl. oz. *OTC.*
Use: Nutritional supplement.

2-Tone Disclosing Solution. (Young Dental) Dropper Bot. 2 oz.
Use: Disclosing solution.

Twynsta. (Boehringer Ingelheim) Amlodipine besylate/telmisartan. 5 mg/40 mg, 10 mg/40 mg, 5 mg/80 mg, 10 mg/ 80 mg. Sorbitol. Tab. Blisters. 30s, 90s. *Rx.*
Use: Antihypertensive.

•**tybamate.** (TIE-bam-ate) USAN.
Use: Anxiolytic.

Ty-Cold. (Major) 30 mg pseudoephedrine, 2 mg chlorpheniramine maleate, 15 mg dextromethorphan HBr, 325 mg acetaminophen. Tab. Pkg. 24s. *OTC.*
Use: Analgesic; antihistamine; antitussive; decongestant.

Tygacil. (Wyeth) Tigecycline 50 mg. Lactose. Preservative free. Pow. for Inj., lyophilized. Single-dose vial. 10 mL. *Rx.*
Use: Anti-infective, glycylcycline.

Tykerb. (GlaxoSmithKline) Lapatinib 250 mg. Film-coated. Tab. 150s. *Rx.*
Use: Tyrosine kinase inhibitor, antineoplastic.

Tylenol Allergy Multi-Symptom. (McNeil Consumer) Phenylephrine hydrochloride 5 mg, chlorpheniramine maleate 2 mg, acetaminophen 325 mg. 24s. **Capl.:** PEG, sucralose. **Gelcaps:** Benzyl alcohol, parabens. *OTC.*
Use: Upper respiratory combination, decongestant, antihistamine, analgesic.

Tylenol Allergy Multi-Symptom Convenience Pack. (McNeil Consumer) **Day:** Phenylephrine hydrochloride 5 mg, chlorpheniramine maleate 2 mg, acetaminophen 325 mg. Sucralose. Capl. 24s. **Night:** Phenylephrine hydrochloride 5 mg, diphenhydramine hydrochloride 25 mg, acetaminophen 325 mg. Sucralose. Capl. 24s. *OTC.*
Use: Upper respiratory combination, decongestant, antihistamine, analgesic.

Tylenol Allergy Multi-Symptom Nighttime. (McNeil Consumer) Phenylephrine hydrochloride 5 mg, diphenhydramine hydrochloride 25 mg, acetaminophen 325 mg. Sucralose. Capl. 24s. *OTC.*
Use: Upper respiratory combination, decongestant, antihistamine, analgesic.

Tylenol Arthritis Pain. (McNeil Consumer) Acetaminophen 650 mg.
ER Capl.: 24s, 50s, 100s, 150s, 225s. **ER Gelltabs:** Parabens. 20s, 40s, 80s. *OTC.*
Use: Analgesic.

Tylenol Chest Congestion. (McNeil Consumer) **Capl.:** Acetaminophen 325 mg, guaifenesin 200 mg. Mannitol, PEG, polyvinyl alcohol, sucralose. Cool burst flavor. 24s. **Liq.:** Acetaminophen 166.67 mg, guaifenesin 66.67 mg per 5 mL. PEG, sorbitol, sucralose, sucrose. Cool burst flavor. Bot. 240 mL. *OTC.*
Use: Upper respiratory combination, analgesic, expectorant.

Tylenol Children's. (McNeil Consumer) Acetaminophen. **Meltaways (Chew. Tab./Dispersible):** 80 mg. Dextrose, sucralose. Bubble gum, grape, and watermelon flavors. 30s. **Susp.:** 160 mg/ 5 mL. Sodium 2 mg/5 mL. Cherry, grape, bubblegum flavors (alcohol free, dye free, butylparaben, corn syrup, sorbitol); strawberry flavor (butylparaben, corn syrup, sorbitol, sucralose); cherry flavor (dye free, parabens, sorbitol, sucralose, sucrose). Bot. 60 mL, 120 mL. *OTC.*
Use: Analgesic.

Tylenol Cold Head Congestion Daytime. (McNeil Consumer) Dextromethorphan 10 mg, phenylephrine hydrochloride 5 mg, acetaminophen 325 mg. Sucralose. Cool burst flavor. Capl. 24s. *OTC.*
Use: Upper respiratory combination, antitussive combination.

Tylenol Cold Head Congestion Nighttime. (McNeil Consumer) Dextromethorphan 10 mg, chlorpheniramine 2 mg, phenylephrine hydrochloride 5 mg, acetaminophen 325 mg. Sucralose. Cool burst flavor. Capl. 24s. *OTC.*
Use: Upper respiratory combination, antitussive combination.

Tylenol Cold Multi-Symptom Daytime. (McNeil Consumer) **Capl.:** Dextromethorphan 10 mg, phenylephrine hydrochloride 5 mg, acetaminophen 325 mg. Sucralose. Cool burst flavor. 24s. **Gelcap:** Dextromethorphan 10 mg, phenylephrine hydrochloride 5 mg, acetaminophen 325 mg. Benzyl alcohol, EDTA, parabens. 24s. **Liq.:** Dextromethorphan 3.33 mg, phenylephrine hydrochloride 1.67 mg, acetaminophen 108.33 mg per 5 mL. Ethanol, sodium 1.67 mg per 5 mL, sorbitol, sucralose. Citrus burst flavor. Bot. 240 mL. *OTC.*
Use: Upper respiratory combination, antitussive combination.

Tylenol Cold Multi-Symptom Nighttime. (McNeil Consumer) **Capl.:** Dextromethorphan 10 mg, chlorpheniramine maleate 2 mg, phenylephrine hydrochloride 5 mg, acetaminophen 325 mg. Sucralose. Cool burst flavor. 24s. **Liq.:** Dextromethorphan 3.33 mg, doxylamine succinate 2.08 mg, phenylephrine hydrochloride 1.67 mg, acetaminophen 108.33 mg per 5 mL. Sodium, sorbitol, sucralose. Cool burst flavor. Bot. 240 mL. *OTC.*
Use: Upper respiratory combination, antitussive combination.

Tylenol Cold Severe Congestion Daytime. (McNeil Consumer) Dextromethorphan HBr 15 mg, guaifenesin 200 mg, pseudoephedrine hydrochloride 30 mg, acetaminophen 325 mg. Mannitol, sodium 3 mg, sucralose. Cool burst flavor. Capl. 100s. *OTC.*
Use: Upper respiratory combination, antitussive and expectorant combination.

Tylenol Cough & Sore Throat Daytime. (McNeil Consumer) Dextromethorphan HBr 5 mg, acetaminophen 166.7 mg per 5 mL. Sodium 3.7 mg per 5 mL, sorbitol, sucrose. Liq. Bot. 240 mL. *OTC.*
Use: Upper respiratory combination, antitussive combination.

Tylenol Cough & Sore Throat Nighttime. (McNeil Consumer) Dextromethorphan HBr 5 mg, doxylamine succinate 2.08 mg, acetaminophen 166.7 mg per 5 mL. Sodium 3.67 mg per 5 mL, sorbitol, sucralose. Cool burst flavor. Liq. Bot. 240 mL. *OTC.*
Use: Upper respiratory combination, antitussive combination.

Tylenol 8 Hour. (McNeil Consumber) Acetaminophen 650 mg. Polyvinyl alcohol, sucralose. ER Capl. 24s, 50s, 100s, 150s. *OTC.*
Use: Analgesic.

Tylenol Extra Strength. (McNeil Consumer) Acetaminophen. **Capl.:** 500 mg. Castor oil, sucralose. Regular and cool flavors. Bot. 50s, 100s. **Chew Tab. (GoTabs):** 500 mg. Acesulfame K, dextrose, sucralose. Spearmint ice flavors. 6s. **Liq.:** 166.6 mg/5 mL. Corn syrup, saccharin, sorbitol. 240 mL with dosage cup. **Rapid Release Tab.:** 500 mg. Benzyl alcohol, parabens. 24s, 50s, 100s, 225s. **Tab. (EZ Tab):** 500 mg. Sucralose. 50s, 100s, 225. *OTC.*
Use: Analgesic.

Tylenol Extra Strength GoTabs. (McNeil Consumer) Acetaminophen 500 mg. Acesulfame, potassium, sucralose. Spearmint ice flavor. Chew. Tab. 6s. *OTC.*
Use: Analgesic.

Tylenol, Infants'. (McNeil Consumer) Acetaminophen 100 mg/mL. Cherry and grape flavors (corn syrup, sorbitol), cherry flavor (dye free, parabens, sorbitol, sucralose). Soln. Conc. Oral. 15 mL, 30 mL with 0.8 mL dropper. *OTC.*
Use: Analgesic.

Tylenol Meltaways, Jr. (McNeil Consumer) Acetaminophen 160 mg. Dextrose, sucralose. Bubble gum and grape punch flavors. Chew. Tab./Dispersible. 24s. *OTC.*
Use: Analgesic.

Tylenol Plus Cold, Children's. (McNeil Consumer) Phenylephrine hydrochloride 2.5 mg, chlorpheniramine maleate 1 mg, acetaminophen 160 mg per 5 mL. Sorbitol, sucrose. Grape flavor. Susp. Bot. 118 mL. *OTC.*
Use: Upper respiratory combination, decongestant, antihistamine, analgesic.

Tylenol Plus Cough & Runny Nose, Children's. (McNeil Consumer) Dextromethorphan HBr 5 mg, chlorpheniramine maleate 1 mg, acetaminophen 160 mg per 5 mL. Acesulfame K, corn syrup, sorbitol. Cherry flavor. Susp.

Bot. 120 mL. *OTC.*
Use: Upper respiratory combination, antitussive combination.

Tylenol Plus Cough & Sore Throat, Children's. (McNeil Consumer) Dextromethorphan HBr 5 mg, acetaminophen 160 mg per 5 mL. Acesulfame K, corn syrup, sorbitol. Cherry flavor. Susp. Bot. 120 mL. *OTC.*
Use: Upper respiratory combination, antitussive combination.

Tylenol Plus Flu, Children's. (McNeil Consumer) Dextromethorphan HBr 5 mg, chlorpheniramine maleate 1 mg, phenylephrine hydrochloride 2.5 mg, acetaminophen 160 mg per 5 mL. Sorbitol, sucrose. Bubble gum flavor. Susp. Bot. 120 mL. *OTC.*
Use: Upper respiratory combination, antitussive combination.

Tylenol Plus Multi-Symptom Cold, Children's. (McNeil Consumer) Dextromethorphan HBr 5 mg, chlorpheniramine maleate 1 mg, phenylephrine hydrochloride 2.5 mg, acetaminophen 160 mg per 5 mL. Sorbitol, sucrose. Grape flavor. Susp. Bot. 120 mL. *OTC.*
Use: Upper respiratory combination, antitussive combination.

Tylenol PM. (McNeil Consumer) Acetaminophen 500 mg, diphenhydramine 25 mg. Tab. Bot. 24s, 50s, 100s, 150s. Gelcap. Parabens. Bot. 50s. Geltab. Parabens. Bot. 50s, 100s. *OTC.*
Use: Upper respiratory combination, analgesic, antihistamine.

Tylenol Regular Strength. (McNeil Consumer) Acetaminophen 325 mg. Tab. 100s. *OTC.*
Use: Analgesic.

Tylenol Severe Allergy. (McNeil Consumer) Diphenhydramine hydrochloride 12.5 mg, acetaminophen 500 mg. Tab. 24s. *OTC.*
Use: Upper respiratory combination, analgesic, antihistamine.

Tylenol Sinus Congestion & Pain Nighttime. (McNeil Consumer) Phenylephrine 5 mg, chlorpheniramine maleate 2 mg, acetaminophen 325 mg. Sucralose. Cool burst flavor. Tab. 24s. *OTC.*
Use: Upper respiratory combination, decongestant, antihistamine, and analgesic combination.

Tylenol Sinus Congestion & Pain Severe Daytime. (McNeil Consumer) Phenylephrine hydrochloride 5 mg, guaifenesin 200 mg, acetaminophen 325 mg. Sucralose. Cool burst flavor. Tab. 24s. *OTC.*

Use: Upper respiratory combination, decongestant and expectorant combination.

Tylenol Sinus Severe Congestion. (McNeil Consumer) Pseudoephedrine hydrochloride 30 mg, guaifenesin 200 mg, acetaminophen 325 mg. Mannitol, sucralose. Cool burst flavor. Tab. 24s. *OTC.*
Use: Upper respiratory combination, decongestant, expectorant, analgesic.

Tylenol Sore Throat Daytime. (McNeil Consumer) Acetaminophen 166.6 mg/ 5 mL. Sucralose, sucrose, sorbitol. Cool burst flavor. Liq. Bot. 240 mL. *OTC.*
Use: Analgesic.

Tylenol Sore Throat Nighttime. (McNeil Consumer) Diphenhydramine hydrochloride 8.3 mg, acetaminophen 166.6 mg per 5 mL. Sodium 3.6 mg per 5 mL, sorbitol, sucralose, sucrose. Cool burst flavor. Liq. 240 mL. *OTC.*
Use: Upper respiratory combination, antihistamine, analgesic.

Tylenol with Codeine. (Ortho-McNeil) **Tab.:** Acetaminophen 300 mg with codeine phosphate. **No. 2:** Codeine phosphate 15 mg. Bot. 100s, 500s. **No. 3:** Codeine phosphate 30 mg. Bot. 100s, 500s, 1000s, UD 100s. **No. 4:** Codeine phosphate 60 mg. Bot. 100s, 500s, UD 500s. *c-III.*
Use: Analgesic combination; narcotic.

Tylenol with Codeine. (Ortho-McNeil) Acetaminophen 120 mg, codeine phosphate 12 mg/5 mL w/alcohol 7%. Elix. Bot. 480 mL. *c-v.*
Use: Analgesic combination; narcotic.

Tylenol with Flavor Creator Children's. (McNeil Consumer Health) Acetaminophen 160 mg/5 mL. Sugar free. Butylparaben, corn syrup, sorbitol, sucralose. Apple, bubble gum, chocolate, and strawberry flavors. Oral Susp. 120 mL. *OTC.*
Use: Analgesic.

Tylosterone. (Eli Lilly) Diethylstilbestrol 0.25 mg, methyltestosterone 5 mg. Tab. Bot. 100s. *Rx.*
Use: Androgen, estrogen combination.

Tylox. (Ortho-McNeil) Oxycodone hydrochloride 5 mg, acetaminophen 500 mg. Cap. Bot. 100s, UD 100s. *c-II.*
Use: Analgesic combination; narcotic.

•**tyloxapol.** (till-OX-ah-pahl) *USP 34.*
Use: Detergent, ophthalmic; cystic fibrosis. [Orphan Drug]
See: Enuclene.

Typhim Vi. (Aventis Pasteur) Typhoid purified Vi polysaccharide vaccine 25 mcg/ 0.5 mL, sodium chloride 4.15 mg, di-

sodium phosphate 0.065 mg, monosodium phosphate 0.023 mg, Sterile Water for Injection 0.5 mL. Inj. Syringes 0.5 mL, vial 20 dose, 50 dose. *Rx.*
Use: Immunization, typhoid.

typhoid vaccine.
Use: Immunization.
See: Vivotif Berna.

typhoid Vi polysaccharide vaccine.
Use: Immunization.
See: Typhim Vi.

Tyrex-2. (Ross) Protein 30 g, fat 15.5 g, carbohydrates 30 g, Na 880 mg, K 1370 mg, Cal 410/100 g. With appropriate vitamins and minerals. Phenylalanine and tyrosine free. Pow. Can 325 g. *OTC.*
Use: Nutritional supplement.

Tyrodone. (Major) Hydrocodone bitartrate 5 mg, pseudoephedrine hydrochloride 60 mg/5 mL, alcohol 5%. Liq. Bot. 473 mL. *c-III.*
Use: Antitussive; decongestant.

Tyromex-1. (Ross) Protein 15 g, fat 23.9 g, carbohydrates 46.3 g, linoleic acid 1800 mg, Fe 9 mg, Na 190 mg, K 675 mg, Cal 480/100 g. With appropriate vitamins and minerals. Phenylalanine, tyrosine, and methionine free. Pow. Can 350 g. *OTC.*
Use: Nutritional supplement.

•**tyropanoate sodium.** (TIE-row-PAN-oh-ate) *USP 34.*
Use: Diagnostic aid (radiopaque medium, cholecystographic).

tyropaque caps. (Sanofi-Synthelabo) Tyropanoate sodium. *Rx.*
Use: Oral cholecystographic medium.

•**tyrosine.** (TIE-row-SEEN) *USP 34.* L-Tyrosine.
Use: Amino acid.

tyrosine hydroxylase inhibitor.
Use: Antihypertensive.
See: Demser.

tyrosine kinase inhibitors.
Use: Antineoplastic.
See: Lapatinib.
  Pazopanib.
  Vandetanib.

Tyrosum Skin Cleanser. (Summers) Isopropanol 50%, polysorbate 80 2%, and acetone 10%. Bot. 120 mL, pt. Towelettes 24s, 50s. *OTC.*
Use: Dermatologic, cleanser.

Tysabri. (Elan) Natalizumab 20 mg/mL. Preservative free. Inj., Soln., Conc. Single-use vials. *Rx.*
Note: Only available through a special restricted distribution program (the TOUCH prescribing program).
Use: Immunologic agent, immunomodulator.

Tyvaso. (United Therapeutics) Treprostinil 0.6 mg/mL. Soln.; Inhal. Ampule. 2.9 mL. *Rx.*
Use: Vasodilator, peripheral vasodilator.

Tyzeka. (Novartis) Telbivudine. **Tab.:** 600 mg. Film-coated. 30s. **Soln.:** 100 mg per 5 mL. Saccharin, sodium 47 mg per 30 mL. Passion fruit flavor. Bot. 300 mL. *Rx.*
Use: Antiretroviral, nucleoside reverse transcriptase inhibitor.

Tyzine. (Kenwood) Tetrahydrozoline hydrochloride 0.1%, benzalkonium chloride, EDTA. Soln. Bot. 30 mL with dropper. Spray bot. 15 mL. *Rx.*
Use: Nasal decongestant, imidazoline.

Tyzine Pediatric. (Kenwood) Tetrahydrozoline hydrochloride 0.05%, benzalkonium chloride, EDTA. Soln. Dropper bot. 15 mL. *Rx.*
Use: Nasal decongestant, imidazoline.

U

UAA. (Econo Med Pharmaceuticals) Methenamine 40.8 mg, phenyl salicylate 18.1 mg, methylene blue 5.4 mg, benzoic acid 4.5 mg, atropine sulfate 0.03 mg, hyoscyamine 0.03 mg. Tab. Bot. 100s, 1000s. *Rx.*
Use: Anti-infective, urinary.

UAD Cream. (Forest) Clioquinol 3%, hydrocortisone 1%, ceresin, glyceryl oleate, propylene glycol, parabens, mineral oil, pramoxine hydrochloride. Cream. Tube. 15 g. *Rx.*
Use: Corticosteroid; anesthetic, local.

UAD Lotion. (Forest) Clioquinol 0.75%, hydrocortisone 0.25%, cetyl alcohol, glyceryl stearate, lanolin, parabens, mineral oil, pramoxine hydrochloride, propylene glycol. Lot. Bot. 20 mL. *Rx.*
Use: Corticosteroid; anesthetic, local.

•**ubidecarenone.** *NF 29.*
Use: Dietary supplement.

UBT. (Biomerica) For detection of blood in the urine.
Use: Diagnostic aid.

UCG-Beta Slide Monoclonal II. (Wampole) Two-minute latex agglutination inhibition slide test for the qualitative detection of B-hCG/hCG (sensitivity 0.5 units hCG/mL) in urine. Kit 50s, 100s, 300s.
Use: Diagnostic aid.

UCG-Beta Stat. (Wampole) One-hour passive hemagglutination inhibition tube test for the qualitative detection and quantitative determination of B-hCG/hCG (sensitivity 0.2 units hCG/mL) in urine. Kit 50s, 300s.
Use: Diagnostic aid.

UCG-Lyphotest. (Wampole) One-hour passive hemagglutination inhibition tube test for the qualitative or quantitative determination of human chorionic gonadotropin (sensitivity 0.5-1 units hCG/mL) in urine. Kit 10s, 50s, 300s.
Use: Diagnostic aid.

UCG-Slide Test. (Wampole) Rapid latex agglutination inhibition slide test for the qualitative detection of human chorionic gonadotropin (Sensitivity: 2 units hCG/mL) in urine. Kit 30s, 100s, 300s, 1000s.
Use: Diagnostic aid.

UCG-Test. (Wampole) Two-hour hemagglutination inhibition tube test for the determination of human chorionic gonadotropin (sensitivity 0.5 units hCG/mL undiluted specimen; 1.5 units hCG/mL 1:3 diluted specimen) in urine and serum. Kit 10s, 25s, 100s, 300s.
Use: Diagnostic aid.

UCG-Titration Set. (Wampole) Two-hour hemagglutination inhibition tube test for the determination of human chorionic gonadotropin (sensitivity 1 units hCG/mL) in urine or serum. Kit 45s.
Use: Diagnostic aid.

U-cort. (Taro) Hydrocortisone acetate 1%. Urea 10%, alcohol, EDTA. Cream. 28.35 g, 7 g. *Rx.*
Use: Anti-inflammatory.

Udamin. (Kowa Pharm) Vitamins B_{12} 500 mcg, B_6 25 mg, E 150 units (as d-alpha tocopheryl acid succinate) and 34 mg (as d-gamma, d-delta, d-beta tocopheryls), Se, Zn, folic acid 2,000 mcg. Lycopene complex 5 mg. Coconut oil, maltodextrin, polydextrose, PEG, soy protein. Film coated. Tab. 100s. *Rx.*
Use: Multivitamin with minerals (except iron).

Udamin SP. (Kowa Pharm) Vitamins B_{12} 250 mcg, B_6 12.5 mg, E 75 units (as d-alpha tocopheryl acid succinate) and 17 mg (as d-gamma, d-delta, d-beta tocopheryls), Se, Zn, folic acid 1,000 mcg. Lycopene complex 2.5 mcg, saw palmetto extract 320 mg. Maltodextrin, polydextrose, PEG, soy protein. Film coated. Tab. 100s. *Rx.*
Use: Multivitamin with minerals (except iron).

Udderly Smooth. (Redex) Dimethicone, isopropyl myristate, lanolin oil, mineral oil, parabens, PEG-2, urea. Cream 227 g. *OTC.*
Use: Emollient.

•**udenafil.** (ue-DEN-a-fil) USAN.
Use: Erectile dysfunction.

Uendex. Dextran sulfate, inhaled, aerosolized.
Use: Cystic fibrosis treatment. [Orphan Drug]

Ulcerease. (Med-Derm) Liquified phenol 0.6%, glycerin, sugar free. Liq. Bot. 180 mL. *OTC.*
Use: Anesthetic, local.

Ulcerin. (Sanofi-Synthelabo) Aluminum hydroxide. Tab. *OTC.*
Use: Antacid.

Ulcerin P. (Sanofi-Synthelabo) Aluminum hydroxide. Tab. *OTC.*
Use: Antacid.

•**uldazepam.** (ul-DAZ-e-pam) USAN.
Use: Hypnotic; sedative.

•**ulimorelin.** (UE-li-moe-REL-in) USAN.
Use: Gastrointestinal agent.

•**ulimorelin hydrochloride.** (UE-li-moe-REL-in) USAN.
Use: Gastrointestinal agent.

•**ulipristal.** (UE-li-PRIS-tal) USAN.
Use: Contraceptive agent.
•**ulipristal acetate.** (UE-li-PRIS-tal)
USAN.
Use: Contraceptive agent.
Uloric. (Takeda Pharmaceuticals
America) Febuxostat 40 mg, 80 mg.
Lactose. Tab. 30s, 90s (40 mg), 100s
(80 mg), 500s (40 mg), 1000s (80 mg),
UD 100s. *Rx.*
Use: Agent for gout, xanthine oxidase
inhibitor.
Ulpax. (Roche) Ablukast sodium.
Use: Antiasthmatic (leukotriene antago-
nist).
Ultane. (Abbott) Sevoflurane. Bot.
250 mL. *Rx.*
Use: Anesthetic, general, volatile liquid.
Ultiva. (Bionich Pharma Group) Remifen-
tanil hydrochloride (as base) 1 mg
(3 mL vials), 2 mg (5 mL vials), 5 mg
(10 mL vials), preservative free. Glycine
15 mg. Pow. for Inj. *c-II.*
Use: Opioid analgesic.
**UltraBag Dianeal PD-2 w/4.25% Dex-
trose.** (Baxter) Dextrose 4.25 g/L, Na^+
132 mEq/L, Ca^{++} 3.5 mEq/L, Mg^{++}
0.5 mEq/L, Cl^- 96 mEq/L, lactate
40 mEq/L, osmolarity 485 mOsm/L.
Preservative free. Inj., Soln. *UltraBag*
container. 1,500 mL, 2,000 mL,
2,500 mL, 3,000 mL. *Rx.*
Use: Electrolyte, peritoneal dialysis solution.
**UltraBag Dianeal PD-2 w/1.5% Dex-
trose.** (Baxter) Dextrose 1.5 g/L, Na^+
132 mEq/L, Ca^{++} 3.5 mEq/L, Mg^{++}
0.5 mEq/L, Cl^- 96 mEq/L, lactate
40 mEq/L, osmolarity 346 mOsm/L.
Preservative free. Inj., Soln. *UltraBag*
container. 1,500 mL, 2,000 mL,
2,500 mL, 3,000 mL. *Rx.*
Use: Electrolyte, peritoneal dialysis solution.
**UltraBag Dianeal PD-2 w/2.5% Dex-
trose.** (Baxter) Dextrose 2.5 g/L, Na^+
132 mEq/L, Ca^{++} 3.5 mEq/L, Mg^{++}
0.5 mEq/L, Cl^- 96 mEq/L, lactate
40 mEq/L, osmolarity 396 mOsm/L.
Preservative free. Inj., Soln. *UltraBag*
container. 1,500 mL, 2,000 mL,
2,500 mL, 3,000 mL. *Rx.*
Use: Electrolyte, peritoneal dialysis solution.
Ultrabex. (Health for Life Brands) Vitamins B_1 20 mg, C 50 mg, B_2 2 mg, B_6
0.5 mg, niacinamide 35 mg, calcium
pantothenate 0.5 mg, wheat germ oil
30 mg, B_{12} 20 mcg, liver desiccated
150 mg, iron 11.58 mg, calcium 29 mg,
phosphorus 23 mg, dicalcium phos-

phate 100 mg, magnesium 1.11 mg,
manganese 1.3 mg, potassium
2.24 mg, zinc 0.68 mg, choline 25 mg,
inositol 25 mg, pepsin 32.5 mg, diastase 32.5 mg, hesperidin 25 mg, biotin
20 mcg, hydrolyzed yeast 81.25 mg,
protein digest 47.04 mg, amino acids
34.21 mg. Cap. Bot. 50s, 100s, 1000s.
OTC.
Use: Mineral, vitamin supplement.
Ultra B-50. (NBTY) Vitamins B_1 50 mg,
B_2 50 mg, B_3 50 mg, B_5 50 mg, B_6
50 mg, B_{12} 50 mcg, folic acid 0.1 mg,
PABA 50 mg, inositol 50 mg, biotin
50 mcg, choline 50 mg, lecithin 50 mg.
Tab. Bot. 60s, 180s. *OTC.*
Use: Vitamin supplement.
Ultra B-100. (NBTY) Vitamins B_1 100 mg,
B_2 100 mg, B_3 100 mg, B_5 100 mg, B_6
100 mg, B_{12} 100 mcg, folic acid
0.1 mg, PABA 100 mg, inositol 100 mg,
biotin 100 mcg, choline bitartrate
100 mg. TR Tab. Bot. 50s. *OTC.*
Use: Vitamin supplement.
ULTRAbrom. (WE Pharmaceuticals)
Brompheniramine maleate 12 mg,
pseudoephedrine hydrochloride
120 mg. ER Cap. Bot. 100s, dispenser
pack 10s. *Rx.*
Use: Upper respiratory combination, antihistamine, decongestant.
ULTRAbrom PD. (WE Pharmaceuticals)
Brompheniramine maleate 6 mg,
pseudoephedrine 60 mg. ER Cap. Bot.
100s. *Rx.*
Use: Upper respiratory combination, antihistamine, decongestant.
Ultracal. (Bristol-Myers Squibb) Protein
44 g, carbohydrate 123 g, fat 45 g, Na
930 mg, K 1610 mg, mOsm 310 kg
H_2O, 1.06 cal/mL, vitamins A, B_1, B_2,
B_3, B_5, B_6, B_{12}, C, D, E, K, folic acid,
choline, biotin, Ca, P, I, Fe, Mg, Cu,
Zn, Mn, Cl, Se, Cr, Mo. Liq. Can. 8 oz.
OTC.
Use: Nutritional supplement.
Ultra Cap. (Weeks & Leo) Acetaminophen 300 mg, guaifenesin 100 mg,
chlorpheniramine maleate 4 mg,
phenylephrine hydrochloride 10 mg,
dextromethorphan HBr 6 mg. Cap. Vial
18s. *Rx.*
Use: Analgesic; antihistamine; antitussive; decongestant; expectorant.
Ultra-Care. (Allergan) **Disinfecting
Soln.:** Hydrogen peroxide 3%, sodium
stannate, sodium nitrate, phosphate
buffer. Bot. 120 mL, 360 mL. **Neutralizer Tab.:** Catalase, hydroxypropyl
methylcellulose, buffering agents. Pkg.

12s, 36s w/cup. *OTC.*
Use: Contact lens disinfection system.

Ultracet. (Ortho-McNeil) Tramadol hydrochloride 37.5 mg, acetaminophen 325 mg. Film-coated. Tab. Bot. 20s, 100s, 500s, UD 100s. *Rx.*
Use: Nonnarcotic analgesic combination.

Ultracortinol. (Novartis) Agent to suppress overactive adrenal glands. Pending release.

Ultra Freeda. (Freeda) Vitamins A 4166 units, D 133 units, E 66.7 mg, B_1 16.7 mg, B_2 16.7 mg, B_3 33 mg, B_5 33 mg, B_6 16.7 mg, B_{12} 33 mcg, C 333 mg, folic acid 0.27 mg, iron 2 mg, calcium 27 mg, zinc 1.1 mg, choline, inositol, bioflavonoids, PABA, biotin 100 mcg, Cr, I, K, Mg, Mn, Mo, Se. Tab. Bot. 90s, 180s, 270s. *OTC.*
Use: Mineral, vitamin supplement.

Ultra Freeda Iron Free. (Freeda) Vitamins A 4166 units, D 133 units, E_2 66.7 mg, B_1 16.7 mg, B_2 16.7 mg, B_3 33 mg, B_5 33 mg, B_6 16.7 mg, B_{12} 33 mcg, C 333 mg, FA 0.27 mg, Ca 27 mg, Zn 1.1 mg, choline, inositol, bioflavonoids, PABA, biotin 100 mcg, Cr, I, K, Mg, Mn, Mo, Se. Tab. Bot. 90s, 180s, 270s. *OTC.*
Use: Mineral, vitamin supplement.

Ultragesic. (Stewart-Jackson Pharmacal) Acetaminophen 500 mg, hydrocodone bitartrate 5 mg. Cap. Bot. 100s. *c-III.*
Use: Analgesic combination; narcotic.

Ultralan. (Elan) Protein 60 g, fat 50 g, carbohydrates 202 g, Na 1.035 g, K 1.755 g/L. Lactose free. With appropriate vitamins and minerals. Liq. In 1000 mL *New Pak* systems w/ and w/o *ColorCheck. OTC.*
Use: Nutritional supplement.

ultralente insulin.
See: Iletin.

Ultram. (Janssen) Tramadol hydrochloride 50 mg. Lactose, PEG. Film-coated. Tab. Bot. 100s. *Rx.*
Use: Opioid analgesic.

Ultram ER. (Pricara) Tramadol hydrochloride 100 mg, 200 mg, 300 mg. Polyvinyl alcohol. ER Tab. 30s. *Rx.*
Use: Opioid analgesic.

Ultra Mide 25. (Ivax) Bot. 8 oz. *OTC.*
Use: Emollient.

Ultra-Natal. (Ethex) Iron (carbonyl iron) 90 mg, iodine (potassium iodide) 150 mcg, calcium citrate 200 mg, cupric oxide 2 mg, zinc oxide 25 mg, folic acid 1 mg, vitamins A 2700 units, D_3 400 units, E 30 units, C 120 mg, B_1

3 mg, B_2 3.4 mg, B_6 20 mg, B_{12} 12 mcg, niacinamide 20 mg, docusate sodium. Dye free. Tab. UD 100s. *Rx.*
Use: Vitamin, mineral supplement.

Ultra-NatalCare. (Ethex) Ca 200 mg, Fe (as carbonyl iron) 90 mg, vitamin A 2700 units, D_3 400 units, E (dl-alphatocopheryl acetate) 30 units, B_1 3 mg, B_2 3.4 mg, B_3 20 mg, B_6 20 mg, B_{12} 12 mcg, C 120 mg, folic acid 1 mg, Zn 25 mg, Cu, I, docusate sodium 50 mg. Tab. UD 100s. *Rx.*
Use: Vitamin, mineral supplement.

Ultrapred. (Horizon) Prednisolone acetate 1%. Susp. Bot. 5 mL. *Rx.*
Use: Corticosteroid, ophthalmic.

Ultrasone. (Gordon Laboratories) Ultrasound aid. Bot. Qt, gal. Plastic Bot. 8 oz.
Use: Ultrasound contact cream.

Ultra Strength D2000. (Mason Natural) Vitamin D_3 (cholecalciferol) 2000 units. Cap. 60s. *OTC.*
Use: Vitamin, fat-soluble vitamin.

Ultra Strength Vitamin D3. (Nature's Blend) Cholecalciferol 5,000 units per mL. Soybean oil, vitamin E. Gluten free. Drops. 52.5 mL. *OTC.*
Use: Fat-soluble vitamin.

Ultravate. (Ranbaxy) Halobetasol propionate. *Rx.*
Use: Corticosteroid, topical.

Ultravate PAC. (Ranbaxy) Halobetasol propionate 0.05%. Beeswax, petrolatum, propylene glycol. Cream. 50 g w/ 225 g of ammonium lactate 12% lotion. *Rx.*
Use: Anti-inflammatory agent, topical corticosteroid.

Ultravist 150. (Baxter) Iopromide 311.7 mg, iodine 150 mg/mL. EDTA. Inj. Vials. 50 mL. *Rx.*
Use: Radiopaque, parenteral.

Ultravist 300. (Baxter) Iopromide 623.4 mg, iodine 300 mg/mL. EDTA. Inj. Vials. 50 mL, 100 mL, 150 mL. *Rx.*
Use: Radiopaque, parenteral.

Ultravist 370. (Baxter) Iopromide 768.86 mg, iodine 370 mg/mL. EDTA. Inj. Vials. 50 mL, 100 mL, 150 mL. 200 mL fill in 250 mL vial. *Rx.*
Use: Radiopaque, parenteral.

Ultravist 240. (Baxter) Iopromide 498.72 mg, iodine 240 mg/mL. EDTA. Inj. Vials. 50 mL, 100 mL fill in 250 mL vial. *Rx.*
Use: Radiopaque, parenteral.

Ultra Vitamin A & D. (NBTY) Vitamins A 25,000 units, D 1000 units. Tab. Bot. 100s. *OTC.*
Use: Vitamin supplement.

Ultra Vita Time. (NBTY) Iron 6 mg, vitamins A 10,000 units, D 400 units, E 13 units, B_1 25 mg, B_2 25 mg, B_3 50 mg, B_5 12.5 mg, B_6 15 mg, B_{12} 50 mcg, C 150 mg, folic acid 0.4 mg, B, Ca, Cr, Cu, I, K, Mg, Mn, Mo, P, Se, Zn 5 mg, biotin 1 mg, bioflavonoids, bone meal, PABA, choline bitartrate, betaine, inositol, lecithin, desiccated liver, rutin. Tab. Bot. 100s. *OTC.*
Use: Mineral, vitamin supplement.

Ultrazyme Enzymatic Cleaner. (Allergan) Subtilisin A, effervescing, buffering, and tableting agents for dilution in hydrogen peroxide 3%. Tab. Pkg. 5s, 10s, 15s, 20s. *OTC.*
Use: Contact lens care.

Ultrum. (Towne) Vitamins A 5000 units, E 30 units, C 90 mg, folic acid 400 mcg, B_1 2.25 mg, B_2 2.6 mg, niacinamide 20 mg, B_6 3 mg, B_{12} 9 mcg, biotin 45 mcg, D 400 units, pantothenic acid 10 mg, calcium 162 mg, phosphorus 125 mg, iodine 150 mcg, iron 27 mg, magnesium 100 mg, copper 3 mg, manganese 7.5 mg, potassium 7.5 mg, zinc 22.5 mg. Tab. Bot. 100s. *OTC.*
Use: Mineral, vitamin supplement.

Ultrum with Selenium. (Towne) Vitamins A 5000 units, E 30 units, C 90 mg, folic acid 2.25 mg, B_1 2.25 mg, B_2 2.6 mg, niacinamide 20 mg, B_6 3 mg, B_{12} 9 mcg, D 400 units, biotin 45 mcg, pantothenic acid 10 mg, calcium 162 mg, phosphorus 125 mg, iodine 150 mcg, iron 27 mg, magnesium 100 mg, copper 3 mg, manganese 7.5 mg, potassium 7.7 mg, chloride 7 mg, molybdenum 15 mcg, selenium 15 mcg, zinc 22.5 mg. Tab. Bot. 130s. *Rx.*
Use: Mineral, vitamin supplement.

Umecta. (JSJ) Urea. **Emulsion:** 40%. Helianthus annuus oil, EDTA. 113.5 g. **Nail Film:** 40%. EDTA, PEG-6 caprylic/capric glycerides. 18 mL with applicator. **Top. Aerosol:** 40%. Glycine, shea butter oil, sunflower oil. 114 g. **Top. Susp.:** 40%. Helianthus annuus oil, EDTA. 283.4 g. *Rx.*
Use: Emollient.

Umecta 40%. (JSJ) Urea 40%. EDTA, glycerin, PEG-6. Susp. 18 mL with applicator. *Rx.*
Use: Emollient.

Umecta PD. (JSJ) **Emulsion:** Urea 40%. EDTA, shea butter oil, sunflower oil. 142 g, 200 g. **Susp.:** Urea 40%. EDTA, shea butter oil, sunflower oil. 257 g. *Rx.*
Use: Emollient.

•**umirolimus.** (UE-mir-OH-li-mus) USAN.
Use: Prevention of restenosis.

UN-Aspirin, Extra Strength. (Zee Medical) Acetaminophen 500 mg. Castor oil. Tab. 250s. *OTC.*
Use: Analgesic.

Unasyn. (Roerig) Ampicillin sodium 1 g/ sulbactam sodium 0.5 g, ampicillin sodium 2 g/sulbactam sodium 1 g, ampicillin sodium 10 g/sulbactam sodium 5 g. Inj., Pow. for Soln. Vial, bottles. *ADD-Vantage* vials (except 10 g/5 g). Bulk pkg. (10 g/5 g only). *Rx.*
Use: Penicillin, aminopenicillin.

•**undecanoate.** (un-DEK-a-NOE-ate) USAN.
Use: Antifungal.

10-undecenoic acid. Undecylenic acid.
Use: Antifungal, topical.

10-undecenoic acid, zinc (2+) salt. Zinc undecylenate.
Use: Antifungal, topical.

undecoylium chloride-iodine. (Ruson) Virac, preps.
Use: Anti-infective, topical.

•**undecylenic acid.** (un-deh-sill-EN-ik) *USP 34.*
Use: Antifungal, topical.
See: Desenex.
  DiabetiDerm.
  Elon Dual Defense Antifungal Formula.
  Fungi Cure Maximum Strength.
  Gordochom.
W/Zinc Undecylenate.
See: Desenex.

undecylenic acid salts. Calcium, copper, zinc.

Undelenic Ointment. (Gordon Laboratories) Undecylenic acid 5%, zinc undecylenate 20%. Jar oz, lb. *OTC.*
Use: Antifungal, topical.

Undelenic Tincture. (Gordon Laboratories) Undecylenic acid 10%, chloroxylenol 0.5%. Brush Bot. oz. Bot. pt. *OTC.*
Use: Antifungal, topical.

Unguentine. (Lee) Phenol 1% in ointment base. Tube oz. *OTC.*
Use: Dermatologic; counterirritant.

Unguentine Maximum Strength. (Lee) Benzocaine 5%, resorcinol 2%. Alcohols, methylparaben, mineral oil. Cream. 28.3 g. *OTC.*
Use: Local anesthetic, topical.

Unibase. (Gallipot) Proprietary blend of emulsifiers and preservative cream; conc. 500g. *Rx.*
Use: Ointment and Lotion base.

Unicap. (Pfizer) **Cap.:** Vitamins A 5000 units, D 400 units, E 30 units, B_1 1.5 mg, B_2 1.7 mg, B_3 20 mg, B_6 2 mg,

B$_{12}$ 6 mcg, C 60 mg, FA 0.4 mg. Bot. 120s. **Tab.:** Vitamins A 5000 units, D 400 units, E 15 units, B$_1$ 1.5 mg, B$_2$ 1.7 mg, B$_3$ 20 mg, B$_6$ 2 mg, B$_{12}$ 6 mcg, C 60 mg, FA 0.4 mg. Tab. Bot. 120s. OTC.
Use: Vitamin supplement.
Unicap Jr. Chewable. (Pfizer) Vitamins A 5000 units, D 400 units, E 15 units, C 60 mg, folic acid 400 mcg, B$_1$ 1.5 mg, B$_2$ 1.7 mg, B$_3$ 20 mg, B$_6$ 2 mg, B$_{12}$ 6 mcg. Tab. Bot. 120s. OTC.
Use: Vitamin supplement.
Unicap M. (Pfizer) Iron 18 mg, vitamins A 5000 units, D 400 units, B$_1$ 1.5 mg, B$_2$ 1.7 mg, B$_3$ 20 mg, B$_5$ 10 mg, B$_6$ 2 mg, B$_{12}$ 6 mcg, C 60 mg, folic acid 0.4 mg, Ca, Cu, I, K, Mn, P, Zn 15 mg, tartrazine. Tab. Bot. 120s. OTC.
Use: Mineral, vitamin supplement.
Unicap Plus Iron. (Pfizer) Vitamins A 5000 units, D 400 units, E 30 units, C 60 mg, folic acid 0.4 mg, B$_1$ 1.5 mg, B$_2$ 1.7 mg, B$_3$ 20 mg, B$_5$ 10 mg, B$_6$ 2 mg, B$_{12}$ 6 mcg, iron 22.5 mg, Ca. Tab. Bot. 120s. OTC.
Use: Mineral, vitamin supplement.
Unicap Sr. (Pfizer) Iron 10 mg, vitamins A 5000 units, D 200 units, E 15 units, B$_1$ 1.2 mg, B$_2$ 1.4 mg, B$_3$16 mg, B$_5$ 10 mg, B$_6$ 2.2 mg, B$_{12}$ 3 mcg, C 60 mg, folic acid 0.4 mg, Ca, Cu, I, K, Mg, Mn, P, Zn 15 mg. Tab. Bot. 120s. OTC.
Use: Mineral, vitamin supplement.
Unicap T. (Pfizer) Iron 18 mg, vitamins A 5000 units, D 400 units, E 30 units, B$_1$ 10 mg, B$_2$ 20 mg, B$_3$ 100 mg, B$_5$ 25 mg, B$_6$ 6 mg, B$_{12}$ 18 mcg, C 500 mg, folic acid 0.4 mg, Cu, I, K, Mn, Se, Zn 15 mg, tartrazine. Tab. Bot. 60s. OTC.
Use: Mineral, vitamin supplement.
Unicomplex-M. (Rugby) Vitamins A 5,000 units, D 400 units, E 30 units, B$_1$ 1.5 mg, B$_2$ 1.7 mg, B$_3$ 20 mg, B$_5$ 10 mg, B$_6$ 2 mg, B$_{12}$ 6 mcg, C 60 mg, folic acid 0.4 mg, Ca 60 mg, Cu, Fe, I, K, Mn, P, Zn. Maltodextrin, tartrazine. Tab. 90s. OTC.
Use: Mineral, vitamin supplement.
Unicomplex-T & M. (Rugby) Iron 18 mg, vitamins A 5000 units, D 400 units, E 30 mg, B$_1$ 10 mg, B$_2$ 10 mg, B$_3$ 100 mg, B$_5$ 25 mg, B$_6$ 6 mg, B$_{12}$ 18 mcg, C 500 mg, FA 0.4 mg, Ca, Cu, I, K, Mn, Zn 15 mg. Tab. Bot. 60s. OTC.
Use: Mineral, vitamin supplement.
Unicomplex-T with Minerals. (Rugby) Iron 10 mg, vitamins A 5000 units, D 400 units, E 15 mg, B$_1$ 10 mg, B$_2$ 10 mg, B$_3$ 100 mg, B$_5$ 20 mg, B$_6$ 2 mg, B$_{12}$ 4 mcg, C 300 mg, folic acid

0.4 mg, Ca, Cu, I, K, Mg, Mn. Tab. Bot. 60s. OTC.
Use: Mineral, vitamin supplement.
Unifed. (Altaire) Pseudoephedrine hydrochloride 30 mg per 5 mL. Methylparaben, glycerin, sorbitol, sucrose. Liq. 118 mL. OTC.
Use: Nasal decongestant.
Unifiber. (Niche) Powdered cellulose. Pow. Bot. 150 g, 270 g, 480 g. OTC.
Use: Laxative.
• **unifocon A.** (you-nih-FOE-kahn A) USAN.
Use: Contact lens material (hydrophic).
Uniphyl. (Purdue) Theophylline. CR Tab. **400 mg:** 100s, 500s. **600 mg:** 100s. Rx.
Use: Bronchodilator.
Uniretic. (Schwarz Pharma) Moexipril hydrochloride/hydrochlorothiazide 7.5 mg/12.5 mg, 15 mg/12.5 mg, 15 mg/25 mg. Lactose. Film-coated. Tab. Bot. 100s. Rx.
Use: Antihypertensive.
Unisol. (Alcon) Buffered isotonic solution with sodium Cl, boric acid, sodium borate. Bot. 15 mL (25s), 120 mL (2s, 3s). OTC.
Use: Contact lens care.
Unisol 4 Sterile Saline. (Alcon) Buffered isotonic solution with sodium Cl, boric acid, sodium borate. Bot. 120 mL. OTC.
Use: Contact lens care.
Unisol Plus. (Alcon) Buffered isotonic solution w/NaCl, boric acid, sodium borate. Aerosol Bot. 240 mL, 360 mL. OTC.
Use: Contact lens care.
Unisom Nighttime Sleep-Aid. (Chattem) Doxylamine succinate 25 mg. Tab. Blister pack 8s, 16s, 32s, 48s. OTC.
Use: Sleep aid.
Unisom PM Pain. (Chattem) Acetaminophen 325 mg, diphenhydramine hydrochloride 50 mg. Mineral oil. Tab. 30s. OTC.
Use: Nonprescription sleep aid combination.
Unisom SleepGels. (Chattem) Diphenhydramine hydrochloride 50 mg. Cap. 8s, 16s, 32s. OTC.
Use: Antihistamine, nonselective ethanolamine.
Unisom SleepMelts. (Chattem) Diphenhydramine hydrochloride 25 mg. Mannitol, sucralose, sucrose. Cherry flavor. Tab., Orally disintegrating. 24s. OTC.
Use: Nonprescription sleep aid.
Unisom with Pain Relief. (Pfizer) Acetaminophen 650 mg, diphenhydramine hydrochloride 50 mg. Tab. Blister Pack

16s. *OTC.*
Use: Analgesic; sleep aid.
Unithroid Direct. (Lannett) Levothyroxine sodium 0.025 mg, 0.05 mg, 0.075 mg, 0.088 mg, 0.1 mg, 0.112 mg, 0.125 mg, 0.15 mg, 0.175 mg, 0.2 mg, 0.3 mg, lactose. Tab. Bot. 100s, 1000s. *Rx.*
Use: Hormone, thyroid.
Uni-Tussin DM. (United Research Laboratories) Dextromethorphan HBr 10 mg, guaifenesin 100 mg/5 mL. Syr. Bot. 118 mL. *OTC.*
Use: Antitussive; expectorant.
Univasc. (Schwarz Pharma) Moexipril hydrochloride 7.5 mg, 15 mg. Lactose. Film-coated. Tab. Bot. 100s, unit-of-use 90s. *Rx.*
Use: Antihypertensive; renin angiotensin system antagonist; angiotensin-converting enzyme inhibitor.
Unna's boot.
See: Zinc Gelatin.
Unproco Capsules. (Solvay) Dextromethorphan HBr 30 mg, guaifenesin 200 mg. Cap. Bot. 100s. *OTC.*
Use: Antitussive; expectorant.
UpCal D. (Global Health) **Chew. Tab.:** Vitamin D$_3$ 125 units, Ca, Mg. Sucralose. Fruit punch and cinnamon flavors. 120s. **Pow.:** Vitamin D$_3$ 250 units per packet/scoop, Ca. Dextrose. Single-use packet. 454 g, 2.5 g. *OTC.*
Use: Multivitamin with minerals.
Uplex. (Arcum) Vitamins A 5000 units, D 400 units, B$_1$ 3 mg, B$_2$ 3 mg, B$_6$ 1 mg, B$_{12}$ 2.5 mcg, nicotinamide 20 mg, calcium pantothenate 5 mg, C 50 mg. Cap. Bot. 100s, 1000s. *OTC.*
Use: Mineral, vitamin supplement.
Uplex No. 2. (Arcum) Vitamins A palmitate 10,000 units, D 400 units, B$_1$ 5 mg, B$_2$ 5 mg, C 100 mg, B$_6$ 2 mg, B$_{12}$ 3 mcg, E 2.5 units, niacinamide 25 mg, calcium pantothenate 5 mg. Cap. Bot. 100s, 1000s. *OTC.*
Use: Mineral, vitamin supplement.
u-polycosanol 410.
W/Antipyrine, Benzocaine.
See: Treagan.
upper respiratory combinations.
See: Antihistamine and Analgesic Combinations.
Antitussive and Expectorant Combinations.
Antitussive Combinations.
Antitussives with Expectorants.
Decongestant and Analgesic Combinations.
Decongestant and Antihistamine Combinations.

Decongestant, Antihistamine, and Analgesic Combinations.
Decongestant, Antihistamine, and Anticholinergic Combinations.
Decongestant, Antihistamine, and Expectorant Combinations.
Decongestant and Expectorant Combinations.
Expectorants with Analgesics.
Topical Combinations.
Urabeth Tabs. (Major) Bethanechol 5 mg, 10 mg, 25 mg, 50 mg. Tab. **5 mg:** Bot. 100s. **10 mg:** Bot. 250s. **25 mg:** Bot. 250s, 1000s. **50 mg:** Bot. 100s, UD 100s. *Rx.*
Use: Genitourinary.
Uracid. (Wesley) dl-Methionine 0.2 g. Cap. Bot. 100s, 1000s. *Rx.*
Use: Diaper rash preparation.
•**uracil.** (YOUR-ah-sil) USAN.
Use: Potentiator in tegafur therapy.
uradal.
See: Carbromal.
Uramaxin. (Medimetriks Pharmaceuticals) Urea. **Cream:** 45%. Camphor, edetate disodium, eucalyptus oil, menthol. 255 g. **Aer. Foam:** 20%. Cetearyl and cetyl alcohols, ammonium lactate, PEG, petrolatum. 100 g. **Lot.:** 25%. Camphor, edetate disodium, ethyl alcohol, eucalyptus oil, menthol, titanium dioxide. 473 mL. *Rx.*
Use: Emollient.
Uramaxin GT. (Medimetriks) Urea 45%. Camphor, edetate disodium, eucalyptus oil, menthol, propylene glycol. Soln. 20 mL prefilled applicator. *Rx.*
Use: Emollient.
•**urea.** (your-EE-a) *USP 34.*
Use: Topically for dry skin; diuretic.
See: Aluvea.
Aquacare.
Aquacare-HP.
BP-50.
Carmol.
Carmol 40.
Carmol 10.
Carmol 20.
Dermal Therapy Finger Care.
Gormel.
Hydro 40.
Hydro 35.
Kerafoam.
Kerafoam 42.
Keralac.
Keralac Nail Gel.
Keralac Nailstik.
Kerol.
Kerol AD.
Kerol ZX.
Latrix XM.

Nutraplus.
Rea-lo.
RE-U40.
RE Urea 50.
Rinnovi Nail System.
TL 45%.
Umecta.
Umecta PD.
Uramaxin.
Uramaxin GT.
Urea 50%.
Urea 40.
Urea 45%.
Urea 42%.
Urea Nail Gel.
Vanamide.
W/Combinations.
See: Amino-Cerv.
Akne Drying Lotion.
W/Micronized Hydrocortisone Acetate.
See: Carmol-HC.
W/Papain.
See: Pap-Urea.
urea. (Clay Park) Urea 40%. Glycerin, EDTA. Gel. 15 mL. *Rx.*
Use: Emollient.
urea. (Fougera) Urea 50%. Cetyl alcohol, disodium EDTA, glycerin, lactic acid, PEG-6, titanium dioxide, vitamin E. Emulsion. 284 g. *Rx.*
Use: Emollient.
urea. (Hi-Tech) Urea. **Cream:** 40%. Mineral oil, petrolatum, cetyl alcohol. 28.35 g, 198.6 g. **Lot.:** 40%. Mineral oil, petrolatum, cetyl alcohol. 236.6 mL. *Rx.*
Use: Emollient.
urea. (Prasco) Urea. **Emulsion:** 40%. EDTA, glycerin, sunflower oil. 114 g, 228 g. **Susp.:** 40%. EDTA, glycerin, sunflower oil. 285 g. *Rx.*
Use: Emollient.
urea. (River's Edge) Urea 35%. Cetyl alcohol, EDTA, lactic acid. Lot. 207 mL, 325 mL. *Rx.*
Use: Emollient.
urea. (Various Mfr.) Urea 50%. May contain caprylic/capric triglyceride, cetyl alcohol, edetate disodium, glycerin, lactic acid, linoleic acid, PEG-6, propylene glycol, salicylic acid, titanium dioxide, triethanolamine, vitamin E. Susp., Top. Tube. 284 g. *Rx.*
Use: Emollient.
•**urea C 14.** (yoor-EE-a) *USP 34.*
Ureacin-10. (Pedinol Pharmacal) Urea 10%. Lot. Bot. 8 oz. *OTC.*
Use: Emollient.
Ureacin-20 Creme. (Pedinol Pharmacal) Urea 20%. Cream. Jar 2.5 oz. *OTC.*
Use: Emollient.

•**urea C 13.** (yoor-EE-a) *USP 34.*
Urea 50%. (Acella Pharmaceuticals) Urea 50%. Caprylic/capril triglycerides, cetyl alcohol, disodium EDTA, glycerin, lactic acid, linoleic acid, PEG-6, polysorbate 60, propylene glycol, titanium dioxide, triethanolamine, vitamin E, zinc. Emuls. 295 mL. *Rx.*
Use: Emollient.
Urea 50%. (E. Fougera) Urea 50%. Cetyl alcohol, disodium EDTA, glycerin, lactic acid, PEG 6, vitamin E, zinc pyrithione. Oint. 45 g. *Rx.*
Use: Emollient.
Urea 40. (Kylemore) Urea 40%. Disodium EDTA, glycerin, PEG. Gel. 15 mL w/ applicator brush. *Rx.*
Use: Emollient.
Urea 45%. (River's Edge) Urea 45%. Camphor, edentate disodium, ethyl alcohol, eucalyptus oil, menthol, titanium dioxide. Cream. 255 g. *Rx.*
Use: Emollient.
Urea 42%. (River's Edge) Urea (carbamide) 42%. Disodium EDTA, glycerine, lactic acid. Cloth, Top. 30s. *Rx.*
Use: Emollient.
Urea Nail Gel. (A. Aarons) Urea 50%. EDTA. Gel. 18 mL. *Rx.*
Use: Emollient.
Urea Nail Gel. (Kylemore Pharmaceuticals) Urea 45%. Camphor, disodium EDTA, eucalyptus oil, menthol. Gel. 28 mL. *Rx.*
Use: Emollient.
urea peroxide.
See: Gly-Oxide.
Proxigel.
urea topical suspension 50%.
(A. Aarons) Urea 50%. Cetyl alcohol, EDTA, glycerin, lactic acid, PEG, titanium dioxide. Top. Susp. 284 g. *Rx.*
Use: Emollient.
Urecholine. (Barr/Duramed) Bethanechol chloride 5 mg, 10 mg, 25 mg, 50 mg. Lactose. Tab. 100s. *Rx.*
Use: Urinary cholinergic.
•**uredepa.** (YOU-ree-DEH-pah) USAN.
Use: Antineoplastic.
See: Avinar.
p-ureidobenzenearsonic acid.
See: Carbarsone.
Urelief. (Rocky Mtn.) Methenamine 2 g, salol 0.5 g, methylene blue 1/10 g, benzoic acid g, hyoscyamine sulfate g, atropine sulfate g. Tab. Bot. 100s. *Rx.*
Use: Anti-infective, urinary.
Urelle. (Pharmelle) Methenamine 81 mg, sodium phosphate monobasic 40.8 mg, phenyl salicylate 32.4 mg, methylene blue 10.8 mg, hyoscyamine sulfate

0.12 mg, sugar, mineral oil. Tab. 90s. *Rx.*
Use: Anti-infective, urinary.
• **urelumab.** (ue-REL-ue-mab) USAN.
Use: Antineoplastic.
Urese.
See: Benzthiazide.
urethan. Ethyl Carbamate, Ethyl Urethan, Urethane.
Use: Antineoplastic.
Uretron D/S. (Marin) Methenamine 120 mg, sodium biphosphonate 40.8 mg, phenyl salicylate 36.2 mg, methylene blue 10.8 mg, hyoscyamine sulfate 0.12 mg, parabens, sucrose. Tab. 100s. *Rx.*
Use: Anti-infective, urinary.
Urex. (3M) Methenamine hippurate 1 g. Tab. Bot. 100s. *Rx.*
Use: Anti-infective, urinary.
Uric Acid Reagent Strips. (Bayer Consumer Care) *Seralyzer* reagent strip. For uric acid in serum or plasma. Bot. 25s.
Use: Diagnostic aid.
uricosuric agents.
See: Anturane.
Benemid.
Uricult. (Orion) Urine culture test to detect bacteria and identify uropathogens. Bot. 10s.
Use: Diagnostic aid.
uridine. Idoxuridine.
Use: Reagent.
• **uridine triacetate.** (URE-i-deen trye-AS-e-tate) USAN.
Use: Antidote for 5-fluorouracil toxicity.
Urifon-Forte. (T.E. Williams Pharmaceuticals) Sulfamethizole 450 mg, phenazopyridine hydrochloride 50 mg. Cap. Bot. 100s, 1000s. *Rx.*
Use: Anti-infective, urinary.
Urigen. (Fellows) Calcium mandelate 0.2 g, methenamine 0.2 g, phenazopyridine hydrochloride 50 mg, sodium phosphate 80 mg. Cap. Bot. 100s, 1000s. *Rx.*
Use: Anti-infective, urinary.
Urimar-T. (Marnel) Methenamine 120 mg, sodium phosphate monobasic 40.8 mg, phenyl salicylate 36.2 mg, methylene blue 10.8 mg, hyoscyamine sulfate 0.12 mg. Sugar-coated. Tab. Bot. 4s, 100s. *Rx.*
Use: Anti-infective, urinary.
Urimax. (Xanodyne) Methenamine 81.6 mg, sodium biphosphate 40.8 mg, phenyl salicylate 36.2 mg, methylene blue 10.8 mg, hyoscyamine sulfate 0.12 mg. Magenta. Film-coated. DR Tab. 100s. *Rx.*

Use: Treatment of urinary tract infections.
Urinary Antiseptic #3 S.C.T. (Teva) Atropine sulfate 0.06 mg, hyoscyamine sulfate 0.03 mg, methenamine 120 mg, methylene blue 6 mg, phenyl salicylate 30 mg, benzoic acid 7.5 mg. Tab. Bot. 100s, 1000s. *Rx.*
Use: Anti-infective, urinary.
Urinary Antiseptic #2. (Various Mfr.) Atropine sulfate 0.03 mg, hyoscyamine 0.03 mg, methenamine 40.8 mg, methylene blue 5.4 mg, phenyl salicylate 18.1 mg, benzoic acid 4.5 mg. Tab. Bot. 100s, 1000s. *Rx.*
Use: Anti-infective, urinary.
Urinary Antiseptic #2 S.C.T. (Teva) Atropine sulfate 0.03 mg, hyoscyamine sulfate 0.03 mg, methenamine 40.8 mg, methylene blue 5.4 mg, phenyl salicylate 18.1 mg, benzoic acid 4.5 mg. Tab. Bot. 100s, 1000s. *Rx.*
Use: Anti-infective, urinary.
urinary cholinergics.
See: Bethanechol Chloride.
Neostigmine Methylsulfate.
urine sugar test.
See: Clinistix.
urine tests.
See: Diagnostic Agents.
Urin-Tek. (Bayer Consumer Care) Tubes, plastic caps, adhesive labels, collection cups, and disposable tube holder. Package 100 × 5.
Urisan-P. (Sandia) Atropine sulfate 0.03 mg, hyoscyamine 0.03 mg, gelsemium 6.1 mg, methenamine 40.8 mg, salol 18.1 mg, benzoic acid 4.5 mg, methylene blue 5.4 mg, phenylazo diamino pyridine hydrochloride 100 mg. Tab. Bot. 100s, 1000s. *Rx.*
Use: Anti-infective, urinary.
Urisedamine. (PolyMedica) Methenamine mandelate 500 mg, l-hyoscyamine 0.15 mg. Tab. Bot. 100s. *Rx.*
Use: Anti-infective, urinary.
Uriseptic. (SDA Labs) Methenamine 40.8 mg, phenyl salicylate 18.1 mg, methylene blue 5.4 mg, benzoic acid 4.5 mg, atropine sulfate 0.03 mg, hyoscyamine sulfate 0.03 mg. Tab. 100s. *Rx.*
Use: Anti-infective, urinary.
Urispas. (Ortho-McNeil) Flavoxate hydrochloride 100 mg, castor oil. Tab. Bot. 100s, UD 100s. *Rx.*
Use: Anticholinergic.
Uristix. (Siemens Medical) Urine test for glucose and protein. Reagent strips. 100s.
Use: Diagnostic aid.

Uristix 4 Reagent Strips. (Bayer Consumer Care) Urinalysis reagent strip test for glucose, protein, nitrite, leukocytes. Bot. 100s.
Use: Diagnostic aid.

Uristix Reagent Strips. (Bayer Consumer Care) Urinalysis reagent strip test for protein and glucose. Bot. 100s.
Use: Diagnostic aid.

Uritact DS. (Cypress) Hyoscyamine sulfate 0.06 mg, methenamine 81.6 mg, phenyl salicylate 36.2 mg, atropine sulfate 0.06 mg, methylene blue 10.8 mg, benzoic acid 9 mg. Alcohol free and sugar free. Tab. 100s. *Rx.*
Use: Anti-infective, urinary.

Uritin. (Global Source) Methenamine 40.8 mg, atropine sulfate 0.03 mg, hyoscyamine sulfate 0.03 mg, salol 18.1 mg, benzoic acid 4.5 mg, methylene blue 5.4 mg, gelsemium 6.1 mg. Tab. Bot. 1000s. *Rx.*
Use: Anti-infective, urinary.

Uritin Formula. (Various Mfr.) Atropine sulfate 0.03 mg, hyoscyamine 0.03 mg, methenamine 40.8 mg, methylene blue 5.4 mg, phenyl salicylate 18.1 mg, benzoic acid 4.5 mg. Tab. Bot. 1000s. *Rx.*
Use: Anti-infective, urinary.

Urobak. (Shire US) Sulfamethoxazole 500 mg. Tab. Bot. 100s, 1000s. *Rx.*
Use: Anti-infective, sulfonamide.

Uro Blue. (R.A. McNeil) Methenamine 120 mg, sodium phosphate monobasic 40.8 mg, phenyl salicylate 36.2 mg, methylene blue 10.8 mg, hyoscyamine sulfate 0.12 mg, sugar. Tab. 100s. *Rx.*
Use: Anti-infective, urinary.

Urocit-K. (Mission Pharmacal) Potassium citrate 5 mEq, 10 mEq, 15 mEq. ER Tab. 100s. *Rx.*
Use: Genitourinary.

•**urofollitropin.** (YOUR-oh-fahl-ih-TROE-pin) USAN.
Use: Sex hormone, ovulation stimulant.
See: Bravelle.

urogastrone. (Chiron Vision)
Use: Corneal transplant surgery.
[Orphan Drug]

Urogesic. (Edwards) Phenazopyridine hydrochloride 100 mg. Tab. Bot. 100s. *Rx.*
Use: Interstitial cystitis agent.

Urogesic Blue. (Edwards) Methenamine 81.6 mg, monobasic sodium phosphate 40.8 mg, methylene blue 10.8 mg, hyoscyamine (as sulfate) 0.12 mg. Mannitol. Tab. 100s. *Rx.*
Use: Anti-infective, urinary.

urography agents.
See: Iodohippurate Sodium.

Iodopyracet.
Iodopyracet Compound.
Renografin.
Renovist.
Renovue.

•**urokinase.** (YOUR-oh-KIN-ace) USAN.
Use: Plasminogen activator; thrombolytic agent; thrombolytic enzyme.

•**urokinase alfa.** (YOUR-oh-KIN-ace) USAN.
Use: Thrombolytic (plasminogen activator).

Uro-KP-Neutral. (Star) Phosphorus 250 mg, potassium 49.4 mg, sodium 250.5 mg. Film-coated. Tab. Bot. 100s. *Rx.*
Use: Mineral supplement.

Urologic Sol G. (Abbott Hospital Products) Bot. 1000 mL.
Use: Irrigant, ophthalmic.

Uro-Mag. (Blaine) Magnesium oxide 140 mg (elemental Mg 84.5 mg). Cap. Bot. 100s, 1000s, UD 100s. *OTC.*
Use: Mineral.

uronal.
See: Barbital.

Uro-Phosphate. (ECR) Sodium biphosphate 434.78 mg, methenamine 300 mg. Film-coated Tab. Bot. 100s. *Rx.*
Use: Anti-infective, urinary.

Uroplus DS. (Shire US) Trimethoprim 160 mg, sulfamethoxazole 800 mg. Tab. Bot. 100s, 500s. *Rx.*
Use: Anti-infective.

Uroplus SS. (Shire US) Trimethoprim 80 mg, sulfamethoxazole 800 mg. Tab. Bot. 100s, 500s. *Rx.*
Use: Anti-infective.

Uroquid-Acid No. 2. (Beach) Methenamine mandelate 500 mg, sodium acid phosphate monohydrate 500 mg. Tab. Bot. 100s. *Rx.*
Use: Anti-infective, urinary.

urotropin new. (Various Mfr.) Methenamine anhydromethylene citrate.

Urovist Cysto. (Berlex) Diatrizoate meglumine 300 mg, edetate calcium disodium 0.05 mg/mL. Dilution Bot. 500 mL w/300 mL. *Rx.*
Use: Radiopaque agent.

Urovist Cysto Pediatric. (Berlex) Diatrizoate meglumine 300 mg, edetate calcium disodium 0.1 mg/mL. Dilution bot. 300 mL w/100 mL soln. *Rx.*
Use: Radiopaque agent.

Urovist Meglumine DIU/CT. (Berlex) Diatrizoate meglumine 300 mg, edetate calcium disodium 0.05 mg/mL. Soln. Bot. 300 mL. Ctn. 10s. *Rx.*
Use: Radiopaque agent.

Urovist Sodium 300. (Berlex) Diatrizoate sodium 500 mg, edetate calcium disodium 0.1 mg/mL. Soln. Vial 50 mL, Box 10s. *Rx.*
Use: Radiopaque agent.
Uroxatral. (Sanofi-Syntholabo) Alfuzosin hydrochloride 10 mg. Mannitol. ER Tab. 30s, 100s, UD 100s. *Rx.*
Use: Antihypertensive, antiadrenergic.
Ursinus Inlay-Tabs. (Novartis) Pseudoephedrine hydrochloride 30 mg, aspirin 325 mg. Tab. Bot. 24s. *OTC.*
Use: Decongestant; analgesic.
URSO. (Novartis) Ursodiol.
Use: Management and treatment of primary biliary cirrhosis. [Orphan Drug]
ursodeoxycholic acid, buffered.
Use: Primary biliary cirrhosis. [Orphan Drug]
•**ursodiol.** (UR-so-DIE-ol) *USP 34.* Ursodeoxycholic acid.
Use: Anticholelithogenic; urolithic. Management and treatment of primary biliary cirrhosis, gallstone solubilizing agent.
See: Actigall.
URSO.
ursodiol. (Teva) Ursodiol 250 mg, 500 mg. Film-coated. Tab. 100s. *Rx.*
Use: GI agent, gallstone solubilizing agent.
ursodiol. (Watson) Ursodiol 300 mg. Cap. 100s. *Rx.*
Use: Anticholelithogenic; urolithic; gallstone solubilizing agent.
Urso Forte. (Axcan Pharma) Ursodiol 500 mg. Film-coated. Tab. 100s, 500s. *Rx.*
Use: Gallstone solubilizing agent.
Urso 250. (Axcan Pharma) Ursodiol 250 mg. Film-coated. Tab. 100s, 500s. *Rx.*
Use: Gallstone solubilizing agent.
•**usistapide.** (ue-SIS-ta-pide) *USAN.*
Use: Treatment of obesity and type 2 diabetes.
•**ustekinumab.** (US-te-KIN-ue-mab) *USAN.*
Use: Immunomodulator.
See: Stelara.
Ustell. (Biocomp Pharma) Methenamine 120 mg, methylene blue 10 mg, phenyl salicylate 36 mg, sodium phosphate monobasic 40.8 mg, hyoscyamine sulfate 0.12 mg. Ammonium hydroxide, propylene glycol. Cap. 100s. *Rx.*
Use: Anti-infective agent, methenamine combination.

Utac. (Breckenridge) Methenamine mandelate 500 mg, sodium acid phosphate monobasic monohydrate 500 mg. Film-coated. Tab. 100s. *Rx.*
Use: Anti-infective, methenamine.
uterine-active agents.
See: Abortifacients.
Cervical Ripening Agents.
Methylergonovine Maleate.
Oxytocics.
Uterine Relaxant.
uterine relaxant.
See: Ritodrine.
uterine stimulants.
See: Ergonovine Maleate.
Methylergonovine Maleate.
Uticap. (Cypress) Methenamine 120 mg, methylene blue 10 mg, phenyl salicylate 36 mg, sodium phosphate monobasic 40.8 mg, hyoscyamine sulfate 0.12 mg. Cap. 100s. *Rx.*
Use: Anti-infective agent, methenamine.
Utimox. (Parke-Davis) Amoxicillin trihydrate. **Cap.:** 250 mg Bot. 100s, 500s, UD 100s; 500 mg Bot. 100s, UD 100s. **Oral Susp.:** 125 mg or 250 mg/5 mL Bot. 80 mL, 100 mL, 150 mL, 200 mL. *Rx.*
Use: Anti-infective, penicillin.
UTI Relief. (Consumers Choice Systems) Phenazopyridine hydrochloride 97.2 mg. Tab. 12s. *Rx.*
Use: Interstitial cystitis agent.
Utrona-C. (Cypress Pharmaceutical) Hyoscyamine sulfate 0.12 mg, methenamine 81.6 mg, methylene blue 10.8 mg, phenyl salicylate 36.2 mg, sodium phosphate monobasic 40.8 mg. Mineral oil, PEG, sugar. Tab. 100s. *Rx.*
Use: Anti-infective, methenamine combination.
Uvadex. (Therakos) Methoxsalen 20 mcg/mL, alcohol 0.05 mL. Soln. Vial 10 mL. *Rx.*
Use: Cutaneous T-cell lymphoma; sclerosis treatment; cardiac allograft rejection prevention; psoralens.
Uvasal. (Sanofi-Synthelabo) Sodium bicarbonate, tartaric acid. Pow. Bot. *OTC.*
Use: Antacid.
uva ursi. (Sherwood Davis & Geck) Leaves. Fluid extract. Bot. pt, gal.
Uvinul MS-40. (General Aniline & Film)
See: Sulisobenzone.
UV Protective. (Kiehl's) Avobenzone 2%, ecamsule 2%, octocrylene 10%. EDTA, glycerin, parabens, stearyl alcohol. Fragrance free. SPF 15. Cream. 100 g. *OTC.*
Use: Sunscreen.

V

•**vabicaserin hydrochloride.** (va-BIK-a-SER-in) USAN.
Use: Antipsychotic.
vaccine, adenovirus. *Rx.*
Use: Immunization.
See: Adenovirus Vaccine.
vaccine, anthrax. *Rx.*
Use: Immunization.
See: Anthrax Vaccine.
vaccine, BCG. *Rx.*
Use: Immunization.
See: BCG Vaccine.
TheraCys.
Tice BCG.
vaccine, Haemophilus b conjugate. *Rx.*
Use: Immunization.
See: ActHIB.
HibTITER.
Liquid PedvaxHIB.
W/Hepatitis B.
See: Comvax.
vaccine, hepatitis A. *Rx.*
Use: Immunization.
See: Havrix.
Vaqta.
vaccine, hepatitis B, recombinant. *Rx.*
Use: Immunization.
See: Engerix-B.
Recombivax HB.
vaccine, influenza A & B. *Rx.*
Use: Immunization.
See: Fluarix.
FluMist.
Fluvirin.
Fluzone.
vaccine, Japanese encephalitis. *Rx.*
Use: Immunization.
See: JE-Vax.
vaccine, measles. *Rx.*
Use: Immunization.
See: Attenuvax.
W/Mumps and Rubella Vaccines.
See: M-M-R II.
vaccine, meningococcal polysaccharide. *Rx.*
Use: Immunization.
See: Menomune A/C/Y/W-135.
vaccine, mumps. Mumps Virus Vaccine Live.
Use: Immunization.
See: Mumpsvax.
vaccine, papillomavirus. *Rx.*
Use: Immunization.
See: Gardasil.
vaccine, pertussis. Pertussis Vaccine. *Rx.*
Use: Immunization.
See: ActHIB/DTP.
Diphtheria and Tetanus Toxoids, Acel-lular Pertussis and Haemophilus Influenzae Type B Conjugate Vaccine.
Diphtheria and Tetanus Toxoids and Acellular Pertussis Vaccine, Adsorbed.
Tripedia.
vaccine, pneumococcal polyvalent. *Rx.*
Use: Immunization.
See: Pneumovax 23.
vaccine, pneumococcal 7-valent conjugate. *Rx.*
Use: Immunization.
See: Prevnar.
vaccine, poliovirus. *Rx.*
Use: Immunization.
See: IPOL.
Poliovirus Vaccine, Inactivated.
vaccine, rabies. Rabies Vaccine. *Rx.*
Use: Immunization.
See: Imovax Rabies.
RabAvert.
Rabies Vaccine Adsorbed.
vaccines, bacterial.
Use: Immunization.
See: Anthrax Vaccine.
BCG Vaccine.
Haemophilus b Conjugate Vaccine.
Haemophilus b Conjugate Vaccine with Hepatitis B Vaccine.
Meningococcal Vaccine.
Pneumococcal Conjugate Vaccine.
Pneumococcal 7-Valent Conjugate Vaccine.
Pneumococcal Vaccine, Polyvalent.
Typhoid Vaccine.
vaccine, smallpox. *Rx.*
Use: Immunization.
See: Dryvax
vaccine, typhoid. *Rx.*
Use: Immunization.
See: Typhim Vi.
Vivotif Berna.
vaccine, varicella. *Rx.*
Use: Immunization.
See: Varivax.
vaccines, viral. *Rx.*
Use: Immunization.
See: Hepatitis A, Inactivated and Hepatitis B, Recombinant Vaccine.
Hepatitis A Vaccine, Inactivated.
Hepatitis B Vaccine, Recombinant.
H5N1 Influenza Vaccine.
Human Papillomavirus Recombinant Vaccine, Bivalent.
Human Papillomavirus Recombinant Vaccine, Quadrivalent.
Influenza A and B Vaccine.
Influenza Virus Vaccine.
Japanese Encephalitis Virus Vaccine.
Measles, Mumps, and Rubella Virus Vaccine, Live.

Measles, Mumps, Rubella, and Varicella Virus Vaccine, Live, Attenuated.
Poliovirus Vaccine, Inactivated.
Rotavirus Vaccine Live.
Rubella and Mumps Virus Vaccine, Live.
Smallpox Vaccine.
Varicella Virus Vaccine.
Yellow Fever Vaccine.
Zoster Vaccine Live.

vaccine, whooping cough. Pertussis Vaccine. *Rx.*
Use: Immunization.
See: Acel-Imune.
ActHIB/DTP.
Diphtheria and Tetanus Toxoids, Acellular Pertussis and Haemophilus Influenzae Type B Conjugate Vaccine.
Diphtheria and Tetanus Toxoids and Acellular Pertussis Vaccine, Adsorbed.
Tripedia.

vaccine, yellow fever. *Rx.*
Use: Immunization.
See: YF-Vax.

vaccine, zoster. *Rx.*
Use: Immunization.
See: Zostavax.

•**vaccinia immune globulin intravenous.** (vax-IN-ee-ah) *USP 34. Formerly Vaccinia Immune Human Globulin.*
Use: Immunization.

vaccinia immune globulin intravenous (human). (Dynport Vaccine Company LLC) Vaccinia immune globulin 50 mcg/mL (immunoglobulin 2,500 mg/vial). Sucrose 5%, albumin (human) 1%. Soln. for Inj. Vials. *Rx.*
Use: Immunization.

vacocin. Under study.
Use: Anti-infective.

Vademin-Z. (Roberts) Vitamin A 12,500 units, D 50 units, E 50 mg, B_1 10 mg, B_2 5 mg, B_3 25 mg, B_5 10 mg, B_6 2 mg, C 150 mg, Zn 2.6 mg, Mg, Mn. Cap. Bot. 60s. *OTC.*
Use: Mineral, vitamin supplement.

Vagifem. (Novo Nordisk) Estradiol 10 mcg (equiv. to hemihydrate 10.3 mcg), 25 mcg (equiv. to hemihydrate 25.8 mcg). Lactose. Film-coated. Vaginal Tab. Single-use applicator. 8s, 18s. *Rx.*
Use: Estrogen, sex hormone.

Vagi-Gard Advanced Sensitive Formula. (Lake Consumer) Benzocaine 5%, resorcinol, methylparaben, sodium sulfite, EDTA, mineral oil. Cream. Tube 45 g. *OTC.*
Use: Vaginal agent.

Vagi-Gard Maximum Strength. (Lake Consumer) Benzocaine 20%, resorcinol 3%, methylparaben, sodium sulfite, EDTA, mineral oil. Cream. Tube 45 g. *OTC.*
Use: Vaginal agent.

vaginal antifungal agents.
See: Butoconazole Nitrate.
Clotrimazole.
Miconazole Nitrate.
Nystatin.
Terconazole.
Tioconazole.

vaginal preparations.
See: Butoconazole Nitrate.
Chlorhexidine Gluconate
Clindamycin Phosphate.
Clotrimazole.
Metronidazole.
Miconazole Nitrate.
Nystatin.
Sulfonamides.
Terconazole.
Tioconazole.
Vaginal Antifungal Agents.

Vagisec Plus. (Durex) Polyoxyethylene nonylphenol 5.25 mg, sodium edetate 0.66 mg, docusate sodium 0.07 mg, aminoacridine hydrochloride 6 mg. Supp. Box 28s. *Rx.*
Use: Vaginal agent.

Vagisil. (Combe) Benzocaine 5%, resorcinol 2%. Aloe, cetearyl alcohol, corn oil, lanolin alcohol, methylparaben, mineral oil, PEG-100, triethanolamine, trisodium EDTA, vitamins A, D_3, E. Cream. 28 g. *OTC.*
Use: Vaginal agent.

Vagisil Maximum Strength. (Combe) Benzocaine 20%, resorcinol 3%. Aloe, cetearyl alcohol, corn oil, glyceryl, lanolin alcohol, methylparaben, mineral oil, PEG-100, propylene glycol, triethanolamine, trisodium EDTA, vitamins A, D_3, and E. Cream. 28 g. *OTC.*
Use: Vaginal preparation.

Vagisil Powder. (Combe) Cornstarch, aloe, mineral oil, benzethonium chloride, magnesium stearate, silica, fragrance. Pow. 198 g, 312 g. *OTC.*
Use: Vaginal agent.

Vagistat-1. (Novartis Consumer Health) Tioconazole 6.5%, white petrolatum. Vaginal Oint. Prefilled single-dose applicator 300 mg. *OTC.*
Use: Antifungal; vaginal.

Vagistat-3 Combination Pack. (Novartis Consumer Health) Miconazole nitrate. **Top. Cream:** 2%. Mineral oil. 9 g. **Vag. Supp.:** 200 mg. Hydrogenated vegetable oil. 3s with 3 disposable applica-

tors. *OTC.*
Use: Vaginal preparation.
Valacet. (Pal-Pak, Inc.) Hyoscyamus
10.8 mg, aspirin 259.2 mg, caffeine an-
hydrous 16.2 mg, gelsemium extract
0.6 mg. Tab. Cap. Bot. 100s, 1000s,
5000s. *Rx.*
Use: Analgesic; anticholinergic; anti-
spasmodic.
• **valacyclovir hydrochloride.** (val-lay-
SIGH-kloe-vihr) USAN.
Tall Man: valACYclovir
Use: Antiviral, antiherpes virus agent.
See: Valtrex.
valacyclovir hydrochloride. (Ranbaxy)
Valacyclovir hydrochloride 500 mg, 1 g.
Film-coated. PEG 400, PEG 6,000.
Tab. 10s, 30s, 500s. *Rx.*
Use: Antiviral, antiherpes virus agent.
• **valategrast hydrochloride.** (val-A-te-
grast) USAN.
Use: Asthma.
Valcyte. (Roche) Valganciclovir. **Tab.:**
450 mg (equiv. to valganciclovir hydro-
chloride). Film-coated. 60s. **Pow. for
Soln.:** 50 mg/mL. Mannitol, Saccharin.
Tutti-frutti flavor. Glass bot. w/ bot.
adapter and 2 oral dispensers. 100 mL.
Rx.
Use: Antiviral.
Valentine. (BDI) Caffeine 200 mg. Tab.
Bot. 100s, 500s. *OTC.*
Use: CNS stimulant, analeptic.
Valergen 20. (Hyrex) Estradiol Valerate
in oil 20 mg/mL, castor oil, benzyl ben-
zoate, benzyl alcohol. Inj. Multi-dose
vial 10 mL. *Rx.*
Use: Estrogen.
• **valerian.** (va-LAR-ee-an) *NF 29.*
Use: Dietary supplement.
valerian. (Eli Lilly) Tincture, alcohol 68%.
Bot. 4 fl oz, 16 fl oz. *Rx.*
• **valerian extract, powdered.** (va-LAR-
ee-an) *NF 29.*
Use: Pharmaceutical vehicle.
Valertest. (Hyrex) **No. 1:** Estradiol valer-
ate 4 mg, testosterone enanthate
90 mg/mL. Vial 10 mL. **No. 2:** Double
strength. Vial 10 mL. Amp. 2 mL, 10s.
Rx.
Use: Androgen, estrogen combination.
valethamate bromide.
Use: Anticholinergic.
• **valganciclovir hydrochloride.** (val-gan-
SIGH-kloe-veer) USAN.
Tall Man: valGANciclovir
Use: Antiviral.
See: Valcyte.
• **valine.** (VAY-leen) *USP 34.*
Use: Amino acid.

valine, isoleucine, and leucine.
Use: Hyperphenylalaninemia. [Orphan
Drug]
See: VIL.
Valisone. (Schering-Plough) Betamethasone valerate. **Cream:** 1 mg hydrophilic
cream of water, mineral oil, petrolatum, polyethylene glycol 1000 monocetyl ether, cetostearyl alcohol, monobasic sodium phosphate, phosphoric acid,
4-chloro-m-cresol as preservative.
Tube 15 g, 45 g, 110 g. Jar 430 g.
Oint.: 1 mg/g base of liquid and white
petrolatum and hydrogenated lanolin.
Tube 15 g, 45 g. **Lot.:** 1 mg/g w/isopro-
pyl alcohol 47.5%, water slightly thick-
ened w/carboxyvinyl polymer, pH adjusted w/sodium hydroxide. Bot. 20 mL,
60 mL. **Reduced Strength Cream
0.01%:** Hydrophilic cream of water, mineral oil, petrolatum, polyethylene glycol 1000 monocetyl ether, cetostearyl
alcohol, monobasic sodium phosphate,
phosphoric acid, 4-chloro-m-cresol as
preservative. Tube 15 g, 60 g. *Rx.*
Use: Corticosteroid, topical.
Valium. (Roche) Diazepam 2 mg, 5 mg,
10 mg. Lactose. Tab. Bot. 100s, 500s.
c-iv.
Use: Anxiolytic; anticonvulsant.
Valium Injection. (Roche) Diazepam
5 mg/mL, propylene glycol 40%, ethyl
alcohol 10%, sodium benzoate 5%,
benzoic acid, benzyl alcohol 1.5%.
Amp. 2 mL. Vial 10 mL. *Tel-E-Ject.*
(Disposable syringe) 2 mL. *c-iv.*
Use: Anxiolytic; anticonvulsant.
vallergine.
See: Promethazine Hydrochloride.
Valnac Cream. (Alra) Betamethasone
valerate 0.1%. Cream. Oint. Tube 15 g,
45 g. *Rx.*
Use: Corticosteroid, topical.
• **valnoctamide.** (val-NOCK-tah-mid)
USAN.
Use: Anxiolytic.
• **valomaciclovir stearate.** (val-oh-ma-
SYE-kloe-veer) USAN.
Use: Herpes zoster (inhibitor of DNA
polymerase).
• **valopicitabine dihydrochloride.** (val-
OH-pi-SYE-ta-been) USAN.
Use: Hepatitis.
Valorin. (Otis Clapp) Acetaminophen
325 mg, 500 mg. Sugar free. Tab. 300s
(325 mg only), UD 300s (500 mg only).
OTC.
Use: Analgesic.
valproate.
Use: Anticonvulsant.
See: Depacon.

valproate. (Various Mfr.) Valproate 100 mg/mL. May be preservative free. Inj., Conc. Single-dose vials. 5 mL. *Rx.*
Use: Anticonvulsant.

•**valproate sodium.** (VAL-pro-ate) USAN.
Use: Anticonvulsant.
See: Depacon.

•**valproic acid.** (VAL-pro-ik) *USP 34.*
Use: Anticonvulsant; antimigraine.
See: Depakene.
Stavzor.

valproic acid. (Various Mfr.) Valproic acid. **Cap.:** 250 mg. Bot. 10s, 30s, 31s, 100s. **Syrup:** 250 mg/5 mL. Bot. 473 mL. *Rx.*
Use: Anticonvulsant.

•**valrocemide.** (val-ROE-se-mide) USAN.
Use: Antiepileptic, anticonvulsant.

•**valsartan.** (VAL-sahr-tan) USAN.
Use: Renin angiotensin system antagonist, angiotensin II receptor antagonist.
See: Diovan.
W/Amlodipine Besylate.
See: Exforge.
W/Amlodipine/Hydrochlorothiazide.
See: Exforge HCT.
W/Hydrochlorothiazide.
See: Diovan HCT.

•**valspodar.** (VAL-spoh-dar) USAN.
Use: Antineoplastic; multidrug resistance inhibitor.

•**valtorcitabine dihydrochloride.** (val-tore-SITE-ah-been) USAN.
Use: Antifungal.

Valtrex. (GlaxoSmithKline) Valacyclovir hydrochloride (as base) 500 mg, 1 g. Film-coated. Tab. Bot. 21s (1 g only); 30s, UD 100s (500 mg only). *Rx.*
Use: Antiviral, antiherpes virus agent.

Valturna. (Novartis) Aliskiren/valsartan 150 mg/160 mg, 300 mg/320 mg. Film-coated. Tab. 30s, 90s, UD 100s. *Rx.*
Use: Antihypertensive combination.

Valuphed. (H.L. Moore Drug Exchange) Pseudoephedrine hydrochloride 60 mg, triprolidine hydrochloride 2.5 mg. Tab. Pkg. 24s. *OTC.*
Use: Antihistamine, decongestant.

Vamate. (Major) Hydroxyzine pamoate 50 mg. Cap. Bot. 100s, 250s, 500s, UD 100s. *Rx.*
Use: Anxiolytic.

Vanacof Dx. (GM Pharmaceuticals) Chlophedianol hydrochloride 12.5 mg, guaifenesin 100 mg, pseudoephedrine hydrochloride 30 mg per 5 mL. Glycerin, propylene glycol, saccharin, sorbitol. Alcohol free, dye free, and sugar free. Raspberry flavor. Liq.

473 mL. *OTC.*
Use: Upper respiratory combination, antitussive and expectorant combination.

Vanadryx TR. (Vangard Labs, Inc.) Dexbrompheniramine maleate 6 mg, pseudoephedrine sulfate 120 mg. Tab. Bot. 100s, 500s. *Rx.*
Use: Antihistamine, decongestant.

Vanamide. (Dermik) Urea 40%, light mineral oil, cetyl alcohol, petrolatum. Cream. 85 g, 199 g. *Rx.*
Use: Emollient.

Vancocin. (ViroPharma) Vancomycin 125 mg, 250 mg. PEG. Cap. Identi-Dose. 20s. *Rx.*
Use: Anti-infective agent.

•**vancomycin.** (van-koe-MY-sin) *USP 34.*
Use: Anti-infective.

•**vancomycin hydrochloride.** (van-koe-MY-sin) *USP 34.* An antibiotic from *Streptomyces orientalis.*
Use: (IV) Gram-positive (staph.) infection; anti-infective.
See: Vancocin.
Vancoled.

vancomycin hydrochloride. (American Pharmaceutical Partners) Vancomycin 5 g, 10 g. Inj., Pow. for Soln. Pharmacy bulk package. 100 mL. *Rx.*
Use: Anti-infective.

vancomycin hydrochloride. (Baxter) Vancomycin 500 mg, 1 g. Inj., Soln. *Galaxy* container. 100 mL (500 mg only), 200 mL (1 g only). *Rx.*
Use: Anti-infective.

vancomycin hydrochloride. (Various Mfr.) Vancomycin 125 mg, 250 mg. PEG. Cap. Identi-Dose. 20s. *Rx.*
Use: Anti-infective.

Vancor Intravenous. (Pharmacia) Vancomycin hydrochloride 500 mg, 1 g. Pow. for Inj. Vials.
Use: Anti-infective.

Vandazole. (Upsher-Smith Laboratories, Inc.) Metronidazole 0.75%. EDTA, parabens. Vaginal Gel. Tube. 70 g with 5 applicators. *Rx.*
Use: Vaginal preparation, anti-infective.

•**vandetanib.** (van-DET-a-nib) USAN.
Use: Antineoplastic.

vandetanib. (AstraZeneca) Vandetanib 100 mg, 300 mg. Film coated. Tab. 30s. *Rx.*
Use: Tyrosine kinase inhibitor.

Vanex Expectorant. (Jones Pharma) Pseudoephedrine hydrochloride 30 mg, hydrocodone bitartrate 2.5 mg, guaifenesin 100 mg/5 mL. Alcohol 5%, glucose, saccharin, sorbitol, sucrose, tart-

razine. Tropical fruit punch flavor. Liq. Bot. 473 mL. *c-III.*
Use: Antitussive, decongestant, expectorant.

Vanex-HD. (Great Southern Labs) Hydrocodone bitartrate 1.7 mg, chlorpheniramine maleate 2 mg, phenylephrine hydrochloride 5 mg per 5 mL. Benzyl alcohol. Dye free. Cherry flavor. Liq. 473 mL. *c-III.*
Use: Upper respiratory combination, antitussive combination.

Vanicream. (Pharmaceutical Specialties) Oil in water vanishing cream containing white petrolatum, cetearyl alcohol, ceteareth-20, sorbitol, propylene glycol, simethicone, glyceryl monostearate, polyethylene glycol monostearate, sorbic acid. Oint. 1 lb. *OTC.*
Use: Pharmaceutical aid; ointment base.

Vanicream Sunscreen SPF 30. (Pharmaceutical Specialties) Titanium dioxide 5%, zinc oxide 5%, caprylic/capric triglyceride, cetyl alcohol, PEG-12, PEG-30, etrasodium EDTA, vitamin E. PABA free. Cream. 113 g. *OTC.*
Use: Sunscreen.

Vanicream Sunscreen SPF 35. (Pharmaceutical Specialties) Octinoxate 7.5%, zinc oxide 8%, glycerin, PEG-30, castor oil, vitamin E. PABA free. Cream. 113 g. *OTC.*
Use: Sunscreen.

•**vanilla.** (va-NIL-a) *NF 29.*
Use: Pharmaceutic aid (flavor).

vanillal.
See: Ethyl Vanillin.

•**vanilla tincture.** (va-NIL-a) *NF 29.*
Use: Pharmaceutic aid (flavor).

•**vanillin.** (vah-NILL-in) *NF 29.*
Use: Pharmaceutic aid (flavor).

•**vaniprevir.** (van-I-pre-vir) USAN.
Use: Hepatitis C.

Vaniqa. (SkinMedica) Eflornithine hydrochloride monohydrate 150 mg/g, parabens, cetearyl alcohol, mineral oil, stearyl alcohol. Cream. Tube 30 g, 2 × 30 g. *Rx.*
Use: Reduce unwanted facial hair.

vanirome.
See: Ethyl Vanillin.

Vanocin. (ViroPharma) Sodium sulfacetamide 10%, sulfur 5%, benzyl alcohol, cetyl alcohol, EDTA, parabens, stearyl alcohol. Lot. Bot. 30 g, 60 g. *Rx.*
Use: Anti-infective.

Vanos. (Medicis) Fluocinonide 0.1%. Cream. 30 g, 60 g. *Rx.*
Use: Anti-inflammatory agent, topical corticosteroid.

Vanoxide HC. (Summers Laboratories) Benzoyl peroxide 5%, hydrocortisone 0.5%. Cetyl alcohol, lanolin oil, mineral oil, parabens, tetrasodium EDTA. Lot. 25 g and kits with *Benzoyl-Pak* and *ABC Lotion. Rx.*
Use: Dermatologic, acne.

Vanquish. (Bayer Consumer Care) Aspirin 227 mg, acetaminophen 194 mg, caffeine 33 mg, aluminum hydroxide 25 mg, magnesium hydroxide 50 mg. Capl. Bot. 60s, 100s. *OTC.*
Use: Analgesic combination; antacid.

Vantas. (Endo Pharmaceuticals) Histrelin acetate 50 mg. Implant, Subcutaneous. In carton with implantation kit. *Rx.*
Use: Hormone, gonadotropin-releasing hormone analog.

Vantin. (Pharmacia & Upjohn) Cefpodoxime proxetil 100 mg, 200 mg. Lactose. Film-coated. Tab. Bot. 20s, 100s, UD 100s. *Rx.*
Use: Anti-infective.

•**vapiprost hydrochloride.** (VAP-ih-prahst) USAN.
Use: Antagonist (thromboxane A_2).

•**vapitadine dihydrochloride.** (va-PI-ta-deen) USAN.
Use: Atopic dermatitis.

Vapocet. (Major) Hydrocodone 5 mg, acetaminophen 500 mg. Tab. Bot. 100s. *c-III.*
Use: Analgesic combination; narcotic.

Vaponefrin. (Medeva) A 2.25% solution of bioassayed racemic epinephrine as hydrochloride, chlorobutanol 0.5%. Soln. Vial 7.5 mL, 15 mL, 30 mL. *OTC.*
Use: Bronchodilator.

Vaporizer in a Bottle. (Columbia) Wick-dispensed medicated vapors.
Use: Cough, cold, sinus, hay fever preparation.

•**vapreotide.** (vap-REE-oh-tide) USAN.
Use: Antineoplastic.

•**vapreotide acetate.** (vap-REE-oh-tide) USAN.
Use: Esophageal bleeding.

Vaprisol Premixed in Dextrose 5%. (Astellas) Conivaptan hydrochloride 0.2 mg/mL. Dextrose 5 g. Inj., Soln. *Intravia* plastic container. 100 mL. *Rx.*
Use: Vasopressin receptor antagonist.

Vaqta. (Merck) **Adult:** Hepatitis A virus antigen 50 U/mL. **Pediatric/Adolescent:** Hepatitis A virus antigen 25 U/ 0.5 mL, Inj. Single-dose vial, prefilled syringe. *Rx.*
Use: Active immunization agent, viral vaccine.

•**vardenafil dihydrochloride.** (var-DEN-a-fil) USAN.
Use: Erectile dysfunction.
vardenafil hydrochloride.
Use: Impotence agent.
See: Levitra.
Staxyn.
•**varenicline tartrate.** (var-e-NI-kleen) USAN.
Use: Smoking cessation.
See: Chantix.
•**varespladib.** (va-res-PLA-dib) USAN.
Use: Treatment of dyslipidemia.
•**varespladib methyl.** (va-res-PLA-dib) USAN.
Use: Treatment of dyslipidemia.
Varibar Honey. (Bracco Diagnostics) Barium sulfate 40%. Apple flavoring, glycerin, polysorbate 80, potassium sorbate, saccharin, simethicone, sodium benzoate, xylitol. Susp. 250 mL. *Rx.*
Use: Radiopaque agent, miscellaneous GI contrast agent.
Varibar Nectar. (Bracco Diagnostics) Barium sulfate 40%. Apple flavoring, glycerin, maltodextrin, polysorbate 80, potassium sorbate, saccharin, simethicone, sodium benzoate, xylitol. Susp. 240 mL. *Rx.*
Use: Radiopaque agent, miscellaneous GI contrast agent.
Varibar Pudding. (Bracco Diagnostics) Barium sulfate 40%. Glycerin, maltodextrin, polysorbate 80, potassium sorbate, saccharin, simethicone, sodium benzoate, vanilla flavoring, xylitol. Paste. 230 mL. *Rx.*
Use: Radiopaque agent, miscellaneous GI contrast agent.
Varibar Thin Honey. (Bracco Diagnostics) Barium sulfate 40%. Apple flavoring, glycerin, polysorbate 80, potassium sorbate, saccharin, simethicone, sodium benzoate, xylitol. Susp. 250 mL. *Rx.*
Use: Radiopaque agent, miscellaneous GI contrast agent.
Varibar Thin Liquid. (Bracco Diagnostics) Barium sulfate 40%. Apple flavoring, maltodextrin, polysorbate 80, saccharin, simethicone, xylitol. Pow. for Susp. 148 g. *Rx.*
Use: Radiopaque agent, miscellaneous GI contrast agent.
varicella virus vaccine.
Use: Immunization, viral vaccine.
See: Varivax.
Zostavax.
varicella-zoster IgG IFA test system. (Wampole) Test for the qualitative or semi-qualitative detection of VZ IgG antibody in human serum. Test kit 100s.
Use: Diagnostic aid.
•**varicella-zoster immune globulin.** (var-i-SEL-a ZOS-ter) *USP 34.*
Use: Immunization.
Vari-Flavors. (Ross) Flavor packets to provide flavor variety for patients on liquid diets. Dextrose, artificial flavor, artificial color. Packet 1 g, Ctn. 24s. *Rx.*
Use: Flavoring.
Variplex-C. (NBTY) Vitamins B_1 15 mg, B_2 10 mg, B_3 100 mg, B_5 20 mg, B_6 5 mg, B_{12} 10 mcg, C 500 mg. Tab. Bot. 100s. *OTC.*
Use: Vitamin supplement.
Varivax. (Merck & Co.) Varicella virus vaccine. 1350 PFU of Oka/Merck varicella virus (live), sucrose. Pow. for Inj. Single-dose vials 1s, 10s. *Rx.*
Use: Immunization, viral vaccine.
•**varlitinib.** (var-li-TIN-ib) USAN.
Use: Antineoplastic.
•**varlitinib tosylate.** (var-LI-ti-nib) USAN.
Use: Antineoplastic.
Vascunitol. (Apco) Mannitol hexanitrate 0.5 g. Tab. Bot. 100s. *Rx.*
Use: Vasodilator.
Vascused. (Apco) Mannitol hexanitrate 0.5 g, phenobarbital 0.25 g. Tab. Bot. 100s. *Rx.*
Use: Vasodilator.
Vaseline Dermatology Formula Cream. (Chesebrough-Ponds USA) Petrolatum, mineral oil, dimethicone. Jar 3 oz, 5.25 oz. *OTC.*
Use: Emollient.
Vaseline Dermatology Formula Lotion. (Chesebrough-Ponds USA) Petrolatum, mineral oil, dimethicone. Bot. 5.5 oz, 11 oz, 16 oz. *OTC.*
Use: Emollient.
Vaseline First Aid Carboxylated Petroleum Jelly. (Chesebrough-Ponds USA) Petrolatum, chloroxylenol. Plastic Jar 1.75 oz, 3.75 oz. Plastic Tube 1 oz, 2.5 oz. *OTC.*
Use: Medicated anti-infective.
Vaseline Intensive Care Active Sport. (Chesebrough-Ponds USA) Ethylhexyl p-methoxycinnamate, oxybenzone. PABA free. **SPF 8:** Lot. Bot. 120 mL. **SPF 15:** Lot. Bot. 120 mL. *OTC.*
Use: Sunscreen.
Vaseline Intensive Care Baby SPF 15. (Chesebrough-Ponds USA) Titanium dioxide. PABA free. Waterproof. Lot. Bot. 120 mL. *OTC.*
Use: Sunscreen.
Vaseline Intensive Care Baby SPF 30. (Chesebrough-Ponds USA) Ethylhexyl

p-methoxycinnamate, oxybenzone, 2-ethylhexyl salicylate, titanium dioxide, C12-15 alkyl benzoate, glycerin, aloe vera gel, vitamin E, cetyl alcohol, parabens, EDTA. Lot. Bot. 118 mL. *OTC.*
Use: Sunscreen.

Vaseline Intensive Care Blockout SPF 40+. (Chesebrough-Ponds USA) Padimate O, ethylhexyl p-methoxycinnamate, oxybenzone, 2-ethylhexyl salicylate, titanium dioxide. Waterproof. Lot. Bot. 120 mL. *OTC.*
Use: Sunscreen.

Vaseline Intensive Care Blockout SPF 30. (Chesebrough-Ponds USA) Ethylhexyl p-methoxycinnamate, oxybenzone, 2-ethylhexyl salicylate, titanium dioxide. Waterproof. Lot. Bot. 120 mL. *OTC.*
Use: Sunscreen.

Vaseline Intensive Care Moisturizing Sunscreen. (Chesebrough-Ponds USA) Ethylhexyl p-methoxycinnamate, oxybenzone, C12-15 alkyl octanoate, glycerin, aloe vera gel, cetyl alcohol, petrolatum, vitamin E, parabens, EDTA. SPF 4, SPF 8: Lot. Bot. 117 mL. *OTC.*
Use: Sunscreen.

Vaseline Intensive Care No Burn No Bite SPF 8. (Chesebrough-Ponds USA) Ethylhexyl p-methoxycinnamate, oxybenzone. PABA free. Waterproof. Lot. Bot. 180 mL. *OTC.*
Use: Sunscreen.

Vaseline Intensive Care Sport Sunblock. (Chesebrough-Ponds USA) Ethylhexyl p-methoxycinnamate, oxybenzone, C12-15 alkyl benzoate, aloe vera gel, vitamin E, EDTA. Lot. Bot. 118 mL. *OTC.*
Use: Sunscreen.

Vaseline Intensive Care Sunblock. (Chesebrough-Ponds USA) Ethylhexyl p-methoxycinnamate, oxybenzone, 2-ethylhexyl salicylate. PABA free. Waterproof. SPF 4: Lot. Bot. 180 mL; SPF 8: Lot. Bot. 120 mL, 180 mL; SPF 15: Lot. Bot. 120 mL, 180 mL; SPF 25: Lot. Bot. 120 mL, 180 mL. *OTC.*
Use: Sunscreen.

Vaseline Intensive Care Ultra Violet Daily Defense. (Chesebrough-Ponds USA) Ethylhexyl p-methoxycinnamate, oxybenzone, vitamin E, cetyl alcohol, acetylated lanolin, alcohol, parabens, EDTA. SPF 15. Lot. Bot. 118 mL. *OTC.*
Use: Sunscreen.

Vaseline Pure Petroleum Jelly Skin Protectant. (Chesebrough-Ponds USA) White petrolatum. Tube 1 oz, 2.5 oz. Jar 1.75 oz, 3.75 oz, 7.75 oz, 13 oz. *OTC.*
Use: Dermatologic; counterirritant.

Vaseretic. (Valeant) Enalapril maleate/hydrochlorothiazide 10 mg/25 mg. Lactose. Tab. 100s. *Rx.*
Use: Antihypertensive.

Vasimid.
See: Tolazoline Hydrochloride.

vasoactive intestinal polypeptide. (Research Triangle Pharmaceuticals)
Use: Treatment of acute esophageal food impaction. [Orphan Drug]

Vasoderm. (Taro) Fluocinonide 0.05%, anhydrous glycerin base. Cream. Tube 15 g, 30 g, 60 g. *Rx.*
Use: Corticosteroid, topical.

Vasoderm-E. (Taro) Fluocinonide 0.05%, emollient mineral oil and white petrolatum base. Cream. Tube 15 g, 30 g, 60 g, 120 g. *Rx.*
Use: Corticosteroid, topical.

Vasodilan. (Mead Johnson) Isoxsuprine hydrochloride 10 mg, 20 mg. Tab. 100s, 1000s, UD 100s (10 mg only). *Rx.*
Use: Vasodilator.

vasodilator combinations.
See: Isosorbide Dinitrate/Hydralazine Hydrochloride.

vasodilator combinations, peripheral.
See: Lipo-Nicin.

vasodilators.
See: Amyl Nitrite.
Endothelin Receptor Antagonists.
Human B-Type Natriuretic Peptides.
Nitrates.
Prostacyclin Analog.
Vasodilator Combinations.
Vasodilator Combinations, Peripheral.
Vasodilators, Peripheral.

vasodilators, coronary.
See: Glyceryl Trinitrate.
Isordil.
Khellin.
Papaverine Hydrochloride.
Pentaerythritol Tetranitrate.
Peritrate.

vasodilators, peripheral.
See: Epoprostenol Sodium.
Ethaverine Hydrochloride.
Hydralazine Hydrochloride.
Isoxsuprine Hydrochloride.
Minoxidil.
Papaverine Hydrochloride.
Treprostinil Sodium.
Vasodilator Combinations, Peripheral.

Vasoflo. (Roberts) Papaverine hydrochloride 150 mg. Cap. Bot. 100s. *Rx.*
Use: Vasodilator.

Vasolate. (Parmed Pharmaceuticals, Inc.) Pentaerythritol tetranitrate 30 mg.

Cap. Bot. 100s, 1000s. *Rx.*
Use: Antianginal.
Vasolate-80. (Parmed Pharmaceuticals, Inc.) Pentaerythritol tetranitrate 80 mg. Cap. Bot. 100s, 1000s. *Rx.*
Use: Antianginal.
Vasolex. (Stratus) Balsam peru 87 mg, castor oil 788 mg, trypsin 90 units. White petrolatum. Oint. 5 g, 60 g. *Rx.*
Use: Dermatologic, enzyme preparation.
•**vasopressin.** (VAY-so-PRESS-in) *USP 34.*
Use: Posterior pituitary hormone.
See: Pitressin Synthetic.
vasopressin. (Various Mfr.) Vasopressin 20 pressor units/mL. Chlorobutanol 0.5%. Inj. Vial. 0.5 mL, 1 mL, 10 mL. *Rx.*
Use: Posterior pituitary hormone.
vasopressin receptor antagonist.
See: Conivaptan Hydrochloride.
Tolvaptan.
vasopressors.
See: Dobutamine.
Dobutamine Hydrochloride in 5% Dextrose Injection.
Dopamine Hydrochloride.
Ephedrine.
Epinephrine.
Isoproterenol Hydrochloride.
Metaraminol.
Midodrine Hydrochloride.
Norepinephrine Bitartrate.
Phenylephrine Hydrochloride.
Vasotec. (Biovail) Enalapril maleate 2.5 mg, 5 mg, 10 mg, 20 mg. Lactose. Tab. Bot. 100s, 1000s, 10,000s, unit-of-use 90s, UD 100s. *Rx.*
Use: Renin angiotensin system antagonist, angiotensin-converting enzyme inhibitor.
Vasotus. (Sheryl) Codeine phosphate ⅛ g, phenylephrine hydrochloride, prophenpyridamine maleate. Liq. Bot. 473 mL. *c-v.*
Use: Antihistamine, antitussive, decongestant.
Vaxsyn HIV-1. (MicroGeneSys) T-Lymphotropic Virus Type III GP 160 Antigen.
Use: AIDS. [Orphan Drug]
VaZol. (WraSer) Brompheniramine tannate 2 mg/5 mL. Bubble gum flavor. Liq. 472 mL. *Rx.*
Use: Antihistamine.
VaZol-D. (WraSer) Phenylephrine hydrochloride 7.5 mg, brompheniramine maleate 4 mg per 5 mL. Maltitol, saccharin, sorbitol. Bubble gum flavor. Liq. 474 mL. *Rx.*

Use: Upper respiratory combination, decongestant and antihistamine combination.
Vazosan. (Sandia) Papaverine hydrochloride 150 mg. Tab. Bot. 100s, 1000s. *Rx.*
Use: Vasodilator.
Vazotab. (Wraser Pharmaceuticals) Brompheniramine maleate 6 mg, phenylephrine hydrochloride 15 mg. Mannitol, saccharin, sucrose. Grape flavor. Chew. Tab. 60s. *Rx.*
Use: Upper respiratory combination, decongestant and antihistamine combination.
Vazotan. (Gentex Pharma) Phenylephrine hydrochloride 10 mg, brompheniramine maleate 6 mg, carbetapentane citrate 25 mg per 5 mL. Methylparaben, phenylalanine 8.419 mg/5 mL. Bubble gum flavor. Oral Susp. 120 mL. *Rx.*
Use: Antitussive combination.
Vazotan Tannate. (WraSer) Carbetapentane citrate 25 mg (as carbetapentane tannate 50 mg), brompheniramine maleate 6 mg (brompheniramine tannate 12 mg), phenylephrine hydrochloride 10 mg (as phenylephrine tannate 2 mg). Acesulfame K, aspartame, methylparaben, phenylalanine 8.419 mg/5 mL. Bubble gum flavor. Susp. 118 mL. *Rx.*
Use: Upper respiratory combination, antitussive combination.
VCF. (Apothecus) Contraceptive film: nonoxynol-9 28%, glycerin, and polyvinyl alcohol. Pkg. 3s, 6s, 12s. *OTC.*
Use: Contraceptive; spermicide.
V-Cillin K. (Eli Lilly) Penicillin V potassium 125 mg, 250 mg, 500 mg. Tab. **125 mg:** Bot. 100s. **250 mg:** Bot. 100s, 500s. **500 mg:** Bot. 24s, 100s, 500s. *Rx.*
Use: Anti-infective; penicillin.
V-Cillin K for Oral Solution. (Eli Lilly) Penicillin V potassium 125 mg, 250 mg/5 mL. **125 mg:** Bot. 100 mL, 150 mL, 200 mL, UD 5 mL. **250 mg:** Bot. 100 mL, 150 mL, 200 mL. *Rx.*
Use: Anti-infective; penicillin.
V-Cof. (Macoven Pharmaceuticals) Brompheniramine maleate 6 mg, carbetapentane citrate 25 mg, phenylephrine hydrochloride 10 mg per 5 mL. Acesulfame, aspartame, glycerin, methylparaben, sodium benzoate. Bubble gum flavor. Susp. 118 mL. *Rx.*
Use: Upper respiratory combination, antitussive combination.

V-Dec-M. (Seatrace) Pseudoephedrine hydrochloride 120 mg, guaifenesin 500 mg. SR Tab. Bot. 12s, 100s. *Rx.*
Use: Upper respiratory combination; decongestant, expectorant.

VDRL Antigen. (Laboratory Diagnostics) VDRL antigen with buffered saline. Blood test in diagnosis of syphilis. **Vial:** Sufficient for 500 tests. **Amp.:** 10 × 0.5 mL sufficient for 500 tests.
Use: Diagnostic aid.

VDRL Slide Test. (Laboratory Diagnostics) VDRL antigen. Slide flocculation and spinal fluid test for syphilis. Vial 5 mL Complete kit, reactive control, nonreactive control, 5 mL.
Use: Diagnostic aid.

Vectibix. (Amgen) Panitumumab 20 mg/mL. Preservative free. Sodium acetate, sodium chloride. Soln. for Inj. Single-use vials. 5 mL, 10 mL, 20 mL. *Rx.*
Use: Monoclonal antibody.

Vectical. (Galderma) Calcitriol 0.0003%. Mineral oil, white petrolatum. Oint. Tube. 5 g, 100 g. *Rx.*
Use: Antipsoriatic agent.

Vectrin. (Warner Chilcott) Minocycline 50 mg, 100 mg. Cap. Bot. 50s (100 mg only), 100s (50 mg only), 1000s. *Rx.*
Use: Anti-infective.

• **vecuronium bromide.** (veh-CUE-row-nee-uhm) *USP 34.*
Use: Neuromuscular blocker.

vecuronium bromide. (Marsam) Vecuronium bromide 10 mg, 20 mg. Inj. Vial 10 mL (with and without diluent), 20 mL (without diluent). *Rx.*
Use: Neuromuscular blocker.

vecuronium bromide. (Various Mfr.) Vecuronium bromide 10 mg, 20 mg. May contain mannitol. Pow. for Inj. Vials. 10 mL (10 mg only), 20 mL (20 mg only). *Rx.*
Use: Neuromuscular blocker.

• **vedolizumab.** (VE-doe-LIZ-ue-mab) USAN.
Use: Immunomodulator.

• **vedotin.** (ve-DOE-tin) USAN.
Use: Antineoplastic.

VE-400. (Western Research) Vitamin E 400 units. Cap. Bot. 1008s. *OTC.*
Use: Vitamin supplement.

• **vegetable oil, hydrogenated.** *NF 29.*
Use: Pharmaceutical aid (tablet/capsule lubricant).

vehicle/n and vehicle/n mild. (Neutrogena) Topical vehicle system for compounding. *Appliderm* Applicator Bot. oz. *OTC.*
Use: Pharmaceutical aid.

velacycline.
Use: Anti-infective; tetracycline.

• **velafermin.** (VEL-a-FER-min) USAN.
Use: Mucositis.

• **velaglucerase alfa.** (VEL-a-GLOO-ser-ase) USAN.
Use: Endocrine and metabolic agent.
See: VPRIV.

Velban. (Lilly) Vinblastine sulfate 10 mg. Pow. for Inj. Vial. *Rx.*
Use: Antineoplastic.

Velcade. (Millenium) Bortezomib 3.5 mg. Mannitol 35 mg. Preservative free. Pow. for Inj., lyophilized. Single-dose vials. *Rx.*
Use: Proteasome inhibitor.

• **veliflapon.** (VEL-i-FLAP-on) USAN.
Use: Cardiovascular agent.

• **veliparib.** (veli-PAR-ib) USAN.
Use: Antineoplastic.

Velivet. (Barr) **Phase 1:** Desogestrel 0.1 mg, ethinyl estradiol 25 mcg. 7 tabs. **Phase 2:** Desogestrel 0.125 mg, ethinyl estradiol 25 mcg. 7 tabs. **Phase 3:** Desogestrel 0.15 mg, ethinyl estradiol 25 mcg. 7 tabs. Tab. 28s with 7 inert tabs. *Rx.*
Use: Sex hormone, contraceptive hormone.

• **velnacrine maleate.** (VELL-NAH-kreen) USAN.
Use: Inhibitor (cholinesterase).

• **velneperit.** (vel-NEP-er-it) USAN.
Use: Treatment of clinical obesity.

• **velusetrag.** (vel-u-SET-rag) USAN.
Use: Treatment of constipation.

• **velusetrag hydrochloride.** (vel-u-SET-rag) USAN.
Use: Treatment of constipation.

Velvachol. (Valeant) Hydrophilic ointment base petrolatum, mineral oil, cetyl alcohol, cholesterol, parabens, stearyl alcohol, purified water, sodium lauryl sulfate. Jar lb. *OTC.*
Use: Pharmaceutical aid; ointment base.

• **vemurafenib.** (VEM-ue-RAF-e-nib) USAN.
Use: Antineoplastic.

Venelex. (Stratus) Balsam peru 87 mg, castor oil 788 mg, white petrolatum. Oint. 60 g. *Rx.*
Use: Emollient.

venesetic.
See: Amobarbital Sodium.

venlafaxine. (Upstate Pharma) Venlafaxine 37.5 mg, 75 mg, 150 mg, 225 mg. May contain lactose and mannitol. ER Tab. 30s, 90s. *Rx.*

Use: Antidepressant, serotonin and nor-epinephrine reuptake inhibitor.
• **venlafaxine hydrochloride.** (VEN-lah-fax-EEN) USAN.
Use: Antidepressant.
See: Effexor XR.
venlafaxine hydrochloride. (Various Mfr.) Venlafaxine. **Tab.:** 25 mg, 37.5 mg, 50 mg, 75 mg, 100 mg. May contain lactose, mannitol, PEG. 30s, 60s, 90s, 100s, 500s, 1,000s, UD 100s **ER Cap.:** 37.5 mg, 75 mg, 150 mg. May contain sugar spheres. 30s, 90s. *Rx.*
Use: Antidepressant.
Venofer. (Fresenius) Elemental iron 20 mg/mL, preservative free, sucrose 300 mg/mL w/v. Inj. Single-dose Vial 5 mL. *Rx.*
Use: Trace element.
Venomil. (Bayer Consumer Care) Freeze-dried venom or venom protein. Vials of 12 mcg or 120 mcg for honey bee, white-faced hornet, yellow hornet, yellow jacket, or wasp. Vials of 36 mcg or 360 mcg for mixed vespids (white-faced hornet, yellow hornet, yellow jacket). Diagnostic 1 mcg/mL. Maintenance 100 mcg/mL. Individual patient kit. *Rx.*
Use: Antivenin.
Venstat. (Seatrace) Brompheniramine maleate 10 mg/mL. Vial 10 mL. *Rx.*
Use: Antihistamine.
Ventavis. (CoTherix) Iloprost 10 mcg/mL, 20 mcg/mL. Ethanol 0.81 mg (10 mcg/mL), 1.62 mg (20 mcg/mL). Preservative free. Soln. for Inh. Single-dose ampules. 1 mL. *Rx.*
Use: Treatment of pulmonary hypertension.
Ventolin. (GlaxoSmithKline) Albuterol. **Syr.:** Albuterol sulfate 2 mg/5 mL, saccharin, strawberry flavor. Bot. 480 mL. **Tab.:** Albuterol sulfate 2 mg, 4 mg. Bot. 100s, 500s. *Rx.*
Use: Bronchodilator, sympathomimetic.
Ventolin HFA. (GlaxoSmithKline) Albuterol sulfate 90 mcg/actuation. Aerosol. Can. 18 g (200 inhalations). Contains no chlorofluorocarbons. *Rx.*
Use: Bronchodilator, sympathomimetic.
Ventolin Inhalation Solution. (GlaxoSmithKline) Albuterol sulfate 0.5%. Bot. 20 mL w/calibrated dropper. *Rx.*
Use: Bronchodilator.
Ventolin Nebules. (GlaxoSmithKline) Albuterol sulfate 0.083%, sulfuric acid. Soln. for Inh. In 3 mL unit-dose nebules. *Rx.*
Use: Bronchodilator.

Ventolin Rotacaps. (GlaxoSmithKline) Microfine albuterol sulfate 200 mg, lactose. Cap. for Inh. Bot. 100s, UD 24s. For use with the *Rotahaler* inhalation device. *Rx.*
Use: Bronchodilator.
• **veradoline hydrochloride.** (VEER-aid-OLE-een) USAN.
Use: Analgesic.
Veramyst. (GlaxoSmithKline) Fluticasone furoate 27.5 mcg/actuation. Dextrose 0.015% w/w benzalkonium chloride, polysorbate 80, EDTA. Spray, Susp. Intranasal. 10 g (120 actuations) brown glass bottles with metering atomizing pump and nasal adaptor. *Rx.*
Use: Intranasal steroid, respiratory inhalant.
• **verapamil.** (veh-RAP-ah-mill) USAN.
Use: Vasodilator (coronary).
• **verapamil hydrochloride.** (veh-RAP-ah-mill) *USP 34.*
Use: Antianginal, antiarrhythmic, antihypertensive, calcium channel blocker.
See: Calan SR.
Covera-HS.
Isoptin SR.
Verelan.
Verelan PM.
W/Trandolapril.
See: Tarka.
verapamil hydrochloride. (Various Mfr.) Verapamil hydrochloride. **40 mg. Tab.:** May contain lactose. Bot. 30s, 100s, 500s, 1000s. **80 mg, 120 mg. Tab.:** May contain lactose. 100s, 250s, 500s, 1000s, 4000s (120 mg only), 7000s (80 mg only), UD 100s. **2.5 mg/mL. Inj.:** May contain sodium chloride. 2 mL, 4 mL vials, amps, and syringes; single-use 2 mL fills; *Carpuject* syringe 2 mL; 2 mL fill in single-use 2 mL *Carpuject Interlink* syringe. **ER Cap.:** 100 mg, 200 mg, 300 mg. May contain maltodextrin, sugar spheres. 30s, 100s, 500s. *Rx.*
Use: Antianginal; antiarrhythmic; antihypertensive; calcium channel blocker.
verapamil hydrochloride extended release. (Various Mfr.) Verapamil hydrochloride. **ER Cap.:** 120 mg, 180 mg, 240 mg. May be pellet-filled. May contain sugar. Bot. 100s, 500s, UD 100s. **ER Tab.:** 120 mg, 180 mg, 240 mg. 100s, 500s. *Rx.*
Use: Antianginal; antiarrhythmic; antihypertensive; calcium channel blocker.
verapamil hydrochloride extended release. (Watson) Verapamil hydrochlo-

ride 360 mg. Pellet-filled. ER Cap. 100s. *Rx.*
Use: Calcium channel blocker.

verapamil hydrochloride SR. (Schein) Verapamil hydrochloride 120 mg, 180 mg, 240 mg, 360 mg, parabens. SR Cap. Bot. 100s. *Rx.*
Use: Antianginal; antiarrythmic; antihypertensive.

Verazeptol. (Femco) Chlorothymol, eucalyptol, menthol, phenol, boric acid, zinc sulfate. Pow. Bot. 3 oz, 6 oz, 10 oz. *OTC.*
Use: Vaginal agent.

Verazinc. (Forest) Zinc sulfate 220 mg. Cap. Bot. 100s, 1000s. *OTC.*
Use: Mineral supplement.

Verdeso. (GlaxoSmithKline) Desonide 0.05%. Cetyl alcohol, light mineral oil, white petrolatum. Foam. 100 g. *Rx.*
Use: Topical corticosteroid, antiinflammatory agent.

Veregen. (Doak Dermatologics) Kunecatechins 15%. Gallic acid, caffeine, and theobromine constitute ≈ 2.5% of the product. Isopropyl myristate, oleyl alcohol. Oint. Tube. 15 g. *Rx.*
Use: Catechin, treatment of external genital and perianal warts.

Verelan. (Schwarz Pharma) Verapamil hydrochloride 120 mg, 180 mg, 240 mg, 360 mg. Sugar, parabens. Pellet-filled. ER Cap. Bot. 100s. *Rx.*
Use: Calcium channel blocker.

Verelan PM. (Schwarz Pharma) Verapamil hydrochloride 100 mg, 200 mg, 300 mg. Sugar. Pellet-filled. ER Cap. Bot. 100s. *Rx.*
Use: Calcium channel blocker.

Vergo. (Daywell Laboratories, Inc.) Calcium pantothenate 8%, ascorbic acid 2%, starch. Oint. Tube 0.5 oz. *Rx.*
Use: Keratolytic.

•**verilopam hydrochloride.** (veh-RILL-OH-pam) USAN.
Use: Analgesic.

Veripred 20. (Hawthorn Pharmaceuticals) Prednisolone 20 mg per 5 mL. Equiv. to prednisolone sodium phosphate 26.9 mg. Corn syrup, edetate disodium, methylparaben, saccharin. Grape flavor. Soln., Oral. 237 mL. *Rx.*
Use: Adrenocortical steroid, glucocorticoid.

•**verlukast.** (ver-LOO-kast) USAN.
Use: Antiasthmatic (leukotriene antagonist).

Verluma. (NeoRx; DuPont) Nofetumomab merpentan 10 mg for conjugation w/technetium 99m. Kit. *Rx.*
Use: Radioimmunoscintigraphy agent.

Vermox. (Janssen) Mebendazole 100 mg. Tab. Box 12s. *Rx.*
Use: Anthelmintic.

vernamycins. Under study.
Use: Anti-infective.

vernolepin. A sesquiterpene dilactone. Under study.
Use: Antineoplastic.

•**verofylline.** (VER-OH-fill-in) USAN.
Use: Antiasthmatic; bronchodilator.

veronal sodium.
See: Barbital Sodium.

•**verpasep caltespen.** (VER-pa-sep kal-TES-pen) USAN.
Use: Human papillomavirus.

Versa Alcohol Base. (Humco) Aloe, ethylhexylglycerin, SD alcohol 40, polyacrylamide, laureth-7, phenoxyethanol. Fragrance, oil, and dye free. Gel. 1 lb, 10 lb, 20 lb, 40 lb. *OTC.*
Use: Ointment and lotion base.

Versa Aqua Base. (Humco) DMDM hydantoin, iodoproyl butylcarbamate, PEG-18 palmitate, PPG-18 butyl ether, propylene glycol, SD alcohol 40, triethanolamine. Fragrance and dye free. Gel. 1 lb, 10 lb, 20 lb, 40 lb. *OTC.*
Use: Ointment and lotion base.

Versacaps. (Seatrace) Pseudoephedrine hydrochloride 60 mg, guaifenesin 300 mg, benzyl alcohol, EDTA, parabens, sucrose. SR. Cap. Bot. 100s. *Rx.*
Use: Upper respiratory combination; decongestant, expectorant.

Versa HRT Base Botanical. (Humco) Almond, aloe, carbomer, cetyl alcohol, folic acid, glycerin, glyceryl stearate, grape, MSM, PEG-100 stearate, phenoxyethanol, primrose, red clover, salicylic acid, selenium, stearic acid, triethanolamine, wheat, and vitamins A,C,D, and E. Cream. 1 lb, 10 lb, 20 lb, 40 lb. *OTC.*
Use: Ointment and lotion base.

Versa HRT Base Heavy. (Humco) Almond, C12–15 alkyl benzoate, caprylic/capric triglyceride, carbomer, cetyl alcohol, dimethicone, glyceryl stearate, olive, PEG-100 stearate, propylene glycol, stearic acid, triethanolamine, wheat, and vitamins A and E. Cream. 1 lb, 10 lb, 20 lb, 40 lb. *OTC.*
Use: Ointment and lotion base.

Versa HRT Base Natural. (Humco) Almond, carbomer, cetyl alcohol, glycerin, glyceryl stearate, PEG-100 stearate, phenoxyethanol, salicylic acid, stearic acid, triethanolamine, wheat, and vitamins A, C, and E. Cream. 1 lb, 10 lb, 20 lb, 40 lb. *OTC.*
Use: Ointment and lotion base.

Versal. (Suppositoria Laboratories, Inc.) Bismuth subgallate, balsam peru, zinc oxide, benzyl benzoate. Supp. Box 12s, 100s, 1000s. *OTC.*
Use: Anorectal preparation.

Versa LipoBase Heavy. (Humco) Ceteareth-12, ceteareth-20, cetearyl alcohol, cetearyl isononanoate, cetyl palmitate, glycerin, glyceryl stearate, lecithin, honeysuckle, perilla, polyquaternium-37, PPG-1, trideceth-7, propylene glycol dicaprylate/dicaprate, tea tree, vitamin E. Water and oil soluble. Cream. 1 lb, 10 lb, 20 lb, 40 lb. *OTC.*
Use: Ointment and lotion base.

Versa LipoBase Regular. (Humco) Almond, aloe, C12-15 alkyl benzoate, cetearyl alcohol, cetearyl glucoside, cetyl alcohol, dimethicone, glycerin, glyceryl stearate, grape, hydroxymethylglycinate, lecithin, perilla, phenoxyethanol, polyacrylamide, silicate, wheat, xanthan, and vitamins A, C, and E. Water and oil soluble. Cream. 1 lb, 10 lb, 20 lb, 40 lb. *OTC.*
Use: Ointment and lotion base.

Versa PLO20. (Humco) Isopropyl palmitate, pluronic lecithin 20%, poloxamer 407. Gel. In flowable (with SD alcohol 40) and regular. 1 lb. *OTC.*
Use: Ointment and lotion base.

Versa VaniBase. (Humco) Caprylic/capric triglyceride, ceteareth-20, cetearyl alcohol, dimethicone, ethylhexylglycerin, glyceryl stearate, isopropyl palmitate, octydodecanol, PEG-100 stearate, phenoxyethanol, propylene glycol, triethanolamine. Fragrance and dye free. Cream. 1 lb. *OTC.*
Use: Ointment and lotion base.

versenate, calcium disodium.
See: Calcium Disodium Versenate.

versenate disodium.
See: Disodium Versenate.

•**versetamide.** (ver-SET-ah-mide) USAN.
Use: Pharmaceutical aid.

Versiclear. (Hope) Sodium thiosulfate 25%, salicylic acid 1%, isopropyl alcohol 10%, propylene glycol, menthol, EDTA. Lot. 120 mL. *Rx.*
Use: Anti-infective, topical.

versidyne.
Use: Analgesic.

Verstran. (Parke-Davis) Prazepam.
Use: Anxiolytic.

•**verteporfin.** (ver-teh-PORE-fin) USAN.
Use: Antineoplastic; ophthalmic phototherapy.
See: Visudyne.

•**verubulin.** (VER-ue-BUE-lin) USAN.
Use: Antineoplastic.

•**verubulin hydrochloride.** (VER-ue-BUE-lin) USAN.
Use: Antineoplastic.

•**verucerfont.** (VER-ue-SER-font) USAN.
Use: CNS agent.

Verukan-20. (Syosset Laboratories Co., Inc.) Salicylic acid 16.7%, lactic acid in flexible collodion 16.7%. Bot. 15 mL. *OTC.*
Use: Keratolytic.

Verv Alertness. (A.P.C.) Caffeine 200 mg. Cap. Vial 15s. *OTC.*
Use: CNS stimulant.

VESIcare. (Astellas) Solifenacin succinate 5 mg, 10 mg. Film-coated. Tab. 30s, 90s, UD 100s. *Rx.*
Use: Anticholinergic.

•**vesnarinone.** (VESS-nah-rih-NOHN) USAN.
Use: Cardiovascular agent.

•**vestipitant mesylate.** (ves-tee-PIT-ant) USAN.
Use: CNS agent.

Vexol. (Alcon) Rimexolone 1%. Benzalkonium chloride 0.01%, polysorbate 80, EDTA, sodium chloride. Ophth. Susp. *Drop-Tainers.* 5 mL, 10 mL. *Rx.*
Use: Corticosteroid, ophthalmic.

Vfend. (Roerig) Voriconazole. **Tab.:** 50 mg, 200 mg. Lactose. Film-coated. Bot. 30s. **Pow. for Inj., lyophilized:** 200 mg, sulfobutyl ether beta-cyclodextrin sodium 3200 mg. Preservative free. Single-use vials. **Pow. for Oral Susp.:** 45 g (40 mg/mL after reconstitution). Sodium benzoate, sucrose. Orange flavor. 100 mL w/5 mL oral dispenser. *Rx.*
Use: Antifungal.

Viacaps. (Manne) Vitamins A (soluble) 45,000 units, C 500 mg. Cap. Bot. 60s, 120s, 1000s. *OTC.*
Use: Vitamin supplement.

Viactiv Multi-Vitamin Flavor Glides. (McNeil Nutritionals) Biotin 30 mcg, calcium 200 mg, chromium 12 mcg, copper 2 mg, iodine 38 mcg, iron 18 mg, lutein 250 mg, magnesium 40 mg, manganese 2 mg, molybdenum 75 mcg, pantothenic acid 10 mg, potassium 40 mg, selenium 55 mcg, vitamin A 2,500 units, vitamin B_1 1.5 mg, vitamin B_2 1.7 mg, vitamin B_3 15 mg, vitamin B_6 2 mg, folic acid 400 mcg, vitamin B_{12} 6 mcg, vitamin C 60 mg, vitamin D 400 units, vitamin E 33 units, vitamin K 20 mcg, zinc 15 mg. Glucose, maltodextrin, polydextrose, sucralose. Berry flavor. Tab. 50s. *OTC.*
Use: Nutritional supplement.

Viagra. (Pfizer) Sildenafil citrate 25 mg, 50 mg, 100 mg (except 25 mg), lactose. Film-coated. Tab. Bot. 30s, 100s. *Rx.*
Use: Anti-impotence.

Vianain. (Genzyme) Ananain, comosain. *Use:* Burn treatment. [Orphan Drug]

Vi antigen.
Use: Immunization.
See: Typhim Vi.

Vibativ. (Astellas) Telavancin 250 mg, 750 mg. Hydroxypropyl-beta-cyclodextrin 2,500 mg (250 mg), 7,500 mg (750 mg), mannitol 312.5 (250 mg), 937.5 mg (750 mg). Preservative free. Inj., lyophilized Pow. for Soln. Single-dose vial. *Rx.*
Use: Anti-infective agent, lipoglycopeptide.

vibesate. Polvinate 9.3%, molrosinol 3.1% with propellant.

Vibramycin. (Pfizer) **Cap.:** Doxycycline hyclate 100 mg. Bot. 50s. **Pow. for Oral Susp.:** Doxycycline monohydrate 25 mg/5 mL. Parabens, sucrose. Raspberry flavor. Bot. 60 mL. **Syrup:** Doxycycline calcium 50 mg/5 mL. Parabens, sodium metabisulfite, sorbitol. Apple-raspberry flavor. Bot. 473 mL. *Rx.*
Use: Anti-infective; tetracycline.

Vibramycin IV. (Pfizer) Doxycycline (as hyclate) 200 mg. Powder for Inj. Vial. *Rx.*
Use: Anti-infective; tetracycline.

Vibra-Tabs. (Pfizer) Doxycycline hyclate 100 mg. Film-coated. Tab. Bot. 50s. *Rx.*
Use: Anti-infective; tetracycline.

Vicam IV. (Keene Pharmaceuticals) Vitamins B_1 50 mg, B_2 5 mg, B_{12} 1000 mcg, B_6 5 mg, dexpanthenol 6 mg, niacinamide 125 mg, C 50 mg/mL, benzyl alcohol 1% as preservative in water for injection. Vial, multiple-dose. *Rx.*
Use: Nutritional supplement; parenteral.

Vicks Children's NyQuil Cold & Cough Relief. (Procter & Gamble) Dextromethorphan HBr 5 mg, chlorpheniramine maleate 0.67 mg per 5 mL. Alcohol free. Sucrose, sodium 23.7 mg/5 mL. Liq. 118 mL. *OTC.*
Use: Upper respiratory combination; antitussive combination.

Vicks Cough Drops. (Procter & Gamble) **Menthol flavor:** Menthol 3.3 mg. Eucalyptus oil, corn syrup, sucrose. **Cherry flavor:** Menthol 1.7 mg. Eucalyptus oil, corn syrup, sucrose, citric acid. Loz. Pkg. 20s. *OTC.*
Use: Mouth and throat preparation.

Vicks DayQuil Mucus Control. (Proctor & Gamble) Guaifenesin 66.7 mg per 5 mL. Corn syrup, propylene glycol, saccharin, sodium benzoate, sodium 8.3 mg. Liq. 295 mL. *OTC.*
Use: Respiratory agent, expectorant.

Vicks DayQuil Multi-Symptom Cold/Flu Relief. (Procter & Gamble) **Liq.:** Dextromethorphan HBr 3.33 mg, phenylephrine hydrochloride 1.67 mg, acetaminophen 108.33 mg per 5 mL. Alcohol free. Disodium EDTA, glycerin, propylene glycol, saccharin, sodium 50 mg, sorbitol, sucralose. Original and cherry flavors. Liq. 177 mL, 295 mL. **Liquid-filled Cap.:** Dextromethorphan HBr 10 mg, phenylephrine hydrochloride 5 mg, acetaminophen 325 mg. Sorbitol. 12s, 20s. *OTC.*
Use: Upper respiratory combination, antitussive combination.

Vicks DayQuil Sinex. (Proctor & Gamble) Acetaminophen 325 mg, phenylephrine hydrochloride 5 mg. Glycerin, PEG, sorbitol. Cap., liquid filled. 20s. *OTC.*
Use: Upper respiratory combination, decongestant and analgesic combination.

Vicks Formula 44D Cough & Head Congestion Relief. (Procter & Gamble) Dextromethorphan HBr 6.67 mg, phenylephrine hydrochloride 3.33 mg per 5 mL. Alcohol, saccharin, sorbitol, sucrose, sodium 11 mg/5 mL. Liq. 118 mL, 236 mL. *OTC.*
Use: Upper respiratory combination; antitussive combination.

Vicks Formula 44E Cough & Chest Congestion Relief. (Procter & Gamble) Dextromethorphan HBr 6.67 mg, guaifenesin 66.7 mg/5 mL. Alcohol, corn syrup, saccharin. Liq. Bot. 118 mL, 236 mL. *OTC.*
Use: Upper respiratory combination; antitussive with expectorant.

Vicks Formula 44e Pediatric Cough & Chest Congestion Relief. (Procter & Gamble) Dextromethorphan HBr 3.3 mg, guaifenesin 33.3 mg/5 mL. Corn syrup, saccharin, sodium 27 mg/15 mL. Alcohol free. Cherry flavor. Syrup. 118 mL. *OTC.*
Use: Upper respiratory combination, antitussive with expectorant.

Vicks Formula 44M Cough, Cold & Flu Relief. (Procter & Gamble) Dextromethorphan HBr 7.5 mg, chlorpheniramine maleate 1 mg, acetaminophen 162.5 mg per 5 mL. Alcohol 10%, corn syrup, saccharin, sodium 9.3 mg/5 mL.

Liq. 236 mL. *OTC.*
Use: Upper respiratory combination; antitussive combination.

Vicks Formula 44m Pediatric Cough & Cold Relief. (Procter & Gamble) Chlorpheniramine maleate 0.67 mg, dextromethorphan HBr 5 mg per 5 mL. Corn syrup, saccharin, sodium 9 mg/5 mL. Liq. 118 mL. *OTC.*
Use: Upper respiratory combination, antitussive combination.

Vicks 44 Cough Relief. (Procter & Gamble) Dextromethorphan hydrobromide 10 mg/5 mL. Sodium 28 mg/15 mL, alcohol, corn syrup, saccharin. Liq. Bot. 118 mL. *OTC.*
Use: Nonnarcotic antitussive.

Vicks NyQuil Cold/Flu Relief. (Procter & Gamble) **Liq.:** Dextromethorphan HBr 5 mg, doxylamine succinate 2.08 mg, acetaminophen 166.67 mg per 5 mL. Alcohol 10%, corn syrup, saccharin, sodium 6 mg/5 mL. Regular and cherry flavors. Liq. 180 mL, 300 mL, 420 mL. **Liquid-filled Cap.:** Dextromethorphan HBr 15 mg, doxylamine succinate 6.25 mg, acetaminophen 325 mg. Sorbitol. 12s, 20s. *OTC.*
Use: Upper respiratory combination; antitussive combination.

Vicks NyQuil Cough. (Procter & Gamble) Dextromethorphan HBr 5 mg, doxylamine succinate 2.08 mg per 5 mL. Alcohol, corn syrup, saccharin, sodium 6 mg/5 mL. Liq. 177 mL, 295 mL. *OTC.*
Use: Upper respiratory combination; antitussive combination.

Vicks NyQuil Sinex. (Proctor & Gamble) Acetaminophen 325 mg, doxylamine succinate 6.25 mg, phenylephrine hydrochloride 5 mg. Glycerin, PEG, sorbitol. Cap., liquid filled. 20s. *OTC.*
Use: Upper respiratory combination; decongestant, antihistamine, and analgesic combination.

Vicks NyQuil Sinus. (Procter & Gamble) Phenylephrine hydrochloride 5 mg, doxylamine succinate 6.25 mg, acetaminophen 325 mg. Sorbitol. Liquid-filled Cap. 20s. *OTC.*
Use: Upper respiratory combination; decongestant, antihistamine, analgesic.

Vicks Sinex. (Procter & Gamble) Phenylephrine hydrochloride 0.5%, camphor, menthol, eucalyptol, EDTA, benzalkonium chloride, tyloxapol. Soln. Spray Bot. 14.7 mL. *OTC.*
Use: Nasal decongestant, arylalkylamine.

Vicks Sinex 12 Hour. (Procter & Gamble) Oxymetazoline hydrochloride 0.05%, camphor, menthol, eucalyptol, EDTA, benzalkonium chloride, chlorhexidine, gluconate, sodium chloride, tyloxapol. Soln. Spray Bot. 15 mL. *OTC.*
Use: Nasal decongestant, imidazoline.

Vicks Sinex 12 Hour UltraFine Mist for Sinus Relief. (Procter & Gamble) Oxymetazoline hydrochloride 0.05%, aromatic vapors (camphor, eucalyptus, menthol), tyloxapol, disodium EDTA, benzalkonium chloride, sodium chloride. Soln. Spray Bot. 15 mL. *OTC.*
Use: Nasal decongestant, imidazoline.

Vicks Sinex UltraFine Mist for Sinus Relief. (Procter & Gamble) Phenylephrine hydrochloride 0.5%, camphor, benzalkonium chloride, EDTA, eucalyptol, menthol, tyloxapol. Soln. Spray Bot. 15 mL. *OTC.*
Use: Nasal decongestant, arylalkylamine.

Vicks Vapor Inhaler. (Procter & Gamble) Levmetamfetamine 50 mg, menthol, camphor, lavender oil. Inhaler. Single plastic inhaler. *OTC.*
Use: Nasal decongestant, imidazoline.

Vicks VapoRub. (Procter & Gamble) **Oint.:** Camphor 4.8%, menthol 2.6%, eucalyptus oil 1.2%. Cedarleaf oil, nutmeg oil, petrolatum, turpentine oil. 50 g. **Cream:** Camphor 5.2%, menthol 2.8%, eucalyptus oil 1.2%. EDTA, glycerin, cetyl alcohol, parabens, stearyl alcohol, cedarleaf oil, nutmeg oil, turpentine oil. Jar 85 g. *OTC.*
Use: Upper respiratory topical combination.

Vicks VapoSteam. (Procter & Gamble) Eucalyptus oil 1.5%, camphor 6.2%, menthol 3.2%, alcohol 74%, cedar leaf oil, nutmeg oil. Bot. 4 oz, 8 oz. *OTC.*
Use: Antitussive, decongestant.

Vicks Vitamin C Drops. (Procter & Gamble) Vitamin C (as sodium ascorbate and ascorbic acid) 25 mg. Sucrose, corn syrup. Orange flavor. Loz. Pkg. 20s. *OTC.*
Use: Water-soluble vitamin.

Vicodin. (Abbott) Hydrocodone bitartrate 5 mg, acetaminophen 500 mg. Tab. Bot. 100s, 500s, UD 100s. *c-III.*
Use: Analgesic combination; narcotic.

Vicodin ES. (Abbott) Hydrocodone bitartrate 7.5 mg, acetaminophen 750 mg. Tab. Bot. 100s, UD 100s. *c-III.*
Use: Analgesic combination; narcotic.

Vicodin HP. (Abbott) Hydrocodone bitartrate 10 mg, acetaminophen 660 mg. Tab. Bot. 100s, 500s. *c-III.*
Use: Analgesic combination; narcotic.

Vicon Forte. (UCB) Vitamins A 8000 units, E 50 units, C 150 mg, B_3 25 mg, B_1 10 mg, B_5 10 mg, B_2 5 mg, B_6 2 mg, B_{12} 10 mcg, folic acid 1 mg, zinc sulfate 18 mg, Mg, Mn. Lactose. Cap. Bot. 60s, 500s, UD 100s. *Rx.*
Use: Mineral, vitamin supplement.

Vicon Plus. (UCB) Vitamins A 4000 units, E 50 units, C 150 mg, B_3 25 mg, B_1 10 mg, B_5 10 mg, B_2 5 mg, zinc sulfate 18 mg, Mg, Mn, B_6 2 mg. Lactose. Cap. Bot. 60s. *OTC.*
Use: Mineral, vitamin supplement.

Vicoprofen. (Abbott) Hydrocodone bitartrate 7.5 mg, ibuprofen 200 mg. Tab. Bot. 100s, 500s, UD 100s. *c-III.*
Use: Analgesic; narcotic.

•**vicriviroc maleate.** (VI-kri-VIR-ok) USAN.
Use: Antiviral.

Victors. (Procter & Gamble) Special Vicks Medication (menthol, eucalyptus oil) in a soothing Vicks sugar base. Regular or cherry flavor drops. Stick-Pack 10s, Bag 40s. *OTC.*
Use: Anesthetic, local.

Victoza. (Novo Nordisk) Liraglutide 6 mg/mL. Propylene glycol 14 mg, phenol 5.5 mg. Inj., Soln. Prefilled, multidose pen. *Rx.*
Use: Antidiabetic agent, glucagon-like peptide 1 receptor agonist.

Victrelis. (Merck) Boceprevir 200 mg. Cap. 12s. *Rx.*
Use: Anti-infective agent, antiviral agent.

•**vidarabine.** (vih-DAR-ah-BEAN) *USP 34.*
Use: Antiviral.

•**vidarabine sodium phosphate.** (vih-DAR-ah-BEAN) USAN.
Use: Antiviral.

Vi-Daylin ADC Drops. (Ross) Vitamins A 1500 units, C 35 mg, D 400 units/mL. Bot. 30 mL, 50 mL w/dropper. *OTC.*
Use: Vitamin supplement.

Vi-Daylin ADC Vitamin + Iron Drops. (Ross) Vitamins A 1500 units, C 35 mg, D 400 units, Fe 10 mg/mL. Methylparaben. Bot. 50 mL. *OTC.*
Use: Mineral, vitamin supplement.

Vi-Daylin Chewable. (Ross) Vitamins A 2500 units, D 400 units, E 15 units, C 60 mg, folic acid 0.3 mg, B_1 1.05 mg, B_2 1.2 mg, niacin 13.5 mg, B_6 1.05 mg, B_{12} 4.5 mcg. Tab. Bot. 100s. *OTC.*
Use: Vitamin supplement.

Vi-Daylin Chewable w/Fluoride. (Ross) Fluoride 1 mg, vitamins B_1 1.05 mg, B_2 1.2 mg, niacinamide 13.5 mg, B_6 1.05 mg, C 60 mg, A 2500 units, B_{12} 4.5 mcg, E 15 units, folic acid 0.3 mg, D 400 units. Tab. Bot. 100s. *Rx.*
Use: Dental caries agent; mineral, vitamin supplement.

Vi-Daylin Drops. (Ross) Vitamins A 1500 units, D 400 units, E 5 units, C 35 mg, B_1 0.5 mg, B_2 0.6 mg, niacin 8 mg, B_6 0.4 mg, B_{12} 1.5 mcg/mL. Bot. 50 mL. *OTC.*
Use: Vitamin supplement.

Vi-Daylin/F ADC + Iron Drops. (Ross) Vitamins A 1500 units, C 35 mg, D 400 units, Fe 10 mg, fluoride 0.25 mg/mL. Methylparaben. Bot. 50 mL. *Rx.*
Use: Dental caries agent; mineral, vitamin supplement.

Vi-Daylin/F ADC Vitamins Drops. (Ross) Vitamins A 1500 units, D 400 units, C 35 mg, fluoride 0.25 mg/mL. Alcohol ≈ 0.3%, parabens. Bot. 50 mL. *Rx.*
Use: Dental caries agent; vitamin supplement.

Vi-Daylin/F Drops. (Ross) Vitamins A 1500 units, D 400 units, E 5 units, C 35 mg, B_1 0.5 mg, B_2 0.6 mg, B_3 8 mg, B_6 0.4 mg, fluoride 0.25 mg/mL. Methylparaben. Bot. 50 mL. *Rx.*
Use: Dental caries agent; vitamin supplement.

Vi-Daylin/F Multivitamin + Iron. (Ross) Fluoride 0.25 mg, vitamins A 1500 units, D 400 units, E 4.1 mg, B_1 0.5 mg, B_2 0.6 mg, B_3 8 mg, B_6 0.4 mg, C 35 mg, Fe 10 mg/mL. Alcohol < 0.1%, methylparaben. Drops. Bot. 50 mL. *Rx.*
Use: Dental caries agent; mineral, vitamin supplement.

Vi-Daylin Liquid. (Ross) Vitamins A 2500 units, B_1 1.05 mg, B_2 1.2 mg, B_6 1.05 mg, B_{12} 4.5 mcg, C 60 mg, D 400 units, E 20.4 mg (as d-alpha tocopheryl acetate), niacin 13.5 mg/5 mL. Bot. 8 oz, 473 mL. *OTC.*
Use: Vitamin supplement.

Vi-Daylin Multivitamin Drops. (Ross) Vitamins A 1500 units, D 400 units, E 5 mg, B_1 0.5 mg, B_2 0.6 mg, B_3 8 mg, B_6 0.4 mg, B_{12} 1.5 mcg, C 35 mg/mL. Alcohol < 0.5%. Bot. 50 mL. *OTC.*
Use: Vitamin supplement.

Vi-Daylin Multivitamin Liquid. (Ross) Vitamins A 2500 units, D 400 units, E 15 mg, B_1 1.05 mg, B_2 1.2 mg, B_3 13.5 mg, B_6 1.05 mg, B_{12} 4.5 mcg, C 60 mg/5 mL. Alcohol < 0.5%. Bot. 240 mL, 480 mL. *OTC.*
Use: Vitamin supplement.

Vi-Daylin Multivitamin Plus Iron Chewable. (Ross) Vitamins A 2500 units, D 400 units, E 15 mg, C 60 mg, folic acid

0.3 mg, B₁ 1.05 mg, B₂ 1.2 mg, B₃ 13.5 mg, B₆ 1.05 mg, B₁₂ 4.5 mcg, iron 12 mg. Tab. Bot. 100s. *OTC.*
Use: Mineral, vitamin supplement.

Vi-Daylin Multivitamin + Iron Drops. (Ross) Fe 10 mg, vitamins A 1500 units, D 400 units, E 5 mg, B₁ 0.5 mg, B₂ 0.6 mg, B₃ 8 mg, B₆ 0.4 mg, C 35 mg. Alcohol < 0.5%, methylparaben. Bot. 50 mL. *OTC.*
Use: Mineral, vitamin supplement.

Vi-Daylin Multivitamin Plus Iron Liquid. (Ross) Vitamins A 2500 units, D 400 units, C 60 mg, E 15 units, B₁ 1.05 mg, B₂ 1.2 mg, B₃ 13.5 mg, B₆ 1.05 mg, B₁₂ 4.5 mcg, Fe 10 mg/tsp. ≤ 0.5% alcohol, glucose, sucrose, parabens. 237 mL, 473 mL. *OTC.*
Use: Mineral, vitamin supplement.

Vidaza. (Celgene) Azacitidine 100 mg. Mannitol 100 mg. Preservative free. Pow. for Inj., lyophilized. Single-use vials. *Rx.*
Use: DNA demethylation agent.

Videcon. (Vita Elixir) Vitamin D 50,000 units. Cap. *Rx.*
Use: Vitamin supplement.

Vi-Derm Soap. (Arthrins) Extract of Amaryllis 10%. Cake. Pkg. 1s. Bar 3.5 oz. *OTC.*
Use: Dermatologic; cleanser.

Videx. (Bristol-Myers Squibb) Didanosine 2 g, 4 g. Pow. for Oral Soln. 4 oz (2 g), 8 oz (4 g). *Rx.*
Use: Antiretroviral, nucleoside reverse transcriptase inhibitor.

Videx EC. (Bristol-Myers Squibb) Didanosine 125 mg, 200 mg, 250 mg, 400 mg. DR Cap. (with enteric-coated beadlets) 30s. *Rx.*
Use: Antiretroviral, nucleoside reverse transcriptase inhibitor.

• **vidupiprant.** (vye-DUE-pi-prant) USAN.
Use: Treatment of asthma.

• **vifilcon A.** (vie-FILL-kahn A) USAN.
Use: Contact lens material (hydrophilic).

• **vifilcon B.** (vie-FILL-kahn B) USAN.
Use: Contact lens material (hydrophilic).

Vifluorineed. (Hanlon) Vitamins A 5000 units, D 400 units, C 75 mg, B₁ 2 mg, B₂ 3 mg, niacinamide 20 mg, fluoride 1 mg. Chew. Tab. Bot. 100s. *Rx.*
Use: Mineral, vitamin supplement.

• **vigabatrin.** (vie-GAB-at RIN) USAN.
Use: Anticonvulsant (tardive dyskinesia).
See: Sabril.

Vigamox. (Alcon) Moxifloxacin hydrochloride 0.5% (5 mg/mL). Boric acid, sodium chloride, purified water. Soln.

Drop-Tainer 3 mL. *Rx.*
Use: Antibiotic, ophthalmic.

Vigomar Forte. (Marlop) Fe 12 mg, vitamins A 10,000 units, D 400 units, E 15 units, B₁ 10 mg, B₂ 10 mg, B₃ 100 mg, B₅ 20 mg, B₆ 5 mg, B₁₂ 5 mcg, C 200 mg, I, Mg, Mn, Cu, Zn 1.5 mg. Tab. Bot. 100s. *OTC.*
Use: Mineral, vitamin supplement.

Viibryd. (Trovis Pharmaceuticals) Vilazodone hydrochloride 10 mg, 20 mg, 40 mg. Lactose, PEG. Tab. 30s, 90s, 500s, UD 100s. *Rx.*
Use: Selective serotonin reuptake inhibitor, 5-HT₁ₐ receptor agonist.

Viibryd Patient Starter Kit. (Trovis Pharmaceuticals) Vilazodone hydrochloride 10 mg, 20 mg, 40 mg. Lactose, PEG. Tab. UD 30s (30-tablet blister card containing seven 10 mg tablets, seven 20 mg tablets, and sixteen 40 mg tablets). *Rx.*
Use: Selective serotonin reuptake inhibitor, 5-HT₁ₐ receptor agonist.

VIL. (Leas Research)
Use: Hyperphenylalaninemia. [Orphan Drug]

• **vilanterol.** (vye-LAN-ter-ol) USAN.
Use: Respiratory agent.

• **vilanterol trifenatate.** (vye-LAN-ter-ol trye-FEN-a-tate) USAN.
Use: Respiratory agent.

• **vilazodone.** (vil-AZ-oh-done) USAN.
Use: Antidepressant.

• **vilazodone hydrochloride.** (vil-AZ-oh-done) USAN.
Use: Antidepressant.
See: Viibryd.
Viibryd Patient Starter Kit.

• **vildagliptin.** (VIL-da-GLIP-tin) USAN.
Use: Antidiabetic.

Vilex. (Oxypure) Vitamin B₁ 100 mg, riboflavin phosphate sodium 1 mg, B₆ 10 mg, panthenol 5 mg, niacinamide 100 mg/mL. Amp. 30 mL. *Rx.*
Use: Vitamin supplement.

Viliva. (Vita Elixir) Ferrous fumarate 3 g. *OTC.*
Use: Mineral supplement.

ViloFane-Dp. (Seton Pharmaceuticals) L-methylfolate 7.5 mg. Tab. 30s, 90s. *Rx.*
Use: Water-soluble vitamin.

• **viloxazine.** (vih-LOX-ah-zeen) USAN.
Use: Antidepressant.
See: Catatrol.

Viminate. (Various Mfr.) Vitamins B₁ 2.5 mg, B₂ 1.25 mg, B₃ 25 mg, B₅ 5 mg, B₆ 0.5 mg, B₁₂ 0.5 mcg, Fe 7.5 mg, Zn 1 mg, choline, I, Mg, Mn 5 mL. Alco-

hol 18%. Liq. Bot. 480. *OTC.*
Use: Mineral, vitamin supplement.
Vi-Min-for-All. (Barth's) Vitamins A 3 mg,
D 10 mcg, C 120 mg, B₁ 35 mg, B₁₂
15 mcg, biotin, niacin 2.33 mg, E
30 units, B₆, pantothenic acid, Ca
375 mg, P 180 mg, Fe 20 mg, I 0.1 mg,
rutin 10 mg, hesperidin-lemon bioflavonoid complex 10 mg, choline, inositol
2.4 mg, Cu 10 mcg, Mn 2 mg, Zn
110 mcg, silicone 210 mcg. Tab. Bot.
100s, 500s. *OTC.*
Use: Mineral, vitamin supplement.
Vimovo. (AstraZeneca) Naproxen/
esomeprazole 375 mg/20 mg (as
esomeprazole magnesium trihydrate
22.3 mg), 500 mg/20 mg (as esomeprazole magnesium trihydrate 22.3 mg).
Enteric-coated. Glyceryl monostearate,
polydextrose, polyethylene glycol, polysorbate 80, propylparaben. Tab., delayed release. 60s, 500s, UD 100s
(500 mg/20 mg only). *Rx.*
Use: Nonnarcotic analgesic combination.
Vimpat. (Schwarz Pharma) Lacosamide.
Soln., oral: 10 mg/mL. Acesulfame K,
aspartame, glycerin, parabens, PEG,
phenylalanine 0.016 mg/mL, propylene
glycol, sorbitol. Strawberry flavor.
465 mL. **Tab.:** 50 mg, 100 mg, 150 mg,
200 mg. PEG. Film-coated. 60s, 180s.
Inj., Soln.: 10 mg/mL. Single-use glass
vial. 20 mL. *c-v.*
Use: Anticonvulsant.
Vinactane Sulfate. (Novartis) Viomycin
Sulfate.
•**vinafocon A.** (VIE-nah-FOE-kahn A)
USAN.
Use: Contact lens material (hydro-
phobic).
**Vinate Good Start Chewable Prenatal
Formula.** (Breckenridge) Ca 200 mg,
Fe 29 mg, vitamin A 1000 units, D
400 units, E 30 units, B₁ 3 mg, B₂ 3 mg,
B₃ 15 mg, B₅ 7 mg, B₆ 20 mg, B₁₂
12 mcg, C 100 mg, folic acid 1 mg,
Zn 20 mg. Chew. Tab. 100s. *Rx.*
Use: Prenatal vitamin.
Vinate GT. (Breckenridge) Ca 200 mg,
Fe 90 mg, vitamin A 2700 units, D₃
400 units, E 10 units, B₁ 3 mg, B₂
3.4 mg, B₃ 15 mg, B₅ 6 mg, B₆ 20 mg,
B₁₂ 12 mcg, C 120 mg, folic acid 1 mg,
biotin 30 mcg, docusate sodium 50 mg,
Zn 15 mg, Cu, Mg. Tab. UD 90s. *Rx.*
Use: Vitamin supplement.
vinbarbital.
Use: Hypnotic, sedative.
vinbarbital sodium.
Use: Hypnotic, sedative.

•**vinblastine sulfate.** (vin-BLAST-een)
USP 34. Vincaleukoblastine. Alkaloid
extracted from *Vinca rosea* Linn.
Tall Man: vinBLAStine
Use: Antineoplastic.
See: Velban.
vinblastine sulfate. (Various Mfr.) Vin-
blastine sulfate. **Pow. for Inj.:** 10 mg.
Vial. **Inj.:** 1 mg/mL, benzyl alcohol
0.9%. Vial 10 mL, 25 mL. *Rx.*
Use: Antineoplastic.
vinca alkaloids.
Use: Antimitotic agent.
See: Vinblastine Sulfate.
Vincristine Sulfate.
Vinorelbine Tartrate.
**vincaleukoblastine, 22-oxo-sulfate
(1:1) (salt).** Vincristine Sulfate.
Vincasar PFS. (Gensia Sicor) Vincristine
sulfate 1 mg/mL. Vial 1 mL. *Rx.*
Use: Antineoplastic.
•**vincofos.** (VIN-koe-foss) USAN.
Use: Anthelmintic.
•**vincristine sulfate.** (vin-KRISS-teen)
USP 34.
Tall Man: vinCRIStine
Use: Antineoplastic.
See: Oncovin.
Vincasar PFS.
•**vindesine.** (VIN-deh-seen) USAN.
Use: Antineoplastic.
•**vindesine sulfate.** (VIN-deh-seen)
USAN.
Use: Antineoplastic.
•**vinepidine sulfate.** (VIN-eh-pih-DEEN)
USAN.
Use: Antineoplastic.
•**vinflunine ditartrate.** (vin-FLOO-neen)
USAN.
Use: Treatment of cancer.
•**vinglycinate sulfate.** (vin-GLIE-sin-ate)
USAN.
Use: Antineoplastic.
•**vinleurosine sulfate.** (vin-LOO-row-
seen) USAN. Sulfate salt of an alkaloid
extracted from *Vinca rosea* Linn. Also
see Vinblastine.
Use: Antineoplastic.
•**vinorelbine tartrate.** (vih-NORE-ell-
bean) USAN. Sulfate salt of an alkaloid
extracted from *Vinca rosea* Linn.
Use: Antineoplastic.
See: Navelbine.
vinorelbine tartrate. (Gensia Sicor) Vinorelbine tartrate 10 mg/mL. Inj. Vials. 1 mL, 5 mL. *Rx.*
Use: Antineoplastic.
•**vinpocetine.** (VIN-poe-SEH-teen) USAN.
Use: Antineoplastic.

•**vinrosidine sulfate.** (vin-ROW-sih-deen) USAN. Sulfate salt of an alkaloid extracted from *Vinca rosea* Linn.
Use: Antineoplastic.
See: Vinblastine.

vinyl ether. (VYE-nil)
Use: Anesthetic, general.

vinyzene. Bromchlorenone.
Use: Fungicide.

•**vinzolidine sulfate.** (VIN-ZOLE-ih-deen) USAN.
Use: Antineoplastic.

Vio-Bec. (Solvay) Vitamins B$_1$ 25 mg, B$_2$ 25 mg, niacinamide 100 mg, calcium pantothenate 40 mg, B$_6$ 25 mg, C 500 mg. Cap. Bot. 100s. *OTC.*
Use: Mineral, vitamin supplement.

Viodo HC. (Alra) Iodochlorhydroxyquin 3%, hydrocortisone 1% in cream base. Tube 20 g. *OTC.*
Use: Antifungal; corticosteroid, topical.

Viogen-C. (Ivax) Vitamins B$_1$ 20 mg, B$_2$ 10 mg, B$_3$ 100 mg, B$_5$ 20 mg, B$_6$ 5 mg, C 300 mg, Mg, zinc sulfate 50 mg. Tartrazine. Cap. Bot. 100s. *OTC.*
Use: Mineral, vitamin supplement.

•**vipadenant.** (vye-PA-de-nant) USAN.
Use: Parkinson disease.

•**viprostol.** (vie-PRAHST-ole) USAN.
Use: Hypotensive; vasodilator.

Vi-Q-Tuss. (Vintage) Hydrocodone bitartrate 5 mg, guaifenesin 100 mg per 5 mL. Sugar, alcohol, and dye free. Menthol, parabens, saccharin, sorbitol. Cherry flavor. Syrup. 30 mL, 120 mL, 473 mL, 3785 mL. *c-III.*
Use: Antitussive with expectorant.

Virac. (Ruson) Undecoylium Cl-iodine. Iodine complexed with a cationic detergent. Surgical Soln. Bot. 2 oz, 8 oz, 1 gal. *OTC.*
Use: Antiseptic.

Viracept. (Pfizer) Nelfinavir mesylate. **Tab.:** 250 mg. Bot. 270s, 300s. **Pow.:** 50 mg. Aspartame (11.2 mg phenylalanine), sucrose. Multi-dose bottles. 144 g Pow. w/1 g scoop. *Rx.*
Use: Antiviral.

Viracil. (Health for Life Brands) Phenylephrine hydrochloride 5 mg, hesperidin 50 mg, thenylene hydrochloride 12.5 mg, pyrilamine maleate 12.5 mg, vitamin C 50 mg, salicylamide 2.5 g, caffeine 0.5 g, sodium salicylate 1.25 g. Cap. Bot. 16s, 36s. *OTC.*
Use: Analgesic, antihistamine, decongestant, vitamin supplement.

Viramisol. (Seatrace) Adenosine phosphate 25 mg/mL. Vial 10 mL. *OTC.*
Use: Relief of varicose vein complications.

Viramune. (Boehringer Ingelheim) Nevirapine. **Tab.:** 200 mg. Lactose. 60s. **Oral Susp.:** 50 mg/5 mL (as nevirapine hemihydrate), parabens, sorbitol, sucrose. 240 mL. *Rx.*
Use: Antiviral.

Viranol. (Aventis) Salicylic acid in collodion gel w/lactic acid, camphor, pyroxylin, ethyl alcohol, ethyl acetate. Gel. Tube 8 g. *OTC.*
Use: Dermatologic; wart therapy.

Virasal. (Elorac) Salicylic acid 27.5%. Isopropyl alcohol. Liq. 10 mL w/brush applicator. *Rx.*
Use: Keratolytic agent.

ViraTan-DM B.I.D. (Ani) **Chew. Tab.:** Dextromethorphan tannate 25 mg, pyrilamine tannate 30 mg, phenylephrine tannate 25 mg. Dye free. Mannitol, sucralose, sugar. Grape flavor. 100s. **Susp.:** Dextromethorphan tannate 25 mg, pyrilamine tannate 30 mg, phenylephrine tannate 12.5 mg per 5 mL. Dye free. Methylparaben, sucralose, sucrose. Grape flavor. 473 mL. *Rx.*
Use: Upper respiratory combination, antitussive combination.

Viravan-DM. (PediaMed) **Chew. Tab.:** Dextromethorphan tannate 25 mg, pyrilamine tannate 30 mg, phenylephrine tannate 25 mg. Sugar, sucralose. Dye free. Grape flavor. 100s. **Susp.:** Dextromethorphan tannate 25 mg, pyrilamine tannate 30 mg, phenylephrine tannate 12.5 mg per 5 mL. Methylparaben, sucralose, sucrose. Grape flavor. 473 mL. *Rx.*
Use: Pediatric antitussive.

Viravan-PDM. (Tiber Laboratories) Dextromethorphan hydrobromide 15 mg, pseudoephedrine hydrochloride 15 mg, pyrilamine maleate 15 mg per 5 mL. Methylparaben, sucralose, sucrose. Grape flavor. Susp. 473 mL. *Rx.*
Use: Upper respiratory combination, antitussive combination.

Viravan-P Suspension. (Tiber) Pseudoephedrine hydrochloride 15 mg, pyrilamine maleate 15 mg per 5 mL. Methylparaben, sucralose, sucrose. Cherry bubble gum flavor. Susp. 473 mL. *Rx.*
Use: Upper respiratory combination, decongestant, antihistamine.

Viravan-T. (PediaMed) Phenylephrine tannate 25 mg, pyrilamine tannate 30 mg. Sugar, saccharin. Dye free. Grape flavor. Chew. Tab. 100s. *Rx.*
Use: Decongestant and antihistamine.

Virazole. (ICN) Ribavirin 6 g per vial. Contains 20 mg/mL when reconstituted

w/300 mL sterile water. Pow. for Soln., Lyophilized, Inh. Vials. *Rx.*
Use: Antiviral.

Viread. (Gilead Sciences) Tenofovir disoproxil fumarate 300 mg (equivalent to tenofovir disoproxil 245 mg). Lactose. Film-coated. Tab. Bot. 30s. *Rx.*
Use: Antiretroviral, nucleoside analog reverse transcriptase inhibitor.

• **virginiamycin.** (vihr-JIH-nee-ah-MY-sin) USAN. An antibiotic produced by *Streptomyces virgina.*
Use: Anti-infective.

• **viridofulvin.** (vih-RID-oh-FULL-vin) USAN.
Use: Antifungal.

Virilon. (Star) Methyltestosterone 10 mg. Cap. Bot. 100s, 1000s. *c-III.*
Use: Sex hormone, androgen.

Virogen Herpes Slide Test. (Wampole) Latex agglutination slide test for the detection of herpes simplex virus antigens directly from lesions or cell culture. Test kit 100s.
Use: Diagnostic aid.

Virogen Rotatest. (Wampole) Latex agglutination slide test for the qualitative detection of rotavirus in fecal specimens. Test kit 50s.
Use: Diagnostic aid.

Virogen Rubella Microlatex Test. (Wampole) Latex agglutination microlatex test for the detection of rubella virus antibody in serum. Test kit 500s, 5000s.
Use: Diagnostic aid.

Virogen Rubella Slide Test. (Wampole) Latex agglutination slide test for the detection of rubella virus antibody in serum. Test kit 100s, 500s, 5000s.
Use: Diagnostic aid.

Virogen Rubella Slide Test with Fast Trak Slides. (Wampole) Latex agglutination slide test for the detection of rubella virus antibody in serum.
Use: Diagnostic aid.

Viroptic. (Monarch) Trifluridine 1%, thimerosal 0.001%. Soln. Drop-Dose 7.5 mL. *Rx.*
Use: Antiviral; ophthalmic.

• **viroxime.** (vie-ROX-eem) USAN.
Use: Antiviral.

Virozyme Injection. (Marcen) Sodium nucleate 2.5%, phenol 0.5%, protein hydrolysate 2.5%, benzyl alcohol 0.2%. Vial 5 mL, 10 mL. *Rx.*
Use: Immunomodulator.

Virugon. Under study. Anhydro bis-(beta-hydroxyethyl) biguanide derivative.
Use: Treatment of influenza, mumps, measles, chickenpox, and shingles.

Viscoat. (Alcon) Sodium chondroitin sulfate 40 mg, sodium hyaluronate 30 mg, sodium dihydrogen phosphate hydrate 0.45 mg, disodium hydrogen phosphate 2 mg, sodium chloride 4.3 mg/mL. Soln. Disposable Syr. 0.5 mL. *Rx.*
Use: Viscoelastic.

viscum album, extract. Visnico.
Use: Vasodilator.

Visicol. (Salix) Sodium phosphate monobasic monohydrate 1.102 g, sodium phosphate dibasic anhydrous 0.398 g. Gluten free. Tab. 40s, 100s. *Rx.*
Use: Bowel cleansing agent.

• **visilizumab.** (vye-si-loo-zoo-mab) USAN.
Use: Treatment of organ transplantation rejection and other T lymphocyte-mediated diseases and disorders.

Visine. (J & J Healthcare) Tetrahydrozoline hydrochloride 0.05%. Benzalkonium chloride, boric acid, EDTA, sodium borate. Ophth. Soln. 15 mL, 30 mL. *OTC.*
Use: Ophthalmic decongestant.

Visine-A. (J & J Healthcare) Naphazoline hydrochloride 0.025%, pheniramine maleate 0.3%. EDTA. Soln., Ophth. 15 mL. *OTC.*
Use: Ophthalmic decongestant/antihistamine combination.

Visine A.C. (J & J Healthcare) Tetrahydrozoline hydrochloride 0.05%. Benzalkonium chloride, boric acid, edetate disodium, sodium chloride, sodium citrate, zinc 0.25%. Soln., Ophth. 15 mL, 30 mL. *OTC.*
Use: Ophthalmic and otic agent, ophthalmic antihistamine.

Visine Advanced Relief. (J & J Healthcare) Tetrahydrozoline hydrochloride 0.05%. Dextran 70 0.1%, 1% of polyethylene glycol 400, povidone 1%, benzalkonium chloride, boric acid, EDTA, sodium borate. Ophth. Soln. 30 mL. *OTC.*
Use: Ophthalmic decongestant.

Visine All Day Eye Itch Relief. (J & J Healthcare) Ketotifen 0.025% (as ketotifen fumarate). May contain glycerol, sodium hydroxide and/or hydrochloric acid, benzalkonium chloride 0.01%. Soln., Ophth. 5 mL. *OTC.*
Use: Ophthalmic and otic agent, ophthalmic antihistamine.

Visine Allergy Relief. (Pfizer) Tetrahydrozoline hydrochloride 0.05%. Benzalkonium chloride 0.01%, EDTA, zinc sulfate 0.25%. Soln., Ophth. 15 mL, 30 mL. *OTC.*
Use: Ophthalmic decongestant.

Visine LR. (J & J Healthcare) Oxymetazoline hydrochloride 0.025%. Benzalkonium chloride, boric acid, sodium borate, sodium chloride, EDTA. Ophth. Soln. 15 mL. *OTC.*
Use: Mydriatic; vasoconstrictor; ophthalmic decongestant.

Visine Maximum Redness Relief. (J & J Healthcare) Tetrahydrozoline hydrochloride 0.05%. Benzalkonium chloride, boric acid, edetate disodium, glycerin, hypromellose 0.36%, PEG, sodium chloride, sodium citrate. Soln., Ophth. 15 mL. *OTC.*
Use: Ophthalmic and otic agent, ophthalmic decongestant.

Visine Tears. (J & J Healthcare) Glycerin 0.2%, hypromellose 0.2%, 1% of polyethylene glycol 400. Soln., Ophth. 15 mL, 30 mL. *OTC.*
Use: Artificial tears.

Visine Tears Dry Eye Relief. (J & J Healthcare) Glycerin 0.2%, hypromellose 0.2%, 1% of polyethylene glycol 400. Drops. Single-drop dispenser. 15 mL, 30 mL. *OTC.*
Use: Artificial tears.

Visine Tired Eye Relief. (J & J Healthcare) Glycerin 0.2%, hypromellose 0.36%, 1% of polyethylene glycol 400. PEG, benzalkonium chloride, boric acid, glycine, magnesium chloride, potassium chloride, sodium borate, sodium chloride, sodium citrate, sodium lactate, sodium phosphate dibasic. Soln., Ophth. 15 mL. *OTC.*
Use: Artificial tears.

Visine Totality Multi-Symptom Relief. (J & J Healthcare) Tetrahydrozoline hydrochloride 0.05%. Benzalkonium chloride, boric acid, edetate disodium, glycerin, hypromellose 0.36%, PEG, sodium chloride, sodium citrate, zinc sulfate 0.25%. Soln., Ophth. 15 mL. *OTC.*
Use: Ophthalmic and otic agent, ophthalmic decongestant.

VisionBlue. (Dutch Ophthalmic) Trypan blue 0.06%. Ophthalmic Soln. 0.5 mL in 2.25 mL single-use *Luer Lok* syringe. *Rx.*
Use: Ophthalmic surgery aid.

Visipaque 320. (Nycomed Amersham) Iodixanol 652 mg, iodine 320 mg/mL, EDTA. Inj. Vial 50 mL. Bot. 50 mL, 100 mL, 200 mL, 150 mL fill in 200 mL bot. Flexible containers 100 mL, 150 mL, 200 mL. *Rx.*
Use: Radiopaque agent, parenteral.

Visipaque 270. (Nycomed Amersham) Iodixanol 550 mg, iodine 270 mg/mL, EDTA. Inj. Vial 50 mL. Bot. 50 mL, 100 mL, 200 mL, 150 mL fill in 200 mL bot. Flexible containers 100 mL, 150 mL, 200 mL. *Rx.*
Use: Radiopaque agent, parenteral.

Visken. (Novartis) Pindolol 5 mg, 10 mg. Tab. Bot. 100s. *Rx.*
Use: Antiadrenergic/sympatholytic, beta-adrenergic blocker.

•**vismodegib.** (VIS-moe-DEG-ib) USAN.
Use: Antineoplastic.

Visonex. (Vision) Phenylephrine hydrochloride 30 mg, guaifenesin 900 mg. Film-coated. ER Tab. 100s. *Rx.*
Use: Upper respiratory combination, decongestant and expectorant combination.

Vistacon. (Roberts) Hydroxyzine hydrochloride 50 mg/mL. Inj. 25 mg/mL, 50 mg/mL, benzyl alcohol. Vial 10 mL; UD Vial 1 mL, 2 mL (50 mg/mL only). *Rx.*
Use: Antihistamine; anxiolytic.

Vistaril. (Pfizer) Hydroxyzine pamoate equivalent to hydroxyzine hydrochloride 25 mg, 50 mg, 100 mg. Sucrose. Cap. Bot. 100s. *Rx.*
Use: Anxiolytic; antihistamine, nonselective piperazine.

Vistide. (Gilead Sciences) Cidofovir 75 mg/mL. Preservative free. Inj. Single-use vial 5 mL. *Rx.*
Use: Antiviral.

Visudyne. (QLT Phototherapeutics/Novartis Ophthalmics) Verteporfin 15 mg (reconstituted to 2 mg/mL), egg phosphatidylglycerol. Lyophilized Cake for Inj. Single-use Vial. *Rx.*
Use: Ophthalmic phototherapy.

Vita-Bee with C Caplets. (Rugby) Vitamins B_1 15 mg, B_2 10.2 mg, B_3 50 mg, B_5 10 mg, B_6 5 mg, C 300 mg. TR Cap. Bot. 100s, 1000s. *OTC.*
Use: Vitamin supplement.

Vitabix. (Spanner) Vitamins B_1 100 mg, B_2 2 mg, B_6 5 mg, B_{12} 30 mcg, niacinamide 100 mg, panthenol 10 mg/mL. Vial 10 mL. Multiple-dose vial 30 mL. *Rx.*
Use: Vitamin supplement.

Vita-Bob Softgel Capsules. (ScotTussin) Vitamins A 5000 units, D 400 units, E 30 mg, B_1 1.5 mg, B_2 1.7 mg, B_3 20 mg, B_6 2 mg, B_{12} 6 mcg, C 60 mg, folic acid 0.4 mg. Cap. Bot. 100s. *OTC.*
Use: Vitamin supplement.

Vita-C. (Freeda) Ascorbic acid 1000 mg/¼ tsp. Sugar free. Crystals. Can. 120 g, 1 lb. *OTC.*
Use: Water-soluble vitamin.

Vitacarn. (McGaw) L-carnitine 1 g/10 mL. UD Box 50s, 100s. *Rx.*
Use: L-carnitine supplement.

Vit-A-Drops. (Vision Pharmaceuticals) Vitamin A 5000 units, polysorbate 80. Bot. 10 mL, 15 mL. *OTC.*
Use: Lubricant; ophthalmic.

Vitadye. (AstraZeneca) FD&C yellow No. 5, FD&C red No. 40, FD&C blue No. 1 dyes and dihydroxyacetone 5%. Bot. 0.5 oz, 2 oz. *OTC.*
Use: Cosmetic for hyperpigmentation.

Vitafol Caplets. (Everett) Fe 65 mg, vitamins A 6000 units, D 400 units, E 30 mg, B_1 1.1 mg, B_2 1.8 mg, B_3 15 mg, B_6 2.5 mg, B_{12} 5 mcg, C 60 mg, folic acid 1 mg, calcium. Tab. Bot. 100s, 1000s. *Rx.*
Use: Mineral, vitamin supplement.

Vitafol-PN. (Everett) Ca 125 mg, Fe 65 mg, vitamins A 1700 units, D 400 units, C 60 mg, E 30 mg, folic acid 1 mg, B_1 1.6 mg, B_2 1.8 mg, B_6 2.5 mg, B_{12} 5 mcg, B_3 15 mg, Mg 25 mg, Zn 15 mg. Tab. UD 100s. *Rx.*
Use: Mineral, vitamin supplement.

Vitafol Syrup. (Everett) Fe 90 mg, B_3 39.9 mg, B_6 6 mg, B_{12} 25.02 mcg, folic acid 0.75 mg. Bot. 473 mL. *Rx.*
Use: Mineral, vitamin supplement.

Vitagen Advance. (Midlothian) Vitamin B_{12} 10 mcg, desiccated stomach substance 50 mg, Fe 70 mg (from ferrous asparto glycinate), medium chain triglycerides, succinic acid 75 mg, vitamin C 152 mg (as calcium ascorbate and calcium threonate). Lactose, maltodextrin, polydextrose. Film-coated. Tab. 90s. *Rx.*
Use: Trace element, iron.

Vita-Iron Formula. (Barth's) Fe 120 mg, vitamins B_1 5 mg, B_2 10 mg, C 20 mg, niacin 2 mg, B_{12} 25 mcg, lysine, desiccated liver 200 mg, bromelains. Tab. Bot. 100s, 500s. *OTC.*
Use: Mineral, vitamin supplement.

Vita-Kaps Filmtabs. (Abbott) Vitamins A 5000 units, D 400 units, B_1 3 mg, B_2 2.5 mg, nicotinamide 20 mg, B_6 1 mg, C 50 mg, B_{12} 3 mcg. Bot. 100s, 1000s. *OTC.*
Use: Vitamin supplement.

Vitakaps-M. (Abbott) Vitamins A 5000 units, D 400 units, B_1 3 mg, B_2 2.5 mg, nicotinamide 20 mg, B_6 1 mg, B_{12} 3 mcg, C 50 mg, Fe 10 mg, Cu 1 mg, I 0.15 mg, Mn 1 mg, Zn 7.5 mg. Filmtab. Bot. 100s. *OTC.*
Use: Mineral, vitamin supplement.

Vita-Kid Chewable Wafers. (Solgar) Vitamins A 10,000 units, D 400 units, E 10 mg, B_1 2 mg, B_2 2 mg, B_3 10 mg, B_6 2 mg, B_{12} 5 mcg, C 100 mg, FA 0.3 mg, orange flavor. Bot. 50s, 100s.

OTC.
Use: Vitamin supplement.

Vitalax. (Vitalax) Candy base, gumdrop flavor. Pkg. 20s. *OTC.*
Use: Laxative.

Vital B-50. (Ivax) Vitamins B_1 50 mg, B_2 50 mg, B_3 50 mg, B_5 50 mg, B_6 50 mg, B_{12} 50 mcg, folic acid 0.1 mg, biotin 50 mcg, PABA, choline bitartrate, inositol. TR Tab. Bot 60s. *OTC.*
Use: Vitamin supplement.

Vitalets. (Freeda) Fe 10 mg, vitamins A 5000 units, D 400 units, E 5 mg, B_1 2.5 mg, B_2 0.9 mg, B_3 20 mg, B_5 3 mg, B_6 2 mg, B_{12} 5 mcg, C 60 mg, biotin 25 mcg, Mn, Ca. Chew. Tab. Bot 100s, 250s. *OTC.*
Use: Mineral, vitamin supplement.

VitalEyes. (Allergan) Vitamins A 10,000 units, C 200 mg, E 100 units, Zn 40 mg, Cu, Se, Mn. Cap. Bot. 60s. *OTC.*
Use: Mineral, vitamin supplement.

Vital High Nitrogen. (Ross) Amino acids, partially hydrolyzed whey, meat, and soy, hydrolyzed corn starch, sucrose, safflower oil, MCT mono- and diglycerides, soy lecithin, vitamins A, B_1, B_2, B_3, B_5, B_6, B_{12}, C, D, E, K, folic acid, biotin, choline, Ca, P, Mg, Fe, Cu, Zn, Mn, I, Cl. Packet 80 g. *OTC.*
Use: Nutritional supplement.

Vitalize SF. (Scot-Tussin) Fe 66 mg, B_1 30 mg, B_6 15 mg, B_{12} 75 mcg, l-lysine 300 mg. Liq. Bot. 120 mL. *OTC.*
Use: Mineral, vitamin supplement.

Vitamel with Iron. (Eastwood) Drops 50 mL. Chew. Tab. Bot. 100s. *OTC.*
Use: Mineral, vitamin supplement.

•**vitamin A.** (VYE-ta-min) *USP 34.* Formerly Oleovitamin A.
Use: Antixerophthalmic vitamin; emollient.
See: Aquasol A.
W/Combinations.
See: Advanced Formula Zenate.
Advera.
Bonamil Infant Formula with Iron.
Boost.
Choice DM.
Fosfree.
Neocate One +.
Nepro.
Ocuvite.
Ocuvite Extra.
Ocuvite PreserVision.
Oncovite.
Ondrox.
Prenatal H.P.
Prenatal Plus.
Prenatal Rx.

Prenatal Z Advanced Formula.
StuartNatal Plus 3.
Theragran AntiOxidant.
Tri-Flor-Vite with Fluoride.
vitamin A. (Various Mfr.) Vitamin A 10,000 IU, 15,000 IU, 25,000 IU. Cap. Bot. 100s, 250s (except 25,000 IU), 500s (10,000 units IU). *Rx-OTC.*
Use: Antixerophthalmic vitamin; emollient.
vitamin A acid.
See: Tretinoin.
vitamin A, alphalin. (Eli Lilly) Vitamin A 50,000 units. Gelseal. Bot. 100s. *Rx.*
Use: Vitamin supplement.
vitamin A, water miscible or soluble.
Water-miscible vitamin A.
Use: Vitamin supplement.
vitamin Bc.
See: Folic Acid.
vitamin B combinations.
Use: Nutritional products.
See: Calafol.
  Cardiotek Rx.
  ComBgen.
  DexFol.
  Folpace.
W/Vitamin C.
See: Dialyvite Multi-Vitamins for Dialysis Patients.
  Dialyvite 3000.
  Full Spectrum B.
vitamin B complex. Concentrated extract of dried brewer's yeast and extract of corn processed w/*Clostridium acetobutylicum.*
See: Advanced Formula Zenate.
  Advera.
  Bonamil Infant Formula with Iron.
  Boost.
  Fosfree.
  Neocate One +.
  Nephplex Rx.
  Nephron FA.
  Nepro.
  Ocuvite Extra.
  Oncovite.
  Prenatal H.P.
  Prenatal Plus.
  Prenatal Rx.
  Prenatal Z Advanced Formula.
  StuartNatal Plus 3.
Vitamin B Complex, Betalin Complex, Elixir. (Eli Lilly) Vitamins B_1 2.7 mg, B_2 1.35 mg, B_{12} 3 mcg, B_6 0.555 mg, pantothenic acid 2.7 mg, niacinamide 6.75 mg, liver fraction 500 mg/5 mL, alcohol 17%. Bot. 16 oz. *OTC.*
Use: Vitamin supplement.
Vitamin B Complex, Betalin Complex Pulvules. (Eli Lilly) Vitamins B_1 1 mg,

B_2 2 mg, B_6 0.4 mg, pantothenic acid 3.333 mg, niacinamide 10 mg, B_{12} 1 mcg. Cap. Bot. 100s. *OTC.*
Use: Vitamin supplement.
Vitamin B Complex No. 104. (Century) Vitamins B_1 100 mg, B_2 2 mg, B_6 2 mg, d-panthenol 10 mg, niacinamide 125 mg. Vial, benzyl alcohol 1%, gentisic acid ethanolamide 2.5%. Vial 30 mL. *Rx.*
Use: Vitamin supplement.
Vitamin B Complex 100. (McGuff) Vitamin B_1 100 mg, B_2 2 mg, B_3 100 mg, B_5 2 mg, B_6 2 mg/mL. Inj. Vial 10 mL, 30 mL. *Rx.*
Use: Vitamin supplement.
Vitamin B Complex w/Vitamin C. (Century) Vitamins B_1 25 mg, B_2 5 mg, B_6 5 mg, niacinamide 50 mg, panthenol 5 mg, Ca 50 mg, propethylene glycol 300 10%, gentisic acid ethanolamide 2.5%, benzyl alcohol 2%. Vial 30 mL. *Rx.*
Use: Mineral, vitamin supplement.
vitamin B_8.
See: Adenosine Phosphate.
vitamin B_5. Calcium pantothenate.
Use: Vitamin supplement.
See: Calcium Pantothenate.
vitamin B_{15}.
Use: Alleged to increase oxygen supply in blood. Not approved by FDA as a vitamin or drug. Illegal to sell Vitamin B_{15}.
vitamin B_1. Thiamine hydrochloride.
Use: Vitamin supplement.
See: Thiamilate.
  Thiamine Hydrochloride.
vitamin B_1 mononitrate. Thiamine mononitrate.
Use: Vitamin supplement.
vitamin B_6. Pyridoxine hydrochloride.
Use: Water-soluble vitamin.
See: Aminoxin.
  Pyridoxine Hydrochloride.
vitamin B_6. (Various Mfr.) Vitamin B_6 50 mg, 100 mg, 250 mg, 500 mg. Tab. Bot. 100s, 250s (50 mg, 100 mg only), 1000s (50 mg only). *OTC.*
Use: Water-soluble vitamin.
vitamin B_3. Niacinamide, Nicotinamide.
Use: Vitamin supplement.
See: Niacor.
  Niaspan.
  Nicotinic Acid (Niacin).
  Slo-Niacin.
vitamin B_{12}. Cyanocobalamin. Cobalamine. Vial. Amp.
See: Bedoce.
  B-12.
  Nascobal.

Sigamine.
Twelve Resin-K.
W/Thiamine, Vitamin B$_6$.
See: Orexin.
vitamin B$_{12}$. (Freeda) Vitamin B$_{12}$
50 mcg (sorbitol, mannitol), 100 mcg,
250 mcg, 500 mcg. Loz. Bot. 100s,
250s (250 mcg, 500 mcg only). *OTC.*
Use: Water-soluble vitamin.
vitamin B-12. (Mason) Vitamin B$_{12}$
1000 mcg (dextrose), 5000 mcg (mannitol). Tab., Sublingual. 20s, (5000 mcg
only), 100s (1000 mcg only). *OTC.*
Use: Water-soluble vitamin.
vitamin B$_{12}$. (Nature's Blend) Cyanocobalamin 2,500 mcg. Sorbitol. Tab., sublingual. Gluten
free and preservative free. Tab., sublingual. *OTC.*
Use: Water-soluble vitamin.
vitamin B$_{12}$. (Various Mfr.) Cyanocobalamin. **Tab.:** 100 mcg, 500 mcg,
1,000 mcg. 100s. **Inj.: 100 mcg/mL:**
Vials 30 mL. **1,000 mcg/mL:** Multidose
vials. 10 mL, 30 mL. *Rx.*
Use: Water-soluble vitamin.
vitamin B$_{12}$ a & b.
See: Hydroxocobalamin.
vitamin B$_2$. Riboflavin.
Use: Vitamin supplement.
See: Riboflavin.
vitamin B$_2$. (Nature's Blend) Riboflavin
25 mg. Polydextrose, sorbitol. Gluten
free and preservative free. Tab. 100s.
OTC.
Use: Water-soluble vitamin.
vitamin C. Ascorbic acid, sodium ascor-
bate, calcium ascorbate.
See: Ascorbic Acid.
Calcium Ascorbate.
Cecon.
Cenolate.
Cevi-Bid.
Chewable Vitamin C.
Chew-C.
Dull-C.
N'ice with Vitamin C Drops.
SunKist Vitamin C.
Vicks Vitamin C Orange Drops.
Vita-C.
W/Combinations.
See: Advanced Formula Zenate.
Advera.
Allbee-C.
Allbee C-800.
Allbee-T.
Antiox.
Bonamil Infant Formula with Iron.
Boost.
Choice DM.
Chromagen FA.
Chromagen Forte.

C-Max.
Fosfree.
Fruit C 500.
Fruit C 100.
Fruit C 200.
Neocate One +.
Nephplex Rx.
Nephron FA.
Nepro.
Nialexo-C.
Ocuvite.
Ocuvite Extra.
Ocuvite Lutein.
Ocuvite PreserVision.
Oncovite.
Prenatal H.P.
Prenatal Plus.
Prenatal Rx.
Protegra Softgels.
StuartNatal Plus 3.
Theragran Antioxidant.
Thex Forte.
Tri-Flor-Vite with Fluoride.
Vicon-C.
Vicon Forte.
Vicon Plus.
Vi-Zac.
Z-BEC.
W/Vitamin B.
See: Dialyvite Multi-Vitamins for Dialy-
sis Patients.
W/Zinc, Glutathione.
See: Sucrets Defense Kid's Formula.
vitamin C, cevalin. (Eli Lilly) Ascorbic
acid 250 mg, 500 mg. Tab. Bot. 100s.
OTC.
Use: Vitamin supplement.
vitamin D. Cholecalciferol.
Use: Vitamin D supplement.
See: Ergocalciferol.
W/Combinations.
See: Advanced Formula Zenate.
Advera.
Bonamil Infant Formula with Iron.
Boost.
Caltrate Plus.
Caltrate 600 + D.
Choice DM.
Desert Pure Calcium.
Fosfree.
Neocate One +.
Nepro.
Oesto-Mins.
Oncovite.
Ondrox.
Prenatal Plus.
Prenatal Rx.
StuartNatal Plus 3.
Tri-Flor-Vite with Fluoride.
vitamin D. (Pliva) Vitamin D$_2$
50,000 units. Soybean oil. Cap. 100s,

1000s. *Rx.*
Use: Vitamin supplement.
vitamin D. (Various Mfr.) Ergocalciferol (D₂) 50,000 units. Cap. Bot. 100s, 1000s. *Rx.*
Use: Vitamin supplement.
vitamin D₁.
See: Dihydrotachysterol.
vitamin D₂. Activated ergasterol, Ergocalciferol.
See: Calciferol.
  Drisdol.
  Ergocalciferol Drops.
  Viosterol.
vitamin D₃.
See: Advanced D5000.
  Baby Ddrops.
  Ddrops.
  D3-50.
  D₃ Healthy Kids.
  Delta-D.
  Super Strength D-2000 IU.
  Ultra Strength D2000.
vitamin D₃. (Freeda) Cholecalciferol (D₃) 1000 IU. Sugar free. Tab. Bot. 100s, 500s. *OTC.*
Use: Vitamin supplement.
vitamin D-3-cholesterol. Compound of crystalline vitamin D-3 and cholesterol.
vitamin D, synthetic.
See: Activated 7-Dehydro-Cholesterol.
  Calciferol.
• **vitamin E.** (VYE-ta-min) *USP 34.*
Use: Vitamin E supplement.
See: Aqua-E.
  Aquasol E.
  Aquavit-E.
  Chantel Vitamin E.
  E-Oil.
  Lactinol-E.
  Mixed E 400 Softgels.
  Mixed E 1000 Softgels.
  Natural E 200.
  Natural Vitamin E.
  Nutr-E-Sol.
  One-A-Day Extras Vitamin E.
  Soft Sense.
  Vitamin E with Mixed Tocopherols.
  Vita-Plus E.
  Wheat Germ Oil.
W/Combinations.
See: Advanced Formula Zenate.
  Advera.
  Antiox.
  Bonamil Infant Formula with Iron.
  Boost.
  Choice DM.
  Neocate One +.
  Nepro.
  Ocuvite.
  Ocuvite Extra.

  Ocuvite Lutein.
  Ocuvite PreserVision.
  Oncovite.
  Ondrox.
  Prenatal Plus.
  StuartNatal Plus 3.
  Theragran AntiOxidant.
vitamin E. (Freeda) Vitamin E 15 IU/ 30 mL. Liq. Bot. 30 mL, 60 mL, 120 mL. *OTC.*
Use: Vitamin supplement.
vitamin E. (Various Mfr.) Vitamin E. **Tab.:** d-alpha tocopherol 100 IU, 200 IU, 400 IU, 500 IU, 800 IU. Bot. 100s, 250s (except 800 IU), 500s (200 IU, 400 IU only). **Cap.:** 100 IU, 200 IU, 400 IU, 1000 IU. Bot. 50s (1000 IU only), 100s, 250s (400 IU only). *OTC.*
Use: Vitamin supplement.
vitamin E, eprolin. (Eli Lilly) Alpha-tocopherol 100 units. Gelseal. Bot. 100s. *OTC.*
Use: Vitamin supplement.
• **vitamin E polyethylene glycol succinate.** (VYE-ta-min E POL-ee-ETH-i-leen GLYE-kol SUX-i-nate) *NF 29.*
Use: Vitamin supplement.
vitamin E with mixed tocopherols. (Freeda) Vitamin E 100 IU, 200 IU, 400 IU. Tab. Bot. 100s, 250s, 500s (400 IU only). *OTC.*
Use: Vitamin supplement.
vitamin, fat-soluble.
See: Fat-Soluble Vitamins.
vitamin G.
See: Riboflavin.
vitamin K.
See: Mephyton.
  Phytonadione.
W/Combinations.
See: Advera.
  Bonamil Infant Formula with Iron.
  Choice DM.
  Neocate One +.
vitamin K. (Nature's Blend) Phytonadione 0.1 mg. Gluten free and preservative free. Tab. 100s. *OTC.*
Use: Fat-soluble vitamin.
vitamin K₁.
See: Phytonadione.
vitamin K₃.
See: Menadione.
vitamin K oxide. Not available, but usually K-1 is desired.
vitamin M.
See: Folic Acid.
vitamin, maintenance formula.
See: Stuart Formula.
vitamin-mineral-supplement liquid. (Morton Grove) Vitamins B₁ 0.83 mg, B₂ 0.42 mg, B₃ 8.3 mg, B₅ 1.67 mg,

B_6 0.17 mg, B_{12} 0.17 mcg, I, Fe 2.5 mg, Mg, Zn 0.3 mg, Mn, choline, alcohol 18%. Liq. 473 mL. OTC.
Use: Mineral, vitamin supplement.
vitamin P. Bioflavonoids.
See: Amino-Opti-C.
  Bio-Flavonoid Compounds.
  C Factors "1000" Plus.
  Ester-C Plus 500 mg Vitamin C.
  Ester-C Plus 1000 mg Vitamin C.
  Ester-C Plus Multi-Mineral.
  Flavons.
  Flavons-500.
  Hesperidin.
  Pan C Ascorbate.
  Pan C-500.
  Peridin-C.
  Quercetin.
  Rutin.
  Span C.
  Super Flavons.
  Super Flavons 300.
  Tri-Super Flavons 1000.
vitamins.
See: Fat-Soluble Vitamins.
  Water-Soluble Vitamins.
vitamins, fat soluble.
See: Calcitriol.
  Cholecalciferol.
  Dihydrotachysterol.
  Doxercalciferol.
  Ergocalciferol.
  Paricalcitol.
  Phytonadione.
  Vitamin E.
  Vitamin K.
vitamins, stress formula.
See: Probec-T.
  Stress Formula with Iron.
  Stresstabs 600.
  Thera-Combex H-P.
vitamins, water soluble.
See: Aminobenzoate Potassium.
  Ascorbic Acid.
  Ascorbic Acid Combinations.
  Bioflavonoids.
  Calcium Ascorbate.
  Cyanocobalamin.
  Levoleucovorin.
  L-methylfolate.
  Niacin.
  Niacinamide.
  Pantothenic Acid.
  Pyridoxine Hydrochloride.
  Riboflavin.
  Sodium Ascorbate.
  Thiamin.
vitamins with liver and lipotropic agents.
See: Metheponex.
vitamin T. Sesame seed factor, termite factor.

Use: Claimed to aid proper blood coagulation and promote formation of blood platelets. Not approved by FDA as an active vitamin.
vitamin U. Present in cabbage juice.
Vita Natal. (Scot-Tussin) Folic acid 1 mg. Tab. Bot. 100s. Rx.
Use: Vitamin supplement.
Vitaneed. (Biosearch Medical Products) P-beef, Ca and Na caseinates, CHO-maltodextrin. F-partially hydrogenated soy oil, mono- and diglycerides, soy lecithin. Protein 35 g, CHO 125 g, fat 40 g, Na 500 mg, K 1250 mg/L, 1 Cal/mL, 375 mOsm/kg H_2O. Liq. Ready-to-use 250 mL. OTC.
Use: Nutritional supplement.
Vitaon. (Vita Elixir) Vitamin B_{12} 25 mcg, thiamine hydrochloride 10 mg, ferric pyrophosphate 250 mg/5 mL. OTC.
Use: Vitamin supplement.
Vita-Plus B12. (Scot-Tussin) Vitamin B_{12} 1000 mcg/mL. Inj. Rx.
Use: Vitamin supplement.
Vita-Plus E. (Scot-Tussin) Vitamin E 400 IU as d-alpha tocopheryl acetate. Sugar free. Cap. Bot. 50s. OTC.
Use: Vitamin supplement.
Vita-Plus G. (Scot-Tussin) Vitamins A 10,000 units, D 400 units, E_2 2 mg, B_1 5 mg, B_2 2.5 mg, B_3 40 mg, B_6 1 mg, B_{12} 2 mcg, pantothenic acid 4 mg, C 75 mg, Fe, Ca, Zn 0.5 mg, K, Mg, Mn, P. Softgel Cap. Bot. 100s. OTC.
Use: Mineral, vitamin supplement.
Vita-Plus H Liquid Sugar Free. (Scot-Tussin) Vitamins B_1 30 mg, l-lysine monohydrochloride 300 mg, B_{12} 75 mcg, B_6 15 mg, iron pyrophosphate soluble 100 mg/5 mL. Bot. 4 oz, 8 oz, pt, gal. OTC.
Use: Mineral, vitamin supplement.
Vita-Plus H Softgel. (Scot-Tussin) Fe 13.4 mg, vitamins A 5000 units, D 400 units, E 3 units, B_1 3 mg, B_2 2.5 mg, B_3 20 mg, B_5 5 mg, B_6 1.5 mg, B_{12} 2.5 mcg, C 50 mg, Ca, K, Mg, Mn, P, Zn 1.4 mg. Cap. Bot. 100s. OTC.
Use: Mineral, vitamin supplement.
Vita-PMS. (Bajamar Chemical) Vitamins A 2083 units, E 16.7 units, D_3 16.7 units, folic acid 33 mcg, B_1 4.2 mg, B_2 4.2 mg, B_3 4.2 mg, B_5 4.2 mg, B_6 50 mg, B_{12} 10.4 mcg, biotin, C 250 mg, Ca, Mg, I, Fe, Cu, Zn 4.2 mg, Mn, K, Se, Cr, betaine. Tab. Bot. 100s. OTC.
Use: Mineral, vitamin supplement.
Vita-PMS Plus. (Bajamar Chemical) Vitamins A 667 units, E 16.7 units, D_3 16.7 units, folic acid 33 mcg, B_1 4.2 mg, B_2 4.2 mg, B_3 4.2 mg, B_5 4.2 mg, B_6

16.7 mg, B_{12} 10.4 mcg, biotin, C
250 mg, Mg, I, Ca, Fe, Cu, Zn 4.2 mg,
Mn, K, Se, Cr, betaine. Tab. Bot. 100s.
OTC.
Use: Mineral, vitamin supplement.

Vita-Ray Creme. (Gordon Laboratories)
Vitamins E 3000 units, A 200,000 units/
oz w/aloe 10%. Jar 0.5 oz, 2.5 oz. OTC.
Use: Emollient.

Vitarex. (Taylor Pharmaceuticals) Vitamins A 10,000 units, D 200 units, B_1
15 mg, B_2 10 mg, B_6 5 mg, B_{12} 5 mcg,
C 250 mg, B_3 100 mg, E
15 mg, Fe 15 mg, Ca, Cu, I, K, Mg, Mn,
P, Zn 10 mg. Tab. Bot. 100s. OTC.
Use: Mineral, vitamin supplement.

Vitazin. (Mesemer) Ascorbic acid
300 mg, niacinamide 100 mg, thiamine
mononitrate 20 mg, d-calcium pantothenate 20 mg, riboflavin 10 mg, pyridoxine hydrochloride 5 mg, magnesium
sulfate 70 mg, Zn 25 mg. Cap. Bot.
100s. OTC.
Use: Mineral, vitamin supplement.

Vitazol. (Rochester Pharmaceuticals)
Metronidazole 0.75%. Benzyl alcohol,
emulsifying wax, glycerin, lactic acid.
Cream. 60 g. Rx.
Use: Topical anti-infective, antibiotic
agent.

Vita-Zoo. (Towne) Vitamins A 2500 units,
D 400 units, E 15 units, C 60 mg, folic
acid 0.3 mg, B_1 1.05 mg, B_2 1.2 mg,
niacin 13.5 mg, B_6 1.05 mg, B_{12}
4.5 mcg. Tab. Bot. 100s. OTC.
Use: Vitamin supplement.

Vita-Zoo Plus Iron. (Towne) Vitamins A
2500 units, D 400 units, E 15 units, C
60 mg, folic acid 0.3 mg, B_1 1.05 mg, B_2
1.2 mg, niacin 13.5 mg, B_6 1.05 mg,
B_{12} 4.5 mcg, Fe 15 mg. Tab. Bot. 100s.
OTC.
Use: Mineral, vitamin supplement.

Vitec. (Pharmaceutical Specialties) Dl-
alpha tocopheryl acetate in a vanishing cream base. Cream. 120 g. OTC.
Use: Emollient.

Vitelle Irospan. (Fielding) Iron 65 mg
(from ferrous sulfate exsiccated), ascorbic acid 150 mg. Sugar. Cap. 60s. OTC.
Use: Vitamin and mineral supplement.

Vitelle Lurline PMS. (Fielding) Acetaminophen 500 mg, pamabrom 25 mg,
pyridoxine hydrochloride 50 mg. Tab.
Bot 50s. OTC.
Use: Analgesic combination.

Vitelle Nesentials. (Fielding) Vitamin A
5000 units, D_2 400 units, E 30 units,
B_1 3 mg, B_2 3 mg, B_3 25 mg, B_6 2 mg,
B_{12} 6 mcg, C 120 mg, Ca, P, Zn. Tab.
Bot. 60s. OTC.

Use: Vitamin, mineral supplement.

Vitelle Nestabs OTC. (Fielding) Vitamins
A 5000 units, C 120 mg, D 400 units, E
30 units, thiamin 3 mg, riboflavin 3 mg,
niacinamide 20 mg, B_6 3 mg, folic acid
800 mcg, B_{12} 8 mcg, Ca 200 mg, Fe
29 mg, I, Zn 15 mg. Tab. Bot. 100s.
OTC.
Use: Vitamin, mineral supplement.

●**vitespen.** (vi-TES-pen) USAN.
Use: Antineoplastic.

Vitrase. (ISTA Pharmaceuticals) Hyaluronidase (ovine source). **Pow. for Inj.,**
lyophilized: 6,200 units. Lactose
5 mg. Preservative free. Single-use
5 mL vials with 1 mL syringe and 5 mcg
filter needle. **Soln. for Inj.:** 200 units/
mL. Lactose 0.93 mg. Preservative free.
Single-use 2 mL vials. Rx.
Use: Physical adjunct.

Vitrasert. (Chiron Vision) Ganciclovir
4.5 mg (released over 5 to 8 months).
Intravitreal implant. Box 1. Rx.
Use: Antiviral; cytomegalovirus.

Vitron-C. (Heritage Consumer Products)
Iron (from ferrous fumarate) 66 mg,
ascorbic acid 125 mg. Tab. Bot. 60s.
OTC.
Use: Mineral and vitamin supplement.

Vivactil. (Barr/Duramed) Protriptyline
hydrochloride 5 mg, 10 mg. Lactose.
Film-coated. Tab. Bot. 100s, UD 100s
(10 mg only). Rx.
Use: Antidepressant.

Viva-Drops. (Vision Pharmaceuticals)
Polysorbate 80, sodium chloride, EDTA,
retinyl palmitate, mannitol, sodium cit-
rate, pyruvate. Soln. Bot. 10 mL, 15 mL.
OTC.
Use: Artificial tears.

Vivaglobin. (ZLB Behring LLC) Immune
globulin subcutaneous (human). Protein solution 16% (160 mg/mL). Glycine
2.25%, sodium chloride 0.3%. Preservative free. Inj. Single-use vials. 3 mL,
10 mL, 20 mL. Rx.
Use: Immune globulin.

Vivarin. (GlaxoSmithKline) Caffeine
200 mg, dextrose. Tab. Bot. 16s, 24s,
40s, 80s. OTC.
Use: CNS stimulant, analeptic.

Vivelle. (Novartis) Estradiol 3.28 mg
(0.0375 mg/day), 4.33 mg (0.05 mg/
day), 6.57 mg (0.075 mg/day), 8.66 mg
(0.1 mg/day). Transdermal system.
Calendar pack (8 and 24 systems). Rx.
Use: Estrogen, sex hormone.

Vivelle-Dot. (Novartis) Estradiol 0.39 mg
(0.025 mg/day), 0.585 mg (0.0375 mg/
day), 0.78 mg (0.05 mg/day), 1.17 mg
(0.075 mg/day), 1.56 mg (0.1 mg/day).

Transdermal system. Calendar pack (8 and 24 [0.39 mg only] systems). *Rx.*
Use: Estrogen, sex hormone.

Vivikon. (AstraZeneca) Vitamins B_1 5 mg, B_2 2 mg, B_6 10 mg, d-panthenol 5 mg, niacinamide 10 mg, procaine hydrochloride 2%/mL. 100 mL. *OTC.*
Use: Vitamin supplement.

Vivitrol. (Alkermes) Naltrexone hydrochloride 380 mg per vial. Carboxymethylcellulose sodium salt, sodium chloride. Susp., ER Inj. Single-use vials. *Rx.*
Use: Antidote, detoxification agent.

Vivonex Flavor Packets. (Procter & Gamble) Nonnutritive flavoring for *Vivonex* diets when consumed orally. Orange-pineapple, lemon-lime, strawberry, and vanilla. Pkg. 60s. *OTC.*
Use: Flavoring.

Vivonex, Standard. (Procter & Gamble) Free amino acid/complete enteral nutrition. Six packets provide kcal 1800, available nitrogen 5.88 g as amino acids 37 g, fat 2.61 g, carbohydrate 407 g, and full day's balanced nutrition. Calorie:nitrogen ratio is 300:1. Unflavored pow. Packet 80 g. Pkg. 6s. *OTC.*
Use: Nutritional supplement.

Vivonex T.E.N. (Procter & Gamble) Free amino acid, high nitrogen/high branched chain amino acid complete enteral nutrition. Ten packets provide kcal 3000, available nitrogen 17 g, amino acids 115 g, fat 8.33 g, carbohydrate 617 g, and full day's balanced nutrition. Calorie:nitrogen ratio is 175:1. Unflavored pow. Packet 80 g. Pkg. 10s. *OTC.*
Use: Nutritional supplement.

Vivotif Berna. (Berna) Typhoid vaccine (oral). *Salmonella typhi* Ty21a (viable) 2 to 6 × 10^9 colony-forming units and *S. typhi* Ty21a (non-viable) 5 to 50 × 10^9 colony-forming units, sucrose 26 to 130 mg, ascorbic acid 1 to 5 mg, amino acid mixture 1.4 to 7 mg, lactose 100 to 180 mg, magnesium stearate 3.6 to 4.4 mg. EC Cap. Blister pack 4s. *Rx.*
Use: Immunization.

Vi-Zac. (UCB) Vitamins A 5,000 units, E 50 units, C 500 mg, Zn 18 mg. Lactose. Bot. 60s. *OTC.*
Use: Mineral, vitamin supplement.

Vlemasque. (Dermik) Sulfurated lime topical solution 6% (Vleminck's Soln.), alcohol 7% in drying clay mask. Jar 4 oz. *OTC.*
Use: Dermatologic, acne.

VM. (Last) Vitamins B_1 6 mg, B_2 4 mg, niacinamide 40 mg, Fe 100 mg, Ca

188 mg, P 188 mg, Mn 4 mg, alcohol 12%. Bot. 16 oz. *OTC.*
Use: Mineral, vitamin supplement.

• **vofopitant dihydrochloride.** (voe-FOE-pi-tant) USAN.
Use: Antimetic.

volatile liquids.
Use: Anesthetic, general.
See: Sevoflurane.
Ultane.

• **volazocine.** (voe-LAY-zoe-SEEN) USAN. Under study.
Use: Analgesic.

Volitane. (Trent) Parethoxycaine 0.2%, hexachlorophene 0.025%, dichlorophene 0.025%. Aerosol spray can 3 oz. *OTC.*
Use: Counterirritant; antiseptic.

• **volociximab.** (voe-loe-SIX-i-mab) USAN.
Use: Antineoplastic.

Vol-Tab Rx. (Trigen Labs) Vitamins A 4,000 units, C 120 mg, D 400 units, E 30 units, B_1 3 mg, B_2 3 mg, B_3 20 mg, B_5 7 mg, B_6 3 mg, B_{12} 8 mcg, biotin 30 mcg, folic acid 1 mg, Ca 200 mg, Fe 29 mg, I, Zn, Mg, Cu. PEG, vegetable oil, polysorbate 80. Tab. 90s. *Rx.*
Use: Prenatal vitamin.

Voltaren. (Endo Pharmaceuticals) Diclofenac sodium 1% (1 g contains diclofenac sodium 10 mg). Isopropyl alcohol, mineral oil. Gel. Tubes. 20 g, 100 g.
Use: Antineoplastic.

Voltaren. (Novartis) Diclofenac sodium. **DR Tab.:** 75 mg. Lactose. Enteric-coated. Bot. 60s, 100s, 1000s, UD 100s. **Ophth. Soln.:** 0.1%. EDTA 1 mg/mL, boric acid, polyoxyl 35 castor oil, sorbic acid 2 mg/mL, tromethamine. 2.5 mL, 5 mL w/dropper. *Rx.*
Use: NSAID; ophthalmic.

Voltaren-XR. (Novartis) Diclofenac sodium 100 mg. Sucrose, cetyl alcohol. ER Tab. Bot. 100s, UD 100s. *Rx.*
Use: Analgesic; NSAID.

Voluven. (Hospira) Hydroxyethyl starch 6 g/100 mL. Sodium chloride 900 mg/100 mL. Inj., Soln. 500 mL. *Rx.*
Use: Plasma expander.

vonedrine hydrochloride. Vonedrine (phenylpropylmethylamine) hydrochloride. *OTC.*
Use: Decongestant.

von Willebrand factor complex/antihemophilic factor.
Use: Antihemophilic agent.
See: Humate-P.

Vopac. (Athlon) Codeine phosphate 30 mg, acetaminophen 650 mg. Tab. 100s, 500s. *c-III.*
Use: Narcotic analgesic.

• **vorapaxar.** (VOR-a-PAX-ar) USAN.
Use: Thrombosis.
• **vorapaxar sulfate.** (VOR-a-PAX-ar)
USAN.
Use: Thrombin receptor antagonist.
• **voreloxin.** (vor-el-OX-in) USAN.
Use: Antineoplastic.
• **voriconazole.** (vor-i-KON-a-zole) USAN.
Use: Antifungal.
See: Vfend.
voriconazole. (Various Mfr.) Voricona-
zole 50 mg, 200 mg. May include lac-
tose. Tab. 30s. *Rx.*
Use: Antifungal, triazole antifungal.
• **vorinostat.** (vore-IN-oh-stat) USAN.
Use: Antineoplastic; histone deacety-
lase inhibitor.
See: Zolinza.
• **vorozole.** (VORE-oh-zole) USAN.
Use: Antineoplastic.
• **vosaroxin.** (VOE-sa-ROX-in) USAN.
Use: Antineoplastic.
VōSoL HC. (ECR Pharmaceuticals)
Hydrocortisone 1%, acetic acid 2%,
benzethonium chloride 0.02%, propylene glycol diacetate 3%. Soln., Otic.
10 mL. *OTC.*
Use: Miscellaneous otic preparation.
VoSpire ER. (Dava) Albuterol (as sul-
fate) 4 mg, 8 mg. ER Tab. 100s. *Rx.*
Use: Bronchodilator; sympathomimetic.
Votrient. (GlaxoSmithKline) Pazopanib
200 mg (equiv. to pazopanib hydro-
chloride 216.7 mg). Film-coated. Tab.
30s, 90s, 120s. *Rx.*
Use: Kinase inhibitor, tyrosine kinase in-
hibitor.
• **votumumab.** (vah-TOOM-uh-mab)
USAN.
Use: Monoclonal antibody.
Voxsuprine. (Major) Isoxsuprine hydro-
chloride 10 mg, 20 mg. Tab. Bot. 100s,
250s, 1000s, UD 100s. *Rx.*
Use: Vasodilator.
VPRIV. (Shire Human Genetic Therapies)
Velaglucerase alfa 200 units, 400 units.
Sucrose 100 mg (200 units), 200 mg
(400 units). Preservative free. Single-
use vial. *Rx.*
Use: Endocrine and metabolic agent.
VSL#3 The Living Shield. (Sigma-Tau)
Lyophilized lactic acid. **Pow.:** ≥ 450 bil-
lion units. *Streptococcus thermophi-
lus, Bifidobacterium breve, Bifidobacterium longum, Bifidobacterium infantis,
Lactobacillus acidophilus, Lactobacillus
phantarum, Lactobacillus paracasei,
Lactobacillus delbrueckii.* Maltose. Gluten free. Lemon flavor. 10s, 30s. **Cap.:**
≥ 225 billion units. *Streptococcus ther-*

*mophilus, Bifidobacterium breve, Bifido-
bacterium longum, Bifidobacterium infantis, Lactobacillus acidophilus, Lactobacillus phantarum, Lactobacillus paracasei, Lactobacillus delbrueckii.* Gluten
free. 60s. *OTC.*
Use: Oral nutritional supplement, probiotic.
VSL#3 DS Double Strength. (Sigma-
Tau) Lyophilized lactic acid ≥ 900 billion
units. *Streptococcus thermophilus, Bifidobacterium breve, Bifidobacterium
longum, Bifidobacterium infantis, Lactobacillus acidophilus, Lactobacillus plantarum, Lactobacillus paracasei, Lactobacillus delbrueckii.* Maltose. Gluten
free. Pow. 20s. *OTC.*
Use: Oral nutritional supplement, probiotic.
V-Tuss Expectorant. (Vangard Labs,
Inc.) Hydrocodone bitartrate 5 mg,
pseudoephedrine hydrochloride 60 mg,
guaifenesin 200 mg/5 mL, alcohol
12.5%. *c-III.*
Use: Antitussive, decongestant, expectorant.
Vumon. (Bristol-Myers Squibb Oncology/
Virology) Teniposide 50 mg (10 mg/mL),
benzyl alcohol 30 mg, *Cremophor EL*
(polyoxyethylated castor oil), dehydrated alcohol 42.7%. Inj. Amp. 5 mL.
Rx.
Use: Antineoplastic.
Vusion. (GlaxoSmithKline) Miconazole
nitrate 0.25%, zinc oxide 15%, white
petrolatum 81.35%. Oint. Tube. 30 g.
Rx.
Use: Diaper rash combination product.
Vytone. (Sanofi-Aventis) Hydrocortisone
1%, iodoquinol 1%, greaseless base.
Cream. Bot. 30 g. *Rx.*
Use: Anti-infective; corticosteroid,
topical.
Vytorin. (Merck/Schering-Plough) Ezeti-
mibe/simvastatin 10 mg/10 mg, 10 mg/
20 mg, 10 mg/40 mg, 10 mg/80 mg.
Lactose. Tab. 30s, 90s, 500s (10 mg/
40 mg, 10 mg/80 mg only), 1,000s
(10 mg/10 mg, 10 mg/20 mg only),
2500s (10 mg/80 mg only), 5000s
(10 mg/40 mg only), 10,000s (10 mg/
10 mg, 10 mg/20 mg only), UD 50s
(10 mg/40 mg, 10 mg/80 mg only),
UD 100s (10 mg/10 mg, 10 mg/20 mg
only). *Rx.*
Use: Antihyperlipidemic.
Vyvanse. (Shire US) Lisdexamfetamine
dimesylate 20 mg, 30 mg, 40 mg,
50 mg, 60 mg, 70 mg. Cap. 100s. *c-II.*
Use: Central nervous system stimulant, amphetamine.

VZIG. (American Red Cross; Mass. Public Health Bio. Lab.) Varicella-Zoster immune globulin human globulin fraction of human plasma, primarily IgG 10% to 18% in single-dose vials containing 125 units varicella-zoster virus antibody in 2.5 mg or less. Inj.
Use: Immunization.

W

Wade Gesic Balm. (Wade) Menthol 3%, methyl salicylate 12%, petrolatum base. Tube oz, Jar lb. *OTC.*
Use: Analgesic, topical.

Wade's Drops. Compound benzoin tincture.

Wakespan. (Weeks & Leo) Caffeine 250 mg. TR Cap. Pkg. 15s. *Rx.*
Use: CNS stimulant.

Wal-Finate Allergy. (Walgreen) Chlorpheniramine maleate 4 mg. Tab. Bot. 50s. *OTC.*
Use: Antihistamine.

Wal-Finate Decongestant. (Walgreen) Chlorpheniramine maleate 4 mg, pseudoephedrine sulfate 60 mg. Tab. Bot. 50s. *OTC.*
Use: Antihistamine, decongestant.

Wal-Formula Cough Syrup with D-Methorphan. (Walgreen) Dextromethorphan HBr 15 mg, doxylamine succinate 7.5 mg, sodium citrate 500 mg/ 10 mL. Syr. Bot. 6 oz, 8 oz. *OTC.*
Use: Antihistamine, antitussive, expectorant.

Wal-Formula M Cough Syrup. (Walgreen) Dextromethorphan HBr 30 mg, pseudoephedrine hydrochloride 60 mg, guaifenesin 200 mg, acetaminophen 500 mg/20 mL. Syr. Bot. 8 oz. *OTC.*
Use: Analgesic, antitussive, decongestant, expectorant.

Wal-Frin Nasal Mist. (Walgreen) Phenylephrine hydrochloride 0.5%, pheniramine maleate 0.2%. Soln. Bot. 0.5 oz. *OTC.*
Use: Antihistamine, decongestant.

Walgreen Artificial Tears. (Walgreen) Hydroxypropyl methylcellulose 0.5%. Soln. Bot. 0.5 oz. *OTC.*
Use: Artificial tears.

Walgreen's Finest Iron. (Walgreen) Iron 30 mg. Tab. Bot. 100s. *OTC.*
Use: Mineral supplement.

Walgreen's Finest Vit B$_6$. (Walgreen) Pyridoxine hydrochloride 50 mg. Tab. Bot. 100s. *OTC.*
Use: Vitamin supplement.

Walgreen Soda Mints. (Walgreen) Sodium bicarbonate 300 mg. Tab. Bot. 100s, 200s. *OTC.*
Use: Antacid.

Wal-Phed. (Walgreen) Pseudoephedrine hydrochloride. **Syr.:** 30 mg/5 mL. Bot. 4 oz. **Tab.:** 30 mg. Bot. 50s, 100s. *OTC.*
Use: Decongestant.

Wal-Phed Plus. (Walgreen) Pseudoephedrine hydrochloride 60 mg, chlorpheniramine maleate 4 mg. Tab. Bot. 50s. *OTC.*
Use: Antihistamine, decongestant.

Wal-Tussin. (Walgreen) Guaifenesin 100 mg/5 mL. Bot. 4 oz. *OTC.*
Use: Expectorant.

Wampole One-Step hCG. (Wampole) For in vitro detection of hCG in serum and urine. Test. In 3, 24, 96, 500 test kits.
Use: Diagnostic aid, pregnancy.

•**warfarin sodium.** (WORE-fuh-rin) *USP 34.*
Use: Anticoagulant.
See: Coumadin.
Jantoven.

warfarin sodium. (Various Mfr.) Warfarin sodium 1 mg, 2 mg, 2.5 mg, 3 mg, 4 mg, 5 mg, 6 mg, 7.5 mg, 10 mg. Tab. Bot. 100s, 1000s, 5000s (except 7.5 mg, 10 mg), UD 100s. *Rx.*
Use: Anticoagulant.

Wart Fix. (Last) Castor oil 100%. Bot. 0.3 fl oz. *OTC.*
Use: Dermatologic; wart therapy.

Wart-Off. (Pfizer) Salicylic acid 17% in flexible collodion, alcohol 20.5%, ether 54.2%. Bot. 0.5 oz. *OTC.*
Use: Keratolytic.

wasp venom.
Use: Immunization.
See: Albay.
Pharmalgen.
Venomil.

•**water.** (WA-ter) *USP 34.*
Use: Pharmaceutic aid.

Water Babies Little Licks by Coppertone. (Schering-Plough) SPF 30, ethylhexyl p-methoxycinnamate, oxybenzone, 2-ethylhexyl salicylate, cherry flavor. Lot. Tube 4.8 g. *OTC.*
Use: Sunscreen.

Water Babies UVA/UVB SPF 15 Sunblock. (Schering-Plough) Ethylhexyl p-methoxycinnamate, oxybenzone in lotion base. Lot. Bot. 120 mL. *OTC.*
Use: Sunscreen.

Water Babies UVA/UVB SPF 45 Sunblock. (Schering-Plough) Ethylhexyl p-methoxycinnamate, 2-ethylhexyl salicylate, otocrylene oxybenzone, benzyl alcohol. PABA free, waterproof. Lot. Bot. 120 mL. *OTC.*
Use: Sunscreen.

Water Babies UVA/UVB SPF 30 Sunblock. (Schering-Plough) Ethylhexyl p-methoxycinnamate, 2-ethylhexyl salicylate, homosalate, oxybenzone, benzyl alcohol. PABA free, waterproof. Lot. Bot. 120 mL, 240 mL. *OTC.*
Use: Sunscreen.

Water Babies SPF 25 Sunblock.
(Schering-Plough) Ethylhexyl p-
methoxycinnamate, 2-ethylhexyl salicylate, homosalate, oxybenzone, benzyl alcohol. PABA free, waterproof.
Cream. Bot. 90 g. *OTC.*
Use: Sunscreen.

• **water for hemodialysis.** (WA-ter)
USP 34.
Use: Hemodialysis.

• **water for injection.** (WA-ter) *USP 34.*
Use: Pharmaceutic aid (solvent).

watermelon seed extract.
See: Citrin.

W/Phenobarbital, Theobromine.
See: Cithal.

• **water, purified.** (WA-ter) *USP 34.*
Use: Pharmaceutic aid (solvent).

water-soluble vitamins.
Use: Vitamin supplement.
See: Aminobenzoate Potassium.
Ascorbic Acid.
Ascorbic Acid Combinations.
Bioflavonoids (Vitamin P).
Calcium Ascorbate.
Cyanocobalamin (B_{12}).
Folic Acid and Derivatives.
Leucovorin Calcium.
Levoleucovorin.
Hydroxocobalamin.
Niacin (B_3; Nicotinic Acid).
Niacinamide (Nicotinamide).
Pyridoxine Hydrochloride (B_6).
Riboflavin (B_2).
Sodium Ascorbate.
Thiamin (B_1).
Vitamin B_{12}.
Vitamin C (Ascorbic Acid).

• **wax, carnauba.** (wax kar-NOE-ba)
NF 29.
Use: Pharmaceutic aid (tablet coating
agent).

• **wax, emulsifying.** *NF 29.*
Use: Pharmaceutic aid (emulsifying,
stiffening agent).

• **wax, microcrystalline.** (wax MYE-kroe-
KRIS-ta-lin) *NF 29.*
Use: Pharmaceutic aid (stiffening, tab-
let coating agent).

Waxsol. Docusate sodium.

• **wax, white.** *NF 29.*
Use: Pharmaceutic aid (stiffening
agent).

• **wax, yellow.** (wax YEL-oh) *NF 29.*
Use: Pharmaceutic aid (stiffening
agent).

Wayds. (Wayne) Docusate sodium
100 mg. Cap. Bot. 100s. *OTC.*
Use: Laxative.

Wayds-Plus. (Wayne) Docusate w/
casanthranol. Cap. Bot. 50s. *OTC.*
Use: Laxative.

Wayne-E. (Wayne) Vitamin E. Cap.
100 units, 200 units: Bot. 1000s.
400 units: Bot. 100s. *OTC.*
Use: Vitamin supplement.

Wee Care. (Centurion Labs) Carbonyl
iron 15 mg per 1.25 mL. Acesulfame K,
glycerin, parabens, potassium sorbate,
propylene glycol, sucralose. Wild
cherry flavor. Susp. 118 mL. *OTC.*
Use: Trace element.

Wehless. (Roberts) Phendimetrazine tartrate 35 mg. Cap. Bot. 100s. *c-III.*
Use: Anorexiant.

Wehless-105 Timecelles. (Roberts)
Phendimetrazine tartrate 105 mg. SA
Cap. Bot. 100s. *c-III.*
Use: Anorexiant.

Wehydryl. (Roberts) Diphenhydramine
hydrochloride 50 mg/mL. Vial 10 mL.
Rx.
Use: Antihistamine.

Welchol. (Daiichi Sankyo) Colesevelam
hydrochloride. **Tab.:** 625 mg. Film-
coated. 180s. **Pow. for Susp.:** 1.875 g,
3.75 g. Aspartame, pheylalanine 24 mg
(1.875g), 48 mg (3.75 g). Citrus flavor.
Single-dose packet. *Rx.*
Use: Antihyperlipidemic; bile acid sequestrant.

Welders Eye. (Weber) Tetracaine, potassium Cl, boric acid, camphor, glycerin,
disodium edetate, benzalkonium Cl as
preservatives. Lot. Bot. oz. *OTC.*
Use: Burn therapy.

Wellbutrin. (GlaxoSmithKline) Bupropion
hydrochloride 75 mg, 100 mg. Film-
coated. Tab. 100s. *Rx.*
Use: Antidepressant.

Wellbutrin SR. (GlaxoSmithKline) Bupropion hydrochloride 100 mg, 150 mg,
200 mg. Film-coated. ER Tab (12 hour).
60s. *Rx.*
Use: Antidepressant.

Wellbutrin XL. (BTA Pharmaceuticals)
Bupropion hydrochloride 150 mg,
300 mg. Polyvinyl alcohol. ER Tab
(24 hour). 30s, 90s (150 mg only). *Rx.*
Use: Antidepressant.

WellTuss EXP. (Prasco) Dihydrocodeine
bitartrate 7.5 mg, guaifenesin 100 mg,
pseudoephedrine hydrochloride 15 mg
per 5 mL. Sugar, alcohol, and dye free.
Menthol, saccharin, sorbitol. Syr.
473 mL. *c-III.*
Use: Antitussive and expectorant combination.

Wernet's Adhesive Cream. (Block Drug)
Carboxymethylcellulose gum, ethylene

oxide polymer, petrolatum in mineral oil base. Cream. Tube 1.5 oz. *OTC.*
Use: Denture adhesive.

Wernet's Powder. (Block Drug) Karaya gum, ethylene oxide polymer. Bot. 0.63 oz, 1.75 oz, 3.55 oz. *OTC.*
Use: Denture adhesive.

Wes-B/C. (Western Research) Vitamins B_1 15 mg, B_2 10 mg, B_6 5 mg, niacinamide 50 mg, calcium pantothenate 10 mg, C 300 mg. Cap. Bot. 1000s. *OTC.*
Use: Mineral, vitamin supplement.

Wesmatic Forte Tablets. (Wesley) Phenobarbital 1/8 g, ephedrine sulfate 0.25 g, chlorpheniramine maleate 2 mg, guaifenesin 100 mg. Tab. Bot. 100s, 1000s. *Rx.*
Use: Antihistamine, decongestant, expectorant, hypnotic, sedative.

Westcort. (Ranbaxy) Hydrocortisone valerate 0.2% in a hydrophilic base with white petrolatum. **Cream:** Tube. 15 g, 45 g, 60 g, 120 g. **Oint.:** Mineral oil. Tube. 15 g, 45 g, 60 g. *Rx.*
Use: Corticosteroid, topical.

Westhroid. (RLC Labs) Thyroid 16.25 mg (1/4 gr) (lactose), 32.5 mg (1/2 gr), 48.75 mg (3/4 gr) (lactose), 65 mg (1 gr), 81.25 mg (1 1/4 gr) (lactose), 97.5 mg (1 1/2 gr) (lactose), 113.75 mg (1 3/4 gr) (lactose), 130 mg (2 gr), 146.25 mg (2 1/4 gr) (lactose), 162.5 mg (2 1/2 gr) (lactose), 194.4 mg (3 gr), 260 mg (4 gr) (lactose), 325 mg (5 gr) (lactose). Note: 1 grain (gr) = 64.8 mg. Tab. 100s; 30s, 60s, 90s, 990s, 1,000s, 1,008s (16.25 mg, 48.75 mg, 81.25 mg, 97.5 mg, 113.75 mg, 146.25 mg, 162.5 mg, 260 mg, 325 mg). *Rx.*
Use: Thyroid hormone.

Wesvite. (Western Research) Vitamins B_1 10 mg, B_2 5 mg, B_6 2 mg, pantothenic acid 10 mg, niacinamide 30 mg, B_{12} 3 mcg, C 100 mg, E 5 units, A 10,000 units, D 400 units, Fe 15 mg, Cu 1 mg, I 0.15 mg, Mn 1 mg, Zn 1.5 mg. Tab. Bot. 1000s. *OTC.*
Use: Mineral, vitamin supplement.

Wetting and Soaking. (Bausch & Lomb) Chlorhexidine gluconate 0.006%, EDTA 0.05%, cationic cellulose derivative polymer. Soln. Bot. 118 mL. *OTC.*
Use: Contact lens care.

Wetting and Soaking. (PBH Wesley Jessen) Buffered, isotonic. Chlorhexidine gluconate 0.005%, EDTA 0.02%, sodium chloride, octylphenoxy (oxyethylene) ethanol, povidone, polyvinyl alcohol, propylene glycol, hydroxyethyl-

cellulose. Soln. Bot. 120 mL. *OTC.*
Use: Contact lens care.

wheat germ oil. (Various Mfr.)
Use: Vitamin supplement

wheat germ oil concentrate. (Thurston) Wheat germ oil concentrate. Perles. 6 min. Bot. 100s. *OTC.*
Use: Cardiovascular agent.

whey protein concentrate (bovine).
See: Bovine Whey Protein Concentrate.

Whirl-Sol. (Sween) Moisturizing bath additive. Bot. 2 oz, 8 oz, 16 oz, 21 oz, gal, 5 gal, 30 gal, 55 gal. *OTC.*
Use: Emollient.

white-faced hornet venom.
Use: Immunization.
See: Albay.
   Pharmalgen.
   Venomil.

white lotion. Lotio alba.
Use: Astringent.
See: Zinc Sulfide Topical Suspension.

Whitfield's Ointment. (Various Mfr.) Benzoic acid 6%, salicylic acid 3%. Oint. Tube. *OTC.*
Use: Anti-infective, topical.

•**whooping cough vaccine.** *USP 34.*
See: ActHIB/DTP, Set of DTwP Vial Plus Hib.
   Diphtheria and Tetanus Toxoids with Pertussis Vaccine.
   Infanrix.
   Pertussis Vaccine.
   Tripedia.

Whorto's Calamine Lotion. (Whorton Pharmaceuticals, Inc.) Calamine, zinc oxide, glycerin (U.S.P. strength) in carboxymethylcellulose lotion vehicle. Lot. Bot. 4 oz, gal. *OTC.*
Use: Dermatologic; counterirritant.

Wibi. (Galderma) Purified water, SD alcohol 40, glycerin, PEG-4, PEG-6-32 stearate, PEG-6-32, glycol stearate, carbomer 940, PEG-75, methylparaben, propylparaben, triethanolamine, menthol, fragrance. Lot. Bot. 8 oz, 16 oz. *OTC.*
Use: Emollient.

widow spider species antivenin (Latrodectus mactans). (Merck & Co.) Antivenin, *Lactrodectus mactans.*
Use: Immunization.

Wilate. (Octapharma USA) Antihemophilic factor /von Willebrand factor complex. **450 units/450 units per vial:** Heat treated. Upon reconstitution with the volume of diluent provided (water for injection with 0.1% polysorbate 80), each vial contains VWF:RCo 450 units, factor VIII 450 units, and total protein 7.5 mg or less. Each vial also contains

glycine 50 mg, sucrose 50 mg, sodium chloride 117 mg, sodium citrate 14.7 mg, and calcium chloride 0.8 mg. Preservative free. **900 units/900 units per vial:** Heat treated. Upon reconstitution with the volume of diluent provided (water for injection with 0.1% polysorbate 80), each vial contains VWF:RCo 900 units, factor VIII 900 units, and total protein ($\leq$ 15 mg). Each vial also contains glycine 100 mg, sucrose 100 mg, sodium chloride 234 mg, sodium citrate 29.4 mg, and calcium chloride 1.5 mg. Preservative free. Inj., lyophilized Pow. For Soln. Single-dose vial and a vial of diluents, transfer device, and infusion set. *Rx.*
Use: Hematological agent, antihemophilic factor combination.

wild cherry.
Use: Flavored vehicle.

Wilpor-Clear. (Foy Laboratories) Phentermine hydrochloride 30 mg. Cap. Bot. 1000s. *c-IV.*
Use: Anorexiant.

Wilpowr. (Foy Laboratories) Phentermine hydrochloride 30 mg. Cap. Bot. 100s, 500s, 1000s. *c-IV.*
Use: Anorexiant.

WinRho SDF. (Baxter) RH$_o$(D) immune globulin IV human 1,500 units (300 mcg), 2,500 units (500 mcg), 5,000 units (1,000 mcg), 15,000 units (3,000 mcg). Maltose 10%, polysorbate 80 0.03%. Preservative free. Inj. Soln. Single-dose vial. *Rx.*
Use: Immune globulin.

Wintergreen Sucrets. (GlaxoSmithKline) Dyclonine hydrochloride 0.1%, alcohol 10%, sorbitol. Spray. Bot. 90 mL. *OTC.*
Use: Mouth and throat preparation.

•**witch hazel.** (WICH HAY-zel) *USP 34.*
Use: Astringent.

witch hazel. (Various Mfr.) Hamamelis water (witch hazel). Bot. 120 mL, 240 mL, 280 mL, 480 mL, 960 mL, gal. *OTC.*
Use: Astringent.

Within. (Bayer Consumer Care) Vitamins A 5000 units, E 30 units, C 60 mg, folic acid 0.4 mg, B$_1$ 1.5 mg, B$_2$ 1.7 mg, niacin 20 mg, B$_6$ 2 mg, B$_{12}$ 6 mcg, pantothenic acid 10 mg, D 400 units, Fe 27 mg, Ca 450 mg, Zn 15 mg. Tab. Bot. 60s, 100s. *OTC.*
Use: Mineral, vitamin supplement.

WNS. (Sanofi-Synthelabo) Sulfamylon hydrochloride. Supp. *Rx.*
Use: Anorectal preparation.

Women's Gentle Laxative. (Goldline Consumer) Bisacodyl 5 mg, lactose, sugar. EC Tab. Pkg. 30s. *OTC.*
Use: Laxative.

Women's Tylenol Multi-Symptom Menstrual Relief. (McNeil Consumer) Acetaminophen 500 mg, pamabrom 25 mg. Tab. Bot. 24s. *OTC.*
Use: Analgesic.

Wonderful Dream. (Kondon) Phenylmercuric nitrate 1:5000, oils of tar, turpentine, olive and linseed, rosin, burgundy pitch, camphor, beeswax, mutton tallow. Salve. 34 g. *OTC.*
Use: Topical.

Wonder Ice. (Pedinol Pharmacal) Menthol in a specially formulated base. Gel. Tube 113 mL. *OTC.*
Use: Liniment.

Wondra. (Procter & Gamble) Petrolatum, lanolin acid, glycerin, stearyl alcohol, cyclomethicone, EDTA, hydrogenated vegetable glycerides phosphate, cetyl alcohol, isopropyl palmitate, stearic acid, PEG-100 stearate, carbomer 934, dimethicone, titanium dioxide, imidazolidinyl urea, parabens. Lot. Bot. 180 mL, 300 mL, 450 mL. *OTC.*
Use: Emollient.

wood charcoal. (Cowley) Wood charcoal. 5 g, 10 g. Tab. Bot. 1000s. *OTC.*

wood creosote.
See: Creosote.

wool fat. Lanolin, Anhydrous.

Wyanoids Relief Factor. (Wyeth) Cocoa butter 79%, shark liver oil 3%, corn oil, EDTA, parabens, tocopherol. Supp. 12s. *OTC.*
Use: Anorectal preparation.

Wydase Lyophilized. (Wyeth) Purified bovine testicular hyaluronidase. Vial 150 units/mL, 1500 units/10 mL with lactose and thimerosal. *Rx.*
Use: Absorption facilitator; hypodermoclysis; urography.

Wydase Stabilized Solution. (Wyeth) Purified bovine testicular hyaluronidase 150 units/mL in sterile saline soln. with sodium Cl, EDTA, thimerosal. Vial 1 mL, 10 mL. *Rx.*
Use: Absorption facilitator; hypodermoclysis; urography.

Wymox. (Wyeth-Ayerst) Amoxicillin trihydrate. **Cap.:** 250 mg Bot. 100s, 500s; 500 mg Bot. 50s, 500s. **Pow. for Oral Susp.:** 125 mg/5 mL (as trihydrate) when reconstituted; 250 mg/5 mL (as trihydrate) when reconstituted. Bot. 100 mL, 150 mL. Sucrose. *Rx.*
Use: Anti-infective, penicillin.

Wytensin. (Wyeth) Guanabenz acetate 4 mg, 8 mg, 16 mg. Tab. Bot. 100s; 500s, *Redipak* 100s (4 mg only). *Rx.*
Use: Antihypertensive.

X

Xalatan. (Pfizer) Latanoprost 0.005%, benzalkonium chloride 0.02%, sodium chloride. Soln. In 2.5 mL fill dropper bottles. *Rx.*
Use: Agent for glaucoma.

•**xaliproden.** (ZAL-ip-roe-den) USAN.
Use: Nootrope.

•**xamoterol.** (ZAM-oh-ter-ole) USAN.
Use: Cardiovascular agent.

•**xamoterol fumarate.** (ZAM-oh-ter-ole) USAN.
Use: Cardiovascular agent.

Xanax. (Pfizer) Alprazolam 0.25 mg, 0.5 mg, 1 mg, 2 mg. Lactose. Tab. 100s, 500s, 1000s (except 2 mg), UD 100s (0.25 mg, 0.5 mg only). *c-iv.*
Use: Anxiolytic.

Xanax XR. (Pfizer) Alprazolam 0.5 mg, 1 mg, 2 mg, 3 mg. Lactose. ER Tab. 60s. *c-iv.*
Use: Anxiolytic.

•**xanomeline.** (zah-NO-meh-leen) USAN.
Use: Cholinergic agonist (for Alzheimer disease).

•**xanomeline tartrate.** (zah-NO-meh-leen) USAN.
Use: Cholinergic agonist (for Alzheimer disease).

•**xanoxate sodium.** (ZAN-ox-ate) USAN.
Use: Bronchodilator.

•**xanthan gum.** (ZAN-than) *NF 29.*
Use: Pharmaceutic aid, suspending agent.

xanthine combinations.
Use: Antiasthmatic combinations.
See: Dyphylline and Guaifenesin.
Theophylline and Guaifenesin.

xanthine derivatives.
See: Aminophylline.
Caffeine.
Dyphylline.
Theobromine.
Theophylline.

•**xanthinol niacinate.** (ZAN-thih-nahl NYE-ah-SIN-ate) USAN.
Use: Vasodilator, peripheral.

xanthiol hydrochloride.
Use: Antinauseant.

xanthotoxin. Methoxsalen.

Xclair. (Align) Isohexadecane, Butyrospermum parkii, ethylhexyl palmitate, glycyrrhetinic acid, cera alba, PEG-30 dipolyhydroxystearate, bisabolol, polyglyceryl-6, polyricinoleate, tocopheryl acetate (antioxidant), castor oil, sodium hyaluronate nylon 12, butylene glycol, magnesium sulfate, piroctone olamine, allantoin, magnesium

stearate, disodium EDTA, vitis vinifera, ascorbyl tetraisopalmitate, propyl gallate, telmesteine. Cream. 75 mL. *Rx.*
Use: Dermatological agent, miscellaneous topical combination.

Xeloda. (Roche) Capecitabine 150 mg, 500 mg. Lactose. Film-coated. Tab. Bot. 60s (150 mg only), 120s (500 mg only). *Rx.*
Use: Antimetabolite, pyrimidine analog.

•**xemilofiban hydrochloride.** (ZEM-i-loe-FYE-ban) USAN.
Use: Treatment of unstable angina; prevention of post-recanalization reocclusion of coronary vessels.

Xenaderm. (Healthpoint) Balsam peru/castor oil/trypsin 87 mg/788 mg/ 90 units, 87 mg/788 mg/250-700 units. Safflower oil. Oint. 30 g, 60 g. *Rx.*
Use: Enzyme preparation.

•**xenalipin.** (ZEN-ah-LIH-pin) USAN.
Use: Hypolipidemic.

Xenazine. (Prestwick) Tetrabenazine 12.5 mg, 25 mg. Lactose. Tab. 112s. *Rx.*
Use: CNS agent.

•**xenbucin.** (ZEN-BYOO-sin) USAN.
Use: Antihyperlipidemic.

Xenical. (Roche) Orlistat 120 mg. Cap. Bot. 90s. *Rx.*
Use: Antiobesity agent; lipase inhibitor.

•**xenon Xe 133.** (ZEE-non) *USP 34.*
Use: Radiopharmaceutical.

•**xenon Xe 127.** (ZEE-non) *USP 34.*
Use: Diagnostic aid; medicinal gas; radiopharmaceutical.

Xeomin. (Merz Pharma) IncobotulinumtoxinA 50 units, 100 units. Albumin (human) 1 mg, sucrose 4.7 mg. Preservative free. Inj., lyophilized Pow. for Soln. Single-use vial. *Rx.*
Use: Botulinum toxin.

Xerac AC. (Person and Covey) Aluminum Cl hexahydrate 6.25% in anhydrous ethanol 96%. Bot 35 mL, 60 mL. *Rx.*
Use: Dermatologic, acne.

Xerese. (Meda Pharmaceuticals) Acyclovir 5%, hydrocortisone 1%. Cetostearyl alcohol, mineral oil, propylene glycol, white petrolatum. Cream. 2 g, 5 g. *Rx.*
Use: Topical anti-infective, antiviral combination.

Xeroform 3%. (Various Mfr.) Pow. 0.25 lb, 1 lb. Jar 1 lb, 5 lb.
Use: Wound care.

Xero-Lube. (Scherer) Monobasic potassium phosphate, dibasic potassium phosphate, magnesium Cl, potassium Cl, calcium Cl, sodium Cl, sodium fluo-

ride, sorbitol, sodium carboxymethyl-cellulose, methylparaben. Soln. Bot. 6 oz. *OTC.*
Use: Mouth and throat preparation.

Xgeva. (Amgen) Denosumab 70 mg/mL. Preservative free. Inj., Soln. Single-use vial. *Rx.*
Use: Monoclonal antibody.

Xiaflex. (Auxilium) Collagenase clostridium histolyticum 0.9 mg. Sucrose 18.5 mg. Preservative free. Inj., lyophilized Pow. for Soln. Single-use vial w/ diluent (contains 3 mL of calcium chloride dihydrate 0.3 mg/mL in sodium chloride 0.9%). *Rx.*
Use: Enzyme preparation, injectable enzyme combination.

Xibrom. (Ista Pharm) Bromfenac 0.09%. Benzalkonium chloride 0.05 mg/mL, EDTA 0.2 mg/mL, povidone 20 mg/mL, sodium sulfite 0.2 mg/mL, boric acid, sodium borate, sodium hydroxide. Ophth. Soln. Dropper bottles. 5 mL. *Rx.*
Use: Nonsteroidal anti-inflammatory drug, ophthalmic.

Xifaxan. (Salix) Rifaximin 200 mg, 550 mg. EDTA. Film-coated. Tab. 30s, 100s, UD 100s (200 mg); 60s, UD 60s (550 mg). *Rx.*
Use: Anti-infective.

Xigris. (Eli Lilly) Drotrecogin alfa (activated) 5 mg (sodium chloride 40.3 mg, sucrose 31.8 mg), 20 mg (sodium chloride 158.1 mg, sucrose 124.9 mg). Preservative free. Inj., Lyophilized, Pow. for Soln. Single-use vials. *Rx.*
Use: Thrombolytic agent, human protein C.

•**xilobam.** (ZIE-low-bam) USAN.
Use: Muscle relaxant.

•**ximelagatran.** (zye-mel-a-GAT-ran) USAN.
Use: Investigational antithrombotic.

•**xipamide.** (ZIP-ah-mide) USAN.
Use: Antihypertensive; diuretic.

XiraHist DM Pediatric. (Hawthorn) Dextromethorphan HBr 3 mg, carbinoxamine maleate 2 mg, phenylephrine hydrochloride 2 mg per 1 mL. Sugar, alcohol, and dye free. Saccharin, sorbitol. Peach flavor. Drops, Oral. 30 mL with dropper.
Use: Upper respiratory combination, antitussive combination.

XiraHist Pediatric. (Hawthorn) Phenylephrine hydrochloride 2 mg, carbinoxamine maleate 2 mg per 1 mL. Alcohol, sugar, and dye free. Saccharin, sorbitol. Strawberry flavor. Drops. 30 mL with dropper. *Rx.*

Use: Upper respiratory combination, decongestant and antihistamine combination.

XiraTuss. (Hawthorn) Carbetapentane tannate 60 mg, chlorpheniramine tannate 5 mg, phenylephrine tannate 10 mg. Tab. 60s. *Rx.*
Use: Upper respiratory combination, antitussive combination.

Xodol. (Victory) Hydrocodone bitartrate/ acetaminophen 7.5 mg/300 mg, 10 mg/ 300 mg. Tab. 100s, 500s (except 7.5 mg/300 mg). *c-iii.*
Use: Narcotic analgesic.

Xolair. (Genentech) Omalizumab 202.5 mg (delivers 150 mg/1.2 mL). Preservative free. Sucrose. Inj., Lyophilized Pow. for Soln. Single-use vials. *Rx.*
Use: Monoclonal antibody.

Xolegel. (GlaxoSmithKline) Ketoconazole 2%. Dehydrated alcohol 34%, glycerin. Gel. Tubes. 2 g, 15 g. *Rx.*
Use: Topical anti-infective, antifungal agent.

Xolegel CorePak. (Barrier Therapeutics) Gel. **Xolegel:** Ketoconazole 2%. Alcohol 34%, glycerin. 45 g. **Xebcort:** Hydrocortisone 1%. Castor oil, menthol, SD alcohol 40-B 20%. 22.7 g. *Rx.*
Use: Antiseborrheic combination.

Xolegel Duo Convenience Pack. (Barrier) **Gel:** Ketoconazole 2%. Alcohol 34%. 15 g. **Shampoo:** Pyrithione zinc 1%. Benzyl alcohol, cetyl alcohol. 120 mL. *Rx.*
Use: Antiseborrheic product.

Xolox. (WraSer) Acetaminophen 500 mg, oxycodone hydrochloride 10 mg. Tab. 50s, 100s. *c-ii.*
Use: Opioid analgesic combination.

Xopenex. (Sepracor) Levalbuterol. **Soln. for Inhalation:** As levalbuterol hydrochloride. 0.31 mg/3 mL, 0.63 mg/3 mL, 1.25 mg/3 mL. Preservative free, sulfuric acid. UD Vials. 3 mL. **Soln. for Inhalation, concentrate:** 1.25 mg/ 0.5 mL. Preservative free. UD vials. 0.5 mL. *Rx.*
Use: Bronchodilator, sympathomimetic.

Xopenex HFA. (Sepracor) Levalbuterol (as tartrate) 45 mcg/actuation. Contains no chlorofluorcarbons. Aer. Inh. 15 g (200 inhalations). *Rx.*
Use: Bronchodilator, sympathomimetic.

•**xorphanol mesylate.** (ZOR-fa-nol) USAN.
Use: Analgesic.

Xoten Pain Relief. (MenChem) Methyl salicylate 6.25%, menthol 12.5%, alcohol, aloe, camphor, eucalyptus, grape

seed oil. Lot. 118 mL. *OTC.*
Use: Rub and liniment.

Xpect-AT. (Hawthorn) Carbetapentane citrate 60 mg, guaifenesin 600 mg. ER Tab. 100s. *Rx.*
Use: Upper respiratory combination, antitussive with expectorant.

Xpect-HC. (Hawthorn) Hydrocodone bitartrate 5 mg, guaifenesin 600 mg. ER Tab. 100s. *c-III.*
Use: Antitussive with expectorant.

X-Ray Contrast Media.
See: Iodine Products, Diagnostic.

X•Seb T. (Ivax) Coal tar soln. 10%, salicylic acid 4%. Soln. Bot. 4 oz. *OTC.*
Use: Antiseborrheic.

X•Seb T Plus. (Ivax) Coal tar solution 10%, salicylic acid 0.4%, EDTA. Shampoo. Bot. 118 mL. *OTC.*
Use: Antiseborrheic.

Xtracare. (Sween) Bot. 2 oz, 4 oz, 8 oz, 21 oz, gal. *OTC.*
Use: Emollient.

Xtra-Vites. (Barth's) Vitamins A 10,000 units, D 400 units, C 150 mg, B_1 5 mg, B_2 1 mg, niacin 3.33 mg, pantothenic acid 183 mcg, B_6 250 mcg, B_{12} 215 mcg, E 15 units, rutin 20 mg, citrus bioflavonoid complex 15 mg, choline 6.67 mg, inositol 10 mg, folic acid 50 mcg, biotin, aminobenzoic acid. Tab. Bot. 30s, 90s, 180s, 360s. *OTC.*
Use: Vitamin supplement.

X-Trozine. (Shire US) Phendimetrazine tartrate 35 mg. Cap. Tab. Bot. 1000s. *c-III.*
Use: Anorexiant.

X-Trozine S.R. (Shire US) Phendimetrazine tartrate 105 mg. Cap. Bot. 100s, 200s, 1000s. *c-III.*
Use: Anorexiant.

•**xylamidine tosylate.** (zie-LAM-ih-deen TAH-sill-ate) USAN.
Use: Serotonin inhibitor.

•**xylazine hydrochloride.** (ZYE-la-zeen) USAN.
Use: Analgesic.

•**xylitol.** (ZIE-lih-tahl) *NF 29.*
Use: Pharmaceutic aid, vehicle, sweetened.

Xylocaine. (APP Pharmaceutical) Lidocaine hydrochloride. **Jelly:** 2%. Parabens. 5 mL, 30 mL. **Top. Soln.:** 4%. Parabens. 50 mL. *Rx-OTC.*
Use: Topical local anesthetic, amide local anesthetic.

Xylocaine. (APP Pharmaceutical) **0.5%:** Multidose vial 50 mL, methylparaben. **1%:** Amp. 20 mL. **2%:** Multidose vial 10 mL, 20 mL, 50 mL, methylparaben.

Cartridge 1.8 mL. **0.5% w/epinephrine 1/200,000:** Multidose vial. 50 mL, methylparaben. **1% w/epinephrine 1/100,000:** Multidose vial. 10 mL, 20 mL, 50 mL, methylparaben. **2% w/epinephrine 1/50,000:** Dental cartridge 1.8 mL, sodium metabisulfite. **2% w/epinephrine 1/100,000:** Multidose vial 10 mL, 20 mL, 50 mL, sodium metabisulfite. Cartridge 1.8 mL, sodium bisulfite. **1.5% w/dextrose 7.5%:** Amp. 2 mL. *Rx.*
Use: Anesthetic, local amide.

Xylocaine Hydrochloride 4%. (AstraZeneca) Lidocaine 4%. Soln. Bot. 50 mL. *Rx.*
Use: Anesthetic, local topical.

Xylocaine Hydrochloride IV for Cardiac Arrhythmias. (APP Pharmaceutical) Lidocaine 2% (20 mg/mL). Inj. (for direct IV administration). Amp 5 mL. *Rx.*
Use: Antiarrhythmic agent.

Xylocaine MPF. (APP Pharmaceutical) Lidocaine. **0.5%:** Single-dose vial 50 mL. **1%:** Amp. 2 mL, 5 mL, 30 mL. *PolyAmp DuoFit* 10 mL, 20 mL. Single-dose vial 2 mL, 5 mL, 10 mL, 30 mL. **1.5%:** Amp. 20 mL. *PolyAmp DuoFit* 10 mL, 20 mL. Single-dose vial 5 mL, 10 mL. **2%:** Amp. 2 mL, 10 mL. *PolyAmp DuoFit* 10 mL. Single-dose vial 2 mL, 5 mL, 10 mL. **4%:** Amp. 5 mL. Syr. 5 mL w/laryngotracheal cannula. **1% w/epinephrine 1:200,000:** Amp. 30 mL. Single-dose vial 5 mL, 10 mL, 30 mL, sodium metabisulfite. **1.5% w/epinephrine 1:200,000:** Amp. 5 mL, 30 mL. Single-dose vial 5 mL, 10 mL, 30 mL, sodium metabisulfite. **2% w/epinephrine 1:200,000:** Amp. 20 mL. Single-dose vial 5 mL, 10 mL, 20 mL, sodium metabisulfite. **1.5% w/dextrose 7.5%:** Amp. 2 mL. **5% w/dextrose 7.5%:** Amp. 2 mL. *Rx.*
Use: Anesthetic, local amide.

Xylocaine Ointment. (AstraZeneca) Lidocaine 2.5%, water soluble carbowaxes. Oint. Tube 35 g *OTC.*
Use: Anesthetic, local.

•**xylofilcon A.** (ZILE-oh-FILL-kahn A) USAN.
Use: Contact lens material (hydrophilic).

•**xylometazoline hydrochloride.** (ZYE-loe-me-TAZ-oh-leen) *USP 34.*
Use: Nasal decongestant, imidazoline.
See: 4-Way Moisturizing Relief.
Otrivin.
Otrivin Pediatric Nasal.

•**xylose.** (ZIE-lohs) *USP 34.*
Use: Diagnostic aid, intestinal function determination.

Xyntha. (Wyeth) Antihemophilic factor 250 units, 500 units, 1,000 units, 2,000 units, 3,000 units. L-histidine, sucrose. Preservative free and plasma/albumin free. Solvent/detergent treated, nanofiltrated. Inj., lyophilized Pow. for Soln. Kits w/single-use vial and diluent (sodium chloride 0.9% 4 mL). *Rx.*
Use: Antihemophilic agent.

Xyralid. (Auriga) Lidocaine hydrochloride 3%, hydrocortisone acetate 1%. Cetyl alcohol, mineral oil, parabens, stearyl alcohol, white petrolatum. Cream. 85 g. *Rx.*
Use: Anti-inflammatory agent, topical corticosteroid.

Xyralid RC. (Auriga) Hydrocortisone acetate 1%, lidocaine hydrochloride 3%. Cetyl alcohol, glycerin, mineral oil, parabens, stearyl alcohol, urea, white petrolatum. Cream. 7 g w/applicator and cleansing wipes. *Rx.*
Use: Anorectal preparation, steroid-containing product.

Xyrem. (Jazz Pharmaceuticals) Sodium oxybate 500 mg/mL. Sodium 91 mg/mL. Oral Soln. 180 mL with syringe and dosing cups. *c-III.*
Note: Available only through the Xyrem Success Program. Call 1-866-997-3688 for more information.
Use: Psychotherapeutic agent, miscellaneous.

Xyzal. (Sanofi-Aventis) Levocetirizine dihydrochloride. **Oral Soln.:** 2.5 mg/5 mL. Maltitol, parabens, saccharin. 150 mL. **Tab.:** 5 mg. Lactose. Film-coated. 90s, 180s, UD 30s. *Rx.*
Use: Antihistamine, peripherally selective piperazine.

Y

Yager's Liniment. (Yager) Oil of turpentine and camphor w/clove oil fragrance, emulsifier, emollient, ammonium oleate (less than 0.5% free ammonia) penetrant base. *OTC.*
Use: Rubefacient.

Yasmin. (Bayer Healthcare) Ethinyl estradiol 30 mcg, drospirenone 3 mg. Lactose. Film-coated. Tab. Blister pack 28s with 7 inert tabs. *Rx.*
Use: Sex hormone, contraceptive hormone.

yatren.
See: Chiniofon.

YAZ. (Bayer) Drospirenone 3 mg/ethinyl estradiol 0.02 mg. Lactose. Film-coated. Tab. 24s. 4 inert tables. Blister-pack 28s. *Rx.*
Use: Sex hormone, estrogen and progestin combined.

Y-Cof DM Extended-Release. (Larken) Dextromethorphan hydrobromide 30 mg, dexbrompheniramine maleate 6 mg, phenylephrine hydrochloride 20 mg. ER Tab. 100s. *Rx.*
Use: Upper respiratory combination, antitussive combination.

YDP Lice. (Youngs Drug) Synthetic pyrethroid in aerosol. Spray. Can. 5 oz. *OTC.*
Use: Pediculicide, inanimate objects.

yeast adenylic acid. An isomer of adenosine 5-monophosphate, has been found inactive.

yeast, dried.
Use: Protein and vitamin B Complex source.

Yeast-Gard Medicated Disposable Douche. (Lake Consumer) Povidone-iodine 0.3% when reconstituted. Soln. 180 mL twin-pack w/two 5.4 mL medicated douche concentrate packets. *OTC.*
Use: Douche.

Yeast-Gard Medicated Disposable Douche Premix. (Lake Consumer) Octoxynol 9, lactic acid, sodium lactate, sodium benzoate, aloe vera. Soln. 180 mL twin-pack. *OTC.*
Use: Douche.

Yeast-Gard Medicated Douche. (Lake Consumer) Povidone-iodine 10%. Soln. Concentrate. 240 mL. *OTC.*
Use: Douche.

yeast tablets, dried.
Use: Supplementary source of B complex vitamins.
See: Brewer's Yeast.

yeast, torula.
See: Torula Yeast.

Yeast-X. (C.B. Fleet) Pulsatilla 28x. Supp. Pkg. 12s w/applicator. *OTC.*
Use: Vaginal agent.

Yelets. (Freeda) Iron 20 mg, vitamins A 10,000 units, D 400 units, E 10 units, B_1 10 mg, B_2 10 mg, B_3 25 mg, B_5 10 mg, B_6 10 mg, B_{12} 10 mcg, C 100 mg, folic acid 0.1 mg, PABA, lysine, glutamic acid, Ca, I, Mg, Mn, Se, Zn 4 mg. Tab. Bot. 100s, 250s. *OTC.*
Use: Mineral, vitamin supplement.

yellow enzyme.
See: Riboflavin.

•**yellow fever vaccine.** (YEL-oh FEE-ver) *USP 34.*
Use: Immunization.
See: YF-Vax.

yellow hornet venom.
Use: Desensitizing agent.
See: Albay.
  Pharmalgen.
  Venomil.

yellow jacket venom.
Use: Desensitizing agent.
See: Albay.
  Pharmalgen.
  Venomil.

yellow mercuric oxide 1%. (Various Mfr.) Yellow mercuric oxide 1% Oint. Tube 3.5, 3.75, 30 g. *OTC.*
Use: Antiseptic.

yellow mercuric oxide 2%. (Various Mfr.) Yellow mercuric oxide 2%. Oint. Tube 3.5, 3.75, 30 g. *OTC.*
Use: Antiseptic.
See: Stye.

yellow ointment.
Use: Pharmaceutic aid. (ointment base).

yellow wax.
Use: Pharmaceutic aid. (stiffening agent).

Yervoy. (Bristol-Myers Squibb) Ipilimumab 5 mg/mL. Mannitol, polysorbate 80. Preservative free. Inj., Soln.; concentrate. Single-use vial. 10 mL, 40 mL. *Rx.*
Use: Antineoplastic agent, monoclonal antibody.

YF-Vax. (Aventis Pasteur) Yellow fever vaccine not less than 4.74 $\log_{10}$ plaque-forming units (PFU) per 0.5 mL dose when reconstituted. Gelatin, sorbitol. Pow. for Inj., lyophilized. Single-dose vials with 0.6 mL diluent. 5-dose vials with 3 mL of diluent. *Rx.*
Use: Immunization.

Yocon. (Glenwood) Yohimbine hydrochloride 5.4 mg. Tab. Bot. 100s, 1000s. *Rx.*
Use: Anti-impotence agent.

Yodora Deodorant. (Numark) Cream. Jar 2 oz. *OTC.*
Use: Deodorant.

Yodoxin. (Glenwood) Iodoquinol. **Pow.:** Bot. 25 g. **Tab.:** 210 mg, 650 mg. Bot. 100s, 1,000s. *Rx.*
Use: Amebicide.

•**yohimbine hydrochloride.** (yoe-HIM-been) *USP 34.*
Use: Yohimbine has no FDA-sanctioned indications.
See: Aphrodyne.

yohimbine hydrochloride. (Various Mfr.) Indolalkylamine alkaloid. 5.4 mg. Tab. Bot. 100s, 500s, 1000s. *Rx.*
Use: Yohimbine has no FDA-sanctioned indications.

Yohimex. (Kramer) Yohimbine hydrochloride 5.4 mg. Tab. Bot. 100s. *Rx.*
Use: Antiimpotence agent.

ytterbium Yb 169 pentetate injection.
Use: Radiopharmaceutical.

•**yttrium Y 90 clivatuzumab tetraxetan.** (IT-ree-um KLYE-va-TUE-zue-mab) USAN.
Use: Radiopharmaceutical.

•**yttrium Y 90 epratuzumab.** (IT-ree-um e-pra-TOO-zoo-mab) USAN.
Use: Radiopharmaceutical.

•**yttrium Y 90 ibritumomab.** (IT-ree-um ib-ri-TYOO-mo-mab) *USP 34.*
Use: Radiopharmaceutical.

•**yttrium Y 90 labetuzumab.** (IT-ree-um la-be-TOO-zoo-mab) USAN.
Use: Radiopharmaceutical.

•**yttrium Y 90 tacatuzumab.** (IT-ree-um tak-a-TUE-zoo-mab) USAN.
Use: Radiopharmaceutical.

Yutopar. (AstraZeneca) Ritodrine hydrochloride 10 mg/mL. Amp. 5 mL. 15 mg/mL. Vial 10 mL, Inj. syringe 10 mL. *Rx.*
Use: Uterine relaxant.

Z

●**zacopride hydrochloride.** (ZAK-oh-pride) USAN.
Use: Antiemetic; stimulant (peristaltic).

Zaditor. (Novartis Ophthalmics) Ketotifen fumarate 0.025%, glycerol, sodium hydroxide/hydrochloric acid, purified water, benzalkonium chloride 0.01%. Soln. 5 mL. *OTC.*
Use: Antiallergic.

●**zafirlukast.** (zah-FEER-loo-kast) USAN.
Use: Antiasthmatic (leukotriene antagonist).
See: Accolate.

zafirlukast. (Various Mfr.) Zafirlukast 10 mg, 20 mg. May contain lactose, PEG. Tab. 30s, 60s, 100s, 500s, UD 100s. *Rx.*
Use: Leukotriene receptor antagonist.

●**zalcitabine.** (zal-SYE-ta-been) *USP 34.*
Use: Antiretroviral.

●**zaleplon.** (ZAL-eh-plahn) USAN.
Use: Nonbarbiturate sedative and hypnotic, pyrazolopyrimidine.
See: Sonata.

zaleplon. (Corepharma) Zaleplon 5 mg, 10 mg. Lactose. Cap. 100s. *c-iv.*
Use: Nonbarbiturate sedative and hypnotic, pyrazolopyrimidine.

●**zalospirone hydrochloride.** (zal-OH-spy-rone) USAN.
Use: Anxiolytic.

●**zaltidine hydrochloride.** (ZAHL-tih-deen) USAN.
Use: Antiulcerative.

●**zalutumumab.** (ZAL-ue-TOOM-ue-mab) USAN.
Use: Antineoplastic.

Zamicet. (Hawthorn Pharmaceuticals) Acetaminophen 108.3 mg, hydrocodone bitartrate 3.3 mg per 5 mL. Alcohol 6.7%, edetate disodium, glycerin, methylparaben, saccharin, sorbitol, sucrose. Fruit flavor. Soln., Oral. 473 mL. *c-iii.*
Use: Opioid analgesic combination.

Zanaflex. (Acorda Therapeutics) Tizanidine (as base). **Cap.:** 2 mg (equivalent to tizanidine hydrochloride 2.29 mg), 4 mg (equivalent to tizanidine hydrochloride 4.58 mg), 6 mg (equivalent to tizanidine hydrochloride 6.87 mg). Sugar spheres. 150s. **Tab.:** 2 mg (equivalent to tizanidine hydrochloride 2.29 mg), 4 mg (equivalent to tizanidine hydrochloride 4.58 mg). Lactose. 150s. *Rx.*
Use: Skeletal muscle relaxant.

●**zanamivir.** (zan-AM-ih-veer) USAN.
Use: Antiviral; influenza virus neuraminidase inhibitor.
See: Relenza.

Zanfel. (Zanfel Labs) Polyethylene granules, nonoxynol-9, disodium EDTA, triethanolamine. Cream. Tube. 30 g. *OTC.*
Use: Dermatitis.

Zanfel Wash. (Zanfel Labs) Polyethylene granules, sodium lauroyl sarcosinate, nonoxynol-9, EDTA, triethanolamine. Wash. 30 mL. *OTC.*
Use: Poison ivy treatment.

●**zankiren hydrochloride.** (zan-KIE-ren) USAN.
Use: Antihypertensive.

●**zanolimumab.** (zan-oh-LIM-ue-mab) USAN.
Use: Isoantibody.

Zanosar. (Gensia Sicor) Streptozocin 1 g (100 mg/mL). Pow. for Inj. Vial. *Rx.*
Use: Antineoplastic.

●**zanoterone.** (zan-OH-ter-ohn) USAN.
Use: Antiandrogen.

Zantac. (GlaxoSmithKline) Ranitidine (as base). **Inj.:** 1 mg/mL, sodium chloride 0.45%. Preservative free. Premixed single-dose plastic containers. 50 mL. 25 mg/mL. Phenol 5 mg/mL. Single-dose vials. 2 mL. Multidose vials. 6 mL. **Syrup:** 15 mg/mL. Alcohol 7.5%, saccharin, sorbitol, parabens. Peppermint flavor. Bot. 480 mL. **Tab.:** 150 mg, 300 mg. Film-coated. 30s (300 mg only), 60s (150 mg only), 180s (150 mg only), 250s (300 mg only), 500s (150 mg only), 1,000s (150 mg only), UD 100s. *Rx.*
Use: Histamine H_2 antagonist.

Zantac EFFERdose. (GlaxoSmithKline) Ranitidine (as base) 25 mg. Aspartame, phenylalanine 2.81 mg, sodium 30.52 mg. Effervescent Tab. 60s. *Rx.*
Use: Histamine H_2 antagonist.

Zantac 150 Maximum Strength. (Boehringer Ingelheim) Ranitidine (as base) 150 mg. Sugar free. Tab. 8s, 24s, 50s, 65s. *OTC.*
Use: Histamine H_2 antagonist.

Zantac 75. (Boehringer Ingelheim) Ranitidine (as base) 75 mg. Sugar free. Tab. Pkg. 4s, 10s, 20s, 30s, 60s, 80s, 100s. *OTC.*
Use: Histamine H_2 antagonist.

Zantine. (Lexis Laboratories) Dipyridamole 25 mg, 50 mg, 75 mg. Tab. Bot. 1000s. *Rx.*
Use: Coronary vasodilator.

Zarontin. (Parke-Davis) Ethosuximide. **Cap.:** 250 mg. Bot. 100s. **Syr.:** 250 mg/5 mL. Bot. Pt. *Rx.*
Use: Anticonvulsant.

Zaroxolyn. (UCB Pharma) Metolazone 2.5 mg, 5 mg. Tab. Bot. 100s, 1000s, UD 100s. *Rx.*
Use: Diuretic.

• **zatosetron maleate.** (ZAT-oh-SEH-trahn) USAN.
Use: Antimigraine.

Zavesca. (Actelion) Miglustat 100 mg. Sodium starch glucollate, gelatin. Cap. 90s, blister card 18s. *Rx.*
Use: Gaucher disease.

Z-BEC. (Wyeth) Vitamins E 45 mg, C 600 mg, B_1 15 mg, B_2 10.2 mg, B_3 100 mg, B_6 10 mg, B_{12} 6 mcg, pantothenic acid 25 mg, Zn 22.5 mg. Tab. Bot. 60s, 100s, 500s. *OTC.*
Use: Mineral, vitamin supplement.

Z-Cof DM. (Zyber) Dextromethorphan HBr 15 mg, guaifenesin 200 mg, pseudoephedrine hydrochloride 40 mg per 5 mL. Grape flavor. Alcohol free, sugar free. Syrup. Bot. 473 mL. *Rx.*
Use: Upper respiratory combination, antitussive, expectorant, decongestant.

Z-Cof DMX. (Zyber) Dextromethorphan HBr 15 mg, guaifenesin 200 mg, pseudoephedrine hydrochloride 36 mg per 5 mL. Alcohol free. Menthol, saccharin, sorbitol, glucose, PEG. Grape flavor. Liq. 473 mL. *Rx.*
Use: Upper respiratory combination, antitussive and expectorant combination.

Z-Cof 8 DM. (Zyber) Dextromethorphan hydrobromide 15 mg, guaifenesin 175 mg, pseudoephedrine hydrochloride 30 mg per 5 mL. Acesulfame K, aspartame, methylparaben, phenylalanine 25.26 mg/mL. Alcohol free. Grape flavor. Susp., Oral. 473 mL. *Rx.*
Use: Upper respiratory combination, antitussive and expectorant combination.

Z-Cof I. (Pernix Therapeutics) Dextromethorphan hydrobromide 15 mg, guaifenesin 211 mg, pseudoephedrine hydrochloride 30 mg. Acesulfame K, aspartame, glycerin, methylparaben, phenylalanine 25.26 mg per 5 mL, sodium benzoate. Alcohol free. Grape flavor. Susp. 473 mL. *Rx.*
Use: Upper respiratory combination, antitussive and expectorant combination.

Z-Cof LA. (Zyber) Dextromethorphan HBr 30 mg, guaifenesin 650 mg. SR Tab. 100s. *Rx.*
Use: Upper respiratory combination, antitussive, expectorant.

Z-Cof LAX. (Zyber) Dextromethorphan HBr 30 mg, guaifenesin 835 mg. ER Tab. 100s. *Rx.*
Use: Antitussive with expectorant.

Z-Cof 12 DM. (Zyber) Dextromethorphan hydrobromide 15 mg (as dextromethorphan tannate 30 mg), guaifenesin 175 mg, pseudoephedrine hydrochloride 30 mg (as pseudoephedrine tannate 60 mg) per 5 mL. Alcohol free. Acesulfame K, aspartame, methylparaben. Grape flavor. Susp. 473 mL. *Rx.*
Use: Upper respiratory combination, antitussive and expectorant combination.

Z-Dex. (Trigen Labs) Dextromethorphan hydrobromide 20 mg, guaifenesin 100 mg, phenylephrine hydrochloride 10 mg per 5 mL. Edetate disodium, glycerin, sorbitol. Alcohol free and sugar free. Strawberry flavor. Syr. 473 mL. *Rx.*
Use: Upper respiratory combination, antitussive, expectorant combination.

Z-Dex Pediatric. (Trigen) Dextromethorphan hydrobromide 3 mg, guaifenesin 35 mg, phenylephrine hydrochloride 2.5 mg per 1 mL. Alcohol and sugar free. Parabens, saccharin. Grape flavor. Drops. 30 mL with dropper. *Rx.*
Use: Upper respiratory combination, antitussive and expectorant combination.

Z-Dex 12D. (Trigen Labs) Chlorpheniramine maleate 8 mg, dextromethorphan hydrobromide 30 mg, phenylephrine hydrochloride 20 mg. ER Tab. 100s. *Rx.*
Use: Upper respiratory combination, antitussive combination.

Zeasorb. (Stiefel) Talc, microporous cellulose, acrylamide/sodium acrylate copolymer, chloroxylenol, imidazolidinylurea. Pow. 70.9 g, 312 g. *OTC.*
Use: Dermatologic.

Zeasorb-AF. (GlaxoSmithKline) Miconazole nitrate. **Gel:** 2%. Alcohol. 24 g. **Pow.:** 2%. Can 70 g. *OTC.*
Use: Antifungal, topical.

Zebeta. (Barr) Bisoprolol fumarate 5 mg, 10 mg. Film-coated. Tab. Bot. 30s. *Rx.*
Use: Antiadrenergic/sympatholytic, beta-adrenergic blocker.

Ze Caps. (Everett) Vitamin E 200 mg, Zn 9.6 mg as gluconate. Cap. Bot. 60s. *OTC.*
Use: Mineral, vitamin supplement.

Zee-Seltzer. (Zee Medical) Aspirin 325 mg, citric acid 1000 mg, sodium bicarbonate 1916 mg, sodium 524 mg. Effervescent Tab. 12s. *OTC.*
Use: Antacid.

Zegerid. (Santarus) **IR Cap.:** Omeprazole/sodium bicarbonate 20 mg/1100 mg, 40 mg/1100 mg. 30s. **Pow.**

for Oral Susp.: Omeprazole/sodium bicarbonate 20 mg/1680 mg, 40 mg/1680 mg. Sucrose, sucralose, xanthan gum, xylitol. 30 unit-dose packets. *Rx.*
Use: Proton Pump Inhibitor.

Zegerid OTC. (Schering-Plough) Omeprazole 20 mg/sodium bicarbonate 1,100 mg. Sodium 303 mg. Cap., immediate release. 14s, 42s. *OTC.*
Use: Proton pump inhibitor combination.

•**zein.** (ZEE-in) *NF 29.*
Use: Pharmaceutic aid (coating agent).

Zelapar. (Valeant Pharmaceuticals) Selegiline hydrochloride 1.25 mg. Aspartame, mannitol, phenylalanine 1.25 mg. Grapefruit flavor. Orally Disintegrating Tab. Blister card. 60s. *Rx.*
Use: Antiparkinson agent.

Zelnorm. (Novartis) Tegaserod maleate. **Note:** Available through investigational limited access program.

Zemaira. (Aventis) Alpha$_1$-proteinase inhibitor (human) 1000 mg. Sodium mannitol. Preservative free. Pow. for Inj., lyophilized. Single-dose vial with 20 mL diluent. *Rx.*
Use: Respiratory enzyme.

Zemalo. (Alra) Sulfur, zinc oxide, camphor, titanium oxide. Bot. 4 oz, pt, gal. *OTC.*
Use: Dermatologic, counterirritant.

Zema-Pak 10 Day. (Macoven Pharmaceuticals) Dexamethasone 1.5 mg. Lactose, sucrose. Tab. 35s. *Rx.*
Use: Adrenocortical steroid, glucocorticoid.

Zema-Pak 13 Day. (Macoven Pharmaceuticals) Dexamethasone 1.5 mg. Lactose, sucrose. Tab. 51s. *Rx.*
Use: Adrenocortical steroid, glucocorticoid.

Zemplar. (Abbott) Paricalcitol. **Cap.:** 1 mcg, 2 mcg, 4 mcg. Alcohol, medium chain triglycerides. 30s. **Inj.:** 2 mcg/mL. Single-dose *Fliptop* vials, 1 mL, 2 mL. *Rx.*
Use: Hyperparathyroidism.

Zemuron. (Organon) Rocuronium bromide 10 mg/mL. Inj. Multidose vials. 5 mL, 10 mL. *Rx.*
Use: Muscle relaxant.

Zenate.
See: Advanced Formula Zenate.

•**zenazocine mesylate.** (zen-AZE-oh-seen) *USAN.*
Use: Analgesic.

Zenchent. (Watson) Ethinyl estradiol 35 mcg, norethindrone 0.4 mg. Lactose. Tab. 28s with 7 inert tabs. *Rx.*
Use: Contraceptive hormone, sex hormone.

Zencia. (Stratus) Sodium sulfacetamide 9%, sulfur 4%. Aloe, cetyl alcohol, edetate disodium, glyceryl, green tea, parabens, PEG-100, stearyl alcohol. Soap. 473 mL. *Rx.*
Use: Acne product combination.

Zendium. (Oral-B) Sodium fluoride 0.22%. Tube 0.9 oz, 2.3 oz.
Use: Dental caries agent.

Zenieva. (River's Edge) Glycerin, olive oil, squalane, vegetable oil. Fragrance free. Emuls.; Top. Kit w/*Pure* cleanser. 70 g. *Rx.*
Use: Miscellaneous emollient.

•**zeniplatin.** (zen-ih-PLAT-in) *USAN.*
Use: Antineoplastic.

Zenpep. (Eurand) Lipase/protease/amylase 5,000 units/17,000 units/27,000 units; 10,000 units/34,000 units/55,000 units; 15,000 units/51,000 units/82,000 units; 20,000 units/68,000 units/109,000 units. Enteric-coated beads. Cap., delayed release. 12s, 100s, 500s (20,000 units/68,000 units/109,000 units only). *Rx.*
Use: Digestive enzyme.

Zephiran. (Sanofi-Synthelabo) **Aqueous soln.:** Benzalkonium chloride 1:750. Bot. 240 mL, gal. **Disinfectant concentrate:** 17% in 120 mL, gal. **Tincture:** 1:750 in gal. **Tincture spray:** 1:750 in 30 g, 180 g, gal. *OTC.*
Use: Antiseptic; antimicrobial.

Zephiran Towelettes. (Sanofi-Synthelabo) Moist paper towels with soln. of zephiran Cl 1:750. Box 20s, 100s, 1000s. *OTC.*
Use: Antiseptic; antimicrobial.

Zephrex. (Sanofi-Synthelabo) Pseudoephedrine hydrochloride 60 mg, guaifenesin 400 mg. Film-coated. Tab. Bot. 100s. *Rx.*
Use: Decongestant, expectorant.

Zephrex LA. (Sanofi-Synthelabo) Pseudoephedrine hydrochloride 120 mg, guaifenesin 600 mg. ER Tab. Bot. 100s. *Rx.*
Use: Decongestant, expectorant.

Zepine. (Foy Laboratories) Reserpine alkaloid 0.25 mg. Tab. Bot. 100s, 500s, 1000s. *Rx.*
Use: Antihypertensive.

•**zeranol.** (ZER-ah-nole) *USAN.*
Use: Anabolic.

Zestoretic. (AstraZeneca) Lisinopril/hydrochlorothiazide 10 mg/12.5 mg, 20 mg/12.5 mg, 20 mg/25 mg. Mannitol. Tab. Bot. 100s. *Rx.*
Use: Antihypertensive.

Zestril. (AstraZeneca) Lisinopril 2.5 mg, 5 mg, 10 mg, 20 mg, 30 mg, 40 mg.

Mannitol. Tab. 100s. *Rx.*
Use: Renin angiotensin system antagonist, angiotensin-converting enzyme inhibitor.

Zetar. (Dermik) Coal tar 1%. Shampoo. Bot. 177 mL. *OTC.*
Use: Antiseborrheic.

Zetia. (Merck/Schering-Plough) Ezetimibe 10 mg. Lactose. Tab. Bot. 30s, 90s, 500s, UD 100s. *Rx.*
Use: Antihyperlipidemic agent.

Zevalin. (Cell Therapeutics) Ibritumomab tiuxetan 3.2 mg. Preservative free. Inj. Vial 2 mL. In-111 ibritumomab tiuxetan and Y-90 ibritumomab tiuxetan kits with sodium acetate 50 mM vial, formulation buffer vial, reaction vial, and identification labels. *Rx.*
Use: Monoclonal antibody.

Zflex. (Huckaby Pharmaceuticals) Acetaminophen 500 mg, phenyltoloxamine citrate 55 mg. Tab. 100s. *Rx.*
Use: Nonnarcotic analgesic combination.

Ziac. (Teva) Bisoprolol fumarate/hydrochlorothiazide 2.5 mg/6.25 mg, 5 mg/6.25 mg, 10 mg/6.25 mg. Tab. Bot. 30s, 100s (except 10 mg/6.25 mg). *Rx.*
Use: Antihypertensive.

Ziagen. (ViiV Healthcare) Abacavir sulfate. **Tab.:** 300 mg. Film-coated. Bot. 60s, UD blister packs of 60s. **Oral Soln.:** 20 mg/mL. Parabens, saccharin, sorbitol. Strawberry-banana flavor. Bot. 240 mL. *Rx.*
Use: Antiviral, nucleoside reverse transcriptase inhibitor.

Ziana. (Medicis) Clindamycin phosphate 1.2%, tretinoin 0.025%. EDTA, glycerin, parabens. Gel. 2 g, 30 g, 60 g. *Rx.*
Use: Topical anti-infective.

•**zibotentan.** (zye-boe-TEN-tan) USAN.
Use: Antineoplastic.

•**ziconotide.** (zi-KOE-noe-tide) USAN.
Use: Analgesic.
See: Prialt.

•**zidometacin.** (ZIE-doe-MEH-tah-sin) USAN.
Use: Anti-inflammatory.

•**zidovudine.** (zie-DOE-view-DEEN) USP 34. Formerly Azidothymidine, AZT.
Use: Antiviral; AIDS; HIV infection.
See: Retrovir.
W/Lamivudine.
See: Combivir.

zidovudine. (Aurobindo Pharma) Zidovudine. **Cap.:** 100 mg. 100s, UD 100s. **Oral Soln.:** 50 mg per 5 mL. Sucrose. Strawberry flavor. 240 mL. *Rx.*
Use: Antiretroviral agent.

zidovudine. (Various Mfr.) Zidovudine 300 mg. Tab. 60s. *Rx.*
Use: Antiretroviral agent.

•**zifrosilone.** (zih-FROE-sih-lone) USAN.
Use: Acetylcholinesterase inhibitor.

Ziks. (Nodum) Methyl salicylate 12%, menthol 1%, capsaicin 0.025%, cetyl alcohol. Cream. Tube. 60 g. *OTC.*
Use: Analgesic.

Zilactin. (Blairex) Benzyl alcohol 10%. Salicylic acid, hydroxypropylcellulose. Gel. 7 g. *OTC.*
Use: Mouth and throat preparation.

Zilactin-B Medicated. (Blairex) Benzocaine 10%, alcohol 76%. Gel. Tube. 7.5 g. *OTC.*
Use: Anesthetic, local.

Zilactin-L. (Blairex) Benzyl alcohol 10%. SD alcohol 37. Liq. 539 mL. *OTC.*
Use: Topical local anesthetic, amide local anesthetic.

ZilaDent. (Zila) Benzocaine 6%, alcohol 74.9%. Gel. Tube. 7.5 g, single packs. *OTC.*
Use: Anesthetic, local.

•**zilantel.** (ZILL-an-tell) USAN.
Use: Anthelmintic.

•**zileuton.** (ZIE-loo-tone) USP 34.
Use: Leukotriene formation inhibitor.
See: Zyflo.
Zyflo CR.

•**zimeldine hydrochloride.** (zie-MELL-ih-deen) USAN. Formerly Zimelidine Hydrochloride.
Use: Antidepressant.

Zinacef. (Glaxo Wellcome) Cefuroxime (as sodium). **Pow. for Inj.:** 750 mg, 1.5 g, 7.5 g. Sodium 2.4 mEq/g. Vials and infusion pack (except 7.5 g). Pharmacy bulk pkg (7.5 g only). **Inj.:** 750 mg, 1.5 g. Sodium 2.4 mEq/g. Premixed, frozen. 50 mL. *Rx.*
Use: Anti-infective, cephalosporin.

•**zinc acetate.** (zink) USP 34. Acetic acid, zinc salt, dihydrate.
Use: Pharmaceutic necessity for zinc-eugenol cement; topical poison ivy product; Wilson disease.
See: Benadryl Itch Relief.
Benadryl Itch Relief, Children's.
Benadryl Itch Relief, Maximum Strength.
Benadryl Itch Stopping Children's Formula.
Benadryl Itch Stopping Maximum Strength.
Caladryl Clear.
Galzin.
Ivy-Dry.
Ivy-Dry Super.

Nasal•Ease with Zinc.
W/Antipyrine, Benzocaine, Glycerin.
See: Neotic.
W/Benzethonium Chloride, Diphenhydramine Hydrochloride.
See: Calagel Maximum Strength.
W/Chloroxylenol, Glycerin, Pramoxine Hydrochloride.
See: Zinotic.
Zinotic ES.
W/Chloroxylenol, Pramoxine Hydrochloride.
See: Zinotic ES.
W/Combinations.
See: Anti-Itch.
Zincate. (Paddock) Zinc sulfate 220 mg (elemental zinc 50 mg). Cap. Bot. 100s, 1000s. OTC.
Use: Mineral supplement.
zinc bacitracin. Bacitracin Zinc.
Use: Anti-infective.
•zinc carbonate. (zink) USP 34.
Use: Antiseptic, topical; astringent.
•zinc chloride. (zink) USP 34.
Use: Astringent; dentin desensitizer.
•zinc chloride Zn 65. (zink) USAN.
Use: Radiopharmaceutical.
zinc citrate.
See: Zinc Lozenges.
zinc-eugenol cement.
Use: Dental protectant.
Zincfrin. (Alcon) Phenylephrine hydrochloride 0.12%. Benzalkonium chloride 0.01%, polysorbate 80, zinc sulfate 0.25%. Soln. OTC.
Use: Ophthalmic decongestant.
zinc gelatin.
Use: Topical protectant.
Zinc-Glenwood. (Glenwood) Zinc sulfate 220 mg. Cap. Bot. 100s. OTC.
Use: Mineral supplement.
•zinc gluconate. (zink) USP 34.
Use: Supplement, trace mineral.
See: Nasal•Ease with Zinc Gluconate.
Zinc Lozenges.
zinc gluconate. (Mericon) Zinc gluconate 10 mg. Cocoa powder, fructose, glycyrrhizic acid, powdered milk, sorbitol. Lozenge. 50s. OTC.
Use: Trace element.
zinc insulin.
See: Insulin Zinc.
Zinc Lozenges. (Ivax) Zinc citrate 23 mg, zinc gluconate. Fructose, sorbitol. Bot. 30s. OTC.
Use: Mineral supplement.
Zincon. (Medtech) Pyrithione zinc 1%. Propylene glycol. Shampoo. Bot. 118 mL, 240 mL. OTC.
Use: Dermatologic agent.

•zinc oxide. (zink) USP 34. Flowers of zinc.
Use: Astringent; topical protectant.
See: Calamine.
Delazinc.
W/Combinations.
See: Akne Drying Lotion.
Anusol Ointment.
Balmex.
Bonate.
Columbia Antiseptic Powder.
Desitin.
Dr. Smith's Adult Care.
Dr. Smith's Diaper.
Hemorrhoidal.
Medicated Powder.
Mexsana.
Pazo Hemorrhoid.
Rectal Medicone.
RVPaque.
Saratoga.
Schamberg's.
Soothe & Cool.
Tucks.
Versal.
W/Dimethicone.
See: A & D Zinc Oxide Cream.
W/Menthol.
See: Calmoseptine.
W/Talc.
See: Caldesene.
zinc oxide. (Gallipot) Zinc oxide 25%. Petrolatum. Paste, top. 454 g. OTC.
Use: Dermatological agent, protectant.
zinc phenolsulfonate.
Use: Astringent.
zinc pyrithione.
Use: Bactericide, fungicide, antiseborrheic.
See: Zincon.
•zinc stearate. (zink STEER-ate) USP 34. Octadecanoic acid, zinc salt.
Use: Dusting powder; pharmaceutic aid (tablet/capsule lubricant).
zinc sulfanilate. Zinc sulfanilate tetrahydrate. Nizin, Op-Isophrin-Z, Op-Isophrin-Z-M (Broemmel).
Use: Anti-infective.
•zinc sulfate. (zink) USP 34. Sulfuric acid, zinc salt (1:1), heptahydrate.
Use: Astringent, ophthalmic.
See: Zinc-Glenwood.
W/Boric Acid, Phenylephrine Hydrochloride.
See: Phenylzin.
W/Calcium Lactate.
See: Zinc-220.
W/Vitamins.
See: Vicon-C.
Vicon Forte.
Vicon Plus.

Vi-Zac.

Z-BEC.

zinc sulfate. (American Regent) Zinc sulfate 1 mg/mL (as zinc sulfate 2.46 mg/mL). Preservative free. Inj., Soln. Single-use vial. 10 mL. *Rx.*
Use: Trace metal.

zinc sulfate. (Various Mfr.) **Cap.:** Zinc sulfate 220 mg. Lactose, gelatin. Bot. 100s. **Inj.:** Zinc 1 mg/mL (as sulfate 4.39 mg), 5 mg/mL (as sulfate 21.95 mg). Vial. 5 mL (5 mg/mL only), 10 mL, 30 mL (1 mg/mL only). *Rx-OTC.*
Use: Nutritional supplement, parenteral.

zinc sulfate, concentrated. (American Regent) Zinc sulfate 5 mg/mL (as zinc sulfate 12.32 mg/mL). Preservative free. Inj., Soln.; concentrate. Vial. 5 mL. *Rx.*
Use: Trace metal.

•**zinc sulfide topical suspension.** (zink) USP 34. Formerly *White Lotion.* Synonym Lotio alba.
Use: Astringent.

zinc-10-undecenoate.
See: Zinc Undecylenate.

zinc trace metal additive. (I.M.S., Ltd.) Zinc 4 mg/mL. Inj. Vial. 10 mL. *Rx.*
Use: Nutritional supplement, parenteral.

Zinc-220. (Alto) Zinc sulfate 220 mg. Cap. Bot. 100s, 1000s, UD 100s. *OTC.*
Use: Mineral supplement.

•**zinc undecylenate.** (zink uhn-deh-SILL-en-ate) USP 34.
Use: Antifungal.
See: Blis-To-Sol.
W/Undecylenic acid.
See: Cruex Spray Powder
Desenex.

Zincvit. (Kenwood) Vitamin A 5000 units, D$_3$ 50 units, E 50 units, B$_1$ 10 mg, B$_2$ 5 mg, B$_6$ 2 mg, C 300 mcg, B$_3$ 25 mg, Zn 40 mg, Mg 9.7 mg, Mn 1.3 mg, folic acid 1 mg. Cap. Bot. 60s. *Rx.*
Use: Mineral, vitamin supplement.

•**zindotrine.** (ZIN-doe-TREEN) USAN.
Use: Bronchodilator.

Zinecard. (Pfizer) Dexrazoxane (as dexrazoxane hydrochloride) 250 mg, 500 mg. Inj., Lyophilized, Pow. for Soln. Single-use vials with 25-mL vial (250 mg), 50-mL vial (500 mg) sodium lactate injection. *Rx.*
Use: Cytoprotective agent.

•**zinoconazole hydrochloride.** (zih-no-KOE-nah-zole) USAN.
Use: Antifungal.

•**zinostatin.** (ZEE-no-STAT-in) USAN.
Formerly Neocarzinostatin.
Use: Antineoplastic.

Zinotic. (Arbor) Chloroxylenol 0.1%, pramoxine hydrochloride 0.5%, glycerin 1%, zinc acetate 0.1%. Drops; Otic. 2 mL and 15 mL w/dropper. *Rx.*
Use: Miscellaneous otic preparation.

Zinotic ES. (Arbor Pharmaceuticals) Chloroxylenol 0.1%, pramoxine hydrochloride 1%, glycerin 1%, zinc acetate 1%. Drops; Otic. 1 mL and 15 mL w/dropper. *Rx.*
Use: Miscellaneous otic preparation.

•**zinterol hydrochloride.** (ZIN-ter-ole) USAN.
Use: Bronchodilator.

•**zinviroxime.** (zin-VIE-rox-eem) USAN.
Use: Antiviral.

Zinx Chlor-D. (Auriga Pharmaceuticals) Chlorpheniramine maleate 8 mg, pseudoephedrine hydrochloride 120 mg. ER Cap. 30s, 100s. *Rx.*
Use: Upper respiratory combination, decongestant and antihistamine.

Zinx D-Tuss. (Auriga) Carbetapentane tannate 30 mg, phenylephrine tannate 25 mg per 5 mL. Aspartame, parabens, phenylalanine 7 mg/5 mL. Strawberry flavor. Susp. 118 mL. *Rx.*
Use: Upper respiratory combination, antitussive combination.

Zinx GCP. (Auriga) Carbetapentane citrate 15 mg, guaifenesin 100 mg, phenylephrine hydrochloride 5 mg per 5 mL. Alcohol free. Maltitol, saccharin, sorbitol. Strawberry flavor. Soln. 118 mL. *Rx.*
Use: Upper respiratory combination, antitussive and expectorant combination.

Zinx GP. (Auriga) Phenylephrine hydrochloride 30 mg, guaifenesin 1000 mg. ER Tab. 100s. *Rx.*
Use: Upper respiratory combination, decongestant and expectorant combination.

Zinx PCM. (Auriga) Phenylephrine hydrochloride 10 mg, chlorpheniramine maleate 2 mg, methscopolamine nitrate 1.25 mg per 5 mL. Alcohol, sugar, and dye free. Saccharin, sorbitol. Berry flavor. Oral Susp. 118 mL. *Rx.*
Use: Upper respiratory combination; decongestant, antihistamine, and anticholinergic combination.

•**ziprasidone hydrochloride.** (zih-PRAY-sih-dohn) USAN.
Use: Antipsychotic, benzisoxazole derivative.
See: Geodon.

•**ziprasidone mesylate.** (zih-PRAY-sih-dohn) USAN.
Use: Antipsychotic.

Zipsor. (Xanodyne) Diclofenac 25 mg. Isopropyl alcohol, PEG, sorbitol. Cap. 100s. *Rx.*
Use: CNS agent, nonsteroidal antiinflammatory agent.
zirconium carbonate or oxide.
See: Dermaneed.
Zirgan. (Sirion Therapeutics Inc) Ganciclovir 0.15%. Benzalkonium chloride 0.075 mg. Gel; Ophth. Tube. 5 g. *Rx.*
Use: Ophthalmic antiviral agent.
Zithranol-RR. (Elorac) Anthralin 1.2%. Preservative free. Cream. 15 g, 45 g. *Rx.*
Use: Dermatological agent, antipsoriatic agent.
Zithromax. (Pfizer) Azithromycin. **Tab.:** 250 mg, 500 mg, 600 mg as dihydrate. Lactose. Film-coated. Bot. 30s, UD 50s (except 600 mg), *Z-Pak* 6s (250 mg only), *TRI-PAK* 3s (500 mg only). **Pow. for Inj.:** 500 mg, sucrose. Lyophilized vials 10 mL, vials 10 mL with 1 *Vial-Mate* adapter. **Pow. for Oral Susp.:** 100 mg/5 mL (as dihydrate) when reconstituted, sucrose. Cherry, banana, and creme de vanilla flavors. 15 mL. 200 mg/5 mL (as dihydrate) when reconstituted, sucrose. Cherry, banana, and creme de vanilla flavors. 15 mL, 22.5 mL, 30 mL. 1 g/packet as dihydrate, sucrose. Cherry and banana flavors. Single-dose pack, 3s, 10s. *Rx.*
Use: Anti-infective, macrolide.
Zmax. (Pfizer) Azithromycin 167 mg per 5 mL (as dihydrate) when reconstituted. Extended-release microspheres. Sucrose, sodium 148 mg. Cherry and banana flavors. Pow. for Oral Susp. Single-dose bottles. 2 g. *Rx.*
Use: Macrolide, anti-infective.
ZNG. (Western Research) Zinc gluconate 35 mg. Tab. *Handicount* 28s (36 bags of 28 tab.). *OTC.*
Use: Mineral supplement.
ZNP Bar. (Stiefel) Pyrithione zinc 2%. Alcohol, castor oil, cetearyl alcohol, glycerin, lactic acid, mineral oil, PEG, titanium dioxide, trisodium EDTA. Soap. 119 g. *OTC.*
Use: Dermatological agent.
ZN-Plus Protein. (Miller Pharmacal Group) Zinc in a zinc-protein complex made with isolated soy protein 15 mg. Tab. Bot. 100s. *OTC.*
Use: Mineral supplement.
Zocor. (Merck) Simvastatin 5 mg, 10 mg, 20 mg, 40 mg, 80 mg. Lactose. Film-coated. Tab. Bot. 1000s, 10,000s (10 mg, 20 mg only), UD 100s, unit-of-use 30s, 90s. *Rx.*

Use: Antihyperlipidemic, HMG-CoA reductase inhibitor.
Zodeac-100. (Econo Med Pharmaceuticals) Fe 60 mg, vitamins A 8000 units, D 400 units, E 30 units, B_1 1.7 mg, B_2 2 mg, B_3 20 mg, B_5 11 mg, B_6 4 mg, B_{12} 8 mcg, C 120 mg, folic acid 1 mg, biotin 300 mcg, Ca, Cu, I, Mg, Zn 15 mg. Tab. Bot. 100s. *Rx.*
Use: Mineral, vitamin supplement.
ZoDen DM. (Trigen Laboratories) Chlorpheniramine maleate 1 mg, dextromethorphan hydrobromide 3 mg, phenylephrine hydrochloride 1.5 mg. Parabens, potassium citrate, potassium sorbate, propylene glycol, sorbitol, sucralose. Alcohol free and sugar free. Fruit gum flavor. Liq. Drops. 30 mL w/dropper. *Rx.*
Use: Upper respiratory combination, antitussive combination.
ZoDerm. (Doak) Benzoyl peroxide.
Cleanser: 4.5%, 5.75% (urea 10%, PEG 100, disodium EDTA), 6.5%, 8.5%. Alcohols, EDTA, glycerin, urea. 400 mL (except 5.75%), 473 mL (5.75% only).
Cream: 4.5%, 6.5%, 8.5%. Alcohols, EDTA, urea. 125 mL. **Gel.:** 4.5%, 6.5%, 8.5%. EDTA, glycerin, urea. 125 mL. *Rx.*
Use: Anti-infective.
Zodryl AC 80. (codaDOSE) Chlorpheniramine maleate 1 mg, codeine phosphate 5 mg per 5 mL. Methylparaben, sucralose. Grape flavor. Liq. 236 mL w/oral dispenser. *c-v.*
Use: Upper respiratory combination, antitussive combination.
Zodryl AC 50 . (codaDOSE) Chlorpheniramine maleate 2 mg, codeine phosphate 5 mg per 5 mL. Methylparaben, sucralose. Grape flavor. Liq. 236 mL w/oral dispenser. *c-v.*
Use: Upper respiratory combination, antitussive combination.
Zodryl AC 40. (codaDOSE) Chlorpheniramine maleate 1.11 mg, codeine phosphate 5 mg per 5 mL. Methylparaben, sucralose. Grape flavor. Liq. 118 mL w/oral dispenser. *c-v.*
Use: Upper respiratory combination, antitussive combination.
Zodryl AC 60. (codaDOSE) Chlorpheniramine maleate 1.335 mg, codeine phosphate 5 mg per 5 mL. Methylparaben, sucralose. Grape flavor. Liq. 236 mL w/oral dispenser. *c-v.*
Use: Upper respiratory combination, antitussive combination.
Zodryl AC 30. (codaDOSE) Chlorpheniramine maleate 1.43 mg, codeine phos-

phate 5 mg per 5 mL. Methylparaben, sucralose. Grape flavor. Liq. 118 mL w/oral dispenser. *c-v.*
Use: Upper respiratory combination, antitussive combination.

Zodryl AC 35. (codaDOSE) Chlorpheniramine maleate 1.25 mg, codeine phosphate 5 mg per 5 mL. Methylparaben, sucralose. Grape flavor. Liq. 118 mL w/oral dispenser. *c-v.*
Use: Upper respiratory combination, antitussive combination.

Zodryl AC 25. (codaDOSE) Chlorpheniramine maleate 1.665 mg, codeine phosphate 5 mg per 5 mL. Methylparaben, sucralose. Grape flavor. Liq. 118 mL w/oral dispenser. *c-v.*
Use: Upper respiratory combination, antitussive combination.

Zodryl DAC 80. (codaDOSE) Chlorpheniramine maleate 1 mg, codeine phosphate 5 mg, pseudoephedrine hydrochloride 15 mg. Methylparaben, sucralose. Grape flavor. Liq. 236 mL. *c-v.*
Use: Upper respiratory combination, antitussive combination.

Zodryl DAC 50. (codaDOSE) Chlorpheniramine maleate 2 mg, codeine phosphate 5 mg, pseudoephedrine hydrochloride 30 mg. Methylparaben, sucralose. Grape flavor. Liq. 236 mL. *c-v.*
Use: Upper respiratory combination, antitussive combination.

Zodryl DAC 40. (codaDOSE) Chlorpheniramine maleate 1.11 mg, codeine phosphate 5 mg, pseudoephedrine hydrochloride 16.665 mg. Methylparaben, sucralose. Grape flavor. Liq. 118 mL. *c-v.*
Use: Upper respiratory combination, antitussive combination.

Zodryl DAC 60. (codaDOSE) Chlorpheniramine maleate 1.43 mg, codeine phosphate 5 mg, pseudoephedrine hydrochloride 20 mg. Methylparaben, sucralose. Grape flavor. Liq. 236 mL. *c-v.*
Use: Upper respiratory combination, antitussive combination.

Zodryl DAC 30. (codaDOSE) Chlorpheniramine maleate 1.43 mg, codeine phosphate 5 mg, pseudoephedrine hydrochloride 21.43 mg. Methylparaben, sucralose. Grape flavor. Liq. 118 mL. *c-v.*
Use: Upper respiratory combination, antitussive combination.

Zodryl DAC 35. (codaDOSE) Chlorpheniramine maleate 1.25 mg, codeine

phosphate 5 mg, pseudoephedrine hydrochloride 18.75 mg. Methylparaben, sucralose. Grape flavor. Liq. 118 mL. *c-v.*
Use: Upper respiratory combination, antitussive combination.

Zodryl DAC 25. (codaDOSE) Chlorpheniramine maleate 1.665 mg, codeine phosphate 5 mg, pseudoephedrine hydrochloride 25 mg. Methylparaben, sucralose. Grape flavor. Liq. 118 mL. *c-v.*
Use: Upper respiratory combination, antitussive combination.

Zodryl DEC 80. (codaDOSE) Codeine phosphate 5 mg, guaifenesin 100 mg, pseudoephedrine hydrochloride 15 mg. Methylparaben, sucralose. Grape flavor. Susp. 236 mL. *c-v.*
Use: Upper respiratory combination, antitussive and expectorant combination.

Zodryl DEC 50. (codaDOSE) Codeine phosphate 5 mg, guaifenesin 100 mg, pseudoephedrine hydrochloride 30 mg. Methylparaben, sucralose. Grape flavor. Susp. 236 mL. *c-v.*
Use: Upper respiratory combination, antitussive and expectorant combination.

Zodryl DEC 40. (codaDOSE) Codeine phosphate 5 mg, guaifenesin 100 mg, pseudoephedrine hydrochloride 16.665 mg. Methylparaben, sucralose. Grape flavor. Susp. 118 mL. *c-v.*
Use: Upper respiratory combination, antitussive and expectorant combination.

Zodryl DEC 60. (codaDOSE) Codeine phosphate 5 mg, guaifenesin 100 mg, pseudoephedrine hydrochloride 20 mg. Methylparaben, sucralose. Grape flavor. Susp. 236 mL. *c-v.*
Use: Upper respiratory combination, antitussive and expectorant combination.

Zodryl DEC 30. (codaDOSE) Codeine phosphate 5 mg, guaifenesin 100 mg, pseudoephedrine hydrochloride 21.43 mg. Methylparaben, sucralose. Grape flavor. Susp. 118 mL. *c-v.*
Use: Upper respiratory combination, antitussive and expectorant combination.

Zodryl DEC 35. (codaDOSE) Codeine phosphate 5 mg, guaifenesin 100 mg, pseudoephedrine hydrochloride 18.75 mg. Methylparaben, sucralose. Grape flavor. Susp. 118 mL. *c-v.*
Use: Upper respiratory combination, antitussive and expectorant combination.

Zodryl DEC 25. (codaDOSE) Codeine phosphate 5 mg, guaifenesin 100 mg, pseudoephedrine hydrochloride 25 mg. Methylparaben, sucralose. Grape flavor. Susp. 118 mL. *c-v.*
Use: Upper respiratory combination, antitussive and expectorant combination.

•**zofenoprilat arginine.** (zoe-FEN-oh-PRILL-at AHR-jih-neen) USAN.
Use: Antihypertensive.

•**zofenopril calcium.** (zoe-FEN-oh-PRILL) USAN.
Use: Enzyme inhibitor (angiotensin-converting).

Zofran. (GlaxoSmithKline) Ondansetron hydrochloride. **Tab.:** 4 mg, 8 mg, 24 mg (as hydrochloride dihydrate). Lactose. Bot. 30s, UD 100s, 1 × 3 UD pack (4 mg, 8 mg only); 1 × 1 daily UD pack (24 mg only). **Inj.:** 2 mg/mL (as hydrochloride dihydrate). Parabens (2 mg/mL only). Single-dose vial 2 mL, multidose vial 20 mL (2 mg/mL). **Oral Soln.:** 4 mg/5 mL (5 mg as hydrochloride dihydrate). Sorbitol, strawberry flavor. Bot. 50 mL. *Rx.*
Use: Antiemetic; antivertigo.

Zofran ODT. (GlaxoSmithKline) Ondansetron hydrochloride (as base) 4 mg, 8 mg. Phenylalanine < 0.03 mg, aspartame, mannitol, parabens. Strawberry flavor. Orally Disintegrating Tab. UD 10s (8 mg only), UD 30s. *Rx.*
Use: Antiemetic; antivertigo.

Zoladex. (AstraZeneca) Goserelin acetate 3.6 mg (16-gauge needle), 10.8 mg (14-gauge needle). Implant. Preloaded Syringes. *Rx.*
Use: Hormone, gonadotropin-releasing hormone analog.

•**zolamine hydrochloride.** (zoe-lah-meen) USAN.
Use: Antihistamine; anesthetic, topical.

•**zolazepam hydrochloride.** (zole-AZ-eh-pam) USAN.
Use: Hypnotic; sedative.

•**zoledronate disodium.** (ZOE-leh-droe-nate) USAN.
Use: Bone resorption inhibitor; osteoporosis treatment and prevention.

•**zoledronate trisodium.** (ZOE-leh-droe-nate) USAN.
Use: Bone resorption inhibitor; osteoporosis treatment and prevention.

•**zoledronic acid.** (ZOE-leh-drah-nik) USAN.
Use: Calcium regulator; osteoporosis treatment and prevention; bisphosphonate.

See: Reclast.
Zometa.

•**zolertine hydrochloride.** (ZOE-ler-teen) USAN.
Use: Antiadrenergic; vasodilator.

•**zolimomab aritox.** (zah-LIM-ah-mab a-rih-TOX) USAN.
Use: Monoclonal antibody (antithrombotic).

Zolinza. (Merck) Vorinostat 100 mg. Cap. 120s. *Rx.*
Use: Antineoplastic, histone deacetylase inhibitor.

•**zolmitriptan.** (zohl-mi-TRIP-tan) USAN.
Tall Man: ZOLMitriptan
Use: Antimigraine agent, serotonin 5-HT$_1$ receptor agonist.
See: Zomig.
Zomig ZMT.

Zoloft. (Pfizer) Sertraline hydrochloride (as base). **Tab.:** 25 mg, 50 mg, 100 mg. Film-coated. Bot. 50s (25 mg only); 100s, 500s, 5000s, UD 100s (50 mg and 100 mg only). **Soln., Oral Conc.:** 20 mg/mL. Menthol, alcohol 12%. Bot. 60 mL. Dropper dispenser contains dry natural rubber. *Rx.*
Use: Antidepressant, selective serotonin reuptake inhibitor.

zolpidem. (Various Mfr.) Zolpidem tartrate 5 mg, 10 mg. May contain lactose. Tab. 10s, 30s, 60s, 100s, 250s, 500s, 1000s, UD 30s, UD 100s. *c-iv.*
Use: Nonbarbiturate sedative/hypnotic, imidazopyridine.

•**zolpidem tartrate.** (ZOLE-pih-dem) USAN.
Use: Hypnotic; sedative.
See: Ambien.
Ambien CR.
Edluar.
Tovalt ODT.

•**zomepirac sodium.** (ZOE-mih-PEER-ack) USAN.
Use: Analgesic; anti-inflammatory.

Zometa. (Novartis) Zoledronic acid 4 mg/5 mL (as zoledronic acid monohydrate 4.264 mg). Mannitol 220 mg. Inj. Soln. Concentrate. Vials. 5 mL. *Rx.*
Use: Bisphosphonate.

•**zometapine.** (zoe-MET-ah-peen) USAN.
Use: Antidepressant.

Zomig. (AstraZeneca) Zolmitriptan. **Nasal Spray:** 5 mg. 100 mcL unit-dose spray device. 6s. **Tab.:** 2.5 mg, 5 mg. Lactose. Film-coated. Blister pack 6s (2.5 mg only), 3s (5 mg only). *Rx.*
Use: Antimigraine agent, serotonin 5-HT$_1$ receptor agonist.

Zomig ZMT. (AstraZeneca) Zolmitriptan 5 mg. Phenylalanine 5.62 mg, 2.5 mg (5 mg), 2.81 mg (2.5 mg), mannitol, aspartame. Orange flavor. Orally disintegrating Tab. UD 3s (5 mg), UD 6s (2.5 mg). *Rx.*
Use: Antimigraine agent, serotonin 5-HT$_1$ receptor agonist.

Zonalon. (Medicis Dermatologics) Doxepin hydrochloride 5%. Cetyl alcohol, petrolatum, benzyl alcohol, titanium dioxide. Cream. Tube. 30 g. *Rx.*
Use: Antihistamine, topical.

•**zonampanel.** (zon-AM-pa-nel) USAN.
Use: Ischemic stroke.

Zonatuss. (Atley) Benzonatate 150 mg. Cap. 100s. *Rx.*
Use: Nonnarcotic antitussive.

Zone-A Forte. (Forest) Hydrocortisone 2.5%, pramoxine hydrochloride in a hydrophilic base containing stearic acid 1%, forlan-L, glycerin, triethanolamine, polyoxyl 40 stearate, di-isopropyl adipate, povidone, silicone fluid-200. Paraben free. Lot. Bot. 60 mL. *Rx.*
Use: Corticosteroid; anesthetic, local.

Zone-A Lotion. (Forest) Hydrocortisone acetate 1%, pramoxine hydrochloride 1%. Bot. 2 oz. *Rx.*
Use: Corticosteroid; anesthetic, local.

Zonegran. (Eisai) Zonisamide 25 mg, 50 mg, 100 mg. Cap. Bot. 100s. *Rx.*
Use: Anticonvulsant.

•**zoniclezole hydrochloride.** (zoe-NIH-klih-ZOLE) USAN.
Use: Anticonvulsant.

•**zoniporide mesylate.** (zon-i-POR-ide) USAN.
Use: Cardioprotective agent.

•**zonisamide.** (zoe-NISS-ah-MIDE) USAN.
Use: Anticonvulsant.
See: Zonegran.

zonisamide. (Various Mfr.) Zonisamide 25 mg, 50 mg, 100 mg. May contain lactose (100 mg only). Cap. 30s, 60s, 100s, 250s, 500s, 1000s, UD 100s (100 mg only). *Rx.*
Use: Anticonvulsants.

Zonite Liquid Douche Concentrate. (Menley & James Labs, Inc.) Benzalkonium Cl 0.1%, menthol, thymol, EDTA in buffered soln. Bot. 240 mL, 360 mL. *OTC.*
Use: Vaginal agent.

•**zopolrestat.** (zoe-PAHL-reh-STAT) USAN.
Use: Antidiabetic; aldose reductase inhibitor.

•**zorbamycin.** (zor-ba-MYE-sin) USAN.
Use: Anti-infective.

Zorbtive. (Serono) Somatropin 8.8 mg ($\approx$ 26.4 units). Sucrose, phosphoric acid. Pow. for Inj. Multidose vial with diluent. *Rx.*
Use: Hormone, growth.

ZORprin. (PAR) Aspirin 800 mg. SR Tab. Bot. 100s. *Rx.*
Use: Analgesic.

Zortress. (Novartis) Everolimus 0.25 mg, 0.5 mg, 0.75 mg. Butylated hydroxytoluene, lactose. Tab. UD 60s. *Rx.*
Use: Kinase inhibitor, mTOR inhibitor.

•**zorubicin hydrochloride.** (zoe-ROO-bih-sin) USAN.
Use: Antineoplastic.

Zostavax. (Merck) Oka/Merck varicella-zoster virus (live) 19,400 PFU. Sucrose. Preservative free. Inj., lyophilized. Single-dose vials. 1s, 10s. *Rx.*
Use: Viral vaccine.

zoster vaccine live.
Use: Active immunization agent, viral vaccine.
See: Zostavax.

Zostrix. (Health Care Products) Capsaicin 0.025%. Cream. Tube. 45 g. *Rx.*
Use: Analgesic, topical.

Zostrix Diabetic Foot Pain. (Health Care Products) Capsaicin 0.075%. Benzyl alcohol, cetyl alcohol, glyceryl, PEG-100, white petrolatum. Cream. 56.6 g w/25 applicator pads. *OTC.*
Use: Counterirritant.

Zostrix-HP. (Health Care Products) *Formerly called Axsain, formerly marketed by Galen.*

Zostrix Maximum Strength. (Health Care Products) Capsaicin 0.075%. Benzyl alcohol, cetyl alcohol, glyceryl, PEG-100, white petrolatum. Cream. 56.6 g w/25 applicator pads. *OTC.*
Use: Counterirritant.

•**zosuquidar trihydrochloride.** (zoe-SOO-kwi-dar) USAN.
Use: Treatment of multidrug resistance.

Zosyn. (Wyeth) Piperacillin sodium/tazobactam sodium. **Inj. Soln.:** 2.25 g/ 50 mL (2 g/0.25 g) (sodium 5.58 mEq), 3.375 g/50 mL (3 g/0.375 g) (sodium 8.38 mEq), 4.5 g/100 mL (4 g/0.5 g) (sodium 11.17 mEq). *Galaxy* containers. **Pow. for Soln. Inj.:** 2.25 g (2 g/ 0.25 g) (sodium 5.58 mEq, EDTA 0.5 mg), 3.375 g (3 g/0.375 mg) (sodium 8.38 mEq, EDTA 0.75 mg), 4.5 g (4 g/0.5 g) (sodium 11.17 mEq, EDTA 1 mg), 40.5 g (36 g/4.5 g) (sodium 100.4 mEq). Single-dose vials (except 40.5 g), *ADD-Vantage* vials (except

40.5 g). Bulk vials (40.5 g only). Preservative free. *Rx.*
Use: Extended-spectrum penicillins.

Zotex. (Vertical) Dextromethorphan HBr 20 mg, guaifenesin 100 mg, phenylephrine hydrochloride 10 mg per 5 mL. Parabens, saccharin. Alcohol free, sugar free. Strawberry flavor. Syr. 10 and 473 mL. *Rx.*
Use: Upper respiratory combination; antitussive, expectorant, decongestant.

Zotex-C. (Vertical) Codeine phosphate 10 mg, phenylephrine hydrochloride 5 mg, pyrilamine maleate 5 mg per 5 mL. Saccharin, sorbitol. Alcohol free and sugar free. Cherry flavor. Syr. 473 mL. *c-v.*
Use: Upper respiratory combination, antitussive combination.

Zotex-D. (Vertical) Dextromethorphan hydrobromide 15 mg, guaifenesin 100 mg, phenylephrine hydrochloride 8.5 mg per 5 mL. Glycerin, propylene glycol, saccharin, sodium benzoate, sorbitol. Alcohol free, dye free, and sugar free. Cherry flavor. Syrup. 473 mL. *Rx.*
Use: Upper respiratory combination, antitussive and expectorant combination.

Zotex-EX. (Vertical) Dextromethorphan hydrobromide 15 mg, guaifenesin 350 mg, phenylephrine hydrochloride 10 mg. Maltodextrin. Tab. 100s. *Rx.*
Use: Upper respiratory combination, antitussive and expectorant combination.

Zotex-G. (Vertical) Dextromethorphan HBr 15 mg, guaifenesin 133 mg, phenylephrine hydrochloride 10 mg per 5 mL. Sugar and alcohol free. Parabens, saccharin. Grape flavor. Syrup. 10 mL, 473 mL. *Rx.*
Use: Antitussive and expectorant.

Zotex GPX. (Vertical) Phenylephrine hydrochloride 8.5 mg, guaifenesin 550 mg. ER Tab. 100s. *Rx.*
Use: Upper respiratory combination, decongestant and expectorant combination.

Zotex-PE. (Vertical) Brompheniramine maleate 6 mg, phenylephrine hydrochloride 30 mg. ER Tab. 100s. *Rx.*
Use: Upper respiratory combination, decongestant and antihistamine combination.

Zotex Pediatric. (Vertical) Phenylephrine hydrochloride 2.5 mg/mL, dextromethorphan HBr 3 mg/mL, guaifenesin 35 mg per 1 mL. Sugar and alcohol free. Parabens, saccharin, grape flavor. Drops. 30 mL with dropper. *Rx.*
Use: Upper respiratory combination, antitussive and expectorant combination.

Zoto-HC. (Horizon) Chloroxylenol 1 mg, pramoxine hydrochloride 10 mg, hydrocortisone 10 mg, propylene glycol diacetate 3%. Benzalkonium chloride. Drops. Plastic dropper vials. 10 mL. *Rx.*
Use: Otic preparation.

Zovia 1/50E. (Watson) Ethinyl estradiol 50 mcg, ethynodiol diacetate 1 mg. Lactose. Tab. Pkg. 21s, 28s (with 7 inert tabs.). *Rx.*
Use: Sex hormone, contraceptive hormone.

Zovia 1/35E. (Watson) Ethinyl estradiol 35 mcg, ethynodiol diacetate 1 mg. Lactose. Tab. Pkg. 21s, 28s (with 7 inert tabs.). *Rx.*
Use: Sex hormone, contraceptive hormone.

Zovirax. (Valeant) Acyclovir. **Cap.:** 200 mg. May contain parabens. Bot. 100s, UD 100s. **Tab.:** 400 mg, 800 mg. Bot. 100s, UD 100s (800 mg only). **Cream:** 5% in aqueous cream base, cetostearyl alcohol, mineral oil, white petrolatum. 2 g. **Susp.:** 200 mg/5 mL. Bot. 473 mL. *Rx.*
Use: Antiviral.

Z-Pak.
See: Zithromax.

Z-Pro-C. (Person and Covey) Zinc sulfate 200 mg (elemental zinc 45 mg), ascorbic acid 100 mg. Tab. Bot. 100s. *OTC.*
Use: Mineral, vitamin supplement.

Z-Tuss AC. (Magna) Chlorpheniramine maleate/codeine phosphate 2 mg/9 mg, 2 mg/10 mg. Saccharin, sorbitol. Alcohol free and sugar free. Cherry flavor. Liq. 473 mL. *c-v.*
Use: Upper respiratory combination, antitussive combination.

ZTuss ZT. (Magna) Hydrocodone bitartrate 5 mg, guaifenesin 300 mg. Tab. 100s. *c-iii.*
Use: Antitussive with expectorant.

•**zucapsaicin.** (zoo-cap-SAY-sin) USAN.
Use: Analgesic, topical.

•**zuclomiphene.** (zoo-KLOE-mih-FEEN) USAN. *Formerly Transclomiphene.*

Zuplenz. (Par) Ondansetron 4 mg, 8 mg. Butylated hydroxytoluene, peppermint flavoring, sucralose. Film. 10s. *Rx.*
Use: Antiemetic/antivertigo agent, 5-HT_3 receptor antagonist.

Zurinol. (Major) Allopurinol. Tab. **100 mg:** Bot. 100s, 500s, 1000s, UD 100s. **300 mg:** Bot. 100s, 500s, UD 100s. *Rx.*
Use: Antigout agent.

Z-Xtra. (Magna) Pyrilamine maleate 2.07 mg, benzocaine 2.08 mg, zinc oxide 41.35 mg/mL, apple blossom, silicone, lanolin, and Wysteria oils, isopropanol, camphor, menthol, parabens. Lot. Bot. 118 mL. *OTC.*
Use: Antihistamine, topical.

Zyban. (GlaxoSmithKline) Bupropion hydrochloride 150 mg. Film-coated. ER Tab. 60s. *Rx.*
Use: Smoking deterrent.

Zyclara. (Graceway Pharmaceuticals) Imiquimod 3.75%. Cetyl alcohol, stearyl alcohol, white petrolatum, benzyl alcohol, parabens. Cream. Single-use packet. 28s. *Rx.*
Use: Topical immunomodulator.

Zyderm I. (Inamed) Highly purified bovine dermal collagen 35 mg/mL implant. Sterile syringe 0.1 mL, 0.5 mL, 1 mL, 2 mL.
Use: Collagen implant.

Zyderm II. (Inamed) Highly purified bovine dermal collagen 65 mg/mL implant. Syringe 0.75 mL.
Use: Collagen implant.

Zydone. (DuPont) Hydrocodone bitartrate 5 mg, 7.5 mg, 10 mg, acetaminophen 400 mg. Cap. Bot. 100s, 500s, UD 100s. *c-III.*
Use: Analgesic combination, narcotic.

Zyflo. (Cornerstone Biopharma) Zileuton 600 mg. Film-coated. Tab. 120s. *Rx.*
Use: Leukotriene formation inhibitor.

Zyflo CR. (Cornerstone Biopharma) Zileuton 600 mg. Mannitol. Film-coated. ER Tab. 120s. *Rx.*
Use: Leukotriene formation inhibitor.

Zyloprim. (Faro Pharmaceuticals) Allopurinol 100 mg, 300 mg. Lactose. Tab. Bot. 100s, 500s (300 mg only). *Rx.*
Use: Antigout agent; antimetabolite; purine analog.

Zymacap. (Pharmacia) Vitamins A 5000 units, D 400 units, E 15 mg, C 90 mg, folic acid 400 mcg, B_1 2.25 mg, B_2 2.6 mg, niacin 30 mg, B_6 3 mg, B_{12} 9 mcg, pantothenic acid 15 mg. Cap. Bot. 90s, 240s. *OTC.*
Use: Vitamin supplement.

Zymar. (Allergan) Gatifloxacin 0.3% (3 mg/mL). EDTA, benzalkonium chloride 0.005%. Soln. Dropper Bot. 2.5 mL, 5 mL. *Rx.*
Use: Antibiotic, ophthalmic.

Zymaxid. (Allergan) Gatifloxacin 0.5%. Benzalkonium chloride 0.005%, EDTA. Soln., Ophth. 2.5 mL, 5 mL. *Rx.*
Use: Ophthalmic and otic agent, ophthalmic antibiotic.

Zymine. (Vindex) Triprolidine hydrochloride 1.25 mg/5 mL, apple flavor. Liq. Bot. 15 mL, 473 mL. *Rx.*
Use: Antihistamine, nonselective alkylamine.

Zymine DXR. (Vindex) Pseudoephedrine tannate 45 mg, triprolidine tannate 2.5 mg per 5 mL. Alcohol and sugar free. Aspartame, parabens, phenylalanine 7 mg/5 mL. Berry flavor. Susp. 473 mL. *Rx.*
Use: Upper respiratory combination, decongestant and antihistamine.

Zymine XR. (Vindex) Triprolidine tannate 2.5 mg/5 mL. Aspartame, parabens, phenylalanine 7 mg/5 mL. Apple flavor. Sugar free. Susp. 473 mL. *Rx.*
Use: Antihistamine, nonselective alkylamine.

Zypram. (Vertical Pharmaceuticals) Hydrocortisone acetate 2.35%, pramoxine hydrochloride 1%. Benzyl alcohol, cetearyl alcohol, glycerin, glyceryl, methylparaben, PEG-12, white petrolatum. Cream. 30 g w/2 wipes and 1 applicator. *Rx.*
Use: Anti-inflammatory agent, topical corticosteroid.

Zyprexa. (Eli Lilly) Olanzapine 2.5 mg, 5 mg, 7.5 mg, 10 mg, 15 mg, 20 mg. Lactose. Tab. Bot. 30s, 1000s, UD 100s. *Rx.*
Tall Man: ZyPREXA
Use: Antipsychotic, dibenzapine derivative.

Zyprexa IntraMuscular. (Eli Lilly) Olanzapine 10 mg. Pow. for Inj. Vial. 10 mg. *Rx.*
Tall Man: ZyPREXA
Use: Antipsychotic.

Zyprexa Relprevv. (Eli Lilly) Olanzapine 210 mg, 300 mg, 405 mg. Mannitol. Inj., Pow. for Susp., extended release. Single-use vial w/diluents. *Rx.*
Use: Antipsychotic agent, dibenzapine derivative.

Zyprexa Zydis. (Eli Lilly) Olanzapine 5 mg (phenylalanine 0.34 mg), 10 mg (phenylalanine 0.45 mg), 15 mg (phenylalanine 0.67 mg), 20 mg (phenylalanine 0.9 mg). Aspartame, parabens, mannitol. Orally disintegrating tab. Dose pack 30s. *Rx.*
Tall Man: ZyPREXA
Use: Antipsychotic, dibenzapine derivative.

Zyrtec Allergy. (McNeil Consumer) Cetirizine hydrochloride 10 mg. **Tab.:** Lactose. 30s. **Tab., orally disintegrating:** Mannitol, sucralose. Citrus flavor. 66s. **Cap., liquid filled:** Glycerin, mannitol,

PEG 400, sorbitan, sorbitol. 12s, 25s, 40s, 65s, 70s. *OTC.*
Tall Man: ZyrTEC
Use: Antihistamine, peripherally selective piperazine.
Zyrtec Children's Allergy. (McNeil Consumer) Cetirizine hydrochloride. **Chew. Tab.:** 5 mg, 10 mg. Acesulfame K, maltodextrin, mannitol, sorbitol, lactose. Grape flavor. 5s (5 mg only), 12s (10 mg only). **Syr., Oral:** 1 mg/mL. Parabens, sugar. Grape flavor. Bot. 118 mL. *OTC.*
Tall Man: ZyrTEC
Use: Antihistamine, peripherally selective piperazine.
Zyrtec Children's Hives Relief. (McNeil Consumer) Cetirizine hydrochloride 1 mg/mL. Parabens, sugar. Grape flavor. Syr., Oral. 118 mL. *OTC.*
Tall Man: ZyrTEC
Use: Antihistamine, peripherally selective piperazine.
Zyrtec-D 12 Hour. (McNeil Consumer) Pseudoephedrine hydrochloride 120 mg (extended release), cetirizine hydrochloride 5 mg (immediate release). Lactose. ER Tab. Bot. 100s. *Rx.*
Tall Man: ZyrTEC

Use: Upper respiratory combination, decongestant, antihistamine.
Zyrtec Hives Relief. (McNeil Consumer) Cetirizine hydrochloride 10 mg. Lactose. Tab. Blister pack 14s. *OTC.*
Tall Man: ZyrTEC
Use: Antihistamine, peripherally selective piperazine.
Zyrtec Itchy Eye. (McNeil Consumer) Ketotifen 0.025% (as ketotifen fumarate). May contain glycerol, sodium hydroxide and/or hydrochloric acid, benzalkonium chloride 0.01%. Soln., Ophth. 5 mL. *OTC.*
Tall Man: ZyrTEC
Use: Ophthalmic and otic agent, ophthalmic antihistamine.
Zyvox. (Pfizer) Linezolid. **Tab.:** 600 mg. Film coated. PEG, sodium 0.1 mEq. 20s, 100s, UD 30s. **Pow. for Oral Susp.:** 100 mg/5 mL. Sodium 0.4 mEq/5 mL, sucrose, aspartame, mannitol, phenylalanine 20 mg, orange flavor. Bot. 115 mL fill in 240 mL. **Inj.:** 2 mg/mL. Sodium 0.38 mg/mL, sodium citrate. Single-use, ready-to-use bag 100 mL, 200 mL, 300 mL. *Rx.*
Use: Oxalodinone.

Reference
Information

Standard Medical Abbreviations

Abbreviation	Meaning
≈	approximately equals
Δ	delta
ε	epsilon; molar absorption coefficient
Ω	omega; ohm
5-HIAA	5-hydroxyindoleacetic acid
5-HT	5-hydroxytryptamine (serotonin)
6-MP	6-mercaptopurine
17-OHCS	17-hydroxycorticosteroids
α	alpha
A	ampere(s)
Å	angstrom(s)
aa	of each (ana)
āā	of each (ana)
AA	Alcoholics Anonymous; amino acid
AACP	American Association of Clinical Pharmacy; American Association of Colleges of Pharmacy
AARP	American Association of Retired Persons
Ab	antibody
ABGs	arterial blood gases
abs feb	when fever is absent (absente febre)
ABVD	Adriamycin (doxorubicin), bleomycin, vinblastine, (and) dacarbazine
ac	before meals or food (ante cibum)
ACCP	American College of Clinical Pharmacy
ACD	acid-citrate-dextrose
ACE	angiotensin-converting enzyme
ACEI	angiotensin-converting enzyme inhibitor
ACh	acetylcholine
ACIP	Advisory Committee on Immunization Practices
ACLS	advanced cardiac life support
ACPE	American Council on Pharmaceutical Education
ACS	American Chemical Society
ACT	activated clotting time
ACTH	adrenocorticotropic hormone
a.d.	right ear (aurio dextra)

Abbreviation	Meaning
ad to;	to; up to (ad)
ADE	adverse drug experience
ADH	antidiuretic hormone
adhib	to be administered (adhibendus)
ad lib	as desired, at pleasure (ad libitum)
ADLs	activities of daily living
ADME	absorption, distribution, metabolism, and elimination
admov	apply (admove)
ADP	adenosine diphosphate
ADR	adverse drug reaction
ADRRS	Adverse Drug Reaction Reporting System
ad sat	to saturation (ad saturatum, ad saturandum)
adst feb	when fever is present (adstante febre)
ad us.	for external use (ad usum externum)
adv	against (adversum)
aer	aerosol
Ag	antigen; silver (argentum)
agit. Ante us.	shake before using (agita ante usum)
agit. Bene	shake well (agita bene)
AHA	American Hospital Association
AID	artificial insemination donor
AIDS	acquired immunodeficiency syndrome
AJHP	American Journal of Hospital Pharmacy
ala	alanine
ALL	acute lymphocytic leukemia
ALT	alanine aminotransferase serum (previously SGPT)
alt hor	every other hour (alternis horis)
A.M.	before noon; morning (ante meridiem)
AMA	American Medical Association
AML	acute myelogenous leukemia
AMP	adenosine monophosphate
ANA	antinuclear antibody(ies)
ANC	acid neutralizing capacity
ANDA	abbreviated new drug application

Abbreviation	Meaning
ANOVA	analysis of variance
ANUG	acute necrotizing ulcerative gingivitis
APA	antipernicious anemia
APAP	acetaminophen
APC	antigen presenting cell(s)
APhA	American Pharmaceutical Association
aPTT	activated partial thrombo-plastin time
aq.	water *(aqua)*
aq. dest	distilled water *(aqua destillata)*
ARC	AIDS-related complex
ARDS	adult respiratory distress syndrome
ARF	acute renal failure
Arg	arginine
ARV	AIDS-related virus
as.	left ear *(aurio sinister)*
ASA	American Society of Anes-thesiologists; aspirin
ASHD	arteriosclerotic heart disease
ASHP	American Society of Hospital Pharmacists
Asn	asparagine
Asp	aspartic acid
AST	aspartate aminotransfer-ase, serum (previously SGOT)
atm.	standard atmosphere
ATN	acute tubular necrosis
ATP	adenosine triphosphate
ATPase	adenosine triphosphatase
ATPD	ambient temperature and pressure, saturated
at wt	atomic weight
au.	both ears *(aures utrae)*
AU	gold *(aurum)*
AUC	area under the plasma concentration-time curve
AV	atrioventricular
A-V.	arteriovenous; atrioventri-cular (block, bundle, conduction, dissociation, extrasystole)
AW	atomic weight
AWP	average wholesale price
ax.	axis
β	beta
BAC	blood-alcohol concentration

Abbreviation	Meaning
BADL	basic activities of daily life
BBB	blood brain barrier
BC	blood culture
BDZ	benzodiazepine
bib	drink *(bibe)*
bid	twice daily; two times a day *(bis in die)*
bm	bowel movement
BMR	basal metabolic rate
bp.	boiling point
BP	blood pressure
BPH	benign prostatic hypertrophy
bpm	beats per minute
BSA	body surface area
BT	bleeding time
BUN	blood urea nitrogen
C	centigrade
C.	*clostridium*
c.	gallon *(cong)*
c̄.	with *(cum)*
°C.	degrees Celsius
Ca	calcium
CA	cancer; carcinoma; cardiac arrest; chronologic age; croup-associated
CAD	coronary artery disease
Cal	Calorie (kilocalorie)
cAMP	cyclic adenosine mono-phosphate
caps	capsule *(capsula)*
CAS	Chemical Abstracts Service
CAT	computerized axial tomography
cath	catheterize
CBA	cost-benefit analysis
CBC	complete blood count
CC	chief complaint
cc	cubic centimeter
CCBs	calcium channel blockers
CCU	coronary care unit; critical care unit
CD4	T-helper lymphocytes and macrophages
CDC	Centers for Disease Control and Prevention
CEA	cost effectiveness analysis
CF	cystic fibrosis
CFC	chlorofluorocarbon
CFU	colony-forming units

Abbreviation	Meaning
CHD	coronary heart disease
CHF	congestive heart failure
Ci	curie
CK	creatinine kinase
Cl	chlorine
Cl_{cr}	creatinine clearance
cm	centimeter
Cm	curium
cm^2	square centimeter(s)
cm^3	cubic centimeter
CMA	Certified Medical Assistant
CMC	carpometacarpal
CMI	cell-mediated immunity
CML	chronic myelocytic leukemia
C_{max}	maximum effective plasma concentration
C_{min}	minimum effective plasma concentration
CMT	Certified Medical Transcriptionist
CMV	cytomegalovirus I
CMVIG	cytomegalovirus immune globulin
CN	cranial nerve
CNM	Certified Nurse Midwife
CNS	central nervous system
CO	cardiac output
CO_2	carbon dioxide
CoA	coenzyme A
COG	center of gravity
comp	compound (compositus)
COMT	catecholamine-o-methyl transferase
cont rem	let the medicine be continued (continuetur remedium)
COPD	chronic obstructive pulmonary disease
CPAP	continuous positive airway pressure
CPK	creatine phosphokinase
CPR	cardiopulmonary resuscitation
CQI	continuous quality improvement
Cr	creatinine; chromium
CrCl	creatinine clearance
CRD	chronic respiratory disease
CRF	chronic renal failure
CRH	corticotropin-releasing hormone

Abbreviation	Meaning
crm	cream
CRNA	Certified Registered Nurse Anesthetist
C&S	culture and sensitivity
CSA	Controlled Substances Act; cyclosporin A
CSF	cerebrospinal fluid; colony-stimulating factors
CSP	cellulose sodium phosphate
ct	clotting time
CT	computerized tomography
CTZ	chemoreceptor trigger zone
cu	cubic
Cu	copper (cuprum)
CV	cardiovascular
CVA	cerebrovascular accident
CVP	central venous pressure
CXR	chest x-ray
cyl	cylinder; cylindrical (lens)
cys	cysteine
d	day (dies)
D5W	Dextrose 5% in Water Solution
D10W	Dextrose 10% in Water Solution
D&C	dilation and curettage; designation applied to dyes permitted for use in drugs and cosmetics
D&E	dilation and evacuation
DC	Doctor of Chiropratic
DDS	Doctor of Dental Surgery
DEA	Drug Enforcement Administration
deglut	swallow (degluttiatur)
DERM	dermatologic
det	give (detur)
DHHS	Department of Health and Human Services
DIC	disseminated intravascular coagulation
dieb alt	every other day (diebus alternis)
dil	dilute (dilue)
dim	one-half (dimidius)
dir prop	with proper direction (directione propria)
div in par aeq	divide into equal parts (divide in partes aequales)
DIS	drug information source

Abbreviation	Meaning
disp	dispense (dispensa)
div	divide
DJD	degenerative joint disease
DKA	diabetic ketoacidosis
dL	deciliter (100 mL)
DMD	Doctor of Dental Medicine
DMSO	dimethyl sulfoxide
DNA	deoxyribonucleic acid
DNR	do not resuscitate
DNS	Director of Nursing Service; Doctor of Nursing Services
DO	Doctor of Osteopathy
DOA	dead on arrival
DP	Doctor of Podiatry
DPH	Doctor of Public Health; Doctor of Public Hygiene
DPI	dry powder inhaler
DPM	Doctor of Physical Medicine; Doctor of Podiatric Medicine
DPS	disintegrations per second
DRG	diagnosis-related groups
DRI	Dietary Reference Intakes
drp	drop(s)
DrPh	Doctor of Public Health; Doctor of Public Hygiene
DRR	Drug Regimen Review
DT	delirium tremens
dtd	give of such a dose (dentur tales doses)
DTP	diphtheria, tetanus toxoids & pertussis vaccine
DTRs	deep tendon reflexes
DUB	dysfunctional uterine bleeding
DUE	Drug Usage Evaluations
DUR	Drug Utilization Review
dur dol	while pain lasts (durante dolore)
DVA	Department of Veterans Affairs
DVM	Doctor of Veterinary Medicine
DVT	deep venous thrombosis
E.	Enterococcus; Escherichia
EBV	Epstein-Barr virus
EC	enteric coated
ECG	electrocardiogram
ECT	electroconvulsive therapy

Abbreviation	Meaning
ed.	editor
ED	emergency department; effective dose
ED_{50}	median-effective dose
EDTA	ethylenediamine tetra-acetic acid
EEG	electroencephalogram
EENT	eye, ear, nose, and throat
EF	ejection fraction
eg.	for example (exempli gratia)
EIA	enzyme immunoassay
EKG	electrocardiogram
el	elixir
ELISA	enzyme-linked immunosorbent assay
elix	elixir
EMIT	enzyme-multiplied immunoassay test
emp	as directed
ENL	erythema nodosum leprosum
ENT	ear, nose, throat
EPA	Environmental Protection Agency
EPAP	expiratory positive airway pressure
EPO	erythropoietin
EPS	extrapyramidal syndrome (or symptoms)
ER	emergency room; estrogen receptor; extended release; endoplasmic reticulum
ESR	erythrocyte sedimentation rate; electron spin resonance
ESRD	end-stage renal disease
et	and
ET	via endotracheal tube
et al.	for 3 or more coauthors or coworkers (et alii)
ex aq	in water
ext rel	extended release
F	fluorine
f	make; let be made (fac, fiat, fiant)
°F	degress Fahrenheit
Fab	fragment of immuno-globulin G involved in antigen binding
FAO	Food and Agriculture Organizations

Abbreviation	Meaning
FAS	fetal alcohol syndrome
FBS	fasting blood sugar
FDA	Food and Drug Administration
FD&C	designation applied to dyes permitted for use in foods, drugs, and cosmetics; Food, Drug and Cosmetic Act
Fe	iron (ferrum)
FEF	forced expiratory flow
FET	forced expiratory time
FEV_1	forced expiratory volume in 1 second
fl oz	fluid ounce(s)
Fru	fructose
FSH	follicle-stimulating hormone
ft.	foot (feet)
ft^2	square foot (feet)
FTC	Federal Trade Commission
FTI	free-thyroxine index
FUO	fever of unknown origin
FVC	forced vital capacity
γ	gamma
g.	gram (gramma)
G-6-P	glucose-6-phosphate
G-6-PD	glucose-6-phosphate dehydrogenase
GABA	gamma-aminobutyric acid
Gal	galactose
gal	gallon
G-CSF	granulocyte colony-stimulating factor
GERD	gastroesophageal reflux disease
GFR	glomerular filtration rate
GGTP	gamma glutamyl transpeptidase
GH	growth hormone
GHRF	growth hormone-releasing factor
GHRH	growth hormone-releasing hormone
GI	gastrointestinal
GLC	gas-liquid chromatography
gln	glutamine
glu	glutamic acid; glutamyl
gly	glycine
Gm	gram (gramma)
gr	grain (granum)
grad	gradually (gradatim)

Abbreviation	Meaning
gran	granule(s)
GRAS	generally regarded as safe
gtt.	a drop (gutta)
GU	genitourinary
Gyn	gynecology
H.	Haemophilus; Helicobacter
h.	hour (hora)
H_2	histamine 2
H_2O	water
HA	hyaluronic acid
Hb	hemoglobin
HbF	fetal hemoglobin
HBIG	hepatitis B immune globulin
HCFA	Health Care Financing Administration
HCG	human chorionic gonadotropin
HCl	hydrochloride
HCN	hydrogen cyanide
Hct	hematocrit
hd.	bedtime (hora decubitus)
HDL	high-densitiy lipoprotein
HEMA	hematologic
HEME	hematologic
hep	hepatic
HEPA	high efficiency particulate air
Hg	mercury (hydragyrum)
Hgb	hemoglobin
HGH	human pituitary growth hormone
Hib.	Haemophilus influenzae
His.	Haemophilus influenzae type b
HIV	human immunodeficiency virus
HLA	human leukocyte antigen
HMG-CoA	3-hydroxy-3-methylglutaryl coenzyme A
HMO	health maintenance organization
hor decub	at bedtime (hora decubitus)
hor som	at bedtime (hora somni)
HPA	hypothalamic-pituitary-adrenocortical (axis)
HPLC	high performance liquid chromatography
HPLC/MS	high performance liquid chromatography/mass spectrometry

Abbreviation	Meaning
HPMC	hydroxypropylmethylcellulose
HPV	human papillomavirus
HR	heart rate
hr	hour
hs	at bedtime *(hora somni)*
HSA	human serum albumin
HSV-1	herpes simplex virus type 1
HSV-2	herpes simplex virus type 2
Hz	hertz
I	iodine
IADL	instrumental activities of daily living
I/O	intake/output
IBW	ideal body weight
IC	intracoronary
ICD	International Classification of Diseases of the World Health Organization
ICF	intracellular fluid
ICP	intracranial pressure
ID	intradermal; infective dose
IDDM	insulin-dependent diabetes mellitus (type 1 diabetes)
IDU	idoxuridine
IFN	interferon
Ig	immunoglobulin
IL	interleukin
Ile	isoleucine
IM	intramuscular
in	inch(es)
in²	square inch(es)
IND	Investigational New Drug
in d.	daily *(in dies)*
INDA	Investigational New Drug Application
Inh	inhaled
INH	isoniazid
Inhal	inhalation
Inj	injection
INR	International Normalized Ratio
int cib	between meals *(inter cibos)*
IOP	intraocular pressure
IP	intraperitoneal(ly)
IPA	International Pharmaceutical Abstracts
IPPB	intermittent positive pressure breathing

Abbreviation	Meaning
IPV	poliovirus vaccine inactivated
IQ	intelligence quotient
ISA	intrinsic sympathomimetic activity
ISF	interstitial fluid
ISI	Institute for Scientific Information
ISO	International Organization for Standardization
IT	intrathecal(ly)
IU	international unit(s)
IUD	intrauterine device
IV	intravenous
IVF	intravascular fluid
IVP	intravenous piggyback
J	joule(s)
JCAH	Joint Commission on Accreditation of Hospitals
JCAHO	Joint Commission on Accreditation of Healthcare Organizations
K	potassium *(kalium)*; kelvin
kcal	kilocalorie(s)
keV	kiloelectronvolt(s)
kg	kilogram
kJ	kilojoule(s)
Kleb.	*Klebsiella*
KVO	keep vein open
L	liter
L.	*Legionella*; *Listeria*
lb	pound
LBW	low body weight
LD	lethal dose
LD-50	a dose lethal to 50% of the specified animals or microorganisms
LDH	lactate dehydrogenase
LDL	low-density lipoprotein
LE	lupus erythematosus
Leu	leucine
LFT	liver function test
LH	luteinizing hormone
liq	liquid *(liquor)*
LM	Licentiate in Midwifery
LOC	level of consciousness
Lot	lotion
LPN	Licensed Practical Nurse
Lr	lawrencium
LSD	lysergic acid diethylamide

Abbreviation	Meaning
LTCF	long-term care facility
LTM	long-term memory
LUQ	left upper quadrant (of abdomen)
LVEDP	left ventricular end-diastolic pressure
LVET	left ventricular ejection time
LVF	left ventricular function
LVN	Licensed Visiting Nurse; Licensed Vocational Nurse
LVP	large-volume parenterals
Lw	former symbol for lawrencium (see Lr)
Lys	lysine
μm	micrometer
μg.	microgram
m	meter
M	mix *(misce)*; molar (strength of a solution)
M.	*Moraxella*; *Mycobacterium*; *Mycoplasma*
m²	square meter (of body surface area)
m³	cubic meter(s)
MA	mental age
MAC	maximum allowable cost
MADD	Mothers Against Drunk Driving
man pr	early morning; first thing in the morning *(mane primo)*
MAO.	monoamine oxidase
MAOI	monoamine oxidase inhibitor
MAP	mean arterial pressure
max	maximum
MBC	minimum bactericidal concentration
MBD	mimimal brain dysfunction
mcg	microgram
MCH	mean corpuscular hemoglobin
MCHC	mean corpuscular hemoglobin concentration
mCi	millicurie
MCT	medium-chain triglyceride
MCV	mean corpuscular volume
MD	Doctor of Medicine *(Medicinae Doctor)*
MDI	metered-dose inhaler
m dict	as directed *(more dictor)*
MDR	minimum daily requirements
MEC	minimum effective concentration
MEDLARS	Medical Literature Analysis and Retrieval System
MEDLINE	National Library of Medicine medical database
mEq	milliequivalent
Met	methionine
MeV	megaelectronvolt(s)
Mg	magnesium
mg	milligram
MHC	major histocompatibility complex
MI	myocardial infarction
MIA	metabolite bacterial inhibition assay
MIC	minimum inhibitory concentration
MID	minimal inhibitory dose
min	minute; minimum
MIP	maximum inspiratory pressure
mixt	a mixture *(mixtura)*
MJ	mejajoule(s)
mL	milliliter
mm	millimeter
mm²	square millimeter(s)
mm³	cubic millimeter(s)
mmHg	millimeters of mercury
mmol	millimole
MMR	measles, mumps and rubella virus vaccine, live
MMWR	Morbidity and Mortality Weekly Report
Mn	manganese
Mo	molybdenum
mo	month
mol	mole(s)
mor dict	in the manner stated *(more dicto)*
mor sol	as usual; as customary *(more solito)*
mOsm	milliosmole
MPH	Master of Public Health
MRI	magnetic resonance imaging
mRNA	messenger RNA
MS	mass spectrometry; mitral stenosis; multiple sclerosis

Abbreviation	Meaning
MW	molecular weight
N	normal (strength of a solution)
N.	*Neisseria*
NA	sodium *(natrium)*
NABP	National Association of Boards of Pharmacy
NABPLEX	National Association of Boards of Pharmacy Licensing Exam
NAD	nicotinamide-adenine dinucleotide phosphate
NADH	reduced form of nicotine adenine dinucleotide
NADP	nicotinamide-adenine dinucleotide phosphate
NADPH	nicotinamide-adenine dinucleotide phosphate (reduced form)
NAPA	*N*-acetyl procainamide
NARD	National Association of Retail Druggists - Now NCPA; National Association of Community Pharmacists
nb	note well *(nota bene)*
nCi	nanocurie(s)
NCPA	National Association of Community Pharmacists
ND	Doctor of Naturopathic Medicine
NDA	new drug application
NF	National Formulary'
ng	nanogram
NG	nasogastric
NK	natural killer (cells); killer T cells
NIDDM	non-insulin-dependent diabetes mellitus (type 2 diabetes)
NIH	National Institutes of Health
NLM	National Library of Medicine
nm	nanometer(s)
NMS	neuroleptic malignant syndrome
NMT	not more than (on prescriptions)
no.	number *(numerus)*
noc	in the night *(nocturnal)*
noc maneq	at night and in the morning *(nocte maneque)*
non rep	do not repeat; no refills *(non repetatur)*

Abbreviation	Meaning
NPN	nonprotein nitrogen
NPO	nothing by mouth
NS	normal saline (as in solution)
NSAIA	nonsteroidal antiinflammatory agent
NSAID	nonsteroidal antiinflammatory drug
NTD	neural tube defect
O	a pint *(octarius)*
OB/GYN	obstetrics and gynecology
OBRA	Omnibus Budget Reconciliation Act of 1990
OBS	organic brain syndrome
OC	oral contraceptive
Oct	a pint *(octarius)*
od.	right eye *(oculus dexter)*
OD	Doctor of Optometry; overdose
Oint	ointment
ol	left eye *(oculus laevus)*
omn hor	at every hour *(omni hora)*
Ophth	ophthalmic
os.	left eye *(oculus sinister)*
OSHA	Occupational Safety and Health Administration
OT	occupational therapy
OTC	over-the-counter (nonprescription)
OPV	oral polioviurs vaccine, live
ou.	each eye *(oculo uterque)*
o/w	oil-in-water (emulsion)
oz.	ounce
P	phosphorus
P	probability
P&T	pharmacy and therapeutics (committee)
Pa	pascal(s)
PA	Physician Assistant; Physician's Assistant
PABA	para-aminobenzoic acid
PAC	premature atrial contraction
$PaCO_2$	arterial plasma partial pressure of carbon dioxide
PAD	premature atrial depolarization
PAF	platelet-activating factor
PaO_2	partial alveolar oxygen
part aeq	equal parts/amounts *(partes aequales)*
part vic	in divided doses *(partitis vicibus)*

Abbreviation	Meaning
PAS	para-aminosalicylic acid
PAW	pulmonary arterial wedge
PAWP	pulmonary arterial wedge pressure
Pb	lead (plumbum)
PBP	penicillin-binding protein
pc	after meals (post cibum; post cibos)
PCA	patient-controlled analgesia
pCO_2	plasma partial pressure of carbon dioxide
PCP	phencyclidine
PCR	polymerase chain reaction
PDGF	platelet-derived growth factor
PDLL	poorly differentiated lymphocytic lymphoma
PE	pulmonary embolism
PEEP	positive and expiratory pressure
PEG	polyethylene glycol
PERLA	pupils equal, react to light and accommodation
PET	positron emission tomography
pg	picograms(s)
PG	prostaglandin
PGA	prostaglandin A
PGB	prostaglandin B
PGE	prostaglandin E
PGF	prostaglandin F
pH	the negative logarithm of the hydrogen ion concentration
PharmD	Doctor of Pharmacy (Pharmaciae Doctor)
PhD	Doctor of Philosophy (Philosophiae Doctor)
Phe	phenylalanine
PhG	German Pharmacopeia (Pharmacopoeia Germanica)
PHS	Public Health Service
pKa	the negative logarithm of the dissociation constant
PKU	phenylketonuria
PMA	Pharmaceutical Manufacturers Association
PMH	past medical history
PMI	posterior myocardial infarction
PMN	polymorphonuclear leukocyte

Abbreviation	Meaning
PMR	patient medication record
PMS	premenstrual syndrome
PND	paroxysmal nocturnal dyspnea
po	by mouth; orally (per os)
pO_2	oxygen pressure (tension)
POR	problem-oriented medical record
POS	point of service
post cib	after meals (post cibos); pc
PPD	purified protein derivative of tuberculin
PPI	patient package insert
ppm	parts per million
PPO	preferred provider organization
pr	per rectum
Pr.	Proteus
prn	as needed; when required (pro re nata)
Pro	proline
pro rat. Aet.	According to patient's age (pro ratione aetatis)
Ps.	Pseudomonas
PSA	prostate-specific antigen
PSP	phenolsulfonphthalein
PSVT	paroxysmal supraventricular tachycardia
pt	pint
PT	prothrombin time; pharmacy and therapeutics; physical therapy
PTH	parathyroid hormone
PTT	partial thromboplastin time
PUD	peptic ulcer disease
pulv	a powder (pulvis)
PUVA	oral administration of psoralen and subsequent exposure to ultraviolet light of A wavelenghts (UVA)
PVC	premature ventricular contraction; polyvinyl chloride
PVD	peripheral vascular disease; premature ventricular depolarizations
pwdr	powder
q	every
Q	volume of blood flow
QA	quality assurance
qad	every other day (quoque alternis die)
QC	quality control

Abbreviation	Meaning
qd.	every day *(quaque die)*
qh.	every hour *(quaque hora)*
q hr	every hour
qid	four times daily *(quarter in die)*
ql	as much as desired *(quantum libet)*
qod.	every other day
q 2 hr	every 2 hours
qs	a sufficient quantity *(quantum sufficiat)*; as much as is enough *(quantum satis)*
qs ad	a sufficient quantity to make
qt	quart
qv	as much as you wish *(quam volueris)*
R&D	research and development
RA	rheumatoid arthritis
RAI.	radioactive iodine
RAS	renin-angiotension system; reticular-activating system
RAST	radioallergosorbent test
RBC.	red blood (cell) count
RDA	Recommended Dietary (Daily) Allowance
RDS	respiratory distress
RDW	red-cell distribution width
RE	reticuloendothelial
rem.	radio equivalent man
REM.	rapid eye movement
rep	let it be repeated *(repetatur)*
RES	reticuloendothelial system
RF	releasing factor
Rh	Rhesus (RH blood group)
RIA.	radioimmunoassay
RN	Registered Nurse
RNA	ribonucleic acid
ROM	range of motion
RPh	registered pharmacist
rpm.	revolutions per minute
rps	revolutions per second
RR	respiratory rate
RT_3U	total serum thyroxine concentration
RUL	right upper lobe (of lung)
RUQ.	right upper quadrant (of abdomen)

Abbreviation	Meaning
Rx	prescription only; take; a recipe *(recipe)*
S.	*Salmonella; Serratia*
s.	second; without *(sine)*
s̄.	without *(sine)*
S&S	signs and symptoms
S-A.	sinoatrial
sa.	according to art *(secundum artem)*
sat	saturated *(sataratus)*
Sb	antimony *(stibium)*
SBE	self breast examination; subacute bacterial endocarditis
SC	subcutaneous(ly)
S_{cr}	serum creatinine
SD	standard deviation; streptodornase
Se	selenium
sec	second
Ser	serine
sf	sugar free
SGGT.	serum gamma-glutamyl transferase
SGOT.	(see AST)
SGPT.	(see ALT)
Sh.	*Shigella*
SIADH	syndrome of inappropriate secretion of antidiuretic hormone
SIDS	sudden infant death syndrome
Sig	label; let it be printed *(signa)*
SI units.	International System of Units
SK	streptokinase
SL	sublingual(ly)
SLE	systemic lupus erythematosus
SMA.	sequential multiple analysis
Sn	tin *(stannum)*
SNF	skilled nursing facility
sol	solution *(solutio)*
soln	solution
solv	dissolve
sp.	species
SPECT.	single photon emission computerized tomography
sp gr.	specific gravity

Abbreviation	Meaning
SPF	sun protection factor
sq.	square
SR	sedimentation rate; sustained release
ss	one-half (semis)
s̄s̄	one-half (semis)
SSRI	selective serotonin reuptake inhibitors
Staph.	Staphylococcus
stat	immediately; at once (statim)
STM	short-term memory
STP	standard temperature and pressure
Str.	Streptococcus
STD	sexually transmitted disease
supp	suppository (suppositorium)
suppl	supplement(s)
susp	suspension
SV	stroke volume
syr	syrup (syrupus)
$t_{1/2}$	half-life
T_3	triiodothyronine
T_4	thyroxine
tab	tablet (tabella)
tal	such
tal dos	such doses
TB	tuberculosis
TBC	thyroxine-binding globulin
TBP	thyroxine-binding proteins
TBPA	thyroxine-binding prealbumin
TBW	total body weight
TCA	tricyclic antidepressant
TD_{50}	median toxic dose
TEEC	transesophageal echocardiography
TEN	toxic epidermal necrolysis
TENS	transcutaneous electrical nerve stimulation
TG	total triglycerides
THC	tetrahydrocannabinol
Thr	threonine
TIA	transient ischemic attack
tid	three times daily (ter in die)
tbsp	tablespoonful
tinct	tincture

Abbreviation	Meaning
TLC	total lung capacity; thin layer chromatography
T_{max}	time to maximum concentration
TMJ	temporomandibular joint
TNF	tumor necrosis factor
TNM	tumor, node, metastasis (tumor staging)
top	topical(ly)
TOPV	trivalent oral polio vaccine
tPA	tissue plasminogen activator
TPN	total parenteral nutrition
TPR	temperature, pulse, respirations
TQM	total quality management
tr	tincture
trit.	triturate (tritura)
tRNA	transfer RNA
Trp	tryptophan
TSA	tumor-specific antigens
TSH	thyroid-stimulating hormone
tsp	teaspoonful
TSS	toxic shock syndrome
TSTA	tumor-specific transplantation antigen
TT	thrombin time
TV	tidal volume
Tyr	tyrosine
U	unit
ud.	as directed
UD	unit-dose package
UK	United Kingdom
ung.	ointment (unguentum)
URI	upper respiratory infection
USAN	United States Adopted Name(s)
USP	United States Pharmacopeia
USPHS	United States Public Health Service
ut dict	as directed (ut dictum)
UTI	urinary tract infection
UVA	ultraviolet A wave
V	volt
VA	Veterans Administration
vag.	vaginal(ly)
Val	valine
var	variety
VC	vital capacity

Abbreviation	Meaning
V_c	volume of distribution of the central compartment
V_d	volume of distribution (one compartment)
$V_{d\beta}$	volume of distribution of the β phase
V_{dss}	steady-state apparent volume of distribution
VHDL	very high-density lipoprotein
VLDL	very low-density lipoprotein
VMA	vanillylmandelic acid
vol	volume
VS	vital signs
v/v	volume in volume
v/w	volume in weight
wa	while awake

Abbreviation	Meaning
WBC	white blood (cell) count
WBCT	whole blood clotting time
WDLL	well-differentiated lymphocytic lymphoma
WFI	water for injection
WHO	World Health Organization
wk	week
WNL	within normal limits
w/o	water in oil
wt	weight
w/v	weight in volume
w/w	weight in weight
y/o	years old
yr	year
ZE	Zollinger-Ellison
Zn	zinc

Calculations

To calculate milliequivalent weight:

$$mEq = \frac{\text{gram molecular weight/valence}}{1000}$$

$$mEq = \frac{mg}{eq\ wt} \qquad \text{equivalent weight or eq wt} = \frac{\text{gram molecular weight}}{valence}$$

Commonly Used mEq Weights			
Chloride	35.5 mg = 1 mEq	Magnesium	12 mg = 1 mEq
Sodium	23 mg = 1 mEq	Potassium	39 mg = 1 mEq
Calcium	20 mg = 1 mEq		

To convert temperature:

Fahrenheit to Celsius: $(°F - 32) \times 5/9 = °C$

Celsius to Fahrenheit: $(°C \times 9/5) + 32 = °F$

Celsius to Kelvin: $°C + 273 = °K$

Temperature Equivalents

$°C = 5 \div sec \times (°F - 32)$

$°F = 9 \div 5 \times (°C) + 32$

$°K = °C + 273$

To calculate creatinine clearance (Ccr) from serum creatinine (mL/min):

Male: $Ccr = \frac{\text{weight (kg)} \times (140 - age)}{72 \times \text{serum creatinine (mg/dL)}}$ for males $\qquad$ Female: $Ccr = 0.85 \times$ calculation

---

To calculate ideal body weight (IBW) (kg) in adults:

IBW (kg) (Males) = 50 + (2.3 × Height in inches over 60 inches)

IBW (kg) (Females) = 45.5 kg + (2.3 × Height in inches over 60 inches)

To calculate absolute neutrophil count (ANC):

WBC × (% Segs + % Bands)

To calculate aninon gap:

$Na^+ - (Cl^-\ HCo_3^-)$

Elevated anion gap usually indicates unmeasured anions in the extracellular fluid due to any of the following: methanol, uremia, diabetes, paraldehyde, ischemia, ethylene glycol, salicylates.

To calculate daily fluid requirements (based on patient's weight):

Weight from 0 to 10 kg: 100 kg

Weight from 10 to 20 kg: 50 mL/kg

Weight > 20 kg: 20 mL/kg

To calculate LDL cholesterol:

$LDL_{chol} = (Total_{chol} - HDL_{chol}) - [\text{Triglycerides (must be} < 400)/5]$

To calculate volume status:

BUN: Serum Creatine ratio

* If > 20:1, Patient is volume depleted and requires fluid replacement.

$$\text{Chem 7} \quad \frac{Na^+}{K^+} \bigg| \frac{Cl^-}{HCO_3^-} \bigg| \frac{BUN}{SrCr} \; / \; \text{Glucose} \qquad WBC \underset{Hct}{\overset{Hgb}{\times}} Plt$$

* Glucose: add 1.6 mEq/L Na^+ for every 100 mg/dL glucose is above normal.

To calculate total calcium corrected for albumin:

[Normal albumin – patient's albumin] $\times$ 0.8 patient's calcium = corrected calcium

Common Systems of Weights and Measures

The listing of common systems of weights and measures is included to aid the practitioner in calculating dosages.

METRIC SYSTEM

Metric Weight			Metric Liquid Measure		
1 femtogram (fg)	= 0.001	pg	1 femtoliter (fL)	= 0.001	pL
1 picogram (pg)	= 0.001	ng	1 picoliter (pL)	= 0.001	nL
1 nanogram (ng)	= 0.001	mcg	1 nanoliter (nL)	= 0.001	μL
1 microgram* (μg [mcg])	= 0.001	mg	1 microliter (μL)	= 0.001	mL
1 milligram (mg)	= 0.001	g	1 milliliter (mL)	= 0.001	L
1 centigram (cg)	= 0.01	g	1 centiliter (cL)	= 0.01	L (= 10 mL)
1 decigram (dg)	= 0.1	g	1 deciliter (dL)	= 0.1	L (= 100 mL)
1 gram (g)	= 1.0	g	1 liter (L)	= 1.0	L (= 1000 mL)
1 dekagram (dag)	= 10.0	g	1 dekaliter (daL)	= 10.0	L
1 hectogram (hg)	= 100.0	g	1 hectoliter (hL)	= 100.0	L
1 kilogram (kg)	= 1000.0	g	1 kiloliter (kL)	= 1000.0	L

* The abbreviation μg or mcg is used for microgram in pharmacy rather than gamma (γ) as in biology.

APOTHECARY SYSTEM*

Apothercary Weight Equivalents			Apothecary Volume Equivalents		
1 grain† (gr)	= 1 gr		1 minim (♏)	= 1 ♏	
1 scruple (℈)	= 20 gr		1 fluidram (fl ʒ)	= 60 ♏	= 8 fl ʒ
1 dram (ʒ)	= 60 gr	= 3 ℈	1 fluid ounce (fl ℥)	= 480 ♏	= 8 fl ʒ
1 ounce (℥)	= 480 gr	= 8 ʒ	1 pint (pt or O)	= 7680 ♏	= 16 fl ℥
1 pound (lb)	= 5760 gr	= 12 ℥	1 quart (qt)	= 15630 ♏	= 32 fl ℥
			1 gallon (gal or cong)	= 61440 ♏	= 128 fl ℥

* Used in preparation of pharmaceuticals.

† The grain in each of the above systems has the same value, and thus serves as a basis for the interconversion of the other units.

AVOIRDUPOIS SYSTEM*

Avoirdupois Equivalents		
1 ounce (oz)	= 437.5 grains (gr)	
1 pound (lb)	= 16 ounces (oz)	= 7000 grains (gr)

* Used by manufacturers and wholesalers.

Approximate Practical Equivalents

The listing of approximate practical equivalents is included to aid the practitioner in calculating and converting dosages among the various systems.

Weight Equivalents

1 grain	=	1 gr	=	65 milligrams
1 milligram	=	1 mg	=	0.017 grains
1 gram	=	1 g	=	15.432 grains
1 gram	=	1 g	=	0.035 ounces
1 ounce avoirdupois	=	1 oz	=	28.35 grams
1 ounce apothecary	=	1 ℥	=	31.1 grams
1 pound avoirdupois	=	1 lb	=	454.0 grams
1 pound avoirdupois	=	1 lb	=	0.45 kilograms
1 kilogram	=	1 kg	=	2.20 pounds avoirdupois (lb)

Measure Equivalents

1 milliliter	=	1 mL	=	16.23 minims (♏,)
1 cubic centimeter*	=	1 cc	=	1.0 mL
1 fluidram†	=	1 f ℨ	=	3.4 mL
1 teaspoonful†	=	1 tsp	=	5.0 mL
1 tablespoonful	=	1 tbsp	=	15.0 mL
1 fluid ounce	=	1 fl ℨ	=	29.57 mL
1 wineglassful	=	2 fl ℨ	=	60.0 mL
1 teacupful	=	4 fl ℨ	=	120.0 mL
1 tumblerful	=	8 fl ℨ	=	240.0 mL
1 pint	=	1 pt or O or Oct	=	473.0 mL
1 quart	=	1 qt	=	946.0 mL
1 liter	=	1 L	=	33.8 fluid ounces (fl ℨ)
1 gallon	=	1 gal or C or Cong	=	3785.0 mL

* Cubic centimeter and milliliter are equivalent.

† On prescription a fluidram is assumed to contain a teaspoonful, which is 5 mL.

Weight to Volume Equivalents

1 mg/dL	=	10 μ/mL
1 mg/dL	=	1 mg %
1% solution	=	10 mg per mL
1 ppm	=	1 mg/L

Linear Equivalents

1 millimeter	=	1 mm	=	0.04 inches
1 inch	=	1 in	=	25.4 millimeters
1 inch	=	1 in	=	2.54 centimeters
1 meter	=	1 meter	=	39.37 inches
1 inch	=	1 in	=	0.025 meters

International System of Units

The *Système international d 'unités* (International System of Units) or *SI* is a modernized version of the metric system. The primary goal of the conversion to SI units is to revise the present confused measurement system and to improve test-result communications.

The SI has 7 basic units from which other units are derived:

Base Units of SI		
Physical quantity	Base unit	SI symbol
length	meter	m
mass	kilogram	kg
time	second	s
amount of substance	mole	mol
thermodynamic temperature	kelvin	K
electric current	ampere	A
luminous intensity	candela	cd

Combinations of these base units can express any property, although, for simplicity, special names are given to some of these derived units.

Representative Derived Units		
Derived unit	Name and symbol	Derivation from base units
area	square meter	m^2
volume	cubic meter	m^3
force	newton (N)	$kg \cdot m \cdot s^{-2}$
pressure	pascal (Pa)	$kg \cdot m^{-1} \cdot s^{-2}$ (N/m^2)
work, energy	joule (J)	$kg \cdot m^2 \cdot s^{-2}$ ($N \cdot m$)
mass density	kilogram per cubic meter	kg/m^3
frequency	hertz (Hz)	1 cycles/s^{-1}
temperature degree	Celsius (°C)	$°C = °K - 273.15$
concentration		
mass	kilogram/liter	kg/L
substance	mole/liter	mol/L
molality	mole/kilogram	mol/kg
density	kilogram/liter	kg/L

Prefixes to the base unit are used in this system to form decimal multiples and submultiples. The preferred multiples and submultiples listed below change the quantity by increments of 10^3 or 10^{-3}. The exceptions to these recommended factors are within the middle rectangle.

Prefixes and Symbols for Decimal Multiples and Submultiples		
Factor	Prefix	Symbol
10^{18}	exa	E
10^{15}	peta	P
10^{12}	tera	T
10^{9}	giga	G
10^{6}	mega	M
10^{3}	kilo	k
10^{2}	hecto	h
10^{1}	deka	da
10^{-1}	deci	d
10^{-2}	centi	c
10^{-3}	milli	m
10^{-6}	micro	µ
10^{-9}	nano	n
10^{-12}	pico	p
10^{-15}	femto	f
10^{-18}	atto	a

To convert drug concentrations to or from SI units:

Conversion factor (CF) = $1000/_{mol\ wt}$

Conversion *to* SI units: µg/mL × CF = µmol/L

Conversion *from* SI units: µmol/L ÷ CF = µg/mL

Normal Laboratory Values

In the following tables, normal reference values for commonly requested laboratory tests are listed in traditional units and in SI units. The tables are a guideline only. Values are method dependent and "normal values" may vary between laboratories.

Blood, Plasma or Serum		
	Reference Value	
Determination	Conventional units	SI units
Alpha-fetoprotein	Adult: < 15 ng/mL Pregnant (16-18 wk): 38-45 ng/mL	Adult: < 15 mcg/L Pregnant (16-18 wk): 38-45 mcg/L
Ammonia (NH_3) - diffusion	20-120 mcg/dL	12-70 mcmol/L
Ammonia nitrogen	15-45 µg/dL	11-32 µmol/L
Amylase	20-100 units/dL	37-185 U/L
Anion gap ($Na^+-[Cl^- + HCO_3^-]$) (P)	7-16 mEq/L	7-16 mmol/L
Antinuclear antibodies	negative at 1:10 dilution of serum	negative at 1:10 dilution of serum
Antithrombin III (AT III)	80-120 U/dL	800-1200 U/L
Bicarbonate: Arterial Venous	21-28 mEq/L 22-29 mEq/L	21-28 mmol/L 22-29 mmol/L
Bilirubin: Conjugated (direct) Total	≤ 0.2 mg/dL 0.1-1 mg/dL	≤ 4 mcmol/L 2-18 mcmol/L
Calcitonin: Female Male	≤ 20 pg/mL ≤ 40 pg/mL	≤ 20 ng/L ≤ 40 ng/L
Calcium: Total Ionized	8.6-10.3 mg/dL 4.4-5.1 mg/dL	2.2-2.74 mmol/L 1-1.3 mmol/L
Carbon dioxide content (plasma)	21-32 mmol/L	21-32 mmol/L
Carcinoembryonic antigen	< 3 ng/mL	< 3 mcg/L
Chloride	95-110 mEq/L	95-110 mmol/L
Coagulation screen: Bleeding time Prothrombin time Partial thromboplastin time (activated) Protein C Protein S	3-9.5 min 10-13 sec 22-37 sec 0.7-1.4 µ/mL 0.7-1.4 µ/mL	180-570 sec 10-13 sec 22-37 sec 700-1400 U/mL 700-1400 U/mL
Copper, total	70-160 mcg/dL	11-25 mcmol/L
Corticotropin (ACTH [adrenocorticotropic hormone]) - 0800 hr	< 60 pg/mL	< 13.2 pmol/L
Cortisol: 0800 hr 1800 hr 2000 hr	5-30 mcg/dL 2-15 mcg/dL ≤ 50% of 0800 hr	138-810 nmol/L 50-410 nmol/L ≤ 50% of 0800 hr
Creatine kinase: Female Male	20-170 IU/L 30-220 IU/L	0.33-2.83 mckat/L 0.5-3.67 mckat/L
Creatinine kinase isoenzymes, MB fraction	0-12 IU/L	0-0.2 mckat/L
Creatinine	0.5-1.7 mg/dL	44-150 mcmol/L
Fibrinogen (coagulation factor I)	150-360 mg/dL	1.5-3.6 g/L
Follicle-stimulating hormone (FSH): Female Midcycle Male	2-13 mIU/mL 5-22 mIU/mL 1-8 mIU/mL	2-13 IU/L 5-22 IU/L 1-8 IU/L
Glucose, fasting	65-115 mg/dL	3.6-6.3 mmol/L

Glucose tolerance test (oral)	mg/dL		mmol/L	
	Normal	Diabetic	Normal	Diabetic
Fasting	70-105	> 140	3.9-5.8	> 7.8
60 min	120-170	≥ 200	6.7-9.4	≥ 11.1
90 min	100-140	≥ 200	5.6-7.8	≥ 11.1
120 min	70-120	≥ 140	3.9-6.7	≥ 7.8

Blood, Plasma or Serum		
	Reference Value	
Determination	Conventional units	SI units
(γ) - Glutamyltransferase (GGT): Male	9-50 units/L	9-50 units/L
Female	8-40 units/L	8-40 units/L
Haptoglobin	44-303 mg/dL	0.44-3.03 g/L
Hematologic tests:		
Fibrinogen	200-400 mg/dL	2-4 g/L
Hematocrit (Hct), female	36%-44.6%	0.36-0.446 fraction of 1
male	40.7%-50.3%	0.4-0.503 fraction of 1
Hemoglobin A_{1C}	4%-6%	0.053-0.075
Hemoglobin (Hb), female	12-16 g/dL	7.49-9.9 mmol/L
male	14-18 g/dL	8.7-11.2 mmol/L
Leukocyte count (WBC)	3800-9800/mcL	$3.8-9.8 \times 10^9$/L
Erythrocyte count (RBC), female	$3.5-5 \times 10^6$/mcL	$3.5-5 \times 10^{12}$/L
male	$4.3-5.9 \times 10^6$/mcL	$4.3-5.9 \times 10^{12}$/L
Mean corpuscular volume (MCV)	80-97.6 mcm^3	80-97.6 fl
Mean corpuscular hemoglobin (MCH)	27-33 pg/cell	1.66-2.09 fmol/cell
Mean corpuscular hemoglobin concentrate (MCHC)	33-36 g/dL	20.3-22 mmol/L
Erythrocyte sedimentation rate (sedrate, ESR)	≤ 30 mm/hr	≤ 30 mm/hr
Erythrocyte enzymes:		
Glucose-6-phosphate dehydrognase (G-6-PD)	250-5000 units/10^6 cells	250-5000 mcunits/cell
Ferritin	10-300 ng/mL	10-300 pmol/L
Folic acid: normal	> 3.1-12.4 ng/mL	7-28.1 nmol/L
Platelet count	150-450 x 10^3/mcL	150-450 x 10^9/L
Reticulocytes	0.5%-1.5% of erythrocytes	0.005-0.015
Vitamin B_{12}	223-1132 pg/mL	165-835 pmol/L
Iron: Female	30-160 mcg/dL	5.4-31.3 mcmol/L
Male	45-160 mcg/dL	8.1-31.3 mcmol/L
Iron binding capacity	220-420 mcg/dL	39.4-75.2 mcmol/L
Isocitrate dehydrogenase	1.2-7 units/L	1.2-7 units/L
Isoenzymes		
Fraction 1	14%-26% of total	0.14-0.26 fraction of total
Fraction 2	29%-39% of total	0.29-0.39 fraction of total
Fraction 3	20%-26% of total	0.20-0.26 fraction of total
Fraction 4	8%-16% of total	0.08-0.16 fraction of total
Fraction 5	6%-16% of total	0.06-0.16 fraction of total
Lactate dehydrogenase	100-250 IU/L	1.67-4.17 mckat/L
Lactic acid (lactate)	6-19 mg/dL	0.7-2.1 mmol/L
Lead	≤ 20 mcg/dL	≤ 2.41 mcmol/L
Lipase	10-150 IU/L	10-150 IU/L
Lipids:		
Total Cholesterol		
Desirable	< 200 mg/dL	< 5.2 mmol/L
Borderline-high	200-239 mg/dL	< 5.2-6.2 mmol/L
High	> 239 mg/dL	> 6.2 mmol/L
LDL		
Desirable	< 130 mg/dL	< 3.36 mmol/L
Borderline-high	130-159 mg/dL	3.36-4.11 mmol/L
High	> 159 mg/dL	> 4.11 mmol/L
HDL		
Low	< 40 mg/dL	
High	≥ 60 mg/dL	
Triglycerides		
Desirable	< 150 mg/dL	
Borderline-high	150-199 mg/dL	
High	200-499 mg/dL	
Very high	> 500 mg/dL	
Magnesium	1.3-2.2 mEq/L	0.65-1.1 mmol/L
Osmolality	280-300 mOsm/kg	280-300 mmol/kg

Blood, Plasma or Serum		
	Reference Value	
Determination	Conventional units	SI units
Oxygen saturation (arterial)	94%-100%	0.94-1 fraction of 1
PCO_2, arterial	35-45 mm Hg	4.7-6 kPa
pH, arterial	7.35-7.45	7.35-7.45
PO_2, arterial: Breathing room air[1] On 100% O_2	80-105 mm Hg > 500 mm Hg	10.6-14 kPa
Phosphatase (acid), total at 37°C	0.13-0.63 IU/L	2.2-10.5 IU/L or 2.2-10.5 mckat/L
Phosphatase alkaline[2]	20-130 IU/L	20-130 IU/L or 0.33-2.17 mckat/L
Phosphorus, inorganic,[3] (phosphate)	2.5-5 mg/dL	0.8-1.6 mmol/L
Potassium	3.5-5 mEq/L	3.5-5 mmol/L
Progesterone Female Follicular phase Luteal phase Male	0.1-1.5 ng/mL 0.1-1.5 ng/mL 2.5-28 ng/mL < 0.5 ng/mL	0.32-4.8 nmol/L 0.32-4.8 nmol/L 8-89 nmol/L < 1.6 nmol/L
Prolactin	1.4-24.2 ng/mL	1.4-24.2 mcg/L
Prostate specific antigen	0-4 ng/mL	0-4 ng/mL
Protein: Total Albumin Globulin	6-8 g/dL 3.6-5 g/dL 2.3-3.5 g/dL	60-80 g/L 36-50 g/L 23-35 g/L
Rheumatoid factor	< 60 IU/mL	< 60 kIU/L
Sodium	135-147 mEq/L	135-147 mmol/L
Testosterone: Female Male	6-86 ng/dL 270-1070 ng/dL	0.21-3 nmol/L 9.3-37 nmol/L
Thyroid Hormone Function Tests: Thyroid-stimulating hormone (TSH) Thyroxine-binding globulin capacity Total triiodothyronine (T_3) Total thyroxine by RIA (T_4) T_3 resin uptake	0.35-6.2 mcU/mL 10-26 mcg/dL 75-220 ng/dL 4-11 mcg/dL 25%-38%	0.35-6.2 mU/L 100-260 mcg/L 1.2-3.4 nmol/L 51-142 nmol/L 0.25-0.38 fraction of 1
Transaminase, AST (aspartate aminotrans- ferase, SGOT)	11-47 IU/L	0.18-0.78 mckat/L
Transaminase, ALT (alanine aminotransfer- ase, SGPT)	7-53 IU/L	0.12-0.88 mckat/L
Transferrin	220-400 mg/dL	2.20-4.00 g/L
Urea nitrogen (BUN)	8-25 mg/dL	2.9-8.9 mmol/L
Uric acid	3-8 mg/dL	179-476 mcmol/L
Vitamin A (retinol)	15-60 mcg/dL	0.52-2.09 mcmol/L
Zinc	50-150 mcg/dL	7.7-23 mcmol/L

[1] Age dependent
[2] Infants and adolescents up to 104 U/L
[3] Infants in the first year up to 6 mg/dL

Urine		
	Reference value	
Determination	Conventional units	SI units
Calcium[1]	50-250 mcg/day	1.25-6.25 mmol/day
Catecholamines: Epinephrine Norepinephrine	< 20 mcg/day < 100 mcg/day	< 109 nmol/day < 590 nmol/day
Catecholamines, 24-hr	< 110 µg	< 650 nmol
Copper[1]	15-60 mcg/day	0.24-0.95 mcmol/day
Creatinine: Child	8-22 mg/kg	71-195 µmol/kg
Adolescent	8-30 mg/kg	71-265 µmol/kg
Female	0.6-1.5 g/day	5.3-13.3 mmol/day
Male	0.8-1.8 g/day	7.1-15.9 mmol/day
pH	4.5-8	4.5-8
Phosphate[1]	0.9-1.3 g/day	29-42 mmol/day
Potassium[1]	25-100 mEq/day	25-100 mmol/day
Protein Total At rest	1-14 mg/dL 50-80 mg/day	10-140 mg/L 50-80 mg/day
Protein, quantitative	< 150 mg/day	< 0.15 g/day
Sodium[1]	100-250 mEq/day	100-250 mmol/day
Specific gravity, random	1.002-1.030	1.002-1.030
Uric acid, 24-hr	250-750 mg	1.48-4.43 mmol

[1] Diet Dependent

Drug Levels*		
	Reference value	
Drug determination	Conventional units	SI units
Aminoglycosides		
Amikacin		
(trough)	1-8 mcg/mL	1.7-13.7 mcmol/L
(peak)	20-30 mcg/mL	34-51 mcmol/L
Gentamicin		
(trough)	0.5-2 mcg/mL	1-4.2 mcmol/L
(peak)	6-10 mcg/mL	12.5-20.9 mcmol/L
Kanamycin		
(trough)	5-10 mcg/mL	nd[1]
(peak)	20-25 mcg/mL	nd
Netilimicin		
(trough)	0.5-2 mcg/mL	nd
(peak)	6-10 mcg/mL	nd
Streptomycin		
(trough)	< 5 mcg/mL	nd
(peak)	20-30 mcg/mL	nd
Tobramycin		
(trough)	0.5-2 mcg/mL	1.1-4.3 mcmol/L
(peak)	6-10 mcg/mL	12.8-21.8 mcmol/L
Antiarrhythmics		
Amiodarone	0.5-2.5 mcg/mL	1.5-4 mcmol/L
Bretylium	0.5-1.5 mcg/mL	nd
Digitoxin	9-25 mcg/L	11.8-32.8 nmol/L
Digoxin	0.8-2 ng/mL	0.9-2.5 nmol/L
Disopyramide	2-8 mcg/mL	6-18 mcmol/L
Flecainide	0.2-1 mcg/mL	nd
Lidocaine	1.5-6 mcg/mL	4.5-21.5 mcmol/L
Mexiletine	0.5-2 mcg/mL	nd
Procainamide	4-8 mcg/mL	17-34 mcmol/mL
Propranolol	50-100 ng/mL	190-390 nmol/L
Quinidine	2-6 mcg/mL	4.6-9.2 mcmol/L
Tocainide	5-12 mcg/mL	22-52 mcmol/L
Verapamil	50-200 ng/mL	100-420 nmol/L
Anticonvulsants		
Carbamazepine	4-12 mcg/mL	17-51 mcmol/L
Phenobarbital	10-40 mcg/mL	43-172 mcmol/L
Phenytoin	10-20 mcg/mL	40-80 mcmol/L
Primidone	5-15 mg/mL	23-69 mcmol/L
Valproic Acid	50-100 mcg/L	346-693 mcmol/L
Antidepressants		
Amitriptyline	110-250 ng/mL[2]	500-900 nmol/L
Amoxapine	200-500 ng/mL	637-1594 nmol/L
Bupropion	50-100 ng/mL	nd
Clomipramine	80-100 ng/mL	nd
Desipramine	115-300 ng/mL	281-1125 nmol/L
Doxepin	30-250 ng/mL	107-537 nmol/L
Imipramine	100-300 ng/mL	nd
Maprotiline	200-300 ng/mL	nd
Nortriptyline	50-150 ng/mL	190-665 nmol/L
Protriptyline	70-250 ng/mL	266-950 nmol/L
Trazodone	800-1600 ng/mL	nd

Drug Levels[*]			
		Reference value	
Drug determination		Conventional units	SI units
Antipsychotics	Chlorpromazine	50-300 ng/mL	157-942 nmol/L
	Fluphenazine	5-20 ng/mL	nd
	Haloperidol	5-20 ng/mL	10-30 nmol/L
	Perphenazine	2-6 ng/mL	nd
	Thiothixene	2-57 ng/mL	nd
Miscellaneous	Amantadine	300 ng/mL	nd
	Amrinone	3.7 mcg/mL	nd
	Chloramphenicol	10-20 mcg/mL	31-62 mcmol/L
	Cyclosporine[3]	250-800 ng/mL (whole blood, RIA)	nd
		50-300 ng/mL (plasma, RIA)	nd
	Ethanol[4]	0 mg/dL	0 mmol/L
	Hydralazine	100 ng/mL	nd
	Lithium	0.6-1.2 mEq/L	0.6-1.2 mmol/L
	Salicylate	100-300 mg/L	724-2172 mcmol/L
	Sulfonamide	5-15 mg/dL	nd
	Theophylline	10-20 mcg/mL	55-110 mcmol/L
	Vancomycin		
	(trough)	5-15 ng/mL	nd
	(peak)	20-40 mcg/mL	nd

[*] The values given are generally accepted as desirable for treatment without toxicity for most patients. However, exceptions are not uncommon.
[1] nd = No data available.
[2] Parent drug plus N-desmethyl metabolite.
[3] 24-hour trough values.
[4] Toxic: 50-100 mg/dL (10.9–21.7 mmol/L).

The following table is adopted from the Seventh Report of the Joint National Committee on Prevention, Detection, Evaluation, and Treatment of High Blood Pressure, National Institutes of Health.

Classification of Blood Pressure[*]			
	Reference value		
Category	Systolic (mm Hg)		Diastolic (mm Hg)
Normal[1]	< 120	and	< 80
Prehypertension	120-139	or	80-89
High Blood Pressure			
Stage 1 Hypertension	140-159	or	90-99
Stage 2 Hypertension	≥ 160	or	≥ 100

[*] For adults age 18 and older who are not taking antihypertensive drugs and not acutely ill. When systolic and diastolic blood pressures fall into different categories, the higher category should be selected to classify the individual's blood pressure status. In addition to classifying stages of hypertension on the basis of average blood pressure levels, clinicians should specify presence or absence of target organ disease and additional risk factors.
[1] Unusually low readings should be evaluated for clinical significance.

FDA Pregnancy Categories

The rational use of any medication requires a risk vs benefit assessment. Among the myriad of risk factors which complicate this assessment, pregnancy is one of the most perplexing.

The FDA has established five categories to indicate the potential of a systemically absorbed drug for causing birth defects. The key differentiation among the categories rests upon the degree (reliability) of documentation and the risk vs benefit ratio. Pregnancy Category X is particularly notable in that if any data exists that may implicate a drug as a teratogen and the risk vs benefit ratio does not support use of the drug, the drug is contraindicated during pregnancy. These categories are summarized below:

FDA Pregnancy Categories	
Pregnancy Category	**Definition**
A	Controlled studies show no risk. Adequate, well-controlled studies in pregnant women have failed to demonstrate risk to the fetus.
B	No evidence of risk in humans. Either animal findings show risk, but human findings do not; or if no adequate human studies have been done, animal findings are negative.
C	Risk cannot be ruled out. Human studies are lacking, and animal studies are either positive for fetal risk or lacking. However, potential benefits may justify the potential risks.
D	Positive evidence of risk. Investigational or post-marketing data show risk to the fetus. Nevertheless, potential benefits may outweigh the potential risks. If needed in a life-threatening situation or a serious disease, the drug may be acceptable if safer drugs cannot be used or are ineffective.
X	Contraindicated in pregnancy. Studies in animals or humans, or investigational or post-marketing reports have shown fetal risk that clearly outweighs any possible benefit to the patients.

Regardless of the designated pregnancy category or presumed safety, no drug should be administered during pregnancy unless it is clearly needed and potential benefits outweigh potential hazards to the fetus.

Controlled Substances

The Controlled Substances Act of 1970 regulates the manufacturing, distribution, and dispensing of drugs that have abuse potential. The Drug Enforcement Administration (DEA) within the US Department of Justice is the chief federal agency responsible for enforcing the act.

DEA schedules: Drugs under jurisdiction of the Controlled Substances Act are divided into five schedules based on their potential for abuse and physical and psychological dependence. All controlled substances listed in *American Drug Index* are identified by schedule as follows:

Schedule I *(c-i)*: High abuse potential and no accepted medical use (eg, heroin, marijuana, LSD).

Schedule II *(c-ii)*: High abuse potential with severe dependence liability (eg, narcotics, amphetamines, dronabinol, some barbiturates).

Schedule III *(c-iii)*: Less abuse potential than schedule II drugs and moderate dependence liability (eg, nonbarbiturate sedatives, nonamphetamine stimulants, limited amounts of certain narcotics).

Schedule IV *(c-iv)*: Less abuse potential than III drugs and limited dependence liability (eg, some sedatives, antianxiety agents, nonnarcotic analgesics).

Schedule V *(c-v)*: Limited abuse potential. Primarily small amounts of narcotics (codeine) used as antitussives or antidiarrheals. Under federal law, limited quantities of certain *c-v* drugs may be purchased without a prescription directly from a pharmacist if allowed under state statutes. The purchaser must be at least 18 years of age and must furnish suitable identification. All such transactions must be recorded by the dispensing pharmacist.

Registration: Prescribing physicians and dispensing pharmacies must be registered with the DEA, PO Box 28083, Central Station, Washington, DC 20005.

Inventory: Separate records must be kept of purchases and dispensing of controlled substances. An inventory of controlled substances must be made every 2 years.

Prescriptions: Prescriptions for controlled substances must be written in ink and include: Date; name and address of the patient; name, address and DEA number of the physician. Oral prescriptions must be promptly committed to writing. Controlled substance prescriptions may not be dispensed or refilled more than 6 months after the date issued or be refilled more than 5 times. A written prescription signed by the physician is required for schedule II drugs. In case of emergency, oral prescriptions for schedule II substances may be filled; however, the physician must provide a signed prescription within 72 hours. Schedule II prescriptions cannot be refilled. A triplicate order form is necessary for the transfer of controlled substances in schedule II. Forms are available for the individual prescriber at no charge from the DEA.

State Laws: In many cases, state laws are more restrictive than federal laws and therefore impose additional requirements (eg, triplicate prescription forms).

Medical Terminology Glossary

abduction – the act of drawing away from a center.

abstergent – a cleansing application or medicine.

acaricide – an agent lethal to mites.

achlorhydria – the absence of hydrochloric acid from gastric secretions.

acidifier, systemic – a drug used to lower internal body fluid pH in patients with systemic alkalosis.

acidifier, urinary – a drug used to lower the pH of the urine.

acidosis – an accumulation of acid in the body.

acne – an inflammatory disease of the skin accompanied by the eruption of papules or pustules.

active immunity – see Immunity, Active.

acute – a short-term, intense health effect.

acute Hepatitis C – newly acquired symptomatic hepatitis C virus (HCV) infection.

Addison disease – a condition caused by adrenal gland destruction.

adduction – the act of drawing toward a center.

adenitis – a gland or lymph node inflammation.

adjuvant – an agent added to a product formulation that complements or accentuates the active ingredient.

adrenergic – a sympathomimetic drug that activates organs innervated by the sympathetic branch of the autonomic nervous system.

adrenocortical steroid, anti-inflammatory – an adrenal cortex hormone that participates in regulation of organic metabolism and inhibits the inflammatory response to stress; a glucocorticoid.

adrenocortical steroid, salt-regulating – an adrenal cortex hormone that maintains sodium-potassium electrolyte balance by stimulating and regulating sodium retention and potassium excretion by the kidneys.

adrenocorticotropic hormone – an anterior pituitary hormone that stimulates and regulates secretion of the adrenocortical steroids.

adsorbent – an agent that binds chemicals to its surface, thus reducing the bioavailability of toxic substances.

adverse events – undesirable experiences occurring after immunization that may or may not be related to the vaccine.

alkalizer, systemic – a drug that raises internal body fluid pH in patients with systemic acidosis.

allergen – a specific substance that causes an unwanted reaction in the body.

amblyopia – pertaining to a dimness of vision.

amebiasis – an infection with a pathogenic amoeba.

amenorrhea – an abnormal discontinuation of the menses.

amphiarthrosis – a joint in which the surfaces are connected by discs of fibrocartilage.

anabolic – an agent that promotes conversion of a simple substance into more complex compounds; a constructive process for the organism.

analeptic – a potent central nervous system stimulant used to maintain vital functions during severe central nervous system depression.

analgesic – a drug that selectively suppresses pain perception without inducing unconsciousness.

ancyclostomiasis – a disease characterized by the presence of hookworms in the intestine.

androgen – a hormone that stimulates and maintains male secondary sex characteristics.

anemia – a deficiency of red blood cells.

anesthetic, general – a drug that eliminates pain perception by inducing unconsciousness.

anesthetic, local – a drug that eliminates pain perception in a limited area by local action on sensory nerves; a topical anesthetic.

angina pectoris – a sharp chest pain starting in the heart, often spreading down the left arm. A symptom of coronary artery disease.

angiography – visualization of blood vessels upon x-ray following an injection of contrast media.

anhidrotic – a drug that checks perspiration flow from sweat glands; an antidiaphoretic.

anodyne – a drug that acts on the sensory nervous system, either centrally or peripherally, to produce relief from pain.

anorexiant – a drug that reduces appetite.

anorexigenic – an agent that promotes appetite reduction.

antacid – a drug that locally neutralizes excess gastric acid secretions.

antiadrenergic – a drug that prevents response to sympathetic nervous system stimulation and adrenergic drugs; a sympatholytic or sympathoplegic drug.

antiamebic – a drug that kills or inhibits the pathogenic protozoan *Entamoeba histolytica*, the causative agent of amebic dysentery.

antianemic – an agent that treats or prevents anemia.

antiasthmatic – an agent that relieves the symptoms of asthma.

antibacterial – a drug that kills or inhibits pathogenic bacteria, the causative agents of many systemic gastrointestinal and superficial infections.

antibiotic – an agent produced by or derived from living cells of molds, bacteria, or other plants that destroy or inhibit the growth of microbes.

antibody – a protein found in the blood that is produced in response to foreign substances (eg, bacteria or viruses) invading the body. Antibodies protect the body from disease by binding to these organisms and destroying them.

anticholesteremic – a drug that lowers blood cholesterol levels.

anticholinergic – a drug that prevents response to parasympathetic nervous system stimulation and cholinergic drugs; a parasympatholytic or parasympathoplegic drug.

anticoagulant – a drug that inhibits blood clotting.

anticonvulsant – a drug that selectively prevents epileptic seizures.

antidepressant – a psychotherapeutic drug that induces mood elevation, useful in treating depressive neuroses and psychoses.

antidiabetic – a drug used to lower blood sugar or counteract diabetes.

antidote – a drug that prevents or counteracts the effects of poisons or drug overdoses by adsorption in the gastrointestinal tract (general antidotes) or by specific systemic action (specific antidotes).

antieczematic – a topical drug that aids in the control of exudative inflammatory skin lesions.

antiemetic – a drug that prevents or controls vomiting.

antifibrinolytic – a drug that decreases fibrin breakdown.

antifilarial – a drug that kills or inhibits pathogenic filarial worms of the superfamily *Filarioidea*, the causative agents of diseases such as loaiasis.

antiflatulent – an agent that inhibits the excessive formation of gas in the stomach or intestines.

antifungal – a drug that kills or inhibits pathogenic fungi; antimycotic.

antigens – foreign substances (eg, bacteria or viruses) in the body that are capable of causing disease. The presence of antigens in the body triggers an immune response, usually the production of antibodies.

antihelmintic – a drug that kills or expels worm infestations such as pinworms and tapeworms (eg, nematodes, cestodes, trematodes).

antihemophilic – a blood derivative containing the clotting factors absent in the hereditary disease hemophilia.

antihistaminic – a drug that prevents response to histamine, including histamine released by allergic reactions.

antihypercholesterolemic – a drug that lowers blood cholesterol levels, especially elevated levels sometimes associated with cardiovascular disease.

antihypertensive – a drug that lowers blood pressure.

anti-infective, local – a drug that kills a variety of pathogenic microorganisms and is suitable for sterilizing the skin or wounds.

anti-inflammatory – a drug that counteracts or suppresses inflammation.

antileishmanial – a drug that kills or inhibits pathogenic protozoa of the genus *Leishmania*, the causative agents of diseases such as kala azar.

antileprotic – an agent used against leprosy.

antilipemic – an agent that reduces the amount of circulating lipids.

antimalarial – a drug that prevents malaria or inhibits the causative agent (ie, malarial parasites).

antimetabolite – a substance that competes with or replaces a certain metabolite.

antimethemoglobinemic – an agent that reduces the production of methemoglobin.

antimycotic – an agent that inhibits the growth of fungi.

antinauseant – a drug that suppresses nausea.

antineoplastic – a drug that is selectively toxic to rapidly multiplying cells and is useful in destroying malignant tumors.

antioxidant – an agent used to reduce decay or transformation of a material from oxidation.

antiperiodic – a drug that prevents the regular recurrence of a disease or symptom.

antiperistaltic – a drug that inhibits intestinal motility, especially for the treatment of diarrhea.

antipruritic – a drug that prevents or relieves itching.

antipyretic – a drug used to reduce fever; antifebrile; febrifugal.

antirheumatic – a drug that suppresses symptoms of rheumatic disease (eg, reduces the inflammation of rheumatic arthritis).

antirickettsial – a drug that kills or inhibits pathogenic microorganisms of the genus *Rickettsia*, the causative agents of diseases such as typhus (eg, chloramphenicol).

antischistosomal – a drug that kills or inhibits pathogenic flukes of the genus *Schistosoma*, the causative agents of schistosomiasis.

antiseborrheic – a drug that aids in the control of seborrheic dermatitis ("dandruff"); prevents or relieves excessive sebum secretion.

antiseptic – a substance that prevents the growth and development of microorganisms that may lead to infection.

antisialagogue – a drug that diminishes the flow of saliva.

antispasmodic – an agent used to quiet the spasms of voluntary and involuntary muscles; calmative; antihysteric.

antisyphilitic – a remedy used in the treatment of syphilis.

antitoxin – a biological drug containing antibodies against the toxic principles of a pathogenic microorganism, used for passive immunization against the associated disease.

antitrichomonal – a drug that kills or inhibits the pathogenic protozoan *Trichomonas vaginalis*, the causative agent of trichomonal vaginitis.

antitrypanosomal – a drug that kills or inhibits pathogenic protozoa of the genus *Trypanosoma*, the causative agents of diseases such as West African trypanosomiasis.

antitussive – a drug that suppresses coughing; antibechic.

antivenin – a biological drug containing antibodies against the venom of a poisonous animal or insect; an antidote for a venomous bite.

antiviral – literally "against virus;" any medicine capable of destroying or weakening a virus.

anxiety – a feeling of apprehension, uncertainty and fear.

aperient – a mild laxative.

aphasia – the inability to use or understand written and spoken words due to language center injuries in the brain.

aphonia – loss of voice due to disease of the larynx or its innervation.

apnea – the absence of breathing.

areola – a pigmented/depigmented zone surrounding a neoplasm.

arsenical – an agent containing arsenic.

arteriosclerosis – a hardening of the arteries.

arthritis – the inflammation of a joint.

ascariasis – a condition caused by roundworms in the intestine.

ascaricide – an agent that kills roundworms of the genus *Ascaris*.

Aspergillus – a genus of fungi.

astasia – the inability to stand up without help.

asthma – a disease characterized by recurring breathing difficulty due to bronchial muscle constriction.

astringent – an agent that causes tissue contraction, arrests secretion, or controls bleeding.

ataractic – an agent that has a quieting, tranquilizing effect.

ataxia – incoordination, especially of gait.

atheroma – lipid deposits on the inner surface of arteries; a characteristic of atherosclerosis.

atrophy – a wasting away.

avitaminosis – a pathologic state or dysfunction resulting in the body lacking one or more vitamins.

axilla – the armpit.

bacteria – tiny one-celled organisms present throughout the environment that require a microscope to be seen. While not all bacteria are harmful, some cause disease. Examples of bacterial disease include diphtheria, pertussis, tetanus, *Haemophilus influenzae*, and pneumococcus (pneumonia).

bacteriostatic – an agent that inhibits the growth of bacteria.

Basedow disease – a form of hyperthyroidism, also known as Grave disease and Parry disease.

biliary colic – a sharp pain in the upper right side of the abdomen due to a gallstone impaction.

bilirubin – a red bile pigment.

biliuria – the presence of bile in the urine.

blood calcium regulator – a drug that maintains the blood level of ionic calcium, especially by regulating its metabolic disposition elsewhere.

blood volume supporter – an intravenous solution whose solutes are retained in the vascular system to supplement the osmotic activity of plasma proteins.

bradycardia – a slow heart rate.

Bright disease – a disease of the kidneys, including the presence of edema and excessive urine protein formation.

bromidrosis – foul-smelling perspiration.

bronchitis – an inflammation of the bronchi.

bronchodilator – a drug that dilates the bronchus or bronchial tubes (air passages of the lung).

bruit – an abnormal arterial sound audible with a stethoscope.

Buerger disease – a thromboanglitis obliterans inflammation of the walls and surrounding rise of the veins and arteries.

bursitis – an inflammation of the bursa.

callus – a tissue mass that develops at bone fracture sites.

calmative – a sedative.

candidiasis – an infection by the yeastlike genus *Candida*, especially *Candida albicans*.

carbonic anhydrase inhibitor – an enzyme inhibitor, the therapeutic effects of which are diuresis and reduced formation of intraocular fluid.

carcinoma – a malignant growth.

cardiac depressant – a drug that depresses myocardial function so as to suppress rhythmic irregularities characterized by fast heart rate; antiarrhythmic.

cardiac stimulant – a drug that increases the contractile force of the myocardium, especially in weakened conditions such as congestive heart failure; cardiotonic.

cardiopathy – a disease of the heart.

caries – the decay of the teeth.

carminative – an aromatic or pungent drug that mildly irritates the gastrointestinal tract and is useful in the treatment of flatulence and colic. Peppermint Water is a common carminative.

carrier – a person or animal that harbors a specific infectious agent without visible symptoms of the disease. A carrier acts as a potential source of infection.

caruncle – a small, fleshy projection on the skin.

cathartic – an agent having purgative action.

caudal – pertains to the distal end or tail.

caustic – an agent whose effect resembles that of a burn; used to remove abnormal skin growths.

central depressant – a drug that reduces the functional state of the central nervous system and with increasing dosage may induce sedation, hypnosis, and general anesthesia; degree of respiratory suppression is agent dependent.

central stimulant – a drug that increases the functional state of the central nervous system and with increasing dosage may induce restlessness, insomnia, disorientation, and convulsions; degree of respiratory suppression is agent dependent.

cerebrum – the parts of the brain relating to the telecephalon and includes mainly the cerebral cortex and basal ganglia.

cerumen – earwax.

childhood immunizations – a series of immunizations that are given to prevent disease that pose a threat to children. The immunizations in the United States currently include: hepatitis B, diphtheria, tetanus, acellular pertussis, *Haemophilus influenzae* type b, inactivated polio, pneumococcal conjugate, measles, mumps, rubella, varicella, and hepatitis A.

chloasma – a skin discoloration.

cholagogue – a drug that stimulates the emptying of the gallbladder and the flow of bile into the duodenum.

cholecystitis – an inflammation of the gallbladder.

cholecystokinetic – an agent that promotes emptying of the gallbladder.

cholelithiasis – the presence of calculi (stones) in the gallbladder.

choleretic – a drug that increases the production and secretion of bile by the liver.

chorea – a disorder, usually of childhood, characterized by uncontrolled spasmotic muscle movements; sometimes referred to as St. Vitus' dance.

chronic health condition – a health-related state that lasts for a long period of time (eg, multiple sclerosis, asthma).

chronic hepatitis C – liver inflammation in patients with chronic HCV infection; characterized by abnormal levels of liver enzymes.

chymotrypsin – a proteinase in the gastrointestinal tract; its proposed use has been the treatment of edema and inflammation.

cirrhosis – widespread disruption of normal liver structure (scarring of the liver).

claudication – limping.

climacteric – a time period in women just preceding menopause.

clonus – movements noted by rapid muscle contraction then relaxation.

coagulant – an agent that stimulates or accelerates blood clotting.

coccidiostat – a drug used in the treatment of coccidal (protozoal) infections in animals, especially birds; used in veterinary medicine.

colitis – an inflammation of the colon.

colloid – a disperse system of particles larger than those of true solutions but smaller than those of suspensions (1 to 100 millimicrons in size).

collyrium – an eyewash.

colostomy – the surgical formation of a cutaneous opening into the colon.

combination vaccine – two or more vaccines combined and administered at once in order to reduce the number of shots given. For example, the MMR (measles, mumps, rubella) vaccine.

communicable – capable of spreading disease. Also known as infectious.

contagious – capable of being transmitted from one person to another by contact or close proximity.

corticoid – a term applied to hormones of the adrenal cortex or any substance, natural or synthetic, having similar activity.

corticosteroid – a steroid produced by the adrenal cortex.

coryza – acute rhinitis.

counterirritant – an agent (irritant) that causes irritation of the part to which it is applied, and draws blood away from a deep-seated area.

cranial – pertaining to the skull.

crepitation – a crackling sound.

cryptitis – an inflammation of a follicle or glandular tubule, usually in the rectum.

Cryptococcus – a genus of fungi that does not produce spores, but reproduces by budding.

cryptorchidism – the failure of one or both testes to descend.

cutaneous – pertaining to the skin.

cyanosis – a blue or purple skin discoloration due to oxygen deficiency.

cycloplegia – the loss of light accommodation due to loss of control in the eye 's ciliary muscle.

cycloplegic – a drug that paralyzes accommodation of the eye.

cystitis – an inflammation of the bladder.

cystourethography – the examination by x-ray of the bladder and urethra.

cytostasis – a slowing of the movement of blood cells at an inflamed area, sometimes causing capillary blockage.

debridement – the cutting away of dead or excess skin from a wound.

decongestant – a drug that reduces congestion.

decubitus – the patient's position in bed; the act of lying down.

demulcent – an agent generally used internally to sooth and protect mucous membranes.

dermatitis – an inflammation of the skin.

dermatomycosis – a fungal skin infection caused by dermatophytes, yeasts, and other fungi.

detergent – a cleansing or purging agent; an emulsifying agent useful for cleansing wounds and ulcers as well as the skin.

dextrocardia – a condition when the heart is located on the right side of the chest.

diagnostic Aid – a drug used to determine the functional state of a body organ or the presence of a disease.

diaphoretic – a drug used to increase perspiration; hydroticorsudorfice.

diarrhea – an abnormally frequent defecation of semisolid or fluid fecal matter from the bowels.

digestive enzyme – an enzyme used in digestion.

digitalization – the administration of digitalis to obtain a desired tissue level of drug.

diplopia – double vision.

disease – symptomatic sickness, illness, or loss of health.

disinfectant – an agent that destroys pathogenic microorganisms on contact and is suitable for sterilizing inanimate objects.

distal – farthest from a point of reference.

diuretic – a drug that promotes renal excretion of electrolytes and water, thereby increasing urine volume.

dysarthria – a difficulty in speech articulation.

dysmenorrhea – pertaining to painful menstruation.

dysphagia – a difficulty in swallowing.

dyspnea – a difficulty in breathing.

ecbolic – a drug used to stimulate the gravid uterus to the expulsion of the fetus, or to cause uterine contraction; oxytocic.

eclampsia – a toxic disorder occurring late in pregnancy involving hypertension, edema, and renal dysfunction.

ectasia – pertaining to distension or stretching.

ectopic – out of place; not in normal position.

eczema – an inflammatory disease of the skin with infiltrations, watery discharge, scales, and crust.

effervescent – a bubbling; sparkling; giving off gas bubbles.

embolus – a plug (typically a thrombus, bacteria mass, or foreign body) lodged in a vessel; may obstruct circulation.

emetic – a drug that induces vomiting, either locally by gastrointestinal irritation or systemically by stimulation of receptors in the central nervous system.

emollient – a topical drug, especially an oil or fat, used to soften the skin and make it more pliable.

endemic – the continual, low-level presence of disease in a community.

endometrium – the uterine mucous membrane.

enteralgia – an intestinal pain.

enterobiasis – a pinworm infestation.

enuresis – an involuntary urination, as in bedwetting.

epidemic – the occurrence of disease within a specific geographical area or population that is in excess of what is normally expected.

epidemiology – the study of the spread of diseases. Epidemiologists are often sent to investigate outbreaks.

epidermis – the outermost layer of the skin.

episiotomy – a surgical incision of the vulva when deemed necessary during childbirth.

epistaxis – a nosebleed.

erythema – redness.

erythrocyte – a red blood cell.

escharotic – corrosive.

estrogen – a hormone that stimulates and maintains female secondary sex characteristics and functions in the menstrual cycle to promote uterine gland proliferation.

etiology – the cause of a disease.

euphoria – an exaggerated feeling of well-being.

eutonic – a normal muscular tone.

exfoliation – a scaling of the skin.

exophthalmos – a protrusion of the eye-balls.

expectorant – a drug that increases secretion of respiratory tract fluid by lowering its viscosity and promoting its ejection.

extension – the movement of a joint that increases the angle between the bones of the limb at the joint.

exteroceptors – the receptors on the exterior of the body.

fasciculations – the visible twitching movements of muscle bundles.

fibroid – a tumor of fibrous tissue, resembling fibers.

filariasis – the condition of having roundworm parasites reproducing in the body tissues.

fistula – an abnormal opening between one epithelialized surface to another epithelialized body cavity.

flexion – the movement of a joint that decreases the angle between the bones of the limb at the joint.

fulminant – occurring suddenly, with lightning-like rapidity, and with great intensity or severity.

fungistatic – the inhibition of the growth of fungi.

furunculosis – a condition marked by the presence of boils.

gallop rhythm – a heart condition where three separate beats are heard instead of two.

gastralgia – a stomach pain.

gastritis – an inflammation of the stomach lining.

gastrocele – a hernial protrusion of the stomach.

gastrodynia – a pain in the stomach, a stomach ache.

geriatrics – a branch of medicine caring for medical problems of the aged.

germicidal – an agent that kills germs or other pathogenic microorganisms.

gingivitis – an inflammation of the gums.

glaucoma – a disease of the eye evidenced by an increase in intraocular pressure and resulting in hardness of the eye, atrophy of the retina, and eventual blindness.

glossitis – an inflammation of the tongue.

glucocorticoid – a corticoid that increases gluconeogenesis, thereby raising the concentration of liver glycogen and blood sugar.

glycosuria – an abnormal quantity of glucose and carbohydrates in the urine.

gout – a disorder that is characterized by a high uric acid level and sudden onset of recurrent arthritis.

granulation – the formation of small round fleshy granules on a wound as part of the healing process.

Guillain-Barré syndrome – an inflammation of the nerves of unknown cause characterized especially by muscle weakness and paralysis.

hematemesis – the vomiting of blood.

hematinic – an agent that improves blood quality by increasing the hemoglobin concentration and/or the number of red blood cells.

hematopoietic – a drug that stimulates formation of blood cells.

hemiplegia – a condition in which one side of the body is paralyzed.

hemophilia – a sex-linked hereditary blood defect that occurs almost exclusively in males and is characterized by delayed clotting of the blood and consequent difficulty in controlling hemorrhage even after minor injuries.

hemoptysis – the coughing-up of blood.

hemorrhage – an escape of blood through vessel walls; to bleed.

hemostatic – a locally-acting drug that arrests hemorrhage by promoting clot formation or by serving as a mechanical matrix for a clot.

hepatitis – an inflammation of the liver.

hepatitis A – a liver disease caused by the hepatitis A virus (HAV). HAV does not cause a chronic (long-lasting) illness. The virus is transmitted through close intimate contact with an infected person or through ingestion of contaminated food or water.

hepatitis B – a liver disease caused by the hepatitis B virus (HBV). HBV is found in the blood of infected persons and is most commonly transmitted through unprotected sex.

hepatitis B core antibody (anti-HBc) – appears at the onset of symptoms in acute hepatitis B and persists for life. The presence of anti-HBc indicates previous or ongoing infection with HBV.

hepatitis B e antigen (HBeAg) – a secreted product of the nucleocapsid gene of HBV and is found in serum during acute and chronic hepatitis B. Its presence indicated that the virus is replicating and the infected individual is potentially infectious.

hepatitis B immune globulin (HBIG) – a product available for prophylaxis against hepatitis B virus infection. HBIG is prepared from plasma containing high titers of anti-HBs and provides short-term protection (3 to 6 months).

hepatitis B surface antibody (anti-HBs) – the presence of anti-HBs is generally interpreted as indicating recovery and immunity from HBV infection.

hepatitis B surface antigen (HBsAg) – a serologic marker on the surface of HBV. It can be detected in high levels in serum during acute or chronic hepatitis. The body normally produces antibodies to surface antigen as part of the normal immune response to infection.

hepatitis C – a liver disease caused by the hepatitis C virus (HCV), which is found in the blood of persons who have the disease. HCV is spread by contact with the blood of an infected person, most commonly through injection drug use.

hepatitis D – a liver disease caused by hepatitis delta virus (HDV). HDV is a defective virus that needs HBV to exist. HDV is found in the blood of persons infected with the virus and is transmitted in much the same way as HBV is transmitted; however, the case fatality rate with HDV infection is higher than with hepatitis B.

hepatitis E – a disease of the liver caused by the hepatitis E virus (HEV). HEV is transmitted in much the same way as HAV. Hepatitis E, however, does not often originate in the United States. Mortality is high among pregnant women who have hepatitis E.

hepatocellular carcinoma (HCC) – the most common primary malignant liver tumor.

high-risk group – a group in the community with an elevated risk of disease.

histoplasmosis – a lung infection caused by the inhalation of fungus spores, often resulting in pneumonitis.

HIV – human immunodeficiency virus.

Hodgkin disease – a disease marked by chronic lymph node enlargement that may also include spleen and liver enlargement.

hydrocholeresis – the puffing out of a thinner, more watery bile.

hypercholesterolemia – the condition of having an abnormally large amount of cholesterol in the plasma and cells of circulating blood.

hyperemia – an excess of blood in any part of the body.

hyperesthesia – an increase in sensitivity to sensory stimuli.

hyperglycemic – a drug that increases blood glucose levels, especially for the treatment of hypoglycemic states.

hypertension – blood pressure above the normally accepted limits; high blood pressure.

hypertriglyceridemia – an increased level of triglycerides in the blood.

hypnotic – an agent that promotes sleep.

hypodermoclysis – a subcutaneous injection with a solution.

hypoesthesia – a diminished sensation of touch.

hypoglycemic – a drug that lowers blood glucose levels; useful in the control of diabetes mellitus.

hypokalemia – an abnormally small concentration of potassium ions in the blood.

hyposensitize – to reduce the sensitivity to an agent, referring to allergies.

hypotensive – a drug that diminishes tension or pressure to lower blood pressure.

ichthyosis – an inherited skin disease characterized by dryness and scales.

idiopathic – the denoting of a disease of unknown cause.

IDU – injection drug user.

IgM anti-HBc – detected at onset of acute hepatitis B and persists for 3 to 12 months if the disease resolves. In patients who develop chronic hepatitis B, IgM anti-HBc persists at low levels as long as viral replication persists.

ileostomy – the establishment of an opening from the ileum to the outside of the body.

immune globulin (IG) – proteins found in the blood that function as antibodies that fight infection. Previously known as gamma globulin.

immune serum – a biological drug containing antibodies for a pathogenic microorganism, useful for passive immunization against the associated disease.

immune system – the complex system in the body responsible for fighting disease. Its primary function is to identify foreign substances in the body (bacteria, viruses, fungi, or parasites) and develop a defense against them. This defense is known as the immune response. It involves production of protein molecules called antibodies to eliminate foreign organisms that invade the body.

immunity – protection against a disease. There are two types of immunity, passive and active. Immunity is indicated by the presence of antibodies in the blood and can usually be determined with a laboratory test. See Immunity, Active and Passive.

immunity, active – resistance developed in response to an antigen (infecting agent or vaccine) and usually characterized by the presence of antibody produced by the host.

immunity, passive – immunity conferred by an antibody produced in another host.

This type of immunity can be acquired naturally by an infant from its mother or artificially by administration of an antibody-containing preparation (antiserum or immune globulin).

immunization – the process by which a person or animal becomes protected against a disease.

immunizing agent, active – an antigenic preparation (toxoid or vaccine) used to induce formation of specific antibodies against a pathogenic microorganism that provides delayed but permanent protection against the associated disease.

immunizing agent, passive – a biological preparation (antitoxin, antivenin, or immune serum) containing specific antibodies against a pathogenic microorganism that provides immediate but temporary protection against the associated disease.

immunoprophylaxis – preventing the spread of disease by providing physiological immunity.

immunosuppression – when the immune system is unable to protect the body from disease. This condition can be caused by disease (like AIDS) or by certain drugs (like those used in chemotherapy). Individuals whose immune systems are compromised should not receive live, attenuated vaccines.

impetigo – a contagious inflammatory skin infection with isolated pustules, most commonly occurring on the face of young children.

incidence – the number of new disease cases reported in a population over a certain period of time.

incubation period – the time from contact with infectious agents (bacteria or viruses) to onset of disease.

infection – an invasion of an organism by a pathogen such as bacteria or viruses. Some infections lead to disease.

infectious – capable of spreading disease. Also known as communicable.

infectious agents – organisms capable of spreading disease (eg, bacteria or viruses).

insulin – a hormone that promotes use of glucose, protein synthesis, and the formation and storage of neutral lipids; used in the treatment of diabetes mellitus.

inversion – a turning inward.

irrigating solution – a solution for washing wounds or various body cavities.

jaundice – a yellowing of the skin, whites of the eyes, tissues, and certain body fluids, which can result from certain liver diseases, including hepatitis C, or from excessive breakdown of red blood cells due to internal hemorrhage or various other conditions.

keratitis – an inflammation of the cornea.

keratolytic – a topical drug that softens the superficial keratin-containing layer of the skin to promote exfoliation.

lacrimal – pertaining to tears.

laxative – a gentle purgative medicine; mild cathartic.

leishmaniasis – infections transmitted by sand flies.

leukocyte – a white blood cell.

leukocytopenia – a decrease in the number of white blood cells.

leukocytosis – an increased white blood cell count.

leukoderma – an absence of pigment from the skin.

libido – sexual desire.

lipoma – a benign fatty tumor.

lipotropic – a drug, especially one supplementing a dietary factor, that prevents the abnormal accumulation of fat in the liver.

lochia – a vaginal discharge of mucus, blood, and tissue after childbirth.

lues – a plague; specifically syphilis.

macrocyte – a large red blood cell.

malaise – a general feeling of illness.

mastitis – an inflammation of the breast.

melasma – a darkening of the skin.

melena – black feces or black vomit from altered blood in the higher GI tract.

meninges – the membranes covering the brain and spinal cord.

metastasis – the shifting of a disease or its symptoms from one part of the body to another.

microbes – tiny organisms (including viruses and bacteria) that can only be seen with a microscope.

miotics – agents that constrict the pupil of the eye; a myotic.

moniliasis – an infection with any of the species of monilia types of fungi (*Candida*).

morbidity – any departure, subjective or objective, from a state of physiological or psychological well-being.

mortality – the number of deaths in a given time or place.

mucolytic – an agent that can destroy or dissolve mucous membrane secretions.

myalgia – a pain in the muscles.

myasthenia gravis – a chronic progressive muscular weakness caused by myoneural conduction, usually spreading from the face and throat.

myelocyte – an immature white blood cell in the bone marrow.

myelogenous – originating in bone marrow.

myoclonus – involuntary, sudden, rapid, unpredictable jerks.

mydriatic – a drug that dilates the pupil of the eye, usually by anticholinergic or adrenergic mechanisms.

myoneural – pertaining to muscle and nerve.

myopia – nearsightedness.

narcotic – a drug with effects similar to opium and derivatives that produces analgesic effects and has the potential for dependence and tolerance.

neonatal – pertaining to the first four weeks of life.

neoplasm – an abnormal tissue that grows more rapidly than normal and shows a lack of structural organization.

nephritis – an inflammation of the kidney.

nephrosclerosis – a hardening of the kidney tissue.

neuralgia – a pain extending along the course of one or more nerves.

neurasthenia – a condition accompanying or following depression that is characterized by vague fatigue.

neuroglia – the supporting elements of the nervous system.

neuroleptic – a psychotropic drug used to treat psychosis.

neurosis – a psychological or behavioral disorder characterized by anxiety.

NIH – National Institutes of Health.

nocturia – urination at night.

normocytic – erythrocytes that are normal in size, shape, and color.

nosocomial – referring to an infection acquired by a patient while in a hospital.

nuchal – the back of the neck.

nystagmus – a rhythmic oscillation of the eyes.

oleaginous – oily or greasy.

omphalitis – an inflammation of the navel and surrounding area.

onychomycosis – a fungal infection of the nails.

ophthalmic – pertaining to the eye.

oral – pertaining to the mouth.

organism – any living thing. Organisms include humans, animals, plants, bacteria, protozoa, and fungi.

orthopnea – a discomfort in breathing when lying flat.

ossification – a formation of, or conversion to, bone.

osteomyelitis – an inflammation of the marrow of the bone.

osteoporosis – a reduction in bone quantity; skeletal atrophy.

otalgia – pain in the ear; earache.

otitis – inflammation of the ear.

otomycosis – an ear infection caused by fungus.

otorrhea – a discharge from the ear.

outbreak – sudden appearance of a disease in a specific geographic area (eg, neighborhood or community) or population (eg, adolescents).

oxytocic – a drug that selectively stimulates uterine motility and is useful in obstetrics, especially in the control of postpartum hemorrhage.

Paget disease – a skeletal disease in which bone resorption and formation are increased leading to thickening and softening of bones; a disease characterized by lesions around the nipple and areola found in elderly women.

pallor – paleness.

palpitations – an awareness of one's heart action.

pandemic – an epidemic occuring over a very large area.

parasites – any organism that lives in or on another organism without benefiting the host organism; commonly refers to pathogens, most commonly in reference to protozoans and helminths.

parasympatholytic – See Anticholinergic.

parasympathomimetic – See Cholinergic.

parenteral – pertaining to the administration of a drug by means other than through the intestinal tract; subcutaneous, intramuscular, or intravenous drug administration.

parkinsonism – a group of neurological disorders caused by dopamine deficiency marked by hypokinesia, tremor, and muscular rigidity.

paroxysm – a sharp spasm or convulsion.

passive immunity – see Immunity, Passive.

pathogenic – causing an abnormality or disease.

pathogens – bacteria, viruses, parasites, or fungi that can cause disease.

pediatrics – a branch of medicine caring for the medical problems of children from birth through adolescence.

pediculicide – an agent used to kill lice.

pediculosis – an infestation with lice.

pellagra – characterized by GI disturbances, mental disorders, skin redness, and scaling due to niacin deficiency.

pernicious – particularly dangerous or harmful.

phlebitis – an inflammation of a vein.

pleurisy – an inflammation of the membrane surrounding the lungs and the thoracic cavity.

pneumonia – an infection of the lungs.

poikilocytosis – a condition in which pointed or irregularly shaped red blood cells are found in the blood.

polydipsia – excessive thirst.

posology – the science of dosage.

posterior pituitary hormone(s) – a hormone with oxytocic, vasoconstrictor, antidiuretic, and intestinal stimulant properties.

post-exposure prophylaxis (PEP) – prevention or treatment of disease after a possible exposure.

prevalance – the number of disease cases (new and existing) within a population at a given time.

progestin – a hormone that functions in the menstrual cycle and during pregnancy to promote uterine gland secretion and to reduce uterine motility.

pronation – the body's position when lying face downward; rotation of the forearm so the palm on the hand faces backward when the arm is in anatomical position.

prophylactic – a remedy that tends to prevent disease.

protectant – a topical drug that remains on the skin and serves as a physical, protective barrier to the environment.

proteolytic enzyme – an enzyme used to liquify fibrinous or purulent exudates.

psoriasis – an inflammatory skin disease accompanied by itching.

psychotherapy – therapy utilizing communication and interventions with the patient instead of chemical or physical treatments.

ptosis – a drooping or sagging of a muscle or organ, such as the eyelid.

pulmonary – pertaining to the lungs.

purulent – containing or forming pus.

pyelitis – a local inflammation of renal and pelvic cells due to bacterial infection.

pylorospasm – a spasmodic muscle contraction of the pyloric portion of the stomach.

pyoderma – any fever-producing skin infection.

quarantine – to isolate an individual who has or is suspected of having a disease, in order to prevent spreading the disease to others; alternatively, to isolate a person who does not have a disease during a disease outbreak, in order to prevent that person from catching the disease (this is called reverse isolation). Quarantine can be voluntary or ordered by public health officials in times of emergency.

radiopaque medium – a diagnostic drug, opaque to x-rays, whose retention in a body organ or cavity makes x-ray visualization possible.

Raynaud phenomenon – spasms of the digital arteries with blanching and numbness precipitated by cold temperature.

reflex stimulant – a mild irritant suitable for application to the nasopharynx to induce reflex respiratory stimulation.

rheumatoid – resembling rheumatoid arthritis.

rhinitis – an inflammation of the mucous membrane of the nose.

risk – the likelihood that an individual will experience a certain event.

rubefacient – a topical drug that induces mild skin irritation with erythema, sometimes used to relieve the discomfort of deep-seated inflammation.

rubeola/measles – not to be confused with rubella.

saprophytic – receiving nourishment from dead material.

sarcoma – a malignant tumor derived from connective tissue.

scabicide – an insecticide suitable for the erradication of itch mite infestations in humans (scabies).

schistosomacide – an agent that destroys schistosomes; destructive to the trematodic parasites or flukes.

schistosomiasis – an infection with *Schistosoma haematobium*.

scintillation – a visual sensation manifested by an emission of sparks.

sclerosing agent – an irritant suitable for injection into varicose veins to induce their fibrosis and obliteration.

scotomata – an area of varying size and shape within the visual field in which vision is absent or depressed.

seborrhea – a condition arising from an excess secretion of sebum.

sebum – the fatty secretions of sebaceous glands.

sedative – a drug that calms nervous excitement.

seroconversion – development of antibodies in the blood of an individual who previously did not have detectable antibodies.

serology – measurement of antibodies, and other immunological properties, in the blood serum.

side effect – undesirable reaction resulting from immunization or other medication, treatment, etc.

sinusitis – an inflammation of a sinus membrane lining.

skeletal muscle relaxant – a drug that inhibits contraction of voluntary muscles, usually by interfering with their innervation.

smooth muscle relaxant – a drug that inhibits contraction of involuntary (eg, visceral) muscles, usually by action upon their contractile elements.

sociopath – a person designated to have an antisocial personality disorder.

spasmolytic – an agent that relieves spasms and involuntary contractions of a muscle; antispasmodic.

sputum – expectorated mucus.

STD – sexually transmitted disease.

stenosis – the narrowing of the lumen of a blood vessel.

stomachic – a drug that is used to stimulate the appetite and gastric secretion.

stomatitis – an inflammation of the mucous membranes of the mouth.

subcutaneous – underneath the skin.

sudorific – causing perspiration.

superacidity – excessive acidity.

supination – the body's position when lying face upwards; rotation of the forearm so the palm on the hand faces forward when the arm is in anatomical position.

suppressant – a drug useful in the control, rather than the cure, of a disease; an agent that stops secretion, excretion, or normal discharge.

surfactant – a surface active agent that decreases the surface tension between two miscible liquids; used to prepare emulsions, act as a cleansing agent, etc.

susceptible – unprotected against a certain disease.

synarthrosis (fibrous joint) – a joint in which the bony elements are united by continuous fibrous tissue.

syncope – fainting; loss of consciousness.

synovia – a clear fluid that lubricates the joints; joint oil.

systole – the ventricular contraction phase of a heartbeat.

tachycardia – a rapid contraction rate of the heart.

taeniacide – an agent used to kill tapeworms.

taeniafuge – an agent used to expel tapeworms.

therapeutic – a treatment of disease.

thoracic – pertaining to the chest.

thyroid hormone – a drug containing one or more of the iodinated amino acids that stimulate and regulate the metabolic rate and functional state of body tissues.

thyroid inhibitor – a drug that reduces excessive thyroid hormone production, usually by blocking hormone synthesis.

tics – a repetitive twitching of muscles, often in the face and upper trunk.

tinea – a fungal infection of the skin, hair, or nails.

tonic – continuous muscular contraction.

tonometry – the measurement of tension in some part of the body.

topical – the local external application of a drug to a particular place.

toxoid – a modified toxin, less toxic than the original form, used to induce active immunity to bacterial pathogens.

tranquilizer – a psychotherapeutic drug that promotes tranquility without significant sedation, useful in treating certain neuroses and psychoses.

tremors – involuntary rhythmic tremulous movements.

trichomoniasis – an infection with parasitic flagellate protozoa of the genus *Trichomonas*.

trypanosomiasis – any disease caused by *Trypanosomatidae*.

uricosuric – a drug that promotes renal uric acid excretion; used to treat gout.

urolithiasis – a condition marked by the formation of stones in the urinary tract.

urticaria – a rash or hives.

vaccination – injection of a killed or weakened infectious organism in order to prevent the disease.

vaccine – the preparation of live attenuated or dead pathogenic microorganisms, used to induce active immunity.

vaccine schedule – a chart or plan of vaccinations that are recommended for specific ages and/or circumstances.

vasoconstrictor – an agent used to narrow blood vessels; to constrict blood vessels and reduce tissue congestion in the nose.

vasodilator – a drug that relaxes vascular smooth muscles, especially for the purpose of improving peripheral or coronary blood flow.

vasopressor – an adrenergic drug used systemically to constrict blood vessels and raise blood pressure.

verruca – a wart.

vertigo – dizziness.

vesicant – an agent that, when applied to the skin, causes blistering and the formation of vesicles; an epispastic.

virus – a tiny organism that multiplies within cells and causes disease such as chickenpox, measles, mumps, rubella, pertussis, and hepatitis. Viruses are not affected by antibiotics, the drugs used to kill bacteria.

visceral – pertaining to the internal organs.

vitamin – an organic chemical essential in small amounts for normal body metabolism, used therapeutically to supplement the naturally occurring counterpart in foods.

WHO – World Health Organization.

Oral Dosage Forms That Should Not Be Crushed or Chewed

The purpose of this feature is to alert health care professionals about medications that should not be crushed or chewed because of their special pharmaceutical formulations or characteristics. Oral dosage forms that are sustained release (slow release) comprise the vast majority of this designation. Crushing or chewing such products may substantially alter their intended pharmacokinetics. Additional reasons for not chewing or crushing drugs include poor taste, irritant properties, or carcinogenic potential. Alternative liquid forms of these products are listed if available. Refer to the end of the table for a complete explanation of references.

It is important to understand that the inability to crush or chew drugs with slow-release properties does not always mean the dosage form cannot be divided or halved. Some newer slow-release dosage forms (eg, Toprol XL) are commercially available as scored tablets. This reference addresses those drugs that cannot be crushed or chewed.

Anyone who visits any acute- or long-term care facility can observe personnel meticulously grinding tablets or the contents of capsules in a mortar and pestle. Their rationale is well intentioned: they have an order to administer medication to a patient with a nasogastric tube or who cannot swallow solids and have to incorporate the drug into a liquid vehicle. However, they do so at the risk of changing the pharmacokinetics of the solid dosage formulation. Examples of special formulations include sublingual or buccal, enteric-coated, and extended-release tablets or capsules. Products containing extended-release dosage forms frequently have an abbreviation affixed to their brand name that serves as a clue that crushing may affect the formulation (Table 1). In addition, some medications are inherently corrosive to the oral mucosa and/or upper gastrointestinal tract, remarkably bitter to the taste, or capable of staining the oral mucosa and teeth.

Finally, several medications are potentially carcinogenic and require limited handling by medical personnel. Crushing or breaking of products that have carcinogenic/teratogenic potential (ie, antineoplastics) may not alter the dosage form or delivery mechanisms but may cause aerosolization of particles, exposing health care workers who handle these products. The reader is encouraged to review the American Society of Health-System Pharmacists' (previously the American Society of Hospital Pharmacists) bulletin on handling cytotoxic and hazardous drugs.

A more detailed description of the dosage forms mentioned above has been published in previous versions of this article and is summarized in Table 2.

Alternatives to Crushing

For patients who cannot swallow whole tablets or capsules, the most logical approach is to use liquid suspension forms of the same medication. Table 3 identifies examples of medications that have a liquid form commercially available. In some cases, there must be a dosage adjustment when the liquid is substituted. This is especially true if the tablet or capsule is an extended-release medication. If a liquid or suspension is not commercially available, the pharmacist should be consulted to determine if a liquid formulation could be extemporaneously prepared.

Occasionally, it is possible to substitute the injectable form of the medication by placing the appropriate amount of injection in some suitable fluid, such as juice. This should be done, however, only after consultation with a pharmacist to ensure that there are no problems regarding compatibility, stability, or changes in absorption of the drug. Another alternative is to use a chemically different but clinically similar medication that is available in a liquid form. Some medications that cannot be crushed may be administered in other ways, such as administering the contents of a capsule in soft food. This type of information is provided in Table 3 and indexed in the footnote.

Updates to List

Inherent with a listing of this type is the difficulty in keeping such lists current. The author encourages manufacturers, pharmacist, nurses, and other health professionals to notify us of any changes or updates.

References

1. American Society of Hospital Pharmacists. ASHP technical assistance bulletin on handling cytotoxic and hazardous drugs. *Am J Hosp Pharm.* 1990;47:1033-1049.
2. Mitchell JF. Oral dosage forms that should not be crushed: 2000 update. *Hosp Pharm.* 2000;35:553-567.

Table 1: Common Abbreviations for Extended-Release Products

CD	controlled dose
CR	controlled release
CRT	controlled release tablet
LA	long acting
SA	sustained action
SR	sustained release
TR	time release
TD	time delay
XL	extended release
XR	extended release

Table 2: Summary of Drug Formulations that Preclude Crushing

Type	Reason(s) for the formulation
Enteric coated	Designed to pass through the stomach intact with drug being released in the intestines to:
	(1) prevent destruction of drug by stomach acids
	(2) prevent stomach irritation
	(3) delay onset of action
Extended release	Designed to release drug over an extended period of time. Such products include:
	(1) multiple-layered tablets releasing drug as each layer is dissolved
	(2) mixed release pellets that dissolve at different time intervals
	(3) special matrixes that are themselves inert, but slowly release drug from the matrix
Sublingual	Designed to dissolve quickly in oral fluids for rapid absorption by the abundant blood supply of the mouth.
Miscellaneous	Drugs that:
	(1) produce oral mucosa irritation
	(2) are extremely bitter
	(3) contain dyes or inherently could stain teeth and mucosal tissue
	(4) drugs that, if handled without adequate protection, are potentially carcinogenic

Table 3: Medications That Should Not Be Crushed or Chewed

Drug Product	Dosage Form	Reason/Comments[a]
Aciphex	Tablet	Slow-release
Accutane	Capsule	Mucous membrane irritant
Actiq	Lozenge	Slow-release Note: This lollipop delivery system requires the patient to slowly allow dissolution.
Actonel	Tablet	Irritant Note: Chewed, crushed, or sucked tablets may cause oropharyngeal irritation.
Adalat CC	Tablet	Slow-release
Adderall XR	Capsule	Slow-release[b]
AeroHist Plus	Tablet	Slow-release[i]
Afeditab CR	Tablet	Slow-release
Afinitor	Tablet	Mucous membrane irritant
Aggrenox	Capsule	Slow-release
Alavert Allergy Sinus 12 Hour	Tablet	Slow-release
Allegra-D	Tablet	Slow-release
Allfen Jr	Tablet	Slow-release
	Capsule	Slow-release[b]
Alophen	Tablet	Enteric-coated
Alprazolam ER	Tablet	Slow-release
Altoprev	Tablet	Slow-release
Ambien CR	Tablet	Slow-release
Amibid DM	Tablet	Slow-release
Amitiza	Capsule	Slow-release
Ampyra	Tablet	Slow-release Note: Formerly Fampridine-SR
Amrix	Capsule	Slow-release
Aplenzin	Tablet	Slow-release
Apriso	Capsule	Slow-release[b] Note: Maintain pH at ≤ 6
Aptivus	Capsule	Note: Oil emulsion within spheres; taste
Aquatab C	Tablet	Slow-release[i]
Aquatab D	Tablet	Slow-release[i]
Aricept 23 mg	Tablet	Note: Crushing the 23 mg tablet may significantly increase the rate of absorption; the 5 and 10 mg tablets are not affected
Arthrotec	Tablet	Enteric-coated
Asacol	Tablet	Slow-release
Ascriptin A/D	Tablet	Enteric-coated
Atelvia	Tablet	Slow-release Note: Tablet coating is an important part of the delayed release.
Augmentin XR	Tablet	Slow-release[c,i]
Avinza	Capsule	Slow-release[b] (not pudding)

Drug Product	Dosage Form	Reason/Comments[a]
Avodart	Capsule	Note: Drug may cause fetal abnormalities; women who are or may become pregnant should not handle the capsules; all women should use caution in handling capsules, especially leaking capsules.
Azulfidine EN	Tablet	Enteric-coated
Bayer EC	Caplet	Enteric-coated
Bayer Low Adult	Tablet	Enteric-coated
Bayer Regular	Caplet	Enteric-coated
Bellahist-D LA	Tablet	Slow-release
Biaxin-XL	Tablet	Slow-release
Bidex A	Tablet	Slow-release
Bidhist-D	Tablet	Slow-release
Biltricide	Tablet	Taste[i]
Biohist LA	Tablet	Slow-release[i]
Bisac-Evac	Tablet	Enteric-coated[d]
Bisacodyl	Tablet	Enteric-coated[d]
Bisa-Lax	Tablet	Enteric-coated[d]
Boniva	Tablet	Irritant: Do not chew or suck Note: Potential for oropharyngeal ulceration.
Bromfed PD	Capsule	Slow-release
Budeprion SR	Tablet	Slow-release
Calan SR	Tablet	Slow-release[i]
Carbatrol	Capsule	Slow-release[b]
Cardene SR	Capsule	Slow-release
Cardizem	Tablet	Note: Although not described as slow-release in the package insert, the drug has a coating that is intended to release the drug over a period of approximately 3 hours.
Cardizem CD	Capsule	Slow-release
Cardizem LA	Tablet	Slow-release
Cardura XL	Tablet	Slow-release
Cartia XT	Capsule	Slow-release
Cefaclor ER	Tablet	Slow-release
Ceftin	Tablet	Taste[c] Note: Use suspension for children.
Cefuroxime	Tablet	Taste[c] Note: Use suspension for children.
CellCept	Capsule, Tablet	Teratogenic potential[j]
Charcoal Plus	Tablet	Enteric-coated
Chlor-Trimeton 12-Hour	Tablet	Slow-release[c]
Cipro XR	Tablet	Slow-release
Claritin-D 12 Hour	Tablet	Slow-release
Claritin-D 24 Hour	Tablet	Slow-release
Colace	Capsule	Taste[f]

Drug Product	Dosage Form	Reason/Comments[a]
Colestid	Tablet	Slow-release
Concerta	Tablet	Slow-release
Commit	Lozenge	Note: Integrity compromised by chewing or crushing.
Cotazym-S	Capsule	Enteric-coated[b]
Covera-HS	Tablet	Slow-release
Creon 5, 10, 20	Capsule	Slow-release[b]
Crixivan	Capsule	Taste Note: Capsule may be opened and mixed with fruit puree (eg, banana).
Cymbalta	Capsule	Slow-release[b] Note: May add contents of capsule to apple juice or applesauce but not chocolate
Cytoxan	Tablet	Note: Drug may be crushed but company recommends using injection.
Cytovene	Capsule	Skin irritant
Dallergy	Tablet	Slow-release[c,i]
Dallergy-JR	Capsule	Slow-release
Deconamine SR	Capsule	Slow-release[c]
Depakene	Capsule	Slow-release mucous membrane irritant[c]
Depakote	Tablet	Slow-release
Depakote ER	Tablet	Slow-release
Detrol LA	Capsule	Slow-release
Dexilant	Capsule	Slow-release[b]
Dilacor XR	Capsule	Slow-release
Dilatrate-SR	Capsule	Slow-release
Dilt-CD	Capsule	Slow-release
Dilt-XR	Capsule	Slow-release
Diltia XT	Capsule	Slow-release
Ditropan XL	Tablet	Slow-release
Divalproex ER	Tablet	Slow-release
Doxidan	Tablet	Enteric-coated[d]
DriHist SR	Tablet	Slow-release[i]
Drisdol	Capsule	Liquid filled[e]
Drixoral Cold/Allergy	Tablet	Slow-release
Drixoral Nondrowsy	Tablet	Slow-release
Drixoral Allergy Sinus	Tablet	Slow-release
Droxia	Capsule	Note: Exposure to the powder may cause serious skin toxicities; health care workers should wear gloves to administer.
Drysec	Tablet	Slow-release[i]
Dulcolax	Tablet	Enteric-coated[d]
Dulcolax	Capsule	Liquid-filled
DuraHist	Tablet	Slow-release[i]
DuraHist D	Tablet	Slow-release[i]
DynaCirc CR	Tablet	Slow-release
Duraphen II DM	Tablet	Slow-release[i]

Drug Product	Dosage Form	Reason/Comments[a]
Duraphen Forte	Tablet	Slow-release[i]
Duratuss A	Tablet	Slow-release[i]
Dynex	Tablet	Slow-release[i]
Easprin	Tablet	Enteric-coated
EC-Naprosyn	Tablet	Enteric-coated
Ecotrin Adult Low Strength	Tablet	Enteric-coated
Ecotrin Maximum Strength	Tablet	Enteric-coated
Ecotrin Regular Strength	Tablet	Enteric-coated
Ed A-Hist	Tablet	Slow-release[c]
E.E.S. 400	Tablet	Enteric-coated[c]
Effer-K	Tablet	Effervescent tablet[g]
Effervescent Potassium	Tablet	Effervescent tablet[g]
Effexor XR	Capsule	Slow-release
Embeda	Capsule	Slow-release[b]; do not give via nasogastric tube
E-Mycin	Tablet	Enteric-coated
Enablex	Tablet	Slow-release
Entocort EC	Capsule	Enteric-coated[b]
Equetro	Capsule	Slow-release[b]
Ergomar	Tablet	Sublingual form[h]
Ery-Tab	Tablet	Enteric-coated
Erythrocin Stearate	Tablet	Enteric-coated
Erythromycin Base	Tablet	Enteric-coated
Erythromycin Delayed-Release	Capsule	Enteric-coated pellets[b]
Evista	Tablet	Taste; teratogenic potential[j]
Exalgo	Tablet	Slow-release Note: Breaking, chewing, crushing, dissolving before swallowing or administering could result in overdose
Extendryl JR	Capsule	Slow-release
Extendryl SR	Capsule	Slow-release[c]
Feldene	Capsule	Mucous membrane irritant
Feen-a-mint	Tablet	Enteric-coated[d]
Fentora	Tablet	Note: Buccal tablet; swallow whole.
Feosol	Tablet	Enteric-coated[c]
Feratab	Tablet	Enteric-coated[c]
Fergon	Tablet	Enteric-coated
Fero-Grad 500 mg	Tablet	Slow-release
Ferro-Sequels	Tablet	Slow-release
Flagyl ER	Tablet	Slow-release
Fleet Laxative	Tablet	Enteric-coated[d]
Flomax	Capsule	Slow-release
Focalin XR	Capsule	Slow-release[b]
Fosamax	Tablet	Mucous membrane irritant
Gleevec	Tablet	Taste[i] Note: May be dissolved in water or apple juice.

Drug Product	Dosage Form	Reason/Comments[a]
Glucophage XR	Tablet	Slow-release
Glucotrol XL	Tablet	Slow-release
Glumetza	Tablet	Slow-release
Gralise	Tablet	Slow-release
Guaifed	Capsule	Slow-release
Guaifed-PD	Capsule	Slow-release
Guaifenesin/Pseudoephedrine	Tablet	Slow-release
Guaifenex DM	Tablet	Slow-release[i]
Guaifenex GP	Tablet	Slow-release
Guaifenex PSE	Tablet	Slow-release[i]
GuaiMAX-D	Tablet	Slow-release
Halfprin 81	Tablet	Enteric-coated
Hista-Vent DA	Tablet	Slow-release[i]
Hydrea	Capsule	Note: Exposure to the powder may cause serious skin toxicities; health care workers should wear gloves to administer
Imdur	Tablet	Slow-release[i]
Inderal LA	Capsule	Slow-release
Indocin SR	Capsule	Slow-release[b,c]
InnoPran XL	Capsule	Slow-release
Intelence	Tablet	Note: Tablet should be swallowed whole and not crushed; tablet may be dispersed in water
Intuniv	Tablet	Slow-release
Invega	Tablet	Slow-release
Isochron	Tablet	Slow-release
Isoptin SR	Tablet	Slow-release[i]
Isordil Sublingual	Tablet	Sublingual form[h]
Isosorbide Dinitrate Sublingual	Tablet	Sublingual form[h]
Isosorbide SR	Tablet	Slow-release
Jalyn	Capsule	Note: Women who are, or may become, pregnant should not handle crushed or broken tablets[j]
Jenloga	Tablet	Slow-release
Kadian	Capsule	Slow-release[b] Note: May add contents of capsule to applesauce without crushing contents
Kaletra	Tablet	Film-coated
Kapidex	Capsule	Slow-release[b] Note: Name changed to Dexilant
Kapvay	Tablet	Slow-release
Kaon CL-10	Tablet	Slow-release[c]
K-Dur	Tablet	Slow-release
Keppra	Tablet	Taste Note: Some extemporaneous formulas are pharmacy prepared
Ketek	Tablet	Slow-release[c]
Klor-Con	Tablet	Slow-release[c]

Drug Product	Dosage Form	Reason/Comments[a]
Klor-Con M	Tablet	Slow-release[c,i]
Klotrix	Tablet	Slow-release
Kombiglyze XR	Tablet	Slow-release Note: Tablet matrix may remain in stool
K-Lyte	Tablet	Effervescent tablet[g]
K-Lyte CL	Tablet	Effervescent tablet[g]
K-Lyte DS	Tablet	Effervescent tablet[g]
K-Tab	Tablet	Slow-release[c]
Lamictal XR	Tablet	Slow-release
Lescol XL	Tablet	Slow-release
Letairis	Tablet	Slow-release
Levbid	Tablet	Slow-release[i]
Levsinex Timecaps	Capsule	Slow-release
Lialda	Tablet	Slow-release
Liquibid-PD	Tablet	Slow-release[i]
Lithobid	Tablet	Slow-release
Lodrane 24	Capsule	Slow-release
Lodrane 24 D	Capsule	Slow-release
LoHist 12 Hour	Tablet	Slow-release
Lovaza	Capsule	Note: Contents of capsule may erode walls of Styrofoam or plastic materials
Luvox CR	Capsule	Slow-release
Maxifed DM	Tablet	Slow-release[i]
Maxifed DMX	Tablet	Slow-release[i]
Maxiphen DM	Tablet	Slow-release[i]
Medent-DM	Tablet	Slow-release
Mestinon ER	Tablet	Slow-release[c]
Metadate CD	Capsule	Slow-release[b]
Metadate ER	Tablet	Slow-release
Methylin ER	Tablet	Slow-release
Metoprolol ER	Tablet	Slow-release
Micro K Extendcaps	Capsule	Slow-release[b,c]
Miraphen PSE	Tablet	Slow-release
Modane	Tablet	Enteric-coated[d]
Morphine sulfate extended-release	Tablet	Slow-release
Motrin	Tablet	Taste[f]
Moxatag	Tablet	Slow-release
MS Contin	Tablet	Slow-release[c]
Mucinex	Tablet	Slow-release
Mucinex DM	Tablet	Slow-release
Myfortic	Tablet	Slow-release
Namenda XR	Capsule	Slow-release[b]
Naprelan	Tablet	Slow-release
Nasatab LA	Tablet	Slow-release[i]
Nexium	Capsule	Slow-release[b]

Drug Product	Dosage Form	Reason/Comments[a]
Niaspan	Tablet	Slow-release
Nicotinic Acid	Capsule, Tablet	Slow-release[i]
Nifediac CC	Tablet	Slow-release
Nifedical XL	Tablet	Slow-release
Nitrostat	Tablet	Sublingual route[h]
Norflex ER	Tablet	Slow-release
Norpace CR	Capsule	Slow-release form within a special capsule
Norvir	Tablet	Note: Crushing tablets has resulted in decreased bioavailability of drug[c]
Oleptro	Tablet	Slow-release
Oracea	Capsule	Slow-release
Oramorph SR	Tablet	Slow-release[c]
Orphenadrine Citrate ER	Tablet	Slow-release
OxyContin	Tablet	Slow-release Note: Tablet disruption may cause a potentially fatal overdose of oxycodone.
Pancrease Delayed-Release	Capsule	Slow-release
Pancrease MT	Capsule	Enteric-coated[b]
Pancrecarb	Capsule	Enteric-coated[b]
Pancrelipase	Capsule	Enteric-coated[b]
Panocaps	Capsule	Enteric-coated[b]
Panocaps MT	Capsule	Enteric-coated[b]
Paxil CR	Tablet	Slow-release
Pentasa	Capsule	Slow-release
PhenaVent D	Tablet	Slow-release[i]
PhenaVent LA	Capsule	Slow-release
Plendil	Tablet	Slow-release
Pradaxa	Capsule	Note: Bioavailability increases by 75% when the pellets are taken without the capsule shell
Pre-Hist-D	Tablet	Slow-release[i]
Prevacid	Capsule	Slow-release
Prevacid SoluTab	Tablet	Orally disintegrating Note: Do not swallow; dissolve in water only and dispense via dosing syringe or nasogastric tube.
Prevacid Suspension	Suspension	Slow-release Note: Contains enteric-coated granules; mix with water only; not for use in nasogastric tubes.
Prilosec	Capsule	Slow-release
Prilosec OTC	Tablet	Slow-release
Procardia XL	Tablet	Slow-release
Propecia	Tablet	Note: Women who are or may become pregnant should not handle crushed or broken tablets.
Proquin XR	Tablet	Slow-release

Drug Product	Dosage Form	Reason/Comments[a]
Proscar	Tablet	Note: Women who are or may become pregnant should not handle crushed or broken tablets.
Protonix	Tablet	Slow-release
Prozac Weekly	Tablet	Enteric-coated
QDALL	Capsule	Slow-release
QDALL AR	Capsule	Slow-release
Ralix	Tablet	Slow-release[i]
Ranexa	Tablet	Slow-release
Rapamune	Tablet	Note: Pharmacokinetic NanoCrystal technology may be affected[c]
Razadyne ER	Capsule	Slow-release[c]
Renagel	Tablet	Note: Tablets expand in liquid if broken or crushed.
Requip XL	Tablet	Slow-release
Rescon	Tablet	Slow-release[i]
Rescon JR	Tablet	Slow-release[i]
Rescon MX	Tablet	Slow-release[i]
Respa-1st	Tablet	Slow-release[i]
Respa-DM	Tablet	Slow-release[i]
Respahist	Capsule	Slow-release[b]
Respaire SR	Capsule	Slow-release
Revlimid	Capsule	Note: Teratogenic potential; health care workers should avoid contact with capsule contents/body fluids
Ritalin LA	Capsule	Slow-release[b]
Ritalin SR	Tablet	Slow-release
R-Tanna	Tablet	Slow-release
Rythmol SR	Capsule	Slow-release
Ryzolt	Tablet	Slow-release Note: Crushing may cause overdose
Seroquel XR	Tablet	Slow-release
Sinemet CR	Tablet	Slow-release[i]
SINUvent PE	Tablet	Slow-release[i]
Slo-Niacin	Tablet	Slow-release[i]
Solodyn	Tablet	Slow-release
Somnote	Capsule	Liquid-filled
Sprycel	Tablet	Film-coated Note: Active ingredients are surrounded by a wax matrix to prevent health care exposure; women who are or may become pregnant should not handle crushed or broken tablets.
Strattera	Capsule	Note: Capsule contents can cause ocular irritation.
Sudafed 12-hour	Capsule	Slow-release[c]
Sudafed 24-hour	Capsule	Slow-release[c]
Sular	Tablet	Slow-release
Symax Duotab	Tablet	Slow-release

Drug Product	Dosage Form	Reason/Comments[a]
Symax SR	Tablet	Slow-release
Tasigna	Capsule	Note: Disruption of capsule may yield high blood levels causing enhanced toxicity
Taztia XT	Capsule	Slow-release[b]
Tegretol-XR	Tablet	Slow-release
Temodar	Capsule	Slow-release Note: If capsules are accidently opened or damaged, rigorous precautions should be taken to avoid inhalation or contact of contents with the skin or mucous membranes.[j]
Tessalon Perles	Capsule	Note: Swallow whole; temporary local anesthesia of the oral mucosa and choking could occur.
Theo-24	Capsule	Slow-release Note: Contains beads that dissolve throughout the GI tract.
Theochron	Tablet	Slow-release
Tiazac	Capsule	Slow-release[b]
Topamax	Tablet	Taste
	Capsule	Taste[b]
Toprol XL	Tablet	Slow-release[i]
Touro CC-LD	Tablet	Slow-release[i]
Touro LA-LD	Tablet	Slow-release[i]
Toviaz	Tablet	Slow-release
Tracleer	Tablet	Note: Women who are or may become pregnant should not handle crushed or broken tablets.
Trental	Tablet	Slow-release
Treximet	Tablet	Note: Unique drug matrix enhances rapid drug absorption
Tylenol Arthritis	Tablet	Slow-release
Ultram ER	Tablet	Slow-release Note: Tablet disruption may cause a potentially fatal overdose of tramadol.
Ultrase	Capsule	Enteric-coated
Uniphyl	Tablet	Slow-release
Urocit-K	Tablet	Wax-coated; prevents upper GI release
Uroxatral	Tablet	Slow-release
Valcyte	Tablet	Teratogenic and irritant potential[c,i]
Verapamil SR	Tablet	Slow-release[i]
Verelan	Capsule	Slow-release[b]
Verelan PM	Capsule	Slow-release[b]
VesiCare	Tablet	Enteric-coated
Videx EC	Capsule	Slow-release
Vimovo	Tablet	Slow-release
Voltaren XR	Tablet	Slow-release
VoSpire ER	Tablet	Slow-release
Votrient	Tablet	Note: Crushing significantly increases the AUC and T_{max}

Drug Product	Dosage Form	Reason/Comments[a]
Wellbutrin SR, XL	Tablet	Slow-release
Xanax XR	Tablet	Slow-release
Zegerid OTC	Capsule	Slow-release
Zenpep	Capsule	Slow-release[b]
Zolinza	Capsule	Note: Irritant; avoid contact with skin or mucous membranes; avoid contact with crushed or broken tablets.
ZORprin	Tablet	Slow-release
Zortress	Tablet	Note: Crushed powder may cause dangerous effects to mucous membranes
Zyban	Tablet	Slow-release
Zyflo CR	Tablet	Slow-release

a Two official terms are used to designate special-release medication forms: "extended-release" and "delayed-release." Others such as "sustained-release," "controlled-release," etc are commonly used on package labeling. The term "slow-release" is being used here to signify all such drugs with a special-release mechanism.

b Capsule may be opened and the contents taken without crushing or chewing; soft food such as applesauce or pudding may facilitate administration; contents may generally be administered via nasogastric tube using an appropriate fluid, provided entire contents are washed down the tube.

c Liquid dosage forms of the product are available; however, dose, frequency of administration, and manufacturers may differ from that of the solid dosage form.

d Antacids and/or milk may prematurely dissolve the coating of the tablet.

e Capsule may be opened and the liquid contents removed for administration.

f The taste of this product in a liquid form would likely be unacceptable to the patient; administration via nasogastric tube should be acceptable.

g Effervescent tablets must be dissolved in the amount of diluent recommended by the manufacturer.

h Tablets are made to disintegrate under the tongue.

i Tablet is scored and may be broken in half without affecting release characteristics.

j Skin contact may enhance tumor production; avoid direct contact.

Revised by John F. Mitchell, PharmD, FASHP, from an article that originally appeared in *Hosp Pharm*. 1996;1:27–37.

Drug Names That Look Alike and Sound Alike

This list has been prepared to sensitize health care professionals and their support personnel to the need to properly communicate when writing, speaking, reading, and hearing drug names.

No drug name is without problems. Any name can be written or spoken poorly enough so that it can be mistaken for another.

Listed in the accompanying table are drug names in the United States that can look and/or sound alike. Some are dangerously close; whereas others require incomplete prescribing information, poor communication skills, poor listening, and/or lack of knowledge about the drugs for an error to result.

To reduce errors, practitioners must share the common goal of drug name safety with pharmaceutical manufacturers, the Food and Drug Administration (FDA), the World Health Organization (WHO), the United States Adopted Name Council (USANC), and the United States Pharmacopeia (USP).

The potential errors can be reduced by:

- Pretesting proposed names for error potential
- Careful selection of brand names and generic names by manufacturers, FDA, WHO, and USANC
- Legible handwriting
- Clear oral communications
- Writing complete drug orders:
  - Specifying the dosage form (eg, tablet)
  - Specifying the drug strength (eg, 100 mg)
  - Specifying directions (eg, take one daily with breakfast)
  - Specifying the purpose/indication (eg, take one daily with breakfast to control blood pressure)
- Printing orders for new or rarely prescribed drugs
- For those involved in drug dispensing and administration, being aware of the drugs that are available, paying careful attention to the work at hand, and minimizing distractions
- Knowing the patient's condition/problems to ascertain if the drug name that has been read or heard is indicated
- Double-checking completed prescriptions in the pharmacy
- Educating patients about their drug regimens (serves as another final check that the prescription was properly read and dispensed)

Proprietary names are capitalized; other names are in lower case letters.

Accolate	Accupril	Aciphex	Aricept
Accolate	Aclovate	Aclovate	Accolate
Accupril	Accolate	Acnomel	Actonel
Accupril	Aciphex	Actonel	Acnomel
acebutolol	albuterol	Actonel	Actos
acetazolamide	acetohexamide	Actos	Actonel
acetohexamide	acetazolamide	Adacel	Daptacel
acetylcholine	acetylcysteine	Adderall	Inderal
acetylcysteine	acetylcholine	Adriamycin	Aredia
Aciphex	Accupril	Afrin	aspirin

Aggrastat . . . . .Aggrenox
Aggrastat . . . . .argatroban
Aggrenox . . . . .Aggrastat
Albutein . . . . .albuterol
albuterol . . . . .acebutolol
albuterol . . . . .Albutein
albuterol . . . . .atenolol
Aldactazide . . . . . . .Aldactone
Aldactone . . . . .Aldactazide
Aldara . . . . .Alora
Alesse . . . . .Aleve
Aleve . . . . .Alesse
Alfenta . . . . .Sufenta
alfentanil . . . . .Anafranil
alfentanil . . . . .fentanyl
alfentanil . . . . .sufentanil
Alkeran . . . . .Leukeran
Alora . . . . .Aldara
Alora . . . . .Aloxi
Aloxi . . . . .Alora
alprazolam . . . . .alprostadil
alprazolam . . . . .lorazepam
alprostadil . . . . .alprazolam
Altace . . . . .alteplase
alteplase . . . . .Altace
Altocor . . . . .Advicor
Amaryl . . . . .Amerge
Amerge . . . . .Amaryl
amiloride . . . . .amiodarone
amiloride . . . . .amlodipine
amiodarone . . . . . . .amiloride
amitriptyline . . . . . . .nortriptyline
amlodipine . . . . .amiloride
amoxapine . . . . .amoxicillin
amoxicillin . . . . .amoxapine
Amrix . . . . .Amvisc
Amvisc . . . . .Amrix
Anafranil . . . . .alfentanil
Anafranil . . . . .enalapril
Anafranil . . . . .nafarelin
Anaprox . . . . .Anaspaz
Anaspaz . . . . .Anaprox
Anaspaz . . . . .Antispas
Antivert . . . . .Axert
Anusol . . . . .Anusol-HC
Anusol . . . . .Aplisol
Anusol . . . . .Aquasol
Anusol-HC . . . . .Anusol
Aplisol . . . . .Anusol

Aprodine . . . . .aprotinin
aprotinin . . . . .Aprodine
Aquasol . . . . .Anusol
Aralen . . . . .Aranelle
Aranelle . . . . .Aralen
Aranesp . . . . .Aricept
Aredia . . . . .Adriamycin
argatroban . . . . .Aggrastat
Aricept . . . . .Aciphex
Aricept . . . . .Aranesp
Aricept . . . . .Ascriptin
Aricept . . . . .Azilect
Asacol . . . . .Os-Cal
Ascriptin . . . . .Aricept
asparaginase . . . . . .pegaspargase
aspirin . . . . .Afrin
atenolol . . . . .albuterol
atenolol . . . . .timolol
Atgam . . . . .Ativan
Ativan . . . . .Atgam
Avalide . . . . .Avandia
Avandamet . . . . .Avandia
Avandia . . . . .Avalide
Avandia . . . . .Avandamet
Avandia . . . . .Coumadin
Avandia . . . . .Prandin
Aventyl . . . . .Bentyl
Avinza . . . . .Invanz
Avinza . . . . .Evista
Avonex . . . . .Avelox
Axert . . . . .Antivert
azathioprine . . . . . . .Azulfidine
azelaic acid . . . . . . .Azelex
Azelex . . . . .azelaic acid
azidothymidine . . . . .azathioprine
Azilect . . . . .Aricept
azithromycin . . . . . . .erythromycin
Azulfidine . . . . .azathioprine
bacitracin . . . . .Bactrim
bacitracin . . . . .Bactroban
baclofen . . . . .Bactroban
Bactrim . . . . .bacitracin
Bactrim . . . . .Bactroban
Bactroban . . . . .bacitracin
Bactroban . . . . .baclofen
Bactroban . . . . .Bactrim
Benadryl . . . . .benazepril
Benadryl . . . . .Bentyl
benazepril . . . . .Benadryl

Bentyl............	Aventyl
Bentyl............	Benadryl
Betadine..........	betaine
betaine...........	Betadine
betaxolol..........	bethanechol
bethanechol.......	betaxolol
bupivacaine.......	mepivacaine
bupropion.........	buspirone
buspirone.........	bupropion
buspirone.........	risperidone
butabarbital.......	butalbital
butalbital.........	butabarbital
Cafergot..........	Carafate
Caladryl..........	calamine
calamine..........	Caladryl
Calan............	Colace
calcitonin.........	calcitriol
calcitriol..........	calcitonin
calcium glubionate.......	calcium gluconate
calcium gluconate........	calcium glubionate
Capastat..........	Cēpastat
Capitrol..........	captopril
captopril..........	Capitrol
Carac............	Kuric
Carafate..........	Cafergot
Carbatrol.........	Cartrol
carboplatin........	cisplatin
Cardene..........	Cardura
Cardene..........	codeine
Cardizem CD (LA)............	Cardizem LA (CD)
Cardura..........	Cardene
Cardura..........	Cordarone
Cardura..........	Coumadin
Cardura..........	K-Dur
Cardura..........	Ridaura
carteolol..........	carvedilol
Cartrol..........	Carbatrol
carvedilol.........	carteolol
Casodex..........	Kapidex
Cefol............	Cefzil
Cefotan..........	Ceftin
cefotaxime........	cefoxitin
cefotaxime........	ceftizoxime
cefotaxime........	cefuroxime
cefotetan.........	cefoxitin
cefoxitin..........	cefotaxime
cefoxitin..........	cefotetan

ceftazidime........	ceftizoxime
Ceftin............	Cefotan
ceftizoxime........	cefotaxime
ceftizoxime........	ceftazidime
cefuroxime........	cefotaxime
cefuroxime........	deferoxamine
Celebrex..........	Celexa
Celebrex..........	Cerebyx
Cēpastat..........	Capastat
Cerebyx..........	Celebrex
Cerebyx..........	Cerezyme
Ceredase..........	Cerezyme
Cerezyme..........	Cerebyx
Cerezyme..........	Ceredase
chlorambucil.......	Chloromycetin
Chloromycetin.....	chlorambucil
chlorpromazine.....	chlorpropamide
chlorpromazine.....	clomipramine
chlorpromazine.....	prochlorperazine
chlorpropamide....	chlorpromazine
Cidex............	Lidex
cimetidine.........	simethicone
cinoxacin.........	Ciloxan
cisplatin..........	carboplatin
Citracal..........	Citrucel
Citrucel..........	Citracal
Clarinex..........	Claritin
Claritin..........	Clarinex
Clinoril..........	Clozaril
clomiphene........	clomipramine
clomiphene........	clonidine
clomipramine......	chlorpromazine
clomipramine......	clomiphene
clonazepam.......	clorazepate
clonazepam.......	lorazepam
clonidine..........	clomiphene
clonidine..........	clonazepam
clonidine..........	quinidine
clotrimazole.......	co-trimoxazole
Clozaril..........	Clinoril
Clozaril..........	Colazal
codeine..........	Cardene
Colace..........	Calan
Colazal..........	Clozaril
Combivent........	Combivir
Combivir..........	Combivent
Compazine........	Copaxone
Comvax..........	Recombivax HB
Copaxone.........	Compazine

Cordarone . . . . .Cardura
Coreg . . . . .Corgard
Corgard . . . . .Coreg
Cortef. . . . . .Lortab
corticotropin . . . . . . .Cortisporin
Cortisporin . . . . .corticotropin
co-trimoxazole . . . . .clotrimazole
Coumadin. . . . . .Avandia
Coumadin. . . . . .Cardura
Covera HS . . . . .Provera
Cozaar . . . . .Hyzaar
Cozaar . . . . .Zocor
cyclobenzaprine . . . .cycloserine
cyclobenzaprine . . . .cyproheptadine
cyclophosphamide . .cyclosporine
cycloserine. . . . . . . .cyclobenzaprine
cycloserine. . . . . . . .cyclosporine
cyclosporine . . . . . . .cyclophosphamide
cyclosporine . . . . . . .cycloserine
cyclosporine . . . . . . .Cyklokapron
Cyklokapron . . . . . . .cyclosporine
cyproheptadine. . . . . .cyclobenzaprine
dacarbazine . . . . . . .procarbazine
dactinomycin . . . . . .daptomycin
Dantrium . . . . .Daraprim
Daptacel. . . . . .Adacel
Daraprim . . . . .Dantrium
darunavir . . . . .Denavir
Darvocet-N. . . . . . . .Darvon-N
Darvon . . . . .Diovan
Darvon-N . . . . .Darvocet-N
daunorubicin. . . . . . .dactinomycin
daunorubicin. . . . . . .doxorubicin
daunorubicin. . . . . . .idarubicin
deferasirox . . . . .deferoxamine
deferoxamine . . . . . .cefuroxime
deferoxamine . . . . . .deferasirox
Demerol . . . . .Detrol
Denavir . . . . .darunavir
Depo-Medrol . . . . . . .Solu-Medrol
Dermatop . . . . .Dimetapp
desipramine . . . . . . .disopyramide
desipramine . . . . . . .imipramine
Desogen. . . . . .digoxin
desoximetasone . . . .dexamethasone
Desoxyn. . . . . .digoxin
dexamethasone . . . .desoximetasone
Dexedrine. . . . . .Dextran
Dexedrine. . . . . .Excedrin

Dextran . . . . .Dexedrine
DiaBeta . . . . .Zebeta
diazepam . . . . .diazoxide
diazepam . . . . .Ditropan
diazoxide . . . . .diazepam
diazoxide . . . . .Dyazide
dichloroacetic   trichloracetic
    acid . . . .   acid
diclofenac. . . . . .Diflucan
diclofenac. . . . . .Duphalac
Diflucan . . . . .diclofenac
Diflucan . . . . .Diprivan
Diflucan . . . . .disulfiram
digoxin . . . . .Desogen
digoxin . . . . .Desoxyn
digoxin . . . . .doxepin
Dilantin. . . . . .Dilaudid
Dilaudid . . . . .Dilantin
dimenhydrinate. . . . .diphenhydramine
Dimetapp . . . . .Dermatop
Diovan . . . . .Darvon
diphenhydramine . . . .dimenhydrinate
Diprivan . . . . .Ditropan
Diprosone. . . . . .dapsone
dipyridamole. . . . . . .disopyramide
disopyramide . . . . . .desipramine
disopyramide . . . . . .dipyridamole
disulfiram . . . . .Diflucan
dithranol . . . . .Ditropan
Ditropan . . . . .diazepam
Ditropan . . . . .Diprivan
Ditropan . . . . .dithranol
dobutamine . . . . . . .dopamine
donepezil . . . . .doxepin
dopamine . . . . .dobutamine
dopamine . . . . .Dopram
Dopram . . . . .dopamine
doxapram. . . . . .doxazosin
doxapram. . . . . .doxepin
doxapram. . . . . .doxorubicin
doxazosin. . . . . .doxapram
doxazosin. . . . . .doxepin
doxazosin. . . . . .doxorubicin
doxepin . . . . .digoxin
doxepin . . . . .donepezil
doxepin . . . . .doxapram
doxepin . . . . .doxazosin
doxepin . . . . .Doxidan
Doxidan . . . . .doxepin

Doxil.	.Doxy
Doxil.	.Paxil
doxorubicin.	.dactinomycin
doxorubicin.	.daunorubicin
doxorubicin.	.doxacurium
doxorubicin.	.doxapram
doxorubicin.	.doxazosin
doxorubicin.	.idarubicin
Doxy.	.Doxil
doxycycline	.doxylamine
doxylamine.	.doxycycline
dronabinol	.droperidol
droperidol.	.dronabinol
duloxetine.	.fluoxetine
Duphalac	.diclofenac
Durasal	.Durezol
Durezol	.Durasal
Dyazide	.diazoxide
Dynacin	.DynaCirc
DynaCirc	.Dynacin
Ecotrin	.Edecrin
Edecrin.	.Ecotrin
Efavirenz	.Etravirine
Eldepryl	.enalapril
Eldopaque Forte	.Eldoquin Forte
Eldoquin Forte	.Eldopaque Forte
Elmiron.	.Imuran
Enablex	.Enbrel
enalapril.	.Anafranil
enalapril.	.Eldepryl
Enbrel	.Enablex
enflurane	.isoflurane
Enjuvia.	.Januvia
Entex	.Tenex
ephedrine.	.epinephrine
epinephrine	.ephedrine
Epogen	.Neupogen
erythromycin.	.azithromycin
ethanol.	.Ethamolin
ethanol	.Ethyol
ethosuximide	.methsuximide
Ethyol.	.ethanol
etidronate.	.etomidate
etomidate.	.etidronate
Etravirine	.Efavirenz
Eurax	.Evoxac
Eurax	.Serax
Eurax	.Urex
Evoxac.	.Eurax
Excedrin.	.Dexedrine
Factrel	.Sectral
Fareston.	.Fosrenol
Faslodex	.Fosamax
Femara	.Femhrt
Femhrt	.Femara
Femiron	.Femring
Femring	.Femiron
fentanyl	.Alfentanil
fentanyl	.sufentanil
Fioricet.	.Fiorinal
Fiorinal.	.Fioricet
Fiorinal.	.Florinef
flecainide	.fluconazole
Flexeril	.Floxin
Flomax.	.Floranex
Flomax.	.Fosamax
Floranex.	.Flomax
Florinef.	.Fiorinal
Floxin	.Flexeril
fluconazole.	.flecainide
Fludara.	.FUDR
Flumadine	.flunisolide
Flumadine	.flutamide
flunisolide.	.Flumadine
flunisolide.	.fluocinonide
fluocinolone	.fluocinonide
fluocinonide	.flunisolide
fluocinonide	.fluocinolone
fluoxetine	.duloxetine
fluoxetine	.fluvastatin
flutamide	.Flumadine
fluvastatin.	.fluoxetine
folic acid.	.folinic acid
folinic acid	.folic acid
Fosamax	.Faslodex
Fosamax	.Flomax
fosinopril.	.lisinopril
Fosrenol.	.Fareston
Frova	.Provera
FUDR.	.Fludara
furosemide	.Torsemide
glimepiride	.glipizide
glipizide	.glimepiride
glipizide	.glyburide
Glucotrol.	.glyburide
glyburide	.glipizide
glyburide	.Glucotrol
GoLYTELY	.NuLYTELY

guaifenesin	guanfacine
guanabenz	guanfacine
guanfacine	guaifenesin
guanfacine	guanabenz
guanfacine	guanidine
guanidine	guanfacine
Halcion	Haldol
Haldol	Halcion
Haldol	Stadol
Halog	Haldol
Healon	Hyalgan
heparin	Hespan
Hespan	heparin
Humalog	Humulin
Humulin	Humalog
Hyalgan	Healon
Hycodan	Vicodin
hydralazine	hydroxyzine
hydrochlorothiazide	hydroflumethiazide
hydrocodone	hydrocortisone
hydrocortisone	hydrocodone
hydrocortisone	hydroxychloroquine
hydroflumethiazide	hydrochlorothiazide
hydromorphone	morphine
hydroxychloroquine	hydrocortisone
hydroxyurea	hydroxyzine
hydroxyzine	hydralazine
hydroxyzine	Hydrogesic
hydroxyzine	hydroxyurea
Hytone	Vytone
idarubicin	daunorubicin
idarubicin	doxorubicin
Imdur	Imuran
Imdur	K-Dur
imipramine	desipramine
Imodium	Indocin
Imodium	Ionamin
Imuran	Elmiron
Imuran	Imdur
Imuran	Inderal
indapamide	iopamidol
indapamide	Iopidine
Inderal	Adderall
Inderal	Imuran
Inderal	Isordil
Indocin	Imodium
Indocin	Vicodin
Inspra	Spiriva
interferon 2	interleukin 2
interferon alfa-2a	interferon alfa-2b
interferon alfa-2b	interferon alfa-2a
interleukin 2	interferon 2
interleukin 2	interleukin 11
Invanz	Avinza
Invanz	Invega
Invega	Invanz
iodine	Iopidine
Ionamin	Imodium
iopamidol	indapamide
Iopidine	iodipamide
Iopidine	iodine
Iopidine	Lodine
isoflurane	enflurane
Isordil	Inderal
Isordil	Isuprel
Isuprel	Isordil
Januvia	Enjuvia
Kaletra	Keppra
Kapidex	Casodex
K-Dur	Cardura
Keppra	Kaletra
Klaron	Klor-Con
Klor-Con	Klaron
Kuric	Carac
lactose	lactulose
lactulose	lactose
Lamictal	Lamisil
Lamictal	Lomotil
Lamisil	Lamictal
lamivudine	lamotrigine
lamotrigine	lamivudine
Lasix	Lidex
Lasix	Luxiq
leucovorin	Leukeran
Leukeran	Alkeran
Leukeran	leucovorin
Leukeran	Leukine
Leukine	Leukeran
Leustatin	lovastatin
Levatol	Lipitor
Levbid	Lithobid
Levitra	Levora
Levitra	Lexiva
levocabastine	levocetirizine
levocetirizine	levocabastine
Levora	Levitra
levothyroxine	liothyronine
Lexiva	Levitra

Lidex	Cidex
Lidex	Lasix
Lioresal	lisinopril
liothyronine	levothyroxine
Lipitor	Levatol
lisinopril	fosinopril
lisinopril	Lioresal
Lithobid	Levbid
Lithobid	Lithostat
Lithobid	Lithotabs
Lithostat	Lithobid
Lithostat	Lithotabs
Lithotabs	Lithobid
Lithotabs	Lithostat
Lomotil	Lamictal
Lonox	Loprox
Loprox	Lonox
lorazepam	alprazolam
lorazepam	clonazepam
Lortab	Cortef
Lotensin	lovastatin
Lotrimin	Lotrisone
Lotrisone	Lotrimin
lovastatin	Leustatin
lovastatin	Lotensin
Lovenox	Lotronex
Lunesta	Neulasta
Lustra	Lutera
Lutera	Lustra
Luxiq	Lasix
magnesium sulfate	manganese sulfate
manganese sulfate	magnesium sulfate
Maxidex	Maxzide
Maxzide	Maxidex
Mebaral	Medrol
Medrol	Mebaral
medroxyprogesterone	methylprednisolone
medroxyprogesterone	methyltestosterone
melphalan	Mephyton
mephobarbital	methocarbamol
Mephyton	melphalan
Mephyton	mephenytoin
mepivacaine	bupivacaine
methazolamide	metolazone
methenamine	methionine
methionine	methenamine
methocarbamol	mephobarbital
methsuximide	ethosuximide
methylprednisolone	medroxyprogesterone
methyltestosterone	medroxyprogesterone
metolazone	methazolamide
metolazone	metoprolol
metoprolol	metolazone
metoprolol	misoprostol
metyrapone	metyrosine
metyrosine	metyrapone
miconazole	Micronase
miconazole	Micronor
Micro-K	Micronase
Micronase	miconazole
Micronase	Micro-K
Micronase	Micronor
Micronor	miconazole
Micronor	Micronase
Midrin	Mydfrin
Mifeprex	Mirapex
mifepristone	misoprostol
Minocin	niacin
MiraLax	Mirapex
Mirapex	Mifeprex
Mirapex	MiraLax
Mircera	Mirena
Mirena	Mircera
misoprostol	mifepristone
Monopril	Monurol
Monurol	Monopril
morphine	hydromorphone
Mucinex	Mucomyst
Mucomyst	Mucinex
Myambutol	Nembutal
Mycelex	Myoflex
Mydfrin	Midrin
Myleran	Mylicon
Mylicon	Myleran
Myoflex	Mycelex
nafarelin	Anafranil
Naldecon	Nalfon
Nalfon	Naldecon
naloxone	naltrexone
naltrexone	naloxone
Nasarel	Nizoral
Navane	Norvasc
Navane	Nubain
nelfinavir	nevirapine
Nembutal	Myambutol
Neulasta	Lunesta

Neulasta. . . . . .Neumega
Neumega . . . . .Neulasta
Neumega . . . . .Neupogen
Neupogen . . . . .Epogen
Neupogen . . . . .Neupro
Neupogen . . . . .Nutramigen
Neupro. . . . . .Neupogen
Neurontin . . . . .Noroxin
Nevanac. . . . . .Nexavar
nevirapine . . . . .nelfinavir
Nexavar . . . . .Nevanac
niacin . . . . .Minocin
nicardipine . . . . .nifedipine
Nicorette. . . . . .Nordette
nifedipine . . . . .nicardipine
nifedipine . . . . .nimodipine
nimodipine . . . . .nifedipine
nitroglycerin . . . . . . .nitroprusside
nitroprusside. . . . . . .nitroglycerin
Nitrostat . . . . .Hyperstat
Nitrostat . . . . .Nystatin
Nizoral . . . . .Nasarel
Nordette . . . . .Nicorette
Noroxin . . . . .Neurontin
Norpace . . . . .Norvasc
nortriptyline . . . . .amitriptyline
Norvasc . . . . .Navane
Norvasc . . . . .Norpace
Nubain . . . . .Navane
NuLYTELY . . . . .GoLYTELY
Nutramigen . . . . . . .Neupogen
Nystatin . . . . .Nitrostat
Occlusal-HP. . . . . . .Ocuflox
OctreoScan . . . . . . .octreotide
octreotide . . . . .OctreoScan
Ocufen . . . . .Ocuflox
Ocuflox. . . . . .Occlusal-HP
Ocuflox. . . . . .Ocufen
olanzapine . . . . .olsalazine
olsalazine. . . . . .olanzapine
opium tincture . . . . .camphorated
                         tincture of
                         opium (paregoric)
opium tincture,   opium tincture
  camphorated
  (paregoric) . . . .
Optiray . . . . .Optivar
Optivar . . . . .Optiray
Orazinc . . . . .Orencia
Orencia . . . . .Orazinc
Orencia . . . . .Orinase

Orinase . . . . .Orencia
Ortho-Cept . . . . .Ortho-Cyclen
Ortho-Cyclen . . . . . .Ortho-Cept
Os-Cal . . . . .Asacol
oxybutynin . . . . .OxyContin
OxyContin . . . . .oxybutynin
OxyContin . . . . .oxycodone
oxymetazoline . . . . . .oxymetholone
oxymetholone. . . . . . .oxymetazoline
oxymetholone. . . . . . .oxymorphone
oxymorphone . . . . . . .oxymetholone
Oxytrol . . . . .Roxanol
Oxytrol . . . . .Uroxatral
paclitaxel . . . . .paroxetine
paclitaxel . . . . .Paxil
Pamelor . . . . .Panlor
Panlor . . . . .Pamelor
paregoric . . . . .Percogesic
Parlodel . . . . .pindolol
paroxetine . . . . .paclitaxel
paroxetine . . . . .pyridoxine
Paxil. . . . . .Doxil
Paxil. . . . . .paclitaxel
Paxil. . . . . .Plavix
Paxil. . . . . .Taxol
pegaspargase . . . . .asparaginase
penicillamine . . . . . .penicillin
penicillin. . . . . .penicillamine
penicillin G   penicillin G
  potassium. . . . . . .   procaine
penicillin G   penicillin G
  procaine. . . . .   potassium
pentosan . . . . .pentostatin
pentostatin . . . . .pentosan
Percocet. . . . . .Percodan
Percodan . . . . .Percocet
Percodan . . . . .Percogesic
Percodan . . . . .Periactin
Percogesic . . . . .Paregoric
Percogesic . . . . .Percodan
Perdiem . . . . .Pyridium
Peridex. . . . . .Precedex
phentermine . . . . . . .phentolamine
phentolamine . . . . . .phentermine
pHisoDerm . . . . .pHisoHex
pHisoHex. . . . . .pHisoDerm
Phos-Flur . . . . .PhosLo
PhosLo. . . . . .Phos-Flur
physostigmine . . . . .Prostigmin
physostigmine . . . . .pyridostigmine

pindolol	Parlodel
Pitocin	Pitressin
Pitressin	Pitocin
Plaquenil	Plavix
Plavix	Paxil
Plavix	Plaquenil
Plendil	pindolol
Polocaine	prilocaine
pralidoxime	Pramoxine
pralidoxime	pyridoxine
Pramoxine	pralidoxime
Prandin	Avandia
Pravachol	Prevacid
Pravachol	propranolol
PreCare	Precose
Precedex	Peridex
Precose	PreCare
prednisolone	prednisone
prednisone	prednisolone
prednisone	primidone
Premarin	Primaxin
Premarin	Remeron
Premphase	Prempro
Prempro	Premphase
Prevacid	Pravachol
Prevacid	Prevpac
Prevpac	Prevacid
prilocaine	Polocaine
prilocaine	Prilosec
Prilosec	prilocaine
Prilosec	Prinivil
Prilosec	Prozac
Primaxin	Premarin
Primaxin	Primacor
primidone	prednisone
Prinivil	Prilosec
Prinivil	Proventil
ProAmatine	protamine
probenecid	Procanbid
Procanbid	probenecid
procarbazine	dacarbazine
prochlorperazine	chlorpromazine
propranolol	Pravachol
propylthiouracil	Purinethol
Proscar	ProSom
Proscar	Prozac
Proscar	Psorcon
ProSom	Proscar
ProSom	Prozac

ProSom	Psorcon
Prostigmin	physostigmine
protamine	ProAmatine
protamine	Protonix
protamine	Protopam
Protonix	protamine
Protonix	Protopic
Protopam	protamine
Protopic	Protonix
Proventil	Prinivil
Provera	Covera HS
Provera	Frova
Prozac	Prilosec
Prozac	Proscar
Prozac	ProSom
Psorcon	Proscar
Psorcon	ProSom
Purinethol	propylthiouracil
Pyridium	Perdiem
Pyridium	pyridoxine
pyridostigmine	physostigmine
pyridoxine	paroxetine
pyridoxine	pralidoxime
pyridoxine	Pyridium
quinidine	clonidine
quinidine	quinine
quinine	quinidine
Ranexa	Renova
ranitidine	rimantadine
Recombivax HB	Comvax
Reglan	Renagel
Regranex	Repronex
Remeron	Premarin
Remeron	Zemuron
Remicade	Renacidin
Renacidin	Remicade
Renagel	Reglan
Renova	Ranexa
Renova	Renvela
Renvela	Renova
Repronex	Regranex
reserpine	risperidone
Restasis	Retavase
Restoril	Risperdal
Restoril	Zestril
Retavase	Restasis
retinamide	rufinamide
Retrovir	ritonavir
Ribavirin	riboflavin

riboflavin. . . . . .Ribavirin
rifabutin . . . . .rifampin
Rifadin . . . . .Rifater
Rifadin . . . . .Ritalin
Rifamate. . . . . .rifampin
rifampin . . . . .rifabutin
rifampin . . . . .Rifamate
rifampin . . . . .rifapentine
rifampin . . . . .rifaximin
rifaximin . . . . .rifampin
Rifater . . . . .Rifadin
rifaximin . . . . .rifampin
rimantadine . . . . .ranitidine
Risperdal . . . . .Restoril
risperidone . . . . .reserpine
Ritalin. . . . . .Rifadin
Ritalin LA . . . . .Ritalin SR
Ritalin SR. . . . . .Ritalin LA
ritonavir . . . . .Retrovir
Roxanol . . . . .Oxytrol
Roxanol . . . . .Roxicet
Roxanol . . . . .Uroxatral
Roxicet. . . . . .Roxanol
rufinamide . . . . .retinamide
Rynatan . . . . .Rynatuss
Rynatuss . . . . .Rynatan
Salagen . . . . .selegiline
Sandimmune . . . . . . .Sandostatin
Sandostatin . . . . .Sandimmune
saquinavir. . . . . .Sinequan
Sarafem . . . . .Serophene
Sectral . . . . .Factrel
Sectral . . . . .Septra
selegiline . . . . .Salagen
Serax . . . . .Eurax
Serax . . . . .Xerac
Serophene . . . . .Sarafem
sertraline . . . . .Soriatane
simethicone . . . . . . .cimetidine
Sinequan . . . . .saquinavir
Sinequan . . . . .Singulair
Singulair. . . . . .Sinequan
Solaraze. . . . . .Soliris
Soliris. . . . . .Solaraze
Solu-Medrol . . . . . . .Depo-Medrol
somatostatin. . . . . . .Somatuline
Somatuline . . . . .somatostatin
somatropin . . . . .sumatriptan
Soriatane . . . . .sertraline

sotalol . . . . .Stadol
Spiriva . . . . .Inspra
Stadol. . . . . .sotalol
Sufenta . . . . .Alfenta
Sufenta . . . . .Survanta
sufentanil . . . . .alfentanil
sulfadiazine . . . . . . .sulfasalazine
sulfasalazine . . . . . .sulfadiazine
sumatriptan . . . . . . .somatropin
Surbex . . . . .Surfak
Surfak . . . . .Surbex
Survanta. . . . . .Sufenta
Synalar. . . . . .Synarel
Synarel. . . . . .Synalar
Tacrine . . . . .Tarceva
Tarceva . . . . .Tacrine
Tarceva . . . . .Tarka
Tarka . . . . .Tarceva
Taxol . . . . .Paxil
Taxol . . . . .Taxotere
Taxotere. . . . . .Taxol
Tegretol . . . . .Trental
Tekturna. . . . . .Terak
Tenex . . . . .Entex
Tenex . . . . .Xanax
Terak . . . . .Tekturna
terbinafine . . . . .terbutaline
terbutaline . . . . .terbinafine
terbutaline . . . . .tolbutamide
terconazole . . . . . . .tioconazole
tetrabenazine . . . . . .thiabendazole
tetracycline. . . . . . . .tigecycline
thiabendazole. . . . . .tetrabenazine
thioridazine. . . . . . . .thiothixene
thiothixene . . . . .thioridazine
tiagabine . . . . .tizanidine
Tiazac . . . . .Ziac
ticarcillin. . . . . .tigecycline
tigecycline . . . . .tetracycline
tigecycline . . . . .ticarcillin
timolol . . . . .atenolol
Timoptic . . . . .Viroptic
tioconazole. . . . . . . .terconazole
tiopronin . . . . .tiotropium
tiotropium . . . . .tiopronin
tizanidine . . . . .tiagabine
TobraDex . . . . .Tobrex
tobramycin . . . . .Trobicin
Tobrex . . . . .TobraDex

tocilizumab	tositumomab
tolazamide	tolbutamide
tolbutamide	terbutaline
tolbutamide	tolazamide
Torsemide	furosemide
tositumomab	tocilizumab
Tracleer	Tricor
tramadol	Trandate
Trandate	tramadol
Trandate	Trental
Travatan	Xalatan
trazodone	tramadol
Trental	Tegretol
Trental	Trandate
tretinoin	trientine
triamterene	trimipramine
trichloracetic acid	dichloroacetic acid
Tricor	Tracleer
trientine	tretinoin
trimipramine	triamterene
Trimox	Tylox
Trobicin	tobramycin
Tykerb	Tyzeka
Tylenol	Tylox
Tylox	Trimox
Tylox	Tylenol
Tyzeka	Tykerb
Ultane	Ultram
Ultram	Ultane
Urex	Eurax
Uroxatral	Oxytrol
Uroxatral	Roxanol
Valcyte	Valium
Valcyte	Valtrex
Valium	Valcyte
Valtrex	Valcyte
Vaniqa	Viagra
Vasocidin	Vasodilan
Vasodilan	Vasocidin
Verelan	Virilon
Verelan	Vivarin
Verelan	Voltaren
Viagra	Vaniqa
Vicodin	Hycodan
Vicodin	Indocin
Vigamox	Vigomar
Vigomar	Vigamox
vinblastine	vincristine
vinblastine	vinorelbine
vincristine	vinblastine
vinorelbine	vinblastine
Virilon	Verelan
Viroptic	Timoptic
Vivarin	Verelan
Voltaren	Verelan
Vytone	Hytone
Wellbutrin SR	Wellbutrin XL
Xalatan	Travatan
Xanax	Tenex
Xanax	Xenazine
Xanax	Xopenex
Xanax	Zantac
Xeloda	Xenical
Xenazine	Xanax
Xenical	Xeloda
Xerac	Serax
Xopenex	Xanax
Zantac	Xanax
Zantac	Zofran
Zantac	Zyrtec
Zarontin	Zaroxolyn
Zaroxolyn	Zarontin
Zebeta	DiaBeta
Zestril	Restoril
Zestril	Zetia
Zestril	Zostrix
Zetia	Zestril
Ziac	Tiazac
Zocor	Cozaar
Zofran	Zantac
Zofran	Zosyn
Zolinza	Zonalon
Zonalon	Zolinza
ZORprin	Zyloprim
Zostrix	Zestril
Zosyn	Zofran
Zosyn	Zyvox
Zyloprim	ZORprin
Zymar	Zymine
Zymine	Zymar
Zyprexa	Zyrtec
Zyrtec	Zantac
Zyrtec	Zyprexa
Zyvox	Zosyn

This list was compiled by Neil M. Davis, MS, PharmD, FASHP, President, Safe Medication Practices Consulting, Inc., Huntingdon Valley, PA. The list was originally developed by Benjamin Teplitsky, retired Chief Pharmacist of Veterans Administration Hospitals in Albany, NY and Brooklyn, NY.

Discontinued Drugs

The following is a list of products no longer available in the United States because they were discontinued by the manufacturer or withdrawn from the market.

AA-HC Otic
Abarelix
Abbokinase
Absorbine Footcare Spray Liquid
Absorbine Power Gel
Acetest
AccuHist LA
AccuHist DM Pediatric Drops
AccuHist Pediatric Drops
Accutane
Accuzyme
Accuzyme SE
Accuzyme Topical Spray
Acetazolamide Tablets
Acetohexamide
Aci-Jel Vaginal Gel
Aclaro
Acova
Actisite
Activella Tablets
Acular PF
Adapettes
Adeflor M Tablets
ADEKs
Adenosine Phosphate Injection
Adsorbonac
Advanced-RF NatalCare
ADVIA Centaur HBc IgM
Advicor Tablets
Advil Junior Strength Chewable Tablets
Aeroaid
AeroBid
AeroBid-M
Aerocaine
Afrin Children's
Afrin No-Drip Sinus with Vapornase
Afrin No-Drip 12-Hour Severe Congestion
    With Menthol
Afrin Saline, Extra Moisturizing Solution
Afrin Sinus with Vapornase
Agenerase
Airet
AK-Dex
Akineton Tablets
AK-Nefrin
AK-Pred
AK-Rinse
AK-Spore H.C. Otic
AK-Tracin Ointment
AK-Trol Ophthalmic Ointment
AK-Trol Ophthalmic Suspension

Akwa Tears
Alacol DM Drops
Alacol DM Syrup
Albay
Alcon Saline Solution for Sensitive Eyes
Aldoclor 150
Aldoclor 250
Aldoril D50
Aldoril D30
Aldoril-15
Aldoril-25
Alfenta
Alkets, Extra Strength Antacid, Chewable
    Tablets
Allanderm-T
AllanEnzyme
AllanfillEnzyme
AllanHist PDX
All Clear
All Clear AR
Allercreme Skin Lotion
Allercreme Ultra Emollient Cream
Allerfrim Tablets
Allergan Enzymatic
Allergen Ear Drops
Allergy Drops
AllerTan
Allfen Jr
Allres Pd
Almora Tablets
Alor 5/500 Tablets
Aloxi Capsules
Alpha-Keri Moisturizing Soap Bar
Alphatrex Cream
Altace Tablets
Altazine
Alu-Cap
Alupent Aerosol
Alupent Solution for Inhalation
Alu-Tab
Ambi 10 Cream
Ambi 10 Soap
Amcort Injection
Americaine
Americaine Anesthetic Lubricant
Americaine First Aid Burn
Americaine Hemorrhoidal
Americaine Otic Solutions
Amevive Powder for Injection
Amicar Injection
Aminess

Aminess 5.2%
Aminosyn II 5% in 25% Dextrose
Aminosyn II 7% w/Electrolytes
Aminosyn II 3.5% in 25% Dextrose
Amitone Antacid Chewable Tablets
AmLactin AP Topical Cream
AMO Endosol
AMO Endosol Extra
AMO Vitrax
Amoxil Capsules
Amoxil Pediatric Drops
Amphocin
AmVaz
Anaplex DMX
Anaplex HD Liquid
Anaspaz
Ancef Injection
Ancef Powder for Injection
Andehist DM NR
Andehist-DM Syrup
Andehist Drops
Andehist NR
Andehist Syrup
Android
Andryl 200
Anemagen Capsules
Anemagen OB
Anexsia Tablets
Anextuss Tablets
Ansaid
Antilirium Injection
Antiminth Oral Suspension
Antispas
Antivenin (Crotalidae) Polyvalent Injection
Anturane Capsules
Anturane Tablets
Apatate Tablets
Apresazide 50/50
Apresazide 100/50
Apresazide 25/25
AquaBalm Cream
Aquachloral Supprettes
AquaMEPHYTON Injection
Aquaphyllin Syrup
AquaSite Solution
Aquatensen Tablets
Aralast
Aramine Injection
Arduan Powder for Injection
Arfonad
Argesic Cream
Aristocort
Aristocort A
Aristocort Forte Injection

Aristocort Intralesional Injection
ArthriCare Double Ice Gel
ArthriCare Odor Free Rub
ArthriCare Triple Medicated Gel
Arthropan
Articaine Hydrochloride
Ascriptin A/D
Ascriptin Extra Strength
A-Spas S/L
Aspergum
Aspirin/Pravastatin
Astepro
Atarax Syrup
Atolone
Atropine-1
Atuss EX Syrup
Atuss G
Atuss HC
Atuss HD
Atuss HS
Atuss HX
Atuss MS
A-200
Auralgan Otic
Aurothioglucose Injection
Auroto Otic
Auroto Otic Solution
Autoplex T
Aveeno Cleansing for Acne-Prone Skin
Aventyl Solution
Bactine Pain Relieving Cleansing Wipes
Bactrim IV Infusion
Balacet 325
Baltussin HC
Banalg
Banalg Hospital Strength Liniment
Barbidonna Tablets
Barbidonna #2 Tablets
BarnesHind Saline for Sensitive Eyes
Baros Granules
BayRab
BayTet
B-C Bid Tablets
Be-Flex Plus
Belladonna Tincture
Bellamine
Bel-Phen-Ergot SR
Benadryl Maximum Strength Cream
Benadryl Maximum Strength Solution
    (Spray)
Bengay SPA Cream
Benoquin
Ben-Tann
Benylin Adult Liquid

Benylin Pediatric Liquid
Benzac AC 2.5
Benzac AC Wash 2.5
Benzac W 5
Benzac W 10
Benzac W 2.5
Benzthiazide
Bepridil Hydrochloride
Betadine First Aid Antibiotics Plus Moisturizer Ointment
Betadine Plus First Aid Antibiotics and Pain Reliever Ointment
Betadine Vaginal Gel
Betagen Ointment
Betagen Solution
BetaTan
Betaxon Ophthalmic Suspension
Betoptic
Bextra Tablets
Biavax II Powder for Injection
Bicitra Solution
Bicozene
Bidex-DMI Tablets
Bidhist
Big Shot B-12
Bili-Labstix Reagent Strips
Biocef
Bioclate
Biotel Kidney
Biperiden
Bitolterol Mesylate
B-Ject-100
Blairex Lens Lubricant
Blinx
Bluboro
Bo-Cal
Bonine Chewable Tablets
Boric Acid
Borofair Otic
Borofax Skin Protectant
Boropak Powder Packets
Bottom Better
BP New Allergy DM
BranchAmin 4%
Breezee Mist Antifungal
Brethine Injection
Brethine Tablets
Bretylium Tosylate
Bricanyl
Bromatan-DM
Bromfenex
Bromfenex PD
Bromhist PDX Drops
Bromphenex HD Liquid

Bromplex HD
Bronchial
Brondelate
Bucet Capsules
Bucladin-S Softabs
Buclizine
Bumex
B-Vex D
Byclomine
Calan
Calcifediol
Calciferol Injection
Calcium Caseinate
Cal-Nate Tablets
Capitrol
Capozide
Carbastat
Carbetapentane Tannate
Carbinoxamine Compound Drops (Pediatric)
Carbinoxamine Compound Syrup
Carbofed DM Syrup
Carboptic
Cardec
Cardec DM Oral Drops
Cardene Capsules
Cardizem SR Capsules
Cascara Sagrada Tablets
Casec Powder
Cefadyl
Cefamandole Nafate
Cefazolin Sodium
Cefobid
Cefol Filmtab
Cefonicid Sodium
Cefotan
Cefzil
Celestone Phosphate Injection
Cenogen-OB Capsules
CenogenUltra
Cenolate
Centrum Jr. + Extra C
Centrum Jr. + Extra Calcium
Centrum Jr. + Iron
Cēpacol Dual Relief Spray Sore Throat & Cough
Cēpacol Sore Throat Dual Relief Spray
Cēpacol Sore Throat From Post Nasal Drip
Cēpacol Sore Throat Maximum Numbing
Cephadrine Oral
Cephalexin Hydrochloride Monohydrate
Cephapirin Sodium
Ceron-DM Drops
Ceron Oral Drops

Certagen Senior Tablets
Certa-Vite
Certa-Vite Golden
Cerumenex Drops (Solution)
Cetamide Ophthalmic Ointment
Ceta-Plus
Charcoal and Simethicone
Chardonna-2
Chemstrip bG
Chemstrip 8
Chemstrip 4 the OB
Chemstrip 6
Chemstrip uG
Chigger-Tox+
Children's Advil Chewable Tablets
Chloramphenicol
Chloresium Ointment
Chloresium Solution
Chloresium Tablets
Chlorex-A Tablets
Chlorex-A 12 Suspension
Chloromycetin Powder for Solution
Chloromycetin Sodium Succinate I.V.
Chloroptic S.O.P. Ointment
Chlorpheniramine Maleate/Phenylephrine
    Hydrochloride ER Capsules
Cholac
Choledyl SA Tablets
Chorex-5
Choron 10
Chromagen
Chroma-Pak
Ciclopirox Cream
Cidex Solution
Cinoxacin
Cipro XR
Citracal Creamy Bites
Citracal Liquitab
Claripel
Clean-N-Soak Solution
Clearplan Easy Kit
Clinacort Injection
Clindets
Clinistix Reagent Strips
Clinitest
Clofazimine
Codal-DH
Codeine Phosphate Solution
Codiclear DH
Codimal DH Syrup
Codimal PH
Colfed-A Capsules
Colfosceril Palmitate
Collastin Oil Free Moisturizer

Collyrium Fresh
ComBgen Tablets
Combiflex
Combiflex ES Tablets
Combipres
Combunox
Comfort Eye Drops
Compazine Injection
Compazine Spansules
Compazine Suppositories
Compazine Syrup
Compazine Tablets
Complete
Complete All-In-One
Complete Weekly Enzymatic Cleaner
Computer Eyes
Comtussin HC
Conceive Ovulation Predictor Cassettes
Confide Reagent Kit for HIV Blood Tests
Cordron-HC
Cordron-HC NR
Cortamox
Cortatrigen Ear
Cortatrigen Modified Ear Drops
Cortisporin Ophthalmic Suspension
Cortisporin Otic
Cortizone•5 Cream
Cotrim Pediatric
Cotuss EX
Cotuss HD
Cotuss MS
Coughtuss Liquid
Cough-X Lozenges
CP DEC
CP DEC-DM Drops
Creamy Tar Shampoo
Crolom
Crysti 1000
C-Tan D
Cuticura Medicated Shampoo
Cuticura Medicated Soap
Cyclocort
Cyklokapron Tablets
Cysto-Conray
Cysto-Conray II
Cystospaz-M Capsules
Cytadren
Cytosar-U Powder for Injection
Cytovene Capsules
Cytoxan
Cytoxan Lyophilized
Cytuss HC
Cytuss-HC NR
Dacriose

Dalalone DP
Danocrine Capsules
Dapiprazole Hydrochloride
Daranide
Darpaz
Darvocet A500
Darvocet-N 50
Darvocet-N 100
Darvon Compound 32
Darvon-N
Darvon Pulvules
Dayalets Filmtabs Tablets
Dazamide Tablets
Debrisan
Decadron Tablets
Decaject-L.A.
De-Chlor HC
De-Chlor MR
De-Chlor NX
Deconamine SR
Defen-LA Tablets
Defy
Degas
Degest 2
Delatest
Delcort Cream
Deltasone
Demadex Intravenous Solution
Demecarium Bromide
Demulen 1/50
Demulen 1/35
DentiPatch
depMedalone 80
depMedalone 40
Deponit Transdermal Patch
Depopred-80
Depopred-40
Dep-Test
Dermacoat Aerosol
Dermal-Rub Balm
Derma Viva Lotion
Desenex Antifungal, Maximum Strength
Desenex Max
Desenex Powder
Despec Drops
Desquam-E 5 Gel
Desquam-X 5
Desquam-X 10 Gel
Desyrel
Desyrel Dividose
Detussin
Dexacine Ophthalmic Ointment
Dexasol
Dexasone L.A. Injection

Dexedrine
Dexone LA
Dextran 75 Injection
Diabinese Tablets
Diamox Tablets
Diastix Reagent Strips
Diatrizoate Sodium 50%
Diazoxide, Parenteral
Dibent
Dical-D
Dicel
Dicel DM Suspension
Dichlorphenamide
Dicomal DH
Didronel IV Injection
Diethylcarbamazine Citrate
Diflucan Injection
Digitek Tablets
Dihistine DH
Dilacor XR
Dilantin Kapseals
Dilomine
Dilor Elixir
Dilor Injection
Diltiazem Hydrochloride Tablets
Dimaphen
Dinate
Diocto C
DiphenMax D
Diphtheria and Tetanus Toxoids, Acellular
    Pertussis, Haemophilus Influenzae
    Type B Conjugate Vaccine
Dipivefrin Hydrochloride Ophthalmic
    Solution
Di-Spaz
Ditropan Syrup
Ditropan Tablets
Diucardin Tablets
Diurigen
Diurigen w/Reserpine 500
Diurigen w/Reserpine 250
Diuril Sodium Intravenous
Diutensen-R
Dobutrex Injection
Dolobid
Dolorac
Dolsed
Donatussin DC
Dopar
Dostinex
Doxacurium Chloride
Dramamine, Children's
Dramamine Liquid
Dristan Fast Acting Formula

Drixomed Tablets
Drotic
DroTuss
Dry Eyes Solution
Dryvax
D-Test 100
D-Test 200
Duadacin Extra Strength Cold and Flu
    Tablets
DURAcare II
Duradrin
Duradryl JR Capsules
Durahist
Durahist D
Duraphen II
DuraTan DM
DuraTan Forte
DuraTan PE
Durathate-200 Injection
Duratuss AC 12 Tannate
Duratuss DM
Duratuss HD
Duratuss PE Tablets
Durese Tablets
Duricef
Dyclone
Dyclonine Hydrochloride
Dyline-GG Liquid
Dynabac
DynaCirc
Dynatuss DF
Dytan-CD Suspension
Dytan-D Chewable Tablets
Ear Drops
Ear-Eze
Econopred
Econopred Plus
Ed A-Hist Tablets
ED-TLC
ED Tuss HC
E.E.S. 200
Effervescent Potassium
Effexor
Efudex Occlusion Pack
Elixomin
Elixophyllin GG
Elixophyllin-KI
Embeline
Embeline E
EMLA Anesthetic Disc
EndaCof
EndaCof-DH
EndaCof DM
EndaCof-PD

EndaCof XP
Endagen-HD
Endal HD
Endal HD Plus
Endal (Nasal Decongestant) Tablets
Endrate Injection
Enduronyl
Enlon Injection
Enlon Plus
Entex HC
EntroEase
EntroEase Dry
Entuss
Enzymatic Cleaner for Extended Wear
Ephedrine Sulfate
Epifrin Solution
Epinal Solution
Epinephrine Hydrochloride Ophthalmic
    Solution
Epinephrine Hydrochloride Solution
Epinephryl Borate
Ergamisol Tablets
Eryc
Erygel Gel
Eryzole
Esclim Transdermal System
Esidrix Tablets
Eskalith Tablets
Estar Gel
Estrostep 21
Ethaquin
Ethatab
Ethaverine
Ethavex-100
EtheDent Chewable Tablets
Ethezyme
Ethezyme 830
Ethiodol
Ethmozine
ETH-Oxydose
Etrafon (2-10)
Eulexin Capsules
Exact Solution
Excedrin Aspirin Free
ExeClear-DM
Ex-Histine
Exna Tablets
Exocaine Plus
Exosurf Neonatal
Extendryl JR
Extendryl SR
Extra Strength Alenic Alka
Extra Strength Dynafed EX
Exubra

Eye Irrigating Wash
Factrel
Fansidar
FemBack Caplets
Femiron Multivitamin and Iron Tablets
Fem-1
Fentanyl Iontophoretic Transdermal System
Feostat Tablets, Chewable
Fer-Gen-Sol
Ferrex 150 Forte Plus
Ferumoxsil
Fe-Tinic 150
Flagyl IV
Flagyl IV RTU Injection
Flatulex Tablets
Fleet Phospho-Soda
Fleet Prep Kit 1
Fleet Prep Kit 2
Flexaphen
Flex-Care Especially for Sensitive Eyes
Flovent Aerosol
Flovent Diskus
Flovent Rotadisk
Floxin Injection
Fluorescein Sodium Ophthalmic Solution
Fluori-Methane Spray
Fluor-Op
Fluothane
Flu-Oxinate
Flurate
Flurosyn Ointment
FluTuss HC Liquid
Foamicon
Foille
Foille Plus
Fomivirsen Sodium
Fortovase
Foscavir
Fostril Lotion
4-Way Long Acting Nasal Spray
FreAmine III 8.5% w/Electrolytes
Fungizone Intravenous
Furacin Soluble Dressing Ointment
Furacin Topical Solution
Furoxane
Gamimune N Injection
Gammar-P I.V.
Gantrisin
Gantrisin Pediatric
Garamycin Injection
Garamycin Ointment
Garamycin Solution
Gas Permeable Daily Cleaner
GastroMARK

Genahist Tablets
Genapap, Children's Elixir
Genapap Extra Strength Tablets
Genapap Infants' Drops
Genasoft
Genebs
Genebs Extra Strength
GenESA
Geneye Extra
Geneye Ophthalmic Solution
Genoptic
Genoptic S.O.P.
Genotropin Powder for Injection
Genpril
Gentacidin
Gentex HC
Gentlax Tablets
Geocillin
Geref
Gerivite Tablets
Gevral Protein
GFN 550/PSE 60/DM 30
Gladase
Gladase-C
Glaucon Solution
Glutethimide
Glyceryl-T
Gonic
Gonioscopic
GP-500
Granul-Derm
Griseofulvin Microsize
Guaifenex G Tablets (Sustained-release)
Guaifenex LA Tablets (Extended-release)
Guanethidine Monosulfate
Guiatuss CF Syrup
Guiatuss PE Liquid
Gynol II Contraceptive
Haldol Decanoate 50
Halenol Children's
Halfan Tablets
Halofantrine Hydrochloride
Halog Cream
Halotestin Tablets
Halotussin AC Liquid
Halotussin DAC Syrup
Haltran
Hamamelis Water
Healon Yellow Solution
Hemotene
Hepatic-Aid II Instant Drink Powder
Hexadrol Phosphate
Hibiclens
Hibiclens Sponge Brush

HibTITER
Histacol DM Pediatric Syrup
Hista-Vent DA
Histex HC
Histinex-D
Histinex PV
Histolyn-CYL
Histussin D
Histussin HC
Hivid
HMS
Human Albumin Microspheres
Humibid DM Tablets
Humorsol
Humulin L
Humulin U
Hyate:C (Porcine)
Hycodan
Hycotuss Expectorant
Hydase
Hydeltrasol Injection
Hydergine LC Capsules
Hydergine LC Liquid
Hydex PD
Hydrap-ES
Hydrate
Hydrocet Capsules
Hydro Cobex Injection
Hydrocodone Bitartrate and Guaifenesin
Hydrocortone Phosphate Injection
Hydro-Crysti-12 Injection
Hydro-DP
HydroFed
Hydroflumethiazide
Hydro GP
Hydromal
Hydron CP Syrup
Hydron EX
Hydron KGS
Hydron PSC
Hydro-PC II
Hydro-Serp
Hydroserpine
Hydro-Tussin DM Liquid
Hydro-Tussin HC
Hydro-Tussin HD Liquid
Hydro-Tussin HG
Hydro-Tussin XP
Hydroxocobalamin Crystalline
Hydroxyethylcellulose
Hydroxyprogesterone Caproate in Oil
Hygroton
Hy-KXP
Hylaform

Hylorel Tablets
Hylutin Injection
Hypaque-Cysto
Hypaque Meglumine 60%
Hypaque Sodium
Hypaque Sodium 50%
Hyperstat IV Injection
Hyphed
HypoTears PF
Hytakerol Capsules
HyTan Suspension
Hytinic Capsules
Hytone Lotion
Hytuss
Hytuss 2X
Iberet
Iberet-500 Filmtab
Iberet-Folic-500 Filmtab
Icy Hot Stick
Ilotycin
Imovax Rabies I.D.
Imuran Injection
Inapsine
Inderide
Inderide LA Capsules
Indocin Capsules
Indocin SR
Indocin Suppositories
Indocyanine Green
Inflamase Forte
Inflamase Mild
Influenza A (H1N1) 2009 Monovalent
    Vaccine
Insulin Zinc (Pork)
Intrauterine Progesterone Contraceptive
    System
Intropin Injection
Inversine
Iodotope
Ionil-T Plus Shampoo
Ionsys
Iopanoic Acid Iodine
Iophylline
Iothalamate Meglumine
Iplex Injection
Iquix
Ircon-FA
Ismotic
Isoetharine Hydrochloride
Isordil Tembid Tablets
Isuprel Injection
Iveegam EN
J-Tan D HC Liquid
Kantrex Capsules

Kapectolin Suspension
Kay Ciel Liquid
Kay Ciel Packets
Keftab
Kemadrin Tablets
Kenaject-40
Kenalog-H
Keri Crème Cream
Keri Light Lotion
Keto-Diastix Reagent Strips
Ketostix Reagent Strips
Key-Plex Injection
Key-Pred 50
Key-Pred-SP
Key-Pred 25
K-Lease Capsules
Kleen-Handz
K-Lyte/Cl 25
K-Norm Capsules
Kolyum Liquid
Kovia 6.5
K-Pek
K + Care
K + Care ET
K + 8
K-Tan
K-Tan 4
Kuric
Kutapressin Injection
Kutrase
Ku-Zyme Capsules
Ku-Zyme HP Capsules
Kwelcof
LactiCare-HC
Lactinol-E Creme
Lactrex 12%
Lamprene
Lanoxicaps
Larodopa Tablets
LA-12
LC-65 Solution
Lens Drops
Lens Lubricant
Lens Plus Daily Cleaner
Lens Plus Rewetting Drops
Lente Iletin II Injection
Levall 5.0
Levamisole Hydrochloride
Levlen
Levlite
Levobetaxolol Hydrochloride
Levobupivacaine Hydrochloride
Levocabastine Hydrochloride Ophthalmic
    Suspension

Levo-Dromoran
Levomethadyl Acetate Hydrochloride
Lexxel Extended-Release Tablets
Librium Capsules
Librium Powder for Injection
Lidosense 4
Lid Wipes-SPF
Lipomul
Lipram
Lipram 4500 Delayed-Release Capsules
Lipram-PN16 Delayed-Release Capsules
Lipram-PN10 Delayed-Release Capsules
Lipram-PN20 Delayed-Release Capsules
LiQUADD
Liquibid-D 1200 Tablets
Liquifilm Tears
Liquifilm Wetting Solution
Liquiprin
Liver Derivative Complex
LiveTan DM
Livostin
Lobac Capsules
Lodine Capsules
Lodine XL Tablets
LoHist-PD Pediatric
Lomefloxacin Hydrochloride
Long Acting Neo-Synephrine II Nose Drops
    and Nasal Spray
Long Acting Neo-Synephrine II Vapor Spray
Loniten Tablets
Lorabid
Lorcet-HD
Lortab ASA
Lortab 2.5/500
Lortuss DM Liquid
Lortuss HC Liquid
Lozol
Lubriderm Bath Oil
Lubriderm Cream
Lucidex Tablets
Lufyllin Elixir
Lufyllin-GG Tablets
Lufyllin Injection
Lunelle Injection
Lupron
Maalox Antacid/Calcium Supplement
    Tablets, Chewable
Maalox Antacid Caplets
Maalox Antidiarrheal Tablets
Maalox Antigas Extra Strength Liquid
Maalox Extra Strength Suspension
Maalox Extra Strength Tablets
Maalox Maximum Strength Quick Dissolve
    Chewable Tablets

Maalox Plus Extra Strength Chewable Tablets
Maalox Plus Tablets
Maalox Quick Dissolve Chewable Tablets
Maalox Suspension
Maalox Tablets
Maalox TC Suspension
Maalox Therapeutic Concentrate Suspension
Mag-Cal Tablets
Mag-Caps Capsules
Maginex DS Powder
Maginex Tablets, Enteric-coated
Magnaprin
Magnaprin Arthritis Strength
Magsal
Mallamint Chewable Tablets
Mallazine Eye Drops
Maltsupex Liquid
Maltsupex Tablets
Mandol
Maolate
Maranox
Marax-DF Syrup
Marax Tab
Marcof Expectorant
Marlin Salt System
Maxaquin Tablets
Maxiflu G Tablets
Maximum Strength Allergy Drops
Maximum Strength Anbesol Gel
Maximum Strength Desenex Antifungal
Maxiphen G Tablets
Maxipime
Maxi-Tuss HCG
Maxi-Tuss HCX
Maxivate Lotion
Maxolon
MD-Gastroview Solution
Mecasermin Rinfabate
Meda Cap
Medacote
Meda Tab
MED-DM Tablets
Medent-DM
Medicone Ointment
Medicone Suppositories
Medigesic
Mediquell
Medroxyprogesterone Acetate/Estradiol Cypionate
Mefenamic Acid
Mefoxin
Megaton Elixir

Mellaril (all products)
Mandelamine Tablets
M-End Liquid
M-End Max Liquid
Meni-D
Mephentermine
Mephenytoin
Mercurochrome Solution
Mersol Tincture
Meruvax II
Mescolor Tablets
Mesoridazine Besylate
Mestinon Injection
Metahydrin Tablets
Metalone T.B.A.
Metaproterenol Sulfate Solution for Inhalation
Metaraminol Bitartrate
Metatensin
Methalgen
Methenamine Mandelate
Methitest Tablets
Methocarbamol Injection
Methoxyflurane
Methyclodine
Meticorten
Metoclopramide Intensol Concentrated Solution
Metreton Ophthalmic Solution
Miconazole 7
Micro-K LS
Micronase Tablets
microNefrin
Mini Two Way Action Tablets
Minizide
Minocin Powder for Injection
Mintezol
MiraSept Disinfecting Solution
MiraSept Rinse and Neutralizer
MiraSept Step 2
Mivacron
Moban
Mobigesic Tablets
Moctanin Infusion
Molypen
Monarc-M
Monistat-Derm Cream
Monistat-Derm Lotion
Mono-Chlor Liquid
Monochloroacetic Acid
Monocid
Monoctanoin
MouthKote P/R (all products)
MSTA Injection

M.T.E.-5
M.T.E.-5 Concentrated
M.T.E.-4
M.T.E.-4 Concentrated
M.T.E.-7
M.T.E.-6
M.T.E.-6 Concentrated
Mucomyst
Mucosil-10 Solution
Mucosil-20 Solution
Mudrane
Mudrane GG
Mudrane GG-2
MulTE-PAK-5
MulTE-PAK-4
Multistix SG Reagent Strips
Mumps Skin Test Allergen
Mumpsvax
Murocoll-2
Mutamycin
Mylanta Double Strength Liquid
Mylanta Double Strength Tablets
Mylanta Gas Chewable Tablets
Mylanta Lozenges
Mylanta Tablets
Mylocel Tablets
Mylotarg
Mytrex (all products)
Nafazair
Nalex DH Liquid
Nalex Expectorant
Nalmefene Hydrochloride
Naphazoline Plus
Naphcon Forte
Naqua Tablets
Narcan Injection
Nasarel
Nasofed
Nasop Orally Disintegrating Tablets
NatalCare Plus
Natalizumab
NataTab CFe
NataTab Rx
Natru-Vent
Naturetin
Nazarin
Nazarin HC
Nebcin Injection
Nebcin Powder for Injection
NegGram
Nembutal Elixir
NeoDecadron Ophthalmic Solution
Neo-Dexameth
Neo HC

Neoloid Emulsion
Neopap
Neosar Injection
Neosporin Ophthalmic Ointment
NeoStrata Skin Lightening
Neo-Synephrine
Neo-Synephrine 12-Hour
Nephro-Fer
Nephro-Vite + Fe Tablets
Netilmicin Sulfate
Neupro
Neutra-Phos-K Powder Packets
Neutra-Phos Powder Packets
Neutrexin
Nicomide
Nicosyn Lotion
Nilstat Cream
Nilstat Ointment
Nimotop Capsules
Nitrofurazone Ointment
Nitrofurazone Topical Solution
Nitroglyn Capsules
Nitrong Tablets
NitroQuick
NitroTab
Nizoral Tablets
N-Multistix Reagent Strips
N-Multistix SG
Nolahist Tablets
Nolvadex
Norel DM
Normodyne Injection
Norplant
Notuss-Forte
Novacet Lotion
Novamine 15%
Novasal Tablets
Novasus
Novocain Solution
NovoLog Mix 70/30 Injection
NPH Iletin II
Nucofed Expectorant
Nucofed Pediatric Expectorant
Nucofed Syrup
Numorphan
Numzident
Numzit Teething Gel
Nupercainal Cream
Nuprin
Nuprin Backache
Nuromax Injection
Nutropin Depot Injection
Octagam
Octamide PFS

Octicair
OcuClear
OcuCoat PF Solution
OcuCoat Solution
Ocupress Solution
Ocusert Pilo-40
Ocusert Pilo-20
Ocusulf-10
Ogen Tablets
Ogen Vaginal
OncoScint
Ony-Clear Solution
Ophthaine
Opti-Clean Solution
Opti-Clean II
Opti-Soft
Optison
Opti-Tears
Opti-Zyme Enzymatic Cleaner Especially for
    Sensitive Eyes
Orabase Gel
Orasone
Oretic Tablets
Organidin NR
Orinase
Orinase Diagnostic
ORLAAM
Ortho-Est
Or-Tyl
Orudis
Orudis KT Tablets
Oruvail
Osmoglyn
Otic-Care
Oti-Med
OtiTricin
Otobiotic Otic
Otocalm Ear
Otocort
Otomycin-HPN
Ovrette
OvuGen Kit
OvuKIT Self-Test Kit
OvuQuick Self-Test Kit
Oxacillin Sodium Oral Solution
Oxysept Disinfecting Solution
Oxysept Neutralizer Tablets
Oxysept 2
P_4E_1 Solution
P_1E_1 Solution
P_6E_1 Solution
P_2E_1 Solution
Pacis Powder for Suspension
Packer's Pine Tar

Pain-X
Palcaps 20
Palladone
Palmitate-A 5000
Pamelor Oral Solution
Panacet 5/500 Tablets
Panadol, Children's
Panafil
Panafil SE
Panalgesic Cream
Panasal 5/500 Tablets
Panasol-S
Panatuss DX Liquid
Pan C Ascorbate
Pancof-HC Syrup
Pancof PD Syrup
Pancrease
Pancrecarb MS-8
Pancrecarb MS-4
Pancrecarb MS-16
Pancrelipase Tablets
Pangestyme CN 10 Delayed-Release
    Capsules
Pangestyme CN 20 Delayed-Release
    Capsules
Pangestyme EC Delayed-Release Capsules
Pangestyme MT 16 Delayed-Release
    Capsules
Pangestyme UL 18 Delayed-Release
    Capsules
Pangestyme UL 12 Delayed-Release
    Capsules
Pangestyme UL 20 Delayed-Release
    Capsules
Panlor SS
Pannaz
Pannaz S
Panocaps
Panocaps MT 16
Panocaps MT 20
Panokase Tablets
PanOxyl 5
PanOxyl 10
PAN-2400
Papain-Urea-Chlorophyllin
Papfyll
Pap-Urea Ointment
Paraldehyde
Paral Liquid
Paraplatin
Paredrine
PCM Allergy
PD-Cof Drops
PD-Cof Syrup

PD-Hist • D
Pedameth Liquid
Pediaflor Fluoride Drops
PediaTan
PediaTan D
Pediatric Bear-E-Bag
Pediatric Triban
Pediazole Granules for Oral Suspension
Pedi-Boro Soak Paks
Pediotic
Pemoline
Pentobarbital Sodium Capsules
Pentothal Injection
Pepcid Injection
Perchloracap
Percodan-Demi
Perdiem Overnight Relief
Periactin
Permax
Perphenazine Oral Concentrate
Persantine IV
Pfizerpen Injection
PhenaVent Capsules
PhenaVent LA
PhenaVent PED
Phenerbel-S
Phenergan Suppositories
Phenindamine Tartrate
Phenoptic
Phenyl-T Oral Suspension
pHisoDerm Cleansing Bar
Phosphocol P 32
Phrenilin
Pilocar
Pilocarpine and Epinephrine Solutions
    (Ophthalmic Agents for Glaucoma)
Pipecuronium Bromide
Pitressin Injection
Plaquenil
Plaretase 8000
Platinol-AQ Injection
Plenaxis Powder for Injection
Plendil Extended-Release Tablets
Pneumotussin 2.5 Cough
Pnu-Imune 23 Injection
Polocaine With Levonordefrin Injection
Polycitra-K Solution
Polycitra-LC Oral Solution
Polycitra Syrup
Polygam S/D
Poly-Hist HC
Poly-Histine
Polymyxin B Ophthalmic
Polymyxin B Sulfate Sterile Powder for
    Solution

Polysorb Hydrate
Polysporin Ophthalmic
Polysporin Ointment
Polysporin Powder
Poly Tan D
Polythiazide Potassium Perchlorate
Poly-Tussin HD
Poly-Tussin XP
Polyvitamins w/Fluoride 0.5 mg and Iron
Potassium Perchlorate
Pramoxine HC
Pravigard PAC
Predalone 50 Injection
Predcor-50
Prednicen-M
Prednisol
Prednisol TBA
Prefrin Liquifilm
Pre-Hist-D
Prelone Syrup
PremesisRx
Prenatal-H Capsules
Prenatal MR 90
Prenatal-1 + Iron
Prenatal Plus Improved
Prenatal Plus w/Betacarotene
Prenatal Rx 1
Prenatal Z Advanced Formula
Prenate GT Tablets
Pre-Pen
Pretz-D Solution
Prevacid IV
Prevacid NapraPAC 500
Prevacid NapraPAC 375
Preven
Primacor Injection
Pro-Banthine
Procainamide Hydrochloride Capsules
Procainamide Hydrochloride Extended-
    Release Tablets
Procaine Hydrochloride Solution
Procanbid
Prochieve
ProctoFoam
Procyclidine
Profasi
Pro-Fast SA Tablets
Profenal
ProFree/GP Weekly Enzymatic Cleaner
Progestasert Intrauterine System
Prolex DH
Prolixin Decanoate
Promit
ProMod Powder

Pronestyl
Propine Sterile Ophthalmic
Proplex T Injection
Pro-Red
ProSom
Protirelin
Protropin Powder for Injection
Protuss-D Liquid
Protuss DM Tablets
Protuss Liquid
Proventil Aerosol
Proventil Repetabs Tablets
Proventil Tablets
Pseudovent Capsules
Pseudovent-PED Capsules
Psoriatec
PsoriGel Gel
P-Tanna 12 Suspension
P-Tann D Suspension
P.T.E.-5
P.T.E.-4
Pulmicort Turbuhaler
Puralube Ophthalmic Ointment
Purge Liquid (castor oil)
P-V-Tussin Syrup
P-V-Tussin Tablets
Pyrelle H.B.
Pyridiate
QTest Ovulation Kit
Q-Tussin CF Liquid
Quadra-Hist D
Quadra-Hist D PED
Quad Tann Pediatric Oral Suspension
Qualaquin
Qual-Tussin DC
Qual-Tussin Pediatric Oral Solution Drops
Quibron
Quibron-T Dividose
Quibron-300
Quibron-T/SR Dividose
Quick CARE Disinfecting Solution
Quick CARE Rinse and Neutralizer
Quinidex Extentabs Tablets
Raptiva
Rauzide
Rebetron
RE DCP
Redness Reliever
Redur-PCM
Redutemp
Regular Iletin II Injection
Regular Insulin (Pork)
Regulax SS
Relacon-HC NR

Relafen
Relasin-HC
Relefact RTH
Relief Ophthalmic Solution
Renacidin
RenAmin
Renese-R
Renese Tablets
Reno-Dip
Reno-60
Reno-30
ReNu Effervescent Enzymatic Cleaner
ReNu Thermal Enzymatic Cleaner
Replens Gel
Repliva 21/7
Rescula Solution
Resectisol
Respbid Tablets
Respi-Tann G Suspension
Retin-A Solution
Revex
Rēv-Eyes Lyophilized Powder
Rexolate
R-Gel
Rheaban Maximum Strength Tablets
Ridenol
RID Mousse
Rinade-B.I.D. Capsules
Rindal HD Plus Syrup
Rindal HPD Syrup
Riopan
Ritodrine Hydrochloride
Robitussin Cough & Allergy
Rofecoxib
Roferon-A
Rondec
Rondec DM Drops
Rondex
Rosac
Rosets
Rosula Cleanser
R-Tannic-S A/D Suspension
Rubella and Mumps Virus Vaccine, Live
Rulox #1 Tablets
Rulox #2 Tablets
Rum-K
Ryna-C Liquid
Ryna Liquid
Ryna-12 S
Ryneze
Sal-Acid
Salutensin
Salutensin-Demi
SecreFlo Intravenous Solution

Sele-Pak
Selepen
Senna Concentrate
Septi-Soft
Septisol
Septocaine Injection
Septra
Septra IV
Ser-Ap-Es
Serax
Serentil Tablets
Sermorelin Acetate
Servira
Serzone Tablets
SFC
Silfedrine, Children's
Silver Nitrate
Simethicone-Coated Cellulose Suspension
Simuc-HD
Simuc Sustained-Release Tablets
Sinequan Oral Concentrate
Sinutab Sinus Allergy, Maximum Strength
Skelaxin Tablets
Slo-Phyllin GG Capsules
Slo-Phyllin GG Syrup
Slo-Phyllin Gyrocaps Capsules
Slow-K Tablets
SLT Lotion
Sno Strips Test
Soac-Lens Solution
Sodium Bicarbonate and Tartaric Acid
Sodium Bicarbonate Injection
Sodium Hyaluronate and Fluorescein
    Sodium
Sodium Phosphate P 32 Injection
Sodium Thiosalicylate
Sofenol 5 Lotion
Solagé
Solganal Injection
Solotuss Suspension
Soltamox
Solurex
Solurex LA
Soluvite-F Drops
Soma Compound
Soma Compound w/Codeine
Somatrem
SonoRx
Soothe Solution
Sorbitrate Chewable Tablets
Sorbitrate Sublingual Tablets
Sorbitrate Tablets
Soriatane CK
Sparfloxacin

Spectinomycin
Spectrocin Plus Ointment
Spherulin
Stadol NS Solution
Statuss Green
Stay-Wet 4
Stay-Wet 3
Sterapred
Sterapred DS
Sterapred-Unipak
SteriNail
Strema
Streptase
Sublimaze
Suby's Solution G
Succus Cineraria Maritima Solution
Sudafed Children's Non-Drowsy Cold &
    Cough
Sudafed PE Quick-Dissolve Strips
Sudafed Sinus & Cold Non-Drowsy
Sudal 60/500 Tablets
Sudex
Sudodrin
Sulfinpyrazone
Sulfoil Liquid
Sulfoxyl Strong
Sulster Solution
SulZee
Summer's Eve Anti-Itch
Super Flavons
Super Flavons 300
Supprelin Injections
Suprax Tablets
Susano Elixir
Sustaire Tablets
Su-Tuss DM
Su-Tuss HD
Swim-Ear Liquid
Synagis Lyophilized Powder For Injection
Synalar
Synalar-HP Cream
Synophylate-GG
Syntest DS Tablets
Syntest HS Tablets
Synthroid Powder for Injection
Tac-40
Talwin Compound Tablets
Talwin NX
TanDur DM
Tannate DMP-DEX
Tannate 12 S
Tannate-V-DM
Tavist ND
TearGard

Teargen
Teargen II
Tears Renewed
Teczem
Tedrigen
Tempra
Tencon Capsules
Tensilon
Tequin
Terramycin
Teslac
Teslascan
Tesone
Tesone L.A.
Testoderm Transdermal System
Testoject
Testred Cypionate 200
Testrin-P.A.
Tetanus Toxoid, Adsorbed
Tetanus Toxoid, Adsorbed, Purogenated
Tetanus Toxoid Injection
Tetracycline Hydrochloride Fiber
Tetrasine
Tetrasine Extra
T-Gen
Thalitone Tablets
Theobid Duracaps Capsules
Theoclear-80 Syrup
Theoclear L.A. Capsules
Theodrine
Theo-Dur
Theolair Solution
Theolair S.R. Tablets
Theolate
Theomax DF
Theo-Sav Tablets
Theovent Capsules
Theo-X Tablets
Therac Lotion
Theraflu Daytime Severe Cold Packets
Theraflu Nighttime Severe Cold Powder
Theragran-M Caplets
Therapeutic B Complex with Vitamin C
Thiethylperazine Mesylate
Thorazine
Thrombogen
Thypinone
Thyrel TRH
Tibamine LA
Ticarcillin Disodium
Ticar Powder for Injection
Tilade
Timolide 10-25
TI-Screen SPF 15 Lotion

TI-Screen SPF 30 Lotion
Titan
Tocainide Hydrochloride
Tolazoline Hydrochloride
Tolectin DS Capsules
Tolectin 600
Tolectin 200
Tolinase Tablets
Tonocard Tablets
Toothache Gel
Toradol
Torecan Injection
Tornalate
Torsemide
Total Solution
Touro Allergy Tablets
Touro EX Tablets
Trac Tabs 2X
Tramadol Hydrochloride Tablets
Trandate Injection
Tranxene-SD
Tranxene-SD Half Strength
TraumaCal
Travasol 5.5%
Travasol 3.5% w/Electrolytes
Travatan
Trellium Plus Tablets
Triamcinolone Diacetate
Triaminic Cold & Allergy
Triamonide 40
Triant-HC
Triavil Tablets
Triban
Trichlormethiazide
Tricodene Cough and Cold
Tridesilon
Tridil Injection
TriHIBit Injection
Tri-Kort
Tri-Levlen
Trilog
Trilone Injection
Tri-Lo-Sprintec
Trimazide
Trimethaphan Camsylate
Trinalin Repetabs Tablets
Tri-Otic
Triplex AD
Tri Vit w/Fluoride
Trizivir
Trobicin Powder for Injection
Trovafloxacin Mesylate/Alatrofloxacin
    Mesylate
Trovan

T-Stat Pads
T-Stat Solution
Tubocurarine Chloride Injection
Tucks Clear Gel
Tucks Pads
Tusana-D
Tusdec-HC
Tusnel-HC Liquid
Tussafed HC
Tussafed-HCG
Tussafed-LA
Tuss-DM Tablets
Tussex Cough Syrup
Tussiden DM
Tussi-Organidin-DM NR Liquid
Tussi-Organidin-S NR Liquid
Tussizone-12 RF Tablets
Tusso-HC
Tuss-Tan
Tuss-Tan Pediatric
Twin-K
Tympagesic
Tysabri Injection
UAD Otic
Ultra Derm Bath Oil
Ultra Derm Lotion
Ultralytic 2
Ultrase
Ultrase MT 18
Ultrase MT 12
Ultrase MT 20
Ultra Tears
Unibase
Uni-Tex 120/10 ER
Unoprostone Isopropyl
Urealac
Ureaphil
Uridon Modified
Urised
UriSym
Urolene Blue
Vaginex Cream
Valdecoxib
Valrubicin
Valstar Solution
Vantin Granules for Suspension
Vaprisol
Varicella-Zoster Immune Globulin (Human)
Vascor Tablets
VasoClear
Vasocon Regular
Vasosulf Solution
VasoTuss HC Tannate Suspension
Veetids

Velosulin BR (rDNA) Injection
Venoglobulin-S Powder for Injection
Versed Injection
Versed Syrup
Vesanoid
Viactiv Calcium Flavor Glides
Viadur
Vibramycin Capsules
Vicam Injection
Vicon-C
Vidarabine
Vigortol
Viokase 8
Viokase 16
Viokase Powder
Vioxx Suspension
Vioxx Tablets
Vira-A Ointment
Viravan-S
Virilon IM Injection
Visine Allergy Relief
Visine Moisturizing
Vision Care Enzymatic Cleaner
Vision Clear
Visual-Eyes
Vitelle Nestrex
Vitussin
VoSol-HC Solution
VoSol Solution
V-Tann Suspension
WellTuss HC Liquid
Wet-N-Soak
Wet-N-Soak Plus
Wetting Solution
WHF Lubricating Gel
Wigraine Tablets
Wyamine Sulfate
Wygesic Tablets
Xedec Tablets
Xedec II Tablets
X-Prep Bowel Evacuant Kit-1
X-Prep Liquid
Xylocaine Jelly
Xylocaine Viscous
Yeast-Gard
Your Choice Non-Preserved Saline Solution
Your Choice Sterile Preserved Saline
    Solution
Yutopar Injection
Zagam
Zazole
Z-Cof HCX
Zelnorm
Zenapax

Zerit XR Capsules
Zetacet
Zetacet Wash
Zinca-Pak
Zincfrin
Zingo Intradermal Injection

Ziox 405
ZNP Bar Soap
Zostrix Neuropathy
Zovirax Powder for Injection, Lyophilized
ZTuss Expectorant
Zymine HC

Common Abbreviations of Chemotherapy Regimens

5 + 2
Use: Acute myelogenous leukemia (AML; reinduction). *Cycle:* 7 days. Regimen given once after an induction regimen has been used.
Regimen: Cytarabine 100 to 200 mg/m^2/day continuous IV infusion, days 1 through 5
with
Daunorubicin 45 mg/m^2/day IV, days 1 and 2
or
Mitoxantrone 12 mg/m^2/day IV, days 1 and 2

---

7 + 3
Use: Acute myelogenous leukemia (AML; induction). *Cycle:* 7 days. Give 1 cycle only.
Regimen: Cytarabine 100 to 200 mg/m^2/day continuous IV infusion, days 1 through 7
with
Daunorubicin 30 or 45 mg/m^2/day IV, days 1 through 3
or
Idarubicin 12 mg/m^2/day IV, days 1 through 3
or
Mitoxantrone 12 mg/m^2/day IV, days 1 through 3

---

7 + 3 + 7
Use: Acute myelogenous leukemia (AML; induction—adults).
Cycle: 21 days. Give 1 cycle. If patient has persistent leukemia at day 21, give 1 to 2 additional cycles.
Regimen: Cytarabine 100 mg/m^2/day continuous IV infusion, days 1 through 7
Daunorubicin 50 mg/m^2/day IV, days 1 through 3
Etoposide 75 mg/m^2/day IV, days 1 through 7

"8 in 1"
Use: Brain tumors (pediatrics). *Cycle:* 14 days
Regimen: Methylprednisolone 300 mg/m^2/dose PO every 6 hours for 3 doses, day 1, starting at hour 0
Vincristine 1.5 mg/m^2 (2 mg maximum dose) IV, day 1, hour 0
Lomustine 100 mg/m^2 PO, day 1, hour 0
Procarbazine 75 mg/m^2 PO, day 1, hour 1
Hydroxyurea 3,000 mg/m^2 PO, day 1, hour 2
Cisplatin 90 mg/m^2 IV, day 1, starting at hour 3 (6-hour infusion)
Cytarabine 300 mg/m^2 IV, day 1, hour 9
Dacarbazine 150 mg/m^2 IV, day 1, hour 12

ABV
Use: Kaposi sarcoma. *Cycle:* 28 days
Regimen: Doxorubicin 40 mg/m^2 IV, day 1
Bleomycin 15 units IV, days 1 and 15
Vinblastine 6 mg/m^2 IV, day 1

Use: Kaposi sarcoma. *Cycle:* 28 days, continue until disease progression or intolerable toxicity
Regimen: Doxorubicin 10 mg/m^2 IV, days 1 and 15
Bleomycin 15 units IV, days 1 and 15
Vincristine 1 mg (dose is not in mg/m^2) IV, days 1 and 15

---

continued on next page

ABV (cont.)

Use: Kaposi sarcoma. *Cycle:* 28 days for up to 6 cycles
Regimen: Doxorubicin 20 mg/m^2 IV, days 1 and 15
 Bleomycin 10 units/m^2 IV, days 1 and 15
 Vincristine 1 mg (dose is not in mg/m^2) IV, days 1 and 15

ABVD

Use: Lymphoma (Hodgkin). *Cycle:* 28 days for up to 6 cycles
Regimen: Doxorubicin 25 mg/m^2 IV, days 1 and 15
 Bleomycin 10 units/m^2 IV, days 1 and 15
 Vinblastine 6 mg/m^2 IV, days 1 and 15
 with
 Dacarbazine 375 mg/m^2 IV, days 1 and 15
 or
 Dacarbazine 150 mg/m^2/day IV, days 1 through 5

AC (CY/A)

Use: Breast cancer. *Cycle:* 21 days for up to 4 cycles
Regimen: Doxorubicin 60 mg/m^2 IV, day 1
 Cyclophosphamide 600 mg/m^2 IV, day 1

Use: Sarcoma (bone). *Cycle:* 21 to 28 days for up to 6 cycles
Regimen: Doxorubicin 30 mg/m^2/day continuous IV infusion, days 1 through 3
 Cisplatin 100 mg/m^2 IV, day 4

Use: Sarcoma (bone). *Cycle:* 21 days for 6 cycles
Regimen: Doxorubicin 25 mg/m^2/day IV, days 1 through 3
 Cisplatin 100 mg/m^2 IV, day 1

Use: Neuroblastoma (pediatrics). *Cycle:* 21 to 28 days for up to 5 cycles
Regimen: Cyclophosphamide 150 mg/m^2/day PO, days 1 through 7
 Doxorubicin 35 mg/m^2 IV, day 8

Use: Endometrial cancer. *Cycle:* 21 days for up to 8 cycles
Regimen: Doxorubicin 60 mg/m^2 IV, day 1
 Cyclophosphamide 500 mg/m^2 IV, day 1

AC/Docetaxel, Sequential

Use: Breast cancer. *Cycle:* 21 days
Regimen: Give 4 cycles of AC regimen for breast cancer
 followed by
 Docetaxel 100 mg/m^2 IV, day 1 for 4 cycles

AC/Paclitaxel, Dose Dense

Use: Breast cancer. *Cycle:* 14 days. Give 4 cycles of Treatment A, followed by 4 cycles of Treatment B.
Regimen: **Treatment A** (cycles 1 through 4)
  Doxorubicin 60 mg/m^2 IV, day 1
  Cyclophosphamide 600 mg/m^2 IV, day 1
  Filgrastim 5 mcg/kg/day subcutaneously (rounded to 300 or 480 mcg), days 3 through 10
 Treatment B (cycles 5 through 8)
  Paclitaxel 175 mg/m^2 IV over 3 hours, day 1 for 4 cycles
  Filgrastim 5 mcg/kg/day subcutaneously (rounded to 300 or 480 mcg), days 3 through 10

AC/Paclitaxel, Sequential
Use: Breast cancer. *Cycle:* 21 days
Regimen: Give 4 cycles of AC regimen for breast cancer
             followed by
             Paclitaxel 175 mg/m^2 IV over 3 hours, day 1 for 4 cycles

AC/Paclitaxel + Trastuzumab, Sequential
Use: Breast cancer. *Cycle:* 21 days
Regimen: Give 4 cycles of AC regimen for breast cancer
             followed by
             Trastuzumab 4 mg/kg IV, day 1 for first week only (loading dose);
               then trastuzumab 2 mg/kg IV, day 1 of each week for 51 weeks
               (52 weeks total)
             with
             Paclitaxel 175 mg/m^2 IV over 3 hours, every 3 weeks for 12 weeks
             or
             Paclitaxel 80 mg/m^2 IV, day 1 of each week for 12 weeks

ACE (CAE)
Use: Lung cancer (small cell). *Cycle:* 21 to 28 days
Regimen: Doxorubicin 45 mg/m^2 IV, day 1
             Cyclophosphamide 1,000 mg/m^2 IV, day 1
             Etoposide 50 mg/m^2/day IV, days 1 through 5

ACe
Use: Breast cancer. *Cycle:* 21 to 28 days
Regimen: Doxorubicin 40 mg/m^2 IV, day 1
             Cyclophosphamide 200 mg/m^2/day PO, days 3 through 6

AD
Use: Sarcoma (bone, soft tissue). *Cycle:* 21 days
Regimen 1: Patients younger than 65 years of age, or patients without extensive prior radiation therapy:
               Doxorubicin 60 mg/m^2 IV, day 1
               Dacarbazine 250 mg/m^2/day IV, days 1 through 5
Regimen 2: Patients 65 years of age and older, or patients with extensive prior radiation therapy:
               Doxorubicin 45 mg/m^2 IV, day 1
               Dacarbazine 200 mg/m^2/day IV, days 1 through 5

Use: Sarcoma (bone, soft tissue). *Cycle:* 21 days
Regimen: Doxorubicin 15 mg/m^2/day continuous IV infusion, days 1 through 4
             Dacarbazine 250 mg/m^2/day continuous IV infusion, days 1 through 4

ADOC
Use: Thymoma. *Cycle:* 21 to 28 days, delay subsequent cycles until hematologic recovery
Regimen: Doxorubicin 40 mg/m^2 IV, day 1
             Cisplatin 50 mg/m^2 IV, day 1
             Vincristine 0.6 mg/m^2 IV, day 3
             Cyclophosphamide 700 mg/m^2 IV, day 4

Advanced Stage Burkitt or B-Cell ALL Pediatric Protocol (SNCCL/B-ALL)

Use: Lymphoma (Burkitt or B-cell ALL—pediatrics). *Cycle:* 18 to 25 days, based on hematologic recovery. Give Treatment A, then follow with Treatment B after hematologic recovery; repeat alternating treatments a total of 4 times over 5 to 6 months.

Regimen: **Treatment A**

Methotrexate 10 mg/m^2 intrathecal, hours 0 and 72 for first cycle; then hour 0 only of subsequent cycles

Cytarabine 50 mg/m^2 intrathecal, hours 0 and 72 for first cycle; then hour 0 only of subsequent cycles

Cyclophosphamide 300 mg/m^2/dose IV, every 12 hours for 6 doses, given at hours 0, 12, 24, 36, 48, and 60

Vincristine 1.5 mg/m^2 IV, hour 72 (first cycle only: give an additional dose at day 11)

Doxorubicin 50 mg/m^2 IV, hour 72

Treatment B (give after hematologic recovery)

Methotrexate 12 mg/m^2 intrathecal, hour 0

Methotrexate 200 mg/m^2 IV, hour 0 (on day 1)

then

Methotrexate 800 mg/m^2/day continuous IV infusion over 24 hours, begin hour 0 (on day 1)

Cytarabine 50 mg/m^2 intrathecal, hour 24 (on day 2, give at end of methotrexate infusion)

Cytarabine 200 mg/m^2/day continuous IV infusion, days 2 and 3 for first cycle. Increase to 400 mg/m^2/day continuous IV infusion, days 2 and 3 for second cycle; 800 mg/m^2/day continuous IV infusion, days 2 and 3 for third cycle; and 1,600 mg/m^2/day continuous IV infusion, days 2 and 3 for final cycle.

Leucovorin 30 mg/m^2/dose IV, every 6 hours for 2 doses at hours 36 and 42

then

Leucovorin 3 mg/m^2/dose IV, every 12 hours for 3 doses at hours 54, 66, and 78

Use: Lymphoma (Burkitt or B-cell ALL—pediatrics). *Cycle:* Repeat based on hematologic recovery. Give Treatment A, then follow with Treatment B after hematologic recovery; repeat alternating treatments a total of 3 times over 4 to 6 months.

Regimen: **Treatment A**

Cyclophosphamide 300 mg/m^2/dose IV, every 12 hours for 6 doses, given at hours 0, 12, 24, 36, 48, and 60

Cytarabine 50 mg/m^2 (50 mg maximum dose) intrathecal, days 1, 2, and 11

Doxorubicin 50 mg/m^2 IV, day 4

Vincristine 1.5 mg/m^2 (2 mg maximum dose) IV, days 4 and 11

Methotrexate 12 mg/m^2 (12 mg maximum dose) intrathecal, days 4 and 11

Filgrastim 10 mcg/kg/day IV or subcutaneously, from day 5 until the absolute neutrophil count (ANC) is at least 1,500 cells/mm^3 for at least 2 days

continued on next page

Advanced Stage Burkitt or B-Cell ALL Pediatric Protocol (SNCCL/B-ALL)
(cont.) **Treatment B** (give after hematologic recovery)
Methotrexate 12 mg/m² (12 mg maximum dose) intrathecal, hour 0
Methotrexate 200 mg/m² IV, hour 0 (on day 1)
then
Methotrexate 800 mg/m²/day continuous IV infusion over 24 hours, begin hour 0 (on day 1)
Cytarabine 3,000 mg/m²/dose IV, every 12 hours for 4 doses, days 2 and 3
Leucovorin 30 mg/m²/dose IV for 1 dose, hour 42
then
Leucovorin 3 mg/m²/dose IV, every 12 hours for 3 doses at hours 54, 66, and 78
Filgrastim 10 mcg/kg/day IV or subcutaneously, from day 5 until the ANC is at least 1,500 cells/mm³ for at least 2 days

---

AIDA
Use: Acute promyelocytic leukemia (APL; induction). *Cycle:* Give a single induction cycle
Regimen 1: Patients 20 years of age and younger:
Tretinoin 25 mg/m²/day PO, days 1 through 90, or until complete remission, whichever occurs earlier
Idarubicin 12 mg/m² IV, days 2, 4, 6, and 8
Regimen 2: Patients older than 20 years of age:
Tretinoin 45 mg/m²/day PO, days 1 through 90, or until complete remission, whichever occurs earlier
Idarubicin 12 mg/m² IV, days 2, 4, 6, and 8

AP
Use: Ovarian cancer, endometrial cancer. *Cycle:* 21 to 28 days for up to 8 cycles
Regimen: Doxorubicin 50 to 60 mg/m² IV, day 1; consider decreasing initial dose by 25% in patients with radiation therapy during 6 months prior to chemotherapy
Cisplatin 50 to 60 mg/m² IV, day 1

Use: Mesothelioma. *Cycle:* 21 to 28 days for up to 8 cycles
Regimen: Doxorubicin 60 mg/m² IV, day 1
Cisplatin 60 mg/m² IV, day 1

Use: Thyroid cancer. *Cycle:* 21 days
Regimen 1: Patients without extensive prior radiation therapy:
Doxorubicin 60 mg/m² IV, day 1
Cisplatin 40 mg/m² IV, day 1
Regimen 2: Patients with extensive prior radiation therapy:
Doxorubicin 45 mg/m² IV, day 1
Cisplatin 40 mg/m² IV, day 1

Ara-C-DNR
Use: Acute myelogenous leukemia (AML). *Cycle:* 14 days. Give 1 cycle. If patient has persistent leukemia on day 14, give 1 to 2 additional cycles as described below.
Regimen: Cytarabine 100 mg/m²/day continuous IV infusion, days 1 through 7
Daunorubicin 30 or 45 mg/m²/day IV, days 1 through 3
If leukemia is persistent on day 14, additional doses are given: cytarabine on days 1 through 5 and daunorubicin on days 1 and 2, both at same dose as previous cycle.

Ara-C-Doxorubicin

Use:	Acute myelogenous leukemia (AML; induction). *Cycle:* 14 days. Give 1 cycle. If patient has persistent leukemia on day 14, give 1 to 2 additional cycles as described below.
Regimen:	Cytarabine 100 mg/m²/day continuous IV infusion, days 1 through 7
	Doxorubicin 30 mg/m²/day IV, days 1 through 3
	If leukemia is persistent on day 14, additional doses are given: cytarabine on days 1 through 5 and doxorubicin on days 1 and 2, both at same dose as previous cycle.

AT (also see Docetaxel-Doxorubicin)

Use:	Breast cancer. *Cycle:* 21 days for up to 8 cycles
Regimen:	Doxorubicin 50 mg/m² IV, day 1
	Paclitaxel 220 mg/m² IV over 3 hours, day 2 (given 24 hours after doxorubicin)

Use:	Breast cancer. *Cycle:* 21 days for up to 8 cycles
Regimen:	Doxorubicin 50 mg/m² IV, day 1
	Paclitaxel 150 mg/m² continuous IV infusion over 24 hours, day 1 (start 3 hours after doxorubicin)
	Filgrastim 5 mcg/kg/day subcutaneously, from day 3 until neutropenia resolves (start 24 hours after completing paclitaxel infusion)

Use:	Endometrial cancer. *Cycle:* 21 days for up to 7 cycles
Regimen 1:	Patients aged 65 years and younger, or patients with no prior pelvic radiation therapy:
	Doxorubicin 50 mg/m² IV, day 1
	Paclitaxel 150 mg/m² continuous IV infusion over 24 hours, day 1 (start 4 hours after doxorubicin)
	Filgrastim 5 mcg/kg/day subcutaneously, days 3 through 12 or until white blood cell count (WBC) is at least 10,000 cells/mm³
Regimen 2:	Patients older than 65 years of age, or patients with prior pelvic radiation therapy:
	Doxorubicin 40 mg/m² IV, day 1
	Paclitaxel 120 mg/m² continuous IV infusion over 24 hours, day 1 (start 4 hours after doxorubicin)
	Filgrastim 5 mcg/kg/day subcutaneously, days 3 through 12 or until WBC is at least 10,000 cells/mm³

ATC, Sequential, Dose Dense

Use:	Breast cancer. *Cycle:* 14 days. Give 4 cycles of Treatment A, followed by 4 cycles of Treatment B, followed by 4 cycles of Treatment C.
Regimen:	**Treatment A** (cycles 1 through 4)
	Doxorubicin 60 mg/m² IV, day 1
	Filgrastim 5 mcg/kg/day subcutaneously (rounded to 300 or 480 mcg), days 3 through 10
	Treatment B (cycles 5 through 8)
	Paclitaxel 175 mg/m² IV, over 3 hours, day 1 for 4 cycles
	Filgrastim 5 mcg/kg/day subcutaneously (rounded to 300 or 480 mcg), days 3 through 10
	Treatment C (cycles 9 through 10)
	Cyclophosphamide 600 mg/m² IV, day 1
	Filgrastim 5 mcg/kg/day subcutaneously (rounded to 300 or 480 mcg), days 3 through 10

ATRA-Arsenic
Use: Acute promyelocytic leukemia (APL; induction and consolidation).
   Cycle: Give 1 induction cycle followed by 1 consolidation cycle after hematologic recovery

Regimen: **Induction.** *Cycle:* 85 days. Give 1 cycle.
   Tretinoin 22.5 mg/m^2/dose (45 mg/m^2/day) PO twice daily, days 1 through 85, or until complete remission, whichever occurs earlier
   Arsenic trioxide 0.15 mg/kg/day IV, days 10 through 85

Consolidation. *Cycle:* 28 weeks. Give 1 cycle.
   Tretinoin 22.5 mg/m^2/dose (45 mg/m^2/day) PO twice daily, give for 2 weeks followed by 2 weeks of rest, on days 1 through 14, days 29 through 42, days 57 through 70, days 85 through 98, days 113 through 126, days 141 through 154, and days 169 through 182
   Arsenic trioxide 0.15 mg/kg/day IV, for 5 days each week (ie, Monday through Friday), give every other month through week 28, on days 1 through 28, days 57 through 84, days 113 through 140, and days 169 through 196

ATRA + CT—see DA + ATRA

Augmented BFM
Use: Acute lymphocytic leukemia (ALL; consolidation and intensification—pediatrics).

Regimen: **Consolidation.** *Cycle:* 9 weeks. Give a single cycle.
   Cyclophosphamide 1,000 mg/m^2/day IV, days 1 and 29
   Cytarabine 75 mg/m^2/day IV or subcutaneously, days 2 through 5, days 9 through 12, days 30 through 33, and days 37 through 40
   Mercaptopurine 60 mg/m^2/day PO, days 1 through 14 and days 29 through 42
   Vincristine* 1.5 mg/m^2 IV, days 15, 22, 43, and 50
   Asparaginase 6,000 units/m^2/dose IM, days 15, 17, 19, 22, 24, 26, 43, 45, 47, 50, 52, and 54
   Methotrexate intrathecal (dose is based on patient's age, as shown below)[†]:
   Patients without CNS involvement at diagnosis: Give on days 2, 9, 16, and 23
   Patients with CNS involvement at diagnosis: Give on days 2 and 9
   used in conjunction with
   Radiation therapy

Interim Maintenance I. *Cycle:* 8 weeks. Give a single cycle.
   Vincristine* 1.5 mg/m^2 IV, days 1, 11, 21, 31, and 41
   Methotrexate 100 mg/m^2 IV, day 1
   Methotrexate 150 mg/m^2 IV, day 11
   Methotrexate 200 mg/m^2 IV, day 21
   Methotrexate 250 mg/m^2 IV, day 31
   Methotrexate 300 mg/m^2 IV, day 41
   Asparaginase 15,000 units/m^2/dose IM, days 2, 12, 22, 32, and 42

Delayed Intensification I. *Cycle:* 8 weeks. Give a single cycle.
   Dexamethasone 10 mg/m^2/day PO, days 1 through 21, then taper off over next 7 days
   Vincristine* 1.5 mg/m^2 IV, days 1, 15, 22, 43, and 50
   Doxorubicin 25 mg/m^2 IV, days 1, 8, and 15
   Asparaginase 6,000 units/m^2/dose IM for 6 doses each month, days 4, 6, 8, 11, 13, 15, 43, 45, 47, 50, 52, and 54

continued on next page

ATRA + CT—see DA + ATRA (cont.)

Delayed Intensification I (cont.)

Cyclophosphamide 1,000 mg/m^2 IV, day 29

Thioguanine 60 mg/m^2/day PO, days 29 through 42

Cytarabine 75 mg/m^2/day IV or subcutaneously, days 30 through 33 and days 37 through 40

Methotrexate intrathecal (dose is based on patient's age, as shown below),[†] days 30 and 37

Interim Maintenance II. *Cycle:* 8 weeks. Give a single cycle.

Vincristine* 1.5 mg/m^2 IV, days 1, 11, 21, 31, and 41

Methotrexate 100 mg/m^2 IV, day 1

Methotrexate 150 mg/m^2 IV, day 11

Methotrexate 200 mg/m^2 IV, day 21

Methotrexate 250 mg/m^2 IV, day 31

Methotrexate 300 mg/m^2 IV, day 41

Asparaginase 15,000 units/m^2/dose IM, days 2, 12, 22, 32, and 42

Methotrexate intrathecal (dose is based on patient's age, as shown below),[†] days 1, 21, and 41

Delayed Intensification II (same as Delayed Intensification I; doses shown below). *Cycle:* 8 weeks. Give a single cycle.

Dexamethasone 10 mg/m^2/day PO, days 1 through 21, then taper off over next 7 days

Vincristine* 1.5 mg/m^2 IV, days 1, 15, 22, 43, and 50

Doxorubicin 25 mg/m^2 IV, days 1, 8, and 15

Asparaginase 6,000 units/m^2/dose IM, days 4, 6, 8, 11, 13, 15, 43, 45, 47, 50, 52, and 54

Cyclophosphamide 1,000 mg/m^2 IV, day 29

Thioguanine 60 mg/m^2/day PO, days 29 through 42

Cytarabine 75 mg/m^2/day IV or subcutaneously, days 30 through 33 and days 37 through 40

Methotrexate intrathecal (dose is based on patient's age, as shown below),[†] days 30 and 37

Maintenance. *Cycle:* 84 days, continue until 24 months after first interim maintenance in females and until 36 months after first interim maintenance in males.

Vincristine* 1.5 mg/m^2 IV, days 1, 29, and 57

Prednisone 60 mg/m^2/day PO, days 1 through 5, days 29 through 33, and days 57 through 61

Mercaptopurine 75 mg/m^2/day IM, days 1 through 84

Methotrexate 20 mg/m^2/dose PO weekly except for first week, days 8, 15, 22, 29, 36, 43, 50, 57, 64, 71, and 78

Methotrexate intrathecal (dose is based on patient's age, as shown below),[†] day 1

*Note: The vincristine dose is not capped in this protocol. Consult the prescriber if there is any question about the intended vincristine dose.

[†]Note: Dose of intrathecal methotrexate is based on patient's age as follows:

Age 1 to 2 years: Methotrexate 8 mg

Age 2 to 3 years: Methotrexate 10 mg

Age 3 years and older: Methotrexate 12 mg

B-CAVe

Use:	Lymphoma (Hodgkin). *Cycle:* 28 days
Regimen:	Bleomycin 5 units/m^2 IV, days 1, 28, and 35
	Lomustine 100 mg/m^2 PO, day 1
	Doxorubicin 60 mg/m^2 IV, day 1
	Vinblastine 5 mg/m^2 IV, day 1

BCVPP

Use:	Lymphoma (Hodgkin). *Cycle:* 28 days for at least 6 cycles
Regimen:	Carmustine 100 mg/m^2 IV, day 1
	Cyclophosphamide 600 mg/m^2 IV, day 1
	Vinblastine 5 mg/m^2 IV, day 1
	Procarbazine 50 mg/m^2 PO, day 1
	Procarbazine 100 mg/m^2/day PO, days 2 through 10
	Prednisone 60 mg/m^2/day PO, days 1 through 10

BEACOPP

Use:	Lymphoma (Hodgkin). *Cycle:* 21 days for up to 8 cycles
Regimen:	Etoposide 100 mg/m^2/day IV, days 1 through 3
	Doxorubicin 25 mg/m^2 IV, day 1
	Cyclophosphamide 650 mg/m^2 IV, day 1
	Vincristine 1.4 mg/m^2 (2 mg maximum dose) IV, day 1
	Procarbazine 100 mg/m^2/day PO, days 1 through 7
	Prednisone 40 mg/m^2/day PO, days 1 through 14
	Bleomycin 10 units/m^2 IV, day 8
	Filgrastim 300 mcg/day (patients weighing less than 70 kg) to 480 mcg/day (patients weighing 70 kg or more) subcutaneously, starting on day 8, give for 3 days or more or until leukocytes exceed 2,000 cells/mm^3 for 3 days

BEACOPP Escalated

Use:	Lymphoma (Hodgkin). *Cycle:* 21 days for up to 8 cycles
Regimen:	Etoposide 200 mg/m^2/day IV, days 1 through 3
	Doxorubicin 35 mg/m^2 IV, day 1
	Cyclophosphamide 1,200 to 1,250 mg/m^2 IV, day 1
	Vincristine 1.4 or 2 mg/m^2 (2 mg maximum dose) IV, day 1 or 8
	Procarbazine 100 mg/m^2/day PO, days 1 through 7
	Prednisone 40 mg/m^2/day PO, days 1 through 14
	Bleomycin 10 units/m^2 IV, day 8
	Filgrastim 300 mcg/day (patients weighing less than 70 kg) to 480 mcg/day (patients weighing 70 kg or more) subcutaneously, starting on day 8, give for at least 3 days or until leukocytes exceed 2,000 cells/mm^3 for 3 days

BEP (PEB)

Use:	Testicular cancer, germ cell tumors. *Cycle:* 21 days for up to 4 cycles
Regimen:	Etoposide 100 mg/m^2/day IV, days 1 through 5
	Cisplatin 20 mg/m^2/day IV, days 1 through 5
	Bleomycin 30 units IV, days 2, 9, and 16
Use:	Adenocarcinoma (unknown primary). *Cycle:* 21 days for up to 4 cycles
Regimen:	Bleomycin 30 units IV, days 1, 8, and 15
	Etoposide 100 mg/m^2/day IV, days 1 through 5
	Cisplatin 20 mg/m^2/day IV, days 1 through 5

Bevacizumab-Interferon alfa
Use: Renal cell carcinoma. *Cycle:* 14 days, continue until disease progression or intolerable toxicity
Regimen: Bevacizumab 10 mg/kg IV, day 1
Interferon alfa-2a* 9 million units/dose subcutaneously 3 times weekly, throughout entire course
*Note: Interferon alfa-2a is no longer available in the United States. The manufacturer discontinued this product in October 2007 for commercial reasons, not for safety or efficacy reasons.

BIC
Use: Cervical cancer. *Cycle:* 28 days for up to 6 cycles
Regimen: Bleomycin 30 units IV, day 1
Ifosfamide 2,000 mg/m^2/day IV, days 1 through 3
Carboplatin 200 mg/m^2 IV, day 1
Mesna 400 mg/m^2/dose IV, given 15 minutes before and 4 hours after ifosfamide, days 1 through 3
Mesna 800 mg/m^2/dose PO, given 8 hours after ifosfamide, days 1 through 3

Bicalutamide + LHRH-A
Use: Prostate cancer. *Cycle:* Ongoing
Regimen: Bicalutamide 50 mg PO daily
with
Goserelin acetate 3.6 mg/dose implant subcutaneously, every 28 days
or
Leuprolide depot 7.5 mg/dose IM, every 28 days

Bio-Chemotherapy—see Interleukin 2-Interferon alfa 2

BIP
Use: Cervical cancer. *Cycle:* 21 days
Regimen: Bleomycin 30 units/day continuous IV infusion over 24 hours, day 1
Cisplatin 50 mg/m^2 IV, day 2
Ifosfamide 5,000 mg/m^2/day continuous IV infusion over 24 hours, day 2
Mesna 6,000 mg/m^2/cycle continuous IV infusion over 36 hours, day 2 (start with ifosfamide)

BOMP
Use: Cervical cancer. *Cycle:* 6 weeks
Regimen: Bleomycin 10 units IM weekly, days 1, 8, 15, 22, 29, and 36
Vincristine 1 mg/m^2 (2 mg maximum dose) IV, days 1, 8, 22, and 29
Mitomycin 10 mg/m^2 IV, day 1
Cisplatin 50 mg/m^2 IV, days 1 and 22

Bortezomib + Liposomal Doxorubicin
Use: Multiple myeloma. *Cycle:* 21 days for up to 8 cycles
Regimen: Bortezomib 1.3 mg/m^2 IV, days 1, 4, 8, and 11
Liposomal doxorubicin 30 mg/m^2 IV, day 4 (after bortezomib)

BV
Use: Kaposi sarcoma. *Cycle:* 28 days, continue for 2 cycles after maximal response
Regimen: Bleomycin 10 units/m^2 IV, days 1 and 15
Vincristine 1.4 mg/m^2 (2 mg maximum dose) IV, days 1 and 15

C-MOPP—see COPP

CA
Use: Acute myelogenous leukemia (AML; induction—pediatrics).
Cycle: 7 days. Give 2 cycles. If patient has persistent blasts at day 15, give a third cycle.
Regimen: Cytarabine 3,000 mg/m^2/dose IV every 12 hours for 4 doses, days 1 and 2
Asparaginase 6,000 units/m^2 IM, at hour 42

CA-VP16
Use: Lung cancer (small cell). *Cycle:* 21 days for up to 10 cycles
Regimen: Cyclophosphamide 1,000 mg/m^2 IV, day 1
Doxorubicin 45 mg/m^2 IV, day 1
Etoposide 80 mg/m^2/day IV, days 1 through 3

CABO
Use: Head and neck cancer. *Cycle:* 21 days for up to 3 cycles
Regimen: Methotrexate 40 mg/m^2 IV, days 1 and 15
Bleomycin 10 units/dose IV, days 1, 8, and 15
Vincristine 2 mg/dose (dose is not in mg/m^2) IV, days 1, 8, and 15 of first 2 cycles
Cisplatin 50 mg/m^2 IV, day 4

CAE—see ACE

CAF
Use: Breast cancer. *Cycle:* 28 days
Regimen: Cyclophosphamide 100 mg/m^2/day PO, days 1 through 14
Doxorubicin 30 mg/m^2 IV, days 1 and 8
Fluorouracil 500 mg/m^2 IV, days 1 and 8

Use: Breast cancer. *Cycle:* 21 days for 9 to 10 cycles
Regimen: Cyclophosphamide 500 mg/m^2 IV, day 1
Doxorubicin 50 mg/m^2 IV, day 1
Fluorouracil 500 mg/m^2 IV, day 1

CAF, Dose Dense
Use: Breast cancer. *Cycle:* 28 days for up to 4 cycles
Regimen: Cyclophosphamide 600 mg/m^2 IV, day 1
Doxorubicin 60 mg/m^2 IV, day 1
Fluorouracil 600 mg/m^2 IV, day 1

CAL-G—see Larson Regimen

CALGB 8811—see Larson Regimen

CAMP
Use: Lung cancer (non-small cell). *Cycle:* 28 days
Regimen: Cyclophosphamide 300 mg/m^2 IV, days 1 and 8
Doxorubicin 20 mg/m^2 IV, days 1 and 8
Methotrexate 15 mg/m^2 IV, days 1 and 8
Procarbazine 100 mg/m^2/day PO, days 1 through 10

CAP
Use: Lung cancer (non-small cell). *Cycle:* 28 days
Regimen: Cyclophosphamide 400 mg/m^2 IV, day 1
Doxorubicin 40 mg/m^2 IV, day 1
Cisplatin 60 mg/m^2 IV, day 1

continued on next page

CAP (cont.)

Use: Mesothelioma. *Cycle:* 21 days, continue until disease progression or intolerable toxicity

Regimen: Cyclophosphamide 500 mg/m^2 IV, day 1
Doxorubicin 50 mg/m^2 IV, day 1
Cisplatin 80 mg/m^2 IV, day 1 for first 3 cycles; decrease to cisplatin 50 mg/m^2 IV, day 1 for subsequent cycles

Capecitabine-Docetaxel (X + T)

Use: Breast cancer. *Cycle:* 21 days, continue until disease progression or intolerable toxicity

Regimen: Capecitabine 1,250 mg/m^2/dose PO twice daily, days 1 through 14
Docetaxel 75 mg/m^2 IV, day 1

CapeOx-B, Modified (also see XELOX + Bevacizumab)

Use: Metastatic colorectal cancer. *Cycle:* 21 days

Regimen: Capecitabine 850 mg/m^2/dose PO twice daily, days 1 through 14
Oxaliplatin 130 mg/m^2 IV, day 1
Bevacizumab 7.5 mg/kg IV, day 1

CAPIRI

Use: Colorectal cancer. *Cycle:* 21 days

Regimen: Capecitabine 1,000 mg/m^2/dose PO twice daily, days 1 through 14
Irinotecan 80 to 100 mg/m^2 IV, days 1 and 8

Carbo-Tax (also see CaT)

Use: Ovarian cancer. *Cycle:* 21 days for up to 8 cycles

Regimen: Paclitaxel 175 mg/m^2 IV over 3 hours, day 1
Carboplatin IV dose by Calvert equation to AUC 5 to 7.5 mg/mL/min, day 1 (after paclitaxel)

Use: Ovarian cancer. *Cycle:* 21 days

Regimen: Paclitaxel 185 mg/m^2 IV over 3 hours, day 1
Carboplatin IV dose by Calvert equation to AUC 6 mg/mL/min, day 1 (after paclitaxel)

Use: Adenocarcinoma (unknown primary). *Cycle:* 21 days for up to 8 cycles

Regimen: Carboplatin IV dose by Calvert equation to AUC 6 mg/mL/min, day 1
Paclitaxel 200 mg/m^2 IV over 3 hours, day 1 (after carboplatin)
Filgrastim 300 mcg/day subcutaneously, days 5 through 12

Use: Breast cancer. *Cycle:* 21 days, continue until disease progression or intolerable toxicity

Regimen: Paclitaxel 200 mg/m^2 IV over 3 hours, day 1
Carboplatin IV dose by Calvert equation to AUC 6 mg/mL/min, day 1 (after paclitaxel)

Carboplatin-Docetaxel

Use: Breast cancer, lung cancer (non-small cell). *Cycle:* 21 days for up to 6 cycles or until disease progression or intolerable toxicity

Regimen: Docetaxel 75 mg/m^2 IV, day 1
Carboplatin IV dose by Calvert equation to AUC 6 mg/mL/min, day 1 (after docetaxel)

Use: Lung cancer (non-small cell). *Cycle:* 21 to 28 days, continue until disease progression or intolerable toxicity.

Regimen: Carboplatin IV dose by Calvert equation to AUC 6 mg/mL/min, day 1
Docetaxel 60 to 70 mg/m^2 IV, day 1 (after carboplatin)

Carboplatin-Fluorouracil—see CF

CaT (also see Carbo-Tax)

Use:	Adenocarcinoma (unknown primary), lung cancer (non-small cell), ovarian cancer. *Cycle:* 21 days for up to 6 cycles
Regimen:	Paclitaxel 175 mg/m² IV over 3 hours, day 1
	or
	Paclitaxel 135 mg/m²/day continuous IV infusion over 24 hours, day 1
	with
	Carboplatin IV dose by Calvert equation to AUC 7.5 mg/mL/min, day 1 or 2 (give after paclitaxel infusion)

Use:	Lung cancer (non-small cell). *Cycle:* 21 days for 4 to 9 cycles, or until disease progression or intolerable toxicity
Regimen:	Paclitaxel 175 to 225 mg/m² IV over 3 hours, day 1
	Carboplatin IV dose by Calvert equation to AUC 6 mg/mL/min, day 1 (give after paclitaxel)

Use:	Lung cancer (non-small cell). *Cycle:* 7 days for 7 cycles
Regimen:	Carboplatin IV dose by Calvert equation to AUC 2 mg/mL/min, day 1 (administration sequence not specified in protocol)
	Paclitaxel 50 mg/m² IV over 1 hour, day 1
	used in conjunction with
	Radiation therapy, days 1 through 48
	followed by 1 additional day of chemotherapy given 3 weeks after the end of radiation therapy
	Paclitaxel 200 mg/m² IV over 3 hours, day 1
	Carboplatin IV dose by Calvert equation to AUC 6 mg/mL/min, day 1 (give after paclitaxel)

CAV (VAC)

Use:	Lung cancer (small cell). *Cycle:* 21 days for up to 6 cycles
Regimen:	Cyclophosphamide 1,000 mg/m² IV, day 1
	Doxorubicin 40 to 50 mg/m² IV, day 1
	Vincristine 1 to 1.4 mg/m² (2 mg maximum dose) IV, day 1

Use:	Sarcoma (bone). *Cycle:* 21 days for up to 1 year
Regimen:	Cyclophosphamide 1,200 mg/m² IV, day 1
	with
	Doxorubicin 75 mg/m² IV, day 1 for first 5 to 6 cycles (up to maximum cumulative dose of doxorubicin 375 to 450 mg/m²)
	or
	Dactinomycin 1.25 mg/m² IV, day 1 for subsequent cycles after maximum cumulative doxorubicin dose is reached
	with
	Vincristine 1.4 or 2 mg/m² (2 mg maximum dose) IV, day 1
	Mesna 240 mg/m²/dose IV, given before and 4 and 8 hours after cyclophosphamide, day 1

CAV/EP

Use:	Lung cancer (small cell). *Cycle:* 42 days for 3 cycles
Regimen:	Cyclophosphamide 1,000 mg/m² IV, day 1
	Doxorubicin 50 mg/m² IV, day 1
	Vincristine* 1.2 mg/m² IV, day 1
	Etoposide 100 mg/m²/day IV, days 22 through 24
	Cisplatin 25 mg/m²/day IV, days 22 through 24
	*Note: The vincristine dose is not capped in this protocol. Consult the prescriber if there is any question about the intended vincristine dose.

CAV/IE
Use: Sarcoma (bone). *Cycle:* 21 days for up to 1 year
Regimen: Alternate CAV and IE regimens every 21 days

CAV + P/VP
Use: Neuroblastoma (pediatrics). *Cycle:* Repeat based on hematologic recovery, usually every 20 to 31 days for 7 cycles. Delay subsequent cycles until hematologic recovery.
Regimen: **Treatment A** —CAV (cycles 1, 2, 4, and 6)
     Cyclophosphamide 70 mg/kg/day IV, days 1 and 2
     Doxorubicin 25 mg/m^2/day continuous IV infusion, days 1 through 3
     Vincristine* 0.033 mg/kg/day (dose is not in mg/m^2) continuous IV infusion, days 1 through 3
     Vincristine* 1.5 mg/m^2 IV, day 9
     Treatment B —P/VP (cycles 3, 5, and 7)
     Cisplatin 50 mg/m^2/day IV, days 1 through 4
     Etoposide 200 mg/m^2/day IV, days 1 through 3
     used in conjunction with antimicrobial prophylaxis[†]
     Cotrimoxazole (either 80/400 or 160/800 strength) 1 tablet PO daily, throughout entire course
     *Note: The vincristine dose is not capped in this protocol. Consult the prescriber if there is any question about the intended vincristine dose.
     [†]Note: Antimicrobial prophylaxis doses not specified in original article; the dose given here is derived from the *Infectious Diseases Handbook*, 6th edition, a tertiary resource.

CAVE
Use: Lung cancer (small cell). *Cycle:* 21 days for up to 5 cycles
Regimen: Cyclophosphamide 1,000 mg/m^2 IV, day 1
     Doxorubicin 50 mg/m^2 IV, day 1
     Vincristine 2 mg (dose is not in mg/m^2) IV, day 1
     Etoposide 100 mg/m^2/day IV, days 2 through 4

CC
Use: Ovarian cancer. *Cycle:* 28 days for up to 6 cycles
Regimen: Cyclophosphamide 600 mg/m^2 IV, day 1
     Carboplatin 300 to 350 mg/m^2 IV, day 1

CCG 1891 – Double-Delayed Intensification
Use: Acute lymphoblastic leukemia (ALL; consolidation, intensification, and maintenance—pediatrics).
Regimen: **Consolidation.** *Cycle:* 4 weeks. Give a single cycle.
     Mercaptopurine 75 mg/m^2/day PO, days 1 through 28
     Vincristine* 1.5 mg/m^2 IV, day 1
     Methotrexate intrathecal (dose is based on patient's age, as shown below) weekly,[†] days 1, 8, 15, and 22
     may be used in conjunction with
     Radiation therapy
     Interim Maintenance and Delayed Intensification.
     Cycle: 8 weeks. Repeat cycles ABAB for 4 cycles total.
     Treatment A: Interim Maintenance (cycles 1 and 3)
     Prednisone 40 mg/m^2/day PO, days 1 through 5 and days 29 through 33
     Mercaptopurine 75 mg/m^2/day PO, days 1 through 56
     Methotrexate 20 mg/m^2/dose PO weekly, days 1, 8, 15, 22, 29, 36, 43, and 50
     Vincristine* 1.5 mg/m^2 IV, days 1 and 29
     continued on next page

CCG 1891 – Double-Delayed Intensification (cont.)
> **Treatment A (cont.)**
>> Methotrexate intrathecal (dose is based on patient's age as shown below),[†] day 1
>
> **Treatment B:** Delayed Intensification (cycles 2 and 4)
>> Dexamethasone 10 mg/m^2/day PO or IV, days 1 through 21, then taper off over next 7 days
>>
>> Vincristine* 1.5 mg/m^2 IV, days 1, 8, and 15
>>
>> Doxorubicin 25 mg/m^2 IV, days 1, 8, and 15
>>
>> Asparaginase 6,000 units/m^2/dose IM 3 times weekly for 6 doses (eg, days 2, 5, 7, 9, 12, and 14)
>>
>> Cyclophosphamide 1,000 mg/m^2 IV, day 29
>>
>> Cytarabine 75 mg/m^2/day IV or subcutaneously, days 30 through 33 and days 37 through 40
>>
>> Thioguanine 60 mg/m^2/day PO, days 29 through 42
>>
>> Methotrexate intrathecal (dose is based on patient's age as shown below),[†] days 29 and 36

Maintenance. *Cycle:* 84 days, continue until 24 months after first interim maintenance in females and until 36 months after first interim maintenance in males.
> Prednisone 40 mg/m^2/day PO, days 1 through 5, days 29 through 33, and days 57 through 61
>
> Vincristine* 1.5 mg/m^2 IV, days 1, 29, and 57
>
> Mercaptopurine 75 mg/m^2/day PO, days 1 through 84
>
> Methotrexate 20 mg/m^2/dose PO weekly, days 1, 8, 15, 22, 29, 36, 43, 50, 57, 64, 71, and 78
>
> Methotrexate intrathecal (dose is based on patient's age as shown below),[†] day 1

*Note: The vincristine dose is not capped in this protocol. Consult the prescriber if there is any question about the intended vincristine dose.

†Note: Dose of intrathecal methotrexate is based on patient's age as follows:
> Age 1 to 2 years: Methotrexate 8 mg
>
> Age 2 to 3 years: Methotrexate 10 mg
>
> Age 3 years and older: Methotrexate 12 mg

CCG 1922 – OD, Induction

Use: Acute lymphocytic leukemia (ALL—pediatrics)

Regimen: **Induction.** *Cycle:* 28 days. Give a single cycle.
> Dexamethasone 2 mg/m^2/dose (6 mg/m^2/day) PO 3 times daily, days 1 through 28
>
> Vincristine* 1.5 mg/m^2 IV weekly, days 1, 8, 15, and 22
>
> Asparaginase 6,000 units/m^2/dose IM 3 times weekly for 9 doses, starting between days 2 and 4 (eg, days 3, 5, 7, 10, 12, 14, 17, 19, and 21)
>
> Methotrexate intrathecal (dose is based on patient's age, as shown below):[†]
>> Patients without CNS involvement at diagnosis: Give on days 1 and 15
>>
>> Patients with CNS involvement at diagnosis: Give on days 1, 8, 15, and 22

Consolidation. *Cycle:* 84 days. Give a single cycle.
> Dexamethasone 2 mg/m^2/dose (6 mg/m^2/day) PO 3 times daily, days 29 through 33 and days 57 through 61
>
> Vincristine* 1.5 mg/m^2 IV, days 1, 29, and 57

continued on next page

CCG 1922 – OD, Induction (cont.)
    Consolidation (cont.)
        Mercaptopurine 75 mg/m^2/day PO, days 1 through 71
        Methotrexate 20 mg/m^2/dose PO, days 29, 36, 43, 50, 57, 64, and 71
        Methotrexate intrathecal (dose is based on patient's age, as shown below):[†]
            Patients without CNS involvement at diagnosis: Give on days 1, 8, 15, and 22
            Patients with CNS involvement at diagnosis: Give on days 1 and 15

Delayed Intensification. *Cycle:* 56 days. Give a single cycle.
    Dexamethasone 10 mg/m^2/day PO, days 1 through 21, then taper off over next 7 days
    Vincristine* 1.5 mg/m^2 IV, days 1, 8, and 15
    Asparaginase 6,000 units/m^2/dose IM 3 times weekly for 6 doses total, given between days 3 and 17 (eg, days 3, 6, 8, 10, 13, and 15)
    Doxorubicin 25 mg/m^2 IV, days 1, 8, and 15
    Cyclophosphamide 1,000 mg/m^2 IV, day 29
    Thioguanine 60 mg/m^2/day PO, days 29 through 42
    Cytarabine 75 mg/m^2/day IV, days 30 through 33 and days 37 through 40
    Methotrexate intrathecal (dose is based on patient's age, as shown below)[†], day 29

Maintenance. *Cycle:* 84 days, continue until 26 months after diagnosis in females and until 38 months after diagnosis in males.
    Dexamethasone 6 mg/m^2/day PO for 5 days each month, days 1 through 5, days 29 through 33, and days 57 through 61
    Mercaptopurine 75 mg/m^2/day PO, days 1 through 84
    Vincristine* 1.5 mg/m^2 IV, days 1, 29, and 57
    Methotrexate 20 mg/m^2/dose PO weekly except for first week, days 8, 15, 22, 29, 36, 43, 50, 57, 64, 71, and 78
    Methotrexate intrathecal (dose is based on patient's age, as shown below),[†] day 1

*Note: The vincristine dose is not capped in this protocol. Consult the prescriber if there is any question about the intended vincristine dose.

[†]Note: Dose of intrathecal methotrexate is based on patient's age as follows:
    Age 1 to 2 years: Methotrexate 8 mg
    Age 2 to 3 years: Methotrexate 10 mg
    Age 3 years and older: Methotrexate 12 mg

CCG 1962, Induction

Use: Acute lymphocytic leukemia (ALL; induction—pediatrics).
Cycle: 28 days. Give a single cycle.

Regimen: Vincristine* 1.5 mg/m^2 IV weekly, days 1, 8, 15, and 22
Prednisone 40 mg/m^2/day PO daily, days 1 through 28, then taper off over next 10 days
with
Pegaspargase 2,500 units/m^2 IM, day 4
or
Asparaginase 6,000 units/m^2/dose IM for 9 doses, days 4, 6, 9, 11, 13, 16, 18, 20, and 23
used in conjunction with
Intrathecal chemotherapy
*Note: The vincristine dose is not capped in this protocol. Consult the prescriber if there is any question about the intended vincristine dose.

CD

Use: Hepatoblastoma (pediatrics). *Cycle:* 21 days for up to 6 cycles

Regimen 1: Patients weighing less than 10 kg:
Cisplatin 2.67 mg/kg IV, day 1
Doxorubicin 1 mg/kg/day continuous IV infusion, days 2 through 3

Regimen 2: Patients weighing at least 10 kg:
Cisplatin 80 mg/m^2/day continuous IV infusion, day 1
Doxorubicin 30 mg/m^2/day continuous IV infusion, days 2 through 3

CDB

Use: Melanoma. *Cycle:* 21 days, continue until disease progression or intolerable toxicity

Regimen: Cisplatin 25 mg/m^2/day IV, days 1 through 3
Dacarbazine 220 mg/m^2/day IV, days 1 through 3
Carmustine 150 mg/m^2 IV, day 1 of odd-numbered cycles only (eg, cycle 1, 3, 5)

CDB + Tamoxifen (Dartmouth Regimen)

Use: Melanoma. *Cycle:* 21 days, continue until disease progression or intolerable toxicity

Regimen: Tamoxifen 10 mg PO twice daily, throughout entire course, started 1 week prior to cytotoxic chemotherapy
Carmustine 150 mg/m^2 IV, day 1 of odd-numbered cycles only (eg, cycle 1, 3, 5), given before cisplatin and dacarbazine
Cisplatin 25 mg/m^2/day IV, days 1 through 3
Dacarbazine 220 mg/m^2/day IV, days 1 through 3

CDDP/VP-16

Use: Brain tumors (pediatrics). *Cycle:* 21 days for up to 4 cycles

Regimen: Cisplatin 90 mg/m^2 IV, day 1
Etoposide 150 mg/m^2/day IV, days 3 and 4

CDE
Use: Lymphoma (HIV-related, non-Hodgkin—adults). *Cycle:* 28 days for up to 6 cycles
Regimen: Cyclophosphamide 200 mg/m^2/day continuous IV infusion, days 1 through 4
Doxorubicin 12.5 mg/m^2/day continuous IV infusion, days 1 through 4
Etoposide 60 mg/m^2/day continuous IV infusion, days 1 through 4
Filgrastim 5 mcg/kg/day subcutaneously starting on day 6, at least 24 hours after the end of the continuous infusions, and ending when the absolute neutrophil count (ANC) is 10,000 cells/mm^3 or higher

CEF (also see FEC)
Use: Breast cancer. *Cycle:* 28 days for up to 6 cycles
Regimen: Cyclophosphamide 75 mg/m^2/day PO, days 1 through 14
Epirubicin 60 mg/m^2 IV, days 1 and 8
Fluorouracil 500 mg/m^2 IV, days 1 and 8
Cotrimoxazole 2 tablets (strength not specified) PO twice daily, days 1 through 28

CEPP(B)
Use: Lymphoma (non-Hodgkin). *Cycle:* 28 days
Regimen: Cyclophosphamide 600 to 650 mg/m^2 IV, days 1 and 8
Etoposide 70 to 85 mg/m^2/day IV, days 1 through 3
Prednisone 60 mg/m^2/day PO, days 1 through 10
Procarbazine 60 mg/m^2/day PO, days 1 through 10
may or may not give with
Bleomycin 15 units/m^2 IV, days 1 and 15

CetIri—see Cetuximab-Irinotecan

Cetuximab-Cisplatin
Use: Head and neck cancer. *Cycle:* 28 days for up to 6 cycles or until disease progression or intolerable toxicity
Regimen: Cetuximab 400 mg/m^2 IV, day 1 of first cycle only (loading dose)
Cetuximab 250 mg/m^2 IV weekly, days 1, 8, 15, and 22, except for day 1 of first cycle
Cisplatin 100 mg/m^2 IV, day 1

Cetuximab-Gemcitabine
Use: Pancreatic cancer. *Cycle:* 56 days, continue until disease progression or intolerable toxicity
Regimen: Cetuximab 400 mg/m^2 IV, day 1 of first cycle only (loading dose)
Cetuximab 250 mg/m^2 IV weekly, days 1, 8, 15, 22, 29, 36, 43, and 50, except for day 1 of first cycle
Gemcitabine 1,000 mg/m^2 IV, weekly for 7 weeks for first cycle. During subsequent cycles, give weekly for 3 weeks followed by 1 week of rest, on days 1, 8, 15, 29, 36, and 43

Cetuximab-Irinotecan (CetIri)
Use: Metastatic colorectal cancer. *Cycle:* 42 days, continue until disease progression or intolerable toxicity
Regimen: Cetuximab 400 mg/m^2 IV, day 1 of first cycle only (loading dose)
Cetuximab 250 mg/m^2 IV weekly, days 1, 8, 15, 22, 29, and 36, except for day 1 of first cycle
with
Irinotecan 125 mg/m^2 IV, days 1, 8, 15, and 22
or
Irinotecan 180 mg/m^2 IV, days 1, 15, and 29
continued on next page

Cetuximab-Irinotecan (CetIri) (cont.)
or
Irinotecan 350 mg/m² IV, days 1 and 22; reduce each dose to irinotecan 300 mg/m² IV in patients 70 years of age and older

Use: Colorectal cancer. *Cycle:* 14 days, continue until disease progression or intolerable toxicity
Regimen: Cetuximab 500 mg/m² IV, day 1
Irinotecan 180 mg/m² IV, day 1

CEV
Use: Lung cancer (small cell). *Cycle:* 21 days, continue until disease progression or intolerable toxicity
Regimen: Cyclophosphamide 1,000 mg/m² IV, day 1
Vincristine 1.4 mg/m² (2 mg maximum dose) IV, day 1
Etoposide 50 mg/m² IV, day 1
Etoposide 100 mg/m²/day PO, days 2 through 5

CF (also see Cisplatin-Fluorouracil; also see FUP)
Use: Adenocarcinoma, head and neck cancer. *Cycle:* 21 to 28 days for up to 3 cycles or until disease progression or intolerable toxicity
Regimen: Cisplatin 100 mg/m² IV, day 1
Fluorouracil 1,000 mg/m²/day continuous IV infusion, days 1 through 4 or days 1 through 5

Use: Head and neck cancer. *Cycle:* 21 to 28 days for up to 3 cycles or until disease progression or intolerable toxicity
Regimen: Carboplatin 300 or 400 mg/m² IV, day 1
Fluorouracil 1,000 mg/m²/day continuous IV infusion, days 1 through 4 or days 1 through 5

Use: Gastric cancer. *Cycle:* 28 days
Regimen: Cisplatin 100 mg/m² IV, day 1
Fluorouracil 1,000 mg/m²/day continuous IV infusion, days 1 through 5

CFM—see CNF

CHAMOCA (Modified Bagshawe)
Use: Gestational trophoblastic neoplasm. *Cycle:* 18 days or longer, as toxicity permits
Regimen: Hydroxyurea 500 mg/dose PO every 6 hours for 4 doses, day 1 (start at 6 am)
Dactinomycin 0.2 mg/day (dose is not in mg/m²) IV, days 1 through 3 (give at 7 pm)
Vincristine 1 mg/m² (2 mg maximum dose) IV, day 2 (give at 7 am)
Methotrexate 100 mg/m² IV push, day 2 (give at 7 pm)
Methotrexate 200 mg/m² IV over 12 hours, day 2 (give after IV push dose)
Leucovorin 14 mg/dose IM every 6 hours for 6 doses, days 3 through 5 (begin at 7 pm on day 3)
Cyclophosphamide 500 mg/m² IV, days 3 and 8 (give at 7 pm)
Dactinomycin 0.5 mg/day (dose is not in mg/m²) IV, days 4 and 5 (give at 7 pm)
Doxorubicin 30 mg/m² IV, day 8 (give at 7 pm)

CHAP

Use:	Ovarian cancer. *Cycle:* 28 days for up to 12 cycles
Regimen:	Cyclophosphamide 400 mg/m² IV, day 1
	or
	Cyclophosphamide 150 mg/m²/day PO, days 2 through 8
	with
	Doxorubicin 30 mg/m² IV, day 1
	Cisplatin 50 to 60 mg/m² IV, day 1
	Altretamine 150 mg/m²/day PO, days 2 through 8

ChIVPP

Use:	Lymphoma (Hodgkin). *Cycle:* 28 days, continue for 2 cycles after achieving remission
Regimen:	Chlorambucil 6 mg/m²/day (10 mg/day maximum dose) PO, days 1 through 14
	Vinblastine 6 mg/m² (10 mg/day maximum dose) IV, days 1 and 8
	Procarbazine 100 mg/m²/day (150 mg/day maximum dose) PO, days 1 through 14
	Prednisone 40 to 50 mg/day PO, days 1 through 14*

*Note: Prednisolone is recommended in the British literature. In the United States, prednisone is the preferred corticosteroid. The doses of these 2 corticosteroids are equivalent (ie, prednisone 40 mg PO = prednisolone 40 mg PO).

ChIVPP/EVA

Use:	Lymphoma (Hodgkin). *Cycle:* 28 days for up to 8 cycles
Regimen:	Chlorambucil 10 mg/day PO, days 1 through 7
	Vinblastine 10 mg (dose is not in mg/m²) IV, day 1
	Procarbazine 150 mg/day PO, days 1 through 7
	Prednisone 50 mg/day PO, days 1 through 7*
	with
	Etoposide 200 mg/m² IV, day 8
	Vincristine 2 mg (dose is not in mg/m²) IV, day 8
	Doxorubicin 50 mg/m² IV, day 8

*Note: Prednisolone is recommended in the British literature. In the United States, prednisone is the preferred corticosteroid. The doses of these 2 corticosteroids are equivalent (ie, prednisone 40 mg PO = prednisolone 40 mg PO).

CHOP

Use:	Lymphoma (non-Hodgkin), HIV-related lymphoma. *Cycle:* 21 to 28 days for 4 to 6 cycles, or for 3 cycles after achieving remission
Regimen:	Cyclophosphamide 750 mg/m² IV, day 1
	Doxorubicin 50 mg/m² IV, day 1
	Vincristine 1.4 mg/m² (2 mg maximum dose) IV, day 1
	Prednisone 100 mg/day PO, days 1 through 5

Use:	Lymphoma (non-Hodgkin; induction and consolidation—pediatrics)
Regimen:	**Induction.** *Cycle:* Give 1 cycle only (6 weeks)
	Cyclophosphamide 750 mg/m² IV, days 1 and 22
	Doxorubicin 40 mg/m² IV, days 1 and 22
	Vincristine 1.5 mg/m² (2 mg maximum dose) IV weekly, weeks 1 through 6
	Prednisone 40 mg/m²/day PO, days 1 through 28
	may be used in conjunction with
	Radiation therapy

continued on next page

CHOP (cont.)

Consolidation therapy. *Cycle:* 21 days
Cyclophosphamide 750 mg/m² IV, day 1
Doxorubicin 40 mg/m² IV, day 1
Vincristine 1.5 mg/m² (2 mg maximum dose) IV, day 1
Prednisone 40 mg/m²/day PO, days 1 through 5
Note: CHOP refers to induction and consolidation phase. Protocol also
includes maintenance and central nervous system prophylaxis.

CHOP-14

Use: Lymphoma (non-Hodgkin). *Cycle:* 14 days for up to 6 cycles
Regimen: Cyclophosphamide 750 mg/m² IV, day 1
Doxorubicin 50 mg/m² IV, day 1
Vincristine 2 mg (dose is not in mg/m²) IV, day 1
Prednisone 100 mg/day PO, days 1 through 5
Filgrastim 300 mcg/day (patients weighing less than 75 kg) to
480 mcg/day (patients weighing 75 kg or more) subcutaneously,
days 4 through 13

CHOP-Bleo

Use: Lymphoma (non-Hodgkin). *Cycle:* 21 to 28 days for at least
2 cycles
Regimen: **Add to CHOP:** Bleomycin 15 units/day IV, days 1 through 5

CHOP + Rituximab (R-CHOP)

Use: Lymphoma (B-cell). *Cycle:* 21 days for up to 8 cycles
Regimen: **Add to CHOP:** Rituximab 375 mg/m² IV, day 1

Use: Lymphoma (B-cell). *Cycle:* 21 days for up to 8 cycles
Regimen: Rituximab 375 mg/m² IV, day 1
Cyclophosphamide 750 mg/m² IV, day 3
Doxorubicin 50 mg/m² IV, day 3
Vincristine 1.4 mg/m² (2 mg maximum dose) IV, day 3
Prednisone 100 mg/day PO, days 3 through 7

CISCA

Use: Bladder cancer. *Cycle:* 21 to 28 days
Regimen 1: Patients without extensive prior radiation therapy, or patients with-
out tumor in bone marrow:
Cyclophosphamide 650 mg/m² IV, day 1
Doxorubicin 50 mg/m² IV, day 1
Cisplatin 100 mg/m² IV, day 2
Regimen 2: Patients with extensive prior radiation therapy, or patients with tu-
mor in bone marrow:
Cyclophosphamide 550 mg/m² IV, day 1, first cycle only
Cyclophosphamide 650 mg/m² IV, day 1, except for first cycle
Doxorubicin 40 mg/m² IV, day 1, first cycle only
Doxorubicin 50 mg/m² IV, day 1, except for first cycle
Cisplatin 100 mg/m² IV, day 2

CISCA II/VB IV

Use: Germ cell tumors. *Cycle:* Individualized based on duration of myelosup-
pression, continue for 2 cycles after response or remission
Regimen: Cyclophosphamide 500 mg/m²/day IV, days 1 and 2
Doxorubicin 40 to 45 mg/m²/day IV, days 1 and 2
Cisplatin 100 to 120 mg/m² IV, day 3
alternating with
Vinblastine 3 mg/m²/day continuous IV infusion, days 1 through 5
Bleomycin 30 units/day continuous IV infusion, days 1 through 5

Cisplatin-Docetaxel

Use: Bladder cancer. *Cycle:* Every 7 days for 8 weeks
Regimen: Cisplatin 30 mg/m^2 IV, day 1
Docetaxel 40 mg/m^2 IV, day 4
used in conjunction with
Radiation therapy

Use: Bladder cancer. *Cycle:* 21 days for up to 8 cycles
Regimen: Cisplatin 75 mg/m^2 IV, day 1
Docetaxel 75 mg/m^2 IV, day 1

Cisplatin-Doxorubicin-Etoposide-Cyclophosphamide, High Risk Neuroblastoma

Use: High-risk neuroblastoma (pediatrics). *Cycle:* 28 days for 5 cycles
Regimen: Cisplatin 60 mg/m^2 IV, day 1
Doxorubicin 30 mg/m^2 IV, day 3
Etoposide 100 mg/m^2 IV, days 3 and 6
Cyclophosphamide 1,000 mg/m^2/day IV, days 4 and 5

Cisplatin-Doxorubicin-Mitomycin, Chemoembolization Protocol

Use: Hepatocellular cancer, hepatic metastases. *Cycle:* May give a single cycle, or repeat every 4 to 8 weeks, depending on the protocol
Regimen: Cisplatin 50 to 100 mg intraarterially, day 1*
Doxorubicin 50 mg intraarterially, day 1*
Mitomycin 10 mg intraarterially, day 1*
all mixed in same infusion bag to a total volume of 10 to 20 mL with
Radiopaque contrast media, quantity sufficient to provide final volume of 10 to 20 mL
either of the following may be mixed with the other agents or given subsequently as a separate injection, depending on the protocol
Gelfoam powder, mixed to 25 to 30 mg/mL, and given intraarterially, day 1
or
Polyvinyl alcohol
*Note: All agents are mixed together in the same infusion bag. This regimen is usually administered by the Interventional Radiology staff to ensure delivery into the hepatic artery.

Cisplatin-Fluorouracil (also see CF; also see FUP)

Use: Cervical cancer. *Cycle:* 21 days for up to 3 cycles
Regimen: Cisplatin 75 mg/m^2 IV, day 1
followed by
Fluorouracil 1,000 mg/m^2/day continuous IV infusion, days 1 through 4 (for 96 hours total)
used in conjunction with
Radiation therapy

Use: Cervical cancer. *Cycle:* 28 days for up to 2 cycles
Regimen: Cisplatin 50 mg/m^2 IV, day 1 starting 4 hours *before* external beam radiotherapy
Fluorouracil 1,000 mg/m^2/day continuous IV infusion, days 2 through 5
used in conjunction with
Radiation therapy

---

continued on next page

Cisplatin-Fluorouracil (also see CF; also see FUP) (cont.)

Use: Head and neck cancer, esophageal cancer. *Cycle:* 21 days for 3 cycles

Regimen: Cisplatin 100 mg/m^2 IV, day 1

Fluorouracil 1,000 mg/m^2/day continuous IV infusion, days 1 through 5 (for 120 hours total)

Use: Esophageal cancer. *Cycle:* 32 days. Give a single cycle prior to surgery.

Regimen: Cisplatin 100 mg/m^2 IV, day 1

Fluorouracil 1,000 mg/m^2/day continuous IV infusion, days 1 through 4 and days 29 through 32

used in conjunction with

Radiation therapy

Use: Esophageal cancer. *Cycle:* 28 days for 2 cycles

Regimen: Cisplatin 75 mg/m^2 IV, day 1

Fluorouracil 1,000 mg/m^2/day continuous IV infusion, days 1 through 4 (for 96 hours total)

used in conjunction with

Radiation therapy

followed by 4 to 6 weeks of rest then

Repeat chemotherapy for 2 cycles

Use: Anal cancer. *Cycle:* 7 days for 6 cycles

Regimen: Cisplatin 4 mg/m^2/day continuous IV infusion, days 1 through 5

Fluorouracil 250 mg/m^2/day continuous IV infusion, days 1 through 5

used in conjunction with

Radiation therapy

Cisplatin-Irinotecan

Use: Cervical cancer, lung cancer (small cell). *Cycle:* 28 days for up to 4 to 6 cycles

Regimen: Irinotecan 60 mg/m^2 IV, days 1, 8, and 15

Cisplatin 60 mg/m^2 IV, day 1 (after irinotecan)

Use: Esophageal cancer. *Cycle:* 42 days for at least 3 cycles or until disease progression or intolerable toxicity

Regimen: Cisplatin 30 mg/m^2 IV, days 1, 8, 15, and 22

Irinotecan 65 mg/m^2 IV, days 1, 8, 15, and 22

Use: Gastric cancer. *Cycle:* 28 days, continue until disease progression or intolerable toxicity

Regimen: Cisplatin 80 mg/m^2 IV, day 1

Irinotecan 70 mg/m^2 IV, days 1 and 15

Cisplatin-Mitotane

Use: Adrenal cancer. *Cycle:* 21 days for 18 months or until disease progression or intolerable toxicity

Regimen 1: Patients younger than 65 years of age, patients without intolerable adverse effects from prior chemotherapy, or patients without extensive prior radiation therapy:

Cisplatin 100 mg/m^2 IV, day 1

Mitotane 1,000 mg/dose (4,000 mg/day) PO 4 times daily, throughout entire course

used in conjunction with mineralocorticoid and glucocorticoid supplementation

Hydrocortisone 10 to 30 mg/day PO in divided doses, throughout entire course*

Fludrocortisone 0.1 mg/day PO, throughout entire course*

continued on next page

Cisplatin-Mitotane (cont.)

Regimen 2: Patients 65 years of age and older, patients with intolerable adverse effects from prior chemotherapy, or patients with extensive prior radiation therapy:

    Cisplatin 75 mg/m^2 IV, day 1

    Mitotane 1,000 mg/dose (4,000 mg/day) PO 4 times daily, throughout entire course

    used in conjunction with mineralocorticoid and glucocorticoid supplementation

        Hydrocortisone 10 to 30 mg/day PO in divided doses, throughout entire course*

        Fludrocortisone 0.1 mg/day PO, throughout entire course*

*Note: Mineralocorticoid and glucocorticoid doses not specified in original article; the dose given here is derived from *AHFS 2008 Drug Information*, a tertiary resource.

Cisplatin-Topotecan

Use: Cervical cancer. *Cycle:* 21 days for 6 cycles or until disease progression or intolerable toxicity

Regimen: Cisplatin 50 mg/m^2 IV, day 1
Topotecan 0.75 mg/m^2/day IV, days 1 through 3

Cisplatin-Vincristine-Cyclophosphamide

Use: Brain tumor (pediatrics). *Cycle:* 6 weeks for up to 8 cycles

Regimen: Cisplatin 75 mg/m^2 IV, day 1
Vincristine 1.5 mg/m^2 (2 mg maximum dose) IV, days 2, 8, and 15
Cyclophosphamide 1,000 mg/m^2 IV, days 22 and 23

Cisplatin-Vinorelbine (also see Vinorelbine-Cisplatin)

Use: Cervical cancer, head and neck cancer. *Cycle:* 21 days for up to 6 to 8 cycles

Regimen: Cisplatin 80 mg/m^2 IV, day 1
Vinorelbine 25 mg/m^2 IV, days 1 and 8

Use: Lung cancer (non-small cell). *Cycle:* 28 days for 4 cycles

Regimen: Cisplatin 50 mg/m^2 IV, days 1 and 8
Vinorelbine 25 mg/m^2 IV weekly, days 1, 8, 15, and 22

CLD-BOMP

Use: Cervical cancer. *Cycle:* 21 days, continue until disease progression or intolerable toxicity

Regimen: Bleomycin 5 units/day continuous IV infusion, days 1 through 7
Cisplatin 10 mg/m^2/day IV, days 1 through 7
Vincristine* 0.7 mg/m^2 IV, day 7
Mitomycin 7 mg/m^2 IV, day 7

*Note: The vincristine dose is not capped in this protocol. Consult the prescriber if there is any question about the intended vincristine dose.

CMC

Use: Chronic lymphocytic leukemia (CLL, B-cell), lymphoma (non-Hodgkin). *Cycle:* 28 days for up to 3 cycles or until disease progression or intolerable toxicity

Regimen: Cladribine 0.12 mg/kg/day IV, days 1 through 3*
Mitoxantrone 10 mg/m^2 IV, day 1
Cyclophosphamide 650 mg/m^2 IV, day 1

*Note: Investigators compared cladribine for 3 days with cladribine for 5 days at the same daily dose. Response rates were similar with both regimens. Because toxicity increased with cladribine for 5 days, the 3-day cladribine regimen is recommended.

CMF

Use:	Breast cancer. *Cycle:* 28 days for up to 12 cycles
Regimen 1:	Patients 65 years of age and younger:

Methotrexate 40 mg/m^2 IV, days 1 and 8
Fluorouracil 600 mg/m^2 IV, days 1 and 8
with
Cyclophosphamide 100 mg/m^2/day PO, days 1 through 14
or
Cyclophosphamide 750 mg/m^2 IV, day 1

Regimen 2: Patients older than 65 years of age:
Methotrexate 30 mg/m^2 IV, days 1 and 8
Fluorouracil 400 mg/m^2 IV, days 1 and 8
Cyclophosphamide 100 mg/m^2/day PO, days 1 through 14

CMF-IV

Use: Breast cancer. *Cycle:* 21 days for up to 12 cycles
Regimen: Cyclophosphamide 600 mg/m^2 IV, day 1
Methotrexate 40 mg/m^2 IV, day 1
Fluorouracil 600 mg/m^2 IV, day 1

CMFP

Use: Breast cancer. *Cycle:* 28 days
Regimen: Cyclophosphamide 100 mg/m^2/day PO, days 1 through 14
Methotrexate 30 to 40 mg/m^2 IV, days 1 and 8
Fluorouracil 400 to 600 mg/m^2 IV, days 1 and 8
Prednisone 40 mg/m^2/day PO, days 1 through 14

CMFVP

Use: Breast cancer. *Cycle:* 28 days for up to 6 cycles
Regimen: Cyclophosphamide 400 mg/m^2 IV, day 1
Methotrexate 30 mg/m^2 IV, days 1 and 8
Fluorouracil 400 mg/m^2 IV, days 1 and 8
Vincristine 1 mg (dose is not in mg/m^2) IV, days 1 and 8
Prednisone 20 mg/dose PO, given 4 times daily, days 1 through 7

CMV

Use: Bladder cancer. *Cycle:* 21 days for at least 2 cycles
Regimen: Methotrexate 30 mg/m^2 IV, days 1 and 8
Vinblastine 4 mg/m^2 IV, days 1 and 8
Cisplatin 100 mg/m^2 IV, day 2 (at least 12 hours after methotrexate and vinblastine)

Use: Bladder cancer. *Cycle:* 28 days for 2 cycles prior to radiation therapy
Regimen: Methotrexate 30 mg/m^2 IV, days 1, 15, and 22
Cisplatin 70 mg/m^2 IV, day 2
Vinblastine 3 mg/m^2 IV, days 2, 15, and 22

CNF (CFM, FNC)

Use: Breast cancer. *Cycle:* 21 days, continue until disease progression or intolerable toxicity
Regimen: Cyclophosphamide 500 mg/m^2 IV, day 1
Mitoxantrone 10 mg/m^2 IV, day 1
Fluorouracil 500 mg/m^2 IV, day 1

Use: Breast cancer. *Cycle:* 21 days for up to 10 cycles
Regimen: Cyclophosphamide 600 mg/m^2 IV, day 1
Mitoxantrone 12 mg/m^2 IV, day 1
Fluorouracil 600 mg/m^2 IV, day 1

CNOP

Use: Lymphoma (non-Hodgkin). *Cycle:* 21 to 28 days for up to 8 cycles

Regimen: Cyclophosphamide 750 mg/m^2 IV, day 1
Mitoxantrone 10 or 12 mg/m^2 IV, day 1
Vincristine 1.4 mg/m^2 (2 mg maximum dose) IV, day 1
Prednisone 50 mg/m^2/day PO, days 1 through 5

COB

Use: Head and neck cancer. *Cycle:* 21 days for 2 to 3 cycles

Regimen: Cisplatin 100 mg/m^2 IV, day 1
Vincristine 1 mg (dose is not in mg/m^2) IV, days 2 and 5
Bleomycin 30 units/day continuous IV infusion, days 2 through 5

CODE

Use: Lung cancer (small cell). *Cycle:* 9-week regimen (give a single cycle)

Regimen: Cisplatin 25 mg/m^2 IV, every week for 9 weeks
Vincristine* 1 mg/m^2 IV weekly, weeks 1, 2, 4, 6, and 8
Doxorubicin 40 mg/m^2 IV weekly, weeks 1, 3, 5, 7, and 9
Etoposide 80 mg/m^2 IV, day 1 of weeks 1, 3, 5, 7, and 9
Etoposide 80 mg/m^2/day PO, days 2 and 3 of weeks 1, 3, 5, 7, and 9
used in conjunction with
Prednisone 50 mg PO daily for 5 weeks, then alternate days until chemotherapy completion, then taper off over 2 weeks
used in conjunction with antimicrobial prophylaxis
Cotrimoxazole double-strength (160/800) 1 tablet PO twice daily, starting on day 8 and continued throughout chemotherapy
Ketoconazole 200 mg PO daily, starting on day 8 and continued throughout chemotherapy
*Note: The vincristine dose is not capped in this protocol. Consult the prescriber if there is any question about the intended vincristine dose.

CODOX-M/IVAC*

Use: Lymphoma (advanced B-cell). *Cycle:* Give 4 cycles as myelosuppression permits. Give next cycle when granulocyte count is above 1,000 cells/mm^3 and platelet count is above 50,000 cells/mm^3.

Regimen: **Treatment A** —CODOX-M (cycles 1 and 3)
Cyclophosphamide 800 mg/m^2 IV, day 1
Cyclophosphamide 200 mg/m^2/day IV, days 2 through 5
Vincristine 1.5 mg/m^2 (2 mg maximum dose) IV, days 1 and 8
Doxorubicin 40 mg/m^2 IV, day 1
Methotrexate 1,200 mg/m^2 IV over 1 hour, day 10
Methotrexate 240 mg/m^2/hour continuous IV infusion over 23 hours, day 10 (begin after 1,200 mg/m^2 dose)
Leucovorin 192 mg/m^2 IV, day 11, given 36 hours after the start of the methotrexate infusion
Leucovorin 12 mg/m^2/dose IV every 6 hours, day 11, beginning 42 hours after the start of the methotrexate infusion and continued until the methotrexate concentration is below 0.05 microMol/L
Cytarabine 70 mg intrathecal, days 1 and 3
Methotrexate 12 mg intrathecal, day 15
Filgrastim 5 mcg/kg/day subcutaneously, starting on day 13 and continuing until granulocyte count is above 1,000 cells/mm^3
continued on next page

CODOX-M/IVAC* (cont.)

    Treatment B —IVAC (cycles 2 and 4)

        Ifosfamide 1,500 mg/m^2/day IV, days 1 through 5

        Mesna 1,500 mg/m^2/day continuous IV infusion, days 1 through 5

        Etoposide 60 mg/m^2/day IV, days 1 through 5

        Cytarabine 2,000 mg/m^2/dose IV every 12 hours for 4 doses, days 1 and 2

        Methotrexate 12 mg intrathecal, day 5

        Filgrastim 5 mcg/kg/day subcutaneously, starting on day 7 and continuing until granulocyte count is above 1,000 cells/mm^3

    *Note: These 2 regimens are normally used in combination with each other and are rarely given alone. Patients with malignant pleocytosis receive additional intrathecal drugs:

        Cycle 1 (CODOX-M): Cytarabine 70 mg intrathecal on day 5 and methotrexate 12 mg intrathecal on day 15

        Cycle 2 (IVAC): Cytarabine 70 mg intrathecal on days 7 and 9

COMLA

Use: Lymphoma (non-Hodgkin). *Cycle:* 78 to 85 days for up to 3 cycles

Regimen: Cyclophosphamide 1,500 mg/m^2 IV, day 1

        Vincristine 1.4 mg/m^2 (2 mg maximum dose) IV, days 1, 8, and 15

        Methotrexate 120 mg/m^2 IV, days 22, 29, 36, 43, 50, 57, 64, and 71

        Leucovorin 25 mg/m^2/dose PO every 6 hours for 4 doses, beginning 24 hours after each methotrexate dose, days 23, 30, 37, 44, 51, 58, 65, and 72

        Cytarabine 300 mg/m^2 IV, days 22, 29, 36, 43, 50, 57, 64, and 71

COMP

Use: Lymphoma (non-Hodgkin—pediatrics)

Regimen: **Induction.** *Cycle:* Give 1 cycle only

        Cyclophosphamide 1,200 mg/m^2 IV, day 1

        Vincristine 2 mg/m^2 (2 mg maximum dose) IV, days 3, 10, 17, and 24

        Prednisone 15 mg/m^2/dose (60 mg/day maximum dose) PO 4 times daily, days 3 through 30, then taper for 7 to 10 days

        Methotrexate 300 mg/m^2 IV, day 12 or 17

        used in conjunction with

        Intrathecal chemotherapy

    Maintenance therapy. *Cycle:* 28 days for 15 cycles

        Cyclophosphamide 1,000 mg/m^2 IV, day 1

        Vincristine 1.5 mg/m^2 (2 mg maximum dose) IV, days 1 and 15

        Prednisone 15 mg/m^2/dose (60 mg/day maximum dose) PO 4 times daily, days 1 through 5, cycles 2 through 15

        Methotrexate 300 mg/m^2 IV, day 15

        used in conjunction with

        Intrathecal chemotherapy

Cooper Regimen
Use: Breast cancer. *Cycle:* 36 weeks (give a single cycle)
Regimen: Cyclophosphamide 2 mg/kg/day PO, weeks 1 through 36
Methotrexate 0.7 mg/kg IV weekly, weeks 1 through 8
Methotrexate 0.7 mg/kg IV every other week, weeks 10, 12, 14, 16, 18, 20, 22, 24, 26, 28, 30, 32, 34, and 36
Fluorouracil 12 mg/kg IV weekly, weeks 1 through 8
Fluorouracil 12 mg/kg IV every other week, weeks 10, 12, 14, 16, 18, 20, 22, 24, 26, 28, 30, 32, 34, and 36
Vincristine* 0.035 mg/kg IV weekly, weeks 1 through 5
Vincristine* 0.035 mg/kg IV monthly, weeks 8, 12, 16, 20, 24, 28, 32, and 36
Prednisone 0.75 mg/kg/day PO, days 1 through 10, then taper off over next 40 days
*Note: The vincristine dose is not capped in this protocol. Consult the prescriber if there is any question about the intended vincristine dose.

COP
Use: Lymphoma (non-Hodgkin). *Cycle:* 14 to 28 days for up to 12 cycles
Regimen: Cyclophosphamide 800 to 1,000 mg/m^2 IV, day 1
Vincristine 2 mg (dose is not in mg/m^2) IV, day 1
Prednisone 60 mg/m^2/day (or 100 mg/day) PO, days 1 through 5, then taper off over next 3 days

COPE
Use: Lung cancer (small cell). *Cycle:* 21 days for up to 4 cycles
Regimen: Cyclophosphamide 750 mg/m^2 IV, day 1
Etoposide 100 mg/m^2/day IV, days 1 through 3
Cisplatin 50 mg/m^2 IV, day 2
Vincristine 2 mg (dose is not in mg/m^2) IV, day 14

COPE (Baby Brain I)
Use: Brain tumors (pediatrics). *Cycle:* 28 days for up to 24 months
Regimen: Alternate cycles AABAAB.
Cycle A: Vincristine 0.065 mg/kg (1.5 mg maximum dose) IV, days 1 and 8
Cyclophosphamide 65 mg/kg IV, day 1
Cycle B: Cisplatin 4 mg/kg IV, day 1
Etoposide 6.5 mg/kg/day IV, days 3 and 4

COPP (C-MOPP)
Use: Lymphoma (non-Hodgkin or Hodgkin). *Cycle:* 28 days for up to 6 cycles
Regimen: Cyclophosphamide 450 to 650 mg/m^2 IV, days 1 and 8
Vincristine 1.4 to 2 mg/m^2 (2 mg maximum dose) IV, days 1 and 8
Procarbazine 100 mg/m^2/day PO, days 1 through 14
Prednisone 40 mg/m^2/day PO, cycles 1 and 4,* days 1 through 14
*Note: Some clinicians give prednisone with every cycle of COPP. The original clinical trials gave prednisone only with the first and fourth cycles.

CP
Use: Chronic lymphocytic leukemia (CLL). *Cycle:* 14 days for up to 18 months
Regimen: Chlorambucil 30 mg/m^2 PO, day 1
Prednisone 80 mg/day PO, days 1 through 5

continued on next page

CP (cont.)

Use: Ovarian cancer. *Cycle:* 21 to 28 days for 6 to 12 cycles
Regimen: Cyclophosphamide 600 to 1,000 mg/m² IV, day 1
Cisplatin 60 to 80 mg/m² IV, day 1

Use: Ovarian cancer. *Cycle:* 28 days for up to 6 cycles
Regimen: Cyclophosphamide 600 mg/m² IV, day 1
Cisplatin 100 mg/m² IV, day 1

CT

Use: Ovarian cancer. *Cycle:* 21 days for at least 6 cycles
Regimen: Paclitaxel 175 mg/m² IV infusion over 3 hours, day 1
or
Paclitaxel 135 mg/m²/day continuous IV infusion over 24 hours, day 1
with
Cisplatin 75 mg/m² IV, day 1 or 2 (given immediately after paclitaxel infusion)

Use: Cervical cancer. *Cycle:* 21 days for up to 6 cycles
Regimen: Paclitaxel 135 mg/m²/day continuous IV infusion over 24 hours, day 1
Cisplatin 50 mg/m² IV, day 2 (given immediately after paclitaxel infusion)

Use: Lung cancer (non-small cell). *Cycle:* 21 days
Regimen: Paclitaxel 135 mg/m²/day continuous IV infusion over 24 hours, day 1
Cisplatin 75 mg/m² IV, day 2 (given after paclitaxel)

CT - Intraperitoneal

Use: Ovarian cancer. *Cycle:* 21 days for 6 cycles
Regimen: Paclitaxel 135 mg/m²/day continuous IV infusion over 24 hours, day 1
Cisplatin 100 mg/m² intraperitoneal, day 2 (given after paclitaxel infusion)
Paclitaxel 60 mg/m² intraperitoneal, day 8

CVD

Use: Malignant melanoma. *Cycle:* 21 days for at least 2 cycles
Regimen: Vinblastine 1.6 mg/m²/day IV, days 1 through 5
Dacarbazine 800 mg/m² IV, day 1
Cisplatin 20 mg/m²/day IV, days 2 through 5

Use: Malignant melanoma. *Cycle:* 21 days for at least 2 cycles
Regimen: Cisplatin 20 mg/m²/day IV, days 1 through 4
Vinblastine 2 mg/m²/day IV, days 1 through 4
Dacarbazine 800 mg/m² IV, day 1

CVD + IL-2I

Use: Malignant melanoma. *Cycle:* 21 days for 6 to 7 cycles
Regimen: Cisplatin 20 mg/m²/day IV, days 1 through 4
Vinblastine 1.6 mg/m²/day IV, days 1 through 4
Dacarbazine 800 mg/m² IV, day 1
Aldesleukin 9 million units/m²/day continuous IV infusion, days 1 through 4
Interferon alfa 5 million units/m²/day subcutaneously, days 1 through 5, and days 7, 9, 11, and 13

continued on next page

CVD + IL-2I (cont.)
Use: Malignant melanoma. *Cycle:* 42 days for up to 3 cycles
Regimen: Cisplatin 20 mg/m^2/day IV, days 1 through 4 and days 22 through 25
Vinblastine 1.5 mg/m^2/day IV, days 1 through 4 and days 22 through 25
Dacarbazine 800 mg/m^2 IV, days 1 and 22
Aldesleukin 9 million units/m^2/day continuous IV infusion, days 5 through 8, days 17 through 20, and days 26 through 29
Interferon alfa-2b 5 million units/m^2/day subcutaneously, days 5 through 9, days 17 through 21, and days 26 through 30

CVD + IL-2I, Modified
Use: Malignant melanoma. *Cycle:* 21 days for up to 4 cycles
Regimen: Cisplatin 20 mg/m^2/day IV, days 1 through 4
Vinblastine 1.2 mg/m^2/day IV, days 1 through 4
Dacarbazine 800 mg/m^2 IV, day 1
Aldesleukin 9 million units/m^2/day continuous IV infusion, days 1 through 4
Interferon alfa-2b 5 million units/m^2/day subcutaneously, days 1 through 5, and days 8, 10, and 12
Filgrastim 5 mcg/kg/day subcutaneously (rounded to 300 or 480 mcg), days 7 through 16
*used in conjunction with antimicrobial prophylaxis**
Ciprofloxacin 500 mg PO twice daily, days 1 through 14
or
Cephalexin 500 mg PO twice daily, days 1 through 14
*Note: Antimicrobial prophylaxis doses not specified in original article; the dose given here is derived from *AHFS 2008 Drug Information*, a tertiary resource.

CVI (VIC)
Use: Lung cancer (non-small cell). *Cycle:* 28 days for up to 6 cycles
Regimen: Carboplatin 300 to 350 mg/m^2 IV, day 1
Etoposide 60 to 100 mg/m^2 IV, days 1, 3, and 5
Ifosfamide 1,500 mg/m^2 IV, days 1, 3, and 5
Mesna 400 mg/m^2 IV, given before ifosfamide, days 1, 3, and 5
Mesna 1,600 mg/m^2/day continuous IV infusion, days 1, 3, and 5 (give after mesna bolus)

CVP
Use: Lymphoma (non-Hodgkin), chronic lymphocytic leukemia (CLL). *Cycle:* 21 days
Regimen: Cyclophosphamide 300 to 400 mg/m^2/day PO, days 1 through 5
Vincristine 1.2 to 1.4 mg/m^2 (2 mg maximum dose) IV, day 1
Prednisone 40 to 100 mg/m^2/day PO, days 1 through 5

CVP + Rituximab (R-CVP)
Use: Lymphoma (non-Hodgkin). *Cycle:* 21 days for up to 8 cycles
Regimen: Cyclophosphamide 750 mg/m^2 IV, day 1
Vincristine 1.4 mg/m^2 (2 mg maximum dose) IV, day 1
Prednisone 40 mg/m^2/day PO, days 1 through 5
Rituximab 375 mg/m^2 IV, day 1

CVPP

Use:	Lymphoma (Hodgkin). *Cycle:* 28 days for up to 6 cycles
Regimen:	Lomustine 75 mg/m^2 PO, day 1
	Vinblastine 4 mg/m^2 IV, days 1 and 8
	Procarbazine 100 mg/m^2/day PO, days 1 through 14
	Prednisone 40 mg/m^2/day PO, cycles 1 and 4, days 1 through 14

CY/A—see AC

Cyclophosphamide-Fludarabine

Use:	Chronic lymphocytic leukemia (CLL). *Cycle:* 28 days for up to 6 cycles
Regimen:	Cyclophosphamide 250 mg/m^2/day IV, days 1 through 3
	Fludarabine 25 to 30 mg/m^2/day IV, days 1 through 3

Cyclophosphamide-Topotecan—see Topo/CTX

CYVADIC

Use:	Sarcoma (bone, soft tissue). *Cycle:* 21 days for up to 8 cycles
Regimen:	Cyclophosphamide 500 mg/m^2 IV, day 1
	Vincristine 1 mg/m^2 (2 mg maximum dose) IV, days 1 and 5
	Doxorubicin 50 mg/m^2 IV, day 1
	Dacarbazine 250 mg/m^2/day IV, days 1 through 5

Use:	Sarcoma (bone, soft tissue). *Cycle:* 21 days
Regimen:	Cyclophosphamide 500 mg/m^2 IV, day 1
	Vincristine 1.5 mg/m^2 (2 mg maximum dose) IV, day 1
	Doxorubicin 50 mg/m^2 IV, day 1 (total cumulative dose 550 mg/m^2)
	Dacarbazine 750 mg/m^2/day IV, day 1

D + P—see Docetaxel-Prednisone

DA

Use:	Acute myelogenous leukemia (AML; induction—pediatrics). *Cycle:* 14 days. Give 1 cycle. If patient has persistent leukemia on day 14, give 1 to 2 additional cycles as described below.
Regimen:	Daunorubicin 45 to 60 mg/m^2/day IV, days 1 through 3
	Cytarabine 100 mg/m^2/day continuous IV infusion, days 1 through 7
	If leukemia is persistent on day 14, additional doses are given: cytarabine on days 1 through 5 and daunorubicin on days 1 and 2, both at same dose as previous cycle.

DA + ATRA (ATRA + CT)

Use:	Acute promyelocytic leukemia (APL; induction and consolidation)
Regimen:	Tretinoin 45 mg/m^2/day PO, days 1 through 90, or until complete remission, whichever occurs earlier
	Induction. *Cycle:* Give 1 induction cycle followed by 2 consolidation cycles after hematologic recovery.
	Daunorubicin 60 mg/m^2/day IV, days 3 through 5
	Cytarabine 200 mg/m^2/day continuous IV infusion, days 3 through 9
	First consolidation. *Cycle:* Give 1 cycle.
	Daunorubicin 60 mg/m^2/day IV, days 1 through 3
	Cytarabine 200 mg/m^2/day continuous IV infusion, days 1 through 7
	Second consolidation. *Cycle:* Give 1 cycle. Do not give to patients older than 65 years of age.
	Daunorubicin 45 mg/m^2/day IV, days 1 through 3
	Cytarabine 1,000 mg/m^2/dose IV every 12 hours for 8 doses, days 1 through 4

Dartmouth Regimen—see CDB + Tamoxifen

DAT

Use: Acute myelogenous leukemia (AML; induction—pediatrics).
Cycle: 14 to 21 days for up to 3 cycles

Regimen: Cytarabine 100 mg/m^2/dose IV every 12 hours for 14 doses, days 1 through 7
Thioguanine 100 mg/m^2/dose PO every 12 hours for 14 doses, days 1 through 7
Daunorubicin 60 mg/m^2/day continuous IV infusion, days 5 through 7

Use: Acute myelogenous leukemia (AML; induction—pediatrics)

Regimen: **Remission induction.** *Cycle:* Give 1 cycle only
Daunorubicin 45 mg/m^2/day IV, days 1 through 3
Cytarabine 100 mg/m^2/day continuous IV infusion, days 1 through 7
Thioguanine100 mg/m^2/day PO, days 1 through 7
Second induction. *Cycle*: Give a single cycle 14 days after initial remission induction course; delay until hematologic recovery in patients with remission or with hypoplastic marrow.
Daunorubicin 45 mg/m^2/day IV, days 1 and 2
Cytarabine 100 mg/m^2/day continuous IV infusion, days 1 through 5
Thioguanine 100 mg/m^2/day PO, days 1 through 5
used in conjunction with
Intrathecal chemotherapy

DAV

Use: Acute myelogenous leukemia (AML; induction—pediatrics).
Cycle: Give a single cycle

Regimen: Cytarabine 100 mg/m^2/day continuous IV infusion, days 1 through 2
Cytarabine 100 mg/m^2/dose IV every 12 hours for 12 doses, days 3 through 8
Daunorubicin 60 mg/m^2/day IV, days 3 through 5
Etoposide 150 mg/m^2/day IV, days 6 through 8

DCF

Use: Gastric cancer. *Cycle:* 21 days, continue until disease progression or intolerable toxicity

Regimen: Docetaxel 75 mg/m^2 IV, day 1
Cisplatin 75 mg/m^2 IV, day 1
Fluorouracil 750 mg/m^2/day continuous IV infusion, days 1 through 5 (for 120 hours total)

DCT

Use: Acute myelogenous leukemia (AML; induction—adults).
Cycle: 7 days. Give once. May be given a second time based on individual response. Time between cycles not specified.

Regimen: Daunorubicin 40 mg/m^2/day IV, days 1 through 3
Cytarabine 100 mg/m^2/dose IV every 12 hours for 14 doses, days 1 through 7
Thioguanine 100 mg/m^2/dose PO every 12 hours for 14 doses, days 1 through 7

DCTER

Use: Acute myelogenous leukemia (AML; induction and consolidation—pediatrics). *Cycle:* 10 to 14 days. Give 4 cycles.

Regimen 1: Patients younger than 3 years of age:

Dexamethasone 0.067 mg/kg/dose (0.2 mg/kg/day) PO given 3 times daily, days 1 through 4

Cytarabine 6.7 mg/kg/day continuous IV infusion, days 1 through 4*

Thioguanine 1.65 mg/kg/dose (3.3 mg/kg/day) PO given twice daily, days 1 through 4

Etoposide 3.3 mg/kg/day continuous IV infusion, days 1 through 4*

Daunorubicin 0.67 mg/kg/day continuous IV infusion, days 1 through 4*

used in conjunction with

Cytarabine intrathecal, day 1 (dose is based on patient's age):

Age up to 1 year: Cytarabine 20 mg

Age 1 to 2 years: Cytarabine 30 mg

Age 2 to 3 years: Cytarabine 50 mg

Regimen 2: Patients 3 years of age and older:

Dexamethasone 2 mg/m^2/dose (6 mg/m^2/day) PO given 3 times daily, days 1 through 4

Cytarabine 200 mg/m^2/day continuous IV infusion, days 1 through 4*

Thioguanine 50 mg/m^2/dose (100 mg/m^2/day) PO given twice daily, days 1 through 4

Etoposide 100 mg/m^2/day continuous IV infusion, days 1 through 4*

Daunorubicin 20 mg/m^2/day continuous IV infusion, days 1 through 4*

used in conjunction with

Cytarabine 70 mg intrathecal, day 1

*Note: Cytarabine, etoposide, and daunorubicin may be mixed and administered in the same infusion bag.

DHAOx

Use: Lymphoma (non-Hodgkin). *Cycle:* 21 days

Regimen: Oxaliplatin 130 mg/m^2 IV, day 1

Dexamethasone 40 mg/day PO or IV, days 1 through 4

Cytarabine 2,000 mg/m^2/dose IV every 12 hours for 2 doses (total dose 4,000 mg/m^2), day 2

Filgrastim 5 mcg/kg/day subcutaneously, starting on day 3 and continued until granulocyte count is above 500 cells/mm^3

DHAP

Use: Lymphoma (non-Hodgkin). *Cycle:* 21 to 28 days for 6 to 10 cycles

Regimen: Cisplatin 100 mg/m^2/day continuous IV infusion, day 1

Dexamethasone 40 mg/day PO or IV, days 1 through 4

Cytarabine 2,000 mg/m^2/dose IV every 12 hours for 2 doses (total dose 4,000 mg/m^2), day 2

DI

Use:	Sarcoma (soft tissue). *Cycle:* 21 days, continue until disease progression or intolerable toxicity
Regimen:	Doxorubicin 50 mg/m^2 IV, day 1
	Ifosfamide 5,000 mg/m^2/day continuous IV infusion, day 1 (after doxorubicin)
	Mesna 600 mg/m^2 IV bolus infusion, day 1 (before ifosfamide)
	Mesna 2,500 mg/m^2/day continuous IV infusion over 36 hours, day 1 (give after mesna bolus)

Use:	Sarcoma. *Cycle:* 21 days
Regimen:	Doxorubicin 25 mg/m^2/day continuous IV infusion, days 1 through 3
	Ifosfamide 2,000 mg/m^2/day IV, days 1 through 5
	Mesna 400 mg/m^2 IV bolus at same time as first ifosfamide dose, day 1
	Mesna 1,200 mg/m^2/day continuous IV infusion, days 1 through 5 (start after mesna bolus on day 1)

Use:	Sarcoma. *Cycle:* 21 days
Regimen:	Doxorubicin 30 mg/m^2/day continuous IV infusion, days 1 through 3
	Ifosfamide 2,500 mg/m^2/day IV, days 1 through 4
	Mesna 500 mg/m^2 IV bolus at same time as first ifosfamide dose, day 1
	Mesna 1,500 mg/m^2/day continuous IV infusion, days 1 through 4 (start after mesna bolus on day 1)
	Filgrastim 5 mcg/kg/day subcutaneously (rounded to 300 or 480 mcg), starting on day 5, continued until absolute neutrophil count (ANC) is at least 10,000 cells/mm^3

Docetaxel-Carboplatin

Use:	Ovarian cancer. *Cycle:* 21 days for 6 cycles
Regimen:	Docetaxel 75 mg/m^2 IV, day 1
	Carboplatin IV dose by Calvert equation to AUC 5 mg/mL/min, day 1 (after docetaxel)

Use:	Ovarian cancer. *Cycle:* 21 days for 6 cycles
Regimen:	Docetaxel 60 mg/m^2 IV, day 1
	Carboplatin IV dose by Calvert equation to AUC 6 mg/mL/min, day 1 (administration sequence not specified in protocol)

Docetaxel-Cisplatin

Use:	Lung cancer (non-small cell). *Cycle:* 21 days for up to 6 cycles
Regimen:	Docetaxel 75 mg/m^2 IV, day 1
	Cisplatin 75 mg/m^2 IV, day 1 (after docetaxel)

Docetaxel-Doxorubicin

Use:	Breast cancer. *Cycle:* 21 days
Regimen:	Doxorubicin 50 mg/m^2 IV, day 1
	Docetaxel 75 mg/m^2 IV, day 1 (after doxorubicin)
	used in conjunction with antimicrobial prophylaxis
	Ciprofloxacin 500 mg PO twice daily, days 5 through 14 (10 days total)

Docetaxel-Estramustine

Use: Prostate cancer. *Cycle:* 21 days for up to 6 cycles
Regimen: Estramustine 280 mg/dose (1,120 mg/day) PO every 6 hours for
         5 doses, day 1
         Docetaxel 70 mg/m^2 IV, day 1 (given 12 hours after first estra-
         mustine dose)

Use: Prostate cancer. *Cycle:* 21 days for up to 12 cycles
Regimen: Estramustine 280 mg/dose (840 mg/day) PO 3 times daily, days 1
         through 5
         Docetaxel 60 mg/m^2 IV, day 2

Use: Prostate cancer. *Cycle:* 21 days, continue until disease progres-
         sion or intolerable toxicity
Regimen: Estramustine 420 mg/dose (1,260 mg/day) PO 3 times daily for
         4 doses, on days 1 (give in morning, afternoon, and evening) and
         2 (give in morning only)
         Estramustine 280 mg/dose (840 mg/day) PO 3 times daily for
         5 doses, days 2 (give in afternoon and evening) and 3 (give in
         morning afternoon, and evening)
         Docetaxel 35 mg/m^2 IV, days 2 and 9
         Estramustine 420 mg/dose (1,260 mg/day) PO 3 times daily for
         4 doses, on days 8 (give in morning, afternoon, and evening) and
         9 (give in morning only)
         Estramustine 280 mg/dose (840 mg/day) PO 3 times daily for
         5 doses, days 9 (give in afternoon and evening) and 10 (give in
         morning afternoon, and evening)

Docetaxel-Prednisone (D + P)

Use: Prostate cancer. *Cycle:* 21 days for up to 10 cycles
Regimen: Docetaxel 75 mg/m^2 IV, day 1
         Prednisone 5 mg/dose PO twice daily, throughout entire course

Use: Prostate cancer. *Cycle:* 42 days for up to 5 cycles
Regimen: Docetaxel 30 mg/m^2 IV, days 1, 8, 15, 22, and 29
         Prednisone 5 mg/dose PO twice daily, throughout entire course

Dox ➤ CMF, Sequential

Use: Breast cancer. *Cycle:* 21 days
Regimen: Doxorubicin 75 mg/m^2 IV, day 1 for 4 cycles
         followed by
         CMF-IV for 8 cycles

Doxorubicin-Streptozocin

Use: Islet-cell carcinoma. *Cycle:* 42 days, continue until disease progres-
         sion or intolerable toxicity
Regimen: Doxorubicin 50 mg/m^2 IV, days 1 and 22
         Streptozocin 500 mg/m^2/day IV, days 1 through 5

DTIC/Tamoxifen

Use: Malignant melanoma. *Cycle:* 21 days, continue until disease pro-
         gression or intolerable toxicity
Regimen: Dacarbazine 250 mg/m^2/day IV, days 1 through 5
         Tamoxifen 20 mg/m^2/day PO, days 1 through 5

DTPACE

Use: Multiple myeloma. *Cycle:* 28 to 42 days for up to 6 cycles, delay each subsequent cycle until hematologic recovery

Regimen: Dexamethasone 40 mg/day PO, days 1 through 4
Thalidomide 400 mg/day PO, throughout entire course
Cisplatin 10 mg/m^2/day continuous IV infusion, days 1 through 4*
Doxorubicin 10 mg/m^2/day continuous IV infusion, days 1 through 4
Cyclophosphamide 400 mg/m^2/day continuous IV infusion, days 1 through 4*
Etoposide 40 mg/m^2/day continuous IV infusion, days 1 through 4*
Filgrastim 300 mcg/day subcutaneously, from day 5 until the absolute neutrophil count (ANC) is at least 1,000 cells/mm^3 for 2 consecutive days; increase dose to filgrastim 10 mcg/kg/day subcutaneously during first cycle in patients undergoing peripheral blood stem cell mobilization
used in conjunction with antimicrobial prophylaxis
    Fluconazole 200 mg/dose PO 4 times daily, from day 1 until neutropenia resolves
    Levofloxacin 250 mg/dose PO 4 times daily, from day 1 until neutropenia resolves
    Acyclovir 400 mg PO twice daily, from day 1 until neutropenia resolves
    Cotrimoxazole double-strength (160/800) 1 tablet PO twice daily, from day 1 until neutropenia resolves
*Note: Cisplatin, cyclophosphamide, and etoposide may be mixed and administered in the same infusion bag.

DVd

Use: Multiple myeloma. *Cycle:* 28 days, continue until complete remission, disease progression, or intolerable toxicity

Regimen: Liposomal doxorubicin 40 mg/m^2 IV, day 1
Vincristine 1.4 mg/m^2 (2 mg maximum dose) IV, day 1
Dexamethasone 40 mg/day PO, days 1 through 4

DVP

Use: Acute lymphocytic leukemia (ALL; induction—pediatrics). *Cycle:* 35 days. Give a single cycle.

Regimen: Daunorubicin 25 mg/m^2 IV, days 1, 8, and 15
Vincristine 1.5 mg/m^2 (2 mg maximum dose) IV, days 1, 8, 15, and 22
Prednisone 60 mg/m^2/day PO, days 1 through 28, then taper off over next 14 days
used in conjunction with
Intrathecal chemotherapy

EAP

Use: Gastric cancer, small bowel cancer. *Cycle:* 21 to 28 days for up to 6 cycles

Regimen: Doxorubicin 20 mg/m^2 IV, days 1 and 7
Cisplatin 40 mg/m^2 IV, days 2 and 8
Etoposide 100 to 120 mg/m^2/day IV, days 4 through 6

EC

Use: Lung cancer. *Cycle:* 21 to 28 days for up to 4 to 6 cycles

Regimen: Etoposide 100 to 120 mg/m^2/day IV, days 1 through 3
with
Carboplatin 300 to 350 mg/m^2 IV, day 1
or
Carboplatin IV dose by Calvert equation to AUC 6 mg/mL/min, day 1

ECF
Use: Gastric cancer. *Cycle:* 21 days for up to 8 cycles
Regimen: Epirubicin 50 mg/m² IV, day 1
Cisplatin 60 mg/m² IV, day 1
Fluorouracil 200 mg/m²/day continuous IV infusion, days 1 through 180

EDP-Mitotane
Use: Adrenal cancer. *Cycle:* 28 days for up to 6 cycles
Regimen: Doxorubicin 20 mg/m² IV, days 1 and 8
Cisplatin 40 mg/m² IV, days 1 and 9
Etoposide 100 mg/m²/day IV, days 5 through 7
Mitotane 1,000 mg/dose (4,000 mg/day) PO 4 times daily, throughout entire course
some patients may require mineralocorticoid or glucocorticoid supplementation
Hydrocortisone 10 to 30 mg/day PO in divided doses, throughout entire course*
Fludrocortisone 0.1 mg/day PO, throughout entire course*
*Note: Mineralocorticoid and glucocorticoid doses not specified in original article; the dose given here is derived from *AHFS 2008 Drug Information*, a tertiary resource

EFP
Use: Gastric cancer, small bowel cancer. *Cycle:* 21 to 28 days
Regimen: Etoposide 80 to 100 mg/m² IV, days 1, 3, and 5
Fluorouracil 800 to 900 mg/m²/day continuous IV infusion, days 1 through 5
Cisplatin 20 mg/m²/day IV, days 1 through 5

ELF
Use: Gastric cancer. *Cycle:* 21 to 28 days for up to 9 cycles
Regimen: Etoposide 120 mg/m²/day IV, days 1 through 3
with
Leucovorin 300 mg/m²/day IV, days 1 through 3
or
Levoleucovorin 150 mg/m²/day IV, days 1 through 3
plus
Fluorouracil 500 mg/m²/day IV, days 1 through 3 (after leucovorin or levoleucovorin)

EM-V—see Estramustine/Vinblastine

EMA 86
Use: Acute myelogenous leukemia (AML; induction—adults). *Cycle:* Give a single cycle
Regimen: Mitoxantrone 12 mg/m²/day IV, days 1 through 3
Cytarabine 500 mg/m²/day continuous IV infusion, days 1 through 3 and days 8 through 10
Etoposide 200 mg/m²/day continuous IV infusion, days 8 through 10

EP
Use: Testicular cancer. *Cycle:* 21 days for 2 cycles
Regimen: Etoposide 100 mg/m²/day IV, days 1 through 5
Cisplatin 20 mg/m²/day IV, days 1 through 5

Use: Thymoma. *Cycle:* 21 days for up to 8 cycles
Regimen: Etoposide 120 mg/m²/day IV, days 1 through 3
Cisplatin 60 mg/m² IV, day 1

continued on next page

EP (cont.)
Use: Lung cancer, adenocarcinoma. *Cycle:* 21 to 28 days for 2 to 6 cycles
Regimen: Etoposide 80 to 120 mg/m²/day IV, days 1 through 3
Cisplatin 80 to 100 mg/m² IV, day 1

Use: Neuroendocrine tumor. *Cycle:* 28 days, continue until disease progression or intolerable toxicity
Regimen: Etoposide 130 mg/m²/day continuous IV infusion, days 1 through 3
Cisplatin 45 mg/m²/day continuous IV infusion, days 2 through 3

EP + Docetaxel, Sequential
Use: Lung cancer (non-small cell). *Cycle:* See below, cycle length varies throughout protocol. Give 2 cycles of EP + Radiation, followed by 3 cycles of docetaxel alone.
Regimen: EP + Radiation. *Cycle:* 28 days for 2 cycles
Etoposide 50 mg/m²/day IV, days 1 through 5
Cisplatin 50 mg/m² IV, days 1 and 8
used in conjunction with
Radiation therapy
followed after 4 to 6 weeks by
Docetaxel alone. *Cycle:* 21 days for 3 cycles
Docetaxel 75 mg/m² IV, day 1 for the first cycle; may increase to docetaxel 100 mg/m² IV, day 1 for subsequent cycles if tolerated

EPOCH
Use: Lymphoma (non-Hodgkin). *Cycle:* 21 days for at least 6 cycles
Regimen: Etoposide 50 mg/m²/day continuous IV infusion, days 1 through 4
Prednisone 60 mg/m²/day PO, days 1 through 6
Vincristine* 0.4 mg/m²/day continuous IV infusion, days 1 through 4[†]
Doxorubicin 10 mg/m²/day continuous IV infusion, days 1 through 4[†]
Cyclophosphamide 750 mg/m² IV, day 5
Cotrimoxazole double-strength (160/800) 1 tablet PO twice daily, given for 3 consecutive days each week
*Note: The vincristine dose is not capped in this protocol. Consult the prescriber if there is any question about the intended vincristine dose.
[†]Note: Vincristine and doxorubicin may be mixed and administered in the same infusion bag, if diluted with 0.9% Sodium Chloride Injection. Etoposide is usually infused in a separate line.

EPOCH, Dose-Adjusted
Use: Lymphoma (non-Hodgkin) associated with HIV infection.
Cycle: 21 days for up to 6 cycles
Regimen: Etoposide 50 mg/m²/day continuous IV infusion, days 1 through 4
Prednisone 60 mg/m²/day PO, days 1 through 5
Vincristine* 0.4 mg/m²/day continuous IV infusion, days 1 through 4[†]
Doxorubicin 10 mg/m²/day continuous IV infusion, days 1 through 4[†]
with
Cyclophosphamide dose based on cell counts for first and subsequent cycles:
Patients with baseline CD4+ cell counts at least 100 cells/mm³:
Cyclophosphamide 375 mg/m² IV, day 5 for the first cycle; adjust dose for subsequent cycles based on nadir
continued on next page

EPOCH, Dose-Adjusted (cont.)

Patients with baseline CD4+ cell counts less than 100 cells/mm^3: Cyclophosphamide 187 mg/m^2 IV, day 5 for the first cycle; adjust dose for subsequent cycles based on nadir

Nadir absolute neutrophil count (ANC) above 500 cells/mm^3 after first cycle: May increase dose in increments of 187 mg/m^2 (up to 750 mg/m^2 maximum) for subsequent cycles

Nadir ANC less than 500 cells/mm^3 or platelet nadir less than 25,000 cells/mm^3 after first cycle: Decrease dose in increments of 187 mg/m^2 for subsequent cycles

plus

Filgrastim 5 mcg/kg/day subcutaneously, from day 6 until ANC is at least 5,000 cells/mm^3

used in conjunction with antimicrobial prophylaxis[‡]

Cotrimoxazole (either 80/400 or 160/800 strength) 1 tablet PO daily, throughout entire course

plus

Azithromycin 1,200 mg PO once weekly, throughout entire course

or

Clarithromycin 500 mg PO twice weekly, throughout entire course

[*]Note: The vincristine dose is not capped in this protocol. Consult the prescriber if there is any question about the intended vincristine dose.

[†]Note: Vincristine and doxorubicin may be mixed and administered in the same infusion bag, if diluted with 0.9% Sodium Chloride Injection. Etoposide is usually infused in a separate line.

[‡]Note: Antimicrobial prophylaxis drugs and doses not specified in original articles; the doses given here are derived from the *Infectious Diseases Handbook*, 6th edition, a tertiary resource.

EPOCH-R

Use: Lymphoma (B-cell, mantle cell). *Cycle:* 21 days for at least 6 cycles, delay subsequent cycles until hematologic recovery

Regimen: Rituximab 375 mg/m^2 IV, day 1

Etoposide 50 mg/m^2/day continuous IV infusion, days 1 through 4

Vincristine[*] 0.4 mg/m^2/day continuous IV infusion, days 1 through 4[†]

Doxorubicin 10 mg/m^2/day continuous IV infusion, days 1 through 4[†]

Prednisone 60 mg/m^2/day PO, days 1 through 5

Cyclophosphamide 750 mg/m^2 IV, day 5

Filgrastim 5 mcg/kg/day subcutaneously, starting on day 6 and continued until granulocyte count exceeds 5,000 cells/mm^3

Cotrimoxazole double-strength (160/800) 1 tablet PO twice daily, given on Monday, Wednesday, and Friday of each week

[*]Note: The vincristine dose is not capped in this protocol. Consult the prescriber if there is any question about the intended vincristine dose.

[†]Note: Vincristine and doxorubicin may be mixed and administered in the same infusion bag, if diluted with 0.9% Sodium Chloride Injection. Etoposide is usually infused in a separate line.

ESHAP

Use: Lymphoma (non-Hodgkin). *Cycle:* 21 to 28 days for up to 6 to 8 cycles

Regimen: Etoposide 40 to 60 mg/m^2/day IV, days 1 through 4

Methylprednisolone 250 to 500 mg/day IV, days 1 through 4 or days 1 through 5

Cisplatin 25 mg/m^2/day continuous IV infusion, days 1 through 4

Cytarabine 2,000 mg/m^2 IV, day 5 (after etoposide and cisplatin are completed)

Estramustine-Etoposide

Use: Prostate cancer. *Cycle:* 28 days, continue until disease progression or intolerable toxicity

Regimen: Estramustine 3.75 mg/kg/dose (15 mg/kg/day) PO 4 times daily, days 1 through 21

Etoposide 25 mg/m^2/dose (50 mg/m^2/day) PO twice daily, days 1 through 21

Estramustine/Vinblastine (EM-V)

Use: Prostate cancer. *Cycle:* 8 weeks, continue until disease progression or intolerable toxicity

Regimen: Vinblastine 4 mg/m^2 IV weekly, weeks 1 through 6

with

Estramustine 3.33 mg/kg/dose (10 mg/kg/day) PO 3 times daily, days 1 through 42

or

Estramustine 600 mg/m^2/day PO given in 2 to 3 divided doses, days 1 through 42

EVA

Use: Lymphoma (Hodgkin). *Cycle:* 28 days for up to 6 cycles

Regimen: Etoposide 100 mg/m^2/day IV, days 1 through 3

Vinblastine 6 mg/m^2 IV, day 1

Doxorubicin 50 mg/m^2 IV, day 1

F-CL (FU/LV), Biweekly Regimen (de Gramont)

Use: Colorectal cancer. *Cycle:* 14 days, continue until disease progression or intolerable toxicity

Regimen: Leucovorin 200 mg/m^2/day IV, days 1 and 2

Fluorouracil 400 mg/m^2/day IV bolus, days 1 and 2 (after starting leucovorin)

then

Fluorouracil 600 mg/m^2/dose continuous IV infusion for 22 hours, days 1 and 2

F-CL (FU/LV), Mayo Clinic Regimen

Use: Colorectal cancer. *Cycle:* 4 to 5 weeks

Regimen: Low-dose leucovorin:

Leucovorin 20 mg/m^2/day IV, days 1 through 5

Fluorouracil 370 to 425 mg/m^2/day IV, days 1 through 5 (after starting leucovorin)

or

High-dose leucovorin:

Leucovorin 200 mg/m^2/day IV, days 1 through 5

Fluorouracil 370 mg/m^2/day IV, days 1 through 5 (after starting leucovorin)

F-CL (FU/LV), Post-Gastrectomy

Use: Gastric cancer. *Cycle:* Give a single cycle after gastrectomy

Regimen: Fluorouracil 425 mg/m^2/day IV, days 1 through 5

Leucovorin 20 mg/m^2/day IV, days 1 through 5

followed by

Radiation therapy, 5 days per week for 5 weeks, days 29 through 33, days 36 through 40, days 43 though 47, days 50 through 54, and days 57 through 61

Fluorouracil 400 mg/m^2/day IV, days 29 through 32 and days 59 through 61

Leucovorin 20 mg/m^2/day IV, days 29 through 32 and days 59 through 61

followed 1 month later by

Fluorouracil 425 mg/m^2/day IV, days 85 through 89 and days 113 to 117

Leucovorin 20 mg/m^2/day IV, days 85 through 89 and days 113 to 117

F-CL (FU/LV), Roswell Park Regimen

Use: Colorectal cancer. *Cycle:* 8 weeks

Regimen: Leucovorin 500 mg/m^2 IV, weekly for 6 weeks, then 2 weeks of rest

Fluorouracil 600 mg/m^2 IV, weekly for 6 weeks (after starting leucovorin), then 2 weeks of rest

F-CL (FU/LV), Weekly Regimen (German Schedule)

Use: Metastatic colorectal cancer. *Cycle:* Ongoing, continue until disease progression

Regimen: Leucovorin 20 mg/m^2 IV, weekly

Fluorouracil 500 mg/m^2 IV, weekly (after starting leucovorin)

FAC

Use: Breast cancer. *Cycle:* 21 to 28 days

Regimen: Fluorouracil 500 mg/m^2 IV, days 1 and 8

Doxorubicin 50 mg/m^2 IV, day 1

Cyclophosphamide 500 mg/m^2 IV, day 1

FAM

Use: Adenocarcinoma, gastric cancer, pancreatic cancer. *Cycle:* 8 weeks, continue until disease progression or intolerable toxicity

Regimen: Fluorouracil 600 mg/m^2 IV, days 1, 8, 29, and 36

Doxorubicin 30 mg/m^2 IV, days 1 and 29

Mitomycin 10 mg/m^2 IV, day 1

FAMTX

Use: Gastric cancer. *Cycle:* 28 days

Regimen: Methotrexate 1,500 mg/m^2 IV, day 1

Fluorouracil 1,500 mg/m^2 IV, day 1 (give after methotrexate)

Leucovorin 15 mg/m^2/dose PO every 6 hours for 8 doses (start 24 hours after methotrexate); increase dose to 30 mg/m^2/dose PO every 6 hours for 16 doses if 24-hour methotrexate level is 2.5 mol/L or higher

Doxorubicin 30 mg/m^2 IV, day 15

FAP

Use: Gastric cancer. *Cycle:* 5 weeks, continue until disease progression or intolerable toxicity

Regimen: Fluorouracil 300 mg/m^2/day IV, days 1 through 5

Doxorubicin 40 mg/m^2 IV, day 1

Cisplatin 60 mg/m^2 IV, day 1

FAS
Use: Islet cell carcinoma. *Cycle:* 28 days, continue until disease progression or intolerable toxicity
Regimen: Fluorouracil 400 mg/m^2/day IV, days 1 through 5
Doxorubicin 40 mg/m^2 IV, day 1
Streptozocin 400 mg/m^2/day IV, days 1 through 5

FC (also see Fludarabine-Cyclophosphamide)
Use: Lymphoma (non-Hodgkin). *Cycle:* 28 days for up to 8 cycles
Regimen: Fludarabine 20 mg/m^2/day IV, days 1 through 5
Cyclophosphamide 1,000 mg/m^2 IV, day 1
*used in conjunction with antimicrobial prophylaxis**
Cotrimoxazole double-strength (160/800) 1 tablet PO daily, throughout entire course
plus
Acyclovir 200 mg PO 3 times daily, throughout entire course
or
Acyclovir 400 mg PO twice daily, throughout entire course
*Note: Antimicrobial prophylaxis doses not specified in original article; the doses given here are derived from the *Infectious Diseases Handbook*, 6th edition, and *2008 Drug Information*, both tertiary resources.

FCR
Use: Chronic lymphocytic leukemia (CLL). *Cycle:* 28 days for up to 6 cycles. Delay each subsequent cycle until absolute neutrophil count (ANC) is greater than 1,000 cells/mm^3 and platelet count is at least 80,000 cells/mm^3.
Regimen: Fludarabine 25 mg/m^2/day IV, days 1 through 3, except for day 1 of first cycle
Fludarabine 25 mg/m^2 IV, day 4 first cycle only
Cyclophosphamide 250 mg/m^2/day IV, days 1 through 3, except for day 1 of first cycle
Cyclophosphamide 250 mg/m^2 IV, day 4 first cycle only
Rituximab 375 mg/m^2 IV, day 1 first cycle only
Rituximab 500 mg/m^2 IV, day 1 except for first cycle
used in conjunction with antimicrobial prophylaxis
Valacyclovir 500 mg/day PO, throughout entire course
plus
Cotrimoxazole (either 80/400 or 160/800 strength) 1 tablet PO daily, throughout entire course*
or
Pentamidine 300 mg inhaled once monthly, throughout entire course*
*Note: Pneumocystis prophylaxis doses not specified in original articles; the dose given here is derived from the *Infectious Diseases Handbook*, 6th edition, a tertiary resource.

FEC (also see CEF)
Use: Breast cancer. *Cycle:* 21 days for 4 to 6 cycles
Regimen: Fluorouracil 500 mg/m^2 IV, day 1
Epirubicin 100 mg/m^2 IV, day 1
Cyclophosphamide 500 mg/m^2 IV, day 1

FED

Use:	Lung cancer (non-small cell). *Cycle:* 21 days for up to 3 cycles
Regimen:	Cisplatin 100 mg/m^2 IV, day 1
	Fluorouracil 960 mg/m^2/day continuous IV infusion, days 2 through 4
	Etoposide 80 mg/m^2/day IV, days 2 through 4

FL

Use:	Prostate cancer. *Cycle:* Ongoing
Regimen:	Flutamide 250 mg/dose PO every 8 hours
	with
	Leuprolide acetate 1 mg subcutaneously daily
	or
	Leuprolide depot 7.5 mg/dose IM, every 28 days
	or
	Leuprolide depot 22.5 mg/dose IM, every 3 months

FLAG

Use:	Acute myelogenous leukemia (AML; remission induction). *Cycle:* Give a single cycle
Regimen:	Filgrastim 300 mcg/day subcutaneously, from day 1 until neutropenia resolves
	Fludarabine 30 mg/m^2/day IV, days 2 through 6
	Cytarabine 2,000 mg/m^2/day IV, days 2 through 6 (begin 4 hours after starting fludarabine)

FLAG-Ida

Use:	Acute myelogenous leukemia (AML; remission induction). *Cycle:* Give a single cycle. May be given a second time based on individual response. Time between cycles not specified.
Regimen:	Filgrastim 300 mcg/day subcutaneously, from day 1 until neutropenia resolves
	Fludarabine 30 mg/m^2/day IV, days 2 through 6
	Cytarabine 2,000 mg/m^2/day IV, days 2 through 6 (begin 4 hours after starting fludarabine)
	Idarubicin 8 mg/m^2/day IV, days 2 through 4

Fle

Use:	Colorectal cancer. *Cycle:* 1 year
Regimen:	Fluorouracil 450 mg/m^2/day IV, days 1 through 5
	Fluorouracil 450 mg/m^2/week IV, weeks 5 through 52
	Levamisole 50 mg/dose PO every 8 hours, days 1 through 3 of every other week for 1 year*
	*Note: Levamisole is no longer available in the United States. The manufacturer discontinued this product in October 2000 for commercial reasons, not for safety or efficacy reasons.

FLOX

Use:	Colorectal cancer. *Cycle:* 8 weeks for 3 cycles
Regimen:	Leucovorin 500 mg/m^2 IV, days 1, 8, 15, 22, 29, and 36
	Fluorouracil 500 mg/m^2 IV, days 1, 8, 15, 22, 29, and 36 (after starting leucovorin)
	Oxaliplatin 85 mg/m^2 IV, days 1, 15, and 29

Fludarabine-Cyclophosphamide (also see FC)

Use:	Chronic lymphocytic leukemia (CLL). *Cycle:* 4 to 6 weeks based on recovery of myelosuppression. Give up to 6 cycles.
Regimen:	Fludarabine 30 mg/m^2/day IV, days 1 through 3
	Cyclophosphamide 300 mg/m^2/day IV, days 1 through 3

continued on next page

Fludarabine-Cyclophosphamide (also see FC) (cont.)

Use: Chronic lymphocytic leukemia (CLL). *Cycle:* 28 days for up to
         6 cycles

Regimen: Fludarabine 20 mg/m²/day IV, days 1 through 5
             Cyclophosphamide 600 mg/m² IV, day 1
             Filgrastim 5 mcg/kg/day subcutaneously, from day 8 until hemato-
             logic recovery
             used in conjunction with antimicrobial prophylaxis*
                Cotrimoxazole (either 80/400 or 160/800 strength) 1 tablet PO
                daily, throughout entire course, starting 1 day prior to first
                chemotherapy dose
                or
                Pentamidine 300 mg inhaled once monthly, throughout entire
                course, starting 1 day prior to first chemotherapy dose
                plus
                Acyclovir 200 mg PO 3 times daily, throughout entire course,
                starting day 8 of first chemotherapy cycle
                or
                Acyclovir 400 mg PO twice daily, throughout entire course, start-
                ing day 8 of first chemotherapy cycle
             *Note: Antimicrobial prophylaxis doses not specified in original ar-
             ticle; the doses given here are derived from the Infectious Dis-
             eases Handbook, 6th edition, and AHFS 2008 Drug Information,
             both tertiary resources.

Fluorouracil-Gemcitabine

Use: Renal cell carcinoma. *Cycle:* 28 days for at least 2 cycles
Regimen: Fluorouracil 150 mg/m²/day continuous IV infusion, days 1 through 21
             Gemcitabine 600 mg/m² IV, days 1, 8, and 15

Fluorouracil-Interferon

Use: Hepatocellular cancer. *Cycle:* 28 days for at least 2 cycles
Regimen: Fluorouracil 200 mg/m²/day continuous IV infusion, days 1 through 21
             Interferon alfa-2b 4 million units/m²/dose subcutaneously 3 times
             weekly, weeks 1, 2, and 3 (during fluorouracil therapy)

Use: Hepatocellular cancer. *Cycle:* 28 days for at least 3 cycles
Regimen: Fluorouracil 300 mg/m²/day continuous intraarterial infusion,
             days 1 through 5 and days 8 through 12
             Interferon alfa-2b 5 million units/dose subcutaneously 3 times
             weekly, throughout entire course*
             *Note: Interferon dose is in units not units/m².

Fluorouracil-Mitomycin

Use: Head and neck cancer. *Cycle:* 49 days. Give a single cycle.
Regimen: Fluorouracil 600 mg/m²/day continuous IV infusion, days 1 through 5
             Mitomycin 10 mg/m² IV, days 5 and 36
             used in conjunction with
             Radiation therapy

Use: Anal cancer. *Cycle:* 32 days. Give a single cycle prior to surgery.
Regimen: Fluorouracil 1,000 mg/m²/day continuous IV infusion, days 1
             through 4 and days 29 through 32
             Mitomycin 15 mg/m² IV, day 1
             used in conjunction with
             Radiation therapy

continued on next page

Fluorouracil-Mitomycin (cont.)

Use: Anal cancer. *Cycle:* 35 days. Give a single cycle prior to surgery.
Regimen: Fluorouracil 750 mg/m^2/day continuous IV infusion, days 1 through 5 and days 29 through 33
Mitomycin 15 mg/m^2 IV, day 1
used in conjunction with
Radiation therapy

Use: Anal cancer. *Cycle:* 28 days for 2 cycles
Regimen: Fluorouracil 1,000 mg/m^2/day (2,000 mg/day maximum dose) continuous IV infusion, days 1 through 4
Mitomycin 10 mg/m^2 (20 mg maximum dose) IV, day 1
used in conjunction with
Radiation therapy

Fluorouracil-Streptozocin

Use: Islet cell carcinoma. *Cycle:* 42 days, continue until disease progression or intolerable toxicity
Regimen: Fluorouracil 400 mg/m^2/day IV, days 1 through 5
Streptozocin 500 mg/m^2/day IV, days 1 through 5

FMD—see FND

FNC—see CNF

FND (FMD)

Use: Lymphoma (non-Hodgkin). *Cycle:* 28 days for up to 8 cycles
Regimen: Fludarabine 25 mg/m^2/day IV, days 1 through 3
Mitoxantrone 10 mg/m^2 IV, day 1
Dexamethasone 20 mg/day IV or PO, days 1 through 5
Cotrimoxazole double-strength (160/800) 2 tablets PO daily for 2 consecutive days each week (usually given every Saturday and Sunday)

FND-R—see FND + Rituximab, Concurrent

FND + Rituximab, Concurrent (FND-R)

Use: Lymphoma (non-Hodgkin). *Cycle:* 28 days for up to 8 cycles
Regimen: Rituximab 375 mg/m^2 IV, days 1 and 8 for first cycle only; then rituximab 375 mg/m^2 IV, day 1 for cycles 2 through 5
Fludarabine 25 mg/m^2/day IV, days 2 through 4
Mitoxantrone 10 mg/m^2 IV, day 2
Dexamethasone 20 mg/day IV or PO, days 2 through 4
Cotrimoxazole double-strength (160/800) 1 tablet PO twice daily for 2 consecutive days each week (usually given every Saturday and Sunday)

FOLFIRI

Use: Colorectal cancer. *Cycle:* 14 days, continue until disease progression or intolerable toxicity
Regimen: Leucovorin 400 mg/m^2 IV, day 1
or
Levoleucovorin 200 mg/m^2 IV, day 1
with
Irinotecan 180 mg/m^2 IV, day 1 (begin with leucovorin or levoleucovorin)
then
Fluorouracil 400 mg/m^2 IV bolus, day 1
then
continued on next page

FOLFIRI (cont.)

Fluorouracil 2,400 mg/m²/dose continuous IV infusion over 46 hours for 2 cycles, starting on day 1. Increase to 3,000 mg/m²/dose for remaining cycles if tolerated.

FOLFIRI + Bevacizumab

Use: Colorectal cancer. *Cycle:* 14 days, continue until disease progression or intolerable toxicity

Regimen: Bevacizumab 5 mg/kg IV, day 1
Leucovorin 400 mg/m² IV, day 1
Irinotecan 180 mg/m² IV, day 1 (begin with leucovorin)
then
Fluorouracil 400 mg/m² IV bolus, day 1
then
Fluorouracil 2,400 mg/m²/dose continuous IV infusion over 46 hours, starting day 1

FOLFOX-2

Use: Colorectal cancer. *Cycle:* 14 days, continue until disease progression or intolerable toxicity

Regimen: Oxaliplatin 100 mg/m² IV, day 1 (begin with leucovorin)
Leucovorin 500 mg/m²/day IV, days 1 and 2
then
Fluorouracil 1,500 mg/m²/dose continuous IV infusion over 22 hours, days 1 and 2, for 2 cycles. Increase to 2,000 mg/m²/dose for remaining cycles if toxicity was below WHO grade 2 during first 2 cycles.

FOLFOX-3

Use: Colorectal cancer. *Cycle:* 14 days, continue until disease progression or intolerable toxicity

Regimen: Oxaliplatin 85 mg/m² IV, day 1 (begin with leucovorin)
Leucovorin 500 mg/m²/day IV, days 1 and 2
then
Fluorouracil 1,500 mg/m²/dose continuous IV infusion over 22 hours, days 1 and 2, for 2 cycles. Increase to 2,000 mg/m²/dose for remaining cycles if toxicity was below WHO grade 2 during first 2 cycles.

FOLFOX-4

Use: Colorectal cancer. *Cycle:* 14 days
Regimen: Oxaliplatin 85 mg/m² IV, day 1 (begin with leucovorin)
Leucovorin 200 mg/m²/day IV, days 1 and 2
then
Fluorouracil 400 mg/m²/day IV bolus, days 1 and 2
then
Fluorouracil 600 mg/m²/dose continuous IV infusion over 22 hours, days 1 and 2

FOLFOX-4 + Bevacizumab

Use: Colorectal cancer. *Cycle:* 14 days for up to 48 weeks, or until disease progression or intolerable toxicity

Regimen: Bevacizumab 5 or 10 mg/kg IV, day 1
Oxaliplatin 85 mg/m² IV, day 1 (begin with leucovorin)
Leucovorin 200 mg/m²/day IV, days 1 and 2
then
Fluorouracil 400 mg/m²/day IV bolus, days 1 and 2
then
Fluorouracil 600 mg/m²/dose continuous IV infusion over 22 hours, days 1 and 2

FOLFOX-6

Use: Colorectal cancer. *Cycle:* 14 days, continue until disease progression or intolerable toxicity

Regimen: Oxaliplatin 100 mg/m^2 IV, day 1 (begin with leucovorin)
Leucovorin 400 mg/m^2 IV, day 1
then
Fluorouracil 400 mg/m^2 IV bolus, day 1
then
Fluorouracil 2,400 mg/m^2/dose continuous IV infusion over 46 hours for 2 cycles, starting on day 1. Increase to 3,000 mg/m^2/dose for remaining cycles if tolerated.

FOLFOX-7

Use: Colorectal cancer. *Cycle:* 14 days for up to 8 cycles

Regimen: Leucovorin 400 mg/m^2 IV, day 1
or
Levoleucovorin 200 mg/m^2 IV, day 1
with
Oxaliplatin 130 mg/m^2 IV, day 1 (begin with leucovorin or levoleucovorin)
then
Fluorouracil 400 mg/m^2 IV bolus, day 1
then
Fluorouracil 2,400 mg/m^2/dose continuous IV infusion over 46 hours, starting on day 1

FOLFOXIRI

Use: Metastatic colorectal cancer. *Cycle:* 14 days for up to 12 cycles

Regimen: Irinotecan 165 mg/m^2 IV, day 1
Oxaliplatin 85 mg/m^2 IV, day 1
Levoleucovorin 200 mg/m^2 IV, day 1
Fluorouracil 1,600 mg/m^2/day continuous IV infusion, days 1 and 2 (for 48 hours total)

FP

Use: Chronic lymphocytic leukemia (CLL). *Cycle:* 28 days for up to 6 cycles

Regimen: Fludarabine 30 mg/m^2/day IV, days 1 through 5
Prednisone 30 mg/m^2/day PO, days 1 through 5

FR

Use: Chronic lymphocytic leukemia (CLL). *Cycle:* 28 days for 6 cycles

Regimen: Fludarabine 25 mg/m^2/day IV, days 1 through 5
Rituximab 375 mg/m^2 IV, day 1
Rituximab 375 mg/m^2 IV, day 4 first cycle only (loading dose)
or
Fludarabine 25 mg/m^2/day IV, days 1 through 5
Rituximab 50 mg/m^2 IV, day 1 first cycle only (incremental loading dose)
Rituximab 325 mg/m^2 IV, day 3 first cycle only (incremental loading dose)
Rituximab 375 mg/m^2 IV, day 5 first cycle only (loading dose)
Rituximab 375 mg/m^2 IV, day 1, except for day 1 of first cycle

FU/LV—see F-CL

FU/LV/Bevacizumab
Use: Metastatic colorectal cancer. *Cycle:* 8 weeks
Regimen: Fluorouracil 600 mg/m^2 IV, weekly for 6 weeks
Leucovorin 500 mg/m^2 IV, weekly for 6 weeks
Bevacizumab 5 mg/kg IV, days 1, 15, 29, and 43

FU/LV/CPT-11 (IFL Douillard Regimen)
Use: Metastatic colorectal cancer. *Cycle:* 14 days, continue until disease progression or intolerable toxicity
Regimen: Fluorouracil 400 mg/m^2 IV bolus, day 1
then
Fluorouracil 600 mg/m^2/dose continuous IV infusion over 22 hours, day 1
Leucovorin 200 mg/m^2/day IV, days 1 and 2
Irinotecan 180 mg/m^2 IV, day 1
or
Fluorouracil 2,300 mg/m^2/day continuous IV infusion, days 1 and 8
Leucovorin 500 mg/m^2 IV, days 1 and 8
Irinotecan 80 mg/m^2 IV, days 1 and 8

FU/LV/CPT-11 (IFL Saltz Regimen)
Use: Metastatic colorectal cancer.* *Cycle:* 42 days, continue until disease progression or intolerable toxicity
Regimen: Fluorouracil 500 mg/m^2 IV, days 1, 8, 15, and 22
Leucovorin 20 mg/m^2 IV, days 1, 8, 15, and 22
Irinotecan 125 mg/m^2 IV, days 1, 8, 15, and 22
*Note: A study analysis found an increased risk of early deaths (within 60 days of initiating treatment) with use of this regimen. Specific risk factors that may have contributed to death were not identified. Intensive patient monitoring and dosage modification are recommended to reduce the risk of severe adverse effects.

FU/LV/CPT-11, Modified (Modified IFL Saltz Regimen)
Use: Metastatic colorectal cancer. *Cycle:* 21 days, continue until disease progression or intolerable toxicity
Regimen: Fluorouracil 500 mg/m^2 IV, days 1 and 8
Leucovorin 20 mg/m^2 IV, days 1 and 8
Irinotecan 125 mg/m^2 IV, days 1 and 8

FUFOX
Use: Metastatic colorectal cancer. *Cycle:* 35 days, continue until disease progression or intolerable toxicity
Regimen: Oxaliplatin 50 mg/m^2 IV, days 1, 8, 15, and 22
then
Leucovorin 500 mg/m^2 IV, days 1, 8, 15, and 22
Fluorouracil 2,000 mg/m^2/dose continuous IV infusion over 22 hours, days 1, 8, 15, and 22

FUOX
Use: Metastatic colorectal cancer. *Cycle:* 14 days for up to 18 cycles
Regimen: Fluorouracil 1,125 mg/m^2/day continuous IV infusion, days 1 and 2 (for 48 hours total), and days 8 and 9 (for 48 hours total)
Oxaliplatin 85 mg/m^2 IV, day 1

FUP (also see CF for adenocarcinoma)
Use: Gastric cancer. *Cycle:* 28 days
Regimen: Fluorouracil 1,000 mg/m^2/day continuous IV infusion, days 1 through 5
Cisplatin 100 mg/m^2 IV, day 2

FZ

Use:	Prostate cancer. *Cycle:* Ongoing
Regimen:	Flutamide 250 mg/dose PO every 8 hours
	with
	Goserelin acetate 3.6 mg/dose implant subcutaneously every 28 days
	or
	Goserelin acetate 10.8 mg/dose implant subcutaneously every 12 weeks

G + V (also see Gemcitabine-Vinorelbine)

Use:	Lung cancer (non-small cell). *Cycle:* 21 days for up to 6 cycles
Regimen:	Gemcitabine 1,000 to 1,200 mg/m^2 IV, days 1 and 8
	Vinorelbine 25 to 30 mg/m^2 IV, days 1 and 8

GCP

Use:	Adenocarcinoma (unknown primary). *Cycle:* See below, cycle length varies throughout protocol. Give 4 cycles of GCP, followed by 3 cycles of paclitaxel alone.
Regimen:	GCP. *Cycle:* 21 days for 4 cycles
	Gemcitabine 1,000 mg/m^2 IV, days 1 and 8
	Carboplatin IV dose by Calvert equation to AUC 5 mg/mL/min, day 1 (administration sequence not specified in protocol)
	Paclitaxel 200 mg/m^2 IV over 1 hour, day 1
	followed by
	Paclitaxel alone. *Cycle:* 56 days for 3 cycles
	Paclitaxel 70 mg/m^2 IV weekly for 6 weeks then 2 weeks of rest, days 1, 8, 15, 22, 29, and 36

Gemcitabine-Bevacizumab

Use:	Pancreatic cancer. *Cycle:* 28 days, continue until disease progression or intolerable toxicity
Regimen:	Gemcitabine 1,000 mg/m^2 IV, days 1, 8, and 15
	Bevacizumab 10 mg/kg IV, days 1 and 15 (after gemcitabine)

Gemcitabine-Capecitabine

Use:	Pancreatic cancer. *Cycle:* 21 days, continue until disease progression or intolerable toxicity
Regimen:	Gemcitabine 1,000 mg/m^2 IV, days 1 and 8
	Capecitabine 650 mg/m^2/dose PO twice daily, days 1 through 14

Gemcitabine-Carboplatin

Use:	Lung cancer (non-small cell). *Cycle:* 28 days for up to 6 cycles
Regimen:	Gemcitabine 1,000 or 1,100 mg/m^2 IV, days 1 and 8
	Carboplatin IV dose by Calvert equation to AUC 5 mg/mL/min, day 8

Use:	Mesothelioma. *Cycle:* 28 days for up to 6 cycles
Regimen:	Gemcitabine 1,000 mg/m^2 IV, days 1, 8, and 15
	Carboplatin IV dose by Calvert equation to AUC 5 mg/mL/min, day 1

Use:	Ovarian cancer. *Cycle:* 21 days for up to 6 cycles
Regimen:	Gemcitabine 1,000 mg/m^2 IV, days 1 and 8
	Carboplatin IV dose by Calvert equation to AUC 4 mg/mL/min, day 1 (after gemcitabine)

Gemcitabine-Cis (also see Gemcitabine-Cisplatin)

Use:	Lung cancer (non-small cell). *Cycle:* 28 days for up to 6 cycles
Regimen:	Gemcitabine 1,000 to 1,200 mg/m^2 IV, days 1, 8, and 15
	Cisplatin 100 mg/m^2 IV, day 15*
	*Note: Some references state that a single dose of cisplatin may be given on day 1, 2, or 15 of each cycle. However, the best results are seen when cisplatin is given on day 15.

Use:	Lung cancer (non-small cell). *Cycle:* 21 days for up to 6 cycles
Regimen:	Cisplatin 100 mg/m^2 IV, day 1 (before gemcitabine)
	Gemcitabine 1,250 mg/m^2 IV, days 1 and 8

Use:	Mesothelioma. *Cycle:* 28 days for up to 6 cycles
Regimen:	Cisplatin 100 mg/m^2 IV, day 1 (before gemcitabine)
	Gemcitabine 1,000 mg/m^2 IV, days 1, 8, and 15

Gemcitabine-Cisplatin (also see Gemcitabine-Cis)

Use:	Metastatic bladder cancer. *Cycle:* 28 days for up to 6 cycles
Regimen:	Gemcitabine 1,000 mg/m^2 IV, days 1, 8, and 15
	Cisplatin 70 mg/m^2 IV, day 2

Use:	Biliary tract cancer. *Cycle:* 21 days, continue until disease progression or intolerable toxicity
Regimen:	Gemcitabine 1,250 mg/m^2 IV, days 1 and 8
	Cisplatin 75 mg/m^2 IV, day 1

Use:	Cervical cancer. *Cycle:* 21 days for up to 6 cycles
Regimen:	Gemcitabine 1,250 mg/m^2 IV, days 1 and 8
	Cisplatin 50 mg/m^2 IV, day 1 (after gemcitabine)

Use:	Ovarian cancer. *Cycle:* 21 days
Regimen 1:	Patients treated with less than 2 prior chemotherapy regimens:
	Cisplatin 30 mg/m^2 IV, days 1 and 8
	Gemcitabine 750 mg/m^2 IV, days 1 and 8 (after cisplatin)
Regimen 2:	Patients treated with 2 or more prior chemotherapy regimens:
	Cisplatin 30 mg/m^2 IV, days 1 and 8
	Gemcitabine 600 mg/m^2 IV, days 1 and 8 (after cisplatin)

Use:	Pancreatic cancer. *Cycle:* 28 days, continue until disease progression or intolerable toxicity
Regimen:	Gemcitabine 1,000 mg/m^2 IV, days 1, 8, and 15
	Cisplatin 50 mg/m^2 IV, days 1 and 15 (after gemcitabine)

Gemcitabine-Docetaxel

Use:	Lung cancer (non-small cell). *Cycle:* 21 days for up to 6 cycles or until disease progression or intolerable toxicity
Regimen:	Gemcitabine 1,100 mg/m^2 IV, days 1 and 8
	Docetaxel 100 mg/m^2 IV, day 8 (after gemcitabine)
	Filgrastim 150 mcg/m^2/day subcutaneously, days 9 through 15

Use:	Sarcoma. *Cycle:* 21 days for up to 6 cycles
Regimen 1:	Patients with no prior radiation therapy:
	Gemcitabine 900 mg/m^2 IV, days 1 and 8
	Docetaxel 100 mg/m^2 IV, day 8 (after gemcitabine)
	Filgrastim 150 mcg/m^2/day subcutaneously (rounded to 300 or 480 mcg), days 9 through 15
Regimen 2:	Patients with prior radiation therapy:
	Gemcitabine 675 mg/m^2 IV, days 1 and 8
	Docetaxel 75 mg/m^2 IV, day 8 (after gemcitabine)
	Filgrastim 150 mcg/m^2/day subcutaneously (rounded to 300 or 480 mcg), days 9 through 15

Gemcitabine-Erlotinib

Use: Pancreatic cancer. *Cycle:* 56 days, continue until disease progression or intolerable toxicity

Regimen: Gemcitabine 1,000 mg/m² IV weekly for 7 weeks for first cycle; for subsequent cycles, give weekly for 3 weeks followed by 1 week of rest, on days 1, 8, 15, 29, 36, and 43

Erlotinib 100 mg/day PO, throughout entire course

Gemcitabine-Irinotecan

Use: Pancreatic cancer. *Cycle:* 21 days for at least 6 cycles

Regimen: Gemcitabine 1,000 mg/m² IV, days 1 and 8

Irinotecan 100 mg/m² IV, days 1 and 8 (after gemcitabine)

Gemcitabine-Liposomal Doxorubicin

Use: Ovarian cancer. *Cycle:* 21 days

Regimen: Gemcitabine 1,000 mg/m² IV, days 1 and 8

Liposomal doxorubicin 30 mg/m² IV, day 1

Gemcitabine-Vinorelbine (also see G + V)

Use: Lung cancer (non-small cell). *Cycle:* 28 days for up to 6 cycles

Regimen: Gemcitabine 800 or 1,000 mg/m² IV, days 1, 8, and 15

Vinorelbine 20 mg/m² IV, days 1, 8, and 15

GEMOX

Use: Biliary tract adenocarcinoma, pancreatic cancer. *Cycle:* 14 days for up to 6 cycles or until disease progression or intolerable toxicity

Regimen: Gemcitabine 1,000 mg/m² IV, day 1

Oxaliplatin 100 mg/m² IV, day 2

GT

Use: Breast cancer. *Cycle:* 21 days, continue until disease progression or intolerable toxicity

Regimen: Gemcitabine 1,250 mg/m² IV, days 1 and 8

Paclitaxel 175 mg/m² IV over 3 hours, day 1

Use: Lung cancer (non-small cell). *Cycle:* 21 days for up to 6 cycles

Regimen: Paclitaxel 200 mg/m² IV over 3 hours, day 1 (before gemcitabine)

Gemcitabine 1,000 mg/m² IV, days 1 and 8

GTX

Use: Pancreatic cancer. *Cycle:* 14 days

Regimen: Capecitabine 500 to 750 mg/m²/dose PO twice daily, days 1 through 14

Gemcitabine 750 mg/m² IV, days 4 and 11

Docetaxel 30 mg/m² IV, days 4 and 11 (after gemcitabine)

HDCA (High-Dose Cytarabine)

HDMTX

Use: Sarcoma (bone). *Cycle:* 1 to 4 weeks

Regimen: Methotrexate 8,000 to 12,000 mg/m² (20,000 mg maximum dose) IV, day 1

Leucovorin 15 mg/m²/dose PO or IV every 6 hours for 10 doses, beginning 20 to 30 hours after beginning of methotrexate infusion

HEC

Use: Breast cancer. *Cycle:* 21 days for up to 8 cycles

Regimen: Epirubicin 100 mg/m² IV, day 1

Cyclophosphamide 830 mg/m² IV, day 1

Hexa-CAF

Use: Ovarian cancer. *Cycle:* 28 days for at least 6 cycles

Regimen: Altretamine 150 mg/m^2/day PO, days 1 through 14
Cyclophosphamide 100 to 150 mg/m^2/day PO, days 1 through 14
Methotrexate 40 mg/m^2 IV, days 1 and 8
Fluorouracil 600 mg/m^2 IV, days 1 and 8

Hi-C DAZE

Use: Acute myelogenous leukemia (AML; induction—pediatrics).
Cycle: Give a single cycle

Regimen: Cytarabine 3,000 mg/m^2/dose IV every 12 hours for 8 doses,
days 1 through 4
Daunorubicin 30 mg/m^2/day IV, days 1 through 3
Etoposide 200 mg/m^2/day IV, days 1 through 3 and days 6 through 8
Azacitidine 150 mg/m^2/day IV, days 3 through 5 and days 8 through 10

HIDAC (High-Dose Cytarabine)

Hyper-CVAD/HD MTX Ara-C*

Use: Lymphoma (mantle cell). *Cycle:* 21 days, delay subsequent cycles
until hematologic recovery. Give up to 4 cycles.

Regimen: **Treatment A** —Hyper-CVAD (cycles 1 and 3)
Cyclophosphamide 300 mg/m^2/dose IV every 12 hours for
6 doses, days 1 through 3
Dexamethasone 40 mg/day IV or PO, days 1 through 4 and
days 11 through 14
Vincristine 2 mg (dose is not in mg/m^2) IV, day 4 (given 12 hours
after last cyclophosphamide dose) and day 11
Doxorubicin 25 mg/m^2/day continuous IV infusion, days 4 and 5
Filgrastim 5 mcg/kg/day subcutaneously, starting on day 6 and
continued until granulocyte count exceeds 4,500 cells/mm^3
Treatment B —HD MTX Ara-C (cycles 2 and 4)
Methotrexate 200 mg/m^2 IV bolus, day 1
then
Methotrexate 800 mg/m^2/day continuous IV infusion, day 1
Cytarabine dose based on age and renal function:
Patients aged 60 years and younger, or patients with serum
creatinine no more than 1.5 mg/dL: Cytarabine 3,000 mg/
m^2/dose IV every 12 hours for 4 doses, days 2 and 3
Patients older than 60 years of age, or patients with serum
creatinine greater than 1.5 mg/dL: Cytarabine 1,000 mg/
m^2/dose IV every 12 hours for 4 doses, days 2 and 3
Leucovorin 50 mg PO, day 3, given 24 hours after methotrexate
infusion is completed
Leucovorin 15 mg/dose PO every 6 hours for 8 doses, days 3
through 5, starting 30 hours after methotrexate infusion is
completed
Filgrastim 5 mcg/kg/day subcutaneously, starting on day 6 and
continued until granulocyte count exceeds 4,500 cells/mm^3
used in conjunction with
Autologous stem cell transplantation
*Note: These 2 regimens are normally used in combination with
each other and are rarely given alone.

continued on next page

Hyper-CVAD/HD MTX Ara-C* (cont.)

Use: Acute lymphocytic leukemia (ALL; induction—adults).

Cycle: 21 days, delay subsequent cycles until hematologic recovery. Give 8 cycles.

Regimen: **Treatment A** —Hyper-CVAD (cycles 1, 3, 5, and 7)

Cyclophosphamide 300 mg/m^2/dose IV every 12 hours for 6 doses, days 1 through 3

Mesna 600 mg/m^2/day continuous IV infusion, days 1 through 3 (begin with cyclophosphamide)

Dexamethasone 40 mg/day IV or PO, days 1 through 4 and days 11 through 14

Doxorubicin 50 mg/m^2 IV, day 4

Vincristine 2 mg (dose is not in mg/m^2) IV, days 4 and 11

Filgrastim 10 mcg/kg/day subcutaneously, starting day 5 and continued until granulocyte count exceeds 3,000 cells/mm^3

Treatment B —HD MTX Ara-C (cycles 2, 4, 6, and 8)

Methotrexate 200 mg/m^2 IV bolus, day 1

then

Methotrexate 800 mg/m^2/day continuous IV infusion, day 1

Cytarabine dose based on age and renal function:

Patients 60 years of age and younger, or patients with serum creatinine no more than 1.5 mg/dL: Cytarabine 3,000 mg/m^2/dose IV every 12 hours for 4 doses, days 2 and 3

Patients older than 60 years of age, or patients with serum creatinine greater than 1.5 mg/dL: Cytarabine 1,000 mg/m^2/dose IV every 12 hours for 4 doses, days 2 and 3

Leucovorin 15 mg/dose PO or IV every 6 hours for 8 doses, beginning on day 3, starting 24 hours after methotrexate infusion is completed and continued until methotrexate concentration is less than 0.1 microMol/L; increase dose to 50 mg/dose PO or IV every 6 hours if the methotrexate concentration is greater than 20 microMol/L at the end of the infusion or greater than 1 microMol/L 24 hours after the end of the infusion, or greater than 0.1 microMol/L 48 hours after the end of the infusion.

Methylprednisolone 50 mg/dose IV twice daily, days 1 through 3

Filgrastim 10 mcg/kg/day subcutaneously, starting day 4 and continued until granulocyte count exceeds 3,000 cells/mm^3

used in conjunction with

CNS prophylaxis: Give for cycles 1 and 2 for low-risk patients, cycles 1 through 4 for unknown risk, and all 8 cycles for high-risk patients.

Methotrexate 12 mg intrathecal, day 2

Cytarabine 100 mg intrathecal, day 8

used in conjunction with antimicrobial prophylaxis

Fluconazole 200 mg/day PO, throughout entire course

plus

Ciprofloxacin 500 mg PO twice daily, throughout entire course

or

Levofloxacin 500 mg/day PO, throughout entire course

plus

Acyclovir 200 mg PO twice daily, throughout entire course

or

Valacyclovir 500 mg/day PO, throughout entire course

*Note: These 2 regimens are normally used in combination with each other and are rarely given alone.

Hyper-CVAD/HD MTX Ara-C + Rituximab*

Use: Lymphoma (mantle cell). *Cycle:* 21 days, delay subsequent cycles until hematologic recovery. Give up to 8 cycles.

Regimen: **Treatment A** —R-Hyper-CVAD (cycles 1, 3, 5, and 7)

Rituximab 375 mg/m^2 IV, day 1

Mesna 600 mg/m^2/day continuous IV infusion, days 2 through 5 (start 1 hour before cyclophosphamide and continue for 12 hours after last cyclophosphamide dose)

Cyclophosphamide 300 mg/m^2/dose IV every 12 hours for 6 doses, days 2 through 4

Dexamethasone 40 mg/day IV or PO, days 2 through 5 and days 12 through 15

Vincristine 1.4 mg/m^2 (2 mg maximum dose) IV, day 5 (given 12 hours after last cyclophosphamide dose) and day 12

Doxorubicin 16.7 mg/m^2/day continuous IV infusion, days 5 through 7 (start 12 hours after last cyclophosphamide dose)

Filgrastim 5 mcg/kg/day subcutaneously, starting on day 8 and continued until white blood cell count (WBC) is at least 3,000 cells/mm^3

Treatment B —R-HD MTX Ara-C (cycles 2, 4, 6, and 8)

Rituximab 375 mg/m^2 IV, day 1

Methotrexate 200 mg/m^2 IV bolus, day 2

then

Methotrexate 800 mg/m^2 continuous IV infusion over 22 hours, day 2

Cytarabine dose based on age and renal function

Patients 60 years of age and younger, or patients with serum creatinine no more than 1.5 mg/dL: Cytarabine 3,000 mg/m^2/dose IV every 12 hours for 4 doses, days 3 and 4

Patients older than 60 years of age, or patients with serum creatinine greater than 1.5 mg/dL: Cytarabine 1,000 mg/m^2/dose IV every 12 hours for 4 doses, days 3 and 4

Leucovorin 50 mg PO, day 3, given 24 hours after methotrexate infusion is completed

Leucovorin 15 mg/dose PO every 6 hours for 8 doses, days 4 through 6, starting 30 hours after methotrexate infusion is completed

Filgrastim 5 mcg/kg/day subcutaneously, starting on day 6 and continued until WBC is at least 3,000 cells/mm^3

used in conjunction with antimicrobial prophylaxis

Fluconazole 100 mg/day PO, days 8 through 17

Valacyclovir 500 mg/day PO, days 8 through 17

plus

Ciprofloxacin 500 mg PO twice daily, days 8 through 17

or

Levofloxacin 500 mg/day PO, days 8 through 17

*Note: These 2 regimens are normally used in combination with each other and are rarely given alone.

ICE—see MICE

ICE + Autologous Stem Cell Transplantation

Use: Lymphoma (non-Hodgkin—adults). *Cycle:* 14 days for 3 cycles

Regimen: Etoposide 100 mg/m^2/day IV, days 1 through 3

Ifosfamide 5,000 mg/m^2/day continuous IV infusion, day 2*

Mesna 5,000 mg/m^2/day continuous IV infusion, day 2*

Carboplatin IV dose by Calvert equation to AUC 5 mg/mL/min (800 mg maximum dose), day 2

Filgrastim 5 mcg/kg/day subcutaneously, days 5 through 12; increased in third cycle to 10 mcg/kg/day subcutaneously, from day 5 until leukapheresis

used in conjunction with

Autologous stem cell transplantation

*Note: Ifosfamide and mesna may be mixed and administered in the same infusion bag.

ICE Protocol—see Idarubicin, Cytarabine, Etoposide

ICE + Rituximab (R-MICE, RICE)

Use: Lymphoma (non-Hodgkin—adults). *Cycle:* 14 days for 3 cycles

Regimen: Rituximab 375 mg/m^2 IV, day −1 of first cycle only

Rituximab 375 mg/m^2 IV, day 1

Etoposide 100 mg/m^2/day IV, days 3 through 5

Ifosfamide 5,000 mg/m^2/day continuous IV infusion, day 4*

Mesna 5,000 mg/m^2/day continuous IV infusion, day 4*

Carboplatin IV dose by Calvert equation to AUC 5 mg/mL/min (800 mg maximum dose), day 4

Filgrastim 5 mcg/kg/day subcutaneously, days 7 through 14 for first 2 cycles; increased in third cycle to 10 mcg/kg/day subcutaneously, from day 7 until leukapheresis

used in conjunction with

Autologous stem cell transplantation

*Note: Ifosfamide and mesna may be mixed and administered in the same infusion bag.

ICE-T

Use: Breast cancer, sarcoma, lung cancer (non-small cell).

Cycle: 28 days

Regimen: Ifosfamide 1,250 mg/m^2/day IV, days 1 through 3

Carboplatin 300 mg/m^2 IV, day 1

Etoposide 80 mg/m^2/day IV, days 1 through 3

Paclitaxel 175 mg/m^2 IV over 3 hours, day 4

with

Mesna 20% of ifosfamide dose IV before ifosfamide, then mesna 40% of ifosfamide dose PO 4 and 8 hours after ifosfamide, days 1 through 3

or

Mesna 1,250 mg/m^2/day IV, days 1 through 3

IDA-Based BF12—see Idarubicin, Cytarabine, Etoposide

Idarubicin, Cytarabine, Etoposide (ICE Protocol)

Use: Acute myelogenous leukemia (AML; induction—adults).

Cycle: Give a single cycle

Regimen: Idarubicin 6 mg/m^2/day IV, days 1 through 5

Cytarabine 600 mg/m^2/day IV, days 1 through 5

Etoposide 150 mg/m^2/day IV, days 1 through 3

Idarubicin, Cytarabine, Etoposide (IDA-Based BF12)

Use:　　Acute myelogenous leukemia (AML; induction—adults).

　　　　　Cycle: Usually 1 cycle is given. A second cycle may be considered for patients with partial response. Time between cycles not specified.

Regimen:　Idarubicin 5 mg/m^2/day IV, days 1 through 5

　　　　　Cytarabine 2,000 mg/m^2/dose IV every 12 hours for 10 doses, days 1 through 5

　　　　　Etoposide 100 mg/m^2/day IV, days 1 through 5

IDMTX

Use:　　Acute lymphocytic leukemia (ALL; intensification—pediatrics).

　　　　　Cycle: 14 days, for 12 cycles

Regimen:　Methotrexate 1,000 mg/m^2/day continuous IV infusion, day 1 (24-hour infusion)

　　　　　Mercaptopurine 1,000 mg/m^2 IV over 6 hours following methotrexate, day 2

　　　　　Leucovorin 5 mg/m^2/dose IV every 6 hours for at least 5 doses, days 3 and 4, starting 48 hours after the start of the methotrexate infusion and continued until methotrexate concentration is less than 0.1 microMol/L

　　　　　Methotrexate 20 mg/m^2 IM, day 8

　　　　　Mercaptopurine 50 mg/m^2/day PO, days 8 through 14

IDMTX/6-MP

Use:　　Acute lymphocytic leukemia (ALL; consolidation—pediatrics).

　　　　　Cycle: 2 weeks for up to 12 cycles

Regimen:　**Week 1:** Methotrexate 200 mg/m^2 IV bolus, day 1

　　　　　Mercaptopurine 200 mg/m^2 IV bolus, day 1

　　　　　then

　　　　　Methotrexate 800 mg/m^2/day continuous IV infusion, day 1

　　　　　Mercaptopurine 800 mg/m^2 IV over 8 hours, day 1

　　　　　Leucovorin 5 mg/m^2/dose PO or IV every 6 hours for 5 to 13 doses, beginning 24 hours after methotrexate infusion is completed

　　　　　Week 2: Methotrexate 20 mg/m^2 IM, day 8

　　　　　Mercaptopurine 50 mg/m^2/day PO, days 8 through 14

IE (also see IfoVP)

Use:　　Sarcoma (soft tissue). *Cycle:* 21 days for up to 6 cycles

Regimen:　Ifosfamide 1,800 mg/m^2/day IV, days 1 through 5

　　　　　Etoposide 100 mg/m^2/day IV, days 1 through 5

　　　　　with

　　　　　Mesna 1,800 mg/m^2/day IV, days 1 through 5

　　　　　or

　　　　　Mesna 20% of ifosfamide dose IV before, then 4 and 8 hours after each ifosfamide infusion, days 1 through 5

IFL—see FU/LV/CPT-11

IFL + Bevacizumab

Use:　　Colorectal cancer. *Cycle:* 42 days, continue until disease progression or intolerable toxicity

Regimen:　Irinotecan 125 mg/m^2 IV, days 1, 8, 15, and 22

　　　　　Fluorouracil 500 mg/m^2 IV, days 1, 8, 15, and 22

　　　　　Leucovorin 20 mg/m^2 IV, days 1, 8, 15, and 22

　　　　　Bevacizumab 5 mg/kg IV, days 1, 15, and 29

IFN + DTIC
Use: Malignant melanoma. *Cycle:* 28 days for at least 2 to 3 cycles, or
     until disease progression or intolerable toxicity

Regimen: Interferon alfa-2b 15 million units/m²/day IV, days 1 through 5,
     days 8 through 12, and days 15 through 19 of first cycle only

     Interferon alfa-2b 10 million units/m²/dose subcutaneously 3 times
     weekly throughout entire course, except for first cycle

     Dacarbazine 200 mg/m²/day IV, days 22 through 26

Ifosfamide-Paclitaxel
Use: Endometrial cancer. *Cycle:* 21 days for up to 8 cycles

Regimen: Ifosfamide dose based on history of radiation therapy:
     Patients without prior radiation therapy: Ifosfamide 1,600 mg/m²/
     day IV, days 1 through 3

     Patients with prior radiation therapy: Ifosfamide 1,200 mg/m²/
     day IV, days 1 through 3

     Paclitaxel 135 mg/m²/day IV over 3 hours, day 1
     with

     Mesna 2,000 mg/dose continuous IV infusion over 12 hours,
     days 1 through 3 (start 15 minutes before ifosfamide each day)
     or

     Mesna 1,330 mg/dose PO, given 1 hour before, then 4 and 8 hours
     after each ifosfamide infusion, days 1 through 3 (for 3 doses to-
     tal each day)
     with

     Filgrastim 5 mcg/kg/day subcutaneously, from day 4 until granulo-
     cyte count is at least 2,000 cells/mm³

IfoVP (also see IE)
Use: Sarcoma (osteosarcoma—pediatrics). *Cycle:* 21 days for up to
     6 cycles

Regimen: Ifosfamide 1,800 mg/m²/day IV, days 1 through 5
     Etoposide 100 mg/m²/day IV, days 1 through 5
     Mesna 1,800 mg/m²/day IV, days 1 through 5

Interferon-Cytarabine-Hydroxyurea
Use: Chronic myelogenous leukemia (CML). *Cycle:* 28 days for at least
     6 cycles

Regimen: Interferon alfa-2b 5 million units/day subcutaneously, throughout en-
     tire course; adjust dose to white blood cell count (WBC)

     Hydroxyurea 50 mg/kg/day PO, throughout entire course; adjust
     dose to WBC

     Cytarabine 20 mg/m²/day subcutaneously, days 15 through 24
     (therapy modified based on WBC and therapeutic response)

Interleukin 2-Interferon alfa 2
Use: Renal cell carcinoma. *Cycle:* 56 days, continue until disease pro-
     gression or intolerable toxicity

Regimen: Aldesleukin 20 million units/m²/dose subcutaneously 3 times
     weekly, weeks 1 and 4

     Aldesleukin 5 million units/m²/dose subcutaneously 3 times weekly,
     weeks 2, 3, 5, and 6

     Interferon alfa 6 million units/m²/dose subcutaneously once weekly,
     weeks 1 and 4

     Interferon alfa 6 million units/m²/dose subcutaneously 3 times
     weekly, weeks 2, 3, 5, and 6

continued on next page

Interleukin 2-Interferon alfa 2 (cont.)
Use: Renal cell carcinoma
Regimen: **Remission induction.** *Cycle*: 11 days for 2 cycles
    Aldesleukin 18 million units/m^2/day continuous IV infusion, days 1 through 5
    Interferon alfa-2a* 6 million units/dose subcutaneously, days 1, 3, and 5
    Maintenance. *Cycle*: 26 days for 4 cycles
    Aldesleukin 18 million units/m^2/day continuous IV infusion, days 1 through 5
    Interferon alfa-2a* 6 million units/dose subcutaneously, days 1, 3, and 5
    *Note: Interferon alfa-2a is no longer available in the United States. The manufacturer discontinued this product in October 2007 for commercial reasons, not for safety or efficacy reasons.

Interleukin 2-Interferon alfa 2-Fluorouracil
Use: Renal cell carcinoma. *Cycle:* 8 weeks for up to 2 cycles
Regimen: Aldesleukin 20 million units/m^2/dose subcutaneously 3 times weekly, weeks 1 and 4
    Aldesleukin 5 million units/m^2/dose subcutaneously 3 times weekly, weeks 2 and 3
    Interferon alfa-2a* 6 million units/m^2/dose subcutaneously once weekly, weeks 1 and 4
    Interferon alfa-2a* 6 million units/m^2/dose subcutaneously 3 times weekly, weeks 2 and 3
    Interferon alfa-2a* 9 million units/m^2/dose subcutaneously 3 times weekly, weeks 5 through 8
    Fluorouracil 750 mg/m^2/dose IV bolus once weekly, weeks 5 through 8
    *Note: Interferon alfa-2a is no longer available in the United States. The manufacturer discontinued this product in October 2007 for commercial reasons, not for safety or efficacy reasons.

Use: Renal cell carcinoma. *Cycle:* 8 weeks for up to 3 cycles
Regimen: Aldesleukin 10 million units/m^2/dose subcutaneously twice daily, days 3 through 5, of weeks 1 and 4
    Aldesleukin 5 million units/m^2 subcutaneously once daily, days 1, 3, and 5, of weeks 2 and 3
    Interferon alfa-2a* 5 million units/m^2/dose subcutaneously, day 1, of weeks 1 and 4
    Interferon alfa-2a* 5 million units/m^2 subcutaneously once daily, days 1, 3, and 5, of weeks 2 and 3
    Interferon alfa-2a* 10 million units/m^2 subcutaneously once daily, days 1, 3, and 5, of weeks 5 through 8
    Fluorouracil 1,000 mg/m^2/dose IV, day 1, of weeks 5 through 8
    *Note: Interferon alfa-2a is no longer available in the United States. The manufacturer discontinued this product in October 2007 for commercial reasons, not for safety or efficacy reasons.

IPA
Use: Hepatoblastoma (pediatrics). *Cycle:* 21 days for up to 4 cycles
Regimen: Ifosfamide 500 mg/m^2 IV bolus, day 1
    Ifosfamide 1,000 mg/m^2/day continuous IV infusion, days 1 through 3
    Cisplatin 20 mg/m^2/day IV, days 4 through 8
    Doxorubicin 30 mg/m^2/day continuous IV infusion, days 9 and 10

IROX

Use:	Metastatic colorectal cancer. *Cycle:* 21 days, continue until disease progression or intolerable toxicity
Regimen:	Irinotecan 200 mg/m² IV, day 1
	Oxaliplatin 85 mg/m² IV, day 1

ITP

Use:	Bladder cancer. *Cycle:* 21 to 28 days for up to 6 cycles
Regimen:	Paclitaxel 200 mg/m² IV over 3 hours, day 1
	Cisplatin 70 mg/m² IV, day 1 (after paclitaxel)
	Ifosfamide 1,500 mg/m²/day IV, days 1 through 3 (after cisplatin and paclitaxel)
	Mesna 20% of ifosfamide dose IV, given 30 minutes before, then 4 and 8 hours after each ifosfamide infusion, days 1 through 3 (for 3 doses total each day)
	Filgrastim 5 mcg/kg/day subcutaneously, days 6 through 17, or until white blood cell count (WBC) exceeds 10,000 cells/mm³ for 2 days (whichever occurs earlier)

Lapatinib-Capecitabine

Use:	Breast cancer. *Cycle:* 21 days, continue until disease progression or intolerable toxicity
Regimen:	Lapatinib 1,250 mg PO daily, throughout entire course
	Capecitabine 1,000 mg/m²/dose PO twice daily, days 1 through 14

Larson Regimen (CAL-G, CALGB 8811)

Use:	Acute lymphoblastic leukemia (ALL; adults)
Regimen:	**Remission induction.** *Cycle:* 28 days. Give a single cycle.

Patients 60 years of age and younger:
Cyclophosphamide 1,200 mg/m² IV, day 1
Daunorubicin 45 mg/m²/day IV, days 1 through 3
Vincristine 2 mg (dose is not in mg/m²) IV weekly, days 1, 8, 15, and 22
Prednisone 60 mg/m²/day PO or IV, days 1 through 21
Asparaginase 6,000 units/m²/dose subcutaneously for 6 doses, days 5, 8, 11, 15, 18, and 22

Patients older than 60 years of age:
Cyclophosphamide 800 mg/m² IV, day 1
Daunorubicin 30 mg/m²/day IV, days 1 through 3
Vincristine 2 mg (dose is not in mg/m²) IV weekly, days 1, 8, 15, and 22
Prednisone 60 mg/m²/day PO, days 1 through 7
Asparaginase 6,000 units/m²/dose subcutaneously for 6 doses, days 5, 8, 11, 15, 18, and 22

Early intensification. *Cycle:* 28 days. Give 2 cycles.
Methotrexate 15 mg intrathecally, day 1
Cyclophosphamide 1,000 mg/m² IV, day 1
Mercaptopurine 60 mg/m²/day PO, days 1 through 14
Cytarabine 75 mg/m²/day subcutaneously, days 1 through 4 and days 8 through 11
Vincristine 2 mg (dose is not in mg/m²) IV, days 15 and 22
Asparaginase 6,000 units/m²/dose subcutaneously for 4 doses, days 15, 18, 22, and 25

continued on next page

Larson Regimen (CAL-G, CALGB 8811) (cont.)

CNS prophylaxis and interim maintenance. *Cycle*: 84 days. Give a single cycle.

Methotrexate 15 mg intrathecally, days 1, 8, 15, 22, and 29

Methotrexate 20 mg/m^2/dose PO, days 36, 43, 50, 57, and 64

Mercaptopurine 60 mg/m^2/day PO, days 1 through 70

used in conjunction with

Cranial irradiation

used in conjunction with antimicrobial prophylaxis*

Cotrimoxazole (either 80/400 or 160/800 strength) 1 tablet PO daily, throughout entire course

or

Pentamidine 300 mg inhaled once monthly, throughout entire course

Late intensification. *Cycle*: 56 days. Give a single cycle.

Doxorubicin 30 mg/m^2/dose IV, days 1, 8, and 15

Vincristine 2 mg (dose is not in mg/m^2) IV, days 1, 8, and 15

Dexamethasone 10 mg/m^2/day PO, days 1 through 14

Cyclophosphamide 1,000 mg/m^2 IV, day 29

Thioguanine 60 mg/m^2/day PO, days 29 through 42

Cytarabine 75 mg/m^2/dose subcutaneously, days 29 through 32 and days 36 through 39

used in conjunction with antimicrobial prophylaxis*

Cotrimoxazole (either 80/400 or 160/800 strength) 1 tablet PO daily, throughout entire course

or

Pentamidine 300 mg inhaled once monthly, throughout entire course

Prolonged maintenance. *Cycle*: 28 days, continue until 24 months after diagnosis

Vincristine 2 mg (dose is not in mg/m^2) IV, day 1

Prednisone 60 mg/m^2/day PO, days 1 through 5

Methotrexate 20 mg/m^2/dose PO weekly, days 1, 8, 15, and 22, for first cycle only

Mercaptopurine 60 mg/m^2/day PO, days 1 through 28, for first cycle only

used in conjunction with antimicrobial prophylaxis*

Cotrimoxazole (either 80/400 or 160/800 strength) 1 tablet PO daily, throughout entire course

or

Pentamidine 300 mg inhaled once monthly, throughout entire course

*Note: Antimicrobial prophylaxis doses not specified in original articles; the dose given here is derived from the *Infectious Diseases Handbook*, 6th edition, a tertiary resource.

Lenalidomide-Dexamethasone

Use: Multiple myeloma. *Cycle:* 28 days, continue until disease progression or intolerable toxicity

Regimen: Lenalidomide 25 mg/day PO, days 1 through 21

Dexamethasone 40 mg/day PO, days 1 through 4 of all cycles

Dexamethasone 40 mg/day PO, days 9 through 12 and days 17 through 20 of cycles 1 through 4

Linker Protocol

Use: Acute lymphocytic leukemia (ALL; induction and consolidation)

Regimen: **Remission induction.** *Cycle*: Give 1 cycle only
Daunorubicin 50 mg/m^2/day IV, days 1 through 3
Vincristine 2 mg (dose is not in mg/m^2) IV, days 1, 8, 15, and 22
Prednisone 60 mg/m^2/day PO, days 1 through 28
Asparaginase 6,000 units/m^2/day IM, days 17 through 28
If residual leukemia in marrow on day 14:
Daunorubicin 50 mg/m^2 IV, day 15
If residual leukemia in marrow on day 28:
Daunorubicin 50 mg/m^2/day IV, days 29 and 30
Vincristine 2 mg (dose is not in mg/m^2) IV, days 29 and 36
Prednisone 60 mg/m^2/day PO, days 29 through 42
Asparaginase 6,000 units/m^2/day IM, days 29 through 35
Consolidation therapy. *Cycle*: 28 days
Treatment A (cycles 1, 3, 5, and 7)
Daunorubicin 50 mg/m^2/day IV, days 1 and 2
Vincristine 2 mg (dose is not in mg/m^2) IV, days 1 and 8
Prednisone 60 mg/m^2/day PO, days 1 through 14
Asparaginase 12,000 units/m^2/dose IM 3 times weekly for
6 doses, days 2, 4, 7, 9, 11, and 14
Treatment B (cycles 2, 4, 6, and 8)
Teniposide 165 mg/m^2 IV, days 1, 4, 8, and 11
Cytarabine 300 mg/m^2 IV, days 1, 4, 8, and 11
Treatment C (cycle 9)
Methotrexate 690 mg/m^2 IV over 42 hours
Leucovorin 15 mg/m^2/dose IV every 6 hours for 12 doses
(start at end of methotrexate infusion)

M-2

Use: Multiple myeloma. *Cycle:* 5 weeks, continue until disease progression or intolerable toxicity

Regimen: Vincristine 0.03 mg/kg (2 mg maximum dose) IV, day 1
Carmustine 0.5 mg/kg IV, day 1
Cyclophosphamide 10 mg/kg IV, day 1
Prednisone 1 mg/kg/day PO, days 1 through 7, tapered over next
14 days
with
Melphalan 0.25 mg/kg/day PO, days 1 through 4
or
Melphalan 0.1 mg/kg/day PO, days 1 through 7 or days 1 through 10

---

m-BACOD (also see M-BACOD)*

Use: Lymphoma (non-Hodgkin). *Cycle:* 21 days for at least 4 cycles

Regimen: Bleomycin 4 units/m^2 IV, day 1
Doxorubicin 45 mg/m^2 IV, day 1
Cyclophosphamide 600 mg/m^2 IV, day 1
Vincristine 1 mg/m^2 (2 mg maximum dose) IV, day 1
Dexamethasone 6 mg/m^2/day PO, days 1 through 5
Methotrexate 200 mg/m^2 IV, days 8 and 15
Leucovorin 10 mg/m^2/dose PO every 6 hours for 8 doses, begin
24 hours after each methotrexate dose, days 9 through 10 and
days 16 through 17
Sargramostim 5 mcg/kg/day subcutaneously, days 4 through 13
continued on next page

m-BACOD (also see M-BACOD)* (cont.)

used in conjunction with
Intrathecal chemotherapy
*Note: m-BACOD and M-BACOD differ in the dose and timing of the methotrexate dose. Leucovorin dose not specified in original articles; the dose given here is derived from *The Chemotherapy Source Book*, 3rd edition, a tertiary resource.

m-BACOD (Reduced Dose)*

Use: Lymphoma (non-Hodgkin) associated with HIV infection.
Cycle: 21 days for at least 4 cycles
Regimen: Bleomycin 4 units/m^2 IV, day 1
Doxorubicin 25 mg/m^2 IV, day 1
Cyclophosphamide 300 mg/m^2 IV, day 1
Vincristine 1.4 mg/m^2 (2 mg maximum dose) IV, day 1
Dexamethasone 3 mg/m^2/day PO, days 1 through 5
Methotrexate 200 mg/m^2 IV, day 15
Sargramostim 5 mcg/kg/day subcutaneously, days 4 through 13 (added during subsequent cycles), for granulocyte count less than 500 cells/mm^3 at any time during the cycle or less than 1,000 cells/mm^3 on day 22 of any chemotherapy cycle
used in conjunction with
Intrathecal chemotherapy
*Note: m-BACOD (reduced dose) has decreased doses of cyclophosphamide and dexamethasone, and decreased number of methotrexate doses compared with m-BACOD.

M-BACOD (also see m-BACOD)*

Use: Lymphoma (non-Hodgkin). Cycle: 21 days
Regimen: Bleomycin 4 units/m^2 IV, day 1
Doxorubicin 45 mg/m^2 IV, day 1
Cyclophosphamide 600 mg/m^2 IV, day 1
Vincristine 1 mg/m^2 (2 mg maximum dose) IV, day 1
Dexamethasone 6 mg/m^2/day PO, days 1 through 5
Methotrexate 3,000 mg/m^2 IV, day 15
Leucovorin 10 mg/m^2/dose PO every 6 hours for 8 doses, begin 24 hours after each methotrexate dose, days 16 and 17
Sargramostim 5 mcg/kg/day subcutaneously, days 4 through 13
*Note: m-BACOD and M-BACOD differ in the dose and timing of the methotrexate dose. Leucovorin dose not specified in original articles; the dose given here is derived from *The Chemotherapy Source Book*, 3rd edition, a tertiary resource.

M-VAC

Use: Bladder cancer. Cycle: 28 days
Regimen: Methotrexate 30 mg/m^2 IV, days 1, 15, and 22
Vinblastine 3 mg/m^2 IV, days 2, 15, and 22
Doxorubicin 30 mg/m^2 IV, day 2
Cisplatin 70 mg/m^2 IV, day 2

MAC III

Use: Gestational trophoblastic neoplasm (high-risk). Cycle: 21 days
Regimen: Methotrexate 1 mg/kg IM, days 1, 3, 5, and 7
Leucovorin 0.1 mg/kg IM, days 2, 4, 6, and 8 (give 24 hours after each methotrexate dose)
Dactinomycin 0.012 mg/kg/day IV, days 1 through 5
Cyclophosphamide 3 mg/kg/day IV, days 1 through 5

MACC
Use: Lung cancer (non-small cell). *Cycle:* 21 days
Regimen: Methotrexate 30 to 40 mg/m^2 IV, day 1
Doxorubicin 30 to 40 mg/m^2 IV, day 1 (total cumulative dose 550 mg/m^2)
Cyclophosphamide 400 mg/m^2 IV, day 1
Lomustine 30 mg/m^2/day PO, day 1

MACOP-B
Use: Lymphoma (non-Hodgkin). *Cycle:* Give only a single cycle
Regimen: Methotrexate 400 mg/m^2 IV weekly, weeks 2, 6, and 10
Leucovorin 15 mg/dose PO every 6 hours for 6 doses, begin 24 hours after each methotrexate dose, during weeks 2, 6, and 10
Doxorubicin 50 mg/m^2 IV weekly, weeks 1, 3, 5, 7, 9, and 11
Cyclophosphamide 350 mg/m^2 IV weekly, weeks 1, 3, 5, 7, 9, and 11
Vincristine 1.4 mg/m^2 (2 mg maximum dose) IV weekly, weeks 2, 4, 6, 8, 10, and 12
Prednisone 75 mg/day PO for 12 weeks, tapered over last 2 weeks
Bleomycin 10 units/m^2 IV weekly, weeks 4, 8, and 12
used in conjunction with
Intrathecal chemotherapy
used in conjunction with antimicrobial prophylaxis
Ketoconazole 200 mg/day PO, throughout entire course
Cotrimoxazole double-strength (160/800) 2 tablets PO twice daily, throughout entire course

MAID
Use: Sarcoma (bone, soft tissue). *Cycle:* 21 days, continue until disease progression or intolerable toxicity
Regimen: Mesna 2,000 mg/m^2/day continuous IV infusion, days 1 through 4*
Doxorubicin 15 mg/m^2/day continuous IV infusion, days 1 through 4
Ifosfamide 2,000 mg/m^2/day continuous IV infusion, days 1 through 3*
Dacarbazine 250 mg/m^2/day continuous IV infusion, days 1 through 4
*Note: Ifosfamide and mesna may be mixed and administered in the same infusion bag.

MBC
Use: Head and neck cancer. *Cycle:* 21 days for up to 2 cycles
Regimen: Methotrexate 40 mg/m^2 IV, days 1 and 14
Bleomycin 10 units/m^2 IM or IV, days 1, 7, and 14
Cisplatin 50 mg/m^2 IV, day 4

MC
Use: Acute myelogenous leukemia (AML; induction—adults). *Cycle:* Give a single cycle
Regimen: Mitoxantrone 12 mg/m^2/day IV, days 1 through 3
Cytarabine 100 to 200 mg/m^2/day continuous IV infusion or IV, days 1 through 7

MCF
Use: Gastric cancer. *Cycle:* 42 days for up to 4 cycles
Regimen: Mitomycin 7 mg/m^2 (14 mg maximum dose) IV, day 1
Cisplatin 60 mg/m^2 IV, days 1 and 22
Fluorouracil 300 mg/m^2/day continuous IV infusion, days 1 through 180

MF
Use: Breast cancer. *Cycle:* 28 days for up to 12 cycles
Regimen: Methotrexate 100 mg/m^2 IV, days 1 and 8
Fluorouracil 600 mg/m^2 IV, days 1 and 8, given 1 hour after methotrexate
Leucovorin 10 mg/m^2/dose IV or PO every 6 hours for 6 doses, starting 24 hours after each methotrexate dose, days 2 through 3 and days 9 through 10

MICE (ICE)
Use: Sarcoma (adults), osteosarcoma (pediatrics), lung cancer. *Cycle:* 21 to 28 days
Regimen: Ifosfamide 1,250 to 1,500 mg/m^2/day IV, days 1 through 3
Carboplatin 300 to 635 mg/m^2 IV, once on day 1 or 3
Etoposide 80 to 100 mg/m^2/day IV, days 1 through 3
with
Mesna 1,250 mg/m^2/day IV, days 1 through 3
or
Mesna 20% of ifosfamide dose IV before, then 4 and 8 hours after each ifosfamide infusion, days 1 through 3

MidAC
Use: Acute myelogenous leukemia (AML; consolidation—pediatrics). *Cycle:* Give a single cycle
Regimen: Mitoxantrone 10 mg/m^2/day IV, days 1 through 5
Cytarabine 1,000 mg/m^2/dose IV every 12 hours for 6 doses, days 1 through 3
used in conjunction with
Autologous stem cell transplantation

MINE
Use: Lymphoma (non-Hodgkin). *Cycle:* 21 days for up to 6 cycles
Regimen: Ifosfamide 1,330 mg/m^2/day IV, days 1 through 3
Mesna 1,330 mg/m^2/day IV, days 1 through 3, given with ifosfamide
Mesna 500 mg/dose PO, 4 hours after ifosfamide, days 1 through 3
Mitoxantrone 8 mg/m^2 IV, day 1
Etoposide 65 mg/m^2/day IV, days 1 through 3

MINE-ESHAP
Use: Lymphoma (non-Hodgkin). *Cycle:* 21 days
Regimen: Give MINE for 6 cycles, then give ESHAP for 3 to 6 cycles

mini-BEAM
Use: Lymphoma (Hodgkin). *Cycle:* 4 to 6 weeks
Regimen: Carmustine 60 mg/m^2 IV, day 1
Etoposide 75 mg/m^2/day IV, days 2 through 5
Cytarabine 100 mg/m^2/dose IV every 12 hours for 8 doses, days 2 through 5
Melphalan 30 mg/m^2 IV, day 6

MOBP
Use: Cervical cancer. *Cycle:* 6 weeks for up to 2 cycles
Regimen: Bleomycin 30 units/day continuous IV infusion, days 1 through 4
Vincristine* 0.5 mg/m^2 IV, days 1 and 4
Cisplatin 50 mg/m^2 IV, days 1 and 22
Mitomycin 10 mg/m^2 IV, day 2
*Note: The vincristine dose is not capped in this protocol. Consult the prescriber if there is any question about the intended vincristine dose.

MOP

Use:	Brain tumors (pediatrics). *Cycle:* 28 days, continue until patient is 2 years of age
Regimen:	Mechlorethamine 6 mg/m^2 IV, days 1 and 8
	Vincristine 1.5 mg/m^2 (2 mg maximum dose) IV, days 1 and 8
	Procarbazine 100 mg/m^2/day PO, days 1 through 14

MOPP

Use:	Lymphoma (Hodgkin—adults). *Cycle:* 28 days for up to 6 cycles
Regimen:	Mechlorethamine 6 mg/m^2 IV, days 1 and 8
	Vincristine 1.4 mg/m^2 (2 mg maximum dose) IV, days 1 and 8
	Procarbazine 100 mg/m^2/day PO, days 1 through 14
	Prednisone 40 mg/m^2/day PO, cycles 1 and 4,* days 1 through 14
	*Note: Some clinicians give prednisone with every cycle of MOPP. The original clinical trials gave prednisone only with the first and fourth cycles.

Use:	Lymphoma (Hodgkin—pediatrics). *Cycle:* 28 days for up to 6 cycles
Regimen:	Mechlorethamine 6 mg/m^2 IV, days 1 and 8
	Vincristine 1.4 mg/m^2 (2 mg maximum dose) IV, days 1 and 8
	Procarbazine 50 mg PO, day 1
	Procarbazine 100 mg/m^2/day PO, days 2 through 14
	Prednisone 40 mg/m^2/day PO, cycles 1 and 4,* days 1 through 14
	*Note: Some clinicians give prednisone with every cycle of MOPP. The original clinical trials gave prednisone only with the first and fourth cycles.

Use:	Brain cancer (medulloblastoma). *Cycle:* 28 days for up to 12 cycles
Regimen:	Mechlorethamine 3 mg/m^2 IV, days 1 and 8
	Vincristine 1.4 mg/m^2 (2 mg maximum dose) IV, days 1 and 8
	Prednisone 40 mg/m^2/day PO, days 1 through 10
	Procarbazine 50 mg PO, day 1
	Procarbazine 100 mg PO, day 2
	Procarbazine 100 mg/m^2/day PO, days 3 through 10

MOPP/ABV

Use:	Lymphoma (Hodgkin). *Cycle:* 28 days for up to 10 cycles
Regimen:	Mechlorethamine 6 mg/m^2 IV, day 1
	Vincristine 1.4 mg/m^2 (2 mg maximum dose) IV, day 1
	Procarbazine 100 mg/m^2/day PO, days 1 through 7
	Prednisone 40 mg/m^2/day PO, days 1 through 14
	Doxorubicin 35 mg/m^2 IV, day 8
	Bleomycin 10 units/m^2 IV, day 8
	Vinblastine 6 mg/m^2 IV, day 8

MOPP/ABVD

Use:	Lymphoma (Hodgkin). *Cycle:* 28 days for up to 12 cycles (6 MOPP cycles and 6 ABVD cycles)
Regimen:	Alternate MOPP and ABVD regimens every month

MP

Use:	Multiple myeloma. *Cycle:* 21 to 28 days, continue for 6 to 12 months
Regimen:	Melphalan 8 mg/m^2/day PO, days 1 through 4
	Prednisone 60 mg/m^2/day PO, days 1 through 4

Use:	Multiple myeloma. *Cycle:* 42 days
Regimen:	Melphalan 10 mg/m^2/day PO, days 1 through 4
	Prednisone 60 mg/m^2/day PO, days 1 through 4

continued on next page

MP (cont.)
Use: Prostate cancer. *Cycle:* 21 days
Regimen: Mitoxantrone 12 mg/m^2 IV, day 1
Prednisone 5 mg/dose PO twice daily, throughout entire course

MTX/6-MP
Use: Acute lymphocytic leukemia (ALL; continuation—pediatrics).
Cycle: Ongoing, weeks 25 through 130
Regimen: Methotrexate 20 mg/m^2 IM weekly
Mercaptopurine 50 mg/m^2/day PO
used in conjunction with
Intrathecal therapy once every 12 weeks

MTX/6-MP/VP
Use: Acute lymphocytic leukemia (ALL; continuation—pediatrics).
Cycle: Ongoing, 2 to 3 years
Regimen: Methotrexate 20 mg/m^2/dose PO weekly
Mercaptopurine 75 mg/m^2/day PO
Vincristine* 1.5 mg/m^2 IV, once monthly
Prednisone 40 mg/m^2/day PO for 5 days each month
*Note: The vincristine dose is not capped in this pediatric protocol.
Consult the prescriber if there is any question about the intended
vincristine dose.

MTX-CDDPAdr
Use: Osteosarcoma (pediatrics). *Cycle:* 28 days for 2 to 4 cycles
Regimen: Methotrexate 12,000 mg/m^2 IV, days 1 and 8
Leucovorin 20 mg/m^2/dose IV every 3 hours for 8 doses, then give
PO every 6 hours for 8 doses (begin 16 hours after end of each
methotrexate infusion)
Cisplatin 75 mg/m^2 IV, day 15 of cycles 1 through 7
Doxorubicin 25 mg/m^2/day IV, days 15 through 17 of cycles 1
through 7
Cisplatin 120 mg/m^2 IV, day 15 of cycles 8 through 10

MV
Use: Breast cancer. *Cycle:* 6 to 8 weeks
Regimen: Mitomycin 20 mg/m^2 IV, day 1
Vinblastine 0.15 mg/kg IV, days 1 and 21

Use: Acute myelogenous leukemia (AML; induction). *Cycle:* Give
1 cycle. Second cycle may be considered if complete response
not achieved (eg, persistent blasts present on day 21).
Regimen: Mitoxantrone 10 mg/m^2/day IV, days 1 through 5
Etoposide 100 mg/m^2/day IV, days 1 through 5

MVP
Use: Lung cancer (non-small cell). *Cycle:* 6 weeks for up to 6 cycles
Regimen: Mitomycin 8 mg/m^2 IV, day 1
Vinblastine 6 mg/m^2 IV, days 1 and 22
Cisplatin 50 mg/m^2 IV, days 1 and 22

MVPP

Use: Lymphoma (Hodgkin). *Cycle:* 6 weeks for 6 to 8 cycles

Regimen: Mechlorethamine 6 mg/m^2 (10 mg maximum dose) IV, days 1 and 8

Vinblastine 4 to 6 mg/m^2 (10 mg maximum dose) IV, days 1 and 8

Procarbazine 100 mg/m^2/day (150 mg maximum dose) PO, days 1 through 14

Prednisone 40 mg/m^2/day (50 mg maximum dose) PO, cycles 1 and 4,* days 1 through 14

*Note: Some clinicians give prednisone with every cycle of MVPP. The original clinical trials gave prednisone only with the first and fourth cycles. Prednisolone is recommended in the British literature. In the United States, prednisone is the preferred corticosteroid. The doses of these 2 corticosteroids are equivalent (ie, prednisone 40 mg PO = prednisolone 40 mg PO).

NA—see Vinorelbine-Doxorubicin

NFL

Use: Breast cancer. *Cycle:* 21 days for 6 to 8 cycles

Regimen: Mitoxantrone 12 mg/m^2 IV, day 1

Leucovorin 300 mg/day IV, days 1 through 3

Fluorouracil 350 mg/m^2/day IV, days 1 through 3 after leucovorin

---

Use: Breast cancer. *Cycle:* 21 days for at least 2 cycles

Regimen: Mitoxantrone 10 mg/m^2 IV, day 1

Leucovorin 100 mg/m^2/day IV, days 1 through 3, give before fluorouracil on day 1

Fluorouracil 1,000 mg/m^2/day continuous IV infusion, days 1 through 3

NOVP

Use: Lymphoma (Hodgkin). *Cycle:* 21 days for up to 3 cycles

Regimen: Mitoxantrone 10 mg/m^2 IV, day 1

Vinblastine 6 mg/m^2 IV, day 1

Prednisone 100 mg/day PO, days 1 through 5

Vincristine 1.4 mg/m^2 (2 mg maximum dose) IV, day 8

OPA

Use: Lymphoma (Hodgkin—pediatrics). *Cycle:* 15 days for up to 2 cycles. Time between cycles not specified.

Regimen: Vincristine 1.5 mg/m^2 (2 mg maximum dose) IV, days 1, 8, and 15

Prednisone 20 mg/m^2/dose PO 3 times daily, days 1 through 15

Doxorubicin 40 mg/m^2 IV, days 1 and 15

OPPA

Use: Lymphoma (Hodgkin—pediatrics). *Cycle:* 15 days for up to 2 cycles. Time between cycles not specified.

Regimen: **Add to OPA:** Procarbazine 100 mg/m^2/day PO in 2 to 3 divided doses, days 1 through 15

P6

Use: Sarcoma (bone). *Cycle:* Repeat for 7 cycles based on hematologic recovery, delay subsequent cycles until neutrophil count is greater than 500 cells/mm³ post-nadir and platelet count is at least 100,000 cells/mm³ after cycles 1 through 3 or platelet count is at least 75,000 cells/mm³ after cycles 4 through 7.

Regimen: **Treatment A** (cycles 1, 2, 3, and 6)

Patients younger than 10 years of age:

Cyclophosphamide 70 mg/kg/day IV, days 1 and 2

Mesna 70 mg/kg/day continuous IV infusion, days 1 and 2

Doxorubicin 25 mg/m²/day continuous IV infusion, days 1 through 3*

Vincristine 0.67 mg/m²/day (0.67 mg maximum/day, or 2 mg maximum/cycle) continuous IV infusion, days 1 through 3*

Filgrastim 5 mcg/kg/day subcutaneously, from day 5 until hematologic recovery (start at least 24 hours after completion of chemotherapy infusions)

Patients 10 years of age and older:

Cyclophosphamide 2,100 mg/m²/day IV, days 1 and 2

Mesna 2,100 mg/m²/day continuous IV infusion, days 1 and 2

Doxorubicin 25 mg/m²/day continuous IV infusion, days 1 through 3*

Vincristine 0.67 mg/m²/day (0.67 mg maximum/day, or 2 mg maximum/cycle) continuous IV infusion, days 1 through 3*

Filgrastim 5 mcg/kg/day subcutaneously, from day 5 until hematologic recovery (start at least 24 hours after completion of chemotherapy infusions)

Treatment B (cycles 4, 5, and 7)

Ifosfamide 1,800 mg/m²/day IV, days 1 through 5†

Etoposide 100 mg/m²/day IV, days 1 through 5†

with

Mesna 1,800 mg/m²/day IV, days 1 through 5

or

Mesna 20% of ifosfamide dose IV before, then 4 and 8 hours after each ifosfamide infusion, days 1 through 5

plus

Filgrastim 5 mcg/kg/day subcutaneously, from day 6 until hematologic recovery (start at least 24 hours after completion of chemotherapy infusions)

used in conjunction with antimicrobial prophylaxis‡

Cotrimoxazole (either 80/400 or 160/800 strength) 1 tablet PO daily, throughout entire course

or

Pentamidine 300 mg inhaled once monthly, throughout entire course

*Note: Vincristine and doxorubicin may be mixed and administered in the same infusion bag, if diluted with 0.9% Sodium Chloride Injection.

†Note: Ifosfamide and mesna may be mixed and administered in the same infusion bag.

‡Note: Antimicrobial prophylaxis doses not specified in original articles; the dose given here is derived from the *Infectious Diseases Handbook*, 6th edition, a tertiary resource.

PA-CI
Use:	Hepatoblastoma (pediatrics). *Cycle:* 21 days for up to 4 cycles
Regimen:	Cisplatin 90 mg/m² IV, day 1
	Doxorubicin 20 mg/m²/day continuous IV infusion, days 2 through 5

PAC
Use:	Ovarian, endometrial cancer. *Cycle:* 28 days for up to 6 cycles
Regimen:	Cisplatin 50 mg/m² IV, day 1
	Doxorubicin 50 mg/m² IV, day 1
	Cyclophosphamide 500 mg/m² IV, day 1

Use:	Thymoma. *Cycle:* 21 days for up to 8 cycles
Regimen:	Cisplatin 50 mg/m² IV, day 1
	Doxorubicin 50 mg/m² IV, day 1
	Cyclophosphamide 500 mg/m² IV, day 1

PAC-I (Indiana Protocol)
Use:	Ovarian cancer. *Cycle:* 21 days for up to 6 cycles
Regimen:	Cisplatin 50 mg/m² IV, day 1 (total cumulative dose 300 mg/m²)
	Doxorubicin 50 mg/m² IV, day 1
	Cyclophosphamide 750 mg/m² IV, day 1

PACA
Use:	Ovarian cancer. *Cycle:* 28 days for up to 9 cycles
Regimen:	Liposomal doxorubicin 30 mg/m² IV, day 1
	Carboplatin IV dose by Calvert equation to AUC 5 mg/mL/min, day 1 (after liposomal doxorubicin)

Paclitaxel-Bevacizumab
Use:	Breast cancer. *Cycle:* 28 days, continue until disease progression or intolerable toxicity
Regimen:	Paclitaxel 90 mg/m² IV, days 1, 8, and 15
	Bevacizumab 10 mg/kg IV, days 1 and 15

Paclitaxel-Carboplatin (also see PC)
Use:	Endometrial cancer. *Cycle:* 28 days for up to 6 cycles
Regimen:	Paclitaxel 175 mg/m² IV over 3 hours, day 1
	Carboplatin IV dose by Calvert equation to AUC 5 to 7 mg/mL/min, day 1 (give after paclitaxel)

Use:	Head and neck cancer. *Cycle:* 28 days
Regimen:	Paclitaxel 200 mg/m² IV over 3 hours, day 1
	Carboplatin IV dose by Calvert equation to AUC 7 mg/mL/min, day 1 (after paclitaxel)
	Filgrastim 5 mcg/kg/day subcutaneously, days 2 through 12

Paclitaxel-Carboplatin-Bevacizumab
Use:	Lung cancer (non-small cell). *Cycle:* 21 days for up to 6 cycles
Regimen:	Paclitaxel 200 mg/m² IV, day 1
	Carboplatin IV dose by Calvert equation to AUC 6 mg/mL/min, day 1 (give after paclitaxel)
	Bevacizumab 15 mg/kg IV, day 1

Paclitaxel-Carboplatin-Etoposide
Use:	Adenocarcinoma (unknown primary), lung cancer (small cell). *Cycle:* 21 days for up to 4 cycles
Regimen:	Paclitaxel 200 mg/m² IV over 1 hour, day 1
	Carboplatin IV dose by Calvert equation to AUC 6 mg/mL/min, day 1 (give after paclitaxel)
	Etoposide 50 mg/day PO alternated with 100 mg/day PO, days 1 through 10

Paclitaxel-Carboplatin-Fluorouracil

Use: Esophageal cancer. *Cycle:* 21 days for 2 cycles prior to surgery

Regimen: Paclitaxel 200 mg/m^2 IV over 1 hour, day 1

Carboplatin IV dose by Calvert equation to AUC 6 mg/mL/min, day 1 (administration sequence not specified)

Fluorouracil 225 mg/m^2/day continuous IV infusion, days 1 through 21 *used in conjunction with*

Radiation therapy

Paclitaxel-Herceptin

Use: Breast cancer. *Cycle:* 7 days, continue until death or intolerable toxicity

Regimen: Trastuzumab 4 mg/kg IV, day 1 for first cycle only (loading dose); then trastuzumab 2 mg/kg IV, day 1 for subsequent cycles

Paclitaxel 70 to 90 mg/m^2 IV over 1 hour, day 1 (give after trastuzumab)

Paclitaxel-Vinorelbine

Use: Breast cancer. *Cycle:* 28 days, continue until disease progression or intolerable toxicity

Regimen: Vinorelbine 30 mg/m^2 IV, days 1 and 8

Paclitaxel 135 mg/m^2 IV over 3 hours, day 1 (after vinorelbine infusion)

Use: Lung cancer (non-small cell). *Cycle:* 14 days for 9 cycles

Regimen: Paclitaxel 135 mg/m^2 IV over 3 hours, day 1

Vinorelbine 25 mg/m^2 IV, day 1

PC (also see Paclitaxel-Carboplatin)

Use: Lung cancer (non-small cell). *Cycle:* 21 days for 6 cycles

Regimen: Paclitaxel 135 mg/m^2/day continuous IV infusion over 24 hours, day 1

Carboplatin IV dose by Calvert equation to AUC 7.5 mg/mL/min, day 2 (after paclitaxel)

Filgrastim 5 mcg/kg/day subcutaneously (rounded to 300 or 480 mcg), days 3 through 17, of cycles 2 through 6

Use: Lung cancer (non-small cell). *Cycle:* 21 days for up to 6 cycles

Regimen: Paclitaxel 175 mg/m^2 IV over 3 hours, day 1

Cisplatin 80 mg/m^2 IV, day 1 (after paclitaxel)

Use: Head and neck cancer. *Cycle:* 21 days for at least 6 cycles

Regimen: Paclitaxel 175 mg/m^2 IV over 3 hours, day 1

Cisplatin 75 mg/m^2 IV, day 1 (administration sequence not specified in protocol)

Use: Bladder cancer, esophageal cancer. *Cycle:* 21 days for up to 8 cycles, or until disease progression or intolerable toxicity

Regimen: Paclitaxel 200 or 225 mg/m^2 IV over 3 hours, day 1

Carboplatin IV dose by Calvert equation to AUC 5 to 6 mg/mL/min, day 1 (after paclitaxel)

PCG

Use: Bladder cancer. *Cycle:* 21 days

Regimen: Paclitaxel 200 mg/m^2 IV over 3 hours, day 1

Carboplatin IV dose by Calvert equation to AUC 5 mg/mL/min, day 1 (after paclitaxel)

Gemcitabine 800 mg/m^2 IV, days 1 and 8

PCR

Use: Chronic lymphocytic leukemia (CLL). *Cycle:* 21 days for 6 cycles
Regimen: Pentostatin 2 mg/m^2 IV, day 1
Cyclophosphamide 600 mg/m^2 IV, day 1
Rituximab 100 mg/m^2 IV, day 1 of first cycle only
Rituximab 375 mg/m^2 IV, days 3 and 5 of first cycle only (loading dose)
Rituximab 375 mg/m^2 IV, day 1, except for day 1 of first cycle
Filgrastim 5 mcg/kg/day subcutaneously, days 3 through 12 or until absolute neutrophil count (ANC) is greater than 1,000 cells/mm^3 for 2 consecutive days
used in conjunction with antimicrobial prophylaxis*
Cotrimoxazole (either 80/400 or 160/800 strength) 1 tablet PO daily, days 1 through 365
plus
Acyclovir 200 mg PO 3 times daily, days 1 through 365
or
Acyclovir 400 mg PO twice daily, days 1 through 365
*Note: Antimicrobial prophylaxis doses not specified in original article; the doses given here are derived from the *Infectious Diseases Handbook*, 6th edition, and *AHFS 2008 Drug Information*, both tertiary resources.

PCV

Use: Brain tumor. *Cycle:* 6 to 8 weeks, continue for 1 year or until disease progression
Regimen: Lomustine 110 mg/m^2 PO, day 1
Procarbazine 60 mg/m^2/day PO, days 8 through 21
Vincristine 1.4 mg/m^2 (2 mg maximum dose) IV, days 8 and 29

Use: Advanced brain tumor. *Cycle:* 8 weeks for up to 6 cycles
Regimen: Lomustine 130 mg/m^2 PO, day 1
Procarbazine 75 mg/m^2/day PO, days 8 through 21
Vincristine* 1.4 mg/m^2 IV, days 8 and 29
*Note: The vincristine is not capped in this protocol. Consult the prescriber if there is any question about the intended vincristine dose.

PE

Use: Prostate cancer. *Cycle:* 21 days, continue until disease progression or intolerable toxicity
Regimen: Paclitaxel 30 mg/m^2/day continuous IV infusion over 24 hours, days 1 through 4
Estramustine 600 mg/m^2/day PO given in 2 to 3 divided doses (start 24 hours before first paclitaxel infusion)

PEB—see BEP

Pemetrexed-Cisplatin

Use: Mesothelioma. *Cycle:* 21 days
Regimen: Pemetrexed 500 mg/m^2 IV, day 1
Cisplatin 75 mg/m^2 IV, day 1 (after pemetrexed)
used in conjunction with vitamin B supplementation
Folic acid 0.35 to 1 mg/day PO throughout entire course, starting 7 to 21 days before first chemotherapy dose and continued for 21 days after the last pemetrexed dose
Cyanocobalamin 1 mg/dose IM every 9 weeks, starting 7 to 21 days before first chemotherapy dose and continued throughout entire chemotherapy course

PFL
Use: Head and neck, gastric cancer. *Cycle:* 28 days for 2 to 3 cycles
Regimen: Cisplatin 25 mg/m^2/day continuous IV infusion, days 1 through 5
Leucovorin 500 mg/m^2/day continuous IV infusion, days 1 through 6
Fluorouracil 800 mg/m^2/day continuous IV infusion, days 2 through 6

Use: Head and neck, gastric cancer. *Cycle:* 21 days, continue until disease progression or intolerable toxicity
Regimen: Cisplatin 100 mg/m^2 IV, day 1
Fluorouracil 600 to 800 mg/m^2/day continuous IV infusion, days 1 through 5
Leucovorin 50 mg/m^2/dose PO every 4 to 6 hours, days 1 through 6

PIAF
Use: Hepatocellular cancer. *Cycle:* 21 days for up to 6 cycles
Regimen: Cisplatin 20 mg/m^2/day IV, days 1 through 4
Interferon alfa-2b 5 million units/m^2/day subcutaneously, days 1 through 4
Doxorubicin 40 mg/m^2 IV, day 1
Fluorouracil 400 mg/m^2/day IV, days 1 through 4

PNET-3 Protocol
Use: Brain tumors (pediatrics). *Cycle:* 21 days for 4 cycles
Regimen: Alternate cycles ABAB.
Cycle A: Vincristine* 1.5 mg/m^2 IV, days 1, 7, and 14
Etoposide 100 mg/m^2/day IV, days 1 through 3
Carboplatin 500 mg/m^2/day IV, days 1 and 2
Cycle B: Vincristine* 1.5 mg/m^2 IV, days 1, 7, and 14 of first Cycle B (ie, cycle 2), then day 1 of next Cycle B (ie, cycle 4)
Etoposide 100 mg/m^2/day IV, days 1 through 3
Cyclophosphamide 1,500 mg/m^2 IV, day 1
Mesna 750 mg/m^2/dose IV given 15 minutes before, and 4 and 8 hours after cyclophosphamide, day 1
*Note: The vincristine dose is not capped in this protocol. Consult the prescriber if there is any question about the intended vincristine dose.

POC
Use: Brain tumors (pediatrics). *Cycle:* 6 weeks for up to 8 cycles
Regimen: Prednisone 40 mg/m^2/day PO, days 1 through 14
Vincristine 1.5 mg/m^2 IV (2 mg maximum dose), days 1, 8, and 15
Lomustine 100 mg/m^2 PO, day 1

ProMACE
Use: Lymphoma (non-Hodgkin). *Cycle:* 28 days for up to 6 cycles
Regimen: Prednisone 60 mg/m^2/day PO, days 1 through 14
Doxorubicin 25 mg/m^2 IV, days 1 and 8
Cyclophosphamide 650 mg/m^2 IV, days 1 and 8
Etoposide 120 mg/m^2 IV, days 1 and 8
Methotrexate 750 mg/m^2 IV, day 14
Leucovorin 50 mg/m^2/dose IV every 6 hours for 5 doses, starting on day 15 (start 24 hours after methotrexate)

ProMACE/cytaBOM

Use: Lymphoma (non-Hodgkin). *Cycle:* 21 days for at least 6 cycles
Regimen: Prednisone 60 mg/m^2/day PO, days 1 through 14
Doxorubicin 25 mg/m^2 IV, day 1
Cyclophosphamide 650 mg/m^2 IV, day 1
Etoposide 120 mg/m^2 IV, day 1
Cytarabine 300 mg/m^2 IV, day 8
Bleomycin 5 units/m^2 IV, day 8
Vincristine 1.4 mg/m^2 (2 mg maximum dose) IV, day 8
Methotrexate 120 mg/m^2 IV, day 8
Leucovorin 25 mg/m^2/dose PO every 6 hours for 4 doses, starting on day 9 (start 24 hours after methotrexate dose)
Cotrimoxazole double-strength (160/800) 2 tablets PO twice daily, days 1 through 21

ProMACE/MOPP

Use: Lymphoma (non-Hodgkin). *Cycle:* 28 days for at least 6 cycles
Regimen: Prednisone 60 mg/m^2/day PO, days 1 through 14
Doxorubicin 25 mg/m^2 IV, day 1
Cyclophosphamide 650 mg/m^2 IV, day 1
Etoposide 120 mg/m^2 IV, day 1
Mechlorethamine 6 mg/m^2 IV, day 8
Vincristine 1.4 mg/m^2 (2 mg maximum dose) IV, day 8
Procarbazine 100 mg/m^2/day PO, days 8 through 14
Methotrexate 500 mg/m^2 IV, day 15
Leucovorin 50 mg/m^2/dose PO every 6 hours for 4 doses, starting on day 16 (start 24 hours after methotrexate dose)

Pt/VM

Use: Neuroblastoma (pediatrics). *Cycle:* 21 to 28 days for up to 5 cycles
Regimen: Cisplatin 90 mg/m^2 IV, day 1
Teniposide 100 mg/m^2 IV, day 3

PVA

Use: Acute lymphocytic leukemia (ALL; induction—pediatrics).
Cycle: 28 days. Give a single cycle.
Regimen: Prednisone 13.33 mg/m^2/dose (40 mg/m^2/day, or 60 mg/day maximum dose) PO, 3 times daily, days 1 through 28
Vincristine 1.5 mg/m^2 (2 mg maximum dose) IV weekly, days 1, 8, 15, and 22
with
Asparaginase 6,000 units/m^2/dose IM, 3 times weekly for 6 doses total (eg, days 2, 5, 7, 9, 12, and 14)
or
Asparaginase 6,000 units/m^2/dose IM twice weekly for 6 doses total, days 2, 5, 8, 12, 15, and 19
or
Asparaginase 5,000 units/m^2/dose IM twice weekly for 6 doses total, days 2, 5, 8, 12, 15, and 18
used in conjunction with
Intrathecal therapy

PVB

Use: Testicular cancer, adenocarcinoma. *Cycle:* 21 days for up to 4 cycles

Regimen: Cisplatin 20 mg/m^2/day IV, days 1 through 5
Vinblastine 0.15 mg/kg/day IV, days 1 and 2
Bleomycin 30 units IV, days 2, 9, and 16

PVDA

Use: Acute lymphocytic leukemia (ALL; induction—pediatrics). *Cycle:* 28 days. Give a single cycle.

Regimen: Prednisone 40 mg/m^2/day PO, days 1 through 28
Vincristine 1.5 mg/m^2 (2 mg maximum dose) IV weekly, days 1, 8, 15, and 22
Daunorubicin 25 mg/m^2 IV weekly, days 1, 8, 15, and 22
Asparaginase 10,000 units/m^2/dose IM, 3 times weekly for 12 doses, beginning on day 1
used in conjunction with
Intrathecal therapy
Cotrimoxazole 2.5 mg/kg/dose (as trimethoprim) PO twice daily, days 1 through 28

Use: Acute lymphocytic leukemia (ALL; induction—pediatrics). *Cycle:* 28 days. Give a single cycle.

Regimen: Prednisone 40 mg/m^2/day PO, days 1 through 28
Vincristine 1.5 mg/m^2 (2 mg maximum dose) IV, days 2, 8, 15, and 22
Daunorubicin 25 mg/m^2 IV, days 2, 8, 15, and 22
Asparaginase 5,000 units/m^2/dose IM twice weekly for 6 doses, days 2, 5, 8, 12, 15, and 19
used in conjunction with
Intrathecal therapy

R-CHOP—see CHOP + Rituximab

R-CVP—see CVP + Rituximab

R-MICE—see ICE + Rituximab

RICE—see ICE + Rituximab

RTOG 93-10

Use: Lymphoma (central nervous system). *Cycle:* Give a single cycle

Regimen: Methotrexate 2,500 mg/m^2/dose IV, days 1, 15, 29, 43, and 57
Leucovorin 20 mg PO every 6 hours for 12 doses, starting 24 hours after each IV methotrexate dose, days 2, 3, 4, days 16, 17, 18, days 30, 31, 32, days 44, 45, 46, and days 58, 59, 60
Vincristine 1.4 mg/m^2 (2.8 mg maximum dose) IV, days 1, 15, 29, 43, and 57
Procarbazine 100 mg/m^2/day PO once daily, days 1 through 7, days 29 through 35, and days 57 through 63
Dexamethasone 16 mg/day PO, days 1 through 7; then dexamethasone 12 mg/day PO, days 8 through 14; then dexamethasone 8 mg/day PO, days 15 through 21; then dexamethasone 6 mg/day PO, days 22 through 28; then dexamethasone 4 mg/day PO, days 29 through 35; then dexamethasone 2 mg/day PO, days 36 through 42
Methotrexate 12 mg intrathecal via Ommaya reservoir, days 8, 22, 36, 50, and 64
continued on next page

RTOG 93-10 (cont.)

Leucovorin 10 mg PO twice daily for 8 doses, beginning the evening after each intrathecal methotrexate dose, days 9 through 12, days 23 through 26, days 37 through 40, days 51 through 54, and days 65 through 68

followed by

Radiation therapy

followed by

Cytarabine 3,000 mg/m²/day IV, days 106, 107, 127, and 128

*used in conjunction with antimicrobial prophylaxis**

Cotrimoxazole (either 80/400 or 160/800 strength) 1 tablet PO daily, throughout entire course

plus

Clotrimazole lozenge 10 mg PO 3 times daily, throughout entire course

*Note: Antimicrobial prophylaxis doses not specified in original article; the doses given here are derived from the *Infectious Diseases Handbook*, 6th edition, and *AHFS 2008 Drug Information*, both tertiary resources.

Sequential AC/Paclitaxel—see AC/Paclitaxel, Sequential

Sequential Dox ➡ CMF—see Dox ➡ CMF, Sequential

SMF

Use: Pancreatic cancer. *Cycle:* 8 weeks
Regimen: Streptozocin 1,000 mg/m² IV, days 1, 8, 29, and 36
Mitomycin 10 mg/m² IV, day 1
Fluorouracil 600 mg/m² IV, days 1, 8, 29, and 36

Stanford V

Use: Lymphoma (Hodgkin). *Cycle:* 28 days for 3 cycles
Regimen 1: Patients younger than 50 years of age:
Mechlorethamine 6 mg/m² IV, day 1
Doxorubicin 25 mg/m² IV, days 1 and 15
Vinblastine 6 mg/m² IV, days 1 and 15
Vincristine 1.4 mg/m² (2 mg maximum dose) IV, days 8 and 22
Bleomycin 5 units/m² IV, days 8 and 22
Etoposide 60 mg/m²/day IV, days 15 and 16
Prednisone 40 mg/m²/dose PO, every other day continually for 10 weeks, then taper off by 10 mg every other day for next 14 days

used in conjunction with antimicrobial prophylaxis

Cotrimoxazole double-strength (160/800) 1 tablet PO twice daily, throughout entire course
Ketoconazole 200 mg/day PO, throughout entire course
Acyclovir 200 mg PO 3 times daily, throughout entire course

continued on next page

Stanford V (cont.)

Regimen 2: Patients aged 50 years and older:

Mechlorethamine 6 mg/m^2 IV, day 1

Doxorubicin 25 mg/m^2 IV, days 1 and 15

Vinblastine 6 mg/m^2 IV, days 1 and 15 for cycles 1 and 2 only; then vinblastine 4 mg/m^2 IV, days 1 and 15 for cycle 3

Vincristine 1.4 mg/m^2 (2 mg maximum dose) IV, days 8 and 22 for cycles 1 and 2 only; then vincristine 1 mg/m^2 (2 mg maximum dose) IV, days 1 and 15 for cycle 3

Bleomycin 5 units/m^2 IV, days 8 and 22

Etoposide 60 mg/m^2/day IV, days 15 and 16

Prednisone 40 mg/m^2/dose PO, every other day continually for 10 weeks, then taper off by 10 mg every other day for next 14 days

used in conjunction with antimicrobial prophylaxis

Cotrimoxazole double-strength (160/800) 1 tablet PO twice daily, throughout entire course

Ketoconazole 200 mg/day PO, throughout entire course

Acyclovir 200 mg PO 3 times daily, throughout entire course

TAC

Use: Breast cancer. *Cycle:* 21 days for up to 8 cycles

Regimen: Doxorubicin 50 mg/m^2 IV, day 1

Cyclophosphamide 500 mg/m^2 IV, day 1 (after doxorubicin)

Docetaxel 75 mg/m^2 IV, day 1 (after cyclophosphamide)

Ciprofloxacin 500 mg PO twice daily, days 5 through 15

TAD

Use: Acute myelogenous leukemia (AML; induction—adults). *Cycle:* 21 days for 2 cycles

Regimen: Cytarabine 100 mg/m^2/day continuous IV infusion, days 1 and 2

Cytarabine 100 mg/m^2/dose IV every 12 hours for 12 doses, days 3 through 8

Daunorubicin 60 mg/m^2/day IV, days 3 through 5

Thioguanine 100 mg/m^2/dose PO every 12 hours for 14 doses, days 3 through 9

Tamoxifen-Epirubicin

Use: Breast cancer. *Cycle:* 28 days for 6 cycles

Regimen: Tamoxifen 20 mg PO daily, continuously for 4 years

Epirubicin 50 mg/m^2 IV, on days 1 and 8

TAP

Use: Endometrial cancer. *Cycle:* 21 days for up to 7 cycles

Regimen: Doxorubicin 45 mg/m^2 IV, day 1

Cisplatin 50 mg/m^2 IV, day 1

Paclitaxel 160 mg/m^2 IV over 3 hours, day 2

Filgrastim 5 mcg/kg/day subcutaneously, days 3 through 12

TC

Use: Gastric cancer. *Cycle:* 21 days (up to 8 cycles)

Regimen: Docetaxel 85 mg/m^2 IV, day 1

Cisplatin 75 mg/m^2 IV, day 1 (after docetaxel)

TCF

Use:	Esophageal cancer. *Cycle:* 28 days
Regimen:	Paclitaxel 175 mg/m^2 IV over 3 hours, day 1
	Cisplatin 20 mg/m^2/day IV, days 1 through 5 (give after paclitaxel) for first 3 cycles; decrease to cisplatin 15 mg/m^2/day IV, days 1 through 5 for subsequent cycles
	Fluorouracil 750 mg/m^2/day continuous IV infusion, days 1 through 5

TEC

Use:	Prostate cancer. *Cycle:* 28 days for up to 10 cycles
Regimen:	Estramustine 3.33 mg/kg/dose (10 mg/kg/day or 840 mg/day maximum dose) PO 3 times daily, start 2 days before chemotherapy and continue for 2 days after chemotherapy, 5 days total (days −1 to +3 of each cycle)
	Paclitaxel 100 mg/m^2 IV over 1 hour weekly, days 1, 8, 15, and 22
	Carboplatin IV dose by Calvert equation to AUC 6 mg/mL/min (1,000 mg maximum dose), day 1

Temozolomide-Thalidomide

Use:	Malignant melanoma. *Cycle:* 56 days
Regimen 1:	Patients younger than 70 years of age:
	Temozolomide 75 mg/m^2/day PO, days 1 through 42
	Thalidomide 200 mg/day PO, days 1 through 14 first cycle only
	Thalidomide 300 mg/day PO, days 15 through 27 first cycle only
	Thalidomide 400 mg/day PO, days 1 through 56, except for days 1 through 27 of first cycle
Regimen 2:	Patients 70 years of age and older:
	Temozolomide 75 mg/m^2/day PO, days 1 through 42
	Thalidomide 100 mg/day PO, days 1 through 14 first cycle only
	Thalidomide 150 mg/day PO, days 15 through 27 first cycle only
	Thalidomide 200 mg/day PO, days 1 through 56, except for days 1 through 27 of first cycle

Thalidomide-Dexamethasone

Use:	Multiple myeloma. *Cycle:* 28 days for at least 4 cycles
Regimen:	Thalidomide 200 mg/day PO, throughout entire course
	Dexamethasone 40 mg/day PO, days 1 through 4 of all cycles
	Dexamethasone 40 mg/day PO, days 9 through 12 and days 17 through 20 of odd-numbered cycles only (eg, cycle 1, 3, 5)

TIC

Use:	Head and neck cancer. *Cycle:* 21 to 28 days
Regimen:	Paclitaxel 175 mg/m^2 IV over 3 hours, day 1
	Ifosfamide 1,000 mg/m^2/day IV, days 1 through 3
	Mesna 200 mg/m^2/day IV pre-ifosfamide, days 1 through 3
	Mesna 400 mg/m^2/dose IV given 4 hours after ifosfamide, days 1 through 3
	Carboplatin IV dose by Calvert equation to AUC 6 mg/mL/min, day 1

TIP

Use:	Head and neck, esophageal cancer. *Cycle:* 21 to 28 days
Regimen:	Paclitaxel 175 mg/m^2 IV over 3 hours, day 1
	Ifosfamide 1,000 mg/m^2/day IV, days 1 through 3
	Mesna 400 mg/m^2/day IV pre-ifosfamide, days 1 through 3
	Mesna 200 mg/m^2/dose IV given 4 hours after ifosfamide, days 1 through 3
	Cisplatin 60 mg/m^2 IV, day 1 (give after paclitaxel infusion)

continued on next page

TIP (cont.)

Use: Testicular cancer. *Cycle:* 21 days for 4 cycles

Regimen: Paclitaxel 175 to 250 mg/m^2/day continuous IV infusion over 24 hours, day 1

Ifosfamide 1,200 mg/m^2/day IV, days 2 through 6

Mesna 400 mg/m^2/dose IV before, then 4 and 8 hours after each ifosfamide infusion, days 2 through 6

Cisplatin 20 mg/m^2/day IV, days 2 through 6

Use: Testicular cancer. *Cycle:* 21 days for 4 cycles

Regimen: Paclitaxel 250 mg/m^2/day continuous IV infusion over 24 hours, day 1

Ifosfamide 1,500 mg/m^2/day IV, days 2 through 5

Mesna 500 mg/m^2/dose IV before, then 4 and 8 hours after each ifosfamide infusion, days 2 through 5

Cisplatin 25 mg/m^2/day IV, days 2 through 5

Filgrastim 5 mcg/kg/day subcutaneously, days 7 through 18

TIT

Use: Acute lymphocytic leukemia (ALL; CNS prophylaxis—pediatrics).

Regimen: Doses are based on patient's age. Give during weeks 1, 2, 3, 7, 13, 19, and 25 of intensification and every 12 weeks during maintenance.*

Age 1 to 2 years:
Methotrexate 8 mg intrathecal
Cytarabine 16 mg intrathecal
Hydrocortisone 8 mg intrathecal

Age 2 to 3 years:
Methotrexate 10 mg intrathecal
Cytarabine 20 mg intrathecal
Hydrocortisone 10 mg intrathecal

Age 3 to 9 years:
Methotrexate 12 mg intrathecal
Cytarabine 24 mg intrathecal
Hydrocortisone 12 mg intrathecal

Age 9 years and older:
Methotrexate 15 mg intrathecal
Cytarabine 30 mg intrathecal
Hydrocortisone 15 mg intrathecal

*Note: All 3 drugs may be mixed and administered in a single syringe, if diluted with preservative-free 0.9% Sodium Chloride Injection. Regimen used in combination with an induction/maintenance regimen.

Use: Acute lymphocytic leukemia (ALL; CNS prophylaxis—pediatrics).

Regimen: Doses are based on patient's age. Give on day 1 of induction, during weeks 1, 2, 3, 6, 11, 16, 21, and 26 of intensification, during week 31, and every 12 weeks during maintenance.*

Age 1 year:
Methotrexate 10 mg intrathecal
Cytarabine 20 mg intrathecal
Hydrocortisone 10 mg intrathecal

Age 2 years:
Methotrexate 12.5 mg intrathecal
Cytarabine 25 mg intrathecal
Hydrocortisone 12.5 mg intrathecal

continued on next page

TIT (cont.)

Age greater than 3 years:
Methotrexate 15 mg intrathecal
Cytarabine 30 mg intrathecal
Hydrocortisone 15 mg intrathecal

*Note: All 3 drugs may be mixed and administered in a single syringe, if diluted with preservative-free 0.9% Sodium Chloride Injection. Regimen used in combination with an induction/maintenance regimen.

Use:	Acute lymphocytic leukemia (ALL; CNS prophylaxis—adults).
Regimen:	Give on days 1 and 5 of week 1, day 1 of week 4, days 1 and 5 of week 7, day 1 of week 10, days 1 and 5 of week 13, and day 1 of week 16.

Methotrexate 15 mg intrathecal
Cytarabine 40 mg intrathecal
Dexamethasone 4 mg intrathecal*

*Note: No preservative-free product is available; dexamethasone 4 mg/mL injection contains benzyl alcohol 10 mg/mL, a preservative that is unsuitable for intrathecal injection. Because other intrathecal regimens are available that do not include benzyl alcohol-containing products, this regimen should be reserved for use when no other options are available and the benefit to the patient clearly outweighs the risk of benzyl alcohol toxicity. Regimen used in combination with an induction/maintenance regimen.

Topo/CTX (Cyclophosphamide-Topotecan)

Use:	Sarcomas (bone and soft tissue—pediatrics). *Cycle:* 21 days, continue until disease progression or intolerable toxicity
Regimen:	Cyclophosphamide 250 mg/m²/day IV, days 1 through 5

Mesna 150 mg/m²/dose IV before and 3 hours after each cyclophosphamide infusion, days 1 through 5
Topotecan 0.75 mg/m²/day IV, days 1 through 5 after cyclophosphamide
Filgrastim 5 mcg/kg/day subcutaneously, from day 6 until absolute neutrophil count (ANC) is at least 1,500 cells/mm³

TPC

Use:	Breast cancer. *Cycle:* 21 days for 6 cycles
Regimen:	Trastuzumab 4 mg/kg IV, day 1 of first cycle only (loading dose)

Trastuzumab 2 mg/kg IV weekly, days 1, 8, and 15, except for day 1 of first cycle
Paclitaxel 175 mg/m²/dose IV over 3 hours, day 2
Carboplatin IV dose by Calvert equation to AUC 6 mg/mL/min, day 2
followed after 6 cycles by
Trastuzumab 2 mg/kg IV, day 1 of each week until disease progression or unacceptable toxicity

TPF

Use:	Head and neck cancer. *Cycle:* 21 days for up to 4 cycles
Regimen:	Docetaxel 75 mg/m² IV, day 1

Cisplatin 75 mg/m² IV, day 1 (sequence of administration not specified)
Fluorouracil 750 mg/m² IV, days 1 through 5

continued on next page

TPF (cont.)
Use:	Head and neck cancer. *Cycle:* 21 days for up to 3 cycles
Regimen:	Docetaxel 75 mg/m² IV, day 1
	Cisplatin 75 or 100 mg/m² IV, day 1 (give after docetaxel)
	Fluorouracil 1,000 mg/m²/day continuous IV infusion, days 1 through 4 (for 96 hours total)
	used in conjunction with antimicrobial prophylaxis
	Ciprofloxacin 500 mg PO twice daily, days 5 through 15

Trastuzumab-Docetaxel
Use:	Breast cancer. *Cycle:* 28 days, continue until disease progression or intolerable toxicity
Regimen:	Trastuzumab 4 mg/kg IV, day 1 first cycle only (loading dose)
	Trastuzumab 2 mg/kg IV weekly, days 1, 8 and 15, except for day 1 of first cycle
	Docetaxel 35 mg/m²/dose IV, days 1, 8, and 15

Trastuzumab-Paclitaxel
Use:	Breast cancer. *Cycle:* 21 days for at least 6 cycles
Regimen:	Trastuzumab 4 mg/kg IV, day 1 of first cycle only (loading dose)
	Trastuzumab 2 mg/kg IV weekly, days 1, 8, and 15, except for day 1 of first cycle
	Paclitaxel 175 mg/m²/dose IV over 3 hours, day 1

Use:	Breast cancer. *Cycle:* 21 days for 8 cycles
Regimen:	Paclitaxel 175 mg/m²/dose IV over 3 hours, day 1
	Trastuzumab 8 mg/kg IV, day 2 of first cycle only (loading dose)
	Trastuzumab 6 mg/kg IV, day 1, except for first cycle, continued until disease progression or intolerable toxicity

V-TAD
Use:	Acute myelogenous leukemia (AML; induction). *Cycle:* 7 days. Give 1 cycle. Up to 3 cycles have been given, but time between cycles was not specified.
Regimen:	Etoposide 50 mg/m²/day IV, days 1 through 3
	Thioguanine 75 mg/m²/dose PO every 12 hours for 10 doses, days 1 through 5
	Daunorubicin 20 mg/m²/day IV, days 1 and 2
	Cytarabine 75 mg/m²/day continuous IV infusion, days 1 through 5

VAB-6
Use:	Testicular cancer. *Cycle:* 21 to 28 days for 3 to 12 cycles
Regimen:	Cyclophosphamide 600 mg/m² IV, day 1
	Dactinomycin 1 mg/m² IV, day 1
	Vinblastine 4 mg/m² IV, day 1
	Bleomycin 30 units IV push, day 1 (omit from cycle 3)
	Bleomycin 20 units/m²/day continuous IV infusion, days 1 through 3 (omit from cycle 3) (give after IV push dose)
	Cisplatin 120 mg/m² IV, day 4

VAC for lung cancer—see CAV

VAC Pediatric
Use:	Sarcoma (pediatrics). *Cycle:* 21 days
Regimen:	Vincristine 2 mg/m² IV (2 mg maximum dose), day 1
	Dactinomycin 1 mg/m² IV, day 1
	Cyclophosphamide 600 mg/m² IV, day 1

continued on next page

VAC Pediatric (cont.)

Use: Sarcoma (pediatrics). *Cycle:* 21 days

Regimen: Vincristine 1.5 mg/m^2 IV (2 mg maximum dose), days 1, 8, and 15

Dactinomycin 0.015 mg/kg/day (0.5 mg/day maximum dose) continuous IV infusion, days 1 through 5

Cyclophosphamide 2,200 mg/m^2 IV, day 1

Mesna 440 mg/m^2/dose IV given 15 minutes before, and 4 and 8 hours after cyclophosphamide, day 1

Filgrastim 5 mcg/kg/day subcutaneously, from day 6 until hematologic recovery (start at least 24 hours after completion of chemotherapy infusions)

VAC Pulse

Use: Sarcomas. *Cycle:* Give a single cycle

Regimen: Vincristine 2 mg/m^2 (2 mg maximum dose) IV weekly, for 12 weeks

Dactinomycin 0.015 mg/kg/day (0.5 mg/day maximum dose) continuous IV infusion, days 1 through 5, every 3 months for 5 courses

Cyclophosphamide 10 mg/kg/day IV or PO, days 1 through 7, every 6 weeks

---

VAC Standard

Use: Sarcomas. *Cycle:* Give a single cycle

Regimen: Vincristine 2 mg/m^2 (2 mg maximum dose) IV weekly, for 12 weeks

Dactinomycin 0.015 mg/kg/day (0.5 mg/day maximum dose) continuous IV infusion, days 1 through 5, every 3 months for 5 courses

Cyclophosphamide 2.5 mg/kg/day PO, daily for 2 years

VACAdr

Use: Sarcoma (bone and soft tissue—pediatrics). *Cycle:* Give a single cycle

Regimen: Vincristine 1.5 mg/m^2 (2 mg maximum dose) IV, days 1, 8, 15, 22, 29, and 36

Cyclophosphamide 500 mg/m^2 IV, days 1, 8, 15, 22, 29, and 36

Doxorubicin 60 mg/m^2 IV, day 36

followed by 6-week rest period, then

Dactinomycin 0.015 mg/kg/day IV, days 1 through 5

Vincristine 1.5 mg/m^2 (2 mg maximum dose) IV, days 14, 21, 28, 35, and 42

Cyclophosphamide 500 mg/m^2 IV, days 14, 21, 28, 35, and 42

Doxorubicin 60 mg/m^2 IV, day 42 (give on day of final vincristine and cyclophosphamide doses)

VAD

Use: Multiple myeloma. *Cycle:* 3 to 4 weeks, continue for 6 months or indefinitely

Regimen: Vincristine 0.4 mg/day (dose is not in mg/m^2) continuous IV infusion, days 1 through 4*

Doxorubicin 9 mg/m^2/day continuous IV infusion, days 1 through 4*

Dexamethasone 40 mg/day PO, days 1 through 4, days 9 through 12, and days 17 through 20[†]

*Note: Vincristine and doxorubicin may be mixed and administered in the same infusion bag, if diluted with 0.9% Sodium Chloride Injection.

[†]Note: After completing the first 2 cycles of VAD, some clinicians give dexamethasone only on days 1 through 4 of each cycle to reduce the risk of infection. Antibiotic prophylaxis with cotrimoxazole also has been used for this purpose.

---

continued on next page

VAD (cont.)

Use: Acute lymphocytic leukemia (ALL). *Cycle:* 24 to 28 days, may give a single cycle or repeat indefinitely

Regimen: Vincristine 0.4 mg/day (dose is not in mg/m^2) continuous IV infusion, days 1 through 4*

Doxorubicin 9 to 12 mg/m^2/day continuous IV infusion, days 1 through 4*

Dexamethasone 40 mg/day PO, days 1 through 4, days 9 through 12, and days 17 through 20

*Note: Vincristine and doxorubicin may be mixed and administered in the same infusion bag, if diluted with 0.9% Sodium Chloride Injection.

Use: Wilms tumor (pediatrics). *Cycle:* 1 year for 1 cycle only

Regimen 1: Vincristine 1.5 mg/m^2 (2 mg maximum dose) IV, weekly for first 10 to 11 weeks then every 3 weeks for 15 more weeks

Dactinomycin 1.5 mg/m^2 IV every 6 weeks, starting week 1, for 9 doses

Doxorubicin 40 mg/m^2 IV every 6 weeks, starting week 4, for 9 doses

Regimen 2: Vincristine 1.5 mg/m^2 (2 mg maximum dose) IV, given every 6 weeks for 6 to 15 months

with

Dactinomycin 0.015 mg/kg/day IV for 5 doses, given every 6 weeks for 6 to 15 months

or

Dactinomycin 0.06 mg/kg IV, given every 6 weeks for 6 to 15 months

may or may not give with

Doxorubicin 20 mg/m^2 IV, given every 6 weeks for 6 to 15 months

---

VAD/CVAD

Use: Acute lymphocytic leukemia (ALL; induction—adults). *Cycle:* Give 1 cycle only

Regimen: Vincristine 0.4 mg/day (dose is not in mg/m^2) continuous IV infusion, days 1 through 4 and days 24 through 27*

Doxorubicin 12 mg/m^2/day continuous IV infusion, days 1 through 4 and days 24 through 27*

Dexamethasone 40 mg/day PO, days 1 through 4, days 9 through 12, days 17 through 20, days 24 through 27, days 32 through 35, and days 40 through 43

Cyclophosphamide 1,000 mg/m^2 IV, day 24

*Note: Vincristine and doxorubicin may be mixed and administered in the same infusion bag, if diluted with 0.9% Sodium Chloride Injection.

VAD-Liposomal (VLAD)

Use: Multiple myeloma. *Cycle:* 28 days for up to 6 cycles

Regimen: Vincristine 2 mg (dose is not in mg/m^2) IV, day 1

Liposomal doxorubicin 30 to 40 mg/m^2 IV, day 1

Dexamethasone 40 mg/day PO, days 1 through 4, days 9 through 12, and days 17 through 20

VAD, Rapid Infusion
Use: Multiple myeloma. *Cycle:* 28 days for 3 to 4 cycles
Regimen: Vincristine 0.4 mg/day (dose is not in mg/m²) IV over 30 minutes, days 1 through 4*
Doxorubicin 9 mg/m²/day IV over 30 minutes, days 1 through 4*
Dexamethasone 40 mg/day PO, days 1 through 4 of all cycles
Dexamethasone 40 mg/day PO, days 9 through 12 and days 17 through 20 of odd-numbered cycles only (eg, cycle 1, 3, 5)
used in conjunction with antimicrobial prophylaxis
Fluconazole 200 mg PO daily, throughout entire course
Cotrimoxazole double-strength (160/800) PO twice daily, throughout entire course
*Note: Vincristine and doxorubicin may be mixed and administered in the same infusion bag, if diluted with 0.9% Sodium Chloride Injection.

VATH
Use: Breast cancer. *Cycle:* 21 days
Regimen: Vinblastine 4.5 mg/m² IV, day 1
Doxorubicin 45 mg/m² IV, day 1
Thiotepa 12 mg/m² IV, day 1
Fluoxymesterone 10 mg/dose (30 mg/day) PO 3 times daily, throughout entire course

VBAP
Use: Multiple myeloma. *Cycle:* 21 days for 6 to 12 months
Regimen: Vincristine 1 mg/m² (1.5 mg maximum dose) IV, day 1
Carmustine 30 mg/m² IV, day 1
Doxorubicin 30 mg/m² IV, day 1
Prednisone 60 mg/m²/day PO, days 1 through 4

VBCMP
Use: Multiple myeloma. *Cycle:* 35 days for up to 10 cycles
Regimen: Vincristine 1.2 mg/m² (2 mg maximum dose) IV, day 1
Carmustine 20 mg/m² IV, day 1
Cyclophosphamide 400 mg/m² IV, day 1
Melphalan 8 mg/m²/day PO, days 1 through 4
Prednisone 40 mg/m²/day PO, days 1 through 7 of all cycles
Prednisone 20 mg/m²/day PO, days 8 through 14 of first 3 cycles only

VC
Use: Lung cancer (non-small cell). *Cycle:* Ongoing
Regimen: Vinorelbine 30 mg/m² IV, weekly
Cisplatin 120 mg/m² IV, days 1 and 29, then give 1 dose every 6 weeks

Use: Lung cancer (non-small cell). *Cycle:* 28 days for up to 6 cycles, continue until disease progression or intolerable toxicity
Regimen: Vinorelbine 25 mg/m² IV weekly, days 1, 8, 15, and 22
Cisplatin 100 mg/m² IV, day 1

VCAP
Use: Multiple myeloma. *Cycle:* 21 days for 6 to 12 months
Regimen: Vincristine 1 mg/m² (1.5 mg maximum dose) IV, day 1
Cyclophosphamide 125 mg/m²/day PO, days 1 through 4
Doxorubicin 30 mg/m² IV, day 1
Prednisone 60 mg/m²/day PO, days 1 through 4

VCMP—see VMCP

VD

Use:	Breast cancer. *Cycle:* 21 days
Regimen:	Vinorelbine 25 mg/m² IV, days 1 and 8
	Doxorubicin 50 mg/m² IV, day 1

VeIP

Use:	Genitourinary cancer, testicular cancer. *Cycle:* 21 days for up to 4 cycles
Regimen:	Vinblastine 0.11 mg/kg/day IV, days 1 and 2
	Ifosfamide 1,200 mg/m²/day IV, days 1 through 5
	Mesna 1,200 mg/m²/day continuous IV infusion, days 1 through 5
	Cisplatin 20 mg/m²/day IV, days 1 through 5

VIC—see CVI

Vinblastine-Interferon alfa

Use:	Renal cell carcinoma. *Cycle:* 21 days
Regimen:	Vinblastine 0.1 mg/kg IV, day 1
	Interferon alfa-2a* 3 million units/dose subcutaneously 3 times weekly, week 1 of first cycle only
	Interferon alfa-2a* 18 million units/dose subcutaneously 3 times weekly, except for week 1 of first cycle; may decrease to interferon alfa-2a 9 million units/dose subcutaneously 3 times weekly if adverse effects are intolerable
	*Note: Interferon alfa-2a is no longer available in the United States. The manufacturer discontinued this product in October 2007 for commercial reasons, not for safety or efficacy reasons.

Vinblastine-Methotrexate

Use:	Desmoid tumor. *Cycle:* 7 to 10 days for up to 12 months
Regimen:	Vinblastine 6 mg/m² IV, day 1
	Methotrexate 30 mg/m² IV, day 1

Vinorelbine-Carboplatin

Use:	Lung cancer (non-small cell). *Cycle:* 21 days for up to 6 cycles
Regimen:	Vinorelbine 25 mg/m² IV, days 1 and 8
	Carboplatin IV dose by Calvert equation to AUC 6 mg/mL/min, day 1

Vinorelbine-Cisplatin (also see Cisplatin-Vinorelbine)

Use:	Lung cancer (non-small cell). *Cycle:* 42 days, continue until disease progression or intolerable toxicity
Regimen:	Vinorelbine 30 mg/m² IV, weekly
	Cisplatin 120 mg/m² IV, days 1 and 29 for first cycle; then day 1 of subsequent cycles

Vinorelbine-Doxorubicin (NA)

Use:	Breast cancer. *Cycle:* 21 days, for up to 11 cycles
Regimen:	Vinorelbine 25 mg/m² IV, days 1 and 8
	Doxorubicin 50 mg/m² IV, day 1

Vinorelbine-Gemcitabine

Use:	Lung cancer (non-small cell). *Cycle:* 28 days for up to 6 cycles
Regimen:	Vinorelbine 20 mg/m² IV, days 1, 8, and 15
	Gemcitabine 800 mg/m² IV, days 1, 8, and 15

VIP
Use: Genitourinary cancer, testicular cancer, sarcoma (bone).
               Cycle: 21 days for up to 4 cycles
Regimen: Etoposide 75 mg/m^2/day IV, days 1 through 5
             Ifosfamide 1,200 mg/m^2/day IV, days 1 through 5
             Mesna 1,200 mg/m^2/day continuous IV infusion, days 1 through 5
             Cisplatin 20 mg/m^2/day IV, days 1 through 5

Use: Lung cancer (small cell). *Cycle:* 21 to 28 days for up to 4 cycles
Regimen: Ifosfamide 1,200 mg/m^2/day IV, days 1 through 4
             Mesna 120 to 300 mg/m^2 IV, day 1 (give before ifosfamide is
               started)
             Mesna 1,200 mg/m^2/day continuous IV infusion, days 1 through 4
               (after mesna bolus is given)
             Cisplatin 20 mg/m^2/day IV, days 1 through 4
             with
             Etoposide 37.5 mg/m^2/day PO, days 1 through 14
             or
             Etoposide 75 mg/m^2/day IV, days 1 through 4

Use: Lung cancer (non-small cell). *Cycle:* 28 days for up to 4 cycles
Regimen: Ifosfamide 1,000 to 1,200 mg/m^2/day IV, days 1 through 3
             Cisplatin 100 mg/m^2 IV, days 1 and 8
             Etoposide 60 to 75 mg/m^2/day IV, days 1 through 3
             with
             Mesna 300 mg/m^2/dose IV every 4 hours, days 1 through 4 (for
               24 doses total)
             or
             Mesna 20% of ifosfamide dose IV before, then 4 and 8 hours after
               each ifosfamide infusion, days 1 through 4

VLAD—see VAD-Liposomal

VM
Use: Breast cancer. *Cycle:* 6 to 8 weeks
Regimen: Vinblastine 5 mg/m^2 IV, days 1, 14, 28, and 42 for 2 cycles, then
               days 1 and 21 only
             Mitomycin 10 mg/m^2 IV, days 1 and 28 for 2 cycles, then day 1 only

VMCP (VCMP)
Use: Multiple myeloma. *Cycle:* 21 days for 6 to 12 months
Regimen: Vincristine 1 mg/m^2 (2 mg maximum dose) IV, day 1
             Melphalan 6 mg/m^2/day PO, days 1 through 4
             Cyclophosphamide 125 mg/m^2/day PO, days 1 through 4
             Prednisone 60 mg/m^2/day PO, days 1 through 4

VMP
Use: Multiple myeloma.
Regimen: **Induction.** *Cycle:* 42 days. Give 4 cycles.
               Bortezomib 1 or 1.3 mg/m^2 IV, days 1, 4, 8, 11, 22, 25, 29,
                 and 32
               Melphalan 9 mg/m^2/day PO, days 1 through 4
               Prednisone 60 mg/m^2/day PO, days 1 through 4
             Maintenance. *Cycle:* 35 days. Give 5 cycles.
               Bortezomib 1 or 1.3 mg/m^2 IV, days 1, 8, 15, and 22
               Melphalan 9 mg/m^2/day PO, days 1 through 4
               Prednisone 60 mg/m^2/day PO, days 1 through 4

VMPT

Use:	Multiple myeloma. *Cycle:* 35 days for 6 cycles
Regimen:	Bortezomib 1 or 1.3 mg/m^2 IV, days 1, 4, 15, and 22
	Melphalan 6 mg/m^2/day PO, days 1 through 5
	Prednisone 60 mg/m^2/day PO, days 1 through 5
	Thalidomide 50 mg/day PO, throughout entire course

VP

Use:	Lung cancer (small cell). *Cycle:* 21 days for up to 4 cycles
Regimen:	Etoposide 100 mg/m^2/day IV, days 1 through 4
	Cisplatin 20 mg/m^2/day IV, days 1 through 4

X + T—see Capecitabine-Docetaxel

XELIRI

Use:	Metastatic colorectal cancer. *Cycle:* 21 days for up to 12 cycles
Regimen 1:	Patients younger than 65 years of age, patients with creatinine clearance greater than 50 mL/min, or patients without prior pelvic radiation therapy:
	Capecitabine 1,000 mg/m^2/dose PO twice daily, days 1 through 14
	Irinotecan 250 mg/m^2 IV, day 1
Regimen 2:	Patients 65 years of age and older, patients with creatinine clearance of 30 to 50 mL/min, or patients with prior pelvic radiation therapy:
	Capecitabine 750 mg/m^2/dose PO twice daily, days 1 through 14
	Irinotecan 200 mg/m^2 IV, day 1

XELOX

Use:	Colorectal cancer. *Cycle:* 21 days for up to 11 cycles, or until disease progression or intolerable toxicity
Regimen 1:	Patients who have not received prior chemotherapy:
	Capecitabine 1,250 mg/m^2/dose PO twice daily, days 1 through 14
	Oxaliplatin 130 mg/m^2 IV, day 1
Regimen 2:	Patients who have received prior chemotherapy:
	Capecitabine 1,000 mg/m^2/dose PO twice daily, days 1 through 14
	Oxaliplatin 130 mg/m^2 IV, day 1

Use:	Colorectal cancer. *Cycle:* 14 days for up to 12 cycles
Regimen:	Capecitabine 1,750 mg/m^2/dose PO twice daily, days 1 through 7
	Oxaliplatin 85 mg/m^2 IV, day 1

XELOX + Bevacizumab (also see CapeOx-B, Modified)

Use:	Metastatic colorectal cancer. *Cycle:* 21 days, continue until disease progression or intolerable toxicity
Regimen:	Capecitabine 1,000 mg/m^2/dose PO twice daily, days 1 through 14
	Oxaliplatin 130 mg/m^2 IV, day 1
	Bevacizumab 7.5 mg/kg IV, day 1

XELOX-RT

Use:	Rectal cancer. *Cycle:* 42 days. Give a single cycle prior to surgery.
Regimen:	Capecitabine 825 mg/m^2/dose PO twice daily, days 1 through 14 and days 22 through 35
	Oxaliplatin 50 mg/m^2 IV, days 1, 8, 22, and 29
	used in conjunction with
	Radiation therapy

XN

Use:	Breast cancer. *Cycle:* 21 days
Regimen:	Capecitabine 1,000 mg/m^2/dose PO twice daily, days 1 through 14
	Vinorelbine 25 mg/m^2 IV, days 1 and 8

XP

Use:	Breast cancer. *Cycle:* 21 days, continue until disease progression or intolerable toxicity
Regimen:	Capecitabine 825 mg/m^2/dose PO twice daily, days 1 through 14
	with
	Paclitaxel 175 mg/m^2 IV over 3 hours, day 1
	or
	Paclitaxel 80 mg/m^2 IV, days 1 and 8

This section was compiled by the University of Utah Hospitals and Clinics for publication in the *Cancer Chemotherapy Manual.* References are available upon request.

Manufacturer and Distributor Listing

40985
21ST CENTURY HEALTHCARE
480-966-8201
800-530-2178
http://www.21stcenturyvitamins.com

48878
3M ESPE DENTAL PRODUCTS
651-575-5144
800-634-2248
http://www.3m.com

00089
3M PHARMACEUTICALS
See Graceway Pharmaceuticals,
LLC

17518
3M SURGICAL/MEDICAL
800-228-3957
651-733-1110
http://www.3m.com

42549
4UORTHO
888-316-7846
http://www.4udr.com

63801
**7 OAKS PHARMACEUTICAL
CORP**
864-850-1700
http://www.7oakspharma.com

93764
A & D MEDICAL
408-263-5333
888-726-9966
http://www.andmedical.com

18754
A AARONS
973-882-1505
http://www.bradpharm.com

12539
**AG MARIN
PHARMACEUTICALS**
305-593-5333
800-241-4603

**A.H. ROBINS CONSUMER
PRODUCTS**
See Wyeth Consumer Health

A.H. ROBINS INC.
See Wyeth Consumer Health

A.L. LABS
See King Pharmaceuticals, Inc.

A.P. PHARMA, INC.
650-366-2626
http://www.appharma.com

66591
AAI PHARMA
910-254-7350
800-575-4224
http://www.aaipharma.com

50483
**AAPER ALCOHOL &
CHEMICAL CO.**
502-232-7600
800-456-1017
http://www.pharmcoaaper.com

AASTROM BIOSCIENCES, INC.
734-930-5555

60793
**ABANA PHARMACEUTICALS,
INC.**
See King Pharmaceuticals, Inc.

ABBOTT DIABETES CARE
510-749-5400
888-298-4584
http://www.therasense.com

ABBOTT LABORATORIES
847-937-6100
800-323-9100
http://www.abbott.com

**ABBOTT HOSPITAL
PRODUCTS**
224-212-2000
800-615-0187
http://www.hospira.com

00074
**ABBOTT LABORATORIES
PHARMACEUTICAL
DIVISION**
847-937-6100
800-255-5162
http://www.abbott.com

ABBOTT MEDICAL OPTICS
714-247-8200
866-427-8477
http://www.amo-inc.com

ABBOTT NUTRITION
614-624-3191
800-986-8510
http://www.abbottnutrition.com

ABGENIX
See Amgen

63323
ABRAXIS BIOSCIENCE
310-883-1300
http://www.abraxisbio.com

68817
ABRAXIS ONCOLOGY
908-393-8220
http://www.abraxisbio.com

AB SCIENCE
33-1-47-20-10-35

**ACADEMIC
PHARMACEUTICALS, INC.**
847-735-1170

42907
ACCERA, INC.
303-999-3700
877-649-0004
http://www.accerapharma.com

ACCESS DIABETIC SUPPLY
954-975-0036
800-715-5031
http://www.diabeticsupply.com

67404
ACCESS PHARMACEUTICALS
214-905-5100
http://www.accesspharma.com

16729
ACCORD HEALTHCARE
866-941-7875

ACCUMED
609-883-1818
http://www.accumed.org

25356
ACETO PHARMA
516-627-6000
http://www.aceto.com

00924
ACME UNITED CORP.
203-332-7330
800-835-2263
http://www.acmeunited.com

10144
ACORDA THERAPEUTICS
914-347-4300
800-367-5109
http://www.acorda.com

ACTAVIS
973-993-4500
800-432-8534
http://www.actavis.us

ACTAVIS ELIZABETH
973-993-4500
800-432-8534
http://www.actavis.com

ACTAVIS SOUTH ATLANTIC
973-993-4500
800-432-8534
http://www.actavis.us

ACTAVIS TOTOWA
973-993-4500
800-432-8534
http://www.actavis.us

66215
**ACTELION
PHARMACEUTICALS US,
INC.**
650-624-6900
866-228-3546
http://www.actelionus.com

ACURA PHARMACEUTICALS, INC.
847-705-7709
http://www.acurapharm.com

ACURA PHARMACEUTICALS TECHNOLOGIES
574-842-3305
http://www.acurapharm.com

38739
ADAMIS LABORATORIES, INC.
800-223-6837
561-208-2200

63824
ADAMS RESPIRATORY THERAPEUTICS
See Reckitt Benckiser Pharmaceuticals

ADHEREX TECHNOLOGIES, INC.
919-484-8484
http://www.adherex.com

ADOLOR
484-595-1500
866-423-6567
http://www.adolor.com

ADRIA LABORATORIES
See Pfizer US Pharmaceutical Group

ADVANCE BIOFACTURES CORP. BIOSPECIFICS TECHNOLOGIES
516-593-7000
http://www.biospecifics.com

17714
ADVANCE
631-981-4600
http://www.advancepharm.com

08541
ADVANCED BIOHEALING
877-422-4463
858-754-3700
http://www.abh.com

ADVANCED BIOTHERAPY, INC.
818-883-6716

55495
ADVANCED MEDICAL ENTERPRISES
787-436-0666
http://www.ameinc.org

ADVANCED MEDICAL OPTICS
See Abbott Medical Optics

10888
ADVANCED NUTRITIONAL TECHNOLOGY
925-828-2128
800-624-6543
http://www. advancenutritionaltech.com

58790
ADVANCED VISION RESEARCH
781-932-8327
800-579-8327
http://www.theratears.com

11042
ADVANCIS PHARMACEUTICAL CORPORATION
See MiddleBrook Pharmaceuticals

ADVANTAGENE
617-916-5445

ADVENTRX PHARMACEUTICALS
858-552-0866
http://www.adventrx.com

66440
AERO PHARMACEUTICALS, INC.
See Adamis Laboratories, Inc.

AEROVANCE, INC.
510-549-5500

AETERNA ZENTARIS, INC.
418-652-8525

00213
AFFEMANN IMPORTS, INC.
818-348-7767
http://www.affemannimports.com

10572
AFFORDABLE PHARMACEUTICALS
781-848-3062
http://www.affordablepharm.com

08554
AGAMATRIX
603-328-6000
http://www.agamatrix.com

60336
AGI DERMATICS
800-590-4244
516-868-9026
http://www.agiderm.com

AGOURON PHARMACEUTICALS
See Pfizer US Pharmaceutical Group

62584, 68084
AHP
800-707-4621
614-492-8177
http://www.healthpak.com

38206
AID-PACK USA
See NutraMax Products

51709
AIMSCO/DELTA HI-TECH
801-263-0975
http://www.deltahitechinc.com

59196
AIRPHARMA
913-498-0700
http://www.air-pharma.com

17478, 11098
AKORN, INC.
800-932-5676
847-279-6100
http://www.akorn.com

23360
AKORN STRIDES
847-279-6100
800-932-5676
http://www.akorn.com

41383
AKPHARMA
609-645-6100
800-994-4711
http://www.akpharma.com

AKRIMAX PHARMACEUTICALS
908-372-0506
888-383-1733
http://www.akrimax.com

65162
AKYMA PHARMACEUTICALS
See Amneal Pharmaceuticals

68322
ALAMO PHARMACEUTICALS, LLC
See Avanir Pharmaceuticals

68220
ALAVEN PHARMACEUTICAL, LLC
888-317-0001
800-333-7343
http://www.alavenpharm.com

22400
ALBERTO CULVER
708-450-3000
800-333-6666
http://www.alberto.com

20993
ALCON LABORATORIES, INC.
817-293-0450
800-862-5266
http://www.alcon.com

00065, 08065
ALCON SURGICAL
817-293-0450
800-862-5266
http://www.alcon.com

00065
ALCON VISION
817-293-0450
800-862-5266
http://www.alcon.com

43234
ALETHEIA
601-667-3584
http://www.altheialabs.com

25682
ALEXION PHARMACEUTICALS
203-272-2596
http://www.alxn.com

08514
ALIGN PHARMACEUTICALS
908-834-0960
http://www.alignpharma.com

56121, 66177
ALIGON PHARMACEUTICALS
205-663-0521
http://www.aligoninc.com

68611
ALIMERA SCIENCES
678-990-5740
http://www.alimerasciences.com

38697
ALK ABELLO
800-325-7354
512-251-0037
http://www.alk-abello.us

ALK LABORATORIES, INC.
See ALK Abello

67575
ALKERMES
781-609-6000
http://www.alkermes.com

43351
ALLAIRE PHARMACEUTICALS
732-974-6300
414-434-6617

13279
ALLAN PHARMACEUTICAL, LLC.
215-441-9546
877-743-5858
http://www.allanpharmaceutical.com

ALLEGIS PHARMACEUTICALS
601-859-0038
866-468-2419

ALLEN & HANBURYS
See GlaxoSmithKline

ALLENDALE PHARMACEUTICALS, INC.
212-813-2171
888-343-4499
http://www.allendalepharm.com

ALLERCREME
See Carme, Inc.

ALLERDERM LABORATORIES, INC.
800-365-6868
http://www.allerderm.com

00023
ALLERGAN DERMATOLOGICS
714-246-4500
800-347-4500

11980
ALLERGAN, INC.
714-246-4500
800-377-7790
http://www.allergan.com

99965
ALLERGAN OPTICAL
800-433-8871
714-246-4500
http://www.allergan.com

ALLERGY LABORATORIES, INC.
405-235-1451
800-654-3971
http://www.allergylabs.com

49343
ALLERMED
858-292-1060
800-221-2748
http://www.allermed.com

ALLERQUEST
512-251-0037
800-325-7354
http://www.allerquest.com

17355
ALLIANCE LABS
602-276-3434
888-273-9734
http://www.enemeez.com

ALLIANCE PHARMACEUTICAL CORP.
858-410-5200

08462
ALLIANCE TECH MEDICAL
817-326-3183
800-848-8923
http://www.alliancetechmedical.com

68188
ALLIANT PHARMACEUTICALS, INC.
770-817-4500
http://www.alliantpharma.com

ALLIED PHARMACY
817-226-5050

86227
ALLISON MEDICAL
303-795-1618
800-886-1618
http://www.allisonmedical.com

ALLOS THERAPEUTICS
303-426-6262
888-255-6788
http://www.allos.com

54569
ALLSCRIPTS, INC.
847-680-3515
800-654-0889
http://www.allscripts.com

77379, 00311
ALMAY, INC.
919-603-2953
800-992-5629
http://www.almay.com

ALPHA 1 BIOMEDICALS, INC.
See Arriva Pharmaceuticals, Inc.

49669
ALPHA THERAPEUTIC CORP.
See Grifols USA, Inc.

59743
ALPHAGEN LABORATORIES, INC.
770-475-8973

00228
ALPHARMA PUREPAC PHARMACEUTICALS
See Actavis Elizabeth

63857
ALPHARMA USPD, INC.
See King Pharmaceuticals, Inc.

59390
ALTAIRE
631-722-5988
800-258-2471
http://www.otcdruggist.com

ALTANA INC.
973-236-9162
800-645-9833
http://www.altana.com

ALTERNA LLC
973-946-7550
http://www.alternallc.com

91717
ALTERNATIVA NATURAL
631-231-2322
http://www.altnatural.com

00731
ALTO PHARMACEUTICALS, INC.
813-968-0522
800-330-2891
http://www.altopharm.com

ALTUS PHARMA
617-299-2900
888-258-2532

72959
ALVA-AMCO PHARMACAL
COS, INC.
847-663-0700
800-792-2582
http://www.alva-amco.com

47781
ALVOGEN
973-796-3400
http://www.alvogen.com

17314
ALZA CORP.
650-564-5000
800-634-8977
http://www.alza.com

00187
AMARIN PHARMACEUTICALS
See Valeant

66870
AMBI PHARMACEUTICALS,
INC.
352-797-5227

10038
AMBIX LABORATORIES
973-890-9002
http://www.ambixlabs.com

AMCON LABORATORIES
314-961-5758
800-255-6161
http://www.amconlabs.com

61972
AMEND DRUG AND CHEMICAL
CORPORATION
See Ruger Chemical Co.

AMERICAN BIOSCIENCE, INC.
See Abraxis Bioscience

AMERICAN DERMAL CORP.
See Sanofi-Aventis U.S.

62584
AMERICAN HEALTH
PACKAGING
614-492-8177
800-707-4621
http://www.
americanhealthpackaging.com

00008
AMERICAN HOME PRODUCTS
See Wyeth

73930
AMERICAN INTERNATIONAL
INDUSTRIES
323-728-2999
800-621-9585
http://www.aiibeauty.com

AMERICAN LECITHIN
COMPANY
203-262-7100
800-364-4416
http://www.americanlecithin.com

AMERICAN MEDICAL
INDUSTRIES
605-428-5501

63323
AMERICAN
PHARMACEUTICAL
PARTNERS, INC.
See APP Pharmaceutical

52769
AMERICAN RED CROSS
(NATIONAL
HEADQUARTERS)
202-303-5214
800-733-2767
http://www.redcross.org

00517
AMERICAN REGENT, INC.
631-924-4000
800-645-1706
http://www.americanregent.com

41520
AMERICAN SALES COMPANY
716-686-7000
http://www.
americansalescompany.net

63921
AMERIDERM LABORATORIES,
INC.
973-279-5100
800-455-7211
http://www.ameriderm.com

AMERIFIT BRANDS, INC.
860-894-1285
800-722-3476
http://www.amerifit.com

62852
AMERILAB TECHNOLOGIES
763-525-1262
http://www.amerilabtech.com

AMERISOURCEBERGEN
610-727-7000
800-829-3132
http://www.amerisourcebergen.com

AMERSHAM HEALTH
44-0-1494-544000

61470
AMERX HEALTH CARE CORP.
727-443-0530
800-448-9599
http://www.amerigel.com

55513
AMGEN, INC.
805-447-1000
800-772-6436
http://www.amgen.com

AMICUS THERAPEUTICS, INC.
609-662-2000

52152
AMIDE PHARMACAL
See Actavis Totowa

65162
AMNEAL PHARMACEUTICALS
270-629-2956
866-525-7270
http://www.amneal.com

00548
AMPHASTAR
PHARMACEUTICALS, INC.
800-423-4136
http://www.amphastar.com

AMPLIMED CORP.
520-529-1000
http://www.Amplimed.com

00402
AMSCO SCIENTIFIC
See Steris Corp.

68883
AMSINO MEDICAL USA
866-482-1345
http://www.amsinomedusa.com

66780
AMYLIN PHARMACEUTICALS
858-552-2200
http://www.amylin.com

ANABOLIC, INC.
949-863-0340
800-445-6849
http://www.anaboliclabs.com

ANAQUEST
See Baxter Healthcare
Corporation

10370
ANCHEN PHARMACEUTICALS,
INC.
949-837-6178
888-837-6178
http://www.anchen.com

19100
ANDREW JERGENS CO.
See Kao Brands Company

ANDRULIS PHARMACEUTICAL
CORP.
301-419-2400
301-767-1900

ANDRULIS RESEARCH CORP.
301-767-1900

62022
ANDRX LABORATORIES, INC.
See Shionogi Pharma, Inc.

62037
ANDRX PHARMACEUTICALS, INC.
954-382-7600
800-621-7143
http://www.andrx.com

28000
ANESIVA
650-624-9600
http://www.anesiva.com

ANGELINI PHARMACEUTICALS, INC.
201-476-9000

65974
ANGIODYNAMICS
518-798-1215
800-772-6446
http://www.angiodynamics.com

ANI PHARMACEUTICALS
218-634-3500
800-434-1121
http://www.anipharmaceuticals.com

ANIKA THERAPEUTICS
781-932-6616
http://www.anikatherapeutics.com

65781
ANIMAS DIABETES
610-644-8990
877-767-7373
http://www.animascorp.com

ANORMED, INC.
604-530-1057

70907, 14613, 71483
ANSELL HEALTHCARE, INC.
732-345-5400
http://www.ansell.com

55948
ANTARES PHARMA
610-458-6200
http://www.antarespharma.com

ANTHRA PHARMACEUTICALS, INC.
609-514-1060

ANTIBODIES, INC.
530-758-4400
800-824-8540
http://www.antibodiesinc.com

ANTIGENICS INC.
212-994-8200
http://www.antigenics.com

ANTISOMA PLC
44-0-20-8799-8200

ANTISOMA RESEARCH, LTD.
44-2-20-8799-8200

ATRIX LABORATORIES, INC.
970-482-5868
http://www.atrixlabs.com

23601
APEX-CAREX HEALTHCARE PRODUCTS
800-328-2935 (Apex)
800-526-8051 (Carex)
http://www.apex-carex.com

APHTON CORP.
305-374-7338

52380, 18407
APLICARE INC.
203-630-0500
800-760-3236
http://www.aplicare.com

60505
APOTEX
954-384-8007
800-706-5575
http://www.apotexcorp.com

APOTHECA
602-252-5244
800-262-5244

25715
APOTHECARY PRODUCTS, INC.
952-890-1940
800-328-2742
http://www.apothecaryproducts.com

APOTHECON, INC. (BRISTOL-MYERS SQUIBB)
See Bristol-Myers Squibb Co.

48723, 52925
APOTHECUS PHARMACEUTICAL CORP.
516-624-8200
800-227-2393
http://www.apothecus.com

APP PHARMACEUTICAL
847-969-2700
888-391-6300
http://www.appdrugs.com

APPLIED ANALYTICAL INDUSTRIES
910-254-7000
800-575-4224
http://www.aaipharma.com

APPLIED BIOTECH, INC.
858-587-6771
800-257-9525
http://www.abiapogent.com

92896
APPLIED DIABETES RESEARCH
972-241-1884
800-304-7293
http://www. applieddiabetesresearch.org

APPLIED GENETICS INC. DERMATICS
516-868-9026
http://www.agiderm.com

00847
APPLIED NUTRITION CORPORATION
973-734-0023
800-605-0410
http://www.medicalfood.com

16110
AQUA PHARMACEUTICALS
610-644-7000
http://www.aquapharm.com

13310
AR SCIENTIFIC
215-807-1029
877-960-2400
http://www.arscientific.com

ARADIGM CORP.
510-265-9000
http://www.aradigm.com

24338
ARBOR PHARMACEUTICALS
678-334-2420
866-516-4950
http://www.arborphama.com

90401
ARCHON
800-349-1700
http://www.archonvitamin.com

74312
ARCO PHARMACEUTICALS, INC.
See Natures Bounty

ARCOLA LABORATORIES
See Sanofi-Aventis U.S.

ARGINOX PHARMACEUTICALS
888-274-6070

ARIAD PHARMACEUTICALS, INC.
617-494-0400
http://www.ariad.com

24486
ARISTOS PHARMACEUTICALS
866-280-5755
http://www.aristospharm.com

ARK THERAPEUTICS, LTD.
44-20-7388-7722

08317
ARKRAY USA
952-646-3200
800-818-8877
http://www.arkrayusa.com

ARMOUR PHARMACEUTICAL
See CSL Behring

**ARRIVA PHARMACEUTICALS,
INC.**
510-337-1250
http://www.arrivapharm.com

**ARROW INTERNATIONAL
CORP. HEADQUARTERS**
610-378-0131
800-523-8446
http://www.arrowintl.com

**ARTIELLE
IMMUNOTHERAPEUTICS**
503-626-1144
http://www.artielle.com

12870
ARZOL
603-352-5242

65557
ASAFI PHARMACEUTICAL
661-294-9509
http://www.asafi.com

67877
ASCEND LABORATORIES
201-476-1977
http://www.ascendlaboratories.com

17139
ASCEND THERAPEUTICS
703-471-4744
http://www.ascendtherapeutics.com

99207
ASCENT PEDIATRICS, INC.
See Medicis Pharmaceutical
Corporation

46698
ASO LLC
941-379-0300
800-966-8066
http://www.asocorp.com

ASTELLAS PHARMA US, INC.
847-317-8800
800-888-7704
http://www.us.astellas.com

00186
ASTRAZENECA LP
302-886-3000
800-456-3669
http://www.astrazeneca-us.com

38488
**ATHENA FEMININE
TECHNOLOGIES**
866-308-4436
http://www.athenaft.com

59075
**ATHENA NEUROSCIENCES,
INC.**
See Elan Pharmaceuticals

66813
**ATHLON PHARMACEUTICALS,
INC.**
205-986-1111
http://www.athlonpharm.com

59702
**ATLEY PHARMACEUTICALS,
INC.**
804-227-2250
http://www.atley.com

25010
ATON PHARMA
609-671-9010
877-286-6549
http://www.atonrx.com

62107
AUBURN PHARMACEUTICAL
800-222-5609
248-526-3700
http://www.auburnpharm.com

14629
**AURIGA PHARMACEUTICALS,
INC.**
678-282-1600
866-367-8796
http://www.aurigalabs.com

AURIS MEDICAL, INC.
312-283-5633

65862
AUROBINDO PHARMA
732-839-9400
866-850-2876
http://www.aurobindo.com

65504
AURORA HEALTHCARE
414-647-3000
http://www.aurorahelathcare.org

AUTOIMMUNE, INC.
626-792-1235
http://www.autoimmuneinc.com

**AUTOIMMUNITY RESEARCH
FOUNDATION**
805-492-3693

66887
**AUXILIUM
PHARMACEUTICALS, INC.**
484-321-5900
http://www.auxilium.com

68322
**AVANIR PHARMACEUTICALS,
LLC**
949-389-6700
http://www.avanir.com

**AVANT
IMMUNOTHERAPEUTICS,
INC.**
781-433-0771

**AVANTOR PERFORMANCE
MATERIALS**
908-859-2151
800-582-2537
http://www.avantormaterials.com

AVAX TECHNOLOGIES, INC.
913-693-8491
http://www.avax-tech.com

42291
AVKARE
931-292-6222
http://www.avkare.com

AVENTIS BEHRING
See CSL Behring

AVENTIS PHARMACEUTICALS
See Sanofi-Aventis U.S.

AVICENA GROUP, INC.
415-397-2880
http://www.avicenagroup.com

43684
AVIDAS PHARMACEUTICALS
267-895-1755
http://www.avidaspharma.com

AVIGEN, INC.
510-748-1750
http://www.avigen.com

76170
**AVOCET POLYMER
TECHNOLOGIES**
815-609-2170
866-352-7227
http://www.avocetcorp.com

58914
AXCAN PHARMA US, INC.
205-991-8085
800-472-2634
http://www.axcan.com

58914
AXCAN SCANDIPHARM
See Axcan Pharma US, Inc.

18860
AZUR PHARMA
215-832-3752
866-833-3560
http://www.azurpharma.com

63275
B & B PHARMACEUTICALS
303-755-5110
800-499-3100
http://www.bandbpharma.com

00264
B. BRAUN MCGAW
See B. Braun Medical, Inc.

00264
B. BRAUN MEDICAL INC.
800-854-6851
http://www.bbraunusa.com

00225
B. F. ASCHER AND CO.
913-888-1880
800-324-1880
http://www.bfascher.com

44184
BAJAMAR CHEMICAL CO., INC.
314-721-1896
http://www.vesselvite.com

11414
BAKER CUMMINS DERMATOLOGICALS
See Ivax Pharmaceuticals, Inc.

11414
BAKER NORTON PHARMACEUTICALS
See Ivax Pharmaceuticals, Inc.

50770
BALLARD MEDICAL PRODUCTS
801-572-6800
800-528-5591
http://www.kchealthcare.com

63162
BALLAY PHARMACEUTICALS, INC.
512-847-6458

BANNER PHARMACAPS
336-812-8700
800-447-1140
http://www.banpharm.com

BARBEAU PHARMA, INC.
847-441-4142

08011
BARD
See C.R. Bard

49326
BAROLI
305-772-0665

00555
BARR LABORATORIES, INC.
800-222-0190
http://www.barrlabs.com

BARR PHARMACEUTICALS, INC.
845-362-1100
800-222-0190
http://www.barrlabs.com

BARRE-NATIONAL, INC.
See Alpharma

13478
BARRIER THERAPEUTICS
609-945-1200
http://www.barriertherapeutics.com

10116
BARTOR PHARMACAL CO.
914-967-4219

00078
BASEL PHARMACEUTICALS
See Novartis Pharmaceuticals Corp.

BASF CORPORATION
973-245-6000
800-526-1072
http://www.basf.com

00761, 07610
BASIC DRUGS

55458
BASIC ORGANICS
614-863-3004
http://www.basicorganics.com

10119
BAUSCH & LOMB PERSONAL PRODUCTS DIVISION
585-338-6000
800-344-8815
http://www.bausch.com

24208
BAUSCH & LOMB PHARMACEUTICALS INC.
813-975-7770
800-323-0000
http://www.bausch.com

61772
BAUSCH & LOMB SURGICAL
800-338-2020
http://www.bausch.com

17191
BAXA CORPORATION
303-690-4204
800-567-2292
http://www.baxa.com

10019, 60977
BAXTER HEALTHCARE CORPORATION
847-948-4770
800-933-0303
http://www.baxter.com

60977
BAXTER HEALTHCARE CORPORATION - ANESTHESIA CRITICAL CARE PHARMACEUTICALS
908-286-7000
800-667-0959
http://www.baxter.com

00944
BAXTER HEALTHCARE CORPORATION - BAXTER BIOSCIENCE
805-372-3000
800-422-9837
800-423-2090
http://www.baxter.com

00338
BAXTER HEALTHCARE CORPORATION - CLINTEC NUTRITION
800-422-2751
http://www.nutriforum.com

00338
BAXTER HEALTHCARE CORPORATION - MEDICATION DELIVERY
847-948-4770
800-933-0303
http://www.baxter.com

64193
BAXTER HYLAND IMMUNO
See Baxter Healthcare Corporation - Baxter Bioscience

60977
BAXTER PHARM. PRODS., INC. (BAXTER PPI)
See Baxter Healthcare Corporation - Anesthesia Critical Care Pharmaceuticals

00941
BAXTER RENAL
847-948-2000
888-736-2543
http://www.baxter.com

42769
BAY PHARMA
410-281-9450

65044
BAYER ALLERGY PRODUCTS
See Hollister-Stier

BAYER CONSUMER CARE DIVISION
973-254-5000
800-331-4536
http://www.bayercare.com

00026
BAYER CORPORATION
412-777-2000
800-468-0894
http://www.bayerus.com

BAYER DIABETES CARE
800-348-8100
http://www.bayerdiabetes.com

00193
BAYER DIAGNOSTICS
877-229-3711
800-248-2637
http://www.bayerdiag.com

BECTON DICKINSON
201-847-6800
888-237-2762
http://www.bd.com

BD BIOSCIENCES
877-232-8995
http://www.bdbiosciences.com

**BD DIAGNOSTIC SYSTEMS &
 MEDICAL SUPPLIES**
800-675-0908
http://www.bd.com

00486
BEACH
813-839-6565
800-322-8210

BECKMAN COULTER
800-742-2345
http://www.beckmancoulter.com

**BECKMAN COULTER PRIMARY
 CARE DIAGNOSTICS**
714-993-5321
800-526-3821
http://www.beckmancoulter.com

**BD CONSUMER PRODUCTS
 DIVISION**
410-316-4000
800-638-8663
http://www.bd.com

55390
BEDFORD LABORATORIES
440-232-3320
800-562-4797
http://www.bedfordlabs.com

BEIERSDORF JOBST
See BSN Medical

BELL PHARMACEUTICAL
952-873-2288
800-328-5890

24385
**BERGEN BRUNSWIG DRUG
 CO.**
See AmerisourceBergen

50419
BERLEX LABORATORIES, INC.
See Bayer Healthcare Pharma

58337
BERNA
305-443-2900
800-533-5899
http://www.bernaproducts.com

**BERTEK PHARMACEUTICALS,
 INC.**
See Mylan Pharmaceuticals, Inc.

08515
BESTMED
303-271-0300

53062
BETA DERMACEUTICALS, INC.
210-349-9326
800-434-2382
http://www.beta-derm.com

00283
**BEUTLICH
 PHARMACEUTICALS**
847-473-1100
800-238-8542
http://www.beutlich.com

**BI-COASTAL
 PHARMACEUTICAL**
732-530-6606
http://www.bicoastalpharm.com

BIOALLIANCE PHARMA
33-0-1-45-58-76-00
http://www.bioalliancepharma.com

**BIOAXONE THERAPEUTICS,
 INC.**
913-693-8491
http://www.bioaxone.com

04142
BIOCODEX INC.
877-356-7787
650-243-5320
http://www.biocodexusa.com

08216
**BIOCORE MEDICAL
 TECHNOLOGIES**
888-565-5243
888-689-5655
http://www.biocore.com

00093
**BIOCRAFT LABORATORIES,
 INC.**
See Teva Pharmaceuticals USA

**BIOCRYST
 PHARMACEUTICALS, INC.**
205-444-4600
http://www.biocryst.com

BIODEVELOPMENT CORP.
703-006-0290

15594
BIOFILM, INC.
760-727-9030
http://www.astroglide.com

BIOFORM MEDICAL
650-286-4000
866-862-1211
http://www.bioform.com

BIOGEN PHARMACEUTICALS
818-762-7681

59627
BIOGEN IDEC
617-679-2000
800-262-2000
http://www.biogenidec.com

BIOGENEX LABORATORIES
925-275-0550
800-421-4149
http://www.biogenex.com

62436
BIOGLAN PHARMACEUTICALS
See Bradley Pharmaceutical

34061
BIOLIFE, LLC
800-722-7559
http://www.biolife.com

00719
BIOLINE LABS, INC.
888-257-5155
508-880-8990

BIOLITEC PHARMA, LTD.
353-1-463-7415
http://www.biolitecpharma.com

68135
**BIOMARIN PHARMACEUTICAL,
 INC.**
415-506-6700
866-274-0606
http://www.bmrn.com

BIOMEDICAL FRONTIERS, INC.
612-378-0228

83059
BIOMERICA, INC.
949-645-2111
800-854-3002
http://www.biomerica.com

BIOMERIEUX
630-628-6055
800-634-7656
http://www.biomerieux-usa.com

BIOMIRA USA, INC.
780-490-2818
877-234-0444
http://www.biomira.com

17700
BIOMOLECULAR SCIENCES, INC.
818-804-5148
800-260-3587
http://www.
  biomolecularsciences.com

53110
BIONEXUS, LTD
607-266-9492
800-835-0869
http://www.bionxs.com

62086
BIONICHE PHARMA USA
847-739-3246
888-258-4199
http://www.bioniche.com

08539
BIONIME USA CORPORATION
858-481-8485
866-481-8485
http://www.bionime.com

59741
BIOPHARM LABS
215-949-3711
http://www.bio-pharminc.com

BIOPHARMACEUTICS, INC.
See Feminique Corp.

BIOPHYSICA, INC.
858-452-1523
http://www.biophysica.net

BIO PRODUCTS LABORATORY
44-0-208-258-2200
http://www.bpl.co.uk

BIOPURE CORP.
617-234-6500
http://www.biopure.com

BIOSAFE TECHNOLOGIES, INC.
903-463-7321
877-828-4633
http://www.biosafetech.com

BIOSCRIP
952-979-3600
800-444-5951
http://www.bioscrip.com

08611
BIOSENSE MEDICAL DEVICES
877-592-3922

BIOSPECIFICS TECHNOLOGIES CORP.
516-593-7000
http://www.biospecifics.com

BIOSYNEXUS, INC.
301-330-5800
http://www.biosynexus.com

BIO-TECHNOLOGY GENERAL CORP.
732-632-8800

53191
BIO-TECH
479-443-9148
800-345-1199
http://www.bio-tech-pharm.com

55146
BIOTICS RESEARCH
281-344-0909
800-231-5777
http://www.bioticsresearch.com

BIOTRANSPLANT, INC.
617-241-5200

58023
BIOTROL INTERNATIONAL
303-673-0341
800-822-8550
http://www.biotrol.com

64455
BIOVAIL PHARMACEUTICALS, INC.
866-246-8245
908-927-1400
http://www.valeant.com

66658
BIOVITRUM AB
615-213-0343
http://www.biovitrum.com

BIRA CORP.
724-796-1820

50289
BIRCHWOOD LABORATORIES, INC.
952-937-7900
800-328-6156
http://www.birchlabs.com

12136
BIRD PRODUCTS CORP.
760-778-7200
800-232-7633
http://www.viasyscriticalcare.com

00165
BLAINE PHARMACEUTICALS
859-344-9600
800-633-9353
http://www.blainepharma.com

16728
BLAINES RESEARCH LABS
800-307-8818
562-906-4477
http://www.blaineslabs.com

00154
BLAIR LABORATORIES
See Purdue Frederick Co.

50486
BLAIREX LABS, INC.
812-378-1864
800-252-4739
http://www.blairex.com

51674
BLANSETT PHARMACAL
501-758-8635
800-816-9695
http://www.blansett.com

41388
BLISTEX INC.
630-571-2870
800-837-1800
http://www.blistex.com

BLOCK DRUG CO., INC.
See GlaxoSmithKline Consumer
  Healthcare

24658
BLU PHARMACEUTICALS
270-586-6386
877-264-0258
http://www.blurx.us

BLUCOINC.
734-513-4500
http://www.blucoinc.com

99853
BMS MEDIAL IMAGING
800-299-3431
http://www.radiopharm.com

64681
BMS U.S. MEDICINES GROUP
800-332-2056
212-546-4000
http://www.bms.com

08326, 43820, 00904
BOCA MEDICAL PRODUCTS
800-354-8460
http://www.
  bocamedicalproducts.com

64376
BOCA PHARMACAL
954-346-8810
800-354-8460
http://www.bocapharmacal.com

00024
BOCK PHARMACAL CO.
See Sanofi-Aventis U.S.

00597
BOEHRINGER INGELHEIM PHARMACEUTICALS, INC.
203-798-9988
800-520-1631
http://www.boehringer-ingelheim.com

BOERICKE & TAFEL
See Natures Way

00220
BOIRON LABORATORIES
800-264-7661
http://www.boironusa.com

00725
BOLAN PHARMACEUTICALS
516-842-8383
800-872-0159

50051
BONNE BELL
216-221-0800
800-321-1006
http://www.bonnebell.com

00074
BOOTS PHARMACEUTICALS, INC.
See Abbott Laboratories Pharmaceutical Division

BOTANICAL LABORATORIES
360-384-5656
800-232-4005
http://www.botlab.com

00270
BRACCO DIAGNOSTICS
609-514-2200
800-631-5245
http://www.bracco.com

BRADLEY PHARMACEUTICALS, INC.
973-882-1505
800-929-9300
http://www.bradpharm.com

52268
BRAINTREE LABORATORIES, INC.
781-843-2202
800-874-6756
http://www.braintreelabs.com

BRAUN
518-828-0450

00264
BRAUN MEDICAL
See B. Braun Medical, Inc.

51991
BRECKENRIDGE
561-443-3314
800-367-3395
http://www.bpirx.com

58659
BRIDGEPORT WHOLESALE PRODUCTS
425-656-0460

10914
BRIGHTON PHARMACEUTICALS
919-459-3950
866-638-7530
http://www.brightonpharma.com

10007
BRIOSCHI
201-796-4226
http://www.brioschi-usa.com

00015
BRISTOL LABS
609-252-4000
800-468-7746

BRISTOL-MYERS ONCOLOGY/VIROLOGY
609-897-2000
800-426-7644
http://www.bms.com

19810
BRISTOL-MYERS PRODUCTS (OTC/CONSUMER AFFAIRS)
See Novartis Pharmaceuticals Corp.

BRISTOL-MYERS SQUIBB COMPANY
212-546-4000
800-332-2056
http://www.bms.com

15584
BRISTOL-MEYERS SQUIBB/GILEAD
650-574-3000
800-445-3235
http://www.gilead.com

16563,11498
BRONSON PHARMACEUTICALS
800-235-3200
http://www.bronsonvitamins.com

42192
BROOKSTONE PHARMACEUTICALS
678-325-5188
800-541-4802
http://www.acellapharma.com

82161
BROWN MEDICAL INDUSTRIES
712-336-4395
800-843-4395
http://www.brownmed.com

63256.
BRYAN CORPORATION
781-935-0004
800-343-7711
http://www.bryancorp.com

63629
BRYANT RANCH PREPACK
818-764-7225
http://www.byrantranchprepack.com

BSN, JOBST
See BSN Medical

BSN MEDICAL
704-554-9933
http://www.jobst.com

54396
BTG PHARMACEUTICAL CORPORATION
See Savient Pharmaceuticals, Inc.

BUREL PHARMACEUTICALS
601-855-2016
http://www.burelpharmaceuticals.com

BURROUGHS WELLCOME CO.
See GlaxoSmithKline

BIOSAFE LABORATORIES
847-234-8111
http://www.ebiosafe.com

C. B. FLEET CO., INC.
See Fleet Laboratories

08011
C. R. BARD
908-277-8000
800-526-4455
http://www.crbard.com

C.R. BARD, INC. UROLOGICAL DIVISION
770-784-6100
800-526-4455
http://www.crbard.com

10486
C S DENT
859-647-0777

59746
CADISTA PHARMACEUTICALS, INC.
410-860-8500
800-619-9364
http://www.cadista.com

08237, 55559
CALGON VESTAL
See ConvaTec

00799
CALMOSEPTINE, INC.
714-840-3405
800-800-3405
http://www.calmoseptineointment.com

12622
CALWOOD NUTRITIONALS
410-796-5560
800-479-9942
http://www.calwoodnutritionals.com

31722
CAMBER PHARMACEUTICALS
732-377-2029
866-495-1995
http://www.camberpharma.com

CAMBREX BIOSCIENCE
207-594-3400
800-638-8174
http://www.cambrex.com

CAMBRIDGE NEUROSCIENCE
See Baxter Healthcare
   Corporation

43656
**CAMBRIDGE
   NUTRACEUTICALS**
See Baxter Healthcare Corp.

24359
CAMBROOKE FOODS
508-782-2300
866-456-9776
http://www.cambrookefoods.com

38083
CAMPBELL LABS
See Chattem Consumer Products

08396
CAN-AM CARE
678-795-3440
866-202-9067
http://www.canamcare.com

CANGENE
204-275-4200
800-768-2304

42026
**CANOPY ROADS
   PHARMACEUTICALS**
770-664-6050
http://www.crpharma.com

CANYON PHARMACEUTICALS
410-771-8606
888-434-7003
http://www.canyonpharma.com

64543
**CAPELLON
   PHARMACEUTICALS, LTD.**
817-595-5820
http://www.capellon.com

57664, 32247
**CARACO PHARMACEUTICAL
   LABORATORIES**
313-871-8400
800-818-4555
http://www.caraco.com

CARDINAL HEALTH
614-757-5000
800-234-8701
http://www.cardinal.com

08525
CARDIOCOM
952-361-6467
888-243-8881
http://www.cardiocom.com

83076
CARDIOTABS
816-753-4298
800-811-1007
http://www.cardiotabs.com

84841
**CARGILL HEALTH & FOOD
   TECH**
800-221-4455
952-742-7575
http://www.cargill.com

61442,61441
CARLSBAD TECHNOLOGIES
760-431-8284
http://www.
   carlsbadtechnologyinc.com

83078
CARMA LABS INC
414-421-7707
http://www.carma-labs.com

CARME, INC.
707-226-3900
http://www.senetekplc.net

50000
CARNATION
See Nestle Infant Nutrition

00086
CARNRICK LABORATORIES
See Elan Pharmaceuticals

46287
**CAROLINA MEDICAL
   PRODUCTS COMPANY**
252-753-7111
800-227-6637
http://www.carolinamedical.com

**CAROLINA MEDICAL
   PRODUCTS CO.**
800-227-6637
http://www.carolinamedical.com

53303
CARRINGTON
972-518-1300
800-527-5216
http://www.carringtonlabs.com

11411, 41140.
CARTER PRODUCTS
See Church Dwight

22600
CARTER-WALLACE
See Church Dwight

00037
CARTER-WALLACE, INC.
See Meda Pharmaceuticals

15370
CARWIN ASSOCIATES, INC.
205-525-4566
866-525-4566
http://www.carwinassoc.com

18515
CCA INDUSTRIES, INC.
800-524-2720
http://www.ccaindustries.com

64019
**CEBERT PHARMACEUTICALS,
   INC.**
205-981-0201
800-211-0589
http://www.cebert.com

64181
**CEDARBURG
   PHARMACEUTICALS**
262-376-1467
http://www.cedarburgpharma.com

**CELESTIAL SEASONINGS,
   INC.**
303-530-5300
800-525-0347
http://www.
   celestialseasonings.com

59572
CELGENE CORP
908-673-9000
888-423-5436
http://www.celgene.com

65231
CELL PATHWAYS
See OSI Pharmaceuticals

60553
CELL THERAPEUTICS, INC.
206-282-7100
800-215-2355
http://www.ctiseattle.com

**CELLEGY
   PHARMACEUTICALS, INC.**
215-914-0900

**CELLTECH PHARMACEUTICAL
   CO.**
See UCB Pharmaceuticals, Inc.

CENTEON
See CSL Behring

00268
CENTER LABORATORIES
See ALK-Abello

**CENTERS FOR DISEASE
 CONTROL AND PREVENTION**
404-639-3534
800-311-3435
http://www.cdc.gov

99962
**CENTOCOR ORTHO BIOTECH,
 INC.**
888-227-5624
800-457-6399
http://www.
 centocororthobiotech.com

**CENTOCOR ORTHO BIOTECH,
 INC.**
888-227-5624
800-457-6399

38083
**CENTRAL
 PHARMACEUTICALS, INC.**
See Schwarz Pharma

11528
**CENTRIX PHARMACEUTICAL,
 INC.**
205-991-9870
866-991-9870
http://www.cenrx.com

23359
CENTURION LABS, LLC
601-720-0111
http://www.centurionlabs.com

00436
CENTURY
317-849-4210
866-343-2576

63459
CEPHALON
610-344-0200
800-896-5855
http://www.cephalon.com

68330
CEPHAZONE PHARMA
909-392-8900
http://www.cephazone.com

00851
CERA PRODUCTS
843-842-2600
888-237-2598
http://www.ceraproductsinc.com

**CERENEX
 PHARMACEUTICALS**
See GlaxoSmithKline

10223
CETYLITE INDUSTRIES, INC.
865-665-6111
800-257-7740
http://www.cetylite.com

40986, 68016
CHAIN DRUG CONSORTIUM
412-828-2061

63868
**CHAIN DRUG MARKETING
 ASSOCIATION, INC.**
248-449-9300

**CHARLES RIVER
 LABORATORIES
 INTERNATIONAL, INC.**
978-658-6000
877-CRIVER1 (877-274-8371)
http://www.criver.com

54429
CHASE LABORATORIES
See Banner Pharmacaps

41167
**CHATTEM CONSUMER
 PRODUCTS**
423-821-4571
800-366-6833
http://www.chattem.com

**CHESAPEAKE BIOLOGICAL
 LABS., INC.**
See Cangene BioPharma

00521
**CHESEBROUGH-PONDS USA,
 INC.**
See Unilever Home and Personal
Care USA

12462
CHESTER LABS
513-458-3840
800-354-9709
http://www.chester-labs.com

CHEW-RITE CO.
937-746-5509

**CHILDRENS HOSPITAL OF
 COLUMBUS**
614-722-2000

CHILTON LABS., INC.
973-575-1992

67066
CHIRHOCLIN
877-272-4888
301-476-8388
http://www.chirhoclin.com

53905
CHIRON THERAPEUTICS
510-655-8730
800-244-7668
http://www.chiron.com

61772
CHIRON VISION
See Bausch & Lomb Surgical

54993
CHRONIMED INC.
See Bioscrip

96121
CHRONOHEALTH
805-290-4959
866-261-8557

22600
CHURCH DWIGHT
609-683-5900
800-524-1328
http://www.churchdwight.com

00067
CIBA CONSUMER
See Novartis Consumer Health

47113
CIBA VISION CORPORATION
770-476-3937
800-845-6585
http://www.cibavision.com

00078
**CIBA-GEIGY
 PHARMACEUTICALS**
See Novartis Pharmaceuticals
Corp.

CIMA LABS
952-947-8700
http://www.cimalabs.com

52544
**CIRCA PHARMACEUTICALS,
 INC.**
See Watson Laboratories

**CIRRUS HEALTHCARE
 PRODUCTS, L.L.C.**
631-692-7600
800-327-6151
http://www.cirrushealthcare.com

CIS-US, INC.
781-275-7120
800-221-7554
http://www.pharmalucence.com

CITRA ANTICOAGULANTS
781-848-2174
800-299-3411
http://www.
 citraanticoagulants.com

99074
**CLARIS LIFESCIENCES
 LIMITED**
732-422-9100
http://www.clarislifesciences.com

45802
CLAY-PARK LABS, INC.
718-901-2800
800-933-5550
http://www.claypark.com

55553
CLINT PHARMACEUTICALS
615-882-0042
800-677-5022
http://www.
  clintpharmaceuticals.com

CLOSURE MEDICAL CORP.
See Johnson & Johnson

57145
CNS, INC.
952-229-1500
http://www.cns.com

58826
COATS ALOE INTERNATIONAL, INC.
214-340-2563
800-486-2563
http://www.coatsaloe.com

16252
COBALT LABORATORIES, INC.
800-272-5525
239-390-0245
http://www.cobaltlabs.com

43378
CODADOSE
678-866-0172
866-574-8861
http://www.codadose.com

COLGATE-HOYT
See Colgate Oral
  Pharmaceuticals

00126
COLGATE ORAL PHARMACEUTICALS
213-310-2000
800-226-5428
http://www.colgateprofessional.com

35000
COLGATE-PALMOLIVE CO.
212-310-2000
800-221-4607
http://www.colgateprofessional.com

64682, 27280
COLLAGENEX PHARMACEUTICALS
215-579-7388
888-339-5678
http://www.collagenex.com

COLOPLAST
612-337-7800
800-533-0464
http://www.us.coloplast.com

COLORADO BIOLABS, INC.
970-243-4153
888-442-0067
http://www.coloradobiolabs.com

21406, 55056
COLUMBIA LABORATORIES, INC.
973-994-3999
866-566-5636
http://www.columbialabs.com

11509
COMBE, INC.
914-694-5454
800-873-7400
http://www.combe.com

COMPLIMED MEDICAL RESEARCH GROUP
360-384-5656
888-977-8008
http://www.complimed.com

CONAGRA FUNCTIONAL FOODS, INC.
888-828-4242
http://www.culturelle.com

74108
CONAIR INTERPLAX DIVISION
800-726-6247
http://www.interplak.com

08597, 95863
CONCEIVEX
616-642-6917
888-306-6366
http://www.conceptionkit.com

57648
CONCEPTS IN CONFIDENCE
561-369-1700
800-822-4050
http://www.
  conceptsinconfidence.com

CON-CISE CONTACT LENS CO.
510-483-9400
800-772-3911
http://www.con-cise.com

20254
CONCORD LABORATORIES
973-227-6757

49281
CONNAUGHT LABS
See Sanofi Pasteur

63032
CONNETICS CORPORATION
See Stiefel Laboratories

00223
CONSOLIDATED MIDLAND CORP.
845-279-6108

97493
CONSUMERS CHOICE SYSTEMS, INC.
425-883-6310
800-479-5232
http://www.womanswellbeing.com

CONTINENTAL CONSUMER PRODUCTS
248-758-1817
800-542-5903

CONTINENTAL QUEST RESEARCH
317-843-2501
800-451-5773
http://www.continentalquest.com

10267
CONTRACT PHARMACAL CORP.
631-231-4610
http://www.cpc.com

CONVATEC
908-904-2200
800-422-8811
http://www.convatec.com

63535
COOKE PHARMA, INC.
See Unither Pharma (United
  Therapeutics Corp.)

59365
COOPER SURGICAL
203-601-5200
800-480-1985
http://www.coopersurgical.com

59426, 54027
COOPERVISION
949-597-8130
800-538-7850
http://www.coopervision.com

00093
COPLEY PHARMACEUTICAL
See Teva Pharmaceuticals USA

63020
COR THERAPEUTICS, INC.
See Millennium Pharmaceuticals,
  Inc.

64720
COREPHARMA, LLC
732-868-1090
800-850-2719
http://www.corepharma.com

13548
CORIA LABORATORIES
800-548-5100
http://www.corialabs.com

CORIXA
See GlaxoSmithKline

10122
CORNERSTONE THERAPEUTICS
919-678-6611
888-466-6503
http://www.crtx.com

COROMEGA CO., INC.
760-599-6088
877-275-3725
http://www.coromega.com

10148
COTHERIX
650-624-6900
877-483-6828
http://www.cotherix.com

COULTER CORP.
See Beckman Coulter

43199
**COUNTY LINE
PHARMACEUTICALS**
262-439-8109
866-207-5636
http://www.countylinepharma.com

COVIDIEN
508-261-8000
800-722-8772
http://www.covidien.com

11025
**CREATIVE MEDICAL
CORPORATION**
787-714-0100

15310
**CREEKWOOD
PHARMACEUTICAL, INC.**
205-995-7390
http://www.crkrx.com

68734
**CRITICAL THERAPEUTICS,
INC.**
781-402-5700
http://www.criticaltherapeutics.com

37379
CSI PHARM
800-654-5635
http://www.csidesigns.com

00053
CSL BEHRING, LLC
610-878-4000
800-683-1288
800-504-5434
http://www.cslbehring.com

33332
CSL BIOTHERAPIES
888-435-8633
http://www.cslbiotherapies-us.com

67919
**CUBIST PHARMACEUTICALS,
INC.**
781-860-8660
866-793-2786
http://www.cubist.com

66220
**CUMBERLAND
PHARMACEUTICALS, INC.**
615-255-0068
866-423-7259
http://www.cumberlandpharma.com

00869
CUMBERLAND SWAN, INC.
See Vijon Laboratories

66860
CURA PHARMACEUTICALS
888-887-7171
732-982-8300
http://www.curapharma.com

08160
CURAMEDICA, LLC
888-613-0729
http://www.curamedica.com

CURASCRIPT
407-804-6700
800-892-9622
http://www.priorityhealthcare.com

55326
**CURATEK
PHARMACEUTICALS**
See 3M Pharmaceuticals

65628
CUTIS PHARMA, INC.
781-935-8141
http://www.cutispharma.com

67159
CV THERAPEUTICS
See Gilead Sciences

CYANOTECH CORP.
808-326-1353
800-395-1353
http://www.cyanotech.com

53409
**CYCLIN PHARMACEUTICALS
INC.**
800-558-7046
http://www.womenshealth.com

08197
CYGNUS, INC.
650-369-4300
http://www.cygn.com

54799
CYNACON/OCUSOFT
800-233-5469
http://www.ocusoft.com

60258
**CYPRESS PHARMACEUTICAL,
INC.**
601-856-4393
800-856-4393
http://www.cypressrx.com

63004
**CYPROS PHARMACEUTICAL
CORP.**
See Questcor Pharmaceuticals,
Inc.

57902
CYTOGEN CORP.
See Eusa Pharma

23731
CYTOSOL LABORATORIES
781-848-9386
800-288-3858

61534
CYTOSOL OPTHALMICS
828-758-2343
800-234-5166
http://www.cytosol.com

CYTRX CORP.
310-826-5648
http://www.cytrx.com

65759, 10960
**D & K HEALTHCARE
RESOURCES**
314-727-3485
888-727-3485
http://www.dkwd.com
See McKesson

DADE BEHRING
847-267-5300
800-241-0420
http://www.dadebehring.com

63395
**DAIICHI PHARMACEUTICAL
CORP**
See Daiichi Sankyo, Inc.

63395
DAIICHI SANKYO, INC.
973-944-2600
877-437-7763
http://www.dsi.com

00591, 52544
DANBURY PHARMACAL
951-493-5300
800-338-9066
http://www.watson.com

64875
DANCO LABS., LLC
212-424-1950
877-432-7596
http://www.earlyoptionpill.com

60793
**DANIELS PHARMACEUTICALS,
INC.**
See King Pharmaceuticals, Inc.

58869
**DARTMOUTH
PHARMACEUTICALS, INC.**
508-295-2200
800-414-3566
http://www.ilovemynails.com

67253
DAVA PHARMACEUTICALS, INC.
201-947-7442
866-947-3282
http://www.davapharm.com

DAVOL
401-463-7000
800-556-6275
http://www.davol.com

58865
DAWN PHARMACEUTICALS INC.
800-745-3296

52041
DAYTON LABORATORIES
See Propharma

DEGUSSA CORP.
973-541-8000
877-273-2668
http://www.degussa.com

10310
DEL PHARMACEUTICALS
516-844-2020
http://www.dellabs.com

00316
DEL-RAY LABORATORY INC
423-926-4413
800-877-8869
http://www.delrayderm.com

48532
DELMONT LABORATORIES, INC.
610-543-3365
800-562-5541
http://www.delmontlabs.info

53706
DELTA PHARMACEUTICALS
803-407-7733

DEN-MAT CORPORATION
805-922-8491
800-433-6628

00295
DENISON PHARMACEUTICALS
401-723-5500
http://www.hydrolatum.com

DENTAL HERB CO.
561-241-4262
800-747-4372
http://www.dentalherbcompany.com

13913
DEPOMED, INC.
650-462-5900
866-458-6389
http://www.depomedinc.com

DEPOTECH CORP. (SKYEPHARMA)
858-625-2424
http://www.skyepharma.com

99873
DEPUY MITEK
800-382-4682
508-880-8100
http://www.depuymitek.com

25382
DERMA SCIENCES
609-514-4744
800-825-4325
http://www.dermasciences.com

80208
DERMAIDE RESEARCH
312-649-7220
http://www.dermaide.com

10641
DERMALAB
847-266-0000
http://www.dermalab.com

60974
DERMALOGIX PARTNERS
207-883-4103
800-753-0047
http://www.dermalogix.com

61924
DERMARITE
973-569-9000
800-337-6296
http://www.dermarite.com

00066
DERMIK LABORATORIES, INC. (ARCOLA)
See Sanofi-Aventis US

DEROYAL INDUSTRIES, INC.
865-938-7828
888-938-7828
http://www.deroyal.com

08591
DESTAL INDUSTRIES
866-291-2815

16881
DESTON THERAPEUTICS
888-333-1528
http://www.deston.com

08627
DEXCOM, INC.
877-339-2664
http://www.dexcom.com

65430
DEXGEN PHARMACEUTICALS, INC.
732-223-8811
877-339-4361
http://www.dexgen.com

DEXO PHARMA
785-917-9582

49502
DEY L.P.
707-224-3200
800-755-5560
http://www.deyinc.com

DFB PHARMACEUTICALS
800-441-8227
http://www.dfb.com

55887
DHS, INC.
770-751-1787
800-392-7717

94046
DIABETIC SUPPLY OF SUNCOAST
888-469-3579
http://www.pharmasupply.com

DIAGNOSTICS DEVICES
800-366-5901
http://www.prodigymeter.com

17000
DIAL CORPORATION
480-754-3425
800-258-3425
http://www.dialcorp.com

DIAPHARMA GROUP, INC.
513-860-9324
800-526-5224
http://www.diapharma.com

50419
DIATIDE, INC.
See Berlex

10331
DICKINSON BRANDS, INC.
860-267-2279
888-860-2279
http://www.witchhazel.com

59767
DIGESTIVE CARE, INC.
610-882-5950
http://www.digestivecare.com

55392
DINNO PHARMACEUTICALS
617-645-5552

08587
DINORIO
866-354-3449
http://www.dinorio.com

DISCOVERY LABORATORIES, INC.
215-488-9300
http://www.discoverylabs.com

DISCUS DENTAL, INC.
800-422-9448
310-845-8600
http://www.discusdental.com

15630
DISETRONIC MEDICAL SYSTEMS
See Roche Insulin Delivery Systems, Inc.

68258
DISPENSING SOLUTIONS, INC.
888-374-7378
770-751-1787
http://www.
   dispensingsolutionsinc.com

00777
DISTA PRODUCTS CO.
See Eli Lilly and Co.

DIXON-SHANE
See Amneal Pharmaceuticals

64455
DJ PHARMA, INC.
See Biovail Pharmaceuticals, Inc.

10337
DOAK DERMATOLOGICS
See Pharmaderm

DONELL DERMEDEX
See Donell, Inc.

DONELL INC.
212-682-0666
800-324-7455
http://www.donellskin.com

51469
DOVER PHARMACEUTICAL, INC.
781-821-5400
800-777-6847

00514
DOW HICKAM, INC.
See Mylan Pharmaceuticals, Inc.

DOW PHARMACEUTICAL SCIENCES
707-793-2600
877-369-7476
http://www.dowpharm.com

55111
DR. REDDY'S LABORATORIES, INC.
888-375-3784
908-203-4900
http://www.drreddys.com

64061
DREIR PHARMACEUTICALS, INC.
480-607-3584
800-541-4044

58952
DRJ GROUP, INC.
760-635-0174

52316
DSC LABORATORIES
231-777-3012
800-492-5988
http://www.dsclab.com

89411
DSE HEALTHCARE SOLUTIONS, LLC
800-338-8079
732-417-1870
http://www.dsehealth.com

25382
DUMEX
See Derma Sciences

50939
DU-MORE
479-631-1088
http://www.dumoreinc.com

00217, 48878
DUNHALL PHARMACEUTICALS, INC.
See Omnii Pharmaceuticals and See Oxypure

DUPONT PHARMACEUTICALS CO.
See Bristol-Myers Squibb Co.

41333
DURACELL
800-551-2355
http://www.duracell.com

51285
DURAMED PHARMACEUTICALS
See Barr Laboratories, Inc.

02340
DUREX CONSUMER PRODUCTS
770-582-2222
888-566-3468
http://www.durex.com

00145
DURHAM PHARMACAL CORP.
See Stiefel Laboratories, Inc.

67308
DUSA PHARMACEUTICALS, INC.
978-657-7500
877-533-DUSA (877-533-3872)
http://www.dusapharma.com

68803
DUTCH OPHTHALMIC
603-778-6929
800-753-8824
http://www.dorc.nl

47783
DYAX CORPORATION
617-225-2500
800-452-5248
http://www.dyax.com

55516
DYNA PHARM, INC.

00168
E. FOUGERA CO.
631-454-7677
800-645-9833
http://www.fougera.com

E.R. SQUIBB & SONS, INC.
See Bristol-Myers Squibb Co.

EAGLE VISION, INC.
901-380-7000
800-222-7584
http://www.eaglevis.com

EASTMAN KODAK CO.
585-724-4000
800-242-2424
http://www.kodak.com

EATON MEDICAL CORP.
901-274-0000
800-253-5949
http://www.easyeyes.com

ECOLAB
651-293-2233
800-352-5326
http://www.ecolab.com

ECOLOGICAL FORMULAS, INC.
925-827-2636
800-888-4585
http://www.ecologicalformulas.net

38130
ECONO MED PHARMACEUTICALS
336-226-1091
800-327-6007

55053
ECONOLAB
See Breckenridge Pharmaceutical, Inc.

00095
ECR PHARMACEUTICALS
804-527-1950
800-527-1955
http://www.ecrpharma.com

42799
EDENBRIDGE PHARMACEUTICALS
201-292-1292
http://www.
   edenbridgepharma.com

00433
EDWARDS LIFESCIENCE
800-424-3278
800-882-9837
http://www.edwards.com

00485
EDWARDS
662-837-8182
800-543-9560

55806
EFFCON LABORATORIES
770-579-3558
800-722-2428

62856
EISAI, INC.
201-692-1100
888-793-4724
http://www.eisai.com

24477
EKR THERAPEUTICS, INC.
877-435-2524
http://www.ekrtx.com

59075
ELAN PHARMACEUTICALS
800-859-8586
888-638-7605
http://www.elan.com

ELANCO
317-277-3185
800-428-4441
http://www.elanco.com

58298
ELGE
281-232-0463
281-342-8228
http://www.elgeninc.com

00002
ELI LILLY AND COMPANY
317-276-2000
800-545-5979
http://www.lilly.com

42783
ELORAC
847-362-8200

EMD CHEMICALS, INC.
856-423-6300
800-222-0342

EMD SERONO, INC.
781-982-9000
800-283-8088
http://www.emdserono.com

04107, 24155
EMJAY LABORATORIES
See Sheffield Laboratories

91268
EMJOI
212-755-5950
888-310-2493
http://www.emjoi.com

42457
EMMAUS MEDICAL
310-214-0065
877-420-6493
http://www.emmausmedical.com

64068
ENDIT LABORATORIES
910-754-6856
http://www.endit.com

ENDO PHARMACEUTICALS
610-558-9800
800-462-3636
http://www.endo.com

**ENDURANCE PRODUCTS
COMPANY**
503-639-9562
800-964-0876
http://www.endur.com

17433
ENEMEEZ
602-276-3434
888-273-9734
http://www.enemeez.com

62333
**ENVIRODERM
PHARMACEUTICALS, INC.**
310-768-0700
800-624-9659
http://www.enviroderm.com

57665
**ENZON PHARMACEUTICALS,
INC.**
908-541-8600
866-792-5172
http://www.enzon.com

63948
ENZYMATIC THERAPY
800-783-2286
http://www.enzymatictherapy.com

00185
EON LABS
See Sandoz

42806
EPIC PHARMA
718-949-8607
888-374-2791
http://www.epic-pharma.com

62942
EPIEN MEDICAL
952-746-6770
888-884-4675
http://www.epien.com

18270
EQUIDYNE SYSTEMS
714-447-4474
http://www.injex.com

63475
ESCALON MEDICAL CORP
618-688-6830
800-433-8197
http://www.escalonmed.com

67286
ESP PHARMA
See PDL Biopharma

15456
ESPRIT PHARMA
732-828-9950
http://www.espritpharma.com

58177
ETHEX CORP.
314-646-3750
800-321-1705
http://www.ethex.com

63713
**ETHICON, INC. (JOHNSON &
JOHNSON)**
908-218-0707
800-255-2500
http://www.ethicon.com

ETI HOLDING
920-469-1313

EURAND AMERICA, INC.
937-898-9669
http://www.eurand.com

42865
EURAND PHARMACEUTICALS
267-759-9400
888-936-7371
http://www.eurand.com

66521
EVANS VACCINES, LTD.
See Novartis Vaccines and
Diagnostics

42700
EVENFLO COMPANY, INC.
937-415-3300
800-233-5921
http://www.evenflo.com

00642
EVERETT
973-324-0200
800-964-9650
http://www.everettlabs.com

17287
**EVERTON
PHARMACEUTICALS**
877-218-3215

64125
EXCELLIUM
PHARMACEUTICAL
973-276-9600

63807
EXCELSIOR MEDICAL
CORPORATION
732-776-7525
800-487-4276
http://www.excelsiormedical.com

08287,20221
EXEL INTERNATIONAL
800-940-3935
http://www.exelint.com

60843
EYE CARE & CURE
CORPORATION
520-321-1262
800-486-6169
http://www.eyecareandcure.com

68782
EYETECH
PHARMACEUTICALS
See OSI Eyetech

10361
E-Z-EM
See Bracco Diagnostics

94542
FACET TECHNOLOGIES
770-590-6400
800-526-2387
http://www.facettechnologies.com

61314
FALCON PHARMACEUTICALS,
LTD.
800-343-2133
817-293-0450
http://www.falconpharma.com

58892
FALLENE
800-332-5536
http://www.fallene.com

FARMACON, INC.
203-222-8801

60976
FARO PHARMACEUTICALS,
INC.
See Cooper Surgical

61703
FAULDING PHARMACEUTICAL
See Hospira

FDA
301-827-1491
888-463-6332
http://www.fda.gov

50907
FEI PRODUCTS
716-693-6230
877-727-2427
http://www.barrlabs.com

11423
FEMALE HEALTH CO.
312-595-9123
800-884-1601
http://www.
femalehealthcompany.com

08454
FEMCAP
858-481-8837
http://www.femcap.com

00942
FENWAL INTERNATIONAL
847-550-2300
800-333-6925
http://www.fenwalinc.com

48102
FERA PHARMACEUTICALS
414-434-6604
http://www.ferapharma.com

00496
FERNDALE LABORATORIES,
INC.
248-548-0900
800-621-6003
http://www.ferndalelabs.com

31253, 08439
FERRARIS MEDICAL
http://www.ferrarismedical.com

55566
FERRING
PHARMACEUTICALS, INC.
973-796-1600
888-337-7464
http://www.ferringusa.com

08195
FERRIS CORP
630-887-9797
800-765-9636
http://www.polymem.com

FIBERTONE
See Marlyn Neutraceuticals, Inc.

59630
FIRST HORIZON
PHARMACEUTICAL
See Sciele Pharma

90891
FIRST QUALITY PRODUCTS
516-829-3030
800-726-6910
http://www.firstquality.com

FISHER SCIENTIFIC
INTERNATIONAL
603-926-5911
800-640-0640
http://www.fisherscientific.com

FISKE INDUSTRIES
845-398-3340
http://www.cosmeticsolutions.com

54323
FLANDERS, INC.
843-571-3363
http://www.
flandersbuttocksointment.com

78573
FLAVORX
800-884-5771
http://www.flavorx.com

FLEET LABORATORIES
800-999-9711
http://www.cbfleet.com

00256
FLEMING PHARMACEUTICALS
636-343-5306
800-343-0164
http://www.flemingpharma.com

23185
FLENTS PRODUCTS COMPANY
See Apothecary Products, Inc.

FLEX-POWER
510-527-9955
866-353-9769
http://www.flexpower.com

00288
FLUORITAB
231-755-9113

60762
FNC MEDICAL CORPORATION
805-644-7576
800-440-2888
http://www.fncmedical.com

42559
FONTUS PHARMACEUTICALS,
INC.
973-265-2777
http://www.fontuspharma.com

98939
FORA CARE
805-498-8188
http://www.foracare.com

00456
FOREST LABORATORIES
IRELAND, LTD.
See Forest Laboratories, Inc.

00456
FOREST LABORATORIES, INC.
212-421-7850
800-947-5227
800-678-1605
http://www.forestpharm.com

00456
FOREST PHARMACEUTICALS,
INC.
See Forest Laboratories, Inc.

64814
FORTE PHARMA
See Eon Labs Manufacturing, Inc.

00168
FOUGERA
631-454-7677
800-645-9833
http://www.fougera.com

FOURNIER PHARMA
973-683-0024
http://www.
  fournierpharmacorp.com

58487,10432
FREEDA VITAMINS, INC.
718-433-4337
800-777-3737
http://www.freedavitamins.com

90816, 49230
FRESENIUS
781-699-9000
800-662-1237
http://www.fmcna.com

71661
FRUIT OF THE EARTH
972-790-0808
800-527-7731
http://www.fote.com

13551
FSC LABORATORIES
877-387-0021
http://www.fsclabs.com

FUISZ TECHNOLOGIES, LTD.
See Biovail Pharmaceuticals, Inc.

00713
G & W LABS
908-753-2000
800-922-1038
http://www.gwlabs.com

86040
G C AMERICA
800-323-7063
http://www.gcamerica.com

00891
G. HIRSCH & CO.
650-692-8770
800-638-8800
http://www.ghirsch.com

00299
GALDERMA
817-961-5000
866-735-4137
http://www.galdermausa.com

57284
GALEN PHARMA
028-3833-4974
http://www.galen.co.uk

51552
GALLIPOT, INC.
651-681-9517
800-423-6967
http://www.gallipot.com

GAMBRO RENAL PRODUCTS
800-232-6800
800-525-2623
http://www.gambro.com

57844
GATE PHARMACEUTICALS
215-591-3000
800-292-4283
http://www.gatepharma.com

43386
GAVIS PHARMACEUTICALS
908-603-6080
http://www.gavispharma.com

00407
GE HEALTHCARE
262-544-3011
http://www.gehealthcare.com

00386
GEBAUER
216-581-3030
800-321-9348
http://www.gebauerco.com

50242
GENENTECH, INC.
650-225-1000
800-821-8590
http://www.gene.com

GENERAL INJECTABLES &
  VACCINES
276-688-4121
800-521-7468
http://www.giv.com

GENERAL NUTRITION INC.
412-288-4600
888-462-2548
http://www.gnc.com

10139
GENERAMEDIX, INC.
866-436-3721
908-504-1300
http://www.generamedix.com

GENESIS NUTRITION
843-665-6928
800-451-7933
http://www.genesisnutrition.com

00398
GENESIS PHARMACEUTICALS
973-451-9020
800-459-8663

68585
GENESIS PRODUCTS
877-266-8292
http://www.
  genesisproductsinc.com

GENETIC THERAPY, INC.
301-590-2626

00008
GENETICS INSTITUTE
617-876-1170
888-446-3344
http://www.genetics.com

00781
GENEVA DRUGS
See Sandoz
  Pharmaceuticals-Sandoz
  Consumer

82915
GENEXEL-SIEN
480-502-6007

15330
GENPHARM, L.P.
866-436-9155
631-434-2760
http://www.genpharmusa.com

35781
GENSCO LABORATORIES
352-726-6284
http://www.genscolabs.com

00703.
GENSIA SICOR
  PHARMACEUTICALS, INC.
See Teva Pharmaceuticals USA

66657
GENTA INC.
908-286-9800
http://www.genta.com

15014
GENTEX PHARMA LLC
601-201-7231
601-826-0058
http://www.gentexpharma.com

GENVEC, INC.
240-632-5501
240-632-0740
http://www.genvec.com

58468
GENZYME CORPORATION
617-252-7500
800-326-7002
http://www.genzyme.com

63861
GENZYME TRANSPLANT
617-252-7500
800-376-7002
http://www.genzyme.com

GEODESIC MEDITECH, INC.
858-692-0088
http://www.geodesicmeditech.com

72227
**GERBER PRODUCTS
  COMPANY**
231-928-2000
800-443-7237
http://www.gerber.com

54092
**GERIATRIC
  PHARMACEUTICAL CORP.**
See Shire US, Inc.

57896
GERI-CARE
718-382-5000
http://www.gericarepharm.com

92771, 54162
GERITREX CORPORATION
914-668-4003
800-736-3437
http://www.geritrex.com

61958
GILEAD SCIENCES
650-574-3000
800-445-3235
http://www.gilead.com

GILLETTE ORAL CARE
617-421-7000
http://www.gillette.com

47400
GILLETTE PERSONAL CARE
617-421-7000
http://www.gillette.com

36819
GINESIS NATURAL PRODUCTS
256-767-8256
800-492-4818
http://www.ginesis.com

63218, 59366
**GLADES PHARMACEUTICALS,
  LLC**
888-445-2337
http://www.glades.com

GLAXOSMITHKLINE
888-825-5249
215-751-4000
http://www.gsk.com

99929
**GLAXOSMITHKLINE
  CONSUMER HEALTHCARE**
412-200-4000
800-245-1040
http://www.gsk.com

GLAXOSMITHKLINE PHARM.
See GlaxoSmithKline

68462
**GLENMARK
  PHARMACEUTICALS, LTD**
888-721-7115
201-684-8000
http://www.glenmarkpharma.com

41128, 00516
GLENWOOD
201-569-0050
800-542-0772
http://www.glenwood-llc.com

82028
**GLOBAL HEALTH PRODUCTS,
  INC.**
585-235-8818
http://www.globalhp.com

00115
GLOBAL PHARMACEUTICALS
215-933-0323
800-934-6729
http://www.globalphar.com

26893
**GLOBAL PROTECTION
  COMPANY**
617-946-2800
http://www.globalprotection.com

59618
GLOBAL SOURCE
954-747-8977
800-662-7556

33620
GLOVES IN A BOTTLE
818-248-9980
800-600-1881
http://www.glovesinabottle.com

58809
GM PHARMACEUTICALS
888-535-0305
817-303-3800

GML INDUSTRIES, LLC
See Biosafe Technologies, Inc.

60429
**GOLDEN STATE MEDICAL
  SUPPLY**
805-477-9866
800-284-8633
http://www.gsms.us

**GOLDLINE LABORATORIES,
  INC.**
See Ivax Pharmaceuticals, Inc.

10481
GORDON LABORATORIES
610-734-2011
800-356-7870
http://www.gordonlabs.net

13453
**GRACEWAY
  PHARMACEUTICALS, LLC**
423-274-2100
800-328-0255
http://www.gracewaypharma.com

12165
**GRAHAM FIELD HEALTH
  PRODUCTS, INC.**
800-347-5678
http://www.grahamfield.com

10486
GRANDPA BRANDS COMPANY
859-647-0777
800-684-1468
http://www.grandpabrands.com

00034
GRAY PHARMACEUTICAL CO.
See Purdue Frederick Co.

51301
**GREAT SOUTHERN
  LABORATORIES**
281-530-3077
800-747-0783
http://www.greatsouthernlabs.com

**GREEN TURTLE BAY VITAMIN
  CO.**
908-277-2240
800-887-8535
http://www.energywave.com

59762
GREENSTONE
212-733-2323
800-438-1985
http://www.greenstonellc.com

22840
GREER LABORATORIES, INC.
828-754-5327
800-378-3906
http://www.greerlabs.com

68516, 61953
GRIFOLS, INC.
888-474-3657
800-421-0008
http://www.grifolsusa.com

11399
GTX, INC.
901-523-9700
http://www.gtxinc.com

GUARDIAN DRUG COMPANY
609-860-2600
http://www.guardiandrug.com

00327
GUARDIAN LABORATORIES
See United Guardian
Laboratories

62750
GUM-TECH INDUSTRIES, INC.
See Matrixx Initiatives, Inc.

63955
GYNETICS
609-919-1931

54765
GYNOPHARMA

08385
**H&H WHOLESALE SERVICES,
INC.**
248-616-3030
800-995-5750
http://www.hhwholesale.com

52959
H.J. HARKINS COMPANY, INC.
805-929-4060

00839
**H.L. MOORE DRUG
EXCHANGE, INC.**
See Moore Medical Corp.

00556
H R CENCI LABS

64285
HAEMACURE CORPORATION
941-364-3700
http://www.haemacure.com

44411
HALL BIOSCIENCE
770-975-7337
http://www.hallbio.com

12164
**HALOCARBON PRODUCTS
CORPORATION**
800-338-5803
http://www.halocarbon.com

17478
**HAMELN PHARMACEUTICALS
GMBH**
See Akorn, Inc.

41268
HANNAFORD BROTHERS
800-213-9040
http://www.hannaford.com

HARD TO FIND BRANDS, INC.
724-796-0148
888-796-4832
http://www.hardtofindbrands.com

52512
HARMONY LABORATORIES
704-857-0707
800-245-6284
http://www.harmonylabs.com

67405
**HARRIS PHARMACEUTICAL,
INC.**
239-278-4749
800-983-4708
http://www.
 harrispharmaceutical.com

HART HEALTH & SAFETY
800-234-4278
http://www.harthealth.com

00904, 61147
HARVARD DRUG CORP.
800-875-0123
http://www.harvardlink.com
http://www.harvarddrugs.com

67754
**HARVEST
 PHARMACEUTICALS, INC.**
540-633-7976
800-455-5525
http://www.
 harvestpharmaceuticals.com

**HAUSER PHARMACEUTICAL
INC.**
800-441-2309
http://www.
 hauserpharmaceutical.com

66761
HAW PAR HEALTHCARE
510-887-1899
http://www.hawpar.com

63370
HAWKINS CHEMICAL
612-331-6910
612-617-8544
800-375-0009

63717
**HAWTHORN
 PHARMACEUTICALS, INC.**
601-856-4393
800-856-4393
http://www.cypressrx.com

HCD SALES
813-978-3005
800-844-8345
http://www.hcdsales.com

HD SMITH
866-232-1222
800-252-8090
http://www.hdsmith.com

HDC CORPORATION
408-942-7340
800-227-8162
http://www.hdccorp.com

HEALTH ASURE, INC.
831-420-2660
800-635-1233
http://www.healthasure.com

62391
**HEALTH CARE
 LABORATORIES**
281-496-9854
800-909-9854
http://www.bioflexor.com

60569, 61787
HEALTH CARE PRODUCTS
866-263-9003
800-899-3116
http://www.diabeticproducts.com

79573
HEALTH ENTERPRISES
508-695-0727
800-633-4243
http://www.healthenterprises.com

HEALTH PRODUCTS CORP.
914-423-2900

**HEALTHCARE DIRECT
 SERVICES**
See HCD Sales

HEALTHFIRST CORP.
425-771-5733
800-331-1984
http://www.healthfirst.com

00064
HEALTHPOINT MEDICAL
800-441-8227
http://www.healthpoint.com

93595, 55966
HEALTHSTAR
631-273-2630

50114
HEEL INC.
505-293-3843
800-621-7644
http://www.heelusa.com

HELENA LABORATORIES
409-842-3714
800-231-5663
http://www.helena.com

HEMACARE CORP.
818-226-1968
http://www.hemacare.com

HEMAGEN DIAGNOSTICS, INC.
443-367-5500
800-495-2180
http://www.hemagen.com

**HEMISPHERX BIOPHARMA,
INC.**
215-988-0080
http://www.hemispherx.net

HENRY SCHEIN, INC.
631-843-5500
800-472-4346
http://www.henryschein.com

00023, 11980
HERBERT LABORATORIES
See Allergan, Inc.

49730
**HERCON LABORATORIES
CORPORATION**
717-764-1191
http://www.herconlabs.com

23155
**HERITAGE
PHARMACEUTICALS**
732-429-1000
866-901-1230
http://www.heritagepharma.com

10541
HIGH CHEMICAL COMPANY
215-788-3113
800-447-8792
http://www.sarapin.com

HIKMA PHARMACEUTICALS
732-542-1191
http://www.hikma.com

28105
HILL DERMACEUTICALS, INC.
407-323-1187
800-344-5707
http://www.hillderm.com

10542
**HILLESTAD
PHARMACEUTICALS**
800-535-7742
866-358-9773
http://www.hillestadlabs.com

17808
HIMMEL
561-585-0070
800-535-3823
http://www.goliath.ecnext.com

46581
**HISAMITSU
PHARMACEUTICAL CO., INC.**
http://www.salonpas-usa.com

50383
HI-TECH PHARMACAL CO. INC.
631-789-8228
http://www.hitechpharm.com

84160
HMD BIOMEDICAL
321-267-7576
888-446-3246
http://www.hmeproviders.com

HOECHST-MARION ROUSSEL
See Sanofi-Aventis US

95814
**HOGIL PHARMACEUTICAL
CORP.**
914-681-1800
http://www.hogil.com

HOLLES LABORATORIES, INC.
800-356-4015

08380
HOLLISTER
800-323-4060
http://www.hollister.com

42828, 08567
HOLLISTER WOUND CARE
800-323-4060
http://www.hollister.com

65044
**HOLLISTER-STIER
LABORATORIES**
509-489-5656
800-992-1120
http://www.hollisterstier.com

83170
**HOME ACCESS HEALTH
CORPORATION**
847-781-2500
800-448-8378
http://www.homeaccess.com

21292, 56151
HOME DIAGNOSTICS
954-677-9201
800-342-7226
http://www.niprodiagnostics.com

HONEYWELL HOMMED LLC
262-783-5440
888-353-5440
http://www.hommed.com

60267
**HOPE PHARMACEUTICALS,
INC.**
800-755-9595
http://www.hopepharm.com

60904
**HORIZON PHARMACEUTICAL
CORP.**
See Shionigi Pharma, Inc.

61678
HORMEL HEALTHLABS
800-866-7757
http://www.hormelhealthlabs.com

66553
**HOSPAK UNIT DOSE
PRODUCTS**
815-877-6480
815-636-8829

00409
HOSPIRA
224-212-2000
877-946-7747
http://www.hospira.com

00591, 52544
HOUBA (HALSEY DRUG CO.)
See Acura Pharmaceuticals, Inc.

17238
HUB PHARMACEUTICALS
909-476-8394
800-393-3767
http://www.hubrx.com

74312
HUDSON CORP.

65845
HUDSON RCI
951-676-5611
866-246-6990
http://www.hudsonrci.com

44156
**HUMANICARE
INTERNATIONAL**
732-613-9000
800-631-5270
http://www.humanicare.com

03951, 00395
HUMCO HOLDING GROUP, INC.
903-334-6200
800-662-3435
http://www.humco.com

00219
HUMPHREYS PHARMACAL
201-933-7744

00944
HYLAND THERAPEUTICS
See Baxter Healthcare Corp.

75450
HY-VEE
515-267-2800
http://www.hy-vee.com

00186
ICI PHARMACEUTICALS
See AstraZeneca, LP

00187
ICN PHARMACEUTICALS
See Valeant Pharmaceuticals
International

59627
IDEC PHARMACEUTICALS
See Biogen Idec

24108
**IDENIX PHARMACEUTICALS,
INC.**
617-995-9800
http://www.idenix.com

IKARIA
908-238-6600
877-566-9466
http://www.ikaria.com

63861
ILEX ONCOLOGY, INC.
See Genzyme Corp.

24430
IMARX THERAPEUTICS
520-770-1259
800-984-1074
http://www.imarx.com

IMMUCELL CORP.
207-878-2770
800-466-8235
http://www.immucell.com

54129
IMMUNO U.S, INC.
See Baxter Healthcare Corp.

IMMUNOGEN
617-995-2500
http://www.immunogen.com

IMMUNOMEDICS INC.
973-605-8200
http://www.immunomedics.com

28770
IMMUNOTEC RESEARCH LTD.
450-424-9992
888-917-7779
http://www.immunotec.com

00115
IMPAX LABORATORIES, INC.
510-476-2000
http://www.impaxlabs.com

IMS, LTD.
See UCB Pharmaceuticals, Inc.

INAMED CORPORATION
805-683-6761
800-722-2007
http://www.inamed.com

INDEVUS
  PHARMACEUTICALS, INC.
781-861-8444
800-370-4742
http://www.indevus.com

INFLABLOC
  PHARMACEUTICALS, INC.
801-464-6100
866-440-7044
http://www.pharmadigm.com

61607, 66934
INKINE PHARMACEUTICAL
  COMPANY, INC.
See Salix Pharmaceuticals, Inc.

INNER HEALTH GROUP
210-661-9257
800-381-4697
http://www.michaelshealth.com

INNOZEN, INC.
818-593-4880
800-599-8892

INO THERAPEUTICS, INC.
See IKARIA

08489
INPHARMA
877-241-8324

63736
INSIGHT PHARMACEUTICALS
267-852-0505
800-344-7239
http://www.insightpharma.com

16249
INSMED INCORPORATED
804-565-3000
804-565-3079
http://www. insmed.com

58441, 63252
INSOURCE
276-688-0211
800-668-3452
http://www.insourceonline.com

INSPIRE PHARMACEUTICALS,
  INC.
919-941-9777
http://www.inspirepharm.com

08508
INSULET
781-457-5000
800-591-3455
http://www.myomnipod.com

08478, 64895, 08220
INTEGRA LIFESCIENCES
  CORP
800-654-2873
800-931-1709
http://www.integra-ls.com

INTEGRATED THERAPEUTICS
See Integrative Therapeutics

88856
INTEGRATIVE HEALTH
  CONSULTING
See K-Pax Vitamins

INTEGRATIVE THERAPEUTICS
800-917-3696
http://www.integrativeinc.com

10922
INTENDIS, INC.
866-463-3634
http://www.intendis.com

42515
INTERCELL USA, INC.
301-556-4500
http://www.intercell.com

INTERCHEM CORP.
201-261-7333
800-261-7332
http://www.interchem.com

18968
INTERCURE, INC.
201-720-7750
877-988-9388
http://www.intercure.com

54746
INTERFERON SCIENCES
See Hemispherx Biopharma, Inc.

INTERMAX
  PHARMACEUTICALS, INC.
631-777-3318

64116
INTERMUNE
  PHARMACEUTICALS
415-466-2200
http://www.intermune.com

11584
INTERNATIONAL ETHICAL
  LABS
787-765-3510
800-981-5068
http://www.intetlab.com

00665
INTERNATIONAL LABS, INC.
727-327-4094
http://www.internationallabs.com

00548
INTERNATIONAL MEDICATION
  SYSTEMS, LTD.
877-651-2674
800-423-4136
http://www.ims-limited.com

INTERNEURON
  PHARMACEUTICALS, INC.
See Indevus Pharmaceuticals,
  Inc.

53746
INTERPHARM LTD
631-952-0214
http://www.interpharminc.com

00814
INTERSTATE DRUG
  EXCHANGE
See Henry Schein, Inc.

91536
INVACARE CORPORATION
800-333-6900
http://www.invacare.com

49939
INVADO PHARMACEUTICALS
914-715-6232
866-963-8881
http://www.
invadopharmaceuticals.com

INVERESK RESEARCH, INC.
See Charles River Laboratories
International, Inc.

38396
**INVERNESS MEDICAL
INNOVATIONS**
781-647-3900
http://www.invernessmedical.com

16874
INVISION PHARMAEUCTICALS
407-499-2225
800-443-4313

00258
INWOOD LABORATORIES
See Forest Laboratories, Inc.

58768
IOLAB PHARMACEUTICALS
See Ciba Vision Corp.

61646
IOMED
See Iopharm

55532
ION LABS
727-527-1072
877-990-4466
http://www.ionlabs.com

IOP, INC.
714-549-1185
800-535-3545
http://www.iopinc.com

61646
IOPHARM
817-595-5820

54921
IPR PHARMACEUTICALS, INC.
787-750-5353
800-477-6385

55688
IPSEN PHARMACEUTICALS
508-478-8900
http://www.ipsen.com

42211
IROKO PHARMACEUTICALS
267-546-3003
866-916-0576
http://www.iroko.com

ISIS PHARMACEUTICALS
760-931-9200
http://www.isispharm.com

ISO-TEX DIAGNOSTICS, INC.
281-482-1231
800-613-0600
http://www.isotexdiagnostics.com

67425
ISTA PHARMACEUTICALS, INC.
949-788-6000
800-385-7034
http://www.istavision.com

IVAX CORPORATION
949-455-4700
800-545-8800
http://www.tevausa.com

13613
IVAX DERMATOLOGICALS
305-575-4312

**IVAX PHARMACEUTICALS,
INC.**
305-575-6000
800-327-4114
http://www.ivaxpharmaceuticals.com

12126
IVY CORPORATION
973-575-1990
800-443-8856

59291
IYATA PHARMACEUTICAL
813-740-1810

99940,56091
J & J MEDICAL
732-524-0400
888-222-6036
http://www.jnj.com

16837
**J & J MERCK CONSUMER AND
SPECIALTY**
215-273-7000
800-523-3484
http://www.jnj.com

51111
J.B. LABORATORIES
616-738-8500
http://www.jblabs.com

00304
J.J. BALAN, INC.
See HD Smith

**J. R. CARLSON
LABORATORIES**
847-255-1600
888-234-5656
http://www.carlsonlabs.com

10106
J.T. BAKER (MALLINCKRODT)
908-859-2151
800-582-2537
http://www.mallbaker.com

72904
JACKSON-MITCHELL
209-667-2019
800-891-4628
http://www.meyenberg.com

49938
JACOBUS
609-921-7447

10592
JAMOL LABS
201-262-6363

50458
JANSSEN
609-730-2000
800-526-7736
http://www.janssen.com

90011
JARROW FORMULAS
310-204-6936
800-726-0886
http://www.jarrow.com

64661
**JAYMAC PHARMACEUICALS,
LLC**
337-662-5962
800-520-5568
http://www.jaymacpharma.com

**JAZZ PHARMACEUTICALS,
INC.**
650-496-3777
888-867-7426
http://www.
jazzpharmaceuticals.com

68968
JDS PHARMACEUTICALS, LLC
See Noven Pharmaceuticals

50564
JEROME STEVENS
631-567-1113
800-325-9994

42023
JHP PHARMACEUTICALS
877-547-4547
866-923-2547
http://www.jhppharma.com

59841
J-MED PHARMACEUTICALS
617-247-0010

60793
**JMI-CANTON
PHARMACEUTICALS**
See King Pharmaceuticals

00204
JOHNSON & JOHNSON
732-524-0400
http://www.jnj.com

00204
**JOHNSON & JOHNSON
CONSUMER PRODUCTS
COMPANY**
800-526-3967
732-524-0400
http://www.jnj.com

**JOHNSON & JOHNSON
HEALTHCARE**
732-524-0400
http://www.jnj.com

52604
**JONES PHARMA
INCORPORATED**
See King Pharmaceuticals, Inc.

68712
JSJ PHARMACEUTICALS
843-965-8333
800-499-4468
http://www.jsjpharm.com

59746
**JUBILANT
PHARMACEUTICALS**
See Cadista

KABI PHARMACIA
See Pfizer US Pharmaceutical
Group

KABIVITRUM, INC.
See Pfizer US Pharmaceutical
Group

KAO BRANDS COMPANY
513-421-1400
800-742-8798
http://www.jergens.com

42043
KARALEX PHARMA
609-759-1777
866-306-0240
http://www.karalexpharma.com

28785
KAZ
800-477-0457
800-541-8001
http://www.kaz.com

68387
**KELTMAN
PHARMACEUTICALS**
601-936-7533
800-325-0903
http://www.keltman.com

08219, 08881
KENDALL HEALTHCARE
508-261-8000
800-962-9888
http://www.covidien.com

00482
KENWOOD LABORATORIES
See Bradley Pharmaceutical, Inc.

00369
KEY PHARMACEUTICALS
See Schering-Plough Corp.

62291
KIEL LABORATORIES, INC.
678-450-9187
800-538-3146
http://www.kielpharm.com

36000
KIMBERLY-CLARK
972-281-1200
800-544-1847
http://www.kimberly-clark.com

60793
**KING PHARMACEUTICALS,
INC.**
423-989-8000
800-776-3637
http://www.kingpharm.com

**KINGSWOOD LABORATORIES,
INC.**
317-849-9513
800-968-7772
http://www.moi-stir.com

KINRAY
718-767-1234
800-854-6729
http://www.kinray.com

58223
**KIRKMAN LABORATORIES,
INC.**
503-694-1600
800-245-8282
http://www.kirkmanlabs.com

28409
KLI CORP.
317-846-7452
800-308-7452
http://www.entertainers-
secret.com

00074
KNOLL PHARMACEUTICALS
See Abbott Laboratories
Pharmaceutical Division

58472
KODAK DENTAL
585-724-5631
800-933-8031
http://www.kodak.com

62515
KONEC, INC
520-571-9119
http://www.konec-inc.com

00224
KONSYL PHARMACEUTICALS
410-822-5192
800-356-6795
http://www.konsyl.com

60598
KOS PHARMACEUTICS, INC.
See Abbott Laboratories
Pharmaceutical Division

66869
**KOWA PHARMACEUTICALS
AMERICA**
334-288-1288
http://www.kowapharma.com

K-PAX VITAMINS
415-381-7565
877-777-5729
http://www.kpaxpharm.com

55505
**KRAMER LABORATORIES,
INC.**
302-223-1287
800-824-4894
http://www.kramerlabs.com

52083
KRAMER-NOVIS
787-767-2072
787-771-9443
http://www.kramernovis.com

62175
KREMERS URBAN
877-332-1714
609-936-5940
http://www.kremersurbanllc.com

33216
**KRS GLOBAL
BIOTECHNOLOGY**
877-506-0777
http://www.gbtbio.com

68716
KVD PHARMA
908-231-1911
888-477-2220
http://www.gbtbio.com

**KV PHARMACEUTICAL
COMPANY**
314-645-6600
800-234-5874
http://www.kvpharmaceutical.com

10702
KVK TECH, INC.
215-579-1842
http://www.kvktech.com

LABCORP
405-290-4444
800-634-9330
http://www.labcorp.com

LABOPHARM
  PHARMACEUTICALS
609-454-0207
877-345-6177
http://www.labopharm.com

48582
LACLEDE
310-605-4280
877-522-5333
http://www.laclede.com

LACRIMEDICS, INC.
360-376-7095
800-367-8327
http://www.lacrimedics.com

LACTAID, INC.
215-273-7000
800-522-8243
http://www.lactaid.com

10106
LAFAYETTE
  PHARMACEUTICALS, INC.
See J.T. Baker, Inc.

LAKE CONSUMER PRODUCTS
262-677-5007
800-537-8658
http://www.lakeconsumer.com

LAKE ERIE MEDICAL
734-847-3847
800-284-2130
http://www.lakeeriemedical.com

02110
LANE LABS
201-236-9090
800-526-3005
http://www.lanelabs.com

00527
LANNETT
215-333-9000
800-325-9994
http://www.lannett.com

44677
LANSINOH LABORATORIES
703-299-1100
800-292-4794
http://www.lansinoh.com

LANTHEUS MEDICAL IMAGING
800-362-2668
800-299-3431
http://www.radiopharm.com

68047
LARKEN LABORATORIES, INC.
601-855-7678
888-527-5522
http://www.larkenlabs.com

LA ROCHE-POSAY
888-577-5226
800-560-1803
http://www.laroche-posay.us

16477, 00277
LASER PHARMACEUTICALS
864-286-8229
http://www.
  laserpharmaceuticals.com

21247
LCM PHAMACEUTICAL
888-411-5465

LECTEC CORPORATION
903-832-0993
http://www.lectec.com

LEDERLE CONSUMER HEALTH
See Wyeth

00008
LEDERLE LABS
See Wyeth

00008
LEDERLE PHARMACEUTICAL
  DIVISION
See Wyeth

LEDERLE-PRAXIS
  BIOLOGICALS (WYETH)
See Wyeth

23558
LEE PHARMACEUTICALS
626-442-3141
800-950-5337
http://www.leepharmaceuticals.com

25332
LEGERE PHARMACEUTICALS,
  INC.
480-991-4033
800-528-3144

12496
LEHN & FINK
See Reckitt Benckiser
  Pharmaceuticals

05388, 74970, 74980, 59606,
  54499
LEINER HEALTH PRODUCTS
310-835-8400
800-421-1168
http://www.leiner.com

10551
LEITNER PHARMACEUTICALS,
  LLC
866-590-7600
423-989-7238
http://www.leitnerpharma.com

00093
LEMMON CO.
See Teva Pharmaceuticals USA

50222
LEO PHARMA INC.
973-637-1690
877-494-4536
http://www.leo-pharma.us

62991
LETCO MEDICAL
256-350-1297
800-239-5288
http://www.letcomedical.com

49523
LEX PHARMACEUTICAL
305-888-7375

08387
LIBERTY MEDICAL SUPPLY
800-705-5797
866-342-2383
http://www.libertymedical.com

00440
LIBERTY PHARMACEUTICAL
866-836-9936
800-615-0721
http://www.libertymedical.com

72499
LIFE-LINE NUTRITIONAL
  PRODUCTS
520-426-3100
800-662-9862
http://www.nationalvitamin.com

53885
LIFESCAN, INC.
800-227-8862
800-524-7226
http://www.lifescan.com

LIFESIGN LLC
800-526-2125
http://www.lifesignmed.com

LIFESTYLE
732-972-8585
800-622-7376
http://www.purilens.com

64365
LIGAND PHARMACEUTICALS,
  INC.
858-550-7500
800-964-5836
http://www.ligand.com

66715
LIL DRUG STORE PRODUCTS
800-252-0454
319-393-0454
http://www.lildrugstore.com

LINCOLN DIAGNOSTICS
217-877-2531
800-537-1336
http://www.lincolndiagnostics.com

05632
LINE ONE LABORATORIES
818-886-2288
800-222-9848
http://www.lineonelabsusa.com

08566
LIONHEARTED INDUSTRIES
480-502-6007

61799
LIPOSOME CO.
See Elan Pharmaceuticals

16110
LIVERITE PRODUCTS
714-259-1800
888-425-5843
http://www.liverite.com

54859
LLORENS PHARMACEUTICAL
305-716-0595
866-595-5598
http://www.llorenspharm.com

00127
**LOBANA LABORATORIES
(ULMER PHARMACAL)**
218-732-2656
800-848-5637
http://www.lobanaproducts.com

34672
LOBOB LABORATORIES
408-432-0580
800-835-6262
http://www.loboblabs.com

55390
LOCH PHARMACEUTICALS
See Bedford Laboratories

09198
LOGAN PHARMACEUTICALS
859-344-9600
888-644-3478

08429
LOGIMEDIX
800-821-0047
http://www.logimedix.com

61480
LOMA LUX LABORATORIES
918-664-9882
800-316-9636
http://www.lomalux.com

12333
LONGS DRUG
800-865-6647
http://www.longs.com

71249
LOREAL USA
212-818-1500
800-322-2036
http://www.lorealusa.com

00273
LORVIC CORP.
See Young Dental Mfg.

67754
LOTUS BIOCHEMICAL CORP.
See Harvest Pharmaceuticals,
Inc.

LSI AMERICA CORPORATION
800-720-5936
http://www.ondrox.com

61598
LTC PRODUCTS
513-738-5583
http://www.ltcproducts.net

**LUITPOLD
PHARMACEUTICALS, INC.**
631-924-4000
800-645-1706
http://www.Luitpold.com

38673
LUMISCOPE
800-672-8293

67386
LUNDBECK, INC.
866-337-6996
http://www.lundbeckusa.com

10892
LUNSCO, INC.
540-980-4358
800-264-8614

68180
**LUPIN PHARMACEUTICALS,
INC.**
410-576-2000
866-466-1450
http://www.
lupinpharmaceuticals.com

LUYTIES PHARMACAL CO.
800-466-3672
http://www.1-800homeopathy.com

00374
LYNE LABS
508-583-8700
800-525-0450
http://www.lyne.com

LYPHO-MED
See Astellas Pharma US, Inc.

44183
**MACOVEN
PHARMACEUTICALS**
225-644-2494
877-622-6836
http://www.macovenpharma.com

58407
**MAGNA PHARMACEUTICALS,
INC.**
888-206-5525
502-254-5552
http://www.magnaweb.com

43292
**MAGNO-HUMPHRIES
LABORATORIES**
503-684-5464
800-935-6737
http://www.magno-humphries.com

10705
MAJESTIC DRUG
845-436-0011
800-238-0220
http://www.majesticdrug.com

00904
**MAJOR PHARMACEUTICALS,
INC.**
800-616-2471
http://www.
majorpharmaceuticals.com

MALLINCKRODT
314-654-2000
800-778-7898
http://www.mallinckrodt.com

10106
MALLINCKRODT BAKER, INC.
See Avantor Performance
Materials

23635
**MALLINCKRODT BRAND
PHARMA**
314-654-2000
800-554-5343
http://www.mallincrodt.com

MALLINCKRODT CHEMICAL
314-654-2000
800-325-8888
http://www.mallinckrodt.com

99913
**MALLINCKRODT NUCLEAR
MEDICINE**
314-654-2000
888-744-1414
http://www.mallinckrodt.com

99880
**MALLINCKRODT
RESPIRATORY**
800-635-5267

45043
**MANCHESTER
PHARMACEUTICALS**
970-685-4119
866-758-7068
http://www.
manchesterpharma.com

10706
MANNE
843-768-4080
800-517-0228

42998
MARATHON
PHARMACEUTICALS LLC
866-945-7860
866-931-0706
http://www.marathonpharma.com

12539
MARIN PHARMACEUTICALS
See A. G. Marin Pharmaceuticals

MARION MERRELL DOW
See Sanofi-Aventis US

10135
MARLEX PHARMACEUTICALS
302-328-3355
866-820-7381
http://www.marlexpharm.com

MARLIN INDUSTRIES
805-473-2743
800-423-5926

12939
MARLOP PHARM
908-355-8854

MARLYN NUTRACEUTICALS,
INC.
480-991-0200
888-766-4406
http://www.naturally.com

00682
MARNEL PHARMACEUTICALS,
INC.
337-232-1396
800-962-7635

00591, 52544
MARSAM PHARMACEUTICALS
See Watson Pharmaceuticals

52555
MARTEC PHARMACEUTICAL,
INC.
816-241-4144
800-822-6782
http://www.martec-kc.com

11845
MASON VITAMINS
305-428-6861
888-860-5376
http://www.masonvitamins.com

14362
MASS. PUBLIC HEALTH BIO.
LAB.
617-474-3000
800-457-4626

08496
MASTERS PHARMACEUTICAL
513-354-2690
800-982-7922
http://www.mastersrx.com

53905
MATRIX LABORATORIES, INC.
See Chiron Therapeutics

62750
MATRIXX INITIATIVES, INC.
602-385-8888
800-808-4866
http://www.zicam.com

41554
MAYBELLINE
800-944-0730

16169
MAYER LABORATORIES
510-437-8989
800-426-6366
http://www.mayerlabs.com

61703
MAYNE PHARMA (USA) INC.
201-225-5500
866-594-8420
http://www.maynepharma.com

MAYO FOUNDATION
507-284-2511
http://www.mayo.edu

00259
MAYRAND, INC.
See Merz Pharmaceuticals

00264
MCGAW, INC.
See B. Braun Medical, Inc.

49072
MCGUFF PHARMACEUTICALS,
INC.
714-918-7277
800-603-4795
http://www.mcguff.com

63739, 38703, 49348
MCKESSON CORPORATION
415-983-8300
800-482-3784
http://www.mckesson.com

MCKESSON
MEDICAL-SURGICAL
804-264-7500
800-446-3008
http://www.mckgenmed.com

57935
MCNEIL CONSUMER
215-273-7000
800-962-5357
http://www.jnj.com

00045, 00062
MCNEIL PHARMACEUTICAL
See Ortho-McNeil Pharmaceutical

58605
MCR AMERICAN
PHARMACEUTICAL
352-754-8587
http://www.mcramerican.com

53014
MD PHARMACEUTICAL
714-751-5881

58607
ME PHARMACEUTICALS, INC.
765-886-5097
866-578-9637
http://www.mepharmusa.com

MEAD JOHNSON
LABORATORIES
See Bristol-Myers Squibb Co.

MEAD JOHNSON
NUTRITIONALS
812-429-5000
http://www.mjn.com

11883
MEAD-RAYMOND
903-509-0663

00037
MEDA PHARMACEUTICALS
732-564-2200
888-455-8383
http://www.medapharma.us

MEDAREX, INC.
609-430-2880
http://www.medarex.com

53276
MED-CHEM PRODUCTS
781-932-5900
http://www.crbard.com

11940
MEDCO LABS
216-292-7546
http://www.medcolabs.com

60793
MEDCO RESEARCH, INC.
See King Pharmaceuticals, Inc.

08212
MEDCON BIOLAB
TECHNOLOGIES, INC.
508-839-4203
800-443-6332
http://www.ilexpaste.com

45565
MED-DERM
423-926-4413
800-877-8869
http://www.crownlaboratories.com

67112
MEDECOR PHARMA
225-343-9830
http://www.medecorpharma.com

64253
MEDEFIL, INC.
630-682-4600
http://www.medefil.com

MEDEGEN
901-867-2951
800-233-1987
http://www.medegen.com

MEDEVA PHARMACEUTICALS
See UCB Pharmaceuticals, Inc.

MEDI AID CORP.
See Baxa Corp.

MEDICAL ACTION INDUSTRIES
631-231-4600
800-645-7042
http://www.medical-action.com

26974
MEDICAL NUTRITION, INC.
201-569-1188
800-221-0308
http://www.pro-stat.com

08271, 28465
MEDICAL PLASTIC DEVICES
514-694-9835
888-527-2842
http://www.medplas.com

10733
MEDICAL PRODUCTS LABS
800-523-0191
215-677-2700
http://www.
    medicalproductslaboratories.com

00576
**MEDICAL PRODUCTS
    PANAMERICANA**
305-545-6524
305-670-4416

99207
**MEDICIS PHARMACEUTICAL
    CORPORATION**
602-808-8800
888-845-1313
http://www.medicis.com

32671
MEDICORE INC.
305-558-4000
800-324-8894
http://www.medicore.com

25208
MEDICURE
732-584-5231
866-210-1128
http://www.medicurepharm.com

54365
MEDI-FLEX, INC.
913-451-0800
800-523-0502
http://www.medi-flex.com

43538
**MEDIMETRIKS
    PHARMACEUTICALS**
973-882-7512
http://www.medimetriks.com

60574
MEDIMMUNE, INC.
301-398-0000
877-633-4411
http://www.medimmune.com

67150
MEDINICHE
314-542-9539
800-711-4303
http://www.mediniche.com

00095
MEDI-PLEX PHARM., INC.
See ECR Pharmaceuticals

47682
MEDIQUE PRODUCTS CO.
239-790-1962
800-634-7680
http://www.mediqueproducts.com

38779
MEDISCA INC.
518-561-0109
800-932-1039
http://www.medisca.com

MEDISENSE, INC.
See Abbott Diabetes Care

12418
**MEDIX PHARMACEUTICALS
    AMERICAS, INC. (MPA)**
See Johnson & Johnson
    Consumer Products Co.

53329,08327
**MEDLINE/DERMAL
    MANAGEMENT**
800-633-5463
http://www.medline.com

80196
MEDLINE INDUSTRIES
800-MEDLINE
http://www.medline.com

53978
MED-PRO, INC.
308-324-4571
800-447-6060
http://www.med-pro-inc.com

46011
MED-SYSTEMS INC
888-547-5492
http://www.sinucleanse.com

90124, 18122
MEDQUIP
843-815-5301
888-404-5666
http://www.medquip.com

**MEDTECH LABORATORIES,
    INC.**
307-733-1680
800-443-4908
http://www.medtechinc.com

MEDTRONIC INC.
763-514-4000
800-328-2518
http://www.medtronic.com

58281
MEDTRONIC NEUROLOGICAL
800-328-0810
http://www.medtronic.com

66116
MEDVANTX, INC.
858-625-2990
http://www.medvantx.com

41250
MEIJER
616-453-6711
http://www.meijer.com

13143
**MELVILLE BIOLOGICS
    (PRECISION PHARMA
    SERVICES)**
631-752-7314
http://www.precisionpharma.com

MENICON AMERICA
650-378-1424
800-636-4266
http://www.menicon.com

22200
MENNEN CO.
See Colgate-Palmolive Co.

42279
MENPER DISTRIBUTORS, INC.
305-836-0208
800-560-5223

10742
MENTHOLATUM
716-677-2500
800-688-7660
http://www.mentholatum.com

81317
MENTOR UROLOGY
805-879-6000
800-525-0245
http://www.mentorcorp.com

**MERCATOR MEDSYSTEMS,
    INC.**
510-614-4550
http://www.mercatormed.com

00006
MERCK SHARP & DOHME
908-423-1000
800-444-2080
http://www.merck.com

00006
**MERCK HUMAN HEALTH (A
DIVISION OF MERCK & CO.)**
215-652-5000
800-672-6372
http://www.merck.com

66582
**MERCK/SCHERING-PLOUGH
PHARM**
866-637-2501
http://www.msppharma.com

62909
MERETEK DIAGNOSTICS, INC.
720-479-6400
888-637-3835
http://www.meretek.com

00394
MERICON INDUSTRIES, INC.
309-693-2150
800-242-6464
http://www.mericon-industries.com

**MERIDIAN MEDICAL
TECHNOLOGIES**
443-259-7800
800-638-8093
http://www.meridianmeds.com

30727
MERIT PHARMACEUTICALS
323-227-4831
800-696-3748
http://www.meritpharm.com

00259
MERZ PHARMACEUTICALS
336-856-2003
800-637-9872
http://www.merzusa.com

55571
METAGENICS, INC.
800-692-9400
http://www.metagenics.com

64281
METHAPHARM, INC.
954-341-0795
800-287-7686
http://www.methapharm.com

08368
METRIKA, INC.
408-524-2255
877-212-4968
http://www.A1cNow.com

86560
MET-RX USA
800-556-3879
http://www.met-rx.com

61738
METTLER ELECTRONICS
714-533-2221
800-854-9305
http://www.mettlerelectronics.com

58063
MGI PHARMA, INC.
952-346-4700
800-562-5580
http://www.mgipharma.com

**MICHIGAN DEPARTMENT OF
HEALTH**
517-373-3740

MICROGENESYS, INC.
See Protein Sciences Corp.

42632
MICROLIFE
727-451-0484
888-314-2599
http://www.microlife.com

08564
MICROMEDICS
800-624-5662
http://www.micromedics-usa.com

MICRON TECHNOLOGY, INC.
208-368-4000
http://www.micron.com

11042
**MIDDLEBROOK
PHARMACEUTICALS, INC.**
301-944-6600
800-340-3641
http://www.advancispharm.com

15686
**MIDLAND PHARMACEUTICAL,
LLC**
913-233-0054

68308
**MIDLOTHIAN LABORATORIES,
LLC**
334-288-8661
800-344-8661
http://www.midlothianlabs.com

46672
MIKART
404-351-4510
888-4MIKART
http://www.mikart.com

00026
MILES, INC.
See Bayer Corp.

00396
MILEX PRODUCTS, INC.
See Cooper Surgical

63020
**MILLENNIUM
PHARMACEUTICALS**
617-679-7000
800-390-5663
http://www.millennium.com

17204
MILLER
630-871-9557
800-323-2935
http://www.millerpharmacal.com

53118
**MILLGOOD LABORATORIES,
INC.**

18757
**MILLENNIUM
BIOTECHNOLOGIES**
908-604-2500
888-412-9179
http://www.milbiotch.com

81361
MILUPA NORTH AMERICA
877-264-5872
http://www.milupana.com

60307
MINRAD, INC.
716-855-1068
800-832-3303
http://www.minrad.com

00485
**MISEMER
PHARMACEUTICALS, INC.**
See Edwards Pharmaceuticals,
Inc.

00178
MISSION PHARMACAL
210-696-8400
800-531-3333
http://www.missionpharmacal.com

MOLNLYCKE HEALTHCARE
678-250-7900
800-843-8497
http://www.molnlycke.com

04351
**MONAGHAN MEDICAL
CORPORATION**
518-561-7330
800-833-9653
http://www.monaghanmed.com

61570
**MONARCH
PHARMACEUTICALS**
See King Pharmaceuticals

11868
MONTICELLO DRUG CO.
904-384-3666
800-735-0666
http://
monticellocompanies.com

65883
MONTIFF INC.
310-582-8938

00839
MOORE MEDICAL CORP.
800-234-1464
http://www.mooremedical.com

MOREPEN INC.
609-987-1134
http://www.morepen.com

60432
**MORTON GROVE
PHARMACEUTICALS**
800-346-6854
847-967-5600
http://www.mgp-online.com

MORTON INTERNATIONAL
215-592-3000
http://www.rohmhaas.com

MORTON SALT
312-807-2000
http://www.mortonsalt.com

**MOTHERSOY INTERNATIONAL,
INC.**
812-424-5432
888-769-0769
http://www.mothersoy.com

MOUNT SINAI MEDICAL CTR.
212-241-6500
800-637-4624

**MOVA PHARMACEUTICAL
CORPORATION**
905-816-3944
888-728-4366
http://www.patheon.com

66977
MPM MEDICAL, INC.
972-893-4090
800-232-5512
http://www.mpmmedicalinc.com

74676
MUELLER
608-643-8530
800-356-9522
http://www.muellersportsmed.com

00150
MURRAY DRUG CORP.
270-753-6654

53489
**MUTUAL PHARMACEUTICAL
CO., INC. (UNITED
RESEARCH
LABORATORIES)**
215-288-6500
800-523-3684
http://www.urlmutual.com

00378
MYLAN
724-514-1800
800-796-9526
http://www.mylan.com

20694
MYOGEN
See Gilead Sciences

59730
NABI
301-770-3099
800-685-5579
http://www.nabi.com

57459
**NASTECH PHARMACEUTICAL
CO., INC.**
425-908-3600
http://www.nastech.com

08164
**NATIONAL MEDICAL
PRODUCTS, INC.**
949-768-1147
http://www.jtip.com

94688
NATIONAL NUTRITION, INC.
717-569-8561
877-271-3570
http://www.medtritionnni.com

54629
NATIONAL VITAMIN
559-781-8871
800-538-5828
http://www.nationalvitamin.com

NATREN, INC.
805-371-4737
800-992-3323
http://www.natren.com

47469
NATROL, INC.
818-739-6000
800-262-8765
http://www.natrol.com

94604
NAT-RUL HEALTH PRODUCTS
800-628-7855
http://www.natrulhealth.com

NATURALLY VITAMINS CO.
480-991-0200
888-766-4406
http://www.naturallyvitamins.com

93265
NATURES BEST
312-245-2834
800-551-2544
http://www.
naturesbestenzyme.com

74312
NATURES BOUNTY, INC.
800-348-0090
631-567-9500
http://www.naturesbounty.com

**NATURES SUNSHINE
PRODUCTS, INC.**
801-342-4300
800-223-8225
http://www.naturessunshine.com

65203
NATURE'S VISION
269-327-8282
877-740-8180
http://www.naturesvisioninc.com

NATURE'S WAY
801-489-1500
800-926-8883
http://www.naturesway.com

74312
NBTY, INC.
See Nature's Bounty, Inc.

60242
NEIL LABS
609-448-5500
http://www.neillabs.com

05928
NEILMED PHARMACEUTICALS
707-525-3784
877-477-8633
http://www.neilmed.com

72559
**NELLSON NEUTRACEUTICAL
(FORMERLY NCI MEDICAL
FOODS)**
626-812-6522
800-869-1515

NEORX CORP.
206-281-7001
http://www.neorx.com

58414
NEOSTRATA
609-520-0715
800-225-9411
http://www.neostrata.com

51759
NEPHROCEUTICALS
937-281-0123
http://www.nephroceuticals.com

00487
**NEPHRON
PHARMACEUTICALS CORP.**
407-246-1389
800-433-4313
http://www.nephronpharm.com

59528
NEPHRO-TECH
785-883-4108
800-879-4755
http://www.nephrotech.com

99825
**NESTLE HEALTHCARE
NUTRITION**
847-317-2800
877-463-7853
http://www.
nestleclinicalnutrition.com

NESTLE INFANT NUTRITION
800-284-9488
http://www.verybestbaby.com

62860
NEUREX PHARMACEUTICALS
See Elan Pharmaceuticals

NEUROGENESIS
800-345-8912
http://www.neurogenesis.com

14565
NEUROSCI
937-848-9130
http://www.neurosciinc.com

**NEUTRACEUTICAL
SOLUTIONS, INC.**
361-854-0755
800-856-7040
http://www.eliquidsolutions.com

10812
NEUTROGENA CORPORATION
310-642-1150
800-582-4048
http://www.neutrogena.com

**NEUTRON TECHNOLOGY
CORP.**
See Micron Technology, Inc.

NEW WORLD TRADING CORP.
407-566-0608

10530
NEXCO PHARMA
713-896-4949
http://www.nexcopharma.com

00722
NEXGEN PHARMA
949-862-0340
http://www.nexgenpharm.com

61958
**NEXSTAR
PHARMACEUTICALS**
See Gilead Sciences

24478
**NEXTWAVE
PHARMACEUTICALS**
847-996-6200
http://www.nextwavepharm.com

14789
NEXUS PHARMACEUTICALS
888-806-4606
847-996-3789
http://www.nexuspharma.net

45611
NFI CONSUMER PRODUCTS
800-432-9334
http://www.nfiproducts.com

59016
NICHE PHARMACEUTICALS
817-491-2770
800-677-0355
http://www.niche-inc.com

08384,38384
NIPRO DIAGNOSTICS
800-342-7226
http://www.niprodiagnostics.com

38379,41405
**NIPRO MEDICAL
CORPORATION**
305-599-7174
888-647-7698
http://www.nipro.com

12948
NITROMED, INC.
781-266-4000
http://www.nitromed.com

15662
NNODUM CORPORATION
513-861-2329
888-301-0457
http://www.zikspain.com

51801
NOMAX, INC.
314-961-2500
800-397-0012
http://www.nomax.com

NORAMCO INC.
706-353-4400
http://www.noramco.com

50445
NORDISK
609-987-5800
http://www.novonordisk-us.com

59730
**NORTH AMERICAN
BIOLOGICALS, INC.**
See Nabi

76906
NORTH AMERICAN HERBAL
800-836-3095
http://www.
northamericanherbal.com

62448
**NORTH AMERICAN VACCINE,
INC.**
See Baxter Healthcare Corp.

92942
**NORTHERN RESEARCH
LABORATORIES, INC.**
See Epien Medical

16714
NORTHSTAR RX
480-502-6007
800-206-7821
http://www.northstarrxllc.com

29033
**NOSTRUM
PHARMACEUTICALS, INC.**
732-635-0036
http://www.nostrumpharma.com

08548
NOVA BIOMEDICAL
781-894-0800
800-458-5813
http://www.novabiomedical.com

NOVADEL PHARMA
908-203-4640
http://www.novadel.com

99780
NOVAPLUS
See Novation

00067.
**NOVARTIS CONSUMER
HEALTH**
See Novartis Pharmaceuticals
Corp.

00212, 41679
**NOVARTIS MEDICAL
NUTRITION**
862-778-8300
888-669-6682
http://www.novartisnutrition.com

58768
**NOVARTIS OPHTHALMICS,
INC.**
866-393-6336
See Novartis Pharmaceuticals
Corp.

NOVARTIS PHARMA AG
See Novartis Pharmaceuticals
Corp.

00078
**NOVARTIS
PHARMACEUTICALS
CORPORATION**
862-778-8300
888-669-6682
http://www.pharma.us.
novartis.com

NOVATION
888-766-8283
http://www.novationco.com

66500
NOVAVAX
240-268-2000
http://www.novavax.com

68968
NOVEN PHARMACEUTICALS
305-253-5099
888-253-5099
http://www.noven.com

NOVEN THERAPEUTICS, LLC
866-663-2539
800-455-8070
http://www.jdspharma.com

00169, 59060
NOVO NORDISK
  PHARMACEUTICALS
609-987-5800
800-727-6500
http://www.novonordisk-us.com

49197
NOVOGEN
203-966-2556
http://www.novogen.com

00093
NOVOPHARM USA, INC.
See Teva Pharmaceuticals USA

00159, 48932
NOYES
800-522-2469
http://www.pjnoyes.com

NU SKIN ENTERPRISES
801-345-1000
800-487-1000
http://www.nuskinenterprises.com

NUGYN, INC.
763-398-0108
877-774-1442
http://www.eros-therapy.com

08910
NULINE PHARMACEUTICALS
914-939-8881
http://www.nulinepharma.com

55499
NUMARK LABS
732-417-1870
800-338-8079
http://www.numarklabs.com

07249, 00221
NUTRA BALANCE
800-654-3691
317-356-5478
http://www.nutra-balance-
  products.com

NUTRACEA
877-723-1700
http://www.nutracea.com

NUTRACEUTICAL SOLUTIONS
361-854-0755
800-856-7040
http://www.eliquidsolutions.com

02359
NUTRACEUTICS
  CORPORATION
877-664-6684
http://www.neutraceutics.com

55970
NUTRAMAX LABORATORIES,
  INC.
410-776-4000
800-925-5187
http://www.nutramaxlabs.com

NUTRAMAX PRODUCTS
978-282-1800
http://www.nutramax.com

NUTRASAL, LLC
207-856-2222
888-437-5772
http://www.nutrasal.com

NUTRI VENTION
210-661-8589
800-390-7940

49735
NUTRICIA NORTH AMERICA
301-795-2300
800-365-7354
http://www.shsna.com

NUTRITION 21
914-701-4500
800-696-0860
http://www.nutrition21.com

90962
NUTRITIONAL DESIGNS
516-612-4900
888-263-5227
http://www.ndlabs.com

91124
NUVORA, INC.
408-856-2200
877-530-9811
http://www.nuvorainc.com

00407
NYCOMED AMERSHAM
See GE Healthcare

NYCOMED US INC.
631-454-7677
800-645-9833
http://www.nycomedus.com

11169
OAKHURST CO.
516-731-5380
800-831-1135
http://www.oakhurst-medicine.com

62032
OBAGI MEDICAL PRODUCTS
562-628-1007
http://www.obagi.com

68682
OCEANSIDE
  PHARMACEUTICALS
949-461-6199
http://www.
  oceansidepharmaceuticals.com

55515, 80831.
OCLASSEN
  PHARMACEUTICALS, INC.
See Watson Pharmaceuticals

21406, 55056
O'CONNOR, INC.
See Columbia Laboratories, Inc.

68209
OCTAPHARMA USA, INC.
703-766-4860
866-766-4860
http://www.octapharma.com

53152
OCTOGEN PHARMACAL
770-843-7032
800-729-4613
http://www.octogenpharma.com

65473
ODYSSEY
  PHARMACEUTICALS, INC.
877-427-9068
http://www.odysseypharm.com

51660
OHM LABORATORIES, INC.
877-646-5227
http://www.ohmlabs.com

OMNII ORAL
  PHARMACEUTICALS
561-689-1140
800-445-3386
http://www.4oralcare.com

94030
OMNIS HEALTH
877-450-6734
http://www.omnishealth.com

73796
OMRON MANAGED
  HEALTHCARE
877-216-1333
847-680-6200
http://www.omronhealthcare.com

16781
ONSET THERAPEUTICS
888-713-8154
877-702-0532
http://www.onsettx.com

68305, 93286
ONTOS, INC
360-740-0888
888-469-7546
http://www.4myskin.com

ONY
716-636-9096
877-274-4669
http://www.onyinc.com

11916, 64108
OPTICS LABORATORY, INC.
626-350-1926
800-968-6788
http://www.opticslab.com

OPTIKEM INTERNATIONAL
800-525-1752

63369
**OPTIMED CONTROLLED
   RELEASE LAB**
See Quality by Design Packaging

50520
OPTIMOX
310-618-9370
800-223-1601
http://www.optimox.com

00041
ORAL-B LABORATORIES
800-566-7252
http://www.oral-b.com

65976
ORAPHARMA, INC.
215-956-2200
866-273-7846
http://www.orapharma.com

ORASURE TECHNOLOGIES
610-882-1820
800-869-3535
http://www.orasure.com

68820
ORCHID HEALTHCARE
480-502-6007
480-227-7661

ORGANOGENESIS INC.
781-575-0775
http://www.organogenesis.com

00052
ORGANON, INC.
973-325-4500
800-222-7579
http://www.organon-usa.com

66203
ORGANON SANOFI
973-325-4500
http://www.organon-usa.com

ORGANON TEKNIKA CORP.
See Biomerieux

15377
ORIGIN BIOMED
902-423-5745
888-234-7256
http://www.originbiomed.com

62161
ORPHAN MEDICAL, INC.
See Jazz Pharmaceuticals

66607
**ORPHAN PHARMACEUTICALS
   USA**
See Rare Disease Therapeutics

**ORTHO BIOTECH PRODUCTS,
   L.P.**
See Centocor Ortho Biotech, Inc.

00562
**ORTHO-CLINICAL
   DIAGNOSTICS, INC.**
800-828-6316
http://www.orthoclinical.com

99948
ORTHO DERM
800-426-7762
http://www.orthodermatologics.com

00062
**ORTHO-MCNEIL
   PHARMACEUTICAL**
800-682-6532
http://www.ortho-mcneil.com

ORTHO NEUTROGENA
800-426-7762
http://www.orthoneutrogena.com

67707
OSCIENT PHARMACEUTICALS
781-398-2300
http://www.oscient.com

65231
OSI PHARMACEUTICALS
631-962-2000
800-572-1932
http://www.osip.com

10244
OTIS CLAPP & SONS
800-775-5400
http://www.otisclapp.com

15210
OTN GENERICS
650-952-8400
800-482-6700
http://www.lynx2otn.com

59148
OTSUKA AMERICA
301-990-0030
800-562-3974
http://www.otsuka.com

67386
**OVATION PHARMACEUTICALS,
   INC.**
847-282-1000
888-514-5204
http://www.ovationpharma.com

08470, 08214
OWEN MUMFORD
770-977-2226
800-421-6936
http://www.owenmumford.com

64803
**OXFORD PHARMACEUTICAL
   SERVICES**
973-256-0600
http://www.oxfordpharm.com

OXIS INTERNATIONAL
650-212-2568
800-547-3686
http://www.oxisresearch.com

99949
P & G HEALTH
513-983-1100
800-543-7270
http://www.pg.com

99958
P & G PAPER PRODUCTS
513-983-1100
800-543-7270
http://www.pg.com

P & S LABORATORIES, INC.
See Standard Homeopathic Co.

64393
PACIFIC EMERALD CO.
425-485-9208

60758
PACIFIC PHARMA
800-811-4184
714-246-4600

65250
**PACIRA PHARMACEUTICALS,
   INC.**
858-625-2424
858-625-2414
http://www.pacira.com

16571
**PACK PHARMACEUTICALS,
   LLC**
847-229-0153
800-521-5340
http://www.packpharma.com

00574
**PADDOCK LABORATORIES,
   INC.**
763-546-4676
800-328-5113
http://www.paddocklabs.com

38142
PAL MIDWEST, LTD.
815-965-2981
815-332-9405
http://www.rashcream.com

25294
PALCO LABS
831-430-1600
800-346-4488
http://www.palcolabs.com

00516
**PALISADES
PHARMACEUTICALS, INC.**
See Glenwood, Inc.

24518
PALM PHARMACEUTICALS
843-364-3256
http://www.
palmpharmaceuticals.com

16477
**PALMETTO
PHARMACEUTICALS, INC.**
864-286-8229

00525
PAMLAB, LLC
985-893-4097
http://www.pamlab.com

**PAN AMERICAN
LABORATORIES**
See Pamlab, LLC

86679
PAPERPAK
See Attends Healthcare Products

49884
PAR PHARMACEUTICAL, INC.
201-802-4000
800-828-9393
http://www.parpharm.com

66758
**PARENTA
PHARMACEUTICALS, INC.**
803-461-5500
800-898-9948
http://www.parentarx.com

44229,83490
PARI RESPIRATORY
804-253-7274
http://www.pari.com

PARKE-DAVIS - A PFIZER CO.
See Pfizer US Pharmaceutical
Group

64029
**PARKEDALE
PHARMACEUTICALS**
See King Pharmaceuticals, Inc.

00341
PARKER LABORATORIES, INC.
973-276-9500
800-631-8888
http://www.parkerlabs.com

50930
PARNELL
415-256-1800
800-457-4276
http://www.parnellpharm.com

49309
PARTHENON CO., INC.
801-972-5184
800-453-8898
http://www.parthenoninc.com

00418, 11098
PASADENA RESEARCH LABS
See Akorn, Inc.

10866
PASCAL CO., INC.
425-827-4694
800-426-8051
http://www.pascaldental.com

PATHEON
905-821-4001
888-728-4366
http://www.patheon.com

10147
**PATRIOT PHARMACEUTICALS
LLC**
215-325-7676
800-631-5273
http://www.
patriotpharmaceuticals.com

08519
PATTON MEDICAL DEVICES
877-763-7678
http://www.pattonmd.com

PBI
See Upsher-Smith Labs, Inc.

66213
PBM PHARMACEUTICALS
540-832-3282
800-485-9828
http://www.
pbmpharmaceuticals.com

PDK LABS, INC.
631-273-2630
http://www.pdklabs.com

55289
PDRX PHARMACEUTICAL
405-942-3040
800-299-7379
http://www.pdrx.com

66346
**PEDIAMED
PHARMACEUTICALS, INC.**
859-282-8582
866-543-6337
http://www.pediamedpharma.com

**PEDIATRIC
PHARMACEUTICALS**
732-603-7708
http://www.pediatricpharm.com

00884
PEDINOL PHARMACAL, INC.
631-293-9500
800-733-4665
http://www.pedinol.com

10974
PEGASUS
850-478-2770
http://www.pegasuslabs.com

25074
PENEDERM, INC.
See Bertek Pharmaceuticals, Inc.

13893
PENN LABORATORIES
877-300-6153
http://www.pennlaboratories.com

60432
**PENNEX PHARMACEUTICAL,
INC.**
See Morton Grove
Pharmaceuticals, Inc.

**PENTECH
PHARMACEUTICALS, INC.**
847-255-0303
http://www.pentechinc.com

PERNIX THERAPEUTICS, LLC
225-647-2002
800-793-2145
http://www.pernixtx.com

00113, 10768
PERRIGO COMPANY
269-673-8451
800-719-9260
http://www.perrigo.com

00096
PERSON COVEY
818-240-1030
800-423-2341
http://www.personandcovey.com

PERSONAL PRODUCTS CO.
See Johnson&Johnson
Healthcare

00927
PFEIFFER CO.
404-614-0255
800-342-6450
http://www.
pfeifferpharmaceuticals.com

12547
PFIZER CONSUMER HEALTH
973-660-5500
800-762-4675
http://www.pfizer.com

PFIZER US PHARMACEUTICAL GROUP
212-733-2323
800-879-3477
http://www.pfizer.com

PHARMA FRONTIERS
281-775-0609
http://www.pharmafrontier.com

62441
PHARMA MEDICA
905-624-9115
http://www.pharmamedica.com

52959
PHARMA PAC
805-929-1333
800-841-5554
http://www.pharmapac.com

39822
PHARMA-TEK, INC.
See X-Gen Pharmaceuticals, Inc.

00121
PHARMACEUTICAL ASSOCIATES, INC.
864-277-7282
800-845-8210
http://www.pa-inc.net

PHARMACEUTICAL BASICS, INC.
See Upsher-Smith Labs, Inc.

51655
PHARMACEUTICAL CORP OF AMERICA
317-616-4498
800-722-0772

21659
PHARMACEUTICAL LABS, INC.
See Neutraceutical Solutions, Inc.

45334
PHARMACEUTICAL SPECIALTIES, INC.
507-288-8500
800-325-8232
http://www.psico.com

12547
PHARMACIA & UPJOHN CONSUMER HEALTHCARE - A DIVISION OF PFIZER
See Pfizer Consumer Health

PHARMACIA CORP. - A DIVISION OF PFIZER
See Pfizer US Pharmaceutical Group

63704
PHARMACIST PHARMACEUTICAL LLC
540-981-1004

00462
PHARMADERM
678-287-1500
866-337-6457
http://www.pharmaderm.com

55422, 65937
PHARMAKON LABS
813-886-3216
http://www.pharmakonlabs.com

PHARMALUCENCE
781-275-7120
800-221-7554
http://www.pharmalucence.com

15035
PHARMANEX
801-345-9800
http://www.pharmanex.com

51817
PHARMASCIENCE LAB
514-340-9800
800-363-8805
http://www.pharmascience.com

48107
PHARMASSURE, INC.
888-462-2548

31604, 78742
PHARMAVITE
818-221-6200
800-423-2405
http://www.pharmavite.com

PHARMED
800-683-7342
305-592-2324
http://www.pharmed.com

PHARMEDIUM
847-457-2300
800-523-7749
http://www.pharmedium.com

53002
PHARMEDIX
800-486-1811
http://www.pharmedixrx.com

66663
PHARMELLE
See Azur Pharma

00813
PHARMICS, INC.
801-966-4138
800-456-4138
http://www.pharmics.com

67211
PHARMION CORPORATION
See Celgene Corp.

54348
PHARMPAK
415-455-9981
800-541-6315
http://www.pharmpakinc.com

PHOENIX LABORATORIES
516-822-1230

PHOTOCURE ASA
47-22-06-22-10
http://www.photocure.com

PHOTOMEDEX
215-619-3600
http://www.photomedex.com

54868
PHYSICIANS TOTAL CARE
918-254-2273
800-759-3650
http://www.physicianstotalcare.com

PHYTOPHARMICA, INC.
920-469-1313
800-553-2370
http://www.enzymatictherapy.com

60831
PIERRE FABRE PHARMACEUTICALS
973-898-1042
http://www.pierre-fabre.com

44733
PLAINVIEW HEALTHCARE
800-903-3222
http://www.dairycare.com

PLAYTEX CO.
800-222-0453
http://www.playtex.com

50111
PLIVA, INC.
973-386-5566
800-922-0547
http://www.plivainc.com

41100, 11523
PLOUGH, INC.
See Schering-Plough Healthcare Products

37864
PLUS PHARMA
631-543-3334

50991
POLY PHARMACEUTICALS, INC.
601-776-3497
800-882-1041

POLYMEDICA CORPORATION
781-933-2020
800-886-4050
http://www.polymedica.com

**POLYMEDICA
PHARMACEUTICALS**
See Amerifit Brands, Inc.

47144
**POLYMER TECHNOLOGY
CORP.**
978-658-6111
800-323-0000
http://www.polymer.com

08193
**POLYMER TECHNOLOGY
SYSTEMS**
317-870-5610
877-870-5610
http://www.cardiocheck.com

49963
PORTAL PHARMACEUTICALS
787-832-6645

55688
PORTON PRODUCT LIMITED
See Speywood Pharmaceuticals,
Inc.

POWDERJECT VACCINES
See Chiron Therapeutics

POYTHRESS
See ECR Pharmaceuticals

68158
**PRAECIS PHARMACEUTICALS
INCORPORATED**
781-795-4100
877-772-3247
http://www.gsk.com

62263,63370
PRAGMATIC MATERICALS INC.
440-349-1313

66993
PRASCO LABORATORIES
513-618-3333
866-525-0688
http://www.prasco.com

PRATT PHARMACEUTICALS
See Pfizer US Pharmaceutical
Group

68094
PRECISION DOSE, INC
800-397-9228
http://www.precisiondose.com

72058
PRECISION FOODS
800-442-5242
http://www.precisionfoods.com

PREMIER MICRONUTRIENT
615-234-4020
888-606-8883
http://www.premiermicronutrient.com

**PRESS CHEMICAL &
PHARMACEUTICAL
LABORATORIES, INC.**
614-863-2802
http://www.epsal.com

75137
**PRESTIGE BRANDS
INTERNATIONAL**
914-524-6810
800-803-4471
http://www.prestigebrands.com

66378
PRESUTTI LABORATORIES
847-483-6050
http://www.presuttilabs.com

42582
PREVENTION LABORATORIES
800-473-1205
618-252-6922
http://www.preventionlabs.com

00684
PRIMEDICS LABORATORIES
323-770-3005

68040
**PRIMUS PHARMACEUTICALS,
INC.**
480-483-1410
http://www.primusrx.com

39278
PRINCE OF PEACE
800-732-2328
510-887-1799
http://www.popus.com

**PRINCETON PHARM.
PRODUCTS**
See Bristol-Myers Squibb Co.

PRIORITY HEALTHCARE
See Curascript

**PROCTER & GAMBLE
COMPANY**
513-983-1100
800-543-7270
http://www.pgpharma.com

00149
**PROCTER & GAMBLE
PHARMACEUTICALS**
See Warner Chilcott Pharma

PROCYTE CORPORAITON
425-869-1239
http://www.procyte.com

08524
**PROGRESSIVE HEALTH
SUPPLY**
888-887-4772
http://www.
progressivehealthsupply.com

66375
PROMEDICA LABS, INC.
973-925-1001

65483
**PROMETHEUS
LABORATORIES, INC.**
858-824-0895
888-423-5227
http://www.prometheuslabs.com

67857
PROMIUS PHARMA, LLC
866-733-3952
http://www.promiuspharma.com

67555
PRONOVA CORPORATION
305-666-4831
866-703-3508
http://www.pronovacorp.com

50313
PROPHARMA
305-592-9216
800-446-0255

65581
PROPST PHARMACEUTICALS
256-704-6394

PROTEIN DESIGN LABS, INC.
510-574-1400
http://www.pdl.com

PROTEIN SCIENCES CORP.
203-686-0800
800-488-7099
http://www.proteinsciences.com

PROTHERICS INC.
615-327-1027
888-327-1027
http://www.protherics.com

29978
**PROVIDENT
PHARMACEUTICALS, LLC**
719-278-3988
http://www.providentpharma.com

16241
PRX PHARM
See Par Pharmaceutical, Inc.

PSYCHEMEDICS CORP.
978-206-8220
800-628-8073
http://www.psychemedics.com

65005
PTS LABORATORIES, INC.
562-907-3607
http://www.ptsgeolabs.com

65005
**PTS LABS INTERNATIONAL,
INC.**
562-907-3607
http://www.ptsgeolabs.com

00034
PURDUE FREDERICK
203-588-8000
800-877-5666
http://www.purduepharma.com

59011
PURDUE PHARMA L.P.
203-588-8000
800-877-5666
http://www.purduepharma.com

67781
**PURDUE PHARMACEUTICAL
PRODUCTS**
800-877-5666
888-726-7535
http://www.purduepharma.com

PURILENS, INC.
See Lifestyle

PURITANS PRIDE
800-645-9584
http://www.puritan.com

QLT, INC.
604-707-7000
800-663-5486
http://www.qltinc.com

**QLT PHOTOTHERAPEUTICS,
INC.**
See QLT, Inc.

QOL MEDICAL
866-469-3773
http://www.qolmed.com

Q-PHARMA, INC.
609-883-1818

63004
**QUESTCOR
PHARMACEUTICALS, INC.**
510-400-0700
800-411-3065
http://www.questcor.com

QUIDEL CORP.
858-552-1100
800-874-1517
http://www.quidel.com

61941
QUIGLEY CORP.
267-880-1100
http://www.quigley.com

66774
**QUADEX PHARMACEUTICALS,
LLC**
801-453-9614
http://www.viroxyn.com

QUALICAPS, INC.
336-449-3900
800-227-7853
http://www.qualicaps.com

52917
QUALIS, INC.
515-243-3000

00603
QUALITEST
256-859-4011
800-444-4011
http://www.qualitestrx.com

63369
**QUALITY BY DESIGN
PACKAGING**
812-522-9262
http://www.qbdinc.com

49999
QUALITY CARE PHARM, INC.
See Quality Care Products, LLC

49999
**QUALITY CARE PRODUCTS,
LLC**
419-478-0441
http://qcpmeds.com

54391
R & D LABORATORIES, INC.
See Watson Pharmaceuticals

17236
R & S NORTHEAST
215-673-7770
800-262-7770
http://www.rsnortheast.com

12830
R.A. MCNEIL COMPANY
423-493-9170
800-755-3038

54807
R.I.D., INC.
323-268-0635

**R.I.J. PHARMACEUTICAL
CORP.**
845-692-5799
http://www.rijpharm.com

**R.P. SCHERER CARDINAL
HEALTH**
732-537-6200
http://www.cardinal.com

**RAINBOW LIGHT
NUTRITIONAL SYSTEMS**
831-420-2660
800-635-1233

10631
**RANBAXY LABORATORIES
LIMITED**
609-720-9200
http://www.ranbaxy.com

63304
**RANBAXY
PHARMACEUTICALS**
609-720-9200
888-726-2299
http://www.ranbaxyusa.com

67216
RANDAL OPTIMAL NUTRIENTS
707-528-1800
800-966-8874
http://www.randalnutritional.com

30103
**RANDOB LABORATORIES,
LTD.**
845-534-2197

66607
**RARE DISEASE
THERAPEUTICS, INC.**
615-399-0700
http://www.raretx.com

12496
**RECKITT BENCKISER
PHARMACEUTICALS**
973-404-2600
800-333-3899
http://www.reckittbenckiser.com

10952
RECSEI LABS
805-964-2912

67857
REDDY PHARMACEUTICAL
See Promius Pharma, LLC

52380, 18407
REDI-PRODUCTS LABS, INC.
See Aplicare Inc.

00091
REED & CARNRICK
See Schwarz

10956
**REESE PHARMACEUTICAL
CO., INC.**
800-321-7178
http://www.
   reesepharmaceutical.com

**REGENERON
PHARMACEUTICALS**
914-345-7400
http://www.regeneron.com

66779
REGENT LABS, INC.
800-872-1525
http://www.regentlabs.com

65726
RELIANT PHARMACEUTICALS
See GlaxoSmithKline

REMEL, INC.
800-255-6730
http://www.remel.com

67066
REPLIGEN
See Chirhoclin

10961
REQUA, INC.
See W.F. Young, Inc.

00433
RESEARCH INDUSTRIES CORP.
See Edwards

RESEARCH TRIANGLE INSTITUTE
919-541-6000
http://www.rti.org

67492
RESICAL INC
800-204-6434
http://www.resical.com

60575
RESPA PHARMACEUTICALS, INC.
630-543-3333
http://www.respainc.com

47360
RESPIRATORY DELIVERY SYSTEMS
978-970-1947
http://www.rdsusa.com

08373
RESPIRONICS
724-387-4000
800-345-6443
http://www.respironics.com

00122
REXALL GROUP
See Rexall Sundown, Inc.

30768
REXALL SUNDOWN, INC.
561-241-9400
800-327-0908
http://www.rexallsundown.com

54092
REXAR PHARMACEUTICALS
See Shire US, Inc.

RH PHARMACEUTICALS, INC.
See Cangene Corp.

59258
RHODIA
609-860-4000
http://www.rhodia.com

RHONE-POULENC RORER CONSUMER, INC.
See Sanofi-Aventis US

RHONE-POULENC RORER PHARMACEUTICALS, INC.
See Sanofi-Aventis US

RICHARDSON-VICKS, INC.
See Procter & Gamble Pharmaceuticals

RICHIE PHARMACAL, INC.
502-651-6159
800-627-0250
http://www.richiepharmacal.com

00115
RICHLYN LABORATORIES, INC.
See Global Pharmaceuticals, Inc.

54738
RICHMOND PHARMACEUTICALS
804-270-4498

RICOLA USA, INC.
973-984-6811
http://www.ricolausa.com

64980
RISING PHARMACEUTICALS, INC.
201-961-9000
http://www.risingpharma.com

68032
RIVER'S EDGE PHARMACEUTICAL
770-886-3417

54092
ROBERTS PHARMACEUTICAL CORP.
See Shire US, Inc.

50924
ROCHE DIAGNOSTIC SYSTEMS, INC.
See Roche Laboratories

00004
ROCHE LABORATORIES
973-235-5000
800-526-6367
http://www.rocheusa.com

49908
ROCHESTER PHARMACEUTICALS

66358
RODLEN LABORATORIES
847-362-8200

ROERIG
See Pfizer US Pharmaceutical Group

67546
ROMARK LABORATORIES, L.C.
813-282-8544
http://www.romark.com

10802
ROSEDALE THERAPEUTICS
800-247-4896
http://www.rtherapeutics.com

ROSEMONT PHARMACEUTICAL CORP.
See Upsher-Smith Labs, Inc.

64334
ROSE STONE ENTERPRISES
985-892-5939

70074
ROSS PRODUCTS DIVISION, ABBOTT NUTRITIONAL CONSUMER RELATIONS
See Abbott Nutrition

00054
ROXANE LABORATORIES, INC.
800-962-8364
800-562-4797
http://www.roxane.com

00591, 52544
ROYCE LABORATORIES, INC.
See Watson Laboratories

00536
RUGBY LABORATORIES, INC.
678-584-5678
800-645-2158
http://www.watson.com

61972
RUGER CHEMICAL CO
973-926-0331
800-274-7843
http://www.rugerchemical.com

66794, 08367
RX ELITE
208-288-5550
800-414-1901
http://www.rxelite.com

46500
S C JOHNSON
262-260-2000
800-494-4855
http://www.scjohnson.com

12258
S.S.S. COMPANY
404-521-0857
800-237-3843
http://www. ssspharmaceuticals.com

59243
SAGE PHARMACEUTICALS
318-635-1594

53462, 08513
SAGE PRODUCTS
815-455-4700
800-323-2220
http://www.sageproducts.com

64054
SALIENT HCT
847-726-9443

65649
SALIX PHARMACEUTICALS, INC.
919-862-1000
866-669-7597
http://www.salix.com

07411
SALTER LABS
661-854-3166
800-421-0024
http://www.salterlabs.com

66288
SAMSON MEDICAL TECH. LLC
856-751-5051
877-418-3600
http://www.samsonmt.com

00067
SANDOZ CONSUMER
See Novartis Pharmaceuticals
Corp.

00781, 00067
SANDOZ
609-627-8500
800-525-8747
http://www.us.sandoz.com

62053
SANGSTAT MEDICAL CORP.
See Genzyme Transplant

65597
SANKYO
See Daiichi Sankyo, Inc.

00024
SANOFI-AVENTIS U.S.
800-633-1610
800-981-2491
http://www.sanofi-aventis.us

49281
SANOFI PASTEUR
570-839-7187
800-822-2463
http://www.vaccineshoppe.com

SANOFI-SYNTHELABO, INC.
See Sanofi-Aventis U.S.

00024
SANOFI WINTHROP PHARMACEUTICALS
See Sanofi-Aventis U.S.

68012
SANTARUS, INC.
858-314-5700
http://www.santarus.com

65086
SANTEN, INC.
707-254-1750
800-611-2011
http://www.santeninc.com

00281
SAVAGE LABORATORIES
631-454-9071
800-231-0206
http://www.savagelabs.com

54396
SAVIENT PHARMACEUTICALS, INC.
732-418-9300
800-284-2480
http://www.savient.com

SCANDINAVIAN FORMULAS, INC.
215-453-2507
800-688-2276
http://www.
   scandinavianformulas.com

SCHAFFER LABORATORIES
310-325-4200
800-231-6725
http://www.schafferlabs.com

52544
SCHEIN PHARMACEUTICAL, INC.
See Watson Laboratories

00274
SCHERER LABORATORIES, INC.
972-612-6225

00085
SCHERING-PLOUGH CORPORATION
908-298-4000
800-842-4090
http://www.schering-plough.com

41000, 11523
SCHERING-PLOUGH HEALTHCARE PRODUCTS
908-298-4000
800-842-4090
http://www.schering-plough.com

20525
SCHIFF NUTRITION INTERNATIONAL, INC.
801-975-5000
800-435-3948
http://www.schiffnutrition.com

00234, 02340
SCHMID PRODUCTS CO.
See Durex Consumer Products

41000, 11523
SCHOLL, INC.
See Schering-Plough Healthcare
Products

00091
SCHWARZ PHARMA
http://www.schwarzusa.com

SCHWARZKOPF & DEP INC.
800-326-2855
http://www.henkel.com

SCICLONE PHARMACEUTICALS, INC.
650-358-3456
http://www.sciclone.com

59630
SCIELE PHARMA
See Shionogi US, Inc.

66239
SCIENTIFIC LABORATORIES, INC.

65847
SCIOS, INC.
650-564-5000
http://www.sciosinc.com

08589
SCIVOLUTIONS
704-853-0100
http://www.scivolutions.com

00372
SCOT-TUSSIN PHARMACAL, INC.
401-942-8555
800-638-7268
http://www.scot-tussin.com

66424
SDA LABORATORIES, INC.
203-861-0005

08471
SEA-BAND
401-841-5900
http://www.sea-band.com

SEARLE
See Pfizer US Pharmaceutical
Group

15127
SELECT BRAND
501-296-3373
http://www.usadrug.com

63402
SEPRACOR PHARMACEUTICALS
508-481-6700
800-245-5961
http://www.sepracor.com

SEPTODONT, INC.
302-328-1102
800-872-8305
http://www.septodontinc.com

17314
SEQUUS PHARMACEUTICALS, INC.
See Alza Corp.

50694
SERES LABORATORIES
707-526-4526
http://www.sereslabs.com

44087
SERONO LABORATORIES, INC.
See EMD Serono

11026
SEYER PHARMATEC, INC.
787-286-3223
888-782-3585
http://www.spharmatec.com

SHAKLEE CORP.
925-924-2000
800-928-0327
http://www.shaklee.com

49813
SHEAR KERSHMAN LABS
636-519-8900
http://www.shearkershman.com

SHEFFIELD PHARMACEUTICALS
860-442-4451
800-222-1087
http://www.sheffield-pharmaceuticals.com

12772
SHERWOOD

17474, 08219
SHERWOOD DAVIS & GECK
See Kendall Health Care Products

SHIELD MANUFACTURING, INC.
716-694-7100
800-828-7669
http://www.shieldsports.com

45809, 59630
SHIONOGI PHARMA, INC.
800-461-3696
770-442-9790
http://www.shionogipharma.com

45809
SHIONOGI USA, INC.
See Shionogi Pharma, Inc.

54092
SHIRE US, INC.
484-595-8800
800-536-7878
http://www.shire.com

49735
SHS NORTH AMERICA
See Nutricia North America

50111
SIDMAK LABORATORIES, INC.
See Pliva, Inc.

45749, 54482
SIGMA-TAU PHARMACEUTICALS, INC.
301-948-1041
800-447-0169
http://www.sigmatau.com

54838
SILARX PHARMACEUTICALS, INC.
845-352-4020
888-974-5279
http://www.silarx.com

53799, 94841
SIMILASAN
303-539-4060
800-240-9780
http://www.similasanusa.com

98302
SIMPLE DIAGNOSTICS
877-342-2385
http://www.simplediagnostics.com

65880
SIRIUS LABORATORIES, INC.
978-657-7500
877-533-3872
http://www.siriuslabs.com

24839
SJ PHARMACEUTICALS
877-604-7575
http://www.sjpharma.com

67402
SKINMEDICA, INC.
760-448-3600
866-867-0110
http://www.skinmedica.com

SKYEPHARMA, INC.
See Pacira Pharmaceuticals, Inc.

SLATE PHARMACEUTICALS
919-682-8800
http://www.slatepharma.com

08436
SLIM FAST FOODS CO.
561-833-9920
800-726-9866
http://www.slim-fast.com

SMITH & NEPHEW, INC. ENDOSCOPY
978-749-1000
http://www.smith-nephew.com

08363
SMITH & NEPHEW ORTHO
901-396-2121
800-821-5700
http://www.smith-nephew.com

40565, 50484
SMITH & NEPHEW WOUND MANAGEMENT
721-392-1261
800-876-1261
http://www.snwmd.com

58291
SNUVA, INC.
708-725-3783
800-250-4258
http://www.snuva.com

57771
SOLACE NUTRITION
888-876-5223
http://www.solacenutrition.com

SOLGAR CO., INC.
201-944-2311
800-645-2246
http://www.solgar.com

10454
SOLSTICE NEUROSCIENCES
267-620-8000
866-220-5042
http://www.solsticeneuro.com

94922
SOLUBLE SYSTEMS
757-877-8899
http://www.solublesystems.com

00032
SOLVAY PHARMACEUTICALS
770-578-9000
800-241-1643
http://www.solvaypharmaceuticals.com

42847
SOMAXON PHARMACEUTICALS
858-876-6500
www.somaxon.com

63669
SOMBRA COSMETICS
505-888-0288
800-225-3963
http://www.sombrausa.com

39506
SOMERSET PHARMACEUTICALS
813-288-0040
800-892-8889
http://www.somersetpharm.com

58676
SOURCECF
267-759-9400
888-419-8357
http://www.sourcecf.com

45713, 61118
SOUTHWEST TECHNOLOGIES
816-221-2442
800-247-9951
http://www.elastogel.com

58016
**SOUTHWOOD
PHARMACEUTICALS**
800-442-4443
http://www.
southwoodhealthcare.com

**SOVEREIGN
PHARMACEUTICALS**
817-284-0429
http://www.sovpharm.com

66530
**SPEAR DERMATOLOGY
PRODUCTS**
973-895-6447
http://www.speardermatology.com

38415
**SPECIALTY MEDICAL
SUPPLIES**
954-752-5603
http://www.
specialtymedicalsupplies.com

49452
**SPECTRUM CHEMICAL MFG.
CORP.**
310-516-8000
800-813-1514
http://www.spectrumchemical.com

38472
**SPENCO MEDICAL
CORPORATION**
254-772-6000
800-877-3626
http://www.spenco.com

**SPEYWOOD
PHARMACEUTICALS, INC.**
See Ipsen, Inc.

ST. JUDE MEDICAL, INC.
651-483-2000
800-328-9634

67253
**STADA PHARMACEUTICALS,
INC.**
See Dava Pharmaceuticals

99929
STANBACK CO.
See GlaxoSmithKline Consumer
Healthcare, LP

**STANDARD DRUG CO. &
FAMILY PHARMACY**
217-629-9884
800-632-9884

**STANDARD HOMEOPATHIC
CO. & HYL**
310-768-0700
800-624-9659
http://www.hylands.com

00076
**STAR PHARMACEUTICALS,
INC.**
See Esprit Pharma

**STASON PHARMACEUTICALS,
INC.**
949-380-4327
http://www.stasonpharma.com

16590
STAT RX USA
770-227-0065

51318.
STELLAR PHARMACAL CORP.
See Esprit Pharma

STEPHAN COMPANY
954-971-0600
800-327-4963
http://www.thestephanco.com

STERICYCLE
847-367-9493
866-783-7422
http://www.stericycle.com

52544
STERIS CORP.
440-354-2600
800-548-4873
http://www.steris.com

STERLING HEALTH
972-991-9293
http://www.sterlinghealthcenter.com

00024
STERLING WINTHROP
See Sanofi-Aventis US

**STIEFEL CONSUMER
HEALTHCARE**
305-443-3800
http://www.stiefel.com

00145
STIEFEL LABORATORIES, INC.
866-398-5765
http://www.stiefel.com

14168
**STONEBRIDGE
PHARMACEUTICALS**
888-445-2337
http://www.stiefel.com

58980
STRATUS PHARMACEUTICALS
305-254-6793
800-442-7882
http://www.
stratuspharmaceuticals.com

00310
STUART PHARMACEUTICALS
See AstraZeneca, LP

**SUGEN, INC. (INFORMAGEN,
INC.)**
See Pfizer US Pharmaceutical
Group

SUMMA RX LABORATORIES
940-325-0771
800-527-7319
http://www.summalabs.com

11086, 94731
SUMMERS LABS
610-454-1471
800-533-7546
http://www.sumlab.com

SUMMIT INDUSTRIES, INC.
773-588-2444
800-729-9729
http://www.summitindustries.net

00078
SUMMIT PHARMACEUTICALS
See Novartis Pharmaceuticals
Corp.

22252, 22319
SUNBEAM
800-435-1250
http://www.sunbeamhealth.com

14508
**SUN PHARMACEUTICAL
INDUSTRIES**
313-871-8400
800-818-4555
http://www.caraco.com

**SUNOVION
PHARMACEUTICALS**
508-481-6700
800-739-0565
http://www.sunovion.com

33413
SUNRISE MEDICAL
631-435-1515
800-782-0282
http://www.sunriselab.com

41167
SUNSOURCE
423-821-4571

62701
SUPERGEN
925-560-0100
800-353-1075
http://www.supergen.com

48503
SURGICAL APPLIANCE INDUSTRIES
800-888-0458
800-888-0867
http://www.surgicalappliance.com

60232
SWISS-AMERICAN PRODUCTS
972-385-2900
800-633-8872
http://www.elta.net

18867
SWISS BIOCEUTICAL
775-841-7020

SYNCOM PHARMACEUTICALS, INC.
973-787-2405
800-400-0056
http://www.syncom.com

55513
SYNERGEN, INC.
See Amgen, Inc.

00004
SYNTEX LABORATORIES
See Roche Laboratories

66576
SYNTHO PHARMACEUTICALS, INC.
631-755-9898
http://www.synthopharmaceutical.com

63672
SYNTHON PHARMACEUTICALS, INC.
919-493-6006
http://www.synthon-usa.com

SYVA CO.
See Dade Behring

78112, 75137
(THE) DENOREX CO.
866-840-0011
http://www.denorex.com

57464
THE F. C. STURTEVANT COMPANY
914-337-5131
888-871-5661
http://www.columbiapowder.com

11694
(THE) KEY COMPANY
314-965-7629
800-325-9592
http://www.thekeycompanyusa.com

65293
(THE) MEDICINES COMPANY
973-290-6000
800-388-1183
http://www.themedicinecompany.com

00217
T E WILLIAMS
719-687-8770
800-755-7659

64764
TAKEDA PHARMACEUTICALS
224-554-6500
877-825-3327
http://www.tpna.com

13533
TALECRIS BIOTHERAPEUTICS, INC.
919-316-6300
800-243-4153
http://www.talecris.com

75486
TANNING RESEARCH LABS, INC.
386-677-9559
800-874-4844
http://www.htropic.com

TANOX INC.
713-578-4000
http://www.tanox.com

00300
TAP PHARMACEUTICAL PRODUCTS, INC.
847-582-2000
800-621-1020
http://www.tap.com

16730
TARGET
612-696-5941
http://investors.target.com

TARGETED GENETICS CORP.
206-623-7612
800-828-6022
http://www.targen.com

TARGETED MEDICAL PHARMA
310-474-9809
http://www.ptlcentral.com

TARMAC PRODUCTS, INC.
305-557-6423
http://www.tarmacproducts.com

51672
TARO PHARMACEUTICALS USA, INC.
914-345-9001
800-544-1449
http://www.tarousa.com

11098
TAYLOR PHARMACAL (AKORN)
See Akorn, Inc.

67336
TEAMM PHARMACEUTICALS, INC.
919-481-9020
866-481-9020
http://www.teammpharma.com

08605,93573
TECHNOLOGICAL INVESTMENTS, LLC
512-255-2271
http://www.medi-fridge.com

51879, 83626
TEC LABORATORIES, INC.
541-926-4577
800-482-4464
http://www.teclabsinc.com

TEL-TEST, INC.
281-482-2762
800-631-0600
http://www.tel-test.com

TELLURIDE PHARM. CORP.
908-369-1800
http://www.tellpharm.com

68436
TERAL, INC.
787-383-2781

15054
TERCICA
650-624-4900
http://www.tercica.com

08418, 08970
TERUMO MEDICAL CORPORATION
732-302-4900
800-888-3786
http://www.terumomedical.com

TESTPAK, INC.
973-887-4440
http://www.testpak.com

TEVA MARION PARTNERS
816-508-5000
800-221-4026
http://www.tevausa.com

00093
TEVA PHARMACEUTICALS USA
215-591-3000
888-838-2872
http://www.tevausa.com

29273
TG UNITED PHARMACEUTICALS
352-799-9813
http://www.tgunited.com

51672
THAMES PHARMACAL, INC.
See Taro Pharmaceuticals USA, Inc.

08348
THAYER MEDICAL
800-250-3330
http://www.thayermedical.com

64011
THER-RX CORPORATION
314-646-3700
877-567-7676
http://www.ther-rx.com

64067
THERAKOS, INC.
610-280-1000
http://www.therakos.com

**THERAPEUTIC ANTIBODIES,
INC.**
See Protherics, Inc.

THERASENSE
See Abbott Diabetes Care

11926
**THOMPSON MEDICAL CO.,
INC.**
See Chattem Consumer Products

66435
**THREE RIVERS
PHARMACEUTICALS**
724-778-6100
800-405-8506
http://www.3riverspharma.com

23589
TIBER LABORATORIES
770-886-3417
678-208-0388
http://www.tiberlabs.com

66403
TIGER BALM
510-887-1899
http://www.tigerbalm.com

49483
TIME-CAP LABS
631-753-9090
http://www.timecaplabs.com

14654, 54023
TISHCON CORP.
516-333-3050
800-848-8442
http://www.tishcon.com

TOMS OF MAINE, INC.
207-985-2944
800-367-8667
http://www.tomsofmaine.com

36800
TOPCO
847-676-3030
888-423-0139
http://www.topco.com

58211
TOPIX PHARMACEUTICALS
631-226-7979
800-445-2595

38423
TOPOTARGET
866-914-2922
http://www.topotarget.com

13668
**TORRENT
PHARMACEUTICALS**
269-544-2299
http://www.torrentpharma.com

50201
TOWER LABORATORIES
860-767-2127
http://www.towerlabs.com

62511
**TRANSDERMAL
TECHNOLOGIES, INC.**
561-848-2345
800-282-5511
http://www.
transdermaltechnologies.com

TRASK NUTRITION
877-760-9258
800-579-3131
http://www.fibromalic.com

TRI TECH LABORATORIES
434-845-7073
http://www.tritechlabs.com

14290
**TRIAX PHARMACEUTICALS,
LLC**
908-372-0500
866-453-0577
http://www.triaxpharma.com

13811
TRIGEN LABORATORIES
732-721-0070

TRIGEN LABS
See Cadista

68752
TRIMARC LABORATORIES
405-942-3289
http://www.trimarclabs.com

55654
TRIMED LAB, INC.
732-249-6363

61355
TRINITY TECHNOLOGIES
781-235-2223
http://www.trinitytechnologies.com

79511
**TRITON CONSUMER
PRODUCTS, INC.**
847-228-7650
800-942-2009
http://www.mg217.com

10025
TROPICAL PHARMACAL
787-737-8445

50247
TRUTEK CORP
908-685-1111
http://www.trutekcorp.com

00463
TRUXTON
856-933-2333
http://www.truxtonpharma.com

TWEEZERMAN
516-676-7772
800-645-3340
http://www.tweezerman.com

27434
TWINLAB CORP.
631-467-3140
800-645-5626
http://www.twinlab.com

64915
TYLER, INC.
See Integrative Therapeutics

53335
TYSON NUTRACEUTICALS
310-325-5600
http://www.
tysonnutraceuticals.com

00456
UAD LABORATORIES, INC.
See Forest Pharmaceuticals, Inc.

**UCB PHARMACEUTICALS,
INC.**
770-970-7500
866-822-0068
http://www.ucb-usa.com

62592
UCYCLYD PHARMA, INC.
888-829-2593
http://www.medicis.com

51079, 08459
UDL LABORATORIES, INC.
800-848-0462
http://www.udllabs.com

00127
ULMER PHARMACAL CO.
800-848-5637
http://www.lobanaproducts.com

08222, 08474, 57515
ULTIMED
651-291-7909
877-854-3434
http://www.diabetes-care.com

ULURU, INC.
214-905-5145
http://www.uluruinc.com

23535,29300
UNICHEM, INC.
336-578-5476
http://www.unichem.com

60814
UNICITY
800-864-2489
801-226-2600
http://www.makelifebetter.com

59640
UNICO HOLDINGS, INC.
800-367-4477
561-582-3030
http://www.unico-holdings.com

UNIFIRST CORPORATION
800-225-3364
http://www.unifirst.com

62305
UNIGEN PHARMACEUTICAL
410-751-2108
360-486-8200
http://www.unigenpharma.com

UNILEVER HOME AND PERSONAL CARE USA
203-661-2000
800-243-5320
http://www.unilever.com

41785
UNIMED PHARMACEUTICALS
See Solvay Pharmaceuticals

08479
UNIPATH DIAGNOSTICS CO.
See Inverness Medical Innovations

59707
UNIQUEONE PHARMACEUTICAL & MED
See One Pharma & Medical Supply Co

00327
UNITED GUARDIAN LABORATORIES
631-273-0900
800-645-5566
http://www.u-g.com

00677
UNITED RESEARCH LABORATORIES (URL)
See Mutual Pharmaceutical Co., Inc.

63535
UNITHER PHARMA (UNITED THERAPEUTICS CORP.)
301-608-9292
888-808-6838
http://www.unitedtherapeutics.com

59730
UNIVAX BIOLOGICS
See Nabi

UPJOHN CO.
See Pfizer US Pharmaceutical Group

00245
UPSHER-SMITH PHARMACEUTICALS
763-315-2000
800-654-2299
http://www.upsher-smith.com

65580
UPSTATE PHARMA, LLC
770-970-7500
800-477-7877
http://www.ucbpharma.com

92293
UROCARE PRODUCTS, INC.
909-621-6013
800-423-4441
http://www.urocare.com

UROCOR, INC.
See LabCorp

UROLOGIX
763-475-1400
800-475-1403
http://www.urologix.com

US BIOSCIENCE
216-765-5000
800-321-9322
http://www.usbio.com

US DENTEK CORP.
800-433-6835
http://www.usdentek.com

08463
US DIAGNOSTICS
866-216-5303

68728
U.S. FOODS & PHARMACEUTICALS
866-678-4436
http://www.usfp.com

13774
US MEDICAL INSTRUMENTS
619-661-5500
http://www.usmedicalinstruments.com

U.S. NEUTRACEUTICALS, LLC
352-357-2004
877-876-8872
http://www.usnutra.com

52747
US PHARMACEUTICAL CORPORATION
770-987-4745
http://www.uspco.com

63261
UNITED STATES SURGICAL CORP
203-845-1000
800-722-8772
http://www.ussurg.com

00187
VALEANT
800-548-5100
http://www.valeant.com

55592
VALERA PHARMACEUTICALS
See Indevus Pharmaceuticals

30698
VALIDUS PHARMACEUTICALS
866-825-4387
http://www.validuspharma.com

54627
VALMED, INC.
508-845-3438

VALUE IN PHARMACEUTICALS
800-724-3784
http://www.vippharm.com

00615
VANGARD
800-825-4123

67537
VARSITY LABORATORIES
205-986-1111

65199
VATRING PHARMACEUTICALS
276-322-1888

VENTANA MEDICAL SYSTEMS, INC.
520-887-2155
800-227-2155
http://www.ventanamed.com

11391
VENTLAB CORPORATION
336-753-5000
800-593-4654
http://www.ventlab.com

67887
VERACITY PHARMACEUTICALS, INC.
954-426-1919
800-354-8460
http://www.veracitypharma.com

16887
VERNALIS PHARMACEUTICALS
See Ipsen Pharmaceuticals

61748
VERSAPHARM
770-499-8100
800-548-0700
http://www.versapharm.com

VERTEX PHARMACEUTICALS, INC.
617-576-3111
http://www.vpharm.com

67000
VERUM PHARMACEUTICALS
See Victory Pharmaceuticals

13436
VERUS PHARMACEUTICALS, INC.
866-634-8774
http://www.veruspharm.com

78112, 75137
VETCO, INC.
800-754-8853
http://www.littleremedies.com

00702
VHA, INC.
972-830-0626
800-842-5146
http://www.vha.com

VIASYS HEALTHCARE
610-862-0800
866-484-2797
http://www.viasyscriticalcare.com

00149
VICKS HEALTH CARE PRODUCTS
See Procter & Gamble Pharmaceuticals

00149
VICKS PHARMACY PRODUCTS
See Procter & Gamble Pharmaceuticals

67000
VICTORY PHARMA, INC.
858-350-4217
866-427-6819
http://www.victorypharma.com

67204
VINDEX PHARMACEUTICALS, INC.
901-759-4970
http://www.vindexpharm.com

00254
VINTAGE PHARMACEUTICALS, INC.
704-596-9440

53459
VIP INTERNATIONAL
718-390-0490

00187
VIRATEK
See Valeant

VIREXX
See Paladin Labs

66593
VIROPHARMA, INC.
610-458-7300
http://www.viropharma.com

68013
VISION PHARMA
732-974-6300
http://www.visionpharma.com

54891
VISION PHARMACEUTICALS, INC.
605-996-3356
800-325-6789
http://www.visionpharm.com

98669
VISTAKON PHARMACEUTICALS, LLC
904-443-1000
800-843-2020
http://www.vistakonpharmaceuticals.com

66689, 67043
VISTAPHARM, INC.
205-981-1387
877-437-8567
http://www.vistapharm.com

49727
VITA-RX CORP
706-568-1881

08321
VITAL CARE GROUP
305-620-4007
800-392-4547
http://www.vitalcare.com

08166
VITAL SIGNS INC.
973-790-1330
800-932-0760
http://www.vital-signs.com

54022
VITALINE
800-917-3696

VITALITY, INC.
See Vital Care Group

82966
VITAMIN HEALTH
888-890-3937
http://www.vitaminhealthbrands.com

VITAMIN RESEARCH PRODUCT, INC.
775-884-8210
800-877-2447
http://www.vrp.com

62541
VIVUS, INC.
650-934-5200
888-345-6873
http://www.vivus.com

71603
W.E. BASSETT
203-929-8483
http://www.trim.com

11444
W.F. YOUNG
800-628-9653
http://www.absorbine.com

WAKEFIELD PHARMACEUTICALS, INC.
See Ivax Pharmaceuticals, Inc.

40805
WAL-MED, INC.
253-845-6633
877-542-3688
http://www.wallace-medical.com

00017
WAMPOLE LABORATORIES
See Inverness Medical Innovations

00047
WARNER CHILCOTT LABORATORIES
973-442-3200
800-521-8813
http://www.warnerchilcott.com

12546
WARNER LAMBERT AMERICAN CHICLE
973-540-2000
800-524-2624

59930
WARRICK PHARMACEUTICAL, CORP.
See Schering-Plough Corp.

00591, 52544
WATSON LABORATORIES
914-767-2000
800-553-4044
http://www.watsonpharm.com

00591, 52544
WATSON PHARMACEUTICALS
800-272-5525
http://www.watsonpharm.com

55946
WELEDA
800-241-1030
http://www.usa.weleda.com

65197
WELLSPRING PHARMACEUTICAL
941-552-7880
877-273-1396
http://www.wellspringpharm.com

00917
WESLEY PHARMACAL, INC.
215-953-1680

00006
WEST POINT PHARMA
See Merck & Co.

00143
WEST-WARD PHARMACEUTICAL CORPORATION
732-542-1191
800-631-2174
http://www.wwinjectables.com

64727
WESTERN RESEARCH LABORATORIES
See RLC Labs

00072
WESTWOOD SQUIBB PHARMACEUTICALS
See Bristol-Myers Squibb Co.

WHITBY PHARMACEUTICALS, INC.
See UCB Pharmaceuticals, Inc.

72695
WHITE LABS, INC.
858-693-3441
888-593-2785
http://www.whitelabs.com

00317
WHORTON PHARMACEUTICALS, INC.
205-786-2584

35046
WINDMILL CONSUMER PRODUCTS
973-575-6591
800-822-4320
http://www.windmillvitamins.com

51101
WILLIAM LABORATORIES, INC.
860-749-1350
800-767-7643
http://www.williamlabs.com

00427
WINSTON LABORATORIES
847-362-8200
http://www.winstonlabs.com

52047
WINTEC
636-257-5400

12120
WISCONSIN PHARMACAL
262-677-4121
800-558-6614
http://www.pharmacalway.com

WM. WRIGLEY JR. CO.
312-644-2121
800-974-4539
http://www.wrigley.com

64679
WOCKHARDT USA
973-257-4960
800-346-6854
http://www.wockhardtusa.com

WOLLFOAM COMPANY
516-731-5380

64248
WOMEN FIRST HEALTHCARE
See Mutual Pharmaceutical Co., Inc.

64836
WOMENS CAPITAL CORP.
See Barr Laboratories, Inc.

08111, 61168
WOODSIDE BIOMEDICAL
See Abbott Hospital Products

60193
WOODWARD LABORATORIES, INC.
949-362-4600
800-780-6999
http://www.woodwardlabs.com

66992
WRASER PHARMACEUTICALS
601-605-0664
888-252-3901
http://www.wraser.com

00008
WYETH
800-934-5556
800-999-9384
http://www.wyeth.com

WYETH CONSUMER HEALTH
See Pfizer Consumer Health

39822
X-GEN PHARMACEUTICALS, INC.
607-732-4411
866-390-4411
http://www.x-gen.us

XACTDOSE, INC.
See Alpharma

66479
XANODYNE PHARMACEUTICALS, INC.
859-371-6383
877-926-6396
http://www.xanodyne.com

00187
XCEL PHARMACEUTICALS
See Valeant

XOMA LLC/XOMA LTD.
510-204-7200
800-544-9662
http://www.xoma.com

00116
XTTRIUM LABORATORIES
773-268-5800
800-587-3721
http://www.xttrium.com

55212
YASOO HEALTH
919-439-2960
http://www.yasoo.com

YOUNG AGAIN PRODUCTS
910-371-6775
877-950-4400
http://www.younggainproducts.com

00273, 60077
YOUNG DENTAL MFG.
314-344-0010
800-325-1881
http://www.youngdental.com

89901
ZANFEL LABORATORIES, INC.
800-401-4002
http://www.zanfel.com

ZARS PHARMA
801-350-0202
http://www.zars.com

90389
ZEE MEDICAL, INC.
800-841-8417
http://www.zeemedical.com

ZENITH LABORATORIES
See Ivax Pharmaceuticals, Inc.

18011
ZERXIS PHARMA, LLC
985-893-4097
http://www.pamlab.com

51284
ZILA, INC.
602-266-6700
866-945-2776
http://www.zila.com

00053
ZLB BEHRING
See CSL Behring

44206
ZLB BIOPLASMA
See CSL Behring

64909
ZOETICA PHARMACEUTICAL GROUP
See Dava Pharmaceuticals, Inc.

ZONAGEN, INC.
281-719-3400
http://www.zonagen.com

65224
ZYBER PHARMACEUTICALS, INC.
See Pernix Therapeutics, LLC

68382
ZYDUS PHARMACEUTICALS USA, INC.
609-275-5125
877-993-8779
http://www.zydususa.com

23594
ZYLERA PHARMACEUTICALS
http://www.zylera.com

ZYMETX, INC.
405-809-1314
888-817-1314
http://www.zymetx.com

28400
ZYMOGENETICS, INC.
206-442-6600
888-784-7662
http://www.zymogenetics.com